OTHER PMIC TITLES OF INTEREST

CODING AND REIMBURSEMENT TITLES

Collections Made Easy!
CPT Coders Choice®, Thumb Indexed
CPT & HCPCS Coding Made Easy!
CPT Easy Links
CPT Plus!
DRG Plus!
E/M Coding Made Easy!
Getting Paid for What You Do
HCPCS Coders Choice®, Color Coded, Thumb Indexed
Health Insurance Carrier Directory
HIPAA Compliance Manual
ICD-9-CM, Coders Choice®, Thumb Indexed
ICD-9-CM Coding for Physicians' Offices
ICD-9-CM Coding Made Easy!
ICD-9-CM, Home Health Edition
Medical Fees in the United States
Medicare Compliance Manual
Medicare Rules Regulations
Physicians Fee Code
Reimbursement Manual for the Medical Office

PRACTICE MANAGEMENT TITLES

Accounts Receivable Management for the Medical Practice
Achieving Profitability With a Medical Office System
Encyclopedia of Practice and Financial Management
Managed Care Organizations
Managing Medical Office Personnel
Marketing Strategies for Physicians
Medical Marketing Handbook
Medical Office Policy Manual
Medical Practice Forms
Medical Practice Handbook
Medical Staff Privileges
Negotiating Managed Care Contracts
Patient Satisfaction
Performance Standards for the Laboratory
Professional and Practice Development
Promoting Your Medical Practice
Starting in Medical Practice
Working With Insurance and Managed Care Plans

OTHER PMIC TITLES OF INTEREST

RISK MANAGEMENT TITLES
Malpractice Depositions
Medical Risk Management
Preparing for Your Deposition
Preventing Emergency Malpractice
Testifying in Court

FINANCIAL MANAGEMENT TITLES
A Physician's Guide to Financial Independence
Business Ventures for Physicians
Financial Valuation of Your Practice
Personal Money Management for Physicians
Personal Pension Plan Strategies for Physicians
Securing Your Assets

DICTIONARIES AND OTHER REFERENCE TITLES
Drugs of Abuse
Health and Medicine on the Internet
Medical Acronyms and Abbreviations
Medical Phrase Index
Medical Word Building
Medico Mnemonica
Medico-Legal Glossary
Spanish/English Handbook for Medical Professionals

MEDICAL REFERENCE AND CLINICAL TITLES
Advance Medical Directives
Clinical Research Opportunities
Gastroenterology: Problems in Primary Care
Manual of IV Therapy
Medical Care of the Adolescent Athlete
Medical Procedures for Referral
Neurology: Problems in Primary Care
Orthopaedics: Problems in Primary Care
Patient Care Emergency Handbook
Patient Care Flowchart Manual
Patient Care Procedures for Your Practice
Physician's Office Laboratory
Pulmonary Medicine: Problems in Primary Care
Questions and Answers on AIDS

AVAILABLE FROM YOUR LOCAL MED
BOOK STORE OR CALL 1-800-MED-SH

MEDICAL PHRASE INDEX

A Comprehensive Reference to the Terminology of Medicine

Fifth Edition

Jean A. Lorenzini &
Laura Lorenzini Ley

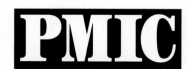

ISBN 1-57066-399-8

Practice Management Information Corporation (PMIC)
4727 Wilshire Blvd.
Los Angeles, California 90010
http://www.pmiconline.com

Printed in China

ABOUT THE EDITORS

Jean A. Lorenzini worked in the medical community for 42 years: 37 years as a medical transcriptionist and 21 of those years as president of Medical Transcript Service. Lorenzini's successful Racine, Wisconsin-based business was one of the first private services to transcribe and translate the dictated/written words of more than 1,000 doctors internationally. Now retired, she enjoys researching new entries for *Medical Phrase Index* on a daily basis.

Laura Lorenzini Ley began her career as a medical transcriptionist at Medical Transcript Service. She now is on staff at All Saints Healthcare in Racine, Wisconsin, enabling her to be aware of new information that will be useful for future revisions of *Medical Phrase Index*.

DISCLAIMER

This publication is designed to offer basic medical terms and phrases. The information presented is based on the experience of the authors. Though all of the information has been carefully checked for accuracy and completeness, neither the editors nor the publisher accepts any responsibility or liability with regard to errors, omissions, misuse, or misinterpretation.

CONTENTS

PREFACE

Transcribing medical dictation can be a frustrating challenge and at the same time a gratifying experience when the challenge is met.

With the diversity of dialects and English-speaking doctors who garble their dictation, a ready reference was needed to assure accuracy in transcription.

Medical Phrase Index is a time-saving, one-step reference for medical transcriptionists, legal secretaries, court reporters, insurance claims adjusters, and anyone responsible for medical records and reports.

This Fifth Edition adds another 6,100 entries to the 277, 000 phrases already catalogued. While all specialties have been included, this edition features additional phrases relating to laser surgery, behavioral sciences, genomics research, geriatrics, cosmetics/plastic surgery, dentistry, cardiology, and hospice and home care. Also lay terms commonly used have been added, e.g., hot tub lung, beauty parlor syncope, and billfold syndrome.

—Jean A. Lorenzini
—Laura Lorenzini-Ley

HOW TO USE THIS BOOK

The *Medical Phrase Index* consists of medical phrases, both formal and informal. The format is essentially the same as that of any standard dictionary. That is, the phrases are listed in alphabetical order. Of necessity, however, it differs from standard dictionaries in some ways. A few special guidelines will help you make the most efficient use of the book.

A major feature of the *Medical Phrase Index* is the cross-indexing of most entries by their major words. For example, the primary entry for the phrase **root canal silver pinning** will be found in alphabetical order under the letter R. The cross-indexed entries for that phrase will be found under C (for **canal**), P (for **pinning**), and S (for **silver**).

Primary entry: root canal silver pinning
Cross-indexed: canal silver pinning, root
                pinning, root canal silver
                silver pinning, root canal

Entries that begin with numerals are listed alphabetically as if the numerals were spelled out.

settling culture, gravity-
#7 NIH angiographic catheter
17-hydroxycorticosteroid test

When a phrase begins with a word that may also be used as the prefix to a compound word, the compound form follows the open form. This is done so that subentries may all be listed in one place.

sun cautery
sun, overexposure to
sunburn
sunflower cataract
sunken acetabulum

Entries in parentheses are disregarded in alphabetizing.

acid phosphate
acid (DNA) polymerase activity ▸ deoxyribonucleic
acid, polyunsaturated fatty

The solid pointer (▸) in the entry above is one of two special symbols used in the *Medical Phrase Index*. The other is the open diamond (◊). The pointer is used to indicate the beginning of a phrase when that phrase may, for some reason, be confusing, or when the phrase itself contains a comma.

Primary entry: ▸ chills, fever and cough
Cross-indexed: fever and cough ▸ chills,
                          cough ▸ chills, fever and

The open diamond is used to indicate that the last word of an entry is part of a compound word.

Primary entry: echocardiogram
Cross-indexed: cardiogram, echo◊

When the same word has two different spellings, both commonly used, the entry for the preferred form will be followed by the parenthetical phrase (*same as*) followed by the other form. The less commonly used word will refer you to the preferred form. In most cases, subentries are listed under the preferred entry.

Primary entry: Haemophilus (*same as* Hemophilus)
Cross-indexed: Hemophilus (*see* Haemophilus)

Sound-alikes appear in italics within brackets:

abductor [*adductor*]
adductor [*abductor*]
tonus [*clonus*]
clonus [*tonus*]

A

A. (Aerobacter)
a (before)
A. (Aerobacter) aerogenes
A, albumin
A and P (anterior and posterior)
A and P (auscultation and percussion)
A, B, AB, O blood group
A, B, AB, O blood type
A B C influenza
A behavior ▸ type
A changes, E to
A. (Aerobacter) cloacae
A. coenzyme
A disc
A globulin (IgA) deficiency, gamma
A, hemoglobin
A, hepatitis virus
A immunoglobulin (IgA) deficiency, gamma
A immunoglobulin (IgA) determination ▸ gamma
A line, Kerley's
a. of esophagus
A, paratyphoid
a., pelvirectal
   a., sphincteral
   a. syndrome, cricopharyngeal
A personality, Type
A, Salmonella paratyphi
A, Shigella arabinotarda Type
A Streptococcus ▸ autopsy-acquired group
A type retroviral particle, human intracisternal
A velocity ▸ peak
A virus, Coxsackie
A virus (HAV), hepatitis
A viruses, serotype
a wave (A wave)
   a. ▸ giant
   A. ▸ precordial
AA (achievement age)
AA (Alcoholics Anonymous)
AA (ascending aorta)
AAA (abdominal aortic aneurysm)
AACD (abdominal aortic counterpulsation device)

AAL (anterior axillary line)
AAMI (Age-Associated Memory Impairment)
Aaron's sign
AARP (American Association of Retired Persons)
Aarskog Syndrome
abacterial thrombotic endocarditis
Abadie's sign
abandoned, patient feels
abandoning patient, caregiver
abandonment
   a., fear of
   a. fears ▸ intense,
   a., feeling of
   a., frantic effort to avoid
   a., imagine
   a., personal
   a., real
   a., rejection and
   a., separation or loss
abarticular gout
abasia
   a. astasia
   a. atactic
   a., choreic
   a., paralytic
   a., paroxysmal trepidant
   a., spastic
   a., trembling
   a. trepidans
abate, symptoms
Abbe
   A. flap
   A., flap repair of lip
   A., lip flap ▸ Stein-
   A., operation
   A. -Zeiss counting chamber
AB-BI (advanced breast biopsy instrumentation)
Abbott
   A. infusion pump
   A. -Lucas operation
   A. -Miller tube
   A. operation
ABC (airway breathing and circulation)
ABD (abdomen)

Abderhalden's dialysis
Abderhalden-Fanconi syndrome
abd. hyst./ab hys (abdominal hysterectomy)
abdomen (ABD)
   a., acute
   a., anterior cutaneous nerve of
   a. ▸ appetite loss from pain in
   a., ascitic fluid in
   a. aspirated
   a., autopsy limited to
   a. bloated
   a., board-like rigidity of
   a., bulge in
   a., cancer of
   a., cecum returned to
   a. ▸ chest tubes present in
   a. closed in layers
   a. contracted
   a., decompression of
   a. distended
   a. distended, patient's
   a. distended, tender, tympanitic
   a. entered
   a. entered and explored
   a., epigastric region of
   a. explored
   a., external oblique muscle of
   a. flat
   a., flat plate of
   a., flexion of thigh on
   a., fluid aspirated from
   a., fluid filled
   a., fluid in
   a., fluid spilling into upper
   a. from Addison's disease ▸ pain in
   a. from appendicitis ▸ pain in
   a. from appendicitis ▸ tenderness in
   a. from colic ▸ pain in
   a. from Crohn's disease ▸ pain in
   a. from diverticulitis ▸ pain in
   a. from diverticulosis ▸ pain in
   a. from diverticulosis ▸ tenderness in
   a. from food poisoning ▸ pain in
   a. from gallstones ▸ pain in
   a. from gastritis ▸ pain in

abdomen—*continued*
a. from gastritis ▸ tenderness in
a. from hepatitis ▸ pain in
a. from hepatitis ▸ tenderness in
a. from hernia ▸ pain in
a. from indigestion ▸ pain in
a. from insect sting ▸ pain in
a. from irritable bowel syndrome ▸ pain in
a. from lactose intolerance ▸ pain in
a. from pancreatitis ▸ pain in
a. from pancreatitis ▸ tenderness in
a. from peritonitis ▸ pain in
a. from peritonitis ▸ tenderness in
a. from proctitis ▸ pain in
a. from ulcers ▸ pain in
a. full of blood
a., fullness in
a., gasless
a., hard
a. ▸ horizontal incision across lower
a., hypogastric region of
a. ▸ in situ examination of
a., internal oblique muscle of
a., itchiness of
a. ▸ large veins on
a., left hypochondriac region of
a., left iliac region of
a., left inguinal region of
a., left lateral region of
a., left lower quadrant (LLQ) of
a., left lumbar region of
a., left upper quadrant (LUQ) of
a., LLQ (left lower quadrant) of
a., lower
a., lump in
a., LUQ (left upper quadrant) of
a., manual exploration of
a. massively dilated
a., normal
a., obese
a. pain ▸ breathing with back, chest or
a., pain in
a. ▸ pain in back and
a., pendulous
a., penetrating wound of the
a., percussion of
a., portable film of
a., pregnant
a., preliminary film of
a. prepped and draped
a. protuberant
a., pubic region of
a., puffiness of

a. ▸ pulsating bulge in
a. radiation therapy, whole
a., rash on
a., right hypochondriac region of
a., right iliac region of
a., right inguinal region of
a., right lateral region of
a., right lower quadrant (RLQ) of
a., right lumbar region of
a., rumbling in
a., right upper quadrant (RUQ) of
a. rigid
a., RLQ (right lower quadrant) of
a. rotund
a., RUQ (right upper quadrant) of
a., scaphoid
a., scrubbed, prepped and draped
a. showed evidence of weight loss
a. soft
a., subcutaneous veins of
a., surgical
a., swelling of
a. taut and distended
a. tender to palpation
a., tenderness of
a. tense
a., transverse muscle of
a., tumor of
a., umbilical region of
a., upper
a., upright film of
a., virginal
a. with back pain ▸ pain in
a. with constipation ▸ pain in
a. with diarrhea ▸ pain in
a. with fever ▸ pain in
a. with nausea ▸ pain in
a. with vaginal discharge ▸ pain in
a. with vomiting ▸ pain in

abdominal (ABD)
a. abscess
a. abscess ▸ intra-
a. adenopathy
a. adhesions
a. adiposity
a. air ▸ free
a. aneurysm
a. aneurysm sac
a. angina
a. aorta
a. aorta atherosclerosed
a. aorta, atherosclerotic
a. aorta ▸ ectasia of
a. aorta ▸ fusiform widening of
a. aorta ▸ infrarenal

a. aorta ▸ saccular aneurysm of
a. aorta thrombotic aneurysm
a. aortic aneurysm (AAA)
a. aortic aneurysm ▸ infrarenal
a. aortic aneurysm ▸ ruptured
a. aortic aneurysm (AAA), reflux dissecting
a. aortic counterpulsation device (AACD)
a. aortic occlusion ▸ acute
a. aortography
a. area, upper
a. arteriosclerotic aneurysm
a. ascites
a. asthma
a. ballottement
a. bandage
a. binder
a. biopsy
a. bleeding ▸ massive intra-
a. bloating
a. body fat
a. breathing
a. bruit
a. bulge
a. calcification, diffuse
a. carcinoma ▸ intra-
a. carcinomatosis
a. cavity
a. cavity ▸ direct drainage (dr'ge) of
a. cavity free of fluid
a. cavity ▸ inflammation lining of
a. circumference
a. complaints, vague
a. compression
a. compression (IAC) ▸ interposed
a. concussion
a. contents
a. counterpulsation ▸ interposed
a. cramping
a. cramping nausea
a. cramping pain
a. cramps
a. crunch
a. crunch/curl-up exercise
a. curl exercises
a. decompression
a. delivery
a. discomfort
a. discomfort, increasing
a. distention
a. distention and tenderness
a. distention ▸ postoperative
a. distress

a. drainage
a. dressing
a. dropsy
a. edema
a. effusion
a. epilepsy
a. escape of gastroduodenal contents ▸ intra-
a. exercises
a. exploration
a. fat
a. fat deposit
a. flap, lower
a. flap, upper
a. foci of infection
a. fullness
a. gas
a. girth
a. girth ▸ increased
a. growls
a. heart
a. hemorrhage ▸ intra-
a. hernia
a. hysterectomy (ab hys/abd. hyst.)
a. hysterectomy ▸ radical
a. hysterectomy ▸ total
a. incision
a. incision ▸ lower transverse
a. infection
a. infection ▸ intra-
a. injury
a. jugular test
a. jump flap
a. laparotomy
a. laser procedure ▸ intra-
a. line
a. lump with Crohn's disease
a. lymph node biopsy
a. lymph nodes
a. lymphangiogram
a. lymphoma ▸ diffuse histiocytic type
a. mass
a. mass ▸ intra-
a. mass ▸ palpable
a. metastases ▸ extensive intra-
a. metastases ▸ intra-
a. migraine
a. muscle guarding
a. muscle injury
a. muscle strength
a. muscle tone
a. muscles, atrophied
a. muscles, atrophy of
a. musculature rigidity

a. nephrectomy
a. nephrotomy
a. obesity
a. obstruction
a. opening
a. organs
a. orifice
a. orifice of uterine tube
a. pain
a. pain and fever ▸ diarrhea,
a. pain and swelling ▸ diarrhea with
a. pain ▸ associated with
a. pain ▸ burning
a. pain, colicky
a. pain ▸ constant
a. pain ▸ cramping
a. pain cramps ▸ cyclic
a. pain, ▸ crampy
a. pain, ▸ dull
a. pain ▸ generalized
a. pain ▸ intermittent episodes of acute
a. pain ▸ intra-
a. pain ▸ lower
a. pain, nausea and vomiting
a. pain, ▸ periodic
a. pain ▸ recurrent
a. pain ▸ vague
a. pain with colitis ▸ recurrent
a. pain with Crohn's disease
a. panniculus
a. paracentesis
a. peristalsis
a. peritoneum
a. pocket
a. port
a. pressure, intra-
a. procedure ▸ intra-
a. pull-through procedure ▸ Soave
a. pulse
a. radiation
a. reflex
a. reflexes, deep
a. reflexes, superficial
a. region
a. region, external
a. region, lateral
a. removal of pregnant uterus
a. respiration
a. ribs
a. rigidity
a. route
a. scars, multiple
a. soft tissue density
a. sonar

a. stalk
a. stimuli
a. stoma
a. straining
a. strength
a. stretch marks from pregnancy
a. striae
a. striae of pregnancy
a. surgery
a. surgery ▸ elective
a. surgery ▸ ileus following
a. surgery, major intra-
a. swelling
a. swelling and pain
a. swelling ▸ breathing with
a. tenderness
a. tenderness, deep
a. tenderness, diffuse
a. tenderness from appendicitis
a. tenderness ▸ gas, bloating and
a. testosterone patch
a. thrust
a. tissue, flap of
a. trauma
a. treatment in radiation therapy ▸ whole
a. tubae uterinae ▸ ostium
a. tumor
a. tumor debulking ▸ intra-
a. ultrasound
a. ultrasound examination
a. uterine exteriorization ▸ extra-
a. varices ▸ intra
a. viscera
a. wall
a. wall closure
a. wall dehiscence
a. wall fascia
a. wall, inner surface of
a. wall musculature
a. wall radiation
a. wall ▸ sagging
a. wall stoma
a. wall surface
a. wall, weakness in
a. wound
a. wound closure
a. wound ▸ penetrating

abdominalis
a., angina
a., aorta
a., ectopia cordis
a., globus
a., purpura

abdominis
- a., diastasis recti
- a., hydrops
- a. muscle ▸ rectus
- a., rectus

abdominocardiac reflex
abdominojugular reflux
abdominoperineal resection
abdominoperineal resection ▸ Miles'
abdominoplasty procedure
abdominothoracic flap
abdominothoracic pump
abducens
- a., alternating
- a., -facial paralysis, congenital
- a. nerve
- a. nerve signs

abducent nerve
abduction [*adduction*]
- a. contraction of hip
- a. exercise ▸ shoulder
- a. exercises
- a. of thumb
- a. position
- a., stress test ▸ external rotation,
- a. test ▸ fabere

abductor [*adductor*]
- a. digiti quinti muscle
- a. muscle of great toe
- a. muscle of little finger
- a. muscle of little toe
- a. muscle of thumb ▸ long
- a. muscle of thumb ▸ short
- a. pollicis brevis muscle
- a. pollicis longus muscle
- a. pollicis longus ▸ musculus
- a. spasmodic dysphonia
- a. tendon ▸ long

abductus, pes
ABE (acute bacterial endocarditis)
Abée's support
Abell-Gilliam suspension
Abell's operation
Abernethy's operation
aberrancy
- a., acceleration dependent
- a., atrial trigeminy with
- a., paradoxical
- a., paroxysmal atrial tachycardia with
- a., postextrasystolic
- a. ▸ tachycardia-dependent

aberrans
- a. of Monokow, fasciculus
- a. of Roth ▸ vas

- a., vas

aberrant [*apparent*]
- a. artery
- a. behavior
- a. bundles
- a. cells
- a. conduction
- a. cycle
- a. duct
- a. endometrial tissue
- a. goiter
- a. pancreas
- a. peripheral innervation
- a. QRS complex
- a. right subclavian artery
- a. sexual behavior
- a. thyroid
- a. umbilical stomach
- a. ventricular conduction
- a. vessel

aberrantis hepatis, vasa
aberration(s)
- a., behavioral
- a., chromatic-type
- a., chromosome
- a., dioptric
- a., distantial
- a., heterosomal
- a., intraventricular
- a., lateral chromatic
- a., longitudinal chromatic
- a., mental
- a., meridional
- a., negative spherical
- a., newtonian
- a. of judgment
- a. of mentation
- a., penta-X chromosomal
- a., positive spherical
- a., sexual
- a., spherical
- a., tetra-X chromosomal
- a. theory, somatic
- a., triple-X chromosomal
- a., zonal

a-beta-lipoproteinemia
A-beta hemolytic streptococci ▸ Group
A-beta streptococcal pharyngitis ▸ Group
ab-externo incision
ab externus
ABG (arterial blood gases)
ABG (arterial blood gases) ▸ deteriorating

ab hys/abd. hyst. (abdominal hysterectomy)
ABI (ankle brachial index)
ability(-ies)
- a. adequate ▸ reasoning
- a. and judgment ▸ mental
- a. and limitations ▸ evaluate
- a. ▸ body's natural healing
- a., body's tumor-killing
- a., bright/normal range of
- a., cancer-killing
- a., cognitive
- a., communication
- a., coping
- a., deceptive
- a. ▸ decline in intellectual
- a. ▸ decline in social
- a. ▸ declining mathematical
- a., expressive
- a., human
- a. ▸ impaired language
- a. ▸ impaired pumping
- a. impairment ▸ mental and physical
- a. ▸ independent functional
- a., intellectual
- a., language
- a., learning
- a. ▸ low average range of
- a. level ▸ difficulty functioning at normal
- a., mechanical
- a., memory
- a., mental
- a. ▸ mentally retarded range of
- a., motor
- a., muscle
- a., numeric
- a. of abstract thinking
- a. of failing heart ▸ pumping
- a. of weakened heart ▸ pumping
- a., overestimates
- a. ▸ patient's cognitive
- a., patient's functional
- a., physical
- a., potential
- a., psychic
- a., reading
- a., recall
- a., replication
- a., reproductive
- a., sensory
- a., sexual
- a., social
- a., spacial

a. test ▸ visual spatial
a. to concentrate, decreased
a. to cope with stress
a. to function ▸ decreased
a. to function independently
a. to hold head up ▸ loss of
a. to perform ▸ patient
a. to perform routine tasks, decline in
a. to react ▸ brain's physical
a. to repeat words
a. to function independently ▸ decreased
a. to sit up ▸ loss of
a. to smell ▸ impaired
a. to smile ▸ loss of
a. to speak ▸ loss of
a. to swallow ▸ impaired
a. to swallow ▸ lose
a. to think or concentrate
a. to understand
a. to walk ▸ loss of
a. to write ▸ loss of
a. ▸ tumor targeting
a., verbal
a., verbal concept formation
Abio-Cor device
abiotrophy, retinal
ablatio placentae
ablatio retinae
ablation [*oblation*]
a. (ACA), accessory conduction
a., adrenal
a., alcohol
a. ▸ alcohol septal
a., androgen
a., AV node
a., bilateral
a., catheter
a., catheter-induced
a. ▸ catheter radiofrequency
a., chemical
a., continuous wave
a., continuous wave laser
a., coronary rotational
a., direct
a., electrical catheter
a., endometrial
a., ethanol
a. ▸ fast pathway radiofrequency
a., His bundle
a., hydrothermal
a. ▸ hysteroscopy and endometrial
a., incision, and excision ▸ tissue
a. ▸ Kent bundle

a., laser
a., laser ▸ rotational
a., marrow
a., operative
a., organ
a., ovarian
a. ▸ parathyroid tumor
a. ▸ percutaneous ethanol
a. ▸ percutaneous tumor
a. ▸ pulsed
a. ▸ pulsed laser
a. (RFA) ▸ radiofrequency
a. ▸ radiofrequency catheter
a. ▸ renal cyst
a., rotational
a., selective
a. ▸ slow pathway
a. ▸ supraventricular tachycardia
a., surgical
a. system ▸ microwave
a. therapy
a. therapy ▸ androgen
a. thermal
a. ▸ thermal balloon
a. threshold
a. ▸ thyroid nodule
a., tissue
a. (TUNA) ▸ transurethral needle
a., tumor
a. ▸ ventricular arrhythmia
ablative
a. cardiac surgery
a. device
a. hormonal therapy
a. laser
a. laser angioplasty
a. pace therapy
a. technique
a. therapy
ABN (abnormal)
abnormal (ABN)
a. accumulation of fluid
a. activity
a. alignment
a. anatomical lesion
a. arterial enlargement
a. behavior
a. behavior, transient
a. bite
a. bladder contraction
a. bleeding
a. blood clotting
a. blood vessels
a. body chemistry
a. body movements

a. bone growth
a. bone growth of spine
a. bone structure
a. brain function
a. brain growth
a. brain tissue
a. brain wave discharges
a. brain wave function
a. calcium level
a. cancerous cells
a. cardiac organogenesis
a. cardiac rhythm
a. cardiac function
a. cell
a. cellular changes
a. chemical activity
a. cholesterol related gene
a. chromosome
a. cleavage of cardiac valve
a. clusters
a. coloration
a. contraction on ventriculogram
a. cytology
a. depression
a. development
a. development of scar tissue
a. development of valve
a. diurnal weight gain
a. dread of school-related activities
a. dreams
a. duration of labor
a. echocardiogram
a. EEG (electroencephalogram)
a. EEG (electroencephalogram) activity
a. electrical activity
a. electrical activity in brain
a. electrical discharges
a. electrical events in heart
a. electrical impulse
a. electrical stimulus
a. electrocardiogram (ECG/EKG)
a. electroencephalogram (EEG)
a. energy metabolism
a. excitation pattern
a. expansion of blood vessels
a. extension
a. eye movements
a. facies
a. facies and ears
a. fatty tissue
a. fetus
a. filament proteins
a. flexion
a. frontal activity

abnormal—*continued*
- a. functioning of the heart
- a. fusion
- a. gait
- a. gait and flexion
- a. gene
- a. gene therapy
- a. genes, suppress
- a. glucose tolerance test
- a. gross changes
- a. growth of neuronal connections
- a. growth process
- a. hair growth
- a. heart activity
- a. heart contractions
- a. heart rhythm
- a. heart valve function
- a. heartbeat ▸ life-threatening
- a. heartbeats
- a. heat pattern
- a. immunologic response
- a. increase in compliance
- a. intolerance to light
- a. intraluminal pressure
- a. karyotype
- a., left axis deviation (LAD)
- a. level
- a. liver enzymes
- a. liver function
- a. lung sound
- a. magnesium level
- a. mass
- a. mass of tissue growth
- a. memory
- a. metabolic activity
- a. metabolism
- a. milk production
- a. motility
- a. motor movements
- a. movement
- a. myocardial blood flow
- a. murmur
- a. muscle movement
- a. muscle tone ▸ persistent
- a. occlusion
- a. ovulation
- a. palmar crease
- a. Pap (Papanicolaou) smear
- a. pattern
- a. peristaltic actions of colon
- a. personality
- a. plaque deposits
- a. position of infant
- a. potassium level
- a. primary function

- a. proliferation of cuboidal cells
- a. proliferation of syncytial cells
- a. pronation
- a. protrusion
- a. protrusion of eyeball
- a. psychology
- a. pulmonary function
- a. red blood cells (RBC)
- a. residual tissue
- a. rhythmic eye movement
- a. right axis deviation (ARAD)
- a. sac containing fluid
- a. sac containing gas
- a. sac containing semisolid material
- a. segment
- a. sexual response
- a. sleep pattern
- a. social play
- a. social play ▸ absent or
- a. sonic appearance
- a. sounds
- a. sperm
- a. stapes
- a. steepening of cornea
- a. stimulation
- a. supination
- a. tangles of filaments
- a. thermogram
- a. thirst
- a. thyroid activity
- a. tissue
- a. tissue mass
- a. tissue swelling
- a. tremor
- a. uterine bleeding
- a. uterine spasm
- a. vaginal bleeding
- a. veins, eradication of
- a. visual field
- a. wakefulness
- a. wave forms

abnormality(-ies)
- a., arterial blood gas
- a., atrioventricular (AV) conduction
- a., autonomic
- a., biochemical
- a., bony
- a., brain
- a., breast
- a., breathing
- a., caliceal
- a., cardiac
- a., cardiopulmonary
- a., cellular

- a., cervicothoracic vascular
- a. characteristic of seizure
- a. ▸ chill with breast
- a., chemical
- a., chromosomal
- a., clotting
- a., conduction
- a., congenital
- a., congenital bladder
- a., congenital ovarian
- a., craniofacial
- a., developmental
- a., diagnostic
- a., diverticulation
- a., ductal
- a. ▸ electrical activation
- a., electrolyte
- a., endocrine
- a., epileptiform
- a., external
- a., extremity
- a., facial
- a. ▸ facial or limb
- a., fetal
- a. ▸ figure-of-8
- a., focal
- a. ▸ focal limb
- a. from antibiotic ▸ tongue
- a. from cranial nerve problem ▸ taste
- a. from dentures ▸ taste
- a., gait
- a., genetic
- a. ▸ genetic metabolic
- a. ▸ genetic underlying lipid
- a., glandular
- a., growth
- a., heart muscle
- a., heart rhythm
- a. ▸ heart valve
- a., hemodynamic
- a., histopathologic
- a. ▸ immune function
- a., immunochemical
- a., immunologic
- a. in brain ▸ chemical
- a. in brain ▸ inherited
- a. in drug abusers ▸ physical
- a. in gas exchange
- a. in heart rate
- a. ▸ inherited genetic
- a., intracranial
- a. ▸ intracranial vascular
- a. (IRMA) ▸ intraretinal microvascular

a., intrinsic colon
a., joint
a., laboratory
a., left atrial
a. ▸ left ventricular (LV) hemodynamic
a. ▸ left ventricular (LV) wall motion
a. ▸ life-threatening heart rhythm
a., limb
a. ▸ limb reduction
a., lipid
a., liver tissue
a., mental
a., metabolic
a., mild
a., mitral valve
a., mucosal
a., mucous membrane
a. (MEA) ▸ multiple endocrine
a., neurogenic
a., nipple
a., no significant
a., nonpalpable
a., nonspecific hepatocellular
a., nuclear
a. ▸ nuclear membrane
a., nutritional
a., ocular
a. of adrenal gland ▸ enzymatic
a. of fetus
a. of respiratory control
a. of structure and function of mitochondria
a., osseous
a. ovaries ▸ enzymatic
a., palpable
a., pathologic
a., physical
a., postural
a., precancerous
a. ▸ protein binding
a., psychological
a., pulmonary
a. ▸ regional wall motion
a., restrictive
a., retrocardiac
a., rhythm
a., right atrial
a., rotator cuff
a. ▸ schizophrenic brain
a., sensory
a. ▸ severe movement
a., sickle cell
a., significant
a., skeletal

a., snowman
a., S-T and T wave
a., structural
a., taste
a., urachal
a., ureteral
a., urinary
a., vascular
a. ▸ ventricular depolarization
a. ▸ vertebral border
a. ▸ vertebral endplate
a., wall motion

abnormally
a. fast activity
a. high concentration of urine
a. high content
a. low content
a. phosphorylated, proteins
a. rapid heart rate
a. sensitive
a. slow heart beat
a. slow rhythm
a. undersized person

ABO
A. blood type
A. erythroblastosis
A. incompatibility

aborted
a. fetus
a. human fetus
a. human fetus ▸ spontaneously
a. paroxysmal atrial tachycardia
a. systole

aborting drug ▸ migraine
abortion(s)
a., afebrile
a., ampullar
a., cervical
a., chemical
a., complete
a., criminal
a., drug induced
a., early
a. ▸ ectopic pregnancy and
a., epizootic
a., habitual
a., imminent
a., incomplete
a., induced
a., inevitable
a., infectious
a., late
a., live births (GPMAL) ▸ Gravida, para, multiple births
a., missed

a. -on-demand
a. ▸ partial birth
a., repeated spontaneous
a., second trimester
a., self-help
a., septic
a., spontaneous
a., suction aspiration
a., surgical
a. (TAB), therapeutic
a., threatened
a., tubal
a., vibrio

abortive
a. clonus
a. pneumonia
a. poliomyelitis abortivenc

abortus
a., Brucella
a. equi, Salmonella
a., gram-negative Brucella

aboulia (*see* abulia)
about
above
a. elbow (AE)
a. elbow (AE) amputation
a. heart level, elevate feet
a. knee (AK)
a. knee (AK) amputation
a. knee (AK) support
a. level of heart

ABP (arterial blood pressure)
ABPM (ambulatory blood pressure monitor)
ABR (auditory brainstem response)
abraded skin
Abrahams' sign
Abrami's disease
Abrams'
A. heart reflex
A. pleural biopsy punch
A. reflex

Abrasio cornea
abrasion(s)
a. and contusions
a. and/or lacerations
a., corneal
a., cortical
a., extremity
a., facial
a., kinetic
a., multiple
a. of bowel
a., pleural
a., scalp

abrasion(s)—*continued*
   a. ▸ subperiosteal cortical
   a., superficial
   a., truncal
abrasive disc
abreaction(s)
   a., completing the
   a., manage
   a., motor
abridged ocular chart (AOC)
Abrikosov's/Abrikossoff's tumor
abrupt
   a. attack of vertigo
   a. cessation
   a. change in vision
   a. closure
   a. convolution
   a. loss of consciousness
   a. mood change
   a. movement
   a. onset
   a. pulse
   a. recurrence
   a. transient
   a. withdrawal
abruptio, placentae
abruptio placentae, marginal
abruption, placental
ABS, Guinea Pig
ABS, Beef cell
abscess(es) [*absence*]
   a., abdominal
   a., acquired
   a., amebic liver
   a., anaerobic lung
   a., anal
   a., annular
   a., anorectal
   a., aortic annulus
   a., apical
   a., appendiceal
   a., aspiration lung
   a., Bezold's
   a., brain
   a., breast
   a., Brodie's
   a., bronchofocal
   a., candidal
   a., caseocavernous
   a. cavity
   a., cerebellar
   a., cerebral
   a., chronic breast
   a., cold
   a., congenital

a., cutaneous
a. ▸ delirium from brain
a., dentoalveolar
a., diverticular
a. drained
a. drained, rectal
a., draining
a., Dubois'
a., embolic
a., epidural
a., esophageal
a., focal
a. formation
a. formation, focal
a. formation, focal serosal
a. formation, pancreatic
a. formation postcesarean section
a. from breastfeeding ▸ breast
a., frontal
a., fungal
a., gram stain of facial
a., gram stain of pelvic
a., granulomatous
a., hepatic
a., I and D (incision and drainage)
   of ischiorectal
a. ▸ iliac fossa
a. in anal canal
a. incised
a., incision and drainage (I and D)
   of
a., intestinal
a. ▸ intra-abdominal
a., intraperitoneal
a. intrascrotal
a., ischiorectal
a. lancet
a., liver
a., loculated
a., lung
a., mediastinal
a., mixed
a., Munro
a., multiple
a., multiple pulmonary
a., myocardial
a., occult
a. of conjunctiva
a. of cornea
a. of foot
a. of frontal sinus, subperiosteal
a. of heel
a. of lung
a. of motion
a. of orbit

a. of toe
a. of vitreous
a., orbital
a., ovarian
a., Paget's
a., pancreatic
a. ▸ papillary muscle
a., parapharyngeal
a., paraspinal
a., parotid
a., Pautrier's
a., pelvic
a., perianal
a., periapical
a., pericholecystic
a., perihepatic
a., perinephric
a., periodontal
a., perirectal
a., peritoneal
a., peritonsillar
a., perivesical
a., pharyngeal
a., postpharyngeal
a. ▸ premassteric space
a., prostatic
a., psoas
a., pulmonary
a., pyogenic
a., rectal
a., renal
a., retropharyngeal
a., ring
a., ruptured peritonsillar
a., scalp
a., scrotal
a., soft tissue
a. ▸ space of Retzius
a., spinal cord
a. ▸ spinal epidural
a., splenic
a., staphylococcal
a., sternal
a., stitch
a., subdiaphragmatic
a., subdural
a., subhepatic
a., subphrenic
a., supralevator
a. testicular
a., throat
a., thyroid
a., tooth
a., traumatic
a., tubo-ovarian

a., tympanomastoid
a., vaginal cuff
a. ▸ ventral epidural
a., wound
abscessed, pseudocysts
abscessus ▸ Mycobacterium
abscission/abscision
abscission, corneal
absence [*abscess*]
    a., congenital
    a. of breast, surgical
    a. of breathing, temporary
    a. of circulation on 4 vessel
        angiography, total
    a. of consciousness ▸ temporary
    a. of depth perception ▸ permanent
    a. of electrical activity
    a. of eyeball
    a. of facial and pubic hair
    a. of fallopian tubes ▸ surgical
    a. of feeling
    a. of friction rub
    a. of heartbeat
    a. of infection
    a. of kidney, congenital
    a. of limb, surgical
    a. of menstrual periods
    a. of movement
    a. of ovaries ▸ surgical
    a. of pedicles
    a. of premonitory symptoms
    a. of pulmonary artery, congenital
    a. of pus cells
    a. of respiration
    a. of seizures
    a. of sense of smell
    a. of sense of touch
    a. of sensibility to pain
    a. of skin ▸ congenital localized
    a. of speech
    a. of ureter, congenital
    a. of urinary bladder ▸ congenital
    a. of uterus, surgical
    a. of vagina, congenital
    a. of voluntary muscle movement
absent
    a. bowel function
    a., breast surgically
    a. breath sounds
    a. breathing ▸ period of
    a., congenitally
    a. corneal reflexes
    a. corneal reflexes, bradycardia
    a. menses
    a. menstrual period from diabetes

a. oculocephalic reflex
a. or abnormal social play
a. pericardium
a. pericardium, congenitally
a., pulse
a. radii (TAR) ▸ thrombocytopenia
    with
a. radius syndrome ▸
    thrombocytopenia-
a., reflex
a. respiration
a. social play
a. spontaneous respiration
a., uterus surgically
absentia epileptica
absentminded, patient
Absidia corymbifera
Absidia ramosa
absolute
    a. accommodation
    a. agraphia
    a. amenorrhea
    a., atmospheric
    a. basophil count
    a. cardiac dullness (ACD)
    a. dehydration
    a. diet
    a. glaucoma
    a. hemianopia
    a. idiocy
    a. intensity
    a. iodine uptake (AIO)
    a. physical measurement
    a. pitch
    a. polycythemia
    a. refractory period (ARP)
    a. scale
    a. scotoma
    a. sterility
    a. strabismus
    a. temperature
    a. viscosity
    a. zero
absorbable
    a. gelatin sponge
    a. surgical suture
    a. suture ▸ monofilament
absorbed
    a. dose, average target
    a. dose, maximum target
    a. dose, minimum target
    a. fraction
    a. ▸ patient self-
    a. poison
    a. radiation

absorbent
    a., antibody
    a. gauze
    a. sterile towels
absorbing and stabilizing ▸ shock-
absorbing quality, ultraviolet
absorptiometry (DEXA) bone density
    test ▸ dual energy x-ray
absorptiometry (DEXA) ▸ dual energy
    x-ray
absorption
    a., alcohol
    a., anesthesia
    a. atelectasis
    a., bone
    a. by radiation, tissue
    a., calcium
    a., carbohydrate
    a. coefficient, linear
    a. coefficient, mass
    a., drug
    a. edges
    a., electromagnetic
    a. enhancer
    a. equivalent thickness (AET)
    a., fantasy proneness and
    a., fat
    a. fever
    a. fluorescent treponemal
    a. in coronary laser angiography
    a. intestinal
    a., iron
    a. ▸ laser energy
    a., light
    a. of cerebrospinal fluid (CSF)
    a. of nicotine
    a. of nutrients
    a., percutaneous
    a., photoelectric
    a. process
    a. process ▸ neutron
    a., protein digestion
    a., radiofrequency
    a., self
    a., shock
    a., small intestine
    a. spectrophotometer
    a. spectrum
    a. studies
    a. studies, fat
    a. study, triolein fat
    a., systemic
    a. test ▸ conglutinating complement
    a. test, d-xylose
    a. test, fat

absorption—*continued*
- a. test ▸ fluorescent treponemal antibody
- a. test, glucose

absorptive mechanisms
abstention vs. moderation of drug use
abstinence(s)
- a., alcohol
- a. -based counseling
- a., cocaine
- a., complete
- a., continued
- a., continuous
- a. from chemicals ▸ periodic
- a. goals
- a., imposed
- a. ▸ initial cocaine
- a., initiating
- a., lifelong
- a., maintain
- a. ▸ maintain sobriety and
- a., methadone
- a., morphine
- a. oriented treatment
- a., periods of
- a., posttreatment
- a. rates ▸ differentials in
- a. ▸ self-imposed
- a. symptom evaluation (ASE)
- a. symptomatology
- a. syndrome
- a. syndrome, acute
- a., total

abstinent
- a. alcoholic
- a. or relapsed
- a., totally

abstract
- a. conceptual memory
- a. conceptual memory, delayed
- a. conceptual memory organization, competent
- a. form
- a. functioning
- a. operational thinking
- a. reasoning
- a. thinking
- a. thinking, ability of
- a. thinking, impaired
- a. thought ▸ decreased capacity for
- a. verbal command

abstractly, think
Abt-Letterer-Siwe syndrome
abulia (*same as* aboulia)
abulia, cyclic

abundant aspirated amnion
abundant leukemic infiltrates
Aburel's operation
abuse(s) (Abuse)
- a. accommodation syndrome, child
- a., adolescent alcohol
- a., adolescent chemical
- a., adolescent drug
- a., adult chemical
- a. ▸ agitation, delusions and tendency to self-
- a., alcohol
- a. ▸ alcohol and substance
- a., alcoholism and drug
- a., alcohol or drug
- a. among men ▸ alcohol
- a. among women ▸ alcohol
- a., amphetamine
- a. ▸ amphetamine or similarly acting sympathomimetic
- a., anabolic steroid
- a. and addiction ▸ treatment of drug
- A. and Neglect (SCAN), Stop Child
- a., antibiotic
- a., antibiotic use and
- a., antisocial behavior and drug
- a., antisocial personality and drug
- a., attachment
- a., autogenic training in drug
- a., barbiturate
- a. behavior
- a. behavior ▸ self-inflicted
- a., behavioral treatment for drug
- a. benefits, substance
- a., cannabis
- a., cardiovascular complications of drug
- a., cardiovascular problems related to drug
- a., cause of drug
- a., child
- a., childhood
- a., childhood sexual
- a., chronic alcohol
- a., chronic child
- a., chronic cocaine
- a., chronic inhalant
- a., chronic opiate
- a., chronic substance
- a., cocaine
- a., cognitive therapy of substance
- a., comorbid alcohol
- a., comorbid cocaine
- a., comorbid opioid

- a., comorbidity of schizophrenia and substance
- a., complications of drug
- a., compulsive
- a., continuous and confirmed memories of
- a. counseling, chemical
- a. counseling, drug
- a. counselor ▸ substance
- a., crack
- a. ▸ cutaneous signs as a screening device for
- a., cutaneous signs of drug
- a., cyclic epidemics of use and
- a. death ▸ drug and alcohol
- a., death due to drug
- a., dermatologic complications of drug
- a. diagnoses, drug
- a., diagnostic tests as a screening device for drug
- a., diagnostic tests in drug
- a. disorder ▸ psychoactive substance
- a. disorder, substance
- a. ▸ dissociation and sexual
- a., domestic
- a., drug
- a. drug testing, alcohol and drug
- a. drugs, treatment of physicians who
- a. during pregnancy ▸ substance
- a. ▸ early intervention in drug
- a., economic costs of drug
- a. education, drug
- a., elder
- a., eliminate alcohol
- a., emotional
- a., endocrinologic complications of drug
- a., endocrinologic problems related to drug
- a., ethanol
- a., ethical
- a., euphoria and drug
- a., fatal child
- a., financial
- a., gastrointestinal (GI) complications of drug
- a., genetic factors in drug
- a., genitourinary (GU) complications of drug
- a., genitourinary (GU) problems related to drug

a., GI (gastrointestinal) problems related to drug
a. group, sexual
a., GU (genitourinary) complications of drug
a., GU (genitourinary) problems related to drug
a., hallucinogen
a., hematopoietic complications of drug
a., hematopoietic problems related to drug
a., hepatic complications of drug
a., hepatic problems related to drug
a. hotline, drug
a., hypnotic
a. ▸ illicit drug
a. ▸ illusory child
a. in alcoholics, prevalence of drug
a. in general patient population, prevalence of drug
a. in physician population, prevalence of drug
a. in pregnancy ▸ polysubstance
a., incestuous
a., incidence of drug
a., inhalant
a., international trends in drug
a. intervention
a., laxative
a., legal restrictions in drug
a. ▸ linking cigarette smoking and drug
a., medical history as screening device for drug
a., memories
a. ▸ memories of child
a., mental
a., monitoring systems in drug
a., multi-drug
a., narcotics
A. (NDA) ▸ National Institute on Drug
a., neonatal complications of drug
a., neuromuscular complications of drug
a., neuromuscular problems related to drug
a., obstetric complications of drug
a. of children, sexual
a. of drugs, acute
a. of drugs, chronic
a. of drugs, nondependent
a. of illicit drug ▸ prenatal
a. of licit drug ▸ prenatal

a. of prescribed drugs
a. of the elderly
a., opioid
a. or neglect, child
a., parent
a., partner
a., patient behavior as a screening device for drug
a., patient education on drug
a., patient had flashback reactions from drug
a., patient interview as a screening device for drug
a., patient questionnaire as a screening device for drug
a., pattern of cannabinoid
a., pattern of depressant
a., pattern of hallucinogen
a., pattern of inhalant
a., pattern of opioid
a., pattern of phencyclidine
a., pattern of stimulant
a. patterns, variety of
a. ▸ perinatal substance
a. ▸ pharmacotherapy of substance
a., phencyclidine (PCP)
a., physical
a., physical effects of cannabinoid
a., physical effects of depressant
a., physical effects of drug
a., physical effects of hallucinogen
a., physical effects of inhalant
a., physical effects of opioid
a., physical effects of phencyclidine
a., physical effects of stimulant
a. ▸ physical examination as a screening device for drug
a., physician drug
a., polysubstance
a., polysubstance use and
a. potential
a. potential of cannabinoids
a. potential of depressants
a. potential of hallucinogens
a. potential of inhalants
a. potential of multiple drugs
a. potential of opioids
a. potential of phencyclidines
a. potential of stimulants
a., preschool sexual
a. ▸ prescription drug
a., prevalence of cannabinoid
a., prevalence of depressant
a., prevalence of drug
a., prevalence of hallucinogen

a., prevalence of inhalant
a., prevalence of opioid
a., prevalence of phencyclidine
a., prevalence of stimulant
a. prevention, drug-
a., prevention of child
a. ▸ primary chemical of
a. problems ▸ children with alcohol
a. problems ▸ men with alcohol
a. problems ▸ women with alcohol
a. program, drug-
a., prolonged
a., propylhexedrine
a., psychiatric complications of drug
a., psychoactive substances
a., psychological
a., psychological effects of cannabinoid
a., psychological effects of drug
a., psychological factors in drug
a., psychological history as a screening device for drug
a., psychological problems related to drug
a., pulmonary complications of drug
a. -reactive behavior
a., recreational drug
a. rehabilitation, substance
a. related depression
a., renal complications of drug
a., renal problems related to drug
a., reproductive complications of drug
A. Resistant Education (DARE) ▸ Drug
a., ritual
a., ritual/cult
a., ritualistic
A. (SRA) Sadistic Ritual
a., screening for drug
a., sedative
a. ▸ sedative, hypnotic, or anxiolytic
a. ▸ self-destructive alcohol
a., septic complications of drug
a., septic problems related to drug
a. services ▸ psychiatric and substance
a. ▸ severe and relentless child
a. ▸ severe trauma and
a., sexual
a., sexual complications of drug
a., social history as a screening device for drug
a., sociological factors in drug
a., spousal

abuse—*continued*
a., spouse
a. statements ▸ makes
a., substance
a. ▸ sudden death due to alcohol
a., survivor of
a. ▸ survivors of sexual
a., surgical complications of drug
a., suspected child
a. ▸ sustained sexual
a., sympathomimetic
a., symptoms as a screening device for drug
a., symptoms of drug
a., system
a., systemic signs of drug
a. threat, drug
a., tobacco
a. treatment, alcohol
a. treatment, alcohol and drug-
a. treatment, cocaine
a. treatment, drug-
a. treatment, drug
a. treatment, family sexual
a. treatment field ▸ substance
A. Treatment (JSAT) Journal of Substance
a. treatment outcome ▸ substance
a. treatment professionals ▸ alcohol and substance
a. treatment program ▸ publicly assisted drug
a. treatment, substance
a., trends in drug
a., verbal
a. victims sexual
a. vulnerability ▸ polysubstance
a. warning, drug
A. Warning Network (DAWN), Drug
a. ▸ warning signs of drug
abused
a. drugs, psychoactive properties of
a. drugs, selection of
a. child
a. children, sexually
a. parent
a. substance
abuser(s)
a., alcohol
a., assessing needs of cannabinoid
a., assessing needs of depressant
a., assessing needs of hallucinogen
a., assessing needs of inhalant
a., assessing needs of multi-drug

a., assessing needs of opioid
a., assessing needs of phencyclidine
a., assessing needs of stimulant
a., attitudes of drug
a., attitudes of physician drug
a., attitudes of society towards drug
a., big H (heroin)
a., cocaine
a. ▸ cocaine free-base
a., confrontation techniques with drug
a., dangerous drug
a., demanding drug
a., hard core drug
a., heroin (big H)
a. ▸ indifferent drug
a. ▸ irresponsible drug
a., IV (intravenous) drug
a. ▸ manipulative drug
a., medical problems in drug
a., methamphetamine
a., obstetrical management of drug
a., physical abnormalities in drug
a., psychiatric disorders in drug
a., psychological problems of drug
a., retention of cocaine
a., risk factors for drug
a. ▸ schizophrenic cocaine
a., sexual complications of drug
a., substance
a., surgical management of drug
abusing
a. mother, drug
a. mothers, substance
a. patients, substance
a. pregnant women ▸ drug
a. women, crack
a. women, opioid
abusive
a. and hostile, patient
a. behavior
a. experience, sexually
a. family system
a., invasive person
a. marriage
a. patient ▸ severely self
a. patterns
a., psychologically
a. relationships
abutment, intermediate
abutment teeth
abutting beams
AC (ac)
A. (acromioclavicular)

A. (air conduction)
A. (axiocervical)
a. (before meals)
A. (accelerator) globulin
A. (alternating current) resistance
A. (acromioclavicular) separation
A. (alternating current) signals, low frequency
A. (alternating current) voltage
AC > BC (air conduction greater than bone conduction)
AC < BC (air conduction less than bone conduction)
AC (BC > AC) ▸ BC greater than
AC (BC < AC) ▸ BC less than
AC (alternating current) ▸ opposition of flow of
ACA (accessory conduction ablation)
Acacia contrast medium, Skiodan
acacia, gum
academic(s)
a. achievement
a. achievement of child
a. achievement ▸ poor
a. inhibition ▸ adjustment disorder with
a. medicine
a. or work inhibition
a. performance ▸ drop in
a. problem
a. progress
a. teaching hospital
a. underachievement disorder
Academy of Child and Adolescent Psychiatry (AACAP) ▸ American
Academy of Neurology ▸ American
acalculous cholecystitis, acute
acanthamoeba (Acanthamoeba)
a. keratitis
A. palestinensis
A. polyphaga
Acanthocheilonema perstans
acantholytic dermatosis ▸ transient
acanthomeatal line
acanthosis nigricans
acanthrotrias, Cysticercus
Acapulco Gold (grade of marijuana)
acardiacus, fetus
acariasis, chorioptic
ACAT (automated computerized axial tomography)
accelerate bone maturation
accelerated
a. atrioventricular (AV) junctional rhythm

a. blockage in arteries
a. breathing, shallow
a. conduction
a. -decelerated breathing ▸ shallow
a. dementia
a. destruction of red blood cells (RBC)
a. fractionation
a. hypertension
a. idionodal rhythm
a. idioventricular rhythm
a. idioventricular tachycardia
a. intraventricular rhythm
a. junctional rhythm
a. liver damage
a. macrovascular disease
a. painless labor
a. pathway
a. peristalsis
a. reaction
a. respiration
a. tissue regeneration
a. treatment
a. ventricular rhythm
accelerating center
accelerating heart rate
acceleration
a., body
a. -dependent aberrancy
a. of blood flow
a. of heart rate, operant
a. time
accelerator (Accelerator)
a., Clinic 18 linear
a. ▸ dual energy linear
a. ▸ dual photon energy
a., dual photon linear
A. (AG) Globulin
a., high energy bent beam linear
a., linear
a. ▸ low energy linear
a., low energy straight beam linear
a. nerves
a., nuclear
a. (SPCA) ▸ serum prothrombin-conversion
a., serum thrombotic
accent syndrome ▸ foreign
accentuated antagonism
accentuated heartbeat
accept or reject medical treatment
acceptable
a. behavior ▸ normal
a. channels, socially
a., morally

acceptance
a. of chemical dependency
a. of death
a. of loss
a., self-
a., social
accepting illness
access
a. atrial pacing
a. bypass procedure ▸ port-
a. catheter ▸ multi-
a., controlled fluid
a. coronary artery bypass grafting ▸ port-
a. coronary artery bypass (PACAB) ▸ port-
a. device-related bacteremia ▸ venous
a., direct
a. in hemodialysis, vascular
a. method
a., portal venous
a., random
a. ▸ side-entry
a. system ▸ peripheral
a. time
a. to fluids, controlled
a., wheelchair
accessibility
a., barrier-free
a., evaluation
a., handicapped
a., maximum
accessible, wheelchair
accessional teeth
accessorium, pancreas
accessory
a. arteriovenous (AV) connection
a. artery
a. atrioventricular (AV) connection
a. atrioventricular (AV) pathways
a. atrium
a. bone
a. cephalic vein
a. chain lymph nodes, spinal
a. conduction ablation (ACA)
a. cramp
a. cuneate nucleus
a. cusp
a. deep peroneal nerve
a. diaphragm
a. -facial neuroanastomosis ▸ spinal
a. fissure, inferior
a. flexor muscle

a. food substance
a. ganglia
a. hemiazygos vein
a. -hypoglossal neuroanastomosis ▸ spinal
a. ligament
a. middle cerebral artery
a. muscles
a. muscles of respiration
a. nerve
a. nerve signs
a. nerve, spinal
a. nerve, vagal
a. nodoventricular fibers
a. pancreas
a. pathway
a. pathway effective refractory period (APERP)
a. phrenic nerves
a. placenta
a. processes
a. saphenous vein
a. sinus
a. spleen
a. thyroid
a. thymic nodules
a. vertebral vein
a. yolk
accident(s)
a. (CVA), acute cerebrovascular
a., alcohol-related
a., auto-pedestrian
a., cardiac
a. (CVA) ▸ cardiovascular
a. (CVA) ▸ cerebrovascular
a., childhood
a. chorea, postcerebrovascular
a. form
a., industrial
a., intracerebrovascular
a. (CVA), lacunar cerebrovascular
a. neurosis
a., nuclear
a. prevention
a. prone
a. prone, patient
a. -related forms
a., treatment of
a., vehicular
accidental
a. amputation
a. burn
a. death
a. death, patient died
a. exposure

accidental—*continued*
- a. hypothermia
- a. image
- a. inhalation
- a. injury
- a. murmur
- a. needle stick
- a. overdose
- a. parasite
- a. positional asphyxia
- a. poisoning
- a. tissue
- a. wound
- a. wound ▸ delayed closure of

accidentally swallowed foreign body
acclimation to heat and work
accommodation(s)
- a., absolute
- a., amplitude of
- a. and compensation
- a., binocular
- a., breadth of
- a., excessive
- a. (L and A) ▸ light and
- a., negative
- a., nerve
- a. of eye ▸ paralysis of
- a., positive
- a. (PERLA) ▸ pupils equal, react to light and
- a. (PERRLA) ▸ pupils equal, round, react to light and
- a. (PRLA) ▸ pupils react to light and
- a., range of
- a., reflex
- a., region of
- a., relative
- a., subnormal
- a. syndrome, child abuse
- a., wheelchair

accommodative
- a. asthenopia
- a. squint
- a. strabismus

accompanying
- a. fever, convulsion
- a. patient on admission ▸ orders
- a. vein
- a. vein of hypoglossal nerve

accomplished
- a., hemostasis
- a., peritoneal closure
- a., reconstruction

accomplishments ▸ inflated judgment of

accomplishments, inflates
according to Greulich and Pyle, bone age
accordion graft
accouchement forcé
accoucheur's hand
accredited psychiatric hospital
accredited sponsor
accreta, placenta
accretio cordis
accretio pericardii
Accu-Chek II
accumulated knowledge
accumulated radiation
accumulating ascites, rapidly
accumulation
- a. and inflammation ▸ fluid
- a. and swelling ▸ fluid
- a., copper
- a. ▸ endobronchial round cell
- a., fluid
- a., focal
- a. in arm ▸ fluid
- a. in legs ▸ fluid
- a. in lung ▸ fluid
- a., lipid
- a. of bile pigments
- a. of blood within joint
- a. of fluid
- a. of fluid, abnormal
- a. of glycogen ▸ excessive
- a. of pus
- a., plaque
- a. test, chlormerodrin

accumulative radiation
accuracy, enhanced
accuracy rate
accurate
- a. digital readout
- a. feedback
- a. information

accusations ▸ retract true
ACD (absolute cardiac dullness)
ACD (active compression-decompression)
ACE (Ace) (ace)
- A. (angiotensin converting enzyme)
- A. (marijuana cigarette)
- A. bandage
- A. (angiotensin converting enzyme) inhibitor
- A. inhibitor ▸ longer acting
- a. of spades sign
- A. wrap

acellular
- a. areas, hyaline
- a. pertussis vaccine ▸ diphtheria, tetanus toxoids, and
- a., specimen

acentric occlusion
Acer plantanoides
Aceraria spiralis
acervulus cerebri
acetabular
- a. angles
- a. asymmetry
- a. bone
- a. cup, Aufranc-Turner
- a. fragments
- a. labrum
- a. notch
- a. region, left
- a. region, right

Acetabularia crenulata
Acetabularia mediterranea
acetabuli, os
acetabulum
- a. of pelvis
- a., pelvic protrusion of
- a., sunken

acetaldehyde levels
acetaminophen, hepatitis and
acetate (DMPA) ▸ depomedroxyprogesterone
acetate, serum
aceti, Acetobacter
aceti, Mycoderma
acetic
- a. acid
- a. acid ▸ aceto▸
- a. acid reaction
- a. acid test
- a. acid test ▸ aceto▸
- a. transaminase (SGOT), serum glutamic-oxalo-

acetoacetic acid
acetoacetic acid test
Acetobacter
- A. aceti
- A. kuetzingianus
- A. melanogenus
- A. oxydans
- A. pasteurianus
- A. rancens
- A. roseus
- A. suboxydans
- A. xylinum
- A. xylinus

acetobutylicum, Clostridium

acetone
- a. extract of cannabis (Smash)
- a., plasma
- a. test
- a., urine

acetosoluble albumin
acetrizoate sodium contrast medium
acetyl choline receptors
acetylating enzyme
acetylsalicylic acid
acetyltransferase activity
acetyltransferase, aminoglycoside
acetyltyrosine ethyl ester
ACF (accessory clinical findings)
achalasia
- a., cricopharyngeal
- a., esophageal

Achard-Thiers syndrome
Achatina fulica
ache(s)
- a. and pains, chronic
- a. and pains ▸ fatigue, muscles
- a. and pains, general
- a. and pains ▸ generalized
- a. and pains ▸ psychosomatic
- a. and pains ▸ vague
- a., back◊
- a., body
- a., ear◊
- a., eye
- a. ▸ generalized muscle
- a., joint
- a., joint and muscle
- a., muscle
- a., neck
- a., pains and stiffness
- a., tooth◊
- a. and pains, general
- a., muscular

achieve high dose
achieve independence ▸ help patient
achievement
- a., academic
- a. age (AA)
- a., creative
- a. level
- a. of child, academic
- a. ▸ poor academic
- a. quotient
- A. Test, Wide Range

achieving tendency
Achillea millefolium
Achilles
- A. bursa
- A. bursitis

A. jerk
A. tendon
A. tendon reflex, timed
A. tendon rupture
A. tendinitis

achillotenotomy, plastic
achiness, general
aching
- a. and burning pain ▸ stiffness,
- a. and numbness
- a. and stiffness
- a. and stiffness ▸ widespread muscle
- a. back, chronic
- a., diffuse
- a. feet
- a. feet, tired
- a., generalized
- a. joints
- a., pain and stiffness ▸ muscle tension,
- a. pain, deep
- a. pain, dull
- a. pain, localized
- a. pain, persistent
- a. pressure discomfort ▸ diffuse, dull,
- a., pulling or itching feeling ▸ fidgeting
- a. sensation, persistent

achlorhydria apepsia
acholangic biliary cirrhosis
Acholeplasma laidlawii
acholuric hemolytic icterus
achondroplasia
- a., heterozygous
- a., homozygous
- a., hyperplastic

achondroplastic dwarfs
Achorion fungi
achrestic anemia
achromatic
- a. lens
- a. mass
- a. objective
- a. vision

achromatin, fascicular
achromic erythrocyte
Achromobacter xylosoxidans
achy feeling in leg ▸ crampy,
achylia gastrica haemorrhagica
achylia pancreatica
achylic anemia
ACI (asymptomatic cardiac ischemia)
acid(s) (Acid)

A. (LSD)
- a., acetic
- a., acetylsalicylic
- a. albumin
- a. alcohol resistance
- a., alpha amino
- a., alpha amino-n-butyric
- a., amino
- a., aminolevulinic
- a., aminopenicillanic
- a., aminosalicylic
- a. analyzer, amino
- a. anemia, folic
- a. antagonist ▸ folic
- a., ascorbic
- a. aspiration syndrome ▸ pulmonary
- a. balance of vagina
- a. base alterations
- a. base balance
- a. base disorder
- a. base disturbance
- a. base imbalance
- a. base physiology
- a. base ratio
- a. base therapy
- a. (BOBA), beta-oxybutyric
- a., bile
- a. binding resin, bile
- a., blood uric
- A. (LSD), Blotter
- a. burn
- a. calculus, uric
- a. content of stomach
- a. contrast medium, iodalphionic
- a. contrast medium, iopanoic
- a. contrast medium, iophenoxic
- a. core, nucleic
- a. crystals, fatty
- a. crystals, uric
- a. deficiency ▸ folic
- a. dehydrase, aminolevulinic
- a., delta-aminolevulinic
- a. (DNA), deoxyribonucleic
- a. (RNA) dependent DNA (deoxyribonucleic acid) polymerase ▸ ribonucleic
- a. depletion, ovarian ascorbic
- a., diacetic
- a. diathesis, uric
- a. diet, low uric
- a. diethylamide (LSD) addict, lysergic
- a. diethylamide (LSD) addiction, lysergic

acid(s)—*continued*

a. diethylamide (LSD) dependency, lysergic
a. diethylamide (LSD) habit, lysergic
a. diethylamide (LSD)-induced psychosis ▸ lysergic
a. diethylamide (LSD) ingested, lysergic
a. diethylamide (LSD) intoxication ▸ lysergic
a. diethylamide (LSD), lysergic
a. diethylamide (LSD) user, lysergic
a. diethylamide (LSD) withdrawal, lysergic
a. digestion
a. diuresis
a. dyspepsia
a. efficiency, lactic
a. effusion
a., essential fatty
a. ethyl ester ▸ fatty
a., excess fatty
a., excess uric
a. -fast
a. -fast bacilli
a. -fast bacillus (AFB)
a. -fast bacteria
a. -fast organism
a. -fast stain
a. -fast stain of sputum
a., fatty
a. (5-HIAA), 5-hydroxyindole-acetic
a. flow
a., folic
a., formiminoglutamic
a., free fatty
a., free hydrochloric
a., fusidic
a. (GABA), gamma aminobutyric
a., gastric
a., gluconic
a., glucuronic
a. heartburn
a., hippuric
a., histamine phosphate
a., homogentisic
a., homovanillic
a. hydrazide, isonicotinic
a., hydrochloric
a., hydroxyindoleacetic
a., hydroxyl aminobutyric
a. in stomach ▸ neutralizing
a. indigestion
a. infarct, uric

a. inhibitor, gastric
a. into esophagus ▸ backwash of stomach
a. intoxication
a. labile
a., lactic
a., leukocyte ascorbic
a. level in blood ▸ high
a. level, isovaleric
a. level, uric
a., long chain fatty
a. (DNA) maker ▸ deoxyribo-nucleic
a., mandelic
a., medium chain fatty
a. (mRNA), messenger ribonucleic
a. ▸ metabolic waste product lactic
a. metabolism, amino
a. metabolism ▸ disorder of amino
a. metabolites, arachidonic
a. (DNA) molecules, deoxyribonucleic
a. mucopolysaccharide
a., neutralization
a., nicotine
a., nucleic
a. output, basal
a. output, maximal
a., oxalic
a., pantothenic
a. (LSD), Paper
a., penicillic
a. (PPA), phenylpyruvic
a. phosphatase
a. phosphatase, prostatic
a. phosphatase (TSPAP) ▸ total serum prestatic
a. phosphate
a. (DNA) polymerase activity deoxyribonucleic
a. (DNA) polymerase ▸ ribonucleic acid (RNA) dependent deoxyribonucleic
a., polyunsaturated fatty
a. production
a. production, free fatty
a., pteroylglutamic
a., pyruvic
a., radioiodinated fatty
a. reaction
a. reaction, acetic
a. (DNA) ▸ recombinant deoxyribonucleic
a. reduction
a. reflux
a. reflux disease

a. -resistant and penicillinase-resistant penicillins
a. -resistant penicillins
a. (RNA) reverse transcriptase ▸ ribonucleic
a. (RNA) ▸ ribonucleic
a., salicylic
a. (HIDA) scan ▸ hepatoiminodiacetic
a. secretion
a. secretion, gastric
a. sequence, amino
A. (DNA) sequencing ▸ deoxyribonucleic
A. sequestrants, bile
a., serum uric
a. (RNA) ▸ soluble ribonucleic
a. stable
a. stain
a., stomach
a. (DNA) switch ▸ deoxyribo-nucleic
a. (DNA) synthesis, deoxyribonucleic
a. synthesis, folic
a., synthesize fatty
a. taste in mouth
a. technology ▸ nucleic
a. test, acetic
a. test, acetoacetic
a. test, ascorbic
a. test, bile
a. test, hippuric
a. test, homogentisic
a. test, lactic
a. test, phosphoric
a. test, uric
a., tetrahydrofolic
a., titers, anti-teichoic
a., total fatty
a. ▸ trans-fatty
a., trichloroacetic
a., triglyceride fatty
a. ulcers
a., unesterified fatty
a., uric
a., uridine diphosphoglucuronic
a., usnic
a., vanillylmandelic
a. (DNA) virus, deoxyribonucleic
a. (RNA) virus, ribonucleic
acidemia, isovaleric
acidemia, methylmalonic
acidic
a. fibroblast growth factor
a. fluid

a. foods
acidifiers, urinary
acidilactici, Bacillus
acidilactici, Pediococcus
acidity
   a., gastric
   a., neutralize stomach
   a., stomach
   a., total
   a., vaginal
acidophil/acidophile
acidophil granules
acidophilic
   a. adenoma
   a. cell
   a. erythroblast
   a. index
acidophilus, Lactobacillus
acidophilus milk
acidosis
   a. and coma, severe metabolic
   a., anion gap metabolic
   a., cannulation-induced metabolic
   a., diabetic
   a., hypercapnic
   a., hyperchloremic
   a., hyperchloremic renal
   a., increasing respiratory
   a., ketotic
   a., lactic
   a., metabolic
   a., methylmalonic
   a., nonrespiratory
   a., renal tubular
   a., respiratory
   a., severe
   a., starvation
   a. test
   a., terminal respiratory
   a., uremic
acidotic and hypoxic ▸ infant
acidulated compound
aciduria
   a., glutaric
   a., orotic
   a. ▸ test for glutaric
acinar
   a. adenocarcinoma
   a. cancer
   a. carcinoma
   a. cells
   a. cells columnar
   a. cells ▸ cuboidal to columnar
   a. connective tissue, overgrowth of inter-

a. connective tissue, overgrowth of intra-
   a. emphysema, central
   a. emphysema ▸ mild centri-
   a. nodule
   a. tissue ▸ atrophy of
Acinetobacter
   A. anitratus
   A. calcoaceticus
   A. calcoaceticus baumannii complex
   A. ▸ gram-negative coccobacilli
   A. lwoffi
   A. parapertussis
   A. species
acini
   a., atrophic
   a., digestive
   a., residual
   a., thyroid
acinic cell adenocarcinoma
acinous cancer
acinous carcinoma
acinus, lung
AC (acromioclavicular) joint
Ackerman's criteria
aclasis, diaphyseal
aclasis, tarsoepiphyseal
ACLS (advanced cardiac life support)
ACLS protocol ▸ (advanced cardiac life support)
acmesthesia/acmaesthesia
acne
   a., adult
   a., aged
   a. areata
   a. blemishes
   a. ciliaris
   a., comedo
   a. conglobata
   a., cystic
   a. cystica
   a. disseminata
   a. excoriée des jeunes
   a., facial
   a. indurata
   a. juvenilis
   a. lancet
   a. mechanica
   a. neonatorum
   a., noncystic
   a. papulosa
   a. pitting
   a. -prone pores
   a., propionibacterium

a. pustulosa
   a. rosacea
   a. rosacea conjunctivitis
   a. rosacea keratitis
   a. scars
   a. sebacea
   a. urticata
   a. varioliformis
   a. vulgaris
acneform eruption
acneiform/acneform
acnes, Corynebacterium
acnes, Propionibacterium
ACOA (Adult Children of Alcoholics)
acollis, uterus
acorn-shaped implant
acorn-tipped catheter
Acosta's disease
acoustic
   a. agnosia
   a. agraphia
   a. and phonetic analysis
   a. aphasia
   a. artery ▸ primitive
   a. chamber
   a. hair cell
   a. imaging
   a. impedance
   a. meatus
   a. meatus, external
   a. meatus, internal
   a. meatus, nerve of external
   a. microscope
   a. nerve
   a. nerve signs
   a. neurinoma
   a. neuritis
   a. neuroma
   a. neuroma ▸ slow-growing
   a. neurotomy
   a. papilla
   a. pressure amplitude
   a. quantification
   a. radiation
   a. reflex testing
   a. shadow
   a. shadowing
   a. shock wave ▸ photo
   a. stimulation (FAS) ▸ fetal
   a. stimulus
   a. striae
   a. trauma
   a. trauma deafness
   a. tubercle
   a. tumor

acoustic—*continued*
- a. window

acoustogram study

ACPE (acute cardiogenic pulmonary edema)

acquaductus fallopi, knee of

acquaintance
- a. rape
- a. rape perpetrator
- a. rape victim

acquired
- a. abscess
- a. agammaglobulinemia
- a. atelectasis
- a. bladder infection, community-
- a. bloodstream infection ▸ hospital-
- a. character
- a. color deficiency
- a. defect of labyrinth
- a. disease, newly
- a. dysmenorrhea
- a. epilepsy
- a. functional megacolon
- a. group A Streptococcus ▸ autopsy-
- a. harelip
- a. hemolytic anemia
- a. hepatitis, autopsy-
- a. hernia
- a. hydrocephalus
- a. hypogammaglobulinemia
- a. immune deficiency syndrome (AIDS)
- a. immune deficiency syndrome (AIDS) antibodies
- a. immune deficiency syndrome (AIDS) antibody
- a. immune deficiency syndrome (AIDS) associated
- a. immune deficiency syndrome (AIDS) carrier, patient
- a. immune deficiency syndrome (AIDS) carrier, patient unknown
- a. immune deficiency syndrome (AIDS) crisis
- a. immune deficiency syndrome (AIDS) dementia complex
- a. immune deficiency syndrome (AIDS) ▸ emotional effects of
- a. immune deficiency syndrome (AIDS) epidemic
- a. immune deficiency syndrome (AIDS), fetal

- a. immune deficiency syndrome (AIDS), heterosexual contact with male carriers of
- a. immune deficiency syndrome (AIDS) illness
- a. immune deficiency syndrome (AIDS) infected child
- a. immune deficiency syndrome (AIDS) mandatory testing
- a. immune deficiency syndrome (AIDS) patient
- a. immune deficiency syndrome (AIDS), patient at risk for
- a. immune deficiency syndrome (AIDS) patients ▸ secretions and spills from
- a. immune deficiency syndrome (AIDS) ▸ prevention
- a. immune deficiency syndrome (AIDS) primary pathogen
- a. immune deficiency syndrome (AIDS) related complex (ARC)
- a. immune deficiency syndrome (AIDS) -related dementia
- a. immune deficiency syndrome (AIDS) -related macular degeneration
- a. immune deficiency syndrome (AIDS) related pneumonia
- a. immune deficiency syndrome (AIDS) residential treatment facility
- a. immune deficiency syndrome (AIDS) -tainted transfusion
- a. immune deficiency syndrome (AIDS) testing
- a. immune deficiency syndrome (AIDS) testing, mandatory
- a. immune deficiency syndrome ▸ transfusion-associated (AIDS)
- a. immune deficiency syndrome (AIDS) ▸ transfusion-transmitted
- a. immune deficiency syndrome (AIDS) transmission
- a. immune deficiency syndrome (AIDS) treatment
- a. immune deficiency syndrome (AIDS) treatment trials ▸ federal
- a. immune deficiency syndrome (AIDS) vaccine, anti-
- a. immune deficiency syndrome (AIDS) victim
- a. immune deficiency syndrome (AIDS) virus ▸ blood products contaminated by

- a. immune deficiency syndrome (AIDS) virus infection
- a. immune deficiency syndrome (AIDS), mother infected with
- a. immune deficiency syndrome (AIDS) virus testing
- a. immunity
- a. immunodeficiency ▸ primary-
- a. infection, community-
- a. infection, hospital-
- a. lobar pneumonia ▸ community-
- a. megacolon
- a. meningitis, community-
- a. organism, hospital-
- a. pneumonia, community-
- a. pneumonia, hospital-
- a. pneumonia protocol ▸ community-
- a. ptosis
- a. reflex
- a. resistance to antibiotic
- a. syndrome, congenital vs.
- a. tolerance
- a. torsades de pointes, source of
- a. tuberculosis, autopsy-
- a. urinary tract infection ▸ hospital-
- a. violence immune deficiency syndrome (AVIDS)
- a. viral hepatitis, hospital-
- a. weakness in arterial wall

acquisita, myotonia

acquisition
- a. (MUGA) blood pool radionuclide scan, multiple gated
- a. computed axial tomography ▸ rapid
- a., continuous volumetric
- a. (MUGA) electrocardiogram (ECG) ▸ stress multiple gated
- a. gate
- a., gradient
- a., language
- a. (MUGA), multiple gated
- a. time

Acremonium kiliense

Acrocomia sclerocarpa

acrodermatitis
- a. chronica atrophicans
- a. continua
- a. enteropathica
- a., Hallopeau's
- a., infantile lichenoid
- a., infantile papular
- a. of childhood (PAC), papular
- a. papulosa infantum

a. perstans
acromegalic
a. gigantism
a. heart disease
acromegaly
a., conventional radiation, therapy in
a. of knees
a., transsphenoidal resection in
acromial bone
acromial bursa
acromicria, pituitary
acromioclavicular (AC)
a. articulation
a. joint
a. joint, meniscus of
a. joint, separated
a. ligament
a. separation
acromiocoracoid ligament
acromion
a., hooked
a. process
a. scapulae
a., tip of
acrosomal cap
acrosomal granule
across lower abdomen ▸ horizontal incision
across orifice ▸ flow
Acrotheca pedrosoi
Acrothesium floccosum
acrylate, cyano◊
acrylic
a. ball implant
a. ball implant material
a. bar
a. cement
a. implant
a. lens
a. partial dentures
a. resin teeth
a. splint
acryocyanosis, prominent
ACSS (acute caretaker's stress syndrome)
ACT (act)(s)
A. (axial computed tomography)
a., aggressive
A., Anatomical Gift
a., antisocial
a. before thinking ▸ patient
A., Catastrophic Health Care Coverage
A. ▸ Drug-Free Workplace
A., Good Samaritan

a. of omission
a. of self-mutilation
a. of swallowing
a. out fantasies
a. ▸ patient repeats ritualistic
A. (PSDA) ▸ Patient Self-Determination
a., repetitive
a., ritualistic
a., self-destructive
a., self-mutilative
a. ▸ senseless, ritualistic
a., skilled
Actaea spicata
ACTH (adrenocorticotropic hormone)
A. (adrenocorticotropic hormone) syndrome, ectopic
A. (adrenocorticotropic hormone) test
A. (adrenocorticotropic hormone) therapy
actifed ▸ nose stuffiness from
actin and myosis molecule ▸ filamentous
acting
a. ace inhibitor ▸ longer
a. anesthetic, long
a. barbiturate, intermediate
a. barbiturate, long-
a. barbiturate, short-
a. calcium blocker ▸ long-
a. dependence ▸ barbiturate similarly
a. dependence ▸ hypnotic similarly
a. dependence ▸ sedative similarly
a. dose, long-
a. hallucinogen, short-
a. in and acting out
a. inappropriately, patient
a. insulin, fast-
a. insulin, long-
a. insulin, short-
a. out
a. out, acting in and
a. out behaviors
a. out, criminal
a. out, impulsive
a. out, patient
a. out, sexual
a. out tendencies ▸ rebellious, aggressive
a. sympathomimetic abuse ▸ amphetamine or similarly
a. sympathomimetic delirium ▸ amphetamine or similarly

a. sympathomimetic dependence ▸ amphetamine or similarly
a. sympathomimetic intoxication ▸ amphetamine or similarly
a. sympathomimetic withdrawal ▸ amphetamine or similarly
a. thyroid-stimulating (LATS) hormone, long-
actinic
a. cheilitis
a. conjunctivitis
a. granuloma
a. keratoses
a. keratitis
a. keratosis, precancerous
a. ray
a. ray ophthalmia
a. reticuloid dermatitis
a. retinitis
actinium emanation
Actinobacillus
A. actinoides
A. actinomycetemcomitans
A. equuli
A. hominis
A. lignieresii
A. mallei
A. pseudomallei
A. suis
A. ureae
A. whitmori
actinoides, Actinobacillus
actinoides, Actinomyces
Actinomadura madurae
Actinomadura pelletierii
Actinomyces
A. actinoides
A. baudetii
A. bovis
A. bovis, gram-positive
A. eriksonii
A. israelii
A. muris
A. muris-ratti
A. necrophorus
A. rhusiopathiae
A. thermophilia
A. vinaceus
actinomycetemcomitans, Actinobacillus
actinomycetes, thermophilic
actinomycosis
a. of bone
a. of cornea
a. of sinus

actinomycosis—*continued*
- a., pulmonary

action(s)
- a., addictive feelings and
- a., aggressive
- a., alkylating
- a., antibacterial
- a., antidiuretic
- a., automatic
- a., cardiac
- a., catecholamine
- a., ciliary
- a., clot dissolving
- a., dose, route and method of administering
- a., drug
- a., faulty valve
- a., heart
- a., heart's pumping
- a. hunger, stimulus
- a., impulsive
- a., inappropriate
- a. ▸ ineffective heart
- a., inhibition of
- a., inhibitory neurotransmitter
- a. ▸ irregular heart
- a., knee
- a., mechanism
- a., metabolic
- a., microbial
- a., mode of
- a., muscular
- a., normal bowel
- a. of blood, clotting
- a. of colon ▸ abnormal peristaltic
- a. of drugs, sedative
- a. of heart (DAH) ▸ disordered
- a. of reflexes ▸ increased
- a. pain, stress
- a. ▸ patient makes deliberate
- a. pattern
- a. pattern, fixed
- a., pharmacological
- a., physiologic
- a. potential
- a. potential, biphasic
- a. potential, cardiac
- a. potential duration
- a. potential duration ▸ monophasic
- a. potential, evoked
- a. potentials (FAP), fibrillating
- a. potentials, individual motor unit
- a. potential, monophasic
- a. potential, motor nerve
- a. potential, motor unit
- a. potential, muscle
- a. potential, nerve
- a. potential, polyphasic
- a. potential (SNAP), sensory nerve
- a. potentials, tetraphasic
- a. potential, triphasic
- a., rapid heart
- a., repetitive
- a., repetitive words and
- a., reflex
- a. rituals
- a., site of
- a. ▸ slowness of mental
- a., stress
- a., sustained
- a. taken, effective
- a., tamponade
- a., therapeutic
- a. therapy
- a. tremor
- a., trigger
- a., vagal
- a., vasoconstriction
- a. ▸ voluntary muscular

activate(s)
- a. chemical impulse in brain
- a. facial expression
- a. graft
- a. immune system
- a. pleasure centers of brain

activated
- a. charcoal
- a. clotting time
- a. coagulation time
- a. computer, voice-
- a. epilepsy
- a. ergosterol
- a. glutaraldehyde
- a. killer (LAK) cell, lymphokine-
- a. monitor ▸ Event
- a. partial thromboplastin time (APTT)
- a. unit, voice

activating
- a. factor ▸ platelet
- a. inhibitory fibers
- a. neurohormones
- a. specific compensatory mechanism
- a. system, reticular

activation
- a. abnormality ▸ electrical
- a. analysis
- a. analysis ▸ neutron
- a. and behavior

- a., cell
- a. ▸ eccentric atrial
- a., epicardial
- a., functional
- a., intracellular
- a. ▸ length dependent
- a. map-guided surgical resection
- a., mapping, atrial
- a. mapping ▸ retrograde
- a. mapping ▸ retrograde atrial
- a., metabolic
- a., motor
- a. ▸ myofilament contractive
- a. of bladder, autonomic
- a. of endogenous pathogens
- a., oncogene
- a. procedure
- a. sequence ▸ intra-atrial
- a. sequence ▸ intracardiac atrial
- a. sequence mapping
- a. time ▸ ventricular
- a. (TPA) ▸ tissue plasminogen

activator
- a. (TPA) ▸ tissue plasminogen
- a. (TPA) infusion ▸ tissue plasminogen
- a. inhibitor ▸ plasminogen
- a., lymphocyte
- a. ▸ urokinase-type plasminogen

active
- a. alcohol use
- a. alcoholic
- a. alcoholism
- a. alignment
- a. and equal bilaterally ▸ deep tendon reflexes (DTR)
- a. antiretroviral therapy (HAART) ▸ highly
- a. assisted exercise
- a. bending exercise
- a. bilaterally ▸ deep tendon reflexes (DTR) equal and
- a. bilaterally ▸ reflexes equal and
- a. bisexual men, sexually
- a. bleeding
- a. bleeding disorder
- a. borborygmi
- a. bowel sounds
- a. bowel tones
- a. brain tissue
- a. carrier, patient
- a. child
- a. compression-decompression (ACD)
- a. congestion

a. contractions
a. cortical nephrogenic zone
a. culture
a. cure treatment
a. death decisions
a. delirium
a. disease
a. disease, no evidence of
a. disease process
a. dorsiflexion
a. drug ▸ cell wall
a. drug user
a. dynamic stiffness
a. ear
a. electrode
a. epileptic process, highly
a. euthanasia
a. euthanasia, condemnation of
a. euthanasia, involuntary
a. euthanasia, nonvoluntary
a. euthanasia, voluntary
a. exercise
a. expansion of lung
a. extension in stroke patients ▸
   increase of
a. fibroblasts
a. finger extension
a. flexion, gentle
a. gastritis, chronic
a. hallucinations
a. head motion
a. hepatitis, chronic
a. homosexual men, sexually
a. hyperemia
a. hyperemia of retina
a. immune response
a. immunity
a. immunization
a. incontinence
a. infant ▸ minimally
a. infection
a. infection ▸ patient admitted with
a. infiltrate
a. infiltration
a. infiltrative process
a. insufficiency
a. intervention
a. invasive infectious process
a. involvement
a. knee flexion
a. labor
a. lesbian, sexually
a. lesions
a. lifestyle
a. lifestyle, resume

a. listening
a. liver disease
a. lung disease
a. lupus kidney disease
a. management of labor program
a. maternal behavior, normal
a. medication
a. mentally
a. microorganisms
a. mobilization, gentle
a. motion
a. movement
a. muscle movement
a. necrosis
a. neurologic disorder
a. oozing from site
a. oozing from wound
a. painkilling ingredients
a. panic attack
a. parenchymal change
a. parenchymal disease
a. ▸ patient physically
a. period
a. peristalsis
a. person, sexually
a. pulmonary disease
a. pulmonary pathology
a. pulmonary tuberculosis
a. quad strengthening exercises
a. range of motion (ROM)
a. relapse prevention, pro-
a. relaxation
a. resistive exercises
a. seizures
a. sexually
a. site
a. sleep
a. sleep state
a. spermatogenesis
a. status, patient regained
a. substance
a. substance, methylene blue
a. tension curve ▸ length
a. therapy, reduced
a. tissue ▸ metabolically
a. treatment
a. treatment period
a. tuberculosis
a. tumor
a. ulcer
a. ulcer crater
a. vaccine
a. vaginal bleeding

actively
a. caused death ▸ doctors

a. chemically dependent
a. hallucinating, patient
a. terminated patient
activists, disability rights
Activitrax rate-responsive unipolar
   ventricular pacemaker ▸ Medtronic
activity(-ies) (Activity)
a., abnormal
a., abnormal chemical
a. ▸ abnormal dread of school-
   related
a., abnormal EEG
   (electroencephalogram)
a., abnormal electrical
a., abnormal frontal
a., abnormal heart
a., abnormal metabolic
a. ▸ abnormal thyroid
a., abnormally fast
a., absence of electrical
a., acetyltransferase
a., aerobic
a., aerobic physical
a., alpha
a., alpha frequency
a. and awareness, muscle
a. and desensitization ▸ headache
a. and emotions, brain wave
a., anterior temporal slow
a., antibacterial
a., anticancer
a., anticarcinogenic
a., antidiabetic
a., antifungal
a., anti-inflammatory
a., antiplatelet
a., antiretroviral
a., antitumor
a., antiviral
a., area of increased
a. ▸ areas of fibroblastic
a., arrhythmic
a., asynthetase
a., atrial
a., attenuation
a., autonomic control by alpha
a., avoidance of
a., background
a., background of slow
a., bacteriostatic
a., balance
a. based therapy
a., bed-mat
a., beta
a., beta endorphin

activity—*continued*

a. between electrodes ▸ electrical
a., bilateral
a., blocking
a., blood granulocyte specific
a., blood pool
a., bone morphogenetic
a., bone scan reveals increased
a., brachial plexus
a., brain
a., brain electrical
a., brain function
a., brains' metabolic
a., build-up of seizure
a., burst
a., burst of rhythmic
a., bursts of alpha
a., bursts of beta
a., bursts of delta
a., bursts of theta
a., cardiovascular
a., catalytic
a., caudate
a. ▸ cell membrane
a., cellular
a., central nervous system (CNS)
a., cerebral
a., cerebral paroxysmal
a., cessation of
a., change in
a., chaotic electrical
a. ▸ chaotic heart muscle
a., child-related
a., cholinergic
a., cognitive
a., complement
a., concentrated mental
a., conscious
a., continuing tumor
a., continuous cerebral
a. ▸ continuous intellectual
a., continuous seizure
a., controlled
a., controlling alpha
a., coordination of mental
a. curve ▸ time
a., daily multidisciplinary
a., daily physical
a., decreased
a., decreased brain
a., decreased brain wave
a., decreased tonic EMG
  (electromyogram)
a. ▸ deficiency of slow brain wave
a. deficit, diversional

a., delta
a., delusional type of
a., deoxyribonucleic acid (DNA)
  polymerase
a., depressed reflex
a., determinations (FAD), fetal
a., diffuse
a., digestive
a., diminished
a., diminished brain
a., diminution of background
a., diminution of recorded
a., discontinuous
a., discrete
a., disease
a., displacement
a., diversionary
a., DNA (deoxyribonucleic acid)
  polymerase
a., downsloping
a., drug-induced
a., dysjunctive motor
a., dysrhythmic
a., ectopic
a., EEG (electroencephalogram)
a., EEG (electroencephalogram)
  alpha
a., eighth nerve
a., electrical
a., electrical cardiac
a., electroencephalogram (EEG)
a., electroencephalogram (EEG)
  alpha
a., emotional
a. ▸ endogenous biotin
a. ▸ endogenous peroxidase
a., endurance
a. ▸ energy for muscle
a., enzymatic
a., enzyme
a., epileptiform
a., erythroid
a., evaluation of resting
a., exceedingly fast
a., excessive
a., excessive brain
a. ▸ excessive fast EEG brain wave
a., excessive functional
a., excessive mental
a. ▸ excessive physical
a., excessively fast
a., exertional
a., family oriented
a., fast
a., feedback of speech muscle

a., fetal
a., fibrin lytic
a., fitness
a., focal moderately slow
a., focal slow
a., focus of slow
a. ▸ forcible sexual
a., frontal intermittent rhythmic delta
a., frontal irregular rhythmic delta
a., frontal slow
a., full
a., functional
a., general gonadotropic
a., generalized bisynchronous delta
a., generalized exceedingly slow
a., generalized fast
a., generalized slightly slow
a., generalized slow
a., genetic
a., group
a., hazardous
a., headache
a., heavy exertional
a., hemispheric
a. ▸ high impact
a. ▸ high risk sexual
a., high voltage
a., high voltage fast
a., high voltage slow wave
a., highest level of
a. ▸ His bundle
a., home-related
a., homosexual
a., hormonal
a., hypersecretory
a. ▸ impaired brain
a. ▸ impaired muscular
a., impaired normal
a. in brain, abnormal electrical
a. in nerve and muscle ▸ electrical
a. ▸ in vitro
a., increase in amplitude of
  electrical
a. ▸ increase in occupational
a. ▸ increase in sexual
a. ▸ increase in social
a. ▸ increase in social, occupational,
  sexual
a., increased
a., increased brain
a., increased physical
a., increased psychomotor
a., increased reflex
a., increased sexual
a., increased thyroid

a., increased tonic EMG (electromyogram)
a. index (SPAI) ▸ steroid protein
a. indicative of brain metastases ▸ seizure
a., inflammatory
a., inhibition of
a., insertion
a., institutional
a., insulin-like
a., intellectually stimulating
a. interests and aptitude
a., interictal paroxysmal
a., intermediate fast
a. intolerance
a. ▸ intrinsic sympathomimetic
a. ▸ involvement in reckless
a., jaw muscle
a., job-related
a., labor
a., latent paroxysmal
a. ▸ legitimate therapeutic
a., leisure
a., leisure time
a. level
a. level, excessive
a. level, increased
a., lifestyle
a., limitations of physical
a., limited
a., limited physical
a. ▸ load-bearing
a., local brain
a., localized brain
a., localized electroencephalogram (EEG)
a., locomotor
a. ▸ loss of interest in
a. ▸ loss of interest in peer social
a. ▸ loss of interest in usual
a., low impact
a., low level of spontaneous
a., low voltage
a., low voltage fast
a., low voltage waking
a., manual
a., mat
a. ▸ mast cell enhancing
a., meaningful
a., medium voltage
a. ▸ membrane stabilizing
a., mental
a. ▸ mentally stimulating
a., midtemporal focus of slow
a. ▸ mild increase in motor

a., mind
a. ▸ mind-clearing repetitious
a., minimum aerobic
a. ▸ moderate aerobic
a. ▸ moderate intensity
a. ▸ moderate physical
a. ▸ moderate recent
a. modification
a., modified
a., monitor patient care
a., monorhythmic sinusoidal delta
a., motor
a., muscle
a. ▸ muscle sympathetic nerve
a., neural
a., neurological
a., neuronal
a., neurotransmitter
a., neutrophil
a., nonrhythmic electroencephalogram (EEG)
a., nonsimultaneous occurrence of electroencephalogram (EEG)
a., nonspecific peripheral
a., nonstrenuous
a., nonvigorous
a., normal
a., normal electroencephalogram (EEG)
a., normal heart
a., normal metabolic
a., normal waking
a., no voluntary
a., nucleotidyltransferase
a., occasional seizure
a. (OIRDA), occipital intermittent rhythmical delta
a., occupational
a. of antibodies, tumor suppressive
a. of anticancer enzymes
a. of both hemispheres
a. of brain, cerebral
a. of brain, electrical
a. of cochlea, electrical
a. of daily living (ADL)
a. of daily living (ADL), independent in
a. of daily living (ADL), verbal cueing for
a. of daily living (ADL) with supervision, patient does
a. of eosinophils, chemotactic
a. of heart, electrical
a. of low amplitude, delta
a. of mesothelial surface ▸ fibrinolytic

a. of pancreas
a. of pancreas, external secretory
a. of radioisotopes
a. of retina, electrical
a. of thyroid gland ▸ excessive
a. of ventricular fibrillation ▸ chaotic
a. of voluntary muscles
a., optical
a., organ
a., osteoblastic
a., paroxysmal
a., paroxysmal cortical
a., paroxysmal slow
a., passive
a., patient independent in bedmatic
a., patient perseverates in motor
a. ▸ patient unable to perform basic
a. pattern
a., peristaltic
a. ▸ peritoneal fibrinolytic
a., persistent alpha
a., phasic
a., phosphotransferase
a., photoconvulsive
a., photomyoclonic
a., photomyogenic
a., photoparoxysmal
a., physical
a. ▸ physical work
a., physiologic
a., plasma insulin
a., plasma renin
a., platelet
a. ▸ platelet monoamine oxidase
a., polyphasic
a., polymorphic
a., polyrhythmic
a., positive
a., posterotemporal slow
a., postheparin lipolytic
a., postictal
a. ▸ potentiation of motor
a. program, physical
a., progression of
a., prolonged
a. ▸ prolonged task-oriented
a., prothrombin
a., psychomotor
a. ▸ psychotherapeutic and educational
a. ▸ pulseless electrical
a., questionable seizure
a., radiation protection
a. range, limited
a. ▸ rapidly pulsing electrical

activity—*continued*
a., RAS (renin-angiotensin system)
a. ▸ receptor kinase
a., reckless
a. ▸ reckless and impulsive
a., recorded electrical brain
a., recording of electrical
a., recreational
a., recruitment pattern of electrical
a., reduced
a. ▸ reduced tolerance for physical
a., reflex
a., reflex vasculospastic
a., reflexive
a., regenerative
a. ▸ regular physical
a. -related heart problem
a., relative specific
a., renal vein renin
a., renewed tumor
a., renin
a., repetitive
a. ▸ repetitive weight bearing, strenuous
a., respiratory
a., resting muscle
a., restricted
a., restricted physical
a. restrictions
a., restrictions in
a. ▸ resume nonthreatening
a., retained alpha
a., retard bone
a., rhythmic
a., rhythmic electroencephalogram (EEG)
a., ruminative
a., runs of slow
a., salaam
a. scale
a., scalp muscle
a., secretary
a., seizure
a., selected physiologic
a., self-care
a., self-nurturing
a. sensing pacemaker
a., sexual
a., shift in direction and pattern of brain electrical
a., shifting brain electrical activity toward sleep
a., simultaneous
a. ▸ sinoaortic baroreflex
a., skeletal muscle

a., skin emotional
a., slow
a., slow waking
a., slow wave
a., social
a., spastic muscle
a., specific
a., spike seizure
a., spikey dysrhythmic
a., spindliform
a., spindling
a., spontaneous
a. ▸ stimulating fetus into
a., strenuous
a. ▸ strenuous physical
a., stressful
A. Study (PAS) ▸ Physicians
A. Study (PAS), Professional
a., subject engaged in mental
a., subjective
a., suppress specific seizure wave electroencephalogram (EEG)
a., suppression of electroencephalogram (EEG)
a., sustained
a., sympathetic
a. ▸ sympathetic nerve
a., synchronous
a., synergistic
a., teenage sexual
a., tertiary peristaltic
a. test, invasive
a., therapeutic
a. therapist
a. therapy
a. thermogenesis (NEAT) ▸ nonexercise
a., theta
a., thought
a., threshold
a., thyroid gland
a., thyroxine specific
a. to emotional situations, reduced
a., tolerance for
a., total
a. toward sleep activity ▸ shifting brain electrical
a., transketolase
a., tumor
a., unconscious
a., undesired motor
a., unilateral
a., unilateral EEG (electroencephalogram)
a., uterine

a., variations in electrical
a., vasomotor
a., ventricular ectopic
a., veto
a., vigorous
a. ▸ vigorous past
a. ▸ vigorous physical
a. ▸ vocal cord
a., voltage
a., voluntary
a., wave lengths of rhythmic
a. ▸ weight bearing
a. ▸ withdrawn from
a. ▸ withdrawal from family, friends or school
a., workaholic
actual
a. behavioral parameters
a. cautery
a. cell proliferation
a. consent
a. events, cognitive distortions of
a. grief
a. immunity
a. or perceived loss
a. pressure
a. sugar
a. suicide attempt
a. tissue damage
actuarial survival curve
actuated learning process, self-
actuation ▸ direct mechanical ventricular
ACU (Ambulatory Care Unit)
acuity
a., auditory
a., central visual
a., decreased
a. (DVA) ▸ distance visual
a., hearing
a. left eye visual
a. level (SAL) ▸ sensory
a. level (SAL) test ▸ sensory
a., loss of
a., mental
a., motor discriminative
a. (NVA) ▸ near visual
a. of color vision
a. right eye, visual
a. screening, hearing
a. screening, visual
a. test, visual
a. (VA), visual
a., visual discriminatory

acuminata
- a., Cephaelis
- a., condylomata
- a., Magnolia
- a., verruca

acuminatum
- a., condyloma
- a., papilloma
- a., perianal condyloma
- a., Trichophyton

acuminatus, lichen

acupressure infusion pump

acupressure point

acupuncture
- a., infertility
- a. instruments
- a., laser
- a., medical
- a. points
- a. technique
- a., therapeutic
- a. therapy
- a. treatment
- a. treatment, long-term

acustica sacculi, macula

acustica utriculi, macula

acute
- a. abdomen
- a. abdominal aortic occlusion
- a. abdominal pain
- a. abdominal pain ▸ intermittent episodes of
- a. abstinence syndrome
- a. abuse of drugs
- a. acalculous cholecystitis
- a. adverse psychological reaction
- a. alcoholic
- a. alcoholic hepatitis
- a. alcoholic intoxication
- a. alcoholic patient
- a. allergic extrinsic alveolitis
- a. allograft rejection
- a. amnionitis
- a. anaphylaxis
- a. and chronic ▸ alcoholic cardiomyopathy: preclinical
- a. and chronic inflammation
- a. and long-term damage
- a. angle closure glaucoma
- a. anterolateral myocardial infarction (MI)
- a. anxiety
- a. anxiety neurosis
- a. anxiety reaction
- a. anxiety state
- a. anxiety tension
- a. aortic dissection
- a. aortic emboli
- a. aortic occlusion
- a. aortic thrombi
- a. appendicitis
- a. arterial embolism
- a. arterial occlusion
- a. ascending myelitis
- a. aseptic meningitis
- a. asthmatic attack
- a. asthmatic bronchitis
- a. ataxia
- a. attack
- a. attack of asthma
- a. back pain
- a. bacterial endocarditis (ABE)
- a. bacterial exacerbation
- a. bacterial meningitis
- a. bacterial myocarditis
- a. bacterial otitis media
- a. bacterial prostatitis
- a. bacterial sinusitis
- a. biliary pain
- a. brain deficiency
- a. brain disturbance
- a. brain syndrome
- a. bronchial pneumonia
- a. bronchitis
- a. bronchopneumonia
- a. bronchopneumonia, focal
- a. bulbar polioencephalitis
- a. bulbospinal poliomyelitis
- a. Campylobacter gastroenteritis
- a. cardiac insufficiency
- a. cardiogenic pulmonary edema (ACPE)
- a. cardiorespiratory arrest
- a. cardiorespiratory failure
- a. cardiovascular disease
- a. care facility
- a. care ▸ geriatric
- a. care hospital
- a. care medical unit
- a. caretaker's stress syndrome (ACSS)
- a. catarrhal inflammation
- a. catarrhal pharyngitis
- a. care, primary
- a. catarrhal tonsillitis
- a. cerebellar ataxia
- a. cerebrovascular accident (CVA)
- a. cheilitis
- a. chest syndrome
- a. childhood leukemia
- a. cholangitis
- a. cholecystitis
- a. chorea
- a. clinical illness
- a. cocaine intoxication
- a. colitis
- a. complications
- a. compression triad
- a. confusion
- a. congestion, marked
- a. congestive glaucoma
- a. conjunctivitis
- a. coronary syndrome
- a. crisis
- a. crystal arthritis
- a. cystitis
- a. dacryocystitis
- a. delirium
- a. detoxification
- a. detoxification unit
- a. disabling vertiginous episodes
- a. disease
- a. disorder
- a. disorientation
- a. dissecting aneurysm
- a. disseminated encephalitis
- a. disseminated encephalo-myelitis
- a. diverticulosis
- a. drug intoxication, acute treatment for
- a. drug intoxication, clinical manifestations of
- a. drug intoxication, differential diagnosis in
- a. drug intoxication, psychological state in
- a. drug intoxication, subacute treatment of
- a. drug intoxication, symptoms of
- a. drug reaction
- a. drug reactions, diagnosis of
- a. drug reactions in violent patients, treatment of
- a. drug reactions, psychological manifestations of
- a. drug reactions, symptoms of
- a. drug reactions to cannabinoids, treatment of
- a. drug reactions to depressants, treatment of
- a. drug reactions to hallucinogens, treatment of
- a. drug reactions to inhalants, treatment of

acute—*continued*

- a. drug reactions to multiple drugs, treatment of
- a. drug reactions to opioids, treatment of
- a. drug reactions to phencyclidines, treatment of
- a. drug reactions to stimulants, treatment of
- a. drug reactions, treatment of
- a. drug reaction withdrawal, treatment of
- a. duodenal ulcer
- a. dyspnea
- a. dystonia
- a. dystonic reaction
- a. ear
- a. edema
- a. endocarditis
- a. endoscopic sclerotherapy
- a. eosinophilic pneumonia ▸ idiopathic
- a. epidemic infectious adenitis
- a. epididymitis
- a. epiglottitis
- a. exacerbation
- a. exacerbation and remission
- a. exacerbation of chronic bronchitis
- a. exacerbation of sinusitis
- a. exacerbation of tonsillitis
- a. exacerbation ▸ schizophrenia, catatonic type, chronic with
- a. exacerbation ▸ schizophrenia, catatonic type, subchronic with
- a. exacerbation ▸ schizophrenia, disorganized type, chronic with
- a. exacerbation ▸ schizophrenia, disorganized type, subchronic with
- a. exacerbation ▸ schizophrenia, paranoid type, chronic with
- a. exacerbation ▸ schizophrenia, paranoid type, subchronic with
- a. exacerbation ▸ schizophrenia, residual type, chronic with
- a. exacerbation ▸ schizophrenia, residual type, subchronic with
- a. exacerbation ▸ schizophrenia, undifferentiated type, chronic with
- a. exacerbation ▸ schizophrenia, undifferentiated type, subchronic with
- a. facial paralysis
- a. fatty liver
- a. febrile polyneuritis
- a. febrile reaction
- a. febrile syndrome
- a. fibrinous pericarditis
- a. flaccid paralysis (AFP)
- a. flank pain
- a. focal glomerulosclerosis
- a. food allergy
- a. fulminant liver failure
- a. fulminating meningococcemia
- a. gastric dilatation
- a. gastritis
- a. gastroduodenal ulcer
- a. gastroenteritis
- a. gastrointestinal hemorrhage
- a. glaucoma
- a. glomerulonephritis
- a. gout
- a. gouty arthritis
- a. granulocytic leukemia
- a. grief
- a. hallucinatory mania
- a. hallucinatory paranoia
- a. hallucinosis
- a. heart attack
- a. heart failure
- a. heart muscle degeneration
- a. hemarthrosis
- a. hematogenous osteomyelitis
- a. hemiplegia
- a. hemorrhagic broncho-pneumonia
- a. hemorrhagic leukoencephalitis
- a. hemorrhagic pancreatitis
- a. hepatic failure
- a. hepatitis
- a. hepatitis C
- a. hepatocellular necrosis
- a. histoplasmosis
- a. homosexual panic
- a. hospital care
- a. hydrocephalus
- a. hypertensive episode
- a. idiopathic polyneuritis
- a. illness
- a. infantile diarrhea
- a. infantile gastroenteritis
- a. infarct
- a. infarct scintigraphy
- a. infection
- a. infection, recent
- a. infectious disease
- a. infectious gastroenteritis
- a. infectious mononucleosis
- a. infectious process
- a. infective endocarditis (AIE)
- a. infective polyneuritis
- a. inflammation
- a. inflammation of portal tracts
- a. inflammation of spinal cord
- a. inflammatory cells
- a. inflammatory episodes ▸ superimposed
- a. inflammatory cells ▸ interstitial
- a. inflammatory infiltration of liver
- a. inflammatory polyradiculoneuropathy
- a. injury
- a. injury to brain
- a. intermittent porphyria (AIP)
- a. interstitial pneumonia
- a. interstitial pneumonitis
- a. intervention
- a. intoxication
- a. intoxication, treatment of
- a. intoxication with cannabinoids
- a. intoxication with depressants
- a. intoxication with hallucinogens
- a. intoxication with inhalants
- a. intoxication with multiple drugs
- a. intoxication with opioids
- a. intoxication with phencyclidines
- a. intoxication with stimulants
- a. intrascrotal pain
- a. intraventricular hemorrhage
- a. ischemia
- a. ischemic heart disease
- a. isolated myocarditis
- a. juxtapapillary chorioretinitis
- a. kidney failure
- a. kidney inflammation
- a. knee injury
- a. labyrinthitis
- a. laryngeal tracheitis
- a. laryngotracheobronchitis
- a. laryngotracheobronchitis virus
- a. left ventricular heart failure
- a. leukemia antigen ▸ common
- a. leukosis
- a. ligation of coronary artery
- a. liver failure
- a. lobar pneumonia ▸ fibrinous
- a. lung injury
- a. lung rejection
- a. lymphoblastic leukemia (ALL)
- a. lymphoblastic leukemia antigen ▸ common
- a. lymphocytic leukemia
- a. lymphocytic leukemia, Burkitt-type

a. macular neuroretinopathy
a. management
a. mania
a. mastitis
a. mastoid osteitis
a. medical care facility ▸ external
a. medical illness
a. medical management/ intervention
a. megacolon
a. melancholia
a. meningitis
a. menopausal symptoms
a. mental disorder
a. mental disturbance
a. mesenteric ischemia
a. MI (myocardial infarction)
a. middle cerebral artery thrombosis
a. middle ear
a. migraine therapy
a. miliary tuberculosis
a. monoblastic leukemia (AMOL)
a. monocytic leukemia (AML)
a. mononucleosis syndrome
a. mountain sickness
a. multiple sclerosis
a. muscle strain
a. myeloblastic leukemia (AML)
a. myelocytic leukemia (AML)
a. myelomonoblastic leukemia (AMMOL)
a. myelomonocytic leukemia (AMML)
a. myocardial infarction (AMI)
a. myocardial infarction (AMI), conduction defects in
a. myocardial infarction (AMI), pathogenesis of
a. myocardial ischemia
a. myocarditis
a. myoglobinuria
a. necrosis, extensive
a. necrotizing encephalitis
a. necrotizing pancreatitis
a. neurologic deficit
a. neurological trauma
a. nonlymphocytic leukemia (ANLL)
a. nonlymphoid leukemia (ANLL)
a. nonperforated ulcers
a. obliterating bronchiolitis
a. occlusion
a. onset
a. onset adult diabetes
a. onset of atrial fibrillation

a. or chronic alcohol ingestion
a. or persistent psychosis
a. orchitis
a. organic brain syndrome
a. otitis
a. otitis media
a. overdosage
a. pain
a. pain state
a. pancreatitis
a. pancreatitis ▸ drug-associated primary
a. pancreatitis ▸ management of
a. panic reaction
a. paralytic strabismus
a. paranoid reaction
a. parenchymatous tonsillitis
a. parotitis
a. passive congestion
a. passive congestion of liver
a. passive congestion ▸ severe
a. pericarditis, focal
a. peritonitis
a. perivascular myelinoclasis
a. pharyngitis
a. pharyngitis syndrome
a. phase
a. phase of treatment
a. pleurisy
a. pleuritis, fibrinous
a. pneumonia
a. pneumonia, focal
a. pneumonia ▸ gelatinous
a. porphyria
a. portal inflammation
a. postinfectious polyneuritis
a. process
a. proliferative
a. progressive myositis
a. promyelocytic leukemia (APL)
a. prostatitis
a. psychiatric disorder
a. psychiatric dysfunction
a. psychotic reaction
a. psychotic state
a. psychotic thought disorder
a. pulmonary edema
a. pulmonary edema ▸ fatal
a. pulmonary embolism
a. pulmonary hemorrhage
a. pulmonary thromboembolism
a. purulent labyrinthitis
a. purulent otitis media
a. pyelonephritis
a. radiation pneumonitis

a. radiculitis
a., rapidly progressive course
a. reaction to radiation therapy
a. reaction to stress
a. rectal hemorrhage
a. rejection
a. renal failure (ARF)
a. renal failure (PTARF) ▸ post-traumatic
a. respiratory disease (ARD)
a. respiratory distress ▸ infant in
a. respiratory distress syndrome (ARDS)
a. respiratory failure (ARF)
a. respiratory infection
a. respiratory syndrome ▸ severe,
a. respiratory tract infection
a. responding vs late responding tissue
a. response
A. Resuscitation (MedSTAR), Medical Shock Trauma
a. retinal necrosis
a. retroviral syndrome
a. rhabdomyolysis
a. rheumatic arthritis
a. rheumatic fever
a. rhinosinusitis
a. right ventricular heart failure
a. salivary adenitis
a. schizophrenic episode
a. sensitivity to light
a. sensitivity to sound
a. septicemia
a. serous otitis media
a. severe hypotension
a. shortness of breath
a. sinusitis
a. situational reaction
a. situational or stress reaction
a. solar cheilitis
a. spleen enlargement
a. stabbing pain
a. stage
a. stage of alcoholism
a. stress reaction
a. subendocardial myocardial infarct
a. suppurative labyrinthitis
a. supraglottitis
a. symptom management
a. symptoms ▸ vivid,
a. syndrome
a. tamponade
a. throat infection

acute—*continued*
- a. throat irritation
- a. thrombosis
- a. thrombotic aneurysm
- a. thyroiditis
- a. thyroiditis with tenderness
- a. toxic disorder
- a. toxic hepatitis
- a. toxoplasmosis infection
- a. tracheobronchitis
- a. transverse myelitis
- a. traumatic seizure
- a. treatment for acute drug intoxication
- a. treatment for flashback reactions
- a. treatment for organic brain syndrome
- a. treatment for overdosing
- a. treatment for panic reactions
- a. treatment for psychotic reactions
- a. treatment for withdrawal
- a. tubular necrosis (ATN)
- a. ulceration ▸ perforating
- a. uncomplicated cystitis
- a. undifferentiated leukemia
- a. urethral syndrome
- a. urinary retention
- a. uveitis
- a. vascular compromise
- a. ventricular assist device (AVAD)
- a. vertigo
- a. vestibular disease
- a. vestibular neuronitis
- a. viral hepatitis
- a. viral infection
- a. warning sign
- a. watery diarrhea
- a. withdrawal medication
- a. withdrawal symptoms
- a. yellow atrophy

acutely
- a. ill
- a. ill patient
- a. inflamed appendix

acutus, Ceratophyllus
acutus, pemphigus
AC (alternating current) voltage
acyl-carrier protein
acyanotic heart disease
ad antrum, aditus
AD (axiodistal)
AD (right ear)
A/D, ADC (analog digital conversion)
adamantine substance of tooth
adamantinoma, pituitary

adamantinoma polycysticum
adamantinum adenoma
adamantinum, odontoma
adamantoblastoma, fibro◊
Adamkiewicz artery
Adamkiewicz's test
Adams(') (Adam's)
- A. apple
- A. clasp
- A. disease
- A. hip arthroplasty ▸ Crawford-
- A. operation
- A. operation, Alexander-
- A. operation ▸ Horwitz-
- A. saw
- A. -Stokes attack
- A. -Stokes disease
- A. -Stokes syncope
- A. -Stokes syndrome
- A. -Stokes syndrome ▸ Morgagni-
- A. syndrome ▸ Stokes-

adaptability, social
adaptation
- a. and stress, behavior
- a., behavior
- a., color
- a., dark
- a., family
- a. ▸ impaired dark
- a., light
- a. ▸ light to dark
- a., minor shoe
- a., retinal
- a. syndrome, general
- a., to environment

adapter
- a., catheter
- a., McReynold's
- a., Y

Adaptic gauze
adaptic pacemaker, Dash single-chamber rate
adaptive (Adaptive)
- a. attitude
- a. behavior
- a. change
- a. colitis
- a. coloration
- a. convergence
- a. coping
- a. devices
- a. devices ▸ rate
- a. ego functions
- a. enzyme
- a. equipment

- a. exhaustion
- a. functioning
- a. growth
- a. hypertrophy
- a. immunity
- a. immunotherapy
- a. measure
- a. mechanism
- a. mechanism ▸ neurogenetic
- a. pacemaker ▸ rate
- a. peak
- A. Phased Array microwave technology
- a. radiation
- a. rate ▸ pacemaker
- a. response
- a. skills
- a. technique
- a. therapy
- a. toys

adaptometer, color
adaptometer, Feldman
ADC (axiodistocervical)
Add-a-line IV
added salt (NAS) diet, no
addict(s) (Addicts)
- A. Anonymous (SAA) ▸ Sex
- a., Big H (heroin)
- a., chloroform
- a., chocolate
- a., computer
- a., crack
- a., detoxification
- a. ▸ detoxification of heroin
- a. ▸ detoxified opiate
- a., drug
- a., fitness
- a. ▸ halfway house for drug
- a., heroin (big H)
- a. ▸ long-term heroin
- a., LSD (lysergic acid diethylamide)
- a., narcotic
- a., nicotine
- a., opiate
- a., pregnant
- a., recovering
- a. ▸ rehabilitation center for drug
- a., relapse-prone
- a., teenage
- a. ▸ treatment of opiate
- a. ▸ tricuspid endocarditis in drug

addicted
- a., dually
- a. mother
- a. mother ▸ narcotic-

a. patient
a. patient ▸ crack
a. person
addicting, psychologically
addiction(s) (Addiction)
a., alcohol
a., anatomy of
a., at risk for
a., barbiturate
a. behavior
a. behavior, cocaine
a., Big H (heroin)
a., caffeine
a., chemical
a., cigarette
a., cocaine
a., comorbid
a., computer
a. concept
a., craving for
a., cross
a. ▸ cultural definition of
a., destructive
a. disease
a. disorder, computed
a., drug
a., dual drug
a., family patterns of
a., full-blown
a., gambling
a., heroin (big H)
A. History form ▸ Diagnostic, Social
   and
a. history of opioid
a. in brain
a. liability of nicotine
a., LSD (lysergic acid diethylamide)
A. Medicine (ASAM) ▸ American
   Society of
a. medicine service ▸ hospital's
a., methamphetamine (Crank)
a., morphine
a., nicotine
a., mental
a., opium
a., permanent
a., pharmacologic
a., physical
a., physically
a., physiological
a., polysurgical
a. ▸ possible psychological
a. potential
a. potential, drug's
a., primary

a. programs ▸ private sector
a. ▸ progression of
a., psychological
a. relationships syndrome
a. research
A. Research and Education
   (NAPARE) ▸ National
   Association for Perinatal
a. severity index (ASI)
a., sexual
a., shame and
a., smoking
a., speed
a. substance
a. syndrome, cocaine
a. to alcohol, severe
a. to drugs, severe
a., tobacco
a. ▸ transpersonal treatment for
a. treatment
a. treatment, cocaine
a. treatment criteria
a. ▸ treatment of cocaine
a. ▸ treatment of drug abuse and
a. treatment resources
a. treatment unit ▸ medically
   managed intensive
a., untreated
a., work
addictionologist, certified
addictive
a. and isolated ▸ highly
a. androgen
a. behavior
a. behavior ▸ psychology of
a. behaviors, comorbid
a. behaviors ▸ treatment of
a. disease
a. disease producing drug
a. disorder
a. drug
a. feelings and actions
a., highly
a. -illicit drugs
a. illness
a. personality
a., physically
a. potential
a. potential, drug's
a., relationships syndrome
a. substances
a. use
a. use of cocaine
a. way, non-

Addis
A. count
A. method
A. test
addisoni, Cercosphaera
addisonian crisis
addisonian syndrome
addisonii, melasma
Addison's
A. anemia
A. disease
A. disease ▸ bleeding injury from
A. disease ▸ blood pressure
   lowered in
A. disease ▸ collapse from
A. disease ▸ dehydration from
A. disease ▸ loss of appetite from
A. disease ▸ pain in abdomen from
A. maneuver
A. plane
additional
a. diagnosis
a. films
a. surgery
additive hormonal therapy
additivity and synergism, therapeutic
adducta, coxa
adduction [*abduction*]
a. contracture of hip
a. exercise ▸ shoulder
a. position
adductocavus, metatarsus
adductor [*abductor*]
a. hallucis muscle
a. longus muscle
a. magnus muscle
a. muscle, great
a. muscle, long
a. muscle of great toe
a. muscle of thumb
a. muscle, short
a. muscle, smallest
a. pollicis muscle
a. reflex
a. reflex of foot
a. spasmodic dysphonia
a. spasticity of hips
a. stretch exercise, hip
a. tendon release
adductovarus, metatarsus
adductus, bilateral metatarsus
adductus, pes
Adelmann's operation
adenasthenia gastrica
adenia, leukemic

adenitis
a., acute epidemic infectious
a., acute salivary
a., cervical
a., mesenteric
a., phlegmonous
a., sclerosing
a., suppurative
a., tuberculous
a., vestibular
adenoassociated virus
adenocarcinoma
a., acinar
a., acinic cell
a., ampullary
a., Barrett's
a. bladder, undifferentiated
a., bronchial
a., bronchiolar
a., bronchioloalveolar
a., bronchogenic
a., cervical
a. ▸ chronic blood loss from an
a., ciliated cell
a., Clara cell
a., clear cell
a., comatoid
a., cylindromatous
a., cyst◊
a., cystic
a. ▸ distal gastric
a. ▸ duct cell
a., duodenal
a., endometrial
a. ▸ endometrial secretory
a., focal
a. gallbladder, primary
a. ▸ gastrointestinal tract
a., hepatoid
a. in head of pancreas
a. in situ
a., intraluminal
a., invasive
a. kidney
a., kinetics of cell
a. lacrimal gland
a. left lung
a. lung
a. ▸ lymphangitic spread of prostatic
a., mesonephric
a., metastatic
a., metastatic papillary
a. ▸ mucin-producing
a., mucinous
a., mucoid

a. of colon
a. of colon ▸ polypoid
a. of duodenum
a. of prostate
a. of rectum
a. pancreas, metastatic
a., pancreatic
a., papillary
a., parotid
a., pleomorphic
a., poorly differentiated
a., recurrent
a., renal
a., renal cell
a., resectable
a. right lung
a., secretory
a., serous
a. ▸ slowly growing invasive
a., staging of
a., stomach
a., undifferentiated
a., unresectable
a. ureter
a. urethra
a. urinary bladder
a., uterine
a. uterus, well differentiated
a. with myometrial invasion
a. with squamous differentiation
adenocystic
a. carcinoma
a. ovary
a. tumor
adenocystoma lymphomatosum, papillary
adenocystoma, papillo◊
adenofibroma ▸ cyst
adenohypersthenia gastrica
adenoid(s)
a. appear enlarged
a. cancer
a. cystic carcinoma
a. cystic carcinoma of pharynx
a., disorder of
a. do not appear enlarged
a., excision of
a., facies
a. function
a., hypertrophic
a., hypertrophied
a. hypertrophy
a. ▸ hypertrophy of tonsils and
a., infected
a., pharyngeal

a. punch
a. punch, Meltzer
a. tissue
adenoidal enlargement
adenoidectomy
a. and tonsillectomy
a., secondary
a., tonsillectomy and
adenoides, carcinoma epitheliale
adenoma
a., acidophilic
a., adamantinum
a., adnexal
a., adrenal
a., adrenal cortex
a., adrenocortical
a., aldosterone-producing
a., apocrine
a., autonomous
a., basal cell
a., basophilic
a., benign
a., benign polypoid
a., bladder neck
a., bronchial
a., bronchoalveolar cell
a. bronchus
a., calcified thyroid
a., carcinoma ex pleomorphic
a., carotid sheath
a., cholangio▸
a., chondromatous
a., chromophilic
a., chromophobic
a., colloid
a., colorectal
a., cortical
a., corticotrophic
a., cyst▸
a., cystic pituitary
a., ductal
a., ectopic
a., ectopic parathyroid
a., embryonal
a. endometrioides ovarii
a., eosinophilic
a., fetal
a., fibro◊
a., fibroid
a., follicular
a., hepatic
a. ▸ hepatocellular
a. ▸ Hürthle cell
a. ▸ islet cell
a., kidney

a., lactating
a., langerhansian
a. ▸ liver cell
a., lymph◊
a., macrocystic
a., macrofollicular
a., mediastinal
a., medullary
a., microcystic
a., microfollicular
a., monomorphic
a., myx◊
a., nephrogenic
a. ▸ null cell
a. of breast
a. of nipple
a. ▸ ovarian tubular
a. ovarii testiculare
a., oxyphilic
a., papillary
a. ▸ papillary cystic
a., parathyroid
a., pedunculated
a., perianal
a., pituitary
a., pleomorphic
a., polypoid
a., prostatic
a. ▸ proximal tubular
a., renal cortical
a., retrotracheal
a., sebaceous gland
a. sebaceum
a., sessile
a., somatrophic
a., sweat gland
a., thyroid
a., tracheal
a., tubular
a., tubulare testiculars ovarii
a., tubulovillous
a. ▸ undifferentiated cell
a., villotubular
a., villous
adenomata, colloid
adenomata, follicular
adenomatosis (MEA) ▸ multiple
   endocrine
adenomatosis, pulmonary
adenomatosum, carcinoma
adenomatous
   a. focus
   a. goiter
   a. hyperparathyroidism
   a. hyperplasia

a. polyp
a. polyp, benign
a. polyp, pedunculated
a. polyposis (FAP) ▸ familial
a. polyps, multiple
a. polyps ▸ small pedunculated
a. prolactin cells
adenomyoma with cystic degeneration
adenomyosis uteri
adenomyosis, uterine
adenopathy (-ies)
   a., abdominal
   a., axillary
   a., cervical
   a., gross
   a., hilar
   a., internal iliac
   a., mediastinal
   a., metastatic
   a. (MEA), multiple endocrine
   a., paratracheal
   a., postinflammatory
   a., pulmonary
   a., regional
   a., retroperitoneal
   a., scalene
   a. ▸ secondary axillary
   a., suppurative
   a., thoracic
   a. ▸ tuberculous mediastinal
adenosarcoma, cyst◊
adenosarcoma, müllerian
adenosine
   a. analog
   a. arabinoside
   a. deaminase deficiency
   a. diphosphate
   a. echocardiography
   a. monophosphate (CAMP), cyclic
   a. radionuclide perfusion imaging
   a. thallium test
   a. triphosphate (ATP)
adenosis, microglandular
adenosis, sclerosing
adenosquamous carcinoma
adenosquamous carcinoma of lung
adenoviral pneumonia
adenovirus
   a. immunization
   a. infection
   a. -mediated gene transfer
   a., mutant
   a. type 3
adenylylating enzyme
adequacy

a. of cardiac competence
a. of intravascular volume
a. of treatment
adequate
   a. affect
   a. airway
   a. bilaterally ▸ chest expansion
   a. blood flow
   a. blood supply
   a. blood volume
   a. calorie intake
   a. cardiac output
   a. clinical trial
   a. collateral
   a. diet
   a. flap developed
   a. flow of blood ▸ preventing
   a. fluid replacement
   a., gait and station
   a. gynecoid pelvis
   a. hemostasis maintained
   a. hydration
   a. literacy skills
   a., lung expansion
   a. nutrition
   a. patient care
   a. range of motion and suppleness
   a. ▸ reasoning ability
   a. rest
   a. spontaneous breathing ▸
      stimulate
   a. stimulus
   a. treatment
adequately
   a. bilaterally ▸ chest expands
   a. evacuated, bowel
   a. expanded, lungs
   a. visualized, orifices
ADG (axiodistogingival)
ADH (antidiuretic hormone)
ADHD (attention deficit hyperactivity
   disorder)
adhere, transplanted skin
adherent
   a. cataract
   a. lens
   a. pericardium
   a. placenta
   a., renal capsules
   a. to esophageal walls ▸ barium
   a. tongue
adhesed ▸ jejunum and ileum
adhesion(s)
   a., abdominal
   a., amniotic

adhesion(s)—*continued*
a., band of
a., banjo-string
a. ▸ bilateral apical fibrous pleural
a., bowel obstructing
a., breaking up
a., capsular
a., chest wall
a., conjunctival
a., dense
a., dense fibrous
a. dissected free
a. division of cortical
a., dry
a., fibrinous
a. ▸ fibrinous intraseptal pleural
a., fibrinous pleural
a., fibrofibrous
a., fibrous
a., fibrous pleural
a., filamentous
a., filmy
a. focal fibrous
a. formation
a. formation ▸ intraperitoneal
a. formation, secondary
a., hepatodiaphragmatic
a., inflammatory
a., intestinal
a., laryngeal
a., lysed
a., lysis pelvic
a., meningeal
a. molecule (ELAM) ▸ endothelial
   leukocyte
a. ▸ multiple apical fibrous
a., multiple fibrinous
a., multiple fibrous
a., multiple pelvic
a., multiple pericardial
a., numerous
a. of cauda equina
a. of pericardium around heart
a., old fibrous
a., omental
a., paratubular
a., parietoperitoneal
a., peritoneal
a., pleural
a., pleural diaphragmatic
a., pleuropericardial
a., retroperitoneal
adhesive
a., Aron Alpha

a. arachnoiditis
a. atelectasis
a. band
a. band, broad
a. band, omental
a. bandages
a. capsulitis
a., denture
a. disease
a. dressing, Kling
a. otitis media
a. pericarditis
a. pericarditis ▸ internal
a. peritendinitis
a. phlebitis
a. platelet, in vivo
a. pleurisy
a. ▸ polymerizing tissue
a. silicone implant
a. silicone implant material
a. silicone implant ▸ Silastic
   medical
a. skin patches ▸ small
a., tissue
adhesiveness, platelet
ADI (axiodistoincisal)
Adie's pupil
Adie's syndrome
adiposa
a. congenita, macrosomatia
a., hernia
a., pseudophakia
a., ptosis
a. renis, capsula
adipose
a. capsule
a. cell
a. ligament
a. tissue
a. tissue extract
a. tissue, subcutaneous
adiposis
a. cardiaca
a. cerebralis
a. dolorosa
a. hepatica
a. orchalis
a. tuberosa simplex
a. universalis
adipositas cordis
adiposity, abdominal
adiposity, cerebral
adiposum
adiposum, hepar
adiposus, ascites

adiposus, panniculus
aditus
a. ad antrum
a. antrum, attic-
a. laryngis
a. orbitae
adjacent
a. electrodes
a. field x-ray beam dosimetry
a. meninges
a. stable teeth
a. tissue
a. to chest wall, using bolus
adjunct(s)
a., airway
a. therapy
a. treatment
adjunctive
a. balloon angioplasty
a. glucocorticoid therapy
a. medication
a. nephrectomy
a. procedure
a. techniques
a. technology
a. therapy
adjust dosage
adjustable
a. anterior guide
a. breast implant
a. cane
a. cushioned heel (WACH) shoe,
   wedge
a. diaphragm
adjusting dosage
adjustment (Adjustment)
a., adolescent
a. assessment ▸ vocational
a., attitude
a., automatic fulcrum height
a., behavioral
a. disorder
a. disorder with academic inhibition
a. disorder with anxious mood
a. disorder with depressed mood
a. disorder with disturbance of
   conduct
a. disorder with mixed disturbance
   of emotions and conduct
a. disorder with mixed emotional
   features
a. disorder with physical complaints
a. disorder with withdrawal
a. disorder with work (or academic)
   inhibition

a., divorce
a., dosage
a., emotional
a., family
a., functional
a., impaired
a., improved psychological
a., long-term
a., marital
a., medication
a., physical
a., poor school
a., postural
a., psychologic
a., psychological
a., psychosocial
a. react with physical symptoms
a. reaction
a. reaction with mixed emotional
features
a. reaction with withdrawal
a. reactions to adulthood
a. scale, cardiac
A. Scale (MSAS) ► Mandel Social
a., school
a. ► secondary cataract membrane
a., sibling
a., social
a., spinal
a. therapy, sexual
a. to death of spouse
a. to environment
a. to illness, family
A. to Illness Scale ► Psychosocial
a. to sobriety
a., to work

adjuvant
a. analgesic
a. chemotherapy
a., complete Freund
a., Freund
a. hormonal or chemotherapy
treatment
a. hyperthermia
a. ► incomplete Freund
a. irradiation
a. medical therapy
a., mycobacterial
a. pulmonary irradiation
a. studies
a. systemic therapy
a. therapy
a. therapy for breast cancer
a. therapy, surgical
a. therapy, systemic

a. treatment
ADL (activities of daily living)
A. (activities of daily living),
independent in
A. (activities of daily living), verbal
cueing for
A. (activities of daily living) with
supervision, patient does
Adler('s)
A. test
A. test, Kapeller-
A. theory
ad lib (as desired)
ad lib, patient up
administer, prescribe and
administered
a., anesthesia
a., drug self-
a. injection, self-
a., oxygen
a. systematic desensitization ► self-
a. treatment, catheter
administering medication ► action,
dose, route and method of
administration
a., blood component
a., contrast
a., drug
a., exogenous steroid
A. (FDA), Food and Drug
a. ► intralymphatic radioactivity
a., intramuscular (IM)
a. ► intraperitoneal drug
a., intraspinal
a. of medication, intravenous (IV)
a. of medication ► self
a. of opioids ► long-term self-
a., parenteral
a., peripheral intravenous (IV)
a., route of
a., vasodilator
a. with cannabinoids, mode of
a. with depressants, mode of
a. with hallucinogens, mode of
a. with inhalants, mode of
a. with opioids, mode of
a. with phencyclidines, mode of
a. with stimulants, mode of
administrative medicine
admiration
a. and envy
a. ► constantly seeking praise or
a. ► demand for constant
admission(s) (Admissions)
a., appropriate

a. approved
a. blood work
a. chest x-ray
a., conditions of
a., costs per
a. criteria
a., detoxification
a. diagnosis
a., elective medical
a., elective/urgent
a. electrocardiogram (ECG/EKG)
a., emergency
a., emergent psychiatric
a. hemoglobin
a., hospital
a., inappropriate
a. information, pre-
a., involuntary
a., multiple
a. of children
A. Office
a., orders accompanying patient on
a., orders mailed in prior to
a. orders sent to Admitting Office
a. orientation
a. paper work
a., patient requesting
a. physical examination
a., potential inpatient
a., potential outpatient
a. practices
a., prior to
a. process
a., refer to previous
a., refused
a., standing orders on routine
a., timely
a. to emergency care center (ECC)
a., total infections vs. total
a. urinalysis
a., voluntary
a. worker
admit, direct
admit observers
► authorization form to
admitted
a. and transfused with fresh frozen
plasma ► patient
a. and transfused with whole blood
► patient
a. as emergency, patient
a. crowning, patient
a. for evaluation and workup ►
patient
a. for medical evaluation ► patient

admitted—*continued*
- a. for medical reassessment ▸ patient
- a. for observation and treatment ▸ patient
- a. for observation ▸ patient
- a. for terminal care ▸ patient
- a. in dazed condition ▸ patient
- a., patient
- a. with active infection ▸ patient
- a. with disguised infection ▸ patient
- a. with miscarriage ▸ patient
- a. with multiple complaints ▸ patient

admitting (Admitting)
- a. diagnosis
- A. Office
- A. Office ▸ admission orders sent to
- a. physician
- a. privileges

admixture, venous

adnata oculi, tunica

adnexa
- a. ▸ lymphoma of ocular
- a. negative
- a., ocular
- a. oculi
- a., pelvic
- a., tenderness in both
- a., transposed
- a. uteri

adnexal
- a. adenoma
- a. area
- a. cortex
- a. malignancy, ocular
- a. mass
- a. region
- a. metastases
- a. tenderness

ADO (axiodisto-occlusal)

adolescence
- a. ▸ avoidant disorder of
- a. ▸ avoidant disorder of childhood or
- a., complex disorder of
- a. ▸ disturbance of emotions specific to
- a. ▸ emancipation disorder of
- a. ▸ mixed emotional disturbances of
- a., nontranssexual type of
- a. or adulthood, nontranssexual type ▸ gender identity disorder of

adolescent(s)
- a. adjustment
- a. alcohol abuse
- a. and preteens
- a. antisocial behavior
- a. behavior problems
- a., behavioral problems of
- a., behavioral problems of pre-
- a. cataract
- a. chemical abuse
- a. communication ▸ parent-
- a. detoxification
- a. development
- a. drug abuse
- a., emotional and behavioral disorders in
- a. ▸ gender identity disorder of
- a. hypertension
- a. in family recovery
- a. insanity
- a. ▸ introverted behavior in
- a. ▸ patient placement program for
- a. polydrug use
- a. population, high risk
- a. psychiatric disorder
- a. psychiatrist
- A. Psychiatry ▸ American Academy of Child and
- a. psychologist ▸ trained
- a. psychotherapy
- a. psychotherapy group ▸ structured
- a. recklessness
- a. rheumatology
- a., runaway
- a. sexual behavior
- a. sexuality
- a., shyness in
- a. stage
- a. suicide
- a., treatment of poisoning of

adoption placement

adoptive
- a. family environment
- a. immunity
- a. immunotherapy
- a. parents

ADP (automatic data processing)

adrenal(s)
- a. ablation
- a. adenoma
- a. angle
- a. artery
- a., autolyzed
- a. axis ▸ hypophyseal pituitary

- a. (HPA) axis ▸ hypothalamic-pituitary-
- a. capsule
- a. cortex
- a. cortex adenoma
- a. cortex, carcinoma of
- a. cortical hormone
- a. cortical hyperplasia
- a. crisis
- a. disease
- a. dysfunction
- a. function, sustained
- a. gland
- a. gland biopsy
- a. gland ▸ enzymatic abnormality of
- a. gland failure
- a. gland ▸ focal metastasis left
- a. gland hormones
- a. gland insufficiency
- a. gland, medulla of
- a. gland tissue transplant
- a. gland tumor
- a. glands ▸ hemorrhagic infarcts of
- a. glands ▸ shrunken
- a. hemorrhage, peri-
- a., hemorrhagic
- a. hormone
- a. hyperplasia
- a. hyperplasia ▸ congenital
- a. hyperplasia ▸ congenital virilizing
- a. hyperplasia ▸ nodular cortical
- a. hypertension
- a. hypoplasia, congenital idiopathic
- a. insufficiency
- a. lesion
- a. ▸ leukemic infiltrates of
- a. lipid depleted
- a., Marchand's
- a. medulla
- a. metastases
- a. shadow
- a. slightly lipid
- a. steroid hormones
- a. steroidogenesis, suppressing
- a. suppression
- a. tissue
- a. transplant
- a. tuberculosis
- a. tumor
- a. vein aldosterone
- a. virilism ▸ congenital

adrenalectomy procedure

adrenalin
- a. and cocaine (TAC), tetracaine
- a. ▸ excess production of

a. rush
a. subcutaneously
a. test
adrenergic
a. agonist, beta
a. antagonist
a. attack ▸ postmicturitional
a. blockers, beta
a. blocking agent, beta
a. nervous system
a. receptor, beta
a. receptors
a. stimulant
a. stimulation, alpha
a. stimulation, beta
adrenoceptor stimulation, beta
adrenocortical
a. adenoma
a. axis (HPAA) ▸
hypothalamicpituitary
a. cancer
a. cells
a. compounds
a. extract
a. inhibition test
a. insufficiency
a. insufficiency ▸ chronic
a. insuffiency ▸ permanent
a. insufficiency ▸ primary
a. insufficiency ▸ secondary
adrenocorticotropic
a. hormone (ACTH)
a. hormone (ACTH) test
a. hormone (ACTH) therapy
a. polypeptide
adrenogenic tissue
adrenogenital syndrome
adrenoleukodystrophy (ALD) diagnosis
adrenoleukodystrophy ▸ patient has
adrenomedullary triad
adrenoreceptor agonist, alpha
adrenoreceptor agonist, beta
Adriamycin, Cytoxan (FAC)
chemotherapy ▸ 5 fluorouracil,
AD7C test
Adson('s)
A. -Coffey scalenotomy
A. maneuver
A. sign
A. suction tube
A. test
adsorption
a., agglutinin
a. column
a., differential

a., selective
adult(s) (Adult)
a. acne
a. alcoholic
a. analysis
a. antisocial behavior
a. bacterial meningitis
a. behavior
a. betrayal
a. betrayal trauma
a. cancer
a. celiac disease
a. chemical abuse
A. Children of Alcoholics (ACOA)
a. children of alcoholics counseling
▸ individual
a. children of dysfunctional families
A. CPR (cardiopulmonary
resuscitation) techniques
a. day care
a. day care center
a. diabetes ▸ acute onset
a. disorder
a., disoriented
a. dosage
a. dwarf
a., emotional and behavioral
disorders in
a. factitious disorder
a. genitalia ▸ normal female
a. genitalia ▸ normal male
a. grief cycle
A. Intelligence Scale (WAIS) Test,
Wechsler
a. life ▸ emancipation disorder of
early
a. life ▸ gender identity disorder of
a. long-term unit
a. maladjustment
a. neuroblastoma
a. nightmares
a. onset
a. onset diabetes
a. onset diabetes mellitus (DM)
A. or Children ▸ Halstead
Neuropsychological Test Battery
for
a. overconvergence
a. patient, institutionalized
a., patient placement program for
a. polycystic kidney disease
(APKD)
a. psychiatry
a. quality vision
a. rehabilitation

a. respiratory distress syndrome
(ARDS)
a. respiration, normal
a. sexual stage
a. situation, depressed
a. situational stress reaction
a. skull
a. stem cells
a. sublimation ▸ latency and
a. teratoma
a. trauma
a. traumatic reaction
a. tuberculosis
a. Wilms' tumor
adulterated drugs
adulthood
a., adjustment reactions to
a., nontranssexual type ▸ gender
identity disorder of adolescence
or
a. ▸ nontranssexual type of
adultorum, scleredema
advance(s)
a. directive
a. notification
a. palliative care
a., phase
a., significant medical
a. syndrome, phase
a., technological
advanced
a. age
a. age-related macular
degeneration (AMD)
a. alcoholism
a. and inflammatory breast
carcinoma, locally
a. aortic atherosclerosis
a. atherosclerotic cardiovascular
disease
a. breast biopsy instrumentation
(AB-BI)
a. breast cancer
a. breast carcinoma
a. bronchogenic carcinoma
a. cancer
a. carcinoma, far
a. cardiac life support (ACLS)
a. cardiac life support (ACLS)
protocol
a., catheter
a. cervical disease
a. cirrhosis
a. dementia
a. diabetes

advanced—_continued_
a. directly into duodenum ▸ scope
a. disease
a. disease, combined treatment in
a. disease, far
a. emphysema
a. exercises
a. fetal monitoring
a. gum disease
a. heart ailment
a. heart disease
a. imaging
a. imaging scan
a. injury
a. instrumentation
a. left ventricular (LV) dysfunction
a. level practitioner
a. life support (ALS)
a. liver damage
a. liver disease
a. lung malignancy
a. malignancy
a. management
a. maternal age
a. medical pain management
a. metastases
a. metastatic carcinoma
a. metastatic disease
a. metastatic disease, palliation in
a. neoplasm
a. nonmetastatic carcinoma
a. proliferative diabetic retinopathy
a. prostate cancer
a. pulmonary disease
a. regional carcinoma
a. retinopathy
a. sleep phrase syndrome (FASPS)
    ▸ familial
a. spurring
a. squamous cell carcinoma, locally
a. stage
a. stage of bacterial shock
a. stage of cancer
a. stage of congestive heart failure
    (CHF)
a. stage terminal cancer
a. state of disease
a. techniques
a. to cardia of stomach ▸ scope
a. transfer
a. trauma life support (ATLS)
a. treatment directive
a. tuberculosis
a. tumor
a. upward, knife

a. uterine mixed mesodermal tumor
a. uterine sarcoma
advancement
a., capsular
a. flap, localized
a. flap, rotation
a. flap ▸ V-Y
a. of external rectus muscle
a. of eye muscle
a. of inferior oblique muscle
a. of inferior rectus muscle
a. of internal rectus muscle
a. of lateral rectus muscle
a. of medial rectus muscle
a. of medicine
a. of ocular muscle
a. of superior oblique muscle
a. of superior rectus muscle
a., patellar tendon
a. procedure, flap
a., technological
a., tendon
advancing
a. age
a. disease
a. disease, rapidly
a. tumor, steadily
a. union of fracture
adventitia
a., aortic tunica
a., esophageal
a., fragments of
a., tunica
adventitial
a. bed
a. cells
a. layer
a. rupture
a. sheath
a. tearing
a. tissue
adventitious
a. albuminuria
a. breath sounds
a. bursa
a. proteinuria
a. sounds
adverse
a. clinical event
a. drug reaction
a. effect
a. effects, long-term
a. epilepsy
a. exercise
a. experiences, clinical

a. factor
a. fetal outcomes
a. influences ▸ relapse-inducing
a. oxidative reaction
a. psychiatric reaction
a. psychological effects
a. psychological reaction, acute
a. reaction
a. reaction after chemotherapy
a. reaction ▸ local
a. reaction to therapy
a. side-effects
a. therapy reaction
adversive therapy
advice
a. (AMA) form signed ▸ against
    medical
a. legal
a., seek medical
advisor, physician
Advisory (advisory)
A. Committee ▸ Fertility Maternal
    Health Drugs
a. committee of FDA
A. Council, AIDS (acquired immune
    deficiency syndrome)
advocate, patient-family
advocates, disability rights
adynamia episodica hereditaria
adynamic fever
adynamic ileus
AE (above elbow)
AE (above elbow) amputation
Aeby's muscle
Aeby's plane
AEC (Atomic Energy Commission)
AECG (ambulatory
    electrocardiography)
AECG (ambulatory
    electrocardiography) monitoring
AED (automatic external defibrillator)
AED (automated external defibrillator) ▸
    SurVivaLink
Aedes
A. aegypti
A. africanus
A. albopictus
A. aldrichi
A. cinereus
A. circumluteolis
A. communis
A. excrucians
A. flavescens
A. leucocelaenus
A. polynesiensis

A. pseudoscutellaris
A. punctor
A. scapularis
A. scutellaris pseudoscutellaris
A. sollicitans
A. spencerii
A. stimulans
A. taeniorhynchus
A. togoi
A. varipalpus
A. vexans
aedoeocephalus
AEG (air encephalogram)
aegophony (see **agophony)**
aegypti, Aedes
aegyptiaca, Hirudo
Aegyptianella pullorum
aegyptius, Haemophilus
aegyptius, Hemophilus
AEM (ambulatory electrocardiographic monitoring)
AEP (average evoked potential)
aequabiliter justo major, pelvis
aequabiliter justo minor, pelvis
AER (auditory evoked response)
aerated
  a. and crepitant ▸ lungs well
  a. blood
  a., lungs well
  a., sinuses well
aeration both lung fields ▸ poor
aeration of lungs
aerial conduction
aerial infection
Aerobacter (A.)
  A. aerogenes
  A. aerogenes, gram-negative
  A. cloacae
aerobes
  a., facultative
  a. ▸ gram-negative
  a., obligate
aerobic(s)
  a. activity
  a. activity, minimum
  a. activity ▸ moderate
  a. -anaerobic infections ▸ mixed
  a. and strength-building experience
  a. aquatic exercise
  a. bacilli ▸ gram-negative
  a. capacity
  a. capacity ▸ loss of
  a. capacity, maximum
  a. coliforms
  a. conditioning

a. dancing
a., elderly
a. exercise
a. exercise, cardiovascular
a. exercise ▸ condition muscles with
a. exercise ▸ high impact
a. exercise, regular
a. exercise stress test
a., eye
a. fitness, enhance
a. for arthritis ▸ water
a. gram-negative rod
a. gram-positive cocci
a., impact
a. infection
a., low impact
a. metabolism
a. oral
a. organism
a. physical activity
a. respiration
a. step
a. streptococci
a. threshold
a., water
a. workout
a. workout ▸ low impact
aerocele, epidural
aerocele, intracranial
Aerococcus viridans
aerofoetidum, Clostridium
aerogenes
  a., Aerobacter
  a., Bacterium
  a. capsulatus, Bacillus
  a., Enterobacter
  a., Escherichia
  a., gram-negative Aerobacter
  a. group, coli
  a., paracolon
  a., Pasteurella
aerogenoides, Paracolobactrum
aerogenic tuberculosis
aeroginosum, sputum
aeromedical transport
Aeromonas
  A. caviae
  A. hydrophila
  A. liquefaciens
  A. punctata
  A. salmonicida
  A. sobria
  A. veronii
aerophagia/aerophagy

aerosol(s)
  a. keratitis
  a. saline solution
  a. therapy
aerosolized treatment
aerosolized vomitus
aerospace medicine
aerotitis/aero-otitis
aerotitis media
aerotympanal conduction
aertrycke, Bacillus
aertrycke, gram-negative Salmonella
aeruginosa
  a., Bacterium
  a., gram-negative Pseudomonas
  a. infections, Pseudomonas
  a., Pseudomonas
  a., sepsis pseudomonas
aeruginosum, Bacterium
aesthesia (see **esthesia)**
aesthetics (see **esthetics)**
AET (absorption equivalent thickness)
AET (atrial etopic tachycardia)
aetiology (see **etiology)**
AFB (acid-fast bacillus)
AFBG (aortofemoral bypass graft)
afebrile [febrile**]**
  a. abortion
  a. delirium
  a., patient
afetal pregnancy
affairs in order ▸ putting
Affairs Medical Center ▸ Veterans
affect [effect**]**
  a., adequate
  a. and emotion
  a., anxious
  a., appropriate
  a., blunted
  a., blunted or flat
  a., depressive
  a. dull, patient's
  a., flat
  a., flattened
  a., inappropriate
  a., labile
  a., lewd
  a. ▸ marijuana-induced
  a. memory
  a., normal
  a. of drug ▸ depressant
  a., patient has flat
  a. ▸ profound change in
  a. self-generation
  a., shallow

affect—*continued*
- a. -starved child
- a., superficial
- a., synergistic

affected
- a. area, apply to
- a. area ▸ inflammation within
- a. area ▸ restore tissue to
- a. bones ▸ swelling deformity of
- a. by stress
- a. ear ▸ ringing in
- a. facial muscle
- a. individual, severely
- a. joint
- a. neurons
- a. parts
- a. patient, severely
- a. side
- a. side, muscles of
- a. side of face ▸ pain on
- a. site

affecting physical condition ▸ psychological factors

affection, express

affection, lack of

affectionate correction

affective
- a. disorder
- a. disorder, bipolar
- a. disorder, depressed ▸ bipolar
- a. disorder ▸ intermittent
- a. disorder, major
- a. disorder, manic ▸ bipolar
- a. disorder, mixed ▸ bipolar
- a. disorder, predominance of major
- a. disorder (SAD), seasonal
- a. disorder syndrome (SADS) seasonal
- a. disturbance
- a. dyscontrol ▸ serious
- a. expression
- a. flattening
- a. functioning
- a. illness
- a. insanity
- a. instability
- a. involvement
- a. lability
- a. melancholia
- a. personality
- a. personality disorder
- a. psychosis
- a. responsiveness
- a., schizo-

- a. syndrome ▸ drug-induced organic
- a. syndrome, organic

affectomotor memory organization

afferens glomeruli, vas

afferent
- a. arteriole
- a. artery
- a. fibers
- a. fibers, blocking vagal
- a. glomerular arterioles
- a. impulse
- a. impulses
- a. loop
- a. nerve
- a. nerve fibers
- a. nerve path
- a. neuron
- a. neurons ▸ primary
- a. pathway
- a. reflex
- a. spinal nerve fibers
- a. tracts
- a. veins
- a. vessels

afferentia
- a. lymphoglandulae ▸ vasa
- a. nodi lymphatici ▸ vasa
- a., vasa

affiliation, church

affinity
- a. antibody ▸ high
- a., chemical
- a. chromatography
- a., drug
- a., dual
- a., elective
- a. maturation
- a., residual
- a., testosterone binding

affirmation, patient

affirmation, personal

affix plate

afflicted joint

affliction(s)
- a., age-related
- a., brain
- a., congenital
- a., debilitating
- a., heart
- a., incurable
- a., interminable
- a., mental
- a., nerve
- a., physical

- a., social

afibrinogenemia, congenital

AFIP (Armed Forces Institute of Pathology)

AFP (acute flaccid paralysis)

African
- A. -Burkitt's lymphoma
- A. cardiomyopathy
- A. endomyocardial fibrosis
- A. histoplasmosis
- A. meningitis
- A. sleeping sickness
- A. tick fever, South
- A. tick typhus
- A. tick typhus, South

africana, Taenia

africanus, Aedes

africanus, Paragonimus

after
- a. -cataract
- a. chemotherapy ▸ adverse reaction
- a. chemotherapy ▸ lip and mouth care before and
- a. damage to nerve fibers, regeneration
- a. death, care of body
- a. -effects, delayed
- a. fatty meal
- a. 48 hours incubation ▸ growth
- a. irradiation, biopsy
- a. -loading colpostat ▸ Fletcher
- a. -loading system
- a. -loading tandem ▸ Fletcher
- a. mastectomy, breast reconstruction
- a. meals (pc)
- a. meals (p.p. or postprandial)
- a. presedation ▸ nausea and vomiting
- a. 72 hours ▸ organism isolated
- a. stain
- a. stroke, rehabilitation
- a. treatment, functioning

afterbirth expelled

afterbirth pains

aftercare
- a. agencies
- a. counseling
- a. plan
- a. planning
- a. planning, complete
- a. programs
- a. treatment, long-term

afterdepolarization (DAD), delayed

afterdepolarization (EAD), early
afterimage, negative
afterimage, positive
afterload
- a. matching
- a. mismatching
- a. reducers
- a. reduction
- a. resistance
- a., ventricular

afterpotential
- a., diastolic
- a., oscillatory
- a. oversensing
- a., pacemaker
- a., positive

afunctional occlusion
AG (axiogingival)
AGA
- A. (appropriate for gestational age)
- A. (appropriate for gestational age) female neonate, term
- A. (appropriate for gestational age) male neonate, term

against (Against)
- a. authority, rebels
- A. Driving Drunk (SADD) ‣ Students
- A. Drunk Driving (MADD) ‣ Mothers
- a. environment, barrier
- a. infection, natural defense
- a. injury, local defense
- a. medical advice (AMA)
- a. medical advice (AMA) form signed
- a. medical advice (AMA) ‣ patient released

agalactia, contagious
agalactiae, Streptococcus
agammaglobulinemia
- a., acquired
- a., Bruton's sex-linked
- a., common variable
- a., congenital
- a., Swiss-type
- a. ‣ X-linked

Agamodistomum ophthalmobium
Agamomermis culicis
Agamonematodum migrans
aganglionic megacolon
aganglionic segment of colon
agar
- a. ‣ eosin methylene blue
- a. nasi

- a. plate, blood

Agaricus campestris
Agaricus muscarius
agate sputum, moss-
AGCT (Army General Classification Test)
age
- a. according to Greulich and Pyle, bone
- a. (AA), achievement
- a., advanced
- a. ‣ advanced maternal
- a., advancing
- a. -appropriate articulation level
- a. -appropriate fantasies
- a. (AGA), appropriate for gestational
- a. assessment ‣ gestational
- A. -Associated Memory Impairment (AAMI)
- a. ‣ benign forgetfulness of old
- a., biological
- a., bone
- a., childbearing
- a. (CA), chronological
- a., debilitating effects of old
- a. ‣ decrepitude with
- a. development ‣ latency
- a. equivalent
- a. equivalent score
- a. (AGA) female neonate, term appropriate for gestational
- a., fetal
- a., gestational
- a. -group average
- a., height
- a., in proportion to
- a. (LGA), large for gestational
- a. limit
- a. (AGA) male neonate, term appropriate for gestational
- a., maternal
- a., menstrual
- a., mental
- a. neonate ‣ large for gestational
- a. neonate ‣ small for gestational
- a., normal atrophy of old
- a. of menarche
- a., old
- a. period ‣ latency
- a., phenomena of old
- a., physiological
- a., premature old
- a., problems of old
- a. ratio, bone

- a. -related affliction
- a. -related ailment
- a. -related cataracts
- a. -related cognitive decline (ARCD)
- a. -related degeneration of valve
- a. -related dementia
- a. -related disease
- a. -related eye disease
- a. -related fear
- a. -related hearing loss
- a. -related loss of muscle
- a. -related loss of nerve cells
- a. -related macular degeneration (ARMD)
- a. -related macular degeneration (AMRD) ‣ advanced
- a. -related macular degeneration (AMRD) ‣ dry
- a. -related macular degeneration (AMRD) ‣ intermediate
- a. -related macular degeneration (AMRD) ‣ wet
- a. -related memory loss
- a. -related muscle malfunction
- a. -related phenomenon
- a. -related tissue shrinkage
- a. -related visual impairment
- a. -related weight problems
- a. relation
- a. (SGA), small for gestational
- a. spots
- a. spots on skin
- a. spread, middle-
- a. -undetermined myocardial infarction

aged acne
agency(-ies)
- a. aftercare
- a., designated assessing
- A., Drug Enforcement (DEA)
- a., health care
- a. ‣ home health care
- a. ‣ referral to community
- a., regulatory

agenda, personal
agenesia corticalis
agenesis
- a., callosal
- a., corpus callosum
- a., gonadal
- a., liver
- a., lumbosacral
- a., nuclear
- a., ovarian

agenesis—*continued*
- a., pulmonary
- a., pure red cell
- a., renal
- a., sacral
- a. syndrome, splenic
- a., thymic
- a. ▸ unilateral pulmonary
- a., uterine
- a., vaginal
- a., vermian
- a. with associated stigmata ▸ patent ductus renal

agenetic fracture

agent(s)
- a., alkylating
- a., alpha blocking
- a., analeptic
- a., analgesic
- a. and techniques, physical
- a., antianxiety
- a., antiarrhythmic
- a., antibacterial
- a., anticancer
- a., antidepressant
- a., antidiabetic
- a., antidiarrheal
- a., antiemetic
- a., antifolic
- a., antifungal
- a., antihypertensive
- a., anti-inflammatory
- a., antimicrobial
- a., antineoplastic
- a., antineoplastic chemotherapeutic
- a., antiparasitic
- a., antiparkinsonian
- a., antiplatelet
- a., antiproliferative
- a., antipruritic
- a., antiresorptive
- a., antiviral
- a., bacteriostatic
- a., beta adrenergic blocking
- a., beta blocking
- a., betamimetic
- a., biologic
- a., blood-borne
- a., blood-borne infectious
- a., blood thinning
- a. B27 ▸ histocompatibility
- a. ▸ calcium channel blocking
- a., cancer causing
- a., cancer chemotherapeutic
- a., cancer destroying

- a., carcinogenic
- a., cardiovascular
- a., causal
- a., causative
- a., chemical
- a., chemotherapeutic
- a., cholinergic
- a., contrast
- a., cytotoxic
- a., diagnostic
- a., dispersing
- a., dissolving
- a., diuretic
- a., dopaminergic
- a., Eaton
- a., etiologic
- a., etiological
- a., exogenous toxic
- a., experimental chemothera-peutic
- a. ▸ fluid embolic
- a. ▸ fluid vascular occluding
- a., ganglionic blocking
- a., gonadotropin releasing
- a. ▸ health care
- a., heat transfer
- a., hormonal
- a., hypertensive
- a., hypoglycemic
- a., hypotensive
- a., imaging
- a., immunizing
- a., immunopotentiating
- a., immunosuppressive
- a., infectious
- a., infective
- a., infusion of chemotherapeutic
- a., ingestion of toxic
- a., inhalation
- a., inotropic
- a., intravascular
- a., intravenous anesthetic
- a., life-threatening infectious
- a. ▸ macrolide antimicrobial
- a., natural anticancer
- a., nephrotoxic
- a., neuroleptic
- a., neuromuscular blocking
- a., neuroprotective
- a. ▸ nonglycoside inotropic
- a., nonsteroidal anti-inflammatory
- a. of infection
- a., oncogenic
- a., oral
- a. ▸ oral antifungal
- a., oral narcotic

- A. Orange
- A. Orange syndrome
- a., ototoxic
- a., ovulatory
- a. ▸ parenteral antimicrobial
- a., pathogenic
- a., pharmacologic
- a., photoreactive
- a., physical
- a., plaque-cleaning
- a. pneumonia, Eaton
- a., polyfunctional alkylating
- a., presumptive diagnosis of etiologic
- a., progestational
- a., prophylactic
- a., protective
- a., psychomimetic
- a., psychotropic
- a., saluretic
- a., sclerosing
- a. ▸ steroid sparing
- a. ▸ superparamagnetic contrast
- a., sympatholytic
- a., targeting
- a. ▸ tetracycline antiulcer
- a., therapeutic
- a., thrombolytic
- a., uricosuric
- a. ▸ urographic contrast
- a., vasodilating
- a., vasodilator
- a., ventilation
- a., viral
- a. (CCA) virus ▸ chimpanzee coryza
- a., virus inactivating

ageusic aphasia

agglomerans, Enterobacter

agglutinable substance

agglutinating
- a. antibodies ▸ sperm
- a. substance
- a. vibrios, non◊

agglutination
- a., bacterial
- a., bacteriogenic
- a. binding, ▸ lentil
- a., chick cell
- a., cold
- a., direct
- a., H
- a., heterophil
- a. inhibition assay
- a. inhibition test ▸ latex

a. inhibition titer
a., intravascular
a., latex
a. ▸ lectin
a., macroscopic
a., mediate
a., microscopic
a., O
a., platelet
a. pregnancy test, direct
a. reaction, mixed cell
a., salt
a. studies
a., T-
a. test
a. test, latex slide
a. titer
a. titer, differential
a., Vi

agglutinative thrombus
agglutinin(s)
a. adsorption
a., alpha
a., anti-Rh
a., beta
a., chief
a., cold
a., complete
a., cross
a. disease, cold
a., febrile
a., flagellar
a., group
a., H
a., haupt
a., heterophilic
a., immune
a., leukocyte
a., O
a., partial
a., platelet
a. pneumonia, cold
a., Rh
a., somatic
a., soybean
a., warm
a. ▸ wheat germ

agglutinoid reaction
aggravated
a. assault
a. by motion, pain
a. by movement, pain

aggregate(s)
a., discrete
a., fibrinoplatelet

a., focal lymphocytic
a., lymphoid
a. measurements
a. nodules

aggregated albumin (human), iodinated
I 131
aggregated albumin kit, Tc (technetium)
99m
aggregating factor ▸ platelet-
aggregation
a. alteration ▸ platelet
a., familial
a. of cells, focal
a. of cells ▸ reversible
a. of white blood cells (WBC)
a. platelet

aggregatum, Chlorochromatium
aggregometry, impedance
aggression
a. and deceit ▸ impulsivity,
a., anticipatory
a., constructive
a., destructive
a. discharge ▸ focus of
a., impulsive
a., inward
a. or rage
a. or rage ▸ outbursts of
a. ▸ physical threatening and
a. ▸ stress-induced
a., violent

aggressive
a. acting-out tendencies ▸
   rebellious,
a. action
a. acts
a. approach
a. behavior
a. behavior ▸ positive paroxysmal
a. behavior ▸ unusually hostile or
a. behavior, violent and
a. care
a. chemotherapy
a. child
a. confusion
a. drive
a. exercise
a. feelings
a. hepatitis, chronic
a. ideation
a. intense therapy
a. laser treatment
a. medical care
a. medical mangement
a. ▸ moody, irritable and

a. or violent behavior
a., passive-
a. patient
a. personality disorder ▸ passive
a. personality, passive-
a., physically
a. rebellious behavior
a. rehabilitation program
a. strategy
a. therapy
a. treatment
a. type ▸ conduct disorder, solitary
a. type ▸ undersocialized conduct
   disorder

aggressiveness ▸ irritability and
aggressivity, drinking-related
agilis, Azotobacter
agility
a., coordination and
a. drills
a., mental

aging
a., anatomy of
a., biological
a. capillaries
a., cellular
a. ▸ color vision deteriorate with
a. diet, anti-
a., dizziness in
a., effects of
a., forgetfulness from
a. gene, anti-
a. ▸ graying hair from
a. ▸ gum problems from
a. ▸ hearing loss from
a., heatstroke in
a., hypothermia in
a. ▸ loss of smell from
a. musculoskeletal soft tissue
a., normal
a. of brain
a. of brain ▸ stress-related
a. of cells ▸ delay
A. (OPTIMA) ▸ Oxford Project to
   Investigate Memory and
a., premature
a., problems of
a. process, natural
a. process, normal
a., process of
a., rapid
a., skin
a. ▸ skin discoloration in
a. skin, prematurely
a. skin spots

aging—*continued*
- a., stress and
- a., stroke and
- a. therapy, anti-
- a., tinnitus and
- a. ▸ tooth yellowing from
- a. ▸ transient ischemic attack
- a. treatment, anti-
- a., trembling in
- a. ▸ vision change in
- a. ▸ voice change in
- a. ▸ weight gain in
- a. ▸ white matter loss due to
- a. ▸ wrinkled ear in

agitans
- a., dystaxia
- a., paralysis
- a., pseudoparalysis

agitata, amentia
agitated
- a. and confused ▸ patient
- a. behavior
- a. ▸ depressed and
- a. depression
- a., irritable and easily annoyed
- a. melancholia
- a. movement ▸ disjointed
- a. movements
- a. patient
- a. ▸ patient aimlessly
- a. ▸ patient combative and
- a. response

agitation
- a., aimless
- a. and irritability
- a., and restlessness ▸ irritability,
- a., delusions and tendency to self-abuse
- a., extreme
- a., fatigue and
- a., intense motor
- a. or confusion
- a., psychomotor
- a., restlessness and pacing

agglomerans, Enterobacter
Agnew's operation
agni, Clostridium
agnogenic myeloid metaplasia
agnosia [*anoxial*]
- a., acoustic
- a., auditory
- a., body-image
- a., finger
- a., ideational
- a., tactile

- a., time
- a., visual

AgNO₃ (silver nitrate)
agonal
- a. clot
- a. expiration
- a. gasping
- a. respirations
- a. rhythm
- a. spinal cord hemorrhage
- a. thrombosis
- a. thrombus

agonist(s)
- a., alpha
- a., alpha adrenoreceptor
- a., beta adrenergic
- a., beta adrenoreceptor
- a., calcium channel
- a., dopamine
- a. drug, beta-
- a. inhalers, beta-
- a., muscarinic
- a. properties, dopamine receptor

agonistic muscle
agophony (*same as* aegophony)
agoraphobia
- a. ▸ panic disorder with
- a. ▸ panic disorder without
- a., patient has
- a. symptoms
- a. with panic attacks
- a. without history of panic disorder
- a. without panic attacks

agouti/agouty
agranulocytic angina
agranulocytica, mucositis necroticans
agranulocytosis, Kostmann's infantile
agraphia
- a., absolute
- a., acoustic
- a. amnemonica
- a. atactica
- a., cerebral
- a., jargon
- a., literal
- a., mental
- a., motor
- a., optic
- a., verbal

A/G (albumin/globulin) ratio
A/G (albumin/globulin) ratio test
agreement, family treatment
agricultural anthrax
agrypnodal coma
ague

- a., brass-founders'
- a., catenating
- a., dumb
- a., quartan
- a., quintan
- a., quotidian
- a., shaking
- a., tertian

AHA (American Heart Association) diet
AHAF (American Health Assistance Foundation)
AHD (atherosclerotic heart disease)
ahead, failure to plan
ahead ▸ impulsivity to plan
AHG (antihemophilic globulin)
AHI (apnea hypopnea index)
A-H interval
Ahlfeld's sign
AHM (ambulatory Holter monitoring)
Ahumada-del Castillo syndrome
AI (aortic insufficiency)
AI (axioincisal)
AICA (anterior inferior communicating artery)
AICD (automatic implantable cardioverter defibrillator)
AICD (automatic internal cardioverter defibrillator)
AID (automatic implantable defibrillator)
aid(s) (Aid)
- a. ▸ analog hearing
- a. and attendance
- a. assessment, bathroom
- a., behind-the-ear hearing
- a., binaural hearing
- a., bioptic
- a., body worn hearing
- a., completely in the canal hearing
- a., diagnostic
- a., digital hearing
- a. ▸ downsizing of hearing
- a. ▸ emotional first
- a., first
- a. group ▸ mutual
- a., hearing
- a. in assessment and diagnosis
- a. in dying
- a. ▸ in-the-canal hearing
- a. ▸ in-the-ear hearing
- a. ▸ low vision
- A. malfunction ▸ (automatic implantable defibrillator)
- a. mattress, rotating
- a., memory
- a. mobility

a., perform first
a. ▸ programmable analog hearing
a. (RMA) ▸ refusal of medical
a., sleep
a. surgery, band-
a. techniques, first
a. ▸ therapeutic sleep
a. to ambulation
a. ▸ traditional hearing
a., visual
a., walking

aide
a., home health
a., nurse's
a., therapy

AIDS (acquired immune deficiency syndrome)
A. Advisory Council
A. antibodies
A. antibody test
A. associated anemia
A. associated transfusion
A. awareness
A. carrier, patient
A. carrier, patient unknown
A. crisis
A. dementia complex
A. education
A. ▸ emotional effects of
A. epidemic
A., fetal
A., heterosexual contact with male carriers of
A. home care programs ▸ specialized
A. illness
A. infected child
A. look-alike case
A. ▸ loss of appetite from
A. mandatory testing
A. patient
A., patient at risk for
A. patients ▸ secretion spills from
A. ▸ physical effects of
A. prevention
A. primary pathogen
A. ▸ problems with central nervous system from
A. related complex (ARC)
A. related dementia
A. related illness
A. related macular degeneration
A. related pneumonia
A. residential treatment facility
A. -tainted transfusion

A. testing
A. testing, mandatory
A. ▸ transfusion-associated
A. transfusion-transmitted
A., transmission of
A. treatment
A. treatment trials ▸ federal
A. vaccine, anti-
A. victim
A. ▸ victims,
A. virus ▸ blood products contaminated by
A. virus infection
A. virus, mother infected with
A. virus testing
A. virus transmission

AIE (acute infective endocarditis)
ailment
a., advanced heart
a., age-related
a., chronic
a., heart
a., incapacitating
a., job-related
a., physical
a., respiratory
a., terminal lung

aimed laser, imprecisely
aimless agitation
aimless wandering
aimlessly agitated ▸ patient
aimlessly, eyes wander
AIO (absolute iodine uptake)
AIOD (aortoiliac obstructive disease)
AIP
A. (acute intermittent porphyria)
A. (autoimmune thrombocytopenic purpura)
A. (average intravascular pressure)

air
a., alternate inspiration and expiration of
a., alveolar
a. alveologram
a., ambient hospital
a. ambulance service
a. and particulates, entrained
a. arthrography
a., average volume of
a. bag
a. bag, Politzer
a. barrier, blood
a., bladder distended with
a. block
a. -block glaucoma

a. -blood barrier
a. bone gap
a. (resting) ▸ breathing
a. (standing) ▸ breathing
a. bronchogram
a. bronchogram sign
a. bubble
a. bubble, gastric
a. bubble instilled in anterior chamber
a. butterfly configuration
a. calorics test
a., capillary blood gas at room
a. cavity
a. cells
a. cells, ethmoid
a. cells, mastoid
a. cells, tubal
a. chamber
a. collection, expired
a., complemental
a. concussion
a. conduction (AC)
a. conduction (BC > AC) ▸ bone conduction greater than
a. conduction (BC < AC) ▸ bone conduction less than
a., contamination from ambient hospital
a. contrast
a. contrast colon examination
a. contrast study
a. control
a. -cuff plethysmography
a. cystoscopy
a. -delivery system
a. dome sign
a. dose
a. douche
a. -dried, slide
a. -driven artificial heart
a. drying, open-
a. -emboli induced lung injury
a. embolism
a. embolism, cerebral
a. embolism ▸ diving
a. embolism, venous
a. embolization
a. embolus
a. encephalogram (AEG)
a., entrained
a. entry
a., escape of
a. evacuation of trauma patient
a. exchange

air—*continued*
- a. exchange, bilateral
- a. exchange, disturbance in
- a. exchange, poor
- a. exhaled
- a., expiratory trapping of
- a., expressed from ventricle
- a., extrapleural
- a., factitious
- a. -filled cavities
- a. -filled tube
- a., filtered hot
- a. flow during expiration ▸ prolongation of
- a. flow, impairment of
- a. flow (LAF) isolation room ▸ laminar
- a. flow (LAF) ▸ laminar
- a. flow, prolongation of
- a. flow room (LAFR) ▸ laminar
- a. flow unit (LAFU) ▸ laminar
- a. fluid cavity
- a. fluid level
- a. fluid levels ▸ multiple
- a., forced
- a., free
- a., free abdominal
- a., free intraperitoneal
- a., free peritoneal
- a. gap correction
- a. gap correction, isodose shift method for
- a., gasping for
- a., germ-laden
- a., high-efficiency particulate
- a., high viscosity barium and
- a. hunger
- a. in colon ▸ intraluminal
- a. in diaphragm, free
- a. in large bowel ▸ intraluminal
- a. in pleural cavity
- a. inhaled
- a., injection of
- a. injection, perinephric
- a. inspirated, volume of
- a. insufflation
- a., intraperitoneal
- a. kerma rate constant
- a. leak
- a. leak, peripheral
- a., leakage of
- a., liquid
- a., mediastinal
- a. microbes
- a. monitor
- a. movement
- a., normal hospital
- a., obstruct flow of
- a. or gel cushioning
- a. passage
- a. passage ▸ foreign body (FB) in
- a. passages become inflamed
- a. passages, obstruction of
- a. passageway
- a. pathways
- a. pocket
- a. pockets, subpleural
- a. pollutants, toxic
- a. pollution
- a. -powered nebulizer
- a. pressure, equalize
- a. pressure, higher
- a. pressure, lower
- a. pressure, reduced
- a., pressurized
- a. proctoscopic
- a. -puff tonometer
- a. pulmonary embolism
- a. pump
- a. pyelography
- a. ratio, scatter
- a. ratio, tissue
- a., reduction in volume of
- a. rescue
- a., reserve
- a., residual
- a., roentgens delivered in
- a. sacs
- a. sacs, congested
- a. sacs, elasticity of
- a. sacs, enlarged
- a. sacs ▸ vital microscopic
- a. saccules
- a. sickness
- a. sickness, compressed-
- a. sign ▸ intravascular fetal
- a. space
- a. space consolidation
- a. space disease, diffuse
- a. -space disease
- a. spaces, alveolar
- a. spaces, intraparenchymal
- a. spaces, peripheral
- a. spaces, subpleural
- a. study
- a. study, perirenal
- a. study, retrococcygeal
- a. study, retroperitoneal
- a., submucosal
- a. supply
- a., swallowed
- a. swallower
- a. swallowing
- a., tidal
- a., total
- a. transport, critical care
- a. transport of patient
- a., trapping of
- a. trousers
- a. tunnels
- a., vaginal
- a. vaporizer, cold
- a. velocity index (AVI)
- a. ▸ venous alveolar
- a. volume
- a. volume, total

airborne
- a. bacterial concentrations
- a. bacterium
- a. bugs
- a. contaminants
- a. contamination
- a. gap
- a. germs
- a. infection
- a. molds and bacteria
- a. pathogen
- a. route
- a. route of transmission
- a. vibrations

airflow
- a., block
- a., impairment of
- a., laminar
- a., obstruction
- a. obstruction ▸ fixed
- a. ▸ obstruction of
- a., respiratory
- a. restricted
- a. system, negative

airing procedure, de
air-jet insulin injector
airline flight radiation
Airloss Therapy, Flexicair Low
airspace consolidation
airspaces, peripheral
airtight closure
airway(s)
- a., adequate
- a. adjuncts
- a., artificial
- a. bacterial colonization
- a., binasal pharyngeal
- a., blocked
- a., branching

a. breathing, and circulation (ABC)
a., bronchial
a. care
a., chronically inflamed
a., clear
a. clear, nasal
a. clearance
a. clearance ▸ ineffective
a., clearing of
a., clearing of pulmonary
a., clogged
a. closure
a., complete obstruction of
a. constriction
a., continuous positive pressure
a. defect, obstructive
a. defect, restrictive
a., dilated
a. disease
a. disease, chronic obstructive
a. disease, lower obstructive
a. disease, obstructive
a. disease ▸ over-reactive
a. disease, reactive
a. disease ▸ restrictive
a. disease ▸ reversible obstructive
a. disease ▸ small
a. disease syndrome (RADS) ▸ reactive
a. disease, upper
a., disposable
a., emergency
a., esophageal
a. ▸ esophageal obturator
a. established
a., faulty
a., flabby
a., food obstructing
a., foreign body (FB) obstructing
a. ▸ froth in upper
a., full artificial
a. function
a. function test
a., hyperreactive
a., intubation of
a. lesions ▸ synchronous
a. maintenance
a. management
a. muscles ▸ spontaneous spasm of
a. narrowing
a., nasal
a., nasopharyngeal
a. ▸ nonspecific irritant in
a. obstructed

a. obstructed, nasal
a., obstructed upper
a. obstruction
a. obstruction, chronic
a. obstruction disease
a. obstruction ▸ foreign body
a. obstruction, lower
a. obstruction, nasal
a. obstruction ▸ stop-valve
a. obstruction ▸ unconscious
a. obstruction, upper
a. occlusion technique
a., open
a., opening
a., oral
a., oropharyngeal
a., partial artificial
a., patent
a., penetrating injury of major
a. pressure, bi-level positive
a. pressure (CPAP) ▸ continuous positive
a. pressure ▸ expiratory positive
a. pressure ▸ inspiratory positive
a. pressure (NCPAP) ▸ nasal continuous positive
a. pressure (PAP), positive
a. pressure (PEAP), positive end-
a. pressure release ventilation (APRV)
a. pressure ▸ variable positive
a. problems ▸ allergic asthma
a. reactivity index (ARI)
a. receptor ▸ upper
a. reconstruction ▸ Sheen
a. resistance
a. resistance, increasing
a. secured
a. skills, obstructed
a. stenosis
a., suction
a. support
a. tissue ▸ inflamed
a., tongue obstructing
a. unobstructed, nasal
a. walls ▸ swelling of
aitiology (see etiology)
AJ (ankle jerk)
AK (above knee)
AK (above knee) amputation
AK (above knee) support
akamushi
a., Leptus
a., Microtrombidium
a., Rickettsia

a., Trombicula
akari, Rickettsia
Akerlund diaphragm
Akerlund's deformity
akinesia
a., anterior wall
a., Nadbath
a., O'Brien
a. of lids, satisfactory
a., Van Lint
akinesis/akynesis
akinetic
a. apraxia
a. autism
a. epilepsy
a. mania
a. mutism-
Akron artificial heart ▸ University of
AL (axiolingual)
A.La. (axiolabial)
ala
a. auris
a. cerebelli
a. cinerea
a. ilium
a. nasi
a. of nose ▸ levator muscle of upper lip and
a., sacral
ALAD (abnormal left axis deviation)
A.LaG (axiolabiogingival)
A.LaL (axiolabiolingual)
alanine aminotransferase (ALT)
Al-Anon Family Groups
Al-Anon Group
alar
a. bone
a. cartilage
a. chest
a. flaring
a. folds
a. scapula
alarm mattress, apnea
alarm reaction
alaryngeal speech
alata, Ascaris
alata, scapula
Alateen Group
alba (Alba)
a. cervicalis, linea
a. dolens, phlegmasia
a. dolens puerperarum, phlegmasia
a. hernia, linea
a., linea
a., lochia

alba—*continued*
a., pneumonia
A. powder (Pwd) ▸ Pan
Albarran's gland
albedo retinas
Albee('s)
A. -Delbet operation
A. fracture table
A. operation
A. spinal fusion
A. technique
Albers
A. -Schönberg bone
A. -Schönberg disease
A. -Schönberg position
A. -Schönberg syndrome
Albertini-Zellweger syndrome, Fanconi-
Albert's disease
Albert's operation
albescens, retinitis punctata
albicans
a., Candida
a., corpora
a., corpus
a., Endomyces
a., Monilia
a., Saccharomyces
albicantia, corpora
albiceps, Chrysomyia
albida, macula
Albini's nodules
albinism, ocular
albinotic fundus
Albinus' muscle
albopictus, Aedes
Albright('s)
A. disease
A. syndrome
A. syndrome ▸ Forbes-
A. syndrome, Lightwood-
A. syndrome, McCune-
albuginea oculi
albuginea, tunica
albumo, Trichophyton
albumin/albumen
a. A
a., acetosoluble
a., acid
a., alkali
a., blood tested for
a., caseiniform
a. clearance
a., coagulated
a. -coated vascular graft
a., crystalline egg

a., derived
a. /globulin (A/G) ratio
a. /globulin (A/G) ratio test
a., hematin
a. (HSA), human serum
a., iodinated human serum
a. (human), iodinated I 131 aggregated
a. (human), iodinated I 131 serum
a., iodinated I 125 serum
a., iodinated macroaggregated
a., iodinated serum
a. kit, Tc (technetium) 99m aggregated
a. kit, Tc (technetium) 99m serum
a., low serum
a. (MAA), macroaggregated
a. microspheres kit ▸ Tc (technetium) 99m
a., normal human serum
a. of Bence Jones
a., Patein's
a., qualitative
a., quantitative
a., radioactive iodinated human serum
a., radioiodinated serum
a., radioiodinized serum
a. (RISA) scan, radioiodinized serum
a., serum
a., soap
a. (RISA) study, radioactive iodinated serum
a. tannate
a. test
a., triphenyl
a., urine tested for
albuminoid sputum
albuminous
a. granules
a. nephritis
a. swelling
albuminuria
a., adventitious
a., globular
a., nephrogenous
a., postrenal
a., renal
a., residual
albuminuric amaurosis
albumose-free tuberculin
albumosuria
a., Bence Jones
a., Bradshaw's

a., enterogenic
a., pyogenic
albus
a., lichen
a., Saccharomyces tumefaciens
a., Staph
a., Staphylococcus
a., Streptomyces
a., tumor
Albuterol nebulizer
ALC (axiolinguocervical)
alcalescens, Veillonella
Alcaligenes, (alcaligenes)
a., Bacillus faecalis
A. bookerii
A. bronchosepticus
A. faecalis
A. marshallii
A. metalcaligenes
A. piechaudii
A. recti
A. xylosoxidans
A. viscolactis
alcaptonuria (*see* alkaptonuria)
Alcatel pacemaker, Medtronic-Laurens-
alcian blue
alcian blue stain
alco sensor
alcohol (Alcohol)
a. ablation
a. absorption
a. abstinence
a. abuse
a. abuse, adolescent
a. abuse among children
a. abuse among men
a. abuse among women
a. abuse, chronic
a. abuse, comorbid
a. abuse death ▸ drug and
a. abuse, eliminate
a. abuse problems ▸ children with
a. abuse problems ▸ men with
a. abuse problems ▸ women with
a. abuse ▸ self-destructive
a. abuse ▸ sudden death due to
a. abuse treatment
a. abuser
a. addiction
a. amnestic disorder
a. amnestic syndrome
a. and drug abuse testing
a. and drug abuse treatment
a. and drug counseling
a. and drug education

a. and drug treatment issues ▸ impaired employees
a. and drug use
a. and sexuality
a. and substance abuse
a. and substance abuse treatment professionals
a. baby ▸ fetal
a., blood
a. brain damage
a. ▸ cardiovascular effects of
a., cellular effects of
a., cessation of
a., cirrhosis from
a. cleansing, general
a. concentration, blood
a., consume
a. consumption
a. consumption, excessive
a. consumption, heavy
a. consumption ▸ level of
a. consumption, moderating
a. consumption, reduced
a. consumption, sensitive to
a. content (BAC), blood
a. dehydrogenase
a., delirium from
a., delirium induced by
a. ▸ dementia induced by
a. dependence
a. dependence, drug and
a. dependence syndrome
a. dependency
a. dependency program
a. dependent, patient
a., depression from
a. deterioration
a. detox
a. detoxification
a., drowsiness from
a. drug, anti-
a., drug interaction with
a. during pregnancy ▸ drinking
a. effect on brain
a. effect on liver
a. effect on lungs
a. enforcement
a. ▸ ethnic susceptibility to
a., ethyl
a. ▸ excessive consumption of
a. expectancies
a. exposure, chronic
a. exposure ▸ long-term
a. exposure ▸ prenatal
a. ▸ eye puffiness from

a. family systems
a., flushing from
a., forgetfulness from
a., gastritis from
a., gastroenteritis
a., genetic predisposition to
a. group
a., gout from
a. habit
a. habituation
a., hallucinations from
a. hallucinosis
a., headache from
a. heart muscle disease ▸ symptomatic
a. ▸ heat intolerance from
a., heavy consumption of
a. idiosyncratic intoxication
a. impairs cardiac function
a. impairment
a. in blood stream
a., incapacitated by
a. -induced amnestic disorder
a. -induced blackouts
a. -induced cardiomyopathy
a. -induced damage
a. -induced dementia
a. -induced disorder
a. -induced functional impairment
a. -induced injury
a. -induced liver disease
a. -induced pancreatitis
a. -induced sleep disorder
a. industry
a., infertility from
a. ingestion ▸ acute or chronic
A. Inpatient Review System (PAIRS) program ▸ Psychiatric
a., insomnia from
a. intake
a. intake, excessive
a. intake ▸ initial levels of
a. intake, limiting
a. intake withdrawal
a. interactions
a. interventions
a. intoxication
a. intoxication, idiosyncratic
a., isopropyl
a. lamp flame
a., leukoplakia from
a. level, blood
a. level ▸ high blood
a. level, serum
a. maintenance

a. message, anti-
a. metabolism
a. misuse
a., moderate amounts of
a. molecule
a. on breath
a. or drug abuse
a. or drug use ▸ recent
a. or drug use ▸ recovery of
a. overdose
a. pad
a., palpitations and
a., pancreatitis from
a. patch
a., pepper, spicy (CAPS) foods-free diet ▸ caffeine,
a. poisoning, methyl
a., polyvinyl
a., powerless over
a. pneumonia
a. ▸ prenatal effects of
a. prevention
a. prevention strategy
a. problems
a. psychosis
a. -related accident
a. -related behavior
a. -related birth defects
a. -related cerebral disorder
a. -related death
a. -related defects
a. -related dementia
a. -related diseases
a. -related fatalities
a. -related headache
a. -related health hazards
a. -related heart disorders
a. -related hepatitis
a. -related illness
a. -related injuries
a. -related mortality statistics
a. -related offenses
a. -related problems
a. -related skin disorder
a. -related violence
a. -related vitamin deficiency
a. research
a. resistance, acid
a. retardation, fetal
a., seizure from
a. septal ablation
a., severe addiction to
a. skin flushing
a., smell of
a. substance abuse

alcohol—*continued*
- a. swab
- a., swelling from
- a. symptoms ▸ minimization of
- a. syndrome (FAS), fetal
- a. syndrome, full
- a., taste of
- a. test meal, Ehrmann's
- a. testing, breath
- a. tolerance
- a. treatment
- a., ulcers from
- a., urination from
- a. usage, heavy
- a. use, active
- a. use ▸ elderly
- a. use ▸ excessive
- A. Use Inventory (AUI)
- a. use ▸ pattern pathologic
- a. use ▸ post-treatment
- a. user, heavy
- a. withdrawal
- a. withdrawal delirium
- a. withdrawal hallucinosis
- a. withdrawal seizure
- a. withdrawal symptoms, differential diagnosis of
- a. withdrawal syndrome (AWS)
- a. withdrawal syndrome ▸ severe
- a. withdrawal, uncomplicated

alcoholic(s) (Alcoholic)
- a., abstinent
- a., active
- a., acute
- a., adult
- A. (ACOA), Adult Children of
- a. amblyopia
- a. amentia, Steam's
- A. Anonymous (AA)
- a. ataxia
- a., average
- a. beverage
- a. brain syndrome
- a. brain syndrome, chronic
- a. breath
- a. cardiomyopathy
- a. cardiomyopathy: preclinical, acute and chronic
- a., children of
- a., chronic
- a. cirrhosis
- a. coma
- a. counseling ▸ individual adult children of
- a. delirium, chronic

- a. dementia
- a. drug dependent person
- a. encephalopathy
- a. family
- a. fatty liver
- a. gastritis
- a., halfway house for
- a. hallucinosis
- a., hard core
- a. heart muscle disease
- a. heart muscle disease ▸ chronic
- a. hepatitis
- a. hepatitis, acute
- a. hepatitis, clinical
- a. hyaline inclusion bodies
- a. individual
- a. insanity
- a. intake, excessive
- a. intolerance
- a. intoxication, acute
- a. jealousy
- a., juvenile
- a. label
- a. lifestyle
- a. liver disease
- a. liver disease ▸ clinical
- a. liver disease ▸ severe
- a. malnutrition
- a. myocardiopathy
- a. myopathy
- a. ▸ newly recovering
- a. pancreatitis
- a. paranoia
- a. parents ▸ child of
- a. parents ▸ daughter of
- a. parents ▸ son of
- a. patient
- a. patient, acute
- a. ▸ patient functioning
- a. personality
- a. ▸ personality traits in
- a. pneumonia
- a. population
- a., potential
- a., prevalence of drug abuse in
- a. psychiatric outpatient ▸ non-
- a. psychosis
- a., recovering
- a., rehabilitation center for
- A. Screen Testing (CAST) ▸ Children of
- a., Stearns'
- a. stimulant
- a., suffering
- a., teenage

- a., treat
- a., Type I
- a., Type II
- a., typical
- a. user, hard

alcoholism
- a., active
- a. ▸ acute stage of
- a., advanced
- a. and alpha-theta biofeedback
- a. and drug abuse
- a. ▸ cardinal sign of
- a., chronic
- a. -chemical dependency program
- a., cognitive impairment in
- a., comorbid
- a. community treatment
- a. counseling
- a. counselor
- a., crisis counseling for
- a. ▸ dementia associated with
- a., denial of
- a. ▸ depression and
- a. ▸ diagnosis and treatment of
- a. disorder
- a. education
- a. etiology
- a. gene
- a., genetic
- a. ▸ genetic aspects of
- a., genetic component to
- a., geriatric
- a., hepatitis and
- a., hypothermia and
- a., laryngitis and
- a., metabolic aspect of
- a., parental
- a. ▸ persistent injury by chronic
- a., pharmacotherapy for
- a. ▸ problem with central nervous system from
- a. ▸ risk of developing
- a. ▸ ripple effect of
- a. self-testing
- a. susceptibility
- a., therapy for
- a. treatment field
- a., treatment resistant
- a., Types I and II

ALD (adrenoleukodystrophy) diagnosis
ALD (assistive living device) ▸ personal
aldehyde-fuchsin ▸ trypsin,
aldolase test
aldosterone
- a., adrenal vein

a. antagonist
a. cascade ▸ renin angiotensin
a. depression
a. excretion rate
a. -producing adenoma
a. secretion defect
a. secretion rate
a. system ▸ renin angiotensin
a. test
a., urine and plasma
aldosteronism, juvenile
aldosteronism, primary
Aldrich('s)
A. operation
A. scale
A. syndrome
A. syndrome, Wiskott-
aldrichi, Aedes
aleolar/alveolar
aleolar yokes of mandible
alert (Alert)
a. and cooperative ▸ patient
a. and cooperative ▸ patient awake,
a. and oriented ▸ patient
a. awake subject
a. behavior
a. device, emergency
A., Group
A., Life
a. necklace or bracelet ▸ medical
a. patient
a. ▸ patient mentally
a. state of consciousness
a. state, quiet-
a. to space, time and persons ▸
  patient
a. wallet card ▸ medical
alertness
a. and arousal
a. and coordination, reduce
a. and lucidity ▸ periods of
a. and memory
a., decreased
a. ▸ gradual loss of
a., impaired
a. increased
a., increased energy/
a. ▸ lack of awareness and
a., mental
aleukemic myelosis
aleukia, congenital
aleukia hemorrhagica
aleukocythemic leukemia
aleuron/aleurone
aleuronoid granules

Aleutian disease
Alexander('s)
A. -Adams operation
A. operation
A. technique
alexandrinus, Mus
alexandrinus, Rattus rattus
alexandrite laser
alexia, optical
Alexithymia Scale ▸ Toronto
alfreddugesi, Eutrombicula
ALG (axiolinguogingival)
algae, blue-green
algae-like fungus
algebraic reconstruction technique
algera
a., aphagia
a., apraxia
a., cyskinesia
a., dysopia
algica, synesthesia
algid stage
alginolyticus, Vibrio
ALGOL (ALGOrithmic Language)
algorithm
a., bone
a., computer
a. ▸ radix two
ALGOrithmic Language (ALGOL)
aliases ▸ use of
aliasing artifact
aliasing, image
Alibert-Bazin syndrome
Alice in Wonderland syndrome
alienation of others
alienation, parental
aligned, bone
alignment
a., active
a., anatomical position and
a. and apposition
a. and apposition of fracture ▸
  proper
a. and position
a., body
a., bony
a. disorder, knee joint
a., eye
a. ▸ improper foot
a., knee
a. mark
a. of body ▸ vertical
a. of fracture
a. of fracture ▸ position and
a. of tangential beam

a. of temporomandibular joint
  (TMJ) ▸ proper
a. of vertebrae
a., orbicular
a., overall
a., passive
a., position and
a. ▸ restoration of normal anatomic
a., spinal
a., structural
a. system, laser
a., toe
alike case ▸ AIDS look-
alimentary [*elementary*]
a. bolus
a. canal
a. edema
a. hypoglycemia
a. obesity
a. toxemia
a. tract
alimentation, intravenous
alimentation, parenteral
a-line IV ▸ Add-
alisphenoid bone
alive and well
ALK (automated lamellar keratoplasty)
alkalescens, Escherichia
alkalescens, Shigella
alkali
a. albumin
a. denaturation test
a. -soluble nitrogen
a. syndrome ▸ milk
a. test
a. tolerance test
a., volatile
alkaline
a. intoxication
a. phosphatase (ALP)
a. phosphatase ▸ heat stable
a. phosphatase ▸ leukocyte
a. phosphatase ▸ serum
a. phosphatase test
a. phosphatase (LAP) test,
  leukocyte
a. phosphate
a. reaction
a. tuberculin
alkalinization, obligatory
alkaloid
a., cocaine
a., periwinkle
a., plant
a., Rauwolfia

alkaloid—*continued*
- a. test
- a., vinca

alkalosis
- a., altitude
- a., metabolic
- a., primarily respiratory
- a., respiratory

alkaptonuria (*same as* alcaptonuria)
alkylating
- a. action
- a. agent
- a. agent ▸ polyfunctional

all (All)
- A. (acute lymphoblastic leukemia)
- a. extremities ▸ peripheral cyanosis of
- A. -Flex diaphragm
- a. -night electroencephalogram (EEG) recording
- a. -night sleep recording
- a. or none law

allantoic
- a. circulation
- a. fluid
- a. parasite
- a. stalk
- a. vein

allegation of rape
alleged rape
allele, mutant
Allen('s)
- A. -Brown shunt
- A. implant
- A. maneuver
- A. -Masters syndrome
- A. test
- A. test, Corner-
- A. -Thorpe goniolens
- A. vision test

allergen(s)
- a., cerebral
- a., environmental
- a., exposure to
- a., food
- a. -induced asthma
- a. -induced mediator release

allergic
- a. alveolitis
- a. alveolitis, extrinsic
- a. angiitis
- a. arthritis
- a. asthma
- a. asthma airway problems
- a. bronchopulmonary aspergillosis

- a. bronchospasm
- a. condition
- a. conjunctivitis
- a. conjunctivitis ▸ perennial
- a. conjunctivitis ▸ seasonal
- a. contact dermatitis
- a. coryza
- a. cosmetic reactions
- a. diathesis
- a. disorder
- a. eczema
- a. encephalomyelitis, experimental
- a. extrinsic alveolitis, acute
- a. fungal sinusitis
- a. granulomatosis
- a. granulomatous angiitis
- a. medication, anti-
- a. pannus
- a., patient
- a. purpura
- a. reaction
- a. reaction, anaphylaxis
- a. reaction ▸ fatal
- a. reaction ▸ life-threatening
- a. reaction ▸ psychological
- a. reaction ▸ severe
- a. reaction, systemic
- a. reaction to dye
- a. reaction to penicillin ▸ fatal
- a. reaction to stings
- a. rhinitis
- a. rhinitis ▸ congestive, seasonal
- a. rhinitis ▸ nonseasonal
- a. rhinitis ▸ perennial
- a. rhinitis ▸ seasonal
- a. salute
- a. shiners
- a. shock
- a. skin reaction
- a. skin reaction ▸ widespread
- a. stomatitis
- a. symptoms
- a. to aspirin
- a. to insect venom
- a. tubulointerstitial nephritis
- a. -type reactions
- a. vasculitis

allergy(-ies)
- a., acute food
- a. ▸ altitude change, ear stuffiness from
- a. and immunology
- a., bacterial
- a. ▸ bee sting
- a., bronchial

- a., cold
- a., colic and
- a., contact
- a., coughing from
- a., delayed
- a., drug
- a., food
- a. from chemical
- a., house dust
- a., immediate
- a., -immune system
- a., induced
- a., insect sting
- a., iodine
- a. ▸ latex protein
- a., milk lactose
- a., nasal
- a., patch test for
- a., pediatric
- a., problems, sperm
- a. -related bronchitis
- a., respiratory
- a., seasonal
- a., severe latex
- a., shellfish
- a., sneezing from
- a. sufferer, seasonal
- a., sulfite
- a. syndrome ▸ oral
- a. syndrome, total
- a. to chemical
- a. to dairy product
- a. to food
- a. to insect venom
- a. to insulin
- a. to plants

Allescheria boydii
alleviate(s)
- a. pain
- a. panic attack
- a. suffering
- a. symptoms of nicotine withdrawal

alleviating
- a. disease
- a. psychiatric symptoms
- a. symptoms

alleviation of pain
alleviation of symptoms
alliance, therapeutic
allied health professionals
allied reflexes
Allis's sign
Allison hiatal hernia repair
allocate donated organ ▸ procure and
allochiria/allocheiria

allogeneic
- a. graft
- a. marrow transplantation
- a. transplant
- a. transplantation
- a. veins

allograft
- a., artery and vein
- a. atherosclerosis, cardiac
- a., bone chip
- a., bovine
- a., cardiac
- a., cryopreserved heart valve
- a., cryopreserved human aortic
- a., CryoVein saphenous vein
- a., lung
- a., pancreatic
- a. reaction
- a., renal
- a. rejection, acute
- a. survival
- a. survival enhancement
- a. survival, total lymphoid irradiation for
- a. tissue transplantation
- a. valve ▸ stent-mounted
- a. vasculopathy
- a. vasculopathy, cardiac

Allopurinol induced hepatitis
allorhythmic pulse
allosteric site
allotropic type
allowable concentration ▸ maximum
allowance (RDA), recommended daily
allowances (RDA), recommended dietary
allowed beta transition
ALMCA (anomalous left main coronary artery)
ALO (axiolinguo-occlusal)
alobar holoprosencephaly ▸ familial
Aloe reading unit
alone
- a. ▸ fear of being
- a. ▸ intolerance of being
- a. laser treatment ▸ stand-

aloneness, fear of
along incision site ▸ redness
along skin incision ▸ induration
aloofness, social
alopecia
- a., androgenic
- a. areata
- a., drug-induced
- a., frontal

- a., male
- a., malignant
- a. mucinosa
- a. neurotica
- a. orbicularis
- a., patterned
- a., postpartum
- a., radiation
- a. seborrheica
- a., syphilitic
- a., total
- a. totalis
- a., variable
- a., vertex

Almeica syndrome, Lutz-Splendore-de
alone, patient walks
Alouette's amputation
ALP (alkaline phosphatase)
Alpar's implant
alpha (Alpha)
- a. activity
- a. activity ▸ autonomic control by
- a. activity, bursts of
- a. activity, controlling
- a. activity ▸ electroencephalogram (EEG)
- a. activity, persistent
- a. activity, retained
- a. adhesive, Aron
- a. adrenergic stimulation
- a. -adrenoreceptor agonist
- a. agglutinin
- a. agonist
- a. -alpha homodimer
- a. amino acids
- a. amino-n-butyric acid
- a. amino nitrogen
- a. amino nitrogen test
- a. amylase
- a. antitrypsin
- a. asymmetry ▸ minor
- a. band
- a. beta values
- a. -beta variation
- a. biofeedback
- a. biofeedback and anxiety
- a. biofeedback ▸ colitis and
- a. biofeedback ▸ concepts of
- A. blockers
- a. blocking agent
- a. brain waves
- a. bursts
- a. cells
- a. chain
- a. chamber

- a. coma
- a. conditioning sessions
- a. control
- A. Cradle
- a. decay
- a. -epilepsy research
- a. fetoprotein test
- a. frequency
- a. frequency activity
- a. frequency, rhythm of
- a. frequency, waves of
- a., frequent individual bursts of
- a. fungus
- a. globulin
- a. globulin antibodies
- a. granules
- a. hemolytic
- a. hemolytic streptococcus
- a. homodimer, alpha-
- a. hydroxy acids (AHA)
- a. index
- a., interferon
- a. intrusion
- a. lipoproteins
- a. methyldopa
- a. -methyltyrosine
- a. motoneurons
- A_1 (Alpha$_1$)
- a. -l-antitrypsin deficiency
- a. -l-antitrypsin serum
- a. particles
- a. pattern
- a. procedure, hypnotic-
- a. production
- a. production, control of
- a. radiation
- a. rays
- a. receptors
- a. ▸ recombinant interferon
- a. response
- a. rhythm
- a. rhythm, alternate with
- a. rhythm, intermixed with
- a. rhythm, normal
- a. rhythm, steady
- a. scan
- a. staphylolysin
- a. state
- a. stimulator
- a. streptococcus
- a. substance
- a. synchrony biofeedback ▸ hemispheric
- a. thalassemia

alpha—*continued*
- a. thalassemia X-linked retardation syndrome
- a. therapy ▸ interferon
- a. -theta biofeedback ▸ alcoholism and
- a. -theta electroencephalogram (EEG) frequency range
- a. -theta waves
- a. threshold
- A₂ (Alpha₂)
- a. 2 fat cells
- A. II interferon
- a. 2 receptors
- a. variant
- a. variant rhythm, fast
- a. variant, slow
- a. wave

alphabet
- a. exercise ▸ ankle
- a. keratitic
- a. pointing board
- a., sign language

alphanumeric characters

alphoid rhythm

Alport's syndrome

ALS (advanced life support)

ALS (amyotrophic lateral sclerosis)

ALS (antilymphocyte serum)

Alström-Olsen syndrome

ALT (alanine amino transferase)

alta, patella

ALTE (apparent life-threatening event)

alter(s)
- a. brain chemistry
- a., endless memories ▸ endless
- a. gastric function
- a., managing satanic
- a. personality, violent

alteration(s)
- a., acid base
- a., behavioral
- a., blood gas
- a., cognitive
- a., communication
- a., genetic
- a., gross
- a. immunologic competence
- a. in bladder elimination
- a. in body, physiologic
- a. in cardiac output
- a. in comfort
- a. in diet
- a. in elimination
- a. in endocrine function
- a. in hydration intake
- a. in lifestyle
- a. in mental status
- a. in mood temporary
- a. in normal walk
- a. in nutrition intake
- a. in pattern of urinary elimination
- a. in physical capabilities
- a. in respiratory function
- a. in rest pattern
- a. in sleep pattern
- a. in thought processes
- a. in time perception
- a. in wave form
- a. in wave form ▸ instrumental
- a., inherited gene
- a. mental
- a., mood
- a. of blood brain barrier
- a. of body awareness
- a. of body tone
- a. of cardiovascular function ▸ drug-induced
- a. of consciousness
- a. of media surrounding brain
- a. of memory
- a. of mental function
- a. of muscle tone
- a. of perception
- a. of temperature
- a., pathological
- a. ▸ platelet aggregation
- a., psychotherapy by somatic
- a., pulmonary
- a., sense
- a., sensory
- a. ▸ sensory perceptual
- a., ST
- a. tissue perfusion

altered
- a. body temperature
- a. bowel habits
- a. bowel movements
- a. brain function
- a. by behavior
- a. cells, genetically
- a. cells, ▸ TNF (tumor necrosis factor) gene-
- a. cerebral tissue perfusion
- a. comfort
- a. development
- a. emotions
- a. facial appearance
- a. facial characteristics
- a. family processes
- a. genes
- a. growth and development
- a. health maintenance
- a. level of consciousness
- a. mental state
- a. mentation or physical status
- a. metabolizing enzyme
- a. mood and perceptions
- a. nutrition
- a. oral mucous membrane
- a. orientation in space ▸ sensation of
- a. parenting
- a. patterns of urinary elimination
- a. perceptions
- a. performance
- a. personal behavior
- a. pulmonary surface tensions
- a. renal tissue perfusion
- a. role performance
- a. school performance
- a. sensations
- a. sexuality patterns
- a. somatic sensation
- a. speech
- a. spiritual values
- a. state of conscious awareness
- a. state of consciousness
- a. thought process
- a. time perception
- a. tubular reabsorption
- a. tumor cells ▸ genetically
- a. tumor infiltrating lymphocytes (TIL) ▸ genetically
- a. virus

altering
- a. brain function
- a. capacity, mood
- a. chemical transmitters, mood
- a. chemicals, mood
- a. drug ▸ mind-
- a. drug ▸ mood-
- a. effects, mind-
- a. substances, mood-

alternans
- a., auditory
- a., auscultatory
- a., concordant
- a., cycle length
- a., diabetes
- a., discordant
- a., electrical
- a. of the heart
- a., parvus
- a., pulsus

a., QRS
a. ▸ ST segment
a., systole
a., total
a. ▸ T wave
a. ▸ U wave

alternant, trace
alternate
a. behaviors
a. binaural loudness balance
a. care
a. care nursing facility
a. contractions
a. hemianesthesia
a. hemiplegia
a. inspiration and expiration of air
a. physician ▸ authorization for delivery by
a. physician ▸ consent to delivery by
a. sides of baseline
a. with alpha rhythm

alternately tightening and relaxing muscles
alternating
a. abducens
a. atrial pacemaker
a. bidirectional tachycardia
a. calculus
a. contracting and relaxing of muscles
a. current (AC)
a. current (AC) ▸ opposition of flow of
a. current, range-
a. current (AC) resistance
a. current (AC) signals, low frequency
a. current (AC) voltage
a. douche
a. esophoria
a. esotropia
a. exophoria
a. exotropia
a. hypertropia
a. hypotropia
a. insanity
a. movements (RAM), rapid
a. nystagmus (PAN), periodic
a. oculomotor hemiplegia
a. personality
a. placebo
a. pulse
a. sides of baseline
a. strabismus

a. sursumduction hyperphoria
alternation
a., cardiac
a., concordant
a., cycle length
a., discordant
a., mechanical
a. of heart ▸ electrical
a. of heart ▸ mechanical
alternative(s)
a. approach
a. atrial pacing mode
a., breast preserving
a. diagnosis
a. empiric therapy
a., health care
a. leisure activity
a. lifestyle
a. medications
a. medicine
a. method of treatment
a., nonsurgical
a., positive
a. procedure
a. relaxation technique
a., teaching
a. technology
a. therapies
a. to violent behavior
a. treatment
Althaea officinalis
althea/althaea
altitude
a. alkalosis
a. change, ear stuffiness from allergy
a. hypoxia
a. pulmonary edema, high
a. related disorders, high
a. -related emergency
a. -related illnesses, high
a. sickness
a. sickness, high
a. simulation study
a. simulation test ▸ high
a., stresses of
altitudinal hemianopia
Altmann's
A. fluid
A. granule
A. theory
altruism, reciprocal
altruistic donation
altruistic motivation
alum hematoxylin

aluminosis pulmonum
aluminum
a. equivalent
a. -garnet (Nd:YAG) laser ▸ neodymium: yttrium-
a. hydroxide
a. hydroxide gel
ALVAD (abdominal left ventricular assist device)
Alvarez valve prosthesis
alvei
a., Bacillus
a., Enterobacter
a., Hafnia
alveodental suppuration
alveolabial sulcus
alveolar/aleolar
a. air
a. air spaces
a. air ▸ venous
a. arch
a. asthma
a. bone
a. bronchiole
a. canals
a. cancer
a. capillary bed
a. capillary block
a. capillary membranes
a. capillary thickening
a. capillary unit
a. carbon dioxide (CO_2) pressure
a. carbon dioxide (CO_2) tension
a. carcinoma
a. cavity
a. cell
a. cell carcinoma
a. cell ▸ desquamation of atypical
a. cell, great
a. cell hyperplasia
a. cell ▸ proliferation of atypical
a. cell, squamous
a. cell tumor
a. concentration (MAC) ▸ minimum
a. crown, extra-
a. damage, diffuse
a. damage, typical
a. dead space
a. debris, intra-
a. densities
a. differentiation
a. duct
a. duct emphysema
a. dysplasia, congenital
a. ectasia

alveolar—*continued*
- a. edema
- a. emphysema
- a. epithelium
- a. fibrinous exudate ▸ intra-
- a. fibrinous material, intra-
- a. filling disease ▸ diffuse
- a. filling pattern
- a. flooding
- a. gingiva
- a. hemorrhage
- a. hemorrhage, diffuse
- a. hemorrhage ▸ diffuse pulmonary
- a. hemorrhage, intra-
- a. hemorrhage ▸ pulmonary
- a. hydatid disease
- a. hypertension
- a. hyperventilation
- a. hypoventilation
- a. hypoxia
- a. infiltrate ▸ fluffy
- a. leak
- a. lung disease ▸ diffuse
- a. macrophage
- a. marking ▸ bilateral patchy
- a. microlithiasis, pulmonary
- a. minute ventilation
- a. nerve
- a. nerve, inferior
- a. nerve, superior
- a. neutrophils, intra-
- a. opacification
- a. osteitis
- a. osteitis, localized
- a. oxygen partial pressure (PAO₂)
- a. oxygen (O₂) tension
- a. partial pressure
- a. partial pressure of inhalational anesthetic
- a. phagocyte
- a. proteinosis
- a. proteinosis, pulmonary
- a. pulmonary infiltrates ▸ bilateral
- a. rhabdomyosarcoma
- a. ridge
- a. rupture
- a. saccules
- a. sacs
- a. septal amyloidosis
- a. septum ▸ focal thickening of
- a. sloughing ▸ chronic inflammation with
- a. socket
- a. soft part sarcoma
- a. space

- a. spaces ▸ hyaline membranes lining
- a. ventilation
- a. ventilation per minute
- a. vessels
- a. vessels ▸ extra-
- a. wall
- a. wall, outer layer of
- a. walls ▸ hyalinization of
- a. yokes of mandible
- a. yokes of maxilla

alveolare, periosteum
alveolaris, Echinococcus
alveolaris, pyorrhea
alveolectomy
- a., mandibular recontouring
- a., maxillary
- a., maxillary recontouring

alveoli
- a., clusters of milk-secreting
- a., contracted
- a., emphysematous
- a., dental
- a. dentales mandibulae
- a. dentales maxillae
- a., fluid filled
- a., pulmonary
- a. pulmonis
- a., removal of dental
- a. ▸ squamous cells in

alveolingual sulcus
alveolitis
- a. ▸ acute allergic, extrinsic,
- a., allergic
- a. ▸ chronic diffuse, sclerosing,
- a., chronic extrinsic
- a., chronic fibrosing
- a. (CFA) cryptogenic fibrosing
- a., desquamative
- a., desquamative fibrosing
- a., diffuse sclerosing
- a., extrinsic
- a. ▸ extrinsic allergic
- a., fibrosing
- a., lymphoid
- a. ▸ mural fibrosing
- a. sicca dolorosa

alveoloarterial oxygen (O₂) tension gradient
alveolodental osteoperiostitis
alveolocapillary membrane
alveolocapillary partial pressure gradient
alveologram, air
alveoloplasty, maxillary

alveoloplasty reparative closure
alveolus, removal of dental
alvine dejections
Alzheimer's
- A. cell
- A. dementia
- A. diagnostic assessment services
- A. disease
- A. disease brain cells
- A. disease ▸ brain plaques and tangles of
- A. disease ▸ early onset
- A. disease ▸ early onset familial
- A. disease (FAD) ▸ familial
- A. disease, plaques of
- A. disease-related pattern ▸ non-
- A. Disease Research
- A. disease ▸ support groups for
- A. diseased brain
- A., early onset
- A. patient
- A. sclerosis
- A. senility
- A. stain
- A. syndrome
- A. type, presenile onset, with delirium ▸ primary degenerative dementia of
- A. type, presenile onset, with delusions ▸ primary degenerative dementia of
- A. type, presenile onset, with depression ▸ primary degenerative dementia of
- A. type (SDAT) senile dementia
- A. type, senile onset, uncomplicated ▸ primary degenerative dementia of the
- A. type, senile onset, with delirium ▸ primary degenerative dementia of
- A. type, senile onset, with delusions ▸ primary degenerative dementia of
- A. type, senile onset, with depression ▸ primary degenerative dementia of

AM (axiomesial)
AMA
- AMA (against medical advice)
- AMA (American Medical Association)
- AMA (against medical advice) form signed

AMA (against medical advice) ▸ patient released
amacrine cells
amalgam
  a., dental
  a., emotional
  a., emotional-object
  a. filling
  a. filling, mercury
amalonaticus, Citrobacter
Amanita
  A. muscaria
  A. pantherina
  A. phalloides
  A. rubescens
  A. verna
amantadine hydrochloride
amara, Simaruba
amaurosis
  a., albuminuric
  a., Burns'
  a., cat's eye
  a., central
  a. centralis
  a., cerebral
  a., congenital
  a. crapulosa
  a. cruciata
  a., diabetic
  a. ex anopsia
  a. fugax
  a., hysteric
  a., intoxication
  a., Leber's
  a., nocturnal
  a. partialis fugax
  a., postmarital
  a., quinine
  a., saburral
  a., toxic
  a., traumatic
  a., uremic
amaurotic axonal idiocy, spastic
amaurotic familial idiocy
amazon thorax
AMB (ambulatory)
amber-colored urine
ambient
  a. factor
  a. fissure
  a. hospital air
  a. hospital air ▸ contamination from
  a. pressure
  a. temperature and pressure (ATP)
ambigua, Shigella

ambiguous symptoms ▸ vague and
ambiguus, nucleus
ambiguus, situs
ambition and motivation ▸ loss of
ambivalent feelings
ambivalent patient
Amblyomma
  A. americanum
  A. cajennense
  A. hebraeum
  A. maculatum
  A. ovale
  A. tuberculatum
  A. variagata
  A. variegatum
amblyopia
  a. alcoholica
  a., arsenic
  a., astigmatic
  a. ex anopsia
  a., hysteric
  a., toxic
  a., uremic
ambofaciens, Streptomyces
Ambrosia artemisiaefolia
Ambrosia trifida
Ambu
  A. bag
  A. CardioPump
  A. respirator
  A. resuscitator ▸ infant
ambulance service, air
ambulans, pestis
ambulated, patient
ambulates
  a. on parallel bars, patient
  a. with assistance, patient
  a. with minimal assist
  a. with walker, patient
ambulating, difficulty
ambulating with walker nonweight
  bearing ▸ patient
ambulation [*angulation*]
  a., aids to
  a. balance
  a., contact assistance for patient released
  a., early
  a. goal
  a., gradual
  a., independent
  a., patient independent in
  a., progressive
  a., standby assist with

  a., standby assistance in transfers and
  a., standing
  a. with walker
ambulatory (AMB) (Ambulatory)
  a. basis
  a. blood pressure monitor (ABPM)
  a. care
  a. care, continued
  A. Care Unit (ACU)
  a. clinic
  a. electrocardiographic monitoring (AEM)
  a. electrocardiography (AECG)
  a. electrocardiography (ECG) monitoring
  a. Holter monitoring (AHM)
  a. ischemia monitoring
  a. monitoring system ▸ transtelephonic
  a. nuclear detection
  a. nuclear detector
  a. opiate detoxification
  a. patient
  a. patient, semi◊
  a. peritoneal dialysis (CAPD), continuous
  a. peritoneal dialysis patient
  a. phlebectomy
  a. schizophrenia
  a. surgery
  a. with crutches
Ambulift, patient
ambylopia fugax
amblyopic eye
Ambystoma mexicanum
AMC (axiomesiocervical)
AMD (axiomesiodistal)
ameba
  a., artificial
  a. colitis
  a., coprozoic
amebiasis (*same as* amoebiasis)
  a. cutis
  a., hepatic
  a., intestinal
  a. of bladder
  a., pulmonary
amebic (*same as* amoebic)
  a. appendicitis
  a. colitis
  a. dysentery
  a. granuloma
  a. hepatitis
  a. infection

amebic—*continued*
- a. invasion
- a. liver abscess
- a. meningitis
- a. meningoencephalitis, primary
- a. pericarditis
- a. pneumonia
- a. prevalence rate
- a. ulcer

amebocyte (*same as* amoebocyte)

ameboid (*same as* amoeboid)
- a. cell
- a. glia
- a. movements

amelanotic melanoma

amelanotic nevus

ameliorate pain

ameliorate symptoms

ameliorated, headache

ameloblastic hemangioma

ameloblastic odontoma

ameloblastoma
- a., melanotic
- a., pigmented
- a., pituitary

ameliorate pain

amelodentinal junction

amelogenesis imperfecta

amenorrhea/amenorrhoea
- a., absolute
- a. and hirsutism
- a., dysponderal
- a., functional
- a., hypothalamic
- a., lactation
- a., ovarian
- a., physiologic
- a., pituitary
- a., postpill
- a., premenopausal
- a., primary
- a., relative
- a., secondary

amenorrheal/amenorrhoeal

amenorrheic/amenorrhoeic

amentia
- a. agitata
- a. attonita
- a., nevoid
- a. occulta
- a., paranoides
- a., phenylpyruvic
- a., Stearn's alcoholic

American
- A. Academy of Child and Adolescent Psychology
- A. Academy of Neurology
- A. Association for Partial Hospitalization
- A. Association of Retired Persons (AARP)
- A. blastomycosis, North
- A. blastomycosis, South
- A. Health Assistance Foundation (AHAF)
- A. Heart Association (AHA) diet
- A. hemorrhagic fever, South
- A. Junin virus ▸ South
- A. mountain fever
- A. Psychiatric Association (APA)
- A. Sleep Disorders Association
- A. Society of Addiction Medicine
- A. Society of Laser Medicine and Surgery (ASLMS)
- A. trypanosomiasis

americana
- a., Cochliomyia
- a., Persea
- a., Scopulariopsis

americanum, Amblyomma

americanus, Necator

Ames shunt

amethopterin, 6-mercaptopurine and prednisone (VAMP) ▸vincristine,

ametropia
- a., axial
- a., curvature
- a., index
- a., position
- a., refractive

AMG (axiomesiogingival)

AMI (acute myocardial infarction)

AMI (axiomesioincisal)

Amici's
- A. disk
- A. line
- A. striae

amide synthetase

amidine, insoluble

amidine, tegumentary

Amidostomum anseris

amimia
- a., amnesic
- a., ataxic

amine
- a., aromatic
- a., biogenic
- a., catechol◊

- a. depletion brain
- a., primary
- a., secondary
- a., sympathomimetic
- a., tertiary
- a. type product solution ▸ quaternary-

amino
- a. acid
- a. acid analyzer
- a. acid metabolism
- a. acid metabolism ▸ disorders of
- a. acid sequence
- a. acids, alpha
- a. nitrogen, alpha
- a. nitrogen test, alpha
- a. transferase (ALT), alanine

aminobutyric acid (GABA), gamma-

aminobutyric acid, hydroxyl

aminoglycoside(s)
- a. acetyltransferase
- a. antibiotics
- a. molecules
- a. nucleotidyltransferase
- a. resistant antibiotics
- a. toxicity

aminohippurate clearance, para-

aminolevulinic
- a. acid
- a. acid dehydrase
- a. acid, delta-

amino-n-butyric acid, alpha

aminopenicillanic acid

aminopeptidase
- a., cystine
- a., leucine
- a. test, leucine

aminosalicylate sodium

aminosalicylic acid

aminotransferase
- a., alanine
- a., aspartate
- a., tyrosine

amiodarone-induced hyperthyroidism

Amipaque contrast medium

AML
- AML (acute monocytic leukemia)
- AML (acute myeloblastic leukemia)
- AML (acute myelocytic leukemia)

Ammi, majus

Ammi, visnaga

AMML (acute myelomonocytic leukemia)

AMMOL (acute myelomonoblastic leukemia)

ammonia
a., Blastomycoides
a., blood
a. hemate
a. level
ammoniacum, Dorema
ammonium chloride
ammonium chloride, intravenous
Ammon's horn
Ammon's operation
Ammospermophilus leucurus
amnemonic aphasia
amnemonica, agraphia
amnesia
a., anterograde
a., associated
a., auditory
a., Broca's
a., circumscribed
a., dissociative
a. ▸ disorientation with
a., emotional
a. ▸ emotional numbing and
a., episodic
a. ▸ fractional retrograde
a., global
a., immunologic
a., infantile
a., lacunar
a., localized
a., olfactory
a., organic
a., patchy
a., posthypnotic
a., post-traumatic
a., progressive
a., psychogenic
a., retroactive
a., retrograde
a., short-term
a., source
a., tactile
a. ▸ temporary global
A. Test (GOAT) ▸ Galveston Orientation and
a., total
a. (TGA) ▸ transient global
a., traumatic
a., tropical
a., verbal
a., visual
amnesic
a. amimia
a. aphasia
a. color blindness

a. disorder
a., patient
amnestic
a. aphasia
a. apraxia
a. disorder
a. disorder, alcohol
a. disorder, alcohol-induced
a. disorder, anxiolytic
a. disorder, hypnotic
a. disorder ▸ psychoactive substance
a. disorder, sedative
a. syndrome
a. syndrome, alcohol
a. syndrome ▸ drug-induced
amnii, liquor
amniocentesis indicative of infection
amnion, abundant aspirated
amnion membranes
amnionitis, acute
amniotic
a. adhesions of fetus
a. cavity
a. cavity, outlining
a. cyst
a. ectoderm
a. fluid
a. fluid aspiration
a. fluid at term
a. fluid culture
a. fluid cultured and aspirated
a. fluid drained and preserved
a. fluid embolism
a. fluid, foul smelling
a. fluid ▸ odorous
a. fluid syndrome
a. hernia
a. fluid, meconium stained
a. fold
a. infection syndrome
a. sac
a. saline infusion, intra-
a. umbilicus
a. villus
AMO (axiomesio-occlusal)
A-mode (amplitude modulation)
A. echocardiography
A. echo-tracking device
A. scanning
A. ultrasonography
Amoeba
A. buccalis
A. cachexica
A. coli

A. coli mitis
A. dentalis
A. dysenteriae
A. histolytica
A. limax
A. meleagridis
A. organism
A. proteus
A. urinae granulata
A. urogenitalis
A. verrucosa
amoebiasis (*see* amebiasis)
Amoebobacter
A. bacillosus
A. granula
A. roseus
amoebocyte (*see* amebocyte)
amoeboid (*see* ameboid)
Amoebotaenia sphenoides
amok (*same as* amuck)
AMOL (acute monoblastic leukemia)
among men ▸ alcohol abuse
among women ▸ alcohol abuse
amoral personality
amorphous
a. crystal
a. debris
a. parenchymal opacification
a. phosphate crystals
a. urates
amorphus, fetus
amotio retinae
amotivational syndrome
amount(s)
a. of alcohol, moderate
a. of food, rapid ingestion of large
a. of asbestos exposure ▸ threshold
a. of medication
a. of narcotic ▸ present
AMP (average mean pressure)
amphetamine(s)
a. (Beans)
a. (Bennies)
a. (Black Beauties)
a. (Black Cadillacs)
a. (Black Mollies)
a. (Brown and Clears)
a. (Copilots)
a. (Crank)
a. (Crosses)
a. (Crossroads)
a. (Crystal)
a. (Dexies)
a. (Double Cross)

amphetamine(s)—*continued*
- a. (Footballs)
- a. (Hearts)
- a. (Meth)
- a. (Minibennies)
- a. (Oranges)
- a. (Peaches)
- a. (Pep Pills)
- a. (Rosas)
- a. (Roses)
- a. (Speed)
- a. (Splash)
- a. (Thrusters)
- a. (Truck Drivers)
- a. (Uppers)
- a. (Wake-ups)
- a. (Water)
- a. (Whites)
- a. abuse
- a., blood level of
- a. delirium
- a. delusional disorder
- a. dependence
- a. effect, chronic
- a. hallucinogenic
- a. -induced paranoid psychotic state
- a. (Speed) ingested
- a. (Speed) injected
- a. intoxication
- a. or similarly acting sympathomimetic abuse
- a. or similarly acting sympathomimetic delirium
- a. or similarly acting sympathomimetic dependence
- a. or similarly acting sympathomimetic intoxication
- a. or similarly acting sympathomimetic withdrawal
- a. psychosis
- a. sulfate
- a. toxicity
- a., urine level of
- a., urine screen for
- a. withdrawal

amphidiarthrodial joint
amphibolic stage
Amphileptus branchiarum
Amphimerus noverca
Amphimerus pseudofelineus
amphipathic helix
Amphistoma
- A. conicum
- A. hominis
- A. watsoni

amphophil granules
amphophilic
- a. basophil
- a., gram-
- a. -oxyphil

amphoric
- a. echo
- a. murmur
- a. rale
- a. respiration
- a. voice

amphoteric dipolar ion
amphoteric electrolyte
Amplatz cardiac catheter
Amplatz technique
amplification(s)
- a., automatic
- a. by stimulated emission of radiation (laser) beam, light
- a. by stimulated emission of radiation (MASER) ▸ microwave
- a. factor
- a., gas
- a., gene
- a., light
- a., microwave (mw)
- a., ratio of
- a., reduced
- a., sound

amplified fluoroscopy, image-amplifier
- a., balanced
- a., buffer
- a., chopped
- a., differential
- a., differential electroencephalogram (EEG)
- a., direct coupled
- a., direct current
- a., electroencephalogram (EEG)
- a., image
- a. input frequency
- a., linear
- a., log
- a., nuclear pulse
- a., output
- a. output frequency
- a., pulse
- a. refractory period ▸ pacemaker
- a., resistance-capacitance (R-C) coupled
- a., single-ended
- a., voltage

amplifying factor

amplifying factors ▸ stress-amplitude
- a., acoustic pressure
- a. ▸ apical interventricular septal
- a., atrial pulse
- a., attenuated in
- a., contractile
- a., delta activity of low
- a., extreme lateralized reduction in
- a., frequency and form of
- a., gradient
- a. image
- a. linearity
- a. maximal in proximity of vertex
- a. modulation (A-mode) scanning
- a. modulation (A-mode) ultrasonography
- a. of accommodation
- a. of convergence
- a. of electrical activity ▸ increase in
- a. of electroencephalogram (EEG) waves
- a. of fusion
- a. of signal
- a. of successive responses
- a. of wave, point of maximum
- a. period, peak
- a., pressure
- a., pulse
- a. pulse duration ▸ half
- a. ▸ R wave
- a., reduction in
- a. slowing, bi◊
- a. threshold
- a., unequal
- a., variable
- a., varying
- a. ▸ ventricular pulse
- a., wall
- a. waves
- a., waves of increasing

ampule ampul ampoule
ampulla
- a. canaliculi lacrimalis
- a. ductus deferentis
- a. ductus lacrimalis
- a., Henle's
- a. hepatopancreatica
- a. of gallbladder
- a. of lacrimal duct
- a. of vas deferens
- a. of Vater
- a., phrenic
- a., rectal

a., sphincter muscle of hepatopancreatic
a., Thoma
ampullar abortion
ampullar nerve
  a.n. anterior
  a.n. inferior
  a.n. lateral
  a.n. posterior
  a.n. anterior
ampullares tubae uterinae, plicae
ampullaris, cupula cristae
ampullary adenocarcinoma
ampullary aneurysm
amputated
  a. above ankle
  a., appendix ligated and
  a., forefoot
  a., left lower extremity (LLE)
  a., left upper extremity (LUE)
  a., lower extremities bilaterally
  a., partially
  a., right lower extremity (RLE)
  a., right upper extremity (RUE)
  a. stump
amputation(s)
  a., above elbow (AE)
  a., above knee (AK)
  a., accidental
  a., AE (above elbow)
  a., AK (above knee)
  a. Alouette's
  a. at a joint
  a. bandage, stockinette
  a., BE (below elbow)
  a., Béclard's
  a., below elbow (BE)
  a., below knee (BK)
  a., Bier's
  a., BK (below knee)
  a., Bunge's
  a., Callander's
  a., Camden's
  a., chop
  a., Chopart's
  a., cineplastic
  a., circular
  a., closed
  a., coat-sleeve
  a., complete
  a., congenital
  a., consecutive
  a., cutaneous
  a., diaclastic
  a., double-flap

a., Dupuytren's
a., eccentric
a., elliptic
a., entire lower limb
a., Farabeuf's
a., fingertip
a., flap
a., flapless
a., Forbe's
a., forequarter
a., galvanocaustic
a., Gritti
a., Gritti-Stokes
a., guillotine
a., Guyon's
a., Hancock's
a., Hey's
a., immediate
a., Jaboulay
a., Kirk's
a., Langenbeck's
a., Larrey's
a., LeFort's
a., linear
a., Lisfranc's
a., MacKenzie's
a., Maisonneuve's
a., major
a., mediotarsal
a., minor
a., mixed
a., multiple
a., musculocutaneous
a., natural
a., oblique
a. of cervix
a. of foot at ankle
a. of limb
a., open
a., operative
a., osteoplastic
a., oval
a., partial
a., partial breast
a., pathological
a., periosteoplastic
a., phalangophalangeal
a., Pirogoff's
a., primary
a., quadruple
a., racket
a., rectangular
a., Ricard's
a., root
a., secondary

a. site
a., spontaneous
a., Stokes'
a. stump
a. stump, cone-shaped
a. stump, revision of
a., subastragalar
a., subperiosteal
a., surgical
a., Syme's
a., synchronous
a., Teale's
a., technique
a., tendoplastic
a., tertiary
a., transmetatarsal
a., traumatic
a., Tripier's
a., Wladimiroff-Mikulicz
amputee(s)
  a. ▸ land mine
  a., patient bilateral lower limb
  a., patient bilateral upper limb
AMS (automatic mode switching)
AMSA, prednisone, and chlorambucil (APC) chemotherapy
Amsler Grid Test
Amsler marker, Gonnin-
Amsterdam dwarf
Amtech-Killeen pacemaker
a.m.u. (atomic mass unit)
amuck (*see* amok)
amusia, motor
amusia, sensory
AMX 110 mobile x-ray unit
amyl nitrate
amylase
  a., alpha
  a. clearance
  a. ▸ decrease in serum
  a. ▸ decreased tubular reabsorption of
  a. elevation, serum
  a. excretion, urinary
  a. pancreatic
  a., salivary
  a., serum
  a., serum urine
  a. test
  a., urinary
  a., urine
amyloid
  a. angiopathy, cerebral
  a. arthropathy
  a., beta

amyloid—*continued*
- a. bodies
- a. degeneration
- a., degraded
- a. deposit
- a. fibrils
- a. heart disease
- a. hypothesis, beta
- a. infiltration
- a. kidney
- a. liver
- a. nephrosis
- a. plaques
- a. precursor protein
- a. production, beta
- a. protein
- a. protein, beta
- a. stain
- a. tongue
- a. tumor

amyloidosis
- a., alveolar septal
- a., cardiac
- a., familial
- a., lichen
- a., mediastinal
- a. ▸ nodular pulmonary
- a. of conjunctive
- a. of heart
- a., parenchymal
- a., pleural
- a., primary
- a. ▸ primary systemic
- a. ▸ pseudotumoral mediastinal
- a., pulmonary
- a., renal
- a., secondary
- a., senile
- a., tracheobronchial

amyostatic-kinetic type
amyotonia congenita
amyotrophia, neuralgic
amyotrophia spinalis progressiva
amyotrophic
- a. chorea
- a. lateral sclerosis (ALS)
- a. lateral sclerosis (FALS), familial

amyotrophy, brachial
amyotrophy, diabetic
amythistinum, Chromobacterium
AN region
ANA (antinuclear antibodies)
anabolic
- a. agent, androgenic
- a. effect

- a. nerve
- a. steroid
- a. steroid abuse

anacidity, gastric
anaclitic depression
anaclitic therapy
anacrotic
- a. limb
- a. notch
- a. pulse

anadicrotic pulse
anaemia (*see* anemia)
anaemic (*see* anemic)
anaerobes
- a., facultative
- a., fecal
- a., mouth
- a., obligate

anaerobic
- a. bacillus organisms
- a. bacteria
- a. bacteroides
- a. chamber
- a. culture
- a. cultures of cardiac blood
- a. decomposition
- a. derived energy
- a. empyema
- a. endurance
- a. exercise
- a. gas mixture
- a. glycolysis
- a. gram negative rods
- a. infection
- a. infections ▸ mixed aerobic-
- a. lung abscess
- a. metabolism
- a. organisms
- a. pneumonitis
- a. respiration
- a. respiratory infection
- a. staphylococci
- a. threshold

anaerobius, Peptostreptococcus
anaesthetic (*see* anesthetic)
anaesthetist (*see* anesthetist)
anaesthetize (*see* anesthetize)
Anagnostakis, operation
anal
- a. abscess
- a. canal
- a. canal ▸ abscess in
- a. canal carcinoma
- a. cancer
- a. condyloma

- a. cushion
- a. development
- a. disorders
- a. dysplasia
- a. eroticism
- a. fissure
- a. fissure bleeding
- a. fissures from childbirth
- a. fistula
- a. fistula, chronic
- a. incontinence
- a. intercourse
- a. intercourse, homosexual
- a. irritation
- a. itch
- a. itching
- a. itching and antibiotic
- a. manometry
- a. mucous membrane
- a. opening
- a. orifice
- a. pain
- a. prolapse
- a. protrusion
- a. reflex
- a. region
- a. sinuses
- a. sphincter
- a. sphincter, contract
- a. sphincter ▸ lax
- a. sphincter muscles
- a. sphincterotomy
- a. stenosis
- a. stricture
- a. surgical repair
- a. tears
- a. tone
- a. verge

analeptic agent
analeptic enema
analgesia
- a., epidural
- a. medication
- a., obstetric
- a., patient-controlled
- a., pinprick
- a., postoperative
- a., regional
- a., spinal

analgesic
- a., adjuvant
- a. agent
- a., buffered
- a. drug
- a. effect

a. medication, parenteral
a., mild
a., narcotic
a. nephropathy
a., nonnarcotic
a., nonopioid
a., opioid
a., oral
a. (PCA) ▸ patient-controlled
a. rebound
a. requirements

analog/analogue
a., adenosine
a. computations
a. computer
a. date
a. digital conversion (A/D, ADC)
a. feedback
a. hearing aid
a. hearing aid ▸ programmable
a. (PCPy/PHP), phencyclidine
a. (Rocket Fuel), phencyclidine
a. (TCP/TPCP), phencyclidine
a. photo
a. rate meter
a. scale ▸ visual
a. signal
a. -to-digital converter

analogous
a. data
a. in vitro
a. rhythm
a. tissue

analysis(-es) (Analysis)
a., acoustic and phonetic
a., activation
a., adult
a. and culture, biochemical
A. and Retrieval System
  (MEDLARS) ▸ Medical Literature
a. and synthesis ▸ distributive
a., arterial blood gas
a. at conclusion of clinical trials
a., automatic
a., backscatter
a., bacterial
a., bayesian
a., beat-to-beat
a., behavioral
a., biochemical
a., bivariant
a., body composition
a., body fat
a., bull's eye
a., cell block

a., character
a., checkerboard
a., chemical
a., child
a., cholesterol
a., chromosomal
a., chromosome
a., circumstantial
a., combined
a., compartmental
a., computed
a., computer
a., carotid
a., correlation
a., cumulative
a., cytogenic
a., data
a., decision
a., developmental
a., digital image
a., dimensional
a. ▸ direct immunofluorescence
a., DNA (deoxyribonucleic acid)
a., Doppler
a., Doppler spectral
a., Doppler wave form
a., dose intensity
a., dot blot
a., drawing
a., duodenal fluid
a., ego
a., electrophoretic
a., epidemiological
a., feather
a., fecal
a. ▸ fetal blood
a., fingerprint
a. ▸ flow cytometric
a. ▸ forced vital capacity
a., frequency
a. ▸ frequency domain
a., functional
a., gait
a., gastric
a., genetic
a., heteroduplex
a., histologic
a., hormone
a., image
a. ▸ image display and
a., immunocytochemical
a., immunofluorescence
a., immunogenotypic
a., immunohistochemical
a., immunophenotypic

a., interim
a., joint fluid
a., laboratory
a., least-squares
a., linear displacement
a., linkage
a., lipoprotein
a., live cell
a., microscopic
a., molecular
a. ▸ molecular genetic
a. ▸ multicolor data
a., multicomponent
a. ▸ multilinear regression
a., multivariant
a. ▸ multivariant regressional
a., narrow band frequency
a. ▸ neutron activation
a., nutrient
a., nutrition
a. of hair follicles ▸ segmental
a. of secretion ▸ microscopic
a. of variance
a. of variance ▸ multivariate
a. ▸ optic nerve head
a., pentagastrin stimulated
a., perceptual-motor organization
  and
a., period
a. ▸ phase image
a., post hoc
a. ▸ pressure volume
a., probability
a., prognostic
a., quantitative
a. ▸ quantitative coronary
  angiographic
a., radiometric
a., regression
a., retrospective
a., risk
a., risk-benefit
a., saturation
a., semen
a., sensitivity
a., Simkin
a. ▸ sinoatrial (SA) cell
a. ▸ slot blot hybridization
a. ▸ Southern blot
a. ▸ Southern transfer
a., specific drug
a., spectral
a., Spenco R
a., sputum
a. ▸ standard procedure of rigorous

analysis—*continued*
- a., statistical
- a., test, hair
- a. test, semen
- a. ▸ three-dimensional
- a. ▸ time domain
- a. ▸ transfer function
- a., univariant
- a., univariate
- a., urine
- a., visual
- a. ▸ visual detail
- a. ▸ wall motion
- a. ▸ wave-form
- a. ▸ Western blot
- a. ▸ x-ray diffraction

analyst, health records

analytic
- a. approach ▸ strategic, experiential, and ego
- a. psychology
- a. skills
- a. specificity

analytical
- a. balance
- a. chemistry
- a. immunofiltration
- a. psychotherapy for anxiety
- a. psychotherapy for depression

analyzed ▸ amniotic fluid cultured

analyzed, patient

analyzer(s) (Analyzer)
- a., amino acid
- a., automatic
- a., blood auto-
- A. Computer (SMAC) ▸ Sequential Multiple
- a., cyto▸
- a., gas
- a., multichannel
- a. ▸ pacing system
- a. ▸ pulse height
- a. (SMA-6) test, sequential multiple
- a. (SMA-12) test, sequential multiple
- a. time

analyzes tissue health

analyzing machine, portable

analyzing surgical tissue

anancastic personality disorder

Anamirta cocculus

anamnestic reaction

anamnestic response

anancastic personality

anangioid disk

anaphylactic
- a. antibody
- a. attack
- a. conjunctivitis
- a. crisis
- a. intoxication
- a. reaction
- a. rhinitis
- a. shock
- a. symptoms
- a. transfusion reaction

anaphylactoid purpura

anaphylactoid reaction

anaphylaxis
- a., acute
- a. allergic reaction
- a. emergency treatment
- a. ▸ insect ring
- A. ▸ slow-reacting substance of

Anaplasma
- A. centrale
- A. marginale
- A. ovis

Anaplasmosis centrale

anaplastic
- a. astrocytoma
- A. astrocytoma ▸ multifocal
- a. carcinoma
- a. carcinoma of bladder
- a. carcinoma of kidney
- a. carcinoma, poorly differentiated
- a. disease
- a. infiltrating single cells
- a. sarcoma
- a. thyroid tumor

anaplerotic sequence

anarthria, cortical

anasarca, dyspnea and

anasarca, massive

anastomose artery

anastomosed to duodenum ▸ gallbladder

anastomosed to loop of bowel

anastomosis
- a., aneurysm by
- a., anterocolic
- a., antiperistaltic
- a., aortic
- a., arterial
- a. arteriovenosa
- a., arteriovenous
- a. (BCA), bidirectional cavopulmonary
- a. (BSCA), bidirectional superior cavopulmonary anastomosis

- a., biliary enteric
- a., Billroth I
- a., Billroth II
- a., Braun's
- a., bronchial artery
- a., cavopulmonary
- a., Clado's
- a., cobra-head
- a., colocolic
- a., colorectal
- a., Cooley intrapericardial
- a., Cooley modification of Waterson
- a., crucial
- a., delayed
- a., distal
- a. end of stomach
- a., end-to-end
- a., end-to-side
- a., endogenous
- a., enteric
- a., erosive
- a., esophagojejunal
- a. ▸ Fontan atriopulmonary
- a., Galen's
- a., gastrojejunal
- a., Glenn
- a., graft
- a., hepatojejunal
- a., heterocladic
- a., homocladic
- a., Hyrtl's
- a., ileoanal
- a., ileorectal
- a. intact
- a., intestinal
- a., isoperistaltic
- a., Jacobson's
- a., jejunojejunostomy
- a., Kugel
- a. ▸ laser-assisted vascular
- a., leptomeningeal
- a., Nakayama
- a. of carotid artery
- a. of pancreatic duct, surgical
- a. of retinal and choroidal vessels
- a. of Riolan
- a. ▸ percutaneous portocaval
- a., peristaltic
- a., portacaval
- a., portoportal
- a. ▸ portopulmonary venous
- a., portosystemic
- a., postcostal
- a., Potts
- a. ▸ Potts-Smith

a., precapillary
a., precostal
a., primary
a., pyeloileocutaneous
a., Roux-en-Y
a., side-to-end
a., side-to-side
a. ▸ stenotic esophagogastric
a., stirrup
a., Sucquet-Hoyer
a. ▸ systemic to pulmonary artery
a., terminoterminal
a., transureteroureteral
a., ureteroileocutaneous
a., ureterotubal
a., ureteroureteral
a., vascular
a. ▸ vertebral carotid
a., vessel
a. ▸ Waterston extrapericardial

anastomotic
a. artery ▸ Kugel
a. leak
a. site
a. stricture
a. vein, inferior
a. vein, superior
anastomotica, aneurysm
anastomoticum, vas
anatomic
a. alignment ▸ restoration of normal
a. assessment
a. barrier
a. block
a. bypass ▸ extra-
a. conjugate diameter
a. coronary disease
a. defect
a. diagnosis
a. factors
a. impression
a. layers, chest closed in
a. layers, closed in
a. layers, wound closed in
a. lesion
a. localization
a. location
a. locations, usual
a. measurements of patient, topography and
a. occlusion
a. origin and distribution
a. position, normal
a. position, usual
a. site

a. situation, normal
a. structure
a. teeth
anatomical
a. appearance
a. asplenia
a. closure
a. considerations in radiation therapy
a. crown
a. dead space
a. depression
a. factors
a. gift
A. Gift Act, Uniform
A. Gift card, Uniform
a. gift statement
a. imaging
a. landmarks
a. lesion, abnormal
a. location
a. measurements
a. neck of humerus
a. position
a. position and alignment
a. research
a. rigidity
a. site
a. snuff box
a. theories
anatomically
a., incision closed
a. normal
a. normal, kidneys
anatomy (Anatomy)
a., applied
a., atrial
a., brain
a., cardiovascular
a., comparative
a., coronary
a., coronary vessel
a., dental
a., descriptive
a., developmental
a., ductal
a., general
A., Gray's
a., gross
a., histologic
a. ▸ immune system
a., internal
a., macroscopic
a., medical
a., microscopic

a., minute
a. ▸ native coronary
a. of addiction
a. of aging
a., oncologic
a., pathologic
a., pathological
a., physiognomonic
a., physiological
a. ▸ plantar compartmental
a., plastic
a., radiographic
a., radiological
a., regional
a., skin
a., spinal
a., surface
a., surgical
a., systematic
a., topographic
a., x-ray
a., zonal
anatoxin reaction
anatricrotic pulse
anatum, Salmonella
anchelys, Chlamydophrys
anchor with suture ligatures
anchorage
a., facial
a., mandibular
a., maxillary
anchoring villus
anchylose (*see* ankylose)
anchylosis (*see* ankylosis)
anchylotic (*see* ankylotic)
ancillary dialysis
ancillary health care
anconeus muscle
a.m., lateral
a.m., medial
a.m., short
ancylose (*see* ankylose)
ancylosis (*see* ankylosis)
Ancylostoma
A. brasiliense
A. braziliense
A. caninum
A. duodenale
ancyroid (*same as* ankyroid)
and [*end*]
and-pin sensation, touch-
Andernach's ossicles
Anders' disease
Andersch's nerve
Andersen's disease

Anderson procedure, Kestenbach-
andersoni, Dermacentor
Anderson's operation
Andogsky's syndrome
Andral decubitus
André-Thomas sign
Andresen appliance
Andrews maneuver, Brant-
Andrews operation
androgen
    a. ablation
    a. ablation therapy
    a., addictive
    a. hormones
    a. -secreting thecal cells
    a., synthetic
androgenic alopecia
androgenic anabolic agent
android pelvis
androsterone sulfate
Anectine, Pentothal and
Anel's operation
anemia (*same as* anaemia)
    a., achrestic
    a., achylic
    a., acquired hemolytic
    a., Addison's
    a., AIDS (acquired immune
        deficiency syndrome) associated
    a. and fatigue
    a., aplastic
    a. ▸ appetite loss from pernicious
    a., aregenerative
    a., autoimmune hemolytic
    a., Bagdad Spring
    a., Biermer-Ehrlich
    a., blood loss
    a. ▸ blurred vision from
    a., breast
    a. ▸ breathing difficulty from
    a., cameloid
    a., cancer-associated
    a., cerebral
    a., chlorotic
    a., chronic hemolytic
    a., chronic myelocytic
    a., chronic refractory
    a., Chvostek's
    a., congenital dyserythropoietic
    a., congenital hemolytic
    a., congenital hypoplastic
    a., congenital nonspherocytic
        hemolytic
    a., Cooley's
    a., crescent cell

a., cytogenic
a., Czerny's
a. ▸ dementia from pernicious
a., dimorphic
a., drepanocytic
a., Dresbach's
a. ▸ drug-induced immune hemolytic
a., dyserythropoietic
a., Edelmann's
a., elliptocytotic
a., enzyme deficiency
a., erythroblastic
a., erythronormoblastic
a., factor, antipernicious
a., fainting from
a., familial erythroblastic
a., Fanconi's
a., folic acid
a. from chemical
a. from hookworm
a. ▸ GI (gastrointestinal) bleed with
a., globe-cell
a. ▸ glucose-6-phosphate
    dehydrogenase deficiency
a. ▸ ground itch
a. ▸ heavy menstrual period from
a. ▸ Heinz body hemolytic
a., hemolytic
a., hereditary hemolytic
a., Herrick's
a., hookworm
a., hypersplenic
a., hypochromic
a. hypochromica siderochrestica
    hereditaria
a., hypoplastic
a., iatrogenic
a., icterohemolytic
a., idiopathic
a. ▸ idiopathic hemolytic
a. ▸ idiopathic hypochromic
a. ▸ immune hemolytic
a., inherited
a., iron deficiency
a., Jaksch's
a., jaundice from
a., juvenile pernicious
a., Larzel's
a., Lederer's
a., Leishman's
a., leukoerythroblastic
a. ▸ limp hair from
a., macrocytic
a., Mediterranean
a., megaloblastic

a. ▸ memory loss from
a., microangiopathic hemolytic
a., microcytic
a., miner's
a., mountain
a., myelopathic
a., myelophthisic
a. neonatorum
a., normochromic
a., normocytic
a., nosocomial
a. of childhood, erythroblastic
a. of newborn, congenital
a. of pregnancy, megaloblastic
a. of questionable etiology
a. of undetermined origin
a., ovalocytary
a., pallor from
a., paraneoplastic
a., pernicious
a., physiologic
a., polar
a., pregnancy-related
a., primary
a. ▸ primary aplastic
a., pseudoleukemica infantum
a., pyridoxine-responsive
a., refractory
a. related to chemotherapy
a., reversible
a., scorbutic
a. screening, sickle cell
a., secondary
a. ▸ secondary aplastic
a. secondary to blood loss
a., sickle cell
a., sideroblastic
a., sideropenic
a., spherocytic
a., spherocytosis
a., splenic
a. ▸ spots before eyes from
a. ▸ spur cell
a. syndrome ▸ pulmonary disease
a. (HHA) test ▸ hereditary
    hemolytic
a., thalassemia major
a. therapy
a., thrombopenic
a. ▸ tongue problems from
a. ▸ tropical macrocytic
a., von Jaksch's
a. ▸ weight loss from pernicious
a. ▸ white or pale nails from
a. ▸ white patches from

a. with excess blasts (RAEB) ▸ syndrome of refractory
anemic (*same as* anaemic)
  a. fetus
  a. headache
  a. hypoxia
  a. murmur
  a., patient
  a. phlebitis
  a. polyneuritis
  a. softening
  a. urine
Anemonopsis californica
anephric, patient
anergic, patient
anergic stupor
anergy/energy
aneroid manometer
anesthesia
  a., absorption
  a. administered
  a. awareness
  a., balanced
  a., block
  a., Carbocaine
  a., caudal
  a., chemical
  a., circular block
  a., closed
  a., cocaine
  a., conduction
  a., corneal
  a., Corning's
  a. delivery
  a., digital block
  a., electricity-induced
  a., electro◊
  a., electronic dental
  a., endobronchial
  a., endotracheal
  a., endotracheal general
  a., epidural
  a. equipment, contamination from
  a., ether
  a., (EUA), examination under
  a., extradural
  a. feedback monitoring
  a., field block
  a., general
  a. ▸ general inhalational
  a., gustatory
  a., halothane
  a., Holocaine
  a., induction of
  a., infiltration

a., inhalation
a., inhalational
a., insufflation
a., intercostal
a., intranasal
a., intraoral
a., intraspinal
a., intravenous (IV)
a., intubation
a., IV (intravenous)
a., level of
a., lining
a., local
a., local eye
a. ▸ low spinal
a., modified
a., nasotracheal intubation
a., nerve blocking
a., obstetric
a., ocular
a. of leg muscles
a. of skin
a., open drop
a., Ophthaine
a., oral
a., partial
a., partial rebreathing
a., pelvic examination under
a., Pentothal
a., peridural
a., perineural
a., peridontal
a., preoperative
a., pressure
a., pudendal block
a. recovery area ▸ post◊
a., rectal
a., regional
a. ▸ regional block
a. -related problem
a., room, post-◊
a., sacral
a., sacral block
a., saddle block
a., satisfactory general
a. shock
a., sodium Pentothal
a., spinal
a., standby
a., stellate block
a., surface
a., surgical
a., sympathetic block
a., topical
a., topical cocaine

a. ▸ toxic reaction to local
a., transient
a., transtracheal
a., twilight
a., twilight sleep
anesthesiologist-on-call
anesthetic (*same as* anaesthetic)
  a. agents, intravenous
  a. ▸ alveolar partial pressure of inhalational
  a. augmentation
  a. authorization form
  a. consent form
  a. drug, general
  a. effect ▸ prolonged
  a., epidural
  a. eye drops
  a., general
  a. -induced convulsion
  a., infiltration
  a., liquid
  a., local
  a., long-acting
  a. monoclonal antibodies, anti-
  a., paracervical
  a., regional
  a. -related complications
  a. ▸ respiratory depression inhalation
  a., spinal
  a. surgery
  a., topical
  a. vapor
anesthetist (*same as* anaesthetist)
anesthetize (*same as* anaesthetize)
anesthetized
  a., entire limb
  a., operative field
  a., patient
  a. patient, deeply
  a. ▸ pharynx, larynx and trachea
  a., wound
anesthetizing effect of ice and snow
anestrous/anoestrous
anestrum/anoestrum
aneuploid lesions
aneurismal (*see* aneurysmal)
aneurysm/aneurism
  a., abdominal
  a., abdominal aorta thrombotic
  a. (AAA) ▸ abdominal aortic
  a., acute dissecting
  a., acute thrombotic
  a., ampullary
  a. anastomotica

aneurysm—*continued*

a., anterior wall
a., aortic
a., aortic arch
a., aortic sinusal
a., aortoiliac
a., arterial
a., arteriosclerotic abdominal
a., arteriovenous (AV)
a., arteriovenous (AV) pulmonary
a., atherosclerotic
a., atrial septal
a., AV (arteriovenous)
a., axial
a., axillary
a., bacterial
a., basilar artery
a., Bérard's
a., berry
a., bifurcation
a., brain
a. ▸ bulging eyes from
a. by anastomosis
a., cardiac
a., carotid
a., carotid artery
a., carotid ophthalmic
a., cavernous
a., cavernous sinus
a. cavity
a., celiac artery
a., cerebral
a., Charcot-Bouchard
a., cirsoid
a. clipped
a. clipped, intracranial
a. clipping
a., communicating artery
a., congenital aortic
a., congenital cerebral
a., congenital left ventricular (LV)
a., congenital renal
a., coronary
a., coronary artery
a., Crisp's
a., cylindroid
a., cystogenic
a., descending thoracic aortic
a., discrete
a., dissecting
a., dissecting aortic
a. ▸ dissecting basilar artery
a., dolichoectatic
a., ectatic
a., embolic

a., embolomycotic
a. ▸ endograft exclusion of
a., exogenous
a., false
a., false aortic
a., fusiform
a. ▸ fusiform aortic
a., giant
a. graft, aortic
a. (HEA) ▸ hemorrhages, exudates
and
a. ▸ hepatic artery
a., hernial
a. ▸ iliac artery
a. in orbit
a., infected
a., inflammatory
a. ▸ inflammatory aortic
a. ▸ infrarenal aortic aneurysm
a., innominate
a. ▸ interventricular septum
a. ▸ intracavernous carotid
a., intracranial
a. ▸ intracranial arterial
a., intramural
a., lateral
a. ▸ left ventricular (LV)
a. ▸ lower basilar
a., luetic
a., miliary
a. ▸ mitral valve
a., mixed
a. mortality ▸ ruptured
a., mural
a., mycotic
a. ▸ mycotic aortic
a. of abdominal aorta
a. of artery
a. of pulmonary artery, congenital
a. or vascular malformation
a., orbital
a., osteo▸
a., Park's
a., pelvic
a., phantom
a., PICA (posterior inferior
cerebellar artery)
a., popliteal
a., popliteal artery
a. ▸ portal vein
a. ▸ posterior communicating artery
a., posterior inferior cerebellar
artery (PICA)
a., pseudo ▸
a., Pott's

a. ▸ pulmonary arteriovenous
a. ▸ pulmonary artery
a., pulsating
a., racemose
a., Rasmussen's
a. ▸ recurrent hemorrhage from
a. redundancy
a., reflux dissecting abdominal
aortic
a., renal
a., renal artery
a. repair
a. repair, aortic
a. repair, DeBakey-Creech
a., resected
a., Richet's
a., Rodrigues'
a. rupture, aortic
a., rupture of congenital
a., rupture of syphilitic aortic
a., ruptured
a. ▸ ruptured abdominal aortic
a. ▸ ruptured aortic
a., ruptured brain
a., ruptured cerebral
a., ruptured iliac
a. sac ▸ abdominal
a., saccular
a., sacculated
a., sacral
a., serpentine
a., Shekelton's
a. ▸ sinus of Valsalva
a., splanchnic
a., splenic
a., spurious
a. ▸ supraclinoid carotid
a. ▸ suprarenal aortic
a., suprasellar
a., surgical closure sac of
a., surgical treatment for
a. surgically sealed
a., syphilitic
a., thoracic
a. ▸ thoracic aorta
a. ▸ thoracoabdominal aortic
a. ▸ thrombosed giant vertebral
artery
a., traction
a., traumatic
a., true
a. ▸ true ventricular
a., tubular
a., undetected
a. ▸ unruptured brain

a., varicose
a. ▸ vein of Galen
a., venous
a., ventricular
a. ▸ ventricular patch
a., verminous
a., windsock
a. wrapping

aneurysmal (*same as* aneurismal)
a. bone cyst
a. bruit
a. cough
a. diathesis
a. dilatation
a. dilatation, localized
a. disease, aortic
a. hematoma
a. hemorrhage
a. murmur
a. phthisis
a. sac
a. thrill
a. varix
a. widening
a. widening, fusiform
a. widening of aorta

aneurysmectomy, Matas
ANF (atrial natriuretic factor)
Angel(s)
A. Dust (hallucinogen)
A. Dust (phencyclidine)
A. (phencyclidine), Dust of

Angelchik anti-reflux prosthesis
Angelman's syndrome
Angelucci's syndrome
anger
a. and depression ▸ fear,
a. and frustration
a. and hopelessness ▸ stress,
a. and resentment
a. arousal
a., at death
a. at God
a. ▸ bursts of irritation and
a., child quick to
a. control
a., coping with
a., covert
a., difficulty controlling
a. ▸ diffusing hostility and
a. disorder
a., excessive
a. ▸ expressions of
a. ▸ feeling of
a. ▸ inability to control

a., inappropriate
a. ▸ inappropriate, intense
a. ▸ inappropriate overt
a. ▸ level of
a. management
a. management (IAM) ▸ integrated
a. management relapse prevention
a. management skills
a., managing
a. or hostility
a., panic or despair ▸ periods of
a. ▸ permitting safe expression of
a., persistent
a., rage and resistance
a., tension, and fatigue
a., unprovoked
a., unreasonable

Anghelescu's sign
angiitis (*same as* angitis)
a., allergic
a., allergic granulomatous
a., Churg-Strauss
a., cutaneous
a., endothelio◊
a., hypersensitivity
a., leukocytoclastic
a., necrotizing
a., nonnecrotizing
a. obliterans, thrombo◊
a., pulmonary
a., visceral

angina
a., abdominal
a. abdominalis
a., agranulocytic
a. and breathlessness
a., anxiety
a. attack
a., band-like
a., benign croupous
a., Bretonneau
a., cardiac
a., cervicoprecordial
a. chest pain
a., chronic stable
a., cold-induced
a., cordis
a., coronary spastic
a., crescendo
a. cruris
a. decubitus
a. dyspeptica
a., effort
a. ▸ ergonovine maleate
provocation

a., esophageal
a. ▸ exercise-induced
a., exertional
a., exudative
a., false
a. ▸ first effort
a., food
a. from coldness
a. from spasm of artery
a., fusospirochetal
a. gangrenosa
a. -guided therapy
a., Heberden's
a., hippocratic
a., hypercyanotic
a., hysteric
a. in legs
a., intermittent
a., intestinal
a., inversa
a. ▸ ischemic rest
a., lacunar
a. ▸ life-threatening
a., Ludwig's
a., microvascular
a., mixed
a., monocytic
a. nervosa
a., neurotropic
a., neutropenic
a., nocturnal
a., nonexertional
a., nosocomii
a. notha
a., office
a. ▸ pacing-induced
a. pectoris (AP)
a. pectoris decubitus
a. pectoris, disabling
a. pectoris, variant
a., pectoris vasomotoria
a. phlegmonosa
a., Plaut-Vincent's
a., Plaut's
a., postinfarction
a., postprandial
a., preinfarction
a., Prinzmetal's
a., Prinzmetal's variant
a., pseudomembranous
a. questionnaire ▸ Seattle
a. ▸ rate-dependent
a., rebound
a., recurrent
a., reflex

angina—*continued*
a., rest
a. rheumatica
a. scarlatinosa
a., Schultz's
a. ▸ severe, refractory
a. ▸ severe, unstable
a., sexual
a., silent
a. simplex
a. sine colors
a. ▸ smoking-induced
a. spuria
a., stable
a. streptococcus
a. ▸ stress and
a. ▸ toilet-seat
a. ▸ treadmill-induced
a. ulcerosa
a., unexplained
a., unstable
a. ▸ variable threshold
a., variant
a., vasomotor
a., vasospastic
a., vasotonic
a., Vincent's
a. ▸ walk-through
a. ▸ white coat
anginae, Saccharomyces
anginal
a. attacks, relief and prevention of
a. drug, anti-
a. equivalent
a. perceptual threshold
a. syndrome
a. syndrome, cervical
a. therapy, anti-
anginosa, syncope
anginosus, status
anginosus, Streptococcus
angio-aortic arch study ▸ cardiac-pulmonary
angioblastic lymphadenopathy
angioblastic meningioma
angiocardiogram study
angiocardiography
a., cine◊
a. ▸ exercise radionuclide
a. (ACG) ▸ first-pass radionuclide
a. ▸ gated radionuclide
a., intravenous (IV)
a., radionuclide
a., selective

a. study
a., transseptal
a., venous
angiocentric immunoproliferative lesion
angiocholitis proliferans
Angiocoronary contrast medium
angiodysplasia, intestinal
angiodysplasia of colon
angioedema, idiopathic
angioendotheliomatosis
a., malignant
a. ▸ neoplastic proliferating
a. ▸ reactive proliferating
angiofibroma, juvenile
angiofibroma, nasopharyngeal
angiogenesis
a. factor, anti-
a. factor, tumor
a. inhibitors
a. procedure
a. process
a. treatment
angiogenic breast cancer
angiogram
a. ▸ baseline coronary
a., cerebral
a. ▸ electrocardiogram (ECG) synchronized digital subtraction
a., four vessel
a. ▸ gated nuclear
a., inferior mesenteric
a. (LCA) ▸ left coronary
a., pulmonary
a., radioisotope
a., radionuclide
a., renal
a. (RCA) ▸ right coronary
a., serial
a., splenic system
a. study
a., superior mesenteric
a. ▸ venous digital
angiographic
a. analysis ▸ quantitative coronary
a. assessment
a. assessment ▸ digital
a. catheter
a. catheter, coronary
a. catheter ▸ one hole
a. contrast
a. dilator, French
a. examination
a. instrumentation
a. portography, computed tomography (CT)

a. study
a. study ▸ hemodynamic
angiography
a., absorption in coronary laser
a., aortic arch
a., axial
a., balloon occlusion pulmonary
a., basilar
a., biliary
a., biplane
a., biplane orthogonal
a., bronchial
a., carotid
a. catheter ▸ headhunter
a., celiac
a., cerebral
a., cine ▸
a., color power
a., contrast
a. (carotid MRA) ▸ contrast enhanced carotid magnetic resonance
a., coronary
a., diagnostic
a., diagnostic coronary
a., digital
a. ▸ digital cardiovascular
a. ▸ digital celiac trunk
a. (DSA) ▸ digital subtraction
a. (ERNA) ▸ equilibrium radionuclide
a. ▸ femoral runoff
a. ▸ femorocerebral catheter
a., fluorescein
a. ▸ gated blood pool
a. ▸ gated radionuclide
a., hepatic
a., incomplete
a. ▸ indocyanine green
a. ▸ internal mammary artery graft
a., interventional
a. ▸ intra-arterial digital subtraction
a. ▸ intracranial magnetic resonance (MR)
a., intraoperative
a. (IDSA) ▸ intraoperative digital subtraction
a. (IVA) ▸ intraoperative vascular
a., intravenous
a. ▸ intravenous digital
a. (IVDSA) ▸ intravenous digital subtraction
a. ▸ left aortic
a. ▸ left atrial
a., left coronary artery

a., left ventricular
a., lymph◊
a. (MRA) ▸ magnetic resonance
a., magnification
a., mesenteric
a., multigated
a., noncardiac
a. ▸ noninvasive coronary
a. ▸ nonselective coronary
a., nuclear
a. ▸ pediatric digital
a., peripheral
a. ▸ phase contrast
a., pulmonary
a. ▸ pulmonary wedge
a. (QCA) ▸ quantitative coronary
a., radionuclide
a., renal
a., renovascular
a. ▸ rest and exercise-gated nuclear
a. ▸ rest radionuclide
a., right coronary artery
a., routine
a. ▸ saphenous vein bypass graft
a. (MUGA) scan ▸ multiple-gated
a. scans
a., scinti◊
a., scintigraphic
a., selective
a. ▸ selective arterial magnetic
   resonance (MR)
a. ▸ selective venous magnetic
   resonance (MR)
a. streaks
a., subtraction
a., supra-aortic
a., surveillance
a. ▸ synchroton-based transvenous
a., thermal
a., thoracic
a. ▸ time-of-flight
a., total absence of circulation on
   four vessel
a., ultrasound
a., vascular
a., ventricular
a., vertebral
a., visceral
a. ▸ wedge pulmonary
angioimmunoblastic lymphadenopathy
AngioJet technique
angiolipoma, epidural
angiolipoma ▸ spinal epidural
angiolymphoid hyperplasia
angioma

a., arterial
a. arteriale racemosum
a., capillary
a. cavernosum
a., cavernous
a., cherry
a. cutis
a., encephalic
a. ▸ extracerebral cavernous
a. of brain
a. of lung
a. of meninges
a. of skin
a., pulmonary
a., spider
a., superficial
a., telangiectatic
a. ▸ tibioperoneal trunk
a. venosum
a. venosum racemosum
angiomata, spider
angiomatosis
a. (BA), bacillary
a., cystic
a., encephalotrigeminal
a., epithelioid
a., hemorrhagic familial
a. of bone, cystic
a. of retina
a., retinocerebellar
angioneurotic
a. anuria
a. edema
a. edema, hereditary
a. edema, intermittent
a. edema of vessels
a. hematuria
angioneurotica, purpura
angiopathic retinopathy, Purtscher's
angiopathy, cerebral amyloid
angiopathy of retina
angiophylactic reaction
angiopigtail catheter
angioplasty
a., ablative laser
a., adjunctive balloon
a., balloon
a. (BCA), balloon catheter
a., balloon coarctation
a., balloon coronary
a., balloon laser
a., bootstrap two-vessel
a., brachiocephalic vessel
a., carotid
a., complementary balloon

a., coronary artery
a., coronary artery laser
a., coronary laser
a., direct
a., excimer laser
a. (ELCA) ▸ excimer laser coronary
a., facilitated
a., frozen
a. guiding catheter
a. ▸ high-risk
a. in myocardial infarction ▸ primary
a., infrapopliteal
a. ▸ infrapopliteal transluminal
a. ▸ Kinsey rotation atherectomy
   extrusion
a. ▸ kissing balloon
a., laser
a. (LABA) ▸ laser-assisted balloon
a. ▸ low speed rotational
a., nonsurgical
a. ▸ Osypka rotational
a., patch
a. ▸ patch graft
a. ▸ percutaneous balloon
a. (PCRA) ▸ percutaneous
   coronary rotational
a. (PELCA) ▸ percutaneous
   excimer laser coronary
a. ▸ percutaneous low stress
a. (PTA), percutaneous
   transluminal
a. (PTCA), percutaneous
   transluminal coronary
a., peripheral
a. (PLA) ▸ peripheral laser
a. (PLSA) ▸ physiologic low stress
a. (POBA) ▸ plain old balloon
a. procedure
a. -related vessel
a. -related vessel occlusion
a., renal
a., repeat
a., rescue
a. restenosis ▸ postballoon
a. ▸ salvage balloon
a., subliminal
a. (TPBA) ▸ thermal/perfusion
   balloon
a. ▸ tibioperoneal vessel
a., ultrasonic
a., vibrational
angiopneumogram study
angiosarcoma
a., adeno◊
a., cutaneous

angiosarcoma—*continued*
  a., hepatic
  a., uterine
angiosclerotic gangrene
angiosclerotica
  a., dysbasia
  a. ‣ dysbasia intermittens
  a. intestinalis ‣ dyspragia
    intermittens
angioscopy ‣ percutaneous
  transluminal
angiospastic retinitis, central
angiospastica, dysbasia
angiospastica pseudoanemia
Angiostrongylus cantonensis
angiotensin
  a. aldosterone cascade ‣ renin
  a. aldosterone system ‣ renin
  a. blocker ‣ renin
  a. converting enzyme (ACE)
  a. converting enzyme (ACE)
    inhibitor
  a. ‣ decreased production of
  a. receptor blocker
  a., renin
  a. system (RAS) renin-
  a. II ‣ potent hormone
angiotensinogen gene
angitis (*see* angiitis)
angle(s)('s) (Angle's) [*ankle*]
  a., acetabular
  a., adrenal
  a., antegonial
  a., anterior angulation
  a., basal
  a., blunting costophrenic
  a., blunting costovertebral
  a. board
  a., Boehler's
  a., cardiodiaphragmatic
  a., cardiophrenic
  a., carinal
  a., carpal
  a., cavosurface
  a., cerebellopontile
  a. chest tube ‣ right
  a. -closure glaucoma
  a. -closure glaucoma ‣ acute
  a. concept ‣ solid
  a., conchal mastoid
  a., costal
  a., costophrenic
  a. (CVA) ‣ costovertebral
  a., flip
  a., Gantry

a., gastroesophageal
a. glaucoma, chronic narrow-
a. glaucoma, chronic open
a. glaucoma, closed-
a. glaucoma, narrow-
a. glaucoma, open-
a. glaucoma ‣ primary open
a. glaucoma, wide-
a., hepatic
a., impedance
a., intercept
a., iridocorneal
a., kappa
a., lateral
a., large kappa
a. lens, right-
a., line
a., Louis
a., Ludwig
a., magic
a. ‣ magnetization precession
a. mattress suture, right-
a., medial
a. (ma) ‣ meter-
a. monoplane ultrasound scanner ‣
  Biosound
a. ‣ nail-to-nail bed
a. obliterated, costophrenic
a. of displacement, phase
a. of greatest extension
a. of greatest flexion
a. of incidence
a. of incision
a. of mandible, external
a. of mouth ‣ depressor muscle of
a. of mouth ‣ levator muscle of
a. of scapula, lower
a. of Sylvius
a. of wound, posterior
a., phase
a. port pump
a. ‣ posterior urethrovesical
a., precession
a. ‣ pulse flip
a., QRS
a., QRS-T
a., radiocarpal
a. -recession glaucoma
a., scaphoconchal
a., sphenoid
a., splenic
a., sternal
a., sternoclavicular
a., subcarinal
a. suture

a., talocalcaneal
a. telescope, fight-
a. ‣ tracheal bifurcation
a., triple-
a. tumor, cerebellopontine
a. viewing, wide
a., visual
a., xiphoid
angled pleural tube
angled-vision lens system
Angle's classification
angry
  a. disruptions
  a. outburst
  a., patient
Angström unit
anguish
  a. depression or mental
  a., mental
  a., severe emotional
  a., severe mental
angular
  a. artery
  a. cheilitis
  a. deformity
  a. gyri
  a. incision, Fowler's
  a. junction
  a. junction of eyelids
  a. stomatitis
  a. stress
  a. vein
angularis
  a., blepharitis
  a., gyrus
  a., incisura
angulated multipurpose catheter
angulation [*ambulation*]
  a. angle, anterior
  a., beam
  a., caudal
  a., coronal
  a., palmar
  a. ‣ right anterior oblique (RAO)
  a., volar
angusta, pelvis
angustifolia, Echinacea
anhemolytic streptococcus
anhidrosis/anhydrosis/anidrosis
anhidrotic ectodermal dysplasia
anhidrotic heat exhaustion
anhydrous sugar
ani
  a., crena
  a., levator

a. muscle, levator
a. muscle, sphincter
a., pruritus
a., sphincter
anicteric hepatitis
anicteric leptospirosis
aniline cancer
aniline gentian violet
animal
a. bite injury
a. dander
a. economy
a. life
a. medicine, laboratory
a. parasite
a. pathogen
a. tissue transplant
a. viruses
animatum, virus
anion
a. exchange resin
a. gap
a. gap, low
a. gap metabolic acidosis
Anis Staple implant cataract lens
anisa, Legionella
anisotropic conduction
anisotropic disc
anisotropous disc
anitratus, Acinetobacter
ankle(s) [*angle*]
a. alphabet exercise
a. amputation, above
a., amputation of foot at
a. -arm index
a., bimalleolar fracture of
a. bone
a. -brachial blood pressure
a. -brachial blood pressure ratio
a. -brachial index (ABI)
a. clonus
a. cuffs, weighted
a. dorsiflexion
a. drop
a. edema
a. exercise
a. flexed
a., forced inversion film of
a., fracture of
a. full range of motion (ROM) ▸ left
a. full range of motion (ROM) ▸ right
a. fusion
a. immobilization
a. index, brachial-

a. indices, arm-
a. jerk (AJ)
a. jerk (AJ) ▸ depressed
a. joint
a., long leg brace with free
a. mortice
a. mortise
a. pain
a. ▸ pitting edema of
a. problems
a., puffy
a. pulse
a. reflex
a. replacement
a. restraint
a. ▸ severely swollen
a. splinting
a. sprain
a. sprain ▸ lateral
a. sprain ▸ medial
a. swelling
a., swollen
a., tailors'
a., trimalleolar fracture of
ankyloglossia superior
ankylopoietica, spondylosis chronica
ankylose (*same as* anchylose, ancylose)
ankylosing hyperostosis
ankylosing spondylitis
ankylosis (*same as* anchylosis)
a., bony
a., cricoarytenoid joint
a., fibrous
a., partial
ankylotic (*same as* anchylotic)
ankyroid (*see* ancyroid)
ANLL (acute nonlymphocytic leukemia)
ANLL (acute nonlymphoid leukemia)
Ann (LSD) ▸ Raggedy
Annandale's operation
annealing lamp
annectant gyri
annectentes, gyri
annihilation radiation
anniversary reactor
annoyed, ▸ agitated, irritable, and easily
annoyed, easily
annual
a. checkup
a. digitorectal examination
a. dilated eye examination
a. examination
a. health evaluation
a. mammogram

a. physical examination
a. rescreening
annually ▸ complete gynecologic examination
annually, patient care
annular
a. abscess
a. array transducer
a. calcification
a. calcification, mitral
a. carcinoma
a. dehiscence
a. detachment
a. dilatation
a. fibers
a. hymen
a. lesion
a. ligament
a. mitral valve replacement ▸ supra-
a. pancreas
a. phased array
a. phased array system
a. placenta
a. plexus
a. prosthesis ▸ supra-
a. scleritis
a. sclerosis
a. scotoma
a. staphyloma
a. stomatitis
a. stricture
a. thrombus
annulare, granuloma
annularis, lichen
annularis telangiectodes, purpura
annulatus, Boophilus
annulatus, Margaropus
annuli fibrosi cordis
annulifera, Mansonioides
annulirostris, Culex
annuloaortic ectasia
annuloplasty
a. ▸ prosthetic ring
a. ring, Duran
a. ring prosthesis, Carpentier
a. ring ▸ St. Jude
annulus (see also anulus)
a. abscess, aortic
a., aortic
a., bony
a., bulging
a. ciliaris
a. elevated
a. fibrosus

annulus—*continued*
  a., level of
  a. of Zinn
  a. ovalis
  a., posterior superior
  a. tracheae
  a., tympanic
  a. tympanicus
  a. urethralis
  a., Vieussen's
  a. zinnii
anococcygeal nerves
anodal
  a. closing contraction
  a. closing odor
  a. closing picture
  a. closing sound
  a. closure
  a. closure clonus
  a. closure contraction
  a. closure tetanus
  a. duration
  a. duration contraction
  a. duration tetanus
  a. opening (AC)
  a. opening contraction (AOC)
  a. opening tetanus (AOT)
anode
  a. rays
  a., rotating
  a., stationary
anodyne, Hoffmann's
anoestrous (*see* anestrous)
anoestrum (*see* anestrum)
anogenital pruritus
anogenital warts
anomalies ▸ pneumococcus in vitro fetal
anomalies ▸ unruptured vascular
anomalous
  a. atrioventricular excitation
  a. bronchus
  a. complex
  a. conduction
  a. coronary
  a. first rib thoracic syndrome
  a. left coronary artery
  a. left main coronary artery (ALMCA)
  a. mitral arcade
  a. origin
  a. pulmonary vein
  a. pulmonary venous connection ▸ partial

  a. pulmonary venous connection ▸ total
  a. pulmonary venous drainage ▸ partial
  a. pulmonary venous drainage ▸ total
  a. pulmonary venous return
  a. pulmonary venous return (PAPVR), partial
  a. pulmonary venous return ▸ total
  a. rectification
  a. retinal correspondence (ARC)
  a. veins
  a. vessels of papilla
anomalus, Hoplopsyllus
anomaly(-ies)
  a., anorectal
  a., atrioventricular (AV) junction
  a., cardiac valve
  a., congenital
  a., congenital cardiac
  a., congenital conotruncal
  a., congenital heart
  a., conjoined nerve root
  a., conotruncal
  a., coronary artery
  a., craniofacial
  a., developmental
  a. ▸ double inlet ventricle
  a., duplication
  a., Ebstein's
  a., familial craniofacial
  a., fetal
  a. ▸ fetal cardiac
  a. ▸ fetal chest
  a. ▸ fetal gastrointestinal
  a., Freund's
  a., genital
  a., genitourinary
  a., gross
  a., heart
  a., Heberden's
  a., Hegglin's
  a., infant born with congenital
  a. ▸ jugular bulb
  a., kidney
  a. ▸ limb reduction
  a., May-Hegglin's
  a., metabolic
  a., müllerian duct
  a., multiple congenital
  a. ▸ numerary renal
  a., occipitoatlantoaxial
  a. of mitral valve, congenital
  a. opticociliary vessels

  a. ▸ pediatric venous return
  a., Pelger-Huet
  a., Pelger-Huet nuclear
  a., Peters'
  a., presacral
  a. ▸ pulmonary valve
  a. ▸ pulmonary venous connection
  a. ▸ pulmonary venous return
  a., segmentation
  a., Shone
  a., spinal
  a., structural
  a., structural congenital
  a., Taussig-Bing
  a., Uhl's
  a., Undritz'
  a., unruptured vascular
  a. ▸ urinary tract
  a., uterine
  a., vascular
  a. ▸ vena cava
  a. ▸ viscerobronchial cardiovascular
anomic aphasia
Anon Group, Al-
Anonymous (anonymous)
  A. (AA), Alcoholics
  A. (CA), Cocaine
  A. (CoDA) ▸ Codependents
  A. (GA), Gamblers
  A. (NA), Narcotics
  A. (OA) ▸ Overeaters
  A. (SAA) ▸ Sex Addicts
  A. (SA) ▸ Smokers
  a. veins
Anopheles larvae
Anopheles maculipennis
anopsia
  a., amaurosis ex
  a., amblyopia ex
  a., quadrant
anorectal
  a. abscess
  a. anomaly
  a. atresia
  a. circulation
  a. disease
  a. dressing
  a. fistula
  a. growth
  a. lesion ▸ fibroepithelial polypoid
  a. manometry
  a. orifice
  a. problem from constipation
  a. problem from Crohn's disease
  a. problem from diarrhea

a. stenosis
anorectic, patient
anorexia
a. and bulimia
a. and irritability ▸ restlessness,
a., depression and shyness
a. disorder
a. nervosa
a., pain, nausea and emesis
a., paraneoplastic
a., progressive
a. support group
a., weight loss ▸ weakness
anorexic
a., bingeing behavior of
a. patient
a. ▸ punishing behavior of
a. ▸ purging behavior of
a. ▸ starving behavior of
anoscopic examination
anosmia [*anotia*]
a. gustatoria
a., preferential
a. respiratoria
anosmic aphasia
anosmic conversion reaction
anospinal centers
another mental disorder (nonorganic) ▸
hypersomnia related to
anovular menstruation
anovulatory
a. cycle
a. menses
a. menstruation
anoxemia test
anoxia [*agnosia*]
a., cerebral
a., diffusion
a., global
a., hypoxia and
a., myocardial
a. neonatorum
a., perinatal
a., prolonged period of
a., severe cerebral
a., stagnant
anoxic
a. brain damage
a. brain injury
a. changes
a. changes in brain
a. changes in cortex
a. changes, widespread
a. damage
a. encephalopathy, severe

ansa cervicalis
anserina, Borrelia
anserina bursa tenderness, Borrelia
anserine transfer, pes
anserinus, pes
anseris, Amidostomum
Anspach cement eater
ANT. (anterior)
Antabuse
A. program
A. programming
A. services
A. support
A. therapy
A. treatment
antacid, effervescing
antacid therapy
antagonism
a., accentuated
a., bacterial
a., induced bacterial
a., metabolic
a., salt
antagonist(s)
a., adrenergic
a., aldosterone
a., beta
a., calcium
a., folate
a. ▸ folic acid
a., histamine
a., metabolic
a., opioid
a., pyrimidine
a., serotonin
a. therapy
a. ▸ thromboxane receptor
antagonistic
a. chemotherapy
a. interaction
a. muscle
a. reflexes
antalgic gait
antarctica, Taenia
ante cibum
antebrachial
a. cephalic vein
a. region, anterior
a. region, posterior
a. region, radial
a. region, ulnar
a. region, volar
a. vein, median
antebrachium (*same as* antibrachium)

antecedent (PTA) ▸ plasma
thromboplastin
antecubital
a. approach
a. area
a. cervicodorsal crease
a. ecchymoses, bilateral
a. fossa, left
a. fossa, right
a. space
a. vein
anteflexed/anteverted
anteflexed, uterus
anteflexion of uterus
antegonial angle
antegonial notch
antegrade
a. aortogram
a. approach
a. arteriography ▸ ipsilateral
a. biliary drainage, percutaneous
a. block cycle length
a. conduction
a. internodal pathway
a. pyelography, percutaneous
a. refractory period
a. -retrograde cardioplegia
a. urography, percutaneous
antemortem
a. clot
a. mural thrombi
a. thrombi
a. thrombus
antenatal life
antenatal visit
antepartum
a. death, term delivery
a. fetal death
a. hemorrhage
a. RhoGam
a. testing
anterior (ANT.)
a. ampullar nerve
a. and posterior (A and P)
a. and posterior longitudinal
ligaments, rupture of
a. and posterior opposing portals
a. and posterior (A and P) repair
a. angulation angle
a. antebrachial region
a. aortic cusp, right
a. aspect
a. asynclitism
a. auricular muscle
a. auricular nerves

anterior—*continued*

a. auricular veins
a. axial embryonal cataract
a. axillary line (AAL)
a. basal
a. boundary
a. brachial region
a. bradyrhythmia
a. canal
a. capsule
a. cardiac veins
a. cavity
a. central gyrus
a. centriole
a. cerebellar notch
a. cerebral artery
a. cerebral artery, azygos
a. cerebral bradyrhythmia
a. cerebral vein
a. cerebrospinal fasciculus
a. chamber
a. chamber ‣ air bubble instilled in
a. chamber entered with keratome
a. chamber ‣ fluid released from
a. chamber ‣ foreign body (FB) in
a. chamber irrigated with saline
a. chamber lens, Choyce
a. chamber of eye
a. chamber, seal
a. chest diameter
a. chest ‣ pectus excavatum of
a. chest wall
a. chest wall syndrome
a. choroidal artery
a. cingulate
a. cingulate cortex
a. colliculi
a. column
a. column ‣ gliosis of
a. commissure
a. commissure of cerebrum
a. commissure of labia
a. commissure structure
a. communicating artery
a. compartment compression syndrome
a. component
a. cruciate ligament
a. cruciate ligament ‣ torn
a. crural region
a. crus of stapes
a. cubital region
a. cutaneous nerve of abdomen
a. descending artery
a. descending coronary artery

a. descending (LAD) artery, left
a. descending (LAD) lumen, left
a. dislocation of shoulder joint
a. displacement
a. drawer test
a. ethmoidal nerve
a. external arcuate fibers
a. facial height
a. facial vein, common
a. faucial pillar
a. fontanel, bulging
a. fontanelle
a. fornix
a. fossa
a., fossa cranii
a. fovea
a., frontolaeva
a. gray column
a. gray commissure
a. guide
a. guide, adjustable
a. gyrus centralis
a. head cap
a. heel
a. hemiblock, left
a. horizontal jugular vein
a. horn cell
a. horns of spinal cord
a. hypothalamus
a. hypothalamus (INAH) ‣ interstitial nuclei of
a. infarction
a. inferior communicating artery (AICA)
a. intercostal veins
a. internodal pathway
a. interosseous nerve of forearm
a. intertransverse muscles
a. intertransverse muscles of neck
a. ischemic optic neuropathy
a. jugular vein
a. labial nerves
a. labial veins
a. lacrimal duct
a. lateral myocardial infarct
a. leaflet
a. leaflet, left
a. leaflet, mitral valve
a. ligament
a. ligament of malleus
a. lobe hormone
a. lobe of pituitary gland
a. lobule of pituitary gland
a. luxation
a. lymph node

a. mallear fold of mucous membrane of tympanum
a. mallear fold of tympanic membrane
a. margin
a. median fissure
a. mediastinal lymph nodes
a. mediastinotomy
a. medullary velum
a., mentodextra
a. motion (SAM) ‣ systolic
a. myocardial infarction (AMI)
a. nares
a. neck
a. nephrectomy
a. nerve roots
a. nosebleed
a. oblique
a. oblique (RAO) angulation ‣ right
a. oblique (RAO) equivalent ‣ right
a. oblique (LAO) ‣ left
a. oblique (LAO) position ‣ left
a. oblique (RAO) position ‣ right
a. oblique projection
a. oblique projection, left
a. oblique projection, right
a. oblique (RAO) ‣ right
a., occipitodextra
a., occipitolaeva
a. occlusion
a. palatine nerve
a. palatine suture
a. papillary muscle
a. parotid veins
a. pelvic exenteration
a. ‣ perforated substance,
a. perforation
a. pillar
a. pillar of fauces
a. pillar of fornix
a. pituitary
a. pituitary cells ‣ entrapped
a. pituitary extract
a. pituitary gland
a. polar cataract
a. poliomyelitis
a. -posterior (AP) repair
a. process
a. prominence
a. pyramidal
a. radicular artery, great
a. region of neck
a. resection
a. resection, low
a. rhizotomy

a. sacrococcygeal muscle
a., sacrodextra
a., sacrolaeva
a. sandwich patch technique
a. scalene muscle
a., scapulodextra
a., scapulolaeva
a. scleritis, diffuse
a. scrotal nerves
a. scrotal veins
a. segment of lung
a., serratus
a. serratus muscle
a. sheath of rectus muscle
a. shoulder repair, Mosley method
a. ▸ spina bifida
a. spinal artery
a. splint
a. spurring, degenerative
a. staphyloma
a. subendocardial
a. sulcus
a. superior iliac spine (ASIS)
a. superior spine
a. supraclavicular nerves
a. surface
a. surfaces, concave
a. symblepharon
a. syndrome ▸ scalenus
a. synechia
a. table
a. teeth
a. temporal
a. temporal diploic vein
a. temporal electrode
a. temporal electrodes, true
a. temporal slow activity
a. temporal slow wave focus
a. temporal spike, focal
a. temporal spike focus
a. temporal spiking
a. thalamic nuclei
a. thalamotomy
a. tibial artery
a. tibial compartment
a. tibial compartment syndrome
a. tibial muscle
a. tibial sign
a. tibial vein
a. tibialis
a. transverse temporal gyrus
a., uterus
a. vaginae, paries
a. vertebral vein
a. wall

a. wall akinesia
a. wall aneurysm
a. wall dyskinesis
a. wall infarction (AWI)
a. wall ischemia
a. wall myocardial infarction (AWMI)
a. wall, relaxed
a. white column
a. white commissure
anteriorly directed jet
anterius stapedius, crus
antero-apical segment
anteroapical dyskinesis
anterocolic anastomosis
anterodistal border
anterograde
a. amnesia
a. block
a. conduct
a. flow
a. memory
a. transseptal technique
anteroinferior aspect
anterolateral
a. aspect
a. displacement
a. fontanelle
a. infarction
a. myocardial infarction, acute
a. region
a. sclerosis
a. sulcus
anteromedial joint line
anteromediastinal portal
anteromesial hypokinesis
anteroposterior (AP)
a. and lateral
a. (AP) and lateral films, portable recumbent
a. and lateral views
a. array
a. arrays, longitudinal
a. aspect
a. diameter
a. diameter, uterus normal in
a. film
a. infarction
a. lordotic projection
a., neutral
a. paddles
a. (AP) position
a. projection
a. projection, coned
a. (AP) projection, semiaxial

a. study
a. thoracic diameter
a. vaginal vault repair
a. view
a. (AP) view, normal
anteroposteroseptal infarct
anteroseptal
a. infarct
a. infarction
a. myocardial infarct (ASMI)
a. myocardial infarction (ASMI) ▸ acute
a. wall ▸ fibrosis of
a. wall ▸ scarring of
anterosuperior division left branch ▸ block in
anterotransverse diameter
anteversion neck of femur
anteversion of uterus
anteverted/anteflexed
anteverted position
anthelicis
a., crus
a. crus transversus, sulcus
a. ▸ transversus sulcus
anthelix, prominent
Anthomyia
A. canicularis
A. incisura
A. manicata
A. saltatrix
A. scalaris
Anthomyiidae
A. Fannia
A. Hydrotea
A. Hylemyia
Anthony's compressor
anthracis, Bacillus
anthracis, gram-positive Bacillus
anthracosis, coal workers'
anthracosis linguae
anthracotic
a. hilar nodes
a. lymph nodes
a. tuberculosis
anthrax (Anthrax)
a., agricultural
A. bacillus
a. bacteria
a., cerebral
a., cutaneous
a. cutaneous infection
a., gastrointestinal
a. infection
a., industrial

anthrax—*continued*
- a., inhalational
- a., intestinal
- a., malignant
- a., meningeal
- a. pneumonia
- a., pulmonary
- a., skin
- a. anthrax vaccination ▸ anti-
- a. spores

anthropod venom
anthropoid pelvis
anthropophaga, Cordylobia
anthropophaga, Ochromyia
anthropometric evaluation
anti-aging
- a. gene
- a. therapy
- a. treatment

anti-AIDS (acquired immune deficiency syndrome) vaccine
anti-alcohol drug
anti-alcohol message
anti-allergic medication
anti-anesthetic monoclonal antibodies
anti-angiogenesis factor
anti-G suit
anti-inflammatory protein
anti-inhibitor coagulant complex
anti-metastatic factor
anti-obesity drug
anti-oncogenic factor
anti-reflux drug
anti-tissue sera
anti-virus medication
anti-wrinkle cream
antialdosterone therapy
antianginal
- a. drug
- a. therapy
- a. treatment

antianxiety
- a. agent
- a. and antidepressant medications
- a. drug
- a. medication

antiarrhythmic
- a. agents
- a. device ▸ tiered therapy
- a. drug
- a. therapy
- a. therapy ▸ oral

antibacterial
- a. action
- a. activity

- a. agent
- a. antibody
- a. immunity
- a. regimens

antibasement membrane
antibasement membrane antibody
antibiotic(s)
- a. abuse
- a., acquired resistance to
- a., aminoglycoside
- a., aminoglycoside resistant
- a. ▸ anal itching and
- a., antitumor
- a. -associated diarrhea
- a. -associated enterocolitis
- a., bactericidal
- a., bacteriostatic
- a., beta lactam
- a., broad spectrum
- a., candidiasis from
- a. chemically, destroying
- a. combination therapy
- a. concentration, effective
- a. concentration in serum and tissue
- a. control
- a. destroying enzymes
- a., diarrhea
- a. drug therapy
- a. ▸ hearing loss from
- a., heartburn from
- a. -induced diarrhea
- a., infuse
- a. inhalation, chronic
- a., intravenous (IV)
- a., intrinsic resistance to
- a., IV (intravenous)
- a. ▸ lactose intolerance from
- a. levels, serum
- a. medicine
- a. ointment
- a., oral
- a., precannulation
- a., preoperative
- a., preventive
- a., prophylactic
- a. -related diarrhea
- a. resistance
- a. resistance determinants
- a. -resistant bacteria
- a. -resistant bacteria ▸ harmful
- a. resistant organism
- a. sensitivity
- a. sensitivity pattern
- a. sensitivity testing

- a., suppressive
- a. susceptibility patterns
- a. synergism
- a., systemic
- a. therapy
- a. therapy ▸ empiric
- a. therapy ▸ fever unresponsive to
- a. therapy ▸ intensive topical
- a. therapy, prolonged
- a. tongue
- a. ▸ tongue abnormalities from
- a., topical
- a. toxicity
- a. toxicity risk
- a. -treated lesions
- a. treatment
- a. usage
- a. use and abuse
- a. utilization review
- a. utilization ▸ surgical

antibioticus, Streptomyces
antiblastic immunity
antibody(-ies)
- a. absorbent
- a., acquired immune deficiency syndrome (AIDS)
- a. adsorption test ▸ fluorescent treponemal
- a. after determination
- a., alpha globulin
- a., anaphylactic
- a., anti anesthetic monoclonal
- a., antibasement membrane
- a., antibacterial
- a., antifibrin
- a. antigen complex
- a., antiglomerular basement membrane
- a., antigranulocyte
- a., anti-HCG
- a., antimitochondrial
- a., antineuronal
- a. (ANA), antinuclear
- a. (ASCA) ▸ anti-Saccharomyces cerevisiae
- a., anti-Toxoplasma
- a., antituberculosis
- a., autoimmune
- a., autologous
- a., basement membrane
- a., bifunctional
- a., blocking
- a., cell-bound
- a., cell-fixed
- a., cell-mediated

a., chelated
a., chimeric
a., cold
a., combining site
a., complement fixing
a., core
a., Cytomegalovirus
a., cytophilic
a., cytotoxic
a. darkfield, fluorescent
a. deficiency syndrome
a., direct fluorescent
a. (ENA), extractable nuclear
a., ferritin conjugated
a., fluorescent
a., fluorescent antinuclear
a., fluorescent treponemal
a. fragments
a. ▸ glomerular membrane
a., hemagglutinating
a., hemagglutinating, antipenicillin
a., hemagglutination-inhibition
a. (HBcAb), hepatitis B core
a., hepatitis B
a. (HBeAb), hepatitis B e
a. (HBsAb), hepatitis B surface
a., heterogenetic
a., heterophil
a. ▸ high affinity
a., HIV (human immunodeficiency virus)
a., homogeneous
a. human immunodeficiency virus (HIV)
a. ▸ human insulin
a., humanized
a. ▸ humanized monoclonal
a., humoral
a., idiotype
a. IgM class to Hepatitis B Core Antigen (Anti-HBc Igm)
a. imaging, antifibrin
a. imaging antimyosin
a. immune response
a. indirect fluorescent
a., iodination
a., isotopic linkage of
a., kidney-fixing
a. level
a., low aridity
a. markers
a., maternal
a., mitochondrial
a. molecules
a., monoclonal

a., myoclonal
a., natural
a., nephrotoxic
a., neutralizing
a., opsonizing
a., polyclonal
a. polyreactive
a., prophylactic
a., protective
a., radiation linked
a., radioactive
a., radiobiology and tumor response in
a., radiolabeled
a. reaction, antigen-
a. reaction, heterophil
a. ▸ resistance to
a. response, humoral
a. screen
a. screening
a. sensitivity studies
a., skin sensitizing
a. ▸ sperm agglutinating
a. stain, fluorescent
a., streptococcal
a., streptokinase
a. synthesis
a. test
a. test, AIDS (acquired immune deficiency syndrome)
a. test, Core
a. test, fluorescent
a. test, heterophil
a. tests, standard
a., therapeutic usefulness of
a. therapy ▸ monoclonal
a., thyroid
a. titer, antiheart
a. titer, heterophil
a. titer, microsomal tanned red cell (TRC)
a. titer, Rh (Rhesus)
a. titer ▸ Streptococcal
a. titers ▸ herpes simplex
a. titers, levels of
a. to Hepatitis B Core Antigen (Anti-HBc), Total
A. to Hepatitis B e Antigen, (Anti-HBe)
A. to Hepatitis B Surface Antigen, (Anti-HBs)
a. to human immunodeficiency virus (HIV)
a., tumor suppressive activities of
antibrachium (*see* antebrachium)

anticancer
a. activity
a. agent
a. agent, natural
a. chemotherapy
a. cocktail
a. compound
a. drugs
a. drugs, effective
a. effects
a. gene
a. preparation
a. properties, direct
a. protein
anti-carcinogenic activity
anticholinergic(s)
a. confusion from
a. drug
a. effects
a. medication
a. overdose
a. therapy
anticipated systole
anticipation of misfortune to others
anticipation of misfortune to self
anticipatory
a. aggression
a. anxiety
a. bogus heart rate feedback
a. grief
a. insanity
a. planning
anticlotting medicine
anticoagulant
a. drug
a., lupus
a. medication
a. therapy
a. therapy ▸ intravenous
a. therapy ▸ oral
anticoagulated blood
anticoagulation therapy ▸ long-term
anticoincidence circuit
anticonvulsant drug
anticonvulsant medication
anticonvulsive therapy
anticus
a. muscle, scalenus
a. reflex
a. syndrome, scalenus
antidepressant(s)
a. agent
a., bruising from
a., constipation from
a., cyclic

antidepressant(s)—*continued*
- a., dizziness from
- a. drugs
- a., forgetfulness from
- a. ▸ green urine from
- a. ▸ hair loss from
- a., impotence from
- a. medication
- a. medications ▸ antianxiety and
- a. ▸ nipple discharge from
- a. therapy
- a. treatment
- a. treatment, chronic
- a., tricyclic

antidiabetic
- a. activity
- a. agent
- a. therapy

antidiarrheal agent
antidiarrheal medication
antidiphtheritic globulin
antidiuretic
- a. action
- a. hormone (ADH)
- a. hormone deficiency
- a. hormone (IADH), inappropriate
- a. hormone (SIADH) secretion, syndrome of inappropriate
- a. substance

antidromic
- a. atrioventricular (AV) reciprocating tachycardia
- a. circus movement tachycardia
- a. tachycardia

antiembolic stockings ▸ thigh-high
antiembolism stockings
antiemetic
- a. agent
- a. drug
- a. drug reaction
- a. effectiveness
- a. medication
- a. therapy

antiepileptic drug level
antiepileptic drugs
anti-estrogen receptor
antifibrin antibody
antifibrin antibody imaging
antifibrinolytic therapy
antifoaming inhalant
antifolic agent
antifungal(s)
- a. activity
- a. agent
- a. agent ▸ oral

- a. cream
- a. drug
- a. medication
- a., oral
- a. therapy
- a. therapy ▸ internal

antigen(s)
- A. (Anti-HBc IgM), Antibody IgM class to Hepatitis B Core
- a. -antibody reaction
- A. (Anti-HBe), Antibody to Hepatitis B e
- A. (Anti-HBs), Antibody to Hepatitis B Surface
- a. -antiglobulin reaction
- a., Australia
- a., bacterial
- a., beef heart
- a. binding ▸ fragment
- a., blood group
- a., cancer
- a. capture assay
- a., carbohydrate
- a. (CEA), carcinoembryonic
- a., cell-bound
- a., cell-membrane
- a., cell surface
- a., common
- a., common acute leukemia
- a., common acute lymphoblastic leukemia
- a., common leukocyte
- a. complex, antibody
- a., conjugated
- a., cytokeratin membrane
- a., cytoskeletal
- a., delta
- a., differentiation
- a., diphtheria
- a., E
- a., early
- a., endogenous
- a. ▸ endothelial localization of
- a., epithelial membrane
- a., exogenous
- a., extractable nuclear
- a. ▸ factor VIII-related
- a., factor IX
- a., factor VII
- a., factor X
- a. ▸ fecal carcinoembryonic
- a., Gross virus
- a., hepatitis-associated
- A. (HBeAg), Hepatitis B e
- A. (HBsAg), Hepatitis B Surface

- a., heterogeneic
- a., heterologous
- a., heterophil
- a., histocompatibility
- a., homologous
- A. (HLA), human leukocyte
- a. (HLA), human lymphocyte
- a., idiotypic
- a., incomplete
- a., inhalant
- a., intracellular
- a., isogeneic
- a., isophil
- a., Kveim
- a. ▸ large granular lymphocyte
- a., late
- a. ▸ leukocyte common
- a. ▸ lineage-associated
- a. ▸ lymphocyte function
- a. ▸ lymphogranuloma venereum
- a. ▸ macrophage lineage
- a. ▸ major histocompatibility complex
- a. ▸ mammary serum
- a. ▸ melanoma-associated
- a., membrane-bound
- a. ▸ monocyte lineage
- a. ▸ mumps skin test
- a. ▸ myeloid-associated
- a. ▸ myeloid lineage
- a., myelomonocytic
- a., negative blood
- a., nuclear
- a. ▸ nuclear proliferation
- a. ▸ organ specific
- a. ▸ pan T-cell
- a. ▸ pancreatic oncofetal
- a. ▸ panhematopoietic cell
- a. ▸ plasma cell
- a., pollen
- a. positive blood
- a., private
- a. -producing cancer cells
- a. ▸ progenitor cell
- a. ▸ proliferating cell nuclear
- a. ▸ proliferation-associated
- a. (PSA) ▸ prostate specific
- a. (PSMA) ▸ prostate specific membrane
- a., protein
- a., public
- a., radiolabeled
- a. (HBsAG) reactivity ▸ hepatitis B surface
- a. ▸ red blood cell

a. ▸ Rh (Rhesus) factor
a., Ro
a., rose bengal
a. screen
a., sequestered
a., serodefined
a. ▸ serum hepatitis
a. skin test ▸ Kveim
a. specific lymphocyte transformation
a. studies ▸ hepatitis surface
a., surface
a. ▸ surface membrane
a. test, Australia
a. ▸ thymic lymphocyte
a. ▸ thymus dependent
a. ▸ thymus independent
a. ▸ tissue specific
a. (Anti-HBc), Total Antibody to Hepatitis B Core
a., transplantation
a., tumor
a. ▸ tumor-associated
a., tumor specific transplantation
a. typing ▸ human lymphocyte
a., viral
a., xenogeneic
antigenic
a. determinant
a. determinate site
a. drift
a. site
a. stimulation
a. structural grouping
a. structure
a. structure, viral
a. targets
antigenicity ▸ lowered tumor
antigenicity, tumor
antigens
a., carbohydrate
a., hepatitis-associated
a., incomplete
a., membrane-bound
a., protein
a., viral
antiglare filter
antiglaucoma medication
antiglobulin
a. reaction
a. reaction, antigen-
a. test
antiglomerular basement membrane antibody
antigout drug

antigranulocyte antibody
antigravity muscles
antigravity stimulation
Anti-HBc (Total Antibody to Hepatitis B Core Antigen)
Anti-HBc (Antibody IgM class to Hepatitis B Core Antigen)
Anti-H Be (Antibody to Hepatitis B e Antigen)
Anti-HBs (Antibody to Heptatitis B Surface Antigen)
anti-HCG antibody
antiheart antibody titer
antihelix elastic nodule
antihemophilic factor
antihemophilic globulin (AHG)
antihistamine
a., bruising from
a., confusion from
a., constipation from
a., drowsiness from
a. ▸ dry mouth from
a., fatigue from
a. medication
a., oral
a. ▸ voice change from
antihuman globulin
antihuman-lymphocyte serum
antihyaluronidase titer
antihypertensive
a. agents
a. coronary patients
a. drugs
a. effect
a. medication
a. regimen
a. regimen ▸ stepped-care
a. therapy
anti-immune substance
anti-infective drug
anti-inflammatory(-ies)
a. activity
a. agent
a. agent, nonsteroidal
a. drug
a. drug (NSAID), nonsteroidal
a. medication
a. nonsteroidal
a. steroid
a. therapy
anti-itch medication
antiketogenic ratio, ketogenic-
antileukemic drug
anti-lewisite (BAL) ▸ British
antilymphatic serum

antilymphocyte
a. globulin
a. plasma
a. serum (ALS)
antilymphocytic sera
antimacrophage globulin
antimacrophage serum
antimalaria drug
antimanic drug
antimicrobial
a. agent
a. agent ▸ macrolide
a. agent ▸ parenteral
a. catheter cuff
a. drugs, prophylactic
a. level
a. prophylaxis
a. prophylaxis ▸ perioperative
a. sensitivity patterns
a. susceptibility
a. therapy
a. therapy ▸ intensive
a. therapy ▸ perioperative
a. treatment
antimitochondrial antibody
antimony compound
antimycobacterial chemotherapy
antimyosin antibody imaging
antimyosin infarct avid scintigraphy
antineoplastic agents
antineoplastic therapy
antineuronal antibody
antineutrophic cytoplasmic autoantibody
antineutrophilic serum
antinuclear
a. antibodies (ANA)
a. antibody (ANA) examination
a. antibody, fluorescent
a. factor
antioxidant
a. nutrients
a. research
a. therapy ▸ intravenous
a. vitamin pretreatment
a. vitamins
antiparasitic agent
antiparkinson drug
antiparkinsonian agent
antipathetic symbiosis
antipenicillin antibody, hemagglutinating
antiperistaltic anastomosis
antipernicious anemia factor
antipetit mal substances

antiphase signal
antiphospholipid syndrome
antiphospholipid syndrome therapy
antiplatelet
- a. activity
- a. agent
- a. drug
- a. therapy

antiproliferative agent
antiprotease imbalance ▸ protease-
antipruritic [*antipyretic*] agent
antipruritic, [*antipyretic*] topical
antipseudomonas human plasma
antipsychotic-induced tardive
    dyskinesia
antipsychotic medication
antirabies serum
antirachitic rays
antireflux
- a. procedure, Belsey Mark IV
- a. prosthesis
- a. prosthesis, Angelchik

antirejection
- a. drug
- a. medication
- a. protocol
- a. therapy

antiresorptive agent
antireticular cytotoxic serum
antiretroviral
- a. activity
- a. regimen
- a. resistance testing (GART) ▸
    genotypic
- a. therapy
- a. therapy (HAART) ▸ highly active

anti-Rh agglutinin
antirheumatic drug (DMARD) ▸ disease
    modifying
anti-Saccharomyces cerevisiae
    antibody (ASCA)
antiseizure drug
antiseizure medication
antisepsis ▸ disinfection and
antisepsis, sterilization and disinfection
antiseptic solution
antiseptic technique
antiserum, human thymus
antishock
- a. garment
- a. garment ▸ pneumatic
- a. pants ▸ medical
- a. pants ▸ military
- a. suit ▸ medical
- a. suit ▸ military

- a. trousers (MAST) ▸ medical
- a. trousers, military
- a. trousers (MAST) ▸ pneumatic

antisocial
- a. acts
- a. behavior
- a. behavior, adolescent
- a. behavior, adult
- a. behavior and drug abuse
- a. behavior, childhood
- a. behavior ▸ engaged in
- a. behavior ▸ parental
- a. personality
- a. personality and drug abuse
- a. personality disorder
- a. personality traits
- a. personality traits ▸ inflexible
- a. personality traits ▸ maladapative
- a. personality traits ▸ persistent
- a. tendencies
- a. trait

antispasmodic
- a., biliary
- a. drug
- a. medication

antistreptolysin O (ASO) titer
antistreptolysin titer
antisuicidal contract
antisuicide hotline
antitachycardia
- a. pacemaker
- a. pacing
- a. pacing protocol ▸ Scan

antiteichoic acid titers
antitetanic serum
antitetanus therapy
antithymocyte globulin (ATG)
antithymocyte serum
antithymocytic globulin
antithyroid medication
antitoxic globulin
antitoxic immunity
antitoxin
- a., diphtheria
- a. immunity, toxin
- a. unit

antitoxoid, toxoid-
anti-Toxoplasma antibodies
antitragus, muscle of
antitremor drug
antitrypsin
- a., alpha
- a. deficiency, alpha-1-
- a. serum ▸ alpha-1-

antitryptic reaction

antituberculous
- a. chemotherapy
- a. drug
- a. therapy

antitumor
- a. activity
- a. antibiotic
- a. effect
- a. hormones

antiulcer agent ▸ tetracycline
antiviral
- a. activity
- a. agent
- a. drug
- a. drug ▸ life-saving
- a. drug treatment
- a. effect
- a. factor (CAF), cell
- a. genes
- a. medication
- a. therapy
- a. treatment ▸ poly-
- a. vaccine

Anton-Babinski syndrome
antral
- a. cancer
- a. cells
- a. erosion
- a. floor
- a. folds
- a. gastritis
- a. mucosa
- a. pack
- a. resection
- a. stenosis
- a. ulcer
- a. window

antrectomy, antrosaucerization
antro-aural fistula
antrosaucerization antrectomy
antrotomy, radical frontal
antrotomy, radical maxillary
antrum
- a., aditus ad
- a., attic-aditus
- a. auris
- a., cardiac
- a., distal
- a., ethmoid
- a. ethmoidale
- a., falx of maxillary
- a., focal
- a., frontal
- a., gastric
- a., greater curvature of

a. highmori
a., mastoid
a. mastoideum
a., maxillary
a. of Highmore
a. operation, radical
a., proximal
a., pyloric
a. ▸ retained gastric
a. scarred
a., tympanic
a. tympanicum

anulus (*see also* annulus)
a. conjunctivae
a. iridis major
a. iridis minor
a. of conjunctiva
a. tendineus communis
a. tympanicus

anuresis [*enuresis*]
anuretic [*enuretic*]
anuretic, patient
anuria
a., angioneurotic
a., calculous
a., obstructive
a., postrenal
a., prerenal
a., renal
a., suppressive
a. ▸ trauma-associated

anus
a., bleeding from
a., discharge from
a., ectopic
a., examination of
a., external sphincter muscle of
a., fissure of
a., imperforate
a., internal sphincter muscle of
a., itching in
a., lump in
a., pain in
a., patent
a., plastic repair of
a., tumor of

anvil
a. bone
a., Bunnell's
a. of ear

anxietas presenilis
anxietas tibiarum
anxiety(-ies)
a., acute
a., alpha biofeedback and

a., analytical psychotherapy for
a. and apprehension
a. and beta blockers
a. and depression
a. and depression, crushing
a. and desensitization, phobic
a., and frustration ▸ depression,
a. and irritability
a. and pain ▸ circular interaction between
a. and panic ▸ depression,
a., and suicide ▸ depression,
a. and tension ▸ autogenic training for
a. angina
a., anticipatory
a. associated with depression
a. attack
a. attacks, dream
a. ▸ attention span, shortened from
a., autonomic nervous system and
a., bath
a., behavioral manifestations of
a. ▸ breathing difficulty from
a. ▸ canker sore from
a., castration
a. ▸ cheek biting from
a., chronic
a. ▸ chronic tension and
a., clinical
a., cocaine-induced
a., comorbid generalized
a. components
a. ▸ confront source of
a., confusion and
a., coping with
a., death
a., decrease in
a., decrease tension and
a., decreased
a., decreased signs and symptoms of
a., dental
a. depression
a. depression reaction
a., desensitization for
a., diarrhea from
a. disease
a. disorder
a. disorder, dream
a. disorder, flashbacks and
a. disorder, general
a. disorder ▸ juvenile
a. disorder of childhood
a. disorder, organic

a. disorder, panic
a. disorder ▸ psychoactive substance
a. disorder, separation
a. disorder, social
a. dreams ▸ rapid eye movement (REM) sleep
a. dreams ▸ sleep
a., endogenous
a. episode
a. -evoking stimuli, autonomic response to
a., existential
a., experimental
a. ▸ eye itching from
a., factors influencing
a., fatigue from
a., fear and
a., fear of
a. ▸ fears, phobias, and
a., forgetfulness from
a., free floating
a. from heat exhaustion
a., gastroenteritis from
a., general
a., generalized
a., guilt, or depression
a., high
a. ▸ high level of
a., holiday
a., hyperactivity and irritability
a., hyperactivity from
a., hyperventilation from
a. hysteria
a., image patterns of
a. in elderly ▸ depression and
a., increased
a. -induced pain
a., insomnia from
a. ▸ intense short-term
a. interval
A. Inventory ▸ State Trait
a., irrational
a., irritability or
a., late-life
a. ▸ learning theories of
a. level
a. level, elevated
a., lifelong
a. ▸ loss of appetite from
a. ▸ loss of sexual desire
a., low
a. management
a. management skills
a., managing

anxiety—*continued*
a., maternal
a., menstrual
a., muscle tension and
a., nervousness and
a. neurosis
a. neurosis, acute
a., occasional
a. of children ▸ separation
a. overlay
a., pain and
a., pain determined by level of
a., palpitations from
a., patient
a., patient's level of
a., performance
a. ▸ persistent feelings of
a., phobic
a., physique
a. -producing situations
a., prolonged
a. -provoking choice
a. -provoking situation
a., psoriasis from
a. reaction
a. reaction, acute
a., reduction of
a., reduction of examination
a. -related muscle disorder
a. -related sensation
A. Scale ▸ Thayer Clinical
a., sense
a. sensitivity
a. sensitivity ▸ high
a., separation
a., severe
a. ▸ shortened attention span from
a., situational
a. ▸ source of
a., spasms of
a. state
a. state, acute
a., state-and-trait
a. state, chronic
a., stranger
a. ▸ stress and
a. symptoms
a., systematic desensitization of pervasive
a. tension, acute
a., ▸ tension and headache
a. tension state (ATS)
a. ▸ throat clearing from
a., tinnitus from
a., treatment of chronic

a. treatment, depression-
a., trembling from
a. ▸ trench mouth from
a. triggers
a., urination from
a. ▸ voice change from
a., waking
a. ▸ weight loss from
a. with diarrhea

anxiolytic
a. abuse ▸ sedative, hypnotic, or
a. amnestic disorder
a. dependence ▸ sedative, hypnotic, or
a. intoxication ▸ sedative, hypnotic, or
a. withdrawal delirium

anxious
a. affect
a. and fearful
a. behavior
a., depressed and
a. facies
a., feeling
a. ▸ hostile and
a., intermittently
a. mood
a. mood ▸ adjustment disorder with
a. patient
a. situation ▸ stressful or
a. state

AO
AO (anodal opening)
AO (aortic opening)
AO (axio-occlusal)
AOC (abridged ocular chart)
AOC (anodal opening contraction)
A1 (Alpha1)
A-1 globulins
a-1, 3-glucosidase deficiency
aorta
a., abdominal
a. abdominalis
a. aneurysm ▸ thoracic
a., aneurysmal widening of
a. angiography, supra-
a., arch of
a., arteriosclerotic elongation thoracic
a. ascendens
a. (AA) ▸ ascending
a. atherosclerosed, abdominal
a., atherosclerosis of
a., atherosclerotic abdominal
a., base of

a., buckled
a., button
a. chlorotica
a., coarctation of
a. cross-clamped
a., cross-clamping of
a., cystic medial necrosis of ascending
a., defective
a. descendens
a., descending
a., descending thoracic
a., dextropositioned
a., diseased
a., dissecting
a., distal
a., dorsal
a., double-barreled
a., dynamic
a., ectasia of abdominal
a., ectasia of thoracic
a., elasticity of
a., elongated
a., elongation of thoracic
a., embolectomy of
a., enlargement of
a. ▸ hardening of
a., incision into
a. ▸ infrarenal abdominal
a. ▸ inner layer of
a., insufficiency of
a., junky
a., kinked
a., lumbar
a., lunulae of semilunar valves of
a. ▸ medionecrosis of
a. ▸ multiple sections of
a., narrowing of
a., native
a., overriding
a., palpable
a., patch enlargement of ascending
a., porcelain
a., primitive
a. ▸ pseudocoarctation of
a., pulsating
a., recipients'
a. reclamped
a. ▸ recoarctation of
a., retroesophageal
a., sacrococcygeal
a. ▸ saccular aneurysm of abdominal
a. ▸ severe atheromatous change of
a., stenosis of

a., straddling
a., terminal
a. thoracalis
a., thoracic
a. thoracica
a., throbbing
a. thrombotic aneurysm, abdominal
a. -to-pulmonary artery shunt ▸ ascending
a., tortuous
a. ▸ tulip bulb
a., uncoiling
a., ventral
a., wide tortuous
aortae, bulbus
aortae, lunulae valvularum semilunarium
aortic (A)
a. allograft, cryopreserved human
a. anastomosis
a. aneurysm
a. aneurysm (AAA) ▸ abdominal
a. aneurysm, congenital
a. aneurysm, descending thoracic
a. aneurysm, dissecting
a. aneurysm, false
a. aneurysm ▸ fusiform
a. aneurysm graft
a. aneurysm ▸ inflammatory
a. aneurysm ▸ infrarenal abdominal
a. aneurysm ▸ mycotic
a. aneurysm, reflux dissecting abdominal
a. aneurysm repair
a. aneurysm rupture
a. aneurysm, rupture of syphilitic
a. aneurysm ▸ ruptured
a. aneurysm ▸ ruptured abdominal
a. aneurysm ▸ suprarenal
a. aneurysm ▸ thoracoabdominal
a. aneurysmal disease
a. angiography ▸ left
a. annulus
a. annulus abscess
a. aperture
a. arch
a. arch aneurysm
a. arch angiography
a. arch arteritis
a. arch atresia
a. arch calcification
a. arch, cervical
a. arch, circumflex
a. arch, double
a. arch ▸ interrupted

a. arch interruption
a. arch ▸ right
a. arch study
a. arch study ▸ cardiac-pulmonary angio-
a. arch syndrome
a. arch ▸ tortuous
a. area ▸ secondary
a. arteritis syndrome
a. artery ▸ ruptured
a. atherosclerosis
a. atherosclerosis, advanced
a. atresia
a. balloon counterpulsation, intra-
a. balloon deflation, intra-
a. balloon inflation, intra-
a. balloon, intra-
a. balloon pump
a. balloon pumping (IABP), intra-
a. base
a. bifurcation
a. bifurcation occlusion
a. blood flow
a. blood pressure
a. bodies ▸ para-
a. body tumor
a. bulb
a. bypass ▸ Litwak left atrial
a. calcification
a. closure
a. closure sound
a. coarctation
a. commissure
a. commissurotomy
a. compliance
a. compression
a. contour
a. counterpulsation device (AACD), abdominal
a. cuff
a. cusp
a. cusp, right anterior
a. cusp separation
a. disruption ▸ traumatic
a. dissection
a. dissection, acute
a. dissection, DeBakey-type
a. dissection, right carotid
a. dissection ▸ Stanford-type
a. dissection ▸ thoracic
a. emboli, acute
a. embolism
a. endothelial cells ▸ human
a. envelope
a. facies

a. flow
A. Graft Replacement (AGR)
a. gradient ▸ transvalvular
a. hiatus
a. homograft
a. impedance
a. incompetence
a. incompetent murmur
a. inflammation
a. injury
a. insufficiency
a. (IA), intra-
a. intramural hematoma
a. isthmus
a. jet velocity
a. jugular test
a. knob
a. knuckle
a. knuckle, cervical
a. leaflet
a. left ventricular (LV) tunnel murmur
a. -mitral combined disease murmur
a. motion artifact
a. murmur
a. nipple
a. notch
a. occlusion
a. occlusion, acute
a. occlusion, acute abdominal
a. occlusive emboli
a. opening (AO)
a. orifice
a. override
a. pressure, ascending
a. pressure gradient
a. pressure (MAP) ▸ mean
a. pressure (PSAP) ▸ peak systolic
a. prosthesis
a. prosthesis, discoid
a. prosthesis, trileaflet
a. pullback
a. pullback pressure
a. reblockage
a. reflex
a. regurgitation (AR)
a. regurgitation murmur
a. ring
a. root
a. root dimension
a. root ratio
a. rupture
a. sac
a. saddle embolus

aortic—*continued*
a. sclerosis
a., sclerotic
a. second sound (A2)
a. second sound (A2) accentuated
a. semilunar valves
a. septal defect
a. shadow
a. sinus
a. sinusal aneurysm
a. sound
a. sound (A2) ▸ second
a. stenosis (AS)
a. stenosis, calcific
a. stenosis, calcific nodular
a. stenosis, chronic
a. stenosis, congenital
a. stenosis ▸ discrete subvalvular
a. stenosis, double
a. stenosis infantile hypercalcemia syndrome ▸ supravalvular
a. stenosis jet
a. stenosis murmur
a. stenosis, occult
a. stenosis ▸ senescent
a. stenosis, subvalvular
a. stenosis, supravalvular
a. stenosis syndrome ▸ supravalvular
a. stenosis ▸ valvular
a. tear
a. thrill
a. thrombi, acute
a. thromboembolic disease
a. thrombolysis
a. thrombosis ▸ infrarenal
a. tissue
a. triangle
a. tube graft
a. tumor
a. tunica adventitia
a. tunica intima
a. tunica media
a. valve
a. valve area
a. valve atresia
a. valve, bicommissural
a. valve, bicuspid
a. valve, calcified
a. valve, defective
a. valve, diastolic fluttering
a. valve disease
a. valve disorder
a. valve disorder, congenital
a. valve, ectatic

a. valve, gradient
a. valve leaflet prolapse
a. valve leaflets
a. valve ▸ leaking
a. valve, lunulae of
a. valve ▸ mild leaking of
a. valve ▸ moderate leaking of
a. valve, narrowing of
a. valve, nodules of
a. valve obstruction
a. valve opening
a. valve peak gradient
a. valve prosthesis
a. valve prosthesis, Bjork-Shiley
a. valve prosthesis, Capetown
a. valve prosthesis, Carpentier-Edwards
a. valve prosthesis, Ionescu-Shiley
a. valve prosthesis, Starr-Edwards
a. valve prosthesis ▸ stentless porcine
a. valve prosthesis, St. Jude Medical
a. valve prosthesis ▸ tilting disk
a. valve ▸ prosthetic
a. valve regurgitation
a. valve replacement (AVR)
a. valve resistance
a. valve restenosis
a. valve ▸ scarring of
a. valve ▸ sclerotic
a. valve, stenosed
a. valve stenosis
a. valve stenosis (CAVS), calcific
a. valve thickened
a. valve ▸ thickening of
a. valve vegetation
a. valve velocity profile
a. valvotomy
a. valvotomy, balloon
a. valvular insufficiency
a. valvular stenosis
a. valvulotomy
a. valvulitis
a. valvulitis ▸ syphilitic
a. valvuloplasty
a. valvuloplasty, balloon
a. valvuloplasty ▸ percutaneous balloon
a. vasa vasorum
a. ventricle of heart
a. wall
a. window
aortica, glomera
aorticopulmonary septum

aorticus, sulcus
aortitis
a., bacterial
a., Döhle-Heller
a. ▸ giant cell
a., luetic
a., nummular
a., rheumatic
a., syphilitic
a., Takayasu
aortoannular ectasia
aortobi-iliac bypass
aortocarotid bypass
aortocaval compression
aortocaval fistula
aortocoronary
a. bypass
a. bypass graft
a. saphenous vein bypass
a. vein bypass
aortofemoral
a. arterial runoff
a. artery shunt
a. bypass graft (AFBG)
a. Dacron graft
a. -femoral bypass, descending thoracic
aortogram
a., antegrade
a., flush
a., retrograde
a. study
a., transbrachial arch
a., translumbar
a. with distal runoff
aortography
a., abdominal
a., ascending
a., biplane
a., catheter
a., flush
a., lumbar
a., mycotic
a. procedure
a., retrograde
a., selective
a., selective visceral
a. ▸ single plane
a. ▸ sinus of Valsalva
a. study
a., thoracic
a. ▸ thoracic arch
a., translumbar
a., venous
a., visceral

aortoiliac
- a. aneurysm
- a. bypass
- a. bypass graft
- a. graft, Creech
- a. obstructive disease (AIOD)
- a. stenosis
- a. thrombosis
- a. vascular calcifications

aortoiliofemoral bypass
aortoiliofemoral circuit
aorto-ostial lesion
aortopulmonary
- a. collateral
- a. fenestration
- a. shunt

aortorenal bypass
aorto-subclavian carotid-axilloaxillary bypass
aortovein bypass graft
aortovelography, transvenous
AOT (anodal opening tetanus)
AP
- AP (angina pectoris)
- AP (anterior and posterior)
- AP (anteroposterior)
- AP (arterial pressure)
- AP (axiopulpal)
- AP and lat (anteroposterior and lateral)
- AP (anteroposterior) and lateral films, portable recumbent
- AP (anteroposterior) and lateral views
- AP (anteroposterior) diameter
- AP (anteroposterior) diameter of chest
- AP (anteroposterior) diameter ▸ uterus normal in
- AP (anteroposterior) film
- AP (arterial pressure) line ▸ insertion of
- AP (anteroposterior), neutral
- AP (anteroposterior) position
- AP (anteroposterior) projection
- AP (anteroposterior) projection, coned
- AP (anteroposterior) projection, semi-axial
- AP (anteroposterior) repair
- AP (anteroposterior) study
- AP (anteroposterior) vaginal vault repair
- AP (anteroposterior) view
- AP (anteroposterior) view, normal

apart, spread ribs
apathetic
- a. behavior
- a., emotionally
- a. hyperthyroidism
- a. ▸ listless and
- a., patient
- a. ▸ patient withdrawn, depressed and

apathy
- a. and disorientation ▸ self-neglect,
- a. and irritability
- a. and lack of interest in personal goals
- a. and lack of interest in society
- a., loss of energy, mood changes

apatite [*appetite*]
A-pattern strabismus
APB (atrial premature beat)
APC (atrial premature contraction)
APC (AMSA, prednisone, and chlorambucil) chemotherapy
APDC (atrial premature depolarization contractions)
ape hand
apepsia, achlorhydria
aperiodic waves
A-Person Test, Color-
aperta, rhinolalia
aperta ▸ spina bifida
aperture(s)
- a., aortic
- a., central
- a. imaging, coded-
- a., lateral
- a., medial
- a., multiple
- a., nasal
- a. of frontal sinus
- a. of larynx
- a. of sphenoid sinus
- a., palpebral
- a., piriform
- a., pupillary
- a., pyriform
- a., tympanic

apex (apices)
- a. auriculae
- a. beat
- a., cardiac
- a. cardiogram
- a. cardiogram study
- a. cardiography
- a. cardiography technique
- a. clear to percussion ▸ right

- a. cordis
- a. electrogram ▸ right ventricular (RV)
- a. emphysematous
- a. height
- a. impulse
- a., left pulmonary
- a. ▸ left ventricular (LV)
- a. linguae
- a., lung
- a. murmur
- a. nasi
- a. of bladder
- a. of cochlea
- a. of contraction
- a. of heart
- a. of heart, thrust of
- a. of incision
- a. of left lung
- a. of right lung
- a. of tooth root ▸ excision of
- a. of vagina
- a., petrous
- a. pneumonia
- a. ▸ posterior septum
- a. prostatae
- a. pulse ▸ F point of cardiac
- a. pulse ▸ O point of cardiac
- a. pulse ▸ SF wave of cardiac
- a. ▸ right ventricular (RV)
- a. vesicae urinariae

Apgar
- A., initial
- A. rating
- A. scale
- A. score
- A. score, initial

aphagia algera
aphakia
- a., bilateral
- a. left eye, postsurgical
- a., postsurgical
- a. right eye, postsurgical

aphakic glaucoma
aphasia
- a., acoustic
- a., ageusic
- a., amnemonic
- a., amnesic
- a., amnestic
- a., anomic
- a., anosmic
- a., associative
- a., ataxic
- a., auditory

aphasia—*continued*
- a., Broca's
- a., central
- a., combined
- a., commissural
- a., complete
- a., conduction
- a., cortical
- a., expressive
- a., expressive-receptive
- a., fluent
- a., frontocortical
- a., fontolenticular
- a., functional
- a., gibberish
- a., global
- a., graphomotor
- a., Grashey's
- a., impressive
- a., intellectual
- a., jargon
- a., Kussmaul's
- a., lenticular
- a., Lichtheim's
- a., mixed
- a., motor
- a., motor expressive
- a., nominal
- a., nonfluent
- a., optic
- a., pathematic
- a., pictorial
- a., psychosensory
- a., receptive
- a. ▸ right hemiparesis and
- a., Screening Test ▸ Halstead-Wepman
- a., semantic
- a., sensory
- a. ▸ stroke-like syndrome of
- a., subcortical
- a., syntactical
- a., tactile
- a., temporoparietal
- a., total
- a., transcortical
- a., true
- a., verbal
- a., visual
- a., Wernicke's

aphasic screening test, Reitan-Indiana

aphonia
- a., hysteric
- a. paralytica
- a. paranoica
- a., spastic

aphonic pectoriloquy
aphrophilus, Haemophilus
aphthosa, stomatitis
aphthous
- a. fever
- a. stomatitis
- a. ulcer

apical
- a. abscess
- a. beat, displaced
- a. bleb
- a. bronchus
- a. constriction
- a. cyst
- a. diastolic murmurs
- a. dyskinesia
- a. fibrous adhesions ▸ multiple
- a. fibrous pleural adhesions ▸ bilateral
- a. five-chamber view echocardiogram
- a. foramen
- a. four-chamber view echocardiogram
- a. granuloma
- a. hypertrophy
- a. impulse
- a. impulse, double
- a. impulse, sustained
- a. impulse ▸ systolic
- a. infarction
- a. infection
- a. interventricular septal amplitude
- a. left ventricular (LV) puncture
- a. lesion
- a. lordotic projection
- a. lordotic roentgenogram
- a. lordotic view
- a. mid-diastolic heart murmur
- a. murmur
- a. murmur, systolic
- a. opacifications
- a. pericementitis
- a. pleural fibrosis
- a. pleural thickening
- a. pleurectomy ▸ thorascopic
- a. poles
- a. portion of root
- a. pneumonia
- a. pulse
- a. rate
- a. scarring
- a. segment, antero-
- a. segment of lung

- a. systolic heart murmur
- a. systolic murmur ▸ late
- a. thickening of left ventricle
- a. thrill
- a. two-chamber view echocardiogram

apicalis, Paranthenus
apicis cordis ▸ incisura
apicolysis, extrapleural
apicolysis procedure
apicoposterior segment of lung
apiculatus, Kloeckera
apiculatus, Saccharomyces
apii, Cercospora
apinoid cancer
apiospermum, Monosporium
APKD (adult polycystic kidney disease)
APL (acute promyelocytic leukemia)
aplanatic lens
aplasia
- a. axialis extracorticalis congenita
- a., bone marrow
- a. cutis congenita
- a., dental
- a., fatal bone marrow
- a., germinal
- a., gonadal
- a. ▸ idiopathic megakaryocytic
- a., nuclear
- a., pulmonary
- a. ▸ pure red blood cell
- a., radial
- a. ▸ red cell
- a., retinal
- a., thymic
- a., thymic-parathyroid
- a., uterine

aplastic
- a. anemia
- a. anemia ▸ primary
- a. anemia ▸ secondary
- a. leukemia
- a. lymph node

Apley's sign
Apley's test
apnea
- a. alarm mattress
- a., cardiac
- a., central
- a., central sleep
- a., deglutition
- a. ▸ drowsiness from sleep
- a. /hypopnea index (AHI)
- a. /hypopnea syndrome ▸ sleep
- a., initial

a., late
a., mixed
a. ‣ mixed sleep
a. monitor
a. monitored baby
a. neonatorum
a., neurological
a., obstructive
a., (OSA), obstructive sleep
a., peripheral
a., postanesthetic
a. ‣ problem with central nervous system from sleep
a. ‣ prolonged cerebral
a., sleep
a., symptoms of
a. syndrome, sleep
a., traumatic
a. victim, sleep-
apneic
a. attack
a. attack ‣ recurrent
a. episode
a. episode ‣ silence of
a. infant with decreased heart rate
a., patient
a. periods
apneustic breathing
apneustic respiration
apochromatic lens
apochromatic objective
apocrine
a. adenoma
a. carcinoma
a. gland
a. metaplasia
a. secretions
a. sweat gland
aponeurosis, transverse bundles of palmar
aponeurosis, Zinn's
aponeurotic system (SMAS), superficial musculo-
aponeurotica, galea
apophyseal/apophysial [*epiphyseal*]
a. fracture
a. joint
a. joint, midcervical
apophysis [epiphysis] [Hypothesis]
a., basilar
a., cerebral
a. cerebri
a., genial
a., ring
apophysitis, calcaneo◊

apoplectic
a. coma
a. cyst
a. glaucoma
a. habit
a. retinitis
a. shock
a. type
apoplectiform deafness
apoplexia uteri
apoplexy
a., Broadbent's
a., capillary
a., cerebellar
a., cerebral
a., endometrial
a., fulminating
a., ingravescent
a., meningeal
a., pituitary
a., pontile
a., Raymond's
a., thrombotic
a., uterine
a., uteroplacental
a., verminous
apoptosis ‣ post-heart attack
apoptosis ‣ cellular regeneration and
Aporina delafondi
apostematosa, cheilitis glandularis
apostematosa, pneumonia
apostematous cheilitis
apotu, mania
AP/PA projection, transtabular
apparatus
a., Barany
a., Cloward
a., EOG (electro-oculogram)
a., indirect contact with contaminated laboratory
a., Kirschner's
a., Osteo-Stim
a., procedures and
a., quantitative inhalation challenge
a., Sayre's
a., self-contained underwater breathing
a., skull traction
a. spirometer, Krogh's
a., volutrol
apparent [*aberrant*]
a. death
a. lesion
a. life-threatening event (ALTE)
a. suicide

apparition, visual
appear enlarged
a.e., adenoids
a.e., adenoids do not
a.e., fibroid of uterus does
a.e., heart does
a.e., heart does not
a.e., liver does
a.e., liver does not
a.e., lump in left breast does
a.e., lump in left breast does not
a.e., lump in right breast does
a.e., lump in right breast does not
a.e., spleen does
a.e., spleen does not
a.e., thyroid does
a.e., thyroid does not
a.e., tonsils
a.e., tonsils do not
a.e., uterus does
a.e., uterus does not
appearance
a., altered facial
a., anatomical
a., apple sauce
a., atrophic
a., beaded
a., bubble-like
a., cluster of grapes
a., cobblestone
a., coffee bean
a., coiled-spring
a., coma
a., cords normal in
a., corkscrew
a., cosmetic
a., cushingoid
a., cystic
a., dazed
a., delusions concerning
a., dimensional
a., dirty lung
a., disinterest in personal
a., double-bubble
a., eyes sunken in
a. ‣ finger-in-glove
a. ‣ ground-glass
a., hazy
a., honeycombed
a., inverse comma
a. ‣ inverted-T
a. ‣ jail bars
a. ‣ jelly belly
a. ‣ lace-like
a. ‣ mask-like facial

appearance—*continued*
a., mottled
a., mottled hemorrhagic
a. ▸ neglect of personal
a., newborn
a., normal gross
a. of dye, prompt
a. of liver ▸ histologic
a. ▸ pale facial
a. ▸ peau d'orange
a., pruned tree
a. ▸ railroad track
a., sad or tearful
a., serrated
a., sexually seductive
a., skin mottled in
a. ▸ slapped cheek
a. ▸ spleen had mottled
a., stepladder
a., stippled
a., subnormal sonic
a., sunburst
a., teardrop
a., ulcer crater with target
a., untidy
a., variable
a., waterfall
a., wedge-shaped
a., wineglass

appeared inflamed, mucosa

appearing
a. mass, solid
a. megakaryocytes, atypical
a. nodular density ▸ benign
a. organ, healthy
a. stomach, normal
a. tissue, innocent

appendage(s)
a., atrial
a., auricular
a., cecal
a. electrogram ▸ right atrial
a., epiploic
a., filamentous
a. in embryo, atrial
a. ▸ left atrial
a. of epididymis
a. of eye
a. of fetus
a. of liver, fibrous
a. of skin
a. of testis
a., ovarian
a., right atrial
a., testicular

a., uterine
a., vermicular
a., vesicular

appendectomy
a., incidental
a. performed in routine fashion
a. scar

appendiceal/appendical
a. abscess
a. base
a. fecalith
a. mass
a. mesentery
a. stump
a. stump inverted
a. tissue

appendices epiploicae

appendicitis
a. ▸ abdominal tenderness from
a., acute
a., amebic
a., fulminating
a., gangrenous
a., indigestion from
a. ▸ left-sided
a., nausea from
a. ▸ pain in abdomen from
a., perforated
a., rule out (r/o)
a., suppurative
a. ▸ tenderness in abdomen from
a., vomiting from

appendicular
a. asynergy
a. dyspepsia
a. gastralgia
a. muscles
a. veins

appendix
a., acutely inflamed
a., base of
a. brought into surgical incision
a. brought into surgical wound
a., bury stump of
a., cecal
a. dyspepsia
a. freed up
a., gangrenous
a., hot
a. inflamed
a. ligated and amputated
a., lumen of
a., lymph tissue
a. mass
a., mesentery of

a., Morgagni's
a. perforated
a., removal of vermiform
a., residual
a., retrocecal
a., ruptured
a. ▸ ruptured peritonitis from
a., suppurative
a. swollen
a. uninflamed
a., vermiform
a., virulent
a. visualized

**Apperception Test, Children's
Apperception Test, Thematic**
appetite [*apatite*]
a. and concentration ▸ loss of interest
a. and exercise
a. and increased energy, decreased
a. and weight, loss of
a., change in
a. cravings
a., decrease in
a., decreased
a., depressed
a., depression and
a., diminished
a. disturbance
a., erratic
a., fatigue and loss of
a. from Addison's disease ▸ loss of
a. from AIDS ▸ loss of
a. from anxiety ▸ loss of
a. from Crohn's disease ▸ loss of
a. from depression ▸ insatiable
a. from diabetes ▸ insatiable
a. from flu ▸ loss of
a. from gastritis ▸ loss of
a. from heart failure ▸ loss of
a. from hepatitis ▸ loss of
a. good, patient's
a., inability to control
a., increased
a. ▸ increased sexual
a. ▸ insomnia, hyperactivity and decreased
a. loss from cancer
a. loss from depression
a. loss from pain in abdomen
a. loss from pernicious anemia
a., loss of
a. poor, patient's
a., reduced

a., return of
a., stimulates
a. suppressant
a. suppressant ▸ confusion from
a., voracious
a. with fatigue ▸ loss of
a. with indigestion ▸ loss of
a. with joint swelling ▸ loss of
applanation tonometry, carotid
applanation tonometer, Goldmann's
apple
a., Adam's
a. jelly nodules
a. picker's disease
a. sauce appearance
a. -shaped body
applesauce sign
appliance
a., Andersen
a., Begg
a., Bimler
a., bite-raising
a., craniofacial
a., Crozat
a., dental
a., extra-oral
a. fitting
a., fixed
a., fracture
a., Frankel
a., functional
a., Hawley
a., Johnson twin wire
a., orthodontic
a., prosthetic
a., removable
a., thumb-sucking
a., universal
application
a., clinical
a., electrode
a., facial electrode
a., intracavitary
a., intranasal
a., local
a. of plaster cast
a. of thermography, clinical
a., point of
a. programmer
a. to treatment
a., topical
applicator
a. and sources
a. attenuation
a., cesium

a., cocaine soaked
a., Ernst
a., Ernst radium
a., Fletcher's loading
a., Fletcher-Suit
a., Gifford's
a., intracavitary gynecologic
a., laryngeal
a., nasopharyngeal
a., Plummer-Vinson radium
a., radioactive
a., radioisotope
a., sealed
a., sonic
applied
a. anatomy
a. chemistry
a., dressings and stockinette
a., dry sterile dressings (DSD)
a., electrode
a., eye pad and shield
a., gentle pressure bandage
a. kinesiology
a. microwaves, superficially
a. over cerebral cortex ▸ electrodes
a., pressure
a., pressure dressing
a. psychology
a. relaxation
a., sterile drapes
a., sterile dressing
a. to cast, walker
a. to extremity, traction
a., tourniquet
apply coping strategies
appointed guardian, court
appointment(s)
a., counseling
a., fails to keep
a. system ▸ on-line
Appolionio implant cataract lens
apposition [opposition]
a. and alignment
a., bony
a. fracture
a., margins of wound brought into
a. ▸ mitral-septal
a. of cutaneous margins
a. of fracture ▸ proper alignment
    and
a., stent
a. suture
appraisal arrogant-self
appraisal, health risk

appreciable
a. change, no
a. change, some
a. disease, no
appression
a. anxiety and
a. ▸ stress and
a. underlying
apprehensive
a. and nervous
a. and tense
a. patient
approach(es)
a., aggressive
a., alternative
a., antecubital
a., antegrade
a., arc rotation
a., behavioral
a., brachial artery
a., Caldwell-Luc
a., central
a., cognitive
a., cognitive behavioral
a., common sense
a., conservative
a., Cubbins'
a., disruptive
a., electric
a., empirical
a., family systems
a. ▸ female artery
a., femoral
a., genetic
a., Gibson
a., Gillies'
a., gradient of
a., holistic
a., hospice
a., integrated
a. ▸ integrative neurobehavioral
a., interdisciplinary team
a., Kocher-McFarland
a., logical sequential
a., molecular
a., multidisciplinary
a. ▸ multidisciplinary treatment team
a., multimodality
a., neurobehavioral
a., neurosurgical
a., nonmedical
a., percutaneous
a., posterior
a., primary
a., psychological

approach(es)—*continued*
- a. ▸ retrograde endoscopic
- a. ▸ retrograde femoral
- a., Risdon
- a., self-psychological
- a., short-term therapeutic
- a., shot-gun
- a., Smith-Petersen
- a., Soens
- a. ▸ strategic, experiential and ego-analytic
- a. ▸ supine oblique
- a., surgical
- a., systematic
- a., team
- a., therapeutic
- a., thermal
- a., to pain management, multidisciplinary
- a. to psychotherapy ▸ trauma-focused
- a., transcubital
- a., transgluteal
- a., transvaginal
- a. to treatment, dual
- a., transdural
- a., transthoracic
- a., transvenous
- a., treatment

appropriate
- a. admission
- a. affect
- a. articulation level ▸ age-
- a. behavior
- a. conversation
- a. criteria
- a. educational process
- a. emotional response
- a. fantasies, age-
- a. for gestational age (AGA)
- a. for gestational age (AGA) female neonate, term
- a. for gestational age (AGA) male neonate, term
- a. goals
- a. lengths of stay
- a. level of care
- a. medical attention
- a. nonverbal support, provide
- a. polycythemia
- a. therapy
- a. treatment

appropriateness, discharge
appropriateness for programming
approved, admission

approved medication
approximate
- a. lethal concentration
- a. on phonation
- a. skin edges
- a. wound edges

approximated
- a., edges
- a., pleural edges
- a., skin
- a., subcutaneous tissues
- a. with ties, breast tissue
- a., wound
- a., wound loosely

approximation
- a., healing with
- a. of cutaneous edges
- a. rechecked
- a. suture

apraxia [*ataxia*]
- a., akinetic
- a. algera
- a., amnestic
- a., classic
- a., constructional
- a., cortical
- a., expressive
- a., gait
- a., ideational
- a., ideokinetic
- a., ideomotor
- a., innervation
- a., Leipmann's
- a., limb-kinetic
- a., motor
- a. of eyelid
- a., sensory
- a., transcortical

apraxic, patient is
apron, omental
aptitude, activity interests and
aptitude, clerical
APTT (activated partial thromboplastin time)
AQ (achievement quotient)
aqua jogging
aquacise program
Aquaflo gauze
aquagenic urticaria
Aqua-K pad
aquatic
- a. exercise, aerobic
- a. therapy

aquaticus cancer

aqueduct
- a., cerebral
- a., cochlear
- a., fallopian
- a., gliosis of cerebral
- a. of cochlea
- a. of Cotunnius
- a. of Fallopius
- a. of midbrain
- a. of Sylvius
- a. of the vestibule
- a. of vestibule ▸ vein of
- a., sylvian
- a., ventricular
- a., vestibular

aqueductus
- a. cerebri
- a. cochleae
- a. endolymphaticus
- a. vestibuli

aqueous
- a. barrier, blood
- a. chamber
- a. flare
- a. humor
- a. humor ▸ flow of
- a. humor of eye
- a. penicillin
- a. veins

aquosa, polyemia
AR (aortic regurgitation)
AR (artificial respiration)
arabinoside, adenosine
arabinoside, (ARA-C) cytosine
arabinosus, Lactobacillus
arabinotarda Type A ▸ Shigella
arabinotarda Type B ▸ Shigella
ARA-C (cytosine arabinoside)
arachidic bronchitis
arachidonate metabolism
arachidonic acid metabolites
arachnidism, necrotic
arachnoid
- a., cranial
- a. mater
- a. membrane
- a. of brain
- a. of spinal cord
- a., pia-
- a. pulse
- a. space
- a., spinal
- a. villi

arachnoidal granulations
arachnoidea encephali

arachnoidea spinalis
arachnoiditis
    a., adhesive
    a., cystic
    a., neoplastic
    a. of spine
    a., optochiasmatic
ARAD (abnormal right axis deviation)
Arakawa-Higashi syndrome
Aran
    A. -Duchenne muscular atrophy
    A. -Duchenne muscular disease
    A. muscular atrophy, Duchenne-
araneosus, nevus
Arantius, nodules of
Arantius, ventricle of
arbor virus
arborescens keratitis
arborescent cataract
arborescent white substance of
    cerebellum
arboreus, Argas
arborization heart block
arbovirus, isolated
Arbrus precatorius
ARC (arc)
    ARC (AIDS [acquired immune
      deficiency syndrome] related
      complex)
    ARC (anomalous retinal
      correspondence)
    a. -flash conjunctivitis
    a. lamp
    a. lamp, carbon
    a. lamp, tungsten
    a. laser, xenon (Xe)
    a. light, xenon
    a. rotation approach
    a. rotational technique
    a. simple reflex
    a., simulated radiation
    a. welder lung
arcade
    a., anomalous mitral
    a. collateral
    a., septal
arcanobacterial pharyngitis
ARCD (age-related cognitive decline)
arceau rhythm
arceau, rhythm en
Arcelin's view
arch(es)
    a., alveolar
    a. aneurysm, aortic
    a. angiography, aortic

a., aortic
a. aortogram, transbrachial
a. aortography ▸ thoracic
a. arteritis, aortic
a. atresia, aortic
a., auricular
a., axillary
a., azygos
a. bar
a. bar, custom-made
a. bar, Erich's
a. bar, fixed
a. bar, Jelenko's
a. bar, retainer
a., basal
a., bovine
a., branchial
a. calcification ▸ aortic
a. carcinoma, faucial
a., carotid
a., cervical aortic
a., circumflex aortic
a., circumflex retroesophageal
a., coracoacromial
a., costal
a., crural
a. deformity, high
a., dental
a., digital venous
a., double aortic
a., ductus
a., epiphyseal
a., fallen
a., faucial
a. ▸ fixed lingual
a. flow, palmar
a. fracture ▸ nondisplaced
    zygomatic
a., glossopalatine
a., hemal
a., hyoid
a., hypochordal
a., inflamed
a., inguinal
a. ▸ interrupted aortic
a. interruption, aortic
a. ▸ jugular venous
a. ▸ Lanager's axillary
a., lingual
a., longitudinal
a., malar
a., mandibular
a., maxillary
a., medial
a., metatarsal

a., nasal
a., neural
a. of aorta
a. of Corti
a. of foot ▸ dorsal arterial
a. of foot ▸ dorsal venous
a. of foot ▸ longitudinal
a. of kidney ▸ venous
a. of nose
a. of palate
a. of ribs
a. of thoracic duct
a. of Treitz
a. ▸ open pubic
a., oral
a., osseocartilaginous
a., osseoligamentous
a., paired vertebral
a., palatal
a., palatine
a., palatoglossal
a., palatomaxillary
a., palatopharyngeal
a., palmar
a., paraphyseal
a. ▸ passive lingual
a., pedicle of vertebral
a., pharyngeal
a., pharyngoepiglottic
a., pharyngopalatine
a. photocoagulator, xenon (Xe)
a., plantar
a., popliteal
a., postaural
a., posterior
a., pronated
a., pubic
a., pulmonary
a., residual
a. ▸ residual dental
a., retroesophageal
a., ribbon
a. ▸ right aortic
a., Riolan's
a., Salus'
a. -shaped waves ▸ burst of
a., Shenton's
a. ▸ stationary lingual
a. study, aortic
a. study ▸ cardiac-pulmonary
    angio-aortic
a., subpubic
a., superciliary
a. support, substantial
a. supports

arch(es)—*continued*
- a. syndrome, aortic
- a., systemic
- a., tarsal
- a., tendinous
- a., thyrohyoid
- a. ▸ tortuous aortic
- a. tracing, Gothic
- a., transverse
- a., Treitz's
- a., vertebral
- a., visceral
- a. ▸ V-shaped
- a., Zimmerman's
- a., zygomatic

arched lower back
arched palate, high
architectural barriers to independence
architecture
- a., bony
- a., histologic
- a. ▸ loss of normal
- a., lung
- a., nutmeg
- a., postmenopausal breast
- a., sleep

archoplasmic loop
arciform veins
Arco lithium pacemaker
arcuate
- a. artery
- a. commissure
- a. configuration
- a. fibers, anterior external
- a. ligament
- a. ligament of knee
- a. scotoma
- a. uterus
- a. vein
- a. veins of kidney

arcuatus
- a., nucleus
- a., pes
- a., uterus

arcus
- a., corneal
- a. costarum
- a. glossopalatinus
- a. juvenilis
- a. lipoides corneae
- a. lipoides myringis
- a. palatini
- a. palatoglossus
- a. palatopharyngeus
- a. palpebralis inferior
- a. palpebralis superior
- a. parieto-occipitalis
- a. pharyngopalatinus
- a. senilis
- a. superciliaris
- a. vertebrae, pediculus
- a. vertebrae, radix

ARD (acute respiratory disease)
ardin delteili, Pentatrichomonas
ARDS (acute respiratory distress syndrome)
ARDS (adult resiratory distress syndrome)
area(s)
- a., adnexal
- a., antecubital
- a., aortic valve
- a., asymmetric
- a., atrophy in shoulder
- a., balloon dilated
- a., Bamberger's
- a., body surface
- a., bony
- a., Broca's
- a., Brodmann's
- a., butterfly
- a., cells per unit
- a. ▸ central surface skin
- a., circumscribed
- a., conjunctivotarsal
- a., consolidating
- a., cortical
- a., critical care
- a., crural
- a., damage to Wernicke's
- a. ▸ diverticulosis of cecal
- a. draped free
- a., ecchymotic
- a. ▸ echo-free
- a., echo-spared
- a., echogenic
- a. ▸ end-diastolic
- a., epigastric
- a., Erb
- a. ▸ exercise to rehabilitate injured
- a., facial
- a., fat density
- a., faucial
- a., fibrotic
- a., firing
- a., fixed stenotic
- a., flank
- a., Flechsig's
- a., fluid in scrotal
- a., focal
- a., frontal
- a., frontoparietal
- a., genital
- a., gyrous
- a., hair bearing
- a. hammer ▸ labyrinth
- a., hand-washing in critical care
- a., homologous
- a., hyaline acellular
- a., hyperkeratotic
- a., infected
- a., inflamed
- a. ▸ inflammation within affected
- a., infraclavicular
- a., infrahilar
- a., inguinal
- a. irrigated with saline ▸ operative
- a., Kiesselbach's
- a., Krönig's
- a. lavaged with sterile saline
- a. length method
- a., left central cortical
- a., left subcostal
- a. left wave-spike ▸ parietal
- a., lesion in Broca's
- a., Little's
- a., lytic
- a., malar
- a. ▸ manual percussion of suprapubic
- a., masseteric
- a., midtemporal
- a. (MVA) ▸ mitral valve
- a., motor
- a., mottled
- a., mottled hemorrhagic
- a., necrotic
- a. network ▸ local
- a., neutral or gray
- a., Obersteiner-Redlich
- a., occipital
- a. of atelectasis
- a. of body ▸ tender points specific
- a. of bony destruction
- a. of brain ▸ different
- a. of brain ▸ discrete
- a. of brain ▸ seizure-producing
- a. of bronchiectasis ▸ focal
- a. of bronchopneumonia ▸ patchy
- a. of cardiac dullness
- a. of cerebral cortex, association
- a. of columnar epithelium, circumoral
- a. of consolidation ▸ patchy
- a. of cortex, homologous

a. of density
a. of dermatophytosis
a. of effusion
a. of emphysema ▸ focal
a. of enhancement
a. of erosion
a. of fibroblastic activity
a. of focal scarring
a. of heart muscle, dead
a. of hemorrhage and necrosis
a. of hemorrhage, focal
a. of hyperemia ▸ focal
a. of increased activity
a. of increased pigmentation
a. of increased uptake
a. of infarction ▸ focal
a. of intertrigo
a. of intrapulmonary hemorrhage ▸ focal
a. of local tenderness
a. of lymph nodes, regional node bearing
a. of lymphoid infiltrate ▸ focal
a. of minimal fibrosis ▸ focal
a. of mottling
a. of old fibrosis ▸ patchy
a. of pneumonic consolidation ▸ patchy
a. of recent hemorrhage
a. of scalp ▸ temporal
a. of skin, reddened
a. of squamous metaplasia ▸ focal
a. of strength and weakness
a. of stricture
a. of tenderness
a. of tumefaction
a. on xerogram ▸ suspicious
a., painful
a. ▸ painful, inflamed
a. painted with gentian violet
a., papillary
a., parietal
a. ▸ parieto-occipital
a. patchy
a., patient's perception of problem
a., peak
a., perianal
a., perihilar
a., perineal
a., perispinal
a., persistent, irritated
a., photopenic
a., pilonidal
a., popliteal node
a., portal

a., postanesthesia recovery
a., postauricular
a., postcentral
a. postrema
a., prefrontal
a., premotor
a. prepared sterilely
a. prepared with Septisol
a. prepped and draped
a. prepped and draped in routine manner
a. previously marked ▸ breast
a. ▸ proximal isovelocity surface
a. pterygoidea
a., pubic
a. ▸ pulmonary valve
a., pulmonic
a. ▸ punched-out
a., pupillary
a., radiation therapy perineal
a., radiodensity
a., rarefied
a., raw
a. ▸ regurgitant jet
a., reinforce weakened
a., rejected (TGAR) ▸ total graft
a. ▸ relieve pressure on metatarsal
a. ▸ restore tissue to affected
a., retrocardiac
a., right axillary
a., right central cortical
a., right subcostal
a. right wave-spike ▸ parietal
a., sagittal
a., scapular
a., scar-like
a. scraped vigorously
a., scrotal
a. ▸ secondary aortic
a., sensory
a. sharp wave-spike ▸ parietal
a., silent
a., sloughed
a., Soemmering's
a., somatosensory
a., sonolucent
a., speech
a., spill
a., stimulation of trigger
a., subglottic
a., submitral
a., subsegmental
a., subxiphoid
a., supplementary motor
a., supraclavicular

a., supraorbital
a., surface
a. swabbed with gentian violet
a., sylvian
a. systolic pressure (ASP)
a., tailbone
a. taken, biopsies of
a., temporal
a., trigger
a., ulcerated
a., upper abdominal
a., vagus
a., visual
a., visual association
a. ▸ water density
a., watershed
a., wedge-shaped
a., Wernicke's
areata, acne
areata, alopecia
areatic lesion
aregenerative anemia
areola
a., Chaussier's
a. mammae
a. of mammary gland
a. of nipple
a. papillaris
a., second
a., umbilical
a., vaccinal
areolar
a. choroiditis
a. connective tissue
a. gingiva
a. tissue
Arey's rule
ARF (acute renal failure)
Argamaso-Lewin composite flap
Argas arboreus
Argas hermanni
argentaffin carcinoma
argentaffin stains
argentaffine granules
argentaffinoma syndrome
Argentine hemorrhagic fever
Argentinian hemorrhagic fever
argentipes, Phlebotomus
arginine tolerance test (ATT)
argon
a. ion laser
a. laser
a. laser, balloon-centered
a. laser, green
a. laser surgery

arguing, excessive
Argyll Robertson operation
Argyll Robertson pupil
argyrophil stains
argyrophile plaques
ARI (airway reactivity index)
Arias' syndrome
Arias-Stella phenomenon
aridity antibodies, low
aridosiliculose cataract
aridosiliquate cataract
Aries-Pitanguy mammaplasty
Aries-Pitanguy mammary ptosis
   procedure
A-ring ▸ esophageal
arithmetic disorder, developmental
arithmetic unit
arithmetical disorder
arithmetical reasoning
Arizona organism
arizonae, Paracolobactrum
Arloing-Courmont test
Arlt('s)
   A. disease
   A. -Jaesche operation
   A. operation
   A. operation ▸ Jaesche-
   A. trachoma
arm(s)
   a. -ankle indices
   a., atrophy of
   a., biceps muscle of
   a., blue
   a. cast, long
   a. cast, short
   a. contracted permanently
   a., crook of the
   a. cuff
   a. curl exercises
   a. drift
   a., electric
   a. electrode, left
   a. electrode, right
   a. exercise
   a. extended anteriorly
   a. ▸ dissected tissue
   a. ergometry
   a. ergometry treadmill
   a. exercise stress test
   a. flail wildly
   a. flap, cross-
   a. ▸ fluid accumulation in
   a. flexible
   a., fore◊
   a. hair

a. ▸ hemiparesis left
a. ▸ hemiparesis right
a. ▸ immobilization of injured
a. index, ankle-
a., inferior lateral cutaneous nerve
   of
a. leads ▸ reversed
a., left
a. -leg gradient
a. lift exercises
a. lifts, straight-
a., medial cutaneous nerve of
a. motion
a. movement ▸ outstretched
a. movement ▸ overhead
a. movement ▸ uncoordinated
a. movement ▸ weak
a., myoelectric
a., needle marked
a., needle marks on
a., needle scarred
a. numbness
a. ▸ numbness, weakness and
   paralysis of
a. pain
a. ▸ pain spreading to
a. ▸ paralysis of
a. ▸ patient has swelling of upper
a., posterior cutaneous nerve of
a. raise exercise
a. ratio
a. recumbent, left
a. recumbent, right
a. ▸ red line up
a. ▸ red patch or blister on
a. ▸ repetitive overhead movement
   of
a., right
a. ▸ spasticity of
a. ▸ spider mark on
a. splinting
a. stress test ▸ elevated
a. ▸ sudden numbness of
a. ▸ sudden paralysis of
a. ▸ sudden weakness of
a. ▸ sudden weakness or numbness
   of
a., superior lateral cutaneous nerve
   of
a. support, mobile
a., tingling in
a. -tongue time
a. -tongue time test
a., trembling of
a., triceps muscle of

a., weakness in
a. ▸ weakness or numbness of
armamentarium, medical
Armanni-Ebstein lesion
Armanni-Ehrlich's degeneration
ARMD (age-related macular
   degeneration) ▸ advanced
ARMD intermediate (age-related
   macular degeneration)
Armed Forces Institute of Pathology
   (AFIP)
armillatus, Porocephalus
Armillifer infestation
armored heart
armour heart
armpit, swelling in
armpits, palms ▸ sweating forehead,
   Armstrong unit ▸ King-
Armstrong warmer
Army General Classification Test
   (AGCT)
Arneth's classification
Arneth's syndrome
Arnold-Chiari
   A. -C deformity
   A. -C malformation
   A. -C syndrome
Arnold's
   A. canal
   A. ligament
   A. nerve
Arnoux's sign
aroma therapy
aromatase, enzyme
aromatic
   a. amine
   a. bitter
   a. hydrocarbon, polycyclic
Aron Alpha adhesive
Around
   a. eye ▸ bone cavity
   a. eye ▸ twitching
   a. eyelids, xanthelasma
   a. heart ▸ adhesions of pericardium
   a. him/her ▸ world
   a. infant's neck, cord
   a. lights, glare
   a. lights, halos
   a. lower teeth ▸ pyorrhea
   a. mouth ▸ numbness and tingling
   a. surgery ▸ wrap-
   a. tooth ▸ foul-tasting discharge
   a. upper teeth ▸ pyorrhea
arousability, measure of
arousable, patient

arousal
- a., alertness and
- a., anger
- a., autonomic
- a., confusional
- a., decreased sexual
- a., diminished arousal
- a. disorder ▸ female sexual
- a., early morning
- a. from sleep
- a., full
- a. heart rate
- a., high levels of
- a. in infants ▸ sexual
- a., increased emotional
- a. insomnia, internal
- a., internal emotional
- a., massive
- a., movement
- a., physiological
- a., reducing physical
- a. response
- a., sexual
- a. theory

arouse, patient difficult to
ARP (absolute refractory period)
arrange words properly ▸ inability to
arrangements, funeral home
arrangements, special living
arranging and touching compulsions
array(s) (A)
- a., annular phased
- a., anteroposterior
- a., circumferential
- a., compressed spectral
- a., convex
- a., convex linear
- a., coronal
- a., linear
- a., longitudinal anteroposterior
- A. (APA) microwave technology ▸ Adaptive Phased
- a. of electrodes
- a., phased
- a., research logic linear
- a. sector scanner ▸ phased
- a., sock
- a. study ▸ phased
- a. ▸ symmetrical phased
- a. system, annular phased
- a. system ▸ phased
- a. technology ▸ phased
- a. transducer, annular

arrector muscle(s) of hair
arrectores pilorum muscles

arrest
- a., acute cardiorespiratory
- a., arrhythmias associated with cardiopulmonary
- a. (CA), cardiac
- a., cardiopulmonary
- a., cardiorespiratory
- a., chemical
- a., circulatory
- a., complete sinus
- a., deep hypothermia circulatory
- a., deep transverse
- a., developmental
- a. drugs, cardiac
- a., epiphyseal
- a., field procedure in cardiac
- a. following trauma, cardiac
- a. ▸ full cardiac
- a. ▸ grounds for
- a., growth
- a., heart
- a., heart shocked during cardiac
- a. ▸ hypothermic cardioplegic
- a. ▸ hypothermic fibrillating
- a., maturation
- a. ▸ nontraumatic cardiac
- a. of dilation, secondary
- a. of heartbeat
- a. ▸ patient had respiratory
- a. ▸ patient suffered respiratory
- a., prevention of
- a., respiratory
- a., sinoatrial (SA)
- a., sinus
- a., speech
- a., sudden cardiac
- a., sudden cardiopulmonary
- a. surgery ▸ hypothermic cardiac
- a., sustained cardiac
- a., transient cardiac
- a. ▸ traumatic cardiopulmonary
- a. victim, cardiac

arrested
- a. development
- a. mental development
- a., tuberculosis

arrhythmia(s) (Arrhythmia)
- a. ablation ▸ ventricular
- a. associated with cardiopulmonary arrest
- a., asymptomatic ventricular
- a., atrial
- a., baseline
- a., cardiac
- a. circuit

- a., continuous
- a. control device
- a., controlling
- a., digitalis atrial
- a. ▸ exercise-induced
- a., fatal
- a., fatal heart
- a., fetal
- a. foci
- a. following defibrillation
- a., heart
- a. ▸ hypokalemia-induced
- a., inducible
- a., inotropic
- a., intraoperative
- a., ischemic
- a., junctional
- a., juvenile
- a., lethal
- a., life-threatening
- a. ▸ life-threatening heart
- a. ▸ life-threatening ventricular
- a. ▸ malignant ventricular
- a. ▸ management of cardiac
- a., Mönckeberg
- a. monitoring ▸ transtelephonic
- a., multiple
- a., nodal
- a. ▸ nonphasic sinus
- a. ▸ paroxysmal supraventricular
- a. ▸ pause dependent
- a., pediatric
- a. ▸ peri-infarctional ventricular
- a., perioperative
- a., perpetual
- a. ▸ pharmacological therapy of
- a., phasic
- a. ▸ phasic sinus
- a., postoperative
- a. ▸ primary atrial
- a., reentrant
- a. ▸ refractory supraventricular
- a., reperfusion
- a., respiratory
- a., senile
- a., sinus
- a., specific
- a., sporadic
- a. ▸ stress-related
- A. Suppression Trial (CAST), Cardiac
- a., supraventricular
- a., tachybrady
- a., treatable
- a., vagus

arrhythmia—*continued*
  a., ventricular
  a., warning
arrhythmic
  a. activity
  a. death
  a. review
arrhythmogenic right ventricular (RV)
  dysplasia
arrhythmogenic substrate
arrival
  a. (DOA) ‣ patient dead on
  a. (phencyclidine), DOA/Dead on
  a. (ETA), estimated time of
  a., prior to
arrogant, haughty behavior
arrogant self-appraisal
arrow-shaped graft
Arruga('s)
  A. implant
  A. operation
  A. protector
arsenic amblyopia
arsenic poisoning
arsenicalis, stomatitis
arsenite, potassium
art
  a. medical care ‣ state of the
  a. of reflexology
  a. techniques ‣ state of the
Artane therapy
artefact (*see* artifact)
artefactual density
artemisiaefolia, Ambrosia
arterectomy, carotid
arteriae pulmonalis ‣ lunulae
  vaivularum semilunarium
arterial [*arteriole*]
  a. anastomosis
  a. and arteriolonephro-sclerosis ‣
    mild
  a. aneurysm
  a. aneurysm ‣ intracranial
  a. angioma
  a. arch of foot ‣ dorsal
  a. beds, carotid
  a. bend lesions
  a. bifurcation
  a. bleed
  a. bleeding
  a., bleeding brisk and
  a. blockage
  a. blood
  a. blood clot
  a. blood concentration

a. blood flow
a. blood flow rate
a. blood gas abnormality
a. blood gas analysis
a. blood gases (ABG)
a. blood gases (ABG) ‣
  deteriorating
a. blood, inflow of
a. blood lactate
a. blood pressure (ABP)
a. blood pressure (MABP) ‣ mean
a. blood pressure (ABP) ‣
  monitoring
a. blood samples
a. branches
a. bypass
a. calcification
a. cannulation
a. capillary
a. carbon dioxide (CO$_2$) tension
a. catheter
a. chemotherapy, intra-
a. circulation
a. circulation, poor
a. circulation to the lungs
a. cone
a. constriction
a. counterpulsation ‣ intra-
a. coupling
a. cutdown
a. damage
a. decortication
a. desaturation
a. disease
a. disease ‣ extracranial carotid
a. disease (PAD) ‣ peripheral
a. disease screening ‣ peripheral
a. disorder
a. disorganization ‣ segmental
a. dissection
a. ectasia, diffuse
a. elastance, effective
a. embolectomy catheter
a. embolism
a. embolism, acute
a. embolization ‣ transcatheter
a. enlargement, abnormal
a. entry site
a. filter
a. filter ‣ heparin
a. flow to brain, collateral
a. fluorescence ‣ laser-induced
a. gas samplings
a. graft
a. graft, Dacron

a. graft material,
  polytetrafluoroethylene (PTFE)
a. graft, seamless
a. groove
a. hemorrhage
a. hepatic catheterization ‣ intra-
a. hepatic infusion ‣ intra-
a. hyperemia
a. hypertension
a. hypotension
a. hypoxemia
a. impedance
a. infection ‣ intra-
a. infusion
a. infusion therapy
a. injection of drugs, intra-
a. insufficiency
a. insufficiency ‣ vertebrobasilar
a. (IA), intra-
a. lesion
a. lesion, blunt
a. lesions ‣ penetrating
a. line
a. line insertion
a. line, intra-
a. line monitor catheter placement
a. line placement
a. line, umbilical
a. lining
a. lining ‣ inflammation of
a. lumen
a. magnetic resonance (MR)
  angiography ‣ selective
a. mean
a. mean line
a. measurement of blood pressure
  ‣ intra-
a. media
a. monitoring
a. murmur
a. nephrosclerosis
a. notch
a. obstruction
a. occlusion
a. occlusion, acute
a. occlusive disease
a. occlusive disease ‣ peripheral
a. oxygen saturation (SaO$_2$) ‣ blood
a. partial pressure
a. partial pressure ‣ postanesthetic
a. perfusion
a. peripheral pulsations
a. plaque therapy
a. plaques
a. portography

a. pressure (AP)
a. pressure (AP) line ▸ insertion of
a. pressure (MAP) ▸ mean
a. pressure (PAP) ▸ pulmonary
a. pressure (SAP) ▸ systemic
a. pressure ▸ systemic mean
a. prosthesis
a. prosthesis, Dacron
a. pulsations ▸ spontaneous retinal
a. pulse
a. puncture
a. pyemia
a. reconstruction
a. remodeling
a. repair
a. reserve, coronary
a. rhabdomyolysis
a. rhabdomyolysis ▸ nonocclusive
a. rhabdomyolysis ▸ nontraumatic
a. runoff
a. runoff, aortofemoral
a. samples, umbilical
a. saturation
a. sclerosis
a. sheath
a. spasm
a. spurter
a. stems ▸ transposition of
a. stenosis ▸ symptomatic
    intracranial
a. stick
a. stiffness
a. supply
a. supply, occlusion of
a. switch operation
a. switch probe ▸ Jatene
a. switch procedure
a. system
a. system, carotid
a. systole
a. tension
a. thrill
a. thrombosis
a. thrombosis, major
a. thrombosis ▸ mesenteric
a. tortuosity
a. trauma
a. varix
a. vasculature, pulmonary
a. vasospasm
a. vein
a. vein of Soemmering
a. vessels
a. wall
a. wall balloons out

a. wall ▸ elastic recoil of
a. wall, inherent weakness in
a. wall integrity
a. wall, suture attached to
a. wall, thickened
a. wall, weakness in
a. wave
a. web ▸ pulmonary
a. wedge
arteriale racemosum, angioma
arteriectomy procedure
arteriocapillary fibrosis
arteriocapillary sclerosis
arteriogram
a., brachial
a., carotid
a., cerebral
a., coronary
a., femoral
a., four vessel
a., lumbar
a., pelvic
a., percutaneous
a., pruned-tree
a., retrograde
a., runoff
a., studies
a., subclavian
a., vertebral
a., wedge
arteriograph, coronary
arteriographic evaluation
arteriographic regression
arteriographical imaging studies
arteriography
a. and infusion ▸ infrahepatic
a., bilateral carotid
a., brachiocephalic
a., bronchial
a., carotid
a., carotid cerebral
a., catheter
a., celiac
a., cerebral
a., coronary
a., digital
a., digital subtraction
a., documentary
a., femoral
a. ▸ femoral runoff
a., infrahepatic
a. ▸ ipsilateral antegrade
a., mesenteric
a., percutaneous
a., peripheral

a., pulmonary
a., quantitative
a. ▸ quantitative coronary
a., renal
a., selective coronary
a. ▸ selective renal
a., splenic
a. study
a., visceral
a., vertebral
arteriohepatic dysplasia syndrome
arteriolar
a. compliance
a. hyalinosis
a. light reflex
a. nephrosclerosis
a. nephrosclerosis, hyaline
a. nephrosclerosis, hyperplastic
a. resistance
a. resistance, pulmonary
a. resistance, systemic
a. sclerosis
a. sclerosis, renal
a. thickening
a. vasoconstriction
arteriole(s)
a., afferent
a., afferent glomerular
a., efferent
a., efferent glomerular
a., glomerular
a., Isaacs-Ludwig
a., occlusion of retinal
a. of retina ▸ medial
a. of retina ▸ nasal
a. of retina ▸ temporal
a., postglomerular
a., precapillary
a., preglomerular
a., pulmonary
a., renal
a., spiral
a., splenic
arteriolitis, necrotizing
arteriolonephrosclerosis
a. ▸ mild arterial and
a. ▸ mild arteriolosclerosis with
a. of kidneys
arteriolonephrosclerotic changes
arteriolosclerotic [*arteriosclerotic*]
arteriolovenular bridge
arterionecrosis, hyaline
arterionephrosclerosis, minimal
arteriopathy(-ies)
a., hypertensive

arteriopathy(-ies)—*continued*
- a., occlusive
- a. ▸ plexogenic pulmonary

arterioplasty repair

arteriosclerosis (AS)
- a. and diabetes
- a. ▸ calf pain from
- a., cerebral
- a., coronary
- a., decrescent
- a., diffuse
- a., generalized
- a., hyaline
- a., hyperplastic
- a., hypertensive
- a., infantile
- a., intimal
- a., Mönckeberg's
- a., nodose
- a., nodular
- a. obliterans (ASO)
- a. of eye vessels
- a., peripheral
- a., premature
- a., presenile
- a., senile
- a., severe coronary
- a. ▸ widespread glomerulosclerosis and
- a. with arteriolonephrosclerosis ▸ mild

arteriosclerotic
- a. aneurysm, abdominal
- a. cardiopathy
- a. cardiovascular disease (ASCVD)
- a. dementia, uncomplicated
- a. dementia with delirium
- a. dementia with delusional features
- a. dementia with depressive features
- a. ectasia
- a. elongation thoracic aorta
- a. heart disease (ASHD)
- a. heart disease ▸ hypertensive
- a. kidney
- a. narrowing
- a. nephritis
- a. obliterans
- a. occlusion
- a. occlusive disease
- a. occlusive disease ▸ peripheral
- a. peripheral vascular disease
- a. plaque
- a. retinopathy

- a. vascular disease (ASVD)

arteriosum, cor

arteriosum, ligamentum

arteriosus
- a., bulbus
- a., calcified ductus
- a., closed ductus
- a., ductus
- a. murmur ▸ patent ductus
- a. (PDA), patent ductus
- a. ▸ persistent ductus
- a., persistent truncus
- a., pseudotruncus
- a. ▸ railroad track ductus
- a. ▸ reversed ductus
- a., truncus
- a. umbrella ▸ patent ductus

arteriotomy, brachial

arteriotomy with exploration

arteriovascular malformation

arteriovenosa, anastomosis

arteriovenous (AV)
- a. anastomosis
- a. aneurysm
- a. aneurysm ▸ pulmonary
- a. block
- a. block, first degree
- a. bundle
- a. communication
- a. connection, accessory
- a. crossing
- a. crossing changes
- a. dissociation
- a. fissure
- a. fistula
- a. (AV) fistula, Brescio-Cimino
- a. fistula, pulmonary
- a. fistula ▸ solitary pulmonary
- a. fistula ▸ subclavian
- a. (AV) fistula with good bruits
- a. hemofiltration, continuous
- a. (AV) junctional rhythm
- a. (AV) junctional tachycardia
- a. leaking
- a. malformation (AVM)
- a. malformation ▸ Mondini pulmonary
- a. malformation of brain
- a. malformation ▸ pulmonary
- a. nicking
- a. oxygen difference (AVDO$_2$)
- a. pulmonary aneurysm
- a. pulse
- a. ratio (AVR)
- a. shunt

- a. shunt, Cimino
- a. shunt, Scribner
- a. shunt site
- a. shunt ▸ Vitagraft

arteritis [*arthritis*]
- a., aortic arch
- a., brachiocephalic
- a., carotid artery
- a., coronary
- a., cranial
- a., cranial granulomatous
- a. deformans
- a., fibrinoid
- a. ▸ giant cell
- a., granulomatous
- a., Horton's
- a. hyperplastica
- a., infantile
- a. ▸ localized visceral
- a., mesenteric
- a., necrosing
- a., necrotizing
- a. nodosa
- a. obliterans
- a. of Takayasu ▸ idiopathic
- a., rheumatic
- a., rheumatoid
- a. syndrome, aortic
- a., syphilitic
- a. ▸ Takayasu's
- a., temporal
- a. ▸ temporal granulomatous
- a. umbilicalis
- a. verrucosa

artery(-ies)
- a., aberrant
- a., aberrant right subclavian
- a. ▸ accelerated blockage in
- a., accessory
- a., accessory middle cerebral
- a., Adamkiewicz
- a., adrenal
- a., afferent
- a., anastomose
- a., anastomosis ▸ systemic to pulmonary
- a. and vein allografts
- a. and veins, pericallosal
- a. anastomosis, bronchial
- a., anastomosis of carotid
- a. aneurysm, basilar
- a. aneurysm, carotid
- a. aneurysm, celiac
- a. aneurysm, communicating
- a. aneurysm, coronary

a. aneurysm ▸ dissecting basilar
a. aneurysm ▸ hepatic
a. aneurysm ▸ iliac
a., aneurysm of
a. aneurysm, popliteal
a. aneurysm ▸ posterior communicating
a. (PICA) aneurysm, posterior inferior cerebellar
a. aneurysm ▸ pulmonary
a. aneurysm, renal
a. aneurysm ▸ thrombosed giant vertebral
a. ▸ angina from spasm of
a. angiography ▸ left coronary
a. angiography ▸ right coronary
a. angioplasty, coronary
a., angular
a. (ALMCA), anomalous left main coronary
a. anomaly, coronary
a., anterior cerebral
a., anterior choroidal
a., anterior communicating
a., anterior descending
a., anterior descending coronary
a. (AICA), anterior inferior communicating
a., anterior spinal
a., anterior tibial
a. approach, brachial
a. approach ▸ femoral
a., arcuate
a. arteritis, carotid
a., ascending pharyngeal
a. ▸ asymmetric lesions in coronary
a. atherosclerosis, coronary
a., atherosclerosis in
a. ▸ atherosclerosis of coronary
a., atherosclerotic
a., atherosclerotic, coronary
a., atrial circumflex
a., auricular
a., axillary
a., azygos anterior cerebral
a., balloon-like dilation of
a. band ▸ pulmonary
a. banding ▸ pulmonary
a., basal cerebral
a., basilar
a., basilic
a., bifurcation of basilar
a., bifurcation of common
a. biopsy ▸ temporal
a. block, carotid

a., block coronary
a. blockage
a. blockage, carotid
a., blockage, coronary
a., blockage of renal
a., blocked
a., blocked coronary
a., blocked heart
a. ▸ blocked renal
a. ▸ blood flow from
a., brachial
a., brachiocephalic
a. branches, pulmonary
a., branchial
a., bronchial
a., bulbourethral
a., bulging rectal
a. bypass (CAB), coronary
a. bypass graft
a. bypass graft (CABG), coronary
a. bypass graft ▸ renal
a. bypass graft ▸ subclavian
a. bypass graft ▸ vertebral
a. bypass grafting ▸ endarterectomy and coronary
a. bypass grafting ▸ port-access coronary
a. bypass grafting surgery, coronary
a. bypass, internal mammary
a. bypass (MIDCAB) ▸ minimally invasive direct coronary
a. bypass (OPCAB), off pump coronary
a. bypass (PACAB) ▸ post-access coronary
a. bypass ▸ superior mesenteric
a. bypass (CAB) surgery, coronary
a. bypass surgery ▸ radial
a. bypass (TECAB) ▸ total endoscopic coronary
a. calcification, coronary
a. calcification of
a. ▸ calcification of left coronary
a., callosomarginal
a., candelabra
a. cannulated, femoral
a., caroticotympanic
a., carotid
a. catheter ▸ flow-directed pulmonary
a. catheter ▸ internal mammary
a. catheter, pulmonary
a. catheter, umbilical
a. catheterization, pulmonary

a. catheterization, umbilical
a. catheterized, umbilical
a., caudal branches of
a., cavernous
a., cavernous internal carotid
a., celiac
a., central retinal
a., cephalic
a., cerebellar
a., cerebellolabyrinthine
a., cerebral
a., cervical
a., cervical carotid
a. ▸ cholesterol embolization of
a., choroidal
a., choroidal branches of posterior cerebral
a., cilioretinal
a. circulation, coronary
a. circulation ▸ insufficient coronary
a., circumflex
a., clipping middle cerebral
a., clogged
a., clogged coronary
a., clogged neck
a. -clogging clot
a. -clogging disease
a. -clogging fat
a. -clogging food
a., clogging of
a. -clogging plaque in atherosclerosis patient
a. -clogging thrombus
a., coarctation of pulmonary
a. ▸ collapsed cerebral
a., common carotid
a., common femoral
a., common hepatic
a., common iliac
a., communicating
a., complete transposition of great
a., compression of carotid
a., congenital absence of pulmonary
a., congenital aneurysm of pulmonary
a., constricted coronary
a., constriction
a., constrictor of
a. contusion ▸ superficial femoral
a. (CA), coronary
a., corrected transposition of great
a., cortical
a., cremasteric
a., cricothyroid
a. cutdown, brachial

artery—*continued*
a., cystic
a., deep brachial
a., deep femoral
a., deferential
a., degeneration of
a., degeneration of walls of
a., diagonal
a., diaphragmatic
a., digital
a., dilate coronary
a., dilated pulmonary
a. disease, atherosclerotic carotid
a. disease, atherosclerotic coronary
a. disease, carotid
a. disease (CAD) ▸ coronary
a. disease (CAD) ▸ evaluation of coronary
a. disease ▸ left main coronary
a. disease mortality ▸ coronary
a. disease ▸ peripheral
a. disease ▸ renal
a. disease ▸ silent coronary
a. disease ▸ transplant coronary
a. disease ▸ woven coronary
a., diseased
a. dissection, coronary
a. dissection (SCAD) ▸ spontaneous coronary
a., dominant
a., dorsal
a., dorsalis pedis
a., duodenal
a., dural
a., ectatic
a. ▸ ectatic carotid
a. ectasia
a., efferent
a., elasticity of
a., embolism of
a., embolism of retinal
a. embolization, bronchial
a. embolization ▸ uterine
a., embolized small
a. endarterectomy, carotid
a., epicardial coronary
a., epigastric
a., esophageal
a., ethmoidal
a., excision segment of
a., external carotid
a., external iliac
a. ▸ external mammary
a., facial
a., facioscapulohumeral

a., falx
a., fatty plaques in
a., femoral
a. ▸ first obtuse marginal
a. fistula, coronary
a. flushed
a. ▸ fracture plaque obstructing
a., frontal
a., frontopolar
a., gastric
a., gastroduodenal
a., gastroepiploic
a., genicular
a., giant cell
a., gluteal
a., gonadal
a. graft angiography ▸ internal mammary
a. graft ▸ mammary
a., great
a., great anterior radicular
a., hardening of
a. ▸ hardening of coronary
a., hardening of walls of
a., helicine
a., hepatic
a., hyaloid
a. hypertension (PAH), pulmonary
a., hypogastric
a., iliac
a., ileocolic
a., iliofemoral
a., ilioinguinal
a., imaging of
a. ▸ impaired coronary
a., incision into an
a., inferior epigastric
a. (IMA), inferior mesenteric
a., inflamed
a., inflammation of coronary
a., innominate
a., intercostal
a., interlobar
a., interlobular
a. (ICA), internal carotid
a., internal iliac
a., internal mammary
a., internal thoracic
a., interosseous
a., interventricular
a. ▸ intramural coronary
a. ▸ invisible main pulmonary
a. involvement
a. island flap
a. isolated

a., jejunal
a., kidney
a., Kipp's coronary
a. ▸ Kugel anastomotic
a., laceration middle meningeal
a., lacrimal
a. laser angioplasty, coronary
a., leaky
a., left anterior descending (LAD)
a. ▸ left atrioventricular groove
a. ▸ left circumflex
a., (LCA), left circumflex coronary
a. ▸ left common carotid
a., left coronary
a., left femoral
a. (LIMA) ▸ left internal mammary
a. ▸ left posterior cerebral
a., left pulmonary
a., left subclavian
a., lenticulostriate
a. lesion, coronary
a. ligation (HAL), hemorrhoidal
a., ligation middle meningeal
a. line, mesenteric
a., lingual
a., long posterior ciliary
a., lumbar
a., lumen of
a., lumen of bronchial
a., main pulmonary
a. ▸ malposition of great
a., mammary
a., marginal
a. ▸ marginal circumflex
a., maxillary
a. mean pressure (PAMP) ▸ pulmonary
a., medullary
a., meningeal
a., meningohypophyseal
a., mesenteric
a. (MCA), middle cerebral
a. murmur, bronchial collateral
a. murmur, carotid
a., narrowed
a., narrowed coronary
a., narrowed renal
a. narrowing
a. narrowing, carotid
a., narrowing of
a., narrowing of coronary
a., nodal
a., normal
a., nutrient
a., obstructed

a. ▸ obstructed pulmonary
a., obturator
a. ▸ obtuse marginal
a. (OA), occipital
a., occluded
a. occluded, renal
a. occlusion ▸ central retinal
a. occlusion, coronary
a. occlusion ▸ femoral
a. occlusion ▸ femoropopliteal
a. occlusion ▸ iliac
a. occlusion (ICAO) ▸ internal carotid
a. occlusion ▸ mesenteric
a. ▸ occlusion of
a. ▸ occlusion of intramuscular
a. ▸ occlusion of left carotid
a. ▸ occlusion of right carotid
a. occlusion pressure ▸ pulmonary
a. occlusion ▸ retinal
a. occlusion ▸ temporary unilateral pulmonary
a. occlusive disease ▸ coronary
a. occlusive wedge pressure ▸ pulmonary
a. of brain ▸ constriction of
a. of brain ▸ spasm of
a. of colon ▸ marginal
a. of intracerebral vessels ▸ vertebral
a. of lower extremities ▸ intramuscular
a. of the newborn, Parrot's
a. of upper extremities ▸ intramuscular
a., offending
a., operculofrontal
a., ophthalmic
a., organizing thrombus of basilar
a. ▸ origin of the renal
a., ovarian
a., pancreaticoduodenal
a., parent
a. ▸ parieto-occipital
a. ▸ paroxysm of
a. ▸ partial blockage in
a. ▸ partially clogged
a. patent
a. patent, coronary
a. patient, basilar
a., pelvic
a., penile
a., perforating
a., pericallosal

a., pericardiophrenic
a., perineal
a., periosteal
a., peroneal
a., persistent cilioretinal
a. ▸ persistent primitive trigeminal
a., pharyngeal
a., phrenic
a., Pick's convolutional
a. ▸ pipestem calcification of carotid
a., plugged
a., popliteal
a. ▸ posterior cerebral
a. ▸ posterior circumflex
a. ▸ posterior communicating
a., posterior conjunctival
a. ▸ posterior descending
a. (PICA), posterior inferior cerebellar
a. (PICA), posterior inferior communicating
a., posterior tibial
a., precentral
a., precerebral
a., prefrontal
a., premammillary
a. pressure ▸ elevated pulmonary
a. pressure ▸ increased pulmonary
a. pressure point ▸ facial
a. pressure point ▸ femoral
a. ▸ pressure point on
a. pressure point ▸ popliteal
a. pressure point ▸ radial
a. pressure point ▸ superficial temporal
a. pressure, pulmonary
a., preventricular
a. ▸ primitive acoustic
a. ▸ primitive hypoglossal
a., princeps pollicis
a. probe, coronary
a., profunda brachii
a. ▸ profunda femoris
a., ▸ progressive obstruction of renal
a., pterygoid
a., pudendal
a., pulmonary
a. pulse ▸ radial
a., radial
a., radialis indicis
a. radiation
a., radicular
a. ▸ ramus intermedius
a. ▸ rechannelization of coronary

a. reclogged
a., reconstruction of
a. repair ▸ femoral
a. ▸ repeated narrowing of coronary
a. reperfusion, coronary
a., renal
a., repair of
a., retinal
a. reverse saphenous vein bypass ▸ renal
a. (RCA), right circumflex coronary
a. ▸ right common carotid
a., right coronary
a., right femoral
a., right innominate
a. ▸ right internal mammary
a. ▸ right main coronary
a., right main pulmonary
a. ▸ right posterior cerebral
a., right pulmonary
a., right subclavian
a. right ventricular (RV) fistula, coronary
a., Riolan
a., rolandic
a. ▸ ruptured aortic
a., saphenous
a. scanning, coronary
a. screening ▸ carotid
a. ▸ second obtuse marginal
a., segmental
a. ▸ septal perforating
a. ▸ severe narrowing of
a. ▸ severe narrowing ostia of coronary
a. ▸ severe stenosis left coronary
a. ▸ severe stenosis right coronary
a., short posterior ciliary
a. shunt, aortofemoral
a. shunt ▸ ascending aorta-to-pulmonary
a. shunt, carotid
a. ▸ silver wiring of retinal
a., single umbilical
a. ▸ sinoatrial (SA) node
a. ▸ sinus node
a. slightly thickened
a. sling ▸ pulmonary
a., spasm of coronary
a., spermatic
a., sphenopalatine
a., spinal
a., spinoneural
a., splenic
a., stapedial

artery—*continued*
- a. steal ▸ pulmonary
- a. stenosis, branch pulmonary
- a. stenosis, carotid
- a. stenosis, circumflex
- a. stenosis, coronary
- a. stenosis ▸ pathogenesis of pulmonary
- a. stenosis, pulmonary
- a. stenosis, renal
- a., stenotic femoral
- a., sternocleidomastoid
- a. ▸ stiffness from disease of
- a., subclavian
- a., sulcus of subclavian
- a. ▸ superficial femoral
- a. ▸ superficial temporal
- a. ▸ superior carotid
- a. (SMA), superior mesenteric
- a. ▸ superior thyroid
- a., supernormal
- a., supraorbital
- a., supratrochlear
- a. surgery, coronary
- a., swollen
- a., sylvian
- a. syndrome ▸ epibronchial right pulmonary
- a. syndrome ▸ superior mesenteric
- a. ▸ telencephalic ventriculofugal
- a., temporal
- a., temporooccipital
- a., testicular
- a., thalamoperforating
- a., thoracoacromial
- a., thoracodorsal
- a. ▸ threading catheter into
- a. thrombosis ▸ acute middle cerebral
- a. thrombosis, brachial
- a. thrombosis, cerebral
- a. thrombosis, coronary
- a. thrombosis ▸ femoral
- a. thrombosis, large
- a., thrombosis of
- a. thrombosis ▸ ophthalmic
- a., thyroid
- a., tibial
- a. ▸ tortuous uterine
- a. ▸ total occlusion basilar
- a. transplant, mammary
- a. ▸ transposition of great
- a. tumor, pulmonary
- a. ▸ tumor surrounds carotid
- a., ulnar

- a. ultrasound, carotid
- a., umbilical
- a., unclogged
- a. ▸ unclogging coronary
- a., uterine
- a. ▸ vasoconstriction of coronary
- a. vasospasm, coronary
- a., ventriculofugal
- a., vertebral
- a., vertebrobasilar
- a., vesical
- a., vidian
- a., visceral
- a., volar
- a. wall, ballooning out of
- a. wall permeability
- a. walls
- a. walls, inner
- a., weakened
- a. wedge pressure ▸ mean pulmonary
- a. wedge pressure ▸ pulmonary
- a. wedge, pulmonary
- a. ▸ widely patent ▸ coronary
- a., Zinn's

arthrectomy procedure

arthritic
- a. atrophy
- a. change, degenerative
- a. changes
- a. condition, moderate
- a. deformities, longstanding
- a. degeneration
- a. general pseudoparalysis
- a. joints
- a. knuckle
- a. lipping
- a. overgrowth
- a. pain
- a., patient
- a., patient rheumatoid
- a. ridging
- a. spur
- a. stiffening
- a. tuberculosis

arthritis (Arthritis) [*arteritis*]
- a., acute crystal
- a., acute gouty
- a., acute rheumatic
- a., allergic
- a., Bekhterev's
- a., carcinomatous
- a., cervical
- a. ▸ chronic, painful
- a., coccidioidomycosis

- a., debilitating rheumatoid
- a., degenerative
- a., disseminated
- a., exudative
- a., facet joint
- a. ▸ facial pain from
- a. (RA) factor cell ▸ rheumatoid
- a. factor, rheumatoid
- a., fever from
- a. ▸ foot problem from
- A. Foundation
- a. from Crohn's disease
- a. from gonorrhea
- a., generalized
- a., gonococcal
- a., gonorrheal
- a., gouty
- a. hiemalis
- a., hypertrophic
- a. in hands, carcinomatous
- a. in wrist, carcinomatous
- a., infectious
- a., inflammatory
- a. ▸ inflammatory rheumatoid
- a., inflammatory spine
- a. ▸ joint problems from
- a. (JRA), joint rheumatoid
- a., (JRA) ▸ juvenile rheumatoid
- a. (RA) latex fixation test ▸ rheumatoid
- a., Lyme
- a., Marie-Strümpell
- a. ▸ metatarsophalangeal joint
- a. ▸ mixed rheumatoid and degenerative
- a. mutilans
- a., navicular
- a., nodosa
- a., nonarticular
- a. of knee ▸ degenerative
- a. of the spine
- a., pain from
- a. pain relief
- a., patellar femoral
- a., patellofemoral
- a., patellofemoral degenerative
- a., patient crippled with
- a. ▸ post-traumatic
- a., premature
- a., progressive
- a., psoriatic
- a., pyogenic
- a. quackery
- a., reactive
- a., rheumatoid

a. ▸ self-managing
a., septic
a., spinal
a., stiffness from
a. stop hurting (MASH) ▸ make
a., suppurative
a., temporal
a., total lymphoid irradiation in
a., total lymphoid irradiation in
   rheumatoid
a., traumatic
a., tuberculous
a. -type symptom
a., vertebral
a. ▸ water aerobics for
a. ▸ wear-and-tear
arthrocentesis, joint
arthrocentesis procedure
arthrodesis
  a., Charnley
  a., Lambrinudi triple
  a., McKeever
  a. of hip
  a., shoulder
  a., Steindler's
arthrodial joint
arthrogram, double-contrast
arthrogram study
Arthrographis langeroni
arthrography, air
arthrography, opaque
arthropathy
  a., amyloid
  a., Charcot
  a., cuff
  a., facet
  a., gouty
  a., hemodialysis
  a., hemophilic
  a., Jaccoud
  a., neuropathic
  a., osteo◊
  a. ▸ rotator cuff
  a., secondary hypertrophic
  a., seronegative
arthroplasty
  a., Aufranc-Turner
  a., Austin-Moore endoprosthetic
  a., Charnley-Mueller
  a., Crawford-Adams hip
  a., Girdlestone
  a., hand
  a., joint
  a., Magnuson modified
  a., Magnuson-Stack shoulder

a., McKee-Farrar total hip
a., osteocapsular
a. procedure ▸ hemi-
a., reconstructive
a., reimplantation
a., Schlein-type elbow
a., Stanmore shoulder
a. (TARA), Total Articular
   Replacement
a., total hip
a., total knee
a., wrist
arthropod-borne virus
arthroscopic
  a. debridement
  a. knee surgery
  a. laser microdiscectomy
  a. release of scar tissue
  a. resection
  a. surgery
  a. vision
arthroscopy
  a., diagnostic
  a. procedure
  a., video
arthrosis, Charcot's
arthrosis deformans
articular
  a. calculus
  a. capsule
  a. cartilage
  a. component
  a. cortex
  a. disc
  a. disc, intra-
  a. facet
  a. facet, superior
  a. fracture
  a. fracture, intra-
  a. gout
  a., juxta-
  a. muscle
  a. muscle of elbow
  a. muscle of knee
  a. nerve
  a. nodules, juxta-
  a. osteophytosis, intra-
  a. process
  a. replacement arthroplasty
   (TARA), total
  a. sensation
  a. status, intra-
  a. surface
  a. surface damage
  a. vein, temporomandibular

articularis, meniscus
articularis, pars
articulate, patient
articulated, speech well
articulating femoral (SAF) hip
  replacement, self-
articulating process, superior
articulation(s)
  a., acromioclavicular
  a., brachioulnar
  a., calcaneocuboid
  a., carpal
  a., carpometacarpal
  a., chondrosternal
  a., costocentral
  a., costosternal
  a., costotransverse
  a., costovertebral
  a. delays ▸ severe
  a., difficulty in
  a. disorder, developmental
  a. disorder ▸ severe
  a., ellipsoidal
  a., hinged
  a., humeroradial
  a., humeroulnar
  a., iliosacral
  a., intermetacarpal
  a., intermetatarsal
  a., interphalangeal
  a. level ▸ age-appropriate
  a., metacarpophalangeal
  a., metatarsophalangeal
  a. of auditory ossicles
  a., patellofemoral
  a., phalangeal
  a., poor
  a., radiocarpal
  a., sacrococcygeal
  a., sacroiliac
  a., sternoclavicular
  a., talocalcaneonavicular
  a., talonavicular
  a., tarsometatarsal
  a., tibiofibular
  a., triquestropisiform
  a., trochoidal
articulo mortis
articulorum senilis, malum
artifact (*same as* artefact)
  a., aliasing
  a., aortic motion
  a., barium
  a., baseline
  a., beam hardening

artifact—*continued*
- a., black spot
- a., bone hardening
- a., bowel gas
- a., braces
- a., cable
- a., calibration failure
- a., center line
- a., chemical shift
- a., coin
- a., compression
- a., computer-generated
- a., crescent
- a., crown
- a., data spike detection error
- a., deodorant
- a., edge
- a., electroencephalogram (EEG)
- a., electronic
- a. ▸ end-pressure
- a., equipment
- a., eye movement
- a., eye muscle
- a., eye twitching
- a., ferromagnetic
- a., flow
- a. ▸ foreign material
- a. ▸ glass eye
- a., interfering
- a., lead
- a. ▸ magnetic susceptibility
- a. ▸ main magnetic field inhomogeneity
- a., mercury
- a., metallic
- a., misregistration
- a. ▸ mitral regurgitation
- a., motion
- a., movement
- a., muscle
- a., muscle tension
- a., muscular
- a. ▸ noise spike
- a., ocular tremor
- a., pacemaker
- a., paramagnetic
- a., pellet
- a. ▸ phase shift
- a., pica
- a. potential ▸ asymmetric eyeball movement
- a., pseudofracture
- a., reverberation
- a., rush
- a. ▸ side lobe
- a. ▸ skin fold
- a. ▸ skin lesion
- a. ▸ split image
- a. ▸ stimulated echo
- a., surveillance
- a., T
- a. ▸ temporal instability
- a., tension
- a., truncation
- a., wheelchair
- a., wrinkle
- a., zipper

artifactual bradycardia
artifactually distorted
artificial
- a. airway
- a. airway, full
- a. airway, partial
- a. ameba
- a. blood
- a. blood, Fluosol
- a. cardiac pacemaker
- a. cardiac valve
- a. circulation
- a. cochlea
- a. collapse upper portion of lung
- a. coma
- a. crown
- a. enzyme
- a. eye
- a. feedback signals
- a. feeding
- a. fever
- a. growth hormone
- a. heart
- a. heart, air-driven
- a. heart, Baylor total
- a. heart, Berlin total
- a. heart, CardioWest total
- a. heart ▸ electromechanical
- a. heart ▸ Hershey total
- a. heart implant
- a. heart, implantable
- a. heart ▸ Jarvik-8
- a. heart ▸ Jarvik-7
- a. heart ▸ Jarvik 7-70
- a. heart ▸ Jarvik 2000
- a. heart ▸ Kolff-Jarvik
- a. heart left pump
- a. heart ▸ Liotta total
- a. heart ▸ orthotopic biventricular
- a. heart ▸ orthotopic univentricular
- a. heart, Penn State total
- a. heart, Phoenix total
- a. heart pump device
- a. heart recipient
- a. heart ▸ RTV total
- a. heart, total
- a. heart ▸ University of Akron
- a. heart ▸ Utah total
- a. heart valve
- a. heart valve, defective
- a. heart ▸ Vienna total
- a. immunity
- a. implant
- a. insemination
- a. insemination donor
- a. insemination, homologous
- a. insulin
- a. internal bladder
- a. joint
- a. joint implant
- a. joint implant material
- a. joint parts ▸ wear resistant
- a. joint ▸ silicone-based
- a. kidney
- a. kidney machine
- a. kidney, priming of
- a. kidney (WAK) ▸ wearable
- a. knee
- a. knee joint
- a. knee ligament
- a. larynx
- a. legs
- a. lens
- a. lens implant
- a. lens implantation
- a. lens ▸ soft foldable
- a. life support
- a. life support system
- a. limb
- a. lung
- a. manipulation
- a. means
- a. menopause
- a. nutrition
- a. opening
- a. organ perfusion
- a. pacemaker
- a. palate
- a. pancreas
- a. pneumothorax
- a. prolongation of life
- a. radiation source
- a. respiration (AR)
- a. respiration, excessive
- a. respiration ▸ Schafer method of
- a. replacement teeth
- a. rupture
- a. rupture of membranes

a. saliva
a. scoliosis
a. silk keratitis
a. skin
a. sphincter implant
a. stoma
a. stone
a. sweetener
a. tear pipe
a. tears
a. teeth
a. urinary sphincter
a. valve
a. ventilation

artificially maintained, vital functions
arts ▸ tai-chi martial
aryepiglottic fold
aryepiglottic muscle
arytenoepiglottic/aryepiglottic
arytenoid(s)
a. cartilage
a. cartilage, excision of
a. cartilage of larynx
a. eminence
a., hyperemia of
a. mucosa
a. muscle
a. muscle, oblique
a. muscle, transverse
a. swelling

AS (as)
AS (aortic stenosis)
AS (arteriosclerosis)
AS (left ear)
a. -needed basis

ASA (acetylsalicylic acid)
asaccharolytica, Bacteroides
asaccharolytica, Porphyromonas
asaccharolyticus, Peptostrepto-coccus
asbestos
a. body
a. damage
a. effusions
a. exposure
a. exposure ▸ threshold amount of
a., exposure to
a. ▸ extensive exposure to
a. fibers
a., patient exposed to
a. pneumoconiosis
a. -related disease
a. -related illness

asbestosis
a., pulmonary
a. pulmonary edema

a., scarring of
ASCA (anti-Saccharomyces cerebisiae antibody)
A-scan
Ascaris
A. alata
A. canis
A. equi
A. equorum
A. lumbricoides
A. lumbricoides worm
A. marginata
A. megalocephala
A. mystax
A. ovis
A. suilia
A. suis
A. suum
A. vermicularis
A. vitulorum

Ascarops strongylina
ascendant, Lipiodol
ascendens, aorta
ascending
a. and descending
a. aorta (AA)
a. aorta ▸ cystic medial necrosis of
a. aorta, patch enlargement of
a. aorta-to-pulmonary artery shunt
a. aortic pressure
a. aortography
a. cholangitis
a. colon
a. colon ▸ Dukes C classification of right
a. frontal gyrus
a. hemiplegia
a. loop of Henle
a. lumbar vein
a. mesocolon
a. myelitis, acute
a. paralysis
a. pathway
a. pharyngeal artery
a. polyneuropathy
a. pyelography
a. ramus
a. sensory tract
a. urography
a. vein of Rosenthal

ascensus uteri
ascertainment
a., complete
a., single
a., truncate

Ascher's veins
Aschheim-Zondek test
Aschner's reflex
Aschner's sign
Aschoff('s)
A. body
A. cell
A. node
A. nodule
A. -Rokitansky cyst
A. -Tawara node

ascites
a., abdominal
a. adiposus
a., bile
a., bloody
a. carcinoma, Ehrlich
a., chyliform
a., chylosus
a., chylous
a., exudative
a., fatty
a., fetal
a. fluid
a., gelatinous
a., hemorrhagic
a., hydremic
a., massive
a., milky
a., ovarian carcinoma with
a., pancreatic
a., portal hypertension with
a. praecox
a., preagonal
a., pseudochylous
a., pseudocyst pancreatic
a., purulent
a., rapidly accumulating
a., transudative
a. ▸ yellow-brown serous

ascitic
a. fluid
a. fluid in abdomen
a. fluid tapped daily

ascomycetous fungi
ascorbic
a. acid
a. acid depletion ▸ ovarian
a. acid, leukocyte
a. acid test

ASCVD (arteriosclerotic cardio-vascular disease)
ASCVD (atherosclerotic cardio-vascular disease)
ASD (atrial septal defect)

ASE (abstinence symptom evaluation)
Aselli's pancreas
asemia
- a. graphica
- a. mimica
- a. verbalis

asepsis, isolation and
aseptic
- a. catheterization technique
- a. conditions
- a. fever
- a. meningitis
- a. meningitis, acute
- a. necrosis
- a. necrosis, bone
- a. practice
- a. technique
- a. wound

asexual
- a. cycle
- a. dwarf
- a. trait, (autosomal)

As.H. (hypermetropic astigmatism)
ASH (asymmetrical septal hyper-
    trophy)
ash leaf spots in eye
ashamed and intimidated ▸ guilty
ASHD (arteriosclerotic heart disease)
ashen color skin
Asherman('s)
- A. chest seal
- A. syndrome
- A. syndrome, Fritsch-
- A. syndrome, Fritz-

ashfordi, Parasaccharomyces
Ashley's breast prosthesis
Ashman phenomenon
ASI (addiction severity index)
Asian
- A. flu
- A. flush syndrome
- A. influenza
- A. mosquito-borne hemorrhagic
    fever ▸ Southeast

Asiatic cholera
asiatica, Centella
asiaticae, Vibrio cholerae-
ASIS (anterior superior iliac spine)
asleep, momentary failing
ASLMS (American Society of Laser
    Medicine and Surgery)
As.M. (myopic astigmatism)
ASMI (anteroseptal myocardial infarct)
ASO (arteriosclerosis obliterans)
asocial behavior

asocial withdrawal
ASO (antistreptolysin O) titer
ASP (area systolic pressure)
aspartate aminotransferase
aspect(s)
- a., anterior
- a., anteroinferior
- a., anterolateral
- a., anteroposterior
- a., caudal
- a., cephalad
- a., clinical
- a., contralateral
- a., distal
- a., dorsal
- a., emotional
- a., external
- a., greater curvature
- a. in esophageal atresia ▸
    pulmonary
- a., inferior
- a., inferolateral
- a., inner
- a., ipsilateral
- a., lateral
- a., lesser curvature
- a., medial
- a., median
- a., morphological
- a. of alcoholism ▸ genetic
- a. of alcoholism, metabolic
- a. of cancer, emotional
- a. of cancer ▸ physical
- a. of cancer ▸ physical and
    emotional
- a. of chemical dependency ▸
    cultural
- a. of criminality ▸ genetic
- a. of foot ▸ lateral
- a. of foot ▸ plantar
- a. of health, spiritual
- a. of heart ▸ functional
- a. of heart ▸ physical
- a. of hypothalamus, inferior
- a. of lungs ▸ volumetric
- a. of neurologic function ▸ sensory
- a. of pain ▸ emotional and
    psychological
- a. of program
- a. of resuscitation, legal
- a. of supportive care ▸ emotional
- a. of well being, cognitive
- a., outer
- a., perceptual
- a., peripheral

- a., pharmacologic
- a., physical
- a., plantar
- a., posterior
- a., posteroinferior
- a., posterolateral
- a., posteromedial
- a., psychological
- a., psychosocial
- a., radial
- a., rostral
- a. spinal cord, dorsal
- a., superior
- a., superolateral
- a., terminal
- a., therapeutic
- a., toxicologic
- a., ulnar
- a., ventral
- a., volar

aspera femoris, linea
Asperger's syndrome
aspergillina, otomycosis
aspergilloma formation
aspergillosis
- a., allergic bronchopulmonary
- a., bronchopulmonary
- a., cutaneous
- a. ▸ invasive pulmonary
- a., noninvasive
- a., pleural
- a., primary
- a., pulmonary
- a. ▸ semi-invasive

Aspergillus (aspergillus)
- A. auricularis
- A. barbae
- A. bouffardi
- A. clavatus
- A. concentricus
- A. flavus
- A. fumigatus
- A. fungal infection
- A. giganteus
- A. glaucus
- A. gliocladium
- A. mucoroides
- A. nidulans
- A. niger
- A. ochraceus
- A. parasiticus
- A. pictor
- A. repens
- A. sydowi
- A. ustus

A. versicolor
Asphyxia
a. ▸ accidental positional
a. and death
a., birth
a., blue
a. by neck compression
a., fetal
a. livida
a., local
a., neonatal
a. neonatorum
a. pallida
a., perinatal
a. ▸ repeated partial
a., secondary
a., symmetric
a., traumatic
asphyxial insolation
asphyxial stage
asphyxiant dystrophy (TAD), thoracic
asphyxiant thoracic dystrophy ▸ familial
asphyxiating thoracic dystrophy
Aspicularis tetraptera
aspirant ▸ vomitus or gastric
aspirate(s)
a. culture, tracheal
a., direct lung
a., duodenal
a., endotracheal
a., gastric
a. meconium ▸ newborn
a., nasogastric (NG)
a., needle
a., stomach
a., transtracheal
aspirated
a., abdomen
a. amnion, abundant
a. and flushed
a. and flushed with saline ▸ catheter
a., fluid
a. foreign material
a. from abdomen ▸ fluid
a. from chest ▸ fluid
a. from joint ▸ fluid
a. from knee ▸ fluid
a. into lungs ▸ drug-resistant organisms
a. material
a. meconium
a. thoracentesis
aspiration
a. abortion, suction

a., amniotic fluid
a. and injection of bursae
a. and injection of joints
a. and injection of tendons
a. biopsy
a. biopsy cytology
a. biopsy ▸ fine needle
a. biopsy, thoracic fine needle
a. biopsy ▸ transthoracic needle
a., bone marrow
a., breast cyst
a. bronchopneumonia
a., bronchoscopy with
a., chronic
a., cyst
a. (D and A), dilatation and
a. (FNA), fine needle
a., gastric
a. gastric contents
a. lung abscess
a., meconium
a. ▸ mineral oil
a., needle
a. of blood materials
a. of bone
a. of fluid
a. of food or fluid
a. of food particles
a. of foreign body
a. of gastric contents
a. of gastric contents ▸ terminal
a. of gastrointestinal organisms
a. of lung ▸ needle
a. of newborn
a. of pleural cavity
a. of secretions
a., percutaneous
a., percutaneous needle
a. ▸ pleural fluid
a. pneumonia
a. pneumonia, congenital
a. pneumonia, extensive
a. pneumonia, oil
a. pneumonia, organizing
a. pneumonia ▸ peptic
a. pneumonitis
a. pneumonitis ▸ peptic
a. ▸ preoperative gastric
a. procedure
a., recurrent
a., retromandibular node
a. ▸ shifting vocational
a., skinny needle
a., suprapubic
a. syndrome

a. syndrome ▸ meconium
a. syndrome ▸ pulmonary acid
a., uterine
a. (D and A) uterus ▸ dilatation and
a., vacuum
a., vocational
aspirational biopsy
aspiratory pneumonia
aspirin
a., allergic to
a. and heart attacks
a., bleeding from
a., buffered
a. ▸ burning mouth from
a. ▸ enteric coated
a. gastritis
a. ▸ hearing loss from
a. ▸ heart attack from
a., hypersensitivity to
a. ingestion
a. interaction
a. irritates stomach lining
a., liberal doses of
a. ▸ nasal problem from
a. ▸ patient hypersensitive to
a. poisoning
a. products
a. resistant
a. ▸ Reyes syndrome from
a. -sensitive patient
a. sensitivity
a. sensitivity, asthma-
a. ▸ skin disorder from
a. therapy
a. therapy ▸ chronic
a. therapy, high dose
a. therapy ▸ long-term
a. therapy, low dose
a. therapy ▸ patient intolerant to
a. therapy, preventative
a. ▸ tinnitus from
a. tolerance test
a. tolerance time
a. toxicity
a., ulcer from
a., welt from
asplenia
a., anatomical
a., functional
a. syndrome
asplenic patient
Assam fever
assault(s)
a., aggravated
a. cancer cells

assault(s)—*continued*
a., criminal
a. on staff ▸ patient
a. on tumors, radiation
a., physical
a. ▸ repeated physical
a., sexual
a. treatment center, sexual

assaultive
a. behavior
a. episodes
a., patient

assay(s)
a., agglutination inhibition
a., antigen capture
a., binding
a., bio-
a., cell attachment
a., cholesterol
a., clinical
a., complement
a., C-terminal
a. ▸ dye exclusion
a., erythrocyte enzyme
a., erythropoietin
a., estrogen receptor
a., excision
a. ▸ fluorescent cytoprint
a. ▸ four point
a. ▸ gene transfer transcription
a., gonadotropic hormone
a. ▸ hemolytic complement
a. ▸ hemolytic plaque
a., hormonal
a., immunocytochemical
a., immunoradiometric
a. ▸ in situ
a. ▸ lymphoblast mutation
a. ▸ lymphocyte proliferation
a. medium
a. methodology
a., microbiological
a., microcytotoxicity
a., microencapsulation
a. ▸ mobility shift
a., myoglobin
a., plasma renin
a. ▸ polymerase chain reaction
a. pregnancy blood (Biocept-G),
   radioreceptor
a., radioligand
a., renal venous renin
a. ▸ renin vein
a., sandwich

a. ▸ sandwich enzyme-linked
   immunosorbent
a. ▸ serum Mgb
a. ▸ spleen colony
a. (ELISA) test ▸ enzyme-linked
   immunosorbent
a. test, ER (estrogen receptor)
a. test, Raji cell
a. volume, normal

assembly
a., automated tray
a. language
a. program

assertion ▸ healthy self-
assertion, types of
assertive ▸ patient self-
assertiveness inventory
assertiveness training
assess(es)
a. cardiac metabolism
a. changes
a., clinically
a. functioning of the heart
a. risk
a. the patient

assessing
a. agency, designated
a. and referring patients
a. life stressors
a. needs of cannabinoid abusers
a. needs of depressant abusers
a. needs of hallucinogen abusers
a. needs of inhalant abusers
a. needs of multi-drug abusers
a. needs of opioid abusers
a. needs of phencyclidine abusers
a. needs of stimulant abusers
a. pastoral need
a. patient needs
a. ventricular fashion

assessment (Assessment)
a., anatomic
a. and diagnosis ▸ aid in
a. and diagnosis ▸ nursing
a. and intervention ▸ psychiatric
   nursing
a., angiographic
a., bathroom aids
a., behavioral
a., bereavement
a., bioethical
a., biopsychosocial
a., cardiovascular
a., career
a., causality

a., cell viability
a., clinical
a., cognitive
a., communicative
a. ▸ complete and ongoing
a., comprehensive
a., comprehensive geriatric
a., computerized
a., computerized risk
a., confidential
a., court ordered
a., developmental
a., diagnostic
a. ▸ digital angiographic
a., Doppler
a., echocardiographic
a. evaluation
a., extensive hearing
a., financial
a. findings, personality
a., fitness
a., forensic
a., frequent
a., functional
a. functions
a., gait
a. ▸ gestational age
a., grief
a., health
a., heart
a., heart risk
a., hemodynamic
a., home
a. ▸ in vivo stereologic
a. index, global
a., initial
a. ▸ initial case
a. ▸ initial head
A., Intake
a. interview, risk
a., invasive
a., love
A. Matrix (TRAM) ▸ Treatment
   Rating
A. Matrix (TRAM) ▸ Treatment
   Response
a., medical
a., mental
A. Method (TRAM) ▸ Treatment
   Response
a., microbiologic
a., multicultural
a., multidisciplinary
a. ▸ myocardial function
a., neurobehavioral

a., neurological
a., neuropsychological
a., noninvasive
a., noninvasive cardiac
a. ▸ noninvasive vascular laboratory
a., nutritional
a., objective
a. of effectiveness
a. of function, global
a. of health status
a. of newborn, physical
a. of pain
a. of patient's condition
a. of services
a. of services, Alzheimer's diagnostic
a. of transit times, cinedensitometric
a., outpatient satisfaction
a., patient
a. ▸ patient satisfaction
a., perfusion
a., personality
a. phase, initial
a., physician
a., preoperative
a., pretreatment
a., preventive
a., projective
a., psychiatric
a., psychological
a., psychosocial risk
a. ▸ quantitative risk
a., radiographic
a., radiologic
a. ▸ randomized controlled
a., rapid overall
a., revascularization
a., risk
a., roentgenographic
a., self-
a., sonographic
a. ▸ speech understanding
a., spiritual
a. staff, intake
a., suicide
a., technology
a., types of
a., ultrasound
a., vascular
a. ▸ vocational adjustment
assigned claim
assignment
   a., gender

a., Medicare
a., role
a., sex
assimilation, glucose
assist
   a., ambulates with minimal
   a., contact-standby
   a. device (AVAD), acute-ventricular
   a. device ▸ battery-assisted heart-
   a. device, biventricular
   a. device ▸ left ventricular (LV)
   a. device (VAD), permanently implanted ventricular
   a. device ▸ pulsatile
   a. device ▸ right ventricular (RV)
   a. (EPCA) ▸ external pressure circulatory
   a. pump, heart-
   a. system ▸ implantable left ventricular (LV)
   a. system (LVAS) ▸ left ventricular
   a. ventilation ▸ proportional
   a. with ambulation, standby
   a. with bedpan
   a. with urinal
assistance (Assistance)
   a. and mobility
   a., canine
   a. centers, senior
   a., contact
   a. ▸ continuous mechanical ventilatory
   a. device, walking
   a. for ambulation, contact
   a. for lower body dressing, maximum
   a. for lower body dressing, minimal
   a. for transfers, minimal
   a. for upper body dressing, maximum
   a. for upper body dressing, minimal
   a. for wheelchair mobility, patient needs minimal
   A. Foundation (AHAF) ▸ American Health
   a. (GNA) ▸ general nursing
   a., home care
   a. in transfers and ambulation, standby
   a. in upper body dressing, minimal
   a., life-saving
   a. ▸ long-term mechanical
   a., maximum
   a., minimal
   a., moderate

a., patient ambulates with
a., patient needs
a., patient receiving respiratory
a., patient requires occasional
a., patient transfers with standby
A. Program (EAP), Employee
a., provide medical
a., respiratory
a., robotic
a., set-up and cueing
a., standby
a., total ventilatory
a., ventilatory
a. with walking
assistant
   a., dental
   a., lab
   a., medical
   a., nursing
   a. (PA), physician's
   a. (SHTA) ▸ security hospital treatment
   a. surgeon
   a., surgical
assisted
   a. balloon angioplasty (LABA) ▸ laser-
   a. breathing
   a. circulation
   a. cue-controlled relaxation ▸ biofeedback
   a. design (CAD) prosthesis, computerized
   a. detoxification, medication-
   a. device ▸ motor-
   a. diagnostics, computer-
   a. drug abuse treatment program ▸ publicly
   a. duodenal intubation ▸ endoscopically
   a. exercise, active
   a. in situ keratomileusis (LASIK) correction ▸ laser
   a. in situ keratomileusis (LASIK) ▸ laser-
   a. in situ keratomileusis (LASIK) surgery ▸ laser-
   a. in situ keratomileusis (LASIK) surgery ▸ wavefront-guided laser-
   a. laser surgery, computer
   a. lipectomy ▸ suction-
   a. living
   a. living facility
   a. living ▸ memory impaired

assisted—*continued*
- a. living residence
- a. menu planning ▸ computer
- a. muscular relaxation training, biofeedback
- a. operation, computer
- a. reproductive techniques
- a. respiration
- a. stereotactic laser microsurgery, computer
- a. subepithelial keratectomy (Laser) procedure, laser-
- a. suicide
- a. suicide ▸ ethical validity of
- a. suicide, physician
- a. suicide ▸ police-
- a. surgery ▸ hologram-
- a. thoracic surgery ▸ video-
- a. thorascopic thymectomy ▸ video-
- a. to die, right to be
- a. transfer, maximum
- a. transfer, minimal
- a. uvulopalatoplasty (LAUP) ▸ laser-
- a. vaginal hysterectomy (LAVH) ▸ laparoscopically
- a. vascular anastomosis ▸ laser-
- a. ventilation
- a. ventilation (INPAV) ▸ intermittent negative-pressure

assistive listening device (ALD) ▸ personal
Assmann tuberculous infiltrate Assmann's
associate, research
associated
- a. AIDS (acquired immune deficiency syndrome) ▸ transfusion-
- a. amnesia
- a. anemia, AIDS
- a. anemia, cancer
- a. antigen(s) ▸ hepatitis-
- a. antigen ▸ lineage
- a. antigen ▸ myeloid
- a. antigen ▸ proliferation
- a. antigens ▸ melanoma
- a. antigens ▸ tumor
- a. anuria ▸ trauma
- a. bacteremias ▸ catheter-
- a. bursitis ▸ hip
- a. changes ▸ malignancy
- a. degenerative change
- a. diarrhea, antibiotic
- a. disease, transfusion

- a. enterocolitis, antibiotic-
- a. fatality, drug
- a. features and disorders
- a., gut-
- a. infections ▸ hospital-
- a. infections, IV- (intravenous)
- a. infections ▸ reduce risk of hospital-
- a. infection, transfusion
- a. infectious disease
- a. infertility, endometriosis
- a. lymphoid tissue (GALT) ▸ gut-
- a. memory impairment (AAMI), age-
- a. mismatch ▸ ventilator
- a. motor cognitive disorder ▸ human immunodeficiency virus (HIV)
- a. movement
- a. movement, contralateral
- a. movements, loss of
- a. nystagmus
- a. paralytic polio (VAPP) ▸ vaccine-
- a. pericarditis, drug-
- a. pneumonia ▸ ventilator-
- a. primary acute pancreatitis ▸ drug-
- a. problems
- a. pulmonary fibrosis ▸ rejection-
- a. reaction
- a. respiratory tract infection ▸ hospital-
- a. septicemia, catheter-
- a. stigmata ▸ patent ductus renal agenesis with
- a. symptoms
- a. transfusion, AIDS (acquired immune deficiency syndrome)
- a. valve disease ▸ lupus-
- a. vertigo ▸ migraine-
- a. (CA) virus ▸ croup-
- a. virus ▸ lymphadenopathy-
- a. virus (RAV) ▸ Rous-
- a. with alcoholism ▸ dementia
- a. with blood loss ▸ abdominal pain
- a. with cardiopulmonary arrest, arrhythmias
- a. with depression ▸ anxiety
- a. with drug withdrawal, features
- a. with sepsis ▸ jaundice

association (Association)(s)
- A. (APA), American Psychiatric
- A. ▸ American Sleep Disorders
- a. areas of cerebral cortex
- a. areas, visual

- a. center
- a., clang
- a., controlled
- a., defective
- A. (AHA) diet, American Heart
- a., dream
- a. fibers
- A. for Partial Hospitalization ▸ American
- A. for Perinatal Addiction Research and Education (NAPARE) ▸ National
- a., free
- a., klang
- a., loose
- a., looseness of
- a., negative
- a. nerve
- a. neurosis
- A. (NYHA) ▸ New York Heart
- a., noci◊
- a., noncausal
- A. of Private Psychiatric Hospitals ▸ American
- A. of Retired Persons (AARP), American
- a., perception and
- a. period
- A. (VNA) ▸ Visiting Nurse
- a., word
- A. (WMA), World Medical

associative
- a. aphasia
- a. for patient, quality
- a. in dosimetry, quality
- a. in radiation safety, quality
- a. in simulators, quality
- a. in treatment machines, quality
- a. in treatment planning, quality
- a., quality
- a. reaction
- a. thinking, creative-
- a. thought patterns

assumption of new identity
assured
- a., hemostasis
- a. manner, self-
- a., nonjudgmental attitude ▸ calm,
- a. ▸ patient self-
- a. pressure support ▸ volume-

Ast. (astigmatism)
astasia abasia
astatic diplegia, atonic-
asteatosis cutis
astereognosis, tactile

asterixis noted, early
asternal ribs
Asterococcus canis
Asterococcus mycoides
asteroid body
asteroid hyalitis
asteroides, Nocardia
asteroides, Trichophyton
asthenia
    a. gravis hypophyseogenea
    a., neurocirculatory
    a. ‣ post-viral
asthenia
asthenia,
asthenic [*sthenic*]
    a. chest
    a. diathesis
    a. fever
    a. habit
    a. orthophoria
    a. personality
    a. type
asthenopia
    a., accommodative
    a., muscular
    a., nervous
    a., retinal
asthetic plastic surgery
asthma
    a., abdominal
    a. ‣ acute attack of
    a. airway problems ‣ allergenic
    a., allergen-induced
    a., allergic
    a., alveolar
    a. -aspirin sensitivity
    a., atopic
    a. attack
    a. attack ‣ life-threatening
    a., bacterial
    a. baker's
    a. ‣ breathing difficulty from
    a., bronchial
    a., cardiac
    a., catarrhal
    a., Cheyne-Stokes
    a., chronic
    a., chronic bronchitis with
    a., cigarette smoke
    a., cotton dust
    a., coughing from
    a. crystals
    a., cutaneous
    a. death
    a., dust

    a., Elsner's
    a., EMG (electromyogram)
      biofeedback relaxation in
    a., emphysematous
    a., essential
    a., (EIA), exercise induced
    a., exertional
    a., extrinsic
    a. flare
    a., food
    a., grinders'
    a., Heberden's
    a., horse
    a., humid
    a., infective
    a., intermittent
    a., intrinsic
    a. ‣ late onset
    a. -like symptoms
    a. ‣ meat wrapper's
    a., millers'
    a., miners'
    a., mixed
    a., nasal
    a., nervous
    a., nocturnal
    a., occupational
    a. on lung ‣ effects of
    a. paper
    a., perennial
    a., persistent
    a., pollen
    a. ‣ poorly reversible
    a., potters'
    a., reflex
    a., sexual
    a., spasmodic
    a., steam-fitters'
    a. ‣ steroid-dependent
    a., stone
    a., stone-strippers
    a., subclinical
    a., symptomatic
    a., thymic
    a. trigger
    a., triggers of
    a. triggers ‣ personal
asthmatic
    a. attack
    a. attack, acute
    a. attack subsiding
    a. bronchitis
    a. bronchitis, acute
    a. bronchitis, chronic
    a. bronchitis, infectious

    a. bronchospasm
    a., patient known
    a., pregnant
    a. reaction, delayed
    a. shock
    a. ‣ steroid-dependent
    a. wheeze
    a. wheezing
asthmaticus, status
asthmatoid wheeze
asthmoid respiration
astia, Xenopsylla
astigmatic
    a. amblyopia
    a. keratotomy
    a. keratotomy ‣ radial and
astigmatism (Astigmatism)
    a., compound hypermetropic
    a., compound hyperopic
    a., compound myopic
    a., corneal
    a., corneal irregular
    a. (As.H.) ‣ hypermetropic
    a., hyperopic
    a., irregular
    a., lenticular
    a. ‣ lenticular, irregular
    a., mixed
    a. (As.M.) ‣ myopic
    a., myopic compound
    a., oblique
    a., reduce
Astler-Coller modification
astragaloid bone
astragaloid, calcaneo◊
astragaloscaphoid bone
astragalus, removal of
astral ray
Astrand bicycle exercise stress test
astrocyte, protoplasmic
astrocytic glioma
astrocytoma
    a., cerebellar
    a., cerebral
    a., cystic
    a., fibrillary
    a., gemistocytic
    a. ‣ giant cell
    a. ‣ grade I-IV
    a. ‣ juvenile pilocystic
    a. ‣ macrocystic pilocytic cerebellar
    a., malignant
    a. ‣ microcystic pilocytic cerebellar
    a. ‣ multifocal anaplastic
    a., necrosis in

astrocytoma—*continued*
- a., pilocystic
- a., piloid
- a., protoplasmic
- a. ▸ subependymal giant cell
- a., supratentorial

Astroviridae virus
Astrup blood gas values
ASVD (arteriosclerotic vascular disease)
asylum dysentery
asylum ear
asymmetric
- a. area
- a. eyeball movement artifact potential
- a. lesions in coronary arteries
- a. movement
- a. refraction of lens
- a. septal hypertrophy

asymmetrical septal hypertrophy (ASH)
asymmetry
- a., acetabular
- a., facial
- a. in blood circulation
- a. ▸ minor alpha
- a., reflex
- a., voltage

asymptomatic [*symptomatic*]
- a. bacteriuria
- a. bruit
- a. cardiac ischemia (ACI)
- a. carotid bruit
- a. complex ectopy
- a. cystocele
- a. disease
- a. gallstones
- a. heart attack
- a. heart disease
- a. infection
- a. ischemia
- a. left-ventricular dysfunction
- a. lesion
- a. metabolic disorder
- a. pathogen carrier
- a. patient
- a., patient relatively
- a. pulmonary valve disorder
- a. pyuria
- a. urinary tract infection
- a. ventricular arrhythmias
- a. viral shedding

asynchronous
- a. atrial pacemaker
- a. pacemaker

- a. pacemaker, atrial
- a. pacemaker, external
- a. pacemaker ▸ ventricular
- a. pacing
- a. pulse generator

asynchrony index
asynchrony of motion
asynclitism, anterior
asynclitism, posterior
asynergy
- a., appendicular
- a., axial
- a., axioappendicular
- a., truncal

asynthetase activity
asystole
- a., patient remained in
- a., transient
- a., ventricular

atactica, abasia
atactica, agraphia
ataractic/ataraxic
ataraxia/ataraxy
atavicus, metatarsus
atavistic regression
ataxia [*apraxia*]
- a., acute
- a., acute cerebellar
- a., alcoholic
- a. and intention tremor
- a. and titubation
- a., autonomic
- a., Briquet's
- a., Broca's
- a., central
- a., cerebellar
- a., cerebral
- a. cordis
- a., equilibratory
- a., extremity
- a., family
- a., Fergusson and Critchley's
- a., Friedreich's
- a., frontal
- a., hereditary
- a., hereditary cerebellar
- a., hereditary progressive
- a., hysteric
- a., intrapsychic
- a., kinetic
- a., labyrinthic
- a., Leyden's
- a., locomotor
- a., Marie's
- a., motor

- a., noothymopsychic
- a., ocular
- a., optic
- a., professional
- a., Sanger-Brown's
- a., sensory
- a., severe cerebellar
- a., spinal
- a., spinocerebellar
- a., static
- a. -telangiectasia (AT)
- a., thermal
- a., titubation and tremor
- a., transient
- a., truncal
- a., unilateral cerebellar
- a., vasomotor
- a., vestibular
- a. virus, feline

ataxiagram study
ataxic
- a. amimia
- a. aphasia
- a. gait
- a. gait ▸ diminish excursion of
- a. paraplegia

atelectasis
- a., absorption
- a., acquired
- a., adhesive
- a., areas of
- a., basal pulmonary
- a., basilar
- a., bibasilar
- a., bilateral pulmonary
- a., cicatrizing
- a., compression
- a., compressive
- a., congenital
- a., discoid
- a., focal
- a., focus of
- a. left lung base
- a., linear
- a., lobar
- a., lobular patches of
- a. ▸ lower lobe segmental
- a., mild bibasilar
- a., obstructive
- a., passive
- a., patchy
- a., periaortic
- a. ▸ plate-like
- a., postobstructive
- a., postoperative

a., primary
a., pulmonary
a. ▸ pulmonary immaturity and
a., relaxation
a., resorption
a., resorptive
a. right lung base
a., round
a., rounded
a., secondary
a., segmental
a., subsegmental
atelectatic
a. and edematous lungs
a., firm and
a. lobule
a., lung tissue
a. pneumonitis
a. rales
ateliotic dwarf
ATG (antithymocyte globulin)
atherectomy(-ies)
a. catheter
a., coronary
a., coronary rotational
a. device, directional
a. device, extraction
a. device, rotary
a. device, rotational
a., directional
a. (DCA) ▸ directional coronary
a. extrusion angioplasty ▸ Kinsey
rotation
a. ▸ high speed rotational
a. index
a., percutaneous
a. ▸ percutaneous coronary
rotational
a. procedure
a., pullback
a., rotational
a. ▸ rotational coronary
a. system ▸ peripheral
a. system ▸ rotational
a. technique
a. ▸ transluminal extraction
atheroblation laser
atherogenesis ▸ monoclonal theory of
atherogenesis ▸ response-to-injury
hypothesis of
atherogenic particles
atherogenicity index
atheroma
a., calcified
a., coronary

a., cutis
a., embolized
a., moderate calcified
a., mural
a., severe calcified
a., ulcerated
a., yellow
atheromata, calcified
atheromata, ulcerated
atheromatous
a. change
a. change of aorta ▸ severe
a. cyst
a. emboli
a. lesion
a. material, cores of
a. pattern
a. plaques
a. ulcers
atherosclerosed, abdominal aorta
atherosclerosis
a., advanced aortic
a. and blood flow
a., aortic
a. ▸ burning feet from
a., calcific
a., calcific mural
a., calcified
a., cardiac allograft
a., coronary artery
a., diffuse
a., diffuse calcific
a. ▸ encrustation theory of
a., focal
a., gangrene from
a., graft
a. in artery
a. ▸ lipogenic theory of
a., mild
a., mild systemic
a., moderate
a., occlusive
a. of aorta
a. of coronary arteries
a. of intracerebral vessels
a. patient ▸ artery-clogging plaque in
a., premature
a., problem from
a., progression of
a. scan, coronary
a., stroke and
a., trembling from
a. with calcification ▸ moderate
atherosclerotic
a. abdominal aorta

a. aneurysm
a. aortic disease
a. artery
a. blockage
a. blood vessel
a. build-up
a. cardiovascular disease (ASCVD)
a. cardiovascular disease ▸
advanced
a. carotid artery disease
a., coronary arteries
a. coronary artery disease
a. deposits
a. disease
a. disease ▸ peripheral
a. heart disease
a. heart disease ▸ coronary
a. inflammation
a. lesion
a. narrowing
a. plaque
a. plaque rupture
a. plaques ▸ lipid-filled
a., severely
a. vascular disease
a. vascular disease, calcific
a. vascular disease ▸ mild
athetoid
a. movements
a. movements, choreic
a. movements, periodic spasmodic
a. spasm
athetosic idiocy
athetosis, bilateral
athetosis, congenital
athlete's
a. foot
a. foot ▸ blister from
a. foot ▸ itching from
a. foot ▸ nail breaking from
a. foot ▸ redness and flakiness from
a. foot ▸ skin cracking from
a. foot ▸ skin peeling from
a. heart
a. sickness
athletic(s)
a. heart
a. heart sydrome
a. injury
a. performance
a. type
athreptic immunity
athyreosis/athyrosis
Atkinson-type lid block
Atkinson's technique

atlantoaxial instability
atlas
- a. (C-1 vertebra)
- a., lateral mass of
- a. vertebra

ATLS (advanced trauma life support)
atmosphere
- a., emotionally draining
- a., nonthreatening
- a. of pressure

atmospheric absolute
ATN (acute tubular necrosis)
atom
- a., Na (sodium)
- a. smasher
- a., tagged

atomic (Atomic)
- a. and nuclear structure
- a. binding energy
- a. energy
- A. Energy Commission (AEC)
- a. excitation
- a. force microscope
- a. heat
- a. mass
- a. mass unit (a.m.u.)
- a. number
- a. radiation
- a. spectrum
- a. structure, Bohr model of
- a. volume
- a. weight

atonia (see atony)
atonia of urinary bladder
atonia of uterus
atonic
- a. -astatic diplegia
- a. bladder
- a. constipation
- a. dyspepsia
- a. epilepsy
- a. impotence
- a. labor
- a. neurogenic bladder
- a. pseudoparalysis, congenital

atony (same as atonia)
- a., gastric
- a., intestinal
- a. of bladder
- a., uterine

atopic
- a. asthma
- a. cataract
- a. conjunctivitis
- a. dermatitis

- a. disease
- a. disorder
- a. eczema
- a. erythroderma
- a. reagin

ATP (adenosine triphosphate)
ATP (ambient temperature and pressure)
ATP implantable cardioverter defibrillator▸ Telectronics
atratus, Tabanus
atraumatic chronic sutures
atraumatic suture
atresia
- a., anorectal
- a., aortic
- a., aortic arch
- a., aortic valve
- a., biliary
- a., bronchial
- a., choana
- a., congenital
- a., congenital biliary
- a., congenital intestinal
- a., duodenal
- a., esophageal
- a., glottic
- a. ▸ gross tracheoesophageal
- a., ileal
- a. ▸ inner ear
- a., intestinal
- a. iridis
- a., laryngeal
- a., mitral
- a. of esophagus
- a. of esophagus ▸ congenital
- a. of lacrimal passage
- a. of lacrimonasal duct
- a. ▸ prenatal diagnosis of esophageal
- a., pulmonary
- a. ▸ pulmonary aspects in esophageal
- a., pyloric
- a. ▸ small bowel
- a., tricuspid

atria
- a., cardiac
- a., contraction of
- a. ▸ electrical stimulation of
- a., fibrillating
- a., racing

atrial
- a. abnormality, left
- a. abnormality, right

- a. activation ▸ eccentric
- a. activation mapping
- a. activation mapping ▸ retrograde
- a. activation sequence ▸ intra-
- a. activation sequence ▸ intracardiac
- a. activity
- a. anatomy
- a. angiography ▸ left
- a. aortic bypass ▸ Litwak left
- a. appendage
- a. appendage electrogram ▸ right
- a. appendage ▸ left
- a. appendage, right
- a. appendages in embryo
- a. arrhythmia
- a. arrhythmia ▸ primary
- a. arrhythmias, digitalis
- a. asynchronous pacemaker
- a. axis discontinuity
- a. baffle, intra-
- a. baffle ▸ Mustard
- a. baffle operation
- a. baffle, Senning-type intra-
- a. beat ▸ premature
- a. bigeminy
- a. block, intra-
- a. bolus dynamic computer tomography (CT)
- a. bradycardia
- a. capture threshold
- a. cavities
- a. chambers ▸ chaotic beating of
- a. chaotic tachycardia
- a. circumflex artery
- a. (RA) communication murmur ▸ left ventricular (LV) right
- a. complex ▸ premature
- a. conduction time ▸ intra-
- a. contraction
- a. contraction, effective
- a. contraction ▸ nonconducted premature
- a. contraction (PAC) ▸ premature
- a. (LA) crossover dynamics ▸ left ventricular (LV) left
- a. cuff
- a. defects
- a. defibrillation
- a. defibrillation ▸ implantable
- a. fibrillation ▸ intermittent
- a. defibrillation shocks ▸ QRS synchronous
- a. defibrillation threshold
- a. demand-inhibited pacemaker
- a. demand-triggered pacemaker

a. depression
a. diastole
a. dilatation
a. dilatation, left
a. dimension, left
a. dimension, right
a. dissociation
a. dysrhythmias
a. echoes
a. ectopic tachycardia (AET)
a. ectopy
a. effective refractory period
a. ejection force
a. electrogram
a. electrogram ▸ low septal right
a. emptying index ▸ left
a. enlargement (LAE), left
a. enlargement (RAE), right
a. escape interval
a. escape rhythm
a. extrastimulus method
a. extrasystole
a. fibrillation
a. fibrillation ▸ acute onset of
a. fibrillation, continuous
a. fibrillation, controlled
a. fibrillation ▸ electrical conversion of
a. fibrillation ▸ embolism in
a. fibrillation flutter
a. fibrillation ▸ lone
a. fibrillation, paroxysmal
a. fibrillation ▸ postoperative
a. fibrillation, uncontrolled
a. filling pressure
a. flutter
a. flutter, recurrent
a. flutter with 4:1 conduction
a. flutter with 3:1 conduction
a. foci, ectopic
a. gallop
a. hypertension ▸ left
a. hypertrophy (LAH), left
a. hypertrophy (RAH), right
a. impulses
a. impulses ▸ uncoordinated
a. infarction
a. internodal tracts
a. ischemia ▸ intraoperative
a. isolation procedure ▸ left
a. kick
a. lead
a. lead dislodgement
a. lead impedance
a., left
a. liver pulse

a. malsensing
a. mass, intra-
a. Maze procedure ▸ modified left
a. muscle fiber
a. myocardial infarction (MI)
a. myoma
a. myxoma
a. myxoma ▸ left
a. myxoma ▸ right
a. natriuretic factor (ANF)
a. natriuretic peptide ▸ human
a. natriuretic polypeptide
a. nonsensing
a. notch
a. ostium primum defect
a. overdrive pacing
a. -paced cycle length
a. pacemaker, alternating
a. pacemaker, asynchronous
a. pacemaker, decremental
a. pacemaker ▸ subsidiary
a. pacing, access
a. pacing, burst
a. pacing, decremental
a. pacing, dual-site
a. pacing electrode, temporary
a. pacing ▸ incremental
a. pacing mode
a. pacing mode, alternative
a. pacing, overdrive
a. pacing ▸ rapid
a. pacing stress test
a. pacing ▸ transesophageal
a. pacing wire
a. parasystole
a. paroxysmal tachycardia
a. partitioning ▸ left
a. preferential pathways
a. premature beat (APB)
a. premature complexes
a. premature contraction (APC)
a. premature depolarization
   contractions
a. pressure
a. pressure (LAP) ▸ left
a. pressure (MLAP) ▸ mean left
a. pressure (MRAP) ▸ mean right
a. pressure (RAP) ▸ right
a. pulse amplitude
a. pulse width
a. reentrant tachycardia ▸ intra-
a. reentry tachycardia
a. relaxation
a. repolarization wave
a. rhythm

a. rhythm, normal
a., right
a. ring
a. sensing
a. sensing configuration
a. sensitivity
a. septal aneurysm
a. septal defect (ASD)
a. septal defect, clamshell closure of
a. septal defect ▸ iatrogenic
a. septal defect ▸ primum
a. septal defect ▸ secundum
a. septal defect ▸ sinus venosus
a. septal defect umbrella
a. septostomy, balloon
a. septum
a. shear
a. shunt, ventricular
a., sino◊
a. site ▸ intra-
a. sound
a. spontaneous echo contrast ▸ left
a. standstill
a. stasis
a. stimulation ▸ transesophageal
a. study
a. subendocardial hemorrhages
a. synchronous pacing
a. synchronous pulse generator
a. synchronous ventricular inhibited
   pacemaker
a. synchronous ventricular
   pacemaker
a. synchrony
a. systole
a. tachycardia
a. tachycardia, aborted paroxysmal
a. tachycardia, automatic
a. tachycardia, chaotic
a. tachycardia ▸ ectopic
a. tachycardia ▸ macroreentrant
a. tachycardia (MAT) ▸ multifocal
a. tachycardia (PAT) ▸ paroxysmal
a. tachycardia ▸ reentrant
a. tachycardia with aberrancy,
   paroxysmal
a. tachycardia with high degree
   atrioventricular block
a. tachysystole
a. thrombus
a. thrombus ▸ right
a. tissue
a. to aortic ▸ left
a. tracking pacemaker
a. train pacing

atrial—*continued*
- a. transport function
- a. trigeminy with aberrancy
- a. triggered pulse generator
- a. triggered ventricular-inhibited pacemaker
- a. valve
- a. vector loop
- a. venous pulse
- a. ventricular valve ▸ narrowed
- a. VOO pacemaker
- a. wall
- a. waves
- a. -well technique

atrialized chamber
atrice, substance sensibilis'
Atricor
- A. pacemaker
- A. pacemaker, Cordis
- A. pacemaker, Omni-

atriocarotid interval
atriodextrofascicular tract
atriodigital dysplasia
atriofascicular fiber
atriofascicular tract
atrio-His pathway
atrio-Hisian
- a. bypass tract
- a. connection
- a. fiber
- a. interval

atrionodal bypass tract
atriopressor reflex
atriopulmonary anastomosis ▸ Fontan
atriopulmonary shunt
atrioseptal defects
atrioseptal sign
atriosystolic murmur
atriovenous fistula
atriovenous pulse
atrioventricular (AV)
- a. block
- a. block ▸ atrial tachycardia with high degree
- a. block, congenital complete
- a. block ▸ incomplete
- a. block, second degree (2nd°)
- a. block, third degree (3rd°)
- a. block ▸ Wenckebach
- a. block with intraventricular conduction delay ▸ first degree
- a. branch block
- a. bundle
- a. bundle ▸ lobulated
- a. canal

- a. canal ▸ partial
- a. canal ▸ persistent common
- a. conduction abnormality
- a. conduction defect
- a. conduction delay
- a. conduction disease
- a. conduction disturbance
- a. conduction system
- a. conduction tissue
- a. connection, accessory
- a. connection ▸ univentricular
- a. discordance
- a. dissociation
- a. dissociation, complete
- a. dissociation ▸ incomplete
- a. dissociation, isorhythmic
- a. dissociation with interference, isorhythmic
- a. endothelial cells
- a., excitation anomalous
- a. extrasystole
- a. fistula
- a. flow rumbling murmur
- a. furrow
- a. gradient
- a. groove
- a. groove artery ▸ left
- a. heart block
- a. interval
- a. junction
- a. junction anomaly
- a. junction motion
- a. junctional bigeminy
- a. junctional complex ▸ premature
- a. junctional escape rhythm
- a. junctional heart block
- a. junctional pacemaker
- a. junctional reciprocating tachycardia-
- a. junctional rhythm
- a. junctional rhythm, accelerated
- a. junctional tachycardia
- a. junctional tachycardia▸ nonparoxysmal
- a. malformation (AVM)
- a. nodal (AVN) conduction
- a. nodal extrasystole
- a. nodal pathways
- a. nodal pathways ▸ dual
- a. nodal reentrant paroxysmal tachycardia
- a. nodal reentrant tachycardia ▸ atrial
- a. nodal reentry
- a. nodal rhythm

- a. nodal (AVN) tachycardia
- a. node (AVN)
- a. node (AVN) pathways
- a. node (AVN) reentry
- a. node (AVN) ▸ second
- a. orifice
- a. pacemaker ▸ dual chamber
- a. pathways, accessory
- a. reciprocating tachycardia (AVRT)
- a. reciprocating tachycardia ▸ antidromic
- a. reciprocating tachycardia ▸ orthodromic
- a. refractory period (AVRP)
- a. rhythm
- a. rim
- a. ring
- a. septal defect
- a. septal structures
- a. septation, deficient
- a. septation ▸ normal
- a. septum
- a. sequential pacemaker
- a. sequential pacing
- a. shunt
- a. sulcus
- a. synchrony
- a. synchrony ▸ normal
- a. time
- a. valve
- a. valve, crisscross
- a. valve, incompetent
- a. valve insufficiency
- a. valve ▸ straddling
- a. valves, opening of
- a. ventricularis, truncus fasciculi

atrium (atria)
- a., accessory
- a. ▸ catheter stimulation of right
- a., common
- a., congenital single
- a., contraction of right
- a. cordis
- a. dextrum
- a., emptying of right
- a., filling of right
- a. glottidis
- a. ▸ high right
- a. laryngis
- a. (LA), left
- a. ▸ low septal
- a. meatus medii
- a., oblique vein of left
- a. of glottis
- a. of heart

a. of heart, left
a. of heart, right
a. of larynx
a. of lungs
a. pulmonale
a., pulmonary
a. (RA), right
a., single
a. sinistrum
a., stunned
a. vaginae

atrophic

a. acini
a. appearance
a., breast pendulous and
a. brown skin
a. cardiomyopathy
a. catarrh
a. cervix
a. changes
a. cirrhosis
a. cortex
a. emphysema
a. excavation
a., extremities
a. fracture
a. gastritis
a. gastritis, chronic
a. gingivitis, senile
a. kidney
a. laryngitis
a. left ovary
a. lesion
a., liver
a. macular degeneration
a. menopause
a. mucosal surface
a. muscle
a. muscle fibers
a. muscles of upper extremities
a. omentum and mesentery
a., pancreas
a. papulosis
a. pharyngitis
a. process
a. rhinitis
a., right ovary
a. ▸ spinal cord
a., testes
a. thrombosis
a. ▸ Type I spinal muscular
a. urogenital
a. vaginal wall
a. vaginitis

atrophica, myotonia

atrophica, syringomyelia
atrophicans, acrodermatitis chronica
atrophicans, cancer
atrophicus, lichen sclerosus et
atrophied

a. abdominal muscles
a. cells
a. neurons ▸ shrunken
a. tubules

atrophy

a., acute yellow
a. and cyanosis ▸ muscular
a., Aran-Duchenne muscular
a., arthritic
a., Behr's
a., blue
a., bone
a., brown
a., Buchwald's
a., cardiac
a., cerebral
a., cerebral cortical
a., Charcot-Marie-Tooth
a., compensatory
a., compression
a., concentric
a., convolutional
a., correlated
a., cortical
a., corticostriatal-spinal
a., Cruveilhier's
a. deformity, pressure
a., degenerative
a., Déjerine-Sottas
a., Déjerine-Thomas
a., denervated muscle
a., diffuse
a., disuse
a., Duchenne-Aran muscular
a., eccentric
a., Eichhorst
a., endocrine
a., endometrial
a., Erb's
a., exhaustion
a., facial
a., familial spinal muscular
a., fat replacement
a., fatty
a., Fazio-Londe
a., focal
a. ▸ focal serous fat
a., Fuchs'
a., gastric
a., gastric mucosal

a., glandular
a., gray
a., Gudden's
a., healed yellow
a., hemifacial
a., hemilingual
a., hereditary optic
a., hippocampal
a., Hoffmann's
a., Hunt's
a. in shoulder area
a., idiopathic muscular
a., infantile
a., inflammatory
a., interstitial
a., ischemic muscular
a., juvenile muscular
a., lactation
a., Landouzy-Déjerine
a., leaping
a., Leber's optic
a., linear
a., lobar
a., long lasting muscular
a., macular
a. ▸ moderately prominent generalized
a. ▸ multiple system
a., muscle
a. ▸ muscle disuse
a., muscular
a., myelopathic muscular
a., myopathic
a., neural
a., neuritic muscular
a., neurogenic
a., neurogenic muscular
a., neuromuscular
a., neuropathic
a., neurotic
a., neurotrophic
a., numeric
a. of abdominal muscles
a. of acinar tissue
a. of an endocrine organ
a. of arm
a. of bone ▸ post-traumatic
a. of brain, cerebral
a. of brain ▸ circumscribed
a. of brain ▸ generalized
a. of choroid
a. of disuse
a. of extremity
a. of eyeball
a. of glandular tissue

atrophy—*continued*
- a. of gyri
- a. of iris
- a. of iris ▸ essential
- a. of kidney ▸ granular
- a. of leg
- a. of leg muscles
- a. of liver, cyanotic
- a. of lung ▸ senile
- a. of muscular tissue
- a. of neocortex
- a. of neocortex ▸ severe
- a. of old age ▸ normal
- a. of optic nerve
- a. of pigmented epithelium ▸ senile
- a. of retina
- a. of salivary gland
- a. of skeletal muscle
- a. of tear producing gland
- a. of the newborn, Parrot's
- a. of thenar muscles
- a. of upper extremities ▸ marked
- a., olivopontocerebellar
- a., optic
- a. optic nerve ▸ hereditary
- a., optical nerve
- a., orbicularis
- a., ovarian
- a., pancreatic
- a., parenchymal
- a., pathologic
- a. ▸ permanent optic
- a., peroneal
- a. ▸ peroneal muscular
- a., physiologic
- a., pigmentary
- a. ▸ postinflammatory renal
- a., postmenopausal
- a. ▸ postobstructive renal
- a., pressure
- a., primary optic
- a., progressive
- a., progressive choroidal
- a., progressive muscular
- a., progressive neuromuscular
- a., progressive neuropathic muscular
- a., progressive spinal muscular
- a., progressive unilateral facial
- a., pseudohypertrophic muscular
- a., pulp
- a., quadriceps
- a., receptoric
- a., red
- a., renal

- a., reversionary
- a., rheumatic
- a., Schnabel's
- a., senile
- a., serous
- a., severe disuse
- a., skin
- a., simple
- a., spinal muscular
- a., subacute yellow
- a., subtotal villose
- a., Sudeck's
- a., testicular
- a., thenar
- a., toxic
- a. ▸ toxic optic nerve
- a., trophoneurotic
- a., tubular
- a., unilateral facial
- a., vaginal
- a., vascular
- a., Vulpian's
- a., white
- a., wucher
- a., yellow

atropine
- a. conjunctivitis
- a. stress echocardiography ▸ dobutamine-
- a. test

ATRT (atypical rhabdoid/teratoid tumor)
ATS (anxiety tension state)
ATT (arginine tolerance test)
attached
- a. gingiva
- a. to arterial wall, suture
- a. to skin edges

attachment
- a. abuse
- a. assay, cell
- a. behavior
- a. behavior in dementia
- a. disorder of early childhood ▸ reactive
- a. disorder of infancy or early childhood ▸ reactive
- a. disorder of infancy ▸ reactive
- a. disorder ▸ reactive
- a., electrode
- a., Gottlieb's epithelial
- a., menisculocapsular
- a., muscular
- a., optic nerve
- a., Pierson
- a., scalp electrode

- a., skin electrode
- a. theory
- a. therapy ▸ corrective
- a. to objects ▸ inappropriate
- a. to splint ▸ Pearson
- a., tooth
- a. trauma

attack(s)
- a., active panic
- a., acute
- a., acute asthmatic
- a., acute heart
- a., Adams-Stokes
- a. ▸ agoraphobia with panic
- a. ▸ agoraphobia without panic
- a., alleviate panic
- a., anaphylactic
- a. and aging ▸ transient ischemic
- a., angina
- a., anxiety
- a., apneic
- a. apoptosis ▸ postheart
- a., aspirin and heart
- a., asthma
- a., asthmatic
- a., asymptomatic heart
- a., atypical heart
- a., brain
- a., cannabis-induced panic
- a., cataleptic
- a., clinical
- a., cocaine heart
- a., convulsive
- a., cyanotic
- a. death, sudden heart
- a. ▸ dizziness from heart
- a., dream anxiety
- a., drop
- a., epileptic
- a., epileptoid
- a., exercise induced heart
- a., fatal heart
- a. ▸ fear of panic
- a. frequency
- a. from aspirin ▸ heart
- a. from blood clot ▸ heart
- a., gout
- a., heart
- a., initial
- a., initial heart
- a. ▸ irrepressible sleep
- a., jacksonian
- a. ▸ life-threatening asthma
- a., massive heart
- a., migraine

a. ► Monday morning heart
a. ► nonfatal heart
a. of asthma ► acute
a. of breathlessness
a. of disabling vertigo ► frequent
a. of intense fear
a. of intense terror
a. of severe vertigo ► intermittent
a. of unconsciousness ► spontaneous
a. of vertigo ► abrupt
a. of vertigo ► initial
a. on tumor, radiation
a., pain of heart
a., panic
a., patient candidate for coronary
a. patient depressed ► heart
a. patient ► heart
a. ► postmicturitional adrenergic
a., psychotic
a. rate
a. ► recurrent apneic
a. ► recurrent heart
a. rehabilitation, heart
a., relief and prevention of anginal
a. ► repeat heart
a. risk factor ► heart
a. risk, heart
a. ► risk of first heart
a. ► severity of
a. ► sexual dysfunction after heart
a. shock ► postheart
a., silent
a., silent heart
a., sleep paralysis
a. ► spontaneous panic
a., sporadic
a. strategy
a., subsiding asthmatic
a., sudden
a. ► sudden fatal heart
a. ► suddent vertigo
a. survivor, depressed heart
a. survivor ► heart
a. ► suspected heart
a. symptoms, heart
a., syncopal
a. therapy
a., trance-like
a. ► transient hemispheric
a. (TIA), transient ischemic
a. trigger ► heart
a. ► unprovoked rage
a., vagal
a., vasovagal

a., vertiginous
a. victim, cocaine-related heart
a. victim, heart
a., violent
a., viral disease
a. ► warning signs of heart
a. (TIA) ► warning signs of transient ischemic
attacked ► fear of being
attain [*obtain*]
attainment method, goal
attainment scaling ► goal
attempt(s)
a., actual suicide
a. at suicide, nonfatal
a. ► baby expired following resuscitation
a., failed suicide
a., resuscitation
a., resuscitative
a., suicide
a. ► warning signs of suicide
a., weight loss
attempted
a. cardiopulmonary resuscitation
a. passage of instrument
a. suicide
attend religious services ► loss of desire to
attendance, aid and
attendant self-criticism
attendant side-effects
attending designated treatment team
attending physician
attention
a. and memory ► poor
a. and recent recall ► evaluate orientation,
a., appropriate medical
a., attenuated by
a., blocked by
a. concentration deficit
a., craves
a. deficit disorder (ADD)
a. deficit disorder ► undifferentiated
a. deficit disorder with hyperactivity
a. deficit disorder without hyperactivity
a. deficit hyperactivity disorder (ADHD)
a. ► demand for constant
a. -demanding behavior
a. ► difficulty with
a. disorder (RAD) ► reactive
a., divided

a., focus of
a. ► focus of clinical
a. -getting behavior
a., impaired
a. ► inability to focus
a. ► inability to maintain
a. ► instability to maintain
a. loss
a., orientation, language skills and perception
a. reflex of pupil
a., refocus your
a. seeking
a. -seeking behavior
a. seeking manipulative behavior
a., shift in
a. span
a. span from anxiety ► shortened
a. span in grief
a. span ► increased
a. span, limited
a. span, long
a. span ► low
a. span ► poor
a. span, short
a. span, shortened from anxiety
a. ► spatial skills and
a. test
a. ► verbal memory and
a., visual
attentional deficits
attentive and responsive
attentive ► empathic and
attentiveness, parental over-
attenuated
a. by attention
a. culture
a. dose
a. frequencies
a. in amplitude
a. virus
attenuating factor ► stress-
a. activity
a. and scattering, tissue
a., applicator
a., beam
a., block
a., blocking or
a., broadbend
a. coefficient
a. coefficient, mass
a., decreased
a., digital beam
a., heterogeneous
a. hypothesis

attenuation—*continued*
- a., increased
- a., linear
- a. midbrain and pons, diminished
- a. process
- a., signal
- a., source self-
- a., ultrasonic

attic
- a. -aditus antrum
- a. cavity
- a. perforation
- a. perforation pocket
- a. retraction pocket

atticotomy, transmeatal

attitude
- a., adaptive
- a. adjustment
- a. and behavior
- a. ▸ calm, assured, nonjudgmental
- a., caring
- a., cephalic
- a., combative
- a., contemporary
- a., cultural
- a., curative
- a., demeaning
- a., discobolus
- a., disdainful
- a., dysfunctional
- a. emotion and behavior
- a., emotional
- a., fatalistic
- a., functional
- a., mental
- a., military
- a. ▸ normal behavior and
- a. of drug abusers
- a. of physician drug abusers
- a. of society towards drug abusers
- a., patronizing
- a., pejorative
- a., positive
- a. (PMA), positive mental
- a. pulmonary edema (HAPE) ▸ high
- a., relaxed
- a. scale
- a., snobbish
- a., traditional
- a. ▸ typical behavior and

attitudinal
- a. barrier
- a. goals
- a. reflexes

attonita, amentia

attonita, melancholia

attorney (Attorney)
- a., durable power of
- A. health care document ▸ Power of (POA)
- a., power of

attraction sphere

Attributes Questionnaire (PAQ), Personal

attrition murmur

A₂ (Alpha₂) A_2 (Alpha$_2$)

A₂ (aortic second sound) A_2 (aortic second sound)

A-2 globulins

atypia, esophageal squamous

atypical [*typical*]
- a. alveolar cells ▸ desquamation of
- a. alveolar cells ▸ proliferation of
- a. appearing megakaryocytes
- a. atrioventricular (AV) nodal reentrant tachycardia
- a. cell
- a. cell division
- a. changes, focal
- a. chest pain
- a. child
- a. depressive disorder
- a. ductal hyperplasia
- a. endometrial cells
- a. enterovirus
- a. fibroxanthoma
- a. heart attack
- a. histiocytes, enlarged
- a. hyperplasia
- a. lymphocyte
- a. manic disorder
- a. measles
- a. migraine
- a. mononuclear cells
- a. mycobacteria infection
- a. mycobacterial colonization
- a. Pap smear
- a. pneumonia
- a. pneumonia (PAP), primary
- a. pneumonia syndrome
- a. position
- a. pyelomorphic cells
- a. reactive process
- a. regenerative cells
- a. repetitive spike-and-slow waves
- a. rhabdoid/teratoid tumor (ATRT)
- a. rhabdoid tumor
- a. seizures
- a. sensation
- a. spike waves
- a. tamponade

- a. tuberculosis
- a. verrucous endocarditis

AU (each ear)

Au¹⁹⁸ (gold) Au^{198} (gold)

Auchmeromyia luteola

audible
- a. at bases, rales
- a. grunt
- a. rales
- a. rhonchi
- a. rub
- a. signal
- a. sound

audiclave [*autoclave*]

audio frequency

audiogenic seizure

audiogram, cortical

audiologic evaluation

audiologist, clinical

audiology examination

audiology testing

audiometer, evoked response

audiometric findings

audiometric findings, pure tone

audiometry
- a., Békésy
- a., conditioned orientation reflex
- a., cortical
- A. (ERA), Electric Response
- a., electrodermal
- a., electroencephalic
- a., evoked response
- a., localization
- a., speech
- a. test

audio response unit

audiovestibular dysfunction, central

audiovestibular lesion, central

audio-visual-tactile stimulation

audit, medical

audition
- a., chromatic
- a. colorée
- a., gustatory

audito-oculogyric reflex

auditopsychic center

auditory
- a. acuity
- a. agnosia
- a. alternans
- a. amnesia
- a. and medical evaluation
- a. and olfactory hallucinations ▸ vivid, visual,
- a. and visual signals

a. aphasia
a. awareness
a. brainstem response (ABR)
a. canal
a. canal, blood in
a. canal (EAC) ▸ external
a. canal (IAC) ▸ internal
a. capability
a. capsule
a. cell
a. center
a. comprehension
a. comprehension of language
a. cortex
a. cortex, primary
a. discrimination ▸ gradual loss of
a. disorder
a. division
a. evoked potential
a. evoked potentials (BAEP), brain stem
a. evoked response (AER)
a. evoked response (BAER), brain stem
a. feedback
a. feedback, delayed
a. fremitus
a. function
a. ganglion
a. hairs
a. hallucination
a. hallucinations ▸ occasional
a. illusion
a. impulse
a. (IA), internal
a. interpretation
a. learner
a. listening
a. massage
a. meatus
a. meatus (EAM), external
a. meatus reflex ▸ external
a. memory, immediate
a. nerve
a. nerve ▸ electrical stimulation of
a. nerve ▸ intact
a. ossicle
a. ossicles, articulations of
a. ossicles, muscles of
a. pathway
a. perception of speech sounds
a. processing deficits
a. radiation
a. recall
a. recall, immediate

a. reception
a. recovery function
a. reflex
a. saucer
a. sensation
a. speech center
a. stimulation, visual or
a. stimuli
a. striae
a. suppressions
a. teeth, Huschke's
a. training
a. training sessions
a. tube
a. tube, semicanal of
a. veins, internal
a. verbal language deficits
A. Verbal Learning Test, Rey
a. verbal memory
a. word center
audouinii, Microsporum
Auenbrugger's sign
Auer bodies
Auerbach's ganglion
Auerbach's plexus
Aufranc-Turner arthroplasty
Aufranc-Turner prosthesis
Aufrecht's sign
augenblick diagnosis
Auger effect
Auger electron
augment flow of blood
augment individual's sense of self-worth
augmentation
a., bladder
a., calf
a. cystoplasty
a. ▸ female textured breast
a., iliac
a. mammaplasty
a. mammoplasty, poststatus
a. of intrathoracic blood volume
a. of labor
a. of labor, pitocin
a. or enlargement
a., oxytocin
a. procedure, bilateral
a., reverse
a. ▸ soft tissue
a. surgery, breast
a. therapy
a. with implant
a. with implant material
augmentative communication systems

augmented histamine test
augmented psychological support
Augustine's nail
AUI (Alcohol Use Inventory)
Aujeszky's disease
au lait spots, café
aura
a., classic headache preceded by
a., epigastric
a., kinesthetic
a., migraine
a. of epilepsy
a. of peculiar taste
a., olfactory
a., silent
aural [*oral*]
a. aspergillosis
a. distance, intra-
a. fistula, antro-
a. fullness
a. nystagmus
a. plane, intra-
a. pressure
a. reflex
a. rehabilitation
a. scotoma
auratus, Mesocretus
Aureobasidium pullulans
Aureomycin gauze
aureotope (aurocoloid-198, gold-198)
aurescens, Escherichia
aureus
a. bacteremia ▸ Staphylococcus (Staph)
a. coagulase positive ▸ Staph
a., gram-positive Staphylococcus
a., hemolytic
a., hemolytic Staph
a. (MR-SA) ▸ methicillin-resistant Staphylococcus
a., Micrococcus pyogenes variety
a. penicillinase, Staph
a. prosthetic joint infection ▸ Staph (Staphylococcus)
a., Scopulariopsis
a., Staphylococcus
auricle
a., concha of
a., lobule of
a., oblique muscle of
a., pyramidal muscle of
a. reconstruction, Tanzer's
a. reflex
a., transverse muscle of

auriculae
- a., apex
- a., concha
- a., cymba concha
- a., lobulus

auricular
- a. appendage
- a. arch
- a. artery
- a. beats, premature
- a. block, sino-
- a. branch of vagus nerve
- a. complex
- a. contraction, premature
- a. extrasystole
- a. fibrillation
- a. flutter
- a. ganglion
- a. glaucoma
- a. line
- a. medicine
- a. muscle, anterior
- a. muscle, posterior
- a. muscle, superior
- a. nerve, anterior
- a. nerve, great
- a. nerve, internal
- a. nerve of vagus nerve
- a. nerve, posterior
- a. notch
- a. premature beat
- a. reflex
- a. region
- a. standstill
- a. systole
- a. tachycardia
- a. tachysystole
- a. tags
- a. therapy
- a. tophus
- a. vein, posterior
- a. veins, anterior

auricularis, Aspergillus
auriculocarotid interval
auriculocervical nerve reflex
auriculopalpebral reflex
auriculopressor reflex
auriculotemporal nerve
auriculovenous pulse
auriculoventricular
- a. dissociation
- a. extrasystole
- a. groove
- a. interval
- a. rhythm
- a. valve

auris
- a., ala
- a., antrum
- a. dextra
- a. externa
- a., hematoma
- a. interna
- a. internee, vasa
- a., internal
- a. media
- a. sinistra
- a., vestibulum

aurium, tinnitus
aurocoloid 198 (gold-198, aureotope)
Aurora dual chamber pacemaker
Aurora pulse generator
auscultation
- a. and percussion (A and P)
- a., cardiac
- a. (P and A) ▸ chest clear to percussion and
- a., clear to
- a., direct
- a., immediate
- a., Korányi's
- a., lungs clear on
- a. (P and A) ▸ lungs clear to percussion and
- a., mediate
- a., obstetric
- a. of chest
- a. of heart
- a. of lungs
- a. of neck
- a. (P and A) ▸ percussion and

auscultatory
- a. alternans
- a. gap
- a. percussion
- a. sign
- a. sound

austeni, Culicoides
Austin
- A. -Flint murmur
- A. -Flint respiration
- A. -Flint rumble
- A. -Moore pin
- A. -Moore endoprosthetic arthroplasty
- A. -Moore hip prosthesis

Australia(n)
- A. antigen
- A. antigen test
- A. Q fever
- A. X disease virus

australis, Leptospira
australis, Rickettsia
Austrian syndrome
autacoid substance
authoritarian personality
authoritarian staff behavior
authority(-ies)
- a. figure
- a. figure, parent
- a., medical
- a., physician
- a., rebels against
- a., recognize

authorization
- a. certificate, clinical
- a. for body to be donated for scientific research
- a. for delivery by alternate physician
- a. for treatment of a minor
- a. form, anesthetic
- a. form, autopsy
- a. form, cosmetic surgery
- a. form for operation
- a. form for operation and grafting of tissue
- a. form for recipient of organ transplant
- a. form for removal of tissue for grafting
- a. form for taking and publication of photographs
- a. form for taking of motion pictures of operation
- a. form for televising of operation
- a. form to admit observers
- a. form to use eyes (donor)
- a. form to use eyes (next of kin)
- a. form to use kidney(s) (donor)
- a. form to use kidney(s) (next of kin)
- a., parental

Autima II dual chamber pacemaker
autism
- a., akinetic
- a. disorder
- a., early infantile
- a., infantile

autistic
- a. brain
- a. child
- a. children ▸ stereotyped behavior of
- a. disorder
- a. patient

a. spectrum disorder
a. thinking
autoanalyzer, blood
autobiographical memory
autobiographical recall
autochthonous graft
autochthonous stone
autoclave [*audiclave*]
autoclave gauges
autoclaving, steam
autoclaving sterilization
autocorrelation function
autocorrelation technique ▸ Doppler
autocrine motility factor (AMF)
autodecremental pacing
autodermic graft
autodigestion of connective tissue
autodigestion of pancreatic tissue
autoepidermic graft
autoexacerbating syndrome
autofluoroscope, digital
autogenic
a. feedback training
a. graft
a. relaxation
a. suggestion
a. training
a. training and electroencephalogram (EEG) patterns
a. training and stress-related
problems
a. training, autosuggestion in
a. training for anxiety and tension
a. training for drug abuse
a. training for headache
a. training for hypertension
a. training for insomnia
a. training for migraine headache
a. training in temperature feedback
a. training relaxation exercises
autogenous
a. bone graft
a. graft
a. transplant
a. vein
a. vein graft (VG)
autograft
a., double
a., iliac
a., material
a. ▸ stem cell
autoimmune
a. antibody
a. diabetes
a. disease

a. disease, incurable
a. disorder
a. disorder ▸ chronic
a. hemolytic anemia
a. inner ear disease
a. phenomenon
a. reaction
a. response
a. system disorder
a. thrombocytopenic purpura (ATP)
autoimmunity, beta cell
autoinoculated virus
autologous
a. antibody
a. bland donation
a. blood
a. blood collection
a. blood donations
a. blood transfusion
a. bone marrow transplant
a. chondrocyte implantation
a. clot
a. cultured skin grafting
a. cultured skin transplantation
a. fat graft
a. graft
a. interferon
a. patient donor
a. pericardial patch
a. predeposit donation
a. skin transplantation
a. stem cell transplant
a. transfusion
a. transplant
autolysed, adrenals
autolysis
a., diffuse mucosal
a., focal mucosal
a. of mucosal glands
a. of pancreatic tissue
a., partial
a., postmortem
autolytic, liver
autolytic, pancreas
autolyzed embryo
automated
a. blood pressure cuff
a. border detection
a. border detection ▸
echocardiographic
a. boundary detection system ▸
echocardiographic
a. cervical cell screening system
a. chemistry profile

a. computerized axial tomography
(ACAT)
a. devices, electronic
a. discectomy, percutaneous
a. edge detection
a. exposure
a. external defibrillator (AED)
a. external defibrillator (AED) ▸
SurVivaLink
a. lamellar keratoplasty (ALK)
a. large core breast biopsy
a. monitor
a. multiphasic screening
a. percutaneous lumbar discectomy
a. tray assembly
automatic (Automatic)
a. actions
a. amplification
a. analysis
a. analyzer
a. atrial tachycardia
a. beat
a. behavior
a. bladder
a. BP (blood pressure) monitoring
a. boundary detection
a. bypass
a. chorea
a. collimator
a. data processing (ADP)
a. ectopic tachycardia
a. epilepsy
a. exposure system
a. external defibrillator (AED)
a. fulcrum height adjustment
a. function
a. implantable cardioverter
defibrillator (AICD)
a. implantable defibrillator (AID)
a. implantable defibrillator (AID)
malfunction
a. inflation
a. internal cardioverter defibrillator
(AICD)
a. internal defibrillator
a. interval
a. intracardiac defibrillator
a. mode switching (AMS)
a. movement
a. movement, loss of
a. movements, repetitious
a. oscillometric blood pressure (BP)
monitor
a. pacemaker
a. pacemaker, fully

automatic—*continued*
- a. reflex bladder
- a. repetitive movement
- a. response
- a. resuscitative device (CARD), cardiac
- a. rotating tourniquet
- a. thinking
- a. tomography
- a. ventricular contraction

automatically mediated behavior

automaticity
- a., enhanced
- a., nodal
- a. of performance
- a., pacemaker
- a. ▸ sinus nodal

automatism, epileptic

Auto-MEDI-THERM

autonomic
- a. abnormality
- a. activation of bladder
- a. arousal
- a. ataxia
- a. control by alpha activity
- a. dysfunction
- a. dysreflexia
- a. dysreflexia of bladder
- a. epilepsy
- a. functions
- a. functions ▸ biofeedback hypnotic control of
- a. functions ▸ biofeedback voluntary control of
- a. ganglionic synapse
- a. hyperactivity
- a. hyperreflexia
- a. impairment
- a. innervation of lung
- a. insufficiency
- a. insufficiency, severe
- a. modulation
- a. nerves
- a. nervous system
- a. nervous system and anxiety
- a. nervous system dysfunction
- a. nervous system effect ▸ peripheral
- a. nervous system function ▸ perturbed
- a. nervous system ▸ incomplete development of
- a. nervous system relaxation techniques
- a. neuropathy

- a. parasomnias
- a. reflex
- a. response
- a. response to anxiety-evoking stimuli
- a. sensory innervation
- a. toxicity ▸ peripheral
- a. variables

autonomous
- a. adenoma
- a. depression
- a. ego functioning
- a. induction
- a. plasmid

autonomously, function

autonomy, ego

auto-pedestrian accident

autophagic vacuole

autoplastic graft

autopsy
- a. -acquired group A Streptococcus
- a. -acquired hepatitis
- a. -acquired tuberculosis
- a. anatomic diagnosis
- a. authorization
- a., complete
- a. consent form
- a. denied, permission for
- a. external description
- a. external examination
- a. granted, permission for
- a. gross examination
- a., initial
- a. internal examination
- a. limited
- a. limited to abdomen
- a. limited to brain
- a. limited to heart and lungs
- a. microscopic examination
- a. of brain
- a. permit signed
- a., psychological
- a. report
- a. report cause of death (COD)
- a. requested
- a. studies
- a., total
- a. witness

autoradiographic technique

autoradiography
- a., contract
- a., dip-coating
- a., film-stripping
- a., thick-layer
- a., two-emulsion

autoregulation
- a., heterometric
- a., homeometric
- a., renal

autorhythmic heart muscle cells

autosomal
- a. dominant pattern
- a. dominant polycystic kidney disease (PKD)
- a. dominant transmission
- a. heredity
- a. trait

autosuggestion
- a. in autogenic training
- a. phrases
- a. temperature control

Autosyringe insulin pump

autotoxic cyanosis

autotransferable by conjugation

autotransformer formula

autotransfusion system

autotransfusion unit ▸ Solcotrans

autotransplantation, jejunal

autotransplantation, valve

autumnal catarrh

autumnale, Colchicum

autumnalis
- a., Leptospira
- a., Musca
- a., Trombicula

Auvray incision

auxiliary circulation

auxiliary ventricle

AV (arteriovenous)
- AV aneurysm
- AV block
- AV block, first degree
- AV block ▸ incomplete
- AV block ▸ pseudo-
- AV conduction abnormality
- AV conduction disturbance
- AV conduction tissue
- AV delay interval
- AV discordance
- AV dissociation, complete
- AV endothelial cells
- AV extrasystole
- AV fissure
- AV fistula, Brescio-Cimino
- AV fistula with good bruits
- AV flow rubbing murmur
- AV gradient
- AV junction anomaly
- AV junction motion
- AV junctional bigeminy

AV junctional escape complex
AV junctional escape rhythm
AV junctional extrasystole
AV junctional heart block
AV junctional pacemaker
AV junctional reciprocating tachy-
   cardia
AV junctional rhythm
AV junctional rhythm, accelerated
AV junctional tachycardia
AV leaking
AV nicking
AV nodal conduction
AV nodal extrasystole
AV nodal pathways
AV nodal reentrant paroxysmal
   tachycardia
AV nodal reentrant tachycardia
AV nodal reentry
AV nodal rhythm
AV nodal tachycardia
AV node
AV node ablation
AV node modification
AV node pathway ▸ slow
AV node reentrant
AV orifice
AV reciprocating tachycardia
   (AVRT)
AV reciprocating tachycardia ▸
   antidromic
AV reciprocating tachycardia ▸
   orthodromic
AV reentrant tachycardia ▸
   orthodromic
AV refractory period
AV rim
AV ring
AV septal defect
AV septal structures
AV sequential pacemaker
AV shunt
AV shunt, Cimino
AV shunt, Scribner
AV shunt site
AV (atrioventricular)
AV block, 1st° (first degree)
AV block, 2nd° (second degree)
AV block, 3rd° (third degree)
AV branch block
AV bundle
AV dissociation
AV dissociation, isorhythmic
AV dissociation with interference,
   isorhythmic

AV heart block
AV pacemaker ▸ dual chamber
AV sequential pacemaker
AV synchronous pacemaker
AV synchrony
AV time
AV valve insufficiency
AV Wenckebach biopsy
AVAD (acute ventricular assist device)
availability of health care
available
   a. ▸ donor organs readily
   a. services
   a., treatment resource
avalanche, Townsend's
avascular
   a. graft
   a. necrosis
   a. tissue
AV DO₂ (arteriovenous oxygen
   difference)
Avellis' syndrome
avenger, righteous
average (Average)
   a., age-group
   a. alcoholic
   a. cholesterol level
   a. daily census
   a. daily patient load
   a. deviation
   a. evoked potential (AEP)
   a. evoked response
   a., grade point
   a. intravascular pressure (AIP)
   a. life
   a. mean pressure (AMP)
   a. outcome rate
   a. peak noise
   a. potential
   a. potential electrode
   a. potential reference
   a. pulse magnitude
   a. range of abilities ▸ low
   a. reference
   a. reference electrode, common
   a. remaining lifetime
   a. target absorbed dose
   A. Transients, Computer of
   a. true
   a. volume of air
   a. weight
averaged
   a. echocardiogram ▸ signal-
   a. echocardiography ▸ signal-
   a. electrocardiogram (ECG) ▸ signal

a. electrocardiogram (ECG) ▸ time
   domain signal
a. electrocardiography (ECG) ▸ signal
a. peak velocity ▸ time-
averaging
   a., digital
   a. (EPSA), evoked potential signal
   a., motional
   a., signal
   a. technique, computer
   a. technology
   a., volume
aversion
   a., blunt
   a., chemical
   a. depression
   a. disorder, sexual
   a., electrical
   a., mechanism of taste
   a., shock
   a. therapy
   a. to labor pains ▸ psychogenic
aversive
   a. conditioning
   a. imagery
   a. stimulation, reaction to
   a. stimulus
   a. therapy
   a. therapy, electrical
AVF (arteriovenous fistula)
AVF, Lead
AVI (air velocity index)
avian (Avian)
   a. encephalomalacia
   a. encephalomyelitis
   A. influenza
   a. leukosis
   a. leukosis complex
   a. leukosis virus
   a. tuberculosis
aviation, medicine
aviation sickness
aviator('s)
   a. disease
   a. ear
   a. fracture
   a. stomach
avid
   a. hot spot scintigraphy ▸ infarct
   a. imaging ▸ infarct
   a. myocardial scintigraphy ▸ infarct
   a. scintigraphy, antimyosin infarct
   a. scintigraphy ▸ infarct
AVIDS (acquired violence immune
   deficiency syndrome)

Avila's operation
Avionics scanner, Delmar
avium
- a. complex (MAC) infection ▸ Myco-bacterium
- a. et gallinae, Dermanyssus
- a. intracellulare (MAI), Mycobacterium
- a. intracellulare (MAI) complex ▸ Mycobacterium
- a. intracellulare (MAI) infection ▸ Mycobacterium
- a., Mycobacterium

Avius sequential pacemaker
AVL, Lead
AVM (arteriovenous malformation)
AVM (atrioventricular malformation)
AVN (atrioventricular node)
AVN (atrioventricular node) pathways
AVN (atrioventricular node) reentry
Avogadro's number
avoid(s) [ovoid]
- a. abandonment ▸ frantic effort to
- a. medical care ▸ patient
- a. overuse of muscles
- a. strain in exercise

avoidance
- a. behavior
- a. conditioning in human subjects ▸ escape and
- a. gradient of
- a. of activities
- a. syndrome, school
- a. test, behavioral

avoidant
- a. disorder
- a. disorder of adolescence
- a. disorder of childhood
- a. disorder of childhood or adolescence
- a. personality
- a. personality disorder

AVR
- AVR (arteriovenous ratio)
- AVR (aortic valve replacement)
- AVR Lead

AVRP (atrioventricular refractory period)
AVRT (atrioventricular reciprocating tachycardia)
avulsed
- a. fragment
- a. teeth
- a. teeth, reimplant

avulsing laceration
avulsion [evulsion]

- a. chip fracture
- a., cortex
- a. flap injury
- a. fracture
- a. injury
- a. injury, through-and-through
- a. ▸ lumbar root
- a. of epiphysis
- a. of eyeball
- a. of optic nerve
- a., partial
- a. ▸ peroneus longus muscle
- a., tooth
- a., total
- a., traumatic
- a. ▸ vein ligation and

awake(s)
- a., alert and cooperative ▸ patient
- a. craniotomy
- a. fatigued, patient
- a. recording
- a. state
- a. ▸ struggling to stay
- a. subject, alert

awakening
- a., complete
- a., early morning
- a., forced
- a., momentary
- a., nocturnal
- a., partial
- a., physiological
- a., premature morning
- a. technique

aware of surroundings, patient
awareness (Awareness)
- a., AIDS (acquired immune deficiency syndrome)
- a., alteration of body
- a., altered state of conscious
- a. and alertness ▸ lack of
- a. and change, family
- a. and consciousness
- a. and decrease discomfort ▸ increase
- a., anethesia
- a., auditory
- a., basic
- a., biological
- a., cardiac
- a., concepts of
- a., conscious
- a., drug
- a., emotion
- a. ▸ enhanced sensory

- a., fertility
- a., hazard
- a., health
- a., heart rate control learning and
- a., heightened sense of
- a. in illness, self-
- a., increase
- a., internal
- a., level of
- a. ▸ momentary lapse of
- a., muscle activity and
- a. of illness, length of
- a. of process
- a. of reality
- a. of signal
- a. of touch or taste ▸ heightened
- a., patient safety
- a., patient's
- a., phonemic
- a. process
- a. program
- A., Program, Breast Cancer Detection
- A. Program ▸ Organ Donor
- A., Recognition and Treatment (D/ART) ▸ Depression/
- a., reduced
- a. ▸ reflective self-
- a. relaxation
- A. Resistance Education (DARE) Program ▸ Drug
- a., restful
- a., safety
- a., self-
- a., subjective

away dulling dry, dead cells ▸ flush
away ▸ periosteum stripped
AWI (anterior wall infarction)
awkward motor skills
awl, Wangensteen's
awl, Wilson's
AWMI (anterior wall myocardial infarction)
AWS (alcohol withdrawal syndrome)
Axenfeld
- A. bacillus ▸ Morax-
- A. conjunctivitis ▸ Morax-
- A., diplococcus of Morax-
- A. haemophilus ▸ Morax-
- A. syndrome

Axer's operation
axial
- a. ametropia
- a. aneurysm
- a. angiography

a. asynergy
a. cataract
a. computed tomography (ACT)
a. control
a. embryonal cataract ▸ anterior
a. embryonal cataract ▸ posterior
a. fixation of calcaneus
a. gradient
a. illumination
a. myopia
a. node irradiation, total
a. oblique view ▸ long
a. plane
a. point
a. projection
a. projection, half-
a. projection, inferosuperior
a. projection, lateral oblique
a. projection, medial oblique
a. projection, submento-vertical
a. skeleton
a. stream
a. surface of tooth
a. tomography (ACAT), automated computerized
a. tomography (CAT), computed
a. tomography (CAT) ▸ rapid acquisition computed
a. tomography (CAT) scan, computerized
a. tomography scan ▸ digital holographic (CAT) computerized
a. tomography (CAT) scan ▸ ultrafast computerized
a. tomography (CAT) scanner ▸ helical computerized
a. transverse tomography
axialis extracorticalis congenita ▸ aplasia
axilla [*maxilla*]
axilla, bubonic lymphadenopathy of
axillaris, hidrosadenitis
axillaris, trichomycosis
axillary
a. adenopathy
a. adenopathy ▸ secondary
a. aneurysm
a. arch
a. arch ▸ Lanager's
a. area, right
a. artery
a. block
a. bypass, carotid
a. cataract
a. contents normal ▸ breasts and

a. dissection, radical
a. dissection-radiotherapy (QUART) ▸ quadrantectomy
a. folds
a. fossa
a. hidradenitis
a. line
a. line (AAL) ▸ anterior
a. line (PAL) ▸ posterior
a. lymph node dissection
a. lymph node enlargement ▸ residual
a. lymph node involvement
a. lymph node irradiation
a. lymph node metastasis
a. lymph nodes
a. lymphadenopathy
a. metastases
a. metastases, contralateral
a. muscle, Chassaignac's
a. nerve
a. nerve block
a. nodal metastasis in breast carcinoma
a. nodes
a. projection
a. region
a. site
a. temperature
a. triangle
a. vein
a. view
a. view, Velpeau
axilloaxillary bypass
axilloaxillary bypass ▸ aorto-subclavian carotid-
axillobifemoral bypass
axillofemoral bypass
axioappendicular asynergy
axiodistal (AD)
axiodistocervical (ADC)
axiodistoincisal (ADI)
axiodisto-occlusal (ADO)
axioincisal (AI)
axiolabial (A.La.)
axiolabiogingival (A.La.G)
axiolabiolingual (A.La.L)
axiolingual (AL)
axiolinguogingival (ALG)
axiolinguo-occlusal (ALO)
axiomatic treatment
axiomesial (AM)
axiomesiocervical (AMC)
axiomesiodistal (AMD)
axiomesiogingival (AMG)

axiomesioincisal (AMI)
axiomesio-occlusal (AMO)
axio-occlusal (AO)
axiopulpal (AP)
axis
a. (C-2 vertebra)
a., celiac
a., central
a., cerebrospinal
a., coeliac
a., common
a. cylinder process
a. depth dose of electron beam therapy, central
a. deviation
a. deviation (ALAD), abnormal left
a. deviation (ARAD), abnormal right
a. deviation (LAD) ▸ left
a. deviation, normal
a. deviation (RAD) ▸ right
a. discontinuity, atrial
a., electrical
a., embryonic
a., epistropheus
a. factors, off-
a. ▸ hypophyseal pituitary adrenal
a. ▸ hypothalamic- pituitary-adrenal
a. (HPAA) ▸ hypothalamic pituitary adrenocortical
a. ▸ instantaneous electrical
a. ▸ joule point electrical
a., junctional
a. ligament
a., long
a., long posterior ciliary
a., longitudinal
a. ▸ mean electrical
a. ▸ mean QRS
a. ▸ normal electrical
a. of beam, central
a. of kidney, long
A. I ▸ diagnosis or condition deferred on
a., optic
a. ▸ P wave
a. parasternal view echocardiogram ▸ long
a. parasternal view ▸ short
a. plane ▸ short
a., QRS
a., renal
a., rightward
a., rotation of eye around optical
a. shift
a., short

axis—*continued*
- a., short posterior ciliary
- a. ▸ superior QRS
- a., thoracic
- a., time
- A. II ▸ diagnosis or condition deferred on
- A. two disorder
- a., vertical
- a. view echocardiogram ▸ parasternal long-
- a. view echocardiogram ▸ parasternal short-
- a. view ▸ horizontal long
- a. view, long
- a. view ▸ parasternal long-
- a. view ▸ parasternal short-
- a. view, short
- a. view ▸ vertical long
- a., visual
- a., X
- a., Y
- a., zero isopotential

axodendritic synapse

axon(s)
- a. ▸ dendrites and
- a. hillock
- a. reflex
- a. regenerated

axonal
- a. growth
- a. idiocy spastic amaurotic
- a. reaction

axoplasmic flow

axoplasmic stasis

Ayerza's disease

Ayerza's syndrome

A-Z (Aschheim-Zondek) test

azar (Azar)
- a., canine kala-
- a., infantile kala-
- a., kala-
- a., Mediterranean kala-
- A. Tripod implant cataract lens

azide test, iodine-

azidothymidine (AZT) ▸ medicate patient with

azidothymidine (AZT) treatment

azotemia
- a., extrarenal
- a., nephrosclerosis with
- a., postrenal
- a., prerenal
- a., progressive
- a., renal

azotemic
- a. nephritis
- a. osteodystrophy
- a. uremia

Azotobacter
- A. agilis
- A. chroococcum
- A. indicus

Azotomonas fluorescens

Azotomonas insolita

AZT (azidothymidine) ▸ medicate patient with

AZT (azidothymidine) treatment

Aztec ear

Aztec idiocy

azur granule

azurophil granule

azygoportal interruption

azygos
- a. anterior cerebral artery
- a. arch
- a. lobe
- a. node
- a. vein
- a. vein, left
- a. vein, lesser superior

azygous ganglion

B

B. (bacillus)
B. (borderline)
B antibody, hepatitis
B behavior ▸ type
B Blockers
B carrier, hepatitis
B cell lymphoma
B cells
B core
    Bc. antibody (HBcAb), hepatitis
    Bc. Antigen (Anti-HBc IgM),
        Antibody IgM class to Hepatitis
    Bc. Antigen (Anti-HBc), Total
        Antibody to Hepatitis
B e antibody (HBeAb), hepatitis
B e Antigen (Anti-HBe), Antibody to
    Hepatitis
B e Antigen (HBeAg), Hepatitis
B encephalitis virus ▸ Japanese
B, gastroenteritis paratyphosa
B., hepatitis virus
B (HIB), Hemophilus influenza type
B immune globulin, hepatitis
B infection, hepatitis
B infection, patient immune to
    hepatitis
b knuckle
B (UVB) ▸ light ultraviolet
B line, Kerley's
B, paratyphoid
B personality, Type
B, Salmonella paratyphi
B scan
B., Shigella arabinotarda Type
B surface
    Bs antibody (HBsAB), hepatitis
    Bs Antigen (Anti-HBs), Antibody to
        Hepatitis
    Bs Antigen (HBsAg), Hepatitis
    Bs antigen (HBsAG) reactivity ▸
        hepatitis
B (HIB) vaccine ▸ Hemophilus
    influenza type
B virus(es)
    B.v.
    B.v., Coxsackie
    B.v., (HBV), hepatitis

B.v. infection ▸ chronic hepatitis
B.v., patient has natural immunity to
    hepatitis
B.v., serotype
BA (bacillary angiomatosis)
Ba (barium)
Baastrup's syndrome
Babès-Ernst granules
Babesia equi
Babesia gibsoni
Babinski('s)
    B. downgoing bilaterally
    B. law
    B. reflex
    B. sign
    B. sign, questionable
    B. syndrome
    B. syndrome ▸ Anton-
baby(-ies) ('s)
    b., apnea monitored
    b., blue
    B. Boom
    b., cloud
    b., cocaine
    b., collodion
    b., crack
    b., defective
    b. deteriorated
    b., drug affected
    b., drug exposed
    b., drug-impaired
    b. expired following resuscitation
        attempt
    b. ▸ fetal alcohol
    b. gender selection
    b. grid
    b., high risk
    b. immune system
    b. intubated
    b., knee
    b. syndrome, blue
    b. syndrome, crack
    b. syndrome, gray
    b. syndrome (SBS), shaken
    b. teeth
BABYbird (Bird) respirator
BAC (blood alcohol content)

Baccelli's sign
Bachmann's bundle
bacillary
    b. angiomatosis (BA)
    b. diarrhea, chronic
    b. dysentery
    b. embolism
    b. phthisis
bacille
    b. Calmette-Guërin (BCG)
    b. Calmette-Guërin (BCG)
        immunization
    b. Calmette-Guërin (BCG) vaccine
bacilli
    b., acid-fast
    b., Battey
    b., diphtheroid
    b. ▸ enteric gram-negative
    b., Flexner-Strong
    b., gram-negative
    b. ▸ gram-negative aerobic
    b., gram-negative enteric
    b. ▸ gram's stain negative enteric
    b. infection ▸ gram-negative
    b., influenza
    b., lightly staining gram-negative
        cocco◊
    b., noxious
    b., paracolon
    b., tubercle
bacilliformis, Bartonella
bacillosus, Amoebobacter
bacillus (bacilli) (Bacillus) (B.)
    B. (AFB), acid-fast
    B. acidilactici
    B. aerogenes capsulatus
    B. aertrycke
    B. alvei
    B. anthracis
    B. anthracis, gram-positive
    b., Anthrax
    b., Bang's
    b., Boas-Oppler
    B. botulinus
    B. brevis
    B. bronchisepticus
    B. cereus

bacillus—*continued*
- B. cereus food poisoning
- b. Chauveau's
- B. circulans
- B. coli
- B. diphtheriae
- b., Döderlein's
- b., Ducrey's
- B. dysenteriae
- B. enteritidis
- b., Escherich's
- B. faecalis alcaligenes
- b., Fick's
- b., Flexner
- b., Flexner-Strong
- B. fragilis
- b., Friedländer's
- b., Gärtner's
- b., Ghon-Sachs
- b., glanders
- b., Hansen's
- b., Hofmann's
- b., influenza
- B. influenzae
- b., Johne's
- b., Klebs-Löffler
- b., Klein's
- b., Koch-Weeks
- B. larvae
- B. leprae
- B. licheniformis
- B. mallei
- B. megaterium
- b., Morax-Axenfeld
- b., Morgan's
- b., Newcastle-Manchester
- b., Nocard's
- B. oedematiens
- B. oedematis maligni No. II
- b. organisms, anaerobic
- b., paracolon
- B. pertussis
- B. pestis
- b., Pfeiffer's
- b. pneumonia, Friedländer's
- B. pneumoniae
- B. polymyxa
- b., Preisz-Nocard
- B. proteus
- B. pseudomallei
- B. pseudodiphtheriticum
- B. pumilus
- B. pyocyaneus
- b., rhinoscleroma
- b., Schmitz's

- b., Schmorl's
- b., Shiga's
- b., Sonne-Duval
- B. stearothermophilus
- b., Strong's
- B. subtilis
- B. suipestifer
- b., swine rotlauf
- B. tetani
- b., tetanus
- b., timothy
- b., tubercle
- B. tuberculosis
- b., tularense
- B. typhi
- B. typhosus
- B. welchii
- b., Whitmore's
- B. whitmori

back
- b. and abdomen ▸ pain in
- b. and chest exercises
- b. and in neck ▸ pain in upper
- b., arched lower
- b. -bleeding
- b. brace
- b. brace, Taylor
- b. carrier, hold-
- b., chest or abdomen pain ▸ breathing with
- b., chronic aching
- b. deformity, sway
- b., degenerative disease of
- b. discomfort
- b. discomfort, low
- b. exercise program
- b. extension exercise
- b., eyes rolled
- b., fetal
- b. flattener exerise ▸ low
- b. flow and dilution
- b. from cancer ▸ pain in
- b. from pyelonephritis ▸ pain in
- b. from slipped or ruptured disc ▸ pain in
- b. from TMJ disorder ▸ pain in
- b. from whiplash injury ▸ pain in
- b. ▸ hump in upper
- b., humped
- b., hunched
- b. ▸ inability to straighten
- b. injury ▸ immobilization of
- b. into community ▸ transition
- b. into donor ▸red cells transfused

- b. into normal rhythm ▸ patient shocked
- b. knee
- b. labor
- b., longissimus muscle of
- b., low
- b. mechanism ▸ peeling
- b. muscle spasms ▸ severe
- b. muscles
- b. muscles, strengthen
- b. ▸ nervousness from pain in
- b. nose, saddle-
- b. nose, sway-
- b. ▸ numbness in lower
- b. of tongue ▸ whitish coating
- b. pain
- b. pain, acute
- b. pain after childbirth
- b. pain and weakness
- b. pain ▸ chill with
- b. pain, chronic
- b. pain, chronic intermittent low
- b. pain ▸ cyclic
- b. pain, debilitating
- b. pain extends down legs
- b. pain from disc
- b., pain in
- b. ▸ pain in lower
- b. ▸ pain in middle
- b. pain ▸ intense
- b. pain, low
- b. pain ▸ pain in abdomen with
- b. pain ▸ postpartum low
- b., pain radiating into
- b. pain, severe
- b., patient flexed lower
- b., patient flexed upper
- b. ▸ persistent pain in lower
- b. pressure
- b. problem, postural
- b. problems ▸ reduce risk of
- b. procedure, push-
- b., reposition patient on
- b. rigid
- b., scope drawn
- b. sinew
- b. spasm in
- b. sprain
- b. ▸ stiffness in
- b. strain
- b. strain, chronic low
- b. strain, low
- b. strengthening exercise
- b. stretch exercise ▸ low
- b. stretch exercise ▸ lower

b. stroke
b. surface
b., sway◊
b. syndrome, low
b. syndrome, straight
b. tense
b. type brace ▸chair-
b., urgent symptoms with
b. view ▸ laid
b. with inability to straighten ▸ pain in

backache, chronic low
backache, persistent
backbone, stabilizing the
backfire fracture
backflow
b. of blood
b., pyelolymphatic
b., pyelorenal
b., pyelotubular
b., pyelovenous

background (bg.)
b. activity
b. activity, diminution of
b. count
b. cultural-ethnic
b. density
b., emotional
b. erase
b. form
b. nuclear dust
b. of slow activity
b. pattern
b. program
b., psychophysiological
b. radiation
b. radiation, natural
b. retinopathy
b. signal
b. subtraction technique
b. system

backing IV (intravenous) fluids, piggy-
backscatter
b. analysis
b. factor
b. peak

backstroke injury
backward
b. and upward, displacement of larynx
b. bending exercise
b. flow of blood
b. heart failure
b. into bladder ▸ semen flows

b. movement

backwash of stomach acid into esophagus
bacteremia(s)
b., Bartonella Quintana
b., biliary
b., catheter-associated
b. ▸ catheter-related
b., Enterobacter
b. ▸ gram's stain negative
b., invasive
b., nosocomial
b., Pseudomonas
b., staphylococcal
b. ▸ Staphylococcus aureus (aureus)
b., transient
b. ▸ venous access device-related

bacteremic shock
bacteria
b., acid-fast
b. ▸ airborne molds and
b., anaerobic
b. and fungi
b., anthrax
b., antibiotic-resistant
b. ▸ Bartonella henselae topical
b., body's natural balance
b., botulinum
b., capsulated
b., cellulose breakdown
b., cholera
b., clinical isolates of
b., clumps of
b., cluster of
b., coliform
b., colon
b., colonies of
b., controlling skin
b. diet, low
b. ▸ disease-producing
b., drug resistant
b., encapsulated
b., endogenous
b., enteric
b., facultative
b. ▸ flesh eating
b. ▸ food-borne
b., foot
b. -free environment
b. -free stage of bacterial endocarditis
b., gram-negative
b., gram-positive
b. ▸ harmful antibiotic-resistant

b. in blood smear
b. in feces
b. in urine
b., intracellular
b., invading
b., killer
b., lightly staining coiled
b., Lyme disease
b., microscopic strep
b., odor-causing
b., oral
b., pathogenic
b., plaque
b., pneumococcal
b., pneumococcus
b., predominant resistant
b., pseudomonas
b., pyogenic
b. ▸ resistant strains of
b. resistant to drugs
b., rod
b., rod-shaped
b., salmonella
b., specific strain of
b., spiral shaped
b., streptococcal
b., transmissible lysis of
b., transmission of
b., viable
b. zoonosis

bacteriacea, enteromycosis
bacterial
b. agglutination
b. allergy
b. analysis
b. aneurysm
b. antagonism
b. antagonism, induced
b. antigens
b. aortitis
b. asthma
b. balance in digestive tract
b. blood infection
b. bronchitis
b. cell
b. cell membrane
b. cell unattached to chromosome
b. cell wall
b. chromosome
b. cirrhosis
b. colonies, submucosal
b. colonization
b. colonization, airway
b. colony
b. concentrations, airborne

bacterial—continued
- b. conjunctivitis
- b. contamination
- b. contamination of tissue
- b. content
- b. corneal ulcer
- b. culture
- b. cystitis
- b. disease
- b. encephalitis
- b. endaortitis
- b. endocarditis (BE)
- b. endocarditis (ABE) ▸ acute
- b. endocarditis, bacteria-free stage of
- b. endocarditis (SBE) ▸ subacute
- b. endospores
- b. enteritis
- b. etiology
- b. exacerbation, acute
- b. flora
- b. flora, balance of
- b. flora, mixed
- b. flora, natural
- b. flora ▸ normal
- b. foodborne illness
- b. gene
- b. genera
- b. genetic
- b. genetic variations
- b. genome
- b. growth
- b. growth on feet
- b. heart valve infection
- b. infection
- b. infection ▸ control of nosocomial
- b. infection, mixed
- b. infection of bloodstream
- b. infection of cornea
- b. infection of lung
- b. infection of meninges
- b. infection of skin
- b. infection ▸ prevention of nosocomial
- b. infection, secondary
- b. infection, source of
- b. infection, spread
- b. infiltrate, mixed
- b. keratitis
- b. kinase
- b. labyrinthitis
- b. lesion
- b. meningitis
- b. meningitis, acute
- b. meningitis, adult
- b. meningitis, child
- b. meningitis ▸ meningococcal
- b. morphology
- b. myocarditis
- b. myocarditis, acute
- b. nephritis
- b. nephritis, diffuse
- b. organisms
- b. origin
- b. otitis media, acute
- b. overgrowth
- b. pathogenesis of infection
- b. pathogens
- b. pericarditis
- b. peritonitis
- b. peritonitis (SBP), spontaneous
- b. pharyngitis
- b. phlebitis
- b. plaque
- b. pneumonia
- b. prostatitis
- b. prostatitis, acute
- b. prostatitis, chronic
- b. protein
- b. putrefaction
- b. resistance
- b. ribosome
- b. satellite
- b. sepsis
- b. shock
- b. shock ▸ advanced stages of
- b. shock ▸ complementary therapy of
- b. shock ▸ management of
- b. sinusitis ▸ acute
- b. skin infection
- b. species
- b. spectrum
- b. spores
- b. toxins
- b. vaginitis
- b. vaginosis
- b. vegetations
- b. virus

bactericidal
- b. antibiotic
- b. concentration
- b. concentration, minimal
- b. effect, synergistic
- b. level, minimal
- b. rays
- b. tissue ▸ serum
- b. titer
- b. titer ▸ serum

bacterid/bacteride

bacteriogenic agglutination
bacteriologic diagnosis
bacteriological index
bacteriolytic immunity
bacteriolytic reaction
bacteriophage plaque
bacteriophagic particle
bacteriostatic
- b. activity
- b. agents
- b. antibiotic
- b. soap

bacteriotoxic endometritis
bacterium (Bacterium)
- B. aerogenes
- B. aeruginosa
- B. aeruginosum
- b., airborne
- B. choleraesuis
- B. cloacae
- B. coli
- b., diplococci
- b. diplococcus
- b., donor
- B. dysenteriae
- b., Helicobacter pylori
- B. pestis bubonicae
- b., pneumonia-causing
- b., Proprioni
- B. sonnei
- b., spherical
- b., staphylococcus
- b., streptococcal
- b., streptococcus
- B. tularense
- B. typhosum

bacteriuria
- b., asymptomatic
- b. ▸ nursing home
- b., polymicrobial

Bacteroides (bacteroides)
- b., anaerobic
- B. asaccharolytica
- B. bivius
- B. buccae
- B. corrodens
- B. fragilis
- B. fragilis infections
- B. fragilis isle
- B. funduliformis
- B. fusiformis
- B. gingivalis
- B. intermedius
- B. melaninogenicus
- B. oralis

B. pneumosintes
B. ramosus
bad
   b. breath
   b. breath, chronic
   b. breath from bronchitis
   b. breath from cold
   b. dietary habits
   b. self-talk
   b. taste in mouth
Badal's operation
badge, film
Badgley's operation
Baehr
   B. lesion ▸ Löhlein
   B. -Löhlein lesion
Baelz's syndrome
BAEP (brainstem auditory evoked
   potentials)
BAER (brainstem auditory evoked
   response)
Baer's nystagmus
Baer's vesicle
Baffes transplant
baffle
   b. fenestration
   b. ▸ Gore Tex
   b., intra-atrial
   b. leak
   b. ▸ Mustard atrial
   b. operation, atrial
   b., pericardial
   b., Senning-type intra-atrial
bag(s)
   b., air
   b., Ambu
   b., Champtier de Ribes
   b., colostomy
   b. ▸ fatty eye
   b., Hofmeister drainage (dr'ge)
   b., Hollister drainage (dr'ge)
   b., ice-
   b., ileostomy
   b. of waters
   b. of water bulging
   b. of waters ▸ ruptured
   b., Politzer air
   b., resuscitation
   b. under eyes
   b. with drip chamber ▸ closed
      urinary drainage (dr'ge)
   b. ▸ wrinkles, sags and
Bagdad Spring anemia
BagEasy disposable manual
   resuscitator

baggy eyelids, droopy,
baggy heart
bagpipe sign
bail ▸ hospitalized patients on
baileyi, Cryptosporidium
bailout stenting
bailout valvuloplasty
Bainbridge reflex
Bakamjian flap
baked tongue
Baker('s) (baker)
   b. asthma
   B. cyst
   B. cyst ▸ ruptured
   b., electric
   b. leg
   B. syndrome
Bakwin-Eiger syndrome
BAL (British anti-lewisite)
balance
   b., acid-base
   b. activities
   b., alternate binaural loudness
   b., ambulation
   b., analytical
   b. and coordination
   b. and coordination ▸ gait,
   b. and coordination ▸ lack of
   b. and coordination ▸ loss of
   b. and coordination ▸ maintain
   b. and flexibility ▸ endurance,
      strength,
   b., biochemical
   b., body
   b., body's fluid
   b., brain's delicate
   b., calcium
   b. check, muscle
   b., chemical
   b., chronic disordered water
   b., ▸ deteriorating sense of
   b. disorder
   b. disorder ▸ gait and
   b. ▸ disordered water
   b. ▸ dysmobility rehabilitation and
   b., electrolyte
   b., enzyme
   b. exercise
   b. ▸ feeling off-
   b., fluid
   b. ▸ fluid and electrolyte
   b., genic
   b., hearing and
   b., hormonal
   b., impaired

   b. ▸ impaired posture and
   b. improvement technique
   b. in body, calcium
   b. in digestive tract ▸ bacterial
   b. in neonatal lung ▸ fluid
   b., loss of
   b., maintaining fluid
   b. mechanism
   b. mechanism of inner ear
   b. mechanism to brain
   b., metabolic
   b., mineral
   b., monaural bifrequency loudness
   b. motion clinic
   b. ▸ muscle mass, strength and
   b., muscular
   b. ▸ normal hormonal
   b., normal muscle
   b., occlusal
   b. of bacteria, body's natural
   b. of bacterial flora
   b. of body, salt and water
   b. of heart ▸ metabolic
   b. of vagina, acid
   b., poor
   b. rehabilitation ▸ habituation and
   b. rehabilitation therapy ▸ vestibular
      and
   b. ▸ rest and exercise
   b. restoration, electrolyte
   b., safe standing
   b., sense of
   b. ▸ severe disordered water
   b., sitting
   b. skills
   b., standing
   b. ▸ sudden loss of
   b., sympathovagal
   b. (DWB) ▸ syndrome of disordered
      water
   b. test
   b. test, Fowler loudness
   b., torsion
   b. training
   b., tremor, weakness and rigidity ▸
      poor
   b., water
balanced
   b. alignment
   b. amplifier
   b. anesthesia
   b. bite
   b. circulation
   b. diet
   b. diet, nutritionally

balanced—*continued*
- b. diet, well
- b. exercise program
- b. nutritional planning
- b. occlusion
- b. percent (PB%) ▸ phonetic
- b., phonetically
- b. physical profile
- b. salt solution
- b. skeletal traction
- b. traction

balancing contact
balancing side
balaniceps, Taenia
balanitic epispadias
balanitis
- b., candida
- b. circinata
- b. diabetica
- b., Follmann's
- b. gangraenosa
- b., gangrenous
- b. xerotica obliterans

balanoplasty operation
balantidial colitis
balantidial dysentery
Balantidium coli
bald tongue
bald tongue, Sandwith's
bald spot
balding, frontal
balding process
baldness
- b., crown
- b. ▸ female pattern
- b., male
- b., male pattern
- b., partial
- b., patchy
- b., pattern
- b., prevent
- b., temporary
- b., total
- b. treatment

Baldwin's operation
Baldy's operation
Baldy-Webster operation
Balfour
- B. gastric resection
- B. gastroenterostomy
- B. infective granule

Balint's syndrome
Balkan nephritis
Balkan nephropathy
Balke exercise stress test

Balke-Ware test
ball(s) (Ball's)
- b. -and-cage prosthesis
- b. -and-cage valve ▸ Starr-Edwards
- b. -and-socket joint
- b. - and socket prosthesis
- b. -catcher's projection
- b. clasp
- b., fungus
- b. hemorrhage ▸ eight-
- b. implant, acrylic
- b. implant material ▸ acrylic
- b. implant, meshed
- b. -in-cage prosthetic valve
- b., insertion plastic
- b., keratin
- B. method
- b. of foot
- b. of foot, pain in
- B. operation
- b. osteotomy ▸ cup-and-
- b. ▸ pleural fibrin
- b., polyethylene
- b. prosthesis, caged-
- b. prosthetic valve, caged
- b. pulse, cannon
- b. ▸ renal fungus
- b. roll foot exercise ▸ golf
- b. thrombus
- b. tip electrode
- b. valve
- b. valve, caged
- b. valve prosthesis
- b. valve prosthesis, DeBakey
- b. valve prosthesis ▸ Starr-Edwards
- b. valve, prosthetic
- b. valve ▸ Starr-Edwards prosthetic
- b. valve thrombus
- b. variance
- b. wedge

Ballantyne-Runge syndrome
Ballerup Citrobacter ▸ Bethesda-
ballet (Ballet's)
- b., cardiac
- B. disease
- B. sign

ballistocardiogram examination
ballistocardiogram study
balloon(s)
- b. ablation ▸ thermal
- b. angioplasty
- b. angioplasty, adjunctive
- b. angioplasty, complementary
- b. angioplasty ▸ kissing

- b. angioplasty (LABA) ▸ laser-assisted
- b. angioplasty ▸ percutaneous
- b. angioplasty (POBA) ▸ plain old
- b. angioplasty ▸ salvage
- b. angioplasty (TPBA) ▸ thermal/perfusion
- b. aortic valvotomy
- b. aortic valvuloplasty
- b. aortic valvuloplasty ▸ percutaneous
- b. atrial septostomy
- b. catheter angioplasty (BCA)
- b. catheter, Rashkind
- b. cell melanoma
- b. cells
- b. centered argon laser
- b. coarctation angioplasty
- b. commissurotomy ▸ mitral
- b. commissurotomy ▸ percutaneous mitral
- b. compression
- b. coronary angioplasty
- b. counterpulsation
- b. counterpulsation, intra-aortic
- b. deflation, intra-aortic
- b. dilatation
- b. dilatation, prostatic
- b. dilated area
- b. dilation
- b., esophageal
- b. expandable intravascular stent
- b., inflatable
- b. inflated
- b. inflation
- b. inflation, intra-aortic
- b. inserted, cardiac catheter with
- b., laser
- b. laser angioplasty
- b., latex
- b. lead, endocardial
- b. -like dilation of artery
- b. mitral commissurotomy
- b. mitral valvotomy
- b. mitral valvotomy ▸ repeat
- b. mitral valvuloplasty
- b. mitral valvuloplasty ▸ percutaneous
- b. -occlusion pulmonary angiography
- b. out ▸ arterial wall
- b., prism
- b. pulmonary valvotomy
- b. pulmonary valvuloplasty

b. pulmonic valvuloplasty ▸ percutaneous
b. pump
b. pump, aortic
b. pump, cardiac
b. pumping (IABP), intra-aortic
b. ▸ radiofrequency hot
b. rupture
b. -shaped heart
b. shunt
b. sickness
b., small inflatable
b. tamponade
b. technique ▸ kissing
b. technique ▸ Rashkind
b. therapy ▸ uterine
b., thermal
b. tricuspid valvotomy
b. tuboplasty
b. valve ▸ mitral
b. valvotomy
b. valvotomy, double
b. valvotomy ▸ percutaneous mitral
b. valvotomy ▸ single
b. valvuloplasty
b. valvuloplasty catheterization
b. valvuloplasty, double
b. valvuloplasty ▸ intracoronary thrombolysis
b. valvuloplasty ▸ multiple
b. valvuloplasty ▸ percutaneous
b. valvuloplasty (PMB) ▸ percutaneous mitral
b. valvuloplasty ▸ percutaneous transluminal
b. valvuloplasty ▸ single
b. valvuloplasty ▸ triple
b. videoscope surgery

ballooning
b. mitral cusp syndrome
b. -out of artery wall
b. -out of blood vessel

ballottable patella
ballottement
b., abdominal
b., indirect
b., ocular
b., renal

Balme's cough
balnei granuloma
balsa wood block
Balser's fatty necrosis
Bamatter's syndrome
Bamberger('s)
B. area

B. bulbar pulse
B. fluid
B. -Marie disease
B. sign

bamboo hair
bamboo spine
Bancroft-Plenk operation
bancrofti
b., Filaria
b., microfilaria
b., Wuchereria

Bancroft's filariasis
band(s)
b., adhesive
b. -aid surgery
b., alpha
b., BB
b., beta
b., broad
b., broad adhesive
b. cell
b., contraction
b., delta
b. dense metaphyseal
b. effect, rubber
b., encircling
b. -form granulocyte
b., frequency
b. frequency analysis, broad
b. frequency analysis, narrow
b., germline
b., hymenal
b., iliotibial
b., intratesticular
b. keratitis
b. keratopathy
b. ligation of hemorrhoids ▸ rubber
b. ligation, rubber
b. -like angina
b., MB
b., MM
b., Meckel's
b. metaphyseal
b., monoclonal
b., myocardial
b., narrow frequency
b. necrosis, contraction
b. neutrophil
b. of adhesions
b. of density
b. of muscles ▸ taut
b. of scar tissue
b., oligoclonal
b., omental adhesive
b. operation ▸ gastric

b., Parham
b. procedure ▸ gastric
b. ▸ pulmonary artery
b. saw effect
b., selected frequency
b., theta
b., ventricular
b. -width
b., Z

bandage
b., abdominal
b., Ace
b., adhesive
b. applied, gentle pressure
b., Barton
b., circular
b., compression
b., Desault's
b., elastic
b., Elastoplast
b., Esmarch
b., figure-of-8
b., gauze
b., Gibney's
b., Gibson's
b., immobilizing
b., Kerlix
b., Kling
b., many-tailed
b., plaster
b., pressure
b., Priessnitz
b., protective
b., roller
b., Sayre's
b. scissors
b., scultetus
b., spica
b., stockinette amputation
b., triangular
b., Velpeau's

bandaging and splinting limb
bandaging, circular
bandbox resonance
bandbox sound
banded gastroplasty, Mason vertical
banded gastroplasty, vertical
bandelette, keratitis
banding, chromosome
banding, pulmonary artery
bandpass filter
bandpass filter ▸ triple
bandwidth
b., electroencephalogram (EEG) channel

bandwidth—*continued*
  b., gradient
  b., low
Bang/Bhang (marijuana)
Bang's bacillus
banjo-string adhesions
bank(s) (Bank)
  B., Blood
  B., Bone Graft
  B., Cell
  b., community blood
  b., eye
  B. for Sight Restoration, Eye
  b., gene
  b., hospital-based blood
  b. in brain ▸ memory
  B., Medical Eye
  b., registry and tissue
  B., Skin
  b., skin donor
  b. stress, blood
  b., temporal bone
  B., Tissue
  b. ▸ umbilical cord blood
Bankart('s)
  B. lesion
  B. operation
  B. procedure
  B. procedure for shoulder
    dislocation
banking, cryopreserved tissue
banking, ovarian tissue
Bannister disease
Banter's syndrome
Banti's disease
Banti's syndrome
bar(s) (Bar)('s)
  b., acrylic
  b. appearance ▸ jail
  b., arch
  b., coracoclavicular
  b., cricopharyngeal
  b., custom-made arch
  b., Erich's arch
  b., fixed arch
  b. formation, median
  b., fracture
  b., grab
  B. incision
  b., mandibular arch
  b., outrigger
  b., Passavant's
  b., patient ambulates on parallel
  b., physeal
  b., stabilization

  b., stall
  B. syndrome
  B. syndrome ▸ Louis-
  b., Thronton
  b., trapeze
  b., Winters arch
Barany('s)
  B. apparatus
  B. box
  B. maneuver, Nylen-
  B. pointing test
  B. sign
  B. symptom
  B. syndrome
  B. test
barb-tip lead
barbae, Aspergillus
barbae, Penicillium
barbed epicardial pacing lead
barber surgeon
barber's itch
barbiturate(s) (Barbs)
  b. (Beans)
  b. (Blockbusters)
  b. (Bluebirds)
  b. (Blue Devils)
  b. (Blue Heavens)
  b. (Blues)
  b. (Christmas Trees)
  b. (Downers)
  b. (Foolpills)
  b. (Goofballs)
  b. (Green Dragon)
  b. (Ludes)
  b. (Mexican Reds)
  b. (Nebbies)
  b. (Nimbles)
  b. (Pajao Rojo)
  b. (Pink Ladies)
  b. (Pinks, Reds and Blues)
  b. (Purple Hearts)
  b. (Quads)
  b. (Quas)
  b. (Rainbows)
  b. (Redbirds)
  b. (Red Devils)
  b. (Reds)
  b. (Sleeping Pills)
  b. (Soapers)
  b. (Sopes)
  b. (Stumblers)
  b. (Tooies)
  b. (Trees)
  b. (Yellows)
  b. (Yellow jackets)

  b. abuse
  b. addiction
  b. coma
  b. ingested
  b. injected
  b., intermediate acting
  b., intravenous (IV)
  b., long-acting
  b., nitrous oxide
  b. poisoning
  b., short-acting
  b. similarly acting dependence
  b. therapy
  b. withdrawal
Bard('s)
  B. cardiopulmonary support pump
  B. Clamshell septal umbrella
  B. -Pic syndrome
  B. sign
  B. syndrome
Bardeen's primitive disc
Bardelli's operation
Bardenheuer's extension
bare crown
bariatric surgery
barium (Ba)
  b. adherent to esophageal walls
  b. and air ▸ high viscosity
  b. artifact
  b. burger
  b. column
  b. enema (BE)
  b. enema, double contrast
  b. enema (BE) examination
  b. esophagram
  b. filled esophagus
  b., fleck of
  b. ingestion
  b. meal
  b. meal, dumping of
  b. meal study
  b. mixture
  b., normal evacuation of
  b. passed through esophagus into
    stomach
  b. ▸ pocketing of
  b., reflux of
  b., residual
  b. retained
  b., retrograde flow of
  b. roentgenographic exam
  b. roentgenography
  b. stasis, secondary
  b. sulfate
  b. sulfate contrast medium

b. swallow
b., transient time of
bark cough ▸ seal-
bark disease ▸ maple
Barkan's goniolens
Barkan's operation
Barker classification ▸ Keith-
Wagener-
Barker's operation
barking cough
Barkman's reflex
Barkow, colliculus of
barley sugar
Barlow's syndrome
Barnard mitral valve prosthesis
barometer-maker's disease
barometric pressure
barometric trauma
Baron implant cataract lens
Baron technique
baroreceptor
b., cardiac
b. reflex
b. sensitization
baroreflex activity ▸ sinoaortic
barotitis media
barotrauma, otitic
barotrauma, pulmonary
Barr('s)
B. body
B. chorioretinal disease ▸ Epstein-
B. (EB) disease, Epstein-
B. (EB) syndrome, Epstein-
B. virus (CEBV) ▸ chronic Epstein-
B. virus (EB virus/EBV) ▸ Epstein-
Barré('s)
B. polyneuritis ▸ Guillain-
B. pyramidal sign
B. syndrome ▸ Guillain-
B. syndrome, Landry-Guillain-
B. syndrome ▸ Lieou-
barred teeth
barrel
b. aorta, double-
b. enterostomy ▸ gun-
b. -hooping compression
b. -shaped chest
b. -shaped thorax
barreled colostomy ▸ double-
barreling distortion
Barrels (LSD)
Barrett('s)
B. adenocarcinoma
B. epithelium
B. esophagus

B. syndrome
B. syndrome, Eagle-
B. test ▸ Paul-Bunnell-
barrier(s)
b. against environment
b., air blood
b., alteration of blood-brain
b., anatomic
b., attitudinal
b., blood air
b., blood aqueous
b. (BBB), blood-brain
b., blood cerebrospinal fluid (CSF)
b., blood gas
b., blood retinal
b., blood skin
b., blood thymus
b., cerebrospinal fluid (CSF) brain
b. contraceptive
b. device
b. disruption chemotherapy, blood-
brain
b., emotional
b., endothelial
b., environmental
b. -free accessibility
b. function
b. ▸ gastric component reflex
b., gel
b., integumentary
b., language
b. method
b., mucosal
b., natural
b., physical
b., placental
b. precautions
b., psychological
b. shield
b. ▸ small intestine as defense
b., societal
b. to independence, architectural
b. to recovery
b. to skin transplantation
b., treatment
Barrio's operation
Bársony-Polgár syndrome
Bartholin('s)
B. cyst
B. duct cyst
B. gland
B. gland cyst, marsupialization
B., ▸ urethral and Skene's (BUS)
glands
Barth's hernia

Barton('s)
B. bandage
B. fracture
B. operation
Bartonella
B. bacilliformis
B. henselae topical bacteria
B. Quintana bacteremia
Bart's hemoglobin
Bartter's syndrome
Barwell's operation
basal
b. acid output
b. angle
b., anterior
b. arch
b. body temperature (BBT)
b. cell
b. cell adenoma
b. cell cancer
b. cell carcinoma
b. cell carcinoma of conjunctive
b. cell carcinoma of ear and nose
b. cell carcinoma of eyelid
b. cell carcinoma of lip
b. cell carcinoma, pigmented
b. cell carcinoma, superficial
b. cell epithelioma
b. cell layer
b. cell lesion
b. cell nevus syndrome
b. cell skin cancer
b. cerebral artery
b. cistern
b. crepitations
b. decidua
b. diastolic murmurs
b. drainage (dr'ge)
b. ectoderm
b. electrodes
b. epithelium
b. forebrain
b. forebrain cells
b. ganglia
b. ganglia calcification
b. ganglia ▸ histologic sections of
b. ganglion
b. ganglion disease
b. gastric secretion
b. granule
b. iridectomy
b. joint of thumb
b. joint reflex
b., lateral
b. layer

basal—*continued*
- b. layer of bronchial epithelium
- b., medial
- b. metabolic rate (BMR)
- b. metabolic temperature graph
- b. metabolism
- b. neck fracture
- b., posterior
- b. pulmonary atelectasis
- b. ridge
- b. seat
- b. segment
- b. segmental bronchus
- b. septal hypertrophy
- b. skin resistance
- b. skull fracture
- b. stalk
- b. subarachnoid space
- b. tuberculosis
- b. vein

basalioma syndrome, nevoid
basalis, decidua
basalis of Meynert, nucleus
basaloid carcinoma
base(s) [*basis*]
- b. abusers ▸ cocaine free-
- b. alterations, acid
- b., aortic
- b., appendiceal
- b., atelectasis left lung
- b., atelectasis right lung
- b. balance, acid-
- b., bladder
- b., blood buffer
- b., buffer
- b. carcinoma, tongue
- b., cleavage
- b. cocaine ▸ long-term use of free-
- b. cocaine ▸ smoking free-
- b. crystal, free-
- b. deficit
- b. disorder, acid
- b. disturbance, acid
- b., effusion left
- b., effusion right
- b. element
- b. excess
- b., fluid density in left/right
- b., fluid density in right
- b., fluid left
- b., fluid right
- b. form, free-
- b. (cocaine sulphate), free-
- b., funding
- b. heroin, free-

- b. hospital
- b. imbalance, acid
- b., infiltrate left-right lung
- b., left lung
- b. lesion ▸ benign skull
- b. ▸ malignant skull
- b., lung
- b. management, data
- b. material
- b. of aorta
- b. of appendix
- b. of brain
- b. of fracture site
- b. of left lung
- b. of lung
- b. of neck
- b. of neck, bruit in
- b. of pulmonary trunk
- b. of right lung
- b. of skull
- b. of stapes
- b. of stapes ▸ fixator muscle of
- b. of thumb
- b. of tongue ▸ squamous cell carcinoma
- b. of tumor, painting
- b. pairs
- b. physiology, acid
- b., provide reality
- b., purine
- b., pyrimidine
- b., rales audible at
- b. rates ▸ establishing normative
- b. ratio ▸ acid-
- b., reality
- b., skull
- b. therapy, acid/
- b., total

baseball
- b. finger
- b. finger fracture
- b. pitcher's elbow
- b. suture

based (Based)
- b. artificial joint ▸ silicone-
- b. blood bank, ▸ hospital-
- b., brain-
- b., broad-
- b. cocaine, ▸ free-
- b. cognitive skills ▸ latency-
- b. composite ▸ resin-
- b. conjunctival flap ▸ fornix
- b. counseling, abstinence-
- b. digital imaging ▸ computer
- b. disease ▸ gene-

- b. exercises, land-
- b. gait ▸ wide-
- b. intervention ▸ physician-
- b. intervention ▸ school-
- b. laxative, psyllium-
- b. learning disability ▸ language-
- b. learning problem ▸ language-
- b. mastery fantasy ▸ trauma-
- b. Maze procedure, catheter-
- b. on biopsy, diagnosis
- b. pain control, brain-
- b. physician ▸ hospital-
- b. physician ▸ site-
- b. psychiatry ▸ managed care-
- b. quad cane, patient independent with small
- b. residential program ▸ exercise-
- b. Residential Facility (CBRF) Community
- b. rogaine, minoxidil-
- b. scars, broad
- b. scars ▸ wide broad
- b. stress management ▸ hospital-
- b. therapy ▸ activity
- b. therapy ▸ individual solution-
- b. transvenous angiography ▸ synchronous-
- b. treatment, family
- b. tube feeding, casein
- b. tube feeding, milk
- b. tumor, pleural

basedowificata, struma
Basedow's disease
Basedow's goiter
baseline(s)
- b., alternate sides of
- b. arrhythmia
- b. artifact
- b. behavior
- b. bradycardia
- b. coronary angiogram
- b. cortisol level
- b. data ▸ objective
- b. dyspnea index
- b. echocardiography
- b. EKG (electrocardiogram)
- b. for future problems, studies to serve as
- b. exercise test
- b. infection
- b. level
- b. level, initial
- b. mammogram
- b. mammography
- b. measurement

b. morbidity
b., oscillation of
b. performance
b. procedure
b., Reid's
b. rhythm
b. studies
b. sway
b. swing
b. tachycardia
b. treatment
b. variability
b. variability of fetal heart rate

basement
b. membrane
b. membrane antibody
b. membrane antibody, antiglomerular
b. membrane, capillary
b. membrane, glomerular
b. membrane ▸ myocardial
b. tissue

baseplate gutta-percha
bases [*basis*]
bases, rales audible at
bas-fond
bas-fond formation
bashful bladder
bashing, gay
basic
b. activity ▸ patient unable to perform
b. awareness
b. blood pressure (BP)
b. breastfeeding
b. cardiac diet
b. cardiac life support
b. cycle length
b. diet
b. drive
b. drive cycle length
b. dysphoric mood
b. fibroblast growth factor
b. human functions
b. hygiene
b. immunization
b. kneading maneuver during massage
b. leukemia cell structure
b. life-preserving functions
b. life support
b. magenta
b. mental skills
b. occipital rhythm
b. optional rhythm

b. physical skills
b. research
b. rhythmic frequency
b. sensation
b. stain
b. transfer, patient completes
b. trauma framework
b. variable

basicranial flexure
Basidiobolus haptosporus
basidiomycetous fungi
basihyal bone
basilar
b. aneurysm ▸ lower
b. angiography
b. apophysis
b. artery
b. artery aneurysm
b. artery aneurysm ▸ dissecting
b. artery, bifurcation of
b. artery, organizing thrombus of
b. artery patient
b. artery ▸ total occlusion
b. atelectasis
b. bone
b. cistern
b. extension
b. fracture
b. gliosis
b. hemiplegic migraine
b. impression
b. infiltrate
b. insufficiency
b. insufficiency, vertebro
b. intracerebral vessels
b. membrane
b. meningitis
b. migraine
b. portion of lung
b. projection
b. rales
b. scarring
b. segment
b. skull fracture
b. suture

basilaris cranii
basilaris, sulcus
basilic
b. artery
b. vein
b. vein, median
basilicum, Ocimum
basin
b., emesis
b., pelvic

b., sterile saline
basing, chasing and
basing cocaine, free-
basiotripsy, fetal
basiotripsy operation
basis [*stasis*]
b., ambulatory
b., as-needed
b., biochemical
b. bundles
b., chemotherapy continued on an outpatient
b., congenital
b. crania, foramen ovale
b., empirical
b., experimental
b., genetic
b., limited
b., neurological
b., objective
b. of hyperfractionation, biologic
b. of radiation therapy, biologic
b., outpatient
b., patient followed on outpatient
b., physiologic
b. pontis
b., prophylactic
b., psychogenic
b. pulmonis
b., radiation therapy on prophylactic
b., random
b., treated on an outpatient
b., trial
b., voluntary
b., weekly outpatient

basivertebral vein
basket extraction, blind
basketball heels
basocellulare, carcinoma
basophil/basophile
b., amphophilic
b. cells, vacuolated
b. count, absolute
b. granular leukocytes
b. granules
b. leukopenia
b., polymorphonuclear
basophilia, punctate
basophilic
b. adenoma
b. cell
b. cytoplasm
b. erythroblast
b. erythrocyte
b. hyperpituitarism

basophilic—*continued*
- b. leukemia
- b. leukopenia
- b. myelocytes
- b. normoblast
- b. pleomorphic irregularly shaped nuclei
- b. stippling

basosquamous cell carcinoma
basovertical projection
Bassen-Kornzweig syndrome
Basset's operation
Bassini('s)
- B. inguinal hernia repair
- B. operation
- B. repair
- B. technique
- B. -type hernia repair

bastard measles
Basterra's operation
BAT (bat)
- B. (B-mode Acquisition and Targeting)
- b. ear
- b. wing shadow

bataviae, Leptospira
Bateman('s)
- B. operation
- B. prosthesis
- B. UPF (universal proximal femur) prosthesis

bath(s)
- b. anxiety
- b., bed
- b., blitz
- b., coal tar
- b., complete
- b. ▸ daily warm stiz
- b. ▸ healing power of warm
- b. ▸ iodine-medicated
- b., paraffin
- b., sand
- b., sitz
- b. solution
- b., sponge
- b., tub
- b., vapor
- b., whirlpool

bathe, dress and eat
bathe technique ▸ flush and
bathing
- b., feeding, grooming ▸ dressing,
- b. self-care deficit
- b., sink-side

- b. with cueing, patient independent in

bathroom
- b. aids assessment
- b. privileges (BRP)
- b. safety devices
- b. strategy

bathtub and shower transfer
Batten-Mayou disease
battered
- b. child syndrome
- b. husband
- b. husband syndrome
- b. parent syndrome
- b. spouse syndrome (BSS)
- b. wife syndrome

battering
- b., psychological
- b., sexual
- b. syndrome, child

battery
- b. -assisted-heart-assist device
- b. box, bronchoscopic
- b. cell
- b. change, cardiac pacemaker
- b. ▸ emotional and psychological
- B. for Adults or Children ▸ Halstead Neuropsychological Test
- b., implanted
- b. longevity
- b. pack

Battey bacilli
Battista procedure
Battle('s)
- B. incision
- B. -Jalaguier-Kammerer incision
- b. psychosis
- B. sign

battledore placenta
battlefield trauma
Baudelocque's diameter
Baudelocque's operation
baudetti, Actinomyces
Bauer syndrome
baumannii complex, Acinetobacter calcoaceticus
Baumé's scale
Baumgarten
- B. cirrhosis, Cruveilhier-
- B. murmur, Cruveilhier-
- B. sign, Cruveilhier-
- B. syndrome ▸ Cruveilhier-

bauxite pneumonoconiosis
bay sickness
bayanus, Saccharomyces

Bayes' theorem
bayesian analysis
Bayle's granulations
Baylisascaris procyonis
Bayliss theory
Baylor total artificial heart
Baylor's stump
Bazin syndrome ▸ Alibert-
BB bands
B-B graft
BBB (blood-brain barrier)
BBB (bundle branch block)
BBBB (bilateral bundle branch block)
BBT (basal body temperature)
BC
- BC (bone conduction)
- BC (buccocervical)
- BC > AC (bone conduction greater than air conduction)
- BC < AC (bone conduction less than air conduction)
- BC greater than AC (BC > AC)
- BC less than AC (BC < AC)

BCA (balloon catheter angioplasty)
BCA (bidirectional cavopulmonary anastomosis)
BCG (bacille Calmette-Guérin)
- BCG immunization
- BCG vaccination
- BCG vaccine

BD (buccodistal)
BDD (body dysmorphic disorder)
BE
- BE (bacterial endocarditis)
- BE (barium enema)
- BE (below elbow)
- BE (below elbow) amputation

beach ear
bead(s)
- b. electrode ▸ silver
- b. embolization, Silastic
- b. for radiation beam, lead
- b., immunomagnetic
- b., magnetic
- b., radioactive

beaded
- b. appearance
- b. filaments
- b. hair

beaked nose
beaked pelvis
beak-like protrusion of nose
Beall
- B. disk valve prosthesis
- B. mitral valve

B. mitral valve prosthesis
Beal's
    B. conjunctivitis
    B. disease
    B. syndrome
beam(s) (Beam)
    b., abutting
    b., alignment of tangential
    b. angulation
    b. attenuation
    b. attenuation, digital
    b. -bending magnet
    b., cantilever
    b., central axis of
    b., Cobalt
    b., collimation of radiation
    b. ▸ computer guided laser
    b., cone
    b. computed tomography (EBCT) ▸ electron
    b. computerized tomography (EBCT) ▸ electron
    b., continuous
    b., controlled
    b. CT (computed tomography) ▸ electron
    b., definitive external
    b., deflected
    b., defocused
    B. Digital x-ray ▸ Scanning
    b. direction
    b., direction of radiation
    b. direction therapy
    b., dose and
    b. dosimetry, adjacent field x-ray
    b. dosimetry ▸ cold spots and hot spots with electron
    b. dosimetry ▸ dual x-ray
    b. dosimetry, electron
    b. dosimetry, four field x-ray
    b. dosimetry, large field electron
    b. dosimetry, large field x-ray
    b. dosimetry, rotational electron
    b. dosimetry, rotational x-ray
    b. dosimetry, single electron
    b. dosimetry, single x-ray
    b., electron
    b., exit point of radiation
    b. films
    b. films, fields verified with
    b. film localization, suitable
    b. filtration ▸ x-ray
    b., focused
    b. half-thickness, narrow
    b. hardening artifact

b., high-velocity electron
b. intensity, high
b. intersection point
b. irradiation, external
b. ▸ Jergesen I-
b., laser
b. laser ▸ free
b., lead beads for radiation
b., light amplification by stimulated emission of radiation (laser)
b. linear accelerator, high energy bent
b. linear accelerator, low energy straight
b. localization
b. machine, laser
b., modification of radiation
b. monitor
B. nail ▸ I-
b. of x-rays ▸ high dose
b., opposed parallel
b. overlap in orthogonal fields
b., physical effects of particle
b., pion
b., proton
b., radiation
b. radiation, external
b., restrained
b. ▸ rotating ultrasound
b. scalp irradiation, electron
b. scattering, ▸ broad-
b., secondary shaping blocks for radiation
b., simple
b. splitter
b. study, horizontal
b. surgery, laser
b. therapy, electron
b. therapy ▸ external
b. therapy, eye shields for electron
b. therapy, fast neutron
b. therapy, heavy charged particle
b. therapy, inhomogeneities in electron
b. therapy, intraoral cone for electron
b. therapy in tumors, electron
b. therapy ▸ light-
b. therapy, plastic mask for electron
b. therapy ▸ proton
b. therapy, scattering foils in electron
b. therapy, shielding in electron

b. therapy, skin reactions to electron
b. therapy, total skin electron
b., useful
beaming of microwaves
beamlets, individual
beamlets of radiation
bean appearance, coffee
bean-shaped
    b-s diplococci ▸ gram-negative
    b-s diplococci ▸ gram-negative extracellular
    b-s diplococci ▸ gram-negative intracellular
Beans (amphetamines)
Beans (barbiturates)
Beard('s)
    B. operation, ▸ Collin-
    B. operation, ▸ Cutler-
    B. procedure, ▸ Collin-
    B. syndrome
bearing
    b. activity ▸ load-
    b. activity ▸ weight
    b. area, hair
    b. area of lymph nodes, regional node
    b. as tolerated, weight
    b. brace, ischial weight
    b. brace, nonweight
    b. brace, ▸ weight
    b., complete weight
    b. -down pain
    b. -down sensation
    b. exercises, full weight
    b. exercises ▸ regular weight
    b. exercises, ▸ weight
    b., full weight
    b., gradual weight
    b. graft, hair
    b. joint, weight
    b. nerve fibers ▸ pain
    b., no weight
    b., nonweight
    b., partial weight
    b., patellar tendon
    b. ▸ patient ambulating with walker nonweight
    b. period, child-
    b. ▸ reduced weight
    b., strenuous activity ▸ repetitive weight
    b., weight
    b. with crutches ▸ weight
    b. years, child◊

Bearn-Kunkel syndrome
beat(s)
   b., abnormal heart
   b., abnormally slow heart
   b. analysis, beat-to-
   b., apex
   b. (APB), atrial premature
   b., auricular premature
   b., automatic
   b., capture
   b. ▸ chaotic heart
   b., ciliary
   b., displaced apical
   b., dropped
   b., echo
   b., ectopic
   b., ectopic ventricular
   b., escape
   b., extrasystolic
   b., fascicular
   b., forced
   b. frequency, ciliary
   b., fusion
   b., heart
   b., interference
   b., interpolated
   b., isolated premature
   b. ▸ junctional escape
   b. knee
   b., malignant
   b., missed
   b., mixed
   b., multiple ectopic
   b. (NPB), nodal premature
   b., nodal
   b., occasional premature
   b., paired
   b. per minute
   b., periodic dropped
   b., postextrasystolic
   b., premature
   b. ▸ premature atrial
   b., premature auricular
   b., premature junctional
   b. ▸ premature ventricular
   b., pseudofusion
   b. pulse, dropped
   b., reciprocal
   b., retrograde
   b. ▸ salvo of
   b., sinus premature
   b., skipped
   b., summation
   b. -to-beat analysis
   b. -to-beat variability

   b. -to-beat variability of fetal heart
     rate
   b. variability, beat-to-
   b., ventricular ectopic
   b. (VPB) ▸ ventricular premature
Beath operation ▸ Harris-
beating
   b., child
   b. heart
   b. heart cardiac bypass
   b. heart muscle
   b. heart surgery
   b. of atrial chambers ▸ chaotic
   b. of heart, rapid
   b., spouse
Beatson's operation
Beatty-Bright friction sound
Beau's disease
Beau's syndrome
Beauties (amphetamines), Black
beauty mark
beauty parlor syncope
BEB (benign essential
   bleopharospasm)
Beccaria's sign
Bechtal prosthesis
Bechterew (see Bekhterev)
   B. -Mendel reflex
   B. nucleus
   B. reflex
Beck('s)
   B. cardiopericardiopexy
   B. -Jianu operation
   B. syndrome
   B. triad
Becker-type tardive muscular
   dystrophy
Beckwith's syndrome
Béclard's
   B. amputation
   B. hernia
   B. sign
Bécléres position
Becquerel rays
bed(s)
   b., adventitial
   b., alveolar capillary
   b. angle ▸ nail-to-nail
   b. bath
   b. blocks
   b. capacity, total
   b., capillary
   b., carotid arterial
   b., circOlectric
   B., Clinitron

   b. complement
   b. control, electronic
   b. cradle
   b. cradle, heated
   b. ▸ cyanosis of nail
   b., electric
   b., elevation of head of
   b., fracture
   b., gallbladder
   b., gallbladder shelled out from
     gallbladder
   b., Gatch
   b., hospital
   b., hyperbaric
   b., liver
   b. -mat activities
   b. -mat mobility
   b. mobility
   b. monitoring, multiple-
   b., myocardial
   b., nail
   b. ▸ nail plate of nail
   b. overutilization
   b., pale nail
   b., patient confined to
   b., perfusion
   b. perfusion ▸ splanchnic
   b., pulmonary
   b., radiolucent
   b. rest
   b. rest and traction
   b. rest ▸ hot packs and
   b. rest ▸ patient at complete
   b., Sanders
   b., scleral
   b. sore
   b. ▸ Stress Echo
   b., tissue
   b. utilization
   b., vascular
   b. ▸ venous capacitance
   b., water
   b. wedge
   b. wetting
bedewing of cornea
bedfast patient
bedmatic activities, patient
   independent in
bedpan
   b., assist with
   b., fracture
   b. liner
bedrest ▸ patient at strict
bedrest, prolonged
bedridden, patient

bedside
- b. cabinet, electronic
- b. care
- b. commode
- b. diagnosis
- b. rounds
- b. unit

bedspread restraint

bedtime
- b. bottle
- b. (npo/h.s.) ▸ nothing by mouth at
- b. or hour of sleep (h.s.) ▸ at

bedwetter, patient

bedwetting, childhood

bee
- b. sting
- b. sting allergy
- b. sting hypersensitivity
- b. venom

beechwood sugar

beef (Beef)
- B. cell ABS
- b. heart antigen
- b. insulin
- b. -lung, heparin

beefy red, parenchyma

beefy tongue

beeper, pocket paging

Beer('s) (beer)
- b. and cobalt syndrome, Quebec's
- B. collyrium
- b. -drinkers' cardiomyopathy
- b. heart
- B. operation
- B. position ▸ Löw-
- B. projection ▸ Löw-
- B. view ▸ Löw-

beet sugar

Beevor's sign

before
- b. and after chemotherapy ▸ lip and mouth care
- b. eyes ▸ moving spots
- b. eyes from anemia ▸ spots
- b. eyes ▸ spots
- b. meals (ac)
- b. thinking, patient acts

Begbie's disease

Begg appliance

behaving ▸ negative style of

behavior(s)
- b., aberrant
- b., aberrant sexual
- b., abnormal
- b., abuse

- b., abuse-reactive
- b., abusive
- b., acting out
- b., activation and
- b. adaptation
- b. adaption and stress
- b., adaptive
- b., addictive
- b., adolescent antisocial
- b. adolescent sexual
- b., adult
- b., adult antisocial
- b., agitated
- b., aggressive
- b., aggressive or violent
- b. ▸ aggressive rebellious
- b., alcohol-related
- b., alert
- b., altered personal
- b., alternate
- b., alternatives to violent
- b. and attitude ▸ normal
- b. and attitude ▸ typical
- b. and drug abuse, anti-social
- b. and emotions, muscle
- b. and environment, medication and modification of
- b. and tantrums ▸ repetitious
- b. and thinking
- b., antisocial
- b., anxious
- b., apathetic
- b., appropriate
- b. ▸ arrogant, haughty
- b. as a screening device for drug abuse, patient
- b. as a screening device, patient
- b., asocial
- b., assaultive
- b., attention-demanding
- b., attention getting
- b., attention-seeking
- b., attention-seeking manipulative
- b. ▸ attitude, emotion and
- b., attitudes and
- b., authoritarian staff
- b., automatic
- b., automatically mediated
- b., avoidance
- b., baseline
- b., bizarre
- b., bonding
- b., brash and uninhibited
- b., bruxist
- b. center ▸ sex-

- b. change
- b., change in
- b. change in mood or
- b. change ▸ positive
- b. change, radical
- b. change solution
- b., childhood antisocial
- b., clinical
- b., cocaine addiction
- b., cocaine-seeking
- b., cognitive
- b., comorbid addictive
- b., compulsive
- b., compulsive sexual
- b., confused
- b., contemplative
- b., continued maladapative
- b., contractile
- b., contracts
- b. control
- b., conventional
- b., coping
- b., criminal
- b., decondition pain
- b., defensive
- b., deliberate
- b., delinquent
- b., delusional
- b., destructive
- b., destructive sexual
- b., deviant sexual
- b., deviant social
- b. disorder
- b. disorder, disruptive
- b. disorder, postencephalitic
- b. disorder, severe
- b. disorder ▸ sleep
- b., disorganized
- b., disoriented
- b. ▸ disruptions in previous
- b., disruptive
- b. disturbance
- b., disturbed
- b., drinking
- b., drug-taking
- b., drunken
- b., dynamics of human
- b., dysfunctional
- b., dysfunctional staff
- b., eating
- b., emotional
- b. ▸ engaged in antisocial
- b., erratic
- b., erratic emotional
- b., evolving

behavior(s)—*continued*

b., extinction of drug abusing
b., fine motor
b., goal
b. ▸ goal-oriented
b., habitual
b., harmful
b. ▸ help-seeking
b. ▸ high energy
b., high-risk
b. ▸ high-risk sexual
b., human
b., hyperactive
b., impaired
b., impulsive
b. in adolescent ▸ introverted
b. in child, promiscuous
b. in dementia, attachment
b. ▸ inability to sustain consistent work
b., inappropriate child
b., inappropriate dangerous
b. ▸ inappropriate sexual
b. ▸ inappropriate sexually provocative
b. ▸ inappropriate social
b. increased stereotypical
b., infant exhibits hunger
b., inhibited
b., intellectual
b., intoxicated
b., irrational
b., irresponsible
b. ▸ irresponsible work
b. ▸ jittery, unfocused
b., lawful
b., learned
b., maladaptive
b., manage
b. management
b., manifest
b., manipulative
b. mechanism, compensatory
b., mode of
b., model
b., modification
b. modification technique
b. modification therapy
b. modification treatment, long-term
b., modified
b., moral
b., motivated
b., motor
b., multiple problem
b., muscle

b., nap
b., negative
b., nondrinking
b., nonverbal
b., normal
b. ▸ normal acceptable
b., normal active maternal
b., normal emotional
b., nutritional
b. ▸ obsessive compulsive
b. ▸ odd repetitive
b. of anorexic, bingeing
b. of anorexic ▸ punishing
b. of anorexic ▸ purging
b. of anorexic ▸ starving
b. of autistic children ▸ stereotyped
b. of bulimic, bingeing
b. of bulimic ▸ punishing
b. of bulimic ▸ purging
b. of bulimic ▸ starving
b. of child, classroom
b. of nerve cells
b., oppositional
b., overactive
b., overt
b., pain
b. ▸ parental antisocial
b., parenting
b., patient
b. pattern
b. pattern ▸ self-defeating
b., peculiar
b., personal
b. ▸ positive paroxysmal aggressive
b. ▸ pre-crisis
b., prelatency
b. ▸ present mode of
b., preventive
b. ▸ prior suicidal
b. problem
b. problem, childhood
b. problem, patient
b., problematic
b. ▸ problematic life-threatening
b., problems, adolescent
b. problems, biofeedback in
b. problems, child
b. problems ▸ learning and
b. ▸ profound change in
b., promiscuous
b., provocative
b. ▸ psychology of addictive
b., psychotic
b., purging
b. ▸ random uncontrollable

b., reaching
b., reckless
b. ▸ recurrent suicidal
b. reflex
b., regressive
b., repetitious
b., repetitive
b. ▸ repetitive and persistent pattern of
b. ▸ repetitive ritualized
b. ▸ repetitive stereotyped
b., reproductive
b. response, conditioned
b., risk-taking
b., risky
b., ritual
b., ritualistic
b. role teaming
b., role of proprioception in control of
b., rule-governed
b. ▸ schizophrenia-like
b. ▸ seductive sexual
b. ▸ self-damaging
b., self-defeating
b., self-destructive
b. ▸ self-harming
b. ▸ self-inflicted abuse
b., self-injuring
b., self-mutilating
b., self-mutilative
b., sexual
b., sexually provocative
b. significance
b. skills, defensive
b., sleep
b., smoking
b., social
b. ▸ socially inappropriate
b., solid state electronic
b., spatially oriented
b., specific
b., stereotyped
b., stereotypic
b., subjective
b., suicidal
b., suppress drinking
b. ▸ sustain consistent work
b. syndrome
b. therapist
b. therapy
b. therapy, cognitive
b. therapy, dialectical
b. therapy ▸ iatrogenic effects of
b. therapy ▸ individualized

b. therapy techniques ▸ programmed
b., threatening
b. ▸ trance-like
b., transient abnormal
b. ▸ treatment of addictive
b. ▸ type A
b. ▸ type B
b., uncontrollable manic
b., undirected
b., unfocused
b., uniform
b. ▸ universality of needle sharing
b., unpredictable
b. ▸ unrecognized fluid-seeking
b., unusual
b. ▸ unusual risky
b. ▸ unusual water drinking
b. ▸ unusually hostile or aggressive
b., violent
b., violent and aggressive
b., violent schizophrenic
b. ▸ water-seeking
b. with residual disability ▸ schizophrenic
b., withdrawn

behavioral
b. aberrations
b. adaptation
b. adjustment
b. alterations
b. analysis
b. approach
b. approach, cognitive
b. assessment
b. avoidance test
b. change
b. change, long-term
b. changes ▸ permanent
b. characteristics
b. complication
b. conditioning
b. considerations
b. contagion
b. control
b. coping
b. counseling
b. cues
b. defect
b. deficiency
b. development of children
b. diagnosis
b. difficulties ▸ social and
b. difficulty
b. disorder

b. disorder, childhood
b. disorders in adolescents, emotional and
b. disorders in adults, emotional and
b. disorders in children, emotional and
b. disturbances
b. drowsiness
b. effect
b. emergency
b. event
b. factor
b. family pattern
b. function
b. genes
b. genetic studies
b. genetics
b. health
b. health plans ▸ managed
b. health treatment
b. hypnosis
b. inhibition
b. injury device (SIBID), self-inhibiting
b. intervention
b. intervention, cognitive
b. management
b. management technique
b. manifestations of anxiety
b. medicine
b. methods ▸ evaluation of
b. modification
b. modification program
b. normalcy ▸ socially defined
b. parameters, actual
b. patterns, develop
b. perspective
b. principles
b. problems
b. problems of adolescents
b. problems of pre-adolescents
b. problems, school
b. profile
b. program
b. prone
b. psychological emergency
b. psychological technique
b. reaction
b. rehearsal
b. research
b. response
b. retraining
b. scale, Brazelton
b. science

b. science nursing
b. shyness
b. similarities
b. state
b. strategies
b. support
b. symptoms
b. technique
b. technique, cognitive
b. test
b. theorist
b. therapist
b. therapy
b. therapy (CBT), cognitive
b. therapy ▸ traditional
b. toxicity
b. treatment
b. treatment, broad spectrum
b. treatment, cognitive
b. treatment, effects of
b. treatment for drug abuse
b. treatment for drug dependence
b. typologies
b. visualization
behaviorally disturbed child
behavioristic psychology
Behcet's disease
Behcet's syndrome
Béhier-Hardy sign
behind ear ▸ lump in front of or
behind-the-ear hearing aid
Behnken's unit
beholder's disease
Behring's fluid, von
Behr's
  B. atrophy
  B. disease
  B. pupil
  B. syndrome
BEI (butanol-extractable iodine)
beigelii, Trichosporon
being
  b. alone ▸ fear of
  b. alone ▸ intolerance of
  b. attacked ▸ fear of
  b., cognitive aspect of well-
  b. demeaned ▸ fear of
  b., emotional well-
  b., enhanced well-
  b. ▸ euphoric sense of well-
  b., feeling of well-
  b., general well-
  b., health and well-
  b. index ▸ general well-
  B. Index ▸ Quality of Well-

being—*continued*
b. ▸ individual well-
b. influenced ▸ fear of
b. manipulated ▸ fear of
b. misunderstood ▸ feeling of isolation and
b., patient's well-
b. ▸ periods of well-
b., physical well-
b., sense of well-
Bejel syphilis
Bekesy audiometry
Bekesy test
Bekhterev('s) (*same as* Bechterew)
B. arthritis
B. -Mendel reflex
B. nystagmus
B. reflex
B. reflex ▸ Mendel-
B. spondylitis
B. - (von) Strümpell spondylitis
B. test
belching
b. and indigestion
b., chronic
b. or bloating
Belfield procedure
belief(s)
b. and practices, cultural
b., delusional
b., false
b., false personal
b., irrational
b., religious
b., social
b., spiritual
Bell('s) (bell)
B. crown
B. delirium
B. fracture table
B. law
B. -Magendie law
B. mania
b. -metal resonance
B. muscle
B. nerve
B. palsy
B. palsy ▸ permanent
B. palsy ▸ temporary
B. phenomenon
b. sound
B. spasm
b. tympany
belle indifference, la
Bellevue Test ▸ Wechsler-

belligerency ▸ rage, frustration and
belligerent patient
Bellini's ducts
Bellini's tubules
Bellows (bellows)
b., chest
B. murmur
B. pack
B. sound
belly(-ies)
b. appearance ▸ jelly
b., bloated
b. button surgery
b. stalk
b. syndrome, prune-
b. tap
below
b. elbow (BE)
b. elbow (BE) amputation
b. knee (BK)
b. knee (BK) amputation
Belsey Mark IV antireflux procedure
Belsey's repair
belt(s)
b., lumbosacral
b., Mayo sacroiliac
b., sensory
b. skin transformer
Bem Sex Role Inventory (BSRI)
Benadryl ▸ skin irritation from
Benassi's position
Bence Jones
BJ, albumin of
BJ albumosuria
BJ cylinders
BJ globulin
BJ light chain type
BJ protein method
BJ protein test
BJ proteinuria
BJ urine
bench(es)
b. method
b. press
b. press exercises
b. tub
bend(s)
b., cartilage-wearing knee
b., deep knee
b., diver's
b. exercise ▸ knee
b. exercise ▸ side
b., knee
b. lesions, arterial
Bender-Gestalt Test

bending
b. exercise, active
b. exercise, backward
b. exercise, forward
b. exercise, lateral
b., forward
b. fracture
b., lateral
b., left lateral
b. limitation on
b. magnet, beam-
b. maneuver, forward
b., posterior
b., right lateral
b. twisting and/or
benediction hand
Benedict's test
Benedikt syndrome
beneficial therapeutic nature
beneficial treatment
benefit(s)
b. analysis, risk-
b., chemical dependency
b. estimate, risk-
b. (EOB), explanation of
b., marginal
b., maximum cardiovascular
b. (MHB) ▸ maximum hospital
b., Medicare
b., mental health
b., noncovered
b. of garlic ▸ medicinal
b. of humor ▸ therapeutic
b. of supportive care, potential
b. of treatment ▸ risks
b. of walking ▸ health
b., part A
b., part B
b. (MHB) ▸ patient reached maximum hospital
b., potential risks and
b., radiation
b. ratio, risk-
b., substance abuse
b. threshold, risk-
bengal
b. antigen, rose
b. dye, rose
b. liver scan, rose
b. I 131, sodium rose
b. scan, rose
b. test, rose
benign
b. adenoma
b. adenomatous polyp

b. appearing nodular density
b. brain tumor
b. breast calcifications
b. breast disease
b. breast lump
b. breast tumors
b. calcifying epithelioma
b. calcium particles
b. cells
b. congenital mass
b. cortical defect
b. course
b. croupous angina
b. cystic endometrial hyperplasia
b. cystic epithelioma ‣ multiple
b. disease
b. disease, complex
b. disease ‣ one stage esophagectomy in
b. early repolarization
b. esophageal disease, complex
b. essential blepharospasm (BEB)
b. essential tremor
b. essential tumor
b. febrile convulsion
b. fibrous mesothelioma
b. forgetfulness of old age
b. gastric ulcer
b. glandular tissue, intracranial calcification
b. granuloma, calcified
b. granuloma of thyroid
b. growth
b. gynecological disease
b. heart murmur
b. hereditary tremor
b., histologically
b., hospital course
b. hypertension
b. hypertrophy
b. hypertrophy of prostate
b. inner ear dysfunction
b. intracranial hypertension
b. intraductal papilloma
b. intraepithelial dyskeratosis syndrome, hereditary
b. leptospirosis
b. lesion
b. lesion ‣ excision
b. lesion of bone
b. lesion of eye
b. lesion of soft tissue
b. lichenoid keratoses
b. lipoma
b. lymphadenopathy

b. lymphocytic meningitis
b. lymphoepithelial lesion
b. lymphogranuloma, Schaumann's
b. ‣ malignant metastatic or
b. mass
b. melanoma
b. multinodular goiter
b. multiple sclerosis
b. murmur
b. myalgic encephalitis
b. myalgic encephalomyelitis
b. myocardial tumors
b. neonatal myoclonus
b. nephrosclerosis
b. nodule
b. organism
b. papilloma
b. paroxysmal positional vertigo (BPPV)
b. paroxysmal positional (BPPV) vertigo ‣ recalcitrant
b. pathology
b. pleural fibrous mesothelioma
b. polycythemia
b. polyp
b. polypoid adenoma
b. polyps of large intestine
b. positional vertigo (BPPV)
b. process
b. prostatic hyperplasia
b. prostatic hypertrophy (BPH)
b. pulmonary infections
b. rectal polyps
b. retrovirus
b. rhythm disorder
b. sclerosis
b. senile tremor
b. skull base lesion
b. stupor
b. tertian malaria
b. thyroid tumor
b. thyroid tumor ‣ removal of
b. transformation zone
b. tumor
b. tumors ‣ deep-seated
b. vascular neoplasm
b. viral infection
b. wart ‣ excision
benigna, endocarditis
benignum, empyema
benignum, lymphogranuloma
Bennett's fracture
Bennies (amphetamines)
Benoist's scale
Benson's disease

bent
b. beam linear accelerator, high energy
b. bronchus sign
b. fracture
b. leg crunch exercise
Bentall cardiovascular prosthesis
Bentall inclusion technique
Benton Visual Retention Test
bentonite flocculation test
Bent's operation
Benz sign, Mercedes
benzathine penicillin G
benzidine test
benzin/benzine
benzoate
b., estradiol
b., methyl
b. unit (IBU) ‣ international
benzoin test, colloidal
Bérard's aneurysm
berbera, Borrelia
Berckson's fallacy
bereaved
b. child
b. children
b. friend
b. husband/wife
b. parents
b. person
bereavement
b. assessment
b. counseling
b. followup
b., home care
b. minister
b., natural process of
b., parental
b., period of
b. program, community
b., recent
b. recovery group
b. support
b. support group
b., uncomplicated
Berens(')
B. conical implant
B. implant
B. implant material
B. operation
B. pyramidal implant
B. -Rosa scleral implant
B. sphere implant
Bergenhem implantation
Bergenhem procedure

Berger rhythm
Bergeron's chorea
Berger's paresthesia
Bergh test, van den
Bergmann's hernia, Von
Bergmann's incision
Bergmeister's papilla
beriberi
    b., cerebral
    b., dry
    b., infantile
Berke operation
Berke operation ▸ Krönlein-
Berkeley Boo (grade of marijuana)
Berlin('s)
    B. disease
    B. edema
    B. total artificial heart
Bernard
    B. syndrome
    B. syndrome ▸ Horner-
    B. Soulier disease
Bernays' sponge
Bernheimer's fibers
Bernhardt Disease ▸ Roth-
Bernheim's syndrome
Bernoulli theorem
berolinenis, Mycobacterium
berry aneurysm
berry cell
Bertiella satyri
Bertiella studeri
Bertin('s)
    B. bone
    B. ▸ large column of
    B. ▸ large septum of
    B. ligament
beryllium
    b. disease
    b. granuloma
    b. poisoning
Besnier's disease
Besnier's rheumatism
Bespaloff's sign
Bessey-Lowry unit
best-chance experimental therapy
Best's macular dystrophy
beta [*theta*]
    b. activity
    b. activity, bursts of
    b. adrenergic agonist
    b. adrenergic blockers
    b. adrenergic blocking agent
    b. adrenergic receptor
    b. adrenergic stimulation

b. adrenoceptor stimulation
b. adrenoreceptor agonist
b. agglutinin
b. agonist
b. agonist drug
b. agonist inhalers
b. amyloid
b. amyloid hypothesis
b. amyloid production
b. amyloid protein
b. antagonist
b. bands
b. -beta homodimer
b. blockade in myocardial infarction
b. blockade postmyocardial
    infarction
b. blocker
b. blocker ▸ anxiety and
b. blocker drug
b. blocker therapy
b. blocking agent
b. carotene
b. carotene effect
b. carotene supplement
b. cell autoimmunity
b. cells
b. cells, insulin-producing
b. cells, pancreatic
b. decay
b. detection
b. emitter
b. endorphin
b. endorphin activity
b., epoetin
b. fibers
b. frequencies
b. fungus
b. globulin
b. granules
b. hemolytic
b. hemolytic strains
b. hemolytic streptococci
b. hemolytic streptococci ▸ Group A
b. homodimer, beta-
b. interleukin-1
b. lactam
b. lactam antibiotics
b. lactam ring
b. lactamase inhibitor
b. lactamase penicillinase
b. lactoglobulin
b. lipoprotein
b. lipoprotein ▸ pre-
b. lipoproteinemia ▸ a-
b. -methylcrotonylglycinuria

b. -myosin heavy-chain gene
b. -oxybutyric acids (BOBA)
b. particles
b. pattern
b. propiolactone
b. radiation
b. radiation ▸ millicurie seconds
    (mcs) of
b. ray microscope
b. ray spectrometer
b. rays
b. receptors
b. receptors, stimulation of
b. rhythm
b. rhythm, frontocentral
b. rhythm, variable frontocentral
b., rhythmic
b. staphylolysin
b. streptococcal pharyngitis ▸
    Group A
b. streptococci
b. streptococcus
b. substance
b. subunit radioimmunoassay
b. thalassemia
b. thalassemia intermedia
b. thalassemia major
b. thromboglobulin
b. transition
b. transition, allowed
b. values, alpha
b. variation, alpha
b. waves
Betadine
    B. douche and gel
    B. prep
    B. scrub
    B. soap
betaine diet
betamimetic agent
betanaphthol paste, Lassar's
betatron radiation
betel cancer
Bethea's sign
Bethesda-Ballerup Citrobacter
Bethune's tourniquet
Betke test, Kleihauer-
betrayal
    b., adult
    b. of trust
    b. ▸ sense of
    b., social
    b. trauma
    b. trauma, adult
Bettelheim's granules

better prevention services
betterment ▸ potential for human
between
  b. anxiety and pain ▸ circular
    interaction
  b. donor and recipient ▸ transient
    contact
  b. doses ▸ time interval
  b. electrode and brain ▸ interface
  b. electrode and scalp ▸ interface
  b. electrodes ▸ electrical activity
  b. nerves and muscles ▸ block-in
    normal communication
  b. pairs of electrodes ▸ measured
  b. pairs of electrodes ▸ spacing
  b. shoulders, pain
Beuren syndrome
Beuttner's method
BEV (billion electron volts)
Bevan's incision
bevelled vein
beverage, alcoholic
be with people ▸ patient's need to
bewilderment, mental
Bezold('s)
  B. abscess
  B. ganglion
  B. mastoiditis
  B. perforation
  B. sign
  B. triad
  B. -type reflex
bezziana, Chrysomyia
bezziana, Cochliomyia
BFR (blood flow rate)
BG (buccogingival)
bg. (background)
BH (birth history)
bi amplitude slowing
bi-level positive airway pressure
Bianchi's nodules
bias
  b., detection
  b., selection
  b. ▸ time-to-treatment
biatrial enlargement
biatrial hypertrophy
biatriatum, cor pseudotriculare
biatriatum, cor triloculare
biaxial joint
bibasilar
  b. atelectasis
  b. atelectasis, mild
  b. infiltrate, fluffy
  b. pulmonary infiltrates

  b. rales
Biber-Haab-Dimmer degeneration
bibius, Prevotella
bicarbonate
  b. headache
  b. of soda
  b., sodium
  b. therapy
biceps
  b. brachii muscle
  b. curl exercise
  b. femoris muscle
  b. jerk
  b. muscle of arm
  b. muscle of thigh
  b. reflex
  b. tendon, ruptured
  b. tenosynovitis
bicipital rib
bicipital tendinitis
bicolor guaiac
bicommissural aortic valve
biconcave lens
biconvex lens
bicornis, Ixodes
bicornis, uterus
bicornuate uterus
bicranial vascular headache
bicultural communications skills
bicuspid
  b. aortic valve
  b. teeth
  b. valve
  b. valvotomy
  b. valvulotomy
bicycle
  b. echocardiogram (SBE) ▸ supine
  b. ergometer exercise stress test
  b. ergometer ▸ Gauthier
  b. exercise stress test, Astrand
  b. stress echocardiography ▸
    supine
bicylindrical lens
b.i.d. [t.i.d.]
b.i.d. (twice a day)
bidirectional
  b. cardiac control
  b. cavopulmonary anastomosis
    (BCA)
  b. shunt
  b. shunt calculation
  b. superior cavopulmonary
    anastomosis (BSCA)
  b. tachycardia
  b. tachycardia, alternating

  b. ventricular tachycardia
Biedl syndrome ▸ Laurence-Moon-
bidiscoidal placenta
Biederman's sign
Bieg's sign
Bielschowsky('s)
  B. disease
  B. -Lutz-Cogan syndrome
  B. operation
  B. syndrome ▸ Rot-
  B. test
Biendl syndrome ▸ Laurence-Moon-
Biermer-Ehrlich anemia
Biermer's change
Bier's amputation
Bietti('s)
  B. dystrophy
  B. implant cataract lens
  B. syndrome
bifascicular heart block
bifemoral bypass, axillo-
bifenestratus, hymen
biferious (see bisferious)
biferious pulse
bifermentans, Clostridium
bifid
  b. clitoris
  b. P waves
  b. pelvis
  b. pinna
  b. pulse
  b. thumb
  b. tongue
  b. uvula
bifida
  b. anterior ▸ spina
  b. aperta ▸ spina
  b. cystica ▸ spina
  b. manifesta ▸ spina
  b. occulta, spina
  b. posterior ▸ spina
  b., repair of spina
  b., spina
  b. with meningocele ▸ repair of
    spina
  b. with meningomyelocele ▸ repair
    of spina
  b. with myelodysplasia ▸ spina
bifidus, Lactobacillus
biflexa, leptospira
bifocal
  b. check
  b. contact lens ▸ disposable
  b. contacts
  b. demand pacemaker

bifocal—*continued*
- b. glasses
- b. lens

biforis, hymen
biforis, uterus
bifrequency loudness balance ▸
   monaural
bifrontal headache
bifunctional antibody
bifurcated seamless prosthesis
bifurcated vein graft for vascular
   reconstruction
bifurcatio tracheae
bifurcation
- b. aneurysm
- b. angle ▸ tracheal
- b., aortic
- b., arterial
- b., bronchial
- b., carotid
- b., coronary
- b. graft
- b., iliac
- b. lesion
- b. occlusion, aortic
- b. of basilar artery
- b. of common carotid artery
- b. of foreskin
- b. of pulmonary trunk
- b. of trachea
- b. of vessels
- b. point
- b. prosthesis, Dacron
- b., venous

Big (big)
- B. Chief (Mescaline)
- B. D (LSD)
- B. H (heroin)
- B. H (heroin) abuser
- B. H (heroin) addict
- B. H (heroin) addiction
- B. H (heroin) dependency
- B. H (heroin) habit
- B. H (heroin) user
- B. H (heroin) withdrawal
- b. heel
- b. knee
- b. to pull exercise

Bigelow's
- B. ligament
- B. lithotrite
- B. operation

bigemina, Isospora
bigeminal
- b. bisferious pulse

- b. pregnancy
- b. pulse
- b. rhythm

bigeminum, Coccidium
bigeminy
- b., atrial
- b., atrioventricular (AV) junctional
- b. ▸ escape-capture
- b., junctional
- b., nodal
- b., reciprocal
- b. ▸ rule of
- b., ventricular

Bignami disease ▸ Marchiafava-
Bignami syndrome ▸ Marchiafava-
biischial diameter
bike, ergometric
bikini incision
bilateral
- b. ablation
- b. activity
- b. air exchange
- b. alveolar pulmonary infiltrates
- b. and right serosanguinous pleural
   effusion
- b. antecubital ecchymoses
- b. aphakia
- b. apical fibrous pleural adhesions
- b. athetosis
- b. augmentation procedure
- b. blepharoplasty
- b. bronchopneumonia
- b. bronchopneumonia ▸ patchy
   early
- b. bronchopneumonia ▸ severe
   confluent
- b. bundle branch block (BBBB)
- b. carotid arteriography
- b. carotid bruits
- b. cataracts
- b. centrilobular emphysema
- b. chest tubes
- b. clubfoot
- b. crackles
- b. diffuse necrotizing
   bronchopneumonia
- b. diffuse pulmonary rales
- b. distress syndrome
- b. effusions
- b. emphysema
- b. face movement
- b. ▸ fibrocystic disease of breasts,
- b. fimbrioplasty
- b. fine motor movements
- b. focus

- b. foot drop
- b. gastrectomy
- b. giant cell tumor ▸ familial
- b. hearing loss ▸ rapidly
   progressing
- b. hemianopia
- b. hemianopsia
- b. herniorrhaphy
- b. hilar infiltrates
- b. hydrosalpinx
- b. in-toeing
- b. leg weakness
- b. limb movement
- b. lower limb amputee ▸ patient
- b. lower lobe infiltrates
- b. lung transplant
- b. lung transplant ▸ en bloc
- b. mastectomy
- b. mastectomy scars
- b. metatarsus adductus
- b. nephrectomy
- b. nephrectomy ▸ pretransplant
- b. occipital lobe infarcts
- b. orchiectomy
- b. otitis media
- b. partial salpingectomy
- b. patchy alveolar marking
- b. pleural effusion
- b. pleural rubs
- b. pleuritic chest pain
- b. pneumothoraces
- b. progressive hearing loss
- b. prophylactic oophorectomy
- b. pulmonary atelectasis
- b. pulmonary congestion
- b. pulmonary edema
- b. rales
- b. reduction in voltage
- b. renal function
- b. rhonchi
- b. salpingo-oophorectomy (s-o)
- b. sloughing infiltrates ▸ extensive
- b. strabismus
- b. symmetry
- b. synchrony
- b. synchrony, secondary
- b. tinnitus
- b. tuberculosis
- b. tympanotomy
- b. uncal herniation
- b. vascular congestion
- b. vasodilatation
- b. ventricular dilatation

bilaterally
- b. amputated, lower extremities

b. amputated, upper extremities
b., Babinski downgoing
b., chest expands adequately
b., chest expands equally
b., chest expansion adequate
b., chest expansion equal
b., deep tendon reflexes (DTR) equal and active
b. equal, reflexes
b. functioning
b. in a horizontal plane ▸ fractured
b., incision extended
b. independent
b., peripheral pulses full and equal
b., pleural effusions
b., reflexes equal
b., reflexes equal and active
b., reflexes strong and equal
b. symmetrical
b. symmetrical, chest
b. synchronous
b. synchronously, occur

bile
b. acid
b. acid binding resin
b. acid sequestrants
b. acid test
b. ascites
b., black viscous
b. ▸ block passage of
b., concentrated
b. ▸ dark green viscous
b. drainage, patent opening for
b. duct
b. duct cancer
b. duct carcinoma
b. duct, common
b. duct, dilatation of
b. duct, dilated
b. duct exploration
b. duct, extrahepatic
b. duct obstruction
b. duct opening
b. duct proliferation
b. duct ▸ sphincter muscle of
b. duct stent, occluded common
b. duct stones
b. duct stones ▸ common
b. duct stones, dissolve common
b. duct, stricture of
b. duct tumor
b. flow
b. ▸ high density
b. infarcts
b. mucoid

b. obstruction, chronic
b. outflow of
b. output
b. pigment
b. pigment, accumulation of
b. pigment ▸ produce excess
b. pigment test
b. plugs
b. production
b., reflux of
b., regurgitation of
b. solubility test
b. stasis
b. stasis, extensive
b. stasis, focal
b. stasis ▸ massive centrilobular
b. thrombi
b. ▸ viscid dark green

billford syndrome
bilharzia worm
bilharzial dysentery
biliary
b. angiography
b. antispasmodic
b. atresia
b. atresia, congenital
b. bacteremia
b. calculus
b. cirrhosis
b. cirrhosis, acholangic
b. cirrhosis of children
b. cirrhosis (PBC), primary
b. cirrhosis, secondary
b. cirrhotic liver
b. colic
b. cycle
b. decompression
b. decompression, endoscopic
b. drainage catheter
b. drainage, nonsurgical
b. drainage, percutaneous antegrade
b. duct
b. duct ▸ distension of
b. duct prosthesis
b. duct system
b. duct tolerance
b. dyskinesia
b. dyssynergia
b. encephalopathy
b. enteric anastomosis
b. excretion
b. function
b. function test

b. hypercholesterolemic xanthomatosis
b. imaging
b. lithotripsy
b. obstruction
b. obstruction secondary to carcinoma ▸ extrahepatic
b. outflow tract
b. pain
b. pancreatitis
b. procedure
b. stenosis
b. stone
b. system
b. system ▸ extra-hepatic
b. system patent
b. tract
b. tract cancer
b. tract disease
b. tract obstruction
b. tree
b. tree cannulated
b. tree carcinoma

bili-lite ▸ infant placed under
bilious
b. cholera
b. colic
b. diathesis
b. fever
b. flux
b. headache
b. pneumonia
b. stool

bilirubin
b., cord
b., direct
b., elevated
b. encephalopathy
b. icterus
b., indirect
b. infarcts
b. (MCBR) ▸ minimum concentration of
b., postexchange
b., serial
b., serum
b. test, direct
b. test, indirect
b., total
b., urine
b., volume of distribution of

billion electron volts (BEV)
billowing, cusp
billowing mitral valve syndrome

Billroth('s)
- B., cords of
- B. gastroenterostomy I
- B. gastroenterostomy II
- B. I gastrostomy
- B. II gastrostomy
- B. hypertrophy
- B. I anastomosis
- B. I operation
- B. strands
- B. II anastomosis
- B. II operation

bilobate placenta
bilobed
- b. flap
- b. flap, Zimany's
- b. placenta

bilocular joint
bilocular stomach
biloculare, cor
bilocularis, uterus
Bilopaque contrast medium
bimalleolar fracture of ankle
bimanual
- b. pelvic examination
- b. percussion
- b. precordial palpation

bimastoid coronal incision
bimaxillary dentoalveolar protrusion
Bimler appliance
bimonthly contraceptive injections ▸ monthly/
binary
- b. feedback
- b. instructions
- b. programming
- b. word

binasal
- b. hemianopia
- b. hemianopsia
- b. pharyngeal airway

binaural
- b. hearing aid
- b. loudness
- b. loudness balance ▸ alternate
- b. stethoscope
- b. stimulus

binder
- b., abdominal
- b., obstetrical
- b., scultetus

binding
- b. abnormality ▸ protein
- b. affinity, testosterone
- b. assay

- b. capacity, dye
- b. capacity, iron-
- b. capacity, latent iron-
- b. capacity ▸ oxygen (O₂)
- b. capacity test, iron-
- b. capacity (TIBC) ▸ total iron-
- b. capacity (UIBC) ▸ unsaturated iron-
- b., complement
- b. energy
- b. energy, atomic
- b. ▸ fragment antigen
- b. globulin (CBG) ▸ corticosteroid-
- b. globulin, cortisol
- b. globulin, thyroxine
- b. globulin, unbound thyroxine
- b. ▸ in vivo
- b. index (TBI) ▸ thyroid
- b. index (TBI) ▸ thyroxine
- b. index test ▸ thyroxine
- b., iron
- b. ▸ lentil agglutination
- b. model, receptor
- b., protein-
- b. protein, penicillin
- b. protein, thyroxine
- b., proteoglycan
- b. resin, bile acid
- b. site
- b. site, opiate
- b. sites ▸ receptor
- b. studies, competitive
- b. studies, hormone
- b. ▸ T-lymphocyte

Binelli's styptic
Binet
- B. -Simon test
- B. test
- B. test ▸ Stanford-

Bing
- B. anomaly, ▸ Taussig-
- B. disease ▸ Taussig-
- B. heart ▸ Taussig-
- B. syndrome, ▸ Taussig-
- B. test

binge(s)
- b. and purge syndrome
- b., cocaine
- b. drinking
- b. eating
- b. eating disorder
- b. eating ▸ episodic pattern of
- b. eating syndrome
- b. -purge syndrome

bingeing
- b. and purging
- b. behavior of anorexic
- b. behavior of bulimic

Binkhorst's implant
Binkhorst iridocapsular implant cataract lens
binocular
- b. accommodation
- b. diplopia
- b. dressing
- b. dysfunction
- b. eye dressing
- b. fixation
- b. hemianopia
- b. indirect ophthalmoscopy
- b. instrument
- b. microscope
- b. parallax
- b. shield
- b. strabismus
- b. vision
- b. voluntary movement

Binswanger's dementia
Binswanger's disease
bioabsorbable closure device
bioartificial kidney ▸ Nephros
bioassay, erythropoietin
biobehavioral problems
biobypass procedure
biooccipital headache
biooccipital slowing
Biocclusive transparent dressing
Biocell RTV implant
Biocept-G test
biochemical
- b. abnormality
- b. analysis
- b. analysis and culture
- b. balance
- b. basis
- b. change in brain
- b. changes ▸ postischemic
- b. cycle
- b. defect
- b. deficiency
- b. disturbances
- b. effects, physical and
- b. evaluation
- b. factor
- b. genetics
- b. impairment
- b. metastasis
- b. monitoring
- b. pathway

biologically
- b. depressed
- b. engineered tissues
- b. inactive
- b. vulnerable

biologist, radiation

biology
- b., cell
- b. evolutionary
- b., molecular
- b. specialist, oral
- b., tumor

biomaterial interaction

Biomatrix ocular implant

biomechanical changes

biomedical
- b. electronics
- b. radiography
- b. research

biomolecular reaction

biomolecular structures

bionic ear

bionic pancreas

bioprosthesis
- b. ▸ Mosaic cardiac
- b., porcine
- b. ▸ porcine valve

bioprosthetic heart valve

bioprosthetic valve

biopsy(-ies)
- b. after irradiation
- b. and brushings
- b., aspiration
- b., abdominal
- b., abdominal lymph node
- b., adrenal gland
- b., automated large core breast
- b., A-V Wenckebach
- b., bite
- b., bone marrow
- b., brain
- b., breast
- b., breast core
- b., bronchial brush
- b., bronchoscopic needle
- b., bronchoscopy with
- b., bronchus
- b., brush
- b., cancer
- b., cardiac
- b., catheter-guided
- b., cervical
- b., cervical cone
- b. chest wall ▸ transthoracic
- b. (CVB), chorionic villi

- b., closed needle
- b., closed pleural
- b., colonic
- b., colposcopic directed punch
- b., cone
- b., core
- b., core needle
- b., curette
- b. cytology, aspiration of
- b., cystoscopic
- b., cytological
- b., diagnosis based on
- b., directed
- b., directed cervical punch
- b., endobronchial brush
- b., endometrial
- b., endomyocardial
- b., endoscopic
- b., esophageal
- b., esophagoscopy with
- b., excisional
- b. ▸ excisional breast
- b. excisional surgical
- b., exploratory
- b., fasciotomy wound
- b., fine needle
- b. ▸ fine needle aspiration
- b., followup
- b., four-point
- b., four-quadrant
- b., fractional
- b., gastrointestinal (GI)
- b., heart
- b., hot
- b., iliac crest
- b. ▸ image-guided
- b. ▸ imaging-guided open
- b. incision, healing
- b., incisional
- b. instrumentation (AB-BI) ▸ advanced breast
- b., intestinal
- b., intraocular
- b. investigation, fine needle
- b., laser excisional conization
- b., lesion
- b., lesions accessible for
- b., liver
- b., lung
- b., lymph node
- b., mammotome
- b. ▸ mediastinal lymph node
- b., mediastinal node
- b. method ▸ Stanford
- b., multiple

- b., muscle
- b., myocardial
- b., needle
- b., negative
- b. not deep enough
- b. of area taken
- b. of breast ▸ excision and wedge
- b. of choroid
- b. of liver, needle
- b. of meninges
- b. of nerve
- b. of orbit
- b. of placenta
- b. of skin lesion
- b. of spinal cord
- b. of sternum
- b. of tissue taken
- b. of tumor mass ▸ excisional
- b. of ulcer
- b., open
- b., open lung
- b. ▸ open surgical
- b., pancreatic
- b., percutaneous
- b. ▸ percutaneous liver
- b. ▸ percutaneous needle
- b. ▸ percutaneous peritoneal
- b. perianal wart ▸ excisional
- b., pericardial
- b., peritoneal
- b., permanent
- b., pleural
- b., positive
- b., positive endometrial
- b., premortem bronchial
- b. procedure ▸ minimally invasive breast
- b., prostatic
- b., punch
- b. punch, Abrams' pleural
- b., renal
- b., saucerization and
- b., scalene
- b., scalene fat pad
- b., scalene lymph node
- b., scalene node
- b., scalpel
- b., selected retroperitoneal lymph node
- b. ▸ sentinel node
- b., shaved
- b. site
- b., skin
- b. ▸ small bowel
- b. specimen

b., specimen submitted for
b., sponge
b., stereotactic
b. ▸ stereotactic breast
b. ▸ stereotactic needle
b., sternal
b. submitted for frozen section
b. ▸ supraclavicular lymph node
b., supraclavicular node
b., surface
b., surgical
b. ▸ surgical lung
b. taken, multiple
b. technique ▸ hot
b. technique ▸ minimally invasive
b. ▸ temporal artery
b., testicular
b., thoracic fine needle aspiration
b., thoracoscopy with
b., tissue
b. tissue, inflammation of
b., total
b., tracheal
b., tracheoscopy with
b., tracheotomy with
b., transbronchial
b., transbronchial brush
b., transbronchial lung
b., transrectal needle
b., transthoracic
b. ▸ transthoracic needle aspiration
b., tumor
b., ulcer
b. ▸ ultrasound breast
b. under x-ray control
b., ventricular
b., wedge
b., wedge excisional
b., wide
biopsychological perspective
biopsychosocial disorder
biopsying, brushing and
biopsychosocial assessment
biostatistics, clinical
biosynthetic human growth hormone
biosynthetic human growth
 hormone, Genentech
biotelemetric record
biotelemetry technique
biotherapy, nutritional
bioptic
 b. aid
 b. sampling
 b. telescopes
bioresorbable implant

biosocial theory of development
Biosound wide-angle monoplane
 ultrasound scanner
biosynthesis, porphyrin
biotic energy
biotin activity ▸ endogenous
biotin deficiency
biotransformation, drug
Biotronik pacemaker
Biot('s)
 B. breathing
 B. respiration
 B. sign
biparietal
 b. diameter (BPD)
 b. headache
 b. hump
 b. suture
bipartial measurement
bipartita, placenta
bipartite patella
bipartite placenta
bipartitus, uterus
bipedicle flap
bipedicle mucoperiosteal flap ▸ von
 Langenbeck's
bipennate muscle
biphasic
 b. action potential
 b. illness
 b. pattern
 b. reaction
 b. shock
 b. spikes
 b. stridor
 b. wave
 b. wave form ▸ quasi-sinusoidal
biplanar tomography
biplane
 b. angiography
 b. aortography
 b. fluoroscopy
 b. imaging
 b. orthogonal angiography
 b. projection
 b. ventriculography
bipolar
 b. affective disorder
 b. affective disorder, depressed
 b. affective disorder, manic
 b. affective disorder, mixed
 b. cautery
 b. coagulation
 b. coagulator
 b. depression

b. depth electrode
b. derivation
b. derivations, linked
b. derivations, multiple
b. disease
b. disorder
b. disorder, depressed
b. disorder, depressed, in full
 remission
b. disorder, depressed, in partial
 remission
b. disorder, depressed, mild
b. disorder, depressed, moderate
b. disorder, depressed, severe,
 without psychotic features
b. disorder, depressed, unspecified
b. disorder, depressed, with
 psychotic features
b. disorder, manic, in full remission
b. disorder, manic, in partial
 remission
b. disorder, manic, mild
b. disorder, manic, moderate
b. disorder ▸ manic phase of
b. disorder, manic, severe, without
 psychotic features
b. disorder, manic, unspecified
b. disorder, manic, with psychotic
 features
b. disorder, mixed
b. disorder, mixed, in full remission
b. disorder, mixed, in partial
 remission
b. disorder, mixed, mild
b. disorder, mixed, moderate
b. disorder, mixed, severe without
 psychotic features
b. disorder, mixed, unspecified
b. disorder, mixed, with psychotic
 features
b. disorder ▸ pre-existing
b. disturbance
b. electrocoagulation of
 hemorrhoids
b. electrodes
b. esophageal recording
b. illness
b. lead
b. manic depressive disease
b. Medtronic pacemaker
b. montage
b. montage, circumferential
b. montage, coronal
b. montage, transverse
b. montage, triangular

bipolar—*continued*
- b. myocardial electrode
- b. needle electrode
- b. pacemaker
- b. pacemaker, endocardial
- b. pacing
- b. pacing catheter
- b. placement of electrodes
- b. psychosis
- b. retinal cells
- b. sensing ▸ integrated
- b. staining
- b. version

bipunctata, Macromonas
Birch-Hirschfield lamp
bird('s) (s') (Bird)
- B. (BABYbird) respirator
- b. -breeder's lung
- b. -headed dwarf
- b. -headed dwarf of Seckel
- b. -like face
- b. nest lesions
- b. nest vena cava filter
- B. sign

Birkett's hernia
birminghamensis, Legionella
Birtcher's cautery
birth(s)
- b., abortions, live births (GPMAL) ▸ Gravida, para, multiple
- b. abortion, partial
- b. after Cesarean (VBAC) ▸ vaginal
- b. and early development
- b. asphyxia
- b., breech
- b. canal
- b. canal stretching
- b. center
- b. certificate, hospital
- b., cesarean
- b., child◊
- b., complete
- b., complicated
- b. control
- b. control devices
- b. control pill
- b. control pill ▸ chlamydia from
- b. control pill ▸ fatigue from
- b. control pill ▸ hair loss from
- b. control pill ▸ hepatitis from
- b. control pill ▸ high blood pressure from
- b. control pill ▸ menstrual period with
- b. control pill ▸ migraine headache from
- b. control pill ▸ nipple discharge from
- b. control pill ▸ nose stuffiness from
- b. control pill ▸ phlebitis from
- b. control pill ▸ skin disorder from
- b. control pill ▸ swelling from
- b. control, postcoital
- b. control protection
- b., cross
- b., date of
- b., dead
- B. Dearth
- b. -death ratio
- b. defect
- b. defect ▸ alcohol related
- b. defect, congenital
- b. defect ▸ folate preventable
- b. defect ▸ genetic
- b. defect ▸ spinal cord
- b. defects, prenatal diagnosis of
- b. disorder of vulva
- b. (FTLB), full term living
- b. (GPMAL) ▸ Gravida, para, multiple births, abortions, live
- b., head
- b. history (BH)
- b. index (DBI) ▸ development-at-
- b. injury
- b. (IB) ▸ instrument
- b., live
- b., living child ▸ premature
- b., malformation at
- b. mark
- b. mark, vascular
- b., multiple
- b., neonatal death ▸ premature
- b., normal vaginal
- b. order
- b., post-term
- b., premature
- b., pre-term
- b., prior to
- b. process
- b. rate, low
- b., reduced risks of pre-term
- b. ▸ respiratory distress at
- b. ▸ respiratory distress present at
- b., stress of
- b., surgical
- b., time of
- b., tongue-tie at
- b. trauma
- b., uncomplicated
- b., vaginal
- b. weight
- b. weight infant (LBWI), low
- b. weight (LBW), low
- b. weight, normal

birthing room
bisacodyl ▸ rectal burning from
bisacodyl tannex
bisacromial diameter
Bischoff's
- B. corona
- B. crown
- B. operation

bisected mass
bisexual libido
bisexual men, sexually active
bisferious (*same as* biferious)
bisferious pulse
bisferious pulse, bigeminal
bishop's cap
Bishop's score
bisiliac diameter
bismuth
bismuth ▸ milk of
bispherical lens
bispinous diameter
Bissell's operation
bistoury, Jackson's
bistriata, Trachybdella
bisynchronous delta activity, generalized
bite(s)
- b., abnormal
- b., balanced
- b. biopsy
- b. bite-block
- b. -block, lollipop
- b., brown spider
- b., check-
- b., chigger
- b., closed
- b., cross◊
- b., deep
- b., edge-to-edge
- b., end-to-end
- b. fever ▸ cat-
- b. fever ▸ rat-
- b., human
- b., improper
- b. injury, animal
- b., insect
- b. malocclusion, closed-
- b. malocclusion, open-
- b. of ribs taken
- b. of tissue, deep

b. of tissue, equal
b. of tissue, superficial
b., open
b. opening
b., over
b., poor
b. -raising
b. -raising appliance
b. -raising denture
b. realignment
b., scissors
b., snake
b., stinging insect
b., stork
b., teeth ▸ cross◊
b., tick
b., underhung
b., wax
b. -wing
b. -wing x-rays
b. wound
b., X-
bitemporal
b diameter
b. headache
b. hemianopsia
bitemporalis fugax, hemianopia
biter, patient nail-
biting
b. from anxiety ▸ cheek
b. habit ▸ severe nail-
b. lice
b. louse
b. ▸ nail-
b. of cheek
b. pressure
b. sensation
b., tongue
Bitot spots
bitreous substance of tooth
bitten colony
bitten kidney, flea-
bitter
b., aromatic
b., simple
b., sour taste in mouth
b., styptic
b., Swedish
b. taste in mouth
b. tonic
bitterness and indignation
bitterness ▸ displays enduring
biuret reaction
bivalent
b. conjugate vaccine

b. influenza vaccine
b. vaccine
bivalved, cast
bivariant analysis
biventer, lobulus
biventral lobule
biventricular
b. artificial heart ▸ orthotopic
b. assist device
b. dilatation
b. dilatation and hypertrophy
b. dilatation and hypertrophy ▸ mild
b. endomyocardial fibrosis
b. hypertrophy
b. pacemaker
b. pacing
b. support
biventriculare, cor triloculare
bivius, Bacteroides
bizarre
b. behavior
b. cells
b. delusions
b. dreams
b. eating patterns
b. fixation
b. gait pattern
b. giant plasma cells
b. high frequency potentials
b. incoherent thinking
b. obsessions
b. perceptions
b. private ritual
b. way of thinking
bizygomatic breadth
Bjerrum's
B. scotoma
B. scotometer
B. screen
B. sign
Bjork-Shiley
B. aortic valve prosthesis
B. convexoconcave 60 degree valve prosthesis
B. floating disk prosthesis
B. mitral valve prosthesis
B. valve
BK (below knee)
BK (below knee) amputation
BL (buccolingual)
black (Black)
B. (hashish)
B. Beauties (amphetamines)
B. bowel movement ▸ tarry
B. Cadillacs (amphetamines)

b. cancer
b. cataract
b. death
b. discoloration
b. eye
b. fever
b. fibrotic mass
b. hairy tongue
b. induration
b. lead
b. lung
b. lung disease
b. measles
B. Mollies (amphetamines)
b. phthisis
b. pleura
b. pleura sign
b. reflex
b. sickness
b. silk suture
b. spot artifact
b. spot, Förster-Fuchs'
b. stained sputum
b. stones
b. stool, loose
b. stool ▸ tarry
b. substance
b. sunburst lesion
b. tar
b. tarry stools
b. tongue
b. urine
b. viscous bile
b. widow spider venom
Blackett-Healy position
Blackfan-Diamond Syndrome
Blackfan syndrome, ▸ Josephs-Diamond-
blacking out
blackout(s)
b., alcohol induced
b., history of
b. mentality ▸ total
b., recurring
b. ▸ shallow water
b. spells
Blacky pictures test
bladder
b., adenocarcinoma urinary
b., amebiasis of
b., anaplastic carcinoma of
b. and bowel dysfunction
b. and urethra, inflammation of
b., apex of
b., artificial internal

bladder—*continued*

b., atonia of urinary
b., atonic
b., atonic neurogenic
b., atony of
b. augmentation
b., automatic
b., automatic reflex
b., autonomic
b., autonomic activation
b., autonomic dysreflexia of
b., base of
b., bashful
b. brachytherapy implant, open
b., brain
b. burning during urination
b. calculi ▸ urinary
b. cancer
b. cancer, localized
b. cancer risk
b. cancer ▸ superficial
b. cancer, urinary
b. capacity
b. capacity ▸ reduced
b. capacity, total
b. carcinoma
b. carcinoma, anaplastic
b. carcinoma, metastatic
b. carcinoma ▸ Von Brunn's nests in
b. catheter
b. catheter ▸ indwelling
b. catheterized
b. cell carcinoma, in situ transitional
b. cells
b., complete emptying of
b. congenital abnormality
b., congenital absence of urinary
b. continence, bowel and
b. contour
b. contracted
b. contracted, urinary
b. contraction, abnormal
b. control
b. control muscles
b. control, loss of
b. control, poor
b. control reflex
b., cord
b., defective
b., denervated
b. descends into vagina
b. dilatation
b. disorder, neurogenic

b., distended
b. ▸ distended urinary
b. distended with air
b. distended with water
b. distention
b., diverticulum of
b., dome of
b. drainage (dr'ge)
b dysfunction
b. dysfunction, bowel and
b. dysfunction, postoperative
b., dyssynergic
b. elimination, alteration in
b. emptied
b. emptied completely
b. emptied on voiding
b. empties normally
b. empties reflexively
b. emptying
b. emptying, incomplete
b. evacuation
b. evaluation
b. exploration
b., exstrophy of
b., fasciculated
b., filling of the
b. (KUB) film ▸ kidneys, ureters and
b. flap
b. flap elevated
b. floor
b. function
b. function, disruption of
b. function ▸ loss of control of
b., functions, bowel and
b. fundus
b., fundus of urinary
b., gall◊
b. habit, change in
b. habits
b. ▸ hemorrhage into wall of
b., hernia of the
b. herniation
b. ▸ histologic sections of
b., hyperreflexic
b., hypertonic
b., hyporeflexic
b., hypotonic
b., ileocecal
b. incision
b. ▸ incomplete emptying of
b. incontinence
b. infection
b. infection, community-acquired
b. infections, recurring
b. inflammation

b. inflammation, chronic
b., inflammation of urinary
b., infundibulum of urinary
b. injury
b. ▸ inner lining of
b., intermittent catheterization of
b. ▸ involvement, infection or dysfunction
b. irrigated
b. ▸ irrigation of urinary
b., irritable
b., irritation of
b. (KUB) ▸ kidneys, ureters and
b. lesions
b., level of urinary
b. ▸ malformation of fetal
b. malignancy, inoperable
b., malignant tumor of urinary
b. meridian
b., motor paralytic
b. mucosa
b. mucosa ▸ congestion of
b. mucosa ▸ denuded
b. mucosa, necrotic
b. ▸ mucosa of urinary
b. mucosal hemorrhage
b. muscles
b. muscles contract
b., muscular wall of
b. ▸ muscular weakness of
b. neck
b. neck adenoma
b. neck contracture
b. neck obstruction
b. neck, tight
b., negative filling defects in
b., nervous
b., neuralgia of
b., neurogenic
b., nonreflex
b. ▸ normal motor innervation of
b. obstruction
b. outlet
b. outlet obstruction
b. output
b., overactive
b., overdistention of
b. pain
b., paralytic
b. ▸ partial obstruction of
b. pattern ▸ change in
b., peak flow of urinary
b. peritoneum
b. polyp
b. pressure

b., prolapse of urethra and
b., prolapsed
b. questionnaire
b. reflection
b. reflex
b. repair
b. resection, total
b. retraining
b., rhabdomyosarcoma of urinary
b., ruptured
b., sacculated
b., sagging
b. ▸ semen flows backward into
b., sensory paralytic
b. shadow
b., shadows in urinary
b. shunt
b., sound guided into
b. spasms
b., spastic
b., sphincter muscle of urinary
b., stammering
b., stimulation of urinary
b. stone
b., strangulation of
b., string
b., stripping
b., summit of
b. syndrome ▸ overactive
b. tone
b. training
b. ▸ transitional cell carcinoma of
b., transurethral resection (TUR) of
b., tuberculosis of kidney and
b. tumor
b., TUR (transurethral resection) of
b., uncontrollable
b., undifferentiated adenocarcinoma
  of
b., uninhibited
b., uninhibited neurogenic
b., unstripped
b. untraining
b. urgency
b., urinary
b. urine
b., uvula of
b., vertex of urinary
b. volume and elasticity
b. wall
b. wall, inflammation of
b. ▸ wall of urinary
b. wall thickened
b. wall thin and trabeculated
b. wall trabeculated

b., weakened
b. ▸ weakness of
b. worm
blade(s)
  b. bone, shoulder-
  b., prominent shoulder-
  b. squeeze, shoulder-
  b., tongue
Blainville's ears
Blair('s)
  B. head drape
  B. operation
  B. Brown skin graft
Blaisdell skin pencil
Blake exercise stress test
Blake's discs
Blalock
  B. -Hanlen operation
  B. -Hanlen procedure
  B. -Taussig operation
  B. -Taussig procedure
  B. -Taussig shunt
blame(s)
  b. ▸ parental habits of
  b. self ▸ patient
  b. ▸ symptoms of recantation and
    self-
Blanc syndrome ▸ Bonnet-
  Dechaume
blanch reaction ▸ delayed
blanch test
blanche, tache
blanched, skin
blanching of hands
blanching reaction
Blanco (cocaine), Polvo
bland (Bland)
  b. diet
  b. diet, milk-free
  b. donation, autologous
  b. edema
  b. embolism
  B. -Garland-White syndrome
  b. nonchew diet
  b. nuclei
  b. terms
  b. ulcer diet
blank (Blank)
  b. expressionless face
  b. or downcast stares
  B., Rotter Incomplete Sentence
  b. spots and distortion of lines
  b. stare
blanket
  b., bronchial mucus

b., cooling
b. for hyperthermia, cooling
b., hypothermia
b., hypothermic
b. sutures
b., Therm-O-Rite
b. treatment
b., warming
Blasius' operation
Blaskovics' operation
Blaskovics' operation ▸ Machek-
blast(s)
  b. cell
  b. cell leukemia
  b. chest
  b. crisis
  b. formation
  b. injury
  b. lung
  b. (RAEB) ▸ syndrome of refractory
    anemia with excess
blastema [*blastoma*]
blastic changes, lytic
blastic metastasis
blasting tumors
blastocyst transfer
blastodermic disc
blastodermic ectoderm
blastoma [*blastema*]
  b., amelo◊
  b., astro◊
  b. (*same as* blastema)
  b., chondro◊
  b., endothelio◊
  b., ependymo◊
  b., epithelio◊
  b., erythro ◊
  b., esthesioneuro◊
  b., fibro◊
  b., glio ▸
  b., gynandro◊
  b., hemangio◊
  b., lympho◊
  b., masculinovo◊
  b., medullo◊
  b., meningo◊
  b., meningofibro◊
  b., myelo◊
  b., myo◊
  b., myxo◊
  b., nephro◊
  b., neuro◊
  b., osteo ▸
  b., pheochromo◊
  b., pulmonary

blastoma—*continued*
- b., retino ▸
- b., spongio◊

blastomatosis, erythro◊
blastomatosis, myelo◊
Blastomyces
- B. brasiliensis
- B. coccidioides
- B. dermatitidis
- B. farciminosus

Blastomycoides
- B. ammonia
- B. chemistry
- B. immitis
- B. type
- B. urea

blastomycosis
- b., North American
- b. of cornea
- b., South American

blattae, Endamoeba
Blatt's operation
BLB (Boothby, Lovelace, Buibulian) mask
bleaching fluid
blear eye
bleb(s) [*bled*]
- b., apical
- b., emphysematous
- b. ▸ pinpoint subpleural
- b., pleural
- b. stapling
- b., subpleural
- b., thin-walled

bleed
- b., arterial
- b., esophageal variceal
- b., fetal maternal
- b., initial
- b., large fetal
- b., low pressure
- b., massive intracerebral
- b., massive upper GI (gastrointestinal)
- b., nose◊
- b., recurrent
- b., subchorionic
- b. with anemia ▸ GI (gastrointestinal)

bleeders
- b. clamped
- b. clamped and ligated
- b. clamped and tied
- b. coagulated
- b. electrocoagulated

- b., episcleral
- b. identified
- b. ligated
- b., preperitoneal
- b., subcutaneous
- b., superficial

bleeding [*breathing*]
- b., abnormal
- b., abnormal uterine
- b., abnormal vaginal
- b., active
- b., active vaginal
- b., anal fissure
- b. and cramping
- b. and infection
- b. and oozing
- b., arterial
- b. at site of injection
- b., back
- b. blood vessels
- b. blood vessels, seal
- b., breakthrough
- b. brisk and arterial
- b., cerebral
- b., cessation of
- b. complications
- b., control
- b. controlled
- b. controlled with hemostatic clamps
- b. controlled with ring forceps
- b., copious
- b. diathesis
- b. diffusely
- b., digestive system
- b. disorder
- b. disorder, active
- b. disorder ▸ hereditary
- b. disorder, inherited
- b. disorder, vascular
- b. during pregnancy
- b. during pregnancy ▸ uterine
- b. (DUB), dysfunctional uterine
- b., dysfunctional vaginal
- b. ear
- b., emotional
- b. encountered, excessive
- b., esophageal
- b. esophageal varices
- b. esophageal varices ▸ endoscopic sclerosis of
- b., estrogen withdrawal
- b., excessive
- b., excessive menstrual
- b. factor

- b., fresh
- b. from anus
- b. from aspirins
- b. from chlamydia ▸ vaginal
- b. from ear
- b. from multiple sites
- b. from nose
- b. from rectum
- b., functional
- b., gastric
- b., gastrointestinal (GI)
- b. gastrointestinal lesion, coagulation of
- b., gastrointestinal (GI) ulcers
- b., GI (gastrointestinal)
- b., GI (gastrointestinal) ulcers
- b. gums
- b., implantation
- b. in pregnancy ▸ vaginal
- b. in retina ▸ recent
- b. injury from Addison's disease
- b. inside eye
- b. inside skull
- b., intermenstrual
- b., intermittent
- b., internal
- b., intestinal
- b. into brain tissue
- b. into joints
- b. into lungs
- b. into pericardium
- b. into the brain
- b., intracerebral
- b., intracranial
- b., intramuscular (IM)
- b., intraoperative
- b., intraperitoneal
- b., irregular
- b., irregular uterine
- b., irregular vaginal
- b. laceration
- b. ▸ life-threatening
- b., massive
- b., massive intestinal
- b. ▸ massive intra-abdominal
- b., massive rectal
- b., mediastinal
- b., menstrual
- b. ▸ menstrual-like
- b., midtrimester
- b., minimal
- b., occult
- b. on touch
- b. or perforation ▸ gross
- b., painless

b. ▸ painless intestinal
b. patterns ▸ changes in
b. ▸ perforation and
b., placental
b., pneumatic tourniquet controlled
b. points
b. points coagulated
b. points controlled
b. points electrocoagulated
b. points individually clamped and
    coagulated ▸ muscle
b. points, muscle
b. points secured
b. ▸ possible source of
b., postcoital
b., postextraction
b., postmenopausal
b., postnasal
b., postoperative
b., postpartum
b., post-treatment
b. ▸ pressure to control
b., prevention of re-
b., profuse
b., prolonged uterine
b., pulmonary
b., rectal
b., recurrent
b., recurrent vaginal
b., retinal
b., secondary
b. secondary to hemorrhoids ▸
    rectal
b., site
b. site cauterized
b. ▸ small blood vessel
b. sore
b. ▸ source of intraperitoneal
b., spontaneous
b., stomach
b. stomach ulcer
b., stomatitis with
b., subarachnoid
b. tendencies
b. therapy
b., third trimester
b. time
b. time, Ivy's method
b. time, template
b. ulcer
b. uncontrolled
b., uncontrolled urethral
b., unusual
b., unusual uterine
b., uterine

b. uterine flap
b., vaginal
b., venous
b. vessels
b., voluntary control of
b., withdrawal
blemish(es)
    b., acne
    b., eruptions or pigmentations
    b., skin
blended family
blenderized diet
blenderized tube feeding
blending of stepfamilies
blennorrhagic swelling
blennorrhagica, keratosis
blennorrhagica, vulvitis
blennorrhea, inclusion
blennorrhea neonatorum
blennorrheal conjunctivitis
blepharitis
    b. angularis
    b. ciliaris
    b. marginalis
    b. ▸ recurrent ulcerative
    b. squamosa
    b. ulcerative
    b. ulcerosa
**blepharospasm (BEB) ▸ benign
    essential**
blepharoplasty
    b., bilateral
    b. procedure
    b., transconjunctival
**blepharospasm and oromandibular
    dystonia**
Blessig-Iwanoff cysts
Blessig's cysts
blighted ovum
blind
    b. basket extraction
    b. clinical trial ▸ double-
    b., color
    b. comparison ▸ randomized
        double-
    b. controlled study ▸ double-
    b. coronary dimple
    b. enema
    b. esophageal brushing
    b. experiment, double-
    b. fashion, double-
    b. food challenge ▸ double
    b. gut
    b. headache
    b. loop syndrome

b., mind
b. ▸ patient functionally
b. placebo control prophylactic
    study ▸ double-
b. placebo control study ▸ double-
b. placebo trial, double-
b. procedure, double-
b. spot
b. spot, Mariotte's
b. spots ▸ visual
b. staggers
b. studies ▸ double-
b. study ▸ triple-
b. techniques
b. techniques ▸ controlled double-
b. thoracentesis
blinded
    b., controlled study ▸ randomized,
    b., placebo-controlled, randomized
        study
    b. placebo-controlled trial ▸
        randomized double
    b. serosurvey
    b. trial, double-
blinding
    b. eye disease
    b. head pain
    b. pain
    b. worm
blindness
    b., amnesic color
    b. and paralysis ▸ selective
    b., Bright's
    b., cause of
    b., color
    b., complete foveal
    b., cortical
    b., cortical psychic
    b., eclipse
    b., flight
    b. ▸ irreversible legal
    b., irrevocable
    b., legal
    b., night
    b., nutritional
    b., partial
    b., permanent
    b., progressive
    b., psychic
    b., river
    b., snow
    b., sudden
    b., temporary
    b., total
    b., total color

blindness—*continued*
- b. treatable
- b., twilight
- b., word

blink
- b. reflex
- b. reflex, exaggerated
- b. reflexes, corneal

blinking
- b. and/or staring
- b. and twitching
- b., constant
- b. eyes
- b., infrequent
- b. of eyelids ‣ infrequent
- b. of eyes ‣ frequent
- b. or squinting ‣ involuntary spasmodic
- b. or squinting of eyes ‣ increased winking,
- b., reduce

blip, electrocardiogram (ECG/EKG)
blister(s)
- b., blood
- b., fever
- b. fissuring
- b. ‣ fluid-filled
- b., friction
- b. from athlete's foot
- b. from bromides
- b. from chickenpox
- b. from cold sore
- b. from dyshidrosis
- b. from insect sting
- b. from ringworm
- b., healed
- b. ‣ incision and drainage (I and D) of
- b. on arm ‣ red patch or
- b. on feet, tender
- b. ‣ itchy crop of
- b., painful
- b. ‣ painless, small, intact
- b., poison ivy
- b. -prone feet
- b. puncturing
- b. ‣ pus-filled
- b. ‣ pus-like
- b., rash and
- b. red, scaly and itchy
- b., skin
- b. -type lesion ‣ painful
- b., watery
- b. without infection

blistered skin

blistering
- b. lesions
- b. of skin ‣ cracking, peeling or
- b. rash ‣ painful
- b. skin

blitz (Blitz)
- b. bath
- b., media
- B. technique

bloated
- b. abdomen
- b. belly
- b. cell
- b. feeling
- b., patient
- b. sensation

bloaters, blue
bloating
- b., abdominal
- b. and abdominal tenderness ‣ gas,
- b. and constipation
- b. and cramping
- b. and disruption of evacuation
- b. and gas
- b. and indigestion
- b. and irritable bowel syndrome
- b. and/or diarrhea ‣ cramps, gas,
- b. and regurgitation
- b. from diverticulosis
- b. from gastroenteritis
- b. from lactose intolerance
- b. from malabsorption syndrome
- b. from premenstrual syndrome
- b. or belching
- b. or diarrhea
- b., stomach
- b. ‣ weight gain and

blobs, emphysematous
bloc
- b. bilateral lung transplant ‣ en
- b., en
- b. esophagectomy ‣ en
- b. ‣ heart-lung
- b. no touch technique ‣ en

Bloch-Sulzberger syndrome
blochi, Scopulariopsis
Bloch's scale
block(s)
- b., air
- b. air flow
- b., alveolar capillary
- b. analysis, cell
- b., anatomic
- b. anesthesia

- b. anesthesia, circular
- b. anesthesia, digital
- b. anesthesia, field
- b. anesthesia, pudendal
- b. anesthesia ‣ regional
- b. anesthesia, sacral
- b. anesthesia, saddle
- b. anesthesia, stellate
- b. anesthesia, sympathetic
- b., anterograde
- b., arborization heart
- b., arteriovenous (AV)
- b., Atkinson-type lid
- b. ‣ atrial tachycardia with high degree atrioventricular
- b., atrioventricular (AV)
- b., atrioventricular (AV) branch
- b., atrioventricular (AV) heart
- b., atrioventricular (AV) junctional heart
- b. attenuation
- b., AV (arteriovenous)
- b., axillary
- b., axillary nerve
- b., balsa wood
- b., bed
- b., bifascicular heart
- b. (BBBB), bilateral bundle branch
- b., bite-
- b., blood clot
- b., bone
- b., brachial
- b. (BBB) ‣ bundle branch
- b., bundle branch heart
- b., carotid artery
- b., caudal
- b., cecum
- b., celiac plexus
- b., cell
- b., cervical nerve
- b., cervical plexus nerve
- b. claudication ‣ one-
- b. claudication ‣ three-
- b. claudication ‣ two
- b. (LBBB) ‣ complete left bundle branch
- b. (RBBB) ‣ complete right bundle branch
- b., conduction
- b., congenital complete atrioventricular (AV)
- b., congenital heart
- b. ‣ continuous nerve
- b., cord
- b. coronary arteries

b., cranial nerve
b., critical organ shielding
b. culture ▸ hanging-
b. cycle length
b. cycle length, antegrade
b., desensitization
b. diagram
b., digital nerve
b. dissection
b., disulfiram
b. ▸ diversional heart
b., divisional heart
b. drug, calcium channel
b., dynamic
b., ear
b., electrical current
b., embedded tissue in paraffin
b., entrance
b., epidural
b., extradural
b., facial nerve
b., fascicular
b., fascicular heart
b. ▸ femoral nerve
b., field
b., first degree AV (arteriovenous)
b., first degree heart
b., focal
b. for radiation beam, secondary shaping
b., functional
b. glaucoma ▸ air-
b. glaucoma ▸ vitreous-
b. (HB), heart
b., hemi◊
b., heparin
b. ▸ His bundle branch
b. ▸ His bundle heart
b. in anterosuperior division of left branch
b. in normal communication between nerves and muscles
b. in posteroinferior division of left branch
b. in radiation therapy, humeral
b. in radiation therapy, laryngeal
b. in radiation therapy, spinal cord
b. in radiation therapy, thin liver
b. in radiation therapy, thin lung
b. ▸ incomplete atrioventricular (AV)
b. (BBB) ▸ incomplete bundle branch
b., incomplete heart
b. (LBBB) ▸ incomplete left bundle branch

b. (RBBB) ▸ incomplete right bundle branch
b., infraorbital
b., infranodal
b., intercostal nerve
b. ▸ interscalene nerve
b., interventricular heart
b., intra-atrial
b., intrahepatic
b., intranasal
b., intraspinal
b., intraventricular
b. ▸ intraventricular conduction
b., intraventricular heart
b. (LBBB) ▸ left bundle branch
b., local field
b., lollipop bite-
b., mantle
b., mental
b., Mobitz heart
b. murmur ▸ exit
b., nerve
b. nervous system stimulation
b., neural
b. (NCPB) ▸ neurolytic celiac plexus
b., neurosurgical nerve
b., O'Brien
b. organ shielding
b. osteotomy
b. pain impulses
b., paracervical
b., paraneural
b., parasacral
b., paravertebral
b., partial heart
b. passage of bile
b., peri-infarction
b., perineural
b., peripheral nerve
b. placement in radiation therapy
b., portal
b., presacral
b., protective
b., pudendal
b., regional
b. rejection of transplanted organs
b. resection
b., retrobulbar
b., retrograde
b. (RBBB) ▸ right bundle branch
b., sacral
b., saddle

b. ▸ sciatic nerve
b., 2nd° (second degree) AV (atrioventricular)
b., 2nd° (second degree) heart
b., shock
b., sinoatrial
b. ▸ sinoatrial (SA) exit
b., sinoatrial heart
b., sinoauricular
b., sinoauricular heart
b., sinus
b., sinus exit
b., sphenopalatine
b., spinal
b., spinal cord
b., spinal subarachnoid
b., splanchnic
b., stellate
b., stellate ganglion
b., stellate ganglion nerve
b. ▸ stellate nerve
b., subarachnoid
b., subjunctional heart
b., sun
b. ▸ supraclavicular nerve
b. ▸ supra-Hisian
b., sympathetic
b., sympathetic nerve
b. technique ▸ nerve
b., 3rd° (third degree) (AV) atrioventricular
b., 3:1 heart
b., 3:2 heart
b. ▸ transient heart
b., transsacral
b., trifascicular
b. ▸ trifascicular heart
b., tubal
b., undirectional
b., vagal
b., Van Lint
b. vasoconstriction
b., ventricular
b. ▸ voltage-dependent
b. ▸ Wenckebach atrioventricular (AV)
b., Wenckebach heart
b. ▸ Wenckebach periodicity
b., ▸ Wenckebach with 2:1
b., Wilson
b. with intraventricular conduction delay ▸ first degree atrioventricular

blockade
- ▸ regional sympathetic

blockade therapy ▸ nicotinic receptor

blockage
- b., arterial
- b., artery
- b., atherosclerotic
- b., bowel
- b., carotid artery
- b., circumvent
- b., clot
- b., complete
- b., complete bowel
- b., coronary
- b., coronary artery
- b., blood vessel
- b., bypassed
- b. carotid vessels ▸ major
- b. ▸ eye vessel
- b., fallopian tube
- b. in arteries ▸ accelerated
- b. in artery ▸ partial
- b., intestinal
- b., lung
- b., major
- b., nasal
- b. of light transmission
- b. of plaque
- b. of renal artery
- b. of urethra
- b. ▸ partial bowel
- b. ▸ potential site of
- b., tendon
- b., tubal
- b., urinary
- b., vaporize plaque
- b., vulnerable to

Blockbusters (barbiturates)

blocked
- b. airway
- b. arteries
- b. blood flow
- b. breathing passage
- b. by attention
- b. by infection of ear ▸ eustachian tube
- b. coronary artery
- b. digestive tract
- b. eye vessel
- b. fallopian tubes
- b. fallopian tubes ▸ open
- b. heart artery
- b. kidney
- b. nasal passage
- b. pleurisy

- b. renal artery
- b. sperm duct
- b. tear duct
- b. urinary tract
- b. vessel

blocker(s) (Blocker)
- b., Alpha
- b., angiotensin receptor
- b. ▸ anxiety and beta
- B., B
- b., beta
- b., beta adrenergic
- b., calcium
- b., calcium channel
- b. drug, beta
- b. ▸ long-acting calcium
- b., Proton pump
- b. ▸ renin angiotensin
- b. ▸ slow channel
- b. therapy, beta

blocking
- b. activity
- b. agent, alpha
- b. agent, beta
- b. agent, beta adrenergic
- b. agent ▸ calcium channel
- b. agent, ganglionic
- b. agent, neuromuscular
- b. anesthesia, nerve
- b. antibody
- b. illusion, pain
- b., JV (jugular venous)
- b. medications, cocaine
- b., mental
- b. of electroencephalogram (EEG) rhythms
- b. of passage of cerebrospinal fluid (CSF)
- b. of thought process
- b. oncogene expression
- b. or attenuation
- b. testosterone synthesis
- b. vagal afferent fibers
- b. vagal efferent fibers

Blom-Singer valve

Blom valve ▸ Singer-

Blondlot rays

blood (Blood)
- b. ▸ abdomen full of
- b., aerated
- b. agar plate
- b. -air barrier
- b. alcohol
- b. alcohol concentration
- b. alcohol content (BAC)

- b. alcohol level
- b. alcohol level ▸ high
- b. ammonia
- b. ▸ anaerobic cultures of cardiac
- b. analysis ▸ fetal
- b. and body fluid container
- b. and body fluid secretion
- b. and marrow transplantation
- b. and oxygen to heart, flow of
- b. and secretions
- b. and tissue match
- b. and urine ▸ hypo-osmolarity of
- b., anticoagulated
- b., antigen negative
- b., antigen positive
- b. aqueous barrier
- b., arterial
- b. arterial oxygen saturation (SaO$_2$)
- b., artificial
- b. ▸ augment flow of
- b. auto-analyzer
- b., autologous
- b., backflow of
- b. ▸ backward flow of
- B. Bank
- b. bank, community
- b. bank, hospital-based
- b. bank stress
- b. banks ▸ umbilical cord
- b. barrier, air
- b. blister
- b., blue
- b. -borne agents
- b. -borne disease
- b. -borne infection
- b. -borne infectious agent
- b. -borne irritant
- b. -borne metastases
- b. -borne pathogens
- b. -borne strains
- b. -borne virus
- b. brain barrier (BBB)
- b. brain barrier (BBB), alteration of
- b. brain barrier disruption chemotherapy
- b., bright red
- b., bronchus covered with
- b. buffer base
- b. builder
- b. carbon dioxide (CO$_2$) level
- b., cardiac
- b. cardioplegia
- b. cardioplegia, cold
- b. cardioplegia ▸ whole
- b. cast

b. cataract
b. cell antigen ▸ red
b. cell aplasia ▸ pure red
b. cell count ▸ peripheral
b. cell count (RBC) ▸ red
b. cell count (WBC) ▸ white
b. cell disorder
b. cell (RBC) mass ▸ red
b. cell (RBC) ▸ nucleated red
b. cell (RBC) ▸ red
b. cell (RBC) ▸ spiculed mature red
b. cell (RBC) survival ▸ red
b. cell therapy, cord
b. cell transplant
b. cells
b. cells (RBC) ▸ abnormal red
b. cells (RBC) ▸ accelerated destruction of red
b. cells (WBC) ▸ aggregation of white
b. cells and platelet ▸ produce
b. cells ▸ cancerous growth
b. cells, cord
b. cells (RBC) deficiency ▸ red
b. cells (RBC) ▸ destruction of red
b. cells (WBC) ▸ donor's white
b. cells, immature
b. cells (RBC) loss ▸ red
b. cells, packed human
b. cells, (RBC) ▸ packed red
b. cells per high power field (WBC/hpf) ▸ white
b. cells (RBC) ▸ production of red
b. cells ▸ regenerate
b. cells (RBC) returned to donor ▸ red
b. cells, Rh positive fetal
b. cells (RBC) ▸ sedimentation rate of red
b. cells (WBC) ▸ separate white
b. cells (RBC), transfusion of red
b. cells (RBC) transfusions ▸ packed red
b. cells (WBC) transfusions ▸ white
b. cells ▸ transplanted cord
b. cells (RBC) volume ▸ red
b. cells (WBC) ▸ white
b., central
b. cerebrospinal fluid barrier
b. chemistry
b. cholesterol
b. cholesterol, high
b. cholesterol level
b. cholesterol level ▸ total

b. cholesterol screening
b. circulated to machine for cleansing ▸ patient's
b. circulation, asymmetry in
b. circulation, cerebrovascular
b. circulation, normal
b., circulation of
b. circulation, poor
b. -circulation problems
b. circulation system
b. circulation ▸ venous
b., cleansing
b. clot
b. clot, arterial
b. clot block
b. clot ▸ blue skin from
b. clot, brain
b. clot ▸ bulging eyes from
b. clot, coagulum of
b. clot, dissolve
b. clot ▸ dissolve life-threatening
b. clot, dissolving
b. clot evacuated
b. clot formation
b. clot ▸ heart attack from
b. clot in brain or lung
b. clot in lung
b. clot in phlebitis
b. clot, inhibit
b. clot ▸ life-threatening
b. clot lysis, dilute
b. clot lysis time
b. clot ▸ postmortem
b. clot ▸ pulmonary
b. clot ▸ travel related
b. clot under fingernail
b. clots ▸ pelvic
b. clotted
b. clotting
b. clotting, abnormal
b., clotting action of
b. clotting capacity
b. -clotting cells
b. clotting defect
b. clotting disorder
b. clotting factors
b. clotting factors, purify
b. clotting protein
b. clotting, reduce
b. clotting ▸ slow
b. clotting system
b., coagulated
b. coagulation
b. coagulation factor (I-XIII)

b. coagulation factor ▸ fibrin stabilizing
b. coagulation monitoring
b. coagulation time
b. coating stools
b. collection, autologous
b., compatibility test of
b. component administration
b. component replacement therapy
b. component therapy
b. components
b. components, removal of
b. concentration, arterial
b. condition
b., congealed
b. congestion
b., contaminated
b., contaminated donor
b. contaminated linen
b., cooled
b. ▸ copious bright red
b., cord
b. corpuscle, red
b. corpuscle, white
b. corpuscles
b., coughing up
b. count
b. count (CBC) ▸ complete
b. count, decreasing
b. count, depressed
b. count, differential
b. count drawn ▸ interval
b. count, interval
b. count, low
b. count monitored in office
b. count (WBC) ▸ reduced white
b. count ▸ Schilling
b. count suppression ▸ white
b. count (WBC) ▸ transient depression white
b. count, weekly
b. count (WBC) ▸ white
b. crisis, Lundvall's
b., crossmatching
b. crossmatching interference
b. culture
b. culture, contaminated
b. culture, cord
b. culture drawn
b. culture, positive
b. culture, postmortem
b. culture ▸ postmortem cardiac
b., decontamination of
b. decreases ▸ oxygen content of
b., defibrinated

b. glucose
b. glucose control
b. glucose determinations
b. glucose level
b. glucose levels ▸ erratic
b. glucose levels, maintain
b. glucose meter ▸ home
b. glucose monitor
b. granulocyte pool ▸ total
b. granulocyte specific activity
b., gross
b. group
b. group A, B, AB, O
b. group antigens
b. group, Gonzales
b. group, high frequency
b. group, low frequency
b. group ▸ Rhesus (Rh)
b. group substances
b. group system
b. grouping
b. grouping specific substances
b., gross
b., hazardous
b., heart circulates
b. ▸ hemorrhage and clotted
b., heparinized
b. ▸ hepatitis-tainted
b. ▸ high acid level in
b. histamine
b., HIV (human immunodeficiency virus) tainted
b., human immunodeficiency virus (HIV) infected
b. in auditory canal
b. in brain ▸ leakage of
b. in cerebrospinal fluid (CSF)
b. in duodenum ▸ clotted
b. in feces
b. in feces ▸ endoscopy
b. in nares
b. in nostrils
b. in pleural cavity
b. in semen
b. in seminal fluid
b. in sputum
b. in stomach ▸ freshly clotted
b. in stool
b. in stool, occult
b. in urine
b. in vomit
b. incompatibility
b. ▸ increased pressure of
b. indices, normal
b. ▸ inefficient pumping of

b. infection, bacterial
b. infection, generalized
b., inflow of arterial
b. irradiation, ultraviolet
b., iron-poor
B. Isolation
b. lactate, arterial
b. lactate measurements
b. leakage
b. level
b. level, cholesterol
b. level, magnesium
b. level of amphetamine
b. level of calcium
b. level of cocaine
b. level of depressant
b. level of lead in
b. level of opioids
b. level of phencyclidine
b. level ▸ therapeutic
b. lines
b. lipids
b. localized mass of
b. loss
b. loss ▸ abdominal pain associated with
b. loss anemia
b. loss ▸ anemia secondary to
b. loss, chronic
b. loss (EBL) ▸ estimated
b. loss from an adenocarcinoma ▸ chronic
b. loss ▸ intrapartum
b. loss, minimal
b. loss, negligible
b. loss of gastrointestinal lesion ▸ chronic
b. loss test, ▸ GI (gastrointestinal)
b. loss, total
b., malignant disease of
b. medium culture ▸ charcoal
b., menstrual
b. ▸ mixed venous
b. -monitoring
b. morphology
b., mucous fluid streaked with
b. murmur
b., nostril oozing
b. ▸ nutrients transfer to
b., occult
b. oozing from os
b., oozing of
b. or body fluid, ▸ exposure to
b. or secretion spill
b., osmolarity of

b. oxygen (O₂)
b. ▸ oxygen (O₂) depleted
b. oxygen (O₂) level
b., oxygen-rich
b., oxygenated
b., oxygenating
b. ▸ oxygenation of
b. partrition coefficient, brain-
b., passage of
b. patch injection
b. ▸ patient admitted and transfused with whole
b., patient vomited large quantities of
b., patient vomiting
b. perfusion
b. perfusion monitor
b., peripheral
b. phosphorus level
b. pigment
b. plasma
b. plasma, infectious
b. plate thrombus
b. platelet
b., platelet clumping in
b. platelet disorder
b., platelet-poor
b. platelet thrombus
b. poisoning
b. pool
b. pool activity
b. pool angiography ▸ gated
b. pool imaging
b. pool imaging, cardiac
b. pool imaging ▸ gated
b. pool radionuclide scan ▸ multigated acquisition (MUGA)
b. pool radionuclide scan, multiple gated acquisition (MUGA)
b. pool scan
b. pool scanning ▸ gated
b. pool scintigraphy ▸ gated
b. pool study ▸ equilibrium-gated
b. pool study ▸ gated
b. pools in legs
b., positive occult
b. potassium level ▸ low
b. ▸ predonation of
b. pressure (BP)
b. pressure, ankle brachial
b. pressure, aortic
b. pressure (ABP) ▸ arterial
b. pressure (BP), basic
b. pressure (BP) ▸ borderline high
b. pressure (BP) check

blood—*continued*

b. pressure (BP) ▸ chronic high
b. pressure (BP) clinic
b. pressure (BP) control
b. pressure (BP), controlled high
b. pressure (BP) cuff
b. pressure cuff, automated
b. pressure (BP) cuff deflated
b. pressure (BP), decreased
b. pressure (SBP) ▸ decreased systolic
b. pressure (DBP) ▸ diastolic
b. pressure, differential
b. pressure (BP) ▸ disorder from
b. pressure (BP) ▸ dizziness from
b. pressure (BP) dropped
b. pressure (BP) ▸ elevated
b. pressure (BP) ▸ elevated venous
b. pressure (BP) elevation
b. pressure (BP) fell
b. pressure (FBP) ▸ femoral
b. pressure (BP) fluctuated
b. pressure (BP) fluctuations
b. pressure (BP) from birth control pill ▸ high
b. pressure (BP) ▸ high
b. pressure (BP) ▸ inability to control
b. pressure (BP), increased
b. pressure (BP) ▸ instrumental conditioning of diastolic
b. pressure (BP) ▸ intermittent elevation of
b. pressure ▸ intra-arterial measurement of
b. pressure (BP) ▸ intracranial
b. pressure (BP) labile
b. pressure (LBP) ▸ low
b. pressure (BP) ▸ lowered
b. pressure (BP) lowered in Addison's disease
b. pressure (BP) lowering drug
b. pressure (BP) ▸ marked drop in
b. pressure (MBP) ▸ mean
b. pressure (MABP) ▸ mean arterial
b. pressure (BP) measurement ▸ home
b. pressure (BP), measuring
b. pressure (BP) medication
b. pressure (BP) monitor
b. pressure monitor (ABPM), ambulatory
b. pressure (BP) monitor ▸ automatic oscillometric

b. pressure (BP) monitor ▸ electronic finger
b. pressure (BP) monitoring
b. pressure (ABP) ▸ monitoring arterial
b. pressure (BP) monitoring, automatic
b. pressure (BP) monitoring ▸ home
b. pressure (BP) ▸ monitoring of
b. pressure (BP) ▸ monitoring venous
b. pressure (BP) ▸ normal
b. pressure (BP) ▸ orthostatic
b. pressure (BP) ▸ persistent elevation of
b. pressure ▸ postural
b. pressure ▸ postural low
b. pressure (BP) ▸ primary high
b. pressure ratio, ankle brachial
b. pressure (BP) reaction
b. pressure (BP) reading
b. pressure (BP) ▸ reduce
b. pressure (BP) reduction
b. pressure (BP) reduction ▸ correlates of
b. pressure (BP) rise in
b. pressure (BP) screening
b. pressure (BP) screening, free
b. pressure (BP) ▸ secondary high
b. pressure (BP) ▸ self-monitoring
b. pressure (BP) ▸ sitting
b. pressure (BP) stabilized
b. pressure (SBP) ▸ systemic
b. pressure (SBP) ▸ systolic
b. pressure (BP) test
b. pressure (BP) therapy
b. pressure (BP) track
b. pressure (BP) uncontrolled high
b. pressure (BP), unstable
b. ▸ preventing adequate flow of
b. product transfusion
b. products
b. products contaminated by AIDS (acquired immune deficiency syndrome) virus
b. profusion ▸ Laser Doppler
b., pump
b. purifying process
b. (Biocept-G), radioreceptor assay pregnancy
b. ▸ reabsorption of
b. recipient
b. recipient, potential
b., red venous
b., reflux of

b., re-infuse
b. related diseases
b. relatives
b., reoxygenated
b. replacement
b., reroute
b., retained
b. -retinal barrier
b., Rh negative (Rh-)
b., Rh positive (Rh+)
b., Rh positive (Rh+) fetal
b., safe
b. salicylate
b. sample
b. samples, arterial
b. samples, drawing
b. samples, venous
b. sampling
b. sampling (PUBS), percutaneous umbilical
b. screening
b. screening for drug use
b., screening universal
b. sedimentation rate
b. ▸ semen, hair and
b. serum
b. ▸ shear rate of
b., shrink nasal
b., shunt oozed
b., shunted
b. sinuses
b. skin barrier
b., sludged
b. smear
b. smear, peripheral
b. specimen ▸ routinely drawn
b. specimen, potentially infectious
b. -specked phlegm
b. spill
b. spill, contact with
b. spill, decontamination of
b. spills, contaminated
b. spitting
b., spitting up
b., splanchnic
b., spotting of
b. spun in centrifuge
b. sputum ▸ cough productive of
b. stagnation
b. stained discharge
b. stained fluid, dark
b. stained mucus
b. staining of cornea
b. -starved heart muscle tissue
b. ▸ starved for oxygen (O_2) -rich

b., stool positive for occult
b., storage of
b. streaked discharge
b., streaked with
b. stream
b. studies, peripheral
b., subcutaneous extravasation of
b. substances
b. substitute ▸ Hemopure
b. substitute ▸ recycled human
b. sugar
b. sugar (CBS), capillary
b. sugar control
b. sugar, elevated
b. sugar (FBS) ▸ fasting
b. sugar (FBS) ▸ daily fasting
b. sugar, high
b. sugar, increased
b. sugar ▸ increased level of
b. sugar level
b. sugar, low
b. sugar monitoring
b. sugar monitoring, home
b. sugar, postprandial
b. sugar screening, free
b. sugar, serial
b. sugar, severe low
b. sugar stabilizer
b. sugar stabilizes
b. sugar surge ▸ postmeal
b. sugar test
b. supply
b. supply, adequate
b. supply and matures ▸ develops new
b. supply, decreased
b. supply, deficiency of
b. supply, inadequate
b. supply, insufficient
b. supply, interruption
b. supply ▸ local diminution in
b. supply ▸ loss of
b. supply, nation's
b. supply of brain
b. supply ▸ oxygenated
b. supply safety
b. supply to brain stem
b. supply to heart
b. supply to heart ▸ reduced
b. supply to tissues
b. supply ▸ tumor's
b. syndrome ▸ swallowed
b. systems ▸ cardiac-related vertebrate
b. temperature, reduced

b. test
b., test donated
b. test (FOBT) ▸ fecal occult
b. test, occult
b. test, simple
b. test, stool
b. tested for albumin
b. testing ▸ fecal occult
b. testing, mandatory
b. thinner
b. thinning
b. thinning agents
b. thinning drug
b. thinning medication
b., thinning of
b. thyroid
b. thyroxin(e)
b. -tinged fluid
b. -tinged, fluid content
b. -tinged froth
b. -tinged, mucoid material
b. -tinged sputum
b. -tinged sputum ▸ pinkish,
b. -tinged stool
b. -tinged urine
b. tingling
b. to the brain, lack of
b. ▸ tonometered whole
b. thymus barrier
b. tissue
b. transfusion
b. transfusion, autologous
b. transfusion, contaminated
b. transfusion disease ▸ incompatible hemolytic
b. transfusion ▸ exchange
b. transfusion ▸ form refusing permission for
b. transfusion ▸ heterologous
b. transfusion, incompatible
b. ▸ transfusion of tainted
b. transfusion, periodic
b. transfusion recipients
b. transfusion refusal form
b. transfusion tainted
b. transfusion therapy
b. transfusion, whole
b. transmission
b. transplant, cord
b. triglyceride levels
b., tumor
b., turbulence of flow of
b. type
b. type A, B, AB, O
b., type and crossmatch

b. type factor
b. typing, maternal
b., umbilical cord
b. uncontaminated
b. unit of
b. unoxygenated
b. urea
b. urea clearance
b. urea concentration
b. urea nitrogen (BUN)
b. urea nitrogen (BUN) ▸ elevated
b. urea nitrogen (BUN) fluctuation
b. urea nitrogen (BUN) test
b. uric acid
b. used to prime coil
b., vaginal flow of
b. vessel(s)
b. vessel, abnormal
b. vessel ▸ abnormal expansion of
b. vessel, atherosclerotic
b. vessel, ballooning-out of
b. vessel, bleeding
b. vessel bleeding ▸ small
b. vessel, blockage
b. vessel, capillary
b. vessel cells ▸ tumor
b. vessel ▸ clipping of
b. vessel clot
b. vessel, collateral
b. vessel, constricted
b. vessel, constriction of
b. vessel ▸ constriction or spasm of
b. vessel, contraction
v. vessel, coronary
b. vessel, cut
b. vessel, deterioration of
b. vessel development
b. vessel, dilated
b. vessel, dilating
b. vessel, dilation of
b. vessel dilator
b. vessel disease
b. vessel disease, brain
b. vessel disorder
b. vessel ▸ dissection of
b. vessel elasticity
b. vessel elasticity ▸ impaired
b. vessel, engorged
b. vessel, excision of portion of
b. vessel ▸ expanding
b. vessels, fatty plaque in
b. vessel function
b. vessel, graft
b. vessel ▸ grafted

blood—*continued*
b. vessel growth
b. vessel in vital organs ▸ occlude
b. vessel, incision into
b. vessel inflammation
b. vessel, interlacing
b. vessel, invasion
b. vessel ▸ invasive growth of
b. vessel, large
b. vessel, major
b. vessel ▸ malformation of
b. vessel, mesenteric
b. vessel, microscopic
b. vessel, minuscule
b. vessel, narrowed
b. vessel ▸ narrowing of
b. vessel, occluded
b. vessel of heart ▸
    revascularization of
b. vessel of lung ▸ pressure in
b. vessel of the brain cover ▸ small
b. vessel problem
b. vessel problem in Raynaud's
    disease
b. vessel, reclogged
b. vessel, reconstruction of
b. vessel ▸ renal
b. vessel, repair of
b. vessel, retinal
b. vessel, rupture of
b. vessel, ruptured brain
b. vessel, seal bleeding
b. vessel sealed off
b. vessel ▸ severe spasm of
b. vessel, small
b. vessel, spasm of
b. vessel, spastic
b. vessel, superficial
b. vessel, surface
b. vessel, suture of
b. vessel, swollen
b. vessel ▸ tearing of
b. vessel, thin-walled
v. vessels ▸ transplanted
b. vessel, tumor of
b. vessel, umbilical
b. vessel, uterine
b. vessel, visualization of
b. vessel, wall of
b. vessel, walls dilated
b. vessel walls ▸ weakness in
b. vessel, warmer
b. vessel ▸ weakened
b. vessel, widening
b. vessel with reduced elasticity

b. vessel, workup, cord
b. viscosity
b., viscous
b. volume
b. volume, adequate
b. volume ▸ augmentation of
    intrathoracic
b. volume, central
b. volume changes
b. volume, circulating
b. volume, corrected
b. volume distribution
b. volume, effective circulating
b. volume, measurements
b. volume, placental residual
b. volume, predicted
b. volume, (PBV) ▸ pulmonary
b. volume, regional cerebral
b. volume, studies
b. volume, test
b. volume, total
b., vomiting
b., vomiting up
b. warmer
b. whole
b. with chest pain ▸ coughing up
b. withdrawal
b. within joint ▸ accumulation of
b. work, admission
b. work ▸ liver function
b. workup ▸ full
Bloodgood technique
bloodless
b. field
b. field created
b. phlebotomy
b. surgery
bloodletting, periodic
bloodletting treatment
bloodshot eyes
bloodstream
b., alcohol in
b., bacterial infection of
b. debris
b. infection (BSI)
b. infection, Candida
b. infection ▸ hospital-acquired
b. infection ▸ pneumococcal
b., venous
Bloodwell mitral valve prosthesis,
    Cooley-
bloody
b. ascites
b. diarrhea
b. diarrhea ▸ watery and

b. discharge
b. discharge from breast
b. discoloration
b. effusion
b. expectoration
b. exudate
b. fluid
b. material, aspiration of
b. material, dark
b. mucus
b. nasal discharge
b. peritoneal fluid
b. semen ▸ chill with
b. semen from cancer
b. show
b. sputum
b. sputum ▸ cough productive of
b., stool, dark
b. stools
b. sweat
b. tap
b. vaginal discharge
b. vomitus
Bloom's syndrome
blooming effect
blot (Blot)
b. analysis, dot
b. analysis ▸ Southern
b. analysis ▸ Western
b. dry
b. hybridization analysis ▸ slot
b. test
b. test, ink
b. test ▸ Rorschach ink
B. Test, Western
blotchy complexion
blotchy skin
Blotter Acid (LSD)
blotter squares
Blount
B. disease
B. operation
b. diameter
B. syndrome, Erlacher-
B. staple procedure
blow (B)
B. (cocaine)
b., diastolic
b. -in fracture
b. -out fracture
b. to head
b. to region, sharp
blowing
b. diastolic murmur, soft
b. ejection systolic murmur

b. murmur
b. out ▸ shallow breathing with forced
b. respiration, frequent
b. sound
b. systolic murmur
b. wound

blown
b. addiction ▸ full-
b. compulsion ▸ full-
b. convulsion, ▸ full-
b. dementia ▸ full-
b. infection ▸ full-
b. manic depressive illness ▸ full-
b. panic disorder ▸ full-
b. psychosis ▸ full-
b. stroke, full-
b., symptoms, full-
b. ulcer ▸ full-

blowout view projection
blubbery diastolic murmur
Blue(s) (blue)
B. (barbiturates)
b. active substance ▸ methylene
b. agar, eosin methylene
b., alcian
b. arm
b. asphyxia
b. atrophy
b. baby
b. baby syndrome
b. bloaters
b. blood
b., brilliant cresyl
B. Cap (LSD)
b., carbolic methylene
b. cataract
b. cervix
B. Code
B. Devils (barbiturates)
b., dextran
B., Diagnex
b. disease
b. dome cyst
b. dot cataract
B. Dragon (LSD)
b., dye test ▸ methylene
b. ear lobes
b., eosin methylene
b. fever
b. finger syndrome
b., flaccid and
b. -green algae
b. (morning glory seeds) ▸ heavenly

B. Heavens (barbiturates)
b. histiocyte ▸ sea-
b. insufflation, methylene
b. lips
b. loop intraocular lens (IOL), ▸ Sinskey/Sinskey modified
b., mass
b., methylene
b. moods
b. mouth from coughing
b. mucous membranes
b. nailbeds
b. nevus
b. nevus, cellular
b. O, toluidine
b. ▸ patient feels
b. phlebitis
B., (barbiturates) ▸ Pinks, Reds and
b., portion of foot-plate
b., postoperative
b. sclera
b. skin
b. skin from blood clot
b. stain, alcian
b. -staining cytoplasm
b. stone
b. sweat
B. test, Diagnex
b. tip aspirator
b. toe syndrome
b. tongue
B. (heroin substitute) ▸ Ts and
b. velvet syndrome
b., winter

Bluebirds (barbiturates)
bluish
b. -colored skin
b. fingernails
b. nailbeds
b. -tinge to lips and nailbeds
b. toenails

Blum substance
Blumberg signs ▸ Rovsing and
Blumenau's test
Blumenthal lesion
Blumer's shelf
Blundell-Jones operation
blunt
b. and sharp dissection
b. arterial lesion
b. dissection
b. dissection carried upward
b. dissection, freed by

b. dissection ▸ kidney freed and exposed by
b. eversion
b. eversion carotid endarterectomy
b. force trauma
b. injury
b. injury of major airway
b. injury to heart
b. renal injury
b. trauma

blunted
b. affect
b. ▸ costophrenic sulcus
b., dulled or lessened
b. or flat affect
b., papillae

blunting
b., costal border
b. of costophrenic angle
b. of left calyces
b. of nerve
b. of sulcus

bluntly dissected
blur, indistinct
blurred
b. essential distinctions
b. eyesight
b. or fuzzy vision
b. sensory perceptions
b. vision
b. vision, episode of
b. vision in one eye
b. vision from anemia
b. vision from diabetes

blurring [*burning*]
b. of vision
b. of vision, gradual
b. or dimming of vision
b., visual

blurry, distant objects
blush
b., capillary
b., myocardial
b. phenomenon
b., tumor

blushing, patient
BM (bowel movement)
BM (buccomesial)
BMD (bone mineral density)
BMI (body mass index)
B-mode
B. (brightness modulation)
B, -mode Acquisition and Targeting (BAT)

B-mode—*continued*
- B. ultrasonography
- B. ultrasonography ▸ high resolution
- B. ultrasound

BMR (basal metabolic rate)
BNMSE (Brief Neuropsychological Mental Status Examination)
BO (bucco-occlusal)
board(s) (Board)
- b., alphabet pointing
- b. certification
- b., communication
- b., electrode
- b. ▸ eye gaze
- B. (IRB), Institutional Review
- b. -like rigidity of abdomen

Boas
- B. -Oppler bacillus
- B. -Oppler ▸ lactobacillus of
- B. test
- B. test meal

boastful and pretentious
boat-shaped heart
BOBA (beta-oxybutyric acids)
Bo/Boo (marijuana)
Bobroff's operation
Bocca neck dissection
Bochdalek
- B. foramen
- B. hernia
- B. hernia, foramen of

Bock ganglion
Bock's nerve
Bodansky unit
bodies (*see also*** body)**
- b. ▸ alcoholic hyaline inclusion
- b., amyloid
- b., Aschoff's
- b., Auer
- b., Cabot's ring
- b., colloid
- b., cytoid
- b., cytomegalic inclusion
- b., cytoplasmic inclusion
- b., Donovan's
- b., Elschnig's
- b., fibrin
- b., geniculate
- b., Greeff-Prowazek
- b., Gupta
- b., Heinz
- b., Heinz-Ehrlich
- b., Howell
- b., Howell-Jolly

- b., inclusion
- b., Jolly's
- b., ketone
- b., Landolt's
- b., Leishman-Donovan
- b., loose
- b., Mallory
- b., malpighian
- b., mammillary
- b., Negri
- b., Nissl
- b., opaque foreign
- b., opaque free
- b., pacchionian
- b., pheochrome
- b., polar
- b., Prowazek-Greeff
- b., Prowazek-Halberstaedter
- b., psammoma
- b., rice
- b., sand
- b., Seidelin
- b. test, purine
- b., thoracic vertebral
- b., Todd's

bodily
- b. complaints
- b. fluid
- b. fluids, contaminated with
- b. fluids, potentially infective
- b. functions
- b. functions partially suspended
- b. movements
- b. pain
- b. rejection of organ

Bodo
- B. caudatus
- B. saltans
- B. urinaria

body('s) (*see also*** bodies)**
- b. acceleration
- b. ▸ accidentally swallowed foreign
- b. aches
- b. after death, care of
- b. airway obstruction ▸ foreign
- b. alignment
- b. and brain chemistry
- b. ▸ apple-shaped
- b., asbestos
- b., Aschoff's
- b., aspiration of foreign
- b., asteroid
- b., Auer
- b. awareness, alteration of
- b. balance

- b., Barr
- b. biological clock
- b. brace
- b. building
- b. -building exercises
- b., Cabot's ring
- b., calcified free
- b. calcium balance
- b., cancer ravaged
- b., carotid
- b. cast
- b. cavity
- b., cell
- b. cell mass
- b. cells, undifferentiated
- b., central fibrous
- b. chemistry
- b. chemistry, abnormal
- b., ciliary
- b. circadian pacemaker
- b. ▸ circulatory systems of
- b. clock ▸ internal
- b., colloid
- b. composition
- b. composition analysis
- b. contamination, foreign
- b. contour
- b. contouring
- b. cooling
- b. counter, whole
- b. counting, whole
- b., creola
- b. CT (computerized) scan ▸ full
- b. cyst, ciliary
- b., cytoid
- b., cytomegalic inclusion
- b., cytoplasmic inclusion
- b. ▸ decalcified sections of vertebral
- b., decomposition of
- b. defense mechanism
- b. defense system
- b. density, total
- b., detached loose
- b. disc surface, vertebral
- b. disease ▸ Lewy
- b., disposition of
- b. donated to ▸ patient's
- b., donation of
- b., Donovan's
- b. dressing, independent lower
- b. dressing, independent upper
- b. dressing, lower
- b. dressing, maximum assistance for lower

b. dressing, maximum assistance for upper
b. dressing, minimal assistance for lower
b. dressing, minimal assistance for upper
b. dressing, patient independent in lower
b. dressing, patient independent in upper
b. dressing, upper
b. dysmorphic disorder (BDD)
b., electrically charged
b. (FB) ▸ electromagnetic removal of foreign
b., Elschnig's
b. embalmed
b., elementary
b. encephalitis, subacute inclusion
b. equilibrium, disturbance of
b., esophageal
b. (FB) esophagus ▸ foreign
b. exercise, upper
b. experience (OBE) ▸ out-of-
b. (FB) extraction ▸ foreign
b., falciform
b. fat
b. fat, abdominal
b. fat analysis
b. fat, burning
b. fat deposits
b. fat ▸ gluteal
b. fat ▸ mortality and
b. fat screening
b. fat, total
b., ferruginous
b., fibrin
b., fibrous
b. fluid
b. fluid balance
b. fluid, exposure to blood or
b. fluid, gram stain of
b. fluid, infectious
b. fluid precautions
b. fluid secretion, blood and
b. fluids and secretions
b., flushing of upper
b. for viewing, prepare
b. (FB) ▸ foreign
b., foreign body (FB) in ciliary
b. (FB) from cornea ▸ removal of foreign
b. function
b. function ▸ esophageal
b. function, involuntary

b. functions, various
b. functions ▸ vital
b. ▸ Gamna Gandy
b., generalized irradiation of
b., geniculate
b. (FB) giant cell ▸ foreign
b., golgi
b. ▸ Gordon elementary
b. (FB) granuloma ▸ foreign
b. granulomatous reaction, (FB) ▸ foreign
b., Greeff-Prowazek
b., Gupta
b. body habitus (LBBH) ▸ limited by
b. habitus ▸ patient's
b. hair
b. hair, decreased
b. hair distribution
b. heat
b. heat ▸ excessive loss of
b. heat, internal
b. height, vertebral
b., Heinz
b., Heinz-Ehrlich
b. hematocrit/venous hematocrit ratio
b. hematocrit, whole
b. hemolytic anemia ▸ Heinz
b., Hirano
b., host
b., Howell
b., Howell-Jolly
b., human
b., hyperthermia whole
b. identification
b. image
b. -image agnosia
b. image changes
b. image, cognitive change of
b. image, distorted
b. image distortions
b. image disturbance
b. image ▸ poor
b. image puzzle
b. immersion, full
b. immune response
b., immune system of
b. (FB) ▸ impacted foreign
b. (FB) in air passage ▸ foreign
b. (FB) in anterior chamber ▸ foreign
b. (FB) in bronchus ▸ foreign
b. (FB) in ciliary body ▸ foreign
b. (FB) in cornea ▸ foreign
b. (FB) in ear ▸ foreign

b. in eye ▸ foreign
b. (FB) in iris ▸ foreign
b. in joint, loose
b. (FB) in lacrimal sac ▸ foreign
b. (FB) in lens ▸ foreign
b. (FB) in lung ▸ foreign
b. in lung ▸ neuroepithelial
b. (FB) in nose ▸ foreign
b. (FB) in optic nerve ▸ foreign
b. (FB) in trachea ▸ foreign
b., inclusion
b. infection-fighting immune system
b. infection ▸ systemic
b. (FB) ▸ inhalation of foreign
b. interaction, mind-
b. internal clock
b., internal secretions of
b., intervertebral
b. (FB) ▸ intraocular foreign
b. (FB) ▸ intrauterine foreign
b. ▸ intravascular foreign
b., involuntary trembling of
b. involvement, ciliary
b., iris ciliary
b. irradiation, field size in half-
b. irradiation, total
b. irradiation, whole
b., irregularly shaped
b. irritation, total
b. jacket, Kydex
b. jacket, Royalite
b. jerk, sudden
b., jerking of
b., Jolly's
b., ketone
b., kneading of
b., Lafora
b., Landolt's
b. language
b. language, positive
b., lateral geniculate
b., left side of
b., Leishman-Donovan
b., Lewy
b. lice
b., lifeless
b., lipid
b., locker room odor of
b., loose
b., loss of excretory function of
b. louse
b., lumbar
b., Lyssa
b., malpighian
b., mammillary

body('s)

(*see also* bodies)—*continued*

b. manipulation techniques
b., Maragliano
b. mass
b. mass index (BMI)
b. mass, lean
b. massage ▸ full
b., Masson
b. mechanics
b. mechanics, proper
b., medial geniculate
b. medicine ▸ mind-
b., Medlar
b. membranous cytoplasmic
b. metabolism
b. (MFB) ▸ metallic foreign
b. motility
b. motion
b. movement
b. movement disorder
b. movements, abnormal
b. movements ▸ involuntary
b. movements ▸ major
b. movements ▸ repetitive
b. movements ▸ uncontrollable
b., multilamellar
b. muscles
b., muscular weakness one side of
b., musculature of whole
b. natural balance of bacteria
b. natural defenses
b. natural healing ability
b. natural healing power
b. natural immune defenses
b. negative pressure (LBNP) ▸ lower-
b., Negri
b., nerve cell
b., neuron
b., Nissl
b. ▸ normal chemical reactions in
b. (FB) ▸ nostril obstructed by foreign
b. ▸ numbness one side of
b. (FB) obstructing airway, foreign
b. obstruction, foreign
b. odor
b. of pleura ▸ fibrin
b., olivary
b. (FB) ▸ opaque foreign
b., opaque free
b. or facial contours ▸ normal
b. organs, images of
b., osteocartilaginous

b., overstressed
b. own defense mechanism
b., pacchionian
b. pain, general
b. pain with runny nose
b. (FB) papule ▸ foreign
b. ▸ para-aortic
b., paralysis one side of
b., paranuclear
b. part ▸ liposuction of
b. (FB) passed ▸ foreign
b. ▸ pear-shaped
b., peduncle of pineal
b. phenomenon ▸ mind-
b., pheochrome
b., physiologic alterations in
b. physiology
b., Pick's
b. piercing
b., pineal
b., plane of
b. plethysmograph
b. plethysmography
b., polar
b. position
b. position, frequent change in
b. posture ▸ nonverbal language of
b. posture, relaxed
b. potassium, total
b., preparation of
b. prepare family to view
b. ▸ progressive weakness one side of
b., Prowazek-Greeff
b., Prowazek-Halberstaedter
b., psammoma
b. radiation ▸ full
b. radiation, generalized
b. radiation therapy ▸ total
b. radiation, total
b. reaction, foreign
b., recipient's
b. recontouring
b. recuperative power
b., relaxed perineal
b. (FB) ▸ removal of foreign
b. (FB) removed ▸ foreign
b. reshaping
b. response to pain
b. response to pain ▸ modify
b. (FB) ▸ retained foreign
b. retrieval ▸ intravascular foreign
b. rhythm
b. ▸ rhythmic shaking of part of
b., rice

b., right side of
b. rocking, excessive
b., salt and water balance of
b., sand
b. scanner ▸ computerized tomography (CT)
b. scanner ▸ emission computerized tomographic (ECT)
b. scanner, total
b. scanner, whole
b. scanning technique
b., Schmorl's
b. (FB) ▸ sclerotomy with removal of foreign
b. sculpting
b. sculpturing
b. secretions
b. secretions, direct contact with
b. secretions, exudates and fluids
b. secretions, splashing
b. section radiography
b. section roentgenography
b. (FB) seen on x-ray ▸ foreign
b., Seidelin
b. shape
b. site
b. sites ▸ multiple
b. (FB) ▸ soft tissue foreign
b. solute, total
b. stalk
b. stiffening and shaking
b., stiffening of
b. strength ▸ lower
b. strength ▸ overall
b. strength ▸ upper
b. ▸ sudden weakness one side of
b. ▸ sudden weakness or numbness one side of
b. surface
b. surface area
b. surface burned
b., swaying of
b. symptom whole
b. symptom, whole ▸ urgent
b. systems check
b. temperature
b. temperature, altered
b. temperature (BBT) ▸ basal
b. temperature cooled, patient's
b. temperature ▸ core
b. temperature, elevation of
b. temperature, internal
b. temperature ▸ low
b. temperature mechanism

b. temperature, reduced
b. temperature, regulate
b. temperature, regulation of
b. ▸ temporary weakness one side of
b. ▸ tender points specific areas of
b. tension
b. test, ketone
b. test, purine
b. therapy ▸ mind-
b., thoracic vertebral
b. tissue, fluid in
b. tissues
b. tissues ▸ swelling of
b. to be donated for scientific research ▸ authorization for
b. to be donated for scientific research ▸ consent form for
b., Todd's
b., tomographic images of
b. tone, alteration of
b. toning
b., total
b. toxic wastes
b. (FB) ▸ tracheal foreign
b. transferred to morgue
b., treatment by manipulation of the
b. treatment, total
b. tumor, aortic
b. tumor, carotid
b. tumor-killing ability
b. twitch
b. type
b., ultimobranchial
b., vertebral
b., vertebral surface of
b. ▸ vertical alignment of
b., viewing of
b. vital processes
b., vitreous
b. volume
b. water
b. water, total
b. weakness, generalized
b. weight
b. weight, elevation of
b. weight ▸ full
b. weight gain
b. weight, ideal
b. weight loss
b. weight, normal
b. -weight ratio
b. weight, total
b., whole
b. ▸ whole common disorder of

b., wolffian
b. -worn hearing aid
b., x-irradiation whole
Boeck's
　B. disease
　B. sarcoid
　B. sarcoidosis
Boerema hernia repair
Boerhaave('s)
　B. syndrome
　B. tear
boggy edema
boggy uterus
bogus heart rate feedback ▸ anticipatory
bogus treatment
Bohlman's pin
Böhm's operation
Bohn's nodules
Bohr
　B. equation
　B. model of atomic structure
　B. radius
bois, bruit de
boil on breast
boiling point
boiling water
bois, bruit de
bois, pian
Bolivian hemorrhagic fever
Bollinger's granules
bolster
　b. fingers
　b. muscle strength
　b. suture
Bolt's sign
bolus(es)
　b. adjacent to chest wall, using
　b., alimentary
　b., box
　b., dose of
　b. dynamic computer tomography, atrial
　b. injection
　b. injection of contrast medium, intravenous (IV)
　b. of dye
　b. of food
　b. of food, obstructing
　b. of saline soaked cotton
　b. tie-over graft
bomb, gene
bomb, radium
bombé, iris
Bonaccolto-Flieringa operation

Bonanno's test
Bonchek-Shiley cardiac jacket
bonded ▸ reimplanted, positioned and
bonding
　b. compound, plastic
　b. behavior
　b., human
　b., mother-infant
　b., parent-infant
　b. process
Bondy mastoidectomy (Type I, II, III)
bone(s) (Bone)
　b. absorption
　b., accessory
　b., acetabular
　b., acromial
　b., actinomycosis of
　b. activity, retard
　b. age
　b. age according to Greulich and Pyle
　b. age ratio
　b., alar
　b., Albers-Schönberg
　b. algorithm
　b. aligned
　b., alisphenoid
　b., alveolar
　b. and joint infection
　b. and joints
　b., ankle
　b., anvil
　b. aseptic necrosis
　b., aspiration of
　b., astragaloid
　b., astragaloscaphoid
　b. atrophy
　b., back◊
　B. Bank
　b. bank, temporal
　b., basihyal
　b., basilar
　b., benign lesion of
　b., Bertin's
　b. block
　b. ▸ bone rubbing on
　b., breast
　b., bregmatic
　b., brittle
　b., broken
　b., calcaneal
　b., cancelled
　b., cancellous
　b. cancer

bone(s)—*continued*

b. cancer ▸ primary
b., capitate
b. caries
b., caries of petrous
b., carpal
b. cavity around eye
b., cavity of
b. cell
b. cell formation
b. cells ▸ death of
b. cells, hypermetabolism of
b. cement
b. cement, injecting
b. cement, Surgical Simplex P radiopaque
b., central hyoid
b., cervical vertebrae
b., chalky
b. changes, degenerative
b. chemistry ▸ disorder of normal
b. chip allograft
b. chip ▸ free-floating
b. chips
b. chisel
b. circulation
b., clavicle
b., coccygeal
b., coccygeal vertebrae
b., coccyx
b. collar
b. collar, periosteal
b. ▸ common disorder of
b., compact
b. ▸ compact substance of
b., component
b. concept, ring of
b. conduction (BC)
b. conduction greater than air conduction (BC>AC)
b. conduction less than air conduction (BC<AC)
b. conduction loss
b., condyle
b. constantly breaks down
b., contour of nasal
b., cornu of hyoid
b. corpuscle
b. cortex
b., cortical
b. ▸ cortical substance of
b., costal
b. covered with flap ▸ end of
b., cranial
b. ▸ creeping substitution of

b., crest of iliac
b., cribriform process
b., cuboid
b. cuneiform
b. curetted
b. curetted out of medullary cavity ▸ cancellous
b., cut end of
b. cyst, aneurysmal
b., cystic angiomatosis of
b. deformity
b. degeneration
b. demineralization
b., dense structure of
b. density
b. density, increased
b. density loss
b. density ▸ low
b. density, measure
b. density scan
b. density scan ▸ heel
b. density screening
b. density, small
b. density ▸ spinal
b. density test
b. density test ▸ dual energy x-ray absorptiometry (DEXA)
b., denuded jaw◊
b. deposits, endochondral
b., depression of nasal
b., dermal
b. destruction
b. destruction, localized
b. destructive process
b. deterioration
b., diastasis of cranial
b. disease, brittle
b. disease, crippling
b. disease, debilitating
b. disease ▸ genetic
b. disease ▸ hereditary
b. disease, Köhler's
b. disease, metabolic
b. disease ▸ tissue and
b., diseased
b. disorder
b. donated
b., donation of
b., dorsal vertebrae
b. dysplasia
b. dysplasia, hereditary
b., ectethmoid
b., ectocuneiform
b., endochondral
b. ends, eburnized

b., entocuneiform
b., epactal
b. eroded by cholesteatoma
b. erosion
b., ethmoid
b., ethmoidal notch of frontal
b., exoccipital
b., exostosis
b. exposed
b., facial
b., femoral
b. ▸ fibrous dysplasia of
b., fibular
b., flank
b. flap
b. flap, parietal
b., foot
b. formation
b. formation and resorption
b. formation ▸ extensive new
b. formation ▸ inadequate enchondral
b. formation, new
b. formation rate
b. formation, sparsity of
b. formation ▸ stimulate
b. forming sarcoma
b. fracture
b. fracture, long
b. fracture ▸ pre-existing temporal
b., fracture running length of
b. fracture, shin
b. fracture ▸ temporal
b., fragile
b. fragility
b. fragment
b. fragments, nasal
b., freezing donor
b., frontal
b. gap, air-
b., gladiolus
b. graft
b. graft, autogenous
b. graft, Bonfiglio
B. Graft Bank
b. graft, Brett
b. graft, cancellous-cortical
b. graft, diamond inlay
b. graft donor
b. graft, donor site of
b. graft ▸ dual inlay
b. graft, hemicylindrical
b. graft, homogenous
b. graft, inlay
b. graft, intramedullary

b. graft, medullary
b. graft, onlay
b. graft, osteoperiosteal
b. graft, osteoperiosteal iliac
b. graft, peg
b. graft, Russes
b. graft site
b. graft, sliding inlay
b. graft to femur
b. graft ▸ vascularized
b. grafting
b., greater multangular
b. growth
b. growth, abnormal
b. growth and breakdown
b. growth, disordered
b. growth ▸ faulty
b. growth in ear
b. growth of spine ▸ abnormal
b. growth plates
b. growth, stimulates
b. growth stimulator, implantable
b., hamate
b., hammer
b. hardening artifact
b., haunch
b. head
b. healing method
b., heel
b., hip
b., honeycombed
b., humeral
b., hyoid
b., iliac
b., iliac cancellous
b., ilium
b. imaging
b., immature
b. implant
b. implant material
b., incarial
b., incomplete fracture of
b., incus
b. infection
b. ▸ infection penetrated
b., inferior lamina of sphenoid
b. infusion
b. ingrowth prosthesis
b., inner table frontal
b., innominate
b., interclavicular notch of occipital
b., interclavicular notch of temporal
b., intermaxillary
b., interparietal
b., interruption in continuity of

b., intrachondrial
b., irregular
b., irregularly shaped
b., ischial
b. island
b., ivory
b., jugular notch of occipital
b., jugular notch of temporal
b., knee
b., lacrimal
b., lateral condyle
b., lateral masses of ethmoid
b., lateral meniscus
b., leg
b., lenticular
b. lesion, lytic
b. lesion, metastatic
b., lesser multangular
b., long
b. loss
b. loss, excessive
b. loss ▸ irreversible
b. ▸ loss of
b. loss ▸ rapid
b. loss ▸ severe
b. loss, spinal-
b., lower jaw▸
b., lumbar vertebrae
b. ▸ lump growing in
b., lunate
b., malar
b., malleus
b., mandibular
b., manubrium
b. marrow
b. marrow aplasia
b. marrow aplasia ▸ fatal
b. marrow aspiration
b. marrow biopsy
b. marrow biopsy and aspiration
b. marrow ▸ Buffy layer of
b., marrow, cancerous
b. marrow cavities
b. marrow cells
b. marrow cells ▸ corrected
b. marrow cells ▸ defective
b. marrow, dark red
b. marrow depression
b. marrow depression ▸ late
b. marrow disease, degenerative
b. marrow donor match
b. marrow emboli
b. marrow embolism
b. marrow examination
b. marrow failure

b. marrow harvest
b. marrow, hypocellular
b. marrow, incompatible
b. marrow infection
b. marrow infusion
b. marrow invasion
b. marrow invasion by tumor
b. marrow malfunction
b. marrow malignancy
b. marrow metastases
b. marrow ▸ mildly hyperplastic
b. marrow problem
b. marrow puncture
b. marrow, recipient's
b. marrow, red
b. marrow removed and stored
b. marrow scanning
b. marrow smear
b. marrow stem cells
b. marrow suppression
b. marrow tap
b. marrow toxicity
b. marrow transplant
b. marrow transplant, autologous
b. marrow transplant rejection
b. marrow transplantation
b. marrow, yellow
b. mass
b. mass, density and strength
b. mass, extensive
b. mass ▸ increased
b. mass, loss of
b. mass, peak
b. mass reduction
b. mass, solid
b. mass ▸ spinal
b. mass, strengthening
b., mastoid
b. material, synthetic
b. maturation, accelerate
b. maturation, normal
b., mature
b., maxillary
b. ▸ medullary substance of
b., meniscus
b., mesocuneiform
b. metabolism
b. metabolism ▸ rapid
b., metacarpal
b. metastases
b. metastases, lung and
b. metastases, multiple
b. metastases, painful
b., metatarsal
b., middle ear

bone(s)—*continued*
- b. mineral composition
- b. mineral density (BMD)
- b. mineral density, decreased
- b. -mineral density scan
- b. -mineral loss
- b. mineral test
- b. misalignment
- b. morphogenetic activity
- b. movement, normal
- b., multangular
- b., multiple plasmacytomas of
- b., muscles of hyoid
- b., nasal
- b., navicular
- b., necrosis of
- b. ▸ new column of
- b., occipital
- b. of calvarium
- b. of cranium, cerebral yokes of
- b. of skull ▸ inner table
- b. of skull ▸ outer table
- b. of sternum
- b. or joint pathology
- b., orbital
- b., orbitosphenoidal
- b., osteoporotic
- b., outer table frontal
- b. ▸ Paget's disease of
- b. pain
- b. pain at minimal level
- b. pain, chronic
- b. pain, intractable
- b. pain ▸ radiation therapy for
- b., palatine
- b., palatine notch of palatine
- b., parietal notch of temporal
- b., paste of crushed
- b., patella
- b. pathology
- b., pelvic
- b., percussion of
- b., periosteal
- b., petrous
- b., phalangeal
- b., Pirie's
- b., pisiform
- b. plate
- b. plate and screws
- b. plug
- b., pneumatization of temporal
- b. porosity
- b., porous
- b. porous and spongy
- b., post-traumatic atrophy of

- b. preserving medication
- b. processes
- b. production, optimal
- b. ▸ progressive crushing of vertebral
- b. proliferation of
- b., prominence of
- b. protrusion
- b., pubic
- b. quality
- b., radial
- b., ramus
- b. rasp
- b. rasp, Miltner rotary
- b. rasp, Putti
- b., red ▸ medullary substances of
- b. refractured
- b. regeneration
- b. remodeling
- b. ▸ replaced with new
- b., replacement
- b. resorption
- b. resorption ▸ inhibit
- b., rib
- b., rider's
- b., ring of
- b. rubbing on bone
- b., sacral
- b., sacral vertebrae
- b. sarcoma, primary
- b. saw, Luck
- b. saw, Stryker
- b. scan
- b. scan, isotope
- b. scan negative
- b. scan, normal
- b. scan positive
- b. scan ▸ radioisotope
- b. scan, radionuclear
- b. scan reveals increased activity
- b. scan showed increased activity
- b. scanning
- b., scaphoid
- b., scapular
- b. seeker
- b., semilunar
- b. sensibility
- b., sesamoid
- b. severed surface of
- b., shaft of
- b., shin
- b., short
- b., shoulder blade
- b. shrinkage
- b. skids

- b. sonometer
- b., sphenoid
- b., sphenopalatine notch of palatine
- b. spicules
- b. ▸ splitting breast
- b., spongy
- b., spongy part of
- b. ▸ spongy substance of
- b. spur
- b. spurs ▸ detection of
- b., squamosal
- b., stapes
- b. ▸ stimulate formation and increase mass in
- b. stimulation, temporal
- b., stirrup
- b. storage technique ▸ refine
- b. strength
- b. strength ▸ loss of
- b., strong
- b. structure
- b. structure, abnormal
- b. structure, intact
- b. structure ▸ periapical
- b. structure, small
- b., subperiosteal
- b., supernumerary
- b. ▸ supratrochlear foraminal
- b. surface, debrided
- b. survey
- b. survey, long
- b. ▸ swelling deformity of affected
- b., syphilis of
- b., talus
- b., tarsal
- b., temporal
- b. thickness
- b., thigh
- b. thinning
- b. thinning effects of estrogen loss
- b., thinning process of
- b., thoracic vertebrae
- b., tibia
- b., tiny
- b. tissue
- b. tissue ▸ deterioration of
- b. tissue ▸ gradual loss of
- b. to thicken ▸ cause
- b., toe
- b., tongue of sphenoid
- b. transplant
- b. transplant graft ▸ whole
- b., trapezium
- b., trapezoid
- b. trauma

b., triangular
b., triquetral
b., tuberculosis of
b., tuft of
b., tumor of
b., turbinate
b. turnover
b., tympanic
b., ulna
b., ulnar styloid
b., unciform
b., uncinate
b., upper jaw◊
b., ► upper thigh
b., ► urgent symptom with
b., vesalian
b., vomer
b. wax
b. wax, Horsley's
b. weakening
b. weakening, brittle
b. weakening cavity
b. weakening cyst
b. weakening disease
b. weakening osteoporosis
b., wedge-shaped cut into
b., whettle
b., whorl
b., wrist
b., xiphoid
b., zygomatic
Bonferroni correction
Bonfiglio bone graft
bongkrek intoxication
Bonhoeffer's symptom
bonito fish insulin
Bonnaire's method
Bonner's position
Bonnet('s)
    B. -Dechaume-Blanc syndrome
    b., gluteal
    B. operation
    B. sign
    B. syndrome
Bonnevie-Ullrich syndrome
Bonney's hysterectomy
bony
    b. abnormality
    b. alignment
    b. ankylosis
    b. annulus
    b. apposition
    b. architecture
    b. areas
    b. bridge

b. bridging
b. cage
b. cataract
b. changes of feet
b. choana
b. deformity
b. density
b. deposits
b. destruction
b. destruction, area of
b. destructive change
b. destructive process
b. disease
b. elements
b. encasement
b. enlargement
b. ethmoidal cells
b. excrescence
b. fragment
b. fusion
b. growth
b. hard palate
b. healing
b. heart
b. hump
b. injury
b. insertion
b. island
b. labyrinth
b. landmarks
b. matrix
b. metastases, widespread
b. osteolytic lesions ► widespread
b. outgrowth
b. overgrowth
b. overhang
b. palate
b. pelvis
b. profile
b. projection
b. proliferation
b. prominence
b. protrusion
b. protuberance
b. pyramid
b. reabsorption, subchondral
b. rongeur
b. sclerosis
b. sites
b. socket
b. spur
b. spurring
b. structure, coiled
b. structures demineralized
b. substance of tooth

b. suture
b. swelling
b. table
b. tenderness
b. thoracic cage
b. thorax
b. tissue
b. trauma
b. union
b. union, solid
b. vertebral fractures
b. wall
Bonzel's operation
Boo (grade of marijuana), Berkeley
Boo (marijuana), Bo/
book, controlled substance
bookerii, Alcaligenes
Boom, Baby
booming rumble
Boophilus annulatus
boost
    b. dosage
    b. dose of radiation, small
    b. radiation
booster
    b. heart
    b., immune
    b. phenomenon
    b., ► pneumonia vaccination
    b., tetanus
boosting and rolling, ► patient independent in
boosting drugs, dopamine-
boot
    b. brace, Wilke
    b., compression
    b., gelatin compression
    b. ► intermittent pneumatic compression
    b., knee
    b., plaster
    b. -shaped heart
    b., sheepskin
    b., splint
    b., Unna's
    b. ► Unna's paste
bootees, cover gown and
Boothby, Lovelace, Bulbulian (BLB) mask
bootleg lotion
bootstrap
    b. dilatation
    b. two-vessel angioplasty
    b. two-vessel technique
boozing, sniffing, and smoking

borborygmi, active
border(s) [*quarter*]
- b. abnormality ▸ vertebral
- b., anterodistal
- b. blunting, costal
- b., brush
- b., cardiac
- b. cells
- b., demarcated
- b. detection, automated
- b. detection ▸ echocardiographic automated
- b., elevated rolled
- b. extent, tumor
- b., heart
- b., indistinct
- b., indistinct cell
- b., intestinal brush
- b. irregularity
- b., lateral
- b. (LSB) ▸ left sternal
- b. level
- b. movement
- b. of cardiac dullness
- b. of dullness, cardiac
- b. of esophagus
- b. of inguinal ligament, shelving
- b. of optic disc ▸ nasal
- b. of pupil ▸ lower
- b. of pupil ▸ upper
- b. of wound, inferior
- b., outer
- b., poorly defined
- b., pupillary
- b. rale
- b. rays
- b. reattachment
- b. (RSB) ▸ right sternal
- b. seal
- b., serpiginous
- b., shifting
- b., sternal
- b., superior
- b., vermilion
- b. well outlined ▸ cytoplasmic

bordering on insanity
borderline (B)
- b. cardiac competence
- b. cardiomegaly
- b. case
- b. coarsening
- b. curve
- b. diabetes mellitus (DM)
- b. diabetic
- b. disorder

- b. effectiveness
- b. electrocardiogram (ECG/EKG)
- b. glucose tolerance test
- b. high blood pressure (BP)
- b. hypertension
- b. intellectual functioning
- b. intelligence
- b. left ventricular fullness
- b. low
- b. malignant lesion
- b. normal record
- b., patient
- b. pelvis
- b. personality
- b. personality and depression
- b. personality disorder (BPD)
- b. rays
- b. right ventricular fullness
- b. septal hypertrophy
- b. state
- b. systolic hypertension

Bordet-Gengou
- B-G agar
- B-G bacillus
- B-G culture medium
- B-G phenomenon
- B-G reaction

Bordetella
- B. bronchiseptica
- B. parapertussis
- B. pertussis

bored, easily
boredom
- b. and loneliness
- b., chronic emptiness and
- b. ▸ inability to tolerate

Borg
- B. numerical scale
- B. Perceived Exertion Scale (BPES)
- B. Treadmill Exertion Scale (BTES)

Borges method
boring cancer
boring pain
born with congenital anomalies, infant
Borna sickness
borne
- b. agents, blood-
- b. bacteria ▸ food-
- b. disease, blood-
- b. disease ▸ family-
- b. disease ▸ vector-
- b. encephalitis ▸ tick-
- b. encephalitis virus ▸ tick-

- b. hemorrhagic fever ▸ Southeast Asian mosquito-
- b. illness ▸ pet-
- b. illness ▸ tick-
- b. infection, blood-
- b. infection, food-
- b. infection, insect-
- b. infection ▸ water-
- b. infectious agent, blood-
- b. irritant, blood-
- b. metastases ▸ blood-
- b. parasites, blood-
- b. pathogens, blood-
- b. strains, blood-
- b., tooth-
- b. virus ▸ arthropod-
- b. virus, blood-
- b. virus ▸ tick-

Bornholm's disease
boron counter
Borox therapy
Borrelia
- B. anserina
- B. berbera
- B. buccalis
- B. burgdorferi
- B. carteri
- B. caucasica
- B. duttonii
- B. hermsii
- B. hispanica
- B. kochii
- B. parkeri
- B. persica
- B. recurrentis
- B. refringens
- B. turicatae
- B. venezuelensis
- B. vincentii

borreliosis, Lyme
Borthen operation
boss, parietal
Bossalino's operation
bosselated surface
bosselated uterus
Bostock catarrh
Bosworth's operation
Botallo's duct
both
- b. adnexa, tenderness in
- b. eyes (OU)
- b. hemispheres, activity of
- b. kidneys, tomography of
- b. lung fields ▸ poor aeration
- b. tubes, hydrosalpinx

Bo-Tox (Botulinum Toxin) cosmetic
   surgery
Bo-Tox (Botulinum Toxin) injection
botryomycosis, pulmonary
Botterer score
bottle
  b. baby
  b., bedtime
  b. drainage system, two-
  b., evacuated
  b. -fed infant
  b. heart ▸ water-
  b. neck stenosis
  b. operation, Andrews
  b., prescription
  b., sealed vacuum
  b. sound
  b. stomach, leather
  b. syndrome, nursing
  b. tooth decay ▸ nursing
  b., vacuum culture
  b. warmer
  b., waterseal drainage (dr'ge)
bottlemakers, cataract
bottom
  b. foot, rocker-
  b. hitting
  b. of container ▸ red cells gravitate
    to
  b., weaver's
bottomed out
botulinum (Botulinum)
  b. bacteria
  b., Clostridium
  B. Toxin (Bo-Tox) cosmetic surgery
  B. Toxin (Bo-Tox) injection
botulinus, Bacillus
botulism toxin
botulism, wound
Bouchard('s)
  B. aneurysm, Charcot-
  B. nodes
  B. nodules
bouche de tapir
Bouchet's disease
Bouchut's respiration
boueti, Cimex
boueti, Leptocimex
bouffardi, Aspergillus
bouffardi, Penicillium
bougie tube brachytherapy, cesium
  137
bougienage, esophageal
Bouillaud's
  B. sign

B. syndrome
B. tinkle
Bouilly's operation
Bouilly procedure
Bouin's fluid
Bouin's solution
bounce sign
bouncing exercise
bound(s)
  b. antibody, cell
  b. antigen, cell
  b. antigens ▸ membrane-
  b. down
  b. down, fallopian tube
  b. electron
  b. fat
  b. -free ratio
  b. iodine (PBI) ▸ protein-
  b. iodine, serum-
  b. iodine (SPBI) ▸ serum protein-
  b. iron, high serum-
  b. iron, low serum-
  b. iron, serum-
  b., power
  b. thyroxine (PBT) ▸ protein-
  b., wheelchair
boundary
  b., anterior
  b. detection, automatic
  b. detection system ▸
    echocardiographic automated
  b. electrophoresis, moving
  b., posterior
bounding
  b. heartbeat
  b. pulse
  b. pupil
boundless energy ▸ burst of
bouquet fever
bouquet of vessels
Bourneville's disease
Bourneville's syndrome
Bourns infant ventilator
bout(s)
  b. of coughing
  b. of coughing, severe
  b. of crying ▸ sudden
  b. of dysreflexia
  b. of rejection
boutonniere deformity
Bouveret's syndrome
Bovie
  B. coagulating current
  B. coagulator
  B. current

B. cutting current
B. electrocautery
B., low current
B. needle
B. unit
bovine
  b. allograft
  b. arch
  b. biodegradable collagen
  b. cells
  b. collagen
  b. encephalomyelitis, sporadic
  b. graft
  b. heart
  b. heart valve
  b. heterograft
  b. lavage extract surfactant
  b. orphan (ECBO) virus ▸ enteric
    cytopathic
  b. pericardial valve
  b. pericardium strips
  b. scabies
  b. spongiform encephalopathy
bovinum, cor
bovinus, Tabanus
bovis
  b., Actinomyces
  b., Cysticercus
  b., gram-positive Actinomyces
  b., Haemophilus
  b., Hemophilus
  b., Hypoderma
  b., Miyagawanella
  b., Mycobacterium
  b., Psoroptes
  b., Streptococcus
bow IUD (intrauterine device)
bow-legged, patient is
bowed
  b. drum
  b., legs
  b. vocal cords
bowel(s)
  b., abrasion of
  b. action, normal
  b. adequately evacuated
  b. ▸ anastomosed to loop of
  b. and bladder continence
  b. and bladder dysfunction
  b. and bladder functions
  b. atresia ▸ small
  b. biopsy ▸ small
  b. blockage
  b. blockage ▸ complete
  b. blockage ▸ partial

bowel(s)—*continued*
b., bruising of
b. cancer
b. cancer, lower
b. cleansing
b., clogged
b. constipated
b. contents
b. control
b. control ▸ loss of
b. control ▸ normal
b. ▸ cyclic muscular contractions of
b., dilated loops of
b. disease ▸ extensive inflammatory
b. disease, debilitating
b. disease, functional
b. disease, inflammatory
b. disease ▸ ulcerative
b. ▸ diseased segment of
b. disorder
b. inflammation
b. disorder ▸ inflammatory
b., distal small
b., distended
b. distended, large
b. dysfunction, bladder and
b. evacuated
b. evacuation
b. fills and evacuates satisfactorily
b., fluid filled loop of
b. follow-through (SBFT), small
b. function
b. function, absent
b. function, decreased
b. function, normal
b. functions ▸ normal stomach and
b., gangrene of
b., gangrenous small
b. gas artifact
b. gas pattern
b. gas, superimposed
b., greedy
b. habit, change in
b. habits
b. habits, altered
b. impaction
b. incapacity
b. incontinence
b. ▸ inflammatory disease of
b. ▸ intramural air in large
b., irritable
b. ischemia ▸ small
b., kinking of
b., large

b., layers of
b., lazy
b. loops
b. lumen
b. malabsorption, small
b. malignancy
b. management program
b. movement
b. movement, comfortable
b. movement ▸ fiber and
b. movement, loose
b. movement ▸ straining on
b. movement ▸ tarry black
b. movement ▸ urgent
b. movements ▸ altered
b. movements, diminished
b. movements ▸ frequent
b. movements ▸ irregular
b. movements, watery
b. mucosa
b. mucosa, small
b., multiple loops of small
b. ▸ muscle contraction of
b. ▸ necrosis of
b. obstructing adhesions
b. obstruction
b. obstruction, complete
b. obstruction ▸ intermittent small
b. obstruction, large
b. obstruction, mechanical
b. obstruction, small
b. obstruction with ascites ▸ small
b. pattern
b. pattern ▸ change in
b. perforation
b. peristalsis
b. ▸ petechial hemorrhages of
b. prep
b. preparation ▸ liquid
b. problems ▸ intermittent functional
b., proximal small
b. -related diseases
b. requirement, postsurgical
b. resection ▸ postoperative
b. resection, small
b., segment of
b. series, small
b. shadows, superimposition of
b., sluggish
b., small
b. sounds
b. sounds, active
b. sounds, decreased
b. sounds, hyperactive

b. sounds, hypoactive
b. sounds, normal
b. sounds, normoactive
b. sounds, positive
b., stimulation of lower
b., strangulated small
b. syndrome ▸ bloating and irritable
b. syndrome, functional
b. syndrome, gay
b. syndrome (IBS), irritable
b. syndrome ▸ pain in abdomen from irritable
b. syndrome ▸ short
b. syndrome, spastic
b. syndrome with constipation ▸ irritable
b. tones
b. tones, active
b. tones, hyperactive
b. tones, hypoactive
b. tones, normoactive
b. training
b. training program
b. wall
b. wall hemorrhages
Bowenoid papulosis
Bowen's disease
Bowie's stain
bowing
b. of fracture
b. of mitral valve leaflet
b. of nail
b. of vocal cords ▸ senile
b. tic
bowl, heel
Bowman('s)
B. capsule
B. discs
B. membrane
B. muscle
B. test, Visscher-
B. operation
bows, traction
box
b., anatomical snuff
b., Barany
b. bolus
b., bronchoscopic battery
b., control
b. ▸ digital constant current pacing
b., emergency drug
b. ▸ inflammation of voice
b., jack
b., Stockholm
b., voice

boxer's fracture
Boy (heroin)
Boyce sign
Boyd('s)
- B. implant
- B. incision
- B. operation
- B. operation ▸ Speed-
- B. perforating vein
- B. point
- B. posterior incision
- B. reduction technique ▸ Speed and

Boyden flap, Sewell-
Boyden's test meal
boydii
- b., Allescheria
- b., Pseudallescheria
- b., Shigella

Bozeman operation
bozemanii, Legionella
BP (blood pressure)
- BP, arterial
- BP, basic
- BP check
- BP ▸ chronic high
- BP cuff deflated
- BP, decreased
- BP, decreased systolic
- BP dropped
- BP elevated
- BP elevation
- BP fell
- BP fluctuated
- BP fluctuations
- BP, instrumental conditioning of diastolic
- BP, intermittent elevation of
- BP ▸ intracranial
- BP ▸ lowered
- BP measurement, home
- BP medication
- BP monitor
- BP monitor ▸ automatic oscillometric
- BP monitor ▸ electronic finger
- BP monitoring, automatic
- BP monitoring ▸ home
- BP, monitoring of
- BP normal
- BP ▸ orthostatic
- BP, persistent elevation of
- BP ▸ primary high
- BP reaction
- BP reading

BP reduce
BP reduction
BP reduction, correlates of
BP, rise in
BP screening
BP screening, free
BP ▸ secondary high
BP stabilized
BP test
BP therapy
BP track
BP, unstable
BP (bronchopleural)
BP (buccopulpal)
BPD (biparietal diameter)
BPD (bronchopulmonary dysplasia)
BPES (Borg Perceived Exertion Scale)
BPH (benign prostatic hypertrophy)
BPPV (benign paroxysmal positional vertigo)
BPV (benign positional vertigo)
bra, Jobst's
brace(s)
- b. artifact
- b., back
- b., body
- b., caliper
- b., cervical
- b. ▸ ceramic or plastic
- b., chair-back type
- b., Cook walking
- b., custom knee
- b., dental
- b., drop foot
- b., 49er knee
- b., four-poster cervical
- b., gaiter
- b., head
- b., Hudson's
- b., hyperextension
- b., ischial
- b., ischial weight bearing
- b., Jewett
- b., King cervical
- b., knee
- b., Knight's
- b., Kydex
- b., lingual
- b., long leg
- b., Lyman-Smith
- b., Milwaukee
- b., nonweight bearing
- b., Oppenheim
- b., polyurethane

b., preventive knee
b., prophylactic
b., prophylactic knee
b., protective
b., Schanz collar
b., short leg
b., stirrup
b., Taylor back
b., toedrop
b., traditional metal
b., Warm Springs
b., weight-bearing
b., Wilke boot
b. with drop-lock knee ▸ long leg
b. with free ankle ▸ long leg
b. with large tibial cuff oblong leg
bracelet
- b. ▸ medical alert necklace or
- b., patient identification (ID)
- b., weighted wrist
brachial
[*brachial, bronchial, bronchiole*]
- b. amyotrophy
- b. -ankle index
- b. arteriogram
- b. arteriotomy
- b. artery
- b. artery approach
- b. artery cutdown
- b. artery, deep
- b. artery thrombosis
- b. block
- b. blood pressure, ankle
- b. blood pressure ratio, ankle
- b. bypass
- b. catheter
- b. dance
- b. embolectomy
- b. index (ABI) ▸ ankle
- b. locomotion
- b. muscle
- b. nerve, intercostal
- b. nerve, intercosto◊
- b. neuralgia
- b. neuritis, paralytic
- b. palsy
- b. plexopathy
- b. plexus
- b. plexus activity
- b. plexus involvement
- b. plexus palsy
- b. pressure index ▸ penile-
- b. pulses
- b. region
- b. region, anterior

brachial—*continued*
- b. syndrome
- b. technique ▸ modified
- b. vein

brachii
- b. artery, profunda
- b. muscle, biceps
- b. muscle, triceps

brachioaxillary bridge graft fistula
brachiocephalic
- b. arteriography
- b. arteritis
- b. artery
- b. ischemia
- b. system
- b. trunk
- b. vein
- b. vein, left
- b. vein, right
- b. vessel angioplasty

brachiocephalicus, truncus
brachioradial ligament
brachioradial muscle
brachioulnar articulation
Brachmann-de Lange syndrome
Bracht's maneuver
Bracht-Wachter lesion
brachygnathia and cleft palate
brachypellic pelvis
brachytherapy
- b., breast
- b., cesium 137 bougie
- b. implant, open bladder
- b., interstitial
- b. mold, endolaryngeal
- b., ophthalmic
- b. procedure
- b. radium needle
- b., reoxygenation and
- b., scattering in
- b., transcatheter
- b. treatment

bracing
- b. and rehabilitation ▸ elevation,
- b., prophylactic
- b. vessel walls open

Bradford kidney, Rose-
Bradley Method
Bradshaw's albumosuria
bradyarrhythmia pacing
bradycardia
- b. and absent corneal reflexes
- b. and rigidity ▸ tremor,
- b., artifactual
- b., atrial

- b., baseline
- b., Branham's
- b., cardiomuscular
- b., central
- b., clinostatic
- b., essential
- b., fetal
- b. hypotensive
- b., idiopathic
- b., idioventricular
- b., junctional
- b., nodal
- b. pacing
- b., postinfectious
- b., postinfective
- b., pulseless
- b., relative
- b., sinoatrial
- b., sinus
- b., symptomatic
- b. syndrome ▸ tachycardia-
- b. -tachycardia syndrome
- b., vagal
- b., ventricular

bradykinesia ▸ slow diminished movement of
bradyrhythmia, anterior
bradyrhythmia, anterior cerebral
bradytachycardia syndrome
Bragard's sign
Bragg
- B. curve
- B. fever, Fort
- B. -Paul pulsator
- B. peak
- B. peak, sharp
- B. peak, spread

braided silk suture
braid-like lesion
Braid's strabismus
Brailey operation
Brailey procedure
braille embosser
Brailler, Perkins
brain(s) (Brain)('s)
- b., abnormal electrical activity in
- b. abnormalities ▸ schizophrenic
- b. abnormality
- b. abscess
- b. abscess ▸ delirium from
- b. ▸ activate chemical impulse in
- b., activate pleasure centers of
- b. activity
- b. activity, decreased
- b. activity, diminished

- b. activity, excessive
- b. activity ▸ impaired
- b. activity, increased
- b. activity, local
- b. activity, localized
- b. activity, recorded electrical
- b. ▸ acute injury to
- b., addiction in
- b. affliction
- b., aging of
- b., alcohol effect on
- b., alterations of media surrounding
- b., Alzheimer diseased
- b. amine depletion
- b. anatomy
- b. and nervous system, disorders of
- b. and spinal cord ▸ focal disorders of
- b. aneurysm
- b. aneurysm, ruptured
- b. aneurysm ▸ unruptured
- b., angioma of
- b. ▸ anoxic changes in
- b., arachnoid of
- b., arteriovenous malformation of
- b. attack
- b. atrophy
- b. autistic
- b., autopsy limited to
- b., autopsy of
- b. ▸ balance mechanism to
- b. barrier, alteration of blood
- b. barrier (BBB), blood-
- b. barrier, (CSF) cerebrospinal fluid
- b., base of
- b. -based
- b. -based pain control
- b., biochemical change in
- b. biopsies
- b. bladder
- b., bleeding into the
- b. blood barrier disruption chemotherapy
- b. blood clot
- b., blood flow to
- b. -blood partition coefficient
- b., blood supply of
- b. blood vessel disease
- b. blood vessel, ruptured
- b. bypass ▸ extracranial-intracranial
- b. cancer
- b. cancer treatment
- b. cavity
- b. cell malfunction

b. cell transplant
b., cell within
b. cells
b. cells ▸ Alzheimer's disease
b. cells, damaged
b. cells, death of
b. cells, destruction of
b. cells, fetal
b. cells ▸ irreversible damage to
b. cells misfiring
b. cells ▸ reinvigorate
b. center
b. centers ▸ depression of vital
b. centers, vital
b., cerebral activity of
b., cerebral atrophy of
b. changes, organic
b. changes physically
b. chemical
b., chemical abnormality in
b. chemical changes
b., chemical disruption in
b., chemical systems of
b., chemical transmitters in
b. chemistry
b. chemistry, alters
b. chemistry, body and
b. chemistry, irregularity in
b., chronic inflammation of
b. circuit
b., circulation in
b., circulation to
b., circumscribed atrophy of
b., collateral arterial flow to
b., compression of the
b. concussion
b. ▸ congenital defects of
b. ▸ constriction of arteries of
b. controls
b., contusion of
b., convexes of
b. cortex
b. ▸ cortical necrosis of
b. cortography
b. cover ▸ small blood vessels of
the
b. damage
b. damage, alcohol
b. damage, anoxic
b. damage, fatal
b. damage from cerebral
hemorrhage
b. damage injury
b. damage, irreversible

b. damage, irreversible
catastrophic
b. damage ▸ massive
b. damage, permanent
b. damage ▸ physical
b. damage, severe
b., damaged
b., damaged cell membranes in
b. damaged patient
b. dead, patient
b. death
b. death, clinical
b. death criteria
b. death, criteria for determination
of
b. death, diagnosed
b. death diagnosis
b. death ▸ irreversible
b. death ▸ maternal
b. death, pronouncement of
b. death, traumatic
b. death ▸ whole
b. defect
b. deficiency, acute
b. degeneration
b. degeneration ▸ midlife
b., degenerative disease of
b. 's delicate balance
b., dementia from
b. deposits
b., depth of the
b. destroying disorder
b. deterioration ▸ progressive
b. development
b., different areas of
b., diffuse degeneration of
b., diminished production of protein
in
b., discrete area of
b. disease
b. disease, degenerative
b. disease, focal
b. disease, human
b. disease ▸ incipient degenerative
b. disease, incurable
b. disease ▸ inheritable
b. disease, metastatic
b. disease, organic
b. disease ▸ progressive
b. disease, progressive organic
B. disease, Russell
b. disease ▸ slowly developing
b. disorder
b. disorder ▸ biological
b. disorder, chronic

b. disorder, degenerative
b. disorder, incurable
b. disorder ▸ inherited
b. disorder, organic
b. disorder ▸ progressive
b. disorder, serious
b. ▸ disordered state in
b. disorganization
b., dissection of
b. disturbance
b. disturbance, acute
b., dizziness from
b., dominant side of
b. dose, minimize normal
b. drain
b., dura mater of
b., dural membrane of
b. dysfunction
b. dysfunction (MBD), minimal
d. ▸ dysplastic left hemisphere of
d. ▸ dysplastic right hemisphere of
b. edema
b. edematous
b., electrical activity of
b. electrical activity ▸ shift in
direction and pattern of
b. electrical activity toward sleep
activity ▸ shifting
b. ▸ electrical firings of
b., electrical reactivity of
b., electrical stimulation of
b., electrical stimulation to
b. electrodes, implanting
b., elevated surface of
b. ▸ energy use in
b., epilepsy from
b., excision frontal lobe of
b., excision occipital lobe of
b., excision parietal lobe of
b., excision temporal lobe of
b., excision tumor of
b. excitation, levels of
b. explored
b. exploring cannula, Kanavel
b. extremely degenerated
b., female rat
b. fever
b. ▸ fixation and sectioning of
b. flow
b., fore◇
b. formation ▸ fetal
b., fourth ventricle of
b., frontal lobe of
b., full radiation of
b. function

brain(s)—*continued*

b. function ► abnormal
b. function activity
b. function, altered
b. function, altering
b. function ► diminished heart, kidney and
b. function ► disintegration of cognitive
b. function ► general deterioration of
b. function ► heart, kidney and
b. function, irregular
b. function, meaningful
b. function, mind-
b. function, organically impaired
b., fungating
b., fungus of the
b., generalized atrophy of
b. glistening
b., glucose metabolism in
b. graft surgery
b., gray matter of
b. grossly symmetrical
b. growth ► abnormal
b. gut peptide
b., hallucinations from
b. 's hearing center
b. -heart infusion
b., hemispheres of
b. hemorrhage
b. hemorrhage ► small
b. hemiation
b., hind◊
b., histologic sections of
b., human
b. hypersensitivity
b. ► hypoxic change in
b. imaging
b. imaging scan
b. imaging study
b. imaging technique
b. impairment
b. implant surgery
b. impulse
b. including brain stem, ► irreversible cessation of all functions of entire
b. infarct
b. infection
b. ► inflammation and gliosis in
b., inflammation of
b., inherited abnormality in
b. injury
b. injury, anoxic

b. injury ► irreversible
b. injury, irreversible catastrophic
b. injury, life-threatening
b. injury ► localized
b. injury ► sports-
b. injury ► traumatic
b., inter◊
b., interface between electrode and
b., investigation
b. irradiation, whole
b., isolated
b., isotope scanning studies of
b., labyrinth of
b., lack of blood to the
b., lack of oxygen (O_2) to the
b. ► language center in
b. ► leakage of blood in
b. lesion ► focal
b., left hemisphere of
b., left side of
b. lesion
b., limbic
b., limbic lobe of
b. 's limbic system
b., lining of
b., living
b., lobes of
b. lymphoma
b., male rat
b. malformation
b. malfunction
b. malignancy
b. mapper
b. mantle
b. mapping
b. mass
b. mass, posterior
b. ► memory bank in
b. ► memory loss from
b., mesial surface of occipital lobe of
b. messages
b. 's metabolic activity
b. metabolism
b. metastases
b. metastases ► choriocarcinoma lung with
b. metastases, multiple
b. metastases, palliation in
b. mets (metastases) ► patient has
b., microscopically immature
b. ► micturition reflex center in
b., mid◊
b. ► motor control center of
b. 's motor control system

b. murmur
b. natriuretic peptide
b. natural chemicals
b. natural Dopamine production
b., necrosis of
b. neoplasm
b., nerve cells within
b. nerve fibers
b. ► neuron destroying plaques in
b., neurons of
b. new
b. nutrient
b. occipital lobe of
b., old
b. olfactory
b., olfactory lobe of
b. or lung ► blood clot in
b. ► organic damage to
b., outermost covering of
b. ► oxygen (O_2) starved
b. pacemaker
b. pale white
b. parenchyma
b., parietal lobe of
b. pathology
b. patient, split-
b. ► periodic electrical stimulation to
b., permanent pacemaker for
b. physical ability to react
b., physical change in
b., physical disorder of
b., pia mater of
b. plaques
b. plaques and tangles of Alzheimer's disease
b. ► plaques in
b., pleasure centers in
b. potential ► event-related
b. power
b., pressure on the
b. processing of words
b., protective layer of
b., puncture of
b. radiation therapy ► full
b. radiation therapy ► whole
b. radiation therapy, whole brain vs local
b. radiation, whole
b., rat
b. receptor
b. ► reduce swelling in
b. ► reduced blood flow to
B. reflex
B. reflex, Russell
b. 's regulatory center

b. resets rhythm
b., respirator
b. resuscitation potential
b., reticulum cell sarcoma of
b., retraining
b., right hemisphere of
b., right side of
b. ▸ sagittal sections of
b. sand
b. scan
B. scan, MR (magnetic resonance)
b. scan negative
b. scan positive
b. scan, radioactive
b. scan, rapid flow
b. scanner ▸ Electric and Musical Industries (EMI)
B. scanning
b. science
b., seizure from
b. ▸ seizure-producing areas of
b. ▸ serial coronal section of
b., severely traumatized
b. shrinking medication
b., shrunken
b. sites
b., smell
b., softening of the
b. ▸ spasm of arteries of
b., speech center in
b. ▸ sponge-like holes in
b., stabilize
b. states, shift
b. stem
b. stem auditory evoked potential (BAEP)
b. stem auditory evoked response (BAER)
b. stem, blood effusion
b. stem, blood supply to
b. stem, cancer of
b. stem ▸ chemoreceptors in
b. stem control
b. stem, descending
b. stem disease ▸ severe
b. stem, dorsal surface of
b. stem ▸ Duret's hemorrhage in
b. stem evoked response (BSER)
b. stem functions
b. stem glioma
b. stem hemorrhage
b. stem ▸ impairment of functions of
b. stem, irreversible cessation of all functions of entire brain including

b. stem, lesion of
b. stem, lower
b. stem, massive infarct of
b. stem nuclei
b. stem reflexes
b. stem response (ABR), auditory
b. stem ▸ reticular formation of
b. stem stroke
b. stem stroke syndrome, postoperative
b. stem, tectum of
b. stem, traumatized
b. stem tumor
b. stem, upper
b. stem vascular disease
b., stimulatic dopamine production in
b. stimulation
b. stimulation, deep
b. stimulation, thalamic deep
b. stimulator, deep
b. ▸ stress-related aging of
b. structures
b. substance
b. substance ▸ electrode implanted in
b. sugar
b., sulci in
b. ▸ superior insular gyrus of
b. support
b., supporting tissue of
b. surface
b. surface, fissures on
b. surgery
b. surgery ▸ invasive
b. surgery, minimally invasive
b. surgery, radical
b. surgery ▸ split
b. swell, severe
b. swelling
b. symmetrical
b. ▸ synapses in
b. syndrome
b. syndrome ▸ acute
b. syndrome, acute organic
b. syndrome, acute treatment for organic
b. syndrome, alcoholic
b. syndrome ▸ chronic
b. syndrome, chronic alcoholic
b. syndrome, chronic organic
b. syndrome, clinical manifestations of organic
b. syndrome, differential diagnosis in organic

b. syndrome, drug reactions in organic
b. syndrome ▸ organic
b. syndrome ▸ reversible
b. syndrome ▸ split-
b. syndrome, subacute treatment for organic
b. syndrome, treatment of organic
b. syndrome ▸ wet
b. syndrome with cannabinoids, organic
b. syndrome with depressants, organic
b. syndrome with hallucinogens, organic
b. syndrome with inhalants, organic
b. syndrome with multiple drugs, organic
b. syndrome with opioids, organic
b. syndrome with phencyclidines, organic
b. syndrome with stimulants, organic
b. ▸ tangles in
b. temperature
b., temporal lobe of
b. test, noninvasive
b., third ventricle of
b., thrombosis of vessels of
b. tissue
b. tissue, abnormal
b. tissue, active
b. tissue, bleeding into
b. tissue, bruised
b. tissue, cultured
b. tissue, damaged
b. tissue, death of
b. tissue degenerates
b. tissue, distorted
b. tissue ▸ destroyed
b. tissue implants
b. tissue ▸ necrosis
b. tissue ▸ normal immature
b. tissue, normal
b. to electrical stimulation, response of
b. toxin
b. ▸ tracking blood flow to the
b. ▸ transmitting electrochemical messages to
b. transplantation
b., transverse section of
b. trauma
b. tumor
b. tumor, benign

brain(s)—*continued*
b. tumor, childhood
b. tumor, destroy
b. tumor, inoperable
b. tumor, lower
b. tumor ▸ malignant
b. tumor, massive
b. tumor ▸ metastatic
b. tumor, primary
b. tumor ▸ rapidly growing
b. tumor, recurrent
b. tumor research
b. tumor ▸ surgical treatment for
b. tumor suspects
b. tumor, target
b. tumor treatment
b., tween-
b. ▸ vascular system of
b., ventricles of the
b., ventricular system of
b., vessels ▸ malformation of
b., vessels of
b., visceral
b., visual centers of
b. vs local brain radiation therapy, whole
b. wasting disease
b., water
b. wave
b. wave, abnormal
b. wave activity and emotions
b. wave activity, decreased
b. wave activity ▸ deficiency of slow
b. wave activity ▸ excessive fast EEG
b. wave, alpha
b. wave components
b. wave components ▸ production of various
b. wave discharges, abnormal
b. wave frequency range
b. wave frequency, slow
b. wave function, abnormal
b. wave, high voltage
b. wave index
b. wave, low voltage
b. wave pattern
b. wave pattern, recorded
b. wave responses
b. wave, slow
b. wave, suppression of seizure specific
b. wave, theta
b. ▸ waxy deposit in
b. weight

b., wet
b., white matter of
b. system of neurotransmitters
brainstorming exercise
brake, duodenal
braking radiation (bremsstrahlung)
bran, diarrhea from
branch(es)
b., arterial
b. block, AV (atrioventricular)
b. block (BBBB), bilateral bundle
b. block (BBB) ▸ bundle
b. block (LBBB) ▸ complete left bundle
b. block (RBBB) ▸ complete right bundle
b. block ▸ His bundle
b., block in anterosuperior division of left
b., block in posteroinferior division of left
b. block (BBB) ▸ incomplete bundle
b. block (LBBB) ▸ incomplete left bundle
b. block (RBBB) ▸ incomplete right bundle
b. block (LBBB) ▸ left bundle
b. block (RBBB) ▸ right bundle
b., bronchial
b., bronchus
b., buccal
b., callosal marginal
b., caudal
b. circumflexed
b., cochlear
b. compromise ▸ side
b., conus
b. fibrosis, bundle
b. heart block ▸ bundle
b., left bundle
b. lesion
b. ▸ obtuse marginal
b. occlusion ▸ side
b. of artery, caudal
b. of bronchial tree
b. of posterior cerebral artery, choroidal
b. of radial nerve ▸ superficial
b. of ulnar nerve ▸ dorsal
b. of ulnar nerve ▸ superficial
b. of vagus nerve, auricular
b., patent
b., pulmonary artery
b. pulmonary artery stenosis
b. reentrant tachycardia, bundle

b. reentry, bundle
b. retinal vein occlusion
b., right bundle
b., secondary
b. stenosis, pulmonary
b., superior rectal
b. vessel occlusion
b. vessel pruning
branched chain
branchial [*brachial, bronchial, bronchiole*]
b. arches
b. artery
b. cleft
b. cleft cyst
b. cyst
b. pulse
b. vestige
branchiarum, Amphileptus
branching
b. airways
b. decay
b. fraction
b., multiple
b. of neurons ▸ synaptic
b. ratio
b. technique
branchiogenous cancer
Branchiostoma californiense
Branchiostoma virginiae
brand name drug
Brandt('s)
B. -Andrews maneuver
B. brassiere
B. syndrome
B. technique
B. treatment
brandy nose
Branham('s)
B. sign ▸ Nicoladoni-
B. bradycardia
B. sign
Branhamella catarrhalis
Bras disease ▸ Stuart-
Brasfield chest radiograph
brash
b. and uninhibited behavior
b., water
b., weaning
brasiliense, Ancylostoma
brasiliensis
b., Blastomyces
b., Leishmania
b., Nocardia
b., Paracoccidioides

b., Xenopsylla
brass-founders' ague
brassiere, Brandt's
brassy cough
Brauer operation
Braun('s)
 B. anastomosis
 B. -Fernwald sign
 B. graft
 b. pinch graft technique
 B. sign, Roser-
 b. -Wangensteen graft
brauni, Diplogonoporus
Braunwald's prosthesis
Braunwald's sign
Bravais-jacksonian epilepsy
brawny
 b. edema
 b. edema, Stellwag's
 b. induration
 b. trachoma
Braxton
 B. Hicks contraction
 B. Hicks sign
 B. Hicks version
Brazelton behavioral scale
Brazilian spotted fever
braziliense, Ancylostoma
braziliense, Uncinaria
braziliensis, Leishmania
brazilienseis, Nocardia
bread
 b. -and-butter textbook sign
 b. -and-butter pericardium
 b. exchange
breadth [*breath*], bizygomatic
breadth [*breath*] of accommodation
break(s)
 b. down ▸ bone constantly
 b. ▸ hangman's
 b. in reality contact
 b. in the skin
 b., periodic
 b. shock
breakaway splice
breakbone fever
breakdown
 b. bacteria, cellulose
 b., bone growth and
 b., cartilage
 b., complete
 b., emotional
 b. ▸ gum tissue
 b., muscle
 b., myofibril

b., nervous
b. products, fibrinogen
b., skin
b. syndrome, social
b., tissue
breakfast, oil
breaking
 b. and swallowing ▸ impaired
 b. from athlete's foot ▸ nail
 b. from circulatory problem ▸ nails
 b. up adhesions
breakout, skin
breakthrough pain
breast(s) [*crest*]
 b. abnormality
 b. abnormality ▸ chill with
 b. abscess
 b. abscess, chronic
 b. abscess from breastfeeding
 b., adenoma of
 b. amputation, partial
 b. and axillary contents normal
 b. anemia
 b. architecture, postmenopausal
 b. area previously marked
 b. augmentation
 b. augmentation ▸ female textured
 b. augmentation surgery
 b., bilateral ▸ fibrocystic disease of
 b. biopsy
 b. biopsy, automated large core
 b. biopsy ▸ excisional
 b. biopsy instrumentation (AB-BI) ▸ advanced
 b. biopsy procedure ▸ minimally invasive
 b. biopsy ▸ stereotactic
 b. biopsy, ▸ ultrasound
 b. ▸ bloody discharge from
 b., boil on
 b. bone
 b. bone and ribs inflammation of
 b. bone ▸ splitting
 b. brachytherapy
 b. bridge
 b., caked
 b., caking of
 b. calcifications
 b. calcifications, benign
 b. calcifications ▸ speckled
 b. cancer
 b. cancer ▸ adjuvant therapy for
 b. cancer, advanced
 b. cancer, angiogenic
 b. cancer causing chemical

b. cancer cells
B. Cancer Detection Awareness Program
b. cancer, disseminated
b. cancer ▸ early detection of
b. cancer ▸ early-stage
b. cancer fatality rate
b. cancer genes
b. cancer ▸ hereditary
b. cancer ▸ high risk for
b. cancer ▸ increased risk of
b. cancer, inflammatory
b. cancer, invasive
b. cancer link, potential
b. cancer, metastatic
b. cancer ▸ mole
b. cancer ▸ nonhereditary
b. cancer, operable
b. cancer patient
b. cancer ▸ postmenopausal
b. cancer prevention
b. cancer rate
b. cancer, recurrent
b. cancer research
b. cancer risk
b. cancer therapy, cellular
b. cancer therapy ▸ molecular
b. cancer treatment
b. cancer treatment, experimental
b. carcinoma
b. carcinoma, advanced
b. carcinoma, axillary nodal metastasis in
b. carcinoma, locally advanced and inflammatory
b. carcinoma, peau d'orange in
b. carcinoma ▸ recurrent
b. carcinoma, survival relative to nodal involvement in
b. cells
b. cells ▸ maturation of
b. change, fibrocystic
b., colostrum expressed from
b. ▸ common disorder of
b. condition, fibrocystic
b. conservation surgery
b. conservation therapy
b., contour of
b. core biopsy
b. cyst
b. cyst aspiration
b., cystic
b., cystic disease of
b. deformity, pigeon
b. development ▸ failure of

breast(s)—*continued*

b. dimpling
b., dimpling from
b. ▸ direct injection of silicone into
b. discomfort
b. disease, benign
b. disease, fibrocystic
b. does appear enlarged ▸ lump in left
b. does appear enlarged ▸ lump in right
b. does not appear enlarged ▸ lump in left
b. does not appear enlarged ▸ lump in right
b., dose to contralateral
b. engorgement
b. enhancement
b. enhancement surgery
b. enlargement
b. enlargement ▸ male
b. examination
b. examination ▸ clinical
b., excision and wedge biopsy of
b. -fed, infant
b. feeding
b., female
b. fibroadenosis
b., fibrocystic
b., fibrocystic changes in
b. firmness and discomfort, excessive
b. firmness, excessive
b., fluid-filled cysts in
b., fluid-filled sacs in
b., fullness of
b., giant fibroadenoma
b. heart, thrust
b., heat generation of
b., heat radiated by
b., hyperthermia in
b. hypertrophy
b. imaging
b. imaging technology
b. implant
b. implant, adjustable
b. implant, double lumen
b. implant, expandable
b. implant, Extrafil
b. implant, Heyer-Schulte
b. implant, leaking
b. implant, saline-filled
b. implant, self-sealing
b. implant, silicone
b. implant, silicone-filled

b. implant, silicone gel
b. implant ▸ silicone gel-filed
b. implant, temporary
b. ▸ infiltrating ductal carcinoma of
b., inflammatory carcinoma of
b. injury ▸ nipple discharge from
b., intraductal carcinoma of
b. ▸ intraductal papilloma of
b., invasive carcinoma of
b., lactating
b. lift
b. ▸ localized pain in
b. line
b. lump
b. lump, benign
b. lump, palpable
b. lump pressing
b. lumpiness
b. malignancy
b. ▸ malignant calcifications of
b. mass
b., medial and lateral tangential
b. microcalcifications
b. milk
b. milk ▸ alcohol in
b. nipple, retraction of
b. nodule
b. -ovarian cancer syndrome ▸ hereditary
b., overstimulation of
b. ▸ Paget's disease of
b. pain
b. pain after childbirth
b. pain, cyclical
b. pain from breastfeeding
b. pain from caffeine
b., pain in
b. pain, noncyclical
b., painful swelling of
b. pang
b. pendulous
b. pendulous and atrophic
b., pigeon
b. pocket
b. prosthesis
b., postmenopausal
b. preserving alternatives
b. prosthesis, Ashley's
b. prosthesis fitting
b. ptosis
b. pump
b., quadrant of
b., radiation therapy for intact
b., reconstructed
b. reconstruction

b. reconstruction after mastectomy
b. reconstruction surgery
b. ▸ red and warm
b. ▸ red spot on
b. reduction
b. reduction female
b. reduction male
b. reduction surgery
b. removal preventive
b. ▸ retracted nipple from
b. ropy or granular
b., sagging
b., sclerosis of
B. Screening Program
b. secretion
b. self-examination (BSE)
b. self-examination, concentric circle pattern of
b. self-examination, vertical pattern of
b. self-examination, wedge section pattern of
b. self-exams (BSE) ▸ monthly
b. sensor pad
b. shadow
b. size
b. size, decreased
b. skin, diminution of
b. soreness
b. stimulation
b. stretch marks from pregnancy
b., striae of
b. structures, normal
b. surgery, cosmetic
b. surgery prophylactic
b. surgery, reconstructive
b., surgical absence of
b. swelling
b. symmetrical
b. ▸ tender, swollen
b. tenderness
b. tenderness, premenstrual
b. therapy
b. thermography
b., thickening of
b. tissue
b. tissue approximated
b. tissue cells ▸ invasive
b. tissue cells ▸ normal
b. tissue ▸ dense
b. tissue expander
b. tissue, hardening of
b., tissue, reconstruction of
b. tissue, scarring of
b. tissue, surrounding

b. tumefaction
b. tumor, benign
b. tumor, curable
b. tumor, hot vs cold
b. tumor ▸ localized cancerous
b. tumor recurrence ▸ ipsilateral
b., tumor of
b. tumor, preexisting
b. tumor ▸ vaporizing
b. x-rays ▸ low-dose

breastfeeding
b. basic
b. ▸ breast abscess from
b. ▸ breast pain from
b., diarrhea and
b. ineffective
b., long-term
b., mastitis with
b. ▸ nipple problem from
b., patient

breaststroke injury
breath(s)
b. ▸ acute shortness of
b., alcohol on
b. alcohol testing
b., alcoholic
b., bad
b., chest discomfort with shortness of
b., chronic bad
b. coordination, hand-
b., deep cleansing
b. diffusion ▸ single
b. excretion test
b. (SOB) ▸ exercise induced shortness of
b., four quick
b. (SOB) from anxiety ▸ shortness of
b. from bronchitis ▸ bad
b. from cold ▸ bad
b., gasping for
b. -holding test
b. ▸ increased shortness of
b., liver
b., malodorous
b. nitrogen curve ▸ single
b. nitrogen washout test ▸ single
b. odor
b. on exertion, shortness of
b. (SOB) ▸ palpitations and shortness of
b., patient short of
b. pentane test

b. (SOB) ▸ progressive shortness of
b., recurrent shortness of
b., shortness of
b. sounds
b. sounds, absent
b. sounds, adventitious
b. sounds, bronchial
b. sounds, bronchovesicular
b. sounds, coarse
b. sounds, crowing
b. sounds, decreased
b. sounds, diminished
b. sounds, diminution of
b. sounds ▸ distant
b. sounds, good
b. sounds ▸ lungs revealed diminished
b. sounds ▸ metallic
b. sounds ▸ quiet
b. sounds ▸ tubular
b. (SOB) ▸ sudden shortness of
b. test
b. test ▸ Fowler single
b. test, single
b., three-part
b. (SOB) ▸ weakness fatigue and shortness of
b., yogic complete

breathalyzer results
breathalyzer test
breather, mouth
breathes with mouthpiece
breathing [*bleeding*]
b., abdominal
b. abnormality
b. air (resting)
b. air (standing)
b. and circulation (ABC) ▸ airway
b. and heartbeat, depressed
b. and limpness ▸ rapid
b. and relaxation exercises
b. and relaxation techniques
b. apneustic
b. apparatus ▸ self-contained underwater
b. assisted
b., Blot's
b., bronchial
b. capacity (IMBC) ▸ indirect maximum
b. capacity, maximal
b. capacity, maximum
b., cavernous
b., cease

b., cessation of
b., chest pain on deep
b., Cheyne-Stokes
b. circuit, patient
b., conscious
b. (CPPB) ▸ continuous positive pressure
b., control of
b., controlled
b., deep
b., deep chest
b., deep slow
b., diaphragmatic
b., diaphragmatic and chest
b. difficulty
b. difficulty ▸ chest pain with
b. difficulty from anemia
b. difficulty from anxiety
b. difficulty from asthma
b. difficulty from bronchitis
b., difficulty in
b. ▸ difficulty in nasal
b. difficulty, initial
b. difficulty, temporary
b. difficulty with problem from central nervous system
b., dilatation
b. disorder
b., distress in
b. ▸ dizziness from rapid and deep
b., dyspneic
b. efficiency
b. emergency
b., enhancing normal
b. excessive
b. exercises
b. exercises, deep
b. exercises ▸ stretching and
b., expulsion
b. failure
b., forced
b., frog
b. function
b. function ▸ loss of effective
b., glossopharyngeal
b. in tobacco smoke
b. ▸ increased and labored
b. (IPPB) ▸ intermittent positive pressure
b., irregular
b., Kussmaul's
b., labored
b., laryngitis from
b., minimal spontaneous
b. ▸ momentary lapse in normal

breathing—*continued*
- b., mouth
- b., mouth-to-mouth
- b. muscle
- b., nasal
- b. ► Ondine curse
- b., paced
- b. pacemaker
- b. passage, blocked
- b. passages ► constriction of
- b., patient has labored
- b., patient taught deep
- b. pattern
- b. pattern ► central neurogenic
- b. pattern ► ineffective
- b. pattern, irregular
- b. patterns, monitoring
- b. ► period of absent
- b., periodic
- b. ► periodic cessation of
- b. (PPB) ► positive pressure
- b. problems, chronic
- b. prolonged and deep
- b. ► pursed-lip style of
- b. ► pursed lips
- b., rapid
- b. ► rapid shallow
- b. rate ► increase heart and
- b., relaxed
- b., rescue
- b. reserve
- b. retraining, computerized diaphragmatic
- b. rhythm, decelerate
- b., rhythmical
- b. sensation ► loaded
- b., shallow
- b., shallow accelerated
- b. ► shallow, rapid
- b. ► sign mechanism for ventilator
- b. ► sleep disordered
- b., slow and shallow
- b., sonorous
- b., spontaneous
- b., stertorous
- b., stimulate
- b., stimulate adequate spontaneous
- b. supported by mechanical respirator
- b. technique
- b. technique, deep-
- b., temporary absence of
- b., transition
- b., trouble
- b. tubes

- b., wheezing while
- b. ► whistling in nose while
- b. with abdominal swelling
- b. with back, chest or abdomen pain
- b. with exercise ► coordinate
- b. with forced blowing out ► shallow
- b. with neck swelling
- b. with palpitation
- b., Yoga

breathless
- b., patient
- b. ► patient pulseless and
- b. ► relieve swelling and

breathlessness
- b. and fatigue
- b. ► angina and
- b., attack of
- b., excessive
- b. ► extreme
- b., ► insomnia and orthopnea
- b. ► unexpected
- b. ► unexplained fatigue and

breathy voice
breech
- b. birth
- b., complete vaginal
- b. deformity ► riding
- b. delivery
- b. delivery, partial
- b. delivery, vaginal
- b. extraction
- b. extraction, partial
- b. extraction, total
- b., frank vaginal
- b. position, complete
- b. position, incomplete
- b. postural deformity
- b. presentation
- b. presentation, complete
- b. presentation, footling
- b. presentation, frank
- b. presentation, full
- b. presentation, knee

breeder(s) ('s)
- b. 's disease, pigeon
- b. 's lung, bird-
- b. 's lung, pigeon
- b. reactor

breeding, cross◊
bregmatic bone
bregmatic fontanelle
bregmocardiac reflex
Breisky's disease
Breisky's pelvimeter

bremsstrahlung (braking radiation)
bremneri, Taenia
Brenner('s)
- B. carotid bypass shunt
- B. operation
- B. tumor

Brentano's syndrome
Brent's eyebrow reconstruction
brephoplastic graft
brequinar sodium
Breschet's veins
Brescio-Cimino AV (arteriovenous) fistula
Bretonneau angina
Brett bone graft
Brett's operation
Breuer-Hering inflation reflex
Breuer reflex ► Hering-
Breu's mole
brevia, vasa
breves insulae, gyri
brevicaulis, Scopulariopsis
brevis
- b., Bacillus
- b. muscle, abductor pollicis
- b. muscle, extensor carpi radialis
- b. muscle, extensor digitorum
- b. muscle, extensor hallucis
- b. muscle, extensor pollicis
- b. muscle, flexor digitorum
- b. muscle, flexor hallucis
- b. muscle, flexor pollicis
- b. muscle, palmaris
- b. muscle, peroneus
- b., musculus extensor pollicis
- b., musculus flexor pollicis
- b., Siderobacter
- b. tendon, extensor pollicis
- b. transplant, peroneus

Brewer's infarct
Bricker procedure
Bricker's operation
Brickner position
bridge(s) (Bridge) [*ridge*]
- b., arteriolovenular
- b., bony
- b., breast
- b., broad nasal
- b., cell
- b., cross-
- b., cytoplasmic
- b., dental
- b., dentin
- b., extension
- b., fixed

b. graft fistula, brachioaxillary
b., Iglesias
b. impression
b., intercellular
b., intracellular
b., myocardial
b., nasal
b. of nose
b., permanent
b. prosthesis ▸ Rosi L-type nose
b., removable
b., stationary
B. test ▸ Yerkes-
b., Wheatstone
bridgework, fixed
bridgework, removable
bridging
b., bony
b., muscle
b., myocardial
b. veins
bridle
b. stricture
b. suture
b. suture, superior rectus
brief (Brief)
b. depressive reaction
b. duration, fever of
b. examination
b. exposure to heat stress
b. loss of consciousness
B. Neuropsychological Mental
Status Examination (BNMSE)
b. observation ▸ patient discharged
after
b. progressive relaxation
b. quivering spells
b. reactive psychosis
b. recurrent seizures
b. treatment, detoxification and
Briggs' operation
Briggs Type Indicator (MBTI) test ▸
Myers-
bright (Bright's)
B. blindness
B. disease
b. echo
B. eye
B. friction sound ▸ Beatty-
B. granulation
b. light ▸ sensitivity to
B. murmur
b. /normal range of abilities
b. red blood
b. red blood ▸ copious

brightness modulation (B mode)
brightness modulation B-mode
scanning
Brill-Symmers disease
Brill-Zinsser disease
brilliant
b. cresyl blue
b. green
b. green dye
b. green, outlined with
brim of pelvis
brim, pelvic
brimstone liver
B-ring ▸ esophageal
Brinton's disease
Briquet's ataxia
Briquet's syndrome
brisement force
brisk
b. and arterial, bleeding
b. epistaxis
b. hemorrhage
b. reactive pupils
b. reflexes
b. ▸ reflexes equal and
b. walking
Brissaud('s)
B. dwarf
B. reflex
B. scoliosis
B. -Sicard syndrome
bristle cells
Bristowe's syndrome
Bristow's operation
British anti-lewisite (BAL)
Brittain operation ▸ Dunn-
Brittain's operation
brittle
b. bone disease
b. bone weakening
b. bones
b. diabetes
b. diabetic, patient
b. fingernails
b. nail
b. toenails ▸ misshapen,
broach
b., Harris
b., root canal
b., smooth
broad
b. adhesive band
b. band
b. band frequency analysis
b. -based

b. -based scars
b. -based scars ▸ wide
b. -beam scattering
b. ligament
b. ligament, leaves of
b. -minded
b. nasal bridge
b. range of effects
b. septate hyphae
b. spectrum
b. spectrum antibiotics
b. spectrum behavioral treatment
b. thumbs
broadbend attenuation
Broadbent's apoplexy
Broadbent's sign
Broca's
B. amnesia
B. aphasia
B. area
B. area, lesion in
B. ataxia
B. center
B. convolution
B. fissure
B. gyrus
B. pouch
B. region
B. space
Brock
B. infundibulectomy
B. operation
B. procedure
B. syndrome
B. transseptal commissurotomy
Brockenbrough('s)
B. effect
B. sign
B. transseptal commissurotomy
Brockhurst technique, ▸ Schepens-
Okamura-
Brockman's operation
Brödel's line
Broden's position
Broders' classification
Broders' index
Brodie's
B. abscess
B. disease
B. finger
B. joint
B. knee
B. ligament
Brodmann's area

broken
- b. back
- b. bone
- b. catheter tip
- b. facial capillaries
- b., gross continuity
- b., gross continuity not
- b. heart valves
- b. injury
- b. jaw
- b. neck
- b. ribs
- b. ring, Landolt's
- b. skin

Brom repair

bromhidrosis of feet

bromide(s)
- b., blister from
- b. intoxication
- b. test, Walter's

Brompton('s)
- B. mixture
- B. cocktail
- B. solution

Bromsulphalein test

bronchi
- b., dilatation of
- b. erythematous
- b. erythematous and inflamed
- b., hyparterial
- b., lavage of
- b., lobar
- b. looked erythematous
- b., main
- b. occluded
- b., paries membranaceus
- b. ▸ peripheral dilatation of
- b., segmental
- b., stretched
- b., upper lobe segmental

bronchial [branchial, brachial, bronchiole]
- b. adenocarcinoma
- b. adenoma
- b. airways
- b. allergy
- b. angiography
- b. arteries
- b. arteriography
- b. artery anastomosis
- b. artery embolization
- b. artery, lumen of
- b. asthma
- b. atresia
- b. bifurcation

- b. biopsy, premortem
- b. branch
- b. breathing
- b. breath sounds
- b. brush biopsy
- b. brushing, cytology of
- b. brushings
- b. brushings ▸ double sheath
- b. bud
- b. carcinoma
- b. casts
- b. cells
- b. challenge test
- b. circulation
- b. collateral
- b. collateral artery murmur
- b. congestion
- b. constriction
- b. constriction and spasm
- b. crisis
- b. cyst
- b. dehiscence
- b. drainage (dr'ge)
- b. dysplasia
- b. epithelial cells
- b. epithelium ▸ basal layer of
- b. epithelium, ciliated
- b. epithelium ▸ germinal layer of
- b. epithelium ▸ sloughed
- b. fremitus
- b. glandular cells
- b. hyperreactivity
- b. irritation
- b. lavage
- b. lesions, intrinsic
- b. lining
- b. lumens
- b. lymph nodes
- b. markings
- b. meniscus sign
- b. mucosa
- b. mucosa, edema of
- b. mucosa ▸ extensive hemorrhage
- b. mucous membrane
- b. mucus blanket
- b. mucus inhibitor
- b. murmur
- b. obstruction
- b. orifice
- b. orifice ▸ left lower lobe (LLL)
- b. orifice ▸ left upper lobe (LUL)
- b. orifice ▸ LLL (left lower lobe)
- b. orifice ▸ LUL (left upper lobe)
- b. orifice ▸ right lower lobe (RLL)
- b. orifice ▸ right middle lobe (RML)

- b. orifice ▸ right upper lobe (RUL)
- b. orifice ▸ RLL (right lower lobe)
- b. orifice ▸ RML (right middle lobe)
- b. orifice ▸ RUL (right upper lobe)
- b. passage
- b. pattern, normal
- b. pneumonia
- b. pneumonia, acute
- b. provocation
- b. rales
- b. ramifications
- b. respiration
- b. restriction
- b. secretions
- b. secretions, thick
- b. sleeve resection
- b. smooth muscle
- b. smooth muscle tone
- b. spasm
- b. stenosis
- b. stump
- b. suctioning ▸ endotracheal-
- b. suture
- b. tissue
- b. toilet
- b. tree
- b. tree ▸ branches of
- b. tree, embryo
- b. tree examined
- b. tree, flexibility of
- b. tree, left
- b. tree ▸ mucus plugging of
- b. tree, right
- b. tree, sensitive
- b. tube
- b. tube constrict
- b. tube, dilate
- b. tubes, enlarged
- b. tubes ▸ hyperreactive
- b. tubes ▸ inflammation of
- b. tubes ▸ spasm of
- b. vein
- b. wall
- b. washings
- b. wheezing

bronchiale, septum

bronchic cell

bronchiectasis
- b., capillary
- b. chemical
- b., chronic
- b. congenital
- b., cylindrical
- b., cystic
- b., distal

b. dry
b. ▸ focal areas of
b., follicular
b. fusiform
b., pseudocylindrical
b., saccular
b., severe
b. traction
bronchiectatic rale
bronchiogenic [*bronchogenic*]
bronchiolar adenocarcinoma
bronchiolar carcinoma
bronchiole(s) [*bronchial, branchial, brachial*]
b., alveolar
b., dilation of
b. lack cartilage ▸ tiny
b., lobular
b., respiratory
b., terminal
bronchiolitis
b., acute obliterating
b. exudativa
b. fibrosa obliterans
b. follicular
b. obliterans
b. obliterans organizing pneumonia
b. obliterative
b., vesicular
b., viral
bronchioloalveolar adenocarcinoma
bronchiseptica, Bordetella
bronchiseptica, Brucella
bronchisepticus
b., Bacillus
b., Haemophilus
b., Hemophilus
bronchitis
b., acute
b. ▸ acute exacerbation of chronic
b., acute asthmatic
b., acute laryngotracheal
b. ▸ allergy-related
b., arachidic
b., asthmatic
b., bacterial
b. ▸ bad breath from
b. ▸ breathing difficulty from
b., capillary
b., Castellani
b., catarrhal
b., cheesy
b., chronic
b., chronic asthmatic

b., chronic obstructive
b., chronic subacute
b., croupous
b., dry
b., epidemic capillary
b., ether
b., exudative
b., fibrinous
b., hemorrhagic
b., infectious asthmatic
b., mechanic
b., membranous
b. obliterans
b., phthinoid
b., plastic
b., polypoid
b., productive
b., pseudomembranous
b., putrid
b., secondary
b. sicca
b., smoker's
b., staphylococcal
b., staphylococcus
b., streptococcal
b., streptococcus
b., suffocative
b., tracheal
b., vegetal
b., verminous
b., vesicular
b., viral
b., winter
b. with asthma, chronic
b. with emphysema, chronic
bronchoalveolar
b. carcinoma
b. cell adenoma
b. lavage
b. lavage fluid
b. washings
bronchocavernous respiration
bronchocentric granulomatosis
bronchocutaneous fistula
bronchodilator, inhaled
bronchodilator medication
bronchoesophageal muscle
bronchofocal abscess
bronchogenic [*bronchiogenic*]
b. adenocarcinoma
b. cancer
b. carcinoma
b. carcinoma, advanced
b. carcinoma ▸ small cell variety
b. carcinoma, undifferentiated

b. carcinoma ▸ unknown cell type
b. cyst
b. cyst of mediastinum
b. neoplasm
b. oat cell carcinoma
b. Pancoast-type tumor
b. poorly differentiated squamous cell carcinoma
b. squamous cell carcinoma
b. tumor, small cell
bronchogram
b., air
b. sign, air
b., tantalum
bronchographic examination
bronchography
b. Cope-method
b. inhalation
b., percutaneous
b. ▸ percutaneous transtracheal
bronchophony
b., pectoriloquous
b., sniffling
b., whispered
bronchoplasty repair
bronchopleural (BP)
bronchopleural fistula
bronchopneumonia(e)
b., acute
b., acute hemorrhagic
b., aspiration
b., bilateral
b. ▸ bilateral diffuse necrotizing
b., chronic
b., confluent
b., consolidated
b., diffuse
b., focal
b., focal acute
b., hemorrhagic
b., hypostatic
b., Miyagawanella
b., necrotizing
b. ▸ patchy areas of
b. ▸ patchy early bilateral
b., sequestration
b. ▸ severe confluent bilateral
b., subacute
b., viral
b. virus
bronchopneumonic, infiltrate
bronchoprovocation challenge ▸ methacholine
bronchoprovocation test

bronchopulmonary
- b. aspergillosis
- b. aspergillosis, allergic
- b. cyst
- b. disease
- b. dysplasia (BPD)
- b. dysplasia (BPD) ▸ early
- b. fistula
- b. foregut malformation
- b. histoplasmosis
- b. lymph nodes
- b. segment
- b. spasm
- b. spirochetosis
- b. washings

bronchorrhaphy repair

bronchoscope
- b., fiberoptic
- b. ▸ flexible fiberoptic
- b. inserted through vocal cords with ease
- b. passed
- b. ▸ patient intubated with

bronchoscopic
- b. battery box
- b. evaluation
- b. examination
- b. face shield
- b. lavage
- b. magnet
- b. needle biopsy
- b. spirometry
- b. study

bronchoscopy
- b. and dilatation ▸ operative
- b. examination
- b., fiberoptic
- b. ▸ fiberscopic
- b. ▸ flexible fiberoptic
- b., operative
- b., rigid
- b. ▸ ultrasound-guided
- b. with aspiration
- b. with biopsy
- b. with dilatation
- b. with drainage (dr'ge)
- b. with irrigation

bronchosepticus, Alcaligenes

bronchospasm
- b., allergic
- b., asthmatic
- b. ▸ exercise-induced
- b., recurrent
- b., reversible

bronchospastic component

bronchovesicular
- b. breath sounds
- b. markings
- b. respiration
- b. sound

bronchus
- b., adenocarcinoma of
- b., adenoma of
- b., anomalous
- b., apical
- b. basal segmental
- b., biopsy of
- b. branches
- b., carcinoma of
- b., cardiac
- b. covered with blood
- b., distortion left main stem
- b., diverticulum of
- b., endoscopic examination of
- b., epiarterial
- b., epidermoid carcinoma
- b. ▸ erosion of main stem
- b., esophageal
- b., fistula of
- b., foreign body (FB) in
- b., hyparterial
- b., intermediate
- b. intermedius
- b., left
- b., left main
- b., left stem
- b., lingular
- b., lobar
- b., lower lobe
- b., main stem
- b., middle lobe
- b., occlusion left
- b., occlusion of
- b. ▸ occlusion of main stem
- b., partial occlusion main
- b. pig
- b. plastic reconstruction of
- b., plastic repair of
- b. principalis dexter
- b. principalis sinister
- b., repair of
- b., right
- b., right main stem
- b., right primary
- b., right stem
- b., ruptured
- b., secondary
- b., segmental
- b. sign ▸ bent
- b. sign ▸ open

- b. sign ▸ patent
- b. sign ▸ stretched
- b. sign ▸ thumbprint
- b., stem
- b., stenosis of
- b., stump of
- b. subsegmental
- b., tracheal
- b. transected and closed
- b., ulceration of
- b., upper lobe

bronze diabetes

bronzing, nuclear

Brophy's operation

Brophy's plate

broth
- b. culture
- b., milliliter of nutrient
- b., nutrient
- b. test

Broudie's pain

brought
- b. into apposition ▸ margins of wound
- b. into surgical incision ▸ appendix
- b. into surgical wound ▸ appendix
- b. into view ▸ gently
- b. out near edge of incision
- b. out through stab wound
- b. out through wound ▸ tissue

Brouha's test

Brow(s)
- b. -down position
- b., drooping
- b., hairline of
- b. lift
- b. lift procedure
- b. lift surgery
- b. pang
- b. presentation
- b. ptosis
- b. ptosis repair
- b. -up position

brown (Brown)('s)
- B. (heroin)
- B. and Clears (amphetamines)
- B. ataxia ▸ Sanger
- b. atrophy
- b. cataract
- b. cortex ▸ laminated yellowish-brown
- B. -Dohlman implant
- b. edema
- b. enamel, hereditary
- b. fat

b. fat tissue
B. femoral head replacement ▸ Matchett-
B. graft ▸ Blair-
B. head halter traction ▸ Forrester-
b. induration
b. induration ▸ idiopathic
b. induration of lung
B. -Kelly syndrome ▸ Paterson
b. lung disease
B. (Iranian heroin), Persian
b. pigment laded macrophages
B. prosthesis ▸ Matchett-
B. -Sequard lesion
B. -Sequard syndrome
b. serous ascites ▸ yellow-
B. shunt ▸ Allen-
b. skin, atrophic
b. skin graft ▸ Blair-
b. spider bites
b. sputum
B. sugar (heroin)
B. syndrome
B. syndrome ▸ Sanger-
B. tendon sheath syndrome
b. urine ▸ passage of dark
brownies (hashish) ▸ Hash
Browning's vein
brownish-red discharge
Broyles' tube
BRP (bathroom privileges)
Bruce
B. exercise stress test
B. protocol exercise test
B. protocol ▸ modified
B. protocol ▸ standard
B. treadmill
B. treadmill protocol
brucei, trypanosoma
Brucella
B. abortus
B. abortus ▸ gram-negative
B. bronchiseptica
B. melitensis
B. melitensis ▸ gram-negative
B. suis
B. suis ▸ gram-negative
Bruch's membrane
Brücke('s)
B. fibers
B. lens
B. muscle
B., tunica nervea of
Brudzinski's reflex

Brudzinski's sign
Brueghel's syndrome
Brugia malayi
Brugia timori
Bruhl's disease
bruisability, easy
bruised
b. and puffy face
b. brain tissue
b. forehead
b. muscle
bruise(s)
b., catheter site
b. ▸ devil's pinch
b., easily
b., painful
b., skin
bruising
b. and swelling
b., easy
b., ecchymosis and
b. from antidepressant
b. from antihistamines
b. from bismuth
b. of bowel
b., simple
bruit(s)
b., abdominal
b., aneurysmal
b., arteriovenous (AV) fistula with good
b., asymptomatic
b., asymptomatic carotid
b., bilateral carotid
b., carotid
b., cranial cervical
b. d'airain
b. de bois
b. de canon
b. de choc
b. de clapotement
b. de claquement
b. de craquement
b. de cuir neuf
b. de diable
b. de drapeau
b. de froissement
b. de frolement
b. de frottement
b. de galop
b. de grelot
b. de la roue de moulin
b. de Leudet
b. de lime
b. de moulin

b. de parchemin
b. de piaulement
b. de pot fêlé
b. de rape
b. de rappel
b. de Roger
b. de scie
b. de scie ou de rape
b. de soufflet
b. de tabourka
b. de tambour
b. de triolet
b., epigastric
b., false
b. in base of neck
b., intracranial
b., Leudet's
b., musical
b. placentaire
b., placental
b., prominent
b., renal
b., Roger's
b., seagull
b. skodique
b., supraclavicular
b., systolic
b., thyroid
b., Traube
b., Verstraeten's
brunerri, Taenia
brunescent cataract
Brunfelsia hopeana
Brunhilde virus
Brunn's nests in bladder carcinoma ▸ Von
Bruns' glucose medium
Brunschwig's operation
Bruser's incision
brush(es)
b., Barraquer's
b. biopsy
b. biopsy, bronchial
b. biopsy, endobronchial
b. biopsy, transbronchial
b. border
b. border, intestinal
b. burn
b. discharge
B. electrocardiographic score
b., Haidinger's
brushed and washed, lining
Brushfield-Wyatt disease
Brushfield's spot

brushing(s)
    b. and biopsying
    b. and flossing teeth
    b. and flossing, tooth
    b., biopsy and
    b., blind esophageal
    b., bronchial
    b. ▸ cytology of bronchial
    b. ▸ double sheath bronchial
    b. for malignancy ▸ cytology
    b., lung
    b. of esophageal lesion
    b. ▸ washings and
brusque dilatation of esophagus
brutalization and desensitization
Bruton's agammaglobulinemia
Bruton sex-linked
    agammaglobulinemia
bruxist behavior
Bryan cervical disc
Bryant's sign
Bryant's traction
BSCA (bidirectional superior
    cavopulmonary anastomosis)
B-scan frame
BSE (breast self-examination)
BSER (brain stem evoked response)
BSI (bloodstream infections)
BSP (Bromsulphalein)
BSRI (Bem Sex Role Inventory)
BSS (battered spouse syndrome)
BTES (Borg Treadmill Exertion Scale)
B-12 deficiency, Vitamin
B27 ▸ histocompatibility agent
bubble
    b., air
    b. appearance, double-
    b. chamber
    b. flushing reservoir, double-
    b., gastric
    b. humidifier
    b. instilled in anterior chamber ▸ air
    b. -like appearance
    b. oxgenation
    b. oxygenator
    b. trap
bubbling from mouth ▸ saliva
bubbling rale(s)
bubbly lung syndrome
bubo
    b., chancroidal
    b., gonorrheal
    b., venereal
bubonic
    b. lymphadenopathy of axilla

    b. lymphadenopathy of groin
    b. plague
bubonica, pestis
bubonicae, Bacterium pestis
buccae ▸ Bacteroides
buccae, Prevotella
buccal
    b. branch
    b. cavity
    b. cusps
    b. embrasure
    b. flange
    b. gingiva
    b. lesions
    b. lymph nodes
    b. mucosa
    b. mucosa, squamous cell
        carcinoma
    b. mucosa, ulcerated
    b. nerve
    b. occlusion
    b. region
    b. smear
    b. sulcus
    b. surface of tooth
    b. tablet
    b. teeth
    b. tube
buccalis
    b., Amoeba
    b., Borrelia
    b., Entamoeba
    b., Leptothrix
    b., Leptotrichia
    b., psoriasis
    b., Trichomonas
buccinator
    b. muscle
    b. muscle ▸ feedback training of
        parts of
    b. nerve
buccolingual diameter
buccopharyngeal membrane
buccopharyngeal muscle
Buchwald's atrophy
bucket
    b. -handle fracture
    b. -handle tear
    b. -handle tear of meniscus
Buckholz prosthesis
buckle, scleral
buckle ▸ vitrectomy and scleral
buckled aorta
Bückler disease ▸ Reis-
buckler implant ▸ Silastic scleral

buckling
    b. and/or locking of knee
    b., chordal
    b., cortical
    b., midsystolic
    b. of cortex
    b. of sclera
    b. procedure, scleral
    b., scleral
Buck's
    B. extension
    B. extension traction
    B. operation
    B. traction
Bucky
    B. diaphragm
    B. diaphragm, Potter-
    B. film
    B. grid
    B. grid ▸ Potter-
    B. -Potter diaphragm
    B. rays
    B. studies
    B. technique
Bucy syndrome ▸ Klüver-
bud(s)
    b., bronchial
    b., taste
    b., tongue
Budd-Chiari syndrome
Budd's cirrhosis
Budge's center
Budinger-Ludloff-Laewen disease
Budinger's operation
Budin's joint
Buerger's disease
buffer
    b. amplifier
    b. base
    b. base, blood
buffered
    b. analgesic
    b. aspirin
    b. saline, phosphate
    b. saline solution
buffering, secondary
buffy (Buffy)
    b. coat smear
    b. coated cells
    B. layer of bone marrow
Bugbe electrode
bugs, airborne
Buhl's desquamative
    pneumonia
Buie position

build
- b. -down region
- b. -down region of irradiated medium
- b. muscle
- b. -up ▸ atherosclerotic
- b. -up drain fluid
- b. -up ▸ ear wax
- b. -up ▸ excessive wax
- b. -up ▸ express fluid
- b. -up ▸ fatty plaque
- b. -up, fluid
- b. -up ▸ hyperventilation (HV)
- b. -up implant
- b. -up, mucus
- b. -up of drugs ▸ dangerous
- b. -up of pressure ▸ rapid
- b. -up of scar tissue
- b. -up of seizure activity
- b. -up, plaque
- b. -up region
- b. -up region of irradiated medium
- b. -up, reversing plaque

builder, blood
building(s)
- b., body
- b. drug ▸ muscle-
- b. exercise, body
- b. experience ▸ aerobic and strength-
- b., muscle
- b. positive relationships
- b. resources ▸ reproducible skill
- b. self-esteem
- b. ▸ social skills

built-in sexuality
bulb
- b. and sweep ▸ duodenal
- b. anomaly ▸ jugular
- b. aorta ▸ tulip
- b. aortic
- b. carotid
- b., coarsening of duodenal
- b., deformity of duodenal
- b., duodenal
- b., hair
- b., irritable duodenal
- b. of penis ▸ vein of
- b. of vestibule ▸ vein of
- b., olfactory
- b. scarring, duodenal
- b., suction
- b., thrombosis of jugular

bulbar
- b. conjunctiva
- b. palsy
- b. paralysis
- b. paralysis, infectious
- b. polioencephalitis
- b. polioencephalitis ▸ acute
- b. poliomyelitis
- b. pulse
- b. pulse, Bamberger's
- b. sclerosis
- b. ulcer, duodenal

bulbi
- b., cyanosis
- b., fascia
- b., phthisis
- b., siderosis
- b. urethrae, septum
- b., xanthomatosis

bulbocavernous muscle
bulbocavernous reflex
bulbomimic reflex
bulbospinal poliomyelitis ▸ acute
bulbourethral artery
bulbourethral glands
bulbous
- b. cervix
- b. nose ▸ swollen
- b. turbinates
- b. urethra

bulboventricular
- b. foramen
- b. groove
- b. loop
- b. sulcus
- b. tube

Bulbulian (BLB) mask ▸ Boothby, Lovelace,
bulbulus, Vibrio
bulbus
- b. aortae
- b. arteriosus
- b. caroticus
- b. cordis
- b. oculi
- b. penis
- b. urethrae
- b. venae jugularis

bulgaricus, Lactobacillus
bulge(s)
- b., abdominal
- b. and droops ▸ eye
- b. in abdomen
- b. in abdomen ▸ pulsating
- b., precordial

bulging
- b. annulus
- b. anterior fontanel
- b. ▸ bag of waters
- b., cyst
- b. disc
- b. eye
- b. eyes from aneurysm
- b. eyes from blood clot
- b. fat
- b. fatty infiltration
- b. fontanel
- b. ▸ generalized disc
- b. ▸ infarct
- b. lesion
- b. of minor fissure
- b. rectal arteries
- b. red tympanic membrane
- b. varicose veins
- b., venous
- b. yellow tympanic membrane

Bulimarexia (starvation and purging)
bulimia
- b., anorexia and
- b., exercise
- b. nervosa
- b., patient has

bulimic
- b., bingeing behavior of
- b. ▸ punishing behavior of
- b. ▸ purging behavior of
- b. ▸ starving behavior of

bulk
- b. diet, high
- b. -forming laxative
- b., muscle

bulky
- b. compression dressing
- b. compression dressing, light
- b. diet
- b. dressing
- b. stool

bulla(e)
- b., emphysematous
- b., ethmoid
- b., subpleural
- b., superficial

bullata, Mycoplana
Buller's shield
bullet wound
bullets, magic
bullosa
- b., concha
- b. (EB), epidermolysis
- b., epidermosis
- b., impetigo
- b., keratitis

bullosa—*continued*
- b., myringitis
- b., purpura

bullosis diabeticorum

bullous
- b. disease
- b. emphysema
- b. impetigo
- b. keratopathy
- b. pemphigoid
- b. scleroderma

bull's-eye
- b. analysis
- b. lesion
- b. maculopathy
- b. polar coordinate mapping

bullying ▸ tendency toward

Bumke's pupil

bump(s)
- b., ductus
- b., eyelid
- b. ▸ skin goose
- b., pump

bumper-fender fracture

bumpy skin

BUN (blood urea nitrogen)
- BUN elevated
- BUN fluctuation
- BUN test

bunamiodyl contrast medium

bunching suture

bundle(s)
- b., aberrant
- b. ablation, His
- b. ablation ▸ Kent
- b. activity ▸ His
- b., arteriovenous
- b., atrioventricular (AV)
- b., Bachmann's
- b., basis
- b. branch block (BBB)
- b. branch block (BBBB), bilateral
- b. branch block (LBBB) ▸ complete left
- b. branch block (RBBB) ▸ complete right
- b. branch block ▸ His
- b. branch block (BBB) ▸ incomplete
- b. branch block (LBBB) ▸ incomplete left
- b. branch block (RBBB) ▸ incomplete right
- b. branch block (LBBB) ▸ left
- b. branch block (RBBB) ▸ right
- b. branch fibrosis
- b. branch heart block
- b. branch reentrant tachycardia
- b. branch reentry
- b., Bruce's
- b., commissural
- b. deflection ▸ His
- b. depolarization ▸ His
- b. electrocardiogram (ECG) ▸ His
- b. electrode ▸ His
- b. electrogram ▸ His
- b., extracostal
- b., fundamental
- b., ground
- b. heart block ▸ His
- b., Helweg's
- b., His
- b., image
- b., interwoven
- b., James
- b., Keith's
- b., Kent-His
- b., Kent's
- b. ▸ lobulated atrioventricular (AV)
- b., longitudinal medial
- b. Mahaim
- b., main
- b., medial forebrain
- b., medial neurovascular
- b., Meynert's
- b., Monakow's
- b., muscle
- b., myocardial fiber
- b., nerve
- b. ▸ nerve fiber
- b., neurovascular
- b. of Drualt
- b. of His
- b. of nerve fibers
- b. of nonmyelinated nerve fibers
- b. of Oort
- b., of palmar aponeurosis, transverse
- b. of Rasmussen, olivocochlear
- b. of Stanley-Kent
- b. of tendons ▸ primary
- b. of tonofilaments
- b. of tonofilaments ▸ desosomes with
- b. of Vicq d'Azyr
- b., penetrating
- b., posterior longitudinal
- b., predorsal
- b. recording ▸ His
- b., Schultze's
- b., Schutz's
- b., sinoatrial
- b., thalamomamillary
- b., Thorel's
- b., Türck's
- b., vascular
- b., Weissmann's

Bunge's amputation

bunion
- b. joint
- b., Keller
- b. osteotomy, Keller

bunionectomy
- b., Keller
- b., McBride
- b., Mitchell
- b., silver

Bunker's implant

Bunnell ('s)
- B. flap
- B. operation
- B. suture
- B. tendon transfer
- B. test, Paul

Bunsen burner

Burch's operation

Burdach's tract

burden, ischemic

burdens, emotional

burgdorferi, Borrelia

Burger('s) (burger)
- b., barium
- B. scalene triangle
- B. triangle

buried
- b. cortex
- b., pterygium
- b. suture
- b. suture, interdermal
- b. tonsil

Burkholderia cepacia

Burkitt('s)
- B. lymphoma
- B. lymphoma, African
- B. tumor
- B. -type acute lymphocytic leukemia

burn(s) (Burn)('s)
- b., accidental
- b., acid
- b., brush
- b. cases, flash
- b., cement
- b. center
- b. center, regional
- b., chemical

b. coma
b., contact
b., corneal
b. ▸ corneal scarring from chemical
b., defibrillator
b., depth of
b., electrical
b., fatal
b., first degree
b., flash
b., fourth degree
b., friction
b. from chemical
b. healthy tissue
b., heart◊
b. index
b., infant
b. infections
b. injury
b. marks, paddle
b., minor
b. of cornea
b. off calories
b. off tissue
b. ▸ patient sustained first, second, third or fourth degree
b. present, paddle
b., radiation
b. rate, caloric
b. scar contracture
b. scar, hypertrophic
b. scars, old
b., second degree
b. shock
b., skin
b., summer
b., sun◊
b., thermal
b., third degree
b., tissue
b. to respiratory tract from gases
b. trauma
b. treatment, early
B. Unit
b. victim
b. wound
b., x-ray

burned
b. beyond recognition ▸ patient
b., body surface
b. out germinal centers ▸ hyalinized
burner, Bunsen
burner meridian ▸ triple
burnetii, Coxiella
Burnett's disinfecting fluid

Burnett's syndrome
burning [*blurring*]
b. abdominal pain
b. and frequent urination
b. body fat
b. chest discomfort
b. during urination ▸ bladder
b., epigastric distress and
b. feet
b. feet from atherosclerosis
b. foot sensation
b. foot syndrome
b. from bisacodyl ▸ rectal
b., itching and redness of skin
b. knife-like pain
b. mouth from aspirin
b. mouth from cold sore
b. mouth from dentures
b. mouth from depression
b. mouth from diabetes
b. mouth syndrome
b., nasal
b. ▸ numbness, tingling and
b. of feet ▸ painful
b. on urination
b. or freezing pain
b. pain
b., pain and numbness ▸ cold,
b. pain, intense
b. pain ▸ stiffness, aching and
b., rectal
b. sensation
b. sensation in chest
b. sensation in chest ▸ painful,
b. sensation in eyes
b. sensation in stomach
b. sensation in upper chest
b. sensation ▸ itching or
b. sensation, retrosternal
b. sensation, substernal
b. sensation ▸ tingling and
b. sensation while urinating
b. skin
b., tingling, or prickly feeling
b. tongue
b. tongue syndrome or glossodynia
b., urinary
burnout
b. and heart disease ▸ exhaustion,
b., emotional
b., job
b. ▸ mental
b. ▸ physical
b. symptoms
Burns' amaurosis

Burns ▸ space of
Burow's
B. operation
B. solution
B. vein
burr
b. cell
b. erythrocyte
b. holes
burrowing hair
bursa
b., Achilles
b., acromial
b., adventitious
b., aspiration and injection of
b., calcaneal
b. -equivalent
b. ▸ fluid-filled
b., nasopharyngeal
b., olecranon
b., pharyngeal
b. tenderness, anserine
bursal equivalent tissue
bursata, exostosis
Bursera gummifer
bursitis
b., Achilles
b., Duplay's
b., gluteal
b. ▸ hip-associated
b., ischial
b. of foot
b. of shoulder
b., prepatellar
b., radiation treatment for
b., radiohumeral
b., retrocalcaneal
b., septic
b., subacromial
b., subdeltoid
b., Tornwaldt's/Thornwaldt's
b., traumatic hemorrhagic
b., trochanteric
burst(s) (Burst)
b. activity
b., alpha
b. atrial pacing
B. forming cells
b., fourteen and six hertz (Hz) positive
b., high voltage
b., isolated
b., K complex
b., laser
b. of alpha activity

burst(s)—*continued*
- b. of alpha ▸ frequent individual
- b. of arch-shaped waves
- b. of beta activity
- b. of boundless energy
- b. of creativity
- b. of delta activity
- b. of drowsiness ▸ rhythmic temporal theta
- b. of high voltage, periodic
- b. of irritation and anger
- b. of motivation
- b. of radiation
- b. of rhythmic activity
- b. of theta activity
- b. of theta frequency
- b. of uncontrolled muscle contractions
- b. of ventricular tachycardia
- b. pacing
- b. pacing ▸ pacemaker
- b. pacing ▸ rapid
- b., paroxysmal
- b., periodic slow
- b., respiratory
- b. shock
- b., short
- b. spike and wave
- b. -suppression
- b. -suppression pattern
- b., theta
- b., tone
- b. veins, spider

bursting fracture
bursting spherons
bury stump of appendix
burying the stump
BUS (Bartholin's, urethral and Skene's) glands
Busacca nodules
Buschke
- B. disease ▸ Busse-
- B. -Loewenstein tumor
- B. -Ollendorff syndrome
- B. ▸ scleredema of

bush sickness
bushy stunt virus
buski, Fasciola
buski, Fasciolopsis
Busse-Buschke disease
Busse saccharomyces
buster, clot
busting drug, clot
busulfan lung syndrome
butanol-extractable iodine (BEI)

bütschlii, Entamoeba
bütschlii, Iodamoeba
Bütschli's emulsion
Bütschli's granules
butter pericardium, ▸ bread-and-
butter textbook sign, bread-and-
butterfly
- b. area
- b. configuration, air
- b. dressing
- b. fracture
- b. fragments
- b. shadow
- b. -shaped rash on face, red
- b. stroke injury

Butter's cancer
buttock(s)
- b. claudication
- b. ▸ incision and drainage (I and D) of left
- b. ▸ incision and drainage (I and D) of right
- b. lift
- b. lipectomy
- b. muscles
- b. pain ▸ constant

button(s)
- b. (Mescaline)
- b., call
- b. cautery
- b., cell
- b., Chlumsky's
- b. drainage (dr'ge)
- b. electrode
- b. infuser
- b., Jaboulay's
- b. ▸ Kistner tracheal
- b. lesion collar
- b. -makers' chorea
- b., Moore's tracheostomy
- b. of aorta
- b. of vein tissue ▸ small
- b., Panje voice
- b., polyethylene collar
- b., Reuter
- b., skin
- b. surgery, belly
- b. suture
- b. suture ▸ double-
- b. technique
- b., Teflon
- b., tracheal
- b. tube, collar
- b., walking

buttonhole
- b. deformity
- b. fracture
- b. incision
- b., mitral
- b. mitral stenosis

buttress, fragmatic
buttress ▸ Teflon pledget suture
butyl ether (MTBE) ▸ methyl test-
butyric acid ▸ alpha amino-n-
butyricum, Clostridium
butyricum ▸ gram-positive Clostridium
butyricum, Mycobacterium
butyrocholinesterase level
butyrous colony
buyo cheek cancer
buzzing in ears
Buzzi's operation
B-W graft
by mouth at bedtime (npo/h.s.) ▸ nothing
bypass
- b., aortobi-iliac
- b., aortocarotid
- b., aortocoronary saphenous vein
- b., aortoiliac
- b., aortoiliofemoral
- b., aortorenal
- b., aorto-subclavian carotid-axilloaxillary
- b., arterial
- b., automatic
- b., axilloaxillary
- b., axillobifemoral
- b., axillofemoral
- b. ▸ beating heart cardiac
- b. blockage
- b., brachial
- b., cardiopulmonary
- b., carotid axillary
- b., carotid-carotid
- b., carotid subclavian
- b. circuit
- b. coloplasty ▸ one-stage retrosternal
- b. ▸ conventional cardiac
- b., coronary
- b., coronary artery
- b., cross femoral-femoral
- b., crossover
- b. ▸ descending thoracic aortofemoral-femoral
- b., end-to-side vein
- b. ▸ extra-anatomic

b. ▸ extracranial-intracranial brain
b. ▸ femoral-femoral
b., femoral popliteal
b. ▸ femoral-tibial
b. ▸ femoral-tibial-peroneal
b., femoroaxillary
b. ▸ femorofemoral crossover
b., femoropopliteal
b. ▸ femorotibial
b., gastric
b. graft
b. graft angiography ▸ saphenous vein
b. graft, aortocoronary
b. graft (AFBG), aortofemoral
b. graft, aortoiliac
b. graft, aortovein
b. graft, artery
b. graft, cardiac
b. graft, clogged
b. graft, coronary
b. graft (CABG), coronary artery
b. graft, femoropopliteal
b. graft ▸ lower extremity
b. graft ▸ mesenteric
b. graft ▸ renal artery
b. graft, saphenous vein
b. graft ▸ subclavian artery
b. graft ▸ vein
b. graft ▸ vertebral artery
b. grafting
b. grafting ▸ endarterectomy and coronary artery
b. grafting ▸ port-access coronary artery
b. grafting surgery, coronary artery
b., heart-lung
b. heart surgery, triple
b., iliopopliteal
b., infracubital
b., internal mammary artery
b., intestinal
b., jejunal
b., jejunoileal
b., left heart
b. ▸ Litwak left atrial aortic
b. machine
b. machine, cardiopulmonary
b. (MIDCAB) ▸ minimally invasive direct coronary artery
b., natural
b. occluded segments
b. (OPCAB), off pump coronary artery
b. operation, cardiopulmonary

b. operation ▸ gastric
b., partial
b., partial cardiopulmonary
b. ▸ partial ileal
b. (PCPB) ▸ percutaneous cardiopulmonary
b. ▸ percutaneous left heart
b. (PACB) ▸ port-access coronary artery
b., postcardiopulmonary
b. procedure, coronary
b. procedure, gastric
b. procedure ▸ port-access
b. procedure ▸ robotic partial
b., pulmonary
b. pump ▸ cardiopulmonary
b. pump ▸ left ventricular
b. ▸ renal artery reverse saphenous vein
b., reversed
b., right heart
b. ▸ Roux-en-Y
b., saphenous vein
b. shunt, Brenner carotid
b., side-to-side vein
b. ▸ subclavian carotid
b. ▸ subclavian-subclavian
b. ▸ substernal gastric
b. ▸ superior mesenteric artery
b. support ▸ percutaneous cardiopulmonary
b. surgery
b. surgery ▸ cardiac
b. (CAB) surgery, coronary artery
b. surgery, femoral popliteal
b. surgery ▸ gastric
b. surgery, heart
b. surgery, intestinal
b. surgery ▸ keyhole
b. surgery ▸ quintuple
b. surgery ▸ radial artery
b. surgery ▸ rescue coronary
b., total cardiopulmonary
b. ▸ total duodenal
b. tract
b. tract, atrio-Hisian
b. tract, concealed
b. tract, nodo-Hisian
b. tract, Wolff-Parkinson-White
b. vein graft
b. vein graft ▸ popliteal tibial
Byrd-Dew method
Bywaters' syndrome

C

C (centigrade)
C (cocaine)
c (with)
C acute hepatitis
C and S (culture and sensitivity)
C classification of right ascending
    colon ▸ Dukes
C disease, sickle cell hemoglobin
C, hemoglobin
C infection, chronic hepatitis
C, mosaic trisomy
C, Salmonella paratyphi
C screening ▸ hepatitis
C virus
C virus, hepatitis
C wave
CA (cancer)
CA (carcinoma)
CA (cardiac arrest)
CA (cervicoaxial)
CA (chronological age)
CA (Cocaine Anonymous)
CA (coronary artery)
CA (rule out carcinoma) ▸ r/o
CA (croup-associated) virus
CAB (coronary artery bypass)
CAB (coronary artery bypass) surgery
Caballo (heroin)
CABG (coronary artery bypass graft)
cabin fever
cabinet(s)
    c., electronic bedside
    c., medicine
    c. respirator
cable
    c. artifact
    c. graft
    c. pacing
Cabot's ring bodies
Cabral coronary reconstruction
Cacajao rubicundus
Cacchione syndrome ▸ De Sanctis-
Cache Valley virus
cachectic
    c. diarrhea
    c. endocarditis
    c., extremities

    c. fever
    c., patient
    c., patient severely
cachectica, purpura
cachexia
    c. and dehydration
    c. and nutrition
    c., cancerous
    c., cardiac
    c., exophthalmica
    c., fluoric
    c., hypophyseal
    c., hypophysiopriva
    c., lymphatic
    c., malarial
    c. mercurialis
    c. ovariopriva
    c., pachydermic
    c., pituitary
    c. reaction
    c., saturnine
    c. strumipriva
    c., suprarenalis
    c. thyreopriva
    c., thyroid
    c., tropical
    c., uremic
    c., urinary
    c., verminous
cachexial fever
cachexica, Amoeba
cacti, Coccus
Cactus (Mescaline)
CAD (computer-assisted design)
    prosthesis
CAD (coronary artery disease)
cadaver
    c. donor
    c., elderly
    c. exchange
    c. homografts
    c. kidney
    c. organ
    c. organ donation
    c. organ ▸ transplantable
    c. organs for transplantation ▸
        procurement of

    c. preserved for anatomical study
    c., young
cadaveric
    c. donor transplantation
    c. dura
    c. ecchymoses
    c. graft
    c. kidney
    c. organ
    c. reaction
    c. rigidity
    c. spasm
    c. transplant
caddy stool
Cadence implantable cardioverter
    defibrillator ▸ Ventritex
Cadillacs (amphetamines), Black
cadmium diagnostic laser ▸ helium
cadmium fumes
caecum, punctum
caecutiens, Onchocerca
caesarean (see cesarean)
CAF (cell antiviral factor)
café au lait spots
cafe coronary
caffeine
    c. addiction
    c., alcohol, pepper, spicy (CAPS)
        foods-free diet
    c. ▸ breast pain from
    c. ▸ chapped lip from
    c. ▸ eye twitching from
    c. ▸ fibrocystic disease from
    c., flushing from
    c., headache from
    c., insomnia from
    c. intake
    c. intoxication
    c., nervousness from
    c. or nicotine consumption
    c., palpitation from
    c. poisoning
    c. ▸ restless leg from
    c., trembling from
    c., ulcer from
    c., urination from
    c. withdrawal

Caffey('s)
- C. disease
- C. -Silverman syndrome
- C. -Smyth-Roske syndrome

cage
- c., bony
- c., bony thoracic
- c., chest
- c. ▸ inflammation of cartilage of rib
- c. intact, rib
- c., rib
- c. ▸ splaying open rib
- c., thoracic
- c., titanium
- c. valve ▸ disk
- c. valve ▸ Starr-Edwards ball and

caged-ball
- c. prosthesis
- c. prosthetic valve
- c. valve

Cagot ear
Cairns' operation
cairograph, cardio◊
Caisson disease
caisson sickness
cajennense, Amblyomma
cake kidney
caked breast
caking of breast
Calabar swellings
calamus scriptorius
C$_{alb}$ (albumin clearance)
calcaneal
- c. bone
- c. bursa
- c. region
- c. spur
- c. spur, plantar

calcaneocuboid articulation
calcaneofibular ligament
calcaneonavicular ligament
calcaneovalgus, talipes
calcaneovarus, talipes
calcaneus
- c., axial fixation of
- c., fracture of
- c., pes
- c., talipes
- c., tendon

calcar femorale
calcar pedis
calcarea, peritendinitis
calcareous
- c. cataract
- c. conjunctivitis

- c. deposit
- c. metastasis
- c. nodules

calcarine
- c. fissure
- c. sulcus
- c. tract, ▸ geniculo-

calce, soda cum
calcific
- c. aortic stenosis
- c. aortic valve stenosis (CAVS)
- c. atherosclerosis
- c. atherosclerosis, diffuse
- c. changes, minimal
- c. debris
- c. density
- c. deposits
- c. mitral stenosis
- c. mural atherosclerosis
- c. nodular aortic stenosis
- c. pancreatitis
- c. pancreatitis, chronic
- c. pericarditis
- c. shadows
- c. stenosis
- c. stones, puncta
- c. tendinitis

**calcificans congenita ▸
chondrodystrophia**
calcification(s)
- c., annular
- c., aortic
- c. ▸ aortic arch
- c. ▸ aortoiliac vascular
- c., arterial
- c., basal ganglia
- c., benign breast
- c. benign glandular tissue,
  intracranial
- c., breast
- c., cerebral
- c., coronary artery
- c., curvilinear
- c., diffuse abdominal
- c., dystrophic
- c. intervertebral cartilage
- c., intervertebral disc
- c., intracranial
- c., irregular
- c., ligamentous
- c., lung
- c. mediocollateral ligament of
  knee
- c., mitral annular

- c. ▸ moderate atherosclerosis
  with
- c., mottled
- c., multiple
- c. ▸ napkin ring
- c. necrosis
- c. of arteries
- c. of breast ▸ malignant
- c. of carotid artery ▸ pipestem
- c. of cartilage
- c. of choroid plexus
- c. of costal cartilages, premature
- c. of intervertebral cartilage
- c. of left coronary artery
- c. or cerebral vessels ▸ medial
- c., pancreatic
- c., Pellegrini Stieda
- c., periarticular
- c., pericardial
- c., pineal gland
- c., Raynaud's phenomenon,
  scleroderma, telangiectasia
  (CRST) syndrome
- c., secondary
- c., significant
- c., soft tissue
- c. ▸ speckled breast
- c. spiculated
- c., submitral
- c., tooth-like
- c., tracheal
- c., valvular
- c., vascular

calcified
- c. aortic valve
- c. atheroma
- c. atheroma, moderate
- c. atheroma, severe
- c. atheromata
- c. atherosclerosis
- c. benign granuloma
- c. cartilage
- c. density
- c. ductus arteriosus
- c. epithelioma
- c. fetus
- c. foci
- c. focus
- c. focus of tuberculosis
- c. free body
- c. gallbladder
- c. granuloma
- c. granulomata ▸ multiple focal
- c. hemangioma
- c. hilar nodes

c. leiomyoma of uterus
c. leiomyomas ▸ multiple small
c. lesion
c. lymph node
c. mass
c. material
c. mesenteric node
c. mitral leaflet
c. nodes
c. nodules
c. pericardium
c., pineal gland
c. plaques
c. thrombus
c. thyroid adenoma
c. uterine fibroid
c. valve
c. wall of gallbladder

calcifying
c. cell epithelioma
c. epithelioma
c. epithelioma, benign
c. fascitis, exudative

calcinosis
c. cutis circumscripta
c. interstitialis
c. universalis

calcis, os
calcitonin level
calcitriol, synthetic
calcium
c. absorption
c. antagonists
c. balance
c. balance in body
c. blocker
c. blocker ▸ long-acting
c., blood level of
c. carbonate
c. channel
c. channel agonist
c. channel blocker
c. channel blocking agents
c. channel blocking drug
c. channel ▸ receptor operated
c. channel ▸ voltage-dependent
c. concentration
c. concentration ▸ intracellular
c. concentration, serum
c. concretions
c. content, cholesterol
c. contrast medium, ipodate
c. contrast medium, Oragrafin
c. current ▸ transsarcolemmal
c. deficient diet

c. deficiency
c. depletion
c. deposit
c. deposition ▸ mitochondrial
c. deposits on heart valve
c., endogenous fecal
c. flow, increased
c. flux ▸ transmembrane
c. gluconate
C. gout
c. homeostatic mechanisms
c. in urine
c. intake
c. intake, premenopausal
c. iodide
c. ions
c. level
c. level, abnormal
c. level ▸ urinary
c., low ionized serum
c., lower serum
c. metabolism
c. molecules
c., Oragrafin
c. orthophosphate
c. oxalate
c. oxalate calculus
c. oxalate crystals
c. oxalate stone
c. paradox
c. particles, benign
c. phosphate
c. phosphorus
c. pills
c. plaques
c. product
c. receptors in heart ▸ stimulate
c. removal prophylaxis
c. -rich diet
c. rigor
c. score
c., serum
c. sign
c. stones
c. stones ▸ kidney
c. sufficient diet
c., Sulkowitch's
c. supplement
c. test
c. test, serum
c., transient
c. transport
c., urine
c. ▸ valvular deposits of
Calciviridae virus

calcoaceticus, Acinetobacter
calcoaceticus baumannii complex,
    Acinetobacter
calculated
c. as given dose ▸ dose
c. as mid-depth dose ▸ dose
c. date of confinement (CDC)
c. in a tangential plane, dose
c., premeditated death
calculation
c., computer dose
c., dose
c. factors
c., hemodynamic
c., irregular field technique for dose
c., isocentric technique for dose
c., Johnson's
c., rotation technique for dose
calculosa, pericarditis
calculous anuria
calculous pyelitis
calculus (-i)
c., alternating
c., articular
c., biliary
c., calcium oxalate
c., cardiac
c. cholecystitis, chronic
c., cholesterol
c. cirrhosis
c. control
c., coral
c., cystine
c., decubitus
c., dendritic
c., dental
c., encysted
c., fibrin
c., gallbladder
c., gonecystic
c., hemp seed
c., hepatic
c., indigo
c. lacrimal gland
c., left ureteral
c., lucent
c., lung
c., matrix
c., mulberry
c., nephritic
c., nonopaque
c., opaque
c., ovarian
c., oxalate
c., palatine tonsil

calculus—*continued*
  c., pancreatic
  c., prostatic
  c. removed
  c., renal
  c., right ureteral
  c., salivary
  c., spermatic
  c., staghorn
  c., struvite
  c., tonsil
  c. ▸ tooth discoloration from
  c., urate
  c., ureteral
  c., urethral
  c., uric acid
  c. ▸ urinary bladder
  c., urinary tract
  c., urostealith
  c., uterine
  c., vesical
  c., vesicoprostatic
  c., visible
  c., xanthic
Caldwell('s)
  C. -Luc approach
  C. -Luc operation
  C. -Luc procedure
  C. -Moloy classification
  C. -Moloy method
  C. position
  C. x-ray view
calf(-ves)
  c. augmentation
  c. claudication
  c. cramps, nighttime
  c. -heel stretch exercise
  c., lateral cutaneous nerve of
  c., medial cutaneous nerve of
  c. muscle
  c. muscle, contraction of
  c. muscle, sore
  c. muscle stretches
  c. muscle tenderness
  c. muscle, weakening
  c. muscles ▸ pain in
  c. muscles ▸ tight
  c. pain from arteriosclerosis
  c. raises
  c. stretch exercise
  c., thighs and hamstrings ▸
    stretching
  c., triceps muscle of
caliber vessel, small
calibrate position

calibrated device
calibration
  c., E-dial
  c. factor (N_{gas}), cavity-gas
  c. failure artifact
  c., film density
  c. of urethra
  c. procedure
  c. signal
  c., urethral
calibrator, digital isotope
calibrator, radioisotope
caliceal (*see* calyceal)
caliceal abnormality
calicectasis/caliectasis
calicectomy/caliectomy
caliculus ophthalmicus
caliectasis/calicectasis
caliectasis, minimal
caliectomy/calicectomy
California
  C. disease
  C. encephalitis
  C. encephalitis virus
  C. Sunshine (LSD)
  C. virus
californica, Anemonopsis
californica, Houttuynia
californiense, Branchiostoma
caligo
  c. corneae
  c. lentis
  c. pupillae
calisaya, Cinchona
call
  c., anesthesiologist-on-
  c. button
  c. chaplain, on-
  c., coroner-on-
  c., counselor-on-
  c., doctor-on-
  c., intern-on-
  c., laboratory-technician-on-
  c., nurse-on-
  c., orderly-on-
  c., pathologist-on-
  c., pharmacist-on-
  c., physician-on-
  c., resident-on-
  c., respiratory-care-technician-on-
  c., surgical-nurse-on-
  c., technician-on-
  c., x-ray-technician-on-
Callahan's operation
Callander's amputation

Callaway's test
Callison's fluid
callosa, pericarditis
callosal
  c. agenesis
  c. gyrus
  c. marginal branch
  c. sulcus
  c. syndrome
callosi, genu corporis
callosi of Reil ▸ taeniola corporis
callosomarginal artery
callosotomy, corpus
callosotomy operation, corpus
callosum agenesis, corpus
callosum, corpus
callosus, gyrus
callous(es) (callus) [*talus*]
  c., corns and
  c., cynical and contemptuous
  c., definitive
  c., ensheathing
  c. formation
  c. formation, excessive
  c., infected
  c., intermediate
  c., medullary
  c., myelogenous
  c. on feet
  c. on hands
  c., painful
  c., peripheral
  c., permanent
  c., provisional
  c. trimmed
calm
  c. and relaxed, patient
  c., assured, nonjudgmental
    attitude
  c. ▸ reassuring and
calmed down, patient
Calmette
  C. -Guérin (BCG) ▸ bacille
  C. -Guérin bacillus
  C. -Guérin (BCG) immunization ▸
    bacille
  C. -Guérin (BCG) vaccine ▸ bacille
  C. reaction
calmness, state of untroubled
calomel electrode
calor
  c. febrilis
  c. fervens
  c. innatus
  c. internus

caloric
- c. burn rate
- c. intake
- c. intake, daily
- c. irrigation, cold
- c. nystagmus
- c. ray
- c. restriction
- c. stimulation
- c. stimulation response, Hallpike
- c. stimulation test, Hallpike
- c. test
- c. testing of vestibular function

calorie(s)
- c., burn off
- c. deficiency ▸ protein-
- c. diet, high
- c. diet, low
- c. expenditure, total
- c. food group, negative
- c. (G-cal) ▸ gram-
- c. intake, adequate
- c. intake ▸ optimum
- c. (Kg-cal) ▸ kilogram-
- c. malfunction ▸ protein
- c. malnutrition, protein
- c., restricted
- c. restriction
- c. restriction diet

calvarial lesion, osteolytic
calvarium, bones of
calvarium without palpable lesion
Calvé
- C. -Legg-Perthes syndrome
- C. -Perthes disease
- C. -Waldenstrom disease ▸ Legg-

calyceal (*same as* caliceal)
- c. cups
- c. cyst
- c. dilatation
- c. diverticulum
- c. pattern
- c. sign of hydronephrosis
- c. stone
- c. system

calyces
- c. and ureters ▸ pelves,
- c., blunting of left
- c., central
- c., effacement of
- c., major
- c., minor
- c., pelves and/or
- c. renales minores
- c., superior pole of

calyx, lower pole
calyx, palpable
C$_{am}$ (amylase clearance)
Cam tent
Cambridge electrocardiograph (ECG)
Camden's amputation
Camel (LSD)
cameloid anemia
camera
- c., fiberoptic
- c., gamma
- c. ▸ gamma scintillation
- c., Medx
- c. ▸ multicrystal gamma
- c., positron scintillation
- c., radioisotope
- c., scintillating
- c., scintillation
- c. ▸ single crystal gamma
- c., thermovision
- c., TV light
- c., video display

Cameron photon densitometry ▸ Norland-
Cammann's stethoscope
camouflage, scar
CAMP (computer-assisted menu planning)
CAMP (cyclic adenosine monophosphate)
Camp('s) (camp)
- C. corset
- C. -Coventry position
- c. fever
- C. -Gianturco method
- c. grid cassette
- C. sign, de la

Campbell's operation
campestris, Agaricus
Campylobacter
- C. enteritis
- C. fetus
- C. gastroenteritis, acute
- C. intestinalis
- C. jejuni
- C. jejuni infection
- C. organism
- C. pylori

Camurati-Engelmann syndrome
can scrotum, watering-
canadensis, Hydrastis
canadensis, Mentha
Canadian crutches
canal(s)
- c. ▸ abscess in anal

- c., alimentary
- c., alveolar
- c., anal
- c. and drums
- c., anterior
- c., Arnold's
- c., atrioventricular
- c., auditory
- c., birth
- c., blood in auditory
- c., Braune's
- c. broach, root
- c. carcinoma, anal
- c., carotid
- c. cautery, endocervical
- c., central
- c., cervical
- c., cervical neural
- c. clear, ear
- c., Cloquet's
- c., crural
- c. curettings, lower uterine
- c. curettings, upper uterine
- c. cushion, atrioventricular (AV)
- c., decompression of carpal
- c. defect, atrioventricular (AV)
- c., Dorello's
- c., ear
- c., encroachment on
- c., endocervical
- c., eustachian
- c., external
- c. (EAC) ▸ external auditory
- c., external ear
- c., femoral
- c., fenestration of semicircular
- c., Ferrein's
- c. filling, root
- c., fine root
- c., floor of inguinal
- c., fluid-filled
- c., Guyon's
- c., haversian
- c. hearing aid, completely in-the-
- c. hearing aid ▸ in-the-
- c., His
- c., horizontal
- c., Hunter's
- c., Huschke's
- c., hyaloid
- c. ▸ impacted wax in ear
- c., inflammation of ear
- c., inflammation of external ear
- c. ▸ inflammation of semicircular
- c., inguinal

canal(s)—*continued*
c. inspection ▸ video otoscopic ear
c. (IAC) ▸ internal auditory
c., intramedullary
c., lacrimal
c., lateral
c., membranous
c., medullary
c., muscular
c. ▸ narrowing of spinal
c., nasal
c., nerve
c., nerve of pterygoid
c., neural
c. of Corti
c. of diaphragm, esophageal
c. of Nuck
c. of spinal cord ▸ central
c., palatine
c. ▸ partial atrioventricular
c., pelvic
c., perivascular
c. ▸ persistent common
    atrioventricular
c., Petit's
c., posterior
c., prominence of
c., prominence of facial
c., pulmoaortic
c., pulp
c., pyloric
c. rays
c., rectal
c., Reissner's
c., root
c., Schlemm's
c., semicircular
c. silver pinning, root
c., skin ▸ ear
c., spinal
c., Stensen's
c., Stilling's
c. ▸ stimulation of semicircular
c. stretching, birth
c. therapy, root
c. tomogram, interauditory
c., tortuous root
c. treatment ▸ root
c. tumor, spinal
c., vein of cochlear
c., vein of pterygoid
c., ventricular
c., vertebral
c. vessels, spinal
c., vestibular

c., vidian
c., Volkmann's
c., Walther's
c. work, root
canalicular system
canaliculus(-i) [*colliculus*]
c. chordae tympani
c., cicatricial stenosis of
c. cochleae
c., dental
c., granuloma in
c. lacrimalis
c. lacrimalis, ampulla
c., mastoid
c. mastoideus
c. of chorda tympani
c. of cochlea
c. of cochlea ▸ vein of
c. of eye ▸ slitting of
c., plastic operation on
c., polyp in
c., sporotrichosis of
c., streptotrichosis of
c. tympanicus
canalith repositioning
Cananga odorata
canariensis, Pseudolynchia
Canavan disease
cancellated bone
cancellous
c. bone
c. bone curetted out of medullary
    cavity
c. bone, iliac
c. -cortical bone graft
c. formation
c. graft
c. tissue
cancer (Cancer) (CA)
c., acinar
c., acinous
c., adenoid
c. à deux
c. ▸ adjuvant therapy for breast
c., adrenocortical
c., adult
c., advanced
c., advanced breast
c., advanced prostate
c., advanced stage of
c., advanced stage terminal
c., alveolar
c., anal
c., angiogenic breast
c., aniline

c. antigen
c., antral
c., apinoid
c. ▸ appetite loss from
c., aquaticus
c., areolar
c. -associated anemia
c. atrophicans
c., basal cell
c., basal cell skin
c., betel
c., bile duct
c., biliary tract
c. biopsy
c., black
c., bladder
c. ▸ bloody semen from
c., bone
c., boring
c., bowel
c., branchiogenous
c., breast
c., bronchogenic
c., Butter's
c., buyo cheek
c. cachexia
c. -causing agent
c. -causing chemicals
c. -causing genes
c. -causing tumors
c. cell collector
c. cell membranes
c. cells
c. cells, antigen-producing
c. cells, assault
c. cells, breast
c. cells, destroying
c. cells, foreign
c. cells, heating
c. cells ▸ implanted
c. cells, liver
c. cells, microscopic
c. cells ▸ ovarian
c. cells ▸ prostate
c. cells, residual
c. cells, stray
c. cells ▸ suppress estrogen
    receptors in
c. cells ▸ transformed
c., cellular
c., cerebriform
c., cervical
c. chemotherapeutic agent
c. chemotherapy
c. chemotherapy ▸ colorectal

c., childhood
c., chimney-sweeps'
c., chondroid
c., choroidal
c. classification
c., classification system for
c., claypipe
c., clinical spectrum of
c., colloid
c., colon
c., colonic
c., colorectal
c., contact
c., corset
c. counseling
c., curable
c. cure
c., cystic
c. death
c. ▸ death from cervical
c. death ▸ risk of colon
c., deep-seated
c., dendritic
c. -dependent enzyme
c., dermatomyositis related to
c., dermoid
c. destroying agent
c. detection
C. Detection Awareness Program, Breast
c. detection, cervical
c. detection, early
c. detection methods
c., detection of
c. detection, prevention and screening
c. detection, prevention and treatment
c. detection, prostate
c. detection test
c. diagnosis
c., disseminated breast
c., distant
c. drug ▸ anti◊
c., drug-induced
c., duct
c., Dukes' C colon
c., dye workers'
c., early detection of
c. ▸ early detection of breast
c. ▸ early detection of colorectal
c., early lung
c., early stage
c. ▸ early stage breast
c. ▸ early stage prostate

c. embolus
c. ▸ emotional aspects of
c. en cuirasse
c., encephaloid
c. ▸ end-stage
c., endometrial
c., endothelial
c. enzyme
c., epidermal
c., epidermoid
c., epiesophageal
c., epithelial
c., ethmoid sinus
c., esophageal
c. ▸ extended dissection for thoracic
c., eye
c., eyelid
c. ▸ eyelid skin
c., fallopian tube
c., familial colon
c., familial colorectal
c. ▸ familial polyposis and
c., family history
c. family syndrome
c. fatality rate
c. fatality rate ▸ breast
c. ▸ feces and colonic
c. ▸ fiber and colonic
c. fighting cells
c. fighting drug
c. formation
c. -forming cells
c. -free
c. -free life
c., fungous
c., gallbladder
c., gastric
c., gastrointestinal (GI)
c. gene
c. gene ▸ colon
c. gene screening ▸ colon
c. genes, breast
c., genital
c. genetics
c., genitourinary (GU)
C. GI (gastrointestinal)
c., glandular
c., green
c. growth
c. growth ▸ slow down
c., hard
c., head
c., hematoid
c., hepatitis-induced liver
c., hereditary

c. ▸ hereditary breast
c., hereditary colon
c. (HNPCC) ▸ hereditary nonpolyposis colon
c. ▸ hereditary nonpolyposis colorectal
c. ▸ hereditary prostate
c. ▸ high risk for breast
c. ▸ high risk of developing cervical
c., human pancreatic
c., immune system
c. immunotherapy
c. in remission
c. in situ
c. incidence
c. ▸ increased risk of breast
c., incurable
c. -inducing virus
c., infiltrating lobular
c., inflammatory breast
c. ▸ inherited colon
c., inoperable
c. ▸ inoperable metastatic lung
c., inoperable ovarian
c. ▸ inoperable pancreatic
C. Institute (NCI) ▸ National
c., intraoral
c. ▸ intrathoracic esophageal
c., invasive
c., invasive breast
c., invasive cervical
c. ▸ invasive ductal
c. ▸ invasive lobular
c., jacket
c., jaundice from
c., kang
c., kangri
c., kidney
c. killer
c. -killing ability
c. -killing dye
c., kit, colorectal
c., laryngeal
c., larynx
c., latent
c. link, ▸ fiberglass-
c. link, potential breast
c. -linked microbial infections
c., lip
c., liver
c., Lobstein's
c., local
c., localized
c., localized bladder

cancer—*continued*

c. ▸ localized form of
c. localized in original site
c. ▸ localized prostate
c., lower bowel
c., lung
c., lymphatic
c. ▸ lymphadenectomy of
   intrathoracic esophageal
c. management
c., maxillary sinus
c., medullary
c., melanotic
c. ▸ metachronous lung
c., metastatic
c., metastatic breast
c., metastatic colon
c., metastatic colorectal
c., metastatic mammary
c., metastatic testicular
c., microinvasive cervical
c. ▸ mole breast
c., monitor
c., mouth
c., mule-spinners'
c., multiple
c., musculoskeletal
c. (MCC), mutated colorectal
c., nasal cavity
c., nasal vestibule
c., nasopharyngeal
c., neck
c., nervous system
c., neurologic complications of
   systemic
c. ▸ node negative for
c. ▸ nonhereditary breast
c., noninfiltrating
c., noninvasive
c. ▸ noninvasive cervical
c. ▸ nonmelanoma skin
c., nonoperable
c. ▸ nonsmall cell lung
c., occult
c., occult lung
c. of abdomen
c. of bladder
c. of brain
c. of brain stem
c. of cervix
c. of chest lining
c. of colon
c., colorectal
c. of kidney
c. of larynx

c. of lip, skin
c. of lung ▸ small cell
c. of lymph nodes
c. of male reproductive tract
c. of mouth
c. of pharynx
c. of prostate gland
c. of reproductive system
c. of stomach
c. of the cervix ▸ screening
c. of thyroid
c. of uterus
c., operable
c., operable breast
c., oral
c., oral cavity
c., ovarian
c. ▸ ovarian epithelial
c., pain from
c. ▸ pain in back from
c. pain management
c. pain research
c. pain, terminal
c., pancreas
c., pancreatic
c., paraffin
c., paranasal sinus
c. patient, breast
c. patient, depressed
c. patient ▸ immune system of
c. patient, immunocompromised
c. patients' warrior white cells
c., pattern of local spread in
c., penile
c. ▸ person's susceptibility to
c. personality
c., pharyngeal wall
c., pharynx
c., phlebitis from
c. ▸ physical and emotional aspects
   of
c. ▸ physical aspects of
c., pitch-workers'
c. -positive nodes
c., postcricoid
c. ▸ postmenopausal breast
c., preferred treatment in
c. ▸ prevalence of prostate
c. prevention
c. prevention and early detection
c. prevention, breast
c. prevention, colon-
c., prickle cell
c. ▸ primary bone
c., primary liver

c., produce
c. ▸ proliferation of esophageal
c. -prone
c. -prone families
c., prostate
c., prostatic
c., pyriform sinus
c. quackery
c. ▸ radiation-induced
c. radiation therapy
c., rare
c. rate, breast
c. ravaged body
c. reaction
c., rectal
c., rectum
c., recurrence of
c., recurrent
c., recurrent breast
c. ▸ recurring colon
c., regional
C. Registry
c. -related checkup
c. -related diagnostic services
c. remission
c., renal
c., renal cell
c., renal pelvis
c., reproductive
c. research
c. research, breast
c. research, clinical
C. Research Foundation of Boston
   ▸ Children's
c. responsive to systemic therapy
c., retrograde
c. risk
c. risk, bladder
c. risk, breast
c. risk, uterine
c., rodent
c., roentgenologist's
c., scirrhous
c. screening
C. Screening Center
c. screening, cervical
c. screening, colon
c. screening, colorectal
c. screening, oral
c. screening procedure ▸ prostate
c. screening, routine
c. screening, skin
c., shrink
c., skin
c. ▸ slow spread of

c., small cell lung
c. ▸ small intestine
c. smear
C. Society (ACS) ▸ American
c., soft
c. ▸ soft tissue
c., solanoid
c. ▸ solid tumor
c., soot
c. ▸ sore throat from
c. specialist
c., sphenoid sinus
c., spider
c. ▸ sporadic colon
c. spread ▸ lymphangitic pattern of
c., sputum cytology in lung
c. ▸ squamous cell
c. ▸ squamous cell skin
c., stabilize
c., stomach
c., superficial
c. ▸ superficial bladder
c., surface
c. surgery ▸ radical
c. survivor
c. syndrome ▸ family
c. syndrome ▸ hereditary breast-
ovarian
c. syndrome ▸ inherited
c., systemic
c., tar
c. -targeting cells
c., terminal
c., terminal lung
c., testicle
c., testicular
c. therapy
c. therapy, biological
c. therapy, cellular breast
c. therapy, experimental
c. therapy ▸ molecular breast
c. therapy, radiation necrosis in
skin
c. ▸ thoracic esophageal
c., thyroid
c. ▸ tobacco-related
c., tongue
c. treatment
c. treatment, brain
c. treatment, breast
c. treatment, experimental breast
c. treatment ▸ hormonal
c. treatment, prostate
c. treatment ▸ surgical
c. treatment, undergoing

c. trials
c., tubular
c. ▸ uncontrolled cell growth of
c., unresponsive
c., ureter
c., urinary bladder
c., urinary tract
c., uterine
c. vaccine
c. vaccine, experimental
c., vaginal
c. victim
c., villous duct
c., virulent
c., vocal cord
c. ▸ voice change from
c. vulnerable cells
c., vulvar
c., warning signals of
c. ▸ warning signs of oral
c., water
c. ▸ weight loss from
c., withering
cancericidal/cancerocidal
cancericidal level
cancerous
c. bone marrow
c. breast tumor ▸ localized
c. cachexia
c. cells
c. cells, abnormal
c. gland
c. growth
c. growth of blood cells
c. keratoses ▸ pre-
c. lesion
c. lump
c. mass
c., pre◊
c. region
c. thyroid nodule
c. tissue
c. tumor
c. tumor, thin
c. tumors, vaporize
cancerphobia/cancerophobia
cancrum (*see* canker)
c. nasi
c. oris
candelabra artery
Candida (candida)
C. albicans
C. balanitis
C. bloodstream infection
C. glabrata

c. granuloma
C. guilliermondi
c. infection
C. infection ▸ systemic
C. krusei
C. mesenterica
C. mycosis
C. parakrusei
C. parapsilosis
c. plaquing
C. pneumonia
C. pseudotropicalis
C. stellatoidea
C. tropicalis
c. urinary tract infection
C. vaginitis
C. vulvovaginitis
C. yeast infection
candidal abscess
candidal granuloma infection
candidate
c. for coronary attack ▸ patient
c. for myocardial infarction ▸ patient
c. for surgery ▸ patient
c., high risk
c., organ recipient
c., surgical
c., transplant
c., vital organ donor
Candidemia, nosocomial
Candidemia, systemic
candidiasis
c., chronic mucocutaneous
c., esophageal
c. from antibiotic
c., generalized
c., genital
c., intestinal
c., oral
c., oropharyngeal
c., pharyngeal
c., pulmonary
c., systemic
c., vaginal
candle(s) (Candles)
C. (LSD)
c. (fc) ▸ foot-
c. meter (fcm) ▸ foot-
candidum, Geotrichum
Candy (cocaine), Nose
cane (Cane)
c., adjustable
c., curved-handle
c., English
c., four-pronged

cane—*continued*
- c., large base quad
- c. or walker ▸ weighted
- c., patient independent with small based quad
- c., patient uses
- c., quad
- c., quadripod
- c., quadruped
- c. sugar
- c., swan-neck
- c., tripod
- c. with verbal cueing ▸ patient uses quad

canicola, Leptospira
canicularis, Anthomyia
canicularis, Fannia
canimorsus, Capnocytophaga
canina ▸ Centrocestus cuspidatus variety
canine
- c. assistance
- c. eminence
- c. fossa
- c. hysteria
- c. kala-azar
- c. leptospirosis
- c. muscle
- c. teeth
- c. -to-canine lingual splint
- c. transmissible tumor

caninum, Ancylostoma
caninum, Dipylidium
caninus, risus
canis
- c., Ascaris
- c., Asterococcus
- c., Ctenocephalides
- c., Haemobartonella
- c., Microsporum
- c., Toxocara

canisuga, Ixodes
canker (*same as* cancrum)
canker sore
canker sore from anxiety
cannabinoid(s)
- c. abuse, pattern of
- c. abuse, physical effects of
- c. abuse, potential of
- c. abuse, prevalence of
- c. abuse, psychological effects of
- c. abusers, assessing needs of
- c., acute intoxication with
- c., flashback reactions with
- c., mode of administration with

- c., organic brain syndrome with
- c., panic reactions with
- c., patient OD (overdosed) with
- c., potential tolerance to
- c., psychoactive properties of
- c., psychotic reactions with
- c., therapeutic potential of
- c., tolerance to
- c., topical
- c., toxicity of
- c., treatment of acute drug reactions to
- c., withdrawal from

cannabis (Cannabis) (marijuana)
- c. abuse
- c. (Smash), acetone extract
- c. cigarettes
- c. delusional disorder
- c. dependence
- c. -induced panic attack
- c. intoxication
- c. smoked
- c. usage

cannonball
- c. metastases
- c. metastasis to lung
- c. pulse

Cannon's
- C. endarterectomy loop
- C. ring
- C. sound
- C. theory

cannot be roused, patient
cannula
- c. ▸ femoral perfusion
- c., nasal
- c., oxygen (O_2) by nasal

cannulated
- c., biliary tree
- c., femoral artery
- c., heart
- c. nail
- c. percutaneously
- c., vessels of extremity

cannulation/cannulization
- c. antibiotic ▸ pre◊
- c., arterial
- c., ductal
- c. -induced metabolic acidosis
- c., internal jugular vein
- c., subclavian vein
- c., venous

canon, bruit de
cantering rhythm
canthal ligament
Cantharis vesicatoria

canthomeatal line
canthus
- c. electrode, external
- c., external
- c., inner
- c., left inner
- c., left outer
- c., left-right external
- c., nasal
- c. of eye, outer
- c., outer
- c., right inner
- c., right outer
- c., temporal

cantliei, Saccharomyces
cantilever beam
cantonensis, Angiostrongylus
Cantor tube
cantorum, chorditis
Cantrell's pentalogy
cap (Cap)
- c., acrosomal
- c., anterior head
- c., bishop's
- C. (LSD), Blue
- c., cervical
- c., cradle
- c., cranial
- c. crown
- c. crown ▸ half-
- c. delivery ▸ vacuum
- c., duodenal
- c., dutch
- c., enamel
- c., fibrous
- c., knee◊
- c., metanephric
- c., phrygian
- c., pleural
- c., postnuclear
- c., prosthesis ▸ McKeever patella
- c., prosthesis, McKeever Vitallium
- c. prosthesis ▸ Speed radius
- c., pyloric
- c., root
- c., shell
- c., skull
- c. ▸ thin fibrous
- c., Zinn's

capability(-ies)
- c. ▸ alteration in physical
- c., diagnostic
- c., emotional
- c., inherent
- c., mental

c., palliative
c., physical
c., sensing
c., trance
c., vision
c., wound healing
capable of independent living
capacitance
    c. bed ▸ venous
    c. (R C) coupled ▸ amplifier resistance
    c. factor
    c. vessel
capacitive radiofrequency
capacity
    c., aerobic
    c. analysis ▸ forced vital
    c., bladder
    c., blood clotting
    c., cardiac functional
    c., cardiovascular
    c., cardiovascular work
    c. classification ▸ functional
    c., cranial
    c., decreased diffusion
    c., diffusing
    c., diminished
    c., dye binding
    c., electrical
    c., electrostatic
    c., enzyme secreting-
    c. evaluation ▸ functional
    c., exercise
    C. exercise stress test ▸ Physical Work
    c. for abstract thought ▸ decreased
    c. ▸ forced expiratory
    c. (FIVC) ▸ forced inspiratory vital
    c. (FVC) ▸ forced vital
    c., functional reserve
    c., functional residual
    c. (FVC) ▸ functional vital
    c., heart flow
    c., heat
    c. (IMBC) ▸ indirect maximum breathing
    c., (IC), inspiratory
    c. ▸ inspiratory reserve
    c., intellectual
    c., iron-binding
    c., latent iron-binding
    c. ▸ loss of aerobic
    c., low diffusing
    c., lung
    c., maximal breathing

c. (MSVC) ▸ maximal sustainable ventilatory
c., maximal tubular excretory
c. (MVC) ▸ maximal vital
c., maximum aerobic
c., maximum breathing
c., memory
c., mental
c. ▸ metabolic vasodilatory
c., mood altering
c., natural trance
c., normal
c. ▸ normal vital
c. of lung, diffusing
c., oxygen
c. ▸ oxygen (O_2) binding
c. ▸ oxygen (O_2) carrying
c. ▸ oxygen (O_2) diffusing
c., physical work
c. ▸ problem solving
c., radiation protection
c. ratio ▸ forced vital
c. (RV/TLC) ratio ▸ residual volume to total lung
c. ▸ reduced bladder
c., reduced cranial
c. ▸ reduced lung
c., reproductive
c., (RLC), residual lung
c., respiratory
c. ▸ retraining visual
c., slow vital
c., stomach
c. test, iron-binding
c., testamentary
c., thermal
c. (VC) ▸ timed vital
c. to function
c., total
c., total bed
c., total bladder
c. (TIBC) ▸ total iron-binding
c., total lung
c. (VC) ▸ total vital
c. (TVC) ▸ total volume
c., trypsin-inhibitory
c., tubular excretory
c., unit of heat
c., ventilatory
c., virus neutralizing
c., visual
c. (VC) ▸ vital
c. ▸ weakened pumping
c., work

CAPD (continuous ambulatory peritoneal dialysis)
Cape Town aortic valve prosthesis
Cape Town prosthesis
Capgras delusion
Capgras syndrome
capillare, vas
Capillaria contorta
capillary(-ies) [*papiliary*]
    c. aging
    c. angioma
    c. apoplexy
    c., arterial
    c. basement membrane
    c. bed
    c. bed, alveolar
    c. block, alveolar
    c. ▸ blood flow from
    c. blood gas (CBG)
    c. blood gas at room air
    c. blood sugar (CBS)
    c. blood vessels
    c. blush
    c., broken facial
    c. bronchiectasis
    c. bronchitis
    c. bronchitis, epidemic
    c. cavernous hemangioma, mixed
    c. cordeolum, petechial
    c. drainage (dr'ge)
    c. embolism
    c. engorgement
    c. filtration coefficient
    c. flow, effective
    c. fracture
    c. fragility, Rumpel-Leede's
    c. fragility test
    c. hemangioblastoma
    c. hemangioma
    c. hemorrhage
    c. hemostatic
    c. hydrostatic pressure
    c. leak syndrome
    c. leak, transient
    c., leaking pulmonary
    c., leaky
    c. loop
    c. loop in dermal papilla
    c. loop in hair papilla
    c., lymph
    c., Meigs'
    c. membrane, alveolar
    c. microscope
    c. muscle
    c. permeability, increasing

capillary—*continued*
- c. points of ooze
- c. pressure
- c. pressure, mean
- c. pressure, pulmonary
- c., pulmonary
- c. pulse
- c. pulse, Quincke's
- c. refill
- c. sample
- c. stenosis
- c. thickening, alveolar
- c. unit, alveolar
- c., venous
- c. wall
- c. walls ▸ thickening of
- c. wedge pressure
- c. wedge pressure, monitor pulmonary
- c. wedge pressure ▸ pulmonary
- c. wedge (PCW), pulmonary

capillitii, pediculosis
capillitii, Saccharomyces
capital epiphysis
capital femoral epiphysis
capitate
- c. and hamate
- c. bone
- c. dislocation

capitis
- c., pediculosis
- c., Pediculus
- c., Pediculus humanus
- c., Pediculus humanus var.
- c., tinea

capitular process
capitulum humeri
capitulum of stapes
Caplan's syndrome
Capnocytophaga canimorsus
Capnophagia species
capped
- c. elbow
- c. knee
- c. lead

capping, pulp
capping, Silastic
capre, Damalinia
capricola, Trichostrongylus
CAPS-free diet (caffeine, alcohol, pepper, spicy) foods
capsid layer
capsula
- c. adiposa renis
- c. fibrosa renis

c. glomeruli
c. lentis
capsular
- c. adhesions
- c. advancement
- c. cataract
- c. contraction
- c. contracture
- c. decidua
- c. epithelium
- c. glaucoma
- c. hemiplegia
- c. insufficiency
- c. joint
- c. ligament
- c. nephritis
- c. occlusion
- c. opacities
- c. reefing, medial
- c. rheumatism, MacLeod's
- c. substance, specific
- c. surface
- c. surface smooth and glistening
- c. swelling
- c. thrombosis syndrome
- c. tightness

capsularis, decidua
capsulated bacteria
capsulatum, Histoplasma
capsulatus
- c., Bacillus aerogenes
- c., Cryptococcus
- c., Endomyces
- c., Torula

capsule(s)
- c., adherent renal
- c., adipose
- c., adrenal
- c., anterior
- c., articular
- c., auditory
- c., Bowman's
- c., carbohydrate
- c., Crosby-Kugler
- c. dissected, Tenon's
- c., Ernst radium
- c., exfoliation of lens
- c. exposed
- c. fibers
- c., fibrous
- c. fibrous, liver
- c., gelatin
- c., Gerota's
- c., Glisson's
- c., glomerular

c., hepatic
c., Heyman
c., identified
c., joint
c., knee of internal
c., lens
c., liver
c., malpighian
c., medial
c., millerian
c., nasal
c. of corpora, fibrous
c. of glomerulus
c. of kidney, fatty
c. of kidney, glomerular
c. of Tenon
c. opened
c., otic
c., pelvioprostatic
c., perinephric
c., pills and
c., platinum iridium
c. polisher, posterior
c., posterior
c., radium
c., reefing of medial
c., renal
c., Schweigger's
c., shoulder
c., splenic
c. strip easily
c. stripped
c. stripped easily
c. stripped easily ▸ renal
c., suprarenal
c., synovial
c. tear of
c., Tenon's
c. tumor
c., wireless endoscopy

capsulitis, adhesive
capsulitis joint
capsuloganglionic hemorrhage
capsulolenticular cataract
capsulothalamic syndrome
capsulotome, Darling's
capsulotomy procedure
capture
- c. assay, antigen
- c. beats
- c. bigeminy ▸ escape-
- c. complex
- c. cross section
- c., electron
- c. gamma rays

c., K-
c., pacemaker
c., resonance
c. threshold
c. threshold, atrial
c. threshold ▸ ventricular
c., ventricular
caput
    c. medusae
    c. stapedis
    c. succedaneum
car
    c. seat, infant
    c. seat, lumbar
    c. sickness
Carabello sign
carateum, Treponema
carbamate, hemoglobin
Carbocaine anesthesia
Carbocaine with Neo-Cobefrin
carbohydrase enzyme
carbohydrate
    c. absorption
    c. antigens
    c. capsule
    c. deficiency
    c. diet, high
    c. foods
    c. granules
    c. intolerance
    c. metabolism index (CMI)
    c. moiety
carbolic methylene blue
carbolized, stump
carbon
    c. arc lamp
    c. deposition ▸ subpleural reticulated
    c. deposits
    c. dioxide (CO_2)
    c. dioxide (CO_2) combining power
    c. dioxide (CO_2) ▸ dizziness from
    c. dioxide ($ETCO_2$) ▸ end-tidal
    c. dioxide ($FECO_2$) ▸ fraction of
        expired
    c. dioxide ($FICO_2$) ▸ fraction of
        inspired
    c. dioxide gas laser ▸ (CO_2)
    c. dioxide (CO_2) instilled
    c. dioxide (CO_2), insufflation of
    c. dioxide (CO_2) laser Sharplan 733
    c. dioxide (CO_2) laser skin
        resurfacing
    c. dioxide (CO_2) laser vaporization
    c. dioxide (CO_2) level ▸ blood

c. dioxide (CO_2) levels ▸ oxygen
    (O_2) and
c. dioxide (PCO_2) ▸ partial pressure of
c. dioxide (CO_2) pressure
c. dioxide (CO_2) pressure, alveolar
c. dioxide (CO_2) production
c. dioxide (CO_2) tension
c. dioxide (CO_2) tension, alveolar
c. dioxide (CO_2) tension, arterial
c. dioxide (CO_2) therapy
c. dioxide (CO_2) with oxygen
c. ion therapy
c. monoxide (CO)
c. monoxide (CO) poisoning
carbonate, magnesium
carbonis detergens (LCD), liquor
carbonizing cellular debris
carbonless paper syndrome
carborundum disc
carboxamide (DTIC/DIC) ▸
    dimethyltriazeno imidazole
carbuncular fever
carcinoembryonic antigen (CEA)
carcinoembryonic antigen ▸ fecal
carcinogenesis, radiation induced
carcinogenic agent
carcinogenic substance
carcinogenicity study
carcinogens, chemical
carcinoid
    c. disease
    c. flush
    c. heart disease
    c. ▸ intestinal tract
    c. involving pulmonary valve
    c. malignancy
    c. murmur
    c. plaque
    c. syndrome
    c. syndrome ▸ malignant
    c. syndrome ▸ metastatic
    c. tumor
    c. tumor of intestine
    c. valve disease
carcinoma(s)
    c., acinous
    c., adeno◊
    c., adenocystic
    c. adenoid cystic
    c. adenomatosum
    c., adenosquamous
    c., adrenal cortex
    c., advanced breast
    c., advanced bronchogenic
    c., advanced metastatic

c., advanced nonmetastatic
c. advanced regional
c., alveolar
c., alveolar cell
c., anal canal
c., anaplastic
c., annular
c., apocrine
c., argentaffin
c. axillary nodal metastasis in breast
c., basal cell
c., basaloid
c. base of tongue ▸ squamous cell
c., basocellulare
c., basosquamous cell
c., bile duct
c., biliary tree
c., bladder
c. bladder, anaplastic
c. body of uterus
c., breast
c. breast, inflammatory
c., bronchial
c., bronchiolar
c., bronchoalveolar
c., bronchogenic
c., bronchogenic oat cell
c., bronchogenic poorly
    differentiated squamous cell
c., bronchogenic squamous cell
c. bronchus
c. bronchus, epidermoid
c. buccal mucosa, squamous cell
c. cecum
c., cells consistent with invasive
c., cerebriform
c., cervical
c., cervical lymph node
    classification in squamous cell
c. cervix, squamous cell
c., cholangio◊
c., cholangiocellular
c., chondro◊
c., chorio ▸
c., chorionic
c., choroid plexus
c., circumferential invasive
c., colloid
c. colon
c., colonic
c., colorectal
c., comedo◊
c., corpus
c., cribriform
c. cutaneum

carcinoma(s)—*continued*

c., cylindrical
c., cylindrical cell
c., cylindromatous
c., cysto◊
c., differentiated
c., diffuse
c., disseminated
c. dorsum of hand, squamous cell
c., duct cell
c., ductal cell
c., Duke's
c., Dukes' classification of
c., duodenal
c. durum
c., ear
c. ear and nose, squamous cell
c., Ehrlich ascites
c. ▸ electrodesiccation and
   curettage in squamous cell
c., embryonal
c., encephaloid
c. en cuirasse
c., endocervical
c., endometrial
c., epibulbar
c., epidermoid
c., epithelial
c. epitheliale adenoides
c., erectile
c., esophagectomy for
c. esophagus, epidermoid
c. ex pleomorphic adenoma
c. ex ulcere
c., exophytic
c., extensive inoperable
c., extrahepatic biliary obstruction
   secondary to
c., extrathoracic spread pattern of lung
c., eyelid
c. eyelid, squamous cell
c., fallopian tube
c., far advanced
c., faucial arch
c. fibrosum
c. floor of mouth
c., focus of
c., gastric
c. ▸ gastrointestinal tract
c., gelatiniform
c., gelatinous
c., giant cell
c. gigantocellulare
c. gingiva, squamous cell
c., glandular

c., glottic
c., granulosa theca cell
c., gyriform
c., hair-matrix
c., hand
c., hard palate
c. head of pancreas
c., hematoid
c., hepatic
c. hepatocellular
c., hormonal therapy in endometrial
c., Hürthle cell
c., hyaline
c., hypernephroid
c., hypopharyngeal
c., hystero◊
c. infantile embryonal
c., infectious
c., infiltrating
c., infiltrating ductal cell
c. ▸ infiltrating squamous cell
c., infiltrative ductal
c., inflammatory
c., inoperable gastric
c in situ (CIS)
c. in situ, cells indicative of
c. in situ (DCIS) ▸ ductal
c. in situ (CIS) ▸ lobular
c. in situ of vulva
c., in situ transitional bladder cell
c., in situ, vaginal
c. ▸ inoperable esophageal
c., intra-abdominal
c., intraepidermal
c., intraepithelial
c. ▸ intrathoracic esophageal
c. invading mucosa and
   submucosa
c. invading muscularis
c., invasive
c., invasive cervical
c., invasive vulvar
c., kidney
c., Krompecher's
c., Kulchitzky-cell
c., large cell
c. ▸ large cell undifferentiated
c., laryngeal
c., lenticular
c. lenticulare
c., lip
c., lip, squamous cell
c., lipomatous
c., liver cell
c. liver, metastatic

c., lobular
c., local recurrence of
c., local spread pattern of lung
c., locally advanced and
   inflammatory breast
c., locally advanced squamous cell
c., lung
c. lung, epidermoid
c., lymph node involvement in
   nasopharyngeal
c., lymphangitic
c., lymphatic spread of
   nasopharyngeal
c., lymphatic spread pattern of lung
c., lymphoepithelial
c., macrofolliculoid
c. malignancy metastatic to liver
c. mastitoides
c., masto◊
c. medullare
c., medullary
c., meibomian gland
c. melanodes
c., melanotic
c., metastatic
c., metastatic bladder
c., metastatic endometrial
c. ▸ metastatic large cell
   undifferentiated
c., metastatic lung
c. ▸ metastatic pulmonary
c., microfolliculoid
c., microinvasive
c. molle
c., mucinous
c. muciparum
c. mucocellulare
c., mucoepidermoid
c. mucosum
c., mucous
c., multifocal infiltrated duct cell
c., myometrial invasion in
   endometrial
c. myxomatodes
c. (NPC), nasopharyngeal
c. nigrum
c., noninfiltrating intraductal
c., nonoat cell
c. ▸ nonsmall cell
c., nose
c., oat cell
c., oat seed cell
c. of adrenal cortex
c. of bladder ▸ transitional cell
c. of breast ▸ infiltrating ductal

c. of breast, intraductal
c. of breast, invasive
c. of cecum
c. of cervix
c. of colon, Dukes'
c. of conjunctiva ▸ basal cell
c. of conjunctiva ▸ epidermoid
c. of cornea ▸ epidermoid
c. of duodenum
c. of ear and nose, basal cell
c. of endometrium
c. of esophagus
c. of eyelid, basal cell
c. of kidney ▸ anaplastic
c. of kidney, renal cell
c. of large intestine
c. of larynx
c. of lip, basal cell
c. of liver
c. of lung, adenosquamous
c. of lung, small cell
c. of lung ▸ squamous cell
c. of nasopharynx
c. of ovary
c. of pancreas
c. of penis
c. of renal pelvis ▸ transitional cell
c. of sigmoid colon
c. of testis
c. of thyroid
c. of thyroid ▸ medullary
c. of vagina
c. of vocal cord ▸ squamous cell
c., oral
c., oropharyngeal
c. ossificans
c. ▸ ossified papillary thyroid
c., osteoid
c., ovarian (with ascites)
c. pancreas
c., pancreatic
c., papillary
c., papillary thyroid
c., papillo◊
c., parenchymatous
c., peau d'orange in breast
c., pelvic
c. ▸ perianal squamous cell
c., periportal
c., peritoneal seeding in endometrial
c., periurethral duct
c., pharyngoesophageal (PE)
c., pigmented basal cell
c. ▸ poorly differentiated
c., poorly differentiated anaplastic

c. ▸ poorly differentiated ductal
c. ▸ poorly differentiated large cell
c., poorly differentiated squamous cell
c., preinvasive
c., presumptive
c., prickle cell
c., primary ovarian
c. ▸ primary peritoneal
c., prognosis for
c., prostate
c., prestatic
c., psammo◊
c., pultaceous
c., radiation therapy for
c., rectosigmoid
c. rectum
c., recurrent
c. ▸ recurrent breast
c., renal cell
c., reserve cell
c., salivary gland
c., sarco◊
c. sarcomatodes
c., schneiderian
c., scirrhous
c. scroti
c., sebaceous gland
c., signet-ring cell
c., silent
c. simplex
c., small cell
c., small cell undifferentiated
c., small cell variety ▸ bronchogenic
c., small round cell
c., solanoid
c., spheroidal cell
c., spindle cell
c. splenic flexure
c., soft tissue
c. spongiosum
c., squamous
c., squamous cell
c., squamous cell skin
c. stomach
c., string
c., stump
c., subglottic
c. submandibular gland
c., superficial basal cell
c. ▸ superficial squamous cell
c., supraclavicular node metastasis in lung
c., supraglottic
c., survival relative to nodal involvement in breast

c., sweat gland
c. telangiectaticum
c. telangiectodes
c., terato◊
c., terminal
c., testicular
c., thyroid
c. to be ruled out (r/o CA)
c. tongue
c., tongue base
c. tongue, squamous cell
c., tonsillar fossa
c. trachea, epidermoid
c., transitional cell
c. tuberosum
c., tuberous
c., tumor doubling time in lung
c. ▸ underlying undifferentiated large cell
c., undifferentiated
c., undifferentiated bronchogenic
c., undifferentiated epidermoid
c., undifferentiated large cell
c., undifferentiated renal
c. ▸ undifferentiated small cell
c., unknown cell type ▸ bronchogenic
c. unknown, primary
c., unresectable
c., upper third of esophagus
c., urethral
c., uterine cervical
c. uterine cervical stump
c., verrucous
c. villosum
c., visceral
c. ▸ Von Brunn's nests in bladder
c., vulvar
c. ▸ well differentiated
c. ▸ well differentiated hepatocellular
c., widespread
c. with metastases ▸ primary ovarian
c. with respiratory tract fistula ▸ esophageal
carcinomatosis
c., abdominal
c., leptomeningeal
c., lymphangitic
c., meningeal
c., peritoneal
c. peritonei
carcinomatous
c. arthritis
c. arthritis in hands
c. arthritis in wrist

carcinomatous—*continued*
- c. lesion
- c. pericarditis

carcinosarcoma, embryonal
carcinosis cutis
CARD (cardiac automatic resuscitative device)
card
- c., consent
- c., discharge
- c., donor pledge
- c. ▸ medical alert wallet
- c., organ donor
- c., patient's kardex
- c. test ▸ stool
- c., uniform anatomical gift
- C., Uniform Donor

Cardarelli sign
cardia
- c., gastric
- c., incompetent
- c. of stomach
- c. of stomach ▸ scope advanced to

cardiac (Cardiac)
- c. abnormality
- c. accident
- c. action
- c. action potential
- c. activity, electrical
- c. adjustment scale
- c. allograft
- c. allograft atherosclerosis
- c. allograft vasculopathy
- c. alternation
- c. amyloidosis
- c. aneurysm
- c. angina
- c. anomaly, congenital
- c. anomaly ▸ fetal
- c. antrum
- c. apex
- c. apex pulse ▸ F point of
- c. apex pulse ▸ O point
- c. apex pulse ▸ SF wave of
- c. apnea
- c. arrest (CA)
- c. arrest drugs
- c. arrest, field procedure in
- c. arrest following trauma
- c. arrest ▸ full
- c. arrest, heart shocked during
- c. arrest ▸ nontraumatic
- c. arrest, sudden
- c. arrest surgery ▸ hypothermic
- c. arrest, sustained

- c. arrest, transient
- c. arrest victim
- c. arrhythmia
- C. Arrhythmia Suppression Trial (CAST)
- c. arrhythmias ▸ management of
- c. assessment, noninvasive
- c. asthma
- c. atria
- c. atrophy
- c. auscultation
- c. automatic resuscitative device (CARD)
- c. awareness
- c. ballet
- c. balloon pump
- c. baroreceptor
- c. bioprosthesis ▸ Mosaic
- c. biopsy
- c. blood
- c. blood ▸ anaerobic cultures of
- c. blood culture ▸ postmortem
- c. blood pool imaging
- c. border of dullness
- c. borders
- c. bronchus
- c. bypass ▸ beating heart
- c. bypass ▸ conventional
- c. bypass graft
- c. bypass surgery
- c. cachexia
- c. calculus
- c. care
- c. care, continuing
- c. care, emergency
- c. care ▸ history and symptoms of emergency
- C. Care Unit (CCU)
- c. catheter microphone
- c. catheter with balloon inserted
- c. catheterization
- c. catheterization ▸ interventional
- c. catheterization laboratory
- c. catheterization laboratory ▸ hospital
- c. catheterization, left
- c. catheterization, right
- c. catheterization technique
- c. cell contraction
- c. cells
- c. center
- c. chamber
- c. chamber, enlargement of
- c. chambers
- c. cirrhosis

- c. cocktail
- c. compensation
- c. competence
- c. competence ▸ adequacy of
- c. competence, borderline
- c. complications
- c. compression
- c. compression maneuvers ▸ external
- c. conditioning, operant
- c. conduction
- c. conduction system
- c. confusion
- c. consultation
- c. contractility
- c. contraction
- c. control, bidirectional
- c. cooling jacket
- c. cooling jacket ▸ Medtronic
- c. cripple
- c. cripple, patient
- c. crisis
- c. cushion
- c. cycle (CC)
- c. cycle ▸ isometric period of
- c. cycle (CC) ▸ resting phase of
- c. death
- c. death ▸ risk of
- c. death, sudden
- c. decompensation
- c. decompression
- c. defect
- c. defects, congenital
- c. defibrillation
- c. defibrillator
- c. defibrillator insertion ▸ implantable
- c. defibrillator (ICD), implantable
- c. depressant
- c. depression
- c. depressor reflex
- c. device
- c. device, Cournand
- c. device ▸ Rashkind
- c. diagnostics
- c. diastole
- c. diet
- c. diet, basic
- c. dilatation
- c. disease (CD)
- c. disease, end stage
- c. disease ▸ extracranial
- c. disorder
- c. diuretic
- c. Doppler examination
- c. dropsy

c. drug therapy
c. dullness
c. dullness (ACD) ▸ absolute
c. dullness, area of
c. dullness, border of
c. dullness (RCD) ▸ relative
c. dysfunction
c. dyspnea
c. dysrhythmias
c. echo
c. edema
c. effects
c. effusion
c. electrophysiology
c. emergency
c. endothelial cells
c. enlargement (CE)
c. enlargement (CE) ▸ massive
c. enzyme level
c. enzymes
c. evaluation
c. evaluation ▸ noninvasive
c. event
c. examination
c. failure
c. failure, chronic
c. failure, congestive
c. fibrillation
c. fibroma
c. fluoroscopy
c. follow-up
c. function
c. function, abnormal
c. function ▸ alcohol impairs
c. function, impaired
c. function, marginal
c. functional capacity
c. ganglia
c. gap junction protein
c. gating
c. gene expression
c. gene therapy
c. generator
c. generator, change of
c. glands
c. glucosides
c. glycogenosis
c. glycoside
c. hemodynamic monitoring
c. hemoptysis
c. herniation
c. heterotaxia
c. histiocyte
c. hypertrophy
c. imaging

c. imaging ▸ mask-mode
c. imaging system, digital
c. -imaging technique
c. inflammation
c. impairment
c. impression
c. impulse
c. incisura
c. index (CI)
c. index (MCI) ▸ mean
c. infarction
c. infection
c. injury
c. instability
c. insufficiency (CI)
c. insufficiency (CI), acute
c. insult
c. interstitium
c. intervention
c. invasive procedure (CIP)
c. irregularity
c. ischemia
c. ischemia (ACI), asymptomatic
c. jacket, Bonchek-Shiley
c. jelly
c. lacerations and hemopericardium
c. laser
c. lesion, organic
c. life support (ACLS) ▸ advanced
c. life support, basic
c. life support (ACLS) protocol ▸ advanced
c. limb
c. liver
c. loop
c. lung
c. malfunction
c. mapping
c. mass
c. massage
c. massage, closed chest
c. massage ▸ direct
c. massage, external
c. massage, internal
c. massage ▸ open chest
c. memory
c. metabolism, assess
c. metastasis
c. minute output (CMO)
c. monitor
c. monitoring
c. monocytes ▸ embryonic
c. mortality
c. murmur
c. murmur, functional

c. muscle
c. muscle ▸ embryonic
c. muscle fiber
c. muscle ▸ lack of O_2 to
c. muscle necrosis
c. muscle wrap
c. myocyte
c. myosin
c. myxoma
c. nerve, inferior
c. nerve, inferior cervical
c. nerve, middle
c. nerve, middle cervical
c. nerve, superior
c. nerve, superior cervical
c. nerves, supreme
c. nerves, thoracic
c. neural crest
c. neurosis
c. notch
c. notch of left lung
c. notch of stomach
c. obstruction
c. obstruction in syncope
c. organogenesis
c. organogenesis, abnormal
c. orifice
c. origin
c. output
c. output, adequate
c. output, alteration in
c. output, decreased
c. output, inadequate
c. output index
c. output ▸ low
c. output, marginal
c. output markedly reduced
c. output measurement
c. output, reduced
c. output, resting
c. output, systemic
c. output ▸ thermodilution
c. output ▸ vasodilators increase
c. overloading
c. pacemaker
c. pacemaker, artificial
c. pacemaker battery change
c. pacemaker ▸ dual chamber
c. pacemaker, electric
c. pacemaker ▸ Maestro implantable
c. pacemaker ▸ permanent
c. pacemaker ▸ Relay
c. pacemaker ▸ Stride
c. pacemaker, temporary
c. pacemaker, Versatex

cardiac—*continued*
c. pacing
c. pacing electrode ▸ Stockert
c. pacing lead ▸ permanent
c. pacing systems, permanent
c. patch
c. perforation
c. performance
c. perfusion
c. plexus
c. polyp
c. probe
c. profile
c. proteinuria
c. -pulmonary angio-aortic arch study
c. pulmonary shunt
C. Pulse Generator ▸ Chardack-Greatbatch Implantable
c. puncture
c. puncture, direct
c. rate
c. reflexes
c. refractory periods
c. rehabilitation
c. rehabilitation facilities
c. rehabilitation mental stress
c. rehabilitation program
c. rehabilitation team
c. region
c. -related vertebrate blood systems
c. reserve
c. response
c. resuscitation
c. resuscitation, open chest
c. revascularization procedure
c. resynchronization therapy
c. rhythm
c. rhythm, abnormal
c. rhythm, disturbance in
c. rhythm, reassessment of
c. rhythm, sinus
c. risk factor
c. risk factor modification
c. risk factors ▸ multiple
c. risk index
c. risk index score ▸ Goldman
c. risk, known
c. risk ▸ modified multifactorial index of
c. risk reduction
c. roentgenography
c. rupture
c. rupture, risk of
c. sarcoidosis myocarditis

c. sarcoma
c. scan
c. scan ▸ gated
c. scanning, nuclear
c. section of stomach
c. self-regulation
c. sensory nerve
c. shadow
c. shock
c. shunt
c. shunt detection
c. silhouette
c. size
c. size and function
c. size, small
c. sling
c. sonogram
c. souffle
c. sounds
c. sounds normal
c. spasm
c. spasm, fatal
c. sphincter
c. standstill
c. status
c. status, compensated
c. stepdown unit and telemetry
c. stimulant
c. stimulator
c. stomach
c. stress
c. stress test
c. studies
c. stump
c. stump inverted
c. surgery
c. surgery, ablative
c. surgery ▸ excisional
c. surgery ▸ junctional rhythm after
c. surgery ▸ reparative
c. surgery ▸ substitutional
c. symphysis
c. symptoms
c. syncope
c. Syndrome X
c. systole
c. tagging
c. tamponade
c. tamponade, nontraumatic
c. telemetry
c. thrust
c. tissue, diseased
c. tonic
c. toxicity
c. transplant

c. transplant ▸ heterologous
c. transplant ▸ heterotopic
c. transplant ▸ homologous
c. transplant ▸ orthotopic
c. transplant recipient
c. tumor
c. tumors, metastatic
c. tumor, primary malignant
c. ultrasonography
c. ultrasound
c. ultrasound ▸ Shimadzu
c. valve
c. valve, abnormal cleavage of
c. valve anomaly
c. valve, artificial
c. valve disorder
c. valve leaflets
c. valve prosthesis
c. valve prosthesis ▸ Cutter-Smeloff
c. valve prosthesis ▸ Lillehei-Kaster
c. valve prosthesis ▸ Omniscience single leaflet
c. valve prosthesis ▸ Smeloff
c. valve prosthesis ▸ Starr-Edwards
c. valve ▸ prosthetic
c. valve thrombosis
c. valves ▸ incompetence of the
c. variability
c. vein
c. vein, anterior
c. vein, great
c. vein, middle
c. vein, smallest
c. ventriculography
c. volume
c. volume ▸ relative
c. waist
c. wall hypokinesis
c. wall thickening
c. work index (CWI)
c. workup
c. wound, penetrating
cardiaca
c., adiposis
c., ganglia
c., steatosis
cardial enzymes
cardinal
c. ligament
c. sign of alcoholism
c. symptoms
c. tongue
c. vein
c. vessel
cardioaccelerating center

cardioaccelerator nerve
cardioactive glycoside
cardioangiography, retrograde
cardioarterial interval
cardioauditory syndrome
cardioauditory syndrome ▸ Sanchez-
    Cascos
Cardiobacterium hominis
cardiocentesis procedure
CardioCoil coronary stent
Cardio-Cool myocardial protection
    pouch
Cardio-Cuff, Childs
CardioData MK-3 Holter scanner
cardiodiagnostic procedure
cardiodiaphragmatic angle
cardioembolic stroke
cardioesophageal
    c. junction
    c. junction, tear in mucosa at
    c. reflux
cardiofacial syndrome
cardiogenic
    c. pulmonary edema
    c. pulmonary edema (ACPE), acute
    c. shock
    c. shock ▸ patient in
    c. syncope
Cardiografin contrast medium
cardiogram
    c., apex
    c., ballisto◊
    c., dextro◊
    c. dye
    c., echo◊
    c., ergo◊
    c., esophageal
    c., exercise
    c., myo◊
    c., negative
    c., precordial
    c., roentgeno◊
    c., vector◊
cardiograph, electro◊
cardiograph, myo◊
cardiography
    c., apex
    c., ballisto◊
    c., cineangio◊
    c., Doppler
    c., echo◊
    c. ▸ echo Doppler
    c., echophono◊
    c., electro◊
    c., ergo◊

c., phono◊
c. study
c. technique, apex
c., ultrasonic
c., ultrasound
c., vector◊
Cardio-Green
cardiohepatic sulcus
cardiohepatic triangle
cardioinhibitory
    c. syncope
    c. syncope ▸ vasodepressor
    c. type
cardiolipin
    c. complement fixation
    c. microflocculation
    c. natural lecithin
    c. synthetic lecithin
    c. Wassermann test
Cardiolite scan
Cardiolite stress test ▸ Technetium
cardiologic magnification
cardiology (Cardiology)
    C. Intensive Care Unit (CICU)
    c., pediatric
    c. procedure ▸ nonsurgical
cardiomediastinal silhouette
cardiomegaly
    c., borderline
    c., congestive
    c., false
    c., glycogen
    c., glycogenic
    c., hypertrophy
    c., idiopathic
    c., minimal
    c., moderate
    c., normal
cardiometer center
Cardiometrics cardiotomy reservoir
cardiomuscular bradycardia
cardiomyopathy
    c., African
    c., alcohol induced
    c., alcoholic
    c., atrophic
    c., beer drinkers'
    c., cobalt
    c., concentric hypertrophic
    c., congestive
    c., degenerative idiopathic
    c., dilated
    c., drug-induced
    c., end-stage
    c., false

c., familial hypertrophic
c., familial hypertrophic obstructive
c., fibroplastic
c., focal
c. ▸ genetic hypertrophic
c., hypertensive
c. ▸ hypertensive hypertrophic
c., hypertrophic
c., hypertrophic obstructive
c., idiopathic
c., idiopathic dilated
c. ▸ idiopathic restrictive
c., infectious
c., infiltrative
c., ischemic
c., mitochondrial
c., nephropathic
c. ▸ nonischemic dilated
c., obliterative
c. ▸ obstructive hypertrophic
c., parasitic
c. patient, restrictive
c., pediatric
c., peripartum
c. ▸ pneumatic dilation and
c., postpartum
c.: preclinical, acute and chronic ▸
    alcoholic
c., primary
c. ▸ Quebec beer drinker's
c., restrictive
c., right ventricular
c., secondary
c. ▸ tachyarrhythmias secondary to
c. ▸ tachycardia-induced
c., toxic
c. transplant ▸ rejection
c., viral
cardiomyoplasty, dynamic
cardiomyoplasty procedure
cardiopathia nigra
cardiopathy
    c., arteriosclerotic
    c., endocrine
    c., fatty
    c., hypertensive
    c., infarctoid
    c., nephropathic
    c., thyrotoxic
    c., toxic
    c., valvular
cardiopericardiopexy, Beck
cardiopexy ▸ ligamentum teres
cardiophone, electro-
cardiophonogram, electro-

cardiophonograph, electro-
cardiophrenic angle
cardioplegia
  c., antegrade-retrograde
  c., blood
  c., cold blood
  c., cold crystalloid
  c., cold potassium
  c. cooling
  c., crystalloid potassium
  c., hyperkalemic
  c., normothermic
  c., nutrient
  c. ▸ whole blood
cardioplegic
  c. arrest ▸ hypothermic
  c. solution
  c. solution, crystalloid
cardiopulmonary
  c. abnormality
  c. arrest
  c. arrest, arrhythmias associated
    with
  c. arrest, sudden
  c. arrest ▸ traumatic
  c. bypass
  c. bypass machine
  c. bypass operation
  c. bypass, partial
  c. bypass (PCPB) ▸ percutaneous
  c. bypass pump
  c. bypass support ▸ percutaneous
  c. bypass, total
  c. circulation
  c. disease
  c. disease, end stage
  c. exercise test
  c. failure
  c. murmur
  c. reserve
  c. resuscitation (CPR)
  c. resuscitation (CPR), attempted
  c. resuscitation (CPR) ▸ initiate
  c. resuscitation (CPR), mechanical
  c. resuscitation (CPR), one and two
    rescuer
  c. resuscitation (CPR), one person
  c. resuscitation (CPR), one rescuer
  c. resuscitation (CPR), techniques
  c. resuscitation (CPR) ▸ toilet
    plunger
  c. resuscitation (CPR), two-rescuer
  c. support
  c. support ▸ percutaneous
  c. transplantation

CardioPump, Ambu
cardiorespiratory
  c. arrest
  c. arrest, acute
  c. centers ▸ paralysis of medullary
  c. endurance
  c. failure
  c. failure, acute
  c. fitness
  c. murmur
cardioresuscitation team, emergency
cardioscopy, electro◊
cardiospasm, tropical
CardioTec scan
cardiothoracic ratio (CTR)
cardiothoracic surgery
cardiothymic silhouette
cardiotomy
  c., Intersept
  c. reservoir
  c. reservoir, Cardiometrics
  c. reservoir, Cobe
  c. reservoir ▸ Jostra
  c. reservoir ▸ Polystan
  c. reservoir ▸ Shiley
cardiotonic drug
cardiotoxica, myolysis
cardiotuberculous cirrhosis
cardiovascular
  c. accident (CVA)
  c. activity
  c. aerobic exercise
  c. agent
  c. anatomy
  c. angiography ▸ digital
  c. anomaly ▸ viscerobronchial
  c. assessment
  c. benefit, maximum
  c. biofeedback
  c. capacity
  c. collapse
  c. complication
  c. complications of drug abuse
  c. condition, congenital
  c. conditioning
  c. death
  c. development
  c. development ▸ epigenetic factor in
  c. development ▸ gene regulation of
  c. diagnostic study
  c. disability
  c. disease (CVD)
  c. disease, acute
  c. disease (ASCVD), arteriosclerotic
  c. disease (ASCVD), atherosclerotic

  c. disease ▸ functional
  c. disease (HCVD), hypertensive
  c. disease ▸ Lewis upper limb
  c. disease ▸ premature
  c. disease prevention
  c. disease (CVD) ▸ severity of
  c. disorder
  c. disorder, chronic
  c. disturbance
  c. drug
  c. effects
  c. effects of alcohol
  c. effects of methamphetamine
  c. efficiency
  c. endurance
  c. evaluation
  c. event
  c. excitatory cells
  c. exerciser
  c. exercises
  c. fitness
  c. function
  c. function ▸ drug-induced
    alterations of
  c. implications
  c. inhibitory cells
  c. instability
  c. maldevelopment
  c. malformation, congenital
  c. malformations
  c. medication
  c. morbidity and mortality
  c. mortality
  c. nursing
  c. patch ▸ Gore-Tex
  c. physiology
  c. pressure
  c. problems related to drug abuse
  c. prosthesis, Bentall
  c. renal disease
  c. response
  c. risk
  c. risk factor
  c. shunt
  c. silhouette
  c. silk suture
  c. steady state
  c. stimulation
  c. strain
  c. structures
  c. support
  c. surgery (CVS)
  c. surveillance
  c. symptomatology
  c. syphilis

c. system (CVS)
c. system ‣ perturbation in
c. system ‣ stress responses of
c. therapy
c. work capacity

cardioversion
c., chemical
c., congestive heart failure and
c., defibrillation and electrical
c., direct current
c., elective
c., electrical
c., electro◊
c., high energy
c. ‣ implantable defibrillator in
c., low energy
c. ‣ low energy synchronized
c. paddles
c., pharmacological

cardioverted, patient

cardioverter
c. defibrillator
c. defibrillator (AICD), automatic
   implantable
c. defibrillator (AICD), automatic
   internal
c. defibrillator ‣ external
c. defibrillator (ICD) ‣ implantable
c. defibrillator ‣ internal
c. defibrillator ‣ Medtronic
   external
c. defibrillator ‣ Medtronic PCD
   implantable
c. defibrillator ‣ nonthoracotomy
   implantable
c. defibrillator ‣ nonthoracotomy
   lead implantable
c. defibrillator ‣ pacer
c. defibrillator (PCD) ‣
   programmable
c. defibrillator ‣ subpectoral
   implantation of
c. defibrillator ‣ Telectronics ATP
   implantable
c. defibrillator ‣ Transvene
   nonthoracotomy implantable
c. defibrillator ‣ transvenous
   implantation of
c. defibrillator ‣ Ventritex Cadence
   implantable
c. electrodes ‣ implantable
c., external
c., implantable
c. ‣ Jewell pacer

CardioWest total artificial heart

carditis
c., Coxsackie
c., Lyme
c., peri◊
c., rheumatic
c., Sterges'
c., streptococcal
c., verrucous

care (Care)
c. activities, monitor patient
c. activities ‣ self-
c., acute
c., acute hospital
c., adequate patient
c., adult day
c. ‣ advance palliative
c. agency, health
c. agency ‣ home health
c. agent, health
c., aggressive
c., aggressive medical
c. air transport, critical
c., airway
c., alternate
c. alternative, health
c., ambulatory
c., ancillary health
c. and treatment during pregnancy
c. annually, patient
c. antihypertensive regimen ‣
   stepped-
c., appropriate level of
c. area, critical
c. area ‣ hand-washing in critical
c. assistance, home
c. ‣ availability of health
c. -based psychiatry ‣ managed
c., bedside
c. before and after chemotherapy ‣
   lip and mouth
c. bereavement, home
c., cardiac
c. center (ECC) ‣ admission of
   emergency
c. center, adult day
C. Center (CCC), Continuing
c. center, day
c. center, emergency
C. Center ‣ Same Day
c. center, tertiary
C. Center ‣ Urgent
c., chiropractic
c., clinical patient
c., clinical skin
c. ‣ collaborative patient

c., colostomy
c. community, continuing
c. conference, patient
c., conservative
c. consultant, health
c., continued ambulatory
c., continuing cardiac
c., continuity of
c., continuous home
c., continuum of
C. Coordinator, Home
c. coordinator, patient
c. cost, hospital
c. cost reduction ‣ health
c. costs, health
c. costs ‣ rising health
C. Coverage Act, Catastrophic
   Health
c. coverage, health
c. crisis, elderly
c. criteria ‣ skilled level of
c., critical
c., custodial
c. decision, health
c. decision, informed health
c. decision making, health
c. declaration, health
c., decubitus
c., decubitus skin
c. deficit, bathing self-
c. deficit, dressing self-
c. deficit ‣ feeding self-
c. deficit ‣ grooming self-
c. deficit ‣ hygiene self-
c. deficit, self-
c. deficit ‣ toileting self-
c., definitive medical
c., definitive surgical
c., dental
c., diabetic eye
c., diabetic foot
c., direct patient
c. disciplines
c. document ‣ Power of Attorney
   health
c. documents, health
c. ‣ effective mental health
c., elected palliative
c., emergency cardiac
c., emergency medical
c., emergency room
c. ‣ emotional aspects of supportive
c. ‣ end of life
c., enhance emergency
c., enhanced

care—continued

c. environment ▸ supportive
c. equipment, patient
c. experience, patient
c. facility, acute
c. facility, extended
c. facility ▸ external acute medical
c. facility, health
c. facility, intensive
c. facility, intermediate
c. facility ▸ long-term health
c. facility, residential
c. facility, tertiary
c., follow-up
c., follow-up wound
c., foot
c., foster home
c. function ▸ self-
c. funding, indigent
c., general
c. (GNC) ▸ general nursing
c., geriatric
c., geriatric acute
c. -giver, designated
c. -giver, in-home
c. -giver, primary
c. -givers, program for
c., good prenatal
c., group
c., gynecological
c., hands-on
c., health
c. ▸ high levels of
c., high-quality
c. ▸ high-quality medical
c. ▸ history and symptoms of
    emergency cardiac
c., home
c., home health
c., home nursing
c., hospice
c. hospital, acute
c., immediate patient
c., improper foot
c., in-home
c., incisional
c., increased prenatal
c., independent self-
c., individualized
c., industrial eye
c., industry, health
c., inpatient
c., inpatient psychiatric
c. institution ▸ comprehensive
    health

c. institution, health
c., institutional
c., intensive
c., intensive coronary
c., intensive prenatal
c., intermediate nursing
c. ▸ intermittent skilled nursing
c. intervention ▸ primary
c., intraoperative
c., intravenous (IV) needle site
c., juvenile residential
c. kit, catheter
c. kit, urinary catheter
c., lack of medical
c., level of
c., life-saving medical
c., long-term
c., long-term skilled nursing
c., managed
c. management ▸ self-
c. manager (GCM) ▸ geriatric
c. measures ▸ self-
c., medical
c., medical health
c., medical self-
c. medical unit, acute
c., medicine, critical
c., mental health
c., mouth
c., multidisciplinary
c., multidisciplinary palliative
c., nail infection and
C. (NIC) ▸ Neonatal Intensive
c. network
c., neurological nursing
c., newborn infant
c. nurse, critical
c. nurse, specially
C. Nursery (ICN) ▸ Intermediate
C. Nursery (SCN), Special
c. nursing, coronary
c. nursing facility, alternate
c., nutritional
c. of body after death
c. of child mental retardation
c. of family physician ▸ patient
    discharged to
c. of patient
c. of patient ▸ emergency
c. of patient ▸ optimum
c. of patient ▸ supportive
c. of relatives ▸ patient discharged to
c. of relatives ▸ patient released in
c., one-on-one personal
c., ongoing pastoral

c., optimal
c., orthopedic nursing
c., ostomy
c., outpatient
c., palliative home
c., pastoral
c., patient
c., patient admitted for terminal
c. ▸ patient avoids medical
c., patient discharged to home
c. ▸ patient-centered
c., patient-focused
c., patient responded to
c., patient transferred for custodial
c., patient transfused and treated
    with supportive
c., patient treated with supportive
c., patient under psychiatric
c., pediatric eye
c., perineal
c., periodontal gum
c. person, primary
c., personal
c., personnel health
c., physical/emotional
c., physician
c., physician directed interdisciplinary
c. physician (PCP) ▸ primary
C. Physician ▸ Urgent
c., preconceptional
c., prepaid health
c., preventive dental
c. plan, nursing
c., posthospital
c., postnatal
c., postoperative
c., postpartum
c., potential benefits of supportive
c. practices, patient
c., prehospital emergency
c., prehospital trauma
c., prenatal
c., preoperative
c., preventive
c., primary
c., primary acute
c., private duty
c., primary eye
c. procedures, patient
c. products, health
c. professional, health
C. Program, Coordinated Home
c. program, day
C. Program, Home
c. program, hospice home

C. Program ▸ patient discharged to Coordinated Home
c. program, respite
c. program, terminal
c. programs ▸ specialized AIDS home
c., progressive patient
c., prolonged hospital
c. provider, health
c. provider ▸ primary
c., psychiatric
c., psychiatric nursing
C. Pump, Life
c., quality health
c. questionnaire, health
c. rationing plan ▸ health
c. record, patient
c., refractive
c., residential
c. resources, health
c., respiratory
c., respiratory nursing
c., respite
c., respite and in-home
c., restorative
C. Retirement Community (CCRC), Continuing
c., routine
c., routine foot
c., routine general practitioner
c., routine home
c., routine prenatal
c., self-
c., senior day
C. Service ▸ Urgent
c. services, health
c. services ▸ long-term
c. setting ▸ primary
c., short-term
c., short-term institutional respite
c. ▸ short-term nursing
c., short-term skilled nursing
c., site
c., skilled nursing
c. skills ▸ self-
c., special wound
c. specialist, health
c., specialized nursing
c. staffing, continuing
c., standard inpatient
c., standards of
c., state-of-the-art medical
c. support environment, home
c. support, home
c., supportive

c., supportive home
c. ▸ supportive medical/nursing
c., supportive nursing
c., surgical inpatient
c. system, health
c. system ▸ managed
c. team, health
C. Team, Home
c. technician on-call, respiratory
c. techniques, patient
c. techniques, self-
c. technology, health
c. (TLC) ▸ tender loving
c., terminal
c., terminating
c., total health
c., total patient
c., tracheostomy
c., traditional home
c., transitional
c., 24 hour emergency
c., type of
c., uncompensated
c. ▸ understanding, insight and self-
C. Unit (ACU) ▸ Ambulatory
C. Unit (CCU) ▸ Cardiac
C. Unit (CICU) ▸ Cardiology Intensive
C. Unit, Community
C. Unit (CCU) ▸ Coronary
C. Unit (CICU) ▸ Coronary Intensive
C. Unit (ISCU) ▸ Infant Special
C. Unit (ICU) ▸ Intensive
C. Unit (ICCU) ▸ Intensive Coronary
C. Unit (IMCU) ▸ Intermediate Medical
C. Unit (MICU) ▸ Medical Intensive
C. Unit, Mobile Coronary
C. Unit, Mobile Intensive
C. Unit (NICU) ▸ Neonatal Intensive
C. Unit (PICU), Prenatal Intensive
c. unit (ICU) psychosis ▸ intensive
C. Unit (PICU) ▸ Pulmonary Intensive
C. Unit (RCU) ▸ Respiratory
C. Unit (SCU) ▸ Self-
C. Unit (SICU) ▸ Surgical Intensive
c. unit (ICU) syndrome ▸ intensive
c. utilization, health
c. utilization, medical
c., ventilatory
c. withdrawn, supportive
c. workers (HCW), health
c., wound

career
c. assessment
c. counseling
c. guidance
careful dissection
caregiver(s)
c. abandoning patient
c. ▸ idealize potential
c. neglectful
c. nurtures patient
c. withholding and uncaring
Caretaker's stress syndrome (ACSS) ▸ acute
caretaking, infant
Carey-Coombs murmur
caries
c., dental
c., foul sputum ▸ malnourished multiple
c. of bone
c. of petrous bone
c., rampant dental
carina
c., fixation of
c. fornicis
c. freely movable
c. midline sharp and mobile
c. of trachea
c., primary
c., secondary
c. sharp
c., tertiary
c. urethralis vaginas
c., widening of
carinal angle
carinatum, pectus
caring
c. attitude
c., coping with
c. environment
c. ▸ feeling of dullness and not
c. for self, patient incapable of
c., humane individuals
c. touch
carinii, Pneumocystis
carinii pneumonitis ▸ Pneumocystis
carious lesion
carious teeth
Carlen tube
Carleton's spots
Carlo method, Monte
carlsbergensis, Saccharomyces
C-arm fluoroscopy unit
Carmichael's crown
carmine dye, indigo

carmine test, indigo
carnaria, Sarcophaga
carnis, Sporothrix
carnosus, panniculus
carolinense, Solanum
carolinensis, Pelomyxa
carotene
    c., beta
    c. effect, beta
    c. level
    c. supplement, beta
caroticotympanic artery
caroticotympanic nerves
caroticovertebral stenosis
caroticus, bulbus
caroticus, sinus
carotid [*parotid*]
    c. analysis
    c. anastomosis ▸ vertebral
    c. aneurysm
    c. aneurysm ▸ intracavernous
    c. aneurysm ▸ supraclinoid
    c. angiography
    c. angioplasty
    c. aortic dissection, right
    c. applanation tonometry
    c. arch
    c. arterectomy
    c. arterial beds
    c. arterial disease ▸ extracranial
    c. arterial system
    c. arteriogram
    c. arteriography
    c. arteriography, bilateral
    c. artery
    c. artery, anastomosis of
    c. artery aneurysm
    c. artery arteritis
    c. artery, bifurcation of common
    c. artery block
    c. artery blockage
    c. artery, cavernous internal
    c. artery, cervical
    c. artery, common
    c. artery, compression of
    c. artery disease
    c. artery disease, atherosclerotic
    c. artery, ectatic
    c. artery endarterectomy
    c. artery, external
    c. artery (ICA), internal
    c. artery ▸ left common
    c. artery murmur
    c. artery narrowing
    c. artery occlusion (ICAO), internal

c. artery ▸ occlusion of left
c. artery ▸ occlusion of right
c. artery ▸ pipestem calcification of
c. artery ▸ right common
c. artery screening
c. artery shunt
c. artery stenosis
c. artery ▸ superior
c. artery ▸ tumor surrounds
c. artery ultrasound
c. axillary bypass
c. -axilloaxillary bypass, aorto-subclavian
c. bifurcation
c. body
c. body tumor
c. bruit
c. bruit, asymptomatic
c. bruits, bilateral
c. bulb
c. bypass, carotid-
c. bypass shunt, Brenner
c. bypass ▸ subclavian
c. canal
c. -carotid bypass
c. cavernous fistula
c. cavernous sinus ▸ fistula of
c. cerebral arteriography
c. compression
c. damage ▸ repetitive
c. Doppler
c. duplex scan
c. ejection time
c. endarterectomy
c. endarterectomy, blunt eversion
c. endarterectomy, left
c. endarterectomy, right
c. endarterectomy shunt ▸ Sundt
c. ganglion
c. ganglion, inferior
c. ganglion, superior
c. gland
c. insensitivity
c. magnetic resonance angiography (carotid MRA) ▸ contrast enhanced
c. MRA ▸ contrast enhanced (carotid magnetic resonance angiography)
c. massage
c. nerve, internal
c. nerves, external
c. obstructive disease
c. occlusive disease
c. ophthalmic aneurysm

c. plaque
c. plexus
c. pulsation
c. pulsation ▸ transmitted
c. pulse
c. pulse, effective
c. pulse obtained by massage
c. pulse, palpable
c. pulse tracing
c. pulses equal
c. sheath
c. sheath adenoma
c. shudder
c. shunt, Pruitt-Inahara
c. shunt ▸ Vascu Flo
c. sinus
c. sinus compression
c. sinus hypersensitivity
c. sinus massage
c. sinus nerve
c. sinus reflex
c. sinus reflex ▸ hyperactive
c. sinus sensitivity
c. sinus stimulation
c. sinus syncope
c. sinus syndrome
c. sinus syndrome ▸ hypersensitive
c. sinus test
c. siphon
c. siphon ▸ Moniz
c. steal syndrome
c. stenosis
c. stenosis ▸ stratified by
c. stent
c. stimulation
c. subclavian bypass
c. syncope
c. tracing (CT)
c. triangle
c. ultrasound
c. upstroke, decreased
c. vaso-occlusive disease
c. vein, external
c. vessel
c. vessels ▸ major blockage
c. vessels ▸ major obstruction
c. vessels ▸ occluded

carpal
    c. angle
    c. articulations
    c. bones
    c. canal ▸ decompression of
    c. fracture
    c. ligament, volar
    c. lunate implant, Swanson

c. scaphoid fracture
c. scaphoid implant, Swanson
c. spasm
c. tunnel
c. tunnel decompression
c. tunnel endoscopy
c. tunnel projection, Templeton and Zim
c. tunnel release
c. tunnel syndrome (CTS)

Carpentier
C. annuloplasty ring prosthesis
C. Edwards glutaraldehyde preserved porcine xenograft prosthesis
C. -Rhone-Poulenc mitral ring prosthesis
C. ring

carpet sanitizing
carphology/carphologia
carpi
c. radialis brevis muscle, extensor
c. radialis, flexor
c. radialis longus ▸ extensor
c. radialis muscle, flexor
c. radialis tendon, flexor
c. ulnaris muscle, extensor
c. ulnaris muscle, flexor

Carpoglyphus passularum
carpometacarpal
c. articulations
c. joint
c. ligament

carpopedal contraction
carpopedal spasm
Carpue's rhinoplasty
carpus curvus
Carrel-Dakin fluid
Carrell's operation
Carrel patch
carried down to fracture site ▸ incision
carried upward ▸ blunt dissection
carrier(s)
c., asymptomatic pathogen
c., chronic staph
c. -free
c. -free radioisotope
c., gene
c., hepatitis B
c., hold-back
c., mobile chart
c., obligate
c. of AIDS (acquired immune deficiency syndrome), heterosexual contact with male

c. of human immunodeficiency virus (HIV)
c. of infection, human
c. of virus, lifelong
c., patient active
c., patient AIDS (acquired immune deficiency syndrome)
c., patient chronic
c., patient unknown acquired immune deficiency syndrome (AIDS)
c., potential virus
c., primary
c. protein ▸ acyl-
c., shedding
c., sine wave
c., staphylococcal
c., state
c., streptococcal
c. tube
c., wheelchair

Carrington pneumonia
Carrion penile prosthesis ▸ Small-
carrionii, Cladosporium
carrionii, Hormodendrum
carrying
c. capacity ▸ oxygen (O₂)
c. cell ▸ plasmid-
c. red cells ▸ oxygen (O₂)

Carswell's grapes
cart
c., crash
c., distribution
c., medication
c., metabolic
c., monitoring
c., resuscitation
c., transporter

carteri, Borrelia
Carter's introducer
Carter's operation
cartilage(s)
c., alar
c., articular
c., arytenoid
c. breakdown
c., calcification intervertebral
c., calcification of
c., calcified
c. cells
c., chondritis costal
c., chondritis intervertebral
c., conchal
c., congenital
c., corniculate

c., costal
c., cricoid
c., cuneiform
c. damage
c., deflection septal
c. degeneration
c. destruction
c., dislocation of
c., ear
c., ensiform
c., epiglottic
c., eroded
c., erosion of
c., eustachian
c., excision of arytenoid
c., falciform
c., floating
c., gingival
c. graft
c. graft ▸ Kimura
c. grafts, diced
c. hoops
c., hyaline
c., impaired
c., implant
c., infected
c., inflamed
c., interarticular
c., interosseous
c., intervertebral
c., intrathyroid
c., joint
c., knee
c., lesser alar
c., level of cricoid
c., loss of
c., medial patellar facet
c., nasal
c. of larynx, arytenoid
c. of Luschka, laryngeal
c. of rib cage ▸ inflammation of
c. padding ▸ displacement of
c. particles ▸ loose
c., premature calcification of costal
c., quadrilateral
c., regenerate
c., regeneration
c. repair
c. retracted
c. retracted, cricoid
c. rings
c., Santorini's
c., semilunar
c., septal
c., sesamoid

cartilage—*continued*
  c., soft
  c., softening and swelling of
  c. tear
  c., tendon
  c., thyroid
  c. ▸ tiny bronchioles lack
  c., topical
  c., torn
  c., torn knee
  c., toxicity
  c., tracheal
  c., transplant
  c., transplantation
  c., trimmed, edges of
  c., unossified
  c. ▸ upper ear
  c., vomeronasal
  c., -wearing knee bends
  c., worn
  c., Wrisberg's
  c., xiphoid (xyphoid)
cartilaginea, exostosis
cartilagineum, Gelidium
cartilaginous
  c. discs
  c. exostosis, multiple
  c. growths
  c. joint
  c. portion
  c. pyramid
  c. ring, first
  c. ring, second
  c. ring, third
  c. rings incised
  c. septum
  c. tissue
  c. tube
  c. tumor
  c. vault
cartography, brain
Cartwright heart prosthesis
Cartwright valve prosthesis
caruncle(s)
  c., hymenal
  c., lacrimal
  c., Morgagni's
  c., sublingual
  c., urethral
caruncula lacrimalis
carunculae, trichosis
Carvallo sign
Casanellas' operation
cascade
  c., coagulation

c. phenomenon
c. ▸ renin angiotensin aldosterone
C. Simulator
c. stomach
c., stress
Cascos cardioauditory syndrome ▸ Sanchez-
case(s)
  c. ▸ AIDS look-alike
  c. assessment ▸ initial
  c., borderline
  c. conference, consecutive
  c. -control study
  c., coroner's
  c., flash burn
  c. formulation, clinical
  c. histories
  c. management
  c. management program ▸ psychiatric
  c. method
  c., operable
  c. presentation
  c. prognosis
  c. report
  c. study
  c. worm
caseated tissue
caseating granulomata
caseation, tuberculous
casei, Lactobacillus
casein-based tube feeding
caseiniform albumin
caseocavernous abscess
caseosa
  c., nephritis
  c., rhinitis
  c., vernix
caseous
  c. cataract
  c. lymphadenitis
  c. necrosis
  c. pneumonia
  c. tonsillitis
Casoni's
  C. intradermal test
  C. reaction
  C. test
Caspar's ring opacity
casserian muscle
Casser's fontanelle
Casser's muscle
cassette
  c., camp grid
  c., Sanchez-Perez

c., Schonander
cast(s) (Cast) (CAST)
  C. (Cardiac Arrhythmia Suppression Trial)
  C. (Children of Alcoholic Screen Testing)
  c., application of plaster
  c. bivalved
  c., blood
  c., body
  c., bronchial
  C. Clinic
  c., corrective
  c., Cotrel's
  c., cylinder
  c., epithelial
  c., extremity immobilized in
  c., fat
  c., granular
  c., halo
  c., hanging
  c., hip spica
  c., hyaline
  c., immobilized in plaster
  c. inlay
  c., lightweight
  c., long arm
  c., long leg
  c. metal partial dentures
  c., Pietrie's
  c., plaster
  c., plaster of Paris
  c. reapplication
  c., red cell
  c. removal
  c., Risser localizer
  c., Sarmiento
  c., short arm
  c., short leg
  c., short leg walking
  c., shoulder spica
  c., spica
  c. stare ▸ blank or down
  c., supportive halo
  c., temporary plaster
  c. trimmed
  c., Velpeau
  c., walker applied to
  c., walking
  c., waxy
  c., white cell
  c., window in
  c., window replaced in
Castellanella castellani
Castellani (castellani)

C. bronchitis
c., Castellanella
C. test
Castellino sign
Castelman's disease
Castillo syndrome ▸ Ahumada-Del
casting tape, fiberglass
castration
c. anxiety
c., chemical
c. complex
c., radiation for ovarian
castrensis gravis, icterus
castrensis levis, icterus
casual
c. contact
c. drug users
c. relationship
c. social drinking
CAT (chlormerodrin accumulation test)
CAT (computerized axial tomography)
C. scan
C. scan ▸ digital holographic
C. scan ▸ ultrafast
C. scanner
C. scanner ▸ helical
cat('s)
c. -bite fever
c. ear
c. eye amaurosis
c. eye pupil
c. eye reflex
c. heart, tabby
c. mite dermatitis
c. -scratch disease
c. -scratch fever
c. striation, tabby
c. stroking maneuver during
massage
catacrotic pulse
catacrotic wave
catadicrotic pulse
catadicrotic wave
catalase, hepatic
cataleptic attack
cataleptic systole
catalytic activity
catalytic site
catamenialis, iritis
cataplexie du reveil
cataplexy muscle weakness
cataract(s)
c., adherent
c., adolescent
c., after-

c., age-related
c., anterior axial embryonal
c., anterior polar
c., arborescent
c., aridosiliculose
c., aridosiliquate
c., atopic
c., axial
c., axillary
c., bilateral
c., black
c., blood
c., blue
c., blue dot
c., bony
c., bottlemakers'
c., brown
c., brunescent
c., calcareous
c., capsular
c., capsulolenticular
c., caseous
c., central
c., cerulean
c., cheesy
c., choroidal
c., complicated
c., congenital
c., contusion
c., coralliform
c. coralliformis
c., coronary
c., cortical
c., cryoextraction of
c., cupuliform
c., cystic
c., depression of
c. development
c., diabetic
c., diabetic polar
c., discission of
c. disease
c., double needle operation on
c., dry-shelled
c., electric
c., embryonal nuclear
c., extracapsular extraction of
c. extraction
c. extraction, cryogenic
c. extraction, extracapsular
c. extraction, intracapsular
c., fibroid
c. flap operation
c., floriform
c. floriformis

c., fluid
c., fusiform
c., general
c., glassblowers'
c. glasses
c., glaucomatous
c., gray
c., hard
c., heat-ray
c., hedger's
c., heterochromic
c., hypermature
c., immature
c. implant lens, Lieb and Guerry
c., incipient
c., infantile
c. inspection
c., intracapsular extraction of
c., intumescent
c., irradiation
c., juvenile
c., Koby's
c., lacteal
c., lamellar
c., lamellar zonular perinuclear
c., lens
c. lens, Anis Staple implant
c. lens, Appolionio implant
c. lens, Azar Tripod implant
c. lens, Baron implant
c. lens, Bietti implant
c. lens, Binkhorst iridiocapsular
c. lens, Choyce implant
c. lens implantation
c. lens, Krasnov implant
c. lens, Pearce Tripod implant
c. lens, Platina Clip implant
c. lens, Ridley implant
c. lens, Schachar's implant
c. lens, Scharf's implant
c. lens, Strampelli implant
c., lenticular
c., lightning
c., mature
c. membrane adjustments ▸
secondary
c., membranous
c., milky
c., mixed
c., morgagnian
c., myotonic
c., naphthalinic
c., needling of
c., nuclear
c., O'Brien's

cataract—*continued*
- c., overripe
- c., partial
- c., perinuclear
- c., peripheral
- c., polar
- c., posterior axial embryonal
- c., posterior polar
- c. (PSC), posterior subcapsular
- c., primary
- c. procedure ▸ one-stitch
- c., progressive
- c., puddler's
- c., punctate
- c., pyramidal
- c., reduplication
- c., regrowth
- c., removal
- c., removal, no stitch and no patch
- c., ripe
- c. ▸ ripeness of
- c., rosette
- c., sanguineous
- c., secondary
- c., sedimentary
- c., senile
- c., siliculose
- c., siliquose
- c., snowflake
- c., snowstorm
- c., Soemmering's ring
- c., soft
- c., spindle
- c., spindle-shaped
- c., stationary
- c., stellate
- c., subcapsular
- c., sunflower
- c., surgery for
- c. surgery, left
- c. surgery ▸ no stitch
- c. surgery, right
- c. surgery ▸ small incision
- c. surgery, sutureless
- c. surgery, with implant
- c., sutural
- c., syphilitic
- c., tetany
- c., total
- c., toxic
- c., traumatic
- c. treatment
- c., tremulous
- c., unripe
- c., vision threatening

- c., Vogt's
- c., zapping
- c., zonular

catarrh
- c., atrophic
- c., autumnal
- c., Bostock
- c., hypertrophic
- c., Laennec's
- c., nasal
- c., postnasal
- c., sinus
- c., suffocative
- c., vernal

catarrhal
- c. asthma
- c. bronchitis
- c. cholangitis
- c. conjunctivitis
- c. croup
- c. dysentery
- c. dyspepsia
- c. fever
- c. fever, epidemic
- c. gastritis
- c. gingivitis
- c. inflammation, acute
- c. laryngitis
- c. laryngitis, chronic
- c. nephritis
- c. ophthalmia
- c. pharyngitis
- c. pharyngitis, acute
- c. pneumonia
- c. rhinitis
- c. stomatitis
- c. tonsillitis
- c. tonsillitis, acute
- c. tonsillitis, chronic
- c. vaginitis

catarrhalis
- c., Branhamella
- c., herpes
- c., icterus
- c., Moraxella
- c., Neisseria

catastrophic
- c. brain damage, irreversible
- c. brain injury, irreversible
- c. disease
- c. event
- C. Health Care Coverage Act
- c. health insurance
- c. hemorrhaging
- c. illness

- c. life-threatening illness
- c. reaction
- c. situation

catatonia, coma and convulsions

catatonic
- c. patient,
- c. schizophrenia
- c. schizophrenic disorder
- c. state
- c. state, patient in
- c. stupor
- c. type, chronic ▸ schizophrenia,
- c. type, chronic with acute exacerbation ▸ schizophrenia,
- c. -type schizophrenia
- c. type, subchronic ▸ schizophrenia,
- c. type, subchronic with acute exacerbation ▸ schizophrenia,
- c. type, unspecified ▸ schizophrenia,

catatricrotic pulse

catch
- c., precordial
- c. syndrome ▸ precordial
- c. -up, developmental
- c. urinalysis, clean
- c. urine, clean

catcher's projection, ball-

catechol spillover ▸ jugular venous

catecholamine(s)
- c. action
- c. metabolism
- c., plasma
- c. receptor
- c., serum
- c. test

category(-ies) (Category)
- c., high-risk
- c. in hollow organs, T
- c. patient, ultra low risk
- C. Test, Halstead

catenary system

catenata, Naumanniella

catenating ague

catgut
- c., fine plain
- c., interrupted plain
- c. mattress suture ▸ chromic
- c., periosteum closed with plain
- c., plain
- c. suture
- c. (CCG) suture ▸ chromic
- c. sutures, continuous
- c. sutures, plain
- c., ties of chromic

Catharanthus roseus

catharsis, Freud's
cathartic
c., compound
c. effect
c. method, Freud's
catheter
c. ablation
c. ablation, electrical
c. ablation ▸ radiofrequency
c., acorn-tipped
c. adapter
c. administered treatment
c. advanced
c. angiography ▸ femorocerebral
c., angiopigtail
c. angioplasty (BCA), balloon
c., angioplasty guiding
c., angulated multipurpose
c. aortography
c., arterial
c., arterial embolectomy
c. arteriography
c. aspirated and flushed with saline
c. -associated bacteremias
c. -associated septicemia
c., atherectomy
c., balloon
c. -based Maze procedure
c., biliary drainage
c., bipolar pacing
c., bladder
c., brachial
c., bulb
c., cardiac
c. care kit
c. care kit ▸ urinary
c., cathematic
c. (CVC) ▸ central venous
c., cephalad
c. cholangiogram, nasobiliary
c. cholangiography
c. coiled upon itself
c., coronary angiographic
c. coronary perfusion
c., coronary seeking
c. coudé
c. cuff, antimicrobial
c. culture ▸ intravascular
c., cutdown
c. delivery system ▸ fiberoptic
c. dilatation
c., drainage
c. drainage (dr'ge), indwelling
c., echo
c., electrode

c. electrode ▸ intravascular
c. electrode ▸ multipolar
c. embolism
c. embolus
c. exchange
c., fenestrated
c., filiform
c., flow-directed pulmonary artery
c. gauge
c., guide
c. -guided biopsy
c. -guided endoscopic intubation
c. ▸ headhunter angiography
c., hyperalimentation
c., impedance
c. in place
c. -induced ablation
c. induced spasm
c. ▸ indwelling bladder
c., indwelling urethral
c., indwelling urinary
c. ▸ indwelling vascular
c., indwelling venous
c., infant with umbilical
c. infection, central venous
c. inserted
c. insertion site
c. instability
c., intercostal
c. ▸ internal mammary artery
c. into artery ▸ threading
c., intracardiac
c., intracranial pressure (ICP)
c., intratracheal O$_2$ (oxygen)
c., intrauterine pressure
c. ▸ intravascular ultrasound
c., intravenous (IV)
c., intraventricular
c. introduced
c., IV (intravenous)
c., laser
c., lumbar subarachnoid
c. mapping
c., marker
c. microphone, cardiac
c. ▸ multi-access
c., multilumen
c., multipolar
c., multisensor
c., mushroom
c., nasotracheal
c., nonflotation
c., nonfunctioning
c., nontraumatizing
c., olive tip

c. ▸ one hold angiographic
c. ▸ optical fiber
c. out, patient pulled
c., oximetric
c., pacemaker
c., pacing
c., passage of
c. passed with ease
c. patency
c., peritoneal
c., pigtail
c. placed graft
c. placement
c. placement, arterial line monitor
c. placement, nasobiliary pigtail
c., polyethylene
c. positioned
c. ▸ prolonged indwelling
c., pulmonary artery
c. radiofrequency ablation
c., radiopaque
c., Rashkind balloon
c. -related bacteremia
c. -related infection
c. -related peripheral vessel spasm
c. -related urinary tract infection
c., reperfusion
c., retention
c., return flow hemostatic
c., right-sided subclavian
c., right subclavian vein dialysis
c., Schneider
c., self-retaining
c. sepsis
c., Silastic mushroom
c. site
c. site bruises
c., spiral tip
c. stimulation of right atrium
c. ▸ straight flush percutaneous
c., subclavian
c., subclavian dialysis
c., subclavian venous
c., suction
c., sump
c., three-way irrigating
c. tip, broken
c. tip culture
c. -tip spasm
c., total parenteral nutrition (TPN)
c., triple lumen
c. tube cultures
c., umbilical
c., umbilical artery
c., umbilical vein

catheter—*continued*
- c., ureteral
- c., urethral
- c., urinary
- c., vascular
- c., ventricular
- c., venous
- c., whistle-tip
- c. with balloon inserted, cardiac

catheterization
- c., balloon valvuloplasty
- c., cardiac
- c., combined heart
- c., contrast arterial
- c., coronary
- c., coronary sinus
- c., heart
- c., hepatic
- c., hepatic vein
- c., intermittent
- c., ▸ intermittent self-
- c. ▸ interventional cardiac
- c., intra-arterial hepatic
- c., laboratory, cardiac
- c., laboratory ▸ hospital cardiac
- c., lacrimonasal duct
- c., laryngeal
- c., left cardiac
- c. ▸ left heart
- c. of bladder, intermittent
- c. of duct
- c. of eustachian tube
- c. ▸ percutaneous transhepatic
- c., pulmonary artery
- c., retrograde
- c., retrourethral
- c., right cardiac
- c., right heart
- c. schedule, strict
- c. stylet, heart
- c. technique, aseptic
- c. technique, cardiac
- c. technique, nonsterile
- c., tracheal
- c. ▸ transseptal left heart
- c., umbilical artery
- c., urinary

catheterized
- c., bladder
- c., patient
- c. specimen
- c. specimen of urine
- c., umbilical artery

cathodal
- c. closing

- c. closing contraction
- c. closing tetanus
- c. closure clonus
- c. closure contraction
- c. closure tetanus
- c. duration
- c. duration tetanus
- c. opening clonus
- c. opening contraction

cathode
- c. ray
- c. -ray tube (CRT)
- c. tube, hot-

cati, Toxocara
cationic protein, eosinophil
catodon, Physeter
Cattell Infant Intelligence Scale
Caucasian female, patient
Caucasian male, patient
caucasica, Borrelia
caucasica, Physaloptera
cauda
- c. cerebelli
- c. equina
- c. equina, adhesions of
- c. equina compression
- c. equina syndrome
- c. equinal tumor

caudad tear
caudal
- c. anesthesia
- c. angulation
- c. aspect
- c. block
- c. branches
- c. branches of artery
- c. flap
- c. flexure
- c. helix
- c. ligament
- c. pancreaticojejunostomy
- c. peritoneum
- c. pole
- c. sac
- c. septum

caudamoeba sinensis
caudate
- c. activity
- c. lobe of liver
- c. nucleus
- c. nucleus ▸ head of

caudatum, Uronema
caudatus, Bodo
caudocranial hemiaxial view
cauliflower ear

cauliflower excrescence
Caulobacter vibrioides
Caulophylium thalictroides
causal
- c. agent
- c. relation
- c. role

causality assessment
causation and management, pain
causation of disease
causative
- c. agent
- c. disease
- c. elements
- c. factor
- c. genes ▸ single
- c. organism
- c. organism identified
- c. role

cause(s)
- c. -and-effect
- c. -and-effect relationship
- c. and treatment ▸ symptoms
- c. bones to thicken
- c., constitutional
- c., exciting
- c., fundamental
- c., immediate
- c. ▸ impaired memory of unknown
- c., infectious
- c., local
- c., noninfectious
- c. ▸ obesity-related
- c. of blindness
- c. of death (COD)
- c. of death (COD) ▸ autopsy report
- c. of death ▸ leading
- c. of drug abuse
- c. of heart disease
- c., organic
- c., patient expired due to natural
- c., precipitating
- c., predisposing
- c., primary
- c., proximate
- c., remote
- c., secondary
- c., specific
- c., ultimate
- c., underlying
- c. undetermined (CU)

caused
- c. by disease ▸ fracture
- c. by infection ▸ fever
- c. by light ▸ constriction

c. by malignancy ► fracture
c. by tuberculosis ► knee monarthritis
c. headaches ► tumor-
c. health problems ► stress

causing
c. agent, cancer
c. bacteria, ► odor-
c. bacterium, pneumonia-
c. chemicals, cancer-
c. death, intentionally
c. gene, disease
c. genes, cancer-
c. organism, disease-
c. organism ► pneumonia-
c. plaque ► odor-
c. tumors, cancer-

caustic gastric secretions
caustic strictures of cervical esophagus
caustic strictures of hypopharynx
cauterization
c., cervical
c., electro◊
c., electrosurgical
c., heater probe

cauterize lining of uterus
cauterized
c. ► bleeding site
c. ► spinothalamic tract
c. tissue

cautery
c., actual
c., bipolar
c., Birtcher's
c., button
c., chemical
c., cold
c., Corrigan's
c., electric
c., electro◊
c., endocervical canal
c., galvanic
c., gas
c., Hildreth's
c., Mils'
c., Mira
c., Mueller's
c., nasal tip
c., Paquelin's
c., Percy's
c., potential
c. puncture, retinal
c., Rommel-Hildreth
c., Rommel's
c., Scheie's ophthalmic

c. snare
c., solar
c., Souttar's
c., steam
c., sun
c. unit
c., virtual
c., von Graefe's
c., Wadsworth-Todd
c., wet field
c., wound
c., Ziegler

cava
c. anomaly ► vena
c. clip ► vena
c. filter ► Greenfield vena
c. (IVC) ► inferior vena
c. occlusion ► inferior vena
c. pressure (IVCP) ► inferior vena
c., retraction of vena
c. (SVC) ► superior vena
c. (SVC) syndrome ► superior vena
c. syndrome ► vena
c. (TIVC) ► thoracic inferior vena
c., vena

cavagram, vena
caval
c. compression
c. compression, vena
c. filter
c. fold
c. (IVC) obstruction ► inferior vena
c. obstruction, vena
c. shunt ► Marion-Clatworthy side-to-end vena
c. tumor, vena
c. valve

cavalryman's osteoma
cavamesenteric shunt
Cave (cave)
C. operation
C. -Rowe operation
c. sickness
c. syndrome

cavernomatous changes
cavernosorum clitoridis, septum corporum
cavernosum, angioma
cavernosus clitoridis, plexus
cavernosus plexus of clitoris
cavernous
c. aneurysm
c. angioma
c. angioma ► extracerebral
c. artery

c. breathing
c. fistula, carotid
c. hemangioma
c. hemangioma, mixed capillary
c. hemangioma of skin
c. internal carotid artery
c. nerves of clitoris
c. nerves of penis
c. rale
c. respiration
c. sinus
c. sinus aneurysm
c. sinus ► fistula of carotid
c. sinus ► phlebitis of
c. sinus ► thrombosis of
c. tissue
c. vein of penis
c. voice

caviae, Aeromonas
caviae, Nocardia
Cavin shunt
cavipalpus, Ixodes
cavitary
c. disease
c. lesion
c. mass
c. tuberculosis

cavitas dentis
cavitation of lobe
cavitation, pulmonary
cavity(-ies)
c., abdominal
c., abscess
c., air
c., air-filled
c., air fluid
c., air in pleural
c., alveolar
c., amniotic
c., anterior
c., aneurysm
c, around eye ► bone
c., aspiration pleural
c., atrial
c., attic
c. ► blood fluid in peritoneal
c., blood in pleural
c., body
c., bone marrow
c., bone weakening
c., brain
c., buccal
c., cancellous bone curetted out of medullary
c. cancer, nasal

cavity(-ies)—*continued*
- c. cancer, oral
- c., chest
- c., compound
- c., cotyloid
- c., cranial
- c. curetted, uterine
- c., dental
- c., direct drainage (dr'ge) of abdominal
- c., ear
- c., endometrial
- c., entered, pleural
- c., entering chest
- c., epidural
- c., fenestration
- c., fluid in pleural
- c. free of fluid ▸ abdominal
- c., -gas calibration factor (N_{gas})
- c., general peritoneal
- c., glenoid
- c., incision through wall of
- c. ▸ inflammation of lining of abdominal
- c. insufflated, peritoneal
- c., intracranial
- c., junctional
- c., lesser peritoneal
- c., lining of
- c., marrow
- c., mastoid
- c., Meckel's
- c., mediastinal
- c., medullary
- c., middle ear
- c., nasal
- c., obliteration of
- c. of bone
- c. of eyeball
- c. of optic papilla
- c. opened, chest
- c., oral
- c., orbital
- c., outlining amniotic
- c. packed, mastoid
- c., pelvic
- c., pelvic peritoneal
- c., pericardial
- c., peritoneal
- c., pleural
- c., posterior
- c., pulp
- c., sinus
- c. sounded, endometrial
- c. sounded to depth of _____ ▸ uterine

- c. sounded, uterine
- c., subarachnoid
- c., synovial
- c., thoracic
- c., tympanic
- c., tympanomastoid
- c., uterine
- c., vaporize
- c., vitreous
- c., wall of
- c., watery fluid in pleural
- c., wound

cavocaval shunt
cavopulmonary
- c. anastomosis
- c. anastomosis (BCA), bidirectional
- c. anastomosis (BSCA), bidirectional superior
- c. connection
- c. connection ▸ total

cavosurface angle
cavovalgus, talipes
CAVS (calcific aortic valve stenosis)
cavum
- c. conchae
- c. epidurale
- c. nasi
- c. septi pellucidi
- c. subarachnoideale
- c. subdurale
- c. tympani
- c. uteri
- c. vergae

cavus
- c. feet
- c., pes
- c., talipes

cayenne pepper grains
cayetanensis, Cyclospora
cayor worm
CBC (complete blood count)
CBC (complete blood count) ▸ interval
CBG (capillary blood gas)
CBG (corticosteroid-binding globulin)
CBS (capillary blood sugar)
CBT (cognitive behavioral therapy)
CC (cc)
- CC (cardiac cycle)
- CC (cardiac cycle) ▸ resting phase of
- CC (chief complaint)
- CC (clinical course)
- cc (cubic centimeter)

C-C (Convexo-Concave) lens
C-C (Convexo-Concave) valve
CCA (chimpanzee coryza agent) virus

CCC (Continuing Care Centers)
ccc (continuous chest compressions)
CCPD (continuous cyclical peritoneal dialysis)
C_{cr} (creatinine clearance)
CCRC (Continuing Care Retirement Community)
CCU (Cardiac Care Unit)
CCU (Coronary Care Unit)
CD
- CD (cardiac disease)
- CD (cardiac dullness)
- CD (cardiovascular disease)

CDC (calculated date of confinement)
CDC (Center for Disease Control)
CDH ▸ fetal (congenital diaphragmatic hernia)
CDR (Clinical Data Repository)
CE (cardiac enlargement)
CE (cardiac enlargement) massive
CEA (carcinoembryonic antigen)
cease [*seize*]
cease breathing
ceased to function
cecal [*thecal*]
- c. appendage
- c. appendix
- c. area ▸ diverticulosis of
- c. fold, vascular
- c. folds
- c. hernia
- c. mesocolic lymph nodes
- c. spasms
- c. vault

cecocentral (*see* centrocecal)
cecocolic intussusception
cecum
- c. block
- c., carcinoma of
- c. delivered
- c., distal tip of
- c., emptying
- c., foremen
- c. grasped
- c., hepatic
- c. mobile
- c. mobilized
- c. of cochlear duct, cupular
- c. of cochlear duct, vestibular
- c. returned to abdomen

cecutiens, Chrysops
Cederschiöld's massage
cefazolin sodium
cefmetazole sodium
cefoxitin sodium

Cegka's sign
Ceiba pentandra
ceiling diuretic ► high
Celebes vibrio
celiac (*same as* coeliac)
- c. angiography
- c. arteriography
- c. artery
- c. artery aneurysm
- c. axis
- c. disease
- c. disease, adult
- c. disease, infantile
- c. flux
- c. ganglia
- c. lymph nodes
- c. nerves
- c. plexus block
- c. plexus block (NCPB) ► neurolytic
- c. sprue
- c. trunk angiography ► digital

celiated bronchial epithelium
celiotomy incision
celiotomy, vaginal
cell(s) ('s)
- c., aberrant
- c., abnormal
- c., abnormal cancerous
- c., abnormal proliferation of cuboidal
- c., abnormal proliferation of syncytial
- c. (RBC) ► abnormal red blood
- c. abnormality, sickle
- c. ABS, Beef
- c., absence of pus
- c. ► (RBC) accelerated destruction of red blood
- c. accumulation ► endobronchial round
- c., acidophilic
- c., acinar
- c., acoustic hair
- c. activation
- c., acute inflammatory
- c. adenocarcinoma, acinic
- c. adenocarcinoma, ciliated
- c. adenocarcinoma, Clara
- c. adenocarcinoma, clear
- c. adenocarcinoma ► duct
- c. adenocarcinoma, renal
- c. adenoma, basal
- c. adenoma, bronchoalveolar
- c. adenoma, Hürthle
- c. adenoma, islet
- c. adenoma ► liver

- c. adenoma ► null
- c. adenoma ► undifferentiated
- c., adenomatous prolactin
- c., adipose
- c., adrenocortical
- c. ► adult stem
- c., adventitial
- c., age-related loss of nerve
- c. agenesis ► pure red
- c. agglutination, chick
- c. agglutination reaction ► mixed
- c. (WBC) ► aggregation of white blood
- c., air
- c., alpha
- c., alpha 2 fat
- c., alveolar
- c., Alzheimer's
- c. ► Alzheimer's disease brain
- c., amacrine
- c., ameboid
- c. analysis, live
- c. analysis ► sinoatrial (SA)
- c. ► anaplastic infiltrating single
- c. and platelet ► produce blood
- c. ► androgen-secreting thecal
- c. anemia, crescent
- c. anemia, ► globe-
- c. anemia screening, sickle
- c. anemia, sickle
- c. anemia ► spur
- c., anterior horn
- c. (TRC) antibody titer, ► microsomal tanned red
- c. antigen ► pan T-
- c. antigen ► panhematopoietic
- c. antigen ► plasma
- c., antigen-producing cancer
- c. antigen ► progenitor
- c. antigen ► red blood
- c. antiviral factor (CAF)
- c., antral
- c. aortitis ► giant
- c. aplasia ► pure red blood
- c. arteries, giant
- c. arteritis ► giant
- c., Aschoff's
- c., assault cancer
- c. assay test, Raji
- c. astrocytoma ► giant
- c. astrocytoma ► subependymal giant
- c., atrioventricular (AV) endothelial
- c., atrophied
- c. attachment assay

- c., atypical
- c., atypical endometrial
- c., atypical mononuclear
- c., atypical pyelomorphic
- c., atypical regenerative
- c., auditory
- c. autograft ► stem
- c., autoimmunity, beta
- c., autorhythmic heart muscle
- c., B
- c., bacterial
- c., balloon
- c., band
- c., bank
- c., basal
- c., basal forebrain
- c., basket
- c., basophilic
- c., battery
- c., behavior of nerve
- c., benign
- c., berry
- c., beta
- c. biology
- c., bipolar retinal
- c., bizarre
- c. ► bizarre giant plasma
- c., bladder
- c., blast
- c., bloated
- c. block
- c. block analysis
- c., blood
- c., blood clotting
- c. body
- c. body, nerve
- c., bone
- c., bone marrow
- c., bone marrow stem
- c., bony ethmoidal
- c., border
- c. borders, indistinct
- c. -bound antibody
- c. -bound antigen
- c., bovine
- c., brain
- c., breast
- c., breast cancer
- c. bridges
- c., bristle
- c., bronchial
- c., bronchial epithelial
- c., bronchial glandular
- c., bronchic
- c. bronchogenic tumor ► small

cell—*continued*

c., buffy coated
c., burr
c., burst forming
c. button
c., cancer
c. cancer, basal
c., cancer fighting
c., cancer-forming
c. cancer of lung ▸ small
c., cancer patients' warrior white
c. cancer, prickle
c. cancer, renal
c. cancer, spindle
c. cancer ▸ squamous
c., cancer-targeting
c., cancer vulnerable
c., cancerous
c. ▸ cancerous growth blood
c. carcinoma, alveolar
c. carcinoma, basal
c. carcinoma base of tongue ▸ squamous
c. carcinoma, basosquamous
c. carcinoma ▸ bronchogenic oat
c. carcinoma ▸ bronchogenic poorly differentiated squamous
c. carcinoma ▸ bronchogenic squamous
c. carcinoma buccal mucosa, squamous
c. carcinoma ▸ cervical lymph node classification in squamous
c. carcinoma, cylindrical
c. carcinoma dorsum of hand, squamous
c. carcinoma, duct
c. carcinoma, ductal
c. carcinoma ear and nose, squamous
c. carcinoma ▸ electro-desiccation and curettage in squamous
c. carcinoma eyelid, squamous
c. carcinoma, giant
c. carcinoma gingiva, squamous
c. carcinoma, granulosa
c. carcinoma, granulosa theca
c. carcinoma, Hürthle
c. carcinoma ▸ infiltrating ductal
c. carcinoma ▸ infiltrating squamous cell
c. carcinoma ▸ in situ transitional bladder
c. carcinoma, Kulchitzky
c. carcinoma, large

c. carcinoma lip, squamous
c. carcinoma, liver
c. carcinoma, locally advanced squamous
c. carcinoma, nonoat
c. carcinoma ▸ multifocal infiltrated duct
c. carcinoma ▸ nonsmall
c. carcinoma, oat
c. carcinoma, oat seed
c. carcinoma of bladder ▸ transitional
c. carcinoma of cervix ▸ squamous
c. carcinoma of conjunctive ▸ basal
c. carcinoma of ear and nose, basal
c. carcinoma of eyelid, basal
c. carcinoma of kidney, renal
c. carcinoma of lip, basal
c. carcinoma of lung, small
c. carcinoma of lung ▸ squamous
c. carcinoma of renal pelvis ▸ transitional
c. carcinoma of vocal cord ▸ squamous
c. carcinoma ▸ perianal squamous
c. carcinoma, pigmented basal
c. carcinoma ▸ poorly differentiated large
c. carcinoma ▸ poorly differentiated squamous
c. carcinoma, prickle
c. carcinoma, renal
c. carcinoma, reserve
c. carcinoma ▸ signet-
c. carcinoma, small
c. carcinoma, spheroidal
c. carcinoma, spindle
c. carcinoma, squamous
c. carcinoma, superficial basal
c. carcinoma ▸ superficial squamous
c. carcinoma tongue, squamous
c. carcinoma, transitional
c. carcinoma ▸ underlying undifferentiated large
c. carcinoma ▸ undifferentiated large
c. carcinoma ▸ undifferentiated small
c., cardiac
c., cardiac endothelial
c., cardiovascular excitatory
c., cardiovascular inhibitory
c., cartilage
c. casts, red

c. casts, white
c., change, malignant
c., chemical messenger
c., chicken wire myocardial
c., chief
c., chronic inflammatory
c., ciliated
c., ciliated epithelial
c., Clara
c., clear
c., cleavage
c., clonogenic
c., clue
c., clump
c., cluster of tumor
c. clusters
c., cochlear
c. collector, cancer
c. color ratio
c., columnar
c., columnar acinar
c., columnar epithelial
c., commissural
c., committed stem
c., cone
c., connective tissue
c. consistent with invasive carcinoma
c. content, clonogenic
c., contractile
c. contraction, cardiac
c. contraction ▸ muscle
c., cord blood
c. cords, splenic
c., corneal
c., cornified
c., cornified superficial
c. ▸ corrected bone marrow
c. count ▸ peripheral blood
c. count, plasma
c. count (RBC) ▸ red
c. count (RBC) ▸ red blood
c. count ▸ spinal fluid
c. count (WBC) ▸ white
c. count (WBC) ▸ white blood
c., counting
c., cover
c., crescent
c. crisis, sickle
c., cuboidal
c. ▸ cuboidal to columnar acinar
c. culture
c. ▸ death of bone
c. cultures, kidney
c. ▸ cyanophilic, granular

c. cycle
c. cycle kinetics analysis
c. cycle redistribution
c. cycle redistribution and dose fractionation
c. cycle redistribution and dose hyperfractionation
c. cycle redistribution, radiosensitivity and
c. cycle time
c., cylindric
c. cytoplasm, liver
c., cytoplasm of
c., damaged brain
c., daughter
c., deactivated
c., dead
c., dead skin
c. death
c. death, heart
c. death of brain
c. ▸ death of myocardial
c. death ▸ programmed
c. debris
c., decidual
c., deep petrosal
c. defect ▸ T-
c., defective
c. ▸ defective bone marrow
c., defensive
c. deficiency ▸ red blood
c., degenerated epithelial
c., degenerating
c. degeneration
c. degeneration ▸ nerve
c., degeneration of dopamine-producing nerve
c. ▸ degeneration of muscle
c., degeneration of nerve
c., degeneration of Purkinje
c. degeneration ▸ slow
c. degranulation ▸ goblet
c., Deiters'
c. ▸ delay aging of
c., dendritic
c., depleted, white
c., desquamated
c., desquamated renal epithelial
c. ▸ desquamation of atypical alveolar
c., destroying cancer
c., destroying myeloma
c. destruction by radiation
c. destruction, drug-induced
c., destruction of brain

c., destruction of nerve
c. ▸ destruction of red blood
c. determinant, germ-
c. diameter (MCD) ▸ mean
c. differentiation
c., disease fighting T
c. disease, sickle
c. disorder, blood
c. disorder ▸ nerve
c. disorder, sickle
c., divided
c., dividing
c. division
c. division and growth ▸ uncontrolled
c. division, direct
c. division, indirect
c. division ▸ unrestrained
c., dome
c., donor
c., donor stem
c. (WBC) ▸ donor's white blood
c., dormant
c., Down's syndrome
c. drained, red
c., dust
c. dysfunction
c., eating
c., effector
c., electrochemical
c. electrophysiology ▸ pacemaker
c. elements
c., ellipsoidal
c., elongated contractile fiber
c., elongated linear
c., elongated ovoid
c., embryonal
c., embryonal connective tissue
c., embryonic
c., emigrated
c., encasing
c., endocervical
c., endometrial
c., endothelial
c. engineering ▸ stem
c. enhancing activity ▸ mast
c., enlarged Schwann
c., entrapped
c. ▸ entrapped anterior pituitary
c. envelope
c. enzyme ▸ cancer-
c., ependymal
c., epithelial
c., epithelioid
c. epithelioma, basal
c. epithelioma, calcifying

c., erythroid
c. ▸ estrogen-secreting granulosa
c., ethmoid
c., ethmoid air
c. examination
c., extension of tumor
c., fat
c. fatty granule
c., ferment
c., Ferrata's
c., fetal
c., fetal brain
c., fiber
c. fibers, twisted nerve
c., fibroblast
c., filaments in
c. -fixed antibody
c., fixed-tissue
c., flagellate
c., flame
c., flat
c., flattened epithelial
c., flattened tissue
c. float to top of container ▸ red
c., floor
c. ▸ flush away dulling, dry, dead
c., foam
c., foamy myocardial
c., focal aggregation of
c. ▸ foci of inflammatory
c. folate, red
c., follicular
c., follicular lutein
c., foot
c., foreign body (FB) giant
c., foreign cancer
c. formation, bone
c., formative
c. fragility, red
c., frontal
c., frozen
c., frozen red
c. function
c. function ▸ luteal
c. function ▸ nerve
c. function, normal
c., fusiform
c., ganglion
c., Gaucher's
c. gene ▸ sickle
c., genetically altered
c. ▸ genetically altered tumor
c., genetically engineered
c. ▸ genetically manipulated
c., germ

cell—*continued*

c., germinal
c., ghost
c., giant
c., giant ganglion
c., gitter
c., glandular
c., glial
c., glitter
c., goblet
c., Golgi's
c., grafted
c., granular
c. granulations
c. granuloma, plasma
c., grape
c. gravitate to bottom of container ▸ red
c., great alveolar
c. growth
c. growth, distorted
c. growth, division, and function
c. growth, erratic
c. growth genes
c. growth ▸ inhibit nerve
c. growth of cancer ▸ uncontrolled
c. growth ▸ prostate
c., gustatory
c., gut intestinal
c., hair
c., hair-like
c. ▸ harvested stem
c. ▸ healthy nerve
c., heart
c., heart disease
c., heart failure
c., heart lesion
c., heart muscle
c., heat-killed
c., heating cancer
c., heckle
c., Heidenhain's
c., helper T
c., hematopoietic
c., hematopoietic stem
c. -hemoglobin C disease, sickle
c. -hemoglobin D disease, sickle
c. hemolysin test, ox
c., Henle's
c., hepatic
c. hepatitis, giant
c. hepatitis, neonatal giant
c. hepatitis, plasma
c., hilar
c. ▸ histiocytes and giant

c., Hodgkin's
c., horizontal
c., horn
c., Hortega's
c., host
c. ▸ human aortic endothelial
c. ▸ human fetal
c., human immune
c., Hürthle
c., hybrid
c., hyperchromatic
c. hypermetabolism of bone
c. hyperplasia, alveolar
c. hyperplasia, juxtaglomerular
c. hypoxia, tumor
c., hypoxic
c., IgE sensitized
c., immature
c., immature blood
c. ▸ immature endothelial
c., immune
c., immune system
c. immunity
c., immunocompetent
c. implant ▸ pig
c., implanted
c. ▸ implanted cancer
c. in alveoli ▸ squamous
c. in ear, hair
c., incasing
c. inclusion
c. indicative of carcinoma in situ
c. indicative of mild dysplasia
c. indicative of moderate dysplasia
c. indicative of severe dysplasia
c. indices, red
c., indifferent
c., individual
c., infected
c., infection fighting
c. ▸ infection fighting T-
c. ▸ infection-fighting white
c. infiltrate, plasma
c. ▸ infiltration by tumor
c. infiltration, chronic inflammatory
c. infiltration, lymphocytic
c., inflammatory
c. inhibitor ▸ mast
c., initial
c., inner ear hair
c., inner hair
c. ▸ inner layer of endothelial
c., inner phalangeal
c., inner pillar
c., insulin producing beta

c. integrity
c., intercalary
c., interstitial
c. ▸ interstitial acute inflammatory
c. ▸ invasive breast tissue
c., irradiated
c. ▸ irregular changes in cervical
c., irregular disfigured
c., irregular wandering
c. ▸ irreversible damage to brain
c., islet
c. isolation
c., juvenile
c., juxtaglomerular
c., karyochrome
c., karyopyknotic
c., keratinized
c. killing
c. kinetics
c. kinetics of adenocarcinoma
c. kinetics of tumors
c., Kupffer's
c., Langerhans'
c., Langhans'
c., Langhans' giant
c. layer, basal
c. layer ▸ granular
c. layer ▸ horny
c. layer ▸ spinous
c., layers of compacted dead skin
c., lens
c. lesion, basal
c. leukemia, blast
c. leukemia, hairy
c. leukemia, lymphosarcoma
c. leukemia, mast
c. leukemia, plasma
c. leukemia, Reider
c. leukemia, reticuloendothelial
c. leukemia, stem
c. leukemia, undifferentiated
c. leukodystrophy, globoid
c., Leydig's
c. ▸ light-sensing
c. ▸ light sensitive
c. -like structures
c. lines
c. lining
c. lining, skin-like
c., liver
c., liver cancer
c., living host
c. loss factor
c. loss, hippocampal
c. loss, nerve

c., loss of substantia Nigra
c. loss ▸ red blood
c. lung cancer ▸ nonsmall
c. lung cancer, small
c., lutein
c., luteum
c., lymph
c., lymphadenoma
c. lymphoblastic leukemia, null
c., lymphocytic
c. lymphokine-activated killer (LAK)
c. lymphoma, B
c. lymphoma, cutaneous T-
c. lymphoma, erythrodermic
  cutaneous T-
c. lymphoma, lymph
c. lymphoma ▸ mantle
c. lymphoma ▸ noncleaved
c. lymphoma, stem
c. lymphoma ▸ T-
c. Lymphotropic Virus (HTLV)
  Human T
c. lymphotropic virus type ▸ simian T
c., lysis of
c., M
c., macrophage
c. malfunction ▸ brain
c., malfunctioning
c., malfunctioning insulin-receptor
c., malignant
c. ▸ malignant transformation of
c., malpighian
c., mammalian
c., marginal
c., marrow
c. ▸ marrow stromal
c. mass
c. mass, body
c. mass, fibrous
c. mass, firm
c. mass, inner
c. mass, intermediate
c. mass, movable
c. mass, ovarian
c. mass, red
c. mass, red blood
c. mass transfusion
c., mast
c. mastitis, plasma
c., mastoid
c., mastoid air
c., matrix
c. ▸ maturation of breast
c., mature
c., mature nerve

c. ▸ matured skin
c. mediastinal tumor, malignant
  germ
c. mediated antibody
c. mediated cytotoxicity
c. mediated immune reactions
c. mediated immunity
c., medullary
c., melanin-pigmented
c. melanoma, balloon
c. membrane
c. membrane activity
c. membrane antigen
c. membrane, bacterial
c. membrane, cancer
c. membrane electrical potential
c. membrane, fatty
c. membranes, memory
c. membrane, nerve
c., membrane potential of nerve
c. membranes in brain, damaged
c., memory
c., meningeal
c., mesangial
c., mesenchymal
c., mesenchymal intimal
c. ▸ mesenchymal stem
c., mesothelial
c. metabolism
c. metaplasia ▸ goblet
c., metaplastic mucus-secreting
c. misfiring ▸ brain
c., microbial
c., microfold
c., microglial
c., microscopic cancer
c. ▸ microscopic examination of
c. ▸ microscopic focus of
c. ▸ microscopic tumor
c. ▸ microvilli in mesothelial
c., migratory
c., Mikulicz's
c., milk producing
c. mitogens
c., mitral
c. mixed with plasma ▸ red
c., monocyte
c., monocytoid reticuloendothelial
c., mononuclear
c., morular
c., mossy
c., mother
c. ▸ motion-controlling nerve
c., motor
c., Mott

c., mouse
c., mouth
c., mucoserous
c., mucous
c., mulberry
c., multinucleated
c. ▸ multinucleated giant
c., multinucleated plasma
c., multipotential
c., muscle
c. mutation
c., myeloid
c., myeloma
c. myeloma, giant
c., myocardial
c. myocarditis, giant
c., myoepithelial
c., myoid
c., myosin lacking
c., nasal
c., natural killer (NK)
c., navicular
c. necrosis ▸ muscle
c., necrotic inflammatory
c., neoplastic
c., nerve
c., Neumann's
c., neuroepithelial
c., neuroglial
c., neuromuscular
c., neurosensory
c., neutrophilic
c., neval
c., nevus
c. nevus, spindle
c. nevus syndrome, basal
c., new host
c., niche
c., Niemann-Pick
c., noble
c., nodal
c., nonpacemaking
c., nonphagocytic squamous
c., nonvirus infected
c., normal
c. ▸ normal breast tissue
c., normal nerve
c., nucleated
c., nucleated contractile fiber
c., nucleated fusiform
c., nucleated red
c., nucleated red blood
c. nuclei
c. nuclei, liver
c. nuclei, muscle

cell—*continued*

c. ▸ nuclei of dividing
c. nucleus
c. nucleus, human
c. nucleus, neurilemmal
c., null
c., nurse
c., nursing
c., nutrient
c., oat
c., oat seed
c., oat-shaped
c. of cerebral cortex, nerve
c. of Corti
c. of hearing, receptor
c. of liver, stellate
c. of myocardium ▸ contractile function in
c. of retina ▸ specialized
c., olfactory
c., olfactory receptor
c., oligodendroglial
c., original host
c., osseous
c., outer hair
c., outer phalangeal
c., outer pillar
c., oval
c. ▸ ovarian cancer
c. O$_2$ (oxygen) ▸ carrying red
c., oxyphil
c., oxyphilic
c., pacemaker
c., pacemaking
c., packed
c., packed human blood
c., packed red blood
c., Paget's
c., palatine
c., pale-staining polyhedral
c., pancreas
c., pancreatic
c., pancreatic islet
c., Paneth's
c., Papanicolaou (Pap) study of
c., papilloma, squamous
c., papilloma, transitional
c., parabasal
c., parent
c., parietal
c. ▸ patch quilt degeneration of muscle
c., pathologic
c. pathology, oat
c. pathway ▸ scavenger

c., pattern of
c., pavement
c., pediculated
c., peg
c., Pelger-Huet
c., pen-r
c., pens
c., peptic
c. per high power field (WBC/hpf) ▸ white blood
c. per unit area
c., pericapillary
c., pericellular
c. ▸ peripheral stem
c. periphery
c., perithelial
c., perivascular
c. pertussis vaccine ▸ diphtheria, tetanus toxoids, and whole
c., pessary
c., phage particle infects new host
c., phage particle maturing in donor
c., phagocytic
c. phagocytosis ▸ impaired Kupffer's
c., phalangeal
c., pheochrome
c. phone radiation
c., physical disruption of
c. ▸ physiological function of
c., pi
c., Pick's
c., pigment
c. ▸ pigment-producing
c., pillar
c., plaque-forming
c., plasma
c., plasmacytoid reticulum
c., plasmid-carrying
c. plates
c., pleomorphic
c., pleomorphic rod-shaped
c., pleuripotential
c., pleuripotential stem
c., pneumatic
c. pneumonia, giant
c. pneumonia, interstitial plasma
c. pneumonia ▸ plasma
c. pneumonitis ▸ marked giant
c. poison
c., polar
c., polychromatic
c., polychromatophil
c., polygonal
c., polyhedral
c., polyhedral epithelial

c., polymorphonuclear
c., polyplastic
c., precancerous
c., precornified
c., precornified superficial
c. precursors ▸ red
c. precursors ▸ red and white
c., predominating
c., prefollicle
c., preganglionic
c., pregnancy
c. preparations, red
c., pressure sensitive
c., prickle
c., primary
c., primitive
c., primitive tumor
c., primitive wandering
c., primordial
c., primordial germ
c., principal
c. production, expanded
c. (RBC) ▸ production of red blood
c. ▸ progesterone-producing corpus luteum
c., progressive growth of
c., proliferating plasma
c. proliferation
c. proliferation ▸ actual
c. ▸ proliferation of atypical alveolar
c., prop
c. ▸ prostate cancer
c. protection, white
c. protein, myeloma-
c., protoplasm of a
c., psychic
c. ▸ pulmonary endocrine
c., pulmonary epithelial
c. ▸ pulmonary mast
c., pulpar
c., pup
c. ▸ purified fetal
c., Purkinje's
c., pus
c., pyramidal
c., RA
c. radiation
c., radiation injury of target
c., raphe
c. reaction, giant
c., reactive
c., receptive
c. receptors
c. receptors ▸ damaged hair
c., recipient

c., red
c. (RBC) ▸ red blood
c. ▸ Reed-Sternberg
c. reflex, oculosensory
c. refractibility
c. ▸ regenerate blood
c. regeneration
c. ▸ regrow damaged nerve
c., regrowth of nerve
c. ▸ reinvigorate brain
c. rejected
c., relaxation of
c. remnants ▸ myocardial
c. reparative granuloma ▸ central giant
c. reparative granuloma ▸ giant
c. reparative granuloma ▸ peripheral giant
c. replacement ▸ stem
c. replication ▸ life
c. replication potential
c. reproduction
c., reserve
c., residential
c., residual cancer
c. resistance
c., respiratory
c. respond to estrogen
c. response, polymorphonuclear
c., resting
c., resting wandering
c., reticular
c., reticuloendothelial
c., reticulum
c., retinal
c., retinal pigment
c. returned to donor ▸ red blood
c. ▸ reversible aggregation of
c., rheumatoid arthritis (RA) factor
c., Rh-positive fetal blood
c., Rieder's
c., Rindfleisch's
c., rod
c., rod-like
c., root
c. rosettes
c., rough (R)
c., round
c., S (smooth)
c., Sala
c., sarcogenic
c. sarcoma, lymphosarcoma reticulum
c. sarcoma of brain, reticulum
c. sarcoma of the knee ▸ synovial

c. sarcoma, reticulum
c., satellite
c., scavenger
c., Schwann
c. screening system, automated cervical
c., secretary
c. (RBC) ▸ sedimentation rate of red blood
c., sedimented red
c., segmented (SEG)
c. segregation, ecto/endocervical
c. ▸ selective degeneration of nerve
c., seminal
c. sensitivity to radiation
c. sensitizer
c., sensory
c., sensory epithelial
c., sensory hair
c., sensory nerve
c., sentinel
c., septal
c., serosal
c., serous
c., Sertoli's
c., sexual
c., Sézary
c., shadow
c., sick
c., sickle
c., signet ring
c., silver
c., skein
c., skeletogenous
c., skin
c. skin cancer, basal
c. skin cancer ▸ squamous
c. skin carcinoma, squamous
c., sloughing of
c., slow renewal and nonrenewal systems of
c., Smee
c., smooth muscle
c., smudge
c., solitary pyramidal
c., somatic
c. sorter
c., sound-sensing
c. soupy cytoplasm
c. ▸ sparse infiltration of extramedullary hematopoietic
c., sperm
c., spermatogenic
c., sphenoid
c., spherical

c., spiculed mature red blood
c., spider
c., spindle
c., spindle-shaped
c., spur
c., squamous
c., squamous alveolar
c., squamous epithelial
c. ▸ squamous-like polygonal
c., stab
c., staff
c., star
c., stellate
c., stem
c. stimulating hormone ▸ interstitial
c., stipple
c., storage
c. strain
c. ▸ stray cancer
c. stroma, spindle
c., stromal
c. structure
c. structure, basic leukemia
c., structure of nerve
c. study
c., superficial
c., supporting
c. ▸ suppress estrogen receptors in cancer
c., suppressor
c. surface
c. surface antigen
c. ▸ surface of epithelial
c. survival, red blood
c. suspended in saline solution
c., suspicious
c., sustentacular
c., sympathetic
c., syncytial
c. system
c. system, rapid renewal
c., T
c., tactile
c., tadpole
c. tagged with radioactive material, red
c. taken off top of solution ▸ white
c. (TRC), tanned red
c., target
c., targeted
c., tart
c., taste
c., tegmental
c., tendon
c. test, LE (lupus erythematous)

cell—*continued*

c. test, sickle
c., T-4
c. thalassemia disease, sickle
c., theca
c., theca-lutein
c. therapy
c. therapy, cord blood
c. therapy, dendritic
c. therapy ▸ red
c., Thoma-Zeiss counting
c. thymoma, spindle
c., thymus dependent
c. thyroiditis, giant
c., tissue
c., tissue culture
c. ▸ TNF (tumor necrosis factor) gene-related
c. -to-slide transfer
c., totipotential
c., touch
c., Touton giant
c. trait, sickle
c., transferred
c. ▸ transferring immature muscle
c. ▸ transformed cancer
c. transformers
c. transfused back into donor ▸ red
c. (RBC), transfusion of red blood
c. transfusion, packed
c. transfusion ▸ perioperative red
c. (RBC) transfusions ▸ packed red blood
c. transfusions, white blood
c., transitional
c., transitional epithelial
c. transplant
c. transplant, autologous stem
c. transplant, blood
c. transplant, brain
c. transplant ▸ fetal nerve
c. transplant ▸ fetal pig
c. transplant ▸ fetus-to-fetus stem
c. transplant, islet
c. transplant ▸ limbal stem
c. transplant ▸ nerve
c. transplant procedure ▸ islet
c. transplant technique ▸ pancreatic
c. transplant ▸ Schwann
c. transplantation
c. transplantation, islet
c. transplantation, stem
c., transplanted
c. ▸ transplanted cord blood
c., transplanted fetal

c., trophoblast
c., trophoblastic
c., tubal air
c. tumor
c. tumor alveolar
c. ▸ tumor blood vessel
c. tumor, chromaffin
c. tumor, clear
c. ▸ tumor-derived
c. tumor, embryonal
c. tumor, familial bilateral giant
c. tumor, germ
c. tumor, giant
c. tumor, granular
c. tumor, granulosa
c. tumor, Hürthle
c. tumor, interstitial
c. tumor, islet
c. tumor, mast
c. tumor ▸ microscopic granular
c. tumor, oat
c. tumor, plasma
c. tumor, Sertoli
c. tumor, Sertoli-Leydig
c. tumor, squamous
c. tumor, stromal
c. tumor, sustentacular
c. tumor, theca
c. tumor ▸ well-differentiated squamous
c., tunnel
c., tympanic
c. type
c. type ▸ bronchogenic carcinoma, unknown
c., type I
c., type II
c., typical
c., umbrella
c. unattached to chromosome ▸ bacterial
c., undifferentiated
c., undifferentiated body
c. undifferentiated carcinoma ▸ large
c. undifferentiated carcinoma ▸ metastatic large
c. undifferentiated carcinoma ▸ small
c., undifferentiated mesenchymal
c., unit
c., unit of packed
c. uptake test, triiodothyronine red
c., vacuolated
c., vacuolated basophil

c., vacuolated plasma
c. vacuole, host
c. ▸ vaporizing corneal
c. variety ▸ bronchogenic carcinoma, small
c. variety, oat
c., variety of small
c., vascular
c. ▸ vascular smooth muscle
c., vasofactive
c., vasoformative
c., ventral horn
c. viability assessment
c., Vignal's
c., Virchow
c. ▸ virus infected tumor
c., visual
c. volume
c. volume, packed
c. volume profile
c. volume, red
c. volume, red blood
c. vulvitis, plasma
c. wall active drug
c. wall, bacterial
c. wall of organism
c. wall, outer
c. wall synthesis
c., Walthard's
c., wandering
c., warrior
c., Warthin's
c., washed red
c., water-clear
c., white
c. (WBC) ▸ white blood
c., whorled
c. ▸ whorls of spindle-shaped
c., wing
c. within brain
c. yield, ectocervical
c. yield, endocervical
c. zone ▸ transitional
c., zymogen
celled
c. organism, single-
c. organisms, one-
c. protein, single-
c. parasites
Cellfalcicula
C. fusca
C. mucosa
C. viridis
cellophane rale

cellular
- c. abnormality
- c. activity
- c. aging
- c. blue nevus
- c. breast cancer therapy
- c. cancer
- c. changes, abnormal
- c. content
- c. cytoplasm
- c. death
- c. debris
- c. debris, carbonizing
- c. degeneration
- c. differentiation
- c. effects of alcohol
- c. element
- c. embolism
- c. embolus
- c. energy production ▸ depress
- c. function
- c. granulation
- c. granules
- c. growth
- c. immune response
- c. immune system
- c. immunity
- c. immunity deficiency syndrome
- c. immunologic reactivity
- c. kinetics
- c. lesion
- c. level
- c. life
- c. lining
- c. material
- c. material, necrotic
- c. mediated immune response
- c. membranes
- c. memory
- c. metabolism
- c. morphology
- c. neuroscience
- c. pattern
- c. physiology
- c. population
- c. proliferation
- c. reaction
- c. regeneration
- c. regeneration and apoptosis
- c. respiration
- c. response
- c. senescence
- c. systems, expanding
- c. systems, nonrenewal
- c. Teflon

- c. transducer linkages

cellularity, increased
cellularity of glomeruli
cellule formation
cellulite treatment
cellulitic phlegmasia
cellulitis
- c., indurated
- c. of foot
- c. of heel
- c. of toe
- c., orbital
- c., pelvic
- c., periorbital
- c., peritonsillar
- c., preorbital
- c., staphylococcal

celluloid implant
celluloid implant material
cellulosae, Cysticercus
cellulose
- c. breakdown bacteria
- c. digestion
- c. gauze
- c. oxidized
- c. splitting

Cellvibrio
- C. flavescens
- C. fulvus
- C. ochraceus
- C. vulgaris

CELO (chicken-embryo-lethal orphan)
celomic hernia
celozoic parasite
Celsius scale
Celsus' operation
cement
- c., acrylic
- c., bone
- c. burn
- c. eater, Anspach
- C. Eater drill
- c., inject sterile liquid
- c., injecting bone
- c., methyl methacrylate
- c. substance
- c., Surgical Simplex P radiopaque bone
- c., Zimmer low viscosity

cemented gingival
cemented joint
cementing substance
cementum fracture
cementum hyperplasia
censor, Freudian

censor, psychic
census, average daily
census, daily
cent, volume per◊
Centella asiatica
center(s) (Center)
- c., accelerating
- c., acoustic
- c. (ECC) ▸ admission to emergency care
- c., adult day care
- c., anospinal
- c., apneustic
- c., association
- c., auditopsychic
- c., auditory
- c., auditory speech
- c., auditory word
- c., birth
- c., brain
- c., brain's hearing
- c., brain's pleasure
- c., brain's regulatory
- c., Broca's
- c., Budge's
- c., burn
- c., cardiac
- c., cardioaccelerating
- c., cardioinhibitory
- c., cardiometer
- c., cheirokinesthetic
- c., ciliospinal
- c., community mental health
- C. (CCC), Continuing Care
- c., coordination
- c., correlation
- c., cortical
- C. cough ▸ World Trade
- c., coughing
- c., dark
- c., day care
- c., defecation
- c., deglutition
- c., dentary
- c., depression of vital brain
- c., detoxification
- c. dialysis, in-
- C., Digestive Disease
- c., dominating
- c., drop-in
- C., Drug Rehabilitation
- C., Drug Treatment
- c., ejaculation
- c., emergency care
- c., epiotic

center—*continued*
- c., epiphyseal
- c., erection
- c., eupraxic
- c., facial
- c., Flemming
- c., flotation
- c., follicular germinal
- c. for alcoholics ▸ rehabilitation
- C. for Disease Control (CDC)
- C. for Disease Control ▸ U.S.
- c. for drug addicts ▸ rehabilitation
- c. for physically disabled ▸ rehabilitation
- c. for physically handicapped ▸ rehabilitation
- c., ganglionic
- c., genetic research
- c., genital
- c., genitospinal
- c., germinal
- c., glossokinesthetic
- c., greater oval
- c., gustatory
- c., health
- c., heat-regulating
- c. ▸ hyalinized burned out germinal
- c. ▸ hypothalamic feeding
- c. in brain ▸ language
- c. in brain ▸ micturition reflex
- c. in brain, pleasure
- c. in brain, speech
- c., inhibitory
- c., kinetic
- c., Kronecker's
- c., Kupressoff's
- c., lesion of cortical
- c., limbic
- c. line artifact
- c., Lumsden's
- c., mammography
- c. ▸ medical and diet
- c., medullary respiratory
- c., metacarpal epiphyseal
- c., micturition
- c., motor
- c., motor speech
- c., neonatal
- c., nerve
- c. of brain, activate pleasure
- c. of brain ▸ motor control
- c. of brain, visual
- c. of cerebellum ▸ medullary
- c. of cornea, conical protrusion of
- c. of field of vision

- c., optic
- c., organ transplant
- c., osmoregulatory
- c., ossification
- c., oval lesions with small white
- C., Pain Treatment
- c., panting
- c. ▸ paralysis of medullary cardiorespiratory
- c., parenchymatous
- c., patient discharged to convalescent treatment
- c., pediatric trauma
- c., phalangeal epiphyseal
- c., phrenic
- c., plasmapheresis
- c., pneumotaxic
- c., polypneic
- C., Pritikin Longevity
- c., pteriotic
- c. ratios, off-
- c., reaction
- c., rectovesical
- c., referral transplant
- c., reflex
- c., regional burn
- c., regional trauma
- c., respiratory
- c., respiratory nerve
- C., Retinal Vascular
- c., rotation
- C. ▸ Same Day Care
- c., Sechenoff's
- c., semioval
- c., senior assistance
- c., sensory
- c., Setchenow's
- c., sex-behavior
- c., sexual assault treatment
- c., sleep disorder
- c., somatic
- c., speech
- c., sphenotic
- c. ▸ spinal micturition reflex
- c., splenial
- c., sudorific
- c., swallowing
- c., sweat
- c., taste
- c. technology, sleep
- c., tendinous
- c., tertiary care
- c., thermoregulatory
- c., transplant
- c., transplantation

- c., trauma
- C. ▸ Urgent Care
- c., vasoconstrictor
- c., vasodilator
- c., vasomotor
- c., vesical
- c., vesicospinal
- C. ▸ Veterans Affairs Medical
- c. ▸ visual control
- c., visual word
- c., vital
- c., vital brain
- c., vomiting
- c., Wernicke's

centered
- c. argon laser, balloon-
- c. care ▸ patient-
- c., excessively self-
- c. interaction, child-
- c., self-
- c. skills, culture
- c. therapy, client-

centeredness and suspicion ▸ self-
centeredness ▸ destructive self-
centigrade scale
centigrade thermometer
centimeter(s) (cm)
- c. (cc) ▸ cubic
- c. (g-cm) ▸ gram-
- c. (cm) level
- c. (ng/cc), nanograms per cubic
- c. per second (cmps)

central (Central)
- c. acinar emphysema
- c. amaurosis
- c. angiospastic retinitis
- c. aperture
- c. aphasia
- c. apnea
- c. approach
- c. ataxia
- c. audiovestibular dysfunction
- c. audiovestibular lesion
- c. axis
- c. axis depth dose of electron beam therapy
- c. axis of beam
- c. blood
- c. blood volume
- c. bradycardia
- c. calyces
- c. canal
- c. canal of spinal cord
- c. cataract
- c. chorioretinitis

c. convulsion
c. cord syndrome
c. core disease
c. core wire
c. cortex
c. cortical area ▸ left
c. cortical area ▸ right
c. cyanosis
c. deafness
c. disk-shaped retinopathy
c. dopaminergic and serotinergic nerve terminal
c. dopaminergic function
c. emetic
c. epilepsy
c. excitatory state
c. fibrous body
c. field of vision
c. fields
c. fovea
c. giant cell reparative granuloma
c. gray masses
c. ▸ gray substance of cerebrum
c. gyrus, anterior
c. gyrus, posterior
c. hyoid bone
c. hypoventilation syndrome, congenital
c. illumination
c. implantation
c. incisor
c. inhibitory state
c. ▸ intermediate substance of spinal cord,
c. lesion
c. lobular congestion
c. lobular necrosis
c. lobule of cerebellum
c. motor program
c. necrosis
c. necrosis ▸ liver congested with
c. nervous system (CNS) activity
c. nervous system ▸ breathing difficulty with problem from
c. nervous system ▸ constipation with problem of
c. nervous system (CNS), damage to
c. nervous system (CNS) defect
c. nervous system (CNS) depressant
c. nervous system (CNS) depression
c. nervous system (CNS) deterioration, organic

c. nervous system (CNS) disease
c. nervous system (CNS) disorder
c. nervous system (CNS) dysfunction
c. nervous system from AIDS ▸ problem with
c. nervous system from alcoholism ▸ problem with
c. nervous system from diet pill ▸ problem with
c. nervous system from sleep apnea ▸ problem with
c. nervous system from vomiting ▸ problem with
c. nervous system (CNS) functioning
c. nervous system (CNS) hypersomnolence ▸ idiopathic
c. nervous system (CNS) infarction
c. nervous system (CNS) infection ▸ nosocomial
c. nervous system (CNS), infratentorial parts of
c. nervous system (CNS), intracranial part of
c. nervous system (CNS) lesion ▸ macroscopic
c. nervous system (CNS) lesion ▸ microscopic
c. nervous system (CNS) lymphoma, primary
c. nervous system (CNS) sequelae
c. nervous system (CNS) shunt
c. nervous system (CNS) stimulant
c. nervous system ▸ strep throat and problem with
c. nervous system, supratentorial parts of
c. nervous system (CNS) therapy
c. nervous system (CNS) tolerance to radiation therapy
c. nervous system (CNS) trauma
c. neurogenic breathing pattern
c. neuron
c. nystagmus
c. obesity
c. occlusion
c. or paracentral scotoma
c. origin, pain of
c. pain
c. pain ▸ neuropathic
c. paraphasia
c. pneumonia
c. pontine myelinoclasis
c. processing unit (CPU)

c. pulmonary vasculatures
c. ray
c. recurrence
c. region
c. respiration
c. respiratory depression
c. retina
c. retinal artery
c. retinal artery occlusion
c. retinal vein
c. retinal vein obstruction
c. scotoma
c. serous chorioretinopathy
c. serous retinitis
c. serous retinopathy
C. Service Director
c. sharp wave transient
c. sleep apnea
c. slow wave focus
c. spike focus
c. splanchnic venous thrombosis
c. stimulant
c. structure
c. sulcus
c. summation
C. Supply
c. surface skin area
c. suture incised
c. terminal electrode
c. terminal ▸ Wilson
c. vascular prominence
c. vein
c. vein of hepatic lobules
c. vein of liver
c. vein of suprarenal gland
c. venous
c. venous catheter (CVC)
c. venous catheter (CVC) infection
c. venous lines
c. venous pressure (CVP)
c. venous pressure ▸ increased
c. venous pressure (CVP) monitoring
c. vertigo
c. vision
c. vision loss
c. vision of retina
c. visual acuity
c. voluntary control
centrale, Anaplasma
centrale, Anaplasmosis
centralis
   c., amaurosis
   c. anterior, gyrus
   c. cerebri, sulcus

centralis—*continued*
- c., fovea
- c., pars
- c., placenta previa
- c. posterior, gyrus
- c. retinae, fovea
- c. retinae, vena

centrencephalic epilepsy
centrencephalic seizures
centri-acinar emphysema ▸ mild
centric occlusion
centric relation
centrifugal
- c. flotation, direct
- c. force, relative
- c. nerve

centrifuge, blood spun in
centrifuge microscope
centrifuged sediment
centrilobar pancreatitis
centrilobar emphysema
centrilobular
- c. bile stasis ▸ massive
- c. congestion
- c. emphysema, bilateral
- c. necrosis
- c. necrosis, massive
- c. necrosis of liver

centriole, anterior
centriole, posterior
centripetal
- c. extrusion
- c. nerve
- c. venous pulse

centrocecal (*same as* cecocentral)
centrocecal scotoma
Centrocestus cuspidatus
Centrocestus cuspidatus variety canina
centrolobar sclerosis, familial
centronuclear myopathy
centroparietal regions of scalp
century syndrome, 20th
Cenurus cerebralis
CEP (congenital erythropoietic porphyria)
Cepacia, Burkholderia
cepacia, Pseudomonas
CEPH FLOC (cephalin flocculation)
Cephaelis acuminata
Cephaelis ipecacuanha
Cephalad aspect
Cephalad catheter
cephalalgia/cephalgia
- c., histamine
- c., pharyngotympanic

- c., quadrantal

cephalhematoma deformans
cephalic
- c. artery
- c. attitude
- c. ganglion
- c. index
- c. presentation
- c. vein
- c. vein, antebrachial
- c. version

cephalin
- c. -cholesterol flocculation test
- c. flocculation (CEPH FLOC)
- c. flocculation test

cephalic flexure
cephalic vein, median
cephalocaudad diameter
cephalohematocele, Stromeyer's
cephalometric radiograph
cephalometric roentgenogram
cephalometry
- c., sequential
- c., serial
- c., ultrasonic

cephalopagus twins
cephalopelvic disproportion (CPD)
cephalosporin toxicity
Cephalosporium falciforme
Cephalosporium granulomatis
cephalothin sodium
ceptor
- c., chemical
- c., contact
- c., distance
- c., noci◊

ceramic(s)
- c., dental
- c. microdetector
- c. or plastic braces
- c. total hip

ceratocricoid muscle
ceratopharyngeal muscle
Ceratophyllus
- C. acutus
- C. fasciatus
- C. gallinae
- C. idahoensis
- C. montanus
- C. punjabensis
- C. silantiewi
- C. tesquorum

cerclage
- c., cervical
- c. procedure

- c., Shirodkar
- c., Thiersch

Cercomonas hominis
Cercomonas longicauda
Cercosphaera addisoni
Cercospora apii
Cercosporalla vexans
cerea, flexibilitas
cerebellar
- c. abscess
- c. apoplexy
- c. artery
- c. artery (PICA) aneurysm, posterior inferior
- c. artery (PICA), posterior inferior
- c. astrocytoma
- c. astrocytoma ▸ macrocystic pilocystic
- c. astrocytoma ▸ microcystic pilocytic
- c. ataxia
- c. ataxia, acute
- c. ataxia, hereditary
- c. ataxia, severe
- c. ataxia, unilateral
- c. atrophy
- c. cortex
- c. deficit
- c. degeneration
- c. disturbance
- c. dysfunction
- c. dysfunction ▸ ocular and
- c. fossa
- c. function
- c. gait
- c. gliosis
- c. hemangioblastoma
- c. hemisphere
- c. impairment
- c. incoordination
- c. infarct
- c. malformation
- c. notch
- c. notch, anterior
- c. notch, posterior
- c. pathway
- c. peduncle, inferior
- c. peduncle, middle
- c. peduncle, superior
- c. pontine angle
- c. rigidity
- c. sclerosis
- c. stalk
- c. syndrome
- c. tonsil

c. vein, inferior
c. vein, superior
c. vermis
cerebellaris, oliva
cerebelli
    c., ala
    c., cauda
    c., corpus
    c., cortex
    c., crura
    c., falx
    c., lingula
    c., monticulus
    c., pons
    c., tentorium
    c., vallecula
    c., vermis
cerebellolabyrinthine artery
cerebellomedullary cistern
cerebellopontine angle
cerebellopontine angle tumor
cerebellum
    c. ▸ arborescent white substance of
    c. and pons
    c., central lobule of
    c., contralateral side of
    c. ▸ histologic sections of
    c. ▸ medulla, pons and
    c., quadrangular lobule of
    c., tentorium of
    c., tonsil of
    c., worm of
cerebral
    c. abscess
    c. activities
    c. activity, continuous
    c. activity of brain
    c. adiposity
    c. agraphia
    c. air embolism
    c. allergen
    c. amaurosis
    c. amyloid angiopathy
    c. anemia
    c. aneurysm
    c. aneurysm, congenital
    c. aneurysm, ruptured
    c. angiogram
    c. angiography
    c. anoxia
    c. anoxia, severe
    c. anthrax
    c. apnea ▸ prolonged
    c. apophysis
    c. apoplexy

c. aqueduct
c. aqueduct, gliosis of
c. arteriogram
c. arteriography
c. arteriography, carotid
c. arteriosclerosis
c. artery
c. artery, accessory middle
c. artery, anterior
c. artery, azygos anterior
c. artery, basal
c. artery, choroidal branches of posterior
c. artery ▸ collapsed
c. artery (MCA), clipping middle
c. artery ▸ left posterior
c. artery ▸ posterior
c. artery ▸ right posterior
c. artery thrombosis
c. artery thrombosis ▸ acute middle
c. astrocytoma
c. ataxia
c. atrophy
c. atrophy of brain
c. beriberi
c. bleeding
c. blood flow
c. blood flow ▸ reduced
c. blood flow study
c. blood volume ▸ regional
c. bradyrhythmia ▸ anterior
c. calcification
c. circulation
c. compression
c. concussion
c. contusion
c. convulsion
c. cortex
c. cortex ▸ electrodes applied over
c. cortex ▸ electrodes implanted in
c. cortex ▸ electrodes inserted in
c. cortex ▸ frontal lobes of
c. cortex loss
c. cortex, nerve cells of
c. cortex, nonfunctioning
c. cortex perfusion rate
c. cortex reflex
c. cortical atrophy
c. deafness
c. death
c. decompression
c. discharges, hypersynchronous
c. disease
c. disorder
c. disorder, alcohol-related

c. dysfunction, diffuse
c. dysplasia
c. dysrhythmia
c. dysrhythmia (PCD) ▸ paroxysmal
c. dystaxia
c. edema
c. embolism
c. embolism ▸ paradoxical
c. embolus
c. epidural space ▸ drainage (dr'ge) of
c. event
c. excitement
c. fissure, lateral
c. fissure, longitudinal
c. flexure
c. fossa
c. fossa, lateral
c. function
c. function monitor (CFM)
c. function ▸ progressive loss of
c. fungus
c. gigantism
c. glucose oxygen quotient
c. halves
c. hemianesthesia
c. hemihypoplasia
c. hemiplegia
c. hemisphere
c. hemisphere, left
c. hemisphere, medial surface of
c. hemisphere, right
c. hemispheres, two
c. hemorrhage
c. hemorrhage ▸ brain damage from
c. hemorrhage ▸ stroke due to
c. hypoperfusion
c. hypoxia
c. infarct
c. infarct ▸ extension of
c. infarction
c. infarction ▸ ischemic
c. infection
c. irritation
c. ischemia
c. ischemia, transient
c. ischemic episode ▸ transient
c. lateralization
c. lesion
c. leukodystrophy, hereditary
c. malaria
c. matrix, vacuolization of
c. meningitis
c. metabolic function

cerebral—*continued*
- c. metabolic rate
- c. metabolic rate of glucose
- c. metabolic rate of oxygen
- c. metastases
- c. neoplasias
- c. neoplasm ▸ primary
- c. nerve ganglionectomy
- c. nerves
- c. neurons
- c. origin
- c. palsied child ▸ deaf
- c. palsy (CP)
- c. palsy (CP) ▸ hemiplegic form of
- c. palsy (CP) ▸ paraplegic form of
- c. paraplegia
- c. paresis
- c. paroxysmal activity
- c. peduncle
- c. peduncle, middle
- c. perfusion
- c. perfusion pressure
- c. phenomena, paroxysmal
- c. pneumography
- c. pneumonia
- c. poliomyelitis
- c. protective therapy
- c. respiration
- c. sclerosis, familial
- c. seizure
- c. seizure, focal
- c. shock
- c. sinus, inflammation of
- c. sinusography
- c. spasm
- c. stimulant
- c. structures, deep
- c. swelling
- c. tabes
- c. thrombosis
- c. tissue perfusion, altered
- c. trauma
- c. tuberculosis
- c. tumor, deep
- c. vasculature
- c. vasculitis
- c. vasculopathy
- c. vasoconstriction
- c. vein, anterior
- c. vein, deep middle
- c. vein, great
- c. vein, inferior
- c. vein, internal
- c. vein, superficial middle
- c. vein, superior

- c. vein thrombosis
- c. veins
- c. ventricles
- c. ventriculography
- c. vessels
- c. vessels ▸ medical calcification or
- c. vomiting
- c. yokes of bone of cranium

cerebrale, tache

cerebralis
- c., adiposis
- c., Cenurus
- c., Coenurus
- c., heterotopia
- c. infantilis ▸ dystaxic

cerebration, unconscious

cerebri
- c., acervulus
- c., apophysis
- c., aqueductus
- c., commotio
- c., crura
- c., epiphysis
- c., falx
- c., fornix
- c., fungus
- c., gyri
- c., gyri profundi
- c., gyri transitivi
- c., hernia
- c., hypophysis
- c. lateralis, fossa
- c., pseudomotor
- c., pseudotumor
- c., sulcus centralis
- c., trabecula
- c., velamenta

cerebriform
- c. cancer
- c. carcinoma
- c. tongue

cerebriforme, Trichophyton

cerebritis, saturnine

cerebrobasilar ischemia

cerebromacular degeneration

cerebromedullary tube

cerebro-ocular

cerebrospinal
- c. arteriosclerosis
- c. axis
- c. endarteritis
- c. fasciculus, anterior
- c. fever
- c. fluid (CSF)
- c. fluid (CSF), absorption of

- c. fluid (CSF) barrier, blood
- c. fluid (CSF) ▸ blocking of passage of
- c. fluid (CSF), blood in
- c. fluid (CSF) brain barrier
- c. fluid (CSF) cytology
- c. fluid (CSF) glucose
- c. fluid (CSF) pressure
- c. fluid pressure (CSFP)
- c. fluid (CSF), replacement of
- c. ganglia
- c. meningitis
- c. meningitis, epidemic
- c. otorrhea
- c. pressure (CSP)
- c. rhinorrhea
- c. sclerosis
- c. syphilis
- c. syphilitic
- c. thromboangiitis obliterans

cerebrotendinous xanthomatosis

cerebrovascular
- c. accident (CVA)
- c. accident (CVA), acute
- c. accident (CVA), lacunar
- c. blood circulation
- c. disease (CVD)
- c. event
- c. insufficiency
- c. lesion
- c. obstructive disease (CVOD)
- c. occlusion, severe
- c. resistance
- c. stroke
- c. syncope
- c. thrombosis

cerebrum
- c., anterior commissure of
- c., central ▸ gray substance of
- c., cistern of lateral fossa of
- c., convolutions of
- c. development
- c. disorder
- c., dural covering of
- c., first ventricle of
- c., fourth ventricle of
- c., gyri of
- c., heterotopia
- c., lateral ventricle of
- c., lobes of
- c., longitudinal fissure of
- c., middle commissure of
- c., posterior portion of
- c., second ventricle of
- c., third ventricle of

c., ventricle of
Cerenkov radiation production
cereus, Bacillus
cereus food poisoning ▸ Bacillus
cerevisiae
    c. antibody (ACA) ▸ anti-
       Saccharomyces
    c., Pediococcus
    c., Saccharomyces
Cerithidia cingulata
certain drugs ▸ slowly metabolize
certain foods, intolerance to
certificate(s)
    c., clinical authorization
    c., death
    c., hospital birth
certification, board
certified
    c. addictionologist
    c., commission
    c. for Medicare
    c. hospitals
    c. milk
    c., skilled nursing facility
    c. sleep-disorder facilities
cerulea dolens, phlegmasia
cerulean cataract
ceruleus, locus
cerumen [*serum*]
    c., excessive
    c., impacted
    c., inspissated
ceruminal impaction
ceruminous deafness
ceruminous gland tumor
cervi, Fasciola
cervi, Paramphistomum
cervical
    c. abortion
    c. adenitis
    c. adenocarcinoma
    c. adenopathy
    c. and endocervical) Pap
       (Papanicolaou) smears ▸ Richart
       and VCE (vaginal,
    c. anginal syndrome
    c. aortic arch
    c. aortic knuckle
    c. artery
    c. arthritis
    c. atypism
    c. biopsy
    c. brace
    c. brace, four-poster
    c. brace, King

c. bruits, cranial
c. canal
c. cancer
c. cancer ▸ death from
c. cancer detection
c. cancer ▸ high risk of developing
c. cancer, invasive
c. cancer, microinvasive
c. cancer ▸ noninvasive
c. cancer screening
c. cap
c. carcinoma
c. carcinoma, invasive
c. carcinoma, uterine
c. cardiac nerve ▸ inferior
c. cardiac nerve ▸ middle
c. cardiac nerve ▸ superior
c. carotid artery
c. cauterization
c. cell screening system,
    automated
c. cells
c. cells ▸ irregular changes in
c. cerclage
c. cesarean (C-) section
c. cesarean (C-) section ▸ low
c. chain
c. chain, superior
c. collar
c. collar ▸ soft
c. colliculus of female urethra
c. cone biopsy
c. conization
c. cord injury
c. cord lesion
c. culture
c. curettage
c. curvature
c. curvature, normal
c. curve, reversal of
c. cytology
c. disc ▸ Bryan
c. disc compression
c. disc decompression
c. disc disease
c. disc, hemilaminectomy for
c. disc problem
c. disc, ruptured
c. disc syndrome
c. discharge
c. dissection
c. dysplasia
c. dystocia
c. dystonia
c. ectopia

c. emphysema
c. end, fundal to
c., endocervical) Pap
    (Papanicolaou) smears ▸ Richart
    and VCE (vaginal,
c., endocervical) Pap
    (Papanicolaou) smears ▸ VCE
    (vaginal,
c., endocervical) smear ▸VCE
    (vaginal,
c. epithelium, regeneration of
c. erosion
c. esophagostomy
c. esophagus
c. esophagus, caustic strictures of
c. fascia
c. flexure
c. fusion
c. ganglion, inferior
c. ganglion, middle
c. ganglion of uterus
c. ganglion, superior
c. growths, precancerous
c. heart
c. incision
c. incompetence
c. infection
c. insertion of radium
c. intraepithelial neoplasia (CIN)
c. involvement, microscopic
c. lymph node
c. lymph node classification in
    squamous cell carcinoma
c. lymph nodes ▸ deep
c. lymph nodes ▸ superficial
c. lymphadenectomy
c. lymphatic metastasis
c. mass
c. mediastinotomy
c. mobilization
c. mucous test
c. mucus
c. muscle spasm
c. musculature
c. neoplasia, laser treatment of
c. neoplasm
c. nerve block
c. nerve, descending
c. nerve, transverse
c. nerves
c. neural canal
c. node
c. os
c. os, incompetent
c. os, internal

cervical—*continued*
- c. os ▸ tissue extruding at
- c. osteoarthritis
- c. Pantopaque column
- c. Pap (Papanicolaou) smear
- c. pleura
- c. plexus
- c. plexus nerve block
- c. polyp
- c. polyposis
- c. pregnancy
- c. punch biopsies, directed
- c. radiculitis
- c. radiculopathy
- c. region
- c. region, lower
- c. region, upper
- c. rib
- c. rib formation
- c. rib syndrome
- c. ribs, supernumerary
- c. sclerosis
- c. smear
- c. spinal cord ▸ proximal
- c. spinal lesion
- c. spinal stenosis
- c. spine
- c. spine deformity
- c. spine, Dens view of
- c. spine disease, headache secondary to
- c. spine ▸ dysfunction of
- c. spine injury
- c. spondylolysis
- c. spondylosis
- c. sprain
- c. stenosis
- c. stromal tissue
- c. stump
- c. stump, carcinoma uterine
- c. stump removed
- c. surface of tooth
- c. surgery
- c. suture
- c. swab
- c. sympathectomy
- c. sympathetic nerve
- c. synechiae
- c. tabes
- c. thoracic esophagus
- c. trachea
- c. traction
- c. traction, intermittent
- c. traction, Kuhlmann
- c. trauma

- c. vaginitis
- c. vein, deep
- c. vein, transverse
- c. venous distention
- c. venous hum
- c. vent-dependent quadriplegic
- c. vertebra, damaged
- c. vertebrae (C1-C7)
- c. vertebrae bone
- c. vertigo
- c. x-ray

cervicalis
- c., ansa
- c., linea alba
- c., Onchocerca
- c., Chlamydiae
- c., nongonococcal

cervicis muscle, iliocostalis
cervicitis
- c., chronic
- c., chronic cystic
- c., granulomatous
- c., traumatic

cervicobrachial neuralgia
cervicobregmatic diameter
cervicocolpitis emphysematosa
cervicodorsal crease, antecubital
cervicofacial face lift
cervicoprecordial angina
cervicoprecordial maneuver
cervicothoracic
- c. sympathectomy
- c. vascular abnormality

cervicouterine ganglion
cervigram test
cervix
- c., amputation of
- c., atrophic
- c., blue
- c., bulbous
- c., cancer of
- c., carcinoma of
- c., clean
- c., clefts of
- c., closed
- c. completely dilated
- c., conglutination of
- c., conization of
- c. cyanotic
- c. defacing
- c., dilatation of
- c., dilated
- c., effaced
- c., effacement of
- c., epithelium of

- c., eroded
- c., excisional conization
- c., extirpation of uterus and
- c., fish-mouthed
- c., friable
- c., fully dilated
- c., gram stain of
- c., granular
- c., grasped
- c. grasped with single tooth tenaculum
- c., incompetent
- c., infection of the
- c., irregular
- c., lacerated
- c., lesion of
- c., lip of
- c. long
- c. long, ▸ thick and closed
- c., neck of
- c., parous
- c. partially dilated
- c., polyps of
- c. ripe
- c. ▸ screening cancer of the
- c., squamous cell carcinoma of
- c. stripped
- c. ▸ superficial layer of
- c. ▸ surface layer of
- c., thinning of
- c. unripe
- c. uteri
- c. uteri, discission of
- c. uteri ▸ partial excision mucous membrane of
- c. uteri rigidity
- c., uterine
- c., vaginal

cesarean (*same as* caesarean)
- c. birth
- c. delivery
- c. hysterectomy
- c. section (CS or C-section)
- c. section (CS), cervical
- c. section (CS), classic
- c. section (CS), corporeal
- c. section (CS), delivery
- c. section (CS), emergency
- c. section (CS), extraperitoneal
- c. section (CS), Kerr's
- c. section (CS), Kronig's
- c. section (CS), Latzko's
- c. section (CS), low
- c. section (CS), low cervical
- c. section (CS), lower segment

c. section (CS) ▸ maternal death after

c. section (CS) ▸ paravesical extraperitoneal

c. section (CS) ▸ patient delivered by

c. section (CS), Porro's

c. section (CS), primary

c. section (CS), repeat

c. section (CS) scar, dehiscence of

c. section (CS) scar ▸ rupture of

c. section (CS) ▸ supravesical extraperitoneal

c. section (CS), transperitoneal

c. section (CS), transverse

c. section (CS), vaginal

c. section (CS), Water's

c. (VBAC) ▸ vaginal birth after

cesium (Cs)

c. applicator

c. cylinder

c. insertion

c., intracavitary

c. irradiation

c. mold

c. 137

c. 137 bougie tube brachytherapy

c. 137 teletherapy machine

c. radiation

c. sources

c. therapy, intracavitary

c. tube

c. tube radiation

cessation

c., abrupt

c., intermittent

c. of activity

c. of alcohol

c. of all functions of entire brain including brain stem ▸ irreversible

c. of bleeding

c. of breathing

c. of breathing ▸ periodic

c. of cigarette smoking

c. of circulatory and respiratory functions, irreversible

c. of menstrual cycle

c. of menstrual periods

c. of ovulation

c. of pain

c. of pulmonary ventilation

c. of respiration

c. of therapy

c. program ▸ smoking

c. program, smoking

c. ▸ short-term smoking

c., smoking

c., temporary

c. therapy ▸ smoking

Cestan-Chenais syndrome

cestode infestation

cestodic tuberculosis

CET (coefficient of equal thickness)

Cetraria islandica

Ceylon sore mouth

ceylonensis ▸ Escherichia dispar var.

ceylonensis, Shigella

ceylonica, Haemadipsa

CF (cardiac failure)

CF (complement fixation)

CF (counting fingers)

CF (cystic fibrosis)

CFA (cryptogenic fibrosing alveolitis)

C-fiber

CFM (cerebral function monitor)

CFM (Corometrics Fetal Monitor)

CFS (chronic fatigue syndrome)

CGT (chorionic gonadotropin)

Chaddock's reflex

Chaddock's sign

Chadwick's sign

chafing of feet ▸ flaking and

chafing of thighs

Chagas' disease

chagasic myocardiopathy

chagrin, peau de

Chailletia cymosa

Chailletia toxicaria

chain(s)

c., alpha

c. and tetrads,short

c., branched

c., cervical

c., closed

c. cocci, short-

c. component ▸ lambda light

c. concentration (TLC) ▸ total L-

c. disease, light

c. fatty acid, long

c. fatty acid, medium

c., ganglionated

c. gene, beta myosin heavy

c., gram-positive cocci in pairs and

c. gram-positive cocci ▸ short-

c., iliac

c., imaging

c., internal mammary

c., kappa light

c. ligature

c., light

c. lymph nodes, spinal accessory

c., lymphatic

c. mobility of ossicular

c. ▸ myosin heavy

c. ▸ myosin light

c. of cocci

c., open

c., ossicular

c., palpation of ossicular

c., paratracheal

c., periaortic

c., polypeptide

c. reaction

c. reaction (PCR) assay ▸ polymerase

c. reaction (PCR) machine ▸ polymerase

c. reaction (PCR) ▸ polymerase

c. reaction (PCR) technique ▸ polymerase

c. reaction (PCR) test ▸ reverse transcriptase polymerase

c. reflex

c., respiratory

c. saw

c. smoker

c., superior cervical

c., superior ossicular

c. suture

c., sympathetic

c. ▸ tetrads and short

c. triglyceride diet, medium

c. triglyceride, long

c. triglyceride, medium

c. type ▸ Bence Jones light

chair

c. -back type brace

c., computer-driven rotatory

c. cushion, wheel

c., Gamer's

c. lift

c. pad, geriatric

c., patient lift

c., patient up in

c. scale

c. sit-up exercise

c. stand exercise

c. stretch

c. tub transfer, two-

chalazion, excision of

chalcosis lentis

chalcosis of cornea

chalk stone

chalky bones
chalky gout
challenge(s)
    c. apparatus ▸ quantitative inhalation
    c. ▸ double blind food
    c., emotional
    c., ergonovine
    c., histamine
    c., inhalation
    c., mental
    c. ▸ methacholine bronchoprovocation
    c. of environment
    c., physical
    c. test, bronchial
    c. test (PCT) ▸ progesterone
    c. test ▸ volume-
challenged
    c. children ▸ mentally
    c., developmentally
    c., mentally
    c., physically
chamber(s)
    c., Abbe-Zeiss counting
    c., acoustic
    c., air
    c., air bubble instilled in anterior
    c., alpha
    c., anaerobic
    c., anterior
    c., aqueous
    c., atrialized
    c. atrioventricular (AV) pacemaker ▸ dual
    c., cardiac
    c. cardiac pacemaker ▸ dual
    c. ▸ chaotic beating of atrial
    c., closed urinary drainage (dr'ge) bag with drip
    c. communication, fetal
    c. compliance ▸ left ventricular (LV)
    c., counting
    c., decompression
    c., delayed reformation of
    c., diffusion
    c., dilated, ventricular
    c., drip
    c. enlargement
    c. enlargement of cardiac
    c. entered with keratome ▸ anterior
    c. eye
    c. eye (anterior)
    c. eye (posterior)
    c., flat

c. ▸ fluid filled
c., fluid released from anterior
c., foreign body (FB) in anterior
c., free-air ionization
c., heart
c., heart's pumping
c., high pressure
c., hyperbaric
c., hyperbaric oxygen (HBO)
c., ionization
c. irrigated with saline ▸ anterior
c. lens, Choyce anterior
c., monoplace
c., multiwire proportional
c., nasal
c. of heart
c. of heart, lower
c. of heart, upper
c. of lungs ▸ pumping
c. pacemaker, Aurora dual
c. pacemaker, Autima II dual
c. pacemaker, dual-
c. pacemaker implantation ▸ dual
c. pacemaker ▸ single
c. pacing, dual
c., pocket
c. prominence
c., pulp
c., pumping
c. rate adaptic pacemaker ▸ Dash single-
c. rate responsive ▸ dual
c. rate responsive ▸ single
c., recessive
c., recompression
c. rupture
c., seal anterior
c., shallow
c., spark
c., sterilizing
c. stiffness
c., Thoma-Zeiss counting
c., ventricular
c. view echocardiogram ▸ apical five
c. view echocardiogram ▸ apical four
c. view echocardiogram ▸ apical two
c. view, five
c. view ▸ four
c. view ▸ two
c., vitreous
c., walk-in high pressure
c., Wilson cloud

c., Zappert's
chambered heart, three-
chambered human heart, four-
Chamberlain-Towne x-ray view
Championnière's disease, ▸ Lucas-
Chan wrist rest
chance
    c. experimental therapy ▸ best-
    c. experimental therapy ▸ last-
    c. fracture
    c., survival
chancre/chancrum
chancre sore
chancroid, phagedenic
chancroid, serpiginous
chancroidal bubo
Chandelier sign
Chandler disease
change(s)
    c., abnormal gross
    c., abrupt mood
    c., active parenchymal
    c., adaptive
    c., anoxic
    c. apathy, loss of energy, mood
    c., arteriolonephrosclerotic
    c., arteriovenous crossing
    c., arthritic
    c., assess
    c., associated degenerative
    c., atheromatous
    c., atrophic
    c., behavior
    c., behavioral
    c., Biermer's
    c., biological potential
    c., biomechanical
    c., blood volume
    c., bony destructive
    c., bony image
    c., brain chemical
    c., calcific
    c., cardiac pacemaker battery
    c., cavernomatous
    c., cellular abnormal
    c., chemical
    c., clinical
    c., cognitive and motor
    c., commitment to
    c. compatible with ischemia ▸ ST-T wave
    c., cystic
    c., degenerative
    c., degenerative arthritic
    c., degenerative bone

c., degenerative disc
c., disorientation and personality
c., dressing
c., dysplastic
c., ear stuffiness from allergy ▸ altitude
c., emphysematous
c., environmental
c., E to A
c. ▸ E to I
c., enzyme
c., erythematous
c., family awareness and
c., fibrinoid
c., fibrocystic breast
c., fibrotic
c., focal atypical
c., focal dysrhythmic
c., focal inflammatory
c., focal inflammatory mucosal
c. ▸ frequent mood
c. from aging ▸ voice
c. from antihistamine ▸ voice
c. from anxiety ▸ voice
c. from cancer ▸ voice
c., functional
c., hormonal
c. ▸ hyaline fatty
c. ▸ hydrocephalus ex vacuo
c., hypertrophic
c. in activity
c. in affect ▸ profound
c. in aging ▸ vision
c. in appetite
c. in behavior
c. in behavior ▸ profound
c. in bladder habit
c. in bladder pattern
c. in bleeding patterns
c. in body position, frequent
c. in bowel habit
c. in bowel pattern
c. in brain ▸ anoxic
c. in brain, biochemical
c. in brain ▸ hypoxic
c. in brain, physical
c. in breast, fibrocystic
c. in cervical cells ▸ irregular
c. in cognition
c. in cognition ▸ profound
c. in color and consistency of stool
c. in color of pupils
c. in communications
c. in cortex ▸ anoxic
c. in eating or sleeping habits

c. in emotion ▸ frequent
c. in epithelium ▸ dysplastic
c. in extremities ▸ sensory
c. in food taste
c. in gait
c. in gait and posture
c. in heart rate
c. in heart rhythm
c. in heart structural
c. in joints ▸ structural
c. in judgment
c. in lifestyle, radical
c. in living conditions
c. in mental status ▸ rapid
c. in mood or behavior
c. in mood ▸ severe premenstrual
c. in perception
c. in personality
c. in plans ▸ unavoidable
c. in pressure, monitor
c. in self-image ▸ profound
c. in sexual habits
c. in skin temperature
c. in sleeping patterns
c. in space and time
c. in spiritual values
c. in thoughts
c. in upper extremities ▸ vasomotor
c. in urine flow from constipation
c. in vision, abrupt
c. in vision and hearing
c. in vision, sudden
c. in vision ▸ sudden dizziness, weakness or
c. in wart or mole
c. in weight
c. induced
c., infiltrative
c., inflammatory
c., internal
c., interstitial fibrotic
c., irreversible functional
c., irreversible structural
c. ▸ irritability, depression and personality
c., ischemic
c. ▸ ischemic electrocardiogram (ECG)
c., large magnitude voluntary heart rate
c., learning
c., leukoplakic
c., lifestyle
c., linen

c., long-term behavioral
c., lytic blastic
c., macular
c. ▸ malignancy-associated
c., malignant cell
c., marginal degenerative
c., menstrual
c., metabolic
c. ▸ mental status
c., microscopic
c. ▸ mild hypoxic neuronal
c., minimal calcific
c., minimal degenerative
c., molecular
c., monitor
c., mood
c. ▸ motivation for
c., motor and sensory
c., myxomatous
c., myxomatous degenerative
c., neoplastic
c., no appreciable
c., no significant
c. ▸ nonspecific climatic
c., nonspecific repolarization
c., nonspecific ST-T wave
c., normal hypertrophic
c., nuclear
c., objective
c. of aorta ▸ severe atheromatous
c, of body image, cognitive
c. of cardiac generator
c. of color in fingertips
c. of color in toes
c. of drapes, gowns and instruments ▸complete
c. of dressing
c. of feet, bony
c. of hip ▸ marked degenerative
c. of life
c. of lifestyle
c. of ovaries, involutional
c. of position
c. of skin, color
c. of sound, Gerhardt's
c. of spine, degenerative
c., olfactory perceptual
c., organic brain
c., osteoarthritic
c., parenchymatous
c., passive congestive
c., pathologic
c., pathological
c., perceptual
c. ▸ permanent behavioral

change—*continued*
c., personal lifestyle
c., personality
c. ▸ physical and emotional
c. physically, brain
c., physiological
c., pigmentary
c., pigmentation
c., pleural fluid
c., pleural inflammatory
c. ▸ positive behavior
c., postischemic
c. ▸ postischemic biochemical
c., postoperative
c. ▸ postovulation hormone
c., post-thoracotomy
c., postural
c. ▸ pre-malignant tissue
c., pressure
c., programmatic
c., prohealthy functioning
c., pseudopolypoid
c., psychological
c. ▸ psychotic personality
c., pupillary
c., QRS
c., QRS-T
c., radiation
c. ▸ radiation-induced heart
c., radiation pigmentation
c., radical behavior
c. ▸ rapid mood
c., reactive
c., reflex
c. ▸ resistant to
c., retinal
c. ▸ retinal exudative
c. ▸ retinal vascular
c., rheologic
c., role
c., sarcomatous
c., scattered degenerative
c. ▸ sensitivity to weather
c., sensorial
c., sensory
c., sequence of potential
c., significant
c., skin
c., sleep/wake pattern
c. solution, behavior
c., some appreciable
c., source of potential
c., space occupying
c., stasis
c., structural

c., ST segment
c., subjective
c. ▸ subtle personality
c. ▸ sudden rhythm
c., systemic
c., temperature
c., tissue
c., trophic
c., tumor-induced
c., T-wave
c. ▸ unexplained personality
c. units (LCU) ▸ life
c. ▸ variation in rate of
c., venous stasis
c., venous volume
c., vision
c., voltage
c., weight
c., widespread anoxic

changing
c. decisions, life-
c. habits
c. skills ▸ life
c. social consciousness

channel(s) (Channel) [*panel*]
c. agonist, calcium
c. bandwidth ▸
   electroencephalogram (EEG)
c. blocker, calcium
c. blocker ▸ slow
c. blocking agent ▸ calcium
c. blocking drug, calcium
c., calcium
c. ▸ dilated lymphatic
c., diversion of drugs from licit
   medical
c., electroencephalogram (EEG)
c. electrocardiogram (ECG) ▸ three
c., fast
c., feeder
c. Holter monitor, 3
c. implants, multiple
C. Instrument ▸ Grass Ten
c., ion
c. irrigating bronchoscope, double
c., lymph
c., lymphatic
c., marker
c., membrane
c., microscopic
c., narrow spinal
c., para-aortic lymphatic
c. receiver/stimulator ▸ 22
c. ▸ receptor operated calcium

c., reduction of sensitivity of an
   electroencephalogram (EEG)
c., sensitivity of
   electroencephalogram (EEG)
c., socially acceptable
c., sodium
c. ulcer, pyloric
c., vascular
c., venous
c. ▸ voltage-dependent calcium
Chaoborus lacustris
chaotic
c. activity of ventricular fibrillation
c. atrial tachycardia
c. beating of atrial chambers
c. electrical activity
c. heart
c. heart beat
c. heart muscle activity
c. heart rhythms
c. rhythm
c. tachycardia, atrial
c. thinking and speech ▸ rapid and
c. upbringing
c., useless rhythm
chaplain-on-call
chapped
c. lips
c. lips from caffeine
c. skin ▸ itchy or
Chapple's syndrome
Chaput's method
character(s)
c., acquired
c., alphanumeric
c. analysis
c., compound
c. defense
c. disorder
c., dominant
c., IMViC
c., mendelian
c. neurosis
c. problems, patient has
c., recessive
c. representation
c., sex-conditioned
c., sex-influenced
c., sex-limited
c., sex-linked
c. traits
c. traits, unattractive
c., unit
characteristic(s)
c. ▸ altered facial

c., behavioral
c., clinical
c., codominant
c. disorders ▸ severe
c., dominant
c. facial futures
c., familial
c. features
c., genetic
c. inflammatory reaction
c., mental
c. movement
c., neuromuscular physical
c. of seizure, abnormalities
c., personality
c., physical
c., primary sex
c. ray
c., recessive
c. rhythm
c., secondary sex
c. symptoms, other
c. wheezing sounds

characterological
c. disorders, severe
c. predisposition thesis
c. vulnerability thesis

Charas (marijuana)

charcoal
c., activated
c. blood medium culture
c. yeast extract

Charcot('s)
C. arthropathy
C. arthrosis
C. -Bouchard aneurysm
C. cirrhosis
C. disease
C. disease ▸ Erb-
C. fever
C. foot
C. gait
C. joint
C. -Leyden crystals
C. -Marie-Tooth atrophy
C. -Marie-Tooth disease
C. -Marie-Tooth-Hoffmann
    syndrome
C. pains
C. sign

**Chardack-Greatbatch Implantable
    Cardiac Pulse Generator**

Chardack-Greatbatch pacemaker

charge(s)
c., cytopathological

c., electrical
c., negative
c. nurse
c., positive
c. time
c. to heart, electrical

charged
c. particle beam therapy, heavy
c. particle therapy in eye tumors,
    heavy
c. particles

Charles vacuuming needle

charlesii, Penicillium

Charlson comorbidity index

charm, superficial

Charnley
C. arthrodesis
C. compression fusion
C. -Mueller arthroplasty

charred tissue

Charreter's flap

Charrière scale

chart(s)
c. (AOC) ▸ abridged ocular
c. carrier, mobile
c., computer screen
c., dosage
c., eye
c. holder
c., isodose
c., Jaeger's eye
c., orders on
c., patient
c., reading
c., Reuss's color
c., see dictation on
c., Snellen's
c., Stilling
c., temperature

chartarum, Pithomyces

chasers, heroin

chasing and basing

Chassaignac's axillary muscle

Chassard-Lapiné maneuver

Chassard-Lapiné projection

chat syndrome ▸ cri-du-

chattering of teeth

Chauffard syndrome, Minkowski-

Chauffard syndrome ▸ Troisier-Hanot-

chauffeur's fracture

Chausse's view

Chaussier's areola

Chaussier's tube

Chauveau's bacillus

chauvoei, Clostridium

CHB (complete heart block)

CHD (congenital heart disease)

CHD (congestive heart disease)

CHD (coronary heart disease)

check(s)
c., bifocal
c. -bite
c., blood pressure (BP)
c., body systems
c., craniotomy
c., depth perception
c., glaucoma
c., landmark
c., muscle balance
c., peripheral vision
c., prenatal
c., presbyopia
c., pupil reflex
c., routine
c. valve
c. -valve sheath
c., vital sign

checkerboard analysis

checkup
c., annual
c., cancer-related
c., mammogram

Cheddi, Siamese

Chédiak-Higashi syndrome

cheek(s)
c. appearance ▸ slapped
c. biting from anxiety
c., biting of
c. ▸ cracked mouth corners from
    sagging
c. ▸ facial implant of
c. flap ▸ over-and-out
c., flushed
c. implant
c., loose
c. piercing
c., sagging
c. ▸ skin disorder of
c. teeth

cheese
c. endometrium, Swiss
c. defect ▸ Swiss
c. hyperplasia, Swiss
c. interventricular septum ▸ Swiss
c. -like discharge, cottage
c. worker's lung
c. worker's lung disease

cheesy
c. bronchitis
c. cataract

cheesy—*continued*
c. discharge ▸ white,
c. necrosis
c. nephritis
c. pneumonia
cheilitis
c., actinic
c., actinica
c., acute
c., acute solar
c., angular
c., apostematous
c., commissural
c. exfoliativa
c. glandularis apostematosa
c. granulomatosa
c., impetiginous
c., migrating
c., solar
c. venenata
cheiloplasty repair
cheiralgia paresthetica
cheiro migraine, oro-
cheirokinesthetic center
Chek II ▸ Accu-
chelate, I$_n$
chelated antibody
chelated magnesium
chelating agent
chelating nutrients ▸ oral
chelation therapy
chelation therapy ▸ oral
chelator, iron
chelonae, Mycobacterium
CHEM (chemotherapy)
Chemical (Chemical)
c. ablation
c. abnormality
c. abnormality in brain
c. abortion
c. abuse, adolescent
c. abuse, adult
C. Abuse and Addiction Treatment
   Outcome Registry (CATOR)
c. abuse counseling
c. activity, abnormal
c. addiction
c. affinity
c. agent
c., allergy to
c. analysis
c., anemia from
c. anesthesia
c. aversion
c. balance

c., brain
c., brain's natural
c. bronchiectasis
c. burn
c. burn ▸ corneal scarring from
c., cancer-causing
c. carcinogens
c. cardioversion
c. castration
c. cautery
c. ceptor
c. changes
c. changes, brain
c. clotting factor
c. code
c. conjunctivitis
c., coughing from
c. decortication
c. dependence disorder
c. dependency
c. dependency acceptance of
c. dependency and mental illness
c. dependency benefits
C. Dependency Clinic ▸ Outpatient
c. dependency ▸ cultural aspects of
c. dependency, free of
c. dependency professionals
c. dependency program
c. dependency program,
   alcoholism/
c. dependency skills
c. dependency, stages of
c. dependency treatment
C. Dependency, Women and
c. depilatories
c. depression
c. determination
c. detoxification
c. diabetes
c. disinfection
c. disruption in brain
c. energy
c. enzyme profile
c. equivalent
c., exposure to
c. forces
c. -free living
c. freedom
c. freedom, total
c. gastritis
c. history
c. history, patient's
c. hysterectomy
c., illegal
c. imbalance

c. imbalance in brain
c. impulse
c. impulse in brain ▸ activate
c. incompatibility
c. indicators of ischemia
c., infertility from
c. inhibition
c. injury
c. interaction
c. irritant
c., laryngitis from
c., light-sensitive
c. messenger
c. messenger cells
c. modifiers
c., mood altering
c. neuroanatomy
c., neurotransmitter
c. ▸ occupational exposure to
c. of abuse ▸ primary
c. origin
c. peel
c. ▸ periodic abstinence from
c. pneumonia
c. pneumonitis
c., powerless of
c. pressure
c. profile
c., protective
c. ray
c. reaction
c. reactions in body ▸ normal
c. restraint of patient
c. screening
c. sense
c. sensitivity
c. sensitivity syndrome
c. shift artifact
c. shower
c. similarity
c. snap packs
c. ▸ spooned nail from
c. sterilization
c. stimulation
c. stimulus
c. straitjacket
c. styptic
c. sympathectomy
c. systems of brain
c., targeted
c. therapy
c., toxic
c. transformation
c. transmitters
c. transmitters in brain

c. transmitters, mood altering
c. usage pattern
c. warfare
c. waste dumps

chemically
c. addicted family
c. coated stents
c. dependent, actively
c. dependent family
c. dependent individual
c. dependent patient
c. dependent person
c., destroying antibiotics
c. -free communication
c. -free lifestyle
c. pure
c. unstable oxygen molecules

chemically pure

chemistry(-ies)
c., abnormal body
c., alters brain
c., analytical
c., applied
c., biological
c., Blastomycoides
c., blood
c., body
c., brain
c., colloid
c., dental
c. ▸ disorder of normal bone
c., ecological
c., forensic
c. graph (SCG) ▸ serum
c., industrial
c., inorganic
c., irregularity in brain
c., medical
c., metabolic
c., mineral
c., organic
c. panel
c., pharmaceutical
c., physical
c., physiological
c. profile, automated
c. profile, Hood
c., pyrolytic
c., routine
c., structural
c. studies
c., surface
c., synthetic
c., therapeutic

chemo wafers implanted

chemoprevention therapy
chemoprophylactic regimen
chemoprophylaxis
c., course of
c., primary
c., secondary

chemoreceptor(s)
c., deficient transmission
c. in brain stem
c. in the brain stem
c., peripheral
c. reflex

chemosurgery, Mohs'
chemotactic activity of eosinophils
chemotactic factor
chemotaxis
c., eosinophilic
c., leukocyte
c., negative
c., positive

chemotherapeutic
c. agent
c. agent, antineoplastic
c. agent, cancer
c. agent, experimental
c. agent, infusion
c. drugs
c. index
c. measures
c. modalities
c. protocol
c. regimens
c. support, effective

chemotherapy (Chemotherapy) (CHEM)
c., adjuvant
c., adverse reaction after
c. after mastectomy, radiation and
c., aggressive
c. ▸ AMSA, prednisone, and chlorambucil (APC)
c. and radiation therapy
c., anemia related to
c., antagonistic
c., anticancer
c., antimycobacterial
c., antituberculous
c., brain blood barrier disruption
c., cancer
c., citrovorum rescue
c. ▸ colorectal cancer
c., combination
c. combined with radiotherapy
c. continued on outpatient basis
c., continuing
c., continuing maintenance

c., continuous infusion
c., COPP
c., (first, second, etc.) course of
c. cycles
c., cytotoxic
C. Department
c. dose
c. drug
c., Einhorn regimen of
c. ▸▸ 5-fluorouracil, Adriamycin, Cytoxan (FAC)
c., fractionation with
c., fractionation without
c., high dose
c. immunity
c., in home
c. -induced nausea
c. -induced vomiting
c., induction
c. initiation and management
c. ▸ intense cycle of high dose
c., intensive
c., intensive combination
c., interval
c., intra-arterial
c., intraperitoneal
c., intrapleural
c., intravenous
c., intravesical
c., irradiation and
c., limitations of
c., lip and mouth care before and after
c. ▸ loss of fertility from
c., maintenance
c., massive doses of
c. ▸ mortality and
c., multiple drug
c., nausea-emesis reaction to
c. ▸ neuropathy of
c. ▸ neurotoxicity of
c., optimal dose of
c., oral
c. patient
c., patient on continuing
c. ▸ patient treated with radiation and
c. port
c., preoperative
c. program, combination
c. prophylaxis
c. protocol
c., radiation and
c. /radiation therapy, combined
c. regime

chemotherapy—*continued*
- c., selective
- c., systemic
- c., topical
- c., topical mechlorethamine
- c., traditional
- c. treatment
- c. treatment ▸ adjuvant hormonal or
- c. treatment, inhalation
- c. treatment ▸ intensive
- c., triple drug
- c., tuberculous
- c. waste

Chenais syndrome ▸ Céstan-
cheopis, Pulex
cheopis, Xenopsylla
cheoplastic teeth
Cherenkov counter
Cherney incision
Chernez incision
Cherry (cherry)
- C. angioma
- C. -Crandall units
- c. -picking procedure
- c. red spot

Chesapeake, hemoglobin
chessboard graft
chest
- c., alar
- c. anomaly ▸ fetal
- c., AP diameter of
- c., asthenic
- c., auscultation of
- c. barrel-shaped
- c. bellows
- c. bilaterally symmetrical
- c., blast
- c. breathing, deep
- c. breathing, diaphragmatic and
- c., burning sensation in upper
- c. cage
- c. cardiac massage, closed
- c. cardiac massage ▸ open
- c. cardiac resuscitation, open
- c. cavity
- c. cavity, entering
- c. cavity opened
- c. circumference
- c. clear to percussion and auscultation (P and A)
- c. closed in anatomic layers
- c., cobbler's
- c. commissurotomy, closed
- c. compression

- c. compressions ▸ (CCC) continuous
- c. compression, external
- c. compressions ▸ manual
- c. compressors
- c., computed tomography (CT) of
- c. congestion
- c. constriction
- c., crushing sensation in
- c. cuirass
- c. diameter
- c. diameter, anterior
- c., diminished expansion of
- c. discomfort
- c. discomfort, burning
- c. discomfort, exertional
- c. discomfort, vague
- c. discomfort with fainting
- c. discomfort with lightheadedness
- c. discomfort with nausea
- c. discomfort with shortness of breath (SOB)
- c. discomfort with sweating
- c. disease, nonmalignant
- c. distress
- c. drainage
- c. drainage, cardiotomy reservoir
- c. dressing, jacket-type
- c. dropsy
- c., emphysematous
- c., empyema of
- c. excursion
- c. excursion diminished
- c. exercises, back and
- c. expansion
- c. expansion, good
- c. expansion adequate bilaterally
- c. expansion equal bilaterally
- c. expansion ▸ restricted
- c. ▸ feeling of tightness in
- c. film
- c. film, post-thoracentesis
- c. films, stereoscopic
- c., flail
- c., flat
- c., fluid aspirated from
- c., fluid drained from
- c., fluttering sensation in
- c. for fluid ▸ tapping of
- c., foveated
- c. fullness
- c., funnel
- c. hair
- c. heaviness
- c., hourglass

- c. hyperaerated
- c. injury, crushed
- c., jaw or extremities ▸ pain in
- c. irradiation
- c., keeled
- c. leads
- c. lesion
- c. lesions, nonmalignant
- c. lining, cancer of
- c., long
- c., mass in
- c., massive trauma to
- c. mediastinum
- c. muscles, intact
- c. muscles opened
- c. muscles retracted
- c. muscles, underlying
- c. nodules
- c., noisy
- c. normal
- c. opacity, left
- c. opacity, right
- c. opened
- c. or abdomen pain ▸ breathing with back,
- c. pain
- c. pain and tightness
- c. pain, angina
- c. pain, atypical
- c. pain ▸ bilateral pleuritic
- c. pain, chronic
- c. pain ▸ coughing up blood with
- c. pain, crushing
- c. pain, diminution in
- c. pain ▸ dull
- c. pain, exertional
- c. pain exertional in nature
- c. pain, fleeting
- c. pain from heart problem
- c. pain from pneumonia
- c. pain from TMJ (temporomandibular joint) disorder
- c. pain ▸ gastroesophageal-related
- c. pain ▸ incapacitating
- c. pain ▸ intense, prolonged
- c. pain ▸ noncardiac
- c. pain on deep breathing
- c. pain on exertion
- c. pain, persistent
- c. pain, pleuritic
- c. pain, precordial
- c. pain ▸ prolonged episodes of
- c. pain radiating to jaw and shoulder

c. pain radiation
c. pain, recurrent
c. pain, retrosternal
c. pain ▸ right pleuritis
c. pain, severe
c. pain, stabbing
c. pain ▸ stress-induced
c. pain symptoms ▸ persistent
C. Pain Unit
c. pain, waxing and waning
c. pain with breathing difficulty
c. pain with hoarseness
c. pain with palpitation
c. pain with sweating
c. ▸ painful, burning sensation in
c., paralytic
c. ▸ pectus excavatum of anterior
c. percussion
c. percussion and vibration
c., phthinoid
c. physiotherapy
c., pigeon
c. pneumothorax, closed
c. port
c., portable semi-upright film of
c. position, knee-
c. press exercise
c. pressure
c. pressure ▸ crushing
c. ▸ pressure sensation in
c., pterygoid
c., quiet
c. radiograph, Brasfield
c., rales in
c., rash on
c., restricted expansion of
c., rhythmic compression of
c., rigid
c. roentgenogram
c. roentgenography
c. seal, Asherman
c. sensation ▸ elephant-on-the-
c. ▸ sensation of fullness in
c. shield
c. skeleton, distorted
c. space
c. ▸ squeezing pain in
c. ▸ squeezing sensation in
c. stretch exercise
c., sucking wounds of the
c. suppression
c. symmetrical
c. syndrome, acute
c., tetrahedron
c. therapy, deep

c. thoracostomy, closed
c. thump
c., tight sensation in
c. tightness
c. tomogram, total
c. trauma
c. trauma, severe
c. tube
c. tube drainage
c. tube placement
c. tube, removal of
c. tube ▸ right angle
c. tube ▸ water seal
c. tubes, bilateral
c. tubes present in abdomen
c. wall
c. wall adhesions
c. wall, anterior
c. wall deformity
c. wall, depressed
c. wall disease
c. wall disorder
c. wall, excision portion of
c. wall flap
c. wall ▸ hematoma of
c. wall, interior
c. wall, left lateral
c. wall, malformation of
c. wall manipulation
c. wall metastases
c. wall pain
c. wall, right anterior
c. wall spasm
c. wall syndrome, anterior
c. wall, transthoracic biopsy
c. wall, using bolus adjacent to
c. water seal drainage, closed
c. wound, sucking
c. x-ray
c. x-ray ▸ follow-up
c. x-ray on admission
c. x-ray ▸ repeat
c. x-ray ▸ serial
Chevalier-Jackson tube
chevron incision
chew or swallow, inability to
chewed and swallowed ▸ peyote
chewing
c., difficulty
c. movements ▸ sucking or
c. ▸ pain on
Cheyletiella parasitovorax
Cheyne
C. nystagmus
C. -Stokes asthma

C. -Stokes breathing
C. -Stokes psychosis
C. -Stokes respiration
C. -Stokes sign
CHF (congestive heart failure)
CHF ▸ advanced stage of
CHF natural history of
CHF recurrent
CHF ▸ sudden
CHF (congestive heart failure)
  therapy
C'H₅₀ (total hemolytic complement)
chi
c. martial arts ▸ tai-
c. -square test
c. technique ▸ tai-
c. treatment ▸ tai-
chiaie teeth
Chiari
C. deformity ▸ Arnold-
C. -Frommel syndrome
C. malformation ▸ Arnold-
C. network
C. syndrome
C. syndrome ▸ Arnold-
C. syndrome ▸ Budd-
chiasm
c. of digitus of hand
c. of musculus flexor digitorum
  sublimis ▸ tendinous
c., optic
c., cistern of
c. of flexor sublimis ▸ tendinous
c. opticum
c., sulcus for optic
chiasma syndrome
chiasma tendinum digitorum manus
chiasmal arachnoiditis
chiasmal tumor
chiasmatic cistern
chiasmatic posterior commissure
chichiko dyspepsia
chick cell agglutination
chick disease, crazy
chicken
c. -embryo-lethal orphan (CELO)
c. fat clot
c. lice
c. louse
c. wire myocardial cell
chickenpox
c., blister from
c. incubation period
c. scar
c. vaccine

chickenpox—*continued*
c. virus
c. virus infection
chief (Chief) [*sheaf, sheath*]
c. agglutinin
c. (Mescaline), Big
c. cells
c. complaint (CC)
c. medical examiner
C. of Service
Chiene's operation
Chiene's test
chigger bites
chignon fungus
Chilaiditi's syndrome
chilblain, necrotized
child (Child)
c. abuse
c. abuse accommodation syndrome
c. Abuse and Neglect (SCAN), Stop
c. abuse, chronic
c. abuse, fatal
c. abuse ▸ illusory
c. abuse ▸ memories of
c. abuse or neglect
c. abuse ▸ severe and relentless
c. abuse, suspected
c., acquired immune deficiency syndrome (AIDS) infected
c., active
c., affect-starved
c., aggressive
c. analysis
c. and infant CPR (cardiopulmonary resuscitation) techniques
c., atypical
c., autistic
c. bacterial meningitis
c. battering syndrome
c. -bearing age
c. -bearing period
c. -bearing years
c. beating
c. behavior, inappropriate
c. behavior problems
c., behaviorally disturbed
c., bereaved
c., biological
c. centered interaction
c., classroom behavior of
c. communication
c., deaf cerebral palsied
c., defective

c., defiant
c., dentistry
c., depressed
c., destructive
c. development
c. development, normal
c., developmentally disabled
c. difficult to manage
c. discipline
c., disruptive
c., disturbed
c., drug-impaired
c., exceptional
c. has language disability
c. has sleep problem
c., hyperactive
c., impulsive
c. inattentive
c. interaction evaluation ▸ parent-
c. interaction, parent-
c. issues, inner
c. ▸ learning disabled
c. ▸ learning impaired
C. Life Orthopedic Shoes
c. ▸ low self-esteem
c. ▸ malnutrition of
c. mental retardation, care of
c. neglect
c. of alcoholic parents
c., overactive
c. -parent relationships
c., premature birth of living
c. problem, parent-
c., promiscuous behavior in
c. psychiatry
c. psychology
c. psychopathology
c. psychotherapy
c. quick to anger
c. -rearing difficulties
c. -related activity
c. sexual abuse
c. sexual abuse treatment
c., specially gifted
c., speech-impaired
c. sterility, one-
c. sterility, two-
c., suicidal
c. syndrome, battered
c. syndrome ▸ fragile
c. tent, Croupette
c. ▸ transmit virus to unborn
c., traumatized
childbearing age
childbed fever

childbirth
c. ▸ anal fissure from
c. ▸ back pain after
c., biofeedback techniques of relaxation during
c. ▸ breast pain after
c. education
c., emotional control in
c., incontinence after
c. injury
c., Lamaze method of
c. ▸ male impotence after
c., natural
c. preparation classes
c. techniques
c. without pain (CWP)
childhood
c. abuse
c. accident
c. antisocial behavior
c. anxiety disorder
c. asthma
c. ▸ avoidant disorder of
c. bedwetting
c. behavior problem
c. behavioral disorder
c. brain tumor
c. cancer
c., chronic granulomatous disease of
c. cirrhosis, Indian
c., complex disorder of
c. depression
c. diarrhea
c. diseases
c. diseases (UCD) ▸ usual
c. disintegrative disorder
c. disorder
c. ▸ disturbance of emotions specific to
c. ear infection
c. (EC), early
c. enuresis
c. epilepsy
c., erythroblastic anemia of
c. experiences ▸ traumatic
c. fantasy ▸ normal
c. ▸ gender identity disorder of
c. ▸ granulomatous disease of
c. history
c. ▸ hyperkinetic reaction of
c. hyperkinetic syndrome
c. immunization
c. incest
c. ▸ introverted disorder of

c. learning disorder
c. leukemia, acute
c. migraine headache
c. ▸ mixed emotional disturbances of
c. muscle-wasting disease
c., myoclonic encephalopathy
c. neurodevelopmental dysfunction disorder
c. or adolescence ▸ avoidant disorder of
c. (PAC), papular acrodermatitis of
c. phobia
c. psychiatric disorder
c. psychiatric treatment
c. psychopathology
c. ▸ psychoses with origin specific to
c. psychosis, early
c. ▸ reactive attachment disorder of early
c. ▸ reactive attachment disorder of infancy or early
c. schizophrenia
c. sexual abuse
c. shyness disorder
c. stress
c. ▸ transient tic disorder of
c. trauma
c., traumatic
c. tuberculosis
c. tumors, lethal
c. victimization
childless woman
children('s) (Children)
c., admission of
C. Apperception Test
C., behavioral development of
c., biliary cirrhosis of
c., cognitive development of
c., depressed
c. ▸ depression in preadolescent
c., disabled
c., dissociative
c., dosage for
c., dyslexic
c., emotional and behavioral disorders in
c. ▸ emotional development of
c. ▸ esophagus replacement with colon in
c., gifted
c. grief and mourning
c. ▸ group treatment for
c. ▸ growth retardation in

C. ▸ Halstead Neuropsychological Test Battery for Adults or
c., homeless
c., hormone deficient
c. ▸ kidney tumor in
c. ▸ knock-knee in
c. ▸ language-delayed (LD)
c. ▸ mentally challenged
c., missing and exploited
c., mnemonic
c. of alcoholics
C. of Alcoholics (ACOA), Adult
c. of alcoholics counseling ▸ individual adult
C. of Alcoholics Screen Testing (CAST)
c. of dysfunctional families, adult
c. of incarcerated parents
c., prepubertal
c., problem
c. ▸ school phobia in
c. ▸ separation anxiety of
c., sexual abuse of
c., sexually abused
c. ▸ skills training for
c. ▸ stereotyped behavior of autistic
c. ▸ suicidal tendencies in
c., terminally ill
C. (WISC), Wechsler Intelligence Scale for
c., treatment of poisoning of
c., urinary infection in
c. ▸ vaginal discharge in
C. (WISC) ▸ Wechsler Intelligence Scale for
c. with alcohol abuse problems
c. with regressive potentials
Childs Cardio-Cuff
chiliani, Haemadipsa
chill(s)
c. and fever
c. and fever ▸ intermittent
c. and fever ▸ jaundice,
c. and fever ▸ onset of
c. and night sweats ▸ shaking
c., congestive
c., diabetes with
c., dyspnea ▸ fever, shaking
c., fever and cough
c., fever and jaundice
c., fever and night sweats
c. ▸ fever, shaking
c. from myocardial infarction
c. from shingles
c. ▸ muscle pain and

c., nausea and vomiting
c., nervous
c. ▸ patient has
c., shaking
c. ▸ tremor and
c., urethral
c. with back pain
c. with bloody semen
c. with breast abnormality
c. with flu
c. with genital pain in males
c. with hypothermia
c. with pneumonia
c. with rash
c. with swollen scrotum and pain
c. with vaginal discharge
chilly ambient temperature
chilly sensation
Chilodon dentatus
Chilodon uncinatus
Chilomastix mesnili
chimera
c., heterologous
c., homologous
c., isologous
c., radiation
chimeric antibody
chimney-sweeps cancer
chimpanzee coryza agent (CCA) virus
chin [shin, skin]
c. ▸ facial implant of
c. implant
c. lift
c. lift maneuver ▸ head tilt and
c. ▸ lump or swelling under
c., protuberance
c. reflex
c. reflex, palm-
c. strap
c. tilt
c. tilt, head tilt with
c., transverse muscle of
c. tucks
China diarrhea ▸ Cochin-
China White (opioid)
chinensis, Phlebotomus
Chinese Restaurant Syndrome (CRS)
chink glottic
chip(s)
c. allograft, bone
c., bone
c. fracture
c. fracture, avulsion
c. ▸ free-floating bone
c., ice

chip(s)—continued
  c., silicone
  c. technology, micro-
chipped teeth
Chiracanthium diversium
Chiracanthium inclusum
chiropractic
  c. care
  c. manipulation
  c. orthopedist
chirospinal manipulation
chisel fracture
chi-square
Chiva (heroin)
chlamydia (Chlamydia)
  c. from birth control pill
  C. genitourinary (GU) infection
  c. infection
  C. oculogenitalis
  c. ▸ pelvic inflammatory disease
    from
  c. ▸ penile discharge from
  C. pneumonia
  C. pneumoniae infection
  C. psittaci
  c. ▸ sore throat from
  C. trachomatis
  c. ▸ vaginal bleeding from
Chlamydiae cervicitis
Chlamydiae urethritis
Chlamydophrys anchelys
Chlamydophrys stercorea
chloasma gravidarum
chloasma uterinum
chlorpromazine ▸ heat intolerance from
chloral hydrate
chlorambucil (APC) chemotherapy ▸
  AMSA, prednisone, and
chloride
  c., ammonium
  c. determination, sweat
  c. diarrhea, congenital
  c. diarrhea, familial
  c., intravenous ammonium
  c. ion
  c., magnesium
  c., polyvinyl
  c., potassium
  c., serum
  c., sodium
  c. test ▸ sweat
  c. test, urine
chlorinated soda
chlormerodrin
  c. accumulation test (CAT)

  c. -cysteine
  c. -cysteine complex
  c. Hg 197
  c. Hg 203
chloroazotemic nephritis
Chlorobacterium symbioticum
Chlorobium limicola
Chlorobium thiosulfatophilum
Chlorochromatium aggregatum
chloroform addict
chloropenic azotemia
chlorophenyl, isopropyl
chloroquine retinopathy
chlorosis vulvae
Chlorostigma stuckertianum
chlorotic anemia
chlorotic phlebitis
chlorotica, aorta
chlorpalladium fluid
Chlumsky's button
choana
  c. atresia
  c., bony
  c. narium
  c., primary
  c., secondary
choanal plug, Mackenty's
choanal polyps
Choanotaenia infundibulum
choc, bruit de
choc en dome
chocked reflex
chocolate
  c. addict
  c. cold sore from
  c. cyst
choice(s) (Choice)
  c., anxiety provoking
  c., factor in treatment
  c., mandated
  c. of medical treatment
  C. procedure ▸ Therma
  c., treatment of
choke
  c., ophthalmovascular
  c. spasm
  c., thoracic
  c., water
choked disc
choked to death ▸ patient
choking
  c. ▸ feeling of
  c. from dentures
  c. management
  c. of optic nerve head

  c., relieve
  c. sensation
  c. victim
  c. victim ▸ unconscious
cholangiocarcinoma, metastatic
cholangiocellular carcinoma
cholangiogram
  c., cholecysto◊
  c., cystic duct
  c., endoscopic
  c., endoscopic retrograde
  c., intraoperative
  c. (IVC), intravenous
  c., intravenous (IV)
  c., nasobiliary catheter
  c., operative
  c., percutaneous
  c., percutaneous needle
  c. (PTC), percutaneous
    transhepatic
  c., retrograde
  c. study
  c., transhepatic
  c., T-tube
cholangiography
  c., catheter
  c., cholecysto◊
  c., delayed operative
  c., direct percutaneous
    transhepatic
  c. (FNTC) ▸ fine needle
    transhepatic
  c., intraoperative
  c., intravenous (IV)
  c., operative
  c., percutaneous
  c., percutaneous hepatobiliary
  c., percutaneous transhepatic
  c., postoperative
  c., transabdominal
  c., transhepatic
  c., transjugular
  c., T-tube
cholangiojejunostomy, intrahepatic
cholangiolitic hepatitis
cholangiopancreatography (ERCP),
  endoscopic retrograde
cholangitis
  c., ascending
  c., catarrhal
  c., concomitant
  c. lenta
  c., primary sclerosing
Cholebrine contrast medium
cholecystectomy, laparoscopic

cholecystitis
- c., acute
- c., acute acalculous
- c., chronic
- c., chronic calculus
- c. emphysematosa
- c., emphysematous
- c., follicular
- c., gaseous
- c. glandularis proliferans
- c., pleuro◊
- c., typhlo◊
- c. with lithiasis

cholecystocausis, electro◊
cholecystocholedochectomy,
  cholangio◊
cholecystogastrostomy, status post
cholecystogram (OCG), oral
cholecystogram study
cholecystography
- c., intravenous (IV)
- c., oral
- c., spot

cholecystolithotomy, percutaneous
cholecystosis, hyperplastic
choledochal cyst
choledochogram study
choledochostomy, choledocho◊
choledochus, ductus
cholelithic dyspepsia
cholemia, familial
cholemia, Gilbert's
cholemic nephrosis
cholepathia spastica
cholera
- c., Asiatic
- c. bacteria
- c., bilious
- c., epidemic
- c. group ▸ hog
- c. infantum
- c. morbus
- c. nostras
- c. vaccine reaction

cholerae, Vibrio
cholerae-asiaticae ▸ Vibrio
choleraesuis, Bacterium
choleraesuis, Salmonella
choleraic diarrhea
choleraicus, status
choleriform, enteritis
cholestasis
- c. of liver ▸ extracellular
- c. of liver ▸ intra
- c. syndrome ▸ familial

cholestatic hepatitis
cholestatic jaundice
cholesteatoma
- c., bone eroded by
- c., choroid plexus
- c., congenital
- c. debris
- c., lateral ventricle
- c. matrix
- c. tympani

cholesteremia/cholesterolemia
cholesterol (Cholesterol)
- c. analysis
- c. assay
- c., blood
- c. blood level
- c. calcium content
- c. calculus
- c., circulating
- c. concentration
- c. control
- c. crystals
- c. deposit
- c. deposits, fatty
- c., detrimental
- c. diet ▸ high fat, high
- c. diet, low
- c. diet, low fat
- c. diet ▸ low fat, low
- c., dietary
- C. Education Program (NCEP) ▸
  National
- c. elevated
- c. emboli
- c. emboli, multiple
- c. embolization of arteries
- c. embolization, research
- c. ester storage disease
- c. esters
- c. ▸ familial high
- c., fasting plasma
- c. filled plaque
- c. flocculation
- c. flocculation, cephalin-
- c. flocculation test ▸ cephalin-
- c. fluctuated, serum
- c. food ▸ low fat, low-
- c. granuloma
- c., high blood
- c. in retina
- c. in urine
- c. in vitreous
- c. ▸ inherited high
- c. intake, dietary
- c. laden food

- c. -laden plaque
- c. level
- c. level, average
- c. level, blood
- c. level, high
- c. level ▸ total blood
- c., lipid-like
- c. lodge
- c., low
- c. lowering diet
- c. lowering drugs
- c. lowering drug therapy
- c. lowering medication
- c., oxidation
- c. pericarditis
- c. -phospholipid ratio
- c. plaque
- c. pleurisy
- c. pneumonitis
- c. production, liver
- c. profile
- c. reduction
- c. related gene ▸ abnormal
- c. saturated fat index
- c. screening
- c. screening, blood
- c., serum
- c. stone
- c. synthesis
- c. test
- c. thorax
- c., total
- c., total serum

cholestyramine resin
choline glycerophosphatide
choline receptors, acetyl
cholinergic
- c. activity
- c. agent
- c. effects
- c. innervation of lung
- c., ophthalmic
- c. receptor
- c. response

cholinesterase
- c. deficiency
- c. inhibitor
- c. test

Cholografin contrast medium
Cholografin methylglucamine
Cholmeley operation ▸ Elmslie-
chondritis costal cartilage
chondritis intervertebral cartilage
chondroblastic growth and maturation
  ▸ epiphyseal

chondrocalcinosis of knees
chondrocyte implantation, autologous
chondrodysplasia punctata
chondrodystrophia calcificans
   congenita
chondrodystrophia fetalis calcificans
chondrodystrophic myotonia
chondrodystrophy malacia
chondroectodermal dysplasia
chondrofibrosarcoma, myxo◊
chondroglossus muscle
chondroid cancer
chondroid tissue
chondroma [*chordoma*]
   c., joint
   c., masto◊
   c. of lung
   c., synovial
chondromalacia
   c. fetalis
   c. of patella
   c., systemic
chondromatosis, Reichel's
chondromatosis, synovial
chondromatous adenoma
chondrometaplasia, tenosynovial
chondromyxoid fibroma
chondropharyngeal muscle
chondrosarcoma
   c., mesenchymal
   c., myxo◊
   c. of posterior fossa
chondrosternal articulations
chondrosternal depression ▸ congenital
Chong sandwich flap ▸ Moore and
chop amputation
chop, karate
Chopart's
   C. amputation
   C. fracture
   C. joint
chopper amplifier
chord [*cord*]
chord, condyle
chorda
   c. dorsalis
   c. gubernaculum
   c. saliva
   c. tendineae cordis
   c. tympani
   c. tympani, canaliculus of
   c. tympani nerve
chordae
   c. ▸ fibrous thickening of
   c., flail

   c. tendineae
   c. tendineae rupture
   c. tympani, canaliculus
chordal
   c. buckling
   c. length
   c. rupture
   c. structure
   c. tissue
   c. transfer
chordalis, endocarditis
chorditis
   c. cantorum
   c. fibrinosa
   c. nodosa
   c. tuberosa
   c. vocalis
chordoma [*chondroma*]
chorea
   c., acute
   c., amyotrophic
   c., automatic
   c., Bergeron's
   c., button-makers'
   c., chronic
   c., chronic progressive
   c., chronic progressive hereditary
   c., chronic progressive
      nonhereditary
   c. cordis
   c., dancing
   c., degenerative
   c., diaphragmatic
   c., dimidiata
   c., Dubini's
   c., electric
   c., epidemic
   c., fibrillary
   c. gravidarum
   c., habit
   c., hemilateral
   c., Henoch's
   c., hereditary
   c., Huntington's
   c., hyoscine
   c., hysterical
   c., imitative
   c., insaniens
   c., involuntary movements of
   c., juvenile
   c., laryngeal
   c., limp
   c., local
   c., major
   c., malleatory

   c., maniacal
   c., methodic
   c., mimetic
   c., minor
   c., mollis
   c., Morvan's
   c., nocturna
   c., nutans
   c., one-sided
   c., paralytic
   c., postcerebrovascular accident
   c., posthemiplegic
   c., prehemiplegic
   c., precursive
   c., rheumatic
   c., rhythmic
   c., rotary
   c., saltatory
   c., school-made
   c., Schrötter's
   c. scriptorum
   c., senile
   c., simple
   c., Sydenham's
   c., tetanoid
   c., tic
choreic
   c. abasia
   c. athetoid movements
   c. convulsion
   c. insanity
   c. tic, progressive
   c. tongue
choreiform movements
choreoathetosis of extremities
chores ▸ refusal to do
chorii, liquor
chorioadenoma destruens
chorioallantoic
   c. culture
   c. graft
   c. membrane
   c. placenta
chorioamnionitis, fulminant
chorioepithelioma malignum
chorioidea (*see* choroidea)
chorioidea, taenia
choriomeningitis
   c., lymphatic
   c., lymphocytic
   c., pseudolymphocytic
   c. (LCM) virus ▸ lymphocytic
chorion frondosum
chorion membranes

chorionic
- c. carcinoma
- c. cyst
- c. ectoderm
- c. epithelioma
- c. gonadotropic, human
- c. gonadotropin (CGT)
- c. gonadotropin, human
- c. gonadotropin test
- c. gonadotropin, urinary
- c. growth hormone prolactin
- c. plaque
- c. somatomammotropin ► human
- c. tissue
- c. vesicle
- c. villi
- c. villi biopsy (CVB)
- c. villus sampling (CVS)

chorioptic acariasis
chorioretinal disease
chorioretinal disease ► Epstein-Barr
chorioretinitis, central
chorioretinitis, senile
chorioretinopathy, central serous
choriovitelline placenta
choroid
- c., atrophy of
- c., biopsy of
- c. coat of eye
- c., coloboma of
- c., crescent
- c., detachment of
- c., hemangioma of
- c., infarction of
- c. layer
- c. of eye, vascular layer of
- c. plexus
- c. plexus, calcification
- c. plexus, carcinoma of
- c. plexus, cholesteatoma of
- c. plexus, excision of
- c. plexus of ventricles
- c., reattachment of
- c. tumor

choroidal
- c. artery
- c. artery, anterior
- c. atrophy, progressive
- c. blood flow
- c. branches of posterior cerebral artery
- c. cancer
- c. cataract
- c. hemangioma
- c. hypertensive disease

- c. melanoma
- c. metastasis
- c. new vessel membranes
- c. osteoma
- c. vasculature
- c. vessels ► anastomosis of retinal and

choroidea (same as chorioidea)
choroideae corrugans ► fibrosis
choroiditis
- c., areolar
- c., Doyne's
- c., Förster's
- c. guttata senilis
- c., juxtapapillitic
- c. myopica
- c., Pneumocystis
- c. serosa
- c., syphilitic
- c., Tay's
- c., toxoplasmic

choroidopathy, hypertensive
Chotzen syndrome, Saethre-Choyce('s)
- C. anterior chamber lens
- C. implant
- C. implant cataract lens
- C. implant, Rayner-
- C. Mark VIII implant

chr. PID (chronic pelvic inflammatory disease)
Christ-Siemens-Touraine syndrome
Christian
- C. disease ► Hand-Schüller-
- C. disease ► Schüller-
- C. disease ► Weber-
- C. syndrome ► Hand-Schüller
- C. syndrome, Weber-

Christmas
- C. disease
- C. factor
- C. Trees (barbiturates)

chromaffin cell tumor
chromaffin tissue
chromaffinoma, medullary
chromatic
- c. aberration, lateral
- c. aberration, longitudinal
- c. audition
- c. granules
- c. spectrum
- c. structure
- c. vision

chromatica, trichomycosis
chromatid [chromatin]

chromatid-type aberration
chromatin [chromatid]
- c. clumps and nucleoli
- c. clumps and nucleoli ► coarse
- c., nuclear
- c. test ► sex
- c., visible

chromatographic-fluorometric technique
chromatography
- c., affinity
- c., electric
- c., electro◊
- c., filter paper
- c., gas
- c., gas-liquid
- c., gas-solid
- c., instant thin layer
- c., paper
- c., partition
- c., thin layer

chromic
- c. catgut (CCG) mattress sutures
- c. catgut (CCG) sutures
- c. catgut sutures (CCG), interrupted
- c. catgut (CCG) ► ties of
- c. gut suture
- c. ligature
- c. phosphate P 32
- c. sutures, atraumatic
- c. sutures, interrupted
- c. sutures, running
- c. sutures, surgical

chromidial substance
Chromobacterium
- C. amythistinum
- C. janthinum
- C. marismortui
- C. violaceum

chromocytoma, pheo◊
chromogenic method
chromophil substance
chromophilic adenoma
chromophilic granules
chromophobe adenoma
chromoradiometer, Holzknecht's
chromoretinography study
chromoscopy, gastric
chromosomal
- c. aberration ► penta-X
- c. aberration ► tetra-X
- c. aberration ► triple-X
- c. abnormality
- c. analysis

chromosomal—*continued*
- c. gene
- c. gene mutation
- c. genes, mutant
- c. material
- c. mediated resistance
- c. satellite
- c. segregation

chromosome(s)
- c. aberration
- c. abnormal
- c. abnormalities
- c. analysis
- c., bacterial
- c., bacterial cell unattached to
- c. banding
- c., donor's
- c., 46
- c., host
- c., human
- c., missing
- c., nonsex
- c., parentage of
- c., Philadelphia
- c., segment of
- c., sex
- c. transferred to recipient ▸ donor's
- c. 21

chronic
- c. abuse of drugs
- c. aches and pains
- c. aching back
- c. active gastritis
- c. active hepatitis
- c. adrenocortical insufficiency
- c. aggressive hepatitis
- c. ailment
- c. airway obstruction
- c. alcohol abuse
- c. alcohol exposure
- c. alcohol ingestion ▸ acute or
- c. alcoholic
- c. alcoholic brain syndrome
- c. ▸ alcoholic cardiomyopathy: preclinical, acute and
- c. alcoholic delirium
- c. alcoholic heart muscle disease
- c. alcoholism
- c. alcoholism ▸ persistent injury by
- c. amphetamine effect
- c. anal fistula
- c. and dilute variant
- c. and progressive illness
- c. and widespread, pain
- c. antibiotic inhalation

- c. antidepressant treatment
- c. anxiety
- c. anxiety state
- c. anxiety, treatment of
- c. aortic stenosis
- c. aspiration
- c. aspirin therapy
- c. asthma
- c. asthmatic bronchitis
- c. atrophic gastritis
- c. autoimmune disorder
- c. bacillary diarrhea
- c. back pain
- c. bacterial prostatitis
- c. bad breath
- c. belching
- c. bile obstruction
- c. bladder inflammation
- c. blood loss
- c. blood loss from an adenocarcinoma
- c. blood loss of gastrointestinal lesion
- c. bone pain
- c. brain disorder
- c. brain syndrome
- c. breast abscess
- c. breathing problems
- c. bronchiectasis
- c. bronchitis
- c. bronchitis ▸ acute exacerbation of
- c. bronchitis with asthma
- c. bronchitis with emphysema
- c. bronchopneumonia
- c. calcific pancreatitis
- c. calculus cholecystitis
- c. cardiac failure
- c. cardiovascular disorder
- c. carrier, patient
- c. catarrhal laryngitis
- c. catarrhal tonsillitis
- c. cervicitis
- c. chest pain
- c. child abuse
- c. cholecystitis
- c. chorea
- c. cocaine abuse
- c. cocaine use
- c. condition
- c. congestive heart failure
- c. connective tissue disorder
- c. constipation
- c. constipation or hemorrhoids
- c. constrictive pericarditis

- c. cough
- c. cough disorder
- c. crisis
- c. cyclic pulmonary disorder
- c. cystic cervicitis
- c. cystic gastritis
- c. cystic infarct
- c. cystic mastitis
- c. cystitis
- c. dacryocystitis
- c. debilitating disease
- c. debilitating disorder
- c. debilitating knee pain
- c. debility
- c. degenerative disease
- c. dementia ▸ incurable
- c. depression
- c. depression ▸ moderate
- c. depressive personality disorder
- c. dermatoses
- c. diabetic neuropathic pain
- c. dialysis
- c. diarrhea
- c. diffuse sclerosing alveolitis
- c. digestive disorder
- c. dilation of bronchi
- c. disability
- c. disability in parent
- c. disease
- c. disease ▸ malnourished patient with
- c. disease ▸ severe
- c. dislocation
- c. disordered water balance
- c. disorders
- c. dissociation
- c. dopamine effect
- c. drinking
- c. drug user
- c. dry eyes
- c. dysphonia
- c. dysphoria
- c. dyspnea
- c. dysthymia
- c. ear infection
- c. earache
- c. electrophysiological study
- c. emotional suffering
- c. emphysema
- c. emptiness and boredom
- c. endemic fluorosis
- c. endocarditis
- c. endocervicitis
- c. endometriosis
- c. eosinophilic pneumonia

c. Epstein-Barr virus (CEBV)
c. Epstein-Barr virus (CEBV) syndrome
c. esophageal dysphagia
c. esophageal sclerosis
c. esophagitis
c. external ophthalmoplegia
c. extrinsic alveolitis
c. facial tics
c. factitious illness with physical symptoms
c. false-positive
c. familial nonhemolytic jaundice
c. fatigue
c. fatigue syndrome (CFS)
c. fecal shedding
c. feelings of deep emptiness
c. feelings of emptiness
c. fever
c. fibrosing alveolitis
c. fibrosing myopathy
c. fibrous pneumonia
c. focal encephalitis
c. focal epilepsy
c. gastric ulcer
c. gastritis
c. gastrointestinal (GI) disorder
c. glaucoma
c. glomerulonephritis
c. granulating wound
c. granulocytic leukemia
c. granulomatous disease (CGD)
c. granulomatous disease of childhood
c. grief
c. gum infection
c. habit
c. halitosis
c. headache pain
c. headaches
c. health problem
c. heart disease
c. heart failure
c. hemodialysis
c. hemolytic anemia
c. hepatitis
c. hepatitis B virus infection
c. hepatitis C infection
c. high blood pressure (BP)
c. hydrocephalus
c. hypersomnia
c. hypertensive disease
c. hypertrophic emphysema
c. hyperventilation syndrome (HVS)
c. hypoglycemia

c. hypomanic personality disorder
c. hypoxia
c. idiopathic orthostatic hypotension
c. idiopathic xanthomatosis
c. illness
c. immune disorder
c. impotence
c. incontinence
c. infarct
c. infection
c. infection in prostate gland
c. inflammation
c. inflammation ► acute and
c. inflammation of bladder wall
c. inflammation of brain
c. inflammation of joints
c. inflammation of lamina propria
c. inflammation of pancreas
c. inflammation with alveolar sloughing
c. inflammatory cell infiltration
c. inflammatory cells
c. inflammatory demyelinating polyneuropathy
c. inflammatory disease
c. inflammatory disease of pancreas
c. inflammatory granulomatous process
c. inflammatory hyperplasia
c. inflammatory infiltrate
c. inflammatory infiltrate ► mild focal
c. inflammatory infiltrate ► patchy
c. inflammatory infiltrates ► peribronchial
c. inflammatory infiltrates ► scattered
c. inflammatory infiltration
c. inhalant abuse
c. insomnia
c. insomniac
c. instability
c. intense envy
c. intermittent low back pain
c. interstitial hepatitis
c. interstitial inflammatory infiltrate
c. interstitial lung disease
c. interstitial pulmonary fibrosis
c. interstitial salpingitis
c. irritation
c. irritation or infection
c. ischemia
c. itch-and-scratch syndrome

c. -itching syndromes
c. joint pain
c. kidney disease
c. kidney failure
c. kidney inflammation
c. labyrinthitis
c. laryngitis
c. leg pain
c. lid infection
c. life-threatening disease
c. liver disease
c. lobular emphysema
c. long term illness
c. loss of function
c. low back pain
c. low back strain
c. low backache
c. low self-esteem
c. lung complaints
c. lung disease
c. lung disorder
c. lymphatic leukemia
c. lymphocytic disease
c. lymphocytic leukemia (CLL)
c. lymphocytic leukemia variant
c. lymphocytic thyroiditis
c. lymphocytic thyroiditis ► nonspecific
c. lymphosarcoma cell leukemia
c. maintenance dialysis
c. maintenance therapy
c. mania ► incurable
c. marijuana use
c. mastitis
c. medical condition
c. medical illness
c. medical problem
c. membranous glomerulonephritis
c. mental illness
c. mesenteric ischemia
c. metabolic disorder
c. methamphetamine intoxication
c. methedrine intoxication
c. middle ear infection
c. migraine headaches
c. minor infection
c. mononucleosis
c. motor or vocal tic disorder
c. motor tic (CMT)
c. motor tic disorder
c. mountain sickness
c. mucocutaneous candidiasis
c. mucus-producing cough
c. muscle pain
c. muscle pain syndrome

chronic—*continued*

- c. muscle paralysis
- c. muscle tension
- c. muscular pain
- c. muscular spasm
- c. myelitis
- c. myelocytic anemia
- c. myelocytic leukemia (CML)
- c. myelogenous disease
- c. myelogenous leukemia (CML)
- c. myeloid leukemia
- c. myelomonocytic leukemia
- c. myocarditis
- c. narrow-angle glaucoma
- c. nephritis
- c. nerve pain
- c. nervous degenerative disease
- c. nervous exhaustion
- c. neurologic disorder
- c. neutrophilic leukemia
- c. nonleukemic myelosis
- c. nonprogressive disturbance
- c. nonspecific sialadenitis
- c. nosebleeds
- c. obesity
- c. obstructive airway disease
- c. obstructive bronchitis
- c. obstructive defect
- c. obstructive lung disease
- c. obstructive pulmonary disease (COPD)
- c. obstructive pulmonary emphysema (COPE)
- c. obstructive respiratory disease
- c. occlusion
- c. occlusive disease
- c. open angle glaucoma
- c. opiate abuse
- c. or incurable disease
- c. organic brain syndrome
- c. organizing pneumonitis
- c. orthopedic impairment
- c. orthostatic hypotension
- c. osteomyelitis
- c. otitis media
- c. otorrhea
- c. outlet obstruction
- c. pain
- c. pain control
- c. pain in ligaments
- c. pain in muscles
- c. pain ▸ long-term
- c. pain, management of
- c. pain of tendons
- c. pain patient

- c. pain, patient in
- c. pain ▸ psychological management of
- c. pain response
- c. pain syndrome
- c. pain, treatment of
- c., painful arthritis
- c., painful condition
- c. pancreatic exocrine insufficiency ▸ mild
- c. pancreatic exocrine insufficiency ▸ moderate
- c. pancreatitis
- c. pancreatitis ▸ etiology of
- c. pancreatitis ▸ management of
- c. paranoid schizophrenia
- c. passive congestion
- c. passive congestion of liver
- c. passive congestion of lungs
- c. patellar subluxation
- c. pelvic inflammatory disease (chr. PID)
- c. pelvic pain
- c. perforating hyperplasia of pulp
- c. pericarditis effusion
- c. periodontal infection
- c. peritonitis
- c. persisting hepatitis
- c. petrous osteomyelitis
- c. pharyngitis
- c. phase
- c. pleurisy
- c. pleuritis
- c. pneumonia
- c. polyarthritis, juvenile
- c. polyneuritis
- c. post-traumatic vertigo
- c. postnasal drip
- c. prepyloric ulcer
- c. process
- c. proctitis
- c. progressive chorea
- c. progressive course
- c. progressive headache
- c. progressive hereditary chorea
- c. progressive lung disease
- c. progressive multiple sclerosis (MS)
- c. progressive nonhereditary chorea
- c. prostatitis
- c. pulmonary cystic lymphangiectasis
- c. pulmonary disorder
- c. pulmonary edema

- c. pulmonary emphysema
- c. pulmonary infection
- c. pulmonary insufficiency of prematurity
- c. pulmonary interstitial fibrosis
- c. pulmonic process
- c. pump inefficiency
- c. pyelonephritis
- c. pyelonephritis, bilateral
- c. radiodermatitis
- c. recurring depression
- c. reflex pain syndrome
- c. reflux esophagitis
- c. refractory anemia
- c. refractory osteomyelitis
- c. rejection
- c. relapsing courses
- c. relapsing diseases
- c. relapsing disorder
- c. relapsing pancreatitis
- c. relapsing schizophrenic patient
- c. renal disease
- c. renal failure
- c. respiratory failure
- c. respiratory problem
- c. rhinitis
- c. salpingitis
- c. sarcoidosis
- c. schizophrenia
- c. ▸ schizophrenia, catatonic type,
- c. ▸ schizophrenia, disorganized type,
- c. schizophrenia-like state
- c. ▸ schizophrenia, paranoid type,
- c. ▸ schizophrenia, residual type,
- c. ▸ schizophrenia, undifferentiated type,
- c. secretory diarrhea
- c. serous meningitis
- c. shock
- c. shoulder dislocation
- c. skin condition
- c. simple glaucoma
- c. sinus infection
- c. sinusitis
- c. skin infection
- c. sleep deprivation
- c. sleep schedule disturbance
- c. slurred speech
- c. smoker
- c. spasm
- c. stable angina
- c. stage
- c. staining
- c. staph carrier

c. stimulant
c. stuffy nose
c. subacute bronchitis
c. subacute leukoencephalitis
c. subcortical encephalitis
c. subdural hematoma
c. subinvolution of uterus
c. substance abuse
c. sudden death
c. sun exposure
c. suppressant therapy
c. suppurative otitis media
c. suppurative pericementitis
c. symptomatic disease
c. symptoms
c. syndrome
c. syphilitic infection
c. tachycardia
c. tamponade
c. tension and anxiety
c. therapy
c. thirst
c. thromboembolic pulmonary hypertension
c. thrombophlebitis
c. thyroiditis
c. tinnitus
c. tinnitus ▸ severe
c. toenail fungus
c. tonsillitis
c. toxic effects
c. tracheitis
c. treatment
c. trigonitis
c. ulcerations of skin
c. ulcerative colitis
c. ultraviolet exposure
c. underlying disease
c. undifferentiated schizophrenia
c. unremitting cough
c. urticaria
c. untreatable condition
c. urethritis
c. urinary infection
c. vaginitis
c. valvulitis
c. vegetating salpingitis
c. venous insufficiency
c. vertigo
c. vestibulopathy
c. villous arthritis
c. viremia
c. visual disturbances
c. voice disorder
c. vulvar pain

c. vulvitis
c. wasting disease (CWD)
c. widespread pain
c. with acute exacerbation ▸ schizophrenia, catatonic type
c. with acute exacerbation ▸ schizophrenia, disorganized type
c. with acute exacerbation ▸ schizophrenia, paranoid type
c. with acute exacerbation ▸ schizophrenia, residual type
c. with acute exacerbation ▸ schizophrenia, undifferentiated type
c. yeast infection
c. yeast vaginitis
chronica
c. ankylopoietica, spondylosis
c. atrophicans ▸ acrodermatitis
c., enteritis cystica
c., gastrorrhea continua
chronically
c. exhausted
c. ill
c. ill, patient
c. infected tonsils
c. inflamed airway
c. inflamed cyst
c. inflamed gallbladder
c. inflamed gallbladder with stones
c. mentally ill
c. painful knee
c. sleep deprived
chronicum migrans (ECM) lesion ▸ erythema
chronicum migrans, erythema
chronicus, lichen simplex
chronological age (CA)
chronotropic incompetence
chronotropic response
chronotropism, negative
chronotropism, positive
chroococcum, Azotobacter
Chrysomyia
C. albiceps
C. bezziana
C. macellaria
Chrysops
C. cecutiens
C. dimidiata
C. discalis
C. silacea
chrysorrhoea, Euproctis
church affiliation

church community supportive
Churg-Strauss angiitis
Churg-Strauss syndrome
Chvostek('s)
C. anemia
C. sign
C. symptom
C. syndrome
C. -Weiss sign
chyle fat
chyli, cisterna
chyliform
c. ascites
c. pleural effusion
c. pleurisy
chylomicron
c. emulsion
c. remnant
c. remnant receptor
chylosa, diarrhea
chylosus, ascites
chylous
c. ascites
c. hydrocele
c. hydrothorax
c. pericardial effusion
c. peritonitis
c. pleurisy
c. urine
CI (cardiac index)
CI (cardiac insufficiency)
CI (color index)
CI (coronary insufficiency)
cibum, ante
cicatriceum, ectropion
cicatricial
c. contraction
c. ectropion
c. kidney
c. mass
c. scoliosis
c. stenosis
c. stenosis of canaliculus
c. stenosis of lacrimonasal duct
c. stricture
c. tissue
cicatrix
c., filtering
c., manometric
c. of limbus
c. of limbus ▸ cystoid
c., trophic
c., umbilical
c., vicious
cicatrization index

cicatrizing atelectasis
cicatrizing enteritis
CICU (Cardiology Intensive Care Unit)
CICU (Coronary Intensive Care Unit)
Cicuta maculata
Cicuta virosa
cidal effect
cigar-shaped rods ▸ gram-negative
cigarette(s)
    c. addiction
    c. breakaway hypnosis program
    c., cannabis
    c. cough
    c., craving for
    c. drain
    c. induced lung disease
    c. induced obstructive lung disease
    c., low tar/nicotine (T/N)
    c. (Ace), marijuana
    c. (Doobie), marijuana
    c. (Joint), marijuana
    c. (Number), marijuana
    c. (Smoke), marijuana
    c. (Reefer), marijuana
    c. (Roach) marijuana
    c. (Stick), marijuana
    c. paper patch
    c., Sherman
    c. smoke asthma
    c. smoke ▸ environmental
    c., smokeless
    c. smoker
    c. smoking
    c. smoking and drug abuse ▸ linking
    c. smoking ▸ cessation of
    c. withdrawal symptoms
ciguatera poisoning
Cilco intraocular lens
cilia syndrome ▸ immotile
ciliares, plicae
ciliares, striae
ciliaris
    c., acne
    c., annulus
    c., blepharitis
    c., corona
    c., corpus
    c. muscle
    c., orbicularis
    c., orbiculus
    c., zonula
ciliary
    c. action
    c. artery, long posterior

c. artery, short posterior
c. axis, long posterior
c. axis, short posterior
c. beat
c. beat frequency
c. body
c. body cyst
c. body ▸ foreign body (FB) in
c. body involvement
c. body, iris
c. crown
c. disk
c. dysentery
c. epithelium
c. folds
c. ganglion
c. ligament
c. movement
c. muscle
c. nerves, long
c. nerves, short
c. process
c. reflex
c. region
c. staphyloma
c. vein
c. vessels ▸ anomaly optics◊
c. zonule
ciliate dysentery
ciliated
    c. cell
    c. cell adenocarcinoma
    c. epithelial cell
cilioretinal
    c. artery
    c. artery, persistent
    c. vein
    c. vein, persistent
ciliospinal center
ciliospinal reflex
cilium pacemaker
cimetidine, confusion from
cimetidine therapy
Cimex
    C. boueti
    C. hemipterus
    C. lectularius
    C. pilosellus
    C. pipistrella
Cimicifuga racemosa
Cimino
    C. arteriovenous (AV) shunt
    C. AV (arteriovenous) fistula ▸ Brescio-
    C. fistula

CIN (cervical intraepithelial neoplasia)
C_{in} (insulin clearance)
Cinchona
    C. calisaya
    C. ledgeriana
    C. succirubra
cincinnatiensis, Legionella
cincture [tincture]
cincture sensation
Cinderella syndrome
cine
    c. computed tomography
    c. loop
    c. loop recording
    c. pulse system
cineangiocardiogram study
cineangiocardiography, radionuclide
cineangiography
    c. and densitometric ejection fraction
    c., conventional
    c., coronary
    c., left coronary
    c., right coronary
    c. study
    c., ventricular function and
cinebronchogram study
cinedensitometric assessment of transit times
cinedensitometric transit time
cinefluorography study
cinema eye
cinemagnetic resonance imaging ▸ velocity encoded
cinephonation study
cineplastic amputation
cineradiographic examination
cinerea
    c., ala
    c., Epicauta
    c., taenia
    c., taeniola
    c., trabecula
cinereus, Aedes
cinereus, Scopulariopsis
cingular gyrus herniation
cingulata, Cerithidia
cingulate
    c. cortex
    c. cortex, anterior
    c. gyrus
    c. sulcus
cinguli
    c., gyrus
    c., pars sulci

c., sulcus
cingulotomy procedure
cintus, Paragordius
CIP (cardiac invasive procedure)
circadian
  c. biological rhythms
  c. cycle
  c. desynchronization
  c. event recorder
  c. pacemaker, body's
  c. pattern
  c. quotient
  c. rhythm
  c. rhythm disturbance syndrome
  c. rhythm sleep disorder
  c. variation
circinata, balanitis
circinate retinitis
circinate retinopathy
circinatus, favus
circlage (see cerclage)
circle(s)
  c. concept ▸ leading
  c. hypothesis ▸ leading
  c. of confusion
  c. of Vieussens
  c. of Willis
  c. of Willis ▸ sclerosis
  c. pattern on breast self-examination ▸ concentric
  c., under-eye
  c. under eyes, dark
  c., vicious
  c., Zinn's
circled slides, etched
circlet, Zinn's
circOlectric bed
circon camera
circuit
  c., anticoincidence
  c., aortoiliofemoral
  c., arrhythmia
  c., brain
  c., bypass
  c., coincidence
  c., electrical
  c., input
  c., macroreentrant
  c., magnetic
  c., patient breathing
  c., phototube output
  c., reentrant
circulaire, folie
circulans, Bacillus

circular
  c. amputation
  c. bandage
  c. bandaging
  c. block anesthesia
  c. enterorrhaphy
  c. fibers
  c. flap
  c. fold
  c. hymen
  c. incision
  c. insanity
  c. interaction between anxiety and pain
  c. inverting suture ▸ continuous
  c. lesion
  c. massaging motion
  c. microtron
  c. motion
  c. muscle
  c. patch plasty ▸ endoventricular
  c. pressure maneuver during massage
  c. psychosis
  c. Santorini's muscles
  c. suture
  c. thinking
circularis, sulcus
circularity index ▸ Gibson
circulated to machine for cleaning ▸ patient's blood
circulates blood, heart
circulating
  c. blood volume
  c. blood volume, effective
  c. cholesterol
  c. fat
  c. granulocyte pool
  c. hemoglobin, total
  c. megakaryocytes
  c. nurse
  c. pituitary hormones
  c. platelets
  c. volume, reduce
circulation
  c. (ABC) ▸ airway breathing and
  c., allantoic
  c., anorectal
  c., arterial
  c., artificial
  c., assisted
  c., asymmetry in blood
  c., auxiliary
  c., balanced
  c., blood

  c., bone
  c., bronchial
  c., cardiopulmonary
  c., cerebral
  c., cerebrovascular blood
  c., collateral
  c. ▸ common disorder of
  c., compensatory
  c., coronary
  c., coronary artery
  c., coronary collateral
  c., cross
  c., decreased hand
  c., decreased leg
  c., deficient
  c., derivative
  c. embarrassment, coronary
  c., embryonic
  c., enterohepatic
  c., extracorporeal
  c., fetal
  c., first
  c., fistula
  c., fourth
  c., general hepatic
  c., good peripheral
  c., greater
  c., hepatofugal venous collateral
  c., impaired
  c., improve
  c. in brain
  c. in hands, poor
  c. in toes, poor
  c., inadequacy of systemic
  c., inadequate
  c., inhibit fetal
  c. ▸ insufficient coronary artery
  c., intervillous
  c. ▸ left dominant coronary
  c., leg
  c., lesser
  c., localized interference with
  c., lymph
  c., myocardial
  c., normal blood
  c. of blood
  c., omphalomesenteric
  c. on 4 vessel angiography ▸ total absence of
  c., parumbilical cutaneous
  c., peripheral
  c. ▸ persistent fetal
  c., placental
  c., poor
  c., poor arterial

circulation—*continued*
  c., poor blood
  c., poor peripheral
  c. ▸ poor venous
  c., portal
  c., portoumbilical
  c., primitive
  c. problems, blood-
  c., pulmonary
  c., reduced
  c., renal
  c., sinusoidal
  c., sluggish
  c., small vessel
  c. ▸ spinal fluid
  c., stimulatic
  c. system
  c. system, blood
  c., systemic
  c., thebesian
  c. time
  c. time (MCT) ▸ mean
  c. to brain
  c. to lung
  c. to lungs ▸ arterial
  c. to optic nerve
  c. to the feet, poor
  c., umbilical
  c., venous
  c., venous blood
  c., vitelline
  c. volume
circulatory
  c. and respiratory functions ▸
    irreversible cessation of
  c. arrest
  c. arrest, deep hypothermia
  c. assist ▸ external
  c. assist (EPCA) ▸ external
    pressure
  c. collapse
  c. compromise
  c. congestion
  c. constriction
  c. control
  c. deficiency
  c. disease
  c. disorder
  c. embarrassment
  c. factor
  c. fluid
  c. hematocrit (HCT), mean
  c. hypoxia
  c. overload
  c. problem

  c. problem ▸ clamminess from
  c. problem ▸ foot problem from
  c. problem from diabetes
  c. problem ▸ nails breaking from
  c. problem with cold sensitivity
  c. shock ▸ treatment of
  c. support system
  c. system function
  c. system, peripheral
  c. systems of body
  c. values, peripheral
circumareolar incision
circumcaval ureter
circumcise [*circumscribe***]**
circumcised, patient
circumcised, patient not
circumcision, newborn
circumcision ▸ release form for ritual
circumcorneal incision
circumference
  c., abdominal
  c., chest
  c., head
  c., occipitofrontal
circumferential
  c. arrays
  c. bipolar montage
  c. erosion
  c. fiber shortening
  c. fiber shortening ▸ velocity of
  c. fracture
  c. implantation
  c. incision
  c. invasive carcinoma
  c. lesion, sharply demarcated
  c. wall stress
  c. wiring
circumflex
  c. aortic arch
  c. artery, atrial
  c. artery ▸ left
  c. artery ▸ marginal
  c. artery ▸ posterior
  c. artery stenosis
  c. coronary artery (LCA), left
  c. coronary artery (RCA), right
  c., distal portion main
  c. femoral veins ▸ lateral
  c. femoral veins ▸ medial
  c. iliac vein ▸ deep
  c. iliac vein ▸ superficial
  c. nerve
  c. retroesophageal arch
  c. system, small
circumflexed branch

circumluteolis, Aedes
circumoral
  c. area of columnar epithelium
  c. cyanosis
  c. incision
circumscribed
  c. amnesia
  c. area
  c. atrophy of brain
  c. edema
  c. leptomeningitis
  c. lesion
  c. new growth
  c. nodule ▸ small firm
  c. pleurisy
circumscribing incision
circumscripta
  c., calcinosis cutis
  c. cystica, meningitis serosa
  c., meningitis serosa
  c., neurodermatitis
circumscriptum, lymphangioma
circumstance(s)
  c., family
  c., life-threatening
  c. of death
  c. ▸ other specified family
  c. problem, life
  c., relapse
  c. ▸ sensitive to environmental
circumstantial analysis
circumvallata, placenta
circumvallate papillae
circumvallate placenta
circumvent blockage
circus
  c. movement tachycardia
  c. movement tachycardia,
    antidromic
  c. rhythm
cirrhosis [*sclerosis***]**
  c., acholangic biliary
  c., advanced
  c., alcoholic
  c., atrophic
  c., bacterial
  c., biliary
  c., Budd's
  c., calculus
  c., cardiac
  c., cardiotuberculous
  c., Charcot's
  c., confusion from
  c., congestive
  c., Cruveilhier-Baumgarten

c., fatty
c. from alcohol
c. from hepatitis
c., Glisson's
c., Hanot's
c., hepatic
c., hypertrophic
c., Indian childhood
c., indigestion from
c., jaundice from
c., Laennec's
c., Maixner's
c., malarial
c. mammae
c., metabolic
c., micronodular
c., multilobular
c., nausea from
c. of children ▸ biliary
c. of kidney
c. of liver
c. of lung
c. of stomach
c., periportal
c., peritonitis from
c., pigment
c., pipe stem
c., portal
c., posthepatic
c., postnecrotic
c. (PBC), primary biliary
c., pulmonary
c., secondary biliary
c., severe micronodular
c. ▸ spider marks from
c., stasis
c., suburban
c., syphilitic
c. ▸ tissue scarring or
c., Todd's
c., toxic
c., unilobular
c., vascular
c. ▸ white or pale nails from
cirrhotic
   c. gastritis
   c. liver
   c. liver, biliary
cirrus [serous, scirrhous, scirrhus]
cirsoid
   c. aneurysm
   c. placenta
   c. varix
cirsoides, placenta
CIS (carcinoma in situ)

cistern(s)
   c., basal
   c., basilar
   c., cerebellomedullary
   c., chiasmatic
   c., great
   c., interpeduncular
   c. of chiasm
   c. fossa of Sylvius
   c. of lateral fossa of cerebrum
   c. of Sylvius
   c., Pecquet's
   c., posterior
   c., subarachnoidal
cisterna
   c. chyli
   c. magna
   c., subarachnoid
   c., subsarcolemma
   c., terminal
cisternal puncture
cisternal tap
cisternography
   c., metrizamide
   c., oxygen
   c., radionuclide
cistoplatin, high dose methotrexate and
cite [site, sight]
citreus, Staphylococcus
Citrobacter [*Siderobacter*]
   C. amalonaticus
   C. freundii
   C. freundii urinary tract infection
   C. species
   C., Bethesda-Ballerup
citrovorum
   c. factor
   c. rescue
   c. rescue chemotherapy
   c. rescue factor
citrullus, Cucurbita
city cultures, triad of
city-wide clinics
civil liability exemptions
CJ (phencyclidine)
CK (conductive keratoplasty)
CK/MB fraction
Clado's anastomosis
Cladosporium
   C. carrionii
   C. herbarum
   C. mansoni
   C. trichoides
   C. werneckii
Clagett closure

claim(s)
   c., assigned
   c., insurance
   c., Medicare
   c., paranormal
   c., unassigned
   c., unproven health
clairvoyant dream
clamminess from circulatory problem
clamminess of skin
clammy
   c., patient cold and
   c. skin
   c. skin cold and
   c. skin, cool,
   c. skin ▸ pale and
clamp time, cross-
clamped
   c. and coagulated ▸ muscle bleeding points individually
   c. and cut
   c. and divided ▸ doubly
   c. and ligated
   c. and ligated ▸ bleeders
   c. and tied ▸ bleeders
   c., aorta cross-
   c., bleeders
   c., cord
   c., cut and ligated ▸ mesoappendix serially
   c., divided and tied
   c., doubly
   c., serially
   c., transected and stump ligated ▸ doubly
clamping habit
clamping of the aorta ▸ cross-
clamshell (Clamshell)
   c. closure
   c. closure of atrial septal defect
   c. device
   C. septal umbrella
   C. septal umbrella, Bard
   c. thoracotomy
clandestine myocardial ischemia
clang association
clapotement, bruit de
clapping, hand
claquement, bruit de
Clara cell adenocarcinoma
Clara cells
clarity, cognitive
clarity, mental
Clark('s)
   C. level of malignant melanoma

Clark('s)—*continued*
    C. ▸ nucleus lateralis of LeGros
    C. scale
Clarke-Hadefield syndrome
clasmocytic lymphoma
clasp [rasp, grasp]
    c., ball
    c. guideline
    c. -knife reflex
    c. -knife rigidity
class(es)
    c., childbirth preparation
    c., cognition
    c., drug
    c., expectant parents
    c., functional
    c. medical model ▸ middle-
    c., parenting
    c., postnatal
    c., postpartum
    c., prenatal
    c., sibling
    c., social
    c. stroke education
    c. syndrome, economy
    c. to Hepatitis B Core Antigen
        (Anti-HBc IgM) ▸ Antibody IgM
classic
    c. apraxia
    c. cesarean (C-) section
    c. headache preceded by aura
    c. incision
    c. massage
    c. migraine
    c. push-ups
    c. syndrome
    c. technique
classical
    c. conditioning
    c. dosimetry
    c. incision
    c. scattering
    c. signs of rejection
classification (Classification)
    c., Angle's
    c., Arneth's
    c., Broders'
    c., Caldwell-Moloy
    c., cancer
    c., Denver
    c., diagnostic
    c. ▸ functional capacity
    c. in squamous cell carcinoma,
        cervical lymph node
    c., Jansky's

c., Jensen's
c., Jewett's
c., Keith-Wagener-Barker
c., Kennedy
c., Kraepelin's
c., Lancefield
c., McNeer
c., Migula's
C., Moss'
c., New York Heart Association
    (NYHA)
c. of carcinoma, Dukes'
c. of convergence insufficiency ▸
    Duane
c. of host
c. of malignant tumors
c. of right ascending colon ▸ Dukes
    C
c., pathologic
c., Reese-Ellsworth
c. ▸ round-robin
c., stone density
c., surgical wound
c. system for cancer
C. Test (AGCT) ▸ Army General
c., therapeutic
c. ▸ tumor, nodes, metastases
    (TNM)
c., Wiberg
classroom behavior of child
Clatworthy side-to-end vena caval
    shunt ▸ Marion-
Claude's hyperkinesis sign
Claude's syndrome
claudication
    c., buttock
    c., calf
    c. in the legs
    c., intermittent
    c., intestinal
    c., ischemic
    c., jaw
    c. limb pain
    c., neural
    c. of legs ▸ painful
    c. ▸ one block
    c. ▸ three block
    c. ▸ two block
    c. ▸ two flights of stairs
    c., vascular
    c., venous
Claudius' fossa
clausa rhinolalia
claustrum [*colostrum*]
clavatus, Aspergillus

clavatus, Porocephalus
Claviceps purpurea
clavicle bone
clavicle, dislocated
clavicular
    c. fracture fragments
    c. notch of sternum
    c. region
clavipectoral triangle
claw
    c. deformity, lobster-
    c. hand
    c. hand, lobster-
    c. -like deformity
    c. toe position
clawhand, syringomyelic
clay
    c. -colored stools
    c. -like consistency
    c. -shoveler fracture
claypipe cancer
clean
    c. and dry ▸ incision
    c. and healed ▸ operative wounds
    c. and healed ▸ wound
    c. catch urinalysis
    c. catch urine
    c. cervix
    c. -contaminated wound
    c. -out, pelvic
    c. -voided specimen
    c. wound
cleaned x-ray tables ▸ inadequately
cleaning
    c. agent, plaque-
    c. compulsion
    c. of ear
    c., ▸ patient's blood circulated to
        machine for
    c., skin
cleanliness fixation
cleanliness, personal
cleansed, skin
cleanser, skin wound
cleansing
    c. blood
    c., bowel
    c. breath, deep
    c., colon
    c., emotional
    c. emulsion, hexachlorophene
    c. enema
    c. enema set ▸ disposable
    c., general alcohol
    c. umbilical cord

clear(s) (Clears)
  c. airway
  C. (amphetamines), ▸ Brown and
  c. cell adenocarcinoma
  c. cell carcinoma
  c. cell tumor
  c. cell, water-
  c. cells
  c. fluid
  c. liquid diet
  c. lung fields
  c., lungs
  c., nasal airways
  c. on auscultation ▸ lungs
  c. ▸ patient mentally
  c. pulmonary fields
  c. scans
  c., sclerae and conjunctivae
  c., sensorium is
  c., spinal fluid
  c. surgical diet
  c. throat
  c. to auscultation
  c. to P and A (percussion and auscultation) ▸ chest
  c. to P and A (percussion and auscultation) ▸ lungs
  c. to percussion
  c. to percussion and auscultation (P and A) ▸ chest
  c. to percussion and auscultation (P and A) ▸ lungs
  c. to percussion ▸ right apex
  c. urine
  c. urine, effluxed

clearance
  c., airway
  c., albumin
  c., amylase
  c., blood urea
  c., creatinine
  c., drug
  c., gas
  c. ▸ ineffective airway
  c., insulin
  c., inulin
  c. measurement ▸ gas
  c. method ▸ gas
  c., mucociliary
  c., para-aminohippurate
  c. rate
  c. rate, metabolic
  c., renal
  c. technique
  c. test, creatinine
  c. test, insulin
  c. test, urea
  c., urea
  c., urine creatinine

cleared, urinary tract infection
clearing
  c., evidence of
  c. from anxiety ▸ throat
  c., interval
  c. medium
  c. of airway
  c. of infiltrate
  c. of mental symptoms
  c. of pulmonary airways
  c. of sensorium
  c., partial
  c. repetitious activity ▸ mind
  c., signs of
  c., throat

Clearsby iris spatula
cleavage
  c. base
  c. cell
  c. fracture
  c. line
  c. of cardiac valve, abnormal

Cleaves' position
cleaving, freeze-
Cleeman's sign
cleft(s)
  c. anterior leaflet
  c., branchial
  c. cyst, branchial
  c. foot
  c. hand
  c., interstitial
  c. lip
  c. lip and palate
  c., middle ear
  c. mitral valve
  c. nose
  c. of cervix
  c. palate
  c. palate, brachygnathia and
  c. palate, congenital
  c. palate impression
  c. palate, posterior
  c. palate prosthesis
  c., pharyngeal
  c., Sondergaard's
  c., synaptic
  c. tongue

cleidocranial dysostosis
cleidotomy, fetal
Cleland's ligament

clenched
  c. fist sign
  c., fists
  c., hand
  c. jaw
  c. muscles in head and neck

clenching
  c. and grinding ▸ teeth
  c., extreme jaw
  c. of teeth ▸ gnashing and

Clerembault's syndrome, de
clergy
  c. intervention
  c. person
  c. support

clerical aptitude
Clerk
  C., Surgical
  C., Unit
  C., Ward

click(s)
  c., early
  c., ejection
  c., Hamman's
  c. heard at hip joint
  c., hip
  c., metallic
  c., midsystolic
  c., mitral
  c., multiple
  c. murmur
  c. -murmur syndrome
  c. murmur syndrome ▸ systolic
  c. ▸ nonejection systolic
  c., Ortolani's
  c., rarefaction
  c. syndrome
  c. syndrome ▸ midsystolic
  c., systolic
  c., systolic ejection

clicking
  c. noise
  c. of malfunctioning valve
  c. pneumothorax
  c. rales
  c. sensation
  c. sound

client(s)
  c. -centered therapy
  c. drop-out
  c., drug-dependent
  c., dysfunctional
  c., problem drinking
  c. readiness
  c., treatment-seeking

climacteric insanity
climacterium praecox
climatic change ▸ nonspecific
climax, Trichodectes
climbing ▸ excessive stair
clinging to parents
clinic(s) (Clinic)
    c., ambulatory
    c., balance motion
    c., blood pressure (BP)
    C., Cast
    c., city-wide
    c., community
    C. 18 linear accelerator
    C., Emergency Medicine
    c., fertility
    c., free
    c., free drug treatment
    c., free-standing
    c., geriatric
    c., headache
    c., industrial
    c., methadone detoxification
    c., multidisciplinary pain
    c., no smoking
    C., Outpatient
    C. ▸ Outpatient Chemical
       Dependency
    C. ▸ Outpatient Community
    c., pain control
    c., physician owned
    c. program, pain
    c., quit smoking
    c., rehabilitation
    c., remote
    c., sleep
    c., sports medicine
    c., syncope
    c., vaccination
    C. (VDC) ▸ Venereal Disease
    c., walk-in laser
clinical
    c. adverse experiences
    c. alcoholic hepatitis
    c. alcoholic liver disease
    c. and pharmacological interactions
    c. anxiety
    C. Anxiety Scale ▸ Thayer
    c. application
    c. application of thermography
    c. aspect
    c. assay
    c. assessment
    c. attack
    c. attention ▸ focus of

c. audiologist
c. authorization certificate
c. behavior
c. biostatistics
c. brain death
c. breast examination
c. cancer research
c. case formulation
c. changes
c. characteristics
c. competence
c. complication
c. condition, patient's
c. coordinator
c. course (CC)
c. correlation
c. criteria
c. crown
c. cure
c. data
C. Data Repository (CDR)
c. death
c. decision-making
c. dehydration
c. depression
c. depression ▸ develop symptoms
    of
c. dermatology
c. deterioration
c. deterioration, progressive
c. diagnosis
c. diagnostic staging
c. dietitian
c. disorder
c. drug evaluation program
c. ecology
c. education
c. effects
c. encephalitis
c. entity
c. epileptic disorders
c. epileptic manifestations
c. episode
c. evaluation
c. event, adverse
c. events
c. evidence
c. evidence of metastatic disease
c. examination
c. experience
c. experiment
c. expertise
c. findings
c. follow-through
c. genetics

c. gerontology
c. heart disease
c. hepatitis
c. hepatitis, transient
c. history
c. hypnosis
c. hypnotherapy
c. illness
c. illness, acute
c. implications
c. impression
c. indicators
c. infection syndromes
c. information
c. interaction and detoxification
c. interpretation
c. intervention
c. interview
c. investigation
c. isolates of bacteria
c. issues
c. judgment
c. laboratory testing
c. literature
c. management
c. maneuvers
c. manifestations
c. manifestations of acute drug
    intoxication
c. manifestations of drug reaction
c. manifestations of flashback
    reactions
c. manifestations of organic brain
    syndrome
c. manifestations of panic reactions
c. manifestations of withdrawal
c. manifestations with overdosing
c. material
c. material ▸ stained smear of
c. medicine
c. microscopy
c. mycology data
c. needs
c. neuropsychologist
c. neuropsychology
c. nightmare, perplexing
c. note
c. nurse
c. nurse manager
c. nurse specialist
c. oncologist
c. oncology
c. osteoporosis
c. otosclerosis
c. parameters

c. patient care
c. pattern
c. pediatric psychopharmacology
c. performance score
c. perspectives
c. pharmacology
c. pharmacology patient, irritable
c. physician
c. picture
c. placement
c. placement ▸ rational/empirical
c. population
c. practice
c. practice issues
c. practice, standards of
c. presentation
c. problems
c. procedures
c. profile
c. program development
c. protocol
c. psychiatry
c. psychoanalysis
c. psychological study
c. psychologist
c. psychology
c. psychopharmacology
c., qualified
c. radiation therapy
c. records
c. relationship
c. remission
c. remission, complete
c. research
C. Research Associates (CRA)
c. research program
c. research subject
c. research trial
c. research unit
c. seizure
c. septic shock
c. service, general
c. services, discounted
c. services, uncompensated
c. setting
c. side-effects
c. significance
c. significance, controversial
c. signs
c. signs and symptoms
c. skills
c. skin care
c. social work
c. social worker
c. specialist

c. specimen
c. spectrum of cancer
c. staff member
c. stage
c. staging
c. standpoint
c. status of nodes
c. studies
c. support
c. symptoms
c. syndrome
c. syndrome, multiple
c. testing
c. toxicity
c. toxicologist
c. training
c. treatment
c. trial
c. trial, adequate
c. trial, analysis at conclusion of
c. trial, controlled
c. trial ▸ double-blind
c. trial ▸ multicenter
c. trial, national
c. trial, ongoing
c. trial ▸ placebo-controlled
c. trial ▸ random control
c. trial, randomized
c. trial ▸ randomized controlled
c. trial ▸ short-term
c. trial summary
c. trials, exclusion rate and
c. trials, false-negative results in
c. trials, matched control studies in
c. trials, methodology
c. trials, multi-institutional
c. trials, nonrandomized
c. trials, pilot study in
c. trials, protocol for
c. trials, randomized
c. trials, randomized vs
    nonrandomized
c. use
c. validity
c. value (MCV) ▸ mean
c. virological efficacy ▸ potential
clinically
c. active stage
c. assess
c. depressed
c. diagnosable seizure
c. effective
c., regressed
c. stable, patient
c. undetected fungal infections

clinician(s)
c., emergency
c., psychiatric nurse
c., responsible
c., trained
clinicopathologic conference
clinicopathologic manifestations
Clinitest, urine tested with
Clinitron Bed
clinoid process
clinostatic bradycardia
clip
c., ligation
c., vascular
c. ▸ vena cava
clipped
c., aneurysm
c., intracranial aneurysm
c., speech
clipping
c., aneurysm
c. middle cerebral artery
c. of blood vessel
c., surgical
clitoridis
c., corpus
c., corpus cavernosum
c., crus
c., crus glandis
c., glans
c., plexus cavernosus
c., septum corporum
    cavernosorum
c., smegma
clitoris
c., bifid
c., cavernosus plexus of
c., cavernous nerves of
c., crura of
c., deep dorsal vein of
c., deep vein of
c., dorsal nerve of
c., enlargement of
c., frenulum of
c., glans of
c., horn of
c., prepuce of
c., superficial dorsal veins of
clivogram test
CLL (chronic lymphocytic leukemia)
cloacae
c., Aerobacter
c., Bacterium
c., Enterobacter
cloacal duct, Reichel's

clock
- c., biological
- c., body's biological
- c. -drawing test
- c., internal
- c. ▸ internal body

clockwise rotation

clockwise torque

clogged
- c. airway
- c. artery
- c. artery ▸ partially
- c. bowel
- c. bypass graft
- c. coronary artery
- c. neck artery
- c. shunt
- c. urinary tract
- c. vessel

clogging
- c. clot ▸ artery-
- c. disease, artery-
- c. fat, artery-
- c. food, artery-
- c. of artery
- c. plaque in atherosclerosis patient ▸ artery-
- c. thrombus, artery-

clonic [chronic, tonic]
- c. contraction
- c. convulsion
- c. motor response
- c. movement, tonic-
- c. perseveration
- c. phase
- c. seizure
- c. seizures, localized
- c. seizures, tonic-
- c. seizures ▸ uncontrolled generalized, tonic-
- c. spasm
- c. spasm of voluntary muscles
- c. spasm ▸ tonic-
- c. -tonic

cloning gene

clonogenic
- c. assay
- c. cell
- c. cell content
- c. technique

Clonorchis
- C. endemicus
- C. sinensis
- C. Trematoda

clonus [tonus, conus]

- c., abortive
- c., ankle
- c., anodal closure
- c., cathodal closure
- c., cathodal opening
- c., knee
- c. reflex, wrist
- c., sustained
- c., unsustained

Cloquet's
- C. canal
- C. ganglion
- C. hernia
- C. node

close
- c. eye ▸ inability to
- c. grip bench press
- c. the skin
- c. -up vision

closed
- c. amputation
- c. anatomically, incision
- c. anesthesia
- c. -angle glaucoma
- c. bite
- c. -bite malocclusion
- c., bronchus transected and
- c. cervix
- c. cervix long, thick and
- c. chain
- c. -chain chain
- c. chest cardiac massage
- c. chest commissurotomy
- c. chest pneumothorax
- c. chest thoracostomy
- c. chest water seal drainage
- c., conjuctiva
- c., defect
- c. dislocation
- c. drainage (dr'ge)
- c. drainage (dr'ge) ▸ thoracotomy with
- c. ductus arteriosus
- c. eye procedure
- c., foramen ovale
- c. fracture
- c. head injury
- c. heart surgery
- c. hospital
- c. in anatomic layers
- c. in anatomic layers ▸ chest
- c. in anatomic layers ▸ wound
- c. in layers ▸ abdomen
- c. in layers ▸ incision

- c. in layers without drainage (dr'ge) ▸ wound
- c. in layers ▸ wound
- c. in serial fashion, incision
- c., incision loosely
- c. injury
- c. iris forceps
- c. loop
- c. loop delivery
- c. loop device
- c. loop insulin pumps
- c. loosely, wound
- c., mediastinal pleura
- c. mitral valve
- c. mouth position
- c. musculofascially, incision
- c. needle biopsy
- c. oval foramen
- c. over wound
- c., peritoneum
- c. pleural biopsy
- c. pleural drainage (dr'ge)
- c. pneumothorax
- c. reduction
- c. reduction of fracture
- c., retroperitoneum
- c. segmental fracture
- c., skin incision
- c. skull fracture
- c., subcutaneous tissues
- c. technique
- c. thoracostomy
- c. transventricular mitral commissurotomy
- c. tube drainage (dr'ge)
- c. urinary drainage (dr'ge) bag with drip chamber
- c. vessel
- c. water seal drainage system
- c. with interrupted silk ▸ skin
- c. with plain catgut ▸ periosteum
- c. with running subcuticular suture of nylon ▸ skin
- c. with sutures ▸ defect
- c. with sutures ▸ wound
- c. womb drainage
- c. womb procedure
- c. womb technique

closely spaced electrodes

closing
- c., cathodal
- c. contraction, anodal
- c. contraction, cathodal
- c. force on urethra
- c. odor, anodal

c. of leaflet, delayed
c. picture anodal
c. pressure (CP)
c. snap
c. sound, anodal
c. tetanus, cathodal

clostridial

c. food poisoning
c. gas gangrene
c. myocarditis
c. nephritis
c. species

Clostridium

C. acetobutylicum
C. aerofoetidum
C. agni
C. bifermentans
C. botulinum
C. butyricum
C. butyricum ▸ gram-positive
C. chauvoei
C. cochlearium
C. difficile
C. difficile colitis
C. difficile toxin
C. fellax
C. feseri
C. haemolyticum
C. histolyticum
C. kluyveri
C. multifermentans
C. nigrificans
C. novyi
C. oedematiens
C. ovitoxicus
C. paludis
C. parabotulinum
C. parabotulinum equii
C. pasteurianum
C. pastorianum
C. perfringens
C. septicum
C. septicum ▸ gram-positive
C. sordellii
C. sordellii ▸ gram-positive
C. species
C. sporogenes
C. sticklandii
C. tertium
C. tetani
C. tetani ▸ gram-positive
C. tetanomorphum
C. thermosaccarolyticum
C. tyrosinogenes
C. welchii

C. welchii ▸ gram-positive

closure

c., abdominal
c., abdominal wall
c., abdominal wound
c., abrupt
c. accomplished, peritoneal
c., airtight
c., airway
c., alveoloplasty reparative
c., anatomical
c., anodal
c., aortic
c., Clagett
c., clamshell
c. clonus, anodal
c. clonus, cathodal
c., complete
c. contraction, anodal
c. contraction, cathodal
c., deep
c., defective
c., delayed
c., delayed primary
c., delayed wound
c. device, bioabsorbable
c., double umbrella
c., epiphyseal
c., final
c. ▸ forceful sustained eye
c. glaucoma ▸ acute angle
c. glaucoma, angle
c., imperfect
c. index ▸ mitral valve
c. interatrial septal defect
c., Latzko's
c., layer
c., method of skin
c., mucosa-to-mucosa
c., ▸ multisided Z-plasty
c., nonoperative
c. of accidental wound ▸ delayed
c. of atrial septal defect, clamshell
c. of colostomy
c. of defect, patch
c. of eyelids ▸ involuntary forcible
c. of laceration, tape
c. of operative wound ▸ delayed
c. of peritoneum
c. of sac of aneurysm ▸ surgical
c. of semilunar valves
c. of skin wound
c. of tracheal fistula
c. of wound

c. open ends of stomach and duodenum
c., peritoneal
c., plastic
c., postoperative skin
c., primary
c., prompt surgical
c., pulmonic
c. reflex, eyelid
c. reopened, temporary
c., secondary
c., skin
c. sound, aortic
c. sound ▸ pulmonic
c. sound ▸ pulmonic valve
c. sound ▸ tricuspid valve
c., subacute
c., temporary
c. tetanus, anodal
c. tetanus, cathodal
c., Tom Jones
c., transcatheter
c., umbrella
c., velopharyngeal
c., vessel
c., wound

clot(s)

c., agonal
c., antemortem
c., arterial blood
c. ▸ artery clogging
c., autologous
c. block, blood
c. blockage
c., blood
c., blood vessel
c. ▸ blue skin from blood
c., brain blood
c. ▸ bulging eyes from blood
c. busters
c. busting drug
c., chicken fat
c., coagulum of blood
c., dissolve
c., dissolve blood
c. ▸ dissolve life-threatening blood
c. dissolving action
c., dissolving blood
c. dissolving drug
c. dissolving therapy
c. dissolving thrombolytic drug
c. evacuated
c. evacuated, blood
c., evacuation of
c. expressed from wounds

clot(s)—*continued*
- c., fibrin
- c. formation
- c. formation ▸ increased risk of
- c. formation, inhibiting
- c. formation, reducing
- c., gummy
- c. ▸ heart attack from blood
- c. in brain or lung ▸ blood
- c. in lung ▸ blood
- c. in phlebitis ▸ blood
- c., inhibit blood
- c., laminated
- c. ▸ life-threatening blood
- c. lysed
- c. lysis
- c. lysis, dilute blood
- c. lysis time
- c. lysis time ▸ blood
- c. lysis time ▸ euglobulin
- c. lysis time ▸ streptokinase
- c. particles
- c., passage of
- c., passive
- c. ▸ pelvic blood
- c. ▸ postmortem blood
- c. present
- c. prevention
- c. ▸ pulmonary blood
- c. retraction
- c. retraction test
- c. retraction time
- c. stabilization test
- c. syndrome ▸ white
- c. trapping filters
- c. ▸ travel related blood
- c. under fingernail ▸ blood

cloth disc
clothes lice
clothes louse
clotted
- c. blood
- c. blood, freshly
- c. blood ▸ hemorrhage and
- c. blood in duodenum
- c. blood in stomach ▸ freshly
- c. hemopericardium

clotting
- c., abnormal blood
- c. abnormality
- c. action of blood
- c. capacity, blood
- c. cells, blood
- c. defect, blood
- c. disorder

- c. disorder, blood
- c., excessive
- c. factor, chemical
- c. factors
- c. factors, blood
- c. factors, purify blood
- c., increased
- c. ▸ leg vein
- c. of blood
- c. protein, blood
- c., reduce blood
- c. risk ▸ high
- c. ▸ slow blood
- c. stimulant
- c. system, blood
- c. time
- c. time, activated
- c. time, Dale-Laidlaw's
- c. time method ▸ Lee-White
- c. time, thrombin

cloud baby
cloud chamber, Wilson
clouded
- c. consciousness
- c. cornea
- c. lens
- c. sensorium
- c. vision

clouding
- c., corneal
- c., diffuse
- c., distortion and scarring
- c., hilar
- c., homogeneous
- c., mental
- c. of consciousness
- c. of cornea
- c. of ethmoids
- c. of eye lens
- c. of lens ▸ progressive
- c. of sinuses

cloudy
- c. fluid
- c., fluid grossly
- c. iris
- c. lens
- c., patient mentally
- c. swelling
- c., urine
- c. vision

clove hitch
clover disease ▸ sweet
cloverleaf plate
cloverleaf-type deformity
Cloward's operation

Cloward's procedure
club (Club)
- c. foot
- c. fungus
- c. hair
- c. hand
- c., health
- C., Ostomy

clubbed penis
clubbing
- c. and cyanosis upper extremities
- c., digital
- c., edema or swelling
- c., finger
- c. of distal phalanges
- c. of extremities
- c. of fingers
- c. of toes
- c. or edema ▸ cyanosis,
- c. or tremor

clubfoot, bilateral
clue cells
clump(s)
- c. and nucleoli ▸ chromatin
- c. and nucleoli ▸ coarse chromatin
- c. cells
- c. kidney
- c. of bacteria

clumping
- c. in blood, platelet
- c. of platelets
- c. of tangled fibers
- c. test, staphylococcal

clumsy hand movements
clumsy hand dysarthria
clumsy, patient
clunial
- c. nerves, inferior
- c. nerves, middle
- c. nerves, superior

cluster(s)
- c., abnormal
- c., cell
- c. disorder ▸ dramatic
- c., epidemic
- c., gram-positive cocci in
- c. headache
- c. ▸ multiple symptom
- c. of bacteria
- c. -of-grapes appearance
- c. of infections
- c. of isolates
- c. of milk-secreting alveoli
- c. of seizures ▸ little
- c. of short gram-negative rods

c. of tubercles
c. of tumor cells
c. suicides
clutter stress syndrome
Clutton's joint
Clyde Mood Scale
Clysodrast contrast medium
cm (centimeter)
cm (cubic centimeter) ▸ cu
cm (centimeters) ▸ **liver down** _____
CMF (cyclophosphamide, methotrexate, fluorouracil)
CMF (Cytoxan, methotrexate, 5-fluorouracil)
CMG (cystometrogram)
CMI (carbohydrate metabolism index)
CMID (cytomegalic inclusion disease)
CMID (cytomegalic inclusion disease) of newborn
CMID (cytomegalic inclusion disease) virus
C/min (cycles per minute)
CML (chronic myelocytic leukemia)
CML (chronic myelogenous leukemia)
cmm (cubic millimeter)
CMO (cardiac minute output)
cmps (centimeters per second)
cm/sec (centimeters per second)
cm^3 (cubic centimeter)
CMV (cytomegalovirus) infection
CMV (cytomegalovirus) infection, primary
CNS (central nervous system)
CNS defect
CNS depressant
CNS depression
CNS deterioration, organic
CNS disease
CNS disorder
CNS dysfunction
CNS functioning
CNS hypersomnolence ▸ idiopathic
CNS infarction
CNS, infratentorial parts of
CNS infection, nosocomial
CNS, intracranial part of
CNS lesion ▸ microscopic
CNS lymphoma, primary
CNS ▸ macroscopic
CNS sequelae
CNS shunt
CNS stimulant
CNS therapy
CNS trauma
CNV (contingent negative variation)

CO (carbon monoxide)
c/o (complained of)
CO (carbon monoxide) poisoning
coach in delivery
coagulant complex, anti-inhibitor
coagulant therapy
coagulase
c. enzyme
c. negative
c. negative Staphylococci (Staph)
c. positive
c. positive ▸ Staph aureus
coagulate or vaporize, cut
coagulate tissues
coagulated
c. albumin
c., bleeders
c., bleeding points
c. blood
c., muscle bleeding points individually clamped and
coagulating current, Bovie
coagulation
c., bipolar
c., blood
c. cascade
c. (DIC), diffuse intravascular
c. disorder
c. (DIC) ▸ disseminated intravascular
c., electro◊
c. factor (I-XIII), blood
c. factor ▸ fibrin-stabilizing blood
c. factors (I through XIII), blood
c. (IRC), infrared
c. (IRC), infrared heat
c. inhibitor ▸ lipoprotein-associated
c., light
c. monitoring, blood
c., multipolar
c. of bleeding gastrointestinal (GI) lesion
c. of hemorrhoids ▸ infrared
c. of tissue
c. phenomena
c., photo◊
c. protein
c. reaction
c. screen test
c. syndrome, colon
c. system ▸ plasma
c. test
c. thrombosis
c. time
c. time, activated
c. time, blood

coagulative myocytolysis
coagulative necrosis
coagulopathy
c., consumption
c. (DIC), diffuse intravascular
c., disseminated intravascular
c., intravascular
c. ▸ intravascular consumption
coagulum formation
coal
c. miners' lung
c. tar
c. tar bath
c. tar soap
c. workers' anthracosis
c. workers' pneumoconiosis
coalescing punctuation
coaptation suture
coarctate retina
coarctation
c. angioplasty, balloon
c., aortic
c., juxtaductal
c., native
c. of aorta
c. of pulmonary arteries
c., reversed
coarse [_course_]
c. breath sounds
c. chromatin clumps and nucleoli
c. crepitation
c. cytoplasmic vacuoles
c. folds
c. hand tremors
c. murmur
c. rale
c. rhonchi
c. rhonchi, scattered
c. scalp hair
c. thrill
c. trabeculation
c. tremor
c. tremors of legs
c. wrinkling
coarsely granular, lungs
coarsened mucosal fold pattern
coarsening
c., borderline
c., mucosal
c. of duodenal bulb
c., rugal
coast memory
coaster emotions ▸ roller
coat(s) (Coat) (s')
C. -a-Count radioimmunoassay

coat(s)—*continued*
- c. angina ▸ white
- C. disease
- c. effect ▸ white
- c. hypertension, white
- c. of eye, choroid
- c. phenomenon ▸ white
- c. phobia ▸ white
- c., protein
- C. retinitis
- C. ring
- c. -sleeve amputation
- c. smear, buffy
- c. syndrome ▸ white

coated
- c. aspirin ▸ enteric
- c. cells, buffy
- c., enteric
- c., polyester suture
- c. stent ▸ drug
- c. stents, chemically
- c. stents ▸ physically
- c. tablet, enteric
- c., tongue
- c. tube ▸ drug
- c. vascular graft, albumin-

coating
- c. autoradiography, ▸ dip-
- c. back of tongue ▸ whitish
- c. stool, blood
- c. stool, pus
- c., tongue

coaxial electrode system, magnetic induction
coaxial pressure
cobalt
- c. beam
- c. cardiomyopathy
- c. irradiation, external
- c., large field
- c. radiation
- c. 60 (Co^{60}) eye plaques
- c. 60 (Co^{60}) teletherapy machine
- c. 60 (Co^{60}) therapy
- c. syndrome, beer and

cobbler's chest
cobbler's suture
cobblestone
- c. appearance
- c. degeneration
- c. tongue

Cobb's method
Cobe cardiotomy reservoir
cobra-head anastomosis
Coburn intraocular lenses (IOL)

Coca (cocaine)
coca, Erythroxylon
cocaine (*Cocaine*)
- c. (Blow)
- c. (C)
- c. (Coca)
- c. (Coke)
- c. (Cola)
- c. (Flake)
- c. (Girl)
- c. (Heaven Dust)
- c. (Ice)
- c. (Lady)
- c. (Line)
- c. (Mujer)
- c. (Nose)
- c. (Nose Candy)
- c. (Paradise)
- c. (Perico)
- c. (Peruvian Flake)
- c. (Pharmaceutical Powder)
- c. (Polvo Blanco)
- c. (Rocks)
- c. (Snow)
- c. (Toot)
- c. (White)
- c. abstinence
- c. abstinence ▸ initial
- c. abuse
- c. abuse, chronic
- c. abuse, comorbid
- c. abuse treatment
- c. abuser
- c. abuser ▸ schizophrenic
- c. abusers, retention of
- c. addiction
- c. addiction behavior
- c. addiction treatment
- c. addiction ▸ treatment of
- c. ▸ addictive use of
- c. alkaloid
- c. and crack crisis
- c. anesthesia
- c. anesthesia, topical
- c. addiction syndrome
- C. Anonymous (CA)
- c. baby
- c. binges
- c. -blocking medications
- c., blood level of
- c., crack
- c. /crack economy
- c. delirium
- c. delusional disorder
- c. dependence

- c. dependence ▸ diagnosis of
- c. dependence treatment
- c. dependency
- c. -dependent patient
- c. epidemic
- c. epidemic, crack
- c. -exposed human infants
- c. exposure
- c. exposure ▸ prenatal
- c. free base abusers
- c., free based
- c., free basing
- c. heart attack
- c. high
- c. hydrochloride
- c. -induced
- c. -induced anxiety
- c. -induced death
- c. -induced depression
- c. -induced respiratory failure
- c. ingested
- c. ingestion ▸ crack
- c. ingestion ▸ sudden death due to
- c., inhale
- c. injected
- c. injection
- c. intoxication
- c. intoxication, acute
- c., kicking
- c. ▸ long-term use of free base
- c. metabolism
- c. metabolites
- c. overdose
- c. paste
- c. paste, smoking
- c. (Ice), patient uses
- c. ▸ prenatal effects of
- c. problem
- C. Program, Intensive
- c. ▸ psychosis induced by
- c. -related complications in pregnancy
- c. -related deaths
- c. -related disorder
- c. -related heart attack victim
- c. -related obstetric disorder
- c. -related vascular headache
- c. -related violence
- c. response
- c., rock or crack
- c. rock, pure
- c. -seeking behavior
- c. seizure
- c. smoked
- c. smoker

c. smokers, habitual
c., smoking
c. ▸ smoking free-base
c. sniffed
c. snorted
c., smokeable
c., snorting
c., snorting lines of
c. soaked applicator
c. sulphate (free base)
c. (TAC) ▸ tetracaine, adrenaline and
c. -to-crime connection
c. treatment
c., urine level of
c., urine screen for
c. use, chronic
c. use, crack
c. user
c. user ▸ opioid-dependent
c. ▸ variable effects of
c. withdrawal
coccemia, meningo◊
cocci
c., aerobic gram-positive
c., chains of
c., clusters of gram-positive
c., gram-negative
c., gram-negative rods and
c., gram-positive
c., gram-positive rods and
c. granuloma
c. in clusters ▸ gram-positive
c. in pairs and chains ▸ gram-positive
c., microaerophilic
c., paired
c., short-chain
c., short-chain gram-positive
c. triad ▸ Q fever, psittacosis
Coccidia, Sporozoa
coccidioidal granuloma
coccidioides, Blastomyces
Coccidioides immitis
coccidioidin test
Coccidioidomyces fungi
coccidioidomycosis
c. arthritis
c., primary
c., primary extrapulmonary
c., pulmonary
Coccidium
C. bigeminum
C. hominis
C. tenellum

coccinella, Holothyrus
coccobacilli
c. Acinetobacter ▸ gram-negative
c. ▸ lightly staining gram-negative
c. ▸ pleomorphic gram-negative
c., small gram-negative
cocculus, Anamirta
Coccus cacti
coccus ▸ gram-positive penicillin sensitive
coccygeal
c. bone
c. ganglion
c. muscles
c. nerve
c. vertebra
c. vertebrae bone
coccygeopubic diameter
coccygodynia/coccydynia
coccyx bone
coccyx, incision of
Cochin-China diarrhea
cochlea
c., apex of
c., aqueduct of
c., canaliculus of
c., coiled
c., cupula of
c., damaged
c., dilated vestibule and
c., electrical activity of
c. fenestra
c., scala vestibuli of
c., spiral ganglion of
c., vein of canaliculus of
cochleae
c., aqueductus
c., artificial
c., canaliculus
c., columella
cochlear
c. aqueduct
c. branch
c. canal, vein of
c. cells
c. degeneration
c. duct
c. duct, cupular cecum of
c. duct, vestibular cecum of
c. implant
c. joint
c. labyrinth
c. microphonic
c. nerve
c. nerve ▸ spinal ganglion of

c. nucleus
c. potential
c. reserve
c. transplant
Cochlearia officinalis
cochleariform process
cochlearis ▸ vas prominens ductus
cochlearium, Clostridium
cochleate uterus
cochleo-orbicular reflex
cochleopalpebral reflex
cochleopalpebral reflex ▸ Gault's
cochleopapillary reflex
cochleostapedial reflex
Cochliomyia
C. americana
C. bezziana
C. hominivorax
Cockayne's syndrome
cocktail
c., anticancer
c. Brompton's
c., cardiac
c., frostbite
c., IM (intramuscular)
c., IV (intravenous)
c., lytic
c., McConckey
c., morphine
c., Philadelphia
c., Rivers'
c., scintillation
cocky, patient
coctum, sputum
COD (cause of death)
CoDA (Codependents Anonymous)
code (Code)
C., Blue
c., chemical
c., diagnostic
c., digital computer
c., electrical
c., ethical
C. Four
c., genetic
c. ▸ human genetic
C., Grey
c., Minnesota
c., molecular
c., moral
c., pacemaker
c., pacing
C., Red
c., state
c. system ▸ pacemaker

coded-aperture imaging
coded flow mapping, color-
codependency
    c., cycle of
    c., shame and
    c. skills
    c., stages of
    c., therapy
    c., treatment
codependent(s) (Codependent)(s)
    C. Anonymous (CoDA)
    c. counseling, individual
    c. patient
    c. personality
coding factor, tissue
Codivilla extension
Codivilla operation
Codman('s)
    C. exercises
    C. sign
    C. triangle
codominant characteristics
codominant system
Coe virus
co-effect thesis
coefficient
    c., absorption
    c., attenuation
    c., blood gas partition
    c., brain-blood partition
    c., capillary filtration
    c., conversion
    c. correlation
    c., damping
    c. homogeneity
    c., Lancet
    c., linear absorption
    c., mass absorption
    c., mass attenuation
    c. of diffusion
    c. of equal thickness (CET)
    c. of induction
    c. of variation
    c., partition
    c. ▸ Pearson correlation
    c., regression
    c., sedimentation
    c., Yvon's
coeliac (*see* celiac)
coeliac axis
Coenurus cerebralis
coenzyme A
COEPS (cortically originating
    extrapyramidal system)
coercive control ▸ environment of

coercive treatment
coeur en sabot
coexistent pathology
coexisting
    c. medical condition
    c. medical problems
    c. psychiatric disorders
coffee bean appearance
coffee ground emesis
Coffey scalenotomy, Adson-
Cogan
    C. dystrophy
    C. syndrome
    C. syndrome ▸ Bielschowski
Cogentin (hallucinogen)
cognition
    c. and communication ▸ learning
    c. and muscle control
    c., change in
    c. class
    c., dysfunctional
    c. ▸ mobility and
    c. ▸ profound change in
    c., subliminal
    c., temperature feedback and
cognitive
    c. abilities, patient's
    c. ability
    c. activities
    c. alteration
    c. and motor changes
    c. approach
    c. aspect of well being
    c. assessment
    c. behavior
    c. behavior therapy
    c. behavioral approach
    c. behavioral intervention
    c. behavioral technique
    c. behavioral therapy (CBT)
    c. behavioral treatment
    c. brain function ▸ disintegration of
    c. change of body image
    c. clarity
    c. complex
    c. decline
    c. decline (ARCD), age-related
    c. defect
    c. deficiencies
    c. deficits
    c. dementia
    c. deterioration ▸ progressive
    c. development
    c. development of children
    c. dexterity

    c. disability
    c. disorder ▸ human
      immunodeficiency virus (HIV)
      associated motor
    c. distortion
    c. distortions of actual events
    c. disturbance
    c. dysfunction
    c. effects
    c. environment
    c. evaluation
    c. function
    c. function ▸ level of
    c. function ▸ reduced
    c. functioning
    c. functioning, impaired
    c. functioning, sufficient
    c. functions ▸ common
    c. impairment
    c. impairment in alcoholism
    c. impairment ▸ mild
    c. impairment ▸ normal general
    c. influence
    c. information
    c. learning
    c. maintenance
    c. malfunction
    c. maturation
    c. mechanisms
    c. mediation
    c. milieu
    c. modification
    c. neuroscience
    c. perception
    c. perceptual motor skills
    c. performance
    c. performance, impaired
    c. power
    c. psychology
    c. rehabilitation
    c. reserve
    c. restructuring
    c. restructuring, confrontational
    c. restructuring ▸
      nonconfrontational
    c. retraining
    c. skills
    c. skills ▸ latency-based
    c. skills training approach
    c. slowing
    c. status
    c. strategy
    c. styles
    c. symptoms
    c. technique ▸ standard

c. techniques
c. test
c. therapy
c. therapy group
c. therapy of depression
c. therapy of personality
c. therapy of substance abuse
c. therapy skills
c. thinking, deficient
c. training
c. treatment for depression
c. understanding

cognitively
c. disabled
c. impaired
c. impaired patient
c. intact
c., patient tested

cog-tooth of malleus
cogwheel
c. motion
c. respiration
c. rigidity

cohabitation, long-term
cohabitation, sexual
coherence tomography ▸ optical
coherent
c., patient
c. scattering
c. thinking

cohesion independence
cohort study
coil (Coil)
c., blood used to prime
c. dialyzer
c. electrode
c. embolization
c. flow rate
c., implanted secondary
transformer
c. IUD (intrauterine device)
c. lesion
c., Margulles'
c., paranemic
c., plectonemic
c., primary transformer
c., relational
C., Saf-T-
c., somatic
c. spring diaphragm
c., standard
c. stent
c., ultraflow

coiled
c. bacteria ▸ lightly staining

c. bony structure
c. cochlea
c. -spring appearance
c. upon itself, catheter

coin
c. artifact
c., fracture en
c. lesion
c. lesion of lung
c. percussion
c. sound
c. test

coincidence
c. circuit
c. counting
c. detection
c. loss
c. positron
c. sum peak

co-insurance days
coke-colored stool
Coke (cocaine)
Cola (cocaine)
Colcher-Sussman method
cold(s)
c. abscess
c. agglutination
c. agglutinin
c. agglutinin disease
c. agglutinin pneumonia
c. air vaporizer
c, allergy
c. and clammy ▸ patient
c. and clammy ▸ skin
c. antibody
c. ▸ bad breath from
c. blade biopsy
c. blood cardioplegia
c. breast tumor, hot vs
c., burning, pain and numbness
c. caloric irrigation
c. cautery
c., common
c. compress
c. cone
c. crystalloid cardioplegia
c., deep
c. ▸ ear problem from
c. environment
c. ▸ excessive exposure to
c. exposure
c. ▸ eye pain from
c. feet
c., fever and
c. flashes, hot or

c. flushes, hot and
c. food related headache
c., frequent
c. gangrene
c. hands
c., head
c. hemoglobinuria ▸ paroxysmal
c. hives
c. immersion
c. -induced angina
c. -induced urticaria
c. -induced vasoconstriction
c. injury, localized
c. intolerance
c. knife cone
c. knife cone biopsy
c. knife conization
c. knife conization biopsy
c. lesion
c. light source ▸ fiberoptic
c. liquid diet
c. lysis, hot-
c. mist humidifier
c. moist skin
c., muscle seated
c. nodule
c. ▸ nose problem from
c. or ice whirlpool treatment
c. packs
c. potassium cardioplegia
c. preservative
c. pressor test
c. pressor testing maneuver
c. quartz mercury vapor lamp
c., rhinoviral
c. sensation ▸ hot and
c. sensitivity
c. sensitivity ▸ circulatory problem
with
c. ▸ sinus headache from
c., sneezing from
c. sore
c. sore ▸ blister from
c. sore ▸ burning mouth from
c. sore from chocolate
c. spot
c. spot perfusion scintigraphy ▸
myocardial
c. spots and hot spots with electron
beam dosimetry
c. stage
c. sweats
c. symptoms
c. system ▸ hot-
c. therapy

cold(s)—*continued*
- c. to the opposite, warm to the same (COWS)
- c. tolerance
- c. turkey
- c. turkey ▸ patient quitting
- c. turkey, quit
- c. urticaria
- c. virus
- c. virus ▸ mutant
- c. viruses, common
- c. water

coldness
- c., angina from
- c., emotional
- c., generalized
- c. ▸ light sensitivity from
- c. of extremity
- c. of skin ▸ lividity and
- c., sensitivity to
- c., trembling from

Cole ▸ herpetiform lesion of
colectomy, partial
Cole's operation
Coley's fluid
coli
- c. aerogenes group
- c., Amoeba
- c., Bacillus
- c. bacteremia ▸ E. (Escherichia)
- c., Bacterium
- c., Balantidium
- c., diverticulosis
- c., E (Escherichia)
- c., Entamoeba
- c. ▸ enteropathic E. (Escherichia)
- c., enteropathogenic Escherichia (E.)
- c., Escherichia (E.)
- c., gram-negative Escherichia (E.)
- c., haustrum
- c. infection ▸ gram-positive E. (Escherichia)
- c., melanosis
- c. mitis, Amoeba
- c. organisms ▸ E. (Escherichia)
- c. sepsis, E. (Escherichia)
- c. sepsis peritonitis ▸ E. (Escherichia)
- c. septicemia, E-
- c. syndrome,polyposis
- c., Vibrio

colic
- c. and allergy
- c. artery

- c., biliary
- c., bilious
- c., crapulent
- c., feigned renal
- c., gallstone
- c., gastro◊
- c., hepatic
- c. lymph nodes ▸ left
- c. lymph nodes ▸ middle
- c. lymph nodes ▸ right
- c., mucous
- c. myoneurosis
- c. omentum
- c. ▸ pain in abdomen from
- c., pancreatic
- c., pseudomembranous
- c., renal
- c., saburral
- c., stercoral
- c., ureteral
- c., uterine
- c. vein
- c. vein, left
- c. vein, middle
- c. vein, right
- c., vermicular
- c., verminous

colicinogenic factor
colicky abdominal pain
colicky infant
coliform(s)
- c., aerobic
- c. bacteria
- c. organisms
- c., paracolon

coliforme, Paracolobactrum
colitis
- c., acute
- c., adaptive
- c., ameba
- c., amebic
- c. and alpha biofeedback
- c., balantidial
- c., chronic ulcerative
- c., Clostridium difficile
- c. cystica profunda
- c. cystica superficialis
- c. ▸ diarrhea from ulcerative
- c., fulminating
- c., gastro◊
- c., granulomatous
- c. gravis
- c., hemorrhagic
- c., infectious
- c., ischemic

- c., mucous
- c., myxomembranous
- c., necrotizing
- c. ▸ necrotizing, pseudomembranous
- c. polyposa
- c., pseudomembranous
- c., radiation
- c. ▸ recurrent abdominal pain with
- c., regional
- c., segmental
- c. toxin
- c., transmural
- c., tuberculous
- c., typhlo◊
- c. ulcerativa
- c., ulcerative
- c. with Crohn's disease ▸ ulcerative
- c. ▸ Yersinia enterocolitica

collaborative
- c. patient care
- c. research study
- c. therapies

collagen
- c., bovine
- c., bovine biodegradable
- c. disease
- c. disorder
- c. fibers
- c. fibrils
- c. implant
- c. injection
- c. matrix ▸ extracellular
- c. matrix ▸ myocardial
- c. mutation
- c. network ▸ fibrillary
- c. network ▸ interstitial and perivascular
- c. skin treatment
- c. sugar
- c. suture
- c. synthesis
- c. tape prosthesis
- c. therapy
- c. treatment, zyderm
- c. vascular disease

collagenous
- c. fibers
- c. pneumoconiosis
- c. tissue, dense

collapse
- c., cardiovascular
- c., circulatory
- c., disc
- c. from Addison's disease

c., hemodynamic
c. ▸ loss of muscle tone and
c. ▸ lower lobe
c., lung
c., massive
c., mental
c. ▸ middle lobe
c. of lung ▸ total
c. of vertebrae
c., peripheral vascular
c., pulmonary
c. rale
c., respiratory
c., right lower lobe (RLL) partial
c. ▸ right ventricular (RV) diastolic
c. therapy
c. upper portion of lung ▸ artificial
c., vitreous
c., volitional

collapsed
c. cerebral artery
c., jugular veins
c. lung
c., patient
c. tissue in throat
c. vertebrae of spine

collapsing pulse

collar
c. bone
c. button lesion
c. button, polyethylene
c. button tube
c., cervical
c. crown
c. graft ▸ velour
c. incision
c. incision, Kocher
c., myocervical
c. of Stokes
c. of tissue
c., periosteal bone
c., Philadelphia
c., Plastizote
c. prosthesis
c. ▸ soft cervical

collateral(s) [lateral]
c., adequate
c., aortopulmonary
c., arcade
c. arterial flow to brain
c. artery murmur, bronchial
c. blood vessels
c., bronchial
c. circulation
c. circulation, coronary

c. circulation, hepatofugal venous
c. damage
c. dilatation
c. filling
c. flow
c. hyperemia
c. immunization
c. interview
c., jump
c. ligament, lateral
c. ligament, medial
c. ▸ rain of
c. respiration
c. sources
c., systemic
c. venous
c. vessel ▸ recruitable
c. vessels

collaterale, vas
collected, secretions
collecting
c. duct ▸ medullary
c. ducts
c. structures
c. system
c. system ▸ duplication of left
c. system ▸ duplication of right
c. system, lower
c. system, renal
c. system, upper
c. tubes
c. tubule

collection(s)
c., autologous blood
c., expired air
c., fluid
c., specimen
c., sputum
c., subphrenic
c. tube ▸ sterile vacuum
c., urine

collective decision
collective unconscious
collector, cancer cell
Coller modification, Astler-
Colles' fracture
Colles' mother
Colley operation ▸ Davies-
colli
c., hydrocele
c., melanoleukoderma
c., pterygium

colliculi
c., anterior
c., inferior

c., superior
colliculus [canaliculus]
colliculus of Barkow
colliculus of female urethra, cervical
colliers' phthisis
collimation of radiation beam
collimator
c., automatic
c., converging
c., diverging
c., focusing
c., multi-hole
c. (MLC) ▸ multileaf
c., parallel-hole
c., pin-hole
c., single-hole
c., thick-septa
c., thin-septa

Collin(s)
C. -Beard operation
C. -Beard procedure
C. pelvimeter
C. syndrome ▸ Treacher-

Collings' electrode
colliquative proteinuria
colliquative softening
collision, elastic
collision, inelastic
Collocalia esculenta
collodion
c. baby
c. dressing
c., flexible
c. solution
c. strip
c., surgical wound covered with

colloid
c. adenoma
c. adenomata
c. bodies
c. cancer
c. carcinoma
c. chemistry
c. content uniform
c. contrast medium ▸ polygelin
c. cyst
c. depletion, mild
c. deposits in optic nerves
c. -filled follicles
c. follicle ▸ unencapsulated
c. goiter
c. goiter, diffuse
c. hydrostatic pressure gradient
c. nodules
c. nodules, focal

colloid—continued
- c. nodules of thyroid
- c. oncotic pressure
- c. osmotic pressure (COP)
- c. osmotic pressure (COP) measurement
- c. osmotic pressure (COP) of plasma
- c., radioactive
- c. replacement solution
- c. shock
- c. substance
- c., synthetic
- c. (TSC), technetium sulfur
- c. type carcinoma

colloidal
- c. benzoin test
- c. electrolyte
- c. gold
- c. gold curve
- c. gold test
- c. iron

colloidoclastic shock
Collostat sponge
collum dentis
collusion, passive
Collyer's pelvimeter
collyrium, Beer's
coloboma
- c., Fuchs'
- c. iridis
- c. left iris ▸ postoperative
- c. lentis
- c. lobuli
- c. of choroid
- c. of iris
- c. of optic nerve
- c. of retina
- c. of vitreous
- c. palpebrale
- c. retinae
- c. right iris ▸ postoperative

colocolic anastomosis
colocolic intussusception
colocutaneous fistula
cologastrostomy, esophago◊
Colombian (marijuana)
Colombian tick fever
colon
- c. ▸ abnormal peristaltic actions of
- c. abnormality, intrinsic
- c., adenocarcinoma of
- c., aganglionic segment of
- c. anastomosis
- c., angiodysplasia of

- c., ascending
- c. bacteria
- c. cancer
- c. cancer death ▸ risk of
- c. cancer, Dukes' C
- c. cancer, familial
- c. cancer gene
- c. cancer, hereditary
- c. cancer (HNPCC) ▸ hereditary nonpolyposis
- c. cancer ▸ inherited
- c. cancer, metastatic
- c. cancer prevention
- c. cancer ▸ recurring
- c. cancer screening
- c. cancer ▸ sporadic
- c., carcinoma of
- c., carcinoma of sigmoid
- c. cleansing
- c. coagulation syndrome
- c. deformity, extrinsic
- c., descending
- c., diseased
- c., distal
- c., distended
- c. ▸ diverticula of descending
- c., diverticula of sigmoid
- c. ▸ diverticula of transverse
- c., diverticulosis
- c. ▸ diverticulosis of sigmoid
- c. ▸ diverticulosis of transverse and descending
- c. ▸ Dukes' C classification of right ascending
- c. Dukes' carcinoma of
- c., duplication of
- c. emptied satisfactorily
- c., endometriosis of
- c. examination ▸ air contrast
- c. ▸ feces in the
- c. fills and evacuates satisfactorily
- c., haustra of
- c., hepatic flexure of
- c., hypotonic
- c., iliac
- c., iliac flexure of
- c. in children ▸ esophagus replacement with
- c., inactive
- c., infarcted transverse
- c. inflammation
- c. interposition for esophageal disease
- c., interposition of
- c. ▸ intramural air in

- c. (IC), irritable
- c., large
- c. ▸ large intestinal descending
- c., lead pipe
- c., left flexure of
- c. ▸ leukemic infiltrates of
- c. ▸ marginal artery of
- c. mass ▸ hard, indurated
- c. muscle, thickening of
- c. obstruction, transverse
- c. pathology, organic
- c., pelvic
- c., perforation of
- c. polyp
- c. ▸ polypoid adenocarcinoma of
- c., postsurgical
- c., proximal
- c., redundancy of
- c. relaxant
- c. resection
- c. resection, segmental
- c. resection, wedge
- c., right flexure of
- c., semilunar folds of
- c., sigmoid
- c., sigmoid flexure of
- c., sigmoid folds of
- c. spasm
- c., spastic
- c., splenic flexure of
- c., swelling in
- c. syndrome, irritable
- c. syndrome, small left
- c. syndrome, spastic
- c., transverse
- c. -typhoid dysentery group
- c., unstable
- c. wall

colonic
- c. biopsy
- c. cancer
- c. cancer ▸ feces and
- c. cancer ▸ fiber and
- c. carcinoma
- c. constipation
- c. contraction
- c. dilation ▸ severe
- c. diverticula
- c. hydrotherapy
- c. inertia
- c. irrigation
- c. ischemia
- c. lesions
- c. lining
- c. mucosa

c. mucosal inflammation
c. obstruction, false
c. pancreatitis
c. penetration
c. perforation
c. polyp
c. polyposis
c. ulcer
c. wall

colonization
c., airway bacterial
c., atypical mycobacterial
c., bacterial
c. factor
c. of host
c., stool

Colonna's operation
colonoscope, fiberoptic
colonoscopic
c. evaluation
c. polypectomy
c. polypectomy ▸ perforation in

colonoscopy
c., optical
c. procedure
c., virtual

colony (-ies)
c. assay ▸ spleen
c., bacterial
c., bitten
c., butyrous
c. count
c., D. (dwarf)
c., daughter
c., dysgonic
c., effuse
c. forming units
c. forming units, spleen
c., gonidial
c., H. (Hauch)
c., M. (mucoid)
c., matte
c. /ml (colonies per milliliter)
c., mucoid (M.)
c., nibbled
c., O. (ohne Hauch)
c. of organisms
c. per milliliter (colonies/ml)
c., R. (rough)
c., S. (smooth)
c., satellite
c., smooth (S.)
c. stimulating factor
c. stimulating factor (GM-CSF) ▸
    human granulocytic-macrophage

c., submucosal bacterial
colophony ▸ pine resin
**coloplasty ▸ one-stage retrosternal
bypass**
color(s) (Color)
c. adaptation
c. adaptometer
c. and consistence of stool, change
    in
c. and cry good
c. and space perceptual
    disturbances
c. and texture, normal
C. and Word Test, Stroop
c. blind
c. blindness
c. blindness, amnesic
c. blindness, total
c. change of skin
c. charts, Reuss's
c. -coded flow mapping
c. deficiency, acquired
c. deficiency, inherited
c. discrimination
c. discs
c. Doppler echocardiography
c. Doppler energy
c. enhanced view
c. flow Doppler
c. flow imaging ▸ Doppler
    transesophageal
c. flow mapping
c. flow mapping ▸ Doppler
c. flow ultrasound Doppler
C. -Form Sorting Test
c. ▸ heightened perception of
c. in fingertips ▸ change of
c. in toes ▸ change of
c. index (CI)
c. jet, Doppler
c. perception
c. perception deficiency
c. perception deficiency ▸ red-
    green
c. perception ▸ light and
c. -pigment
c. power angiography
c. ratio, cell
c. recognition
c. scotoma
c. sense
c. skin, ashen
c., spectrum of
c. -translating television
    microscope ▸ ultraviolet

c. variability
c. vision
c. vision, acuity of
c. vision deficiency
c. vision deteriorate with aging
c. vision deviant
c. vision, normal
c. vision, poor
c. vision test

Colorado tick fever virus
coloration, abnormal
coloration, adaptive
colorectal
c. adenoma
c. anastomosis
c. cancer
c. cancer chemotherapy
c. cancer ▸ early detection of
c. cancer, familial
c. cancer ▸ hereditary
    nonpolyposis
c. cancer kit
c. cancer, metastatic
c. cancer (MCC), mutated
c. cancer screening
c. carcinoma
c. organs
c. polyp
c. screening
c. specialist

colored
c. fluid straw-
c. pericardial fluid ▸ straw-
c. plasma, honey
c. serous fluid ▸ straw-
c. skin, bluish
c. stools, clay-
c. stools, light-
c. urine, amber-
c. urine, straw-

colorée, audition
colorimetric determinations
colorless gas
colostomy
c. bag
c. care
c., cholecysto◊
c., diverting
c., divided
c., double-barreled
c., end-to-side
c., end-to-side ileotransverse
c., functioning
c., gastro◊
c., ileotransverse

colostomy—*continued*
- c. irrigation
- c., loop
- c., normal functioning ileal transverse
- c., patient has
- c., permanent
- c. pouch
- c. procedure
- c., resected end-to-end ileal
- c. sac
- c., sigmoid
- c., sigmoid loop
- c. site
- c., temporary
- c., transverse
- c. tube
- c., viable
- c., Wangensteen's

colostrum [*claustrum*]
- c. expressed from breast
- c. gravidarum
- c. puerperarum

colotomy, cholecysto◊
colotomy, ▸ gastro◊
colovesical fistula
colpectomy, skinning
colpitis
- c. emphysematosa
- c., emphysematous
- c. granulosa
- c. mycotica

colpohysterotomy, laparo◊
colporrhaphy, posterior
colposcopic
- c. -directed punch biopsy
- c. examination ▸ screen
- c. lesion

colposcopy, intensive
colposcopy, screen
colpostat ▸ Fletcher afterloading
colpotomy, celio◊
colpotomy, posterior
columbaczense, Simulium
columbae, Haemoproteus
columbae, Trichomonas
columbarum, Trichomonas
Columbia Mental Maturity Scale
Columbia SK virus
columella cochleas
columella nasi
column(s)
- c., adsorption
- c., anterior
- c., anterior gray

- c., anterior white
- c., barium
- c., cervical Pantopaque
- c., external vein of vertebral
- c. ▸ gliosis of anterior
- c. ▸ gliosis of lateral
- c., lateral
- c., lumbar Pantopaque
- c., Morgagni's
- c. of Bertin
- c. of Bertin ▸ large
- c. of bone ▸ new
- c. of spinal cord ▸ ventral gray
- c. ▸ osteoporotic thinning of vertebral
- c., Pantopaque
- c. ▸ plasma exchange
- c., posterior gray
- c., Sertoli's
- c., spinal
- c., stabilize spinal
- c., Stilling's
- c. stimulator (DCS) ▸ dorsa
- c. ▸ thoracic vertebral
- c., tube
- c., ventral
- c., ventral gray
- c., vertebral

columnar
- c. acinar cells
- c. acinar cells ▸ cuboidal to
- c. cell
- c. epithelial cells
- c. epithelioma
- c. epithelium
- c. epithelium, circumoral area of
- c. mucosa
- c. mucosa, endocervical

coma (Coma)
- c., agrypnodal
- c., alcoholic
- c., alpha
- c. and convulsions ▸ catatonia,
- c., and death ▸ emesis,
- c., apoplectic
- c. appearance
- c., artificial
- c., barbiturate
- c., burn
- c., convulsions and
- c., deep hepatic
- c., diabetic
- c. ▸ disorientation, confusion and
- c., encephalitis from
- c., hepatic

- c., hyperosmolar nonketotic
- c. hypochloraemicum
- c., hypoglycemic
- c. ▸ hypotension and
- c., induction of
- c., irreversible
- c., Kussmaul's
- c., lapsing into
- c., metabolic
- c., myxedema
- c., nontraumatic
- c. ▸ patient in
- c., patient lapsed into
- c., prehepatic
- c., prolonged irreversible
- c., psychogenic
- C. Scale ▸ Glasgow
- c. secondary to head trauma
- c., severe metabolic acidosis and
- c. somnolentium
- c., sudden paralysis and
- c., temporary
- c. therapy, insulin
- c., trance
- c. treatment, insulin
- c., uremic
- c. vigil

comatoid adenocarcinoma
comatose
- c. diabetic
- c. patient
- c., patient deeply
- c., patient semi-
- c. senility

comb rhythm
combat
- c., attitude of
- c. exhaustion
- c. fatigue
- c. neurosis
- c. rejection of transplanted organ
- c. support hospital (CSH)

combative
- c. and agitated ▸ patient
- c. and confused
- c. patient
- c. to stimuli, patient

Comberg localization
Comberg method ▸ Pfeiffer-
combination(s)
- c. chemotherapy
- c. chemotherapy, intensive
- c. chemotherapy program
- c., drug
- c. drug therapies

c. electron and photo therapy
c. high and low energy x-ray therapy
c. modality therapy
c. therapy
c. therapy, antibiotic
c. therapy in patient management
combined
c. analysis
c. aphasia
c. chemotherapy/radiation therapy
c. degeneration, subacute
c. disease murmur, aortic-mitral
c. drug and radiation modality
c. effects
c. forms of preexcitation
c. heart catheterization
c. hemorrhoids
c. hyperlipidemia, false
c. hyperthermia and radiation treatment
c. immune deficiency disease
c. immune deficiency syndrome, severe
c. immunodeficiency
c. immunodeficiency, severe
c. immunodeficiency (SCID) ▸ severe
c. immunodeficiency syndrome (SCIDS) ▸ severe
c. mitral stenosis and regurgitation
c. modality therapy
c. modality therapy, independent toxicity in
c. modality therapy, protocol design in
c. modality therapy, research design in
c. modality therapy, response and
c. modality therapy, spatial cooperation in
c. modality therapy, survival rates with
c. modality therapy, temporal consolidation in
c. pregnancy
c. radiation and 5-fluorouracil
c. sclerosis
c. therapy
c. therapy, continuous
c. transmission-emission scintiphoto
c. treatment group
c. treatment in advanced disease
c. ventricular hypertrophy
c. with radiotherapy, chemotherapy

c. with radiotherapy, 5-fluorouracil
combining
c. power
c. power ▸ carbon dioxide (CO_2)
c. site
c. site antibody
combustion equivalent
Comby's sign
comedo acne
comedo, mixed
comedones and sebaceous cysts
comfort
c., alteration in
c., altered
c. food
c. level
c. level, maximal
c. measures
c. only ▸ patient treated for
c. ring, inflatable
c., spiritual
comfortable
c. bowel movement
c., patient kept
c. self-image
comforting, physical
comitant squint
comitant strabismus
comma
c. appearance
c. appearance, inverse
c. ▸ gram-negative Vibrio
c., Vibrio
command(s)
c., abstract verbal
c., concrete functional
c. hallucinations
c., patient obeys
Commando operation
commercial dose computation systems
commercial preparation
comminuted
c. femoral fracture
c. fracture
c. fracture, compound
c. fracture, simple
c., markedly
c. tibial fracture
c. tibial fracture site
comminution, extensive
Commission (AEC), Atomic Energy
commission certified
commissural
c. aphasia
c. bundle

c. cells
c. cheilitis
c. fusion
c. myelotomy
c. splitting
commissure(s)
c., anterior
c., anterior gray
c., anterior white
c., aortic
c., arcuate
c., chiasmatic posterior
c., Forel's
c., fused
c., great transverse
c., Gudden's
c., habenular
c., interthalamic
c., laryngeal
c., Meynert's
c. of cerebrum ▸ anterior
c. of cerebrum ▸ middle
c. of eyelids ▸ lateral
c. of eyelids ▸ medial
c. of fornix
c. of labia ▸ anterior
c. of labia ▸ posterior
c. of lips of mouth
c. of spinal cord ▸ white
c., optic
c., palpebral
c., posterior
c., posterior gray
c. structure, anterior
c., superior
c., supraoptic
c., transverse
commissurotomy
c., aortic
c., balloon mitral
c., Brock transseptal
c., Brockenbrough transseptal
c., closed chest
c., closed transventricular mitral
c., mitral
c. ▸ mitral balloon
c. ▸ mitral valve
c. ▸ percutaneous mitral
c. ▸ percutaneous mitral balloon
c. ▸ percutaneous transatrial mitral
c. ▸ percutaneous transvenous mitral
c., pulmonary
c. ▸ transventricular mitral valve
c., tricuspid

commitment
- c., involuntary
- c., realistic
- c. to change

committed
- c. mode pacemaker
- c., patient
- c. stem cell

committee (Committee)
- c. ▸ Fertility Maternal Health Drugs Advisory
- C. (ICC) ▸ Infection Control
- c. of FDA ▸ advisory

commode, bedside

common
- c. acute leukemia antigen
- c. acute lymphoblastic leukemia antigen
- c. anterior facial vein
- c. antigen
- c. antigen ▸ leukocyte
- c. atrioventricular canal ▸ persistent
- c. atrium
- c. average reference electrode
- c. axis
- c. bile duct
- c. bile duct stent, occluded
- c. bile duct stones
- c. bile duct stones, dissolve
- c. carotid artery ▸ right
- c. carotid artery, bifurcation of
- c. carotid artery ▸ left
- c. cognitive functions
- c. cold
- c. cold viruses
- c. complications
- c. component
- c. core proteins
- c. digital vein of foot
- c. disorder of back
- c. disorder of body ▸ whole
- c. disorder of bone
- c. disorder of breast
- c. disorder of circulation
- c. dissociative symptoms
- c. duct
- c. duct exploration
- c. duct ▸ narrowing of
- c. duct, obstructed
- c. duct stone
- c. duct tumor, distal
- c. electroencephalogram (EEG) input test
- c. extensor muscle of digits
- c. faint

- c. femoral artery
- c. femoral vein
- c. fibular nerve
- c. flora, mixed
- c. hepatic artery
- c. hepatic duct
- c. iliac
- c. iliac artery
- c. iliac lymph nodes
- c. iliac vein
- c. immunodeficiency
- c. integument
- c. leukocyte antigen
- c. migraine
- c. mode amplification
- c. mode rejection
- c. mode rejection ratio
- c. mode signal
- c. organisms ▸ toxin producing
- c. organisms ▸ viral producing
- c. palmar digital nerves
- c. palmar digital nerves of median nerve
- c. palmar digital nerves of ulnar nerve
- c. pathway ▸ final
- c. peroneal nerve
- c. plantar digital nerves of lateral plantar nerve
- c. plantar digital nerves of medial plantar nerve
- c. pneumonia
- c. psychobiological origin
- c. reaction
- c. reference electrode
- c. reference montage
- c. sensation
- c. sense approach
- c. sense factor
- c. sense judgment
- c. sensibility
- c. tendinous ring
- c. tendon
- c. therapeutic dilemmas
- c. variable agammaglobulinemia
- c. wart

commotio
- c. cerebri
- c. retinas
- c., retinal
- c. spinalis

communicable disease

communicate, inability to

communicated insanity

communicating

- c. artery
- c. artery aneurysm
- c. artery aneurysm ▸ posterior
- c. artery, anterior
- c. artery (AICA), anterior inferior
- c. artery ▸ posterior
- c. artery (PICA), posterior inferior
- c. hydrocele
- c. hydrocephalus
- c., patient

communication
- c. ability
- c. alteration
- c., arteriovenous
- c. between nerves and muscles ▸ block in normal
- c. boards
- c., change in
- c., chemically free
- c., child
- c. difficulty
- c., encourage
- c. (FC), facilitated
- c., fetal chamber
- c., impaired
- c. ▸ impaired verbal
- c., institutional
- c., interarterial
- c. ▸ lack of
- c. ▸ learning, cognition and
- c., level of
- c., marital
- c., mode of
- c. murmur ▸ left ventricular (LV) right atrial (RA)
- c., nonverbal
- c., oral
- c. ▸ parent-adolescent
- c. skills
- c. skills, bicultural
- c. skills, effective
- c. system, augmentative
- c. system, functional
- c. techniques, compensatory

communicative
- c. assessment
- c. disorder
- c. patient

communicators, dissection of

communior ▸ gram-negative Escherichia (E.)

communis
- c., Aedes
- c., anulus tendineus
- c. muscle extensor digitorum

c., Ricinus
c., sacculus
c., Siderococcus
c. ▸ vasa sanguinea integumenti
community (Community)
   c. -acquired bladder infection
   c. -acquired infection(s)
   c. -acquired lobar pneumonia
   c. -acquired meningitis
   c. -acquired pneumonia
   c. -acquired pneumonia protocol
   c. agencies ▸ referral to
   C. Based Residential Facility
      (CBRF)
   c. bereavement program
   c. blood bank
   C. Care Unit (CCU)
   c. clinic
   C. Clinic ▸ Outpatient
   c., continuing care
   C. (CCRC), Continuing Care
      Retirement
   c. education
   c. immunity
   c. implications
   c. mental health center
   c. network
   c., nuclear
   c. psychiatry
   c., recovering
   c. reintegration
   c. resource
   c. self-help groups
   c. service work
   c. support group
   c. supportive, church
   c., therapeutic
   c. ▸ transition back into
   c. treatment, alcoholism
Comolli's sign
comorbid
   c. addiction
   c. addictive behaviors
   c. alcohol abuse
   c. alcoholism
   c. cocaine abuse
   c. generalized anxiety
   c. illness
   c. opioid abuse
   c. substance
comorbidity
   c. index, Charlson
   c. of mental disorders
   c. of schizophrenia and substance
      abuse

c., psychiatric
compact [*contact, contract*]
   c. bone
   c. substance of bones
   c. tissue
compacted ▸ dead skin cell layers
compactum, Fonsecaea
compactum, Hormodendrum
companion, homemaker
comparative
   c. anatomy
   c. dental radiography
   c. depth dose curves
   c. effectiveness
   c. embryology
   c. medicine
   c. psychology
   c. study
compared with previous studies
comparison
   c. film
   c. microscope
   c. ▸ randomized double-blind
   c. views
compartment
   c., anterior tibial
   c. compression syndrome,
      anterior
   c., lateral
   c., medial
   c. of knee, medial
   c. procedure
   c. syndrome
   c. syndrome, anterior tibial
   c. system, two-
   c. system, three-
   c., vascular
compartmental
   c. analysis
   c. anatomy ▸ plantar
   c. syndrome
   c. system, linear
compassion fatigue
compassion therapy
compatibility test of blood
compatible
   c. donor
   c., findings
   c. with grand mal
   c. with hypsarrhythmia
   c. with ischemia ▸ ST-T wave
      changes
   c. with petit mal
   c. with petit mal variant
   c. with psychomotor variant

compensated
   c. cardiac status
   c. heart failure
   c. shock
   c., well
compensation
   c., accommodation and
   c., cardiac
   c., depth
   c. ▸ electronic distance
   c. gain ▸ time
   c. neurosis
   c., occupational
   c., temperature
   c., vestibular
compensator, volume
compensatory
   c. atrophy
   c. behavior mechanism
   c. circulation
   c. communication techniques
   c. curvature of spine
   c. emphysema
   c. hypertrophy
   c. hypertrophy of heart muscle
   c. mechanism
   c. pause
   c. polycythemia
   c. skills
   c. smoking
   c. vessel enlargement
Compere('s)
   C. fixation wires
   C. operation
   C. pin
competence, mental
competence, testamentary
competent abstract conceptual memory
   organization
competing sensory stimuli
competition, overt
competition ratio (MCR) ▸ message
competitive situation
compiling surveillance data on
   infection
complainant, patient
complained of (c/o)
complaint(s)
   c. ▸ adjustment disorder with
      physical
   c., bodily
   c. (CC) ▸ chief
   c., chronic lung
   c., entrance
   c., initial

complaint(s)—*continued*
- c., intestinal
- c., memory
- c., multiple
- c., nonspecific
- c., patient admitted with multiple
- c., physical
- c., psychosomatic
- c., somatic
- c., vague abdominal

complement
- c. absorption test ▸ conglutinating
- c. activity
- c. assay
- c. assay ▸ hemolytic
- c., bed
- c. binding
- c. defects
- c. deviation
- c., dominant
- c. endocellular
- c. fixation (CF)
- c. fixation (CF) ▸ cardiolipin
- c. fixation (CF) reaction
- c. fixation (CF) ▸ Reiter protein
- c. fixation (CF) test
- c. fixation titers
- c. fixing antibody
- c. level, serum
- c. system
- c. (C'H$_{50}$), total hemolytic
- c., whole

complemental air

complementary
- c. balloon angioplasty
- c. hypertrophy
- c. induction
- c. medicine
- c. medicine physician
- c. therapies
- c. therapy of bacterial shock

complementophil group

complete(s)
- c. abortion
- c. abstinence
- c. aftercare planning
- c. agglutinin
- c. amputation
- c. and ongoing assessment
- c. aphasia
- c. ascertainment
- c. atrioventricular (AV) block congenital
- c. atrioventricular (AV) dissociation
- c. autopsy

- c. A-V block
- c. awakening
- c. basic transfer, patient
- c. bath
- c. bed rest ▸ patient at
- c. birth
- c. blockage
- c. blood count (CBC)
- c. bowel blockage
- c. bowel obstruction
- c. breakdown
- c. breath, yogic
- c. breech position
- c. breech presentation
- c. change of drapes, gowns and instruments
- c. clinical remission
- c. closure
- c. contact
- c. corneal coverage
- c. cycle
- c. cystectomy
- c. denture
- c. denture impression
- c. dislocation
- c. emptying of bladder
- c. exhaustion
- c. face lift
- c. filling
- c. foveal blindness
- c. fracture
- c. Freund adjuvant
- c. gynecologic examination annually
- c. harelip
- c. heart block (CHB)
- c. hemianopia
- c., hemostasis
- c. hernia
- c. hysterectomy
- c. impairment of conduction
- c. independent transfer, patient
- c. keratectomy
- c. left bundle branch block (LBBB)
- c. lobectomy
- c. loss of sensation
- c. loss of sight
- c. loss of vision
- c. lower denture
- c., mandatory contact tracing
- c. memory loss ▸ partial or
- c. motor paralysis
- c. myocardial infarction
- c. obstruction
- c. obstruction of airway

- c. occlusion
- c. occlusion of right coronary trunk
- c. pacemaker patient testing system
- c. paralysis
- c. paralysis, partial or
- c. physical evaluation
- c. physical examination
- c. plate
- c. pneumonectomy
- c. psychosocial history
- c. relapse, patient in
- c. relaxation
- c. remission
- c. remission, disease in
- c. remission, patient in
- c. resolution
- c. restraints
- c. restraints, patient in
- c. right bundle branch block (RBBB)
- c. simple mastoidectomy
- c. sinus arrest
- c. situs inversus
- c. tear
- c. thoracoplasty
- c. toilet transfer, patient
- c. transposition of great arteries
- c. upper denture
- c. vaginal breech
- c. weight bearing

completed myocardial infarction

completely
- c. dilated, cervix
- c. disabled, patient
- c. emptying bladder
- c., extends knee
- c. in-the-canal hearing aid
- c., obstructed, urethra

completing the abreactions

Completion Test, Sentence

completion, treatment

complex(es)
- c., aberrant QRS
- c., Acinetobacter calcoaceticus baumannii
- c. (ARC), acquired immune deficiency syndrome (AIDS) related
- c., AIDS (acquired immune deficiency syndrome) dementia
- c., anomalous
- c., antibody antigen
- c. antigen ▸ major histocompatibility

c., anti-inhibitor coagulant
c., atrial premature
c., auricular
c., AV (atrioventricular) junctional escape
c., avian leukosis
c. benign disease
c. benign esophageal disease
c. burst, K
c. capture
c., castration
c., chlormerodrin-cysteine
c., cognitive
c. composite odontoma
c. developmental disorder
c., Diana
c., diphasic
c. disease
c. disease ► immune
c. disorder of adolescence
c. disorder of childhood
c. during sleep, K
c. ectopy, asymptomatic
c., EEG (electroencephalogram)
c., EEG (electroencephalogram) waves and
c., Eisenmenger's
c., Electra
c. electrical wave
c., electroencephalogram (EEG)
c., electroencephalogram (EEG) waves and
c., equiphasic
c. fracture
c., fusion
c., Ghon
c., Golgi
c., guilt
c., immune
c., individual
c. (MAC) infection ► Mycobacterium avium
c., inferiority
c. interaction
c. ► iron dextran
c., isodiphasic
c., junctional
c., K
c., Lutembacher's
c., mental
c., monophasic
c. motor organization
c. ► multiform premature ventricular
c., multiple spike
c., multiple spike-and-slow wave

c., multiple spike-and-wave
c. ► Mycobacterium avium intracellulare (MAI)
c., Oedipus
c. oncologic therapy protocols
c., Parkinson's dementia
c. partial seizure
c., period of the
c., persecution
c. ► plasminogen-streptokinase
c. ► pleomorphic premature ventricular
c. ► polymorphic premature ventricular
c. ► polysaccharide iron
c., polyspike
c., polyspike-and-slow wave
c. precipitation, immune
c. ► premature atrial
c. ► premature atrioventricular junctional
c. ► premature ventricular
c., primary
c. problems
c. protein
c., prothrombinase
c. psychophysiological process
c., QRS
c., QRS-T
c., QS
c., Ranke
c. reaction, immune
c. regional pain syndrome
c., regularly repeated EEG (electrocardiogram)
c., repetitive
c. rhythm ► wide
c. ► R-on-T premature ventricular
c. rotational movement
c., R-prime
c., RS
c., sequence of spike-and-slow wave
c., sharp-and-slow wave
c., Shone
c., short QRS
c. simple fracture
c. ► sinoatrial (SA) pacemaker
c. sleep disorder
c. ► sling ring
c. slow spike-and-slow wave
c., slow wave
c., spike-and-dome
c., spike-and-slow wave
c., spike-and-wave

c., Steidele
c. ► streptokinase plasminogen
c., superiority
c., symptom
c. tachycardia ► narrow
c. tics
c., transposition
c. trigger hypothesis ► premature ventricular
c., TU
c. tubes
c., ventricular
c. ► ventricular premature
c. wave form
c. waves, K
c., widening of QRS
complexion
c., blotchy
c., sallow
c. treatment
complexity, grammatical
compliance
c. ► abnormal increase in
c., alteration in diastolic
c., aortic
c., arteriolar
c., consistent medication
c., diminished
c. ► diminished left ventricular
c., effective
c. ► left ventricular (LV) chamber
c. ► left ventricular (LV) muscle
c. of heart
c., pulmonary
c. rate, oxygenation, and pressure (CROP)
c., rate, oxygenation, and pressure index
c. (TLC) ► total lung
c., treatment
c. with drug regimens, patient
c. with medications ► increased
compliant, patient
complicated
c. birth
c. cataract
c. delivery
c. disease
c. dislocation
c. fracture
c. labor
c. myocardial infarction
c. postoperative course
c., recovery

complication(s)
- c., acute
- c., anesthetic-related
- c., behavioral
- c., bleeding
- c., cardiac
- c., cardiovascular
- c., clinical
- c., common
- c., delayed
- c. ▸ diabetes-related
- c., diabetic
- c., drug
- c. ▸ drug-related medical
- c., fatal
- c., groin
- c. in pregnancy, cocaine-related
- c. in radiation therapy ▸ therapy
- c., infection
- c., legal
- c., life-threatening
- c. ▸ life-threatening respiratory
- c., long-term
- c., macrovascular
- c., medical
- c., metabolic
- c., microvascular
- c., neurologic
- c., neurological
- c., ocular
- c. of diabetes ▸ prevent, stop or reverse
- c. of drug abuse
- c. of drug abuse, cardiovascular
- c. of drug abuse, dermatologic
- c. of drug abuse, endocrinologic
- c. of drug abuse, gastrointestinal (GI)
- c. of drug abuse, genitourinary (GU)
- c. of drug abuse, hematopoietic
- c. of drug abuse, hepatic
- c. of drug abuse, neonatal
- c. of drug abuse, neuromuscular
- c. of drug abuse, obstetric
- c. of drug abuse, psychiatric
- c. of drug abuse, pulmonary
- c. of drug abuse, renal
- c. of drug abuse, reproductive
- c. of drug abuse, septic
- c. of drug abuse, sexual
- c. of drug abuse, surgical
- c. of pregnancy
- c. of prematurity
- c. of problem feet ▸ physical

- c. of radiation therapy
- c. of systemic cancer, neurologic
- c., postoperative
- c., postoperative lung
- c., potential
- c., prematurity
- c. probability curves
- c., psychological
- c., pulmonary
- c. rate
- c., shock-like
- c., social
- c. thesis

component(s)
- c. administration, blood
- c., anterior
- c., anxiety
- c., articular
- c., blood
- c. bones
- c., brain wave
- c., bronchospastic
- c., common
- c., dominant frequency
- c., elastic
- c., electroencephalogram (EEG)
- c., electronic
- c., fast
- c., fast and slow
- c., filamentous
- c., genetic
- c., granular
- c., group-specific
- c., harmonic
- c., homogeneous
- c., hormonal
- c., individual
- c., intra-articular
- c. ▸ lambda light chain
- c., late positive
- c., loosening
- c., low frequency
- c., M
- c. ▸ medical, psychological, spiritual, physical and nutritional
- c., neurogenic
- c. of knee ▸ expand internal
- c. of occlusion
- c. of reflex barrier ▸ gastric
- c. parts
- c., (PTC) ▸ plasma thromboplastin
- c., production of various brain wave
- c., psychological
- c., P wave
- c., removal of blood

- c. replacement therapy, blood
- c. ribs
- c., sciatic
- c., slow
- c., somatic motor
- c., somatic sensory
- c., splanchnic motor
- c., splanchnic sensory
- c., stress
- c., strong educational
- c. therapy, blood
- c. therapy, plasma
- c. (TPC) ▸ thromboplastin plasma
- c. to alcoholism, genetic
- c., variable
- c. waves, sharp peaks of

compos mentis, non

composite
- c. cyclic therapy
- c. fracture
- c. flap, Argamaso-Lewin
- c. graft
- c. joint
- c. odontoma
- c. odontoma, complex
- c. odontoma, compound
- c. ▸ resin-based
- c. veneers

composition, pigment

compound(s)
- c., acidulated
- c., adrenocortical
- c., antimony
- c. astigmatism, myopic
- c. cathartic
- c. cavity
- c. character
- c. comminuted fracture
- c. composite odontoma
- c. cyst
- c. dislocation
- c. flap
- c. fracture
- c. ganglion
- c. hypermetropic astigmatism
- c. hyperopic astigmatism
- c. insanity
- c. joint
- c. medicine
- c. melanocytoma
- c. microscope
- c. myopic astigmatism
- c. nevus
- c., paramecia
- c. periodontitis

c., plastic bonding
c. presentation
c. -Q treatment
c., radioactive
c. reaction ▸ rape trauma syndrome,
c., rotifer
c. scanning
c. skull fracture
c. skull fracture ▸ debridement of
c., unsaturated

comprehension
c., impaired
c., language
c. of language, auditory
c., nonverbal social
c. of spoken language ▸ normal
c., reading
c., skills
c., slow

comprehensive
c. assessment
c. breast care
c. diagnosis
c. examination
c. geriatric assessment
c. health care institution
c. health plan
c. inpatient treatment
c. medical history
c. mental health
c. outpatient treatment
c. treatment

compress(es)
c., cold
c., cribriform
c., dry
c., fenestrated
c., graduated
c., hot
c., hot moist
c., moist
c., Priessnitz

compressed
c. -air sickness
c. EEG (electroencephalogram)
  record
c. Ivalon patch graft
c., nasal pyramid
c. nerve root
c. nerves
c. oxygen (O₂)
c. spectral array
c. vertebrae

compressible sugar
compressible volume

compression(s)
c., abdominal
c. and elevation (PRICE) ▸
  protection, rest, ice
c. and percussion
c. and ventilation
c., aortic
c., aortocaval
c. artifact
c. ▸ asphyxia by neck
c. atelectasis
c. atrophy
c., balloon
c. bandage
c., barrel hooping
c. boot
c. boot ▸ gelatin
c. boots ▸ intermittent pneumatic
c., cardiac
c., carotid sinus
c., cauda equina
c., caval
c., cerebral
c., cervical disc
c., chest
c. (CCC) ▸ continuing chest
c., cord
c. cough
c. -decompression (ACD), active
c., deformity
c., digital
c., downward
c. dressing
c. dressing, bulky
c. dressing, eye patch
c. dressing, light
c. dressing, light bulky
c., elevation (RICE) ▸ rest, ice,
c., external
c., external chest
c., extradural cord
c., extrinsic
c. fracture
c. fracture in vertebra
c. fracture of spine
c. fracture, osteoporotic
c. fracture, pathologic
c. fracture, spinal
c. fracture ▸ vertebral
c. fractures, numerous
c. fusion, Charnley
c., gloves
c., head
c. hooks
c. hose

c., icing
c., impending cord
c. injury, soft tissue
c., instrumental
c. ▸ intermittent pneumatic
c. (IAC) ▸ interposed abdominal
c. maneuvers, external cardiac
c. ▸ manual chest
c., median nerve
c., nerve
c., nerve root
c. neuropathy ▸ ulnar
c., neurovascular
c. of carotid artery
c. of chest, rhythmic
c. of liver cords
c. of pulmonary tissue
c. of spinal nerve
c. of the brain
c. paddle
c. reflex, eyeball
c., rhythmic
c., spinal
c., spinal cord
c. stockings
c. stockings, elastic
c. stockings ▸ graduated
c. stockings ▸ pneumatic
c. syndrome, anterior compartment
c. syndrome, cord
c. therapy
c. thrombosis
c., tracheal
c. triad, acute
c. -type deformity
c., ulnar nerve
c. ultrasonography
c., umbilical cord
c., vena caval
c., vertical

compressive
c. atelectasis
c. force on spine
c. neuropathy

compressor
c., Anthony's
c., chest
c. muscle of naris

compressus, fetus
compromise
c., acute vascular
c., circulatory
c., neurovascular
c. ▸ side branch
c., vascular

compromised
- c. host
- c. host, immune
- c. ineffective family coping
- c. renal function

Compton
- C. edge
- C. effect
- C. electron
- C. photon
- C. scattering
- C. wavelength

compulsion(s) [concussion, convulsion]
- c. ▸ arranging and touching
- c., cleaning
- c., destructive
- c. ▸ full-blown
- c., handwashing
- c., mental
- c. neurosis
- c., obsessive
- c. ▸ persistent, intrusive thoughts and
- c., physical
- c., repetition
- c., repetitive
- c. to drink

compulsive [*convulsive*]
- c. abuse
- c. behavior
- c. behavior, obsessive
- c. conduct disorder ▸ obsessive-
- c. disease, destructive
- c. disorder
- c. disorder (OCD) ▸ obsessive,
- c. disorder ▸ treatment-resistant obsessive
- c. drinker
- c. eater
- c. gamblers
- c. gambling
- c. hair pulling
- c. impulse control disorder
- c. insanity
- c. neurosis ▸ obsessive,
- c., obsessive
- c. overeating
- c. overeating ▸ obsessive,
- c. patient
- c., patient highly
- c. personality
- c. personality disorder
- c. personality disorder ▸ obsessive
- c. personality ▸ obsessive,

- c. reaction ▸ obsessive,
- c. repetition
- c. response
- c. ritual
- c. sexual behavior
- c. shopper
- c. spasm
- c. spectrum disorder ▸ obsessive-
- c. symptom
- c. symptoms ▸ obsessional and
- c. talking
- c. tic
- c. traits
- c. urges
- c. work pattern
- c. worker

compulsory psychological evaluation

compulsory treatment

computation(s)
- c., analog
- c. of radiatic doses
- c. systems, commercial dose

computed
- c. axial tomography (CAT)
- c. axial tomography ▸ rapid acquisition
- c. EEG (electroencephalogram) topogram (CET)
- c. tomogram (CT)
- c. tomographic (CT) colonography ▸ three dimensional
- c. tomographic (CT) scanner ▸ ultrafast
- c. tomography (CT)
- c. tomography (CT) angiographic portography
- c. tomography, axial (ACT)
- c. tomography, cine
- c. tomography (EBCT) ▸ electron beam
- c. tomography (CT) ▸ gated
- c. tomography (CT) of chest
- c. tomography, positron
- C. Tomography (QCT), Quantitative
- c. tomography (HRCT) scan ▸ high resolution
- c. tomography (SPECT) scan ▸ single photon emission
- c. tomography (CT) scanning
- c. tomography (SPECT), single photon emission
- c. tomography (CT) ▸ ultrafast
- c. tomography (CT) ▸ xenon-enhanced

computer (Computer)
- c. addict
- c. addiction
- c. addiction disorder
- c. algorithm
- c., analog
- c. analysis
- c. assisted diagnostics
- c. assisted laser surgery
- c. assisted menu planning
- c. assisted operation
- c. assisted stereotactic laser microsurgery
- c. averaging technique
- c. based digital imaging
- c. code digital
- c. controlled laser
- c., digital
- c. dose calculation
- c. -driven rotatory chair
- c., electromechanical slope
- c. enhanced image
- c. enhancement scan
- c. -generated artifact
- c. -generated images
- c. graphics
- c. graphics, 3-D
- c. guided laser beam
- c. imaging
- c. imaging system
- C. of Average Transients
- c., oxygen consumption
- c. screen chart
- C. (SMAC) ▸ Sequential Multiple Analyzer
- c. summation techniques
- c. syndrome
- c. system, laboratory
- c. therapy program
- c. tomography (CT) ▸ atrial bolus dynamic
- c. vision syndrome
- c., voice activated

computerized (Computerized)
- c. assessment
- c., assisted design (CAD) prosthesis
- c. axial tomography (CAT)
- c. axial tomography (ACAT), automated
- c. axial tomography (CAT) scan ▸ digital holographic
- c. axial tomography (CAT) scan ▸ ultrafast
- c. axial tomography (CAT) scanner

c. axial tomography (CAT) scanner ▸ helical
c. diaphragmatic breathing retraining
c. digital mammography
c. display technique
c. edge detection
c. edge tracing
c. image
c. imaging techniques
c. laser
c. muscle-joint evaluation
c. risk assessment
c. scanning equipment
c. tomographic (CT) colonography
c. tomography (ECT) body scanner ▸ emission
c. tomography (EBCT) ▸ electron beam
c. tomography (CT) scan ▸ thin slice
c. tomography (CT) ▸ thin section
c. tomographic (ECT) system ▸ emission
c. tomographic (ECT) system ▸ radionuclide emission
c. tomography (CT)
c. tomography (CT) body scanner
c. tomography ▸ dynamic
C. Tomography (CT) ▸ Fast-Scan
c. tomography ▸ images produced by
c. tomography (CT) scanning, rapid sequential
c. treatment planning
c. visual field machine
conal septum
conative negative variation
concave
c. anterior surfaces
c., double
c. lens
c. microscopic slide
c., periscopic
c. posterior surfaces
C. (C-C) valve, Convexo-
concavity
c. and depression
c. of spine
c. to left ▸ scoliosis with
c. to right ▸ scoliosis with
concavoconcave lens
concavoconvex lens
concealed
c. bypass tract

c. conduction
c. entrainment
c. fusion ▸ entrainment with
c. hemorrhage
c. hernia
c. illness ▸ patient
c. motives
c. reflex
c. rhythm
concentrate
c. ▸ ability to think or
c., decreased ability to
c. deeply
c., inability to
c., intrinsic factor
c., liver
c., platelet
c. radiation
c., vitamin
concentrated
c. bile
c. mental activity
c. smear
c. specimen
concentrating, difficulty
concentrating, trouble
concentration [*consternation*]
c., airborne bacterial
c. and memory
c., approximate lethal
c., arterial blood
c., bactericidal
c., blood alcohol
c., blood urea
c., calcium
c., cholesterol
c., critical micellar
c. deficit, attention
c., difficulty in
c., difficulty with
c., diminished
c. effect relation
c., effective antibiotic
c. ▸ enhanced interest and
c., equal
c., estradiol
c., focused
c. forgetfulness, poor
c., glucose
c., good
c., high
c., high oxygen
c., hydrogen ion
c., hydroxyl
c., impaired

c. ▸ impaired thinking of
c. in serum and tissue ▸ antibiotic
c., intense
c. ▸ intracellular calcium
c., lack of
c., lactate
c., lethal
c. ▸ loss of
c. ▸ loss of interest, appetite and
c., low
c., low magnesium
c., maximum
c., maximum allowable
c. (MPC) maximum permissible
c., maximum urinary
c. (MCC/MCHC) mean corpuscular hemoglobin
c., minimal bactericidal
c. (MIC) ▸ minimal inhibitory
c., minimal medullary
c. (MAC) ▸ minimum alveolar
c. (MIC) ▸ minimum inhibitory
c., minimum mycoplasmacidal
c. ▸ motivation, visualization and
c. of bilirubin (MCBR) ▸ minimum
c. of dye
c. of dye, delayed
c. of dye, faint
c. of urine ▸ abnormally high
c., oxygen
c., oxygen tension/
c., patient has lack of
c., patient has poor
c., peak serum
c., plasma
c. ▸ plasma endothelin
c., plasma sodium
c., poor
c. ▸ prolonged tissue
c., radon
c. ratio
c., reduced
c., renal vein renin
c., serum calcium
c. test
c. test, Fishberg's
c. test ▸ memory and
c. test, urine
c. test, xylose
c. (TLC) ▸ total L-chain
c., trough
c., tumor
c., urine
concentrator, oxygen

concentric
- c. atrophy
- c. circle pattern on breast self-examination
- c. constriction
- c. hypertrophic cardiomyopathy
- c. hypertrophy
- c. left ventricular (LV) hypertrophy
- c. needle electrode
- c. pantomography
- c. remodeling
- c. swabbing

concentricum, Trichophyton
concentricus, Aspergillus
concept(s) (Concept)
- c., addiction
- c., dependency
- c., diagnostic
- c., disease
- c. formation ability ▸ verbal
- c., improved self-
- c. ▸ leading circle
- c., mental
- c., nonmedical
- c. of alpha biofeedback
- c. of awareness
- c. of biofeedback control
- c. of repression ▸ psychoanalytic
- c. ▸ proof of
- c., psychodynamic
- c., radiobiologic
- c., realistic self-
- c., ring of bone
- C. Scale, ▸ Tennessee Self-
- c. ▸ solid angle
- c., team
- c., traditional disease

conception, legal
conception (POC), products of
conceptual
- c. memory, abstract
- c. memory, delayed abstract
- c. memory organization
- c. memory organization, competent abstract
- c. memory organization ▸ verbal
- c. skill
- c. system

concerning appearance, delusions
concerns, human spiritual
concerns person, human
concha
- c. auriculae
- c. bullosa
- c., ethmoidal

- c. nasalis inferior ossea
- c. nasalis media ossea
- c. nasalis superior ossea
- c. nasalis suprema ossea
- c., nasoturbinal
- c. of auricle
- c. of Santorini
- c., sphenoidal
- c. sphenoidalis

conchae
- c. auriculae, cymba
- c., cavum
- c., nasal
- c. nasal turbinates

conchal
- c. cartilage
- c. flap
- c. mastoid angle
- c. portion

concinna, Haemaphysalis
conclusion, etiological
conclusion of clinical trial ▸ analysis at
concomitant
- c. cholangitis
- c. disinfection
- c. sensation
- c. squint
- c. strabismus
- c. therapy

concordance, ventriculoarterial
concordant alternans
concordant alternation
concrete equivalent
concrete functional command
concretio cordis
concretio pericardii
concretions, calcium
concurrent
- c. disinfection
- c. findings
- c. upper respiratory tract infection (URI)
- c. treatment
- c. validity

concussion [convulsion, compulsion]
- c., abdominal
- c., air
- c., brain
- c., cerebral
- c., labyrinthine
- c., mild
- c., myocardial
- c. of brain
- c. of labyrinth
- c. of retina

- c., pulmonary
- c., severe
- c., spinal cord
- c. syndrome

condemnation of active euthanasia
condensans generalisata, osteitis
condensans ilii, osteitis
condensation of connective tissue
condensed milk
condenser electrometer ▸ dynamic-
conditio sine qua non
condition(s)
- c., allergic
- c., aseptic
- c., assessment of patient's
- c., blood
- c., change in living
- c., chronic
- c., chronic medical
- c. ▸ chronic, painful
- c., chronic skin
- c., chronic untreatable
- c., classical
- c., coexisting medical
- c., congenital cardiovascular
- c., controlled
- c., critical
- c., debilitating
- c. deferred on Axis I ▸ diagnosis or
- c. deferred on Axis II ▸ diagnosis or
- c., degenerative
- c. deteriorated
- c., deteriorating
- c., disabling
- c., diseased
- c., distressing
- c., environmental
- c., experimental
- c., fatal lung
- c., fatal medical
- c., fibrocystic breast
- c., genetic
- c., heart
- c., human
- c. improved
- c., incurable
- c. induced by medication
- c., inflammatory
- c., irreversible medical
- c. ▸ irreversible mental or physical
- c., isocapneic
- c., lethal
- c., life-threatening
- c., low oxygen
- c., medical

c., mental
c., moderate arthritic
c. muscles with aerobic exercises
c., normal size and
c. of admission
c. of participation
c., organic psychotic
c., paradoxic
c., pathological
c., patient admitted in dazed
c., patient discharged in good
c., patient in critical
c., patient in stable
c., patient's clinical
c., perinatal
c., physical
c. ▸ physical and mental
c., postnatal
c., potentially fatal
c., precancerous
c. precipitated by external factors ▸
   patient's
c., preexisting
c., prenatal
c. ▸ presenile organic psychotic
c., progressive
c. ▸ progressive and incurable
c., psychiatric
c. ▸ psychological factors affecting
   physical
c. related to stress
c., relevant maternal
c., reversible
c. ▸ senile organic psychotic
c., sleep-like
c., spiritual
c. stabilized
c. stabilized, patient's
c., stabilized psychiatric
c., stable medical
c. stable, patient's
c. ▸ stress-related heart
c., teeth in good dental
c., terminal
c. ▸ transient organic psychotic
c., treatable
c. unimproved
c., various psychiatric
c. ▸ weak, emaciated
conditionability, heart rate
conditional reflex
conditioned
c. behavior response
c. character, sex-
c. fear response

c. insomnia
c. orientation reflex audiometry
c., patient
c. reflex (CR)
c. reflex skills
c. reflex (CR) therapy
c. relaxation
c. response
c. stimulus
conditioning
c., aerobic
c., aversive
c., behavioral
c., cardiovascular
c. drills
c. exercise
c., fear
c., human operant heart rate
c. in human subjects ▸ escape and
   avoidance
c., instrumental
c. of diastolic blood pressure (BP) ▸
   instrumental
c., operant
c., operant cardiac
c., past
c., physical
c. program
c., respondent
c., rigorous
c. sessions, alpha
c. stimuli
c., strength
condom, female
conduct(s)
c. ▸ adjustment disorder with
   disturbance of
c. ▸ adjustment disorder with mixed
   disturbance emotional and
c. and emotions ▸ mixed
   disturbance of
c., anterograde
c. disorder
c. disorder, aggressive type ▸
   undersocialized
c. disorder, group type
c. disorder, hyperkinetic
c. disorder ▸ obsessive-compulsive
c. disorder, socialized
c. disorder, solitary aggressive type
c. disorder, unaggressive type ▸
   undersocialized
c. disorder, undifferentiated type
c., disturbance of

c. ▸ mixed disturbance of emotions
   and
c., negligent
c. ▸ predominant disturbance of
c., sexual
c., unprofessional
conductance
c. response, skin
c. stroke volume
c. vessel
conducted P waves
conducting
c. fibers, light-
c., sound-
c. treatment
conduction
c., aberrant
c., aberrant ventricular
c. ablation (ACA), accessory
c. abnormality
c. abnormality, atrioventricular (AV)
c., accelerated
c., aerial
c., aerotympanal
c. (AC) ▸ air
c. anesthesia
c., anisotropic
c., anomalous
c., antegrade
c. aphasia
c., atrial flutter with 4:1
c., atrial flutter with 3:1
c., AV (atrioventricular) nodal
c. block
c. block ▸ intraventricular
c. (BC) ▸ bone
c. (BC>AC) ▸ bone conduction
   greater than air
c. (BC<AC) ▸ bone conduction less
   than air
c., cardiac
c., complete impairment of
c., concealed
c. deafness
c. deafness, nerve
c., decremental
c. defect
c. defect, atrioventricular
c. defect in acute myocardial
   infarction
c. defect (IVCD), intraventricular
c. defect, nonspecific
   intraventricular
c. defect ▸ right ventricular
c. delay

conduction—*continued*
  c. delay, atrioventricular (AV)
  c. delay ▸ first degree
    atrioventricular block with
    intraventricular
  c. delay ▸ interventricular
  c. delay, intraventricular
  c. delay, rate dependent
  c. disease, atrioventricular (AV)
  c. disturbance
  c. disturbance, atrioventricular (AV)
  c. disturbance ▸ intraoperative
  c., forward
  c. greater than air conduction
    (BC > AC) ▸ bone
  c., His-Purkinje
  c. in heart ▸ electrical
  c., internodal
  c., intraventricular
  c., latency of
  c. less than air conduction
    (BC < AC) ▸ bone
  c. loss, bone
  c., median sensory
  c. of impulses
  c. of nerve impulses
  c. of nerve impulses ▸ interrupting
  c., orthograde
  c., osteotympanic
  c., partial impairment of
  c. pathways
  c. pattern ▸ intraventricular
  c. phenomenon ▸ gap
  c. ratio
  c., retrograde
  c., saltatory
  c., sensory nerve
  c., sinoventricular
  c. studies, nerve
  c. study ▸ motor and sensory nerve
  c., supranormal
  c. system
  c. system, cardiac
  c. system, ventricular
  c. system atrioventricular
  c. time
  c. time ▸ intra-atrial
  c. time ▸ sinoatrial (SA)
  c. tissue, atrioventricular (AV)
  c. velocity
  c. velocity (MNCV) ▸ motor nerve
  c. velocity of nerve, maximum
  c. velocity study ▸ nerve
  c. velocity tests ▸ nerve
  c. velocity ▸ ventricular

  c., ventricular
  c. ▸ ventricular sensing
  c., ventriculoatrial
conductive
  c. coupling
  c. device
  c. hearing loss
  c. heat
  c. keratoplasty (CK)
  c. loss
  c. of sputum, coughing
  c. radiofrequency electric field
  c. rate, ventricular
  c. type deafness
conductivity, thermal
conductor, electrical
conduit
  c., ileal
  c., inflow
  c., outflow
  c., Rastelli
  c. ▸ respiratory syncytial virus
conduplicato corpore
condylar
  c. emissary venin
  c. fossae
  c. fracture
  c. guide inclination
  c., inter◊
condyle
  c. bone
  c. bone, lateral
  c. cord
  c., femoral
  c., medial
  c., medial femoral
  c. metastasis syndrome, occipital
  c. of mandible
  c., tibial
condyloid joint
condyloid process
condyloma
  c. acuminatum
  c. acuminatum, perianal
  c., anal
  c. latum
  c. subcutaneum
condylomata
  c., giant vulvar
  c., venereal
  c., vulvar
Condy's fluid
C-1 vertebra (atlas)
C1-C7 (cervical vertebrae)
cone (Cone)

  c., arterial
  c. beam
  c. biopsy
  c. biopsy, cold knife
  c. cells
  c., cold
  c., cold knife
  c. biopsy cervical
  c. -down projection
  c. for electron beam therapy,
    intraoral
  c. granules
  c., hot
  c., narrow
  c. projection
  c., retinal
  c. -shaped amputation stump
  c. specimen
  c., starch
  c. tongs ▸ Barton-
  c., transvaginal
  c., truncated
coned AP (anteroposterior) projection
coned-down view
confabulans, paraphrenia
confabulation ▸ recent memory
  impairment and
confectioner's sugar
conference
  c., clinicopathologic
  c., consecutive case
  c., patient care
confervarum, Sideromonas
confervoides, Gracilaria
confidence
  c., develop self-
  c., feeling of
  c., foster
  c., increased self-
  c. level
  c., low self-
  c., self-
  c. ▸ sense of
  c. ▸ severe loss of self-
confident, self-
confidential
  c. assessment
  c. counseling
  c. evaluation and treatment
confidentiality
  c. of information
  c. of records
  c. ▸ patient-therapist
  c. regulations

configuration
- c., air butterfly
- c. and size
- c., arcuate
- c., atrial sensing
- c. ▸ dome-and-dart
- c., doughnut
- c., heart
- c., horseshoe
- c., mitral
- c. ▸ normal size and
- c. of uterus
- c., QRS
- c., size and/or
- c. ▸ spade-like
- c. ▸ spike-and-dome
- c., standard

confined plasma, magnetically
confined to bed, patient
confinement
- c. (CDC), calculated date of
- c. (EDC/EDOC) ▸ estimated date of
- c. (EDC/EDOC), expected date of
- c., inertial
- c., period of

confirmation, histologic
confirmation ▸ recovery and
confirmatory incision
confirmatory tests
confirmed memories of abuse,
continuous and
confirmed transmission of viral
hepatitis
conflict(s)
- c. and violence, family
- c., decisional
- c., emotional
- c., extrapsychic
- c., family
- c., hostile
- c., internal
- c. ▸ internal psychological
- c., interpersonal
- c. intervention
- c., intrapsychic
- c. management, healthy
- c., marital
- c., oedipal
- c. ▸ parental role
- c. resolution
- c. ▸ sexual orientation
- c., unconscious
- c. with teachers

conflicting emotions
confluence of nodules

confluent
- c. bilateral bronchopneumonia ▸ severe
- c. bronchopneumonia
- c. measles
- c. myositis
- c. pneumonia
- c. rash
- c. shadows

conformal radiation therapy
conformal radiation therapy ▸ three-dimensional
conformation of the skull
conformational polymorphism (SSCP) ▸ single strand
conformative coping
conformed radiation treatment
conformer
- c., eye implant
- c. for eye
- c., Fox's
- c., medium size

conforms to social norms
confront source of anxiety
confrontation
- c. naming
- c. of visual fields
- c. ▸ realistic nonhostile
- c. techniques with drug abusers

confrontational
- c. cognitive restructuring
- c. tactics
- c. techniques

confrontations, intense
confusa, Taenia
confused [contused]
- c. and combative
- c. and disoriented
- c. and dyspneic, patient
- c. behavior
- c. conversation
- c. delusions
- c. or faulty memories
- c. or impoverished thought and speech
- c., patient
- c. ▸ patient agitated and
- c. ▸ patient forgetful and
- c. perceptions
- c. thinking

confusion [contusion]
- c. about time and place
- c., acute
- c., aggressive
- c., agitation or

- c. and anxiety
- c. and coma ▸ disorientation,
- c. and dementia
- c. and disorientation
- c., and language loss ▸ disorientation
- c. and lethargy
- c. and poor judgment ▸ loss of recent memory,
- c. and suspicion ▸ nervousness,
- c., cardiac
- c., circle of
- c., disorientation and
- c., external
- c. ▸ fear and
- c. from anticholinergics
- c. from antihistamines
- c. from appetite suppressant
- c. from cimetidine
- c. from cirrhosis
- c. from dehydration
- c. from delirium
- c. from epilepsy
- c. from heart failure
- c. from insulin shock
- c. from migraine headache
- c. from stroke
- c., increased
- c., increasing
- c., intermittent
- c., lightheadedness and
- c., marked
- c., memory loss and
- c., mental
- c., nocturnal
- c., occasional
- c. of ideas
- c. or weakness ▸ fever, cough,
- c. ▸ overstimulation and resulting
- c. ▸ patient has forgetfulness, irritability and
- c., periodic
- c. ▸ persistent headache, vomiting or
- c. pneumonia
- c., postictal
- c., reactive
- c., source
- c., sudden
- c., temporary
- c., transient
- c., vague
- c. with head injury
- c. with light sensitivity

confusional arousal

confusional insanity
congealed blood
congenerous muscles
congenita
  c., amyotonia
  c., aplasia axialis extracorticalis
  c., aplasia cutis
  c., chondrodystrophia calcificans
  c., ectopia pupillae
  c., ichthyosis
  c., macrosomatia adiposa
  c., myatonia
  c., myotonia
congenital
  c. abducens-facial paralysis
  c. abnormalities from accutane
  c. abnormality
  c. abnormality, bladder
  c. abscess
  c. absence
  c. absence of kidney
  c. absence of pulmonary artery
  c. absence of ureter
  c. absence of urinary bladder
  c. absence of vagina
  c. adrenal hyperplasia
  c. adrenal virilism
  c. afibrinogenemia
  c. affliction
  c. agammaglobulinemia
  c. aleukia
  c. alveolar dysplasia
  c. amaurosis
  c. amputation
  c. anemia of newborn
  c. aneurysm of pulmonary artery
  c. aneurysm, rupture of
  c. anomalies, infant born with
  c. anomalies, multiple
  c. anomaly
  c. anomaly of mitral valve
  c. anomaly, structural
  c. aortic aneurysm
  c. aortic stenosis
  c. aortic valve disorder
  c. aspiration pneumonia
  c. atelectasis
  c. athetosis
  c. atonic pseudoparalysis
  c. atresia
  c. atresia of esophagus
  c. basis
  c. biliary atresia
  c. birth defect
  c. bronchiectasis

c. cardiac anomaly
c. cardiac defects
c. cardiovascular condition
c. cardiovascular malformation
c. cartilage
c. cataract
c. central hypoventilation syndrome
c. cerebral aneurysm
c. chloride diarrhea
c. cholesteatoma
c. chondrosternal depression
c. cleft palate
c. complete atrioventricular (AV)
  block
c. conotruncal anomaly
c. conus
c. coronary fistula
c. cyst
c. defect
c. defect in footplate of stapes
c. defect interventricular septum of
  heart
c. defect of labyrinth
c. defects, multiple
c. defects of brain
c. deformity
c. deformity repair
c. dermal sinus
c. development
c. diaphragmatic hernia
c. diaphragmatic hernia (CDH) ▸
  fetal
c. disease
c. dislocation
c. dislocation hip
c. disorder
c. displacement of heart
c. dyserythropoietic anemia
c. ectodermal defect
c. emphysema
c. erythropoietic porphyria (CEP)
c. eversion of organ
c. facial diplegia
c. failure
c. fistula, tracheoesophageal
c. glaucoma
c. goiter
c. heart anomaly
c. heart block
c. heart defect
c. heart disease (CHD)
c. heart failure
c. hemolytic anemia
c. hernia
c. hip dislocation

c. hip displacement
c. history
c. hydrocephalus
c. hypogammaglobulinemia
c. hypopituitarism
c. hypoplastic anemia
c. hypothyroidism
c. idiopathic adrenal hypoplasia
c. immune deficiency
c. immunity
c. immunodeficiency
c. infection
c. intestinal atresia
c. lacrimal obstruction
c. laryngeal stridor
c. left ventricular (LV) aneurysm
c. lesion
c. leukopenia
c. lobar overinflation
c. localized absence of skin
c. long QT syndrome
c. macular degeneration
c. malformation
c. malformed esophagus
c. mass, benign
c. megacolon
c. mitral stenosis
c. murmur
c. nephritis
c. nonspherocytic hemolytic
  anemia
c. ovarian abnormality
c. pancytopenia
c. predisposition
c. pseudoarthrosis
c. pseudarthrosis of leg
c. pterygium
c. ptosis
c. pulmonary arteriovenous
c. pulmonary lymphangiectasis
c. pyloric stenosis
c. radioulnar synostosis
c. renal aneurysm
c. retinal disorder
c. rubella syndrome
c. single atrium
c. spinal stenosis
c. subluxation of knees
c. syphilis
c. thymic dysplasia
c. toxoplasmosis
c. tracheoesophageal fistula
c. urinary tract infection
c. valvular defect
c. vertical talus foot deformity

c. viral infection
c. virilizing adrenal hyperplasia
c. vs acquired syndrome
c. weakness in vessel wall
congenitally absent pericardium
congenitally deformed infant ▸ patient delivered
congenitum, megacolon
congested
  c. air sacs
  c. and edematous ▸ lungs
  c. cough
  c. cortical surface
  c. cortices
  c. kidney
  c., liver parenchyma
  c. ▸ lungs edematous and
  c., lung tissue
  c., microscopically
  c. mucosa
  c. on cross section ▸ liver
  c., parenchyma
  c., parenchyma extremely
  c. rugal folds
  c., sinusoids
  c. skin
  c. ▸ spleen enlarged and
  c., spleen grossly
  c., spleen microscopically
  c., thyroid
  c. vascular structures
  c. with central necrosis ▸ liver
congestion
  c., active
  c., acute passive
  c., bilateral pulmonary
  c., bilateral vascular
  c., blood
  c., bronchial
  c., central lobular
  c., centrilobular
  c., chest
  c., chronic passive
  c., circulatory
  c., fluid
  c., functional
  c., hepatic
  c., hypostatic
  c., increasing
  c., interstitial
  c. interstitial vessels ▸ vascular
  c., lung
  c., lung (passive)
  c., marked acute
  c., marked diffuse

c., nasal
c., neuroparalytic
c. of bladder mucosa
c. of glomeruli
c. of liver
c. of liver, acute passive
c. of liver, chronic passive
c. of lungs
c. of lungs, chronic passive
c. of mucosa
c. of mucosa of stomach
c. of renal medulla ▸ marked
c. of spleen
c., passive
c., passive venous
c., physiologic
c., pleuropulmonary
c., pulmonary
c. ▸ pulmonary edema and
c., pulmonary venous
c., rebound
c. ▸ rebound nasal
c. ▸ severe acute passive
c. symptoms
c., upper respiratory
c., vascular
c., venocapillary
c., venous
congestive
  c. cardiac failure
  c. cardiomegaly
  c. cardiomyopathy
  c. change, passive
  c. chill
  c. cirrhosis
  c. dysmenorrhea
  c. edema
  c. enlargement
  c. failure
  c. failure, overt
  c. glaucoma
  c. glaucoma, acute
  c. headache
  c. heart disease (CHD)
  c. heart factor ▸ florid
  c. heart failure and cardioversion
  c. heart failure (CHF)
  c. heart failure (CHF), acute
  c. heart failure (CHF) ▸ advanced stage of
  c. heart failure (CHF), chronic
  c. heart failure ▸ florid
  c. heart failure (CHF) ▸ natural history of
  c. heart failure (CHF), recurrent

c. heart failure (CHF) ▸ sudden
c. heart failure (CHF) therapy
c. pulmonary disease
c. seasonal allergic rhinitis
c. splenomegaly
conglobata, acne
conglobation reaction
conglomerate densities
conglomerate fibrosis
conglutinating complement absorption test
conglutination of cervix
conglutination reaction
congregate housing
congruous hemianopia
conica, Pila
conica, Pirenella
conical
  c. cornea
  c. implant, Berens
  c. protrusion of center of cornea
  c. stump
  c. tip electrode
conicum, Amphistoma
conization
  c. biopsy, cold knife
  c. biopsy, laser excisional
  c., cervical
  c., cold knife
  c., electrocautery
  c., knife
  c., laser
  c., laser vaporization and excisional
  c., microsurgical
  c. of cervix, excisional
  c., postlaser
conjoined
  c. cusp
  c. hearts
  c. manipulation
  c. nerve root anomaly
  c. tendon
  c. twins
conjoint treatment
conjugate
  c. deviation
  c., diagonal
  c. diameter
  c. diameter, anatomic
  c. diameter, diagonal
  c. diameter, external
  c. diameter, internal
  c. diameter, obstetric
  c. diameter of pelvic inlet
  c. diameter, true

conjugate—*continued*
- c. eye movement
- c. gaze
- c. measurements
- c. movement
- c., obstetric
- c. paralysis
- c. vaccine
- c. vaccine ▸ bivalent
- c. vaccine ▸ pneumococcal

conjugated
- c. antibodies, ferritin
- c. antigen
- c. estrogens
- c. linoleic acid (CLA)

conjugation
- c., autotransferable by
- c., genetic
- c. or transduction ▸ transformation,

conjunctiva
- c., abscess of
- c., adhesions of
- c., amyloidosis of
- c., anulus of
- c., basal cell carcinoma of
- c., bulbar
- c. closed
- c., dissection of
- c., emphysema of
- c., epidermoid carcinoma of
- c., fibroma of
- c., flap of
- c., hemangioma of
- c., herpesvirus of
- c., inflammation of
- c., irritation of
- c., left ▸ flapping of
- c., medication injected under
- c., palpebral
- c., petechiae in
- c., right eye ▸ flapping of
- c., semilunar fold of
- c., syphilis of

conjunctivae
- c., anulus
- c. clear ▸ sclerae and
- c., Dirofilaria
- c., Filaria
- c. icteric
- c., injected
- c., leptotrichosis
- c., limbus
- c., lithiasis
- c. (S and C) ▸ sclerae and
- c., siderosis

- c., xerosis

conjunctival
- c. artery, posterior
- c. cul-de-sac
- c. flap
- c. flap, fornix based
- c. flap, Gunderson
- c. flap, Van Lint
- c. fold
- c. fornix
- c. hemorrhage
- c. hyperemia
- c. incision
- c. infection
- c. injection
- c. membrane
- c. papilloma
- c. pocket
- c. reaction
- c. reflex
- c. smear
- c. tumors
- c. vascular injection
- c. vein, posterior
- c. veins
- c. xerosis

conjunctive symbiosis
conjunctivitis
- c., acne rosacea
- c., actinic
- c., acute
- c., allergic
- c., anaphylactic
- c., arc-flash
- c., atopic
- c., atropine
- c., bacterial
- c., Beal's
- c., blennorrheal
- c., calcareous
- c., catarrhal
- c., chemical
- c., croupous
- c., diphtheritic
- c., diplobacillary
- c., eczematous
- c., Egyptian
- c., Elschnig's
- c., epidemic
- c. ▸ eyelid scaling from
- c., follicular
- c. (GPC) ▸ giant papillary
- c., gonococcal
- c., gonorrheal
- c., granular

- c., inclusion
- c., infectious
- c., itching from
- c., Koch-Weeks
- c., larval
- c. medicamentosa
- c., membranous
- c., meningococcus
- c., Morax-Axenfeld
- c., molluscum
- c. necroticans infectiosus
- c., pain from
- c., Parinaud's
- c., Pascheff's
- c. ▸ perennial allergic
- c. petrificans
- c., phlyctenular
- c., prairie
- c., pseudomembranous
- c., purulent
- c., pus from
- c., Samoan
- c., Sanyal's
- c., scrofular
- c. ▸ seasonal allergic
- c., squirrel plague
- c. (TRIC) ▸ trachoma inclusion
- c., trachomatous
- c., tularensis
- c., uratic
- c., vernal
- c., viral
- c. virus, inclusion
- c., welder's
- c., Widmarks
- c. with eyelashes turning in
- c., Wucherer's

conjunctivotarsal area
conjunctivotarsal surface
connate teeth
connected disability (SCD) ▸ service-
connected in parallel, electrodes
connecting
- c. neurons
- c. stalk
- c. systems
- c. tube, sterile

connection(s)
- c., abnormal growth of neuronal
- c., accessory arteriovenous
- c., accessory atrioventricular
- c. anomaly ▸ pulmonary venous
- c., atrio-Hisian
- c., cavopulmonary

c., cocaine-to-crime
c., earth
c., electrode
c., external
c., ground
c., partial anomalous pulmonary venous
c. ▸ pulmonary venous
c., synaptic
c. ▸ total anomalous pulmonary venous
c. ▸ total cavopulmonary
c. ▸ univentricular atrioventricular

connective tissue
c.t., areolar
c.t., autodigestion of
c.t. cells
c.t. cells, embryonal
c.t. ▸ condensation of
c.t. ▸ damaged
c.t. disease
c.t. disease (MCTD) ▸ mixed
c.t. diseases, secondary
c.t. disorder, chronic
c.t. disorder ▸ genetic
c.t. disorders
c.t., elastic
c.t., epivaginal
c.t., fibrous
c.t., inflammation of
c.t. ▸ layer of
c.t. ▸ long fronds of
c.t., loose
c.t. myxomatous soft
c.t. overgrowth of interacinar
c.t., peribronchiolar
c.t., portal
c.t., reticular fibers of
c.t., scarred
c.t., septal
c.t. sheath
c.t. stains
c.t. stalk
c.t., subcutaneous
c.t., submucosal
c.t., thickened
c.t. ▸ underlying

Connell suture
conning others
Conn's operation
Conn's syndrome
conoid
c. lens
c. ophthalmic lens, Volk
c. process

c., Sturm's
Conolly's system
conorii, Rickettsia
conotruncal
c. anomaly
c. anomaly, congenital
c. inversion ▸ isolated
conoventricular fold and groove
Conray
C., Angio-
C. contrast medium
C. -400
C., residual
consanguineous donor
conscientious, excessively
conscientious objection
conscious
c. activities
c. and mentally competent
c. awareness
c. awareness ▸ altered state of
c. breathing
c. control
c. control of motor units
c. distortion
c. exploitation of others
c., health-
c., intellectually
c. memory
c. mental control
c., patient
c. ▸ patient self-,
c. recollection
c., semi◊
c. -subconscious relationships
c. suppression
c. thought
c. victim
c., weight
consciousness
c. ▸ abrupt loss of
c., alert state of
c., alteration of
c., altered level of
c., altered state of
c. and motor control ▸ loss of
c., awareness and
c. ▸ brief loss of
c., changing social
c., clouded
c., clouding of
c., decreased level of
c., depressed level of
c., exhausted
c. ▸ fluctuating level of

c., impaired
c., lack of
c., lapses of
c., liminal
c. (LOC), level of
c., loss of
c., passive volition versus
c., patient regained
c., patient's level of
c. ▸ periodic loss of
c. ▸ predominant disturbance of
c., retention of
c., specific loss of
c. ▸ spell of decreased
c., state of
c. ▸ temporary absence of
c., threshold of
c., total loss of
c., transient loss of
c. ▸ unity and continuity of
consecutive
c. amputation
c. case conference
c. dislocation
c. insanity
consensual
c. light reaction
c. light reflex
c. reaction
c. reflex
consensus panel
consent
c., actual
c. cards
c. for organ donation
c. for surgery, written
c. form
c. form anesthetic
c. form autopsy
c. form cosmetic surgery
c. form for body to be donated for scientific research
c. form, informed
c. form for operation
c. form operation and grafting of tissue
c. form for recipient of organ transplant
c. form for removal of organ for transplant
c. form for removal of tissue for grafting
c. form for taking and publication of photographs

consent—*continued*
- c. form for taking of motion pictures of operation
- c. form for televising of operation
- c. form operation
- c. form to delivery by alternate physician
- c. form to use eyes (donor)
- c. form to use eyes (next of kin)
- c. form to use kidneys (donor)
- c. form to use kidneys (next of kin)
- c., implied
- c., informed
- c., informed waiver and
- c., medication release
- c., option of
- c., parental
- c., presumed
- c., required
- c. requirement, normal
- c. to intervention
- c. transaction
- c., valid

consequences, long-term
consequences, maladaptive
conservation
- c., energy
- c. surgery, breast
- c. therapy ▸ breast

conservative
- c. approach
- c. care
- c. management of patient
- c. measures
- c. nonpharmacologic therapy
- c. observation
- c. surgery and irradiation
- c. therapy
- c. treatment

conservatively, patient treated
considerable difficulty encountered
considerations
- c., behavioral
- c. in palliation ▸ emotional
- c. in palliation, physical
- c. in radiation therapy, anatomical
- c. in radiation therapy, normal use
- c., moral
- c., placement
- c., social
- c., sociocultural

consistency
- c., clay-like
- c., doughy
- c., firm

- c., firm in
- c., nodular
- c. of myocardium
- c. of stool, change in color and
- c. ▸ size, shape and
- c., test-retest
- c., uniform

consistent
- c., findings
- c. form, fairly
- c. irresponsibility
- c. medication compliance
- c. with invasive carcinoma, cells
- c. work behavior ▸ inability to sustain
- c. work behavior ▸ sustain

console (DDC), direct display
console, tomographic control
consolidated bronchopneumonia
consolidating area
consolidation
- c., air space
- c. and healing
- c. in combined modality therapy, temporal
- c. of lungs
- c., patchy area of
- c. ▸ patchy areas of pneumonic
- c., pneumonic
- c. process ▸ memory

consolidative process
consonating rale
conspiracy ▸ delusion with vague
conspiracy ▸ target of
conspiratorial and persecutory delusions
constant(s)
- c. abdominal pain
- c. admiration, demand for
- c., air kerma rate
- c. attention, demand for
- c. blinking
- c. buttock pain
- c. control, time
- c., corpuscular
- c. coupling
- c. current pacing box ▸ digital
- c., decay
- c., dose rate
- c., empiric
- c. esotropia
- c. exophoria
- c., exposure rate
- c. fatigue
- c., filtered exposure rate

- c., gas
- c., Gorlin
- c., harsh pain
- c. hypertrophia
- c. hypotropia
- c. infusion excretory urogram
- c. monitoring
- c. movement, exhibits
- c. nagging pain
- c. nausea
- c. observation
- c. pain
- c., permeability
- c., Planck's
- c. skin irritation and rubbing
- c., specific gamma ray
- c. strabismus
- c. stress, patient under
- c., time
- c., transformation
- c. verbal cueing
- c. visual contact

constantly
- c. breaks down ▸ bone
- c. running nose
- c. seeking praise or admiration
- c., talks

constellation, family
constellatus, Diplococcus
constellatus, Peptococcus
consternation [*concentration*]
constipated, bowels
constipated, patient
constipation [*obstipation*]
- c. and fecal impaction
- c. ▸ anorectal problem from
- c., atonic
- c., bloating and
- c. ▸ change in urine flow from
- c., chronic
- c., colonic
- c. from antidepressant
- c. from antihistamine
- c. from diverticulosis
- c. from intestinal obstruction
- c., functional
- c., gastrojejunal
- c. ▸ hiatal hernia and
- c., incontinence and
- c., indigestion from
- c. ▸ irritable bowel syndrome with
- c. or hemorrhoids ▸ chronic
- c. ▸ pain in abdomen with
- c., spastic
- c. with diarrhea

c. with problem of central nervous system
constitution, ideo-obsessional
constitution, psychopathic
constitutional
  c. cause
  c. delayed growth
  c. dysfunction of liver
  c. hepatic dysfunction
  c. infantile panmyelopathy
  c. influence
  c. obesity
  c. psychology
  c. psychopathic inferiority
  c. psychopathic state
constraint-induced movement therapy
constrict, bronchial tubes
constrict urethra, muscles
constricted
  c. blood vessels
  c. bronchial tubes
  c. by scar tissue
  c. coronary artery
  c. esophagus
  c., pupils
  c., urethra
constricting
  c. esophageal lesion
  c. lesion
  c. pain, severe
constriction
  c. and spasm ▸ bronchial
  c. apical
  c., arterial
  c., artery
  c., bronchial
  c. caused by light
  c., chest
  c., concentric
  c., cyclic
  c. deformity
  c., duodenopyloric
  c., esophageal
  c. of arteries
  c. of arteries of brain
  c. of blood vessels
  c. of breathing passages
  c. of pupil
  c. or spasm of blood vessel
  c. phenomenon, lateral
  c., primary
  c., pupillary
  c., secondary
  c., throat

constrictive
  c. edema
  c. endocarditis
  c. pericarditis
  c. pericarditis, chronic
  c. ring
constrictor
  c. muscle, inferior
  c. muscle of pharynx ▸ superior
  c. muscle, pharyngeal
  c. of artery
constrictum, Pentastoma
constrictus, Porocephalus
construction, verbal sentence
constructional apraxia
constructive
  c. aggression
  c. discharge
  c. support
constructural task ▸ spatial-visual
consultant, health care
consultant, nurse
consultation
  c., cardiac
  c., diagnostic
  c., initial
  c., inpatient psychiatric
  c. -liaison, psychiatry
  c., nutritional
  c., patient seen in
  c., radiotherapy
  c. request
  c. service
  c., surgical
  c., tissue
consulting, corporate
consulting psychologist, licensed
consume alcohol
consumed by rage
consumers, medical
consumption
  c., alcohol
  c. ▸ caffeine or nicotine
  c. coagulopathy
  c. coagulopathy, intravascular
  c. computer, oxygen
  c., dietary fat
  c., drug
  c., excess fluid
  c., excessive alcohol
  c., fluid
  c., food
  c., galloping
  c., heavy alcohol
  c. index ▸ oxygen (O_2)

  c. level
  c. ▸ level of alcohol
  c., limit milk
  c., loss of control
  c. ▸ maximum oxygen (O_2)
  c., moderating alcohol
  c. ▸ myocardial oxygen (O_2)
  c. of alcohol, excessive
  c. of alcohol, heavy
  c., oxygen (O_2)
  c. ▸ peak exercise oxygen (O_2)
  c. per minute ▸ oxygen (O_2)
  c., reduced alcohol
  c., reducing alcohol
  c., salt
  c., sensitive to alcohol
  c., systemic O_2 (oxygen)
  c. time ▸ prothrombin (Pro)
  c. ▸ volume oxygen (O_2)
contact(s) [*compact, contract*]
  c. allergy
  c. assistance
  c. assistance for ambulation
  c. balancing
  c. between donor and recipient ▸ transient
  c. bifocal
  c., break in reality
  c. burn
  c. cancer
  c., casual
  c. ceptor
  c., complete
  c., constant visual
  c. dermatitis
  c. dermatitis, allergic
  c. dermatitis ▸ rubber
  c., direct
  c., direct patient
  c., direct personal
  c. eczema
  c., electrode
  c., eye
  c. ▸ eye-to-eye
  c., heterosexual
  c. illumination
  c., immediate
  c., indirect
  c., indirect personal
  c. infection
  c. inhibition
  c., initial
  c., interpersonal
  c. ▸ lack of eye
  c. lens

contact(s)—*continued*
- c. lens, contaminated
- c. lens ▸ disposable bifocal
- c. lens, extended wear
- c. lens, full
- c. lens, Hydrocurve
- c. lens infection
- c. lens (ICL) ▸ intraocular
- c. lens, opaque
- c. lens prism, Goldmann's
- c. lens, Sauflon PW
- c. lens, Soflens
- c. lens, T lens
- c. lenses, custom
- c. lenses ▸ rigid gas permeable (RGP)
- c. lenses ▸ soft
- c. lenses ▸ soft disposable
- c., local
- c., maintain eye
- c., male homosexual
- c. metastasis
- c., needle
- c., occlusal
- c. of sensors, skin
- c. physician
- c., prolonged
- c., sexual
- c. shell implant ▸ corrected cosmetic
- c. skin rash
- c., social
- c. sports, nonstrenuous
- c. sports, strenuous
- c. -standby assist
- c. stomatitis
- c. substance
- c., supportive therapeutic
- c., surface of
- c. therapy
- c. tracing
- c. tracing ▸ complete, mandatory
- c. tracing, targeted
- c., transient
- c., transmission by
- c. ulcers
- c. unit
- c., weak
- c. with blood spill
- c. with body secretions, direct
- c. with contaminated blood, direct
- c. with contaminated instruments, indirect
- c. with contaminated laboratory apparatus, indirect

- c. with contaminated oral secretions, direct
- c. with contaminated plasma, direct
- c. with contaminated serum, direct
- c. with environment ▸ loss of
- c. with male carriers of AIDS (acquired immune deficiency syndrome), heterosexual
- c. with patient ▸ direct
- c. with reality
- c. with reality, loss of
- c. with skin, good
- c. with skin, poor
- c., working

contacted, funeral director
contagion
- c., behavioral
- c., direct
- c., immediate

contagiosa, impetigo
contagiosum, molluscum
contagious
- c. agalactia
- c. disease
- c. skin disease
- c. suicide syndrome
- c. viral disease
- c. virus

contained
- c., infection
- c., transportable medical unit ▸ self-
- c. underwater breathing apparatus ▸ self-

container
- c., biohazard
- c. placement, intracavitary
- c., puncture-resistant
- c. ▸ red cells float to top of
- c., rigid puncture resistant

containing
- c, dust ▸ spore
- c. fluid, abnormal sac
- c. gas, abnormal sac
- c. semisolid material ▸ abnormal sac

containment cost
containment, crisis
contaminant(s)
- c., airborne
- c., microbial
- c., particulate
- c. surface

contaminated
- c. blood

- c. blood culture
- c. blood, direct contact with
- c. blood spills
- c. blood transfusion
- c. by AIDS (acquired immune deficiency syndrome) virus ▸ blood products
- c. contact lenses
- c. donor blood
- c. dressings
- c. drinking water
- c. drug needles
- c. environment ▸ severely
- c. equipment
- c. food
- c. instruments, indirect contact with
- c. instruments, puncturing of skin by
- c. laboratory apparatus, indirect contact with
- c. linen, blood
- c. nasal secretions ▸ virus
- c. needle
- c. needle, puncturing of skin by
- c. needle stick
- c. needles and syringes
- c. oral secretions, direct contact with
- c. reservoir nebulizer
- c. serum, direct contact with
- c. surgical supplies
- c. tap water
- c. transfusion
- c., urine culture and sensitivity
- c. vehicle, fecally
- c. water
- c. with blood
- c. with bodily fluids
- c. wound
- c. wound, clean-

contamination
- c., airborne
- c., bacterial
- c., cross
- c., direct fecal
- c., eliminate source of
- c., environmental staphylococcal
- c., exogenous
- c., foreign body
- c. from ambient hospital air
- c. from anesthesia equipment
- c. from instruments
- c. from irrigating solutions
- c. from linens
- c. from unsterile needles

c. ▸ gene therapy
c., ground water
c., hematogenous
c., indirect fecal
c. ▸ life-threatening microbial
c., marijuana
c., microbial
c., microorganism
c., nebulizer monitored for
c. of exogenous sources
c. of tissue, bacterial
c., perineal
c., radon
c., seafood
c., skin
c., source of
contemplated suicide, patient
contemplative behavior
contemporary attitudes
content(s)
c., abdominal
c., abnormally high
c., abnormally low
c., aspiration gastric
c., bacterial
c. (BAC), blood alcohol
c. blood-tinged, fluid
c., bowel
c., cellular
c., cholesterol calcium
c. clonogenic cell
c. determination, oxygen
c., exenteration of orbital
c., fecal
c. flat, emotional
c., fluid
c., gastric
c., harmonic
c., intestinal
c., intra-abdominal escape of
    gastroduodenal
c., latent
c., manifest
c., moisture
c., natural sodium
c. normal, breasts and axillary
c. of blood decreases ▸ oxygen
c. of stomach, acid
c., oral
c. ▸ oxygen (O$_2$)
c., peritoneal
c., reflux of gastric
c., stomach
c. ▸ terminal aspiration of gastric
c., thought

c., total sodium and
c. uniform, colloid
c. validity
context, negative emotional
contiguitatem, extension per
contiguous rib
continence
c. bowel and bladder
c., fecal
c. (WOC) nurse ▸ wound, ostomy,
c., urinary
continent, patient
contingency contracting
contingency management
contingent negative variation (CNV)
Contino's epithelioma
Contino's glaucoma
continua
c., acrodermatitis
c. chronica, gastrorrhea
c., epilepsia partialis
continual irritation of eyeball
continuation of medications
continued
c. abstinence
c. ambulatory care
c. deterioration
c. drinking
c. fever
c. fragmentation
c. intoxication
c. maladaptive behavior
c. medical therapy, recommend
c. on outpatient basis ▸
    chemotherapy
continuing (Continuing)
c. cardiac care
C. Care Centers (CCC)
c. care community
C. Care Retirement Community,
    (CCRC)
c. care staffing
c. chemotherapy
c. chemotherapy, patient on
c. education programs
c. maintenance chemotherapy
c. medical education
c. tumor activity
continuitatem, extension per
continuity
c. broken, gross
c. equation
c. equation, Doppler
c., genetic
c. not broken, gross

c. of bone, interruption in
c. of care
c. of consciousness ▸ unity and
c. of fracture, synthesis of
c., restoration of
c., synthesis of
continuous
c. abstinence
c. ambulatory peritoneal dialysis
    (CAPD)
c. and confirmed memories of
    abuse
c. arrhythmia
c. arteriovenous hemofiltration
c. atrial fibrillation
c. beam
c. biofeedback
c. catgut sutures
c. cerebral activity
c. chest compressions (CCC)
c. circular inverting suture
c. combined therapy
c. cuticular suture
c. cyclical peritoneal dialysis
    (CCPD)
c. drainage (dr'ge)
c. drainage (dr'ge) system
c. epilepsy
c. epileptic seizures
c. fever
c. flow culture
c. flow of energy
c. flow ventilation
c. focal seizures
c. heart murmur
c. hemostatic suture
c. home care
c. infusion chemotherapy
c. insulin infusion
c. intellectual activity
c. invasive monitoring
c. inverting suture
c. irrigation
c. locking manner
c. loop exercise echocardiogram
c. loop wire
c. mandatory ventilation
c. mattress suture
c. mechanical ventilatory
    assistance
c. motion
c. monitoring
c. murmur
c. muscular twitchings
c. nerve block

continuous—*continued*
- c. observation
- c. oxygen
- c. passive motion (CPM) machine
- c. pericardial lavage
- c. positive airway pressure (CPAP)
- c. positive airway pressure (NCPAP) ‣ nasal
- c. positive pressure
- c. positive pressure breathing (CPPB)
- c. ramp protocol
- c. remission
- c. running lock suture
- c. running suture
- c. scan thermograph
- c. seizure activity
- c. silk suture
- c. spasms ‣ intermittent
- c. suction drainage (dr'ge) system
- c. suture
- c. suture, U-shaped
- c. tension
- c. tremor
- c. trial
- c. use
- c. venovenous hemofiltration
- c. volumetric acquisition
- c. wave
- c. wave ablation
- c. wave Doppler echocardiogram
- c. wave Doppler echocardiography
- c. wave Doppler imaging
- c. wave Doppler ultrasound
- c. wave laser
- c. wave laser ablation
- c. wound infusion

continuously monitored, fetus
continuously, postures
continuum of care
contorta, Capillaria
contortions, facial
controtum, Trichosoma
contortus, Haemonchus
contour(s)
- c., aortic
- c., bladder
- c., body
- c., distortion of
- c., height of
- c. line
- c., lobulated
- c. ‣ Murgo pressure
- c., nasal
- c. of breast

- c. of heart
- c. of heart, normal
- c. of nasal bones
- c., smooth
- c., stepped
- c., symmetrical in
- c., uneven
- c., uterus symmetrical in
- c., ventricular

contouring, body
contraband drugs
contraception, intrauterine
contraception, surgical
contraceptive
- c., barrier
- c. counseling
- c. device, intrauterine
- c. diaphragm
- c. film (VCF) ‣ vaginal
- c. -induced hypertension ‣ oral
- c. injections ‣ monthly/bimonthly
- c. options
- c., oral
- c. pill
- c. research
- c., sequential type oral
- c. sponges

contract(s)
- c. anal sphincter
- c., antisuicidal
- c. autoradiography
- c., behavior
- c., bladder muscles
- c., diaphragm
- c., muscles
- c., premature ventricular
- c. synchronously

contracted
- c., abdomen
- c., alveoli
- c., bladder
- c., fingers
- c., heart
- c. heel cord
- c., kidney
- c., muscles
- c. pelvis
- c. permanently, arms
- c., pupil
- c. shoulder
- c., urinary bladder

contractile
- c. amplitude
- c. behavior
- c. cells

- c. efficiency, loss of
- c. element
- c. excursion, diminished
- c. fiber cell, elongated
- c. fiber cell, nucleated
- c. force
- c. function
- c. function in cells of myocardium
- c. mechanism
- c. protein
- c. ring dysphagia
- c. stricture
- c. vacuole
- c. work index

contractility
- c., cardiac
- c., electro◊
- c., galvanic
- c., idiomuscular
- c., isovolumetric
- c. ‣ left ventricular (LV)
- c., myocardial
- c., neuromuscular
- c. of heart muscle
- c. of hypertrophied muscle ‣ impaired
- c., ventricular

contracting
- c. and relaxing of muscles ‣ alternating
- c., contingency
- c., muscle

contraction(s)
- c., abnormal bladder
- c., abnormal heart
- c., active
- c., alternate
- c. and relaxation of heart
- c., anodal closure
- c., anodal duration
- c. (AOC), anodal opening
- c., apex of
- c., atrial
- c. (APC), atrial premature
- c. (APDC) ‣ atrial premature depolarization
- c., automatic ventricular
- c. band
- c. band necrosis
- c., Braxton Hicks
- c., burst of uncontrolled muscle
- c., capsular
- c., cardiac
- c., cardiac cell
- c., carpopedal

c., cathodal closure
c., cathodal opening
c., cicatricial
c., clonic
c., closing
c., colonic
c., coordinated
c. coupling (ECC) ▸ electrical
c. coupling ▸ excitation
c. cycle of heart
c. deformities
c., Dupuytren's
c. during labor
c., effective atrial
c., enhance
c. ▸ escape ventricular
c., esophageal
c., expulsion
c. ▸ external sphincter
c., false Dupuytren's
c. ▸ false labor
c., fibrillary
c., focal ectopic ventricular
c. ▸ force of muscle
c. ▸ forceful heart
c., frequency of
c., frequent
c., gallbladder
c., galvanotonic
c., Gowers'
c. headaches, muscle
c., heart
c., Hicks'
c., hourglass
c., idiomuscular
c., improve muscle
c. ▸ inherent strength of myocardial
c., intensity of labor
c., intermittent
c., intermittent tonic muscular
c., intrauterine
c., involuntary
c., involuntary muscle
c., involuntary muscular
c., ipsilateral
c., irregular
c., isometric
c., isotonic
c., isovolumetric
c., isovolumic
c., junctional
c., labor
c., moderate
c., multifocal
c., muscle

c. ▸ muscle cell
c., muscular
c., myotatic
c., nodal premature
c., nonconducted premature atrial
c. ▸ normal ventricular
c. of atria
c. of blood vessel
c. of bowel ▸ cyclic muscular
c. of bowel ▸ muscle
c. of calf muscles
c. of esophagus ▸ muscle
c. of esophagus, tertiary
c. of hand in tetany
c. of heart muscle
c. of muscle, full voluntary
c. of muscle ▸ sudden, involuntary
c. of myocardium
c. of pupil
c. of uterine muscle
c. of uterus
c. of ventricles
c. of voluntary muscles ▸ violent involuntary
c. on ventriculogram ▸ abnormal
c., opening
c. ▸ painful intestinal
c., painful muscle
c., palmar
c., paradoxical
c., paroxysmal
c., passive
c. pattern
c. period ▸ isometric
c. ▸ physiology of heart
c., postural
c., premature
c. (PAC) ▸ premature atrial
c. ▸ pre-term
c., premature auricular
c. (PVC) ▸ premature ventricular
c., premonitory
c. process
c., rapid
c., rare
c., rate and force of
c. reflex, iris
c. -relaxation cycle
c. ▸ repeated muscle
c., respiratory muscular
c., rested state
c., rheumatic
c., rhythmic
c. ▸ rhythmic muscular
c. right atrium

c. right ventricle
c., right ventricular
c. ring, esophageal
c., segmentation
c., spasmodic
c. ▸ spasmodic muscular
c., spastic
c. ▸ stimulation of muscle
c., stomach
c. stress
c., suppress reflex
c., supraventricular premature
c., synchronous forceful
c., systolic
c., tertiary
c., tetanic
c., thenar muscle
c. time
c. time, isovolumic
c., timed
c., tone
c., tonic
c., transition
c., twitch
c., unifocal
c. (UC), uterine
c. ▸ vascular smooth muscle
c., ventricular
c. (VPC) ▸ ventricular premature
c. (VPDC) ▸ ventricular premature depolarization
c., voluntary
c. wave
c. (PVC) with coupling ▸ premature ventricular

contractive activation ▸ myofilament
contractive spasms, painful
contractual diathesis
contractual management
contracture(s)
c. and swelling, joint
c., bladder neck
c., burn scar
c., capsular
c. deformities
c. deformity ▸ flexion
c., digital flexion
c., Dupuytren's
c., flexion
c. formation
c., hand
c., hip
c., intermittent
c., intermittent facial
c., ischemic

contracture(s)—*continued*
- c. ▸ ischemic muscle
- c. ▸ ischemic paralysis and
- c., joint
- c., myocardium
- c. of digits ▸ flexion
- c. of hip, abduction
- c. of hip, adduction
- c. of hip, flexion
- c. of hip, internal rotation
- c. of knee
- c. of knee, flexion
- c. of left ventricle (LV) ▸ ischemic
- c. of ligament
- c., organic
- c., postpoliomyelitic
- c., veratrin
- c., vesical neck
- c., Volkmann's

contradictory, self-

contraindication(s)
- c., medical
- c. to surgery ▸ major
- c. to surgery ▸ preoperative

contralateral
- c. aspect
- c. associated, movement
- c. axillary metastasis
- c. breast, dose to
- c. ear
- c. ear lobe
- c. hemiplegia
- c. limb
- c. movement
- c. radiation
- c. side of cerebellum
- c. sign

contrast
- c. administration
- c. agent
- c. agent ▸ superparamagnetic
- c. agent ▸ urographic
- c., air
- c., angiographic
- c. angiography
- c. angiography ▸ phase
- c. arterial catheterization
- c. arthrogram, double-
- c. barium enema, double
- c. colon examination ▸ air
- c. dyes
- c. echocardiography
- c. echocardiography (MCE) ▸ myocardial

- c. echocardiography ▸ transesophageal
- c. enema
- c. enema double
- c. enhanced carotid magnetic resonance angiography (MRA)
- c. enhanced echocardiogram
- c. enhancement
- c. enhancement ▸ mean
- c. examination, double
- c. laryngography
- c. ▸ left atrial spontaneous echo
- c. material
- c. material, excretion of
- c. material, intrathecal
- c. material, intravenous (IV)
- c. material ▸ low osmolality
- c. material, non-ionic
- c. material ▸ poor excretion of
- c. material ▸ prompt excretion of
- c. material, reaction to
- c. material Renografin-76
- c. material, residual
- c. material, retention of
- c. material ▸ vein filled with
- c. media
- c. media, injection of
- c. media instilled ▸ x-ray
- c. media, iodinated
- c. media, mottling of
- c. media ▸ poor excretion of
- c. medium
- c. medium, acetrizoate sodium
- c. medium, Amipaque
- c. medium, Angio-Conray
- c. medium, barium sulfate
- c. medium, Bilopaque
- c. medium, bunamiodyl
- c. medium, Cardiografin
- c. medium, Cholebrine
- c. medium, Cholografin
- c. medium, Clysodrast
- c. medium, Conray
- c. medium, Cystografin
- c. medium, Cystokon
- c. medium delivery
- c. medium, diatrizoate meglumine
- c. medium, diatrizoate sodium
- c. medium, Diodrast
- c. medium, Dionosil
- c. medium, diprotrizoate
- c. medium, Duografin
- c. medium, Ethiodane
- c. medium, Ethiodol
- c. medium, Gastrografin

- c. medium, Hippuran
- c. medium, Hypaque
- c. medium, Hypaque-Cysto
- c. medium, Hypaque M
- c. medium, Hypaque Meglumine
- c. medium, Hypaque sodium
- c. medium ▸ injection of radiopaque
- c. medium, intravenous (IV) bolus injection of
- c. medium, Intropaque
- c. medium, iodalphionic acid
- c. medium, iodipamide
- c. medium, iodomethamate
- c. medium, iodophthalein sodium
- c. medium, iodopyracet
- c. medium, iopanoic acid
- c. medium, iophdone
- c. medium, iophendylate
- c. medium, iophenoxic acid
- c. medium, iopydol
- c. medium, iothalamate
- c. medium, ipodate calcium
- c. medium, Isopaque
- c. medium, Kinevac
- c. medium, Lipiodol
- c. medium, Liquipake
- c. medium, meglumine diatrizoate
- c. medium, meglumine iodipamide
- c. medium, meglumine iothalamate
- c. medium, metrizamide
- c. medium, metrizoate sodium
- c. medium, neo-lopax
- c. medium ▸ nonionic
- c. medium, Novopaque
- c. medium, Orabilex
- c. medium, oragrafin calcium
- c. medium, oragrafin sodium
- c. medium, Pantopaque
- c. medium, patient ingested
- c. medium, phentetiothalein
- c. medium ▸ polygelin colloid
- c. medium, Priodax
- c. medium, propyliodone
- c. medium, radiopaque
- c. medium, Renografin
- c. medium, Reno-M-Dip
- c. medium, Reno-M-60
- c. medium, Reno-M-30
- c. medium, Renovist
- c. medium, Salpix
- c. medium, Sinografin
- c. medium, Skiodan
- c. medium, Skiodan Acacia
- c. medium, sodium diatrizoate
- c. medium, sodium iodipamide

c. medium, sodium iodohippurate
c. medium, sodium iodomethamate
c. medium, sodium iothalamate
c. medium, sodium ipodate
c. medium, sodium methiodal
c. medium, sodium thorium tartrate
c. medium, sodium tyropanoate
c. medium, Telepaque
c. medium, Thixokon
c. medium, thorium dioxide (Th-O$_2$)
c. medium, Thorotrast
c. microscope, phase-
c., negative
c., Optiray
c. ratio
c. resolution
c. roentgenography, double
c. ▸ spontaneous echo
c. stain
c. study
c. study air
c. study, double
c. study ▸ dual-
c. study, ▸ single-
c. substance, injection of
c., Ultravist
c. venography
c. ventriculography
c. visualization, double

contrasting temperatures ▸ treatment of
contrecoup
   c. contusion
   c. injury
   c., fracture by
contributing factor
control(s) (Control)
   c. ▸ abnormalities of respiratory
   c., air
   c., alpha
   c. and strength, voluntary
   c. and timing ▸ stress
   c., anger
   c. anger ▸ inability to
   c., antibiotic
   c. appetite, inability to
   c. atrial fibrillation
   c., autosuggestion temperature
   c., axial
   c., behavior
   c., behavioral
   c., bidirectional cardiac
   c., biopsy under x-ray
   c., birth
   c., bladder
   c. bleeding

c. bleeding ▸ pressure to
c. blood pressure (BP) ▸ inability to
c. blood sugar
c., bowel
c. box
c., brain
c., brain-based pain
c., brain stem
c. by alpha activity ▸ autonomic
c., calculus
c. ▸ cause, prevention and
c. center of brain ▸ motor
c. center ▸ visual
C. (CDC) ▸ Centers for Disease
c., cholesterol
c., chronic pain
c., circulatory
c. clinic, pain
c. clinical trial ▸ random
c., cognition and muscle
C. Committee, Infection
c., concept of biofeedback
c., conscious
c., conscious mental
c. console, tomographic
c. consumption, loss of
C. Coordinator (ICC) ▸ Infection
c. counseling, weight
c., damping
c. deficiency ▸ impulse
c., delusions of mind
c. dependence on external
c. device, arrhythmia
c., devices, birth
c., diabetes
c. diet, weight-
c., dietary
c. disease process
c. disorder, compulsive impulse
c. disorder, impulse
c. ▸ disorders of impulse
c. -dominated personality
c. domination response (CDR)
c. dose, tumor
c. drinking, inability to
c., effective infection
c., effective pain
c., electronic bed
c., emotional
c. ▸ environment of coercive
c., environmental
c. exercises, muscular
c. exercises, neuromuscular
c. existing infection
c. ▸ fear of losing

c., feedback mechanisms of
   hormonal
c. ▸ feeling out-of-
c., gain
c. gastric secretion
c., genetic
c., glucose
c., glucose level
c., glycemic
c. group
c. group, placebo
c., hand
c., head
c. head movements
c., heart rate
c., high frequency filter
c. ▸ HIV prevention and
c., hormonal
c., hospital infection
c., illusion of
c., impulse
c. in childbirth, emotional
c. in eating ▸ impulse
c. in functional colitis ▸ intestinal
c., individual voluntary
c., infection prevention and
c., infectious disease
c., intent to
c. itching and sneezing
c., lack of coordination and
c., lack of emotional
c. ▸ lack of motor
c., language
c., learned
c. learning and awareness ▸ heart
   rate
c., local
c., local tumor
c., locus of
c. ▸ long-term weight
c., lose
c., loss of
c., loss of bladder
c. ▸ loss of bowel
c. ▸ loss of consciousness and
   motor
c. ▸ loss of emotional
c. ▸ loss of fecal
c. ▸ loss of muscle
c., loss of self-
c., low frequency filter
c. measures
c. mechanism, stress
c. mechanisms, metabolic
c., medication distribution and

c. withdrawal symptoms

controllable
- c. distress
- c. evacuation
- c. risk factor
- c. sensation

controlled
- c. access to fluids
- c. activity
- c. adolescent behavior
- c. analgesia, patient-
- c. analgesic (PCA) ▸ patient-
- c. assessment ▸ randomized
- c. association
- c. atrial fibrillation
- c. auricular fibrillation
- c. beams
- c., bleeding
- c. bleeding, pneumatic tourniquet
- c., bleeding points
- c. breathing
- c. clinical trial
- c. clinical trial ▸ placebo-
- c. clinical trial ▸ randomized
- c. conditions
- c. diabetes
- c., diabetes mellitus (DM)
- c., diabetes well-
- c. diaphragmatic respiration
- c. diet, fat
- c. diet, sodium
- c. double-blind techniques
- c. drain
- c. drinking
- c. drugs
- c. experiment
- c. experiment, placebo
- c. fluid access
- c. heart failure ▸ stable,
- c. heart rhythm disturbance
- c. high blood pressure
- c. intravenous system ▸ self-
- c. inverse ratio ventilation ▸ pressure
- c. investigation
- c. laser, computer
- c. movements ▸ slow,
- c. outcome study
- c., pain well
- c. procedures
- c. randomized study ▸ blinded, placebo-
- c. relaxation
- c. relaxation ▸ biofeedback-assisted cue-

c. release systems
- c. respiration
- c. smoking
- c. studies
- c. study
- c. study, crossover placebo
- c. study ▸ double-blind
- c. study, placebo-
- c. study ▸ randomized, blinded,
- c. substance
- c. substance book
- c. substances, illegal
- c. surgical robot ▸ voice-
- c. trauma
- c. trial
- c., trial placebo
- c. trials, randomized
- c. trial ▸ randomized double-blinded placebo
- c. trial ▸ randomized, placebo-
- c. variable frequency
- c. ventilation
- c. ventricular response
- c. with hemostatic clamps ▸ bleeding
- c. with ring forceps ▸ bleeding

controller, electronic

controlling
- c. alpha activity
- c. anger, difficulty
- c. arrhythmias
- c. eye pressure
- c. fat
- c. fluid formation
- c. ideology
- c. influence
- c. nerve cells ▸ motion-
- c. parent
- c. patient, drug
- c. risk factors
- c. skin bacteria
- c. symptoms

controversial
- c. clinical significance
- c. diagnosis
- c. therapy

controversy ▸ nature-versus-nurture
contused [*confused*]
contused wound
contusion(s) [*confusion*]
- c. and abrasions
- c. cataract
- c., cerebral
- c., contrecoup
- c., myocardial

c. of brain
- c. of head
- c. of heart
- c. of lung
- c. of spinal cord
- c., pulmonary
- c., recent
- c. ▸ superficial femoral artery

conus [tonus, closus]
- c. branch
- c., congenital
- c. cordis
- c. elasticus laryngis
- c., lateral
- c. medullaris
- c. medullaris nerve
- c. musculature
- c., oblique
- c., pulmonary
- c., underlying

convalescence
- c., late
- c., postoperative
- c., uneventful postoperative

convalescent treatment center ▸ patient discharged to
convalescent unit
convalescing, patient
convective heat
convention, polarity
conventional
- c. behavior
- c. cardiac bypass
- c. cineangiography
- c. EEG (electroencephalogram)
- c. magnetic resonance imaging (MRI)
- c. management
- c. medication
- c. medicine
- c. methods
- c. physical therapy
- c. radiation therapy in acromegaly
- c. radiation treatment
- c. reform eye implant
- c. reform implant ▸ Snellen
- c. shell type implant
- c. surgery
- c. therapy
- c. therapy group
- c. treatment

convergence
- c., adaptive
- c., amplitude of

convergence—*continued*
- c. insufficiency ▸ Duane classification of
- c. (NPC) ▸ near point of
- c. of eyes
- c. sign ▸ hilum

convergency reflex

convergent
- c. exercises
- c. ray
- c. squint
- s. strabismus

converging collimator

converging lens

conversant, patient

conversation, appropriate

conversation, confused

conversational skills

conversational voice

conversion
- c. accelerator (SPCA) ▸ serum prothrombin-
- c. (A/D, ADC) analog digital
- c. coefficient
- c. disorder
- c. disorder ▸ hysterical
- c., electrical
- c. hysteria
- c., internal
- c. into nutrients
- c., Mantoux
- c. neurosis
- c. of atrial fibrillation ▸ electrical
- c. of position
- c. pressure
- c. reaction
- c. reaction, anosmic
- c., somatic
- c. syndrome ▸ fibrinogen fibrin
- c. table

conversive heat

convert sensitization

converted rhythm

converter (Converter)
- c., analog-to-digital
- c., digital scan
- c., energy
- c. enzyme (ACE), angiotensin
- c. enzyme inhibitor
- c. enzyme (ACE) inhibitor ▸ angiotensin
- c., image
- c., infrared image-
- C. (OPTACON), Optical Tactile

converting enzyme (ACE), angiotensin

convex
- c. array
- c., double
- c. lens
- c. linear array
- c., periscopic
- c. sole

convexes of brain

convexity
- c. of lens, increased
- c. of spine
- c., outer
- c. to left ▸ scoliosis with
- c. to right ▸ scoliosis with

convexoconcave heart valve ▸ Shiley

conveying system, pneumatic

conveyor, pneumatic tube

convoluted tubule ▸ distal

convoluted tubule ▸ proximal

convolution(s)
- c., abrupt
- c., Broca's
- c., Heschl's
- c., occipitotemporal
- c. of cerebrum
- c. of Gratiolet
- c., Zuckerkandl's

convolutional
- c. artery, Pick's
- c. atrophy
- c. atrophy, Pick's
- c. markings

convolutions of cerebrum

convulsant drugs

convulsing, patient

convulsion(s) [concussion, compulsion]
- c. accompanying fever
- c. and coma
- c. and death ▸ delirium,
- c., anesthetic-induced
- c., benign febrile
- c. ▸ catatonia, coma and
- c., central
- c., cerebral
- c., choreic
- c., clonic
- c., coordinate
- c., crowing
- c., epileptiform
- c., essential
- c., febrile
- c., full-blown
- c. ▸ grand mal

- c., hysterical
- c., hysteroid
- c., induction of
- c., lethal
- c., local
- c., major
- c., mimetic
- c., mimic
- c. ▸ petit mal
- c., pseudoepileptic
- c., puerperal
- c., salaam
- c. ▸ seizures or
- c., static
- c., syncope with
- c., syncope without
- c., tetanic
- c., tonic
- c., trembling
- c., uremic

convulsive
- c. attack
- c. diathesis
- c. disorder
- c., electro◊
- c. movement
- c., patient
- c. reflex
- c. response, photo◊
- c. seizure
- c. seizure, focal
- c. shock therapy
- c. shock, true
- c. syncope
- c. tic

convulsivus, status

Conway technique

co-occurring mood disorder

cooing murmur

cooing sign

cookie, Gelfoam

cool(s) (Cool)
- c. clammy skin
- c. -down exercise
- c. -down period
- c. -down relaxation exercise
- c. -down ▸ warm up and
- c. laser ▸ excimer
- c. mist vaporizer
- C. myocardial protection pouch, Cardio-
- c. therapy
- c. tip laser
- c. working muscles

cooled
- c. blood
- c., kidneys perfused and
- c., patient's body temperature

cooler, dual use water

Cooley
- C. -Bloodwell mitral valve prosthesis
- C. -intrapericardial anastomosis
- C. modification of Waterson anastomosis
- C. woven Dacron graft

cooling
- c. blanket
- c. blanket for hyperthermia
- c., body
- c., cardioplegia
- c., core
- c. jacket, cardiac
- c. jacket ▸ Medtronic cardiac
- c. therapy for stroke
- c., topical

Coombs'
- C. cord
- C., direct
- C. murmur, Carey
- C. test
- C. test, direct
- C. test, indirect

cooperation in combined modality therapy, spatial

cooperative, patient

cooperative, patient alert and

Coopernail's sign

Cooper's
- C. hernia
- C. irritable testis
- C. ligament

Cooper's ligament [*Pourpart's ligament*]

coordinate
- c. breathing with exercise
- c. convulsion
- c. map ▸ polar
- c. mapping, bull's eye polar
- c. muscle movement
- c. system

coordinated (Coordinated)
- c. convulsion
- C. Home Care Program
- C. Home Care Program ▸ patient discharged to
- c. reflex
- c. rhythm

coordinates ▸ X, Y, and Z

coordination
- c. and agility
- c. and control, lack of
- c. and posture
- c. ▸ balance and
- c. center
- c., defective
- c. disorder
- c. disorder, developmental
- c., disorder of muscular
- c., disturbance of equilibratory
- c., eye-hand
- c., failure of muscular
- c., faulty
- c., fine motor
- c., gait and speech ▸ deterioration of
- c. ▸ gait, balance and
- c. ▸ gross and fine motor
- c., hand-breath
- c., hand-eye
- c., impaired
- c. ▸ impaired motor
- c., lack of
- c. ▸ lack of balance and
- c. ▸ lack of motor
- c., loss of
- c. ▸ loss of balance and
- c., loss of control of muscular
- c. ▸ loss of motor
- c. ▸ maintain balance and
- c., motor
- c., motor power and
- c., muscle
- c., muscular
- c. mental activity
- c. of movement
- c. of surveillance procedures
- c. or equilibrium, decrease in
- c., physical
- c., poor
- c., psychomotor
- c., reduce alertness and
- c., slowed
- c. ▸ small muscle
- c., strength and
- c. ▸ sudden loss of
- c., visual-motor
- c. ▸ weakness and loss of

coordinator (Coordinator)
- c., clinical
- c., employee health
- c., family therapist
- C., Home Care
- C., Hospice

C. (ICC) ▸ Infection Control
- c., insurance
- c., organ recovery
- c., patient care
- c., patient education
- c., procurement
- c., transplant

cop ▸ suicide-by-

COP
- COP (colloid osmotic pressure)
- COP (colloid osmotic pressure) measurement
- COP (colloid osmotic pressure) of plasma
- COP (Cytoxan, Oncovin, Prednisone)

COPD (chronic obstructive pulmonary disease)

COPE (chronic obstructive pulmonary emphysema)

cope(s) (Cope)
- c. ▸ inability to
- C. method bronchography
- c., patient unable to
- c. with daily stress
- c. with stress

Copeland's implant

Copilots (amphetamines)

Coping (coping)
- c. ability
- c., adaptive
- c., behavior
- c., behavioral
- c., compromised ineffective family
- c., conformative
- c., creative
- c., defensive
- c., difficulty
- c. ▸ disabling ineffective family
- c., emotional
- c., family
- c., inadequate
- c. ▸ ineffective family
- c. ▸ ineffective individual
- c., intrapsychic
- c. mechanism
- c. mechanism ▸ ineffective
- c. mechanism ▸ natural
- c. pattern
- c. process
- c. reaction
- c. skills
- c. skills, develop
- c. skills therapy
- c. skills ▸ transcendent

coping—*continued*
- c. strategies
- c. strategies, apply
- c. strategies, healthy
- C. Strategies questionnaire
- C. Strategy Enhancement (CSE)
- c. technique
- c. to reduce stress
- c. with anger
- c. with anxiety
- c. with caring
- c. with pain
- c. with problems
- c. with sobriety
- c. with stress

copious
- c. bleeding
- c. bright red blood
- c. drainage (dr'ge)
- c. irrigation
- c. lavage of joint
- c. lavage performed
- c. mucoid material
- c. sputum
- c. vomiting

COPP chemotherapy
COPP therapy
copper (Copper)
- c. accumulation
- c. metabolism
- c., serum
- C. 7 IUD (intrauterine device) inserted
- c. sulfate
- c. ▸ toxic effect of
- c., urine
- c. vapor laser ▸ Metalase
- c. wire effect

coprogenus, Saccharomyces
Copromonas subtilis
coproporphyria, free erythrocyte
coproporphyria, hereditary
coproporphyrin
- c., free erythrocyte
- c. test
- c., urinary

coprozoic ameba
copying, gene
Coquille plano lens
cor (COR) [*core*]
- C. (Coronary Observation Radio)
- c. adiposum
- c. arteriosum
- c. biloculare
- c. bovinum

C. device ▸ Abio-
C. dextrum
c. en cuirasse
c. hirsutum
c. mobile
c. pacemaker, Omni
c. pendulum
c. pseudotriculare biatriatum
c. pulmonale
c. sinistrum
c. taurinum
c. triatriatum
c. triatriatum dexter
c. triloculare
c. triloculare biatriatum
c. triloculare biventriculare
c. venosum
c. villosum

coracoacromial arch
coracoacromial ligament
coracobrachial muscle
coracoclavicular bar
coracoclavicular ligament
coracohumeral ligament
coracoid
- c. notch
- c. process
- c. process drilled ▸ tip of
- c. process of scapula

coral
- c. calculus
- c. eye implant
- c. thrombus

coralliform cataract
coralliformis, cataract
Coratomic pacemaker
Corbin technique
cord(s) [*chord*]
- c. abscess, spinal
- c. activity ▸ vocal
- c., acute inflammation of spinal
- c. and meninges
- c., anterior horns of spinal
- c., arachnoid of spinal
- c. around infant's neck
- c. bilirubin
- c. biopsy, spinal
- c. birth defect ▸ spinal
- c. bladder
- c. block
- c. block in radiation therapy, spinal
- c. block, spinal
- c. blood
- c. blood banks ▸ umbilical
- c. blood cell therapy

c. blood cells
c. blood cells ▸ transplanted
c. blood culture
c. blood elution
c. blood transplant
c. blood, umbilical
c. blood workup
c., bowed vocal
c., cancer, vocal
c., central canal of spinal
c., central ▸ intermediate substance of spinal
c. clamped
c., cleansing umbilical
c. compression
c. compression, extradural
c. compression, impending
c. ▸ compression of liver
c. compression, spinal
c. compression syndrome
c. compression, umbilical
c. concussion, spinal
c., condyle
c., contracted heel
c., Coombs'
c., contusion of spinal
c. culture
c., cutting of umbilical
c. cyst ▸ spinal
c. damage, spinal
c. decompression, spinal
c., degeneration of spinal
c. destruction
c. disc degeneration ▸ spinal
c. disease, spinal
c. disorder ▸ spinal
c. distortion
c., dorsal aspect spinal
c., dorsal horns of spinal
c., drainage (dr'ge) of spinal
c., dura mater of spinal
c. dysfunction, transient spinal
c. dysfunction ▸ vocal
c., electrical stimulation to spinal
c., excision lesion of spinal
c. exploration, spinal
c., false
c., false vocal
c., fetal
c. fluid ▸ umbilical
c. ▸ focal disorders of brain and spinal
c. functions, spinal
c. ▸ gelatinous substance of spinal
c., gray matter of spinal

c. ▸ gray substance of spinal
c., heel
c., hemisection spinal
c. hemorrhage ▸ agonal spinal
c. ▸ impingement on spinal
c., inflammation of spinal
c. injury, cervical
c. injury paralysis ▸ spinal
c. injury, spinal
c. ▸ intact spinal
c. ▸ larynx with vocal
c., lateral horns of spinal
c., lateral ▸ intermediate substance of spinal
c., lateral region of spinal
c. lengthening, heel
c. lesion, cervical
c. lesion, high thoracic
c. lesion ▸ spinal
c., lining of spinal
c. margin
c., medullary
c. mobile
c. moves normally
c., myelitis of
c. necrosis, spinal
c. ▸ neurons in spinal
c. nodule, vocal
c. normal in appearance
c., nuchal
c. of Billroth
c., opposing vocal
c., outermost covering of spinal
c., ovigerous
c., palpable venous
c. paralysis, vocal
c., paralyzed
c. polyp ▸ vocal
c., pressure on spinal
c., prolapsed
c., protective layer of spinal
c. ▸ proximal cervical spine
c. ▸ regenerating nerves in spinal
c. ▸ regeneration of spinal
c., senile bowing of vocal
c. ▸ sensory input from spinal
c. severed, spinal
c., spermatic
c., spinal
c. ▸ spinal nerve
c., splenic cell
c. ▸ squamous cell carcinoma of vocal
c. stimulation ▸ electrical spinal

c. stimulator ▸ spinal
c. stripping
c. stripping, vocal
c. stroke ▸ spinal
c. structures
c. syndrome, central
c. syndrome, tethered
c., terminal ventricle of spinal
c., thoracolumbar spinal
c. tissue ▸ spinal
c. tolerance in radiation therapy, spinal
c. traction
c. traction ▸ umbilical
c. tracts, spinal
c. ▸ transected spinal
c. transection
c. ▸ transection of spinal
c., true vocal
c. tumor
c. tumor, metastatic spinal
c. tumor, paraplegia in spinal
c. tumor, spinal
c., umbilical
c., ventral gray columns of spinal
c. ▸ ventral horns of spinal
c., ventricle of
c., vocal
c., white commissure of spinal
c. ▸ white substance of spinal
c. with ease ▸ bronchoscope inserted through vocal

cordifolia, Tinospora
cordiformis, uterus
cordis (Cordis)
c. abdominalis, ectopia
c., accretio
c., adipositas
c., angina
c., annuli fibrosi
c., apex
c., ataxia
C. Atricor pacemaker
c., atrium
c., bulbus
c., chorda tendineae
c., chorea
c., concretio
c., conus
c., crena
c., delirium
c., diastasis
c., ectasia
C. Ectocor pacemaker
C. fixed rate pacemaker

c., foramen ovale
c., fossa ovalis
C. -Hakim shunt
c., hypodynamia
c., ictus
c. ▸ incisura apicis
c. intermittens, ischemia
c., malum
c., myasthenia
c., myofibrosis
c., myopathia
C. pacemaker
C. pacemaker unit
c., palpitation
c., paracentesis
c., pulsus
C. pump, Hakim-
C. radiopaque tantalum stent
c., sarcoidosis
c., steatosis
c., sulcus coronarius
c., theca
c., tremor
c., trepidatio
c., tumultus
C. Ventricor pacemaker
c., ventriculus
c., ventriculus dexter
c. ventriculus, sinister
c., vitium

Cordonnier ureteroileal loop
cordrolum, petechial capillary
cordy pulse
Cordyceps sinesis
Cordylobia anthropophaga
core(s) [cor]
c. alcoholic, hard
c. biopsy
c. biopsy, breast
c. body temperature
c. breast biopsy, automated large
c. cooling
c. decompression
c. disease, central
c. drug abuser ▸ hard
c. ▸ large lipid
c. lesion, apple
c. memory
c. mindfulness
c. needle biopsy
c., nucleic acid
c. of atheromatous material
c. personality
c. pneumonia
c. proteins, common

core(s)—continued
- c. services
- c. temperature
- C. -Vent implant
- c. window
- c. wire, central

core antibody
- c.a. (HBcAb), hepatitis B
- c.a. antigen (Anti-HBc IgM), antibody IgM class to hepatitis B
- c.a. antigen (Anti-HBc), total antibody to hepatitis B
- c.a. test

corkscrew appearance

corn(s)
- c. and calluses
- c. pads, medicated
- c., painful
- c. -soy milk

cornea(s) ('s)
- c., abnormal steepening of
- c., abrasion of
- c., abscess of
- c., actinomycosis of
- c. and tissues ▸ organs,
- c., bacterial infection of
- c., bedewing of
- c., blastomycosis of
- c., burn of
- c., chalcosis of
- c., clouded
- c., clouding of
- c., conical
- c., conical protrusion of center of
- c., dendritic ulcer of
- c., denudation of
- c., diabetic melanosis of
- c. disorder
- c., distorted
- c., donated
- c., dryness of
- c., dystrophy
- c., ectasia of
- c., endothelial dystrophy of
- c. endothelial layer
- c., epidermoid carcinoma of
- c., epithelial dystrophy of
- c., erosion of
- c. examination
- c., facet of
- c., farinata
- c., fistula of
- c., foreign body (FB) in
- c., fungal infection of
- c., ghost vessels in

- c. globosa
- c., graft of
- c., guttata
- c., haze of
- c., herpes zoster of
- c., hyaline formation in
- c., inflammation of
- c. ▸ inner layer of
- c., irritation of
- c., keloid of
- c., lead incrustation of
- c., lesion of the
- c., limbus of
- c. luster
- c., marginal dystrophy of
- c., moistened
- c., multiple slits in
- c. opaca
- c., periphery of
- c. plana
- c., preserved
- c. problem
- c. ▸ proper substance of
- c., removal foreign body (FB) from
- c., scarred
- c., shrinking
- c., stimulating
- c. stored, excised
- c., stroma of
- c., sugar-loaf
- c., superficial layers of
- c. ▸ surface of
- c., suture of
- c., tattoo of
- c., thin
- c. transplant
- c., unequal curvature of
- c., vertical meridian of
- c., Vogt's
- c., weakened

corneae
- c., abrasio
- c., arcus lipoides
- c., caligo
- c., herpes
- c., limbus
- c., liquor
- c., macula
- c., phthisis
- c. racemosum, staphyloma
- c. senilis, linea
- c., staphyloma
- c., substantia propria
- c., ulcus serpens

corneal
- c. abrasion
- c. abscission
- c. anesthesia
- c. arcus
- c. astigmatism
- c. blink reflexes
- c. burn
- c. cell
- c. cells ▸ vaporizing
- c. clouding
- c. coverage, complete
- c. damage
- c. degeneration
- c. deposits, posterior
- c. disease
- c. dystrophy, Salzmann's nodular
- c. ectasia
- c. edema
- c. edema, subepithelial
- c. electrode
- c. endothelium
- c. epithelium
- c. fissure
- c. flap
- c. graft
- c. implant
- c. implant material ▸ Silastic
- c. implant, Silastic
- c. infiltrate
- c. injury
- c. irregular astigmatism
- c. lip
- c. margins
- c. microscope
- c. opacity
- c. reflex
- c. reflexes, absent
- c. reflexes, bradycardia and absent
- c. rings
- c. scarring
- c. scarring from chemical burn
- c. section
- c. space
- c. staphyloma
- c. surface
- c. suture
- c. swelling
- c. tissue
- c. tissue, fresh
- c. tissue, frozen
- c. tissue transplant
- c. topographer
- c. topography
- c. transplant

c. transplant recipient
c. transplant scissors, Katzin
c. transplant surgery
c. transplantation
c. transplants ▸ eyes donated for
c. trepanation
c. trephining
c. tube
c. ulcer
c. ulcer, bacterial
c. ulceration
c. ulcers, perforated
c. vascularization
c. warpage
c. wound, perforating
c. xerosis
Cornelia de Lange's syndrome
Cornell exercise protocol
corneolus, Siderophacus
corneomandibular reflex
corneomental reflex
corneopterygoid reflex
corneoscleral
c. incision
c. suture
c. wound
corner(s) (Corner)
C. Allen test
c. ▸ down-turned mouth
c. dystrophy, lattice
c. from sagging cheek ▸ cracked mouth
c., superior
C. tampon
cornerstones of treatment
corneum, stratum
corniculate cartilage
corniculum laryngis
cornified cell
cornified superficial cells
Cornil syndrome ▸ Roussy-Corning('s)
C. anesthesia
C. implant, Dow
C. puncture
C. shunt, Dow
C. silicone, Dow
cornpicker's pupil
cornu
c., dorsal
c., ethmoid
c., inferior
c. of hyoid bone
c., ventral

cornual
c. implantation
c. portion of uterus
c. pregnancy
cornuradicular zone
corollary incision
Corometrics Doppler scanner
Corometrics Fetal Monitor (CFM)
corona
c., Bischoff's
c. ciliaris
c. dentis
c. vascularis
c., Zinn's
coronal
c. angulation
c. arc technique
c. arrays
c. bipolar montage
c. cuts
c. incision
c. incision, bimastoid
c. odontoma
c. plane
c. pulp
c. section
c. section of brain ▸ serial
c. section, serial
c. sections ▸ multiple
c. slice
c. substance
c. suture
c. suture lines
coronarius cordis, sulcus
coronary(ies) (Coronary)
c. anatomy
c. anatomy ▸ native
c. aneurysm
c. angiogram ▸ baseline
c. angiogram (LCA) ▸ left
c. angiogram (RCA) ▸ right
c. angiographic analysis ▸ quantitative
c. angiographic catheter
c. angiographic ▸ quantitative
c. angiography
c. angiography, diagnostic
c. angiography ▸ noninvasive
c. angiography ▸ nonselective
c. angiography (PTCA), percutaneous transluminal
c. angiography (QCA) ▸ quantitative
c. angioplasty
c. angioplasty, balloon

c. angioplasty (ELCA) ▸ excimer laser
c. angioplasty (PELCA) ▸ percutaneous excimer laser
c. angioplasty (PTCA) ▸ percutaneous transluminal
c., anomalous
c. arterial reserve
c. arteries ▸ asymmetric lesions in
c. arteries ▸ atherosclerosis of
c. arteries atherosclerotic
c. arteries, blocked
c. arteries, dilate
c. arteries ▸ hardening of
c. arteries, inflammation of
c. arteries ▸ intramural
c. arteries, Kipp's
c. arteries patent
c. arteries ▸ severe narrowing ostia of
c. arteries ▸ spasm of
c. arteries ▸ vasoconstriction of
c. arteries widely patent
c. arteriogram
c. arteriograph
c. arteriography
c. arteriography ▸ quantitative
c. arteriography, selective
c. arteriosclerosis
c. arteriosclerosis, severe
c. arteritis
c. artery (CA)
c. artery aneurysm
c. artery angiography ▸ left
c. artery angiography ▸ right
c. artery angioplasty
c. artery (ALMCA) ▸ anomalous left main
c. artery anomaly
c. artery, anterior descending
c. artery atherosclerosis
c. artery blockage
c. artery, blocked
c. artery bypass (CAB)
c. artery bypass graft (CABG)
c. artery bypass grafting ▸ endarterectomy and
c. artery bypass grafting ▸ port-access
c. artery bypass grafting surgery
c. artery bypass (MIDCAB) ▸ minimally invasive direct
c. artery bypass (OPCAB) ▸ off pump

coronary—*continued*

- c. artery bypassn (PACAB) ▸ port-access
- c. artery bypass (CAB) surgery
- c. artery bypass (TECAB) ▸ total endoscopic
- c. artery calcification
- c. artery ▸ calcification of left
- c. artery, cannula ▸ Silastic
- c. artery circulation
- c. artery circulation ▸ insufficient
- c. artery, clogged
- c. artery, constricted
- c. artery disease (CAD)
- c. artery disease, atherosclerotic
- c. artery disease (CAD) ▸ evaluation of
- c. artery disease ▸ left main
- c. artery disease mortality
- c. artery disease ▸ silent
- c. artery disease ▸ transplant
- c. artery disease ▸ woven
- c. artery, diseased
- c. artery dissection
- c. artery dissection (SCAD) ▸ spontaneous
- c. artery, epicardial
- c. artery, fistula
- c. artery ▸ impaired
- c. artery laser angioplasty
- c. artery, left
- c. artery (LCA), left circumflex
- c. artery lesion
- c. artery, narrowed
- c. artery, narrowing of
- c. artery occlusion
- c. artery occlusive disease
- c. artery probe
- c. artery ▸ rechannelization of
- c. artery ▸ repeated narrowing of
- c. artery reperfusion
- c. artery, right
- c. artery (RCA), right circumflex
- c. artery ▸ right main
- c. artery right ventricular (RV) fistula
- c. artery scanning
- c. artery ▸ severe stenosis left
- c. artery ▸ severe stenosis right
- c. artery spasm
- c. artery stenosis
- c. artery surgery
- c. artery thrombosis
- c. artery ▸ unclogging
- c. artery vasospasm

- c. atherectomy
- c. atherectomy (DCA) ▸ directional
- c. atherectomy ▸ rotational
- c. atheroma
- c. atherosclerotic heart disease
- c. atherosclerosis scan
- c. attack ▸ patient candidate for
- c. bifurcation
- c. blockage
- c. blood flow
- c. blood flow measurement
- c. blood flow velocity
- c. blood vessel
- c. bypass
- c. bypass graft
- c. bypass procedure
- c. bypass surgery
- c. bypass surgery ▸ rescue
- c., cafe
- c. care, intensive
- c. care nursing
- C. Care Unit (CCU)
- C. Care Unit (ICCU) ▸ Intensive
- C. Care Unit, Mobile
- c. cataract
- c. catheterization
- c. cineangiography
- c. cineangiography, left
- c. cineangiography, right
- c. circulation
- c. circulation embarrassment
- c. circulation ▸ left dominant
- c. collateral circulation
- c. constriction
- c. cushion
- c. cusp
- c. dimple, blind
- c. disease
- c. disease, anatomic
- c. disease ▸ pre-existing
- c. disease ▸ premature
- c. disease ▸ reverse
- c. disease ▸ underlying obstructive
- c. disease ▸ untreatable
- c. distribution
- c. drug project
- c. embolism
- c. endarterectomy
- c. event
- c. filling
- c. fistula, congenital
- c. flow
- c. flow reserve
- c. flow reserve technique
- c. flow (TCF) ▸ total

- c. gene therapy
- c. gene therapy program
- c. graft ▸ Perma-Flow
- c. heart disease (CHD)
- c. imaging
- c. insufficiency (CI)
- c. insufficiency syndrome
- C. Intensive Care Unit (CICU)
- c. laser angiography, absorption
- c. laser angioplasty
- c. lesion ▸ discrete
- c. lesion ▸ macrovascular
- c. ligament
- c. macroangiopathy
- c. mastoid-to-mastoid incision
- c. microangioplasty
- c. microcirculation
- c. microvascular disease
- c. nodal rhythm
- C. Observation Radio (COR)
- c. occlusion
- c. occlusive disease
- c. odontoma
- c. opacification
- c. ostial dimple
- c. ostial stenosis
- c. ostium
- c. ostium ▸ solitary
- c. patient, antihypertensive
- c. perfusion catheter, McGoon
- c. perfusion pressure
- c. plaques
- c. prognostic index (CPI)
- c. reconstruction, Cabral
- c. reflex
- c. resistance vessel
- c. revascularization, postoperative
- c. revascularization (PTCR) ▸ percutaneous transluminal
- c. ring
- c. risk
- c. risk factor
- c. risk reduction
- c. roadmapping
- c. rotational ablation
- c. rotational angioplasty (PCRA) ▸ percutaneous
- c. rotational atherectomy
- c. rotational atherectomy ▸ percutaneous
- c. sclerosis
- c. seeking catheter
- c. sinus
- c. sinus blood flow
- c. sinus catheterization

c. sinus electrogram
c. sinus occlusion ▸ intermittent
c. sinus orifice electrogram
c. sinus ▸ proximal
c. sinus retroperfusion
c. sinus rhythm
c. sinus thermodilution
c. sinus, valve of
c. spasm
c. spasm and prolapse
c. spasm induction
c. spastic angina
c. steal
c. steal mechanism
c. steal phenomenon
c. steal syndrome
c. stenosis
c. stenosis ▸ left main
c. stenosis ▸ single vessel
c. stent
c. stent, CardioCoil
c. stent implantation
c. stent placement
c. stenting
c. sulcus
c. syndrome, acute
c. therapy
c. thrombolysis
c. thrombosis
C. (MAGIC) trial ▸ Magnesium in
c. trunk ▸ complete occlusion of
   right
c. vascular reserve
c. vascular reserve ▸ impaired
c. vascular resistance
c. vascular turgor
c. vasculature
c. vasodilation
c. vasodilator
c. vasodilator reserve
c. vasodilator, topical
c. vasomotion
c. vasospasm
c. vein
c. vein, left
c. venous pressure
c. vessel anatomy
c. vessel ▸ stented
c. vessels
c. vessels ▸ occluded
c. vessels, smaller
coronata, Entomophthora
coronata, Siderocapsa
Coronaviridae virus
coroner-on-call

coroner's case
coronoid
   c. fossa
   c. process
   c. process of ramus
corpectomy, lumbar
corpora
   c. albicans
   c. albicantia
   c., fibrous capsule of
corporate consulting
corporate therapy
corpore, conduplicato
corporeal cesarean section (CS)
corporis
   c. callosi, genu
   c. callosi of Reil ▸ taeniola
   c., Pediculus
   c., Pediculus humanus var.
   c. striati, taenia semicircularis
   c., tinea
corporum cavernosorum clitoridis ▸
   septum
corpse fat
corpus
   c. adiposum orbitae
   c. albicans
   c. callosotomy
   c. callosum
   c. callosum agenesis
   c. carcinoma
   c. cavernosum clitoridis
   c. cerebelli
   c. ciliaris
   c. clitoridis
   c. glandulosum
   c. hemorrhagicum
   c. luteum
   c. luteum cells ▸ progesterone-
      producing
   c. luteum, cyst
   c. luteum ▸ formation of
   c. luteum, hemorrhagic
   c. pineale
   c. spongiosum urethrae muliebris
   c. striatum
   c. uteri
   c., uterine
   c. vitreum
corpuscle(s)
   c., blood
   c., bone
   c., Donne's
   c., Drysdale
   c., Hassall's

   c., hyaloid
   c., Krause's
   c., Langerhans' stellate
   c., malpighian
   c., Meissner's
   c., Miescher's
   c., Pacini's
   c., Purkinje's
   c., red blood
   c., Schwalbe's
   c., taste
   c., white blood
corpuscular
   c. constants
   c. diameter (MCD) ▸ mean
   c. hemoglobin concentration
      (MCC/MCHC) ▸ mean
   c. hemoglobin (MCH) ▸ mean
   c. thickness (MCT) ▸ mean
   c. volume
   c. volume (MCV) ▸ mean
correct
   c. for inhomogeneities
   c. optical error
   c. ▸ sponge and needle count
corrected
   c. blood volume
   c. bone marrow cells
   c. cosmetic contact shell implant
   c. dextrocardia
   c. for heart rate, QT
   c. sedimentation rate (SR)
   c. sinus node recovery time
   c. transposition
   c. transposition of great arteries
   c. transposition of great vessels
   c. vision
correction
   c., affectionate
   c., air gap
   c., Bonferroni
   c., elective
   c., hammer toe
   c., isodose shift method for air gap
   c. ▸ laser-assisted in situ
      keratomileusis (LASIK)
   c. ▸ laser vision
   c. ▸ mild eye
   c. of strabismus
   c., orthodontic
   c. ▸ self-evaluation and
   c. shoe
   c. surgery ▸ vision
   c., surgical
   c., vision

correction—*continued*
- c., Yates

correctional group

correctional psychology

corrective
- c. attachment therapy
- c. cast
- c. cosmetics
- c. device
- c. exercise
- c. eyeglasses
- c. lenses
- c. orthotics ▸ foot control of
- c. procedure
- c. surgery
- c. therapy

correlated atrophy

correlated state

correlates(s)
- c. of blood pressure (BP) reduction
- c., pathophysiologic
- c., somatic

correlation
- c. analysis
- c., auto-
- c. center
- c., clinical
- c., coefficient
- c. coefficient ▸ Pearson
- c., cross-
- c., increased
- c. neuron
- c. technique ▸ Doppler auto

correspondence
- c. (ARC) ▸ anomalous retinal
- c., harmonious retinal
- c., normal retinal
- c., retinal

corresponding ray

corridor procedure

Corrigan's
- C. cautery
- C. disease
- C. pneumonia
- C. pulse
- C. respiration
- C. sign

corrin moiety

corroborated memories

corrodens, Bacteroides

corrosive
- c. esophagitis
- c. poison
- c. sublimate

corrugans, fibrosis choroideae

corset
- c., Camp
- c. cancer
- c., surgical

cortex [*vortex*]
- c., accessible
- c. adenoma, adrenal
- c., adrenal
- c. ▸ anoxic changes in
- c., anterior cingulate
- c., articular
- c., atrophic
- c., auditory
- c. avulsion
- c., bone
- c., brain
- c., buckling of
- c., buried
- c., carcinoma of adrenal
- c., central
- c., cerebellar
- c. cerebelli
- c., cerebral
- c., deep layers of
- c., destruction of
- c., direct recording from
- c., dorsolateral prefrontal
- c., electrodes applied over cerebral
- c., electrodes implanted in cerebral
- c., electrodes inserted in cerebral
- c. entered with cutting bur
- c. fire in synchrony ▸ thalamus and
- c., frontal
- c. ▸ frontal lobes of cerebral
- c. ▸ histologic sections of
- c., homologous areas of
- c., irritation of
- c., kidney
- c. ▸ laminated yellowish-brown
- c. ▸ left prefrontal
- c. lentis
- c., local disease of
- c. loss, cerebral
- c., mastoid
- c., medial
- c., motor
- c., nerve cells of cerebral
- c., nonfunctioning cerebral
- c., occipital
- c., orbitofrontal
- c., parahippocampal
- c. perfusion rate ▸ cerebral
- c., prefrontal
- c., primary auditory
- c. reflex, cerebral

- c., renal
- c. ▸ right prefrontal
- c., rolandic
- c., sensorimotor
- c., sensory
- c., somatic sensory
- c., somatosensory
- c. ▸ steroid depletion of
- c., subcapsular
- c., temporal
- c., thinking
- c. thinned
- c., tumor impinging on
- c., visual
- c. watershed, frontal

Corti('s)
- C., arch of
- C., canal of
- C., cells of
- C. ganglion
- C., organ of
- C. organ, pillar of
- C. rods
- C., tunnel of

cortical
- c. abrasion
- c. abrasion ▸ subperiosteal
- c. activity, paroxysmal
- c. adenoma
- c. adenoma, renal
- c. adhesions, division of
- c. adrenal hyperplasia, nodular
- c. anarthria
- c. aphasia
- c. apraxia
- c. area
- c. area, left central
- c. area, right central
- c. artery
- c. atrophy
- c. atrophy, cerebral
- c. audiogram
- c. audiometry
- c. blindness
- c. bone
- c. bone graft, cancellous-
- c. buckling
- c. cataract
- c. center
- c. center, lesion of
- c. cyst
- c. damage, mild
- c. damage, severe
- c. deafness
- c. defect, benign

c. destruction
c. devastation, senile
c. discharges
c. dysfunction
c. dysrhythmia
c. electrode
c. electroencephalogram (EEG)
c. electrogram
c. encephalitis
c. epilepsy
c. evoked responses
c. fatty tumor
c. fracture
c. fragment
c. function
c. function testing
c. fusi
c. graft
c. graft, single onlay
c. granules
c. hemorrhage, superficial
c. hormone, adrenal
c. hyperostosis, infantile
c. hyperplasia, adrenal
c. hyperplasia, diffuse
c. hyperplastic nodules
c. lesions
c. lobules of kidney
c. margin, lateral
c. medullary junction
c. necrosis
c. necrosis of brain
c. neoplasm, slow growing
c. nephrogenic zone ▸ active
c. nodular hyperplasia ▸ mild focal
c. obliteration
c. opacification
c. necrosis, renal
c. paralysis
c. peel
c. process, focal
c. psychic blindness
c. region
c. response
c. scarring
c. scarring of kidneys
c. seizure
c. sensation, defective
c. sensibility
c. spreading depression (CSD)
c. stromal hyperplasia
c. structures, yellow
c. substance of bone
c. substance of kidney
c. substance of lens

c. substance of lymph nodes
c. substance of suprarenal gland
c. surface
c. surface, congested
c. surfaces, smooth
c. thickness
c. thumb
c. tissue
corticalis, agenesia
cortically originating extrapyramidal system (COEPS)
cortices, congested
cortices, femoral
corticoadrenal tumor
corticobulbar tract
corticogram, electro◊
corticography, electro◊
corticomedullary junctions
corticopontine fibers
corticospinal
c. lesion
c. tract
c. tracts ▸ lesions of
corticosteroid(s)
c. binding globulin (CBG)
c. cream
c. drugs
c. hormones
c. injection
c. medication
c., systemic
c. therapy
corticostriatal
c. encephalopathy
c. -spinal atrophy
c. -spinal degeneration
corticotrophic adenoma
corticotropin releasing factor
corticotropin-releasing hormone (CRH)
cortisol
c. binding globulin
c. level, baseline
c. production rate
c. secretion rate
cortisone
c. acetate
c. -glucose tolerance test
c. injection
c. steroids
c. therapy
Corvisart's facies
corylifolia, Psoralea
corymbifer, Mucor
corymbifera, Absidia
corymbifera, Lichtheimia

Corynanthe johimbe
Corynebacterium
C. acnes
C. diphtheriae
C. diphtheriae ▸ gram-positive
C. enzymicum
C. equi
C. haemolyticum
C. hofmannii
C. minutissimum
C. murisepticum
C. mycetoides
C. ovis
C. parvum
C. pseudodiphtheriticum
C. pseudotuberculosis
C. pyogenes
C. renale
C. ulcerans
C. xerosis
coryza
c. agent (CCA) virus ▸ chimpanzee
c., allergic
c. oedematosa
c. virus
Co^{60} (cobalt 60)
Co^{60} eye plaques
Co^{60} teletherapy machine
Co^{60} therapy
Cosgrove mitral valve replacement
Cosman ICM Tele-Sensor
cosmetic(s)
c. and functional purpose
c. appearance
c. breast surgery
c., camouflage
c. contact shell implant ▸ corrected
c. corrective
c. dentistry
c. disease
c. enhancement
c. enlargement
c. eyelid surgery
c. facial surgery
c. implant
c. implant surgery
c. improvement
c. laser
c. laser surgery
c. lens
c. nasal surgery
c. procedure
c. purposes
c. reactions, allergic
c. reactions, irritant

cosmetic(s)—*continued*
- c. reconstruction
- c. result, good
- c. stitch
- c. surgery
- c. surgery authorization form
- c. surgery, Botulinum Toxin (Bo-Tox)
- c. surgery consent form
- c. surgery ▸ facial
- c. surgery ▸ facial rejuvenation
- c. surgery ▸ liposuction
- c. surgery ▸ reconstructive
- c. symptom

cosmic rays

cost(s)
- c. containment
- c., direct treatment
- c. -effective
- c. -effective care
- c. -effective, quality treatment
- c. -effective services
- c., health care
- c., hospital care
- c. of drug abuse, economic
- c. of euthanasia, psychological
- c. per admission
- c. reduction ▸ health care
- c., reduction in
- c. ▸ rising health care
- c. -shift
- c., treatment

Costa operation ▸ Silva-

costal
- c. angle
- c. arch
- c. bone
- c. border blunting
- c. cartilage
- c. cartilage, chondritis
- c. cartilage, premature calcification of
- c. excursion
- c. margin
- c. margin, left
- c. margin, right
- c. notches of sternum
- c. pleura
- c. pleurisy
- c. respiration
- c. stigma

costarum, arcus

Costen's syndrome

costoaxillary vein

costocentral articulation

costochondral
- c. junction
- c. margin
- c. syndrome

costoclavicular
- c. ligament
- c. rib syndrome
- c. space

costocolic fold

costochrondritis pain

costodiaphragmatic recess of pleura

costomediastinal recess of pleura

costophrenic
- c. angle
- c. angle, blunting of
- c. angle obliterated
- c. sinus
- c. sulcus
- c. sulcus, blunted

costosternal articulations

costosternal syndrome

costoversion thoracoplasty

costovertebral
- c. angle (CVA)
- c. angle, blunting
- c. angle tenderness

costotransverse articulation

cot death

Cotard's syndrome

cottage cheese-like discharge

Cotte's operation

cotton (Cotton)
- c., bolus of saline soaked
- c. dust asthma
- c. fibers
- C. fracture
- c. gauze
- c. gauze pad
- c., moist
- c. pledget
- c. plug
- C. procedure
- c. -roll gingivitis
- c. sutures, interrupted

Cottrell operation ▸ Lucas-

Cotunnius, aqueduct of

Cotunnius, nerve of

CO_2 (carbon dioxide)
- CO_2 (carbon dioxide)
- CO_2 (carbon dioxide) combining power
- CO_2 (carbon dioxide) gas laser
- CO_2 (carbon dioxide) instilled
- CO_2 (carbon dioxide) ▸ insufflation of

- CO_2 (carbon dioxide) laser ▸ Sharplan 733
- CO_2 (carbon dioxide) laser skin resurfacing
- CO_2 (carbon dioxide) laser vaporization
- CO_2 pressure ▸ alveolar (carbon dioxide)
- CO_2 production (carbon dioxide)
- CO_2 (carbon dioxide) tension
- CO_2 tension, alveolar (carbon dioxide)
- CO_2 tension ▸ arterial (carbon dioxide)

CO_2T (carbon dioxide therapy)

cotyledon, placental

cotyloid cavity

cotyloid notch

couch potato

coudé, catheter

cough
- c., and disorientation ▸ fever,
- c. and expectoration
- c. and fever ▸ dyspnea,
- c. and/or hemoptysis
- c. and rigors ▸ dyspnea,
- c. and sputum
- c., aneurysmal
- c., Balme's
- c., barking
- c., brassy
- c. ▸ chills, fever and
- c., chronic
- c. ▸ chronic mucus-producing
- c. ▸ chronic unremitting
- c., cigarette
- c., compression
- c., confusion or weakness ▸ fever,
- c., congested
- c. CPR (cardiopulmonary resuscitation) technique
- c., croupy
- c., deep
- c. disorder ▸ chronic
- c., dog
- c., dry
- c. ▸ dry, hacking
- c., dyspnea and headache
- c., ear
- c. expectorant
- c., extrapulmonary
- c., foul sputum ▸ fever, night sweats
- c. fracture
- c., hacking
- c. headache

c. impulse
c., mechanical
c. medicine
c. minute gun
c., Morton's
c., nagging
c., nonproductive
c. or hoarseness ▸ nagging
c. ▸ paroxysm of
c., paroxysmal
c., persistent
c. ▸ persistent hacking
c., pre-eruptive
c., privet
c., productive
c. productive of bloody sputum
c. productive of sputum
c., quad
c., reflex
c. resonance
c., rhonchorous
c. ▸ seal-bark
c., smoker's
c., sputum producing
c., stomach
c. suppressant
c., syncope
c., Sydenham's
c., tea taster's
c. threshold
c., trigeminal
c., unexplained
c., wet
c., whooping
c., winter
c. with expectoration
c. with hemoptysis ▸ persistent
c. ▸ World Trade Center

coughing

c. and expectoration ▸ productive
c. and/or wheezing
c. and straining
c. ▸ blue mouth from
c., bout of
c. center
c. conductive of sputum
c., dizziness from
c. exercises
c., expulsive
c. from allergy
c. from asthma
c. from chemical
c. from measles
c. from pneumonia
c., impulse on

c., incessant
c., quad
c., severe bout of
c. spasm
c. spasm, paroxysmal
c. spells, episodic
c. up blood
c. up blood with chest pain
c. with fever
c. with flatulence
c. with phlegm

coulomb force
Coulter counter
coumarin pulsed dye laser
**Council, AIDS (acquired immune
    deficiency syndrome) Advisory**
Councilman's lesion
counseling

c., abstinence-based
c., aftercare
c., alcohol and drug
c. appointment
c., behavioral
c., bereavement
c., cancer
c., career
c., chemical abuse
c., confidential
c., contraceptive
c. couples
c., crisis
c., divorce
c., drug
c., drug abuse
c., family
c., financial
c. for alcoholism, crisis
c., genetic
c., grief
c., grief and loss
c., group
c., identity and role
c. in drug abuse
c., individual
c. ▸ individual adult children of
    alcoholics
c., individual codependent
c., individual couple's
c., individual dependent
c., long-term individual
c., marital
c., marriage
c., motivational
c. ▸ multi-family group
c., nutritional

c. ▸ one-to-one
c., outplacement
c., pastoral
c., peer
c., preconception
c., premarital
c., psychological
c. psychology
c., rehabilitation
c. resources
c., risk factor
c., separation
c. session
c. session, prenatal
c. session, transitional
c., single parent
c. skills
c., specialized
c. staff
c., supportive
c., Vietnam era vet
c., vocational
c., weight control

counselor(s) ('s)

c., alcoholism
c., drug
c., family
c., genetic
c., grief
c., inpatient
c., nutrition
c. on-call
c., outpatient
c. role
c. ▸ substance abuse
c., vocational
c., vocational rehabilitation

count(s)

c., absolute basophil
c., Addis
c., background
c., blood
c., colony
c. (CBC) ▸ complete blood
c. correct, sponge
c. correct ▸ sponge and needle
c., decreased peripheral lymphocyte
c., decreasing blood
c. density
c., depressed blood
c., differential
c., differential blood
c., direct platelet
c. drawn, interval blood
c. ▸ end-diastolic

count(s)—*continued*
- c. ▸ end-systolic
- c. evaluation, sperm
- c. fingers
- c. ▸ first shock
- c., indirect platelet
- c., interval blood
- c., interval platelet
- c., kick
- c., low blood
- c., low platelet
- c., low sperm
- c. monitored in office ▸ blood
- c. per minute (cpm)
- c., peripheral blood cell
- c., peripheral lymphocyte
- c., plasma cell
- c., platelet
- c., polymorphonuclear leukocyte
- C. radioimmunoassay, Coat-a-
- c. rate
- c. (RBC) ▸ red blood cell
- c., red cell
- c. (WBC) ▸ reduced white blood
- c. ▸ second through fifth shock
- c., shock
- c. ▸ total patient shock
- c. ▸ touch shock
- c., reduction of platelet
- c., reticulocyte
- c., Schilling blood
- c. ▸ second through fifth shock
- c., shock
- c., sperm
- c., spinal fluid cell
- c., sponge and lap
- c., staff
- c. (WBC) suppression ▸ white blood
- c. (TNTC) ▸ too numerous to
- c. (TRC) ▸ total ridge-
- c. ▸ total patient shock
- c. ▸ touch shock
- c., transient depression white blood
- c., weekly blood
- c. (WBC) ▸ white blood
- c. (WBC) ▸ white blood cell
- c., white cell

countenance, flushed

counter
- c. ▸ antihistamines over-the-
- c., boron
- c., Coulter
- c., Cherenkov
- c. current infection
- c. current mechanism
- c. (OTC) drugs, over-the-
- c. electrophoresis
- c., gamma well
- c., Geiger
- c., Geiger-Müller
- c. incision
- c. (OTC) medication ▸ over-the-
- c. medicine, over-the-
- c. products, over-the-
- c., proportional
- c., radiation
- c., scintillation
- c. stain
- c. -transference ▸ transference and
- c., whole body

counteract spasticity

counterattack ▸ reacts with defiant

counterclockwise rotation

counterconditional procedures, electrical

counterconditioning treatment, long-term

counterpressure, external

counterproductive training

counterpulsation
- c., balloon
- c. device (AACD), abdominal aortic
- c., external
- c. (EECP) ▸ enhanced external
- c. ▸ interposed abdominal
- c., intra-aortic balloon
- c. ▸ intra-arterial
- c. (EECP) therapy ▸ enhanced external
- c. unit ▸ enhanced external

countershock, electrical

countertransference reactions

counting
- c. cell
- c. cell, Thoma-Zeiss
- c. chamber
- c. chamber, Abbe-Zeiss
- c. chamber, Thoma-Zeiss
- c., coincidence
- c. fingers (CF)
- c. of pacer spike, double
- c. rate meter
- c., silent
- c. technique, scintillation
- c. test of vision ▸ finger-
- c., whole body

couple(s) ('s)
- c., counseling
- c. counseling, individual
- c., infertile
- c., step-family
- c. therapy
- c. therapy (ICT) ▸ integrative

coupled
- c. amplifier, direct
- c., amplifier ▸ resistance-capacitance (R-C)
- c. pulse
- c. reaction
- c. rhythm
- c. suturing

couplet with fusion, ventricular

couplets, ventricular

coupling
- c., arterial
- c., conductive
- c., constant
- c. (ECC) ▸ electrical contraction
- c., electromechanical
- c. ▸ excitation contraction
- c., fixed
- c. interval, critical
- c. intervals
- c. intercellular
- c. ▸ premature ventricular contractions (PVC) with
- c. ▸ shock wave
- c., variable
- c., ventriculoarterial

courier, drug

Courmont test, Arloing-

Cournand cardiac device

Cournand dip

course [*coarse*]
- c. ▸ acute, rapidly progressive
- c., benign
- c. benign, hospital
- c., chronic progressive
- c. (CC), clinical
- c. complicated postoperative
- c., cyclical
- c., developmental
- c., disease to pursue natural
- c. dose fractionation, split
- c., downhill
- c., hospital
- c., infant's
- c., loading
- c., mutual self-help
- c., neonatal
- c. normal, postoperative
- c. of chemoprophylaxis
- c. of chemotherapy (first, second, etc.)

c. of dialysis
c. of dialysis uneventful
c. of disease
c. of illness
c. of radiation ▸ full
c. of radiation ▸ patient tolerated full
c. of therapy (first, second, etc.)
c. of treatment
c. of ureters
c., patient had steady downhill
c., patient had stormy
c., patient had uneventful postoperative
c., patient pursued rapid downhill
c., postnatal
c., postoperative
c., postoperatively, stormy
c., postpartum
c., postsurgical
c., prenatal
c., progressively downhill
c., prophylactic
c., radiation therapy ▸ full
c., radiation therapy resumed in full
c. regimen, split
c. ▸ relapsing-progressive
c., relapsing-remitting
c., relentless downhill
c., self-help
c., short
c., short intense
c. stabilized
s., surgical
c. technique, split
c. treatment, split
c. turbulent ▸ patient's hospital
c., uncomplicated postoperative
c. uneventful, postoperative
c., uneventful prenatal
c., wheelchair obstacle
court
c. -appointed guardian
c. -ordered assessment
c. -ordered medical treatment
c. referral for incest
Courvoisier-Terrier syndrome
Couvelaire uterus
cove plane
Coventry position, Camp-
cover
c. cell
c. gown and bootees
c. ▸ small blood vessels of the brain
c. test

c. -uncover eye test
coverage (Coverage)
C. Act, Catastrophic Health Care
c., complete corneal
c., health care
c. ▸ mandated mental health
c., Medicaid
c., Medicare
c., Medigap
covered
c. with blood ▸ bronchus
c. with collodion, surgical wound
c. with flap ▸ end of bone
covering
c. of brain, outermost
c. of cerebrum ▸ dural
c. of spinal cord, outermost
covert anger
coving of ST segments
Cowdria ruminantium
Cowper's gland
Cowper's ligament
cow disease, mad
COWS (cold to the opposite, warm to the same)
cow's milk
coxa
c. adducta
c. flexa
c. magna
c. plana
c. valga
c. vara
c. vara luxans
coxae senilis, malum
Coxiella burnetii
coxitis
c. scoliosis
c. fugax
c., senile
Coxsackie (coxsackie)
C. A, B or C virus
C. carditis
c. viral infection
C. virus infection
c. virus myocarditis
CP (cerebral palsy)
CP (closing pressure)
C$_{pah}$ (para-aminohippurate clearance)
CPAP (continuous positive airway pressure)
CPAP (continuous positive airway pressure), nasal
CPB (cardiopulmonary bypass)
CPD (cephalopelvic disproportion)

CPI
CPI (coronary prognostic index)
CPI Maxilith pacemaker
CPI Minilith pacemaker
CPK (creatine phosphokinase)
CPK isoenzymes
cpm (counts per minute)
CPPB (continuous positive-pressure breathing)
CPR (cardiopulmonary resuscitation)
CPR (cardiopulmonary resuscitation), initiate
CPR (cardiopulmonary resuscitation), mechanical
CPR (cardiopulmonary resuscitation), one and two rescuer
CPR (cardiopulmonary resuscitation), one person
CPR (cardiopulmonary resuscitation), one rescuer
CPR (cardiopulmonary resuscitation) technique cough
CPR (cardiopulmonary resuscitation) techniques
CPR (cardiopulmonary resuscitation) techniques, adult
CPR (cardiopulmonary resuscitation) techniques, child and infant
CPR (cardiopulmonary resuscitation) ▸ toilet plunger
CPR (cardiopulmonary resuscitation), two-rescuer
cps or c/sec (cycles per second)
CPU (central processing unit)
CR (conditioned reflex) therapy
crab lice
crab louse
crack(s)
c. abuse
c. -abusing women
c. addict
c. -addicted patient
c. baby
c. baby syndrome
c. cocaine
c. cocaine epidemic
c. cocaine ingestion
c. cocaine, rock or
c. cocaine use
c. crisis ▸ cocaine and
c. dependence ▸ late-onset
c. economy, cocaine/
c. exchange ▸ sex for

crack(s)—*continued*
- c. fracture
- c. fracture, nondisplaced
- c. generation
- c. house drug dealer
- c. kids
- c., smoking

cracked
- c. and itchy hands ▸ dry, red and
- c. heel
- c. lips
- c. mouth corners from sagging cheek
- c. -pot resonance
- c. -pot sound
- c. skin
- c. skin ▸ dry
- c. skin on heel, dry,

cracker ▸ Leveen plaque

cracking
- c. from athlete's foot ▸ skin
- c. from dermatitis ▸ skin
- c. from eczema ▸ skin
- c., knuckle

crackle(s)
- c., bilateral
- c. ▸ end-inspiratory
- c., pleural

crackling
- c. in lung
- c., knee
- c., peeling or blistering of skin
- c. rale
- c. sounds, dry
- c. sounds in lungs

cradle (Cradle)
- C., Alpa
- c., bed
- c. cap
- c., foot
- c., heated bed

Crafoord operation

craft neurosis

Cragg endoluminal graft

Craig's test

cramp(s)
- c., abdominal
- c., accessory
- c. and diarrhea
- c. and spasms ▸ muscle
- c. ▸ cyclic abdominal pain
- c. ▸ diarrhea with menstrual
- c., gas, bloating and/or diarrhea
- c. ▸ heart muscle
- c., heat

- c., intermittent
- c., leg
- c. -like pelvic pain
- c. -like sensation
- c., menstrual
- c., muscle
- c. ▸ muscle spasms and
- c., musician's
- c., night
- c., nighttime calf
- c. ▸ nighttime leg
- c., nocturnal leg
- c. ▸ painful leg
- c., potassium leg
- c., recumbency
- c., stoker's
- c., stomach
- c., sudden severe
- c., writer's

cramping
- c., abdominal
- c. abdominal pain
- c. and bleeding
- c., bloating and
- c., gas
- c. in legs
- c., intense
- c., intermittent spotting and
- c., leg
- c., muscle
- c. nausea, abdominal
- c. of toes
- c. pain
- c. pain, severe
- c., rhythmic
- c., urinary
- c., uterine

Crampton's muscle

crampy abdominal pain

crampy, achy feeling in leg

Crandall units ▸ Cherry-Crane flap

cranial
- c. arachnoid
- c. arteritis
- c. bones, diastasis of
- c. cap
- c. capacity
- c. capacity, reduced
- c. cavity
- c. cervical bruits
- c. diameter, fetal
- c. diameters
- c. flexure
- c. fossa

- c. fossa ▸ middle
- c. fossa, posterior
- c. granulomatous arteritis
- c. hemorrhage
- c. insufflation
- c. irradiation, prophylactic
- c. massage
- c. nerve (first through twelfth)
- c. nerve block
- c. nerve deficit
- c. nerve distribution
- c. nerve impairment
- c. nerve involvement
- c. nerve neurotomy
- c. nerve palsy
- c. nerve problem ▸ taste abnormalities from
- c. nerve signs
- c. nerve, transection
- c. nerves
- c. nerves grossly intact
- c. nerves intact
- c. neuralgia
- c. neuropathies
- c. puncture
- c. radiation
- c. reflex
- c. sanctuary irradiation
- c. segments
- c. separation
- c. sinus, drainage (dr'ge) of
- c. sinus, phlebitis of
- c. sinus, septic phlebitis of
- c. sutures
- c. synostoses
- c. trauma
- c. vault

cranii
- c. anterior, fossa
- c., basilaris
- c., foramen ovale basis
- c., frons
- c., hyperostosis
- c. media, fossa
- c. ossei, vertex
- c. posterior, fossa
- c., trabecula
- c., vertex

craniocardiac reflex

craniocaudad projection

craniocaudad view

craniocaudal view

craniocerebral injury

cranioclasis, fetal

craniodiaphyseal dysplasia

craniofacial
- c. abnormalities
- c. anomaly
- c. anomaly, familial
- c. appliance
- c. dysostosis

craniohypophyseal xanthoma
craniometric diameter
craniopagus twins
craniophagus parasiticus
craniopharyngeal duct tumor
cranioplasty, Curlex
craniosacral division
craniosacral therapy
craniospinal irradiation
craniotomy
- c., awake
- c. checks
- c., depressant
- c., fetal
- c. flap
- c., osteoplastic

cranium
- c., cerebral yokes of bone of
- c., squamous suture of
- c. ▸ subarachnoid hemorrhage in
- c. ▸ subdural hemorrhage in

crank (Crank)
- C. (methamphetamine) (speed)
- C. (methamphetamine) addiction
- C. (methamphetamine), crystal

Crap (heroin)
crapulent colic
crapulosa, amaurosis
craquement, bruit de
crash
- c. cart
- c. diet
- c. ▸ injurious motor vehicle
- c. survivor
- c. technique
- c. victims

crassicauda, Trichosomoides
crassiceps, Taenia
crassicollis, Taenia
crate cushion, egg
crate mattress, egg
crater
- c., active ulcer
- c., ulcer
- c. with target appearance ▸ ulcer

crateriforme, Trichopyton
craves attention
craving(s)
- c. and urges

- c., appetite
- c. drugs ▸ patient
- c., food
- c. for addiction
- c. for cigarette
- c. for sweets
- c. for sweets ▸ increased
- c. for tobacco
- c., inducing
- c. ▸ irritability, restlessness and intense
- c., physical
- c., physiological
- c., psychological
- c., salt

Crawford-Adams hip arthroplasty
Crawford graft inclusion technique
crawling sensation ▸ skin
crawly syndrome of legs ▸ creepy-
craze, exercise
craze, jogging
crazy chick disease
crazy ▸ fear of going
CRE (cumulative radiation effect)
C-reactive protein (CRP)
C-reactive protein (hs-CRP) ▸ high sensitivity
C-reactive protein test
cream
- c., antifungal
- c., anti-wrinkle
- c., corticosteroid
- c., emollient
- c., estrogen
- c. headache, ice
- c., spermicidal
- c., vaginal

creamy vulvitis
crease(s)
- c., abnormal palmar
- c., antecubital cervicodorsal
- c., deep
- c., ear lobe
- c., flexion
- c., inframammary
- c. line
- c., nasolabial
- c. of palm, simian
- c., palmar
- c., simian
- c., skin
- c., sole
- c. ▸ upper eyelid
- c., vaporizing

create physical need
created
- c., bloodless field
- c., groove
- c. opening, surgically
- c. problems, self-
- c. subcutaneously, tunnel

creatine
- c. kinase
- c. kinase, serum
- c. kinase test, serum
- c. phosphokinase
- c. phosphokinase, serum

creatinine
- c. clearance test
- c. clearance, urine
- c., endogenous
- c. level
- c., serum
- c. sulfate
- c. test, serum

creative
- c. achievement
- c. -associate thinking
- c. coping
- c. thinking

creativity
- c., and flexibility ▸ spontaneity,
- c., burst of
- c., personal
- c. ▸ strengths, gifts and

credentials, medical
Crede's
- C. maneuver
- C. method
- C. prophylaxis

Credo's operation
Creech aneurysm repair, DeBakey-
Creech aortoiliac graft
creeping
- c. disease
- c. eruption
- c. sensation in extremity
- c. substitution of bone
- c. thrombosis

creepy-crawly syndrome of legs
Crego traction
cremasteric
- c., artery
- c. fascia
- c. muscle
- c. reflex

cremated [*crenated*]
cremoris, Streptococcus
crena ani

crena cordis
crenated erythrocyte
crenulata, Acetabularia
creola bodies
crepitans, peritendinitis
crepitant
    c. ▸ lungs well aerated and
    c. rale
    c. rales, fine
crepitation, basal
crepitation, coarse
crepitus at fracture site
crepitus of eyeball
crescendo
    c. angina
    c. -decrescendo murmur
    c. murmur
    c. sleep
crescent
    c. artifact
    c. cell anemia
    c. cells
    c. choroid
    c. incision
    c., myopic
    c., scleral
    c. -shaped flap of tissue
    c. -shaped incision
    c. sign of hydronephrosis
crescentic lobule
crest [*breast*]
    c. biopsy, iliac
    c., cardiac neural
    c., iliac
    c., lacrimal
    c. malformation ▸ neural
    c., maxillary
    c. migration ▸ neural
    c., nasal
    c., obturator
    c. of iliac bone
    c. of ilium
    c. of ilium, posterior
    c. palpated, tibial
    c., pyriform
    c., supraventricular
    c. time
    c. tumor ▸ neural
    c. ▸ vagal neural
cresyl blue, brilliant
cresyl violet
cretin dwarf
cretinoid dysplasia
cretinoid idiocy

Creutzfeldt
    C. disease ▸ Jakob-
    C. -Jakob disease
    C. -Jakob syndrome
    C. -Jakob disease (vCJD) ▸ variant
    C. syndrome ▸ Jakob-
Creveld syndrome, Ellis-van
crevice, gingival
CRH (corticotropin-releasing hormone)
crib death
crib, open
cribriform
    c. carcinoma
    c. compress
    c. hymen
    c. plate
    c. plate of ethmoid
    c. process bone
    c. sinus
    c. tissue
Cricetulus larabensis
Cricetus cricetus
cricoarytenoid
    c. joint ankylosis
    c. ligament
    c. muscle, lateral
    c. muscle, posterior
cricoid
    c. cartilage
    c. cartilage, level of
    c. cartilage retracted
cricopharyngeal
    c. achalasia
    c. achalasia syndrome
    c. bar
cricopharyngeus muscle
cricothyroarytenoid ligament
cricothyroid
    c. artery
    c. ligament
    c. membrane
    c. muscle
    c. puncture, needle
cricothyroidotomy and tracheostomy
cricotracheal ligament
cri du chat syndrome
cries easily ▸ patient
Crigler-Najjar syndrome
Crikelair otoplasty
Crile head traction
crime(s)
    c. connection, cocaine-to-
    c., hate
    c. of violence
    c. victim trauma

    c., violent
Crimean-Congo hemorrhagic fever
criminal
    c. abortion
    c. acting out
    c. assault
    c. behavior
    c. evaluation
    c. liability
    c. psychiatrist
    c. psychology
criminally insane
criminality ▸ genetic aspects of
crimped Dacron prosthesis
crinkle line
cripple
    c., cardiac
    c., pain
    c., patient cardiac
crippled, emotionally
crippled with arthritis ▸ patient
crippling
    c. bone disease
    c. disability
    c. disorder
    c. headaches
    c. malady
    c., progressive
crisis(-es)
    c., acquired immune deficiency
      syndrome (AIDS)
    c., acute
    c., Addisonian
    c., adrenal
    c., anaphylactic
    c. behavior ▸ pre-
    c., blast
    c. bronchial
    c., cardiac
    c., chronic
    c., cocaine and crack
    c. containment
    c. counseling
    c. counseling for alcoholism
    c., diabetic
    c., drug-related
    c., elderly care
    c., emotional
    c. ▸ emotional reaction to
    c. event
    c., existential
    c. hotline
    c., hypercalcemic
    c., hypertensive
    c., hypertensive vascular

c., infection-related
c., initial
c. intervention
c. intervention ▸ disaster
c. intervention service
c. intervention skills
c., laryngeal
c. level
c., life
c., life-threatening
c., Lundvall's blood
c., malpractice
c. management
c., medical
c., myasthenic
c., oculogyric
c. onset
c., pain
c., patient in
c., Pel's
c., pharyngeal
c. ▸ potential fetal hypertensive
c. ▸ potential, hypertensive
c. pregnancy
c. ▸ preoccupation with
c. prevention
c. -related feelings
c., sickle cell
c. situation
C., Spelunker's
c., temporary
c., thoracic
c., utricular
c. worker

Crisp's aneurysm
criss-cross
    c-c atrioventricular (AV) valve
    c-c fashion
    c-c heart
    c-c heart malposition
crista
    c. pattern
    c. terminalis
    c. urethralis femininae
    c. urethralis muliebris
cristae ampullaris, cupula
Critchett's operation
Critchley's ataxia ▸ Fergusson and
criteria
    c., Ackerman's
    c., addiction treatment
    c., admission
    c., appropriate
    c., brain death
    c., clinical

c., development of
c., diagnostic
c., donor
c., eligibility
c., exclusion
c. for determination of brain death
c. for discharge
c. for myocarditis ▸ Ratliff
c. for organ donation
c., full
c., identified
c., medical
c., medical generic screening
c., nurse screening
c., patient inclusion
c. ▸ previous treatment experience
c., psychiatric
c. ▸ skilled level of care
c., sonographic
c., strict medical
c., surgical

criterion, pseudodisappearance
critical
    c. care
    c. care air transport
    c. care area
    c. care areas ▸ hand-washing in
    c. care medicine
    c. care nurse
    c. condition
    c. condition, patient in
    c. coupling interval
    c. diarrhea
    c. enzyme
    c. flicker frequency
    c. flicker fusion
    c. flicker fusion test
    c. fusion frequency
    c. illumination
    c. incident review
    c. incident stress management
    c. information
    c. level
    c. list, patient on
    c. mass
    c. micellar concentration
    c. organ shielding blocks
    c. organs ▸ oxygen deprivation in
    c., oxygen supply
    c., patient
    c., patient is self-
    c. problem-solving
    c. rate
    c. stenosis ▸ point of

critically ill
criticism
    c., attendant self-
    c. ▸ intolerance of
    c. ▸ resentment of
CRL (crown rump length)
crochet, main en
crocodile tongue
Crohn's
    C. disease ▸ abdominal lump with
    C. disease ▸ abdominal pain with
    C. disease ▸ anorectal problem
        from
    C. disease ▸ arthritis from
    C. disease ▸ diarrhea from
    C. disease ▸ drug dependency with
    C. disease, flare-up of
    C. disease ▸ lactose intolerance
        with
    C. disease ▸ loss of appetite from
    C. disease ▸ pain in abdomen from
    C. disease ▸ pale stool with
    C. disease ▸ ulcerative colitis with
Crombie's ulcer
Cromie valve prosthesis ▸ Magovern-
Cronin
    C. implant material ▸ Silastic
    C. implant, Silastic
    C. -Matthews eave flap
crook deformity ▸ shepherd's
crook of the arm
crooked teeth
Crookes' lens
CROP (compliance rate, oxygenation
    and pressure) index
crop of blisters ▸ itchy
Crosby-Kugler capsule
cross (Cross)
    c. -addiction
    c. agglutinin
    c. -arm flap
    c. birth
    c. -bite
    c. -bite teeth
    c. -bridges
    c. circulation
    c. -clamp time
    c. -clamped aorta
    c. -clamping of aorta
    c. contamination
    c. -correlation
    c. -cultural issue
    c. -dependence
    c. dialysis
    C. (amphetamines), Double

cross—*continued*
- c. -dressing
- c. -eye
- c. fashion, criss-
- c. femoral-femoral bypass
- c. fiber friction
- c. -finger flap
- c. -fire treatment
- c. generational problems
- c. immunity
- c. infection
- C. -Jones valve prosthesis
- c. -leg flap
- c. -leg graft
- c. -linkage theory
- c. -linking enzyme
- c. -match
- c. -match, RhoGAM
- c. -modal effects
- c. -modal test
- c. -over
- c. -pin teeth
- c. -reacting material
- c. reaction
- c. -reactivation
- c. section
- c. section, capture
- c. section ▸ liver congested on
- c. section view
- c. -sectional electrocardiogram (EKG)
- c. -sectional echocardiography
- c. -sectional plane
- c. -sectional transverse projection
- c. -sectional two-dimensional echocardiogram
- c. -sectional views
- c. -sensitization
- c. -shaped incision
- c. -table lateral position
- c. -talk pacemaker
- c. -temporal processing
- c. -tolerance
- c. union
- c. union, fracture with

crossed
- c. embolism
- c. eyes
- c. hemianesthesia
- c. hemianopia
- c. hemiplegia
- c. jerk
- c. metastasis
- c. parallax
- c. reflex

Crosses (amphetamines)
crosses, Ranvier's
crossing
- c., arteriovenous (AV)
- c. changes, arteriovenous (AV)
- c. of eyes
- c. over
- c. sign ▸ Gunn

crossmatch [*crosshatch*]
crossmatch blood ▸ type and
crossmatching
- c. blood
- c. interference, blood
- c. test

crossover
- c. bypass
- c. bypass ▸ femorofemoral
- c. dynamics ▸ left ventricular left atrial
- c. electrophoresis
- c. placebo controlled study
- c. trials

Crossroads (amphetamines)
Crosti syndrome, Gianotti-
crotaphitic nerve
Croton tiglium
croup
- c. -associated virus (CA virus)
- c., catarrhal
- c., diphtheritic
- c., false
- c., membranous
- c., patient has
- c., pseudomembranous
- c., spasmodic
- c. tent

Croupette child tent
Croupette, patient place in
croupous
- c. angina, benign
- c. bronchitis
- c. conjunctivitis
- c. laryngitis
- c. nephritis
- c. pharyngitis
- c. pneumonia
- c. rhinitis

croupy cough
Crouzon's disease
Crouzon's syndrome
crowing breath sounds
crowing convulsion
crown(s)
- c., anatomical
- c. artifact

- c., artificial
- c. baldness
- c., bare
- c., bell
- c., Bischoff's
- c., cap
- c., Carmichael's
- c., ciliary
- c., clinical
- c., collar
- c., -crimping pliers
- c., Davis
- c., dental
- c., dowel
- c., extra-alveolar
- c., full
- c., full veneer
- c., half-cap
- c., heel-to-
- c., jacket
- c. lengthening
- c., natural
- c., open-face
- c. or inlays
- c., partial veneer
- c., physiological
- c. rump length (CRL)
- c. rump measurement
- c. saw
- c., shell
- c. restoration
- c. -to-heel
- c. -to-rump
- c., veneered
- c., window

crowned, bell-
crowning
- c., infant
- c. of infant's head
- c., patient
- c., patient admitted

crow's foot
Crozat appliance
CRP (C-reactive protein)
CRS (Chinese Restaurant Syndrome)
CRST (calcification, Raynaud's phenomenon, scleroderma, telangiectasis) syndrome
CRT (cathode-ray tube)
crucial
- c. anastomosis
- c. incision
- c. phase

cruciata, amaurosis
cruciata, hemianesthesia

cruciate
- c. incision
- c. instability
- c. ligament
- c. ligament, anterior
- c. ligament, posterior
- c. ligament tear
- c. ligament ▸ torn anterior

cruciferous vegetables

crude
- c. fiber
- c. mortality ratio
- c. urine

crudum, sputum

cruelty ▸ tendency toward

cruenta, cucurbitula

cruenta, lochia

cruentum, sputum

crunch
- c., abdominal
- c. /curl-up exercise, abdominal
- c. exercise, bent leg
- c. exercise ▸ tummy
- c., Hamman's
- c., mediastinal

crunching sound

crunching sound ▸ xiphisternal

crura
- c. anthelicis
- c. cerebelli
- c. cerebri
- c. fractured
- c. of clitoris

crural
- c. arch
- c. area
- c. canal
- c. hernia
- c. hernia, pectineal
- c. ligament
- c. region, anterior
- c. region, posterior

cruris, angina

cruris, tinea

crus
- c. anterius stapedis
- c. anthelicis
- c. breve incudis
- c. cerebri
- c. clitoridis
- c. fornicis
- c. glandis clitoridis
- c. helicis
- c., lateral
- c., long

- c., medial
- c. mediale nasi
- c. of clitoris
- c. of diaphragm
- c. of helix
- c. of stapes, anterior
- c. of stapes, posterior
- c. of the incus ▸ short
- c. olfactoria
- c. penis
- c. posterius stapedis
- c., stapedial

crush
- c. artifact
- c. injuries
- c. injury ▸ infection prevention in
- c. injury renal problem
- c. injury syndrome
- c. kidney
- c. large stones
- c., obturator nerve
- c. syndrome
- c., torus

crushed
- c. bone, paste of
- c. chest injury
- c. muscle
- c., phrenic nerve

crushing
- c. anxiety and depression
- c. chest discomfort
- c. chest pain
- c. chest pressure
- c. fracture
- c. injury
- c. of intervertebral disk
- c. of nerve
- c. of optic nerve
- c. of vertebral bones ▸ progressive
- c. procedure skull of fetus
- c. sensation in chest
- c. turbinate

crust formation

crusta petrosa

crusta petrosa dentis

crustaceum, Penicillium

crustiness of ear

crusting
- c. from dermatitis ▸ skin
- c. from eczema ▸ skin
- c. of eyelid
- c. of skin

crusty eyelids

crutch(es)
- c., ambulatory with

- c., Canadian
- c., forearm
- c., glasses
- c., jocked stand
- c., Loft-Strand
- c., rolling
- c., walking
- c., weight bearing with

Crutchfield
- C. operation
- C. reduction technique
- C. skeletal traction
- C. tong traction
- C. tongs or halo

Cruveilhier
- C. atrophy
- C. -Baumgarten cirrhosis
- C. -Baumgarten murmur
- C. -Baumgarten sign
- C. -Baumgarten syndrome
- C. joint
- C. nodules
- C. sign

crux of heart

Cruz-Kaster prosthesis ▸ Lillehei-cruzi, Trypanosoma

cry
- c. good ▸ color and
- c., infant had weak
- c. response
- c. state

crying
- c. episodes
- c., excessive
- c. ▸ head rolling, rocking and
- c., inconsolable
- c. out
- c., patient
- c. spells
- c. test, sweat
- c. unexpectedly
- c., whining and

cryocataract extraction

cryodestruction procedure

cryoextraction of cataract

cryogenic cataract extraction

cryogenic fluid ▸ sub-zero

cryoglobulinemia (EMC) ▸ essential mixed

cryokinetic treatment

Cryolife valve graft

Cryopexy treatment

cryophake unit, Keeler

cryoprecipitate, transfusion of

cryopreserved
- c. heart valve allograft
- c. homograft valve
- c. human aortic allograft
- c. tissue banking
- c. venous transplantation

cryosurgery
- c. and laser therapy
- c., focused
- c., gynecologic
- c. technique

cryothalamotomy procedure

cryotherapy
- c., freeze-thaw
- c., initial
- c., scleral
- c. treatment

cryounit, Amoils

CryoVein saphenous vein allograft

crypt, Morgagni's

cryptectomy, electro◊

cryptic tonsil

cryptococcal
- c. disease, nonmeningeal
- c. infection
- c. meningitis
- c. myocarditis

Cryptococcus
- C. capsulatus
- C. epidermidis
- C. gilchristi
- C. histolyticus
- C. hominis
- C. meningitidis
- C. neoformans

cryptogenic
- c. epilepsy
- c. fibrosing alveolitis (CFA)
- c. pyemia
- c. stroke

cryptophthalmos syndrome

cryptosporidiosis infection

Cryptosporidiosis organism

Cryptosporidium baileyi

Cryptosporidium parvum

crypts
- c., Lieberkühn's
- c., Luschka's
- c. of palatine tonsil
- c. of pharyngeal tonsil
- c., tonsillar

crystal(s) (Crystal)
- c. (amphetamines)
- C. (crystal methamphetamine)
- c. (phencyclidine)
- c., amorphous
- c., amorphous phosphate
- c., arthritis, acute
- c., asthma
- c., calcium oxalate
- c., Charcot-Leyden
- c., cholesterol
- c. device ▸ liquid
- c., fatty-acid
- c., free-base
- c. gamma camera ▸ single
- c. healing
- c., hematoidin
- c. methamphetamine
- c. methamphetamine (Crank)
- c. methamphetamine (Crystal)
- c. methamphetamine (Glass)
- c. methamphetamine (Ice)
- c. methamphetamine (Meth)
- c. methamphetamine ▸ smoking of
- c. methamphetamine (Speed)
- c., pseudogout
- c. thermogram (LCT), liquid
- c., triple phosphate
- c., urate
- c., uric acid
- c., Zenker's

crystalline
- c. egg albumin
- c. fluid
- c. humor
- c. insulin
- c. lens
- c. powder, white
- c. structure
- c. swelling, Sommerring's

crystallized intelligence

crystalloid
- c. cardioplegia, cold
- c. cardioplegic solution
- c. potassium cardioplegia

CS (cesarean section)
- CS, corporeal
- CS, Krönig's
- CS, Latzko's
- CS, transverse

CSA (compressed spectral array)

Csapody's operation

Cs (Cesium)

CSD (cortical spreading depression)

CSE (Coping Strategy Enhancement)

c/sec (cycles per second) ▸ cps or

C- (cesarean) section delivery

C- (cesarean) section ▸ patient delivered by

C-section (cesarean section)

C-section, post-

CSF (cerebrospinal fluid)
- CSF, absorption of
- CSF brain barrier
- CSF cytology
- CSF glucose

CSFP (cerebrospinal fluid pressure)

CSH (combat support hospital)

CSM (cerebrospinal meningitis)

CSP (cerebrospinal pressure)

CST (central sharp transients)

CT
- CT (cardiothoracic)
- CT (carotid tracing)
- CT body scanner
- CT (computerized tomographic) colonography
- CT ▸ Fast-Scan
- CT of chest
- CT (cardiothoracic) ratio
- CT (computerized tomographic) scan ▸ full body
- CT scan ▸ thin slice
- CT scanner ▸ Imatron Ultrafast
- CT scanning, rapid sequential
- CT ▸ thin section
- CT ▸ ultrafast

Ctenocephalides canis

Ctenopsyllus segnis

C-terminal assay

C-thalassemia disease, hemoglobin

CTR (cardiothoracic ratio)

CTS (carpal tunnel syndrome)

C2 (cervical) vent-dependent quadriplegic

C-2 vertebra (axis)

C$_u$ (urea clearance)

cu (cause undetermined)

cu cm/cc (cubic centimeter)

cu mm/cmm (cubic millimeter)

Cubbins
- C. approach
- C. incision
- C. operation

Cubes, (LSD) (lysergic acid diethylamide)

cube formula ▸ geometric

cubic
- c. centimeter (cc/cu cm)
- c. centimeter (ng/cc) ▸ nanograms per
- c. millimeter (cmm/cu mm)

cubital
- c. lymph nodes

c. nerve
c. region, anterior
c. region, posterior
c. tunnel syndrome
c. vein, median
cubiti, patella
cubitus valgus
cubitus varus
cuboid bone
cuboid cell
cuboidal
c. cell
c. cells, abnormal proliferation of
c. epithelium
c. epithelium, low
c. to columnar acinar cells
cuboideonavicular ligament
cuboideum, os
cuboidodigital reflex
Cucumis sativus
Cucurbita citrullus
Cucurbita pepo
cucurbitina, Taenia
cucurbitula cruenta
cue(s)
c., behavioral
c. -controlled relaxation ▸ biofeedback-assisted
c. exposure
c., facial
c. ▸ nonverbal social
c. of stress ▸ emotional
c. of stress ▸ physical
c., visual
cueing
c. assistance ▸ set-up and
c. ▸ constant verbal
c. for ADL (activities of daily living) ▸ verbal
c., patient independent in bathing with
c., patient uses quad cane with verbal
c., verbal
cuff(s) (Cuff)
c. abnormality, rotator
c. abscess, vaginal
c., antimicrobial catheter
c., aortic
c. arthropathy
c. arthropathy ▸ rotator
c., arm
c., atrial
c., automated blood pressure
c., blood pressure (BP)

C., Childs Cardio-
c. deflated, blood pressure (BP)
c., finger
c., inflatable
c. injury, rotator
c. lesion ▸ rotator
c., long leg brace with large tibial
c. ▸ misalignment of rotator
c., mucosal
c. muscle
c. muscles ▸ rotator
c., musculotendinous
c. neosalpingostomy
c. Pap (Papanicolaou) smear ▸ vaginal
c. pathology, rotator
c. plethysmography
c. plethysmography, air
c., pneumatic
c. -pressure
c. reefed, vaginal
c. repair ▸ rotator
c., rotator
c., rupture of
c. rupture ▸ rotator
c. salpingostomy
c. sign
c. sign ▸ Löwenberg
c. surgery, rotator
c. tear ▸ rotator
c. tendinitis ▸ rotator
c. tendon ▸ rotator
c. test
c., torn rotator
c., tracheostomy
c., vaginal
c., weighted ankle
c., well-suspended vaginal
cuffed
c. endotracheal tube
c. tracheostomy tube
c. tube ▸ fluffy
cuffing, peribronchial
cuir neuf, bruit de
cuirass
c., chest
c. jacket
c. respirator
c. respirator ▸ Emerson
c., tabetic
c. ventilator
cuirasse
c., cancer en
c., carcinoma en
c., cor en

cul-de-sac
c., conjunctival
c., Douglas'
c., dural
c. fluid
c., free fluid in
c., fullness of
c., lower
c., obliteration of
c. of vagina, posterior
c., sacral
c., superior
culdocentesis procedure
culdotomy incision
Culex
C. annulirostris
C. fatigans
C. molestus
C. pipiens
C. quinquefasciatus
C. tarsalis
C. tritaeniorhyncus
C. uvivittatus
culicis, Agamomermis
culicis, Lankesteria
Culicoides austeni
Culicoides grahami
Culiseta inorata
Culiseta melanura
Cullen's sign
culprit lesion
Culp's ureteropelvioplasty
cult
c. abuse, ritual/
c. involvement, religious
c. practices, deceptive
c., satanic
culturable organisms
cultural
c. aspects of chemical dependency
c. attitudes
c. beliefs and practices
c. definition of addiction
c. -ethnic background
c. factors
c. indoctrination
c. influence
c. issue, cross-
c. perspective
c. referral
c. values
culture(s)
c., active
c., amniotic fluid

culture(s)—*continued*
- c., anaerobic
- c. and sensitivity
- c. and sensitivity contaminated ▸ urine
- c. and sensitivity, urine
- c. and smear
- c., attenuated
- c., bacterial
- c., biochemical analysis and
- c., blood
- c. bottle, vacuum
- c., broth
- c., catheter tip
- c., catheter tube
- c., cell
- c. cells, tissue
- c. centered skills
- c., cervical
- c., charcoal blood medium
- c., chorioallantoic
- c., contaminated blood
- c., continuous flow
- c., cord blood
- c., direct
- c. dose, median tissue
- c. dose, tissue
- c. drawn, blood
- c., ear
- c., endocervical
- c., environmental
- c., flask
- c., followup urine
- c., four site GC (gonococcus)
- c., fractional
- c., fungus
- c., gastric
- c., gravity-settling
- c. grew organisms
- c., hanging-block
- c., hanging-drop
- c., infected tissue
- c. infective dose ▸ median tissue
- c. infective dose ▸ tissue
- c., inhibitors
- c. ▸ intravascular catheter
- c., kidney cell
- c., media
- c., medium
- c., medium, tissue
- c., mixed
- c. (MLC), mixed leukocyte
- c., multiple
- c., nasal
- c., nasopharyngeal

- c., needle
- c., negative
- c. negative endocarditis
- c. negative for growth
- c. negative for pathogens
- c. negative for pathogens ▸ stool
- c., Neisserian
- c. of cardiac blood ▸ anaerobic
- c. of nasal washings
- c. of pleural effusion
- c. of specimen
- c. organism
- c., peripheral
- c., plate
- c., positive
- c., positive blood
- c., postmortem
- c., postmortem blood
- c. ▸ postmortem cardiac blood
- c., premortem
- c., premortem sputum
- c., pure
- c., routine
- c., sedentary
- c., sensitized
- c. sent to lab
- c., shake
- c. shock
- c., slant
- c., slope
- c., smear
- c. ▸ Smith, Klein & French (SKF)
- c., sputum
- c., stab
- c., stained smears and
- c., sterility
- c., stock
- c., stool
- c., streak
- c., stroke
- c. studies, tissue
- c. ▸ success-obsessed
- c. techniques
- c., throat
- c., thrust
- c., tissue
- c., tracheal aspirate
- c., triad of city
- c., tube
- c., tuberculosis (TB)
- c., type
- c., urinary
- c., urine
- c., urine midstream
- c., urine sterile on

- c., vaginal
- c., viral

cultured
- c. and analyzed ▸ amniotic fluid
- c. brain tissue
- c., sample filtered and
- c., seropurulent sputum
- c. skin grafting ▸ autologous
- c. skin transplantation ▸ autologous

culturing, environmental
culturing of environmental surfaces
cum calce, soda
cumulative
- c. analysis
- c. dose
- c. effect
- c. effects of trauma
- c. effects of unprotected sun exposure
- c. experience of
- c. radiation effect (CRE) oophorus
- c. radiation effect (CRE), ovarian
- c. radiation effect (CRE), ovaricus
- c. sleep deficit (CSD)
- c. sun damage
- c. trauma disorder

cuneate
- c. nucleus
- c. nucleus, accessory
- c. tubercle

cuneatus, fasciculus
cuneatus, nucleus
cuneiform
- c. bone
- c. cartilage
- c. joint, metatarsal
- c. ligament
- c. osteotomy
- c. tubercle

cuneonavicular ligament
cuniculi
- c., Encephalitozoon
- c., Eutrichomastix
- c., Psoroptes

cup(s)
- c. -and-ball osteotomy
- c. -and-spill stomach
- c., calycea
- c. ear
- c., glaucomatous
- c., impression
- c., large physiologic
- c., ocular
- c., ophthalmic
- c., optic

c., physiologic
c. prosthesis ▸ Smith-Petersen hip
c., suction
Cupcake (LSD)
cupola (*see* cupula)
cupped disc
cupping of disc or nerve
cupping, optic
cuprophane membrane
cupula
    c. cristae ampullaris
    c. ▸ gravity-dependent movement of
    c. of cochlea
    c. of pleura
    c. technique
cupular cecum of cochlear duct
cupuliform cataract
curable
    c. breast tumor
    c. cancer
    c. hypertension
    c. stage
curare-like drug
curarized state
curative
    c. attitude
    c. dose
    c. dose, median
    c. inoculation
    c. measure
    c. option
    c. resection
    c. result
    c. surgery
    c. treatment
curb intravenous use of drugs
curb tenotomy
cure
    c., cancer
    c., clinical
    c., microbiological
    c., miracle
    c., no known
    c. rate
    c. rate, high
    c. rate, low
    c. treatment, active
    c., vital
curettage
    c. and dessication
    c. and irrigation
    c., cervical
    c., diagnostic
    c. (D and C), diagnostic dilatation and

c. (D and C), dilatation and
c., dull
c., electrodesiccation and
c., endocervical
c., endometrial
c., fractional
c. in squamous cell carcinoma ▸ electrodesiccation and
c., medical
c., periapical
c., sharp
c., subgingival
c., suction
c. (D and C), suction dilatation and
c., vacuum
curette biopsy
curetted
    c., bone
    c. out of medullary cavity ▸ cancellous bone
    c., uterine cavity
curettement, uterine
curettings
    c., lower uterine canal
    c., upper uterine canal
    c., uterine
curiosity, and initiative ▸ reduced spontaneity,
curl(s)
    c. exercise, biceps
    c. exercise, leg
    c. exercise ▸ toe
    c. exercise ▸ trunk
    c. exercises, abdominal
    c. exercises, arm
    c., hamstring
    c., stent tube with pigtail
    c. toe exercise ▸ towel
    c. up exercise, abdominal crunch/
curled enamel
Curlex cranioplasty
Curling's ulcer
curly toes
currant jelly sputum
currens, larva
current
    c. (AC), alternating
    c. amplifier, direct
    c., bioelectric
    c. block, electrical
    c., Bovie coagulating
    c., Bovie cutting
    c. Bovie, low
    c. cardioversion, direct
    c., diastolic

c. (DC), direct
c., eddy
c., electric
c., electrical
c. family situation
c., faradic
c., fast sodium
c. fitness level
c. flow
c., galvanic
c., high frequency
c. infection, counter
c., injury
c. into larynx ▸ passing faradic
c., K
c., leakage
c. ▸ low energy direct
c. medical management
c. medication treatment
c. medications
c., membrane
c. of injury, diastolic
c. of injury ▸ systolic
c. (AC) ▸ opposition of flow of alternating
c. (DC) ▸ opposition of flow of direct
c. output
c. pacing box ▸ digital constant
c. pain medication
c., pseudoalternating
c., pulsating
c., pump
c., radiofrequency
c. ▸ range-alternating
c. (AC) resistance, alternating
c. (DC) resistance, direct
c., saturation
c. (AC) signals, low frequency alternating
c., single phase
c. standards of practice
c. stressors
c. studies
c., three-phase
c. ▸ toxin insensitive
c. ▸ transient inward
c. ▸ transsarcolemmal calcium
c., unidirectional
c. (AC) voltage, alternating
c. (DC) voltage, direct
currently infectious, patient
Curschmann's
    C. disease
    C. mask

Curschmann's—*continued*
  C. spirals
curse breathing ▸ Ondine
curse, Ondine's
cursive epilepsy
Curtis syndrome ▸ Fitz-Hugh-
Curtius' syndrome
curvature
  c. ametropia
  c. aspect, greater
  c. aspect, lesser
  c., cervical
  c., dextroscoliotic
  c., flattening of normal lumbar
  c., greater
  c., lesser
  c., lumbar
  c., normal cervical
  c. of antrum, greater
  c. of cornea
  c. of cornea, unequal
  c. of lens
  c. of radius
  c. of radius, progressive
  c. of spine
  c. of spine, compensatory
  c. of spine ▸ excessive
  c. of spine, lateral
  c. of stomach, greater
  c. of stomach, lesser
  c. site, greater
  c. site, lesser
  c., spinal
  c., surface
curve(s)
  c., actuarial survival
  c., borderline
  c., Bragg
  c., colloidal gold
  c., comparative depth dose
  c., complication probability
  c. ▸ dissociation
  c., double major
  c., dye
  c., escargot
  c., expiratory
  c., flat
  c., flattening of lumbar
  c., flattening of lumbosacral
  c., flow volume
  c. for radiation, spectral distribution
  c. ▸ Frank Starling
  c., frequency response
  c., function
  c., gold

c. ▸ green dye
c. ▸ hemoglobin oxygen (O_2) dissociation
c., Hunter-Driffield
c. ▸ indocyanine dilution
c., initial linear survival
c. ▸ intracardiac pressure
c., isodose
c., isoeffect
c., J
c., joule
c. ▸ left ventricular (LV) pressure volume
c. ▸ length active tension
c., lordotic
c., lumbar
c., lumbar lordotic
c., multifraction survival
c. of development, normal
c. of Spee
c. ▸ oxygen (O_2) dissociation
c. ▸ oxyhemoglobin dissociation
c. pressure ▸ natriuresis
c., pressure volume
c., pulse
c., reversal lumbar
c., sensitometric
c. ▸ single breath nitrogen
c., Starling
c., temperature
c. ▸ time activity
c., Traube's
c. ▸ venous return
c. ▸ ventricular function
c. ▸ volume time
curved
  c. downward, incision
  c. -handle cane
  c. incision
  c. periscapular incision
  c. toenails
curvilinear
  c. calcification
  c. flattening
  c. incision
  c. skin incision
Curvularia lunata
curvus, carpus
Cushing('s)
  C. disease
  C. disease, pituitary
  C. law
  C. medulloblastoma
  C. phenomenon
  C. pressure response

C. reaction
C. reflex
C. syndrome
C. syndrome, ectopic
C. triad
C. tumor
cushingoid appearance
cushingoid facies
cushion(s) (Cushion)
  c., anal
  c., atrioventricular (AV) canal
  c., cardiac
  c., coronary
  c. defects, endocardial
  c. distortion, pin-
  c., egg crate
  c., flotation
  c. formation ▸ endocardial
  c. of the epiglottis
  C., Pedifix's Pedic
  c., sac
  c., special
  c., wheel chair
cushioned heel (WACH) shoe ▸ wedge
adjustable
cushioning, air or gel
cushioning sutures
cusp(s)
  c., accessory
  c., aortic
  c. billowing
  c., buccal
  c., conjoined
  c., coronary
  c. degeneration
  c. eversion
  c. fenestration
  c. ▸ fish mouth
  c. height
  c. motion
  c., noncoronary
  c. separation, aortic
  c. syndrome, ballooning mitral
  c. syndrome ▸ redundant
cuspal enamel
cuspid, deciduous
cuspid teeth
cuspidatus, Centrocestus
cuspidatus variety canina Centrocestus
cuspless teeth
custodial care
custodial care ▸ patient transferred for
Custodis' implant
Custodis' operation
custody evaluation

custody, protective
custom
- c. contact lenses
- c. dentures
- c. designed foot orthotic
- c. fit in ear unit
- c. knee brace
- c. orthotics
- c. training

customized joint repair
customized wheelchair
cut(s) [gut]
- c. and ligated ▸ meso-appendix serially clamped,
- c. blood vessels
- c., clamped and
- c., coagulate or vaporize
- c., coronal
- c. down site
- c. down site, healed
- c. edge
- c. end of bone
- c. fibrous strands
- c. films, serial
- c., intercostal nerves
- c. into bone, wedge-shaped
- c. on hand, fresh
- c. osteotomy, Z-
- c., perceptual
- c. point
- c., sagittal
- c. section
- c. section of liver parenchyma
- c., stapedial tendon
- c. surface
- c., tomographic
- c., umbilical cord
- c., visual field

cutanea tarda (PCT) ▸ porphyria
cutanea tarda symptomatica ▸
  porphyria
cutaneous
- c. abscess
- c. amputation
- c. anaphylaxis, passive
- c. angiitis
- c. angiosarcoma
- c. anthrax
- c. aspergillosis
- c. asthma
- c. blood flow, increased
- c. circulation, parumbilical
- c. disorder
- c. edges approximated
- c. effect
- c. eruption
- c. flushing
- c. fungal disease
- c. fungus
- c., gastro◊
- c. geromorphism
- c. helminthiasis
- c. hyperesthesia
- c. infection
- c. infection ▸ anthrax
- c. infection, nosocomial
- c. inoculation
- c. leishmaniasis
- c. lupus
- c. lymphocyte antigen
- c. malignant melanoma
- c. margins, apposition of
- c. mastocytosis, diffuse
- c. muscle
- c. mycosis
- c. myelocytoma
- c. myiasis
- c. nerve
- c. nerve, intermediate dorsal
- c. nerve, lateral femoral
- c. nerve, medial
- c. nerve of abdomen ▸ anterior
- c. nerve of arm ▸ inferior lateral
- c. nerve of arm ▸ medial
- c. nerve of arm ▸ posterior
- c. nerve of arm ▸ superior lateral
- c. nerve of calf ▸ lateral
- c. nerve of calf ▸ medial
- c. nerve of foot ▸ intermediate dorsal
- c. nerve of foot ▸ lateral dorsal
- c. nerve of foot ▸ medial dorsal
- c. nerve of forearm ▸ dorsal
- c. nerve of forearm ▸ lateral
- c. nerve of forearm ▸ medial
- c. nerve of forearm ▸ posterior
- c. nerve of thigh ▸ lateral
- c. nerve of thigh ▸ posterior
- c. pupillary reflex
- c. reaction
- c. schistosomiasis
- c. sensation
- c. sensitization
- c. signs as a screening device for drug abuse
- c. signs of drug abuse
- c. striae
- c. suture
- c. suture of palate
- c. symptomatology
- c. systemic sclerosis
- c. tag
- c. T-cell lymphoma
- c. T-cell lymphoma ▸ erythrodermic
- c. thoracic patch electrode
- c. ureterostomy
- c. vein, ulnar

cutaneum, carcinoma
cutaneum, Trichosporon
cutaway diagram
cutdown
- c., arterial
- c., brachial artery
- c. catheter
- c. technique
- c., vein
- c., venous

cuticle, enamel
cuticular suture
cutirubrum, Halobacterium
cutis
- c., amebiasis
- c., angioma
- c., asteatosis
- c., atheroma
- c., carcinosis
- c. circumscripta, calcinosis
- c. congenita, aplasia
- c. elastica
- c. graft
- c. hyperelastica
- c. laxa syndrome
- c., leukemia
- c., lymphocytoma
- c., pseudoleukemia
- c., tuberculosis
- c., xerosis

Cutler-Beard operation
Cutler's implant
cutout, lead
Cutter (cutter)('s)
- C. SCDK prosthesis
- C. -Smeloff cardiac valve prosthesis
- C. valve prosthesis ▸ Smeloff-
- c. (VISC), vitreous infusion suction

cutters' phthisis, stone
cutting
- c. current, Bovie
- c. disc
- c. edge
- c. mechanism ▸ exposing plaque to
- c. of teeth
- c. of umbilical cord
- c. pain ▸ sharp

cutting—*continued*
    c. umbilical cord
cuttlefish disc
Cuvier, duct of
CV wave of jugular venous pulse
CVA
    CVA (cardiovascular accident)
    CVA (cerebrovascular accident)
    CVA (cerebrovascular accident),
      acute
    CVA (cerebrovascular accident),
      lacunar
    CVA (costovertebral angle)
    CVA (costovertebral angle)
      tenderness
CVB (chorionic villi biopsy)
CVD (cerebrovascular disease)
**CVOD (cerebrovascular obstructive
    disease)**
CVP
    CVP (central venous pressure)
    CVP (cyclophosphamide,
      vincristine, prednisone)
    CVP (Cytoxan, vincristine,
      prednisone)
CVS (cardiovascular surgery)
CVS (cardiovascular system)
CVS (chorionic villus sampling)
CVS (cyclic vomiting syndrome)
CWD (chronic wasting disease)
CWI (cardiac work index)
CWP (childbirth without pain)
cyanophilic, granular cells
cyanosis
    c., acro◊
    c., autotoxic
    c. bulbi
    c., central
    c., circumoral
    c., clubbing or edema
    c., dependent
    c., erythro◊
    c., false
    c. ▸ hereditary methemoglobinemic
    c., late
    c., livid
    c. ▸ muscular atrophy and
    c. of all extremities ▸ peripheral
    c. of ears
    c. of extremities
    c. of fingernails
    c. of fingertips
    c. of lips
    c. of nail beds
    c. of retina

    c., pallor and
    c., peripheral
    c., pulmonary
    c. retinae
    c., shunt
    c., tardive
    c. upper extremities ▸ clubbing and
cyanotic
    c. atrophy of liver
    c. attack
    c., cervix
    c. discoloration of skin
    c. heart defect
    c. heart disease
    c. induration
    c. infant
    c. kidney
    c., nailbeds
    c., patient
    c., patient gasping and
cybernetics, psycho◊
cycle(s)
    c., aberrant
    c., adult grief
    c., anovulatory
    c., asexual
    c., binary
    c., biochemical
    c., biological sleep-wake
    c. (CC) ▸ cardiac
    c., cell
    c., cessation of menstrual
    c., chemotherapy
    c., circadian
    c., codependency
    c., complete
    c., contraction-relaxation
    c., cytoplasmic
    c., daily biological
    c., daily sleep-wake
    c., day-night
    c., decontamination
    c., duration of
    c., emotional
    c., endogenous
    c., endometrial
    c., estrogen
    c., estrous
    c., exercise
    c., exogenous
    c., fear-tension-pain
    c., forced
    c., gastric
    c., genesial
    c., gonotrophic

    c., grief
    c., growth
    c., hair
    c., Hodgkin
    c., hormonal
    c., intellectual
    c., intranuclear
    c. ▸ irregular menstrual
    c., isohydric
    c. ▸ isometric period of cardiac
    c. ▸ itch-scratch
    c. kinetics analysis, cell
    c., Krebs
    c. length
    c. length alternans
    c. length alternation
    c. length, antegrade block
    c. length, atrial-paced
    c. length, basic
    c. length, basic drive
    c. length, block
    c. length, drive
    c. length ▸ flutter
    c. length ▸ paced
    c. length ▸ pacing
    c. length ▸ sinus
    c. length ▸ tachycardia
    c. length ▸ ventricular tachycardia
    c. length window
    c., life
    c., mammary
    c., masticating
    c., menstrual
    c., mood
    c., myometrial
    c., NREM (nonrapid eye movement)
    c., NREM-REM (nonrapid eye
      movement-rapid eye movement)
    c. of codependency
    c. of disease
    c. of emesis
    c. of heart, contraction
    c. of high dose chemotherapy ▸
      intense
    c. of pain and inactivity
    c., onset of
    c., oogenetic
    c., ovarian
    c., ovulation
    c., pain
    c. (PC), pentose
    c. per minute (c/min)
    c. per second (cps or c/sec)
    c. phase, mid-

c. ▸ phase-shift disruption of 24-hour sleep-wake
c., phosphate
c., physical
c. position, sleep
c., pregnancy
c. redistribution and dose fractionation, cell
c. redistribution and dose hyperfractionation, cell
c. redistribution, cell
c. redistribution, radiosensitivity and cell
c., reproductive
c. (cc) ▸ resting phase of cardiac
c., restored
c., returning
c., RR
c., sexual
c. ▸ short-long-short
c., sleep
c., sleep-wake
c. ▸ sound wave
c., temperature
c. time, cell
c., uterine
c., vaginal
c., weight
c., Wenckebach
c., worry

cycled
c. decelerating flow ventilation ▸ volume
c. ventilation ▸ time-
c. ventilator ▸ pressure

cyclic
c. abdominal pain cramps
c. abulia
c. adenosine monophosphate (CAMP)
c. antidepressant
c. back pain
c. constriction
c. disorder
c. edema
c. edema ▸ idiopathic
c. epidemics of use and abuse
c. insanity
c. irregularity
c., monentary paralysis
c. muscular contractions of bowel
c. proteinuria
c. pulmonary disorder ▸ chronic
c. respiration
c. strabismus

c. treatment
c. therapy
c. therapy, composite
c. vomiting
c. vomiting syndrome (CVS)

cyclical
c. breast pain
c. mastalgia
c. nausea
c. pain
c. peritoneal dialysis (CCPD), continuous

cycling, low-tension

cyclitis
c., heterochromic
c., purulent
c., serous

cyclographic tomogram ▸ Siemen's
cycloid personality
Cyclone (phencyclidine)
cyclooxygenase inhibitor
cyclophosphamide, methotrexate, fluorouracil (CMF)
cyclophosphamide, vincristine, prednisone (CVP)
Cyclospora cayetanensis
Cyclospora infection
cyclosporine therapy
cyclothymic disorder
cyclothymic personality
cycloserine, D-

cylinder(s)
c., Bence-Jones
c. cast
c., cesium
c., Jones
c. process, axis

cylindric cell

cylindrical
c. bronchiectasis
c. carcinoma
c. cell carcinoma
c. epithelioma
c. lens

cylindroid aneurysm
cylindromatous adenocarcinoma
cylindromatous carcinoma
cymba conchae auriculae
cymosa, Chailletia
cynical and tempestuous ▸ callous,
cynomulgus, Macaca
Cyon's nerve
Cyriax's syndrome
cyst(s)
c. ablation ▸ renal

c. adenofibroma
c., amniotic
c., aneurysmal bone
c., apical
c., apoplectic
c., Aschoff-Rokitansky
c. aspiration
c. aspiration, breast
c., atheromatous
c., Baker
c., Bartholin duct
c., Bartholin's
c., Blessig-Iwanoff
c., Blessig's
c., blue-dome
c., bone weakening
c., branchial
c., branchial cleft
c., breast
c., bronchial
c., bronchogenic
c., bronchopulmonary
c. bulging
c., calyceal
c., chocolate
c., choledochal
c., chorionic
c., chronically inflamed
c., ciliary body
c., colloid
c., compound
c., congenital
c., corpus luteum
c., cortical
c., degenerative epidermoid
c., dermoid
c. ▸ dermoid versus sebaceous
c. disease ▸ hydatid
c., echinococcal
c., embryonal
c., endodermal
c., endometrial
c., enteric
c., enucleation
c., epidermal inclusion
c., epidermoid
c., epoophoron
c. ▸ excision ganglionic
c., fluid-filled
c. ▸ fluid mucinous
c., follicular
c. formation
c., ganglion
c., ganglionic
c., gartnerian

cyst(s)—*continued*
c., gastroenterogenous
c., granulosa lutein
c., hard
c., hemorrhagic
c., hydatid
c., hymenal
c., implantation
c. in breast, fluid-filled
c., incision and drainage of
c., inclusion
c., infected pilonidal
c., infected sebaceous
c., inflammatory
c. inside out, suturing
c., involution
c. ▸ isolated renal
c., kidney
c., labial
c. lacrimal gland ▸retention
c., locular
c., loculated
c., lutein
c., malignant ovarian
c., marsupialization Bartholin gland
c., meibomian
c. meniscus of knee
c., mesenteric
c., morgagnian
c., mucoretention
c., mucous
c., multilobular
c., multilocular
c., myxoid
c., nabothian
c., Naboth's
c., necrotic
c., neurenteric
c. of iris
c. of iris, implantation
c. of kidney ▸ retention
c. of liver ▸ thin-walled
c. of mediastinum, bronchogenic
c. of meninges
c. of Morgagni
c. of ovary, dermoid
c. of placenta
c. of retina
c. of tentorium
c., omental
c., oophoritic
c., organizing hemorrhagic
c., ovarian
c., pancreatic
c., paroophoritic

c., parovarian
c., pedicled
c., pericardial
c., periosteal
c., peripelvic
c., peritoneal
c., pilonidal
c. ▸ pilonidal, tailbone pain from
c., polycystic
c., popliteal
c., porencephalic
c., radicular
c., renal
c., retention
c. ▸ ruptured Baker's
c., sacrococcygeal
c., Sampson's
c., sarcosporidian
c., saucerize
c., sebaceous
c. shrink
c. ▸ simple renal
c., solid
c. ▸ spinal cord
c., springwater
c. swell
c., synovial
c., tarsal
c., theca-lutein
c., thymic
c., thyroglossal duct
c., Tornwaldt's/Thornwaldt's
c. torsion, ovarian
c., true
c., tubo-ovarian
c., unilocular
c., urachal
c., urinary retention
c., vaginal inclusion
c., vulvar
c., vitelline duct
c. wall
c., wen
c., wolffian
cystadenocarcinoma
c. of ovary
c. ▸ ovarian serous
c. ovary, papillary
c. ovary, papillary serous
c. ovary, pseudomucinous
c., papillary serous
cystadenoma
c., mucinous
c., pseudomucinous
c., serous

cystectomy
c., chole◊
c., complete
c., ovarian
c., pilonidal
c., subtotal
c., total
cysteine, chlormerodrin-
cysteine complex, chlormerodrin-
cystic
c. acne
c. adenocarcinoma
c. adenoma ▸ papillary
c. angiomatosis
c. angiomatosis of bone
c. appearance
c. arachnoiditis
c. artery
c. astrocytoma
c. breast
c. bronchiectasis
c. cancer
c. carcinoma, adenoid
c. cataract
c. cervicitis, chronic
c. change
c. degeneration, adenomyoma with
c. diathesis
c. dilatation
c. disease
c. disease, medullary
c. disease of breast
c. disease of lungs
c. disease, renal
c. duct
c. duct cholangiogram
c. duct, elongated
c. duct, spiral fold of
c. duct, stump
c. emphysema
c. endometrial hyperplasia ▸ benign
c. enlargement
c. epithelioma, multiple benign
c. fibrosis (CF)
c. fibrosis gene
c. fibrosis of pancreas
c. fibrosis regulator
c. gastritis, chronic
c. goiter
c. gray medulla ▸ focally
c. hernia
c. hygroma
c. hyperplasia
c. hyperplasia, early
c. infarct, chronic

c. infarct, old
c. infarct, small
c. infarction
c. infarction, chronic
c. ischemia
c. kidney
c. lesion
c. lymphangiectasis, chronic pulmonary
c. mass
c. mass, fluid-filled
c. mastitis
c. mastitis, chronic
c. mastopathy
c. medial necrosis
c. medial necrosis of ascending aorta
c. membrane
c. ovarian mass
c. pituitary adenoma
c. structure, polypoid
c. teratoma, mature
c. tumor
c. vein

cystica
c., acne
c. chronica, enteritis
c., cystitis
c., mastopathia
c., meningitis serosa circumscripta
c., osteitis fibrosa
c., osteogenesis imperfecta
c. profunda, colitis
c. ▸ pyelitis, urethritis and cystitis
c., pyeloureteritis
c., severe
c. ▸ spina bifida
c. superficialis, colitis
c., urethritis
cystically dilated glands
Cysticercus
C. acanthrotrias
C. bovis
C. cellulosae
C. fasciolaris
C. ovis
C. tenuicollis
cysticum, lymphangioma
cystiform dilatation of kidney
cystiform enlargement of kidney
cystine
c. aminopeptidase
c. calculus
c. stone

cystitis
c., acute
c. ▸ acute uncomplicated
c., bacterial
c., chronic
c. cystica
c. cystica ▸ pyelitis, urethritis and
c., emphysematous
c., focal hemorrhagic
c. ▸ focal hemorrhagic necrotizing
c., hemorrhagic
c., honeymoon
c., interstitial
c., irradiation
c., nonbacterial
c., pancreatic
cystocele [systole]
c., asymptomatic
c. formation
c., protruding
**Cysto contrast medium, Hypaque-
cystogenic aneurysm**
Cystografin contrast medium
cystogram
c. (XC), excretory
c. (PVC), postvoiding
c., retrograde
c., triple voiding
c., voiding
cystography
c., delayed
c., radionuclide
c., triple voiding
c., voiding
cystoid cicatrix of limbus
cystojejunostomy, Roux-en-Y
Cystokon contrast medium
cystoma, myxoid
cystoma serosum simplex
cystometric pattern
cystometric study
cystometrogram (CMG)
cystoplasty augmentation
cystoradium insertion
cystosarcoma phylloides
cystoscopic
c. biopsy
c. electrocautery
c. examination
c. findings
c. fulguration
c. urography
cystoscopy
c. and dilatation

c. and fulguration
c., air
c., preoperative
c., water
cystostomy, tubeless
cystotomy, suprapubic
cystourethral suspension
cystoureterogram
c. (VCUG), voiding
c., micturition
c., retrograde
c., voiding
cystourethrography
c., expression
c., radionuclide voiding
c., retrograde
c., voiding
cythemolytic icterus
cytidine monophosphate
cytoblast [cytoplast]
cytoblastoma, hemo◊
cytogenetic study
cytogenic analysis
cytogenic anemia
cytohistologic diagnosis
cytoid bodies
cytokeratin membrane antigen
cytologic
c. diagnosis
c. examination
c. studies
c. study
cytological
c. biopsy
c. diagnostic tests
c. technique
cytology [sitology]
c., abnormal
c., aspiration biopsy
c. brushings for malignancy
c. ▸ cerebrospinal fluid (CSF)
c., cervical
c., exfoliative
c., gastric
c. in lung cancer, sputum
c., negative
c. of bronchial brushings
c., pancreatic
c., peritoneal
c., positive
c., positive peritoneal
c., sputum
cytolysis prognastic factor
cytoma
c., astro ◊

cytoma—*continued*
  c., fibrocystic
  c., pheochromo◊
  c., plasma◊
cytomegalic
  c. inclusion bodies
  c. inclusion disease (CMID)
  c. inclusion disease (CMID) of
    newborn
  c. inclusion disease (CMID) virus
cytomegalovirus
  c. antibody
  c. (CMV) disease
  c. (CMV) infection
  c. (CMV) infection, primary
  c. pneumonitis
  c. (CMV) retinitis
cytometric analysis ▸ flow
cytometric indirect
  immunofluorescence
cytopathic
  c. bovine orphan (ECBO) virus ▸
    enteric
  c. effect
  c. human orphan (ECHO) virus ▸
    enteric
  c. human orphan (ECHO) virus ▸
    enteric
  c. monkey orphan (ECMO) virus ▸
    enteric
  c. swine orphan (ECSO) virus ▸
    enteric
cytopathological charge
cytopathology, ocular
cytophil group
cytophilic antibody
cytoplasm
  c., basophilic
  c., blue-staining
  c., cell's soupy
  c., cellular
  c., eosinophilic
  c., eosinophilic dense
  c., granular eosinophilic
  c., liver cell
  c., narrow rim of
  c., neurilemmal
  c. ▸ neurons with eosinophilic
  c. of bacteria
  c. of cell
  c. ratio, nucleus-to-
  c., scanty pale
cytoplasmic
  c. autoantibody ▸ anti-neutrophic
  c. body, membranous

  c. borders well outlined
  c. bridge
  c. cycle
  c. glia
  c. granules
  c. inclusion bodies
  c. inclusion, hyalin
  c. lipid
  c. maturation, nuclear and
  c. organoids
  c. ratio
  c. tail, elongated
  c. vacuolation
  c. vacuoles, coarse
cytoplast [*cytoblast*]
cytoprint assay ▸ fluorescent
cytoreductive surgical management
cytoscopy, ultraviolet
cytosine arabinoside (ARA-C)
cytosine, guanine
cytoskeletal antigen
cytoskeleton, myocardial
cytosolic protein
cytosome, multilamellar
cytotoxic
  c. agent
  c. antibody
  c. chemotherapy
  c. drug
  c. effect
  c. reaction
  c. serum, antireticular
  c. testing
cytotoxicity, cell-mediated
cytotoxicity, macrophage-mediated
cytotoxin substance
Cytoxan
  C. (FAC) chemotherapy ▸
    5-fluorouracil, Adriamycin,
  C., Oncovin, prednisone (COP)
  C., methotrexate, 5-fluorouracil (CMF)
  C., vincristine, prednisone (CVP)
cytozoic parasite
Czermak's operation
Czermak's spaces
Czerny('s)
  C. anemia
  C. disease
  C. -Lembert suture
  C. suture

D

D and A (dilatation and aspiration) uterus

D and C

    D and C (dilatation and curettage)

    D and C (dilatation and curettage) ▸ diagnostic

    D and C (dilatation and curettage) ▸ fractional

    D and C (dilatation and curettage) ▸ suction

D and E (diagnosis and evaluation) staffing

D (LSD) ▸ Big

D. (dwarf) colony

D disease, sickle cell-hemoglobin

D echocardiogram ▸ 2-

D factor

D. hemoglobin

D immunoglobulin (IgD) determination ▸ gamma

D immunoglobulin (IgD), gamma

D milk ▸ vitamin

D resistant rickets ▸ Vitamin

D sleep

D syndrome ▸ trisomy

D to E slope

D virus (HDV) ▸ hepatitis

Dacron

    D. arterial graft

    D. arterial prosthesis

    D. bifurcation prosthesis

    D. graft

    D. graft, aortofemoral

    D. graft, Cooley woven

    D. graft, Meadox Microvel

    D. graft, Sauvage

    D. intracardiac patch

    D. patch

    D. pledget

    D. prosthesis

    D. prosthesis, crimped

    D. shield

    D. sleeve graft

    D. suture

    D. traction suture

    D. tube graft

    D. tube graft ▸ woven

    D. valve prosthesis

    D. vascular graft ▸ Velex woven

    D. vessel prosthesis

dacryoadenitis/dacryadenitis

dacryocystitis

    d., acute

    d., chronic

    d., phlegmonous

    d., syphilitic

    d., trachomatous

    d., tuberculous

dacryolith, Desmarres'

dactinomycin, *same as* actinomycin D (Cosmegen)

dactylocostal rhinoplasty

DAD (delayed after depolarization)

Daggett valve prosthesis ▸ Gott and

DAH (disordered action of heart)

daily

    d. allowance (RDA) ▸ recommended

    d. ▸ ascitic fluid tapped

    d. biological cycles

    d. caloric intake

    d. census

    d. census, average

    d. dietary allowance, recommended

    d. dose (MDD) ▸ mean

    d. evaluation

    d. exchanges

    d. exercise program

    d. fasting blood sugars (FBS)

    d. fractionation rate of rad

    d. functioning

    d. group therapy

    d. high fiber supplement

    d. injections

    d. irrigation

    d. ischemia

    d. life, quality of

    d. living (ADL) ▸ activities of

    d. living environment

    d. living (ADL), independent in activities of

    d. living ▸ relearn skills of

    d. living skills

    d. living (ADL), verbal cueing for activities of

    d. living (ADL) with supervision, patient does activities of

    d. medication

    d. moderate exercise

    d. multidisciplinary activities

    d. observation for rejection

    d. oral hygiene

    d. patient load, average

    d. physical activity

    d. preventive therapy

    d. problem solving

    d. relaxation exercises

    d. routine

    d. schedule of medication

    d. sleep-wake cycle

    d. status report

    d. stress, cope with

    d. stressors

    d. supplemental dose

    d. therapy

    d. urine testing

    d. variation

    d. visit

    d. warm sitz baths

    d. weighing

    d. -wear soft lenses

d'airain, bruit

dairensis, Saccharomyces

dairy

    d. product ▸ allergy to

    d. products ▸ digestion of

    d. products ▸ flatulence from

Dakin('s)

    D. fluid

    D. fluid ▸ Carrel-

    D. solution

Dale-Laidlaw's clotting time

Dalen-Fuchs nodules

Dalkon foam

Dalkon shield

Dalrymple's disease

Dalrymple's sign

dam drain, rubber

dam, rubber

damage [*manage*]
- d., accelerated liver
- d., actual tissue
- d. ▸ acute and long-term
- d. ▸ advanced liver
- d., alcohol brain
- d., alcohol-induced
- d., anoxic brain
- d., arterial
- d., articular surface
- d., asbestos
- d., brain
- d., cartilage
- d., collateral
- d., corneal
- d., cumulative sun
- d., debilitating neurological
- d., degenerative
- d., diffuse alveolar
- d., eighth nerve
- d., end-organ
- d., enzymatic organ
- d., eye
- d., fatal brain
- d., fatigue
- d., free-radical
- d. from cerebral hemorrhage ▸ brain
- d. from noise ▸ irreversible ear
- d., frontocortical
- d., genetic
- d., hearing
- d., heart
- d., heart and liver
- d., heart muscle
- d. ▸ heart valve
- d., immune system
- d., incapacitating nerve
- d. injury, brain
- d. ▸ irradiation-induced lung
- d., irreparable heart
- d., irreparable tissue
- d., irreversible
- d., irreversible brain
- d., irreversible catastrophic brain
- d. ▸ irreversible heart
- d. ▸ irreversible neurological
- d., joint
- d., kidney
- d., lethal
- d., light-induced
- d., liver
- d., localized
- d., lung
- d. ▸ massive brain

- d., median nerve
- d., mild cortical
- d., mitochondrial
- d. ▸ multiple organ
- d., myocardial
- d., nerve
- d., neurological
- d., operative
- d., oxidative
- d., ozone layer
- d., pacemaker
- d., peripheral nerve
- d., permanent
- d., permanent brain
- d., permanent joint
- d. ▸ permanent kidney
- d., phrenic nerve
- d. ▸ physical brain
- d. ▸ postfundoplication vagal nerve
- d., potential tissue
- d., preexisting renal
- d., progressive kidney
- d., radiation
- d., renal
- d. repair, sublethal
- d., residual
- d. ▸ right hemispheric parietal
- d., root
- d., severe brain
- d., severe cortical
- d., severe structural
- d. ▸ silent heart
- d., soft tissue
- d., spinal cord
- d., structural
- d., sun
- d. ▸ susceptible to radiation
- d., tissue
- d. to brain cells ▸ irreversible
- d. to brain ▸ organic
- d. to central nervous system
- d. to deep veins ▸ stretching or
- d. to healthy tissue
- d. to heart ▸ ischemic
- d. to nerve fibers
- d. to nerve fibers, regeneration after
- d. to Wernicke's area
- d. ▸ toxic iron
- d. typical alveolar
- d. ▸ vagal nerve

damaged
- d. brain
- d. brain cells
- d. brain tissue

- d. cancer cells
- d. cell membranes in brain
- d. cervical vertebra
- d. cochlea
- d. connective tissue
- d. donor heart
- d. hair cell receptors
- d. heart muscle
- d. heart ▸ rejuvenate
- d. issues
- d. left ventricle
- d. nerve cells ▸ regrow
- d. nerves ▸ regenerate
- d. or blocked fallopian tubes
- d. patient, brain
- d. ▸ patient feels
- d. site
- d. skin, sun-
- d. valve ▸ repair or replace

damaging behavior ▸ self-
damaging disease ▸ nerve
Damalinia
- D. caprae
- D. hermsi
- D. pilosus

D'Amato's sign
Damian graft procedure
dammini, Ixodes
damnosum, Simulium
damp pressure
damping
- d., catheter
- d. coefficient
- d. control

Dana's operation
dance, brachial
dance, hilar
dancer's scoliosis
dancing
- d., aerobic
- d. chorea
- d. mania

dander, animal
dandruff of scalp
dandruff with itching
dandy (Dandy)
- d. fever
- D. -Walker deformity
- D. -Walker syndrome

Danforth's method
Danforth's sign
dangerous
- d. behavior, inappropriate
- d. buildup of drugs
- d. drug abuser

d. drugs
d. lifestyle
d. objects, potentially
d. patient
d. potentially
danielewskyi, Haemoproteus
Daniel's operation
Danis dystrophy ▸ Maeder-
danis, Trichodectes
Danlos' syndrome
Danlos syndrome ▸ Ehlers-
danubicus, Vibrio
Dardik Biograft
DARE (Drug Awareness Resistance
Education)
DARE (Drug Abuse Resistance
Education) Program
Darier-Roussy sarcoid
Darier's disease
d'Arion silicone tube, fil
dark
d. adaptation
d. adaptation ▸ impaired
d. adaptation ▸ light to
d. -adapted eye
d. blood stained fluid
d. bloody material
d., bloody stool
d. brown urine ▸ passage of
d. center
d. circles under eyes
d. discrimination, light-
d. ▸ fear of
d. floaters
d. green bile
d. green bile ▸ viscid
d. green viscous bile
d. -ground illumination
d. pigmentation
d. ratio, light-
d. reaction
d. red bone marrow
d. skin surrounding nipple
d. -skinned patient
d. staining nuclei
d. urine
darkening of nipples
darkening of skin
darkfield
d. examination
d., fluorescent antibody
d. illumination
d. microscopy
darkly staining gram-positive rods ▸
large

darkness tremor
Darkshevich's fibers
Darkshevich's nucleus
Darling's disease
Darrach's
D. operation
D. procedure
D. resection
Darrow-Gamble syndrome
D/ART (Depression/Awareness
Recognition and Treatment)
dart and dome
dart configuration ▸ dome-and-
Dartmouth protocol
dartoid tissue
dartos muscle of scrotum
dartos reflex
Darwin's ear
Darwin's tubercle
Dash single-chamber rate adaptic
pacemaker
dashboard fracture
dashed line
Dasypus novemcincta
data (Data)
d., analog
d. analysis
d. analysis ▸ multicolor
d. base management
d., clinical
d., clinical mycology
d., derived hemodynamic
d., diagnostic
d., digitized
d., epidemiologic
d. evaluation
d., experimental
d., ferrokinetic
d. fusion
d., histopathologic
d., infection
d., intake
d., laboratory
d. ▸ long-term survival
d., nutritional
d. ▸ objective baseline
d. on infection ▸ compiling
surveillance
d., pharmacological
d. processing (ADP), automatic
d., radiodensity
D. Repository (CDR), Clinical
d., safety test
d., scan
d., spacial-perceptual

d. spike detection error artifact
d., stereotactic
d., surveillance
d., theoretical
d., wavelength
date
d., analogous
d., estimated discharge
d. of birth
d. of confinement (CDC),
calculated
d. of confinement (EDC/EDOC) ▸
estimated
d. of confinement (EDC/EDOC),
expected
d. of delivery (EDD/EDOD) ▸
estimated
daughter
d. cell
d. colony
d. element
d. nuclide
d. of alcoholic parents
d. star
daunorubicin, prednisone ▸
vincristine,
Dava (Iranian heroin)
David operation, Vernon-
David's disease
Davidson protocol exercise test
Daviel's operation
Davies
D. -Colley operation
D. endomyocardial fibrosis
D. myocardial fibrosis
Davis
D. graft
D. operation
D. sign
Davy's test
Dawbarn's sign
DAWN (Drug Abuse Warning
Network)
Dawson's encephalitis
daxensis, Spirochaeta
day(s) (Day)
d. care, adult
d. care center, adult
D. Care Center ▸ Same
d. care centers
d. care program
d. care, senior
d., co-insurance
d. educational programs ▸ family
d. (q.i.d.) ▸ four times a

day(s)—*continued*
- d., hospital
- d., inpatient
- D. Intensive Outpatient Program
- d., lifetime reserve
- d. -night cycle
- d., postoperative
- d. sight
- d. sleepiness, mid-
- D. Surgery, Same
- D. syndrome ▸ Riley-
- d. (t.i.d.) ▸ three times a
- d. (b.i.d.) ▸ twice a
- d. (b.i.d.) ▸ two times a
- d. vision

Daya Syphilis Test (DST)
daydreaming, relaxed and
daydreams, patient
daylight vision
daytime
- d. drowsiness
- d. sleep episodes
- d. sleepiness
- d. sleepiness, excessive
- d. sleepiness, severe
- d. somnolence, excessive

dazed
- d. appearance
- d. condition ▸ patient admitted in
- d., patient
- d. relaxation
- d. state, patient in

dazzle reflex
DB (distobuccal)
db (decibel)
DBI (development-at-birth index)
DBO (distobucco-occlusal)
DBP (diastolic blood pressure)
DBP (distobuccopulpal)
DC
- DC (direct current)
- DC (distocervical)

DC (direct current)
- DC electric shock
- DC ▸ opposition of flow of
- DC resistance
- DC voltage

DCA (directional coronary atherectomy)
Dc'd (discontinued)
DCIS (ductal carcinoma in situ)
DCS (dorsal column stimulator)
D-cycloserine
DDC (direct display console)

DDH (developmental dysplasia of hip)
de
- de bois, bruit
- de canon, bruit
- de choc, bruit
- de clapotement, bruit
- de claquement, bruit
- de Clerembault's syndrome
- de craquement, bruit
- de cuir neuf, bruit
- de diable, bruit
- de drapeau, bruit
- de froissement, bruit
- de frolement, bruit
- de frottement, bruit
- de galop, bruit
- de Graaff generator, Van
- de Grandmont's operation
- de grelot, bruit
- de Kleijn neck reflex ▸ Magnus and
- de la roue de moulin, bruit
- de Leudet, bruit
- de lime, bruit
- de mer, mal
- De Morgan's spots
- de moulin, bruit
- de moulin, bruit de la roué
- de novo
- de novo lesion
- de parchemin, bruit
- de piaulement
- de pointes, dorsades
- de polichinelle ▸ voix
- de pot fêlé, bruit
- de Quervain's disease
- de Quervain's syndrome
- de Quervain's tenolysis
- de Quervain's thyroiditis
- de rape, bruit
- de rape, bruit de scie ou
- de rappel, bruit
- de Roger, bruit
- de scie, bruit
- de scie ou de rape, bruit
- de soufflet, bruit
- de tabourka, bruit
- de tambour, bruit
- de Toni Fanconi syndrome
- de triolet, bruit

deactivated cells
dead
- d. area of heart muscle
- d. birth
- d. cell

- d. cells ▸ flush away dulling dry,
- d., declared legally
- d. fetus
- d. fetus in utero
- d. finger
- d. hand
- d. nerve in tooth
- D. on Arrival (phencyclidine), DOA/
- d. on arrival (DOA) ▸ patient
- d., patient brain
- d., patient pronounced
- d. skin
- d. skin cells
- d. skin cell layers ▸ compacted
- d. space
- d. space, alveolar
- d. space, anatomical
- d. space ▸ physiological
- d. space ventilation
- d. time
- d. tissue
- d. tissue sloughing

deadly flu virus
deaf
- d. cerebral palsied child
- d. -mute
- d. mutism
- D. (TDD), Telecommunications Device for the

deafness
- d., acoustic trauma
- d., apoplectiform
- d., central
- d., cerebral
- d., ceruminous
- d., conduction
- d., conductive type
- d., cortical
- d., functional
- d., hysterical
- d., inner ear
- d., labyrinthine
- d., midbrain
- d., middle ear
- d., mixed
- d., nerve
- d., nerve conduction
- d., nerve-type
- d., neural
- d., noise-induced
- d., organic
- d., paradoxic
- d., perceptive
- d., sensorineural
- d., tone

d., total
d., total nerve
d., toxic
d., traumatic
d., vascular
d., vertigo and tinnitus
d. with tinnitus
d., word
de-airing procedure
dealer(s)
   d., crack house drug
   d., dope
   d., drug
   d., major drug
dealing, drug
dealing with discomfort
deaminase deficiency, adenosine
Dearth, Birth
dearth, donor
death (Death)
   d., acceptance of
   d., accidental
   d. after cesarean section ▸ maternal
   d., alcohol-related
   d., anger at
   d., antepartum fetal
   d. anxiety
   d., apparent
   d., arrhythmic
   d., asphyxia and
   d., asthma
   d. (COD) ▸ autopsy report cause of
   d., biological
   d., black
   d., brain
   d. by poisoning
   d. by starvation and dehydration
   d. by suicide
   d. ▸ calculated, premeditated
   d., cancer
   d., cardiac
   d., cardiovascular
   d., care of body after
   d. (COD), cause of
   d., cell
   d., cellular
   d., cerebral
   d. certificate
   d., chronic sudden
   d., circumstances of
   d., clinical
   d., clinical brain
   d., cocaine-induced
   d., cocaine-related

d., cot
d., crib
d. criteria, brain
d. criteria for determination of brain
d. decision
d. decisions, active
d. ▸ delirium and
d. ▸ delirium, convulsions and
d., denial of
d. ▸ diabetes-related
d., diagnosed brain
d., dignified
d., disease-related
d. ▸ doctors actively caused
d. ▸ drug and alcohol abuse
d., drug-induced
d., drug-related
d. due to alcohol abuse ▸ sudden
d. due to cocaine ingestion ▸ sudden
d. due to drug abuse
d. due to strangulation
d. due to suffocation
d. during exercise ▸ sudden
d. during jogging ▸ sudden
d., early fetal
d., early neonatal
d. ▸ emesis, coma, and
d. experience (NDE) ▸ near
d., family present at time of
d., farm-related
d. ▸ fear of imminent
d., fetal
d. from cervical cancer
d., functional
d., genetic
d., heart cell
d., heart muscle
d. imminent
d. in stroke victim ▸ nerve
d., indices of
d., infant
d. instinct
d., intentionally causing
d., intermediate fetal
d., intrauterine
d. ▸ intrauterine fetal
d. ▸ irreversible brain
d. ▸ ischemic sudden
d., Kübler-Ross time frame of
d., late
d., late fetal
d. ▸ leading cause of
d., lightning related
d., liver

d., local
d. mask
d., maternal
d. ▸ maternal brain
d., melanoma
d., methamphetamine-related
d., molecular
d., muscle
d., natural
d., neonatal
d., nonrenal
d. notice
d., notification of
d. of bone cells
d. of brain cells
d. of brain tissue
d. of heart muscle tissue
d. of myocardial cells
d. of spouse, adjustment to
d. on unit
d. or suicide ▸ recurring thoughts of
d. or suicide ▸ talking of
d., painfully slow
d., patient
d., patient choked to
d., patient died accidental
d., patient died natural
d., patient died unnatural
d., perinatal
d., premature
d., premature birth ▸ neonatal
d., preoccupation with
d., preventable
d. ▸ programmed cell
d., prolonging
d., pronouncement of
d., pronouncement of brain
d. rate
d. rate, high
d. rate, spiraling
d. ratio, birth-
d., reality of
d. ▸ recurrent thoughts of
d. ▸ risk of cardiac
d. ▸ risk of colon cancer
d., risk of sudden
d., smoking
d., somatic
d. struggle, life and
d., sudden
d., sudden cardiac
d., sudden heart attack
D. (SSD), Sudden Sniffing
d., sudden unexplained
d., suicidal

death—*continued*
- d. syndrome (SEDS) ▸ sedentary
- D. Syndrome (SIDS), Sudden Infant
- d., term delivery antepartum
- d., term delivery intrapartum
- d., term delivery neonatal
- d., terminal
- d., terminated in
- d., time of
- d., tissue
- d., traumatic
- d., traumatic brain
- d., unexpected
- d., untimely
- d., voodoo
- d. ▸ whole brain
- d. with dignity
- d. worldwide

Deaver incision

DeBakey
- D. ball valve prosthesis
- D. -Creech aneurysm repair
- D. graft
- D. implant
- D. prosthesis
- D. -type aortic dissection
- D. valve prosthesis
- D. Vasculour II vascular prosthesis

Debaryomyces hansenii

debilitated
- d. ▸ exhausted, weak and
- d. individual, severely
- d., patient
- d., patient dehydrated and
- d. patient, severely
- d., physically
- d., socially

debilitating
- d. affliction
- d. back pain
- d. bone disease
- d. bowel disease
- d. condition
- d. dementia
- d. disease
- d. disease, chronic
- d. disorder
- d. disorder, chronic
- d. effects
- d. effects of old age
- d. elements
- d. emphysema
- d. headache
- d. illness

- d., incurable brain disease ▸ progressive,
- d. injury
- d. knee pain, chronic
- d., longstanding fatigue ▸ generalized,
- d. musculoskeletal pain
- d. neurological damage
- d. osteoarthritis
- d. osteoporosis
- d. pain
- d. ▸ painful and
- d. psychosis
- d. pulmonary fibrosis
- d. radiation
- d. rheumatoid arthritis
- d. sleep disorder
- d. symptoms
- d. symptoms ▸ severe
- d. syndrome

debility
- d. and dyspnea ▸ increasing weakness,
- d. and/or pain
- d. and weakness ▸ patient has increasing
- d., chronic
- d., increasing
- d., severe pain and

Debove's disease

Debove's membrane

Debre-Semelaigne syndrome

debrided
- d. bone surfaces
- d. necrotic tissue
- d., wound
- d., wound edge

debridement
- d. and irrigation
- d. and prosthesis retention
- d. and revision
- d., arthroscopic
- d., enzymatic
- d., extensive
- d., joint
- d., mycotic nail
- d. of bruised tissue
- d. of compound skull fracture
- d. of infected skin
- d. of necrotic tissue
- d., surgical
- d. technique, enzymatic
- d., ulcer

debris
- d. amorphous

- d., bloodstream
- d., calcific
- d., carbonizing cellular
- d., cell
- d., cellular
- d., cholesteatoma
- d., desquamating
- d., embedded
- d., grumous
- d., intra-alveolar
- d., myelin
- d., necrotic
- d., otoconial
- d., proteinaceous
- d., pultaceous
- d., valve
- d., word

deBroglie wavelength

debubbling procedure

debulked, tumor

debulking, intra-abdominal tumor

debulking procedure

decade scaler

decalcified lumbar vertebra

decalcified sections of vertebral bodies

decalcifying fluid

decapacitation factor

decapsulation of kidney

decarboxylase, histidine

decarboxylase, urophyrinogen

decay
- d., alpha
- d., beta
- d., branching
- d. constant
- d., dental
- d., exponential
- d., gamma
- d., isomeric
- d. mode
- d. ▸ nursing bottle tooth
- d. ▸ pain in ear from tooth
- d., patient in state of physical
- d., physical
- d., positron
- d., pressure
- d. product
- d., radioactive
- d. scheme
- d. series
- d. test, modified tone
- d. test, tone
- d., tone
- d., tooth

decayed teeth
decease [*decrease*]
deceased, relationship to
deceit ▸ impulsivity, aggression and
deceitful, patient
decelerate breathing rhythm
decelerated breathing ▸ shallow accelerated-
decelerating flow ventilation ▸ volume cycled
deceleration(s)
  d., early
  d., fetal
  d. injury
  d., late
  d. of heart rate ▸ operant
  d. of monitor
  d. time
  d. time ▸ transmitral E wave
  d., variable
decentered lens
decentration of lenses
deception
  d., deliberate
  d., emotional
  d. ▸ malingering and
deceptive
  d. ability
  d. cult practices
  d., patient
decerebrate
  d. epilepsy
  d. posturing
  d. rigidity
Dechaume-Blanc syndrome ▸ Bonnet-
decibel (db)
decibel (db) hearing test
decibel meters
decidua
  d., basal
  d. basalis
  d., capsular
  d. capsularis
  d., menstrual
  d. menstrualis
  d., parietal
  d. parietalis
  d., reflex
  d. reflexa
  d. serotina
  d. vera
decidual [*residual*]
  d. cell
  d. endometritis

d. fragment, retention of
d. pseudoendometrium
d. tissue
d. tissue, degenerating
d. tissue, necrotic
d. umbilicus
deciduous
  d. cuspid
  d. placenta
  d. teeth
  d. tissue
deciliter, lead per
decimal word
decision(s) [*discission*]
  d., active death
  d. analysis
  d., collective
  d., death
  d., diet
  d., DNR (do not resuscitate)
  d. ▸ durable power of attorney
  d., Durham's
  d., emotional
  d., health care
  d. ▸ inability to make
  d. ▸ incapable of making
  d., informed
  d., informed health care
  d., instinctual
  d., life-changing
  d., life-saving
  d. maker, surrogate
  d. making
  d. making, clinical
  d. making ▸ difficulty in
  d. making, health care
  d. making ▸ interference with judgment and
  d. making, personal
  d. -making process
  d. -making skills
  d., medical
  d., objective
  d., subjective
  d., treatment
  d., treatment placement
  d. trees in patient management
  d., ▸ unwilling to make
decisional conflict
Decker's operation
declamping shock syndrome
declarative memory
declared legally dead
decline
  d. (ARCD), age-related cognitive

d., cognitive
d., functional
d. in ability to perform routine tasks
d. in function ▸ progressive
d. in interest of opposite sex
d. in intellectual abilities
d. in intellectual function ▸ permanent
d. in intellectual function ▸ progressive
d. in job performance
d. in mental function
d. in personal grooming
d. in sexual function
d. in social abilities
d. in social relationships
d., incremental
d., intellectual
d., memory
d., mental
declining
  d. mathematical ability
  d., physically
  d. respiratory status
  d. vision
decompensated heart failure
decompensated shock
decompensation
  d., cardiac
  d., emotional
  d., left ventricular
  d., right ventricular
decomposition
  d., anaerobic
  d. of body
  d. of movement
  d., postmortem
  d., protein
decompressant craniotomy
decompressed, stomach
decompression
  d., abdominal
  d. (ACD), active compression-
  d., biliary
  d., cardiac
  d., carpal canal
  d., carpal tunnel
  d., cerebral
  d., cervical disc
  d. chamber
  d., core
  d., endoscopic biliary
  d., explosive
  d., gastric
  d., heart

decompression—*continued*
  d., Heyns'
  d. laminectomy
  d., median lobe
  d., median nerve
  d., nerve
  d. of abdomen
  d. of heart
  d. of orbit
  d. of pericardium
  d. of rectum
  d. of spinal cord
  d., oral
  d., percutaneous laser disk
  d. sickness
  d., suboccipital
  d., subtemporal
  d. surgery
  d. surgery ▸ microvascular
  d., surgical
  d., thoracic outlet
  d., tumor
decompressive lumbar laminectomy
decondition pain behavior
decongestant
  d. medicine
  d., nasal
  d., oral
decontaminate stethoscope
decontamination
  d. cycle
  d., environmental
  d., gastrointestinal (GI)
  d. of blood
  d. of blood spill
  d. of digestive tract ▸ selective
  d. of secretion spill
decoordination, visual
decora, Macrobdella
decorticate posturing
decortication
  d., arterial
  d., chemical
  d., enzymatic
  d. from hypoglycemia, functional
  d. from hypoxia, functional
  d. from trauma, functional
  d. of heart
  d. of lung
decrease(s) [*decease*]
  d. digestion
  d. discomfort
  d. discomfort ▸ increase awareness
    and
  d. in anxiety

  d. in appetite
  d. in coordination or equilibrium
  d. in energy level
  d. in energy or fatigue
  d. in flexibility
  d. in frequency
  d. in mediastinal widening
  d. in mitochondrial metabolism
  d. in neutrophils
  d. in respiratory effort
  d. in sense of smell
  d. in serum amylase
  d. in urine excretion
  d. in voltage, localized moderate
  d. of function
  d. of tolerance
  d. ▸ oxygen content of blood
  d. pain
  d. production of angiotensin
  d. tension and anxiety
decreased
  d. ability to concentrate
  d. ability to function
  d. ability to function independently
  d. activity
  d. acuity
  d. alertness
  d. anxiety
  d. appetite
  d. appetite and increased energy
  d. appetite ▸ insomnia,
    hyperactivity and
  d. attenuation
  d. blood flow
  d. blood pressure (BP)
  d. blood supply
  d. body hair
  d. bone mineral density
  d. bowel function
  d. bowel sounds
  d. brain activity
  d. brain wave activity
  d. breast size
  d. breath sounds
  d. breath sounds ▸ dullness and
  d. capacity for abstract thought
  d. cardiac output
  d. carotid upstroke
  d. consciousness ▸ spell of
  d. diffusion capacity
  d. deep sleep
  d. drug excretion
  d. energy
  d. energy ▸ fatigue, weakness and
  d. excretion

  d. expansion ▸ lungs revealed
  d. fat mass
  d. flow of saliva
  d. flow of tears
  d. function
  d. hand circulation
  d. hearing
  d. heart rate
  d. heart rate ▸ apneic infant with
  d. immune function
  d. in size, gyri
  d. intake
  d. intelligence
  d. judgment
  d. kidney function
  d. leg circulation
  d. level of consciousness
  d. libido
  d. loudness
  d. memory
  d. memory ▸ patient has
  d. mental tension
  d. metabolism
  d. muscle mass
  d. muscle strength
  d. need for sleep
  d., night vision
  d. penile outflow
  d. peripheral lymphocyte count
  d. platelets
  d. position sense
  d. proprioception
  d. protein synthesis
  d. proteinuria
  d. pulse
  d. rebleeding risk
  d. reflexes
  d. renal function
  d., renal output
  d. respiration
  d. respiratory volume
  d. risk of heart disease
  d. SBP (systolic blood pressure)
  d. sense of taste
  d. sensitivity
  d. serum osmolality
  d. sex drive
  d. sexual arousal
  d. sexual interest
  d. signs and symptoms of anxiety
  d. signs and symptoms of
    depression
  d. specific gravity
  d. spinal motion
  d. stamina

d. strength
d. stress
d. stroke volume
d. sweating
d. systolic blood pressure (SBP)
d. tension
d. tolerance
d. tonic EMG (electromyogram) activity
d. triglycerides
d. tubular reabsorption of amylase
d. urinary output
d. urination
d. vasodilation
d. venous return to heart
d. vision
d. visual acuity

decreasing
d. blood count
d. cardiac output
d. hypertension
d. jaundice
d. peripheral vascular resistance
d. tear production

decremental
d. atrial pacemaker
d. atrial pacing
d. conduction

decrementing response
decrepitude with age
decrescendo
d. early systolic murmur
d. murmur, crescendo-
d. murmur, diastolic

decrescent arteriosclerosis
decubital necrosis
decubitus
d., Andral
d., angina
d., angina pectoris
d. calculus
d. care
d. cough
d. cushion
d. elbow
d. film
d. film, lateral
d. heel
d. position
d. position, dorsal
d. position, lateral
d. position, left
d. position, right
d. skin care
d. ulcer

d. ulcer ▸ infected
d. ulcer ▸ large sacral
d. wound

decumanus, Mus
decurtate pulse
decussation
d., Forel's
d., Meynert
d. of Meynert, fountain
d., optic
d., pyramidal

deductive echocardiography
deductive reasoning
DEEG (depth electroencephalogram)
deep
d. abdominal reflexes
d. abdominal tenderness
d. aching pain
d. and regular respiration
d. and stretching massage
d. bite
d. bites of tissue
d. brachial artery
d. brain stimulation
d. brain stimulation, thalamic
d. brain stimulator
d. breathing
d. breathing ▸ chest pain on
d. breathing ▸ dizziness from rapid and
d. breathing exercises
d. breathing, patient taught
d. ▸ breathing prolonged and
d. breathing technique
d. cerebral structures
d. cerebral tumor
d. cervical lymph nodes
d. cervical vein
d. chest breathing
d. chest therapy
d. circumflex iliac vein
d. cleansing breath
d. closure
d. cold
d. coma
d. concentration
d. cough
d. creases
d. Doppler velocity interrogation
d. dorsal vein of clitoris
d. dorsal vein of penis
d. emptiness, chronic feelings of
d. enough, biopsy not
d. epithelialization
d. facial vein

d. femoral artery
d. femoral vein
d. fibular nerve
d. flexor muscle of fingers
d. frostbite
d. heating, regional
d. hepatic coma
d. hypothermia circulatory arrest
d. inguinal lymph nodes
d. inspiration
d. inspiration ▸ prolonged
d. knee bends
d. lamellar transplant
d. layers
d. layers of cortex
d. lingual vein
d. massage
d. middle cerebral vein
d. midline tumor
d. muscle massage
d. muscle relaxation
d. muscle therapy
d. palpation
d. parotid lymph nodes ▸ superficial and
d. penetrating wound
d. percussion
d. peroneal nerve
d. peroneal nerve, accessory
d. petrosal cells
d. petrosal nerve
d. pressure massage
d. puncture wound
d. radial nerve
d. rage, harboring
d. reflex
d. relaxation, feedback technique of
d. relaxation in labor
d. relaxation ▸ progressive
d. relaxation ▸ rapid,
d. respiration
d. roentgen ray therapy
d. scaler
d. -seated benign tumors
d. -seated cancer
d. -seated guilt
d. -seated lesion
d. -seated pain
d. -seated psychopathology
d. sensibility
d. sleep
d. sleep, decreased
d. sleep of short duration
d. sleep, patient in
d. sleep stage

deep—*continued*
- d. slow breathing
- d. structures
- d. temporal nerves
- d. temporal vein
- d. tendon reflex (DTR)
- d. tendon reflexes (DTR) equal and active
- d. tendon reflexes (DTR) hypoactive
- d. tendon reflexes (DTR) ‣ increased
- d. tendon reflexes (DTR) ‣ monitoring of
- d. tendon reflexes (DTR) symmetrical
- d. therapy unit, Picker Vanguard
- d. tissue massage
- d. tissue massage therapist
- d. tissue massage therapy
- d. transverse arrest
- d. transverse fibers
- d. transverse muscle of perineum
- d. tumors
- d. ulceration
- d. vein of clitoris
- d. vein of penis
- d. vein of thigh
- d. vein of tongue
- d. vein thrombophlebitis ‣ migratory
- d. vein thrombosis, iliofemoral
- d. veins ‣ stretching or damage to
- d. venous insufficiency
- d. venous thrombosis (DVT)
- d. vidian nerve
- d. voice
- d. wound exploratory
- d. x-ray therapy

deepened, incision
deepening of voice
deeper stage of sleep
deepest inspiration
deeply
- d. anesthetized patient
- d. comatose, patient
- d. staining nucleus

defacing, cervix
defatted, skin graft
defeat ‣ intolerance of
defeating
- d. personality disorder ‣ self-
- d. personality ‣ self-
- d. way ‣ patient a perfectionist in self-

defecate ‣ inability to

defecate, urge to
defecation [*desquamation, desiccation*]
- d., feces
- d., pain on
- d., rectum
- d. reflex
- d. syncope

defect(s)
- d., alcohol-related
- d. ‣ alcohol-related birth
- d., aldosterone secretion
- d., anatomic
- d., aortic septal
- d., aorticopulmonary septal
- d., atrial
- d., atrial ostium primum
- d. (ASD), atrial septal
- d., atrioventricular (AV) canal
- d., atrioventricular (AV) conduction
- d., atrioventricular (AV) septal
- d., behavioral
- d. benign cortical
- d., biochemical
- d., birth
- d., blood clotting
- d., brain
- d., cardiac
- d., chronic obstructive
- d., clamshell closure of atrial septal
- d. closed
- d. closed with sutures
- d. closure, interatrial septal
- d., CNS (central nervous system)
- d., cognitive
- d., complement
- d., conduction
- d., congenital
- d., congenital birth
- d., congenital cardiac
- d., congenital ectodermal
- d., congenital heart
- d., congenital valvular
- d., cyanotic heart
- d., developmental
- d., donor
- d., dural
- d., ectodermal
- d., endocardial cushion
- d., extradural
- d., extrafusion
- d., extrinsic
- d., eye
- d., filling
- d. ‣ fixed perfusion

- d., focal
- d. ‣ folate preventable birth
- d., fusion
- d., gene
- d., genetic
- d. ‣ genetic birth
- d., Gerbode
- d., gross
- d., hammer toe
- d., hearing
- d. ‣ heart valve
- d., hereditary
- d. ‣ hereditary heart
- d. ‣ humoral immune
- d. ‣ iatrogenic atrial septal
- d. in acute myocardial infarction, conduction
- d. in bladder ‣ negative filling
- d. in footplate of stapes, congenital
- d. ‣ infundibular septal
- d., inherited
- d., inherited genetic
- d., intellectual
- d. (IASD), interatrial septal
- d. (IVSD), interventricular septal
- d. interventricular septum of heart, congenital
- d., intraluminal filling
- d. (IVCD), intraventricular conduction
- d., intrinsic
- d., irradiated surgical
- d., irregular
- d., labyrinthine
- d., localized
- d., lucent
- d., luminal filling
- d., lytic
- d., macrophage
- d., match
- d., memory
- d., mental
- d., metabolic
- d., mild residual
- d., motor
- d., mucosal
- d., multiple congenital
- d., muscle wall
- d., myocardial conduction
- d., napkin-ring
- d., neural arch
- d. (NTD) ‣ neural tube
- d., neurological
- d., neuropsychological
- d., neutrophil

d., nonspecific intraventricular conduction
d. ▸ nonuniform rotational
d., obstructive
d., obstructive airway
d., obstructive ventilatory
d. of brain ▸ congenital
d. of labyrinth
d. of labyrinth, acquired
d. of labyrinth, congenital
d. on lung scan ▸ ventilation
d., organic
d., ostium primum
d., ostium secundum
d. ▸ oval window
d., panconduction
d., patch closure of
d., pelvic support
d., perfusion
d. ▸ perimembranous ventricular septal
d., plasma
d., plastic repair of
d., platelet
d., posterior inferior
d., posture
d., prenatal diagnosis of birth
d., primary
d. ▸ primum atrial septal
d., radiolucent
d., renal tubular
d., repair of
d., restrictive airway
d., restrictive ventilatory
d., retention
d. ▸ reversible ischemic neurologic
d. ▸ right ventricular conduction
d., sac-like
d. ▸ scintigraphic perfusion
d. ▸ secundum atrial septal
d., sensory
d. (SD), septal
d., septic atrial
d., serum
d. ▸ sex-linked
d. ▸ sex-linked genetic
d. shunt ▸ ventricular septal
d., sinus
d. ▸ sinus venosus
d. ▸ sinus venosus atrial septal
d., skeletal muscular
d., skull
d., speech
d. ▸ spinal cord birth
d., splicing

d., structural
d. ▸ structural heart
d. ▸ structural uterine
d. ▸ subcristal ventricular septal
d., subjective
d., surgical
d. ▸ Swiss cheese
d. ▸ T cell
d., temporal field
d., triangular
d. umbrella, atrial septal
d., underlying
d., valve
d., valvular
d. vegetation ▸ ventricular septal
d., ventilation perfusion
d., ventilatory
d., ventral septal
d., ventricular
d. (VSD) ▸ ventricular septal
d., vision
d., visual
d., visual field
d. ▸ X-linked genetic
defection ▸ scintigraphic perfusion
defective
d. aorta
d. aortic valve
d. artificial heart valve
d. association
d. baby
d. bladder
d. bone marrow cell
d. cartilage
d. cells
d. child
d. closure
d. coordination
d. cortical sensation
d. development
d. development, organs with
d. diaphragm
d. ear
d. enamel
d. erythropoiesis
d. gene
d. gene problem
d. generator
d. genes
d. heart valve
d. immune response
d. implant
d. impression
d. memory
d. motor power

d. nerve signals
d. phages
d. recessive gene
d. renal parenchyma
d. retention
d. virus
defense(s)
d. against infection, natural
d. against injury, local
d. barrier ▸ small intestine as a
d., body's natural
d., character
d., ego
d., host
d., immune
d., immunological
d., malpractice
d. mechanism
d. mechanism, body
d. mechanism, body's own
d. mechanism, natural
d. mechanism of denial
d. mechanisms ▸ individual
d., mental
d., muscular
d. of denial ▸ ego
d. process
d., psychological
d. reaction
d. reflex
d. system, body's
d. system, immune
defensive
d. behavior
d. behavior skills
d. cells
d. coping
d. patterns
d. resistances
defensiveness ▸ diminished denial and
deferens
d., ampulla of vas
d., ductus
d., twisting of vas
d., vas
deferent duct
deferential [*differential*]
deferential artery
deferentis, ampulla ductus
deferred
d. fracture
d. on Axis I ▸ diagnosis or condition
d. on Axis II ▸ diagnosis or condition

deferred—*continued*
- d., rectal
- d. shock

defervesced, patient
defervescent stage
defiant
- d. child
- d. counterattack ▸ reacts with
- d. disorder (ODD), oppositional
- d. patient

defibrillated, heart
defibrillated with single shock of _____ **joules ▸ heart**
defibrillating, patient
defibrillation [*defibrination*]
- d. and electrical cardioversion
- d., arrhythmias following
- d., atrial
- d., cardiac
- d., early
- d., electrical
- d., exertional
- d. lead ▸ nonintegrated transvenous
- d. lead syndrome ▸ nonthoracotomy
- d. pad ▸ Littman
- d. paddles
- d. patch
- d. procedure
- d. shocks
- d. shocks ▸ QRS synchronous atrial
- d. technique
- d. threshold
- d. threshold, atrial
- d. threshold testing
- d., ventricular

defibrillator
- d., (AED), automated external
- d., (AED), automatic external
- d., (AID), automatic implantable
- d., (AICD), automatic implantable cardioverter
- d., (AICD), automatic internal cardioverter
- d., automatic intracardiac
- d. burns
- d., cardiac
- d., cardioverter
- d., external
- d. ▸ external cardioverter
- d. ▸ hand-held
- d. implant

- d. implant support device ▸ Medtronic
- d., implantable
- d. (ICD), implantable cardiac
- d. in cardioversion ▸ implantable
- d. insertion ▸ implantable cardiac
- d. ▸ internal cardioverter
- d., IPCO/Partridge
- d. lead ▸ transvenous
- d. (AID) malfunction ▸ automatic implantable
- d. ▸ Medtronic external cardioverter
- d. ▸ Medtronic PCD implantable cardioverter
- d., multifunctional
- d. ▸ nonthoracotomy implantable cardioverter
- d. ▸ nonthoracotomy lead implantable cardioverter
- d. ▸ pacer cardioverter
- d. ▸ paddle marks from
- d. paddles
- d. patch ▸ epicardial
- d., portable
- d. (PCD) ▸ programmable cardioverter
- d., smart
- d. ▸ subpectoral implantation of cardioverter
- d. (AED) ▸ SurVivaLink automated external
- d. ▸ Telectronics ATP implantable cardioverter
- d. ▸ Transvene nonthoracotomy implantable cardioverter
- d. ▸ transvenous implantation of cardioverter
- d. unit ▸ portable
- d., Ventak
- d. ▸ Ventritex Cadence implantable cardioverter

defibrillatory ▸ implantable atrial
defibrillatory shock
defibrinated blood
defibrination [*defibrillation*]
defibrination syndrome
deficiency(-ies)
- d., acquired color
- d., acute brain
- d., adenosine deaminase
- d., alcohol-related vitamin
- d., alpha-1-antitrypsin
- d. anemia, enzyme
- d. anemia ▸ glucose-6-phosphate dehydrogenase

- d. anemia, iron
- d., antidiuretic hormone
- d., a-1,3-glucosidase
- d., biochemical
- d., behavioral
- d., biotin
- d., calcium
- d., carbohydrate
- d., cholinesterase
- d., circulatory
- d., cognitive
- d., color perception
- d., color vision
- d., congenital immune
- d., dietary
- d., disaccharidase
- d. disease
- d. disease, combined immune
- d. disorder, immunologic
- d. disorder (IDD) ▸ iodine
- d., dopamine
- d., emotional
- d., enzymatic
- d., enzyme
- d. ▸ erythrocyte glutathione peroxidase
- d., estrogen
- d., exercise
- d., Factor III
- d., Factor VIII
- d., Factor IX
- d., Factor X
- d. ▸ familial high density lipoprotein
- d., fibrinogen
- d. ▸ folic acid
- d., folate
- d., functional
- d., galactokinase
- d., galactosidase
- d., gamma A immunoglobulin (IgA)
- d., gamma M globulin (IgM)
- d., gamma M immunoglobulin (IgM)
- d. (GRID) ▸ gay-related immune
- d., glucose-6-phosphate dehydrogenase
- d., growth hormone
- d., hexosaminidase
- d., hormonal
- d. ▸ human growth hormone
- d. idiopathic mental
- d., IgA (gamma A globulin)
- d., immune
- d., immunoglobulin
- d., immunologic
- d. ▸ impulse control

d. in judgment
d., inherited color
d. ▸ inherited procoagulant
d., insulin
d., intellectual
d. ▸ intracellular magnesium
d., iodine
d., iron
d., lactase
d., limb
d., magnesium
d., mental
d., neuropsychological
d., nutrient
d., nutritional
d. of blood supply
d. of slow brain wave activity
d., oxygen (O_2)
d. ▸ parathyroid hormone
d., peripheral
d. ▸ postnatal growth
d., potassium
d., protein
d. ▸ protein-calorie
d. ▸ protein S
d. ▸ red blood cell (RBC)
d. ▸ red-green color perception
d., riboflavin
d., selenium
d., serotonin
d., severe oxygen (O_2)
d., somatotropin
d. state, immunity
d., surfactant
d., symptomatic magnesium
d. syndrome (AIDS), acquired immune
d. syndrome (AVIDS) ▸ acquired violence immune
d. syndrome (AIDS), antibodies, acquired immune
d. syndrome, antibody
d. syndrome (AIDS) antibody test, acquired immune
d. syndrome (AIDS) associated transfusion, acquired immune
d. syndrome (AIDS) carrier, patient acquired immune
d. syndrome (AIDS) carrier, patient unknown acquired immune
d. syndrome, cellular immunity
d. syndrome (AIDS) crisis, acquired immune
d. syndrome (AIDS) dementia complex, acquired immune

d. syndrome (AIDS) ▸ emotional effects of acquired immune
d. syndrome (AIDS) epidemic, acquired immune
d. syndrome (AIDS), fetal acquired immune
d. syndrome (AIDS), heterosexual contact with male carriers of acquired immune
d. syndrome (AIDS) illness, acquired immune
d. syndrome (AIDS) infected child, acquired immune
d. syndrome (AIDS) mandatory testing, acquired immune
d. syndrome (AIDS) patient, acquired immune
d. syndrome (AIDS), patient at risk for acquired immune
d. syndrome (AIDS) primary pathogen, acquired immune
d. syndrome (AIDS) related complex (ARC), acquired immune
d. syndrome (AIDS) related dementia ▸ acquired immune
d. syndrome (AIDS) related macular degeneration ▸ acquired immune
d. syndrome (AIDS) related pneumonia, acquired immune
d. syndrome (AIDS) ▸ prevention acquired immune
d. syndrome (AIDS) residential treatment facility, acquired immune
d. syndrome, 17-hydroxylase
d. syndrome, severe combined immune
d. syndrome (AIDS) tainted transfusion ▸ acquired immune
d. syndrome (AIDS) testing, acquired immune
d. syndrome (AIDS) testing, mandatory acquired immune
d. syndrome (AIDS) transfusion-transmitted ▸ acquired immune
d. syndrome (AIDS) transmission ▸ acquired immune
d. syndrome (AIDS) treatment, acquired immune
d. syndrome (AIDS) treatment trials ▸ federal acquired immune

d. syndrome (AIDS) vaccine, anti-acquired immune
d. syndrome (AIDS) victim, acquired immune
d. syndrome (AIDS) virus infection, acquired immune
d. syndrome (AIDS) virus, mother infected with acquired immune
d. syndrome (AIDS) virus testing, acquired immune
d., thiamine
d., thyroid
d., vasopressor
d., vision
d. vitamin
d., vitamin B-12
d., volume

deficient
d. atrioventricular (AV) septation
d. children, hormone
d. circulation
d. cognitive thinking
d. diet, calcium
d. diet, pyridoxine
d. drainage of tears
d. dwarf, thyroid
d., lactose
d. oxygenation of blood
d. sexual development
d. sperm
d. transmission chemoreceptor

deficit(s)
d., acute neurologic
d., attention concentration
d., attentional
d., auditory processing
d., auditory verbal language
d., base
d., bathing self-care
d., cerebellar
d., chronic dopamine
d., cognitive
d. ▸ cranial nerve
d. disorder (ADD), attention
d. disorder (HDD) ▸ humor
d. disorder ▸ undifferentiated attention
d. disorder with hyperactivity ▸ attention
d. disorder without hyperactivity ▸ attention
d. ▸ diversional activity
d. ▸ dressing self-care
d., facial nerve
d. ▸ feeding self-care

deficit(s)—*continued*
  d., fluid
  d. ▸ fluid volume
  d., focal neurologic
  d., focal neurological
  d., functional tendon nerve
  d. ▸ grooming self-care
  d., hand
  d. ▸ hygiene self-care
  d. hyperactivity disorder (ADHD), attention
  d., hypernatremia and fluid
  d. in oxygen transport
  d., intellectual
  d. (JMD) ▸ juvenile memory
  d., knowledge
  d., known
  d., language
  d., left hemisphere
  d., memory
  d., mental
  d., motor
  d. ▸ motor and sensory
  d., motor planning
  d., nerve
  d., neurologic
  d., neurological
  d., neuromuscular
  d., neuropsychological
  d., nutrient
  d., nutritional
  d., oculomotor
  d., oxygen
  d., perceptual
  d., perfusion
  d., physical
  d., potential nutritional
  d., protracted perfusion
  d. psychology ▸ ego
  d., pulse
  d., right hemisphere
  d., self-care
  d., sensory
  d., severe neurological
  d., sleep
  d., spatial
  d., tactile
  d. ▸ toileting self-care
  d., visual
  d., visual field
  d. ▸ visual-motor
  d. ▸ visual-perceptual
definable illness index
defined
  d. behavioral normalcy ▸ socially

  d. borders, poorly
  d. density, ill-
  d., ill-
  d. margin, well-
  d., poorly
  d., well-
definite mass
definite tremor
definition of addiction ▸ cultural
definition ▸ shock wave
definitive
  d. callus
  d. diagnosis
  d. diagnosis by electron microscopy (EM)
  d. erythroblast
  d. external beam
  d. irradiation
  d. medical care
  d. surgery
  d. surgical care
  d. testing
  d. therapy
  d. treatment
deflated
  d. blood pressure cuff
  d. profile
  d. tourniquet
deflation, intra-aortic balloon
deflected beam
deflected, skin flaps
deflection(s)
  d., delta
  d., downward pen
  d. ▸ His bundle
  d., intrinsic
  d., intrinsicoid
  d., mechanical
  d., microvolts mean
  d., negative
  d. of nasal septum
  d. of septum
  d., peak-to-peak
  d., pen
  d., percent reduction of output pen
  d., positive
  d., Q-S
  d., sensory nerve
  d., simultaneous pen
  d., upward pen
  d., vesicouterine
defloration pyelitis
defocused beam
deformans
  d., arteritis

  d., arthrosis
  d., cephalhematoma
  d., dystonia musculorum
  d., endarteritis
  d. juvenilis, osteochondritis
  d., osteitis
  d., osteochondritis
  d., spondylitis
deformation, residual permanent
deformed
  d. ear
  d. fingernails
  d. gnarled joints
  d. infant ▸ patient delivered congenitally
  d. limb
deforming surgery
deformity(-ies)
  d., Akerlund's
  d., angular
  d., Arnold-Chiari
  d., bone
  d., bony
  d., boutonniere
  d., breech postural
  d., buttonhole
  d., cervical spine
  d., chest wall
  d., claw-like
  d., cloverleaf
  d., cloverleaf-type
  d., compression
  d., compression-type
  d., congenital
  d., congenital vertical talus foot
  d., constriction
  d., contraction
  d., contracture
  d., Dandy-Walker
  d., duodenal
  d., duodenal bulb
  d., epicanthus with telecanthus
  d. ▸ external nose
  d., extrinsic colon
  d., facial
  d., fingernail
  d. ▸ flexion contracture
  d., funnel
  d., fusiform
  d., gibbous
  d., gooseneck
  d., gross
  d., Haglund's
  d., hallux valgus
  d., hand

d., high arch
d. ▸ hockey stick
d., Ilfeld-Holder
d., intimal
d., inversion
d., limb
d., lobster-claw
d., longstanding arthritic
d., Madelung's
d., mandibular
d., maxillary
d., maxillary tuberosity
d., metatarsus primus varus
d., Michel
d., Mönckeberg
d., notch
d. of affected bones ▸ swelling
d. of duodenal bulb
d. of gastric outlet
d. of legs ▸ stiffening and
d. of nose, saddle
d. or edema
d., parachute
d., pectus
d., physical
d., pigeon breast
d., pressure atrophy
d. repair, congenital
d., residual
d. ▸ riding breech
d., saddle nose
d., scar
d., seal-fin
d., serosal
d. ▸ shepherd's crook
d., significant
d., silver-fork
d., skeletal
d., slight
d., spinal
d., Sprengel's
d., storkleg
d., swan-neck
d., swayback
d., syndactyly
d., telecanthus
d., ulnar drift
d., valgus
d., varus
d., Velpeau's
d., Volkmann's
defuse stress
degeneracy, stigma of
degenerated

d. blood
d., brain extremely
d. epithelial cell
d. protoplasm
d. tissue
d. tissue disease
degenerates ▸ brain tissue
degenerating
d. cells
d. decidual tissue
d. fibroid mass
d. yolk stalk
degeneration
d. ▸ acute heart muscle
d., adenomyoma with cystic
d. (ARMD) ▸ advanced age-related
macular
d. (AMD), age-related macular
d., amyloid
d., Armanni-Ehrlich's
d., arthritic
d. ▸ atrophic macular
d., Biber-Haab-Dimmer
d., bone
d., brain
d., cartilage
d., cell
d., cellular
d., cerebellar
d., cerebromacular
d., cobblestone
d., cochlear
d., congenital macular
d., corneal
d., corticostriatal-spinal
d., cusp
d., diffuse hepatocellular
d., disc
d. (ARMD) ▸ dry, age-related
macular
d. ▸ dry, macular
d., eighth nerve
d. ▸ exudative macular
d., fibrinoid
d., glassy
d., granulovacuolar
d., hepatolenticular
d., hippocampal
d., Holmes'
d., hyaline
d. in multiple sclerosis (MS) ▸
nerve
d. (ARMD) ▸ intermediate age-
related macular
d., joint

d. ▸ juvenile macular
d., Kozlowski's
d., lattice
d., macular
d., mental
d. ▸ midlife brain
d., Mönckeberg's
d. ▸ mucoid medial
d., myxomatous
d., nerve
d. ▸ nerve cell
d. of arteries
d. of brain, diffuse
d. of dopamine-producing nerve
cells
d. of heart, fatty
d. of heart valve ▸ myxomatous
d. of hippocampal neurons
d. of liver
d. of mitral valve ▸ myxomatous
d. of motor neuron (MN)
d. of muscle cells
d. of muscle cells ▸ patch quilt
d. of myocardium
d. of nerve cells
d. of nerve cells ▸ selective
d. of optic nerve
d. of Purkinje cells
d. of schizophrenia
d. of spinal cord
d. of valve, age-related
d. of vision
d. of walls of arteries
d., partial reaction of
d., paving stone
d., progressive lenticular
d. ▸ progressive mental
d., progressive retinal
d., proximal tubular
d., Quain's
d., reaction of
d., retinal
d., senile macular
d. ▸ skeletal muscle
d. ▸ slow cell
d. ▸ spinal cord disc
d. ▸ spinal disc
d., spinocerebellar
d., striatal nigral
d., subacute combined
d., Terrien's
d., trabecular
d., transsynaptic retrograde
d., vacuolar
d., vitelliform macular

degeneration—*continued*
  d., Vogt's
  d., wallerian
  d. (ARMD) ▸ wet age-related macular
  d. ▸ wet macular
  d., Zenker's
degenerative
  d. anterior spurring
  d. arthritic change
  d. arthritis
  d. arthritis of knee
  d. arthritis ▸ mixed rheumatoid
  d. arthritis, patellofemoral
  d. atrophy
  d. bone changes
  d. bone marrow disease
  d. brain disease
  d. brain disease ▸ incipient
  d. brain disorder
  d. cells
  d. change
  d. change, associated
  d. change, myxomatous
  d. change of hip, marked
  d. changes
  d. changes, marginal
  d. changes, minimal
  d. changes of spine
  d. changes, scattered
  d. chorea
  d. condition
  d. damage
  d. dementia of Alzheimer type, presenile onset, with delirium ▸ primary
  d. dementia of Alzheimer type, presenile onset, with delusions ▸ primary
  d. dementia of Alzheimer type, presenile onset, with depression ▸ primary
  d. dementia of Alzheimer type, senile onset, uncomplicated ▸ primary
  d. dementia of Alzheimer type, senile onset, with delirium ▸ primary
  d. dementia of Alzheimer type, senile onset, with delusions ▸ primary
  d. dementia of Alzheimer type, senile onset, with depression ▸ primary
  d. disc

  d. disc change
  d. disc disease
  d. disease
  d. disease ▸ chronic
  d. disease, chronic nervous
  d. disease of back
  d. disease of brain
  d. disease process, progressive
  d. disease, progressive
  d. disease, spinocerebellar
  d. disorder
  d. disorder of nervous system
  d. epidermoid cyst
  d. genetic disorder
  d. heart disease (DHD)
  d. idiopathic cardiomyopathy
  d. joint disease (DJD)
  d. lateral spurring
  d. liver disease
  d. lumbar spurring
  d. muscle disorder
  d. nature
  d. nephritis
  d. neurologic disease
  d. neuromuscular disease
  d. process
  d. spinal disease (DSD)
  d. spurring
  d. tear
  d. tic
  d. tic, generalized
  d. tic, localized
degenerativus, status
degloving injury
deglutition
  d. apnea
  d. mechanism
  d. murmur
  d. pneumonia
  d. syncope
Degos-Delort-Tricot syndrome
Degos' disease
degradation
  d., mental
  d., physical
  d. product, fibrin
  d. product ▸ fibrinogen
  d. product ▸ fibrinogen fibrin
degraded
  d. amyloid
  d. DNA (deoxyribonucleic acid) sequences
  d., patient feels
  d. photon
degranulation of eosinophils

degranulation ▸ goblet cell
degree(s)
  d. atrioventricular block ▸ atrial tachycardia with high
  d. (1st °) atrioventricular block with intraventricular conduction delay ▸ first
  d. (2nd °) atrioventricular (AV) block, second
  d. (3rd °) atrioventricular (AV) block, third
  d. AV (arteriovenous) block ▸ first
  d. burn ▸ first, second, third or fourth
  d. burn ▸ patient sustained first, second, third or fourth
  d. heart block ▸ first, second or third
  d., meridian
  d. of dexterity
  d. of drug dependence, estimating
  d. of electrode polarization ▸ varying
  d. of extension
  d. of flexion
  d. of freedom
  d. of involution ▸ moderate
  d. of mental illness, level and
  d. of motility
  d. of paralysis ▸ varying
  d. of physical functioning
  d. of risk, high
  d. of scaling
  d. of syncope ▸ varying
  d., prism
  d. sprain ▸ first, second or third
  d. teeth, zero
  d., trace
  d. uterine prolapse ▸ first, second or third
Dehio's test
dehiscence
  d., abdominal wall
  d., annular
  d., bronchial
  d., iris
  d. of cesarean section scar
  d. of uterus
  d., root
  d., sternal
  d., tertiary
  d., wound
dehydrase, aminolevulinic acid
dehydrase, serine
dehydrated [*rehydrated*]

d. and debilitated ▸ patient
d., emaciated and
d., patient rapidly
d., patient severely

dehydration
d., absolute
d. and exhaustion
d., cachexia and
d., clinical
d., confusion from
d., death by starvation and
d. ▸ diarrhea and
d. fever
d. ▸ fever-induced
d. from Addison's disease
d. from diarrhea
d. from gastroenteritis
d., hypernatremic
d. of wound
d., osmolar
d., severe
d., terminal
d., relative
d., voluntary
d., vomiting and

dehydrogenase
d., alcohol
d. deficiency anemia ▸ glucose-6-phosphate
d. deficiency, glucose-6-phosphate
d. (LDH) fraction, lactic
d., glucose phosphate
d., glyceraldehyde phosphate
d., glycerophosphate
d., hydroxybutyrate
d., hydroxybutyric
d., isocitric
d., lactate
d. (LDH), lactic
d., malic
d., phosphate
d., phosphogluconate
d., phosphoglyceraldehyde
d., pyruvate
d., serum hydroxybutyrate
d., serum isocitric
d., serum lactic
d., sorbitol
d., succinic
d. test, lactic
d. virus, lactic

deionized water
Deiters'
D. cells
D. nucleus

D. terminal frame

déjà
d. entendu
d. éprouvé
d. fait
d. pensé
d. raconté
d. vécu
d. voulu
d. vu
d. vu phenomena
d. vu ▸ sense of

Dejean's syndrome
dejected, patient
dejections, alvine
Dëjerine('s)
D. dystrophy, Landouzy-
D. -Roussy syndrome
D. sign
D. -Sottas atrophy
D. syndrome
D. syndrome ▸ Landouzy
D. -Thomas atrophy

Del Castillo syndrome ▸ Ahumada-
Delafield's fluid
Delafield's hematoxylin
delafondi, Aporina
delay(s)
d. aging of cells
d., atrioventricular (AV) conduction
d., conduction
d. disease progression
d. ▸ first degree (1st °) atrioventricular block with intraventricular conduction
d. ▸ hyperkinesis with development
d. in development
d. in development ▸ specific
d. in gastric emptying ▸ secondary
d. in responding to questions
d. interval, AV
d., intraventricular
d., intraventricular conduction
d. of gratification
d., phase
d., rate dependent conduction
d. ▸ severe articulation
d., specific
d., speech
d. syndrome, phase
d., time
d. time, echo
d. urinary incontinence ▸ minimize or

delayed
d. abstract conceptual memory
d. after depolarization (DAD)
d. after-effects
d. allergy
d. anastomosis
d. asthmatic reaction
d. auditory feedback
d. -blanch reaction
d. (LD) children ▸ language-
d. closing of leaflet
d. closure
d. closure of accidental wound
d. closure of operative wound
d. complication
d. concentration of dye
d. conduction
d. cystography
d. development of speech
d. echolalia
d. emptying
d. first pregnancy
d. flap
d. graft
d. growth, constitutional
d. healing
d. healing of fracture
d. hearing loss
d. heat
d. hemolytic reaction
d. hypersensitivity
d. hypersensitivity, tuberculin-
d. images of brain
d. intervention
d. lymph nodal stage radiograph ▸ 24-hour
d. menses
d. menstruation
d. muscle soreness
d. onset muscle soreness
d. operative cholangiography
d. or impaired speech
d. pregnancy
d. primary closure
d. reaction
d. reaction to radiation therapy
d. reaction to transfusion
d. recall
d. recall ▸ immediate and
d. recall ▸ therapeutic limitations of
d. recall ▸ therapeutic potential of
d. recognition ▸ immediate and
d. reflex
d. reformation of chamber
d. response

delayed—*continued*
  d. sensation
  d. sexual development
  d. shock
  d. sleep phase
  d. sleep phase syndrome (DSPS)
  d. speech
  d. stress syndrome
  d. study
  d. sutures
  d. transfer flap
  d. -type hypersensitivity reaction
  d. union
  d. union of fracture
  d. vagotomy
  d. word recall test
  d. wound closure
Delbet operation ▸ Albee-
DeLee-Hillis obstetric stethoscope
DeLee's maneuver
deletion, gene
deletion syndrome, 13q-
Delfen foam
deliberate
  d. actions ▸ patient makes
  d. behavior
  d. deception
  d. hyperventilation (HV)
delicate balance, brain's
delicate structure
Delille syndrome ▸ Rénon-
delimiting keratotomy
delinquent behavior
delinquent status offenders
delirio, delirium sine
delirious, patient
delirium
  d., active
  d., acute
  d., afebrile
  d., alcohol withdrawal
  d. ▸ amphetamine or similarly acting
    sympathomimetic
  d. and death
  d., anxiolytic withdrawal
  d. ▸ arteriosclerotic dementia with
  d., Bell's
  d., chronic alcoholic
  d., cocaine
  d., confusion from
  d., convulsions and death
  d. cordis
  d., drug-induced
  d., exhaustion
  d., febrile

  d. from alcohol
  d. from brain abscess
  d., hypnotic withdrawal
  d. induced by alcohol
  d., low
  d., macromaniacal
  d., macroptic
  d., melancholia with
  d., micromaniacal
  d. ▸ multi-infarct dementia, with
  d. mussitans
  d., muttering
  d. of fever
  d. ▸ patient in
  d. ▸ phencyclidine (PCP)
  d. ▸ primary degenerative dementia
    of Alzheimer type, presenile
    onset, with
  d. ▸ primary degenerative dementia
    of Alzheimer type, senile onset,
    with
  d., psychoactive substance
  d. schizophrenoides
  d., sedative withdrawal
  d., senile
  d. sine delirio
  d., specific febrile
  d., subacute
  d., toxic
  d., traumatic
  d. tremens (DTs)
  d. with high fever
delivered
  d. by cesarean (C-) section ▸
    patient
  d. by tumbling procedure ▸ lens
  d., cecum
  d. congenitally deformed infant ▸
    patient
  d. in air, roentgens
  d., infant
  d. intact, placenta
  d. intracapsularly, lens
  d., lens
  d. macerated fetus, patient
  d. manually, placenta
  d. meals, home
  d. normal infant, patient
  d., patient
  d., placenta
  d. prematurely, patient
  d. stillborn, patient
  d. to skin, roentgens
  d. triplets, patient
  d. twins, patient

delivery
  d., abdominal
  d., anesthesia
  d., antepartum death ▸ term
  d., breech
  d. by alternate physician ▸
    authorization for
  d. by alternate physician ▸ consent
    form to
  d., C (cesarean) section
  d., cesarean
  d., closed loop
  d., coach in
  d., complicated
  d., contrast medium
  d., difficult vaginal
  d., double footling
  d. (EDD/EDOD) ▸ estimated date of
  d., failed forceps
  d., forceps
  d. (FTND), full term normal
  d., high forceps
  d., induced
  d., instant
  d., intrapartum death ▸ term
  d., Leboyer method of
  d., low forceps
  d., midforceps
  d., midforceps operative
  d., natural
  d., neonatal death ▸ term
  d., normal
  d., normal full term
  d. (NSD) ▸ normal spontaneous
  d. (NSVD) ▸ normal spontaneous
    vaginal
  d. of placenta, manual
  d., orthogonal
  d., outlet forceps
  d. ▸ oxygen (O_2)
  d., partial breech
  d., patient given enema prior to
  d. ▸ pregnancy, labor and
  d., premature
  d., prep for
  d., prior to
  d., product of normal pregnancy and
  d., radiofrequency
  d. room
  d. room ▸ footprint taken of infant in
  d. room ▸ footprint taken of
    newborn in
  d. room ▸ infant footprinted in
  d. room ▸ mother thumbprinted in
  d. room ▸ newborn footprinted in

d., rotation operative
d., single footling
d., spontaneous
d., spontaneous vaginal
d., spontaneous vertex
d., surgical
d. system, air-
d. system, drug
d. system ▸ fiberoptic catheter
d. system ▸ mental health
d. system ▸ preprogrammed insulin
d. systems
d., term
d., term normal
d., threatened premature
d., traumatic vaginal
d., uncomplicated
d. ▸ vacuum cap
d., vacuum extraction operative
d., vacuum vaginal
d., vaginal
d., vaginal breech
d., vaginal vertex
d., vertex
d. wire
Delmar Avionics scanner
Delmege's sign
Delore's method
Delorme's operation
Delort-Tricot syndrome, Degos-
Delphian lymph nodes
delta
d. activity
d. activity, bursts of
d. activity ▸ frontal intermittent rhythmic
d. activity ▸ frontal irregular rhythmic
d. activity, generalized bisynchronous
d. activity ▸ monorhythmic sinusoidal
d. activity (OIRDA), occipital intermittent rhythmical
d. activity of low amplitude
d. -aminolevulinic acid
d. antigen
d. band
d. deflection
d. forms, discrete
d. frequencies
d. granules
d. OD$_{450}$
d. rays
d. rhythm

d. sleep
d. sleep stage
d., staphylolysin
d. wave
d. waves, EEG (electroencephalogram)
d. waves, focal
d. waves (SSSDW) ▸ significant sharp, spike or
delteili, Pentatrichomonas ardin
deltoid
d., left
d. ligament
d. muscle
d. palsy
d. region
d., right
deltopectoral groove
deltopectoral incision
DelToro's operation
delusion(s)
d. and fantasy
d. and paranoia ▸ hallucinations,
d. and tendency to self-abuse ▸ agitation
d., bizarre
d., Capgras
d. concerning appearance
d., confused
d., conspiratorial and persecutory
d., depressive
d., erotomanic
d., expansive
d. ▸ fantasy and
d., fixed
d., Fregoli
d. ▸ full scale
d., functional
d. hallucinations and
d., hypochondriacal
d., minor
d., near
d., nihilistic
d., nonbizarre
d. of grandeur
d. of guilt
d. of jealousy and persecution
d. of mind control
d. of negation
d. of persecution
d. of physical unattractiveness
d. of reference
d. of idea of reference
d. or hallucinations
d., paranoid

d., pathological
d., persecutory
d. ▸ primary degenerative dementia of Alzheimer type, presenile onset, with
d. ▸ primary degenerative dementia of Alzheimer type, senile onset, with
d. ▸ psychiatric treatment of
d., psychotic
d. ▸ schizophrenia with prominent
d., schizophrenic
d. ▸ schizophrenic hallucinations and
d., somatic
d. stupor
d., systematized
d., tactile
d., temporary
d., unsystematized
d., visual
d. with vague conspiracy
delusional
d. behavior
d. beliefs
d. disorder
d. disorder, amphetamine
d. disorder, cannabis
d. disorder, cocaine
d. disorder, hallucinogen
d. disorder, organic
d. disorder ▸ persecutory
d. disorder ▸ phencyclidine (PCP)
d. disorder, sympathomimetic
d. features ▸ arteriosclerotic dementia with
d. jealousy
d. mental illness
d. misidentification
d. mood disorder
d. ▸ multi-infarct dementia, with
d., patient
d. syndrome ▸ drug-induced organic
d. syndrome, organic
d. thinking
d. type of activity
demand(s)
d., abortion on-
d. for constant admiration
d. for constant attention
d., increasing
d. inhibited pacemaker, atrial
d. inhibited pacemaker ▸ ventricular
d. low

demand(s)—*continued*
- d. Medtronic pacemaker
- d., metabolic
- d. ▸ myocardial oxygen (O₂)
- d. pacemaker
- d. pacemaker, bifocal
- d. pacemaker, dual
- d. pacemaker, external
- d. pacemaker, Medtronic
- d. pulse generator
- d., situational
- d., therapeutic
- d. triggered pacemaker, atrial
- d. triggered pacemaker ▸ ventricular
- d. ventricular pacing system, malfunction of permanent
- d. ventricular pacing systems, permanent

demanding behavior
demanding drug abuser
demarariensis, Raillietina
demarariensis, Taenia
demarcated
- d. borders
- d. circumferential lesion, sharply
- d. margin, well-

demarcation(s)
- d., line of
- d., no line of
- d., shell-like
- d., sleep stage
- d., structural

Demarquay's sign
demeaned ▸ fear of being
demeaning attitude
demented patients
demented, severely
dementia
- d., accelerated
- d., advanced
- d., age-related
- d., alcohol-induced
- d., alcohol-related
- d., alcoholic
- d., Alzheimer's
- d. ▸ Alzheimer's type (SDAT) senile
- d. associated with alcoholism
- d., attachment behavior in
- d., Binswanger
- d., cognitive
- d. complex, AIDS (acquired immune deficiency syndrome)
- d. complex, Parkinson's
- d. ▸ confusion and

- d., debilitating
- d., dialysis
- d. disorder
- d., drug-induced
- d., epileptic
- d. from brain
- d. from depression
- d. from pernicious anemia
- d., frontotemporal
- d. ▸ full-blown
- d. ▸ incurable chronic
- d. induced by alcohol
- d., irreversible
- d. ▸ mild symptoms of
- d., mnemonic
- d., multi-infarct
- d. myoclonica
- d. of the Alzheimer type, presenile onset, uncomplicated ▸ primary degenerative
- d. of the Alzheimer type, presenile onset, with delirium ▸ primary degenerative
- d. of the Alzheimer type, presenile onset, with delusions ▸ primary degenerative
- d. of the Alzheimer type, presenile onset, with depression ▸ primary degenerative
- d. of the Alzheimer type, senile onset, with delirium ▸ primary degenerative
- d. of the Alzheimer type, senile onset, with delusions ▸ primary degenerative
- d. of the Alzheimer type, senile onset, with depression ▸ primary degenerative
- d., organic
- d., paralytic
- d. paralytica
- d. paranoides
- d., paretic
- d. praecox
- d., presenile
- d., primary
- d., progressive
- d. pugilistica
- d., secondary
- d., semantic
- d., senile
- d., severe
- d. stroke ▸ vascular
- d., tabetic
- d., terminal

- d., toxic
- d., uncomplicated ▸ arteriosclerotic
- d., uncomplicated ▸ multi-infarct
- d., vascular
- d. with delirium ▸ arteriosclerotic
- d., with delirium ▸ multi-infarct
- d., with delusions ▸ multi-infarct
- d. with delusional features ▸ arteriosclerotic
- d., with depression ▸ multi-infarct
- d. with depressive features ▸ arteriosclerotic

dementing illness
Demerol/Pethadol (Cube)
Demianoff's sign
demineralization of bone
demineralization, patchy
demineralized, bony structures
demise
- d., family present at time of
- d., fetal
- d., patient's

demi-vegetarian diet
demodectic mange
Demodex folliculorum
demographic
- d. factors
- d. information
- d. placement
- d. variables

demonstrable evidence
demonstrable excretion
demonstrated, previously
demonstrated, well
demonstration of safety techniques
demoralization ▸ isolation and
demoralized, patient
demoralized ▸ patient feels
Demours' membrane
demucosatio intestini
demyelinated nerve fibers
demyelinated nerve roots
demyelinating disease
demyelinating encephalopathy
demyelinization of nerve roots
den Bergh test, van
denaturation test, alkali
denatured homograft
dendriform keratitis
dendrites and axons
dendritic
- d. calculus
- d. cancer
- d. cell therapy
- d. cells

d. lesion
d. ulcer
d. ulcer of cornea
dendriticum, Dicrocoelium
dendroblastoma, oligo◇
dendrocyte, oligo◇
dendroglia, oligo◇
dendroglioma, oligo◇
denervated
    d. bladder
    d. heart at rest, evaluation of
    d. muscle atrophy
denervation
    d. procedure
    d., radiofrequency
    d. surgery
dengue
    d. fever
    d. hemorrhagic fever
    d. shock syndrome
    d. virus
denial
    d. and defensiveness, diminished
    d. and isolation
    d. ▸ defense mechanism of
    d., diminished
    d. ▸ ego defense of
    d. in fantasy
    d., ineffective
    d. ▸ level of
    d., neurotic
    d. of aloholism
    d. of death
    d. of disorder
    d. of lifesaving medical treatment
    d., overcoming
    d. response
    d., self-
denied, permission for autopsy
Dennett's diet
Dennie-Marfan syndrome
dens in dente
Dens view of cervical spine
dense
    d. adhesions
    d. breast tissue
    d. collagenous tissue
    d. cytoplasm, eosinophilic
    d., electron-
    d. fibrosis
    d. fibrous adhesions
    d. fibrous tissue
    d. hemiplegia
    d. lobar infiltrate
    d. metaphyseal bands

d. structure ▸ echo
d. structure of bone
d. thrill
Densitometer Scanning
densitometric ejection fraction
densitometric ejection fraction,
    cineangiography and
densitometry, Norland-Cameron
    photon
densitometry, video
density(-ies)
    d., abdominal soft tissue
    d., alveolar
    d. and strength of bone mass
    d. area, fat
    d., area of
    d. area ▸ water
    d., artefactual
    d., background
    d., bands of
    d. ▸ benign appearing nodular
    d. bile ▸ high
    d., bone
    d. (BMD), bone mineral
    d., calcific
    d., calcified
    d. calibration, film
    d. classification, stone
    d., conglomerate
    d., count
    d., decreased bone mineral
    d. ▸ diffuse increase in pancreatic
    d., echo
    d. -exposure relationship of film
    d., fluid
    d. function ▸ probability
    d., gradient
    d., homogeneous
    d., hydrogen
    d., idea
    d., ill-defined
    d., increased
    d., increased bone
    d., inherent
    d. in left base, fluid
    d. in right base, fluid
    d., ionization
    d., linear
    d., linear increased
    d. lipoprotein deficiency ▸ familial
       high
    d. lipoprotein (HDL), high
    d. lipoprotein ▸ intermediate
    d. lipoprotein (LDL), low
    d. lipoprotein (VLDL) ▸ very low

d. loss, bone
d. ▸ low bone
d., marked
d., measure bone
d. measurement
d. measurement, physical
d., metallic
d., minimal stringy
d., mottled
d., nodular
d., nutrient
d., optical
d., parenchymal
d. polyethylene (HDPE) ▸ high
d., proton
d., radiographic
d., radiolucent
d., radiopaque
d., relative vertebral
d., REM (rapid eye movement)
d. scan, bone
d. scan, bone-mineral
d. scan ▸ heel bone
d. ▸ scattered fibroglandular
d. screening, bone
d., small bone
d., spin
d. ▸ spinal bone
d. test, bone
d. test ▸ dual energy x-ray
    absorptiometry (DEXA) bone
d., total body
d. ▸ vague increased
d. (OD) values, ocular
d. (OD) values, optical
d., vapor
d., water
d., wedge-shape
dental [*mental*]
    d. alveoli
    d. alveolus, removal of
    d. amalgam
    d. anatomy
    d. anesthesia, electronic
    d. anxiety
    d. aplasia
    d. appliance
    d. arch
    d. arch ▸ residual
    d. assistant
    d. braces
    d. bridge
    d. calculus
    d. canaliculi
    d. care

dental—*continued*

d. care ▸ preventive
d. caries
d. caries, rampant
d. cavity
d. ceramics
d. chemistry
d. condition, teeth in good
d. crown
d. decay
d. diet, soft
d. disc
d. disease
d. disorder
d. elevator
d. emergency
d. enamel dysplasia syndrome
d. engine
d. erosion
d. excavation
d. exostosis
d. extraction
d. filling
d. flange
d. fluorosis
d. furrow
d. germ
d. granuloma
d. hygiene
d. hygiene, poor
d. hygienist
d. impaction
d. implant
d. implant technology
d. implantology
d. impression
d. inclusion
d. injury
d. ledge
d. molds, intraoral
d. nerve, inferior
d. operculum
d. patients ▸ stress reactions in
d. phobia
d. plaque
d. plate
d. plate, vulcanite
d. procedure
d. procedures ▸ surgical and
d. prosthesis
d. pulp
d. radiography ▸ comparative
d. repair, teeth in good
d. repair, teeth in poor
d. restoration

d. senescence
d. shelf
d. stone
d. tophus
d. veneer
dentale(s)
d. mandibulae, alveoli
d. maxillae, alveoli
d., osteoma
dentalis, Amoeba
dentalis, otalgia
dentary center
dentate
d. facisa
d. fissure
d. fracture
d. gyrus
d. ligament
d. line
d. nucleus
d. suture
dentati, hilus nuclei
dentatus, Chilodon
dentatus, gyrus
dente ▸ dens in
denticular hymen
denticulate ligament
denticulatum, ligamentum
denticulatum, Pentastoma
denticulatus, Porocephalus
dentin/dentine
d. bridge
d., globule
d., hypersensitive
dentinal sclerosis
dentinocemental junction
dentinoenamel junction
dentinogenesis imperfecta
dentis
d., cavitas
d., collum
d., corona
d., crusta petrosa
d., gubernaculum
d., pulpa
d., radix
d., substantia ossea
dentistry
d., child
d., cosmetic
d., pediatric
d., reconstructive
d., restorative
dentition
d. in poor repair

d., precocious
d., retarded
**dentitional odontectomies,
mandibular**
dentoalveolar
d. abscess
d. protrusion, bimaxillary
d. trauma
dentriticum, Dicrocoelium
Dents, Stim-U-
dentulous [*edentulous*]
dentulous, patient
denture(s)
d., acrylic partial
d. adhesive
d., bite-raising
d. ▸ burning mouth from
d., cast metal partial
d., choking from
d., complete
d., custom
d. edge
d., false
d., full
d., full mouth
d., full set of
d., ill-fitting
d. ▸ implant supported
d. impression, complete
d. impression, partial
d. ▸ improper fit of
d., leukoplakia from
d. ▸ lichen planus from
d., loose
d., lower
d., partial
d., partial lower
d., partial upper
d. ▸ patient wears
d., poorly fitting
d., porcelain
d., portrait
d. ▸ red gums from
d., relining of
d., removable
d., slipping
d. sores
d. splints
d., standard
d. supporting structures
d. ▸ taste abnormalities from
d. ▸ tongue pain from
d., upper
denudation
d., endothelial

d. of cornea
d. of distal esophagus ▸ extensive
d. of normal mucosa
denuded
d. bladder mucosa
d., epithelial surface
d. jawbone
Denuse's operation
Denver
D. classification
D. peritoneal venous shunt
D. pleuroperitoneal shunt
D. screening
deodorant artifact
deodorant, room
deorsum vergens, strabismus
deorsumduction of left eye
deorsumduction of right eye
deoxygenated blood
deoxyribonucleic acid (DNA)
d. acid (DNA)
d. acid (DNA) maker
d. acid (DNA) molecules
d. acid (DNA) polymerase activity
d. acid (DNA) polymerase ▸
ribonucleic acid (RNA)
dependent
d. acid (DNA) ▸ recombinant
d. acid (DNA) sequences,
degraded
d. acid (DNA) sequencing
d. acid (DNA) strand
d. acid (DNA) switch
d. acid (DNA) synthesis
d. acid (DNA) virus
Depage-Janeway gastrostomy
DePalma hip prosthesis
Department (department)
D., Chemotherapy
D., Emergency
D., Employee Health
d., hospital emergency
D., Housekeeping
D., Medicophysics
d., musculoskeletal
D. of Mental Health
D. (OPD) ▸ Outpatient
D., Pathology
D., Physical Therapy (PT)
D., Radiology
D., Respiratory Therapy
departmental procedure
dependence
d., alcohol
d., amphetamine

d. ▸ amphetamine or similarly acting
sympathomimetic
d. ▸ barbiturate similarly acting
d., behavioral treatment for drug
d., cannabis
d., cocaine
d., cross-
d. ▸ diagnosis of cocaine
d. disorder, chemical
d. disorder ▸ substance
d., drug
d., estimating degree of drug
d., field
d., hallucinogen
d., hostile
d. ▸ hypnotic similarly acting
d., increased emotional
d., inhalant
d. ▸ late-onset crack
d. ▸ morphine tolerance and
d., nicotine
d. on drugs, physical
d. on external controls
d. on hallucinogens
d. on inhalants
d. on nicotine gum ▸ physical
d. on opioids
d. on phencyclidines
d. on stimulants
d., opioid
d., opioid type
d., phencyclidine (PCP)
d., physical
d., physical and psychological
d., physical drug
d., physiological
d., polysubstance
d. -producing substances
d., psychic
d., psychoactive substance
d., psychological
d., psychological drug
d., psychostimulant
d., relationship
d. ▸ sedative, hypnotic, or anxiolytic
d. ▸ sedative similarly acting
d., steroid
d., substance
d. syndrome, alcohol
d., tobacco
d. treatment, cocaine
d. treatment ▸ marijuana
d., use
dependency (Dependency)
d. ▸ acceptance of chemical

d., alcohol
d. benefits, chemical
d., Big H (heroin)
d., chemical
D. Clinic ▸ Outpatient Chemical
d., cocaine
d. concept
d. ▸ cultural aspects of chemical
d., drug
d., free of chemical
d., heroin (big H)
d., hostile
d., laxative
d., level of
d. line
d., LSD (lysergic acid diethylamide)
d. needs
d., physical
d., polydrug
d. professionals, chemical
d. program, alcohol
d. program, alcoholism/chemical
d. program, chemical
d., psychological
d., selfish
d. skills, chemical
d., stages of chemical
d., substance
d. treatment, chemical
d., ventilator
d. with Crohn's disease ▸ drug
D., Women and Chemical
dependent
d. aberrancy, acceleration
d. aberrancy ▸ tachycardia-
d. activation ▸ length
d., actively chemically
d., alcohol
d. angina ▸ rate-
d. antigen ▸ thymus
d. arrhythmia ▸ pause-
d. asthma ▸ steroid-
d. asthmatic ▸ steroid-
d. block ▸ voltage-
d. calcium channel ▸ voltage-
d. cells, thymus
d. clients, drug-
d. cocaine user ▸ opioid-
d. conduction delay, rate
d. counseling, individual
d. cyanosis
d. diabetes mellitus (NIDDM),
noninsulin
d. diabetes mellitus (IDDM), Type I
insulin

dependent—*continued*
- d. diabetes mellitus (NIDDM), Type II noninsulin
- d. DNA (deoxyribonucleic acid) polymerase ▸ ribonucleic acid (RNA)
- d., dose-
- d. drug user
- d. edema
- d. enzyme, cancer-
- d., frequency
- d. illness, drug-
- d. individual, totally
- d., insulin-
- d. lividity, mild
- d., methamphetamine
- d. movement of cupula ▸ gravity-
- d. ▸ multiple drug
- d., narcotic
- d. neoplasia, estrogen
- d., passive-
- d., patient
- d. patient, alcohol
- d. patient, cocaine
- d. patient, drug-
- d. patient, medically
- d. patient ▸ opioid-
- d., patient oxygen (O_2)
- d. patient ▸ pregnant opiate-
- d. patient ▸ psychoactive substance-
- d., patient totally
- d. peripheral edema
- d. person
- d. person, alcoholic drug
- d. person, chemically
- d. personality
- d. personality disorder
- d. personality, passive-
- d. portion
- d. position, head
- d. quadriplegia, ventilator
- d. quadriplegic, cervical vent-
- d. quadriplegic ▸ vent
- d. rubor
- d. strain, thymidine
- d. swelling
- d., thymus-
- d., time
- d. vaginal dryness, estrogen-
- d., ventilator
- d. women, drug-

deperitonealized surface
depersonalization
- d. disorder
- d. ▸ feelings of
- d. neurosis
- d. or derealization
- d. syndrome

dephosphorylation of proteins
depigmentation of skin ▸ patchy
depilatories, chemical
depilatories, wax
depleted
- d., adrenal lipid
- d. blood ▸ oxygen (O_2)
- d. energy
- d. type ▸ Hodgkin's disease of diffuse histiocytic lymphocyte
- d., white cells

depletion
- d., brain amine
- d., calcium
- d., glycogen
- d., lipid
- d., lymphocyte
- d., lymphoid
- d., mild colloid
- d., mineral
- d., neurotransmitter
- d. of cortex ▸ steroid
- d. of follicles ▸ lymphoid
- d. of lymph nodes ▸ lymphoid
- d. of potassium and magnesium
- d., ovarian ascorbic acid
- d., plasma
- d., potassium
- d., severe lymphocytic
- d., steroid
- d. syndrome, salt
- d., thymic
- d., thymocyte
- d., volume

deployment, stent
depolarization
- d. abnormality ▸ ventricular
- d. contractions (APDC) ▸ atrial premature
- d. contractions (VPDC) ▸ ventricular premature
- d., diastolic
- d. ▸ His bundle
- d., myocardial
- d., rapid
- d., rapid dyssynchronous
- d., transient

depolarizing electrode
deposit(s)
- d., abdominal fat
- d., abnormal plaque
- d., amyloid
- d., atherosclerotic
- d., body fat
- d., bony
- d., brain
- d., calcareous
- d., calcific
- d., calcium
- d., carbon
- d., cholesterol
- d., endochondral bone
- d., extensive tumor
- d., fatty
- d., fatty cholesterol
- d., foreign material
- d., hemosiderin
- d. in brains ▸ waxy
- d. in optic nerves ▸ colloid
- d., iron
- d., metastatic
- d., mineral
- d. of calcium
- d. of calcium ▸ valvular
- d. of pigment
- d. on heart valves, calcium
- d. on lens, pigmentary
- d., plaque
- d., uric salt
- d., waxy

deposition
- d., electro◇
- d., fibrin
- d., liver
- d., marked hyaline
- d. ▸ mitochondrial calcium
- d., power
- d. ▸ subpleural reticulated carbon
- d., urate

depot-medroxyprogesterone acetate (DMPA)
depot reaction
depraved indifference
deprecating ▸ patient self-
deprecation ▸ displays self-
depreciation, self-
depress cellular energy production
depressant(s)
- d. (714's)
- d. (sopor)
- d. (THC)
- d. abuse, pattern of
- d. abuse, physical effects of
- d., abuse potential of
- d. abuse, prevalence of
- d. abusers, assessing needs of

d., acute intoxication with
d. affect of drug
d., blood level of
d., cardiac
d., detoxification from
d. drugs
d. effect ▸ EEG
(electroencephalogram)
nonspecific
d. factor, myocardial
d., flashback reactions with
d., mode of administration with
d., organic brain syndrome with
d., panic reactions with
d., patient OD (overdosed) with
d., potential tolerance to
d., psychoactive doses of
d., psychoactive properties of
d., psychological effects of
d., psychotic reactions with
d. substance ▸ myocardial
d., toxicity of
d., treatment of acute drug reactions to
d., urine level of
d., withdrawal from

depressed
d. adolescent
d. adult situation
d. and agitated
d. and apathetic ▸ patient withdrawn,
d. and anxious
d. ankle jerk (AJ)
d. appetite
d., biologically
d. ▸ bipolar affective disorder,
d. ▸ bipolar disorder,
d. blood count
d. breathing and heartbeat
d. cancer patient
d. chest wall
d. child
d. children
d., clinically
d. diastolic pressure
d. ejection fraction
d. feeling
d. fracture
d. function
d. heart attack patient
d. heart attack survivor
d. ▸ hostile and
d., in full remission ▸ bipolar disorder,

d., in partial remission ▸ bipolar disorder,
d. individual
d. level of consciousness
d., mild ▸ bipolar disorder,
d., moderate ▸ bipolar disorder,
d. mood
d. mood ▸ adjustment disorder with
d. newborn, resuscitation of
d. or irritable mood
d., patient
d. patient, immune
d. realism
d. reflex activity
d. reflexes
d., severe, without psychotic features ▸ bipolar disorder,
d., severely
d. skull fracture
d. sternum
d. systolic pressure
d. T waves
d., trigone
d., unspecified ▸ bipolar disorder
d. vision
d., with psychotic features ▸ bipolar disorder

depression (Depression)
d., abnormal
d., abuse-related
d., agitated
d., aldosterone
d., anaclitic
d., analytical psychotherapy for
d., anatomical
d. and alcoholism
d. and anxiety
d. and anxiety in elderly
d. and appetite
d. and despair
d. and fatigue ▸ withdrawal, isolation,
d. and impotence ▸ fatigue,
d. and lethargy, unexplained
d. and mania
d., and personality changes ▸ irritability,
d., and shyness ▸ anorexia
d. ▸ anxiety and
d., anxiety, and frustration
d., anxiety, and panic
d., anxiety, and suicide
d., anxiety associated with
d. ▸ anxiety, guilt or
d. -anxiety treatment

d. ▸ appetite loss from
d., atrial
d., autonomous
d., aversion
D. /Awareness, Recognition and Treatment (D/ART)
d., bone marrow
d., borderline personality and
d. ▸ burning mouth from
d., cardiac
d., cataract
d., central nervous system (CNS)
d., central respiratory
d., chemical
d., childhood
d., chronic
d., chronic recurring
d., clinical
d., cocaine-induced
d., cognitive therapy of
d., cognitive treatment for
d., concavity and
d., congenital chondrosternal
d. (CSD) ▸ cortical spreading
d., crushing anxiety and
d., dementia from
d. ▸ develop symptoms of clinical
d. ▸ downhill ST segment
d. ▸ downsloping ST segment
d., drowsiness from
d., drug-induced postanesthetic
d., drug-induced postanesthetic respiratory
d., elation or
d., emotional
d., endogenous
d., episode of severe
d., exacerbate
d., extreme
d., fatigue and
d., fatigue from
d., feelings of
d., frequent
d. from alcohol
d. from hypothyroidism
d. from premenstrual syndrome
d., functional
d., groove
d., holiday
d. ▸ hostility and
d., impact of
d., in full remission ▸ major
d., in partial remission ▸ major
d. in preadolescent children
d., incapacitating

depression—*continued*
d., increased
d. inhalation anesthetic ‣ respiratory
d. ‣ insatiable appetite from
d., insomnia and fatigue
d., insomnia from
d., intermittent periods of
d., involutional
d., irreversible
d. ‣ irritability and
d., junctional
d., late bone marrow
d. ‣ late life
d., levels of
d., lightening
d., linear
d., lingering
d. ‣ long-term
d., macular
d., major
d. management skills
d., manic
d., marrow
d., mask
d., masked
d., maternal
d., melancholic
d. ‣ memory loss from
d., menopausal
d., mental
d., midlife
d., mild
d., mild ‣ major
d. ‣ mild-to-moderate levels of
d., moderate
d. ‣ moderate chronic
d., moderate ‣ major
d., mood swings and
d. ‣ multi-infarct dementia, with
d., myocardial
d., narcotic-induced respiratory
d., nasal bone
d., nervous
d., nervousness from
d., neurotic
d., nonviolent
d. of jugular venous pulse
d. of vital brain centers
d. or mental anguish
d., otic
d., pacchionian
d., pathological
d., patient in postnatal
d., postactivation

d., postdormital
d., postdrive
d., postictal
d., postmenopausal
d., postpartum
d., poststimulation respiratory
d., poststroke
d. ‣ P-Q segment
d., precordial
d. ‣ primary degenerative dementia of Alzheimer type, presenile onset, with delirium
d. ‣ primary degenerative dementia of Alzheimer type, presenile onset, with delusions
d. ‣ primary degenerative dementia of Alzheimer type, presenile onset, with depression
d. ‣ primary degenerative dementia of Alzheimer type, senile onset, uncomplicated
d. ‣ primary degenerative dementia of Alzheimer type, senile onset, with delirium
d. ‣ primary degenerative dementia of Alzheimer type, senile onset, with delusions
d. ‣ primary degenerative dementia of Alzheimer type, senile onset, with depression
d., profound
d., psychological overlay and
d., psychotic
d., radial
D. Rating Scale (VDRS) ‣ Verdun
d. reaction, anxiety
d., reactive
d. ‣ reactive type of
d. ‣ reciprocal ST
d., recurrent
d., recurrent, in full remission ‣ major
d., recurrent ‣ major
d., recurrent, mild ‣ major
d., recurrent, moderate ‣ major
d., recurrent, severe, without psychotic features ‣ major
d., recurrent, unspecified ‣ major
d., recurrent, with psychotic features ‣ major
d., refractory
d. ‣ relapse in
d., remission of
d., respiratory
d., retarded

d. scale
D. Scale, Geriatric
D. Scale, Zung
d. screening
d., seasonal
d., sense of
d., serious
d., severe
d. ‣ severe, long-term
d., severe, without psychotic features ‣ major
d., single episode in full remission ‣ major
d., single episode, in partial remission ‣ major
d., single episode ‣ major
d., single episode, mild ‣ major
d., single episode, moderate ‣ major
d., single episode, severe without psychotic features ‣ major
d., single episode, unspecified ‣ major
d., single episode, with psychotic features ‣ major
d., situational
d., ST
d. ‣ ST segment
d., sternal
d., success
d. ‣ suffering from
d. ‣ sufficient symptoms of
d., suicidal
d., superimposed
d., supratrochlear
d. ‣ symptoms of
d., systolic
d., textbook
d., traumataic
d., treatable
d. ‣ treatment-resistant
d. triggered by physical illness
d. triggered by stress
d., unipolar
d., ventricular
d. ‣ weight loss from
d. white blood count ‣ transient
d., winter
d. with psychosis, unipolar
d., with psychotic features ‣ major
d., x

depressive
d. affect
d. attitudes, paranoid
d. delusion

d. disease, bipolar manic
d. disorder
d. disorder, atypical
d. disorder (MDD), major
d. disorder, manic-
d. disorder, recurrent episode ▸ major
d. disorder, single episode ▸ major
d. disorder, unipolar
d. drive, strong
d. effect
d. episode
d. episode, major
d. features ▸ arteriosclerotic dementia
d. feelings
d. hallucination
d. illness
d. illness ▸ full-blown manic
d. illness, manic
d. illness ▸ severe
d. insanity, manic-
d. living syndrome (DLS)
d. neurosis
d. patient, manic-
d. personality disorder ▸ chronic
d. personality, manic-
d. phase
d. psychosis
d. psychosis, manic-
d. reaction
d. reaction, brief
d. reaction, localized
d. reaction, mild
d. reaction, nonspecific
d. reaction, prolonged
d. reaction, psychotic
d. reaction, severe
d. symptoms
d. syndrome
d. type psychosis

depressor
d. muscle of angle of mouth
d. muscle of lower lip
d. muscle of septum of nose
d. muscle, superciliary
d. nerve
d. reflex
d. reflex, cardiac
d. septi nasi muscle
d. substance
d., tongue

deprivation
d. ▸ chronic sleep

d., control of heart rate during oxygen
d., dream
d., emotional
d. in critical organs ▸ oxygen
d., maternal
d. neurosis
d. of maternal touch, temporary
d. ▸ oxygen (O_2)
d., paternal
d., sensory
d. ▸ severe sleep
d., sibling
d., sleep
d. syndrome, sensory
d. therapy, sleep-

deprived
d., chronically sleep
d., emotionally
d. leg muscles ▸ oxygen- (O_2)
d. muscles ▸ nerve
d. patient ▸ sleep
d., sleep
d. state, sensory-

deprogramming ▸ unlearning the training and

depth
d. compensation
d. dose
d. dose curves, comparative
d. dose differential
d. dose distribution
d. dose in scanning
d. dose of electron beam therapy, central axis
d. dose, percentage
d. electrode
d. electrode, bipolar
d. electrode, unipolar
d. electroencephalogram (EEG)
d. electroencephalogram (EEG), stereotactic
d. electroencephalography
d. jump
d., maintenance
d. of burn
d. of respiration
d. of the brain
d. of _____ ▸ sounded to a
d. of _____ ▸ uterine cavity sounded to
d. of wound probed
d. perception
d. perception check
d. perception, distorted

d. perception ▸ permanent absence of
d. perspective, in-
d. psychology
d. ▸ radiography invasion
d., respiratory
d. ▸ severe disorder of psychotic
d. study, in-
d., wrinkle

deranged
d., patient
d., patient mentally
d. thinking

derangement
d., electrolyte
d., gastrointestinal (GI)
d. hemodynamic
d., Hey's internal
d., human dynamic
d. in thought process
d., internal
d. of joint, internal
d. of knee, internal
d. of personality
d. of vasomotor nerves
d., pigment
d., temporary mental

derealization, depersonalization or derealization ▸ feelings of
derby, Salmonella
Dercum's disease
derivation(s)
d., bipolar
d., electroencephalogram (EEG)
d., interhemispheric
d., linked bipolar
d., multiple bipolar
d., referential
d., unipolar

Derivative (derivative)(s)
d. circulation
d., ergotamine
d., hematoporphyrin
D. (PPD) intermediate ▸ Purified Protein
d. method ▸ Raff Glantz
d., penicillin
D. (PPD) ▸ Purified Protein
D. (PPD) skin testing ▸ Purified Protein

derived
d. albumin
d. cells ▸ tumor-
d. energy, anaerobic-
d. exercises ▸ Yoga-

derived—*continued*
- d. free radicals ▸ oxygen- (O₂)
- d. from entitlement ▸ problem
- d. growth factor (PDGF) ▸ platelet-
- d. hemodynamic data
- d. hyperpolarizing factor ▸ endothelium-
- d. immunosuppression ▸ tumor-
- d. relaxing factor ▸ endothelium-
- d. tumor ▸ mesenchymal-

dermabrasion and dermaplaning
dermabrasion procedure
Dermacentor
- D. andersoni
- D. occidentalis
- D. variabilis

dermagraphic ▸ macrotherapy
dermal
- d. bone
- d. epidermal junction
- d. graft
- d. hypoplasia syndrome, focal
- d. lymphatic involvement
- d. malignancy
- d. melanocytoma
- d. micropigmentation
- d. myiasis
- d. or oral herpes
- d. papilla ▸ capillary loop in
- d. pedicle
- d. sensation
- d. sheath
- d. sinus, congenital
- d. subcutaneous junction
- d. tissue

Dermalon cuticular suture
Dermalon suture
Dermanyssus avium et gallinae
dermaplaning ▸ dermabrasion and
dermatitidis, Blastomyces
dermatitidis, Mycoderma
dermatitis
- d., actinic reticuloid
- d., allergic contact
- d., atopic
- d., cat mite
- d., contact
- d., dhobie mark
- d., diaper
- d., drug eruption
- d., dyshidrotic
- d., eczematoid infectious
- d., eruptive
- d. excoriativa infantum
- d. exfoliativa infantum

- d., exfoliative
- d., factitial
- d. ▸ flaking skin from
- d., fungal
- d. gangrenosa infantum
- d., gonococcal
- d., head
- d. herpetiformis
- d., hot tub
- d. infectiosa
- d., itching from
- d., Jacquet's
- d., livedoid
- d. medicamentosa
- d. ▸ mycosis fungoides
- d., nickel
- d., nummular eczematous
- d., oozing from
- d. ▸ peeling skin from
- d., perioral
- d. ▸ red ears from
- d. ▸ rubber contact
- d., scalp
- d. ▸ scalp itching from
- d., seborrheic
- d. ▸ skin cracking from
- d. ▸ skin crusting from
- d. ▸ skin hardening from
- d., stasis
- d., treatment of localized
- d. venenata
- d. verrucosa
- d., verrucous
- d., weeping
- d. ▸ work-related

Dermatobia hominis
dermatofibrosarcoma protuberans
dermatologic
- d. complications of drug abuse
- d. emergency
- d. manifestations

dermatological disorder
dermatology, clinical
dermatome level ▸ sensory
dermatomyositis
- d. in hands
- d. in wrist
- d. ▸ lesion in
- d. related to cancer

dermatopathic lymphadenopathy
Dermatophilus penetrans
dermatophyte
- d. infection
- d. infections of hair
- d. infections of nails

- d. infections of scalp
- d. infections of skin

dermatophytosis, area of
dermatophytosis, weeping
dermatorrhagia parasitica
dermatosis
- d., chronic
- d., genital
- d. papulosa nigra
- d., precancerous
- d. ▸ transient acantholytic
- d., widespread

dermic graft
dermis, papillary
dermis, reticular
dermoepidermal junction
dermoid
- d. cancer
- d. cyst
- d. cyst of ovary
- d. tumor
- d. versus sebaceous cyst

dermopathy, diabetic
Dermoplast spray
dermotropic viruses
derogatory hallucinations
derotation osteotomy
DES (diethylstilbestrol)
de-sac
- d., conjunctival cul-
- d., cul-
- d., Douglas' cul-
- d., dural cul-
- d. fluid, cul-
- d., free fluid in cul-
- d. of vagina ▸ posterior cul-

desaturation, arterial
Desault's fracture
Desault's sign
descaling, teeth
Descartes' law
Descemet's membrane
descended, diaphragms
descendens, aorta
descending
- d. aorta
- d. (LAD) artery, left anterior
- d. artery ▸ posterior
- d., ascending and
- d. brain stem
- d. cervical nerve
- d. colon
- d. colon ▸ diverticula of
- d. colon ▸ diverticulosis of transverse and

d. colon ▸ large intestinal
d. coronary artery ▸ anterior
d. (LAD) ▸ left anterior
d. (LAD) lumen, left anterior
d. mesocolon
d. motor tract
d. necrotizing mediastinitis
d. pathway
d. ramus
d. thoracic aorta
d. thoracic aortic aneurysm
d. thoracic aortofemoral-femoral
  bypass
d. tracts
d. urography
descends into vagina ▸ bladder
descensus uteri
descensus, uterine
descent
d. of jugular venous pulse ▸ y
d. ▸ rapid y
d. trough ▸ X-,
d. trough ▸ Y-,
d. wave ▸ y
description
d., autopsy external
d., external
d., gross
d. of treatment
descriptive
d. anatomy
d. embryology
d. psychiatry
desensitization
d. and relaxation, group
d. and reprocessing (EMDR) ▸ eye
  movement
d. block
d., brutalization and
d. ▸ eye movement
d. for anxiety
d., gradual
d., headache activity and
d. injection
d. of pervasive anxiety ▸
  systematic
d. of phobic reactions ▸ systematic
d. procedure
d. procedure, systematic
d., relaxation in systematic
d., self-administered systematic
d., systemic
d. techniques
d. therapy
desensitizing movement exercises

desert fever
desert rheumatism
desiccated, lesion
desiccated thyroid
**desiccation [*defecation,*
  desquamation]**
desiccation, electro◇
design(s)
d., biological
d., experimental
d. in combined modality therapy,
  protocol
d. in combined modality therapy,
  research
d. for immunology, research
d., gestalt
d., medical study
d. (CAD) prosthesis, computerized
  assisted
d., Silastic penile prosthesis
designated
d. assessing agency
d. care-giver
d. donor
d. recipient
d. treatment team ▸ attending
designed foot orthotic ▸ custom
designer
d. diagnosis
d. disease
d. drugs
desirable weight
desire(s)
d. disorder ▸ hypoactive sexual
d. for personal gain
d. from anxiety ▸ loss of sexual
d. ▸ increased sexual
d. ▸ loss of sexual
d. psychosexual dysfunction,
  inhibited sexual
d., repressed
d. revenge
d., sexual
d. to attend religious services ▸
  loss of
Desmarres' law
Desmodus rotundus
desmoid reaction
desmoplastic formation
desmoplastic reaction
**desmosomes with bundles of
  tonofilaments**
Desnos' disease
Desnos' pneumonia

despair
d. ▸ feelings of
d. ▸ level of
d. ▸ periods of anger, panic or
d., sudden
desperate, patient
desperation, emotional
despondency, feelings of
despondent, patient
desquamated
d. alveolitis
d. cells
d. epithelium
d. fibrosing alveolitis
d. renal epithelial cells
desquamating debris
**desquamation [*desiccation,*
  defecation]**
d. of atypical alveolar cells
d., palmar
d., peribronchial
d., periungual
d., plantar
d., superficial
desquamativa otitis
desquamative
d. gingivitis
d. interstitial pneumonia
d. interstitial pneumonitis (DIP)
d. nephritis
d. pneumonia
d. pneumonia, Buhl's
desquamativum, erythroderma
dessication, curettage and
dessication, mucus
destabilizing impact of trauma
destroy
d. brain tumor
d. healthy tissue
d. surrounding tissue
d. tissue
destroyed
d. brain tissue
d. nasal tissue
d. tissue, layer
destroying
d. agent, cancer
d. antibiotics chemically
d. cancer cells
d. disorder ▸ brain
d. enzymes, antibiotic
d. enzymes, receptor
d. myeloma cells
d. plaques in brain ▸ neuron

destruction
  d., area of bony
  d., bone
  d., bony
  d. by radiation, cell
  d., cartilage
  d., cord
  d., cortex
  d., cortical
  d., drug-induced cell
  d. ▸ fever, swelling and tissue
  d., joint
  d., localized bone
  d., means of self-
  d. of brain cells
  d. of intraepithelial neoplasia, laser
  d. of nerve cells
  d. of nerves ▸ viral
  d. of red blood cells (RBC)
  d. of red blood cells (RBC) ▸ accelerated
  d. of rib, neoplastic
  d. of transformation zone, prophylactic
  d. ▸ plasmatic vascular
  d., platelet
  d., recurrent lung
  d., rib
  d., scarring lung
  d., self-
  d., thermal
  d., tissue
  d., tumor
destructive
  d. acts, self-
  d. addiction
  d. aggression
  d. alcohol abuse ▸ self-
  d. behavior
  d. behavior, self-
  d. change, bony
  d. child
  d. compulsion
  d. -compulsive disease
  d. disease, self-
  d. illness
  d. injury
  d., patient is self-
  d. ▸ patient self-
  d. pattern
  d. procedure
  d. process
  d. process, bone
  d. process, immune
  d. seizures

  d. self-centeredness
  d. sexual behavior
  d. thought pattern
destructiveness ▸ lack of self-
destruens, chorioadenoma
destruens suppurativa ▸
  hidrosadenitis
desultory labor
desultory pain
desynchronization, circadian
desynchronization, EEG
  (electroencephalogram)
desynchronized sleep
detached
  d. loose body
  d. manner
  d. retina
  d. retina, photocoagulation repair of
  d. statoconia ▸ traumatically
detachment
  d., annular
  d., feeling of
  d. ▸ floaters, flashes and retinal
  d. ▸ focal retinal
  d. ▸ impending retinal
  d. medial meniscus
  d. of choroid
  d. of ligament
  d. of medial meniscus
  d. (PVD) ▸ posterior vitreous
  d., primary retinal
  d. repair, retinal
  d., retinal
  d., rhegmatogenous
  d., rhegmatogenous retinal
  d. ▸ scar tissue
  d. ▸ traction retinal
  d., vitreous
detail(s)
  d. analysis ▸ visual
  d. discrimination, essential
  d. obscure
  d. ▸ patient fussy about
  d. ▸ preoccupied with
  d., rib
  d. ▸ speech lacking in
detailed
  d. image on screen
  d. medical history (MH)
  d. rituals and routines
detect time
detectability, theory of signal
detection (Detection)
  d., ambulatory nuclear
  d. and management ▸ early

  d., automated border
  d., automated edge
  d., automatic boundary
  D. Awareness Program, Breast Cancer
  d., beta
  d. bias
  d., cancer
  d., cancer prevention and early
  d., cardiac shunt
  d., cervical cancer
  d., coincidence
  d., computerized edge
  d. device ▸ esophageal
  d., early
  d., early cancer
  d. ▸ echocardiographic automated border
  d., edge
  d. error artifact, data spike
  d. ▸ esophageal intubation
  d., fibrillation
  d., gallstone
  d. level, visual
  d. ▸ manual edge
  d. method, edge
  d. methods, cancer
  d. of bone spurs
  d. of breast cancer ▸ early
  d. of cancer
  d. of cancer ▸ early
  d. of colorectal cancer ▸ early
  d. of gamma rays
  d. of motion
  d., polyp
  d., prevention and screening ▸ cancer
  d., prevention and treatment ▸ cancer
  d. program, early
  d., prostate cancer
  d. rate, tachycardia
  d., shunt
  d. ▸ single photon
  d. system ▸ echocardiographic automated boundary
  d. test, heat
  d. tests, early
  d. threshold, median
  d. through mammography, early
  d., ultrasound gallstone
detector
  d., ambulatory nuclear
  d., dielectric track
  d., Doppler flow

d., flame ionization
d., semiconductor
d., tissue-equivalent
d., ultrasound blood flow
detention, emergency
detergens (LCD), liquor carbonis
detergent workers' lung
deteriorate, heart muscle
deteriorate with aging ‣ color vision
deteriorated
d., baby
d., blood gases
d., condition
d. disc
d., patient rapidly
d., severely
d., patient steadily
d., patient's condition
d., patient's endurance
deteriorating
d. arterial blood gases (ABG)
d. blood gases
d. condition
d. effect of medication
d., emotional
d. heart failure
d. kidney infiltrate
d. neurological disorder
d., patient
d., patient rapidly
d. quality of work
d. sense of balance
deterioration
d., alcohol
d., bone
d., continued
d., downhill
d. due to radiation ‣ spinal
d., ethical
d., generalized personality
d., gradual
d. ‣ gradual mental
d. in renal function
d. in sensation
d. in speech
d. in vision
d., intellectual
d., irreversible motor
d., mental
d., nerve
d., neurologic
d. of blood vessel
d. of bone tissue
d. of brain function ‣ general
d. ‣ of coordination, gait and speech

d. of heart muscle
d. of macula
d. of nerve fibers
d. of retina, macular
d. of retina ‣ progressive
d., organic
d., organic CNS (central nervous system)
d., personality
d., physical
d. ‣ prevention of physical
d., progressive
d., progressive clinical
d. ‣ progressive intellectual
d. ‣ progressive cognitive
d., rapid
d. ‣ rapid mental
d., regressive
d., severe mental
determinant(s)
d., antibiotic resistance
d., antigenic
d., genetic
d., germ-cell
d., hidden
d. of pain, interacting
d. of relapse ‣ potential intrapersonal
d., resistance
d., sex
determinate site, antigenic
determination(s) (Determination) [termination]
D. Act (PSDA) ‣ Patient Self-
d., antibody titer
d., blood glucose
d., chemical
d., colorimetric
d. (FAD), fetal activity
d., field uniformity
d., gamma A immunoglobulin (IgA)
d., gamma D immunoglobulin (IgD)
d., gamma E immunoglobulin (IgE)
d., gamma G immunoglobulin (IgC)
d., gamma M immunoglobulin (IgM)
d., interim glucose
d., laboratory
d., medical self-
d. ‣ metabolic parameter
d. of brain death, criteria for
d. of eligibility
d. of medical necessity
d., oxygen content
d., Pali
d., pH

d., sweat chloride
determine source of infection
determined
d. by expectation ‣ pain
d. by level of anxiety ‣ pain
d. by suggestion ‣ pain
d. ‣ disease genetically
d. ejection fraction ‣ light pen-
d., etiology radiographically not
determinism, psychic
detox (detoxification) ‣ rapid
detoxification (detox)
d., acute
d. admission
d., adolescent
d., alcohol
d., ambulatory opiate
d. and brief treatment
d. and sobriety
d. before surgery
d. center
d., chemical
d. clinic, methadone
d., clinical interaction and
d., drug
d., freestanding
d. from depressants
d. from multiple drugs
d. from opioids
d. from pentazocine
d. from propoxyphene
d. from stimulants
d., heroin
d., inpatient
d., managing
d., medical
d., medication-assisted
d., metabolic
d., methadone use in
d. of addict
d. of heroin addict
d., outpatient
d. phase
d., prior
d. profile
d. programs
d. (detox) ‣ rapid
d. regimens
d., rehydration and
d. services ‣ supervision of
d., short-term
d., social setting
d. therapy
d. treatment, long-term
d., unassisted

detoxification (detox)—*continued*
   d. unit, acute
detoxified opiate addict
detrimental cholesterol
detrimental impact of fatigue
detrusor
   d. dyskinesia
   d. function
   d. hypercontractility
   d. hyperreflexia
   d. pattern
   d. sphincter dyssynergia
   d. urinae muscle
deuterium plasma
Deutschländer's disease
deux, folie +133
devastating
   d. disease
   d., emotionally
   d. illness
   d., physically
   d. side-effects
devastation, emotional
devastation, senile cortical
develop(s)
   d. behavioral patterns
   d. coping skills
   d. isolation techniques
   d. mouth ulcers
   d. new blood supply and
     matures
   d. self-confidence
   d. symptoms of clinical
     depression
developed
   d. flap
   d. (w/d), patient well
   d. spike, poorly
developing
   d. alcoholism ▸ risk of
   d. brain disease ▸ slowly
   d. cervical cancer ▸ high risk of
   d. fetus
   d. lungs
   d. pigment gallstones ▸ prone to
   d. treatment plan
development
   d., abnormal
   d., adolescent
   d., altered
   d., altered growth and
   d., anal
   d., arrested
   d., arrested mental
   d. -at-birth index (DBI)

d., biosocial theory of
d., birth and early
d., blood vessel
d., brain
d., cardiovascular
d., cerebrum
d., child
d., clinical program
d., cognitive
d., congenital
d., defective
d., deficient sexual
d., delay in
d., delayed sexual
d. disorder, mixed
d., drug
d., embryo
d., embryonic
d., emotional
d. ▸ epigenetic factor in
   cardiovascular
d. ▸ failure of breast
d., fetal
d. ▸ fetal growth and
d. ▸ fetal kidney
d. ▸ gene regulation of
   cardiovascular
d., hindgut embryonic
d., human
d. ▸ impaired sexual
d., infant
d., intellectual
d., language
d. ▸ latency age
d., level of personality
d., marked retardation of mental
   and physical
d., mental
d., mosaic
d., motivational
d., motor
d. ▸ mouth embryonic
d., muscular
d., normal child
d., normal curve of
d., normal growth and
d., normal human
d., normal resting
   electroencephalogram (EEG)
   pattern
d., normal sexual
d. of autonomic nervous system ▸
   incomplete
d. of cataract
d. of children, behavioral

d. of children, cognitive
d. of children ▸ emotional
d. of criteria
d. of discharge plan
d. of diverticulosis
d. of electroencephalogram (EEG)
   waves ▸ unequal
d. of gene therapy
d. of gut
d. of inflammation
d. of periodontitis
d. of radiculitis
d. of scar tissue ▸ abnormal
d. of speech, delayed
d. of speech ▸ neuromuscular
d. of valve, abnormal
d., organs with defective
d., postnatal
d., prenatal
d., prepsychotic level of
d., psychosexual
d., psychosocial
d., radiculitis
d., rectum
d. ▸ regression and psychosexual
d., regulative
d., skill
d., slow
d. ▸ specific delays in
d. ▸ social and emotional
d. ▸ social skills
d., socioemotional
d., speech
d., transitional
d., tumor
developmental (Developmental)
   d. abnormality
   d. analysis
   d. anatomy
   d. anomalies
   d. arithmetic disorder
   d. arrest
   d. articulation disorder
   d. assessment
   d. catch-up
   d. coordination disorder
   d. course
   d. defect
   d. delay ▸ hyperkinesis with
   d. disability
   d. disorder
   d. disorder ▸ complex
   d. disorder, pervasive
   d. disorder, specific
   d. distortion

d. dyslexia
d. dysphasia
d. dysplasia of hip (DDH)
d. examination, Dubowitz
d. expressive language disorder
d. expressive writing disorder
d. history
d. history, formal
d. homeostasis
d. idiocy
d. language disorder
d. model
d. pediatrician
d. period
d. psychology
d. quotient
d. reading disorder
d. receptive language disorder
D. Scale, Tanner
d. sequence posture
d. speech disorder

developmentally
d. challenged
d. disabled
d. disabled child

Deventer's diameter
Deventer's pelvis
deviant
d., color vision
d., sexual
d. sexual behavior
d. social behavior

deviate sexual intercourse ▸ involuntary
deviated anteriorly, esophagus
deviated nasal septum
deviation(s)
d. (ALAD) ▸ abnormal left axis
d. (ARAD), abnormal right axis
d., average
d., axis
d., complement
d., conjugate
d. disorders
d. from norm
d., immune
d. (LAD) ▸ left axis
d., manifest
d., medial
d., minimum
d., nasoseptal
d., normal axis
d. of the mean (SDM) ▸ standard
d. of trachea
d., partial ulnar

d., primary
d., radial
d., right axis
d., secondary
d., septal
d., sexual
d., skew
d., squint
d., standard
d., strabismic
d., ST-T
d. (SSD), sum of square
d., tongue
d. to the left
d. to the right
d., tracheal
d., ulnar
d. upper trachea

device(s) [*devise*]
d., (AACD) abdominal aortic counterpulsation
d. ▸ Abio-Cor
d., ablative
d., (AVAD), acute ventricular assist
d., adaptive
d., A-mode-echo-tracking (E-T)
d., arrhythmia control
d., barrier
d., bathroom safety
d., bioabsorbable closure
d., birth control
d. (IUD), bow intrauterine
d., calibrated
d., cardiac
d. (CARD), cardiac automatic resuscitative
d., clamshell
d., closed loop
d. (IUD), coil intrauterine
d., conducting
d., contraceptive
d., corrective
d., Cournand cardiac
d., diagnostic imaging (DI)
d. ▸ directional atherectomy
d. (IUD) dislodged, intrauterine
d. ▸ displacement sensing
d., Doppler sound
d., double umbrella
d., ectopic intrauterine
d., electrical stimulation
d., electromagnetic
d., electronic automated

d., electronic monitoring
d., electronic summation
d., emergency alert
d. ▸ esophageal detection
d., exterior pelvic
d. ▸ extraction atherectomy
d. for drug abuse ▸ cutaneous signs as a screening
d. for drug abuse ▸ diagnostic tests as a screening
d. for drug abuse, medical history as screening
d. for drug abuse, patient behavior as a screening
d. for drug abuse, patient interview as a screening
d. for drug abuse, patient questionnaire as a screening
d. for drug abuse, physical examination as a screening
d. for drug abuse, psychological history as a screening
d. for drug abuse, social history as a screening
d. for drug abuse, symptoms as a screening
D. for the Deaf (TDD), Telecommunications
d., heating
d., imagery
d., imaging
d., implantable
d. ▸ implantable pacing
d., implanted
d. ▸ implanted diagnostic
d. ▸ indwelling prosthetic medical
d. infection ▸ intravascular
d. infection ▸ prosthetic
d., input
d. (IUD) inserted, Copper 7 intrauterine
d., intracaval
d., intramedullary fixation
d., intraoral
d. (IUD) ▸ intrauterine
d., intrauterine contraceptive
d. ▸ left ventricular assist
d., Leksell's stereotaxic
d. (IUD), Lippes loop intrauterine
d. ▸ liquid crystal
d., locking
d., manipulation of prosthetic
d., measuring
d., mechanical
d., medical

device(s)—*continued*
    d. ▸ Medtronic defibrillator implant support
    d. ▸ Medtronic-Hall
    d., metallic fixation
    d., mnemonic
    d., monitoring
    d. ▸ motor-assisted
    d. on level surfaces, assistive
    d., orthotic
    d., output
    d., patient behavior as a screening
    d., patient interview as a screening
    d., patient questionnaire as a screening
    d. (VAD), permanently implanted ventricular assist
    d. (ALD) ▸ personal assistive listening
    d., plaque removal
    d., positive pressure infusion
    d., pressure infusion
    d., pressure monitoring
    D. ▸ Prima Total Occlusion
    d., problem-solving
    d., programmable
    d., prosthetic
    d., psychological history as a screening
    d. ▸ pulsatile assist
    d. ▸ pulse oximetry
    d. ▸ radiant heat
    d. ▸ Rashkind cardiac
    d. ▸ rate adaptive
    d. -related bacteremia ▸ venous access
    d. -related infection
    d., respiratory therapy
    d. ▸ right ventricular (RV) assist
    d. ▸ rotary atherectomy
    d. ▸ rotational atherectomy
    d. (SIBID), self-inhibiting behavioral injury
    d., self-testing
    d., spot film
    d. (IUD) spotting, intrauterine
    d., stereotactic
    d., storage
    d. (IUD) string, intrauterine
    d. ▸ subcutaneous tunneling
    d. ▸ surgically implanted
    d., tedding
    d. tether, implanted
    d., therapeutic
    d. therapy

    d. ▸ tiered therapy antiarrhythmic
    d. to restrain hernia ▸ supportive
    d., transvenous
    d., ventilation
    d., walking assistance
    d. ▸ wavefront scanning
Devic's disease
Devic's syndrome
devil(s)('s) (Devils)
    D. (barbiturates), Blue
    D. (barbiturates), Red
    d. grip
    d. pinch bruises
devise [*device*]
devitalization, pulpal
devitalized tissue
devotion to work ▸ excessive
DeVries procedure
Dew method, Byrd
Dew sign
DeWecker operation
Dewees' sign
DEXA (dual energy x-ray absorptiometry)
DEXA (dual energy x-ray absorptiometry) bone density test
dexamethasone suppression test (DST)
Dexies (amphetamines)
dexter
    d., bronchus principalis
    d., cor triatriatum
    d. cordis, ventriculus
dexterity
    d., cognitive
    d., degree of
    d., fine hand
    d., impaired
    d., loss of
    d., manual
    d., mental
    d., verbal
Dexon suture
dextra, auris
dextran
    d. blue
    d. complex ▸ iron
    d., low molecular weight
dextrocardia
    d., corrected
    d., false
    d., isolated
    d., secondary
    d. with situs inversus
dextroduction of left eye

dextroduction of right eye
dextromethorphan hydrobromide
dextroposition of heart
dextropositioned aorta
dextrorotation of uterus
dextrorotatory scoliosis
dextroscoliotic curvature
dextrose
    d. in water (D/W)
    d. in water (D-5-W/D_5W) ▸ 5%
    d. infusion
    d. -nitrogen (D-N) ratio
    d. solution mixture
    d. test
Dextrostix test
dextroversion of heart
dextrum, atrium
dextrum, cor
D-5-W/D_5W (5% dextrose in water)
DHD (degenerative heart disease)
d'Herelle phenomenon ▸ Twort-
DHL (diffuse histiocytic lymphoma)
dhobie itch
dhobie mark dermatitis
DI (diabetes insipidus)
DI (diagnostic imaging)
Di Guglielmo syndrome
Di Guglielmo's disease
diabetes
    d. ▸ absent menstrual period from
    d., acute onset adult
    d., adult onset
    d., advanced
    d. alternans
    d., arteriosclerosis and
    d., autoimmune ▸ mature onset
    d. ▸ blurred vision from
    d., brittle
    d., bronze
    d. ▸ burning mouth from
    d., chemical
    d. ▸ circulatory problem from
    d., controlled
    d., drug-induced
    d., drugs, oral
    d. ▸ foot problems from
    d., gangrene from
    d. ▸ genetically prone to
    d., gestational
    d., gouty
    d., impotence from
    d., incontinence from
    d., infertility from
    d. ▸ insatiable appetite from
    d. insipidus (DI)

d. insipidus, nephrogenic
d., insulin dependent
d., insulin resistant
d., itching from
d., juvenile
d., juvenile-onset
d., Lancereaux's
d., latent
d. ▸ loss of sexual drive from
d. management
d. mellitus (DM)
d. mellitus (DM) ▸ adult-onset
d. mellitus (DM) ▸ borderline
d. mellitus (DM) ▸ controlled
d. mellitus (GDM) ▸ gestational
d. mellitus (IDDM), insulin
   dependent
d. mellitus (DM) ▸ juvenile onset
d. mellitus (DM), longstanding
d. mellitus (NIDM), noninsulin
d. mellitus (NIDDM), noninsulin
   dependent
d. mellitus ▸ nonketotic
d. mellitus (DM) secondary to
   endocrine disease
d. mellitus (DM) secondary to
   pancreatic disease
d. mellitus (IDDM), Type I insulin
   dependent
d. mellitus (NIDDM), Type II
   noninsulin dependent
d. neuritis
d., newly diagnosed
d., overt
d., pancreatic
d. ▸ penile problems from
d. ▸ prevent, stop or reverse
   complication of
d. -related complication
d. -related death
d. self-management
d., subclinical
d. ▸ sweet smelling urine from
d. therapy
d., thirst from
d., tinnitus from
d., toxic
d., treatment of
d., uncontrolled
d., undiagnosed
d., urination from
d. ▸ vaginal itching from
d. ▸ weight loss from
d. well controlled
d. ▸ white patches from

d. with chills
diabetic [*diuretic, dietetic*]
d. acidosis
d. amaurosis
d. amyotrophy
d., borderline
d., brittle
d. cataract
d. coma
d., comatose
d. complications
d. control with diet
d. crisis
d. dermopathy
d. diet
d. dyslipidemia
d. ear
d. emergency
d. eye care
d. eye disease
d. father
d. foot care
d. foot infection
d. gangrene
d. gangrene of lung
d. gastroparesis
d., gestational
d. glomerulosclerosis
d. heart ▸ vascular disease in
d. history, familial
d. hyperosmolar syndrome
d. hypertension
d. hypertriglyceridemia
d. iritis
d. ketoacidosis (DKA)
d., labile
d. laser treatment
d. macular edema
d. melanosis of cornea
d. microangiopathy
d. microvascular disease
d. mother
d. mother (IDM), infant of
d. nephropathy
d. nerve disease
d. nerve pain
d. neuritis
d. neuropathic pain, chronic
d. neuropathy
d. neuropathy improvement
d. neuropathy ▸ painful
d., nonobese
d., patient
d., patient brittle
d., patient juvenile

d., patient latent
d. peripheral neuropathy
d. phthisis
d. polar cataract
d. pregnancy
d. products
d. -related diseases
d. retinal disease
d. retinitis
d. retinopathy
d. retinopathy, advanced
   proliferative
d. retinopathy, early
d. retinopathy (FFDR) ▸ full florid
d. retinopathy, laser therapy of
d. retinopathy (NPDR) ▸
   nonproliferative
d. retinopathy ▸ proliferative
d. shock
d. stomach
d. sugar
d. tabes
d. ulcers
d. urine
d. vulvitis
d. women ▸ premenopausal
d. xanthoma
diabetica, balanitis
diabeticorum
d., bullosis
d., necrobiosis lipoidica
d., xanthoma
diable, bruit
diabolical itch
diacetate, ethynodiol
diacetate, germine
diacetic acid
diacetyl monoxide
diaclastic amputation
diacondylar fracture
diacylglycerol lipase
diadochokinesia rate
Diagnex Blue
Diagnex Blue test
diagnosable disease
diagnosable seizure ▸ clinically
diagnose disease prenatally
**diagnose, patient tends to self-
diagnosed**
d. and treated ▸ patient
d. brain death
d. diabetes, newly
d., dually
d. infectious disease
d. (NYD) ▸ not yet

diagnosis(-es) (DX)
- d., additional
- d., admission
- d., admitting
- d. ▸ adrenoleukodystrophy (ALD)
- d. ▸ aid in assessment and
- d., alternative
- d. and evaluation
- D. and Evaluation (D and E) Staffing
- d. and implementation ▸ prevention,
- d. and localization
- d. and therapeutic outcome
- d. and treatment, initial
- d. and treatment of alcoholism
- d., augenblick
- d., autopsy anatomic
- d. based on biopsy
- d. bedside
- d., behavioral
- d., biological
- d., brain death
- d. by electron microscopy (EM) ▸ definitive
- d., cancer
- d., clinical
- d., comprehensive
- d., controversial
- d., cytohistologic
- d., cytologic
- d., definitive
- d., designer
- d., differential
- d., direct
- d., discharge
- d., disease
- d., drug abuse
- d., dual
- d., electro◇
- d., endoscopic
- d., entrance
- d., equivocal
- d., etiologic
- d., etiological
- d. ▸ eye screening and
- d. ▸ false-negative flu
- d., final
- d., final pathological
- d. groups, dual
- d., histologic
- d., immediate
- d. in acute drug intoxication, differential

- d. in organic brain syndrome, differential
- d. in panic reactions, differential
- d., intercurrent
- d., laboratory
- d., malignant
- d., medical
- d., microscopic
- d., missed
- d., nursing
- d. ▸ nursing assessment and
- d. of acute drug reactions
- d. of alcohol withdrawal symptoms, differential
- d. of birth defects, prenatal
- d. of cocaine dependence
- d. of esophageal atresia ▸ prenatal
- d. of etiologic agent ▸ presumptive
- d. of exclusion
- d. of proctitis
- d. of psychotic reactions, differential
- d. of sarcopenia
- d. of tachycardia, differential
- d. or condition deferred on Axis I
- d. or condition deferred on Axis II
- d., pathological
- d. patient, dual
- d., perioperative
- d., physical
- d., polysomnographic
- d., positive
- d., possible
- d., postmortem
- d., preliminary
- d., prenatal
- d., preoperative
- d., presenting
- d., presumptive
- d., presumptive etiologic
- d., prevention and treatment
- d., primary
- d. ▸ primary presenting psychiatric
- d. -prognosis
- d., provisional
- d., psychiatric
- d., radiological
- D. Related Groups (DRG)
- d., retrospective
- d., roentgen
- d., serum
- d., specific etiologic
- d., stroke
- d., tentative
- d., tentative etiologic

- d., terminal
- d., tissue
- d., transfer
- d., treatment and recovery
- d. undetermined
- d. unequivocal
- d. verified
- d., viral
- d. with overdosing differential
- d., working

diagnostic(s)
- d. abnormality
- d. agents
- d. aid
- d. and prognostic indicators
- d. angiography
- d. arthroscopy
- d. assessment
- d. assessment services, Alzheimer's
- d. capability
- d., cardiac
- d. classification
- d. code
- d., computer-assisted
- d. concept
- d. consultation
- d. coronary angiography
- d. criteria
- d. curettage
- d. D and C (dilatation and curettage)
- d. data
- d. device ▸ implanted
- d. differentiation
- d. entities
- d. equipment
- d. error
- d. evaluation
- d. evaluation, invasive
- d. evaluation, x-ray
- d. hearing evaluation
- d. imaging (DI)
- d. imaging (DI) device
- d. interview ▸ psychiatric
- d. lamp
- d. laparoscopy
- d. laparotomy
- d. laser ▸ helium cadmium
- d. media, instillation of
- d. method
- d. paracentesis
- d. pneumopedtoneum
- d. pneumothorax
- d. procedure

d. procedure and treatment
d. procedure ► immunohematologic
d. procedure, invasive
d. procedure ► noninvasive
d. procedures well ► patient
   tolerated
d. products
d. program
d. program, electrophysiology
d. purposes
d. radiography
d. radiology
d. -related groups (DRG)
d. -related group (DRG) payments
d. scanning
d. screening test
d. sensitivity
d. separation of transudate and
   exudate
d. services
d. services ► cancer-related
D., Social and Addiction History
   form
d. spinal tap
d. staffing
d. staging, clinical
d. studies
d. studies, x-ray
d. study
d. study, cardiovascular
d. summary
d. surgery
d. synthesis
d. technique
d. technique, screening and
d. test
d. test ► noninvasive
d. test, prenatal
d. testing
d. tests and procedures
d. tests as a screening device for
   drug abuse
d. tests, cytological
d. tests in drug abuse
d. therapy
d. tool
d. training
d. treatment
d. ultrasound
d. value
d. workup
d. workup and staging
d., workup not
d. x-rays
diagonal artery

diagonal conjugate diameter
diagram
   d., block
   d., cutaway
   d., Dieuaide
   d., ladder
   d. ► pressure volume
dial calibration, E-
dialect modification
dialectical behavior therapy
Dialister pneumosintes
dialysis (Dialysis)
   d., Abderhalden's
   d., ambulatory peritoneal
   d., ancillary
   d., blood filtered by
   d. catheter, light subclavian vein
   d. catheter, subclavian
   d., chronic
   d., chronic maintenance
   d. (CAPD), continuous ambulatory
      peritoneal
   d. (CCPD), continuous cyclical
      peritoneal
   d., course of
   d., cross
   d. dementia
   d. diet
   d., electro◇
   d. encephalopathy
   d. encephalopathy, progressive
   d. equilibrium syndrome
   d. fluid
   d., gastro◇
   d., hemo◇
   d., home
   d., in-center
   d., kidney
   d., long-term
   d., lymph
   d. machine
   d., maintenance
   d., medications during
   d. patient
   d. patient, ambulatory peritoneal
   d. periods
   d., peritoneal
   d. procedure
   d., renal
   d. retinae
   d., short-term
   d. shunt
   d. shunt, LeVeen
   d. solution, normal
   d. solution, peritoneal

d., STAT
d. therapy
d. time
d. treatment
d. uneventful, course of
d. unit, hemo-
d. unit, portable
D. Unit, Renal
d. waste
dialyzed, patient
dialyzer
   d., coil
   d., Dow hollow fiber
   d., electro◇
   d., hollow fiber
   d., parallel plate
Diamanus montanus
diameter(s)
   d., anatomic conjugate
   d., anterior chest
   d., anteroposterior (AP)
   d., anteroposterior thoracic
   d., anterotransverse
   d., Baudelocque's
   d., biischial
   d. (BPD), biparietal
   d., bisacromial
   d., bisiliac
   d., bispinous
   d., bitemporal
   d., buccolingual
   d., cephalocaudad
   d., cervicobregmatic
   d., chest
   d., coccygeopubic
   d., conjugate
   d., cranial
   d., craniometric
   d., Deventer's
   d., diagonal conjugate
   d., disc
   d., external conjugate
   d., extracanthic
   d., fetal cranial
   d., fiber
   d., frontomental
   d., fronto-occipital
   d., inferior longitudinal
   d., inside
   d., intercanthic
   d., intercristal
   d., internal
   d., internal conjugate
   d., intertuberal
   d. ► left ventricular (LV)

diameter(s)—*continued*
- d. ▸ left ventricular (LV) internal diastolic
- d., Lohlein's
- d., Mantoux
- d. (MCD) ▸ mean cell
- d. (MCD) ▸ mean corpuscular
- d., mento-occipital
- d., mentoparietal
- d. ▸ minimal luminal
- d. obliqua pelvis
- d., obstetric conjugate
- d., occipitofrontal
- d., occipitomental
- d. of chest AP (anteroposterior)
- d. of heart ▸ transverse
- d. of pelvic inlet ▸ conjugate
- d. of pelvis, oblique
- d. of pelvic outlet, transverse
- d. of pelvis, transverse
- d. of pupil
- d., outside
- d., papilla
- d., parietal
- d., pelvic
- d., posterotransverse
- d., pubosacral
- d., pubotuberous
- d., sacropubic
- d., sagittal
- d., stretched
- d., suboccipitobregmatic
- d., temporal
- d. -thickness ratio (MDTR) ▸ mean
- d. ▸ total end-diastolic
- d. ▸ total end-systolic
- d., transthoracic
- d. transversa pelvis
- d., transverse
- d., true conjugate
- d., uterus normal in anteroposterior (AP)
- d., vertebromammary
- d., vertical

diamine oxidase
diamond (Diamond)
- D. -Blackfan syndrome
- D. -Blackfan syndrome ▸ Josephs-
- d. disc
- d. ejection murmur
- d. inlay bone graft
- d. inlay graft
- d. -shaped murmur
- d. -shaped tracing

Diana complex

diaper dermatitis
diaper rash
diaphanography examination
diaphanography procedure
diaphanoscopy procedure
diaphany, electro◇
diaphoresis, prostration and
diaphoretic
- d., patient
- d., skin
- d., skin pale and

diaphragm
- d., accessory
- d., adjustable
- d., Akerlund
- d., All-Flex
- d., Bucky
- d., Bucky-Potter
- d., coil spring
- d., contraceptive
- d. contracts
- d., crus of
- d., defective
- d., descended
- d. disorder
- d., dome of
- d., elevation of
- d., esophageal canal of
- d., eventration of leaf of
- d., excursion of
- d., flattened
- d., free air in the
- d., inflammation of
- d., involuntary spasm of
- d., iris
- d., leaf of
- d., leaves of
- d., left
- d., level of
- d., metastases to
- d. of mouth
- d. of pelvis
- d. of sella turcica
- d., optic
- d., oral
- d., pelvic
- d. pessary
- d. phenomenon
- d., pillars of
- d., polyarcuate
- d., Potter-Bucky
- d., Ramses'
- d., right
- d., rupture of
- d., secondary

- d. sign ▸ Litten
- d., tenting of
- d. transducer
- d., urogenital
- d., vaginal

diaphragma sellae
diaphragmatic
- d. adhesions, pleural
- d. and chest breathing
- d. artery
- d. breathing
- d. breathing retraining, computerized
- d. chorea
- d. elevation
- d. eventration
- d. excursions
- d. flutter
- d. ganglia
- d. hernia
- d. hernia, congenital
- d. hernia (CDH) ▸ fetal congenital
- d. hernioplasty
- d. infarction
- d. injury
- d. muscle
- d. myocardial infarction
- d. nerve
- d. pacing
- d. pericardium
- d. phenomenon
- d. plaques
- d. pleura
- d. pleurisy
- d. pulmonary infarct
- d. respiration
- d. respiration, controlled
- d. shadow
- d. silhouette
- d. stimulator
- d. surface
- d. surface of left lung
- d. surface of right lung
- d. tic

diaphyseal/diaphysial
- d. aclasia
- d. aclasis
- d. dysplasia
- d. -epiphyseal fusion

diaphysis(-es) [*diathesis*]
diaphysitis, tuberculous
diaporica, Rickettsia
diarrhea
- d., abdominal pain and fever
- d., acute infantile

d., acute watery
d. and breastfeeding
d. and dehydration
d. and disorientation
d. ▸ anorectal problems from
d., antibiotic-associated
d., antibiotic-induced
d., antibiotic-related
d., anxiety with
d. ▸ bloating and
d., bloody
d., cachetic
d., childhood
d., choleraic
d., chronic
d., chronic bacillary
d., chronic secretory
d. chylosa
d., Cochin-China
d., congenital chloride
d., constipation with
d., cramps and
d. ▸ cramps, gas, bloating and/or
d., critical
d., dehydration from
d., Dientameba
d., dysenteric
d., E. coli
d., enteral
d., familial chloride
d., fermental
d., fermentative
d., flagellate
d., frequent nausea and
d. from antibiotic
d. from anxiety
d. from bran
d. from Crohn's disease
d. from diverticulosis
d. from food poisoning
d. from gastroenteritis
d. from intestinal obstruction
d. from lactose intolerance
d. from laxatives
d. from toxic shock syndrome
d. from ulcerative colitis
d., functional
d., gastrogenic
d., Giardia parasite
d., hill
d., infantile
d., infectious
d., inflammatory
d., intermittent
d., intractable

d., irritative
d. ▸ lethargy, jaundice
d., lienteric
d., mechanical
d., morning
d., mucous
d. ▸ nausea, vomiting and
d., neonatal
d., noninflammatory
d., nosocomial
d. of newborn, epidemic
d., osmotic
d. ▸ pain in abdomen with
d. pancreatica
d. ▸ pancreatogenous fatty
d., paradoxical
d., parenteral
d., patient has
d., persistent
d., putrefaction
d., secretory
d., serous
d., severe
d., stercoral
d., summer
d., toxigenic
d., traveler's
d., tropical
d., tubercular
d., uncontrollable
d., viral
d., virus
d., volume and frequency of
d., vomiting and
d., watery
d. ▸ watery and bloody
d. ▸ watery, profuse
d., weakness and nausea
d., white
d. with abdominal pain and swelling
d. with menstrual cramps
d. with vomiting
diarrheal disease
diarthrodial joint
diary
d., Event
d., food
d., Holter
d., symptom
diascopic examination
diastase, pancreatic
diastasis
d. cordis
d., iris
d. of cranial bones

d. of muscle
d. recti
d. recti abdominis
diastatic fracture
diastatic skull fracture
diastole
d., cardiac
d., electrical
d., end-
d., heart in
d., internal dimension-
d., late
d., posterior wall thickness-
d., ventricular
diastoler, atrial
diastolic
d. afterpotential
d. area ▸ end-
d. blood pressure (DBP)
d. blood pressure (DBP) ▸
  instrumental conditioning of
d. blow
d. collapse ▸ right ventricular (RV)
d. compliance, alteration in
d. count ▸ end-
d. current
d. current of injury
d. decrescendo murmur
d. depolarization
d. diameter ▸ left ventricular (LV)
  internal
d. diameter ▸ total end-
d. dimension ▸ end-
d. dimension ▸ left ventricular (LV)
  end-
d. dimension ▸ left ventricular
  internal
d. doming
d. dysfunction
d. filling
d. filling period
d. filling pressure
d. filling rate ▸ peak
d. fluttering aortic valve
d. function
d. gallop
d. gallop (VDG), ventricular
d. gradient
d. grunt
d. heart disease
d. heart factor
d. heart murmur ▸ apical mid-
d. hypertension
d. left ventricular (LV) pressure ▸
  end-

diastolic—*continued*
- d. left ventricular (LV) pressure ▸ mean
- d. mitral inflow ▸ turbulent
- d. motion
- d. murmur (DM)
- d. murmur, apical
- d. murmur, basal
- d. murmur, blubbery
- d. murmur, early
- d. murmur, end
- d. murmur, faint
- d. murmur, late
- d. murmur ▸ mid-
- d. murmur ▸ rumbling
- d. murmur, soft blowing
- d. overload
- d. performance ▸ impairment of systolic and
- d. phase index ▸ left ventricular (LV)
- d. pressure (DP)
- d. pressure (DP) ▸ depressed
- d. pressure (EDP) ▸ end-
- d. pressure (LVDP) ▸ left ventricular
- d. pressure (LVEDP) ▸ left ventricular end-
- d. pressure, optimal
- d. pressure ▸ right ventricular (RV)
- d. pressure (RVEDP) ▸ right ventricular end-
- d. pressure time index
- d. pressure ▸ ventricular
- d. pressure volume relation
- d. reading
- d. relaxation
- d. relaxation ▸ left ventricular (LV)
- d. reserve
- d. rumble
- d. rumble ▸ mid-
- d. shock
- d. stiffness
- d. suction
- d., systolic to
- d. thickness
- d. thrill
- d. velocity, end
- d. volume, end-
- d. volume index ▸ end-
- d. volume (LVEDV) left ventricular end-
- d. volume (RVEDV) ▸ right ventricular end-
- d. volume ▸ ventricular end-

- d. wave, early

diastrophic dwarf
diathermal therapy
diathermy
- d. and massage
- d., pelvic
- d. points
- d. puncture
- d., short wave
- d. therapy
- d. tips
- d., ultrashort wave

diathesis [*diaphysis*]
- d., allergic
- d., aneurysmal
- d., asthenic
- d., bilious
- d., bleeding
- d., contractual
- d., convulsive
- d., cystic
- d., fibroplastic
- d., gouty
- d., hemorrhagic
- d., inopectic
- d., lupus
- d., neuropathic
- d., ossifying
- d., oxalic
- d., psychoactive
- d., psychopathic
- d. secondary to hepatic failure ▸ hemorrhagic
- d., spasmodic
- d., spasmophilic
- d., uric acid

diatoric teeth
diatrizoate
- d. contrast medium, meglumine
- d. contrast medium, sodium
- d. meglumine contrast medium
- d. sodium contrast medium

DIC (diffuse intravascular coagulation)
DIC (diffuse intravascular coagulopathy)
DIC or DTIC (dimethyl triazeno imidazole carboxamide)
DIC (disseminated intravascular coagulation)
diced cartilage grafts
dichromatic vision
Dick test
Dick toxin
Dickson-Diveley operation

Dickson's operation
dicloxacillin sodium
Dicrocoelium dentriticum
Dicrocoelium, Tematoda
dicrotic
- d. notch
- d. pulse
- d. wave

dictation on chart ▸ see
didactic information
didactic systems
Diday's law
didelphys, uterine
didelphys, uterus
die
- d. movement, right-to-
- d., right to
- d., right to be assisted to

died
- d. accidental death, patient
- d. in sleep, patient
- d. natural death, patient
- d. suddenly, patient
- d. unexpectedly, patient
- d. unnatural death, patient

Dieffenbach's operation
dielectric radiofrequency electric field
dielectric track detector
diencephalic syndrome
Dienst's test
Dientameba diarrhea
Dientamoeba fragilis
diet
- d., absolute
- d., adequate
- d., alteration in
- d. and exercise
- d. and exercise program
- d. and medication
- d., Andresen
- d., anti-aging
- d., balanced
- d., basic
- d., basic cardiac
- d., betaine
- d., bland
- d., bland nonchew
- d., bland ulcer
- d., blenderized
- d., bulky
- d., calcium deficient
- d., calcium-rich
- d., calcium sufficient
- d., calorie restriction

d. ▸ caffeine, alcohol, pepper, spicy (CAPS) foods-free
d., cardiac
d. center ▸ medical and
d., cholesterol lowering
d., clear liquid
d., clear surgical
d., cold liquid
d., crash
d. decision
d. ▸ demi-vegetarian
d., Dennett's
d., diabetic
d., diabetic control with
d., dialysis
d., Ebstein's
d., elimination
d., exchange
d., fad
d., fasting-type
d., fat controlled
d., fat-free
d., fat in
d., fat restricted
d., Feingold
d. for papillotomy patient, test
d. formula, liquid
d., full liquid
d., galactosemia
d., general
d., Gerson-Herrmannsdorfer
d., Giordano-Giovannetti
d., gluten-free
d., gluten restricted
d., gouty
d., healthy
d. ▸ heart sensible
d., high bulk
d., high calorie
d., high carbohydrate
d., high fat
d. ▸ high fat, high cholesterol
d. ▸ high fat ketogenic
d. ▸ high fat, low fiber
d., high fiber
d., high fracture
d., high protein
d. history
d. in nutrition ▸ elemental
d., Jarotsky's
d., junk food
d., Karen's
d., Kempner's
d. ▸ lacto-ovo vegetarian
d., lactose-free

d., lactose reduced
d., lactose restricted
d., less-restrictive
d., liberal gastrointestinal (GI)
d., light
d., liquid
d. ▸ liquid supplement to
d., low bacteria
d., low calorie
d., low cholesterol
d., low fat
d., low fat cholesterol
d. ▸ low fat, nonacidic
d., low fat vegetarian
d., low fiber
d., low lipid
d. ▸ low methionine
d., low protein
d., low purine
d., low residue
d., low salt
d., low saturated fat
d., low sodium
d. ▸ low sodium, high potassium
d., low uric acid
d., Löwbeer
d., macrobiotic
d., maintenance
d., mechanical soft
d., Mediterranean
d., medium chain triglyceride
d., Meulengracht
d., mild sodium restricted
d., milk-free bland
d., moderate sodium restricted
d., modified
d., Moro-Heisler
d., NAS (no added salt)
d., nonirritating
d., nonresidue liquid
d., nonroughage
d., nutritionally balanced
d., oriental
d., oxalate
d., papillotomy
d., patient to resume
d. ▸ pesco-vegetarian
d. pill ▸ problem with central nervous system from
d. ▸ pollo-vegetarian
d., Portagen
d. program, liquid
d., protein
d., protein restricted
d., prudent

d., pureed
d., purine-free
d., pyridoxine deficient
d., quick fix
d., reduced fat
d., reduction
d., regular
d., renal
d. ▸ restricted tyramine and MAO (monoamine oxidase) inhibitor
d., rheumatic
d., rice
d., salt-free
d., salt restriction
d. ▸ Sauerbruch-Herrmannsdorfer Gerson
d., select
d. ▸ semi-vegetarian
d., Sippy
d., sodium controlled
d., sodium restricted
d., soft
d., soft dental
d. ▸ soft mechanical
d., staged ulcer
D. ▸ Step-One
d., strict sodium restricted
d. supplement
d., surgical soft
d. sweetener
d., therapeutic
d. therapy
d., tonsillectomy
d., TOPS (Take Off Pounds Sensibly)
d. ▸ utilize galactose in
d. ▸ vegen-vegetarian
d., vegetarian
d., weight control
d., weight gain
d., weight loss
d., weight reduction
d., Weight Watcher's
d., well-balanced
d., yo-yo

dietary (Dietary)
d. allowances (RDA), recommended
d. cholesterol
d. cholesterol intake
d. control
d. deficiencies
d. factor
d. fat
d. fat consumption

dietary—*continued*
- d. fat intake
- d. fiber
- d. fiber ▸ soluble
- d. guidelines
- d. habits
- d. habits, bad
- d. habits, healthy
- d. habits, poor
- d. indiscretion
- d. insufficiency
- d. intake
- d. intake, poor
- d. manipulation
- d. modification
- d. pattern
- d. problems
- d. requirements, fiber
- d. restrictions
- D. Services
- d. sodium
- d. supervision
- d. supplement
- d. therapy
- d. therapy ▸ intensive
- d. thermogenesis
- d. thermogenesis reaction
- d. triggers

dietetic [*diabetic, diuretic***]**
dietetic management
diethylamide
- d. (LSD) addict, lysergic acid
- d. (LSD) addiction, lysergic acid
- d. (LSD) dependency ▸ lysergic acid
- d. (LSD) habit, lysergic acid
- d. (LSD)-induced psychosis ▸ lysergic acid
- d. (LSD) ingested, lysergic acid
- d. (LSD) intoxication ▸ lysergic acid
- d. (LSD), lysergic acid
- d. (LSD) user, lysergic acid
- d. (LSD) withdrawal, lysergic acid

diethylstilbestrol (DES)
dieting
- d. ▸ hazards of yo-yo
- d., obsessive
- d., patient
- d., restrictive
- d. stress
- d. with exercise ▸ patient
- d., yo-yo

dietitian, clinical
Dieuaide diagram
Dieuaide's sign

Dieulafoy's erosion
difference(s)
- d. (AV DO₂), arteriovenous oxygen
- d., biological
- d., electrical potential
- d., inborn personality
- d., individual
- d., light
- d., limen
- d., potential
- d., stability of subject

different areas of brain
different stressors
differential [*deferential***]**
- d. adsorption
- d. agglutination titer
- d. amplifiers
- d. blood count
- d. blood pressure
- d. count
- d., depth dose
- d. diagnosis
- d. diagnosis in acute drug intoxication
- d. diagnosis in organic brain syndrome
- d. diagnosis in panic reactions
- d. diagnosis of alcohol withdrawal symptoms
- d. diagnosis of psychotic reactions
- d. diagnosis of tachycardia
- d. diagnosis with overdosing
- d. distortion divergent method, Isaac's
- d. EEG (electroencephalogram) amplifier
- d. effectiveness of electromyographic feedback
- d. electroencephalogram (EEG) amplifier
- d. in abstinence rate
- d., normal
- d., pressure
- d. reflux, urethrovesiculo-
- d. signal
- d. smear
- d. stain
- d. staining
- d. stethoscope
- d. therapy

differentiated
- d. adenocarcinoma of uterus ▸ well
- d. adenocarcinoma, poorly
- d. carcinoma
- d. carcinoma ▸ poorly

- d. carcinoma ▸ well
- d. ductal carcinoma ▸ poorly
- d. hepatocellular carcinoma ▸ well
- d. internal structures
- d. large cell carcinoma ▸ poorly
- d. lymphocytes (NPDL), nodular poorly
- d. lymphocytic lymphoma, poorly
- d., poorly
- d. squamous cell carcinoma ▸ bronchogenic poorly
- d. squamous cell carcinoma, poorly
- d. squamous cell tumor ▸ well
- d., well

differentiation
- d., adenocarcinoma with squamous
- d., alveolar
- d. antigen
- d., cell
- d., cellular
- d., diagnostic
- d., echocardiographic
- d., nuclear
- d. ▸ process of neurobehavioral sexual
- d., regional
- d., roentgenographic
- d., self-

difficile
- d., Clostridium
- d. colitis, Clostridium
- d. toxin, Clostridium

difficult
- d. menstruation
- d. speech, impaired
- d. to arouse, patient
- d. to manage, child
- d. urination
- d. vaginal delivery

difficulty(-ies)
- d. ambulating
- d., behavioral
- d. breathing
- d. ▸ chest pain with breathing
- d. chewing
- d. child-rearing
- d., communication
- d. concentrating
- d. controlling anger
- d. coping
- d., educational
- d., emotional speech
- d. encountered, considerable
- d., feeding
- d. from anemia ▸ breathing

d. from anxiety ▸ breathing
d. from asthma ▸ breathing
d. from bronchitis ▸ breathing
d. functioning
d. functioning at normal ability level
d. ▸ history of interpersonal
d. in articulation
d. in breathing
d. in concentration
d. in decision making
d. in initiating urination
d. in learning
d. in nasal breathing
d. in speaking
d. in starting urinary stream
d. in urinating
d. in voiding
d. in walking ▸ progressive
d., initial breathing
d., instrument passed without
d. learning
d. on urination
d. or inability to speak
d. performing familiar tasks
d., reading
d., respiratory
d. sleeping
d. ▸ social and behavioral
d. speaking
d., speech
d., subjective
d., subtle
d., sucking and swallowing
d. swallowing
d. swallowing ▸ patient has
d. talking
d., temporary breathing
d. urinating
d. voiding
d. walking
d. with attention
d. with concentration
d. with peers
d. with problem from central
  nervous system ▸ breathing
d. with siblings
d. with speech and swallowing
d., writing
diffluent yellow material
diffraction analysis ▸ x-ray
diffusible stimulant
diffuse [*disuse*]
d. abdominal calcification
d. abdominal tenderness
d. aching

d. activity
d. air space disease
d. alveolar damage
d. alveolar filling disease
d. alveolar hemorrhage
d. alveolar lung disease
d. anterior scleritis
d. arterial ectasia
d. arteriosclerosis
d. atherosclerosis
d. atrophy
d. bacterial nephritis
d. bronchopneumonia
d. calcific atherosclerosis
d. carcinoma
d. cerebral dysfunction
d. clouding
d. colloid goiter
d. congestion, marked
d. cortical hyperplasia
d. cutaneous mastocytosis
d. degeneration of brain
d. disease
d., dull, aching pressure discomfort
d. dysrhythmia
d. emphysema
d. encephalopathy
d. enlargement
d. epithelioma
d. esophageal spasm
d. fibrosis
d. ganglion
d. gliosis
d. goiter
d. hepatic softening
d. hepatocellular degeneration
d., histiocytic lymphocyte depleted
  type ▸ Hodgkin's disease of
d. histiocytic lymphoma
d. histiocytic lymphoma of stomach
d. histiocytic type ▸ abdominal
  lymphoma
d. hypokinesis
d. increase in pancreatic density
d. infiltrative lung disease
d. interstitial lung disease
d. interstitial pulmonary fibrosis
d. intimal thickening
d. into heart muscle, blood
d. intravascular coagulation (DIC)
d. intravascular coagulopathy (DIC)
d. jaundice
d. leukemic infiltrate
d. lung disease
d. lung injury

d. lymphocytic lymphoma
d. lymphoid infiltration
d. lymphomatous infiltrate
d. mild dilatation
d. mucosal autolysis
d. muscular rigidity
d. necrotizing bronchopneumonia ▸
  bilateral
d. necrotizing panangiitis
d. nephritis
d. neurological disease
d. neurological disturbance
d. non-Hodgkin's lymphoma
d. parenchymal softening
d. paroxysmal slowing
d. patchy fibrosis
d. pattern
d. peritonitis
d. petechial hemorrhages
d. pleurisy
d. pneumonitis
d. pulmonary alveolar hemorrhage
d. pulmonary disease
d. pulmonary rales ▸ bilateral
d. reticular nodular pattern
d. rhonchi
d. scar tissue
d. sclerosing alveolitis
d. sclerosing alveolitis, chronic
d. sclerosis
d. spike discharges ▸ -nonspecific
d. spikes
d. splenomegaly
d. subcortical dysfunction
d. swelling
d. symmetrical uterine enlargement
d. systemic sclerosis
d. thyroiditis, subacute
d. wheeze
diffused flashes of light
diffusely
d., bleeding
d. enlarged thyroid
d. infiltrated
diffusible tracer technique
diffusing
d. capacity
d. capacity, low
d. capacity of lung
d. capacity ▸ oxygen- (O_2)
d. hostility and anger
diffusion
d. anoxia
d. capacity, decreased
d. chamber

diffusion—*continued*
- d., coefficient of
- d. equation ▸ Fick's
- d. hypoxia
- d., impairment of
- d. method, disc
- d. of metabolic waste
- d. of oxygen and nutrients
- d. ▸ single breath
- d. study, pulmonary
- d. technique, time
- d. weighted MRI (magnetic resonance imaging)

digastric muscle
digastric nerve
DiGeorge syndrome
digest lactose ▸ inability to
digeted food
digestion
- d. absorption, protein
- d., acid
- d., cellulose
- d., decrease
- d., fat
- d., food
- d., normal process of
- d. of dairy products
- d., proteolytic
- d., self-
- d., stomach

digestive (Digestive)
- d. acini
- d. activity
- D. Disease Center
- d. disease
- d. disease ▸ treatment of
- d. disorder
- d. disorder, chronic
- d. disorder ▸ genetic
- d. disturbance
- d. enzymes
- d. enzymes ▸ natural
- d. fever
- d. gastrosuccorrhea
- d. gland
- d. illness
- d. islets
- d. juices ▸ elimination of pancreatic
- d. process
- d. system
- d. system bleeding
- d. system ▸ reroute
- d. system vascular disease
- d. tonic
- d. tract

- d. tract ▸ bacterial balance in
- d. tract, blocked
- d. tract disorder
- d. tract lining
- d. tract ▸ selective decontamination of
- d. tube

digit(s) (Digit)
- d., common extensor muscle of
- d., extra
- d. ▸ flexion contracture of
- d., missing
- d. of foot ▸ first through fifth
- d. of hand, chiasm of
- d. of hand ▸ first through fifth
- d., proper extensor muscle of fifth
- d. ▸ reattached severed
- d. reattached surgically, severed
- D. Span
- d., supernumerary

digital (Digital)
- d. angiogram ▸ venous
- d. angiographic assessment
- d. angiography
- d. angiography ▸ intravenous
- d. angiography ▸ pediatric
- d. arteriography
- d. artery
- d. autofluoroscope
- d. averaging
- d. beam attenuation
- d. biplane angioscope
- d. block anesthesia
- d. calipers
- d. cardiac imaging system
- d. cardiovascular angiography
- d. celiac trunk angiography
- d. clubbing
- d. compression
- d. computer
- d. computer code
- d. constant current pacing box
- d. conversion (A/D, ADC), analog
- d. converter ▸ analog-to-
- d. dilatation
- d. dilation
- d. dissection
- d. endarteropathy
- d. examination
- d. examination of prostate
- d. flexion contractures
- d. fluoroscopic unit
- d. fluoroscopy
- d. gangrene
- d. hearing aid

- d. holographic CAT (computerized axial tomography) scan
- d. image analysis
- d. imaging
- d. imaging ▸ computer based
- d. ischemia
- d. isotope calibrator
- d. mammogram
- d. mammography, computerized
- d. mammography images
- d. necrosis
- d. nerve
- d. nerve block
- d. nerve, common palmar
- d. nerve, proper palmar
- d. nerves of foot ▸ dorsal
- d. nerves of lateral planter nerve ▸ common plantar
- d. nerves of lateral plantar nerve ▸ proper plantar
- d. nerves of lateral surface of great toe ▸ dorsal
- d. nerves of medial plantar nerve ▸ common plantar
- d. nerves of medial plantar nerve ▸ proper plantar
- d. nerves of medial surface of second toe ▸ dorsal
- d. nerves of median nerve ▸ common palmar
- d. nerves of median nerve ▸ proper palmar
- d. nerves of radial nerve ▸ dorsal
- d. nerves of ulnar nerve ▸ common palmar
- d. nerves of ulnar nerve ▸ dorsal
- d. nerves of ulnar nerve ▸ proper
- d. percussion
- d. phase mapping
- d. photoplethysmography
- d. plethysmograph
- d. pressure measurements
- d. ray
- d. readout
- d., readout, accurate
- d. recorded picture
- d. rectal examination
- d. rectal test
- d. reflex
- d. removal of stool
- d. runoff
- d. scan converter
- d. signals
- d. smoothing
- d. stenosing tenosynovitis

d. stimulation
d. subtraction
d. subtraction angiogram ▸ electrocardiogram (ECG) synchronized
d. subtraction angiography (DSA)
d. subtraction angiography ▸ intra-arterial
d. subtraction arteriography
d. subtraction echocardiography
d. subtraction imaging
d. subtraction ▸ intraoperative
d. subtraction technique
d. subtraction ventriculography
d. subtraction ventriculography ▸ exercise
d. syncope
d. temperature
d. temperature autoregulation
d. thermometer, electronic
D. Vascular Imager (DVI)
D. Vascular Imager (DVI) Multicenter
d. vascular imaging
d. vein of foot ▸ common
d. vein of foot ▸ dorsal
d. vein, palmar
d. vein, plantar
d. venous arches
d. ventriculography ▸ pacing
D. x-ray ▸ Scanning Beam
digitalate pulse
digitalis (Digitalis)
d. atrial arrhythmias
d. effect
d. glycoside
d. intoxication
D. lanata
d. leaf
d. overdosage
d., powdered
d., prepared
D. purpura
d. sensitivity
d. therapy
d. toxicity
d. toxicity ▸ sensitize heart muscle to
digitalization of heart
digitalization, oral
digitalized, patient
digiti
d. minimi muscle, extensor
d. quinti muscle, abductor
d. quinti proprius muscle, extensor

digitized data
digitorectal examination
digitorectal examination ▸ annual
digitorum
d. brevis muscle, extensor
d. brevis muscle, flexor
d. communis muscle, extensor
d. longus muscle, extensor
d. longus muscle, flexor
d. manus, chiasma tendinum
d. profundus muscle, flexor
d. profundus tendon, flexor
d. sublimis muscle, flexor
d. sublimis tendon, flexor
d. superficialis muscle, flexor
digitus minimus
digoxin level
digoxin toxicity
dignified death
dignity, death with
diheteroxenic parasite
dihydrochloride, histamine
dihydroxyacetone phosphate
diisopropyl phosphate
dilantin level
dilatable lesion
dilatation(s) [*dilation*]
d., acute gastric
d. and aspiration (D and A) uterus
d. and curettage (D and C)
d. and curettage (D and C), diagnostic
d. and curettage (D and C), suction
d. and hypertrophy ▸ biventricular
d. and transition ▸ effacement,
d., aneurysmal
d., annular
d., atrial
d., balloon
d., bilateral ventricular
d., biventricular
d., bladder
d., bookstrap
d. breathing
d., bronchoscopy with
d., calyceal
d., cardiac
d., catheter
d., collateral
d., cystic
d., cystoscopy and
d., diffuse mild
d., digital
d., ductal
d., effacement and

d., esophageal
d., esophagoscopy with
d. failure
d., fusiform
d., gastric
d., gastric gaseous
d., homatropine
d. hypertrophy ▸ mild biventricular
d., idiopathic
d., left atrial
d., localized aneurysmal
d., marked
d. of bile duct
d. of bronchi
d. of bronchi ▸ peripheral
d. of bronchiole
d. of calyces
d. of cervix
d. of esophagu
d. of esophagus, brusque
d. of esophagus ▸ pneumatic
d. of kidney, cystiform
d. of larynx
d. of left infundibulum
d. of os uteri
d. of pupils
d. of stomach
d. of ureter
d. of ventricular system
d., operative bronchoscopy and
d., periodic
d., poststenotic
d., prognathic
d., pupillary
d., serial
d. thrombosis
d., toxic
d., tracheoscopy with
d., urethral
d., uterine
d., vascular
d., ventricular
dilate
d. blood vessel
d. bronchial tube
d. coronary arteries
d. narrowed duct
dilated
d., abdomen massively
d. airways
d. and hypertrophied ▸ ventricles
d. area, balloon
d. bile ducts
d. blood vessel
d., blood vessel walls

dilated—*continued*
- d. cardiomyopathy
- d. cardiomyopathy, idiopathic
- d. cardiomyopathy ▸ nonischemic
- d. cardiomyopathy ▸ x-l
- d. cervix
- d., cervix completely
- d. cervix, fully
- d., cervix partially
- d. distally, esophagus
- d. ducts
- d. esophagus
- d. eye examination
- d. eye examination, annual
- d. glands, cystically
- d., heart
- d. ▸ heart hypertrophied and
- d. heart, markedly
- d. kidney tubules
- d. loops of bowel
- d. lymphatic channel
- d., markedly
- d. odontoma
- d. pulmonary artery
- d. pupils
- d. pupils and hypothermia
- d. ▸ pupils fixed and
- d. ▸ renal pelvis mildly
- d. stricture
- d. ▸ ureters patent and not
- d., ventricle
- d., ventricular chambers
- d. ventricular system
- d. venule
- d. vestibule and cochlea

dilating blood vessel
dilating pains
dilation [*dilatation*]
- d. and cardiomyopathy ▸ pneumatic
- d. and evacuation
- d., digital
- d., esophageal
- d., finger
- d. of artery, balloon-like
- d. of blood vessels
- d. of punctum
- d. of pupil, sudden
- d. of pupils
- d. of stricture
- d., pneumatic
- d., poststenotic
- d., prostatic balloon
- d., pupillary
- d., reactive
- d., secondary arrest of

- d. ▸ severe colonic
- d. system ▸ Simpson-Robert vascular
- d. technique ▸ static
- d. thrombosis
- d. tracheostomy ▸ percutaneous

dilator
- d. ▸ blood vessel dilator
- d. muscle of nose
- d. muscle of pupil
- d. system ▸ sheath and

Dilaudid (First Line)
dilemma, existential
dilemmas, common therapeutic
dilute
- d. blood clot lysis
- d. intravenous Pitocin (DIVP)
- d. variant, chronic and

diluting fluid ▸ Rees and Ecker
dilution
- d., back flow and
- d. curve ▸ indocyanine
- d. factor
- d. -filtration technique
- d. (MID) ▸ maximum inhibiting
- d., routine test
- d. studies, tube
- d. technique ▸ indocyanine green indicator
- d. test
- d., thermal
- d., urine

dimension
- d., aortic root
- d. diastole, internal
- d. ▸ end-diastolic
- d. ▸ end-systolic
- d., inner
- d., left atrial
- d., left lateral ▸ internal
- d. ▸ left ventricular (LV) end-diastolic
- d. ▸ left ventricular (LV) end-systolic
- d. ▸ left ventricular internal diastolic
- d., maximum
- d. of grief, prophetic
- d. of grief, spiritual
- d., outer
- d. relation ▸ end-systolic stress
- d., right atrial
- d. ▸ right ventricular (RV)
- d., spatial
- d. systole, internal

dimensional

- d. analysis
- d. analysis ▸ three
- d. appearance
- d. computed tomographic (CT) colonography ▸ three
- d. conformal radiation therapy ▸ three-
- d. echocardiogram, cross-sectional two
- d. echocardiography ▸ quantitative two
- d. echocardiography ▸ real time three
- d. echocardiography ▸ three
- d. echocardiography, two-
- d. image, three-
- d. imaging ▸ Fourier two
- d. radiation therapy ▸ three-
- d., three
- d. view, three-
- d. x-ray images ▸ three-

dimethoxyphenyl penicillin
dimethyl sulfoxide (DMSO)
dimethyl triazeno imidazole carboxamide (DTIC/DIC)
dimidiata
- d., chorea
- d., Chrysops
- d., placenta
- d., Trypanosoma

diminish
- d. activity
- d. activity in brain
- d. brain function
- d. excursion of ataxic gait
- d. swelling
- d. tremor and rigidity

diminished
- d. ability to think or concentrate
- d. activity
- d. appetite
- d. arousal
- d. attenuation midbrain and pons
- d. blood flow
- d. bowel movements
- d. brain activity
- d., breath sounds
- d. breath sounds ▸ lungs revealed
- d. capacity
- d., chest excursion
- d. compliance
- d. concentration
- d. contractile excursion
- d. denial
- d. denial and defensiveness

d. exercise
d. expansion of chest
d. flow of tears
d. hearing
d. hearing and sight
d. heart, kidney and brain function
d. inhibition
d. intensity of movement
d. job performance
d. left ventricular compliance
d. levels of drinking
d. motor function
d. movement of bradykinesia ▸ slow
d. perception of pain and temperature
d. production of protein in brain
d. reflexes
d. responsiveness to pain
d. salt intake
d. secretion of saliva
d. self-esteem
d. self-worth
d. sensation to pinprick
d. sense of smell
d. stamina
d. stress
d. vision
diminishing vision
diminuta, Hymenolepsis
diminution
d. in blood supply ▸ local
d. in chest pain
d. of background activity
d. of blood flow
d. of breath sounds
d. of pain
d. of pain sensation
d. of peripheral pulses
d. of recorded activity
d. of vision
diminutus, Triodontophorus
Dimitri disease, ▸ Sturge-Weber-
Dimitri's disease
dimmed vision
dimmed vision in one eye
Dimmer degeneration ▸ Biber-Haab-
Dimmer keratitis
dimming of vision
dimming of vision, blurring or
dimness
d. of vision ▸ sudden
d. or loss of vision
d. or loss of vision ▸ sudden
d., visual

dimorpha, Mycoplana
dimorphic anemia
dimple(s)
d., blind coronary
d., coronary ostial
d., Fuchs'
dimpled skin
dimpling
d., breast
d. of breast skin
d. of eyeball
d. of skin
DIMS (disturbance in maintaining sleep)
dimutase gene ▸ superoxide
dinitrogen monoxide
Diodrast contrast medium
Dionosil contrast medium
diopter(s)
d. (PD) distance, prism
d. of papilledema
d. (PD) ▸ prism
dioptric aberration
dioptric media
Dioscorides' granule
dioxide
d. (CO_2) ▸ carbon
d. (CO_2) combining power ▸ carbon
d. (Th-O_2) contrast medium, thorium
d. (CO_2) ▸ dizziness from carbon
d. (ETCO_2) ▸ end-tidal carbon
d. (FECO_2) ▸ fraction of expired carbon
d. (FICO_2) ▸ fraction of inspired carbon
d. gas laser ▸ (CO_2) carbon
d. (CO_2) instilled, carbon
d. (CO_2), insufflation of carbon
d. (CO_2) laser, Sharplan carbon
d. (CO_2), laser skin resurfacing, carbon
d. (CO_2) laser vaporization, carbon
d. (CO_2) level ▸ blood carbon
d. (CO_2) levels ▸ oxygen (O_2) and carbon
d. (PCO_2) ▸ partial pressure of carbon
d. (CO_2) pressure, alveolar carbon
d. (CO_2) production, carbon
d. (CO_2) tension, alveolar carbon
d. (CO_2) tension ▸ arterial carbon
d. (CO_2) tension ▸ carbon
d. (CO_2) therapy ▸ carbon
d. (Th-O_2), thorium

d. (CO_2) with oxygen ▸ carbon
Dip (dip) (DIP)
D. (desquamative interstitial pneumonitis)
D. (distal interphalangeal)
D. contrast medium, ▸ Reno-M-
d. coating autoradiography
d., Cournand
d., midsystolic
d. phenomenon
d. septal
Dipetalonema reconditum
diphasic
d. complex
d. P wave
d. slow wave ▸ high voltage
d. T wave
d. wave
diphosphate, adenosine
diphosphate, uridine
diphosphoglucose, uridine
diphosphoglucuronic acid ▸ uridine
diphosphoglycyronyl transferase ▸ uridine
diphosphopyridine nucleotide
diphtheria
d. antigen
d. antitoxin
d., laryngeal
d., pertussis, tetanus ▸ (DPT)
d., tetanus toxoids, and acellular pertussis vaccine
d., tetanus toxoids, and whole cell pertussis vaccine
d. toxoid immunization
diphtheriae
d., Bacillus
d., Corynebacterium
d., gram-positive Corynebacterium
diphtherial tonsillitis
diphtheric
d. conjunctivitis
d. croup
d. myocarditis
d. pharyngitis
d. vulvitis
diphtheritic
d. croup
d. laryngitis
d. paralysis
d. vaginitis
d. vulvitis
diphtheroid bacilli
diphtheroidal forms
diphtheroides, Lactobacilli

diphtheroids isolated in urine
Diphyllobothrium
    D. latum
    D. parvum
    D. taenoides
DIPJ (distal interphalangeal joint)
diplegia
    d., atonic-astatic
    d., congenital facial
    d., infantile
    d., spastic
diplegic idiocy
diplobacillary conjunctivitis
diplobacillus, Morax's
diplococci
    d. bacterium
    d., gram-negative bean-shaped
    d., gram-negative extracellular
        bean-shaped
    d., gram-negative extracellular
        kidney-shaped
    d., gram-negative intracellular
    d., gram-negative intracellular bean-shaped
    d., gram-negative intracellular
        kidney-shaped
    d., gram-negative kidney-shaped
    d., helmet-shaped gram-positive
    d., lancet-shaped gram-positive
Diplococcus (diplococcus)
    d., bacterium
    D. constellatus
    D. genus
    D. magnus
    D. morbillorum
    D. mucosus
    D. of Morax-Axenfeld
    d. of Neisser
    D. paleopneumoniae
    D. plagarumbelli
    D. pneumoniae
    D. pneumoniae, gram-positive
    d., Weichselbaum's
Diplogonoporus brauni
Diplogonoporus grandis
diploic vein
    d.v., anterior temporal
    d.v., frontal
    d.v., occipital
    d.v., posterior temporal
diploidea, Sappinia
diplopia
    d., binocular
    d., heteronymous
    d., homonymous

    d., intermittent
    d., Lancaster's red-green test for
    d., monocular
    d., paradoxical
    d. screen, Hess
    d., torsional
dipolar ion, amphoteric
dipole theory
diprotrizoate contrast medium
dipslides, Uricult
Dipylidium caninum
dipyridamole
    d. echocardiography
    d. thallium imaging
    d. thallium scintigraphy
    d. thallium 201 scintigraphy
direct
    d. ablation
    d. access
    d. admit
    d. agglutination
    d. agglutination pregnancy test
    d. angioplasty
    d. anticancer properties
    d. auscultation
    d. bilirubin test
    d. biologic effects
    d. blood donations
    d. cardiac massage
    d. cardiac puncture
    d. cell division
    d. centrifugal flotation
    d. contact
    d. contact with body secretions
    d. contact with contaminated blood
    d. contact with contaminated oral
        secretions
    d. contact with contaminated
        plasma
    d. contact with contaminated serum
    d. contact with patient
    d. contagion
    d. Coombs' test
    d. coronary artery bypass
        (MIDCAB) ▸ minimally invasive
    d. coupled amplifier
    d. culture
    d. current (DC)
    d. current amplifier
    d. current cardioversion
    d. current ▸ low energy
    d. current (DC) ▸ opposition of flow
        of
    d. current (DC) resistance
    d. current (DC) voltage

    d. diagnosis
    d. display console (DDC)
    d. drainage (dr'ge) of abdominal
        cavity
    d. embolism
    d. emetic
    d. excitation
    d. extension of tumor
    d. fecal contamination
    d. field
    d. fluorescent antibody
    d. Fourier transformation imaging
    d. fracture
    d. fulguration
    d. hernia
    d. illumination
    d. immunofluorescence analysis
    d. infection
    d. inguinal hernia
    d. injection of silicone into breast
    d. inoculation
    d. insertion technique
    d. inspection
    d. killing by lethal injection
    d. killing of incompetent individual
    d. laryngoscopy
    d. lead
    d. light reflex
    d. lung aspirate
    d. mapping sequence
    d. mechanical ventricular actuation
    d. metastasis
    d. murmur
    d. myocardial revascularization
    d. ophthalmoscopy
    d. parallax
    d. patient care
    d. patient contact
    d. percussion
    d. percutaneous transhepatic
        cholangiography
    d. personal contact
    d. platelet count
    d. portal
    d. portal, single
    d. portional, posterior
    d. pressure
    d. push of medication
    d. radial sutures
    d. radiation (EDR), effective
    d. ray
    d. recording from cortex
    d. reflex
    d. respiration
    d. revascularization

d. sequelae
d. smear
d. toxicity
d. transfer flap
d. transfusion
d. treatment costs
d. vision
d. vision internal urethrotomy (DVIU)
d. visual examination
d. visualization

directed
d. biopsy
d. blood donation
d. blood donor
d. cervical punch biopsies
d. contracted, funeral
d. donor
d. donor donation
d. donor transfusion
d. forgetting
d. interdisciplinary care, physician
d. jet, anteriorly
d. laser ‣ spectroscopy-
d. organ donation
d. potential for violence ‣ self-
d. pulmonary artery catheter ‣ flow-
d. punch biopsy, colposcopic
d., take as
d. violence ‣ self-

direction
d. and pattern of brain electrical activity ‣ shift in
d. of radiation beam
d. ray
d., receptivity to suggestion and
d. therapy, beam

directional
d. atherectomy
d. atherectomy device
d. coronary atherectomy (DCA)
d. movement
d. preponderance
d. pressure
d. vascular intervention

directive(s)
d., advance
d. ‣ advanced treatment
d. group play therapy
d., implementation of advance
d., medical
d. therapy

directly
d. into duodenum ‣ scope advanced
d. kill patient
d. observed therapy

Director('s) (director)
D., Central Service
d. hold
D., Inservice Education
D., Medical
D. of Nursing
D. of Operating Room
D., Unit

Dirofilaria
D. conjunctivae
D. genus
D. immitis
D. magalhaesi
D. repens

dirty
d. chest
d. film
d. lung appearance
d. necrosis
d. wound

disability(-ies)
d. as result of stroke ‣ rehabilitation of
d., cardiovascular
d., child has language
d., crippling
d., developmental
d., emotional
d., euthanasia and
d. evaluation
d. evaluation, physical
d., functional
d., general
d. impairment
d. in knees
d. in parent, chronic
d., irreversible
d., job-related
d., language
d. ‣ language-based learning
d., late-life
d. (LD), learning
d., life-long
d., linguistic
d., mental
d., movement
d., muscular
d., neurological
d., partial
d., patient's level of

d. pension
d., permanent
d., physical
d., physical or mental
d., presumptive
d., print
d., prolonged
d., reading
d. rights activists
d. rights advocates
d. risk
d. ‣ schizophrenic behavior with residual
d., secondary
d., sensory
d. (SCD) ‣ service-connected
d. (SRD) ‣ service-related
d., severe multiple
d., significant
d., speech
d. status scale
d. syndrome
d. syndrome ‣ traumatic
d., temporary
d., total

disabled
d. child, developmentally
d. child ‣ learning
d. children
d., cognitively
d., developmentally
d. infant
d. organ
d., patient
d., patient completely
d., patient partially
d., patient totally
d. person
d., physically
d., psychologically
d., rehabilitation center for physically
d., socially

disabling
d. angina pectoris
d. condition
d. disease
d. double vision
d. essential tremor
d. eye
d. genetic disorder
d. handicap ‣ severe
d. heartburn
d. illness
d. ineffective family coping

disabling—*continued*
d. irrational fear
d. joint disorder
d. mental illness
d. migraines ▸ painful and
d. pain
d. positioning vertigo
d. rigidity
d. shaking and trembling
d. stiffness
d. stroke
d. symptoms
d. tremors
d. vertiginous episodes, acute
d. vertigo ▸ frequent attacks of

disaccharidase deficiency
disappearance
d., plasma iron
d. rate, plasma glucose
d. time, plasma iron

disapproval, social
disaster
d. crisis intervention
d. ▸ feeling of impending
d., mass
d., natural
d. psychology
d., technological

disbelief ▸ shock, numbness and
disbelief, shock, numbness ▸ sense of
disc(s) (disk)
d., A
d., abrasive
d., Amici's
d., anangioid
d., anisotropic
d., articular
d. ▸ back pain from
d., Bardeen's primitive
d., Blake's
d., blastodermic
d., blood
d., Bowman's
d. ▸ Bryan cervical
d., bulging
d. bulging ▸ generalized
d. calcification, intervertebral
d., carborundum
d., cartilaginous
d. change, degenerative
d., choked
d., ciliary
d., cloth
d. collapse

d., color
d. compression, cervical
d. crushing of intervertebral
d., cupped
d., cutting
d. decompression, cervical
d. degeneration
d. degeneration ▸ spinal cord
d., degenerative
d., dental
d., deteriorated
d., diameters
d., diamond
d. diffusion method
d. disease
d. disease, cervical
d. disease, degenerative
d. disease ▸ intervertebral
d. disease, spinal
d. displacement
d., early
d., ectodermal
d. ▸ edema of optic
d. electrode
d. electrophoresis
d. elevation
d., embryonic
d., emery
d., Engelmann's
d., extruded
d., floppy
d., gelatin
d., germinal
d., hemilaminectomy for cervical
d., Hensen's
d., herniated
d., herniated intervertebral
d. herniation
d. herniation, intervertebral
d. herniation of
d. impingement
d., interarticular
d., intercalated
d., intermediate
d., interpubic
d., intervertebral
d., intra-articular
d., isotropic
d., J
d. kidney
d., M
d., Merkel's
d. metastasis ▸ optic
d., micrometer
d., nasal border of optic

d. ▸ neck and shoulder pain from
d., Newton's
d., optic
d. or nerve, cupping of
d., outline of
d. oxygenation
d. oxygenator
d. ▸ pain in back from slipped or ruptured
d. pain, slipped
d., pallor of
d., Placido's
d., polishing
d., pressure on
d. problem, cervical
d., prolapsed
d., proligerous
d. protrusion, intervertebral
d., protruding lumbosacral
d. protrusion
d. protrusion, lumbosacral
d., Q
d., Ranvier's tactile
d., Rekoss
d., rupture of intervertebral
d., ruptured
d., ruptured cervical
d. ▸ ruptured spinal
d., sandpaper
d., Schiefferdecker's
d. -shaped rash ▸ scaly,
d. -shaped retinopathy ▸ central
d., sharp
d., slipped
d. space
d. space, intervertebral
d. space ▸ narrowed
d. space, narrowing of
d. space ▸ narrowing of intervertebral
d. space, rudimentary
d. spring
d. stamper, optical
d., stenopeic
d., stroboscopic
d. surface, vertebral body
d. syndrome, cervical
d. syndrome, herniated
d., tactile
d., thin
d., transverse
d. valve
d. valve prosthesis
d. valve prosthesis ▸ Kay-Suzuki
d., vertebral

d., well-outlined
d., Z
discalis, Chrysops
discectomy
   d., automated percutaneous lumbar
   d., lumbar
   d., microscopic
discernible mass
discharge(s) (Discharge)
   d., abnormal brain wave
   d., abnormal electrical
   d. appropriateness
   d. around tooth ▸ foul
   d., blood-stained
   d., blood-streaked
   d., bloody
   d., bloody nasal
   d., bloody vaginal
   d., brownish-red
   d., brush
   d. card
   d., cervical
   d. ▸ chills with vaginal
   d., constructive
   d., cortical
   d., cottage cheese-like
   d., criteria for
   d. date, estimated
   d. diagnosis
   d., disruptive
   d., double
   d., epileptic
   d., epileptiform
   d., epileptogenic
   d., excessive hypersynchronous
   d., excessive neuronal
   d. ▸ fecal
   d., focal epileptiform
   d. ▸ focus of aggression
   d. from antidepressant ▸ nipple
   d. from anus
   d. from birth control pill ▸ nipple
   d. from breast ▸ bloody
   d. from breast injury ▸ nipple
   d. from chlamydia ▸ penile
   d. from wound
   d., frontoparietal spike-and-wave
   d., gram stain of purulent
   d., heavy vaginal
   d., home evaluation prior to
   d., hypersynchronous cerebral
   d., immediate
   d. in children ▸ vaginal
   d., indicators, surgical
   d. instruction sheet

d. ▸ itchy, whitish vaginal
d., larval
d., leukorrheal
d. ▸ long, regular
d., malodorous vaginal
d., meconium
d. medication
d., miniature petit mal
d., mitten
d., mucoid
d., mucopurulent
d., mucopurulent vaginal
d., mucous
d., nasal
d., negative
d., nervous
d., neural
d., nipple
d., nonspecific diffuse spike
d. of feces
d. of feces ▸ involuntary
d. of lining
d. of pus from the ear
d. of urine
d. of urine, excessive
d. of urine ▸ involuntary
d. ▸ pain in abdomen with vaginal
d., paroxysmal
d., paroxysmal high voltage
d., patient
d., penile
d. (PLED), periodic lateralized
   epileptiform
d., petit mal
d., petit mal variant
d., pinkish vaginal
d. placement
d. plan, development of
d. planning
d. planning process
d., positive
d. (PND) ▸ postnasal
d. practices
d., premature
d., prior to
d. process
d. protocol
d., pseudo petit mal
d., psychomotor variant
d., purulent
d., purulent malodorous
d., rectal
d., recurring excessive neuronal
d., repetitive

d., repetitive electroencephalogram
   (EEG)
d., seizure
d., seropurulent
d., six per second spike-and-wave
d., spike
d., spike-and-wave
d., spiking
D. Survey (NHDS) ▸ National
   Health
d., systolic
d. teaching
d. tube
d., urethral
d., vaginal
d., watery
d. ▸ white, cheesy
d., whitish
d., yellowish
discharged
   d. after brief observation ▸ patient
   d. after period of observation ▸
      patient
   d. ambulatory, patient
   d. from hospital, patient
   d. improved, patient
   d. in good condition ▸ patient
   d., patient
   d. to care of family physician ▸
      patient
   d. to care of relatives ▸ patient
   d. to convalescent treatment center
      ▸ patient
   d. to coordinated home care
      program ▸ patient
   d. to follow-up ▸ patient
   d. to home care ▸ patient
   d. to home ▸ patient
   d. to nursing home ▸ patient
   d. to office follow-up ▸ patient
   d. to treatment, patient
disciformans, retinitis
disciformis, keratitis
disciplinary approach to pain
   management, multi-
disciplinary problem
discipline(s)
   d., care
   d., child
   d. ▸ inconsistent parental
   d., medical
   d., self-
   d. skills
   d., various
disciplined, patient self-

discission [*decision*]
- d. cataract
- d. cervix uteri
- d. of lens
- d. of pleura
- d., posterior

disclosure of information
discobolus attitude
discogenic disease
discoid
- d. aortic prosthesis
- d. atelectasis
- d. lupus erythematosus (DLE)
- d. placenta
- d. rash

discoidea, placenta
discoides
- d., lupus erythematosus
- d., Trichophyton
- d., Veillonella

discoloration
- d., black
- d., bloody
- d., dusky
- d., ecchymotic
- d. from calculus ▸ tooth
- d., general
- d., heliotrope infraorbital
- d., hemorrhagic
- d. in aging ▸ skin
- d. of gums
- d. of limb
- d. of skin ▸ cyanotic
- d., skin
- d., urine

discolored, pericardial sac
discolored teeth
discomfit [*discomfort, discomfiture*]
discomfort
- d., abdominal
- d. and fever
- d. and pain
- d., back
- d., breast
- d., burning chest
- d., chest
- d., dealing with
- d., decrease
- d. ▸ diffuse, dull aching pressure
- d., distention
- d., epigastric
- d., excessive breast firmness and
- d., exertional chest
- d., extrathoracic
- d., gastrointestinal (GI)

- d., gnawing
- d. in ligaments ▸ stiffness and
- d. in muscles ▸ stiffness and
- d. in tendons ▸ stiffness and
- d., incisional
- d. ▸ increase awareness and decrease
- d., increasing abdominal
- d., infusion site
- d. level, loudness
- d., low back
- d., lower lumbar
- d., minor
- d., minor painful
- d., mouth
- d. ▸ mouth and throat
- d., muscle
- d. of withdrawal ▸ minimizing
- d., pain and/or
- d., patient's
- d., perianal
- d., physical
- d., postoperative
- d., postprandial
- d., postsurgical
- d., psychological
- d., substernal
- d., threshold of
- d., tongue
- d., undue physical
- d., upper respiratory tract
- d., vague chest
- d. with lightheadedness, chest
- d. with nausea, chest
- d. with shortness of breath (SOB), chest
- d. with sweating, chest

disconjugate gaze
disconnected and racing thoughts
disconnection, internal
discontinuation of medication
discontinued (Dc'd)
- d. intravenous (IV)
- d., therapy
- d., treatment

dicontinuing drug therapy
discontinuity, atrial axis
discontinuous activity
discopathy, traumatic
discophora, Leptothrix
discord, family
discord, marital
discordance, atrioventricular (AV)
discordance, ventriculoarterial
discordant alternans

discordant alternation
discounted clinical services
discrepancy, tooth size
discrete [*discreet*]
- d. activity
- d. aggregates
- d. aneurysm
- d. area of brain
- d. coronary lesion
- d. delta forms
- d. jerking musculature of face
- d. lesion
- d. mass
- d. nodulation
- d. nodulation of lung
- d. nodule
- d. post-trial feedback
- d. segment
- d. subvalvular aortic stenosis

discriminant function
discrimination
- d., color
- d., essential detail
- d. ▸ gradual loss of auditory
- d., impaired left
- d., impaired right
- d., in-phase
- d., light
- d., light-dark
- d., prejudice and
- d., proprioceptive
- d., ratio
- d., sensory
- d., shape
- d. (SD) ▸ speech
- d. (SD) test ▸ speech
- d. (TD) ▸ total
- d., two-light

discriminative
- d. acuity ▸ motor
- d. acuity ▸ visual
- d. stimulus

discriminatory and postural sensation ▸ vibratory,
discriminatory, vibratory and position sensation ▸ impaired
discussion, exploration, and feedback
discussion, verbal
disdain for others' sensitivities
disdain ▸ patient reacts with
disdainful attitude
disease(s) (Disease)
- d. ▸ abdominal lump with Crohn's
- d. ▸ abdominal pain with Crohn's

d., Abrami's
d., accelerated macrovascular
d., acid reflux
d., Acosta's
d., acromegalic heart
d., active
d., active liver
d., active lung
d., active lupus kidney
d., active parenchymal
d., active pulmonary
d. activity
d., acute
d., acute cardiovascular
d., acute infectious
d., acute ischemic heart
d. (ARD), acute respiratory
d., acute vestibular
d., acyanotic heart
d., Adams'
d., Adams-Stokes
d., addictive
d., Addison's
d., adhesive
d., adrenal
d., adult celiac
d. (APKD), adult polycystic kidney
d., advanced
d., advanced atherosclerotic
  cardiovascular
d., advanced gum
d., advanced heart
d., advanced liver
d., advanced metastatic
d., advanced pulmonary
d., advanced state of
d., advancing
d., age-related
d. ▸ age-related eye
d., air-space
d., airway
d., airway obstruction
d., Albers-Schönberg
d., Albert's
d., Albright's
d. ▸ alcohol-induced liver
d., alcohol-related
d. ▸ alcoholic heart muscle
d., alcoholic liver
d., Aleutian
d., alleviating
d., alveolar hydatid
d., Alzheimer's
d., amyloid heart
d., anaplastic

d., anatomic coronary
d. and etiology
d. and treatment ▸ physiology,
d., Anders'
d., Andersen's
d. anemia syndrome ▸ pulmonary
d., anorectal
d. ▸ anorectal problem from Crohn's
d., anxiety
d., aortic aneurysmal
d., aortic thromboembolic
d., aortic valve
d. (AIOD), aortoiliac obstructive
d., aortoiliac occlusive
d., apple picker's
d., Aran-Duchenne muscular
d., Arlt's
d., arterial
d., arterial occlusive
d. (ASCVD), arteriosclerotic
  cardiovascular
d. (ASHD) ▸ arteriosclerotic heart
d., arteriosclerotic occlusive
d., arteriosclerotic peripheral
  vascular
d. (ASVD) ▸ arteriosclerotic
  vascular
d. ▸ arthritis from Crohn's
d., asbestos-related
d., associated infecious
d., asymptomatic
d., asymptomatic heart
d., atherosclerotic aortic
d. (ASCVD), atherosclerotic
  cardiovascular
d., atherosclerotic carotid artery
d., atherosclerotic coronary artery
d., atherosclerotic heart
d., atherosclerotic vascular
d., atopic
d., atrioventricular (AV) conduction
d. attacks, viral
d., Aujeszky's
d., autoimmune
d. ▸ autoimmune inner ear
d. (PKD) ▸ autosomal dominant
  polycystic kidney
d., aviators'
d., Ayerza's
d. bacteria, Lyme
d., bacterial
d., Ballet's
d., Bamberger-Marie
d., Bannister
d., Banti's

d., barometer maker's
d., basal ganglion
d., Basedow's
d., Batten-Mayou
d., Beal's
d., Beau's
d., Begbie's
d., Behcet's
d., beholder's
d., Behr's
d., benign
d., benign breast
d., benign gynecological
d., Benson's
d., beriberi heart
d., Berlin's
d., Bernard Soulier
d., beryllium
d., Besnier's
d., Bielschowsky's
d., biliary tract
d., Binswanger's
d., biological progression of
d., bipolar
d., bipolar manic depressive
d., black lung
d. ▸ bleeding injury from
  Addison's
d., blinding eye
d., bloodborne
d. ▸ blood pressure (BP) lowered in
  Addison's
d., blood-related
d., blood vessel
d. ▸ blood vessel problem in
  Raynaud's
d., Blount
d., blue
d., Boeck's
d., Boerhaaves
d., bone weakening
d., bony
d., Bornholm
d., Bouchet's
d., Bourneville's
d., bowel-related
d., Bowen's
d., brain
d., brain blood vessel
d., brain plaques and tangles of
  Alzheimer's
d., brain stem vascular
d., brain wasting
d., Breisky's
d., Bright's

disease(s)—*continued*

d., Brill-Symmers
d., Brill-Zinsser
d., Brinton's
d., brittle bone
d., Brodie's
d., bronchopulmonary
d., brown lung
d., Bruhl's
d., Brushfield-Wyatt
d., Buerger's
d., bullous
d., Busse-Buschke
d., Caffey's
d., caisson
d., calcific atherosclerotic vascular
d., California
d., Calvé-Perthes
d., Canavan
d., cardiac
d., cardiac muscle
d., cardiopulmonary
d. (CD), cardiovascular
d., cardiovascular renal
d., carcinoid
d., carcinoid heart
d., carcinoid valve
d., carotid artery
d., carotid obstructive
d., carotid occlusive
d., carotid vaso-occlusive
d., Castelman's
d., cat scratch
d., cataract
d., catastrophic
d., causation of
d., causative
d., causes of heart
d. -causing bacteria
d. -causing gene
d. -causing organism
d., cavitary
d., celiac
d. cells, heart
D. Center, Digestive
d., central core
d., central nervous system (CNS)
d., cerebral
d. (CVD), cerebrovascular
d. (CVOD) ▸ cerebrovascular
  obstructive
d., cervical disc
d., Chagas'
d., Chandler's
d., Charcot

d., Charcot-Marie-Tooth
d., cheese workers' lung
d., chest wall
d., childhood
d., childhood muscle-wasting
d., cholesterol ester storage
d., chorioretinal
d., choroidal hypertensive
d., Christmas
d., chronic
d. ▸ chronic alcoholic heart muscle
d., chronic debilitating
d. ▸ chronic degenerative
d., chronic granulomatous
d., chronic heart
d., chronic hypertensive
d., chronic inflammatory
d., chronic interstitial lung
d., chronic kidney
d. ▸ chronic life-threatening
d., chronic liver
d., chronic lung
d., chronic lymphocytic
d., chronic myelogenous
d., chronic nervous degenerative
d., chronic obstructive airway
d., chronic obstructive lung
d. (COPD), chronic obstructive
  pulmonary
d., chronic obstructive respiratory
d., chronic occlusive
d., chronic or incurable
d. (chr. PID) ▸ chronic pelvic
  inflammatory
d. ▸ chronic progressive lung
d., chronic renal
d., chronic symptomatic
d., chronic underlying
d. ▸ (CWD) chronic wasting
d. ▸ cigarette-induced lung
d. ▸ cigarette-induced obstructive
  lung
d., circulatory
D. Clinic (VDC) ▸ Venereal
d. ▸ clinical alcoholic liver
d., clinical evidence of metastatic
d., clinical heart
d., CNS (central nervous system)
d., Coats'
d., cold agglutinin
d., collagen
d., collagen vascular
d. ▸ collapse from Addison's
d., colon interposition for
  esophageal

d., combined immune deficiency
d., combined treatment in advanced
d., communicable
d., complex
d., complex benign
d., complex benign esophageal
d., complicated
d. concept
d., concept, traditional
d., congenital
d. (CHD), congenital heart
d. (CHD) ▸ congestive heart
d., congestive pulmonary
d., connective tissue
d., contagious
d., contagious skin
d., contagious viral
D. Control (CDC) ▸ Centers for
D. Control ▸ U.S. Centers for
d. control, infectious
d., control of local and systemic
d., corneal
d., coronary
d. (CAD) ▸ coronary artery
d., coronary artery occlusive
d., coronary atherosclerotic heart
d., (CHD), coronary heart
d., coronary microvascular
d., coronary occlusive
d., Corrigan's
d., cosmetic
d., course of
d., crazy chick
d., creeping
d., Creutzfeldt-Jakob
d., crippling bone
d., Crohn's
d., Crouzon's
d., curing
d., Curschmann's
d., Cushing's
d., cutaneous fungal
d., cyanotic heart
d., cycle of
d., cystic lung
d. (CMID) ▸ cytomegalic inclusion
d., cytomegalovirus (CMV)
d., Czerny's
d., Dalrymple's
d., Darier's
d., Darling's
d., David's
d., debilitating
d., debilitating bone
d., debilitating bowel

d., Debove's
d. ▸ decreased risk of
d., deficiency
d. ▸ degenerated tissue
d., degenerative
d., degenerative bone marrow
d., degenerative brain
d., degenerative disc
d. (DHD), degenerative heart
d. (DJD) ▸ degenerative joint
d., degenerative liver
d., degenerative neurologic
d. ▸ degenerative neuromuscular
d. (DSD) ▸ degenerative spinal
d., Degos'
d. ▸ dehydration from Addison's
d., demyelinating
d. dental
d., de Quervain's
d., Dercum's
d., designer
d., Desnos'
d. ▸ destructive compulsive
d., Deutschländer's
d., devastating
d., Devic's
d., diabetes mellitus (DM)
  secondary to endocrine
d., diabetes mellitus (DM)
  secondary to pancreatic
d., diabetic eye
d. ▸ diabetic microvascular
d., diabetic nerve
d., diabetic-related
d., diabetic retinal
d., diagnosable
d., diagnosed infectious
d. diagnosis
d. ▸ diarrhea from Crohn's
d., diarrheal
d., diastolic heart
d., diffuse
d., diffuse air space
d. ▸ diffuse alveolar filling
d. ▸ diffuse alveolar lung
d. ▸ diffuse infiltrative lung
d. ▸ diffuse interstitial lung
d., diffuse lung
d., diffuse neurological
d., diffuse pulmonary
d., digestive
d. ▸ digestive system vascular
d., DiGuglielmo's
d., Dimitri's
d., disc

d., discogenic
d., disseminated
d., distant
d., distant metastatic
d., diverticular
d., Döhle
d., Down's
d., Dressler's
d. ▸ drug dependency with Crohn's
d., drug-resistant
d., Dubini's
d., Dubois'
d., Duchenne's
d., Ducrey's
d., Duhring's
d., Duplay's
d. ▸ Durand-Nicolas-Favre
d., Duroziez's
d., dust
d., Eales
d. ▸ early onset Alzheimer's
d. ▸ early onset familial Alzheimer's
d., Ebola
d., Ebstein's
d., Economo's
d. ▸ effusive constrictive
d., Eisenmenger's
d., electrical
d., elephant (elephantiasis)
d., elevator
d. emergency, infectious
d., end stage cardiac
d., end stage cardiopulmonary
d., end stage heart and liver
d. ▸ end stage liver
d. ▸ end stage of
d., end stage organ
d. (ESRD), end stage renal
d., enteroviral
d., environmental lung
d., eosinophilic endomyocardial
d., epidemic
d., Epstein-Barr (EB)
d. ▸ Epstein-Barr chorioretinal
d. eradication
d., Erb's
d., Erb-Charcot
d., Erb-Goldflam
d., Erb-Landouzy
d., Erichsen's
d. (CAD) ▸ evaluation of coronary
  artery
d., evolution of
d., exacerbation of
d., exanthematous

d., exfoliative skin
d. ▸ exhaustion, burnout and heart
d., extensive
d. ▸ extensive hyaline membrane
d. ▸ extensive inflammatory bowel
d., extensive metastatic
d., extracranial
d., extracranial cardiac
d. ▸ extracranial carotid arterial
d., extradural metastatic
d., extramammary Paget's
d., extrapelvic
d., eye
d., Fabry's
d. ▸ facial skin
d., fatal neuromuscular
d., fatty liver
d., familial
d., familial Alzheimer's
d. ▸ family-borne
d., far advanced
d., farmer's lung
d., fat-related
d., fatal
d., fatal granulomatous
d., Fauchard
d., Favre's
d., febrile
d., febrile respiratory
d., femoral popliteal occlusive
d., femoroiliac
d., fibrocalcaneous
d., fibrocystic
d., fibrocystic breast
d., fibroplastic
d., fifth
d. fighting molecules
d. fighting T cells
d. ▸ fish meal lung
d., Flajani's
d., flax dresser's
d., flint
d., focal brain
d., food-borne
d., foot and mouth
d., Forestier's
d., Fournier's
d., Fox-Fordyce
d., fracture caused by
d., Franceschetti's
d., Frankl-Hochwart's
d., Franklin's
d. -free
d. -free period
d. -free survival rate

disease(s)—*continued*
- d., Freiberg's
- d., Friedländer's
- d., Friedreich's
- d. from caffeine ▸ fibrocystic
- d. from chlamydia ▸ pelvic inflammatory
- d., full-fledged
- d., fulminant liver
- d., fulminating
- d., functional bowel
- d. ▸ functional cardiovascular
- d., fungal
- d. ▸ fungal nail
- d. ▸ furrier's lung
- d., Fürstner's
- d., fusospirochetal
- d., gallbladder
- d., gallstone
- d., Gamna's
- d., Gandy-Nanta
- d., gannister
- d., (GERD) ▸ gastroesophageal reflux
- d., gastrointestinal (GI)
- d., Gaucher's
- d., gay
- d. ▸ gene-based
- d., general
- d., general metastatic
- d., genetic
- d. ▸ genetic bone
- d. ▸ genetic neurological
- d. genetically determined
- d., genetotrophic
- d., Gerlier's
- d. ▸ gestational trophoblastic
- d., GI (gastrointestinal)
- d., Gilbert's
- d., Gilchrist's
- d., Gilles de la Tourette's
- d., Glanzmann's
- d. ▸ glomerular kidney
- d., glycogen storage
- d., Goldflam's
- d., gonadal
- d. —gonorrhea (VD6), venereal
- d., Gowers'
- d., Graefe's
- d. (GVHD) ▸ graft-versus-host
- d., granulomatous
- d., Graves'
- d., grinders'
- d., Grover's
- d., gum

- d., Gunther's
- d., Halban's
- d., Hamman's
- d. ▸ hand, foot and mouth
- d., Hanot's
- d., Hansen's
- d., Harada's
- d. ▸ hard metal
- d., Hartnup
- d., Hashimoto's
- d., headache secondary to cervical spine
- d., heart
- d., heart muscle
- d., heart valve
- d., heartworm
- d., Heberden's
- d., Heerfordt's
- d., Heller-Döhle
- d., helminthic
- d., hematologic
- d., hematological
- d., hemoglobin C—thalassemia
- d., hemoglobin E—thalassemia
- d., hemolytic
- d., hemorrhoidal
- d., Henoch's
- d., hepatic
- d., hepatobiliary tract
- d., hepatocellular
- d., hepatocellular liver
- d., hepatolenticular
- d., hepatorenal
- d., hereditary
- d. ▸ hereditary bone
- d., hereditary familial
- d., hereditary respiratory
- d., heredoconstitutional
- d., heredodegenerative
- d., herpetic ocular
- d., Hers'
- d. ▸ highest risk for
- d., Hippel's
- d., Hirschfeld
- d., Hirschsprung's
- d. history (HDH), heart
- d. (HD), Hodgkin's
- d., hookworm
- d., Horton's
- d, (TED) hose, thromboembolic
- d., Huchard's
- d., human brain
- d. ▸ humeroperoneal neuromuscular
- d., Huntington's
- d., Hunt's

- d., Hurler's
- d., Hutchinson's
- d., Hutinel's
- d. (HMD) ▸ hyaline membrane
- d., hydatid
- d. ▸ hydatid cyst
- d., hydrocephaloid
- d., hypertensive arteriosclerotic heart
- d. (HCVD), hypertensive cardiovascular
- d. (HHD), hypertensive heart
- d. ▸ hypertensive ocular
- d., hypertensive pulmonary vascular
- d. (HVD), hypertensive vascular
- d., Icelandic
- d. ▸ idiopathic Raynaud's
- d. ▸ immune complex
- d. ▸ immune kidney
- d. ▸ immune-mediated
- d., immunodeficiency
- d., immunological
- d. in complete remission
- d. in diabetic heart ▸ vascular
- d. in relapse, Hodgkin's
- d. in situ
- d., incapacitating
- d. incidence
- d. ▸ incipient degenerative brain
- d., incompatible hemolytic blood transfusion
- d., incurable
- d., incurable autoimmune
- d., incurable brain
- d. ▸ incurable, progressive
- d. -induced pain
- d., industrial
- d., infantile celiac
- d., infantile motor neuron
- d. ▸ infantile polycystic
- d., infectious
- d. ▸ infectious granulomatous
- d., inflammatory
- d., inflammatory bowel
- d., inhalational lung
- d. ▸ inheritable brain
- d., inherited
- d., inherited blood
- d. ▸ inherited iron storage
- d. ▸ inherited neuromuscular
- d., Inman's
- d. ▸ inorganic dust
- d., interstitial
- d., interstitial lung
- d. ▸ interstitial restrictive lung

d. ▸ intervertebral disc
d., intestinal
d., intracranial
d. ▸ intrastent recurrent
d., invasive
d. ▸ invasive pneumococcal
d. ▸ iron metabolism
d. ▸ iron overload
d. ▸ iron storage
d. ▸ irreversible hereditary
d. (IHD), ischemic heart
d., ischemic leg
d., ischemic limb
d. ▸ ischemic myocardial
d. ▸ ischemic vascular
d. ▸ Jakob-Creutzfeldt
d., Jakob's
d., Janet's
d., Jensen's
d., joint
d., Jüngling's
d., juvenile hereditary motor neuron
d., Kalischer's
d., Kartagener's
d., Kashin-Beck
d., Kawasaki
d., Kempf's
d., kidney
d., Kimmelstiel-Wilson
d. ▸ kinky hair
d., Klebs'
d., Koeppe's
d., Köhler's
d., Köhler's bone
d., Koshevnikoff's
d., Krabbe's
d., Kugelberg-Welander
d., Kuhnt-Junius
d., Kümmell's
d., Kümmell-Verneuil
d., Kussmaul
d. ▸ Kussmaul-Maier
d., labyrinth
d., labyrinthine
d. ▸ lactose intolerance with Crohn's
d., Laennec's
d., lambda
d. ▸ large vessel
d., Larsen-Johansson
d., Lasègue's
d., Lauber's
d., Leber's
d. ▸ left main coronary artery
d., left ventricular
d. ▸ left ventricular muscle

d., Legg-Calvé-Waldenström
d., Legionnaires'
d., Leiner's
d., Lenegre's
d., leptomeningeal
d., lethal
d. ▸ lethal neuromuscular
d., Letterer-Siwe
d., Lev's
d., levels of
d. ▸ Lewis upper limb
   cardiovascular
d. ▸ Lewy body
d. ▸ lifelong, relapsing
d., life-threatening
d. (GVHD) ▸ life-threatening graft
   vs. host
d., light chain
d., Lignac-Fanconi
d., Lignac's
d., Lindau-von Hippel
d., Little's
d., liver
d., local
d., localized
d., localized unresectable
d., Löffler's
d. ▸ long-term neurologic
d. ▸ loss of appetite from Addison's
d. ▸ loss of appetite from Crohn's
d., Lou Gehrig
d. ▸ low grade
d., lower obstructive airway
d., lower obstructive lung
d. ▸ lower risk of heart
d., Lucas-Championnière's
d., luetic
d., lung
d. ▸ lupus-associated valve
d., Lutembacher's
d., Lyme
d., lymph node
d. ▸ lymphocytic infiltrative
d., lymphoproliferative
d., mad cow
d., Maher's
d. Maladie-de-Roger
d., malignant
d. ▸ malnourished patient with
   chronic
d. manageable
d. management
d. ▸ maple bark
d. (MSUD), maple syrup urine
d., Marchiafava-Bignami

d., Marek's
d., Marie-Tooth
d., Masuda-Kitahara
d., Mathieu's
d., Mattingly
d., McArdle's
d. ▸ medical student's
d., medullary
d., medullary cystic
d., Meleda
d., mendelian
d., Meniere's
d., meningococcal
d., mental
d., Mentrier's
d., Merzbacher-Pelizaeus
d., metabolic
d., metabolic bone
d., metastatic
d., metastatic brain
d., metastatic lung
d., microvascular
d. ▸ middle ear
d., Mikulicz's
d. ▸ mild atherosclerotic vascular
d., Mills'
d., Milroy's
d. ▸ minimal residual
d. ▸ minimize risk of transfusion-
   related
d., mitochondrial
d., mitral valve
d., mitral valvular
d. (MCTD) ▸ mixed connective
   tissue
d., mixed nodular type ▸
   Hodgkin's
d., Möbius
d. modifying antirheumatic drug
   (DMARD)
d. modifying drugs ▸ suppressive
   or
d., Monday
d., Mondor's
d., Monge's
d., Morel-Kraepelin
d., Morgagni's
d., Morquio's
d. mortality ▸ coronary artery
d., motor neuron
d., moyamoya
d. ▸ multi-infarct
d., multisystem
d. ▸ multisystem occlusive
d., multivalvular

disease(s)—*continued*

d., multivessel
d. murmur, aortic-mitral combined
d. murmur ▸ multivalvular
d. ▸ muscle paralyzing
d., muscle wasting
d., muscular
d., Myà's
d., myeloproliferative
d., myocardial
d., myocardial ischemic
d. ▸ myoclonic epilepsy and ragged red fiber (MERRF)
d., nasal sinus
d., neoplastic
d., nerve
d. ▸ nerve damaging
d., neurodegenerative
d., neuroendocrinological
d., neurologic
d., neurological
d., neuromuscular
d., neuromyopathic
d., Newcastle
d., newly acquired
d., Nicolas-Favre
d., Niemann
d., Niemann-Pick
d., no appreciable
d. (NED), no evidence of
d., no evidence of active
d. (NERD), no evidence of recurrent
d., no significant
d., noninfectious
d. ▸ nonlethal underlying
d., nonmalignant chest
d., nonmeningeal cryptococcal
d. ▸ nontuberculous mycobacterial
d., Norrie's
d. ▸ obesity-related
d., obliterative vascular
d., obstructive
d., obstructive airway
d., obstructive lung
d., obstructive pulmonary
d., occlusive
d., occlusive vascular
d., occult metastatic
d., occupational lung
d., ocular
d. of artery ▸ stiffness from
d. of back, degenerative
d. of blood, malignant
d. of bone ▸ Paget's

d. of bowel ▸ inflammatory
d. of brain, degenerative
d. of breast, cystic
d. of breast ▸ Paget's
d. of breasts, bilateral ▸ fibrocystic
d. of childhood, chronic granulomatous
d. of childhood ▸ granulomatous
d. of cortex, local
d. of diffuse, histiocytic lymphocyte depleted type ▸ Hodgkin's
d. of heart (VDH), valvular
d. of legs, vascular
d. of liver ▸ veno-occlusive
d. of lungs, infectious
d. of nervous system, hereditary
d. (CMID) of newborn ▸ cytomegalic inclusion
d. of newborn (HDN), hemolytic
d. of newborn, hemorrhagic
d. of pancreas ▸ chronic inflammatory
d. of pleura ▸ malignant
d., Ollier's
d. ▸ one stage esophagectomy in benign
d., Oppenheim's
d., opportunistic
d., organic
d., organic brain
d., organic heart
d., Osgood-Schlatter
d., Osler
d., Osler-Vaquez
d., osseous metastatic
d., Otto's
d. outbreaks
d. ▸ over-reactive airway
d. ▸ overt symptom of heart
d., Pabry's
d., Paget's
d. ▸ pain in abdomen from Addison's
d. ▸ pain in abdomen from Crohn's
d. ▸ pale stool with Crohn's
d., palliation in advanced metastatic
d., palliation in early metastatic
d., pancreatic
d., pandemic
d., paralytic
d., parasitic
d., parathyroid
d. ▸ parenchymal lung
d., Parkinson's
d., paroxysmal

d., Parrot's
d., Parry's
d., Parsons'
d., Patella's
d., pathogenesis of the
d., patient had relapse of
d., patient's underlying
d., Pauzat's
d., Pavy's
d., Payr's
d., pediatric
d., Pelizaeus-Merzbacher
d., Pellegrini-Stieda
d. (PID), pelvic inflammatory
d., peptic inflammatory
d. (PUD), peptic ulcer
d., pericardial
d., periodontal
d., peripheral
d. (PAD) ▸ peripheral arterial
d., peripheral arteriosclerotic occlusive
d. ▸ peripheral artery
d. ▸ peripheral atherosclerotic
d. ▸ peripheral nervous system
d. (PVD), peripheral vascular
d., Perrin-Ferraton
d., Perthes
d., Peyronie's
d., physical manifestation of
d., Pick's
d., pigeon breeder's
d., pink
d., pituitary Cushing's
d., plaques of Alzheimer's
d., pleural
d., Plummer
d., pneumococcal
d., pneumoconiosis-type
d. (PKD), polycystic kidney
d. ▸ polycystic ovary
d., polygenic
d., polyradicular joint
d. ▸ polysaccharide storage
d., Pompe's
d., Posada-Wernicke
d., positive end expiratory
d. ▸ postmenopausal heart
d., potentially fatal
d., potentially terminal
d., Pott's
d., Poulet's
d. ▸ preclinical heart muscle
d. ▸ predisposition to
d. ▸ pre-existing coronary

d. ► pre-existing hepatic
d., Preiser's
d., premature
d. ► premature cardiovascular
d. ► premature coronary
d., premature heart
d. ► premature vascular
d. prenatally, diagnose
d., presumptive metastatic
d., prevent heart
d. ► prevent transmission of
d., preventable
d., preventing
d. prevention
d., prevention and control of
d. prevention, cardiovascular
d. preventive lifestyles
d., primary
d., primary hepatic
d. ► primary inflammatory
d., primary lung
d., primary myocardial
d. ► primary pulmonary
   parenchymal
d., primary renal
d., primary thyroid
d. process
d. process, active
d. process ► inflammatory
d. process ► life-threatening
d. process, progressive
   degenerative
d. process, regression of
d. process ► underlying
d. -producing bacteria
d. producing drug ► addictive
D. (ESRD) Program, End Stage
   Renal
d. progressed slowly
d. progression, delay
d., progression of
d., progression of myocardial
d., progressive
d. ► progressive brain
d. ► progressive, debilitating,
   incurable brain
d., progressive degenerative
d. ► progressive idiopathic
   neuromuscular
d., progressive neuromuscular
d., progressive organic brain
d. ► progressive rheumatic
d. -prone personality
d., prostate
d. ► protein loss in hepatic

d., psychiatric
d. ► psychological manifestations of
   physical
d., psychosomatic
d., pulmonary
d., pulmonary thromboembolic
d. ► pulmonary valve
d. ► pulmonary vascular
d. ► pulmonary vascular obstructive
d. ► pulmonary veno-occlusive
d., pulp
d., pulseless
d., Purtscher's
d., Quincke
d., radiation-induced
d., radiation-linked
d. ► radiation lung
d., ragpicker's
d., ragsorter's
d., rapid dissemination of
d., rapidly advancing
d., rapidly disseminating
d., rapidly progressive pulmonary
d., rare
d., rate of progress
d., Raynaud's
d., reactive airway
d., recurrence of
d., recurrent
d., recurrent Hodgkin's
d., refractive
d., Refsum
d., regression of
d., rehabilitation of heart
d., Reichmann's
d., Reis-Bückler
d., Reiter's
d., relapsing
d. -related death
d. -related pattern ► non-
   Alzheimer's
d., remission of
d., remittent
d., renal
d. ► renal artery
d., renal cystic
d., renal parenchymal
d., Rendu-Osler-Weber
d., renovascular
D. Research, Alzheimer's
D. Research Laboratories (VDRL)
   Test, Venereal
d., residual
d., residual lung

d. (PID) residues, pelvic
   inflammatory
d., resistance to
d., respiratory
d. ► respiratory muscle
d., restrictive
d. ► restrictive airway
d. (HD), restrictive heart
d., restrictive lung
d. ► retina vascular lesion
d., retinal
d. ► reverse coronary
d. ► reverse heart
d. ► reversible obstructive airway
d., rheumatic heart
d., rheumatic valvular
d. ► rheumatoid lung
d., rickettsial
d., Riedel's
d., right ventricular
d. risk
d. risk factor ► heart-
d., risk of heart
d. ► risk of infectious
d. ► risk of kidney
d., Roger's
d., Rokitansky's
d., Romberg's
d., Rosenthal's
d., Roth-Bernhardt
d., Roth's
d., Roussy Lëvy
d., Russell Brain
d. ► salivary gland
d. ► San Joaquin Valley
d., Schamberg's
d., Schanz's
d., Schaumann's
d., Scheuermann's
d., Schilder's
d., Schlatter's
d., Schmorl's
d., Scholz's
d., Schüller-Christian
d. screening ► heart
d. screening ► peripheral arterial
d., secondary connective tissue
d., self-destructive
d., Selter's
d. ► sensory motor
d., serious gum
d., serological markers of
D. Service, Infectious
d. ► severe alcoholic liver
d. ► severe brain stem

disease(s)—_continued_

d. ▸ severe chronic
d. ▸ severe mitral valve
d., severe occlusive
d. ▸ severe renal vascular
d. ▸ severe valvular
d. (CVD) ▸ severity of cardiovascular
d., Sever's
d. ▸ sex-linked
d. (STD), sexually transmitted
d. (PID) ▸ sexually transmitted pelvic inflammatory
d., Shaver's
d., Sheehan's
d., Shoshin
d., shuttlemaker's
d., Sichel's
d., sickle cell
d., sickle cell-hemoglobin C
d., sickle cell-hemoglobin D
d., sickle cell thalassemia
d., Siever's
d., silent
d. ▸ silent coronary artery
d. ▸ silent ischemic heart
d., silo filler's
d., Simmonds'
d. ▸ single gene
d. ▸ single vessel
d., sinopulmonary
d., sinus
d. ▸ sinus node
d. site, unsuspected
d., Sjögren's
d., skeletal
d., slim
d. ▸ slowly developing brain
d. ▸ small airway
d., small duct
d. ▸ small vessel
d., smoking-related
d. (TED) socks, thromboembolic
d., Spielmeyer-Vogt
d., spinal cord
d., spinal disc
d., spinocerebellar degenerative
d., Spira's
d., spirochetal
d. staging
d., Starbardt's
d. state
d., Steinert's
d., Sternberg's
d., Still's

d. (TED) stockings, thromboembolic
d., stress of heart
d., stress-related
d., Stuart-Bras
d., Stühmer's
d., Sturge-Weber-Dimitri
d., Sturge's
d., subclinical
d., Sudeck's
d. ▸ support groups for Alzheimer's
d., suppurative oropharyngeal
d., surgical
d., surgical management of metastatic
d. ▸ surgical treatment for Parkinson's
d., suspected infectious
d., Swediaur's
d. ▸ sweet clover
d., symptomatic
d. ▸ symptomatic alcohol heart muscle
d., symptomatic gallbladder
d. ▸ symptomatic progression of
d. syndrome (RADS) ▸ reactive airways
d. syndrome, respiratory
d. synthesis
d. —syphilis (VDS), venereal
d., systemic
d. ▸ Takayasu-Ohnishi
d. ▸ Takayasu's
d., Talma's
d., Tangier
d., target organ
d. ▸ Taussig-Bing
d., Tay-Sachs
d., terminal
d. therapy ▸ heart
d., Thomsen's
d., thoracic
d., Thornwaldt's
d. ▸ three vessel
d. (TED), thromboembolic
d., thyrocardiac
d., thyroid
d. ▸ thyroid eye
d., thyrotoxic heart
d., Tietze's
d., Tillaux's
d. ▸ tissue and bone
d. to pursue natural course
d., Tornwaldt's
d., Tourette's

d., transfer of
d., transfusion associated
d., transfusion-related
d., transfusion transmitted
d. transmission
d., transmitted
d. ▸ transplant coronary artery
d. ▸ traumatic heart
d., traveler's
d., treatable
d., treatable mental
d., treatment of
d. ▸ treatment of digestive
d., treatment of heart
d. ▸ tricuspid valve
d. triggered
d., triple vessel
d., trophoblastic
d., tropical
d. ▸ true-negative undetected
d., tsutsugamushi
d. ▸ ulcerative bowel
d. ▸ ulcerative colitis with Crohn's
d., underlying
d. ▸ underlying obstructive coronary
d., undetected microscopic
d. ▸ undiagnosed thyroid
d., unilateral
d., unknown origin ▸ myocardial
d., unrecognized
d. ▸ untreatable coronary
d., untreated
d., Unverricht's
d., upper airway
d., upper respiratory
d. (UCD) ▸ usual childhood
d. vaccine ▸ Lyme
d., vaccine preventable
d., Valsuani's
d., valvular
d., valvular heart
d., Vaquez
d., Vaquez-Osler
d. (vCJD) ▸ variant Creutzfeldt-Jakob
d., vascular
d. ▸ vascular heart
d. ▸ vector-borne
d. ▸ vector of
d. (VD) ▸ venereal
d., venous
d. ▸ vertebrobasilar occlusive
d., vessel
d., vestibular
d., vibration

d., viral
d., viral hematodepressive
d. virus, Australian X
d. (CMID) virus ▸ cytomegalic inclusion
d. virus, exanthematous
d. virus ▸ fifth
d. virus, Kyasanur Forest
d. virus (NDV) ▸ Newcastle
d., virulent
d., Vogt's
d., Vogt-Spielmeyer
d., Volkmann's
d., von Gierke's
d., von Graefe's
d., von Hippel-Lindau
d., von Recklinghausen's
d., von Rokitansky's
d., von Willebrand's
d., Wagner's
d. ▸ warning signs of eye
d. ▸ warning signs of sexually transmitted
d., wasting
d., Weber-Christian
d., Wegener's
d., Weil's
d., Weir Mitchell's
d., Wenckebach's
d. ▸ Werdnig-Hoffman
d., Werner's
d., Wernicke's
d., Westphal-Strümpell
d. ▸ wheat weevil
d., Whipple's
d., Wilson's
d., Winkelman's
d. ▸ winter vomiting
d., Woillez'
d. ▸ woven coronary artery
d., Ziehen-Oppenheim
d., zoonotic

diseased
d. aorta
d. artery
d. bone
d. brain, Alzheimer's
d. brain cells, Alzheimer's
d. cardiac tissue
d. colon
d. condition
d. coronary artery
d. eye
d. gene
d. heart

d. heart muscle
d. heart valve
d. joint
d. joint with inflammation
d. human heart
d. kidney
d. lobe
d. marrow
d. mitral valve
d. organ
d. portion
d. segment of bowel
d. tissue
d. tissue specimen
d. tissue, vaporizing
d. valve
d. vessel

disembodied heart
disfigured
d., cells, irregular
d. smile
d. tissue
disfigurement, facial
disfigurement, permanent
disguised infection
disguised infection ▸ patient admitted with
disgust ▸ fear, doubt or
dish
d. -pan fracture
d., Petri
d. sorter
disharmonic hearing, double
disillusioned, patient
disinfecting fluid, Burnett's
disinfecting solution
disinfection
d. and antisepsis
d. and antisepsis ▸ sterilization,
d., chemical
d., concomitant
d., concurrent
d., skin
d., terminal
d., wet
disintegrating kidney stones
disintegration(s)
d., family
d. ▸ increased personality
d., monitor stone
d. of cognitive brain function
d. of judgment
d. of muscle
d. of personality
d. per minute (dpm)

d. rate
d., tissue
disintegrative disorder ▸ childhood
disintegrative psychosis
disinterest in personal appearance
disinterested witness
disjointed, agitated movement
disjointed movement
disjunctive nystagmus
disjunctive symbiosis
disk
d., Amici's
d., anangioid
d. aortic valve prosthesis ▸ tilting
d. cage valve
d., ciliary
d., crushing of intervertebral
d. decompression, percutaneous laser
d. degeneration ▸ spinal
d. electrode
d., floppy
d. kidney
d. occluder prosthesis ▸ Rashkind double-
d., optic
d. oxygenation ▸ rotating
d. prosthetic valve ▸ tilting
d., Rekoss
d. -shaped retinopathy, central
d. stamper, optical
d., stroboscopic
d. valve prosthesis, Beall
d. valve prosthesis ▸ Medtronic-Hall tilting
d. valve prosthesis ▸ Omniscience-tilting
d. valve prosthesis ▸ Starr-Edwards
d., vaporize water in herniated
diskectomy(-ies)
d., percutaneous
d., percutaneous automated
d. technique
dislocated
d. clavicle
d. elbow
d. eye lens
d. hip
d. joint, manipulation of
d. medial meniscus
d. otoconia
d. patella
d. shoulder
dislocation
d., Bankart procedure for shoulder

dislocation—*continued*
d., capitate
d., chronic
d., chronic shoulder
d., closed
d., complete
d., complicated
d., compound
d., congenital
d., congenital hip
d., consecutive
d., divergent
d., economic
d., femur
d., fracture-
d., habitual
d. head of radius
d. hip, congenital
d., incomplete
d., intrauterine
d., joint
d., Kienböck's
d., lens
d., lunate
d., Monteggia's
d., Nélaton's
d. of cartilage
d. of joint
d. of knee
d. of lacrimal gland
d. of patella
d. of shoulder joint, anterior
d., old
d., open
d., painful
d., paralunate
d., partial
d., pathologic
d., perilunate
d., recent
d., recurrent
d., simple
d., Smith's
d., social
d., subastragalar
d., subcoracoid
d., subglenoid
d., TMJ (temporomandibular joint)
d., traumatic
d., voluntary
dislodged, intrauterine device (IUD)
dislodgement, atrial lead
disloyalty ▸ guilt over
dismutase (SOD) ▸ superoxide
disomy, human uniparental

disorder(s)
d., academic underachievement
d., acid base
d., active bleeding
d., active neurologic
d., acute
d., acute mental
d., acute psychiatric
d., acute psychotic thought
d., acute toxic
d., addictive
d., adjustment
d., adolescent psychiatric
d., adult
d., adult factitious
d., affective
d., affective personality
d., aggressive type ▸
   undersocialized conduct
d. ▸ agoraphobia without history of
   panic
d., alcohol amnestic
d., alcohol-induced
d., alcohol-induced amnestic
d., alcohol-related cerebral
d., alcohol-related heart
d., alcohol-related skin
d., alcoholism
d., allergic
d., amnestic
d., amphetamine delusional
d., anal
d., anancastic personality
d., anger
d., anorexia
d., antisocial personality
d., anxiety
d. ▸ anxiety-related muscle
d., anxiolytic amnestic
d., aortic valve
d., aphthous
d., arithmetical
d., arterial
d. as reaction to stress ▸ mixed
d., associated features and
D. Association ▸ American Sleep
d. ▸ asymptomatic metabolic
d., asymptomatic pulmonary valve
d., atopic
d. (ADD), attention deficit
d. (ADHD), attention deficit
   hyperactivity
d., atypical depressive
d., atypical manic
d., auditory

d., autistic
d., autistic spectrum
d., autism
d., autoimmune
d., avoidant
d., avoidant personality
d., Axis two
d., balance
d., behavior
d. ▸ benign rhythm
d., binge eating
d., biological
d. ▸ biological brain
d., biopsychosocial
d., bipolar
d., bipolar affective
d., bleeding
d., blood
d., blood-borne
d., blood cell
d., blood clotting
d., blood fat
d., blood platelet
d., blood vessel
d. (BDD), body dysmorphic
d., body movement
d., bone
d., borderline
d. (BPD), borderline personality
d., bowel
d., brain
d. ▸ brain destroying
d., breathing
d., cannabis delusional
d., cardiac
d., cardiac valve
d., cardiovascular
d., catatonic schizophrenic
d. center, sleep
d., central nervous system (CNS)
d., cerebral
d., cerebrovascular
d., character
d., chemical dependence
d. ▸ chest pain from TMJ
d., chest wall
d., childhood
d., childhood anxiety
d., childhood behavioral
d. ▸ childhood disintegrative
d., childhood learning
d., childhood neurodevelopmental
   dysfunction
d., childhood psychiatric
d. ▸ childhood shyness

d., chronic
d. ▸ chronic autoimmune
d., chronic brain
d., chronic cardiovascular
d., chronic connective tissue
d. ▸ chronic cough
d. ▸ chronic cyclic pulmonary
d., chronic debilitating
d. ▸ chronic depressive personality
d., chronic digestive
d., chronic gastrointestinal (GI)
d. ▸ chronic hypomanic personality
d., chronic immune
d., chronic lung
d., chronic metabolic
d. ▸ chronic motor or vocal tic
d. ▸ chronic motor tic
d. ▸ chronic neurologic
d. ▸ chronic pulmonary
d., chronic relapsing
d., chronic voice
d. ▸ circadian rhythm disturbance
d. ▸ circadian rhythm sleep
d., circulatory
d., clinical
d., clinical epileptic
d., clotting
d., CNS (central nervous system)
d., coagulation
d., cocaine delusional
d., cocaine-related
d., cocaine-related obstetric
d., coexisting psychiatric
d., collagen
d., comorbidity of mental
d., communicative
d. ▸ complex developmental
d. ▸ complex sleep
d., compulsive
d., compulsive impulse control
d., compulsive personality
d., computer addiction
d., conduct
d., congenital
d., congenital aortic valve
d. ▸ congenital retinal
d., connective tissue
d. control, impulse
d., conversion
d., convulsive
d., co-occurring mood
d., coordination
d., cornea
d., crippling
d., cumulative trauma

d., cutaneous
d., cyclic
d., cyclothymic
d., debilitating
d., debilitating sleep
d., degenerative
d., degenerative brain
d., degenerative genetic
d., degenerative muscle
d., delusional
d. ▸ delusional mood
d., dementia
d., denial of
d., dental
d., dependent personality
d., depersonalization
d., depressed ▸ bipolar
d., depressed ▸ bipolar affective
d., depressed, in full remission ▸ bipolar
d., depressed, in partial remission ▸ bipolar
d., depressed, mild ▸ bipolar
d., depressed, moderate ▸ bipolar
d., depressed, severe, without psychotic features ▸ bipolar
d., depressed, unspecified ▸ bipolar
d., depressed, with psychotic features ▸ bipolar
d., depressive
d., dermatological
d., deteriorating neurological
d., developmental
d., developmental arithmetic
d., developmental articulation
d., developmental coordination
d. ▸ developmental expressive language
d. ▸ developmental expressive writing
d., developmental language
d., developmental reading
d. ▸ developmental receptive language
d., developmental speech
d., deviations
d., diaphragm
d., digestive
d., digestive tract
d., disabling genetic
d. ▸ disabling joint
d., disorganized schizophrenic
d., disruptive behavior
d., dissociation
d. ▸ dissociation in eating

d., dissociative
d. ▸ dissociative identity
d., distinct psychiatric
d. ▸ dizziness from TMJ
d. ▸ dramatic cluster
d., dream anxiety
d., drug
d. ▸ drug-induced gastrointestinal
d. ▸ drug-induced mental
d., dual
d., dysthymic
d., eating
d., electrolyte
d., emotional
d., endocrine
d., epilepsy and seizure
d., epileptic
d., epileptoid personality
d., esophageal
d., esophageal motility
d., esophageal sphincter
d., esophagus
d. ▸ evaluation treatment of eating
d., exacerbation of preexisting
d., explosive personality
d., expressive
d. ▸ extrapyramidal nerve
d., eye
d. facilities ▸ certified sleep-
d., factitious
d., fatal
d., fatal blood
d., fatal eating
d. ▸ female sexual arousal
d., fetal genetic
d., flashbacks and anxiety
d., foot
d. from aspirin ▸ skin
d. from birth control pill ▸ skin
d. from blood problem
d. ▸ full-blown panic
d., functional
d. ▸ functional gastrointestinal (GI)
d. ▸ gait and balance
d., gastric
d., gastric tract
d., gastroesophageal
d., gastrointestinal (GI)
d., gender identity
d., general anxiety
d., generalized anxiety
d., genetic
d. ▸ genetic connective tissue
d. ▸ genetic digestive
d., Gilles de la Tourette's

disorder(s)—*continued*

d., glandular
d., glomerular
d., glycosphingolipid
d., group type ▸ conduct
d., hallucinogen delusional
d., hallucinogen mood
d. ▸ hallucinogen persisting
  perception
d., hand
d., hearing
d., heart
d., heart rate
d. ▸ heart rhythm
d. ▸ heart valve
d., heat-related
d., hematologic
d., hematological
d., hereditary
d. ▸ hereditary bleeding
d. ▸ heterogeneity of psychiatric
d., high altitude related
d., histrionic personality
d., hormonal
d., hormone
d., human genetic
d. ▸ human immunodeficiency virus
  (HIV) associated motor cognitive
d. (HDD) ▸ humor deficit
d., hyperkinetic conduct
d., hypersensitivity
d. (nonorganic) ▸ hypersomnia
  related to another mental
d., hypnotic amnestic
d. ▸ hypoactive sexual desire
d., hysterical
d. ▸ hysterical conversion
d., iatrogenic
d., identity
d., idiopathic
d., idiopathic seizure
d., immune
d., immune system
d., immunodeficient
d., immunohematologic
d., immunologic
d., immunologic deficiency
d. ▸ impairment from
d., impulse control
d. ▸ impulse dyscontrol in eating
d. in adolescents ▸ emotional and
  behavioral
d. in adults ▸ emotional and
  behavioral

d. in children ▸ emotional and
  behavioral
d. in drug abusers, psychiatric
d., incurable
d., incurable brain
d., incurable mental
d., induced psychotic
d., infectious
d., infective
d., inflammatory
d. ▸ inflammatory bowel
d. ▸ inflammatory intestinal
d. ▸ inflammatory joint
d., inherited
d., inherited bleeding
d. ▸ inherited blood
d. ▸ inherited brain
d. ▸ inherited immune
d. ▸ inherited metabolic
d. ▸ inherited nerve
d. initiating sleep ▸ persistent
d., inner ear
d. (nonorganic) ▸ insomnia related
  to mental
d. ▸ intermittent affective
d., intermittent explosive
d. ▸ intermittent explosive
  personality
d., internal
d., intestinal
d., intraocular
d., involuntary movement
d. (IDD) ▸ iodine deficiency
d., irreversible
d., isolated explosive
d., joint
d. ▸ joint-related
d. ▸ juvenile anxiety
d., kidney
d., kinesthetic
d., knee joint alignment
d., labyrinthine
d., language
d. ▸ late luteal phase dysphoric
d., learning
d., life-threatening
d., life-threatening rhythm
d., lipid
d., liver
d. ▸ long-term mood
d., loss
d., lung
d., lymphatic
d. ▸ lymphocytic infiltrative
d., lymphoproliferative

d., major affective
d. (MDD), major depressive
d., major mental
d. ▸ major mood
d., male erectile
d., malignant blood
d., manic ▸ bipolar affective
d., manic-depressive
d., manic, in full remission ▸ bipolar
d., manic, in partial remission ▸
  bipolar
d., manic, mild ▸ bipolar
d., manic, moderate ▸ bipolar
d. ▸ manic phase of bipolar
d., manic, severe, without psychotic
  features ▸ bipolar
d., manic, unspecified ▸ bipolar
d., manic, with psychotic features ▸
  bipolar
d., medical
d., medical management of eating
d., memory
d., mendelian
d., menstrual
d., menstruation
d., mental
d., metabolic
d. ▸ metatarsophalangeal joint
d., methamphetamine-induced
d. ▸ methamphetamine-induced
  organic mental
d. ▸ mild pulmonary valve
d., misery and unhappiness
d. ▸ mitral valve
d., mixed ▸ bipolar
d., mixed ▸ bipolar affective
d., mixed development
d., mixed, in full remission ▸ bipolar
d., mixed, in partial remission ▸
  bipolar
d., mixed, mild ▸ bipolar
d., mixed, moderate ▸ bipolar
d., mixed seizure
d., mixed, severe, without psychotic
  features ▸ bipolar
d., mixed, unspecified ▸ bipolar
d., mixed, with psychotic features ▸
  bipolar
d. monitor progression of
d., monogenic
d., monoproliferative
d., mood
d., motility
d., motion
d., motor

d. ▸ motor function
d., mouth
d., movement
d., multifaceted personality
d., multiple
d., multiple personality
d. ▸ multiple personality dissociative
d. ▸ multiplex personality
d., multisystem
d., muscle
d., muscular
d., musculoskeletal
d., myeloproliferative
d., myopathic
d., narcissistic personality
d. ▸ negativistic personality
d., neoplastic
d., nerve
d. ▸ nerve cell
d., nervous
d. ▸ neural tube
d., neurodegenerative
d., neurogenic bladder
d., neurologic
d. ▸ neurologic voice
d., neurological
d., neuromuscular
d., neuromyopathic
d., neuropathic
d., neuropsychiatric
d., neurotic
d. (dream anxiety disorder) ▸ nightmare
d. ▸ nonaffective psychotic
d., nonictal psychiatric
d., noninfectious
d. ▸ non-life-threatening
d., nonmalignant
d., nonorganic sleep
d., nonpsychotic mental
d., nonpsychotic psychiatric
d., non-substance-induced
d., nutritional
d. (OCD) ▸ obsessive-compulsive
d. ▸ obsessive-compulsive conduct
d. ▸ obsessive-compulsive personality
d. ▸ obsessive-compulsive spectrum
d., obstetric
d., occupational
d. ▸ occupational lung
d., ocular
d. of adenoids
d. of adolescence ▸ avoidant

d. of adolescence, complex
d. of adolescence ▸ emancipation
d. of adolescence or adulthood, nontranssexual type ▸ gender identity
d. of adolescence ▸ gender identity
d. of adult life ▸ gender identity
d. of amino acid metabolism
d. of body ▸ whole common
d. of bone ▸ common
d. of brain and nervous system
d. of brain and spinal cord ▸ focal
d. of brain, physical
d. of breast ▸ common
d. of cheek ▸ skin
d. of childhood, anxiety
d. of childhood ▸ avoidant
d. of childhood, complex
d. of childhood ▸ gender identity
d. of childhood ▸ introverted
d. of childhood or adolescence ▸ avoidant
d. of childhood ▸ shyness
d. of childhood ▸ transient tic
d. of circulation ▸ common
d. of coordination
d. of drug abusers, sexual
d. of early adult life ▸ emancipation
d. of early childhood ▸ reactive attachment
d. of facial nerve
d. of heartbeat rhythm
d. of hyponatremia
d. of impulse control
d. of infancy or early childhood ▸ reactive attachment
d. of infancy ▸ reactive attachment
d. of infancy ▸ rumination
d. of initiating sleep ▸ transient
d. of initiating wakefulness ▸ persistent
d. of initiating wakefulness ▸ transient
d. of lungs
d. of maintaining sleep ▸ persistent
d. of maintaining sleep ▸ transient
d. of maintaining wakefulness ▸ persistent
d. of maintaining wakefulness ▸ transient
d. of mood
d. of motor power
d. of muscular coordination
d. of nervous system, degenerative

d. of normal bone chemistry
d. of psychosexual identity
d. of psychotic depth ▸ severe
d. of sensation
d. of urinary excretion
d. of uvula, birth
d., oppositional
d. (ODD) ▸ oppositional defiant
d., optic nerve
d., organic
d., organic anxiety
d., organic brain
d., organic delusional
d., organic mental
d. ▸ organic mental syndrome
d., organic mood
d., organic personality
d., overactive thyroid
d., overanxious
d., overeating
d., ovulation
d., pain
d. ▸ pain in back from TMJ
d. ▸ pain in ear from TMJ
d., painful nerve
d., panic
d., painful anxiety
d., pancreatic
d., paranoid
d., paranoid personality
d. ▸ Parkinson's tremor
d. ▸ passive aggressive personality
d. ▸ past psychiatric
d. patient ▸ eating
d. patient ▸ panic
d. patient ▸ seizure
d. patient ▸ stress
d., perceptive
d., perceptual
d., periluteal phase dysphoric
d. (PLMD) ▸ periodic limb movement
d., peripheral nerve
d. ▸ persecutory delusional
d., personality
d., pervasive developmental
d. ▸ phencyclidine (PCP) delusional
d. ▸ phencyclidine (PCP) mood
d. ▸ phencyclidine (PCP) organic mental
d., phobic
d., physical
d., physical stress

disorder(s)—*continued*

d., physiologic
d., pituitary
d., platelet
d., polygenic
d., postencephalitic behavior
d., posthallucinogen perception
d. (PTSD), post-traumatic stress
d. ▸ potentially serious psychosocial
d., predominance of major affective
d. ▸ pre-existing bipolar
d., pregnancy
d. ▸ pre-malignant
d, premenstrual dysphoric
d., previous seizure
d., primary
d. ▸ primary eye
d. ▸ primary generalized seizure
d. ▸ primary headache
d., progressive
d. ▸ progressive brain
d., progressive irreversible
d., progressive mental
d., progressive movement
d. ▸ progressive neurological
d., prolonged eating
d. ▸ prolonged post-traumatic stress
d., psychiatric
d. ▸ psychoactive substance abuse
d. ▸ psychoactive substance
   amnestic
d. ▸ psychoactive substance anxiety
d. ▸ psychoactive substance
   induced organic mental
d. ▸ psychoactive substance mood
d. ▸ psychoactive substance
   organic metal
d. ▸ psychoactive substance
   personality
d. ▸ psychoactive substance use
d., psychogenic
d., psychological
d., psychoneurotic
d., psychophysiologic
d., psychosexual
d., psychosomatic
d., psychospiritual
d. ▸ psychotherapy of post-
   traumatic stress
d., psychotic
d., psychotic thought
d. ▸ pulmonary heart valve
d. ▸ pulmonary interstitial
d. ▸ pulmonary valve
d., pulmonary vascular

d., purging
d., rage
d., range of
d., rare skin
d., reactive
d. ▸ reactive attachment
d. (RAD) ▸ reactive attention
d., reading
d., receptive
d., recurrent episode ▸ major
   depressive
d., related
d., related heart
d., relational
d., renal
d., repetitive motion
d. ▸ repetitive stress
d., respiratory
d., retinal
d. ▸ rhythmic movement
d., rickettsial
d. ▸ road rage
d. ▸ salivary gland
d., schizoaffective
d., schizoid personality
d., schizophrenic
d. ▸ schizophrenic spectrum
d. ▸ schizophrenic thought
d., schizophreniform
d., schizotypal personality
d., seasonal
d. (SAD), seasonal affective
d. ▸ seasonal mood
d., secondary
d., sedative amnestic
d., seizure
d. ▸ self-defeating personality
d. ▸ sensitivity, shyness, social
   withdrawal
d., sensory
d. (SAD) ▸ separation anxiety
d., serious brain
d. ▸ severe articulation
d. ▸ severe behavior
d. ▸ severe characteristic
d., severe characterological
d., severe epileptic
d., severe inherited
d. ▸ severe lung
d. ▸ severe personality
d., severe rhythm
d., sex-linked
d., sexual
d., sexual aversion
d., shaking

d., shared paranoid
d. ▸ shared psychotic
d., sickle cell
d., single episode ▸ major
   depressive
d., single episode ▸ manic
d. ▸ single gene
d. ▸ single symptom
d., sinusitis
d., situational
d., skeletal
d. ▸ skeletal muscle
d., skin
d., sleep
d. ▸ sleep behavior
d., sleep maintenance
d., sleep pattern
d. ▸ sleep related
d., sleep terror
d., sleep-wake
d. ▸ sleep-wake schedule
d., sleeping
d., sleepwalking
d. ▸ slowly progressive hereditary
d., smell
d., smoking-related
d., socialized conduct
d., solitary aggressive type ▸
   conduct
d., somatization
d., somatoform
d., somatoform pain
d., somnambulism
d., specific developmental
d., speech
d. ▸ speech and language
d. ▸ sphincter of Oddi dysmotility
d. ▸ spinal cord
d., static
d., stereotype/habit
d., stomach
d., stress
d., stress-related
d. ▸ stroke-related
d., structural
d., substance abuse
d. ▸ substance dependence
d. ▸ substance-induced
d. ▸ substance-induced organic
   mental
d. ▸ substance-related
d., swallowing
d., sympathomimetic delusional
d. symptoms, eating
d. ▸ symptoms of neurological

d. syndrome (SADS) ▸ seasonal affective
d. syringomyelia (SM)
d., systemic
d. ▸ systemic vascular
d., taste
d., teeth grinding
d. ▸ terminal genetic
d., thought
d., thromboembolic
d., thyroid
d., tic
d., tobacco use
d., tongue
d., Tourette's
d., transient
d. ▸ transient organic mental
d., transient tic
d., transitory mental
d., treatable
d., treatable psychiatric
d. treatment, nervous
d. (OCD) ▸ treatment-resistant obsessive-compulsive
d. ▸ tricuspid valve
d., trigeminal
d., unaggressive type ▸ undersocialized conduct
d., underlying
d. ▸ underlying blood
d. ▸ underlying psychiatric
d. ▸ undifferentiated attention deficit
d., undifferentiated somatoform
d., undifferentiated type ▸ conduct
d., unipolar
d., unipolar depressive
d., unspecified ▸ eating
d. (nonpsychotic) ▸ unspecified mental
d. ▸ upper esophageal sphincter
d. ▸ upper extremity vascular
d. ▸ upper intestinal
d, urinary tract
d., variable
d., vascular
d., vascular bleeding
d., vasospastic
d., vein
d., vision
d., visual
d., voice
d., voiding
d. with agoraphobia ▸ panic
d. with anxious mood ▸ adjustment

d. with depressed mood ▸ adjustment
d. with disturbance of conduct ▸ adjustment
d. with hyperactivity ▸ attention deficit
d. with mixed disturbance of emotions and conduct ▸ adjustment
d. with mixed emotional features ▸ adjustment
d. with physical complaints ▸ adjustment
d. with physical symptoms ▸ factitious
d. with psychological symptoms ▸ factitious
d. with withdrawal ▸ adjustment
d. with work (or academic) inhibition ▸ adjustment
d., withdrawal
d., without agoraphobia ▸ panic
d., without hyperactivity ▸ attention deficit
d., writing
d. ▸ X-linked

disordered
d. action of heart (DAH)
d. bone growth
d. breathing ▸ sleep
d. eating
d. functioning
d. mind function
d. muscle tone
d. muscular movements
d. patient, mentally
d., sexually
d. sleep
d. state in brain
d. thinking
d. water balance (DWB)
d. water balance (DWB), chronic
d. water balance (DWB), severe
d. water balance (DWB) ▸ syndrome of

disorganization
d., brain
d. of neuronal function
d. ▸ segmental arterial

disorganized
d. behavior
d. behavior, grossly
d. dissociative state
d. globe
d. muscle fibers

d. muscular movements
d. schizophrenia
d. schizophrenic disorder
d. state
d. thinking
d. type, chronic ▸ schizophrenia
d. type, chronic with acute exacerbation ▸ schizophrenia,
d. type, subchronic ▸ schizo-phrenia
d. type, subchronic with acute exacerbation ▸ schizophrenia
d. type, unspecified ▸ schizophrenia,

disorientation
d., acute
d. and confusion
d. and fever
d. and hallucinations, patient has
d. and irritability
d. and personality change
d., confusion and
d., confusion and coma
d., confusion, and language loss
d., diarrhea and
d. ▸ fever, cough and
d. in place and time
d. ▸ irritability, irrationality and
d., marked
d., mental
d. of time and space
d. ▸ self-neglect, apathy and
d., spatial
d. with amnesia

disoriented
d. adult
d. and confused
d. and dysfunctional, patient
d. behavior
d. or slow thought process
d., patient
d. ▸ patient sweating and

dispar
d., Escherichia
d., Shigella
d. var. ceylonensis ▸ Escherichia
d. var. madampensis ▸ Escherichia

dispense medication
dispenser, medication
dispensing of drugs
dispensing tablets
disperse medium
dispersing
d. agent
d. electrode

d. lens

dispersion
- d. medium
- d. of light
- d., QT
- d., QT/QTc
- d., temporal

dispersive medium

displaced
- d. apical beat
- d. femoral neck fracture
- d., femur
- d. fracture
- d. slightly, fracture
- d. vertebra

displacement
- d. activity
- d. analysis, linear
- d., anterior
- d., anterolateral
- d., congenital hip
- d., disc
- d., downward
- d., inferior
- d., lateral
- d., macular
- d. of cartilage padding
- d. of eyeball, forward
- d. of fracture
- d. of fracture fragments
- d. of heart, congenital
- d. of larynx backward and upward
- d. of lower fragment
- d. of rectum
- d., phase angle of
- d. placentogram
- d., posterior
- d. reaction
- d. sensing device
- d., subcoracoid type
- d., traumatic
- d., volar

display(s)
- d. and analysis ▸ image
- d. camera, video
- d. console (DDC), direct
- d., ECG (electrocardiogram) tracing
- d. echo ▸ motion
- d. enduring bitterness
- d. extreme sarcasm
- d. hopelessness
- d. ▸ lack of emotional
- d. obscene gestures ▸ patient
- d. passive loneliness
- d. self-deprecation

d. technique, computerized
d. terminal (VDT) screen glare ▸ video
d. terminal (VDT), video
d. verbal outbursts

disposable
- d. airway
- d. bifocal contact lens
- d. cleansing enema set
- d. contact lenses ▸ soft
- d. elbow protector
- d. equipment
- d. examination gown
- d. examination sheet
- d. gloves
- d. heel protector
- d. manual resuscitator ▸ BagEasy
- d. mortuary gown
- d. syringe
- d. thermometer
- d. underpad
- d. washcloth

disposal, environmental waste
disposition, fetal
disposition, jovial
dispositional tolerance
disproportion (CPD) ▸ cephalopelvic
disproportion, fetopelvic
disproportionate growth
disregard
- d. for others ▸ pervasive pattern of
- d. for safety of others ▸ reckless
- d. for safety of self ▸ reckless
- d. for sensitivity of others ▸ relative
- d. rights of others

disrupt patient's rest
disrupted operative wound ▸ resuture
disrupted rhythm
disrupting ward, patient
disruption
- d., angry
- d. chemotherapy, blood-brain barrier
- d., family
- d. in brain, chemical
- d. in normal urination
- d. of bladder function
- d. of blood flow
- d. of cell, physical
- d. of evacuation ▸ bloating and
- d. of motor function
- d. of normal innervation
- d. of pancreatic duct
- d. of 24-hour sleep-wake cycle ▸ phase-shift

d. operative wound
d., pigment
d., plaque
d. ▸ short-term memory
d., sleep
d. ▸ traumatic aortic
d., wound

disruptive
- d. approach
- d. behavior
- d. behavior disorder
- d. child
- d. discharge
- d. effects
- d. levels
- d. mood swings
- d. patient
- d. sleep pattern

dissecans
- d., endometritis
- d., metritis
- d., osteochondritis
- d., pneumonia
- d. superficialis, esophagitis

dissecta, lingua
dissected
- d., bluntly
- d. free
- d. free, adhesions
- d. free ▸ inferior rectus muscle
- d., Tenon's capsule
- d. tissue arm

dissecting
- d. abdominal aortic aneurysm, reflux
- d. aneurysm
- d. aneurysm, acute
- d. aorta
- d. aortic aneurysm
- d. basilar artery aneurysm
- d. hemorrhage of midbrain
- d. metritis

dissection [*resection*]
- d., acute aortic
- d. and snare
- d. and snare tonsillectomy
- d. and stripping
- d., aortic
- d., arterial
- d., axillary lymph node
- d., block
- d., blunt
- d., blunt and sharp
- d., Bocca neck
- d., careful

d. carried upward, blunt
d., cervical
d., coronary artery
d., DeBakey-type aortic
d., digital
d., en bloc
d., epiphenomena of
d., esophageal
d., extended
d., facial nerve
d., finger
d., fixation and
d. for thoracic cancer ▸ extended
d., freed by blunt
d., freed by sharp
d. hematoma
d., kidney freed and exposed by blunt
d. knife and scissors
d. ▸ lymph node
d., node
d. of aorta
d. of blood vessel
d. of brain
d. of communicators
d. of conjunctiva
d. of heart
d. quality image
d., radial neck
d., radical
d., radical axillary
d., radical inguinal node
d., radical neck
d., radical retroperitoneal node
d. -radiotherapy (QUART) ▸ quadrantectomy-axillary
d., right carotid aortic
d., sharp
d., sharp osteotome
d., spiral
d. (SCAD) ▸ spontaneous coronary artery
d., standard radical neck
d. ▸ Stanford-type aortic
d., subperiosteal
d., supraomohyoid neck
d., therapeutic
d. ▸ thoracic aortic
d., transient

disseminata
d., acne
d., neurodermatitis
d. ▸ tuberculosis miliaris

disseminated
d. arthritis

d. breast cancer
d. carcinoma
d. disease
d. encephalitis, acute
d. encephalomyelitis, acute
d. form
d. herpes zoster infection
d. infection
d. intravascular coagulation (DIC)
d. intravascular coagulopathy
d. malignant lymphoma
d. melanoma
d. myelitis
d. polyarteritis
d. sclerosis

disseminating disease, rapidly
disseminating fungal infection
dissemination, hematogenous
dissemination of disease, rapid
disseminatum, xanthoma
disseminatus (LED), lupus erythematosus
disseminatus, pemphigus
dissimilar twins
dissociated
d. experiences
d. fever ▸ Jaccoud
d. vertical divergence (DVD)

dissociation
d. and repression
d. and sexual abuse
d., arteriovenous (AV)
d., atrial
d., atrioventricular (AV)
d., auriculoventricular
d., AV (artrioventricular)
d. by interference
d., chronic
d., complete AV (atrioventricular)
d. curve
d. curve ▸ hemoglobin oxygen (O₂)
d. curve ▸ oxygen (O₂)
d. curve ▸ oxyhemoglobin
d. disorder
d. dyscontrol
d., electrical mechanical
d., electromechanical
d., electromyocardial
d. ▸ feeling of
d. in eating disorder
d. ▸ incomplete atrioventricular (AV)
d. ▸ intracavitary pressure electrogram
d., interference
d., isorhythmic atrioventricular (AV)

d., longitudinal
d., psychological
d. with interference, isorhythmic atrioventricular (AV)

dissociative
d. amnesia
d. children
d. disorder
d. disorders ▸ multiple personality
d. experience
d. identity disorder
d. memory loss
d. patient
d. reaction
d. state
d. state ▸ disorganized,
d. symptoms
d. symptoms, common

dissolution
d. therapy
d. therapy ▸ oral
d. therapy ▸ percutaneous

dissolve
d. blood clots
d. clots
d. common bile duct stones
d. disc material
d. gallstones
d. kidney stones

dissolved, synechiae
dissolving
d. action, clot
d. agent
d. blood clot
d. drug, clot
d. fluoride pills ▸ slow-
d. gallstones
d. sutures
d. therapy ▸ clot
d. thrombolytic drug, clot-

disseminated tuberculosis
distal
d. anastomosis
d. and proximal
d. antrum
d. aorta
d. aspect
d. bronchiectasis
d. colon
d. common duct tumor
d. convoluted tubule
d. ectasia
d. electrode
d. emphysema
d. end

distal—*continued*
- d. esophageal lesion
- d. esophagectomy
- d. esophagus
- d. esophagus ▸ extension denudation of
- d. esophagus ▸ superficial hemorrhage
- d. femoral epiphysis
- d. fibula
- d. fibular shaft
- d. gastric adenocarcinoma
- d. ileitis
- d. ileum
- d. interphalangeal (DIP)
- d. interphalangeal joint (DIPJ)
- d. intestinal obstruction syndrome
- d. ischemia
- d. latencies
- d. occlusion
- d. pancreaticojejunostomy
- d. phalanges, clubbing of
- d. phalanx
- d. portion
- d. portion main circumflex
- d. portion of small intestine
- d. radial epiphysis
- d. radial metaphysis
- d. radius
- d. runoff, aortogram with
- d. runoff, poor
- d. small bowel
- d. splenorenal shunt
- d. stenosis
- d. subungual
- d. surface of tooth onychomycosis
- d. symmetric polyneuropathy
- d. third
- d. third, junction of
- d. tingling on percussion (DTP)
- d. tip of cecum
- d. tuft
- d. ulna
- d. vessel wall

distally, esophagus dilated
distance(s)
- d. ceptor
- d. compensation ▸ electronic
- d., double
- d., focal
- d., focus to skin
- d. glasses
- d. ▸ half-power
- d. (HD) ▸ hearing
- d., inter-electrode

- d. (PD), interpupillary
- d., intra-aural
- d. ▸ judgment of
- d. ▸ keeping emotional
- d., large inter-electrode
- d., long inter-electrode
- d., poor perception of time and
- d., prism diopter (PD)
- d. (PD) ▸ pupillary
- d. runner, long
- d., short inter-electrode
- d., skin to tumor
- d., small inter-electrode
- d., source
- d. (SSD), source to skin
- d. (TSD) ▸ target skin
- d. test
- d., triple
- d., tumor skin
- d. vision
- d. vision ▸ reduced
- d. visual acuity (DVA)

distant
- d. and unfocused ▸ eyes
- d. breath sounds
- d. cancer
- d. disease
- d. events ▸ loss of memory for
- d. flap, Italian
- d. heart sounds
- d. metastases
- d. metastatic disease
- d. objects
- d. objects blurry
- d. objects fuzzy

distantial aberration
distended
- d. abdomen
- d. abdomen taut and
- d. bladder
- d. bowel
- d. colon
- d., large bowel
- d., neck veins
- d., neck veins not
- d., patient's abdomen
- d., pericardial sac
- d., retinal veins
- d., stomach
- d., tender, tympanitic ▸ abdomen
- d. urinary bladder
- d. with air, bladder
- d. with fluid, stomach
- d. with water, bladder

distensibility, ventricular

distention/distension
- d., abdominal
- d. and tenderness, abdominal
- d., bladder
- d., cervical venous
- d. discomfort
- d., gaseous
- d., gastric
- d., hepatic
- d. (JVD) ▸ jugular vein
- d. (JVD) ▸ jugular venous
- d., neck vein
- d. of biliary ducts
- d. of ventricular system
- d. ▸ postoperative abdominal
- d., venous
- d., visceral

distillate poisoning, petroleum
distilled water
distinct margin
distinct psychiatric disorder
distinctions, blurred essential
distinctive symptoms ▸ presence of
distogingival (DG)
Distoma
- D. pulmonale
- D. ringeri
- D. westermani

distomiasis
- d., hemic
- d., hepatic
- d., intestinal

distorted
- d., artifactually
- d. body image
- d. brain tissue
- d. cell growth
- d. chest skeleton
- d. cornea
- d. depth perception
- d. negative thinking
- d. representation
- d. sensation
- d. sense of time and perception
- d. thinking
- d. thinking ▸ nonpsychotic
- d. ▸ time perception
- d. vision
- d. visual images and hallucinations
- d. visual perception
- d. voice

distortion(s)
- d. and scarring ▸ clouding,
- d., barreling
- d., body image

d., cognitive
d., conscious
d., cord
d., developmental
d. divergent method, Isaac's differential
d. endobronchial tree
d., gross
d. ▸ hypnosis, memory and
d. ▸ illusions or perceptual
d. in taste and smell
d., instrumental
d. left main stem bronchus
d., memory
d. of actual events, cognitive
d. of contour
d. of electroencephalogram (EEG) waves
d. of lens
d. of lines ▸ blank spots and
d. of perceptions
d. of reality
d. of senses
d. of sensory perception
d. of sound ▸ gradual
d. of time and space
d. or retraction of nipple
d., paratactic
d., parataxic
d., perceptual
d., pin-cushion
d., sensory
d., thinking
d., time
d., vision
d., visual
distracted, easily
distracted ▸ tendency to be
distractibility, easy
distraction and imagery ▸ relaxation,
distraught, patient
distress
d., abdominal
d., acute respiratory
d. and burning, epigastric
d. at birth ▸ respiratory
d., breathing
d., chest
d., controllable
d., emotional
d., epigastric
d., exaggerated
d., fetal
d., gastric
d., gastrointestinal (GI)

d., gastronomical
d., impending fetal
d. in breathing
d. ▸ infant in acute respiratory
d. ▸ infant in respiratory
d., intra-uterine
d., menopausal
d., menstrual
d., mental
d., moderate respiratory
d., motion
d., neonatal
d. of newborn ▸ idiopathic respiratory
d., patient in extreme
d., patient in great
d. ▸ patient in respiratory
d., perinatal
d., postcoital
d., precordial
d. present at birth ▸ respiratory
d., psychologic
d., reduce tension and
d., respiratory
d. scale ▸ Tennant
d. ▸ serious respiratory
d., severe fatal
d., silent heart muscle
d., spiritual
d. syndrome (ARDS), acute respiratory
d. syndrome (ARDS) ▸ adult respiratory
d. syndrome, bilateral
d. syndrome ▸ early respiratory
d. syndrome (IRDS) ▸ idiopathic respiratory
d. syndrome ▸ infant respiratory
d. syndrome (RDS) ▸ respiratory
d. tolerance
d., transient emotional
d., transient respiratory
d. ▸ ventilatory support in respiratory

distressed, patient
distressing
d. condition
d. psychedelic experience
d. recollection of incident
d. thoughts

distribution
d., anatomic origin and
d. and control, medication

d. and heterogeneity of patient ▸ dose
d., blood volume
d., body hair
d. cart
d., coronary
d. curve for radiation, spectral
d., depth dose
d., dose
d., fat
d., gas
d., gaussian
d., global
d., gynecoid fat
d., isodose
d. law, Doerner-Hoskins
d., maxwellian
d., mean
d., median
d., nerve
d. of bilirubin ▸ volume of
d. of donor organs and tissues
d. of hair, normal
d. of median nerve
d. of ventilation
d., organ
d., pains of generalized
d., pains of localized
d., Paterson and Parker dose
d., Poisson
d., scabetic
d., sciatic nerve
d., spatial dose
d. ▸ stocking glove
d. system, Manchester dose
d. system, Paris dose
d. system, Quimby dose
d. systems, three-dose
d., ulnar nerve
distributive analysis and synthesis
distributive shock
disturbance(s)
d., acid base
d., acute brain
d., acute mental
d., affective
d., appetite
d., atrioventricular (AV) conduction
d., behavior
d., behavioral
d., biochemical
d., bipolar
d., body image
d., brain
d., cardiovascular

disturbance(s)—*continued*
d., cerebellar
d., chronic nonprogressive
d., chronic sleep schedule
d., chronic visual
d., cognitive
d., color and space perceptual
d., conduction
d. ▸ controlled heart rhythm
d., diffuse neurological
d., digestive
d., eating
d., electrolytic
d., emotional
d., episodic sleep
d. ▸ fatal heart rhythm
d., focal
d., gait
d., gastrointestinal (GI)
d., hearing
d., heart
d., heart rhythm
d., hormonal
d., identity
d. in air exchange
d. in cardiac rhythm
d. in maintaining sleep (DIMS)
d. in self-concept
d. in self-image
d. in sleep patterns
d. in smell
d., increased rhythm
d. index ▸ respiratory
d., life-threatening rhythm
d., intestinal
d. ▸ intraoperative conduction
d., memory
d., mental
d., metabolic
d. ▸ metabolic or electrolyte
d., mood
d., motor
d., narcissistic
d., nervous
d., nutritional
d. of adolescence ▸ mixed
   emotional
d. of body equilibrium
d. of childhood ▸ mixed emotional
d. of conduct
d. of conduct ▸ adjustment disorder
   with
d. of conduct and emotions ▸ mixed
d. of conduct ▸ predominant
d. of consciousness ▸ predominant

d. of emotional and conduct ▸
   adjustment disorder with mixed
d. of emotions and conduct ▸ mixed
d. of emotions ▸ predominant
d. of emotions specific to
   adolescence
d. of emotions specific to childhood
d. of equilibratory coordination
d. of gait and stance
d. of mental equilibrium
d. of mental function ▸ episodic
d. of mood
d. of sensation
d. of speech
d. of vision
d. of visual function
d., orientation
d. ▸ Parkinsonian-like
d., perception
d., perceptual
d. ▸ peri-infarctional
d., persistent identity
d., persistent mood
d. ▸ persisting perceptual
d. ▸ personal identity
d., personality
d., physiological
d., pilomotor
d., predominant psychomotor
d., psychological
d., psychosensory
d., respiratory
d., rhythm
d., secondary
d. ▸ self-esteem
d., sensorial
d., sensory
d., sleep
d., somatic
d., station
d. syndrome ▸ circadian rhythm
d., taste
d., thinking and sensorium
d., transient neurologic
d., transient situational
d., vegetative
d., visceral
d., vision
d., visual
d., voice
d., widespread

disturbed
d. behavior
d. child

d. child, behaviorally
d. (ED), emotionally
d. individuals, emotionally
d. individuals, mentally
d. language
d., patient
d. patient, mentally
d. personal relationship
d. sense of time
d. sleep patterns
d., socially
d. thinking

disulfiram
d. blocks
d. implants
d. treatment, oral

disuse [*diffuse*]
d. atrophy
d. atrophy ▸ muscle
d. atrophy, severe
d., osteopenia of
d. osteoporosis
d. syndrome

ditaeniatus, Tabanus
Dittrich's stenosis
diuresed, patient
diuresis
d., acid
d., loop
d., osmotic
d., saline
d., tubular

diuretic(s) [*diabetic, dietetic*]
d. action, anti-
d. agent
d., cardiac
d. drugs
d., fainting from
d. ▸ hearing loss from
d. ▸ heat intolerance from
d. ▸ high ceiling
d. hormone secretion (SIADH) ▸
   syndrome of inappropriate anti-
d., hydragogue
d., indirect
d., injectable
d., intravenous (IV)
d., loop
d., medication
d., osmotic
d., parenteral
d. ▸ potassium-sparing
d. ▸ potassium-wasting
d., rash from
d., refrigerant

d. therapy
d. therapy, intermittent
d., thiazide
d., thirst from
d., tinnitus from
diurna, microfilaria
diurnal
  d. and matutinal variation
  d. enuresis
  d. epilepsy
  d. rhythm
  d. variation
  d. variation, matutinal and
  d. weight fluctuations
  d. weight gain, abnormal
diurnus, pavor
Diveley operation ▸ Dickson-
divergence (DVD), dissociated
  vertical
divergence insufficiency
divergent
  d. dislocation
  d. method, Isaac's differential
    distortion
  d. rays
  d. squint
  d. strabismus
  d. thinking
diverging collimator
divers' bends
diverse psychosomatic problems
diverse symptoms
diversifolium, Sinomenium
diversiloba, Rhus
diversion
  d. of drugs
  d. of drugs from licit medical
    channels
  d. of flow of blood
  d., urinary
diversional activity deficit
diversional heart block
diversionary activities
diversionary tactics
diversium, Chiracanthium
diverticulectomy, Meckel's
diverticula
  d., colonic
  d., noninflamed
  d., pericardial
diverticular
  d. abscess
  d. disease
  d. hernia
diverticulation abnormality

diverticulectomy ▸ Harrington
  esophageal
diverticulitis, fiber and
diverticulitis of colon
diverticulosis
  d., acute
  d., bloating from
  d. coli
  d. colon
  d., constipation from
  d., development of
  d., diarrhea
  d., jejunal
  d. of cecal area
  d. of sigmoid colon
  d. of transverse and descending
    colon
  d. ▸ pain in abdomen from
  d., sigmoid
  d. ▸ tenderness in abdomen from
diver's syncope
diverticulum(-a)
  d., bladder
  d., bronchus
  d., calyceal
  d., colonic
  d., duodenal
  d., epiphrenic
  d., esophageal
  d., false
  d., gastric
  d., Heister's
  d., hepatic
  d., hypopharyngeal
  d., inflamed
  d., inflammation of
  d., jejunal
  d., Meckel's
  d., mid-esophageal
  d., multiple uninflamed
  d. of descending colon
  d. of esophagus
  d. of transverse colon
  d., pharyngeal
  d., pharyngoesophageal
  d., postbulbar
  d., prostatic
  d., questionable
  d., Rokitansky's
  d. rupture, inflamed
  d., scattered
  d., sigmoid
  d., sigmoid colon
  d. ▸ small sacular posterior
    pharyngeal

d., supradiaphragmatic
d., thyroid
d., tracheal
d., traction
d., Zenker's
diverting colostomy
divide in equal parts
divided
  d. and separated, ends
  d. and tied ▸ clamped,
  d. attention
  d. cells
  d. colostomy
  d., doubly clamped and
  d., muscles
  d. respiration
  d. tendon
  d., fascia transversalis
divider, stress
dividing cells ▸ nuclei of
diving
  d. air embolism
  d. goiter
  d. injury
  d. reflex
division(s)
  d. and function cell growth
  d. and growth ▸ uncontrolled cell
  d., auditory
  d., cell
  d., craniosacral
  d., direct cell
  d., equational
  d., indirect cell
  d. left branch ▸ block in
    anterosuperior
  d. left branch ▸ block in
    posteroinferior
  d. line
  d., maturation
  d. of cortical adhesions
  d. of spine
  d., reduction
  d., thoracicolumbar
  d., thoracolumbar
  d. ▸ unrestrained cell
  d. ▸ vascular ring
divisional heart block
divisum, pancreas
divorce
  d. adjustment
  d. counseling
  d. support group
DIVP (dilute intravenous Pitocin)
Dix-Hallpike maneuver

dizygotic twins
dizziness
- d. and faintness
- d. and joint pain ▸ weakness,
- d. and nausea
- d., episode of
- d., extreme
- d. from antidepressant
- d. from blood pressure (BP)
- d. from brain
- d. from carbon dioxide (CO_2)
- d. from coughing
- d. from epilepsy
- d. from heart attack
- d. from heat stroke
- d. from infection of ear
- d. from insect sting
- d. from rapid and deep breathing
- d. from stroke
- d. from tic douloureux
- d. from TMJ (temporomandibular joint) disorder
- d. from toxic shock syndrome
- d., headache and
- d. in aging
- d. or light-headedness
- d., transient
- d., unexplained
- d. ▸ unexplained sudden
- d., weakness, and nausea
- d., weakness, or change in vision ▸ sudden
- d. with double vision
- d. with nervousness

dizzy
- d. and nauseated
- d. patient
- d. spells

dizzying mood swings
DJD (degenerative joint disease)
DKA (diabetic ketoacidosis)
DLA (distolabial)
DLAI (distolabioincisal)
DLI (distolinguoincisal)
DLO (distolinguo-cclusal)
DLP (distolinguopulpal)
DLS (depressive living syndrome)
DM (diabetes mellitus)
- DM, ▸ adult onset
- DM, borderline
- DM, controlled
- DM, juvenile onset
- DM, longstanding
- DM, secondary to endocrine disease

DM, secondary to pancreatic disease
DM (diastolic murmur)
DMARD (disease modifying antirheumatic drug)
DMD (Duchenne's muscular dystrophy)
DMPA (depot-medroxy-progesterone acetate)
DMSO (dmethyl sulfoxide)
D-N (dextrose-nitrogen) ratio
DNA (deoxyribonucleic acid)
- DNA analysis
- DNA fingerprint
- DNA maker
- DNA molecules
- DNA polymerase activity
- DNA polymerase ▸ ribonucleic acid (RNA) dependent
- DNA recombinant
- DNA samples
- DNA sequences ▸ degraded
- DNA sequencing
- DNA strand
- DNA switch
- DNA synthesis
- DNA ▸ target
- DNA technology ▸ recombinant
- DNA testing
- DNA virus

DNR (do not resuscitate)
- DNR decision
- DNR order
- DNR patient

DO (disto-occlusal)
do
- d. chores ▸ refusal to
- d. not appear enlarged ▸ adenoids
- d. not appear enlarged ▸ tonsils
- d. not repeat
- d. not resuscitate (DNR)

do not repeat
DOA or Dead on Arrival
DOA (dead on arrival) ▸ patient
Dobie's globule
dobutamine
- d. -atropine stress echocardiography
- d. echocardiography
- d. holiday
- d. stress echocardiography
- d. stress echocardiography ▸ transesophageal
- d. stress test

Docke's murmur

Dock's test meal
docs, script
doctor(s) (Doctor)
- d. actively caused death
- d., family
- D. of Medicine (MD), primary
- d. -on-call
- d., patient has fear of
- d. -patient relationship
- d., referring

document(s)
- d. ▸ legal
- d. ▸ Power of Attorney (POA) health care
- d. ▸ health care

documentary arteriogram
documentation, medical record
documented silent ischemia
Döderlein's bacillus
Doderlein's operation
DOE (dyspnea on exercise)
DOE (dyspnea on exertion)
Doerner-Hoskins distribution law
does appear enlarged
- d.a.e., fibroid of uterus
- d.a.e., heart
- d.a.e., liver
- d.a.e., lump in left breast
- d.a.e., lump in right breast
- d.a.e., spleen
- d.a.e., thyroid
- d.a.e., uterus

does not appear enlarged
- d.n.a.e., heart
- d.n.a.e., liver
- d.n.a.e., lump in left breast
- d.n.a.e., lump in right breast
- d.n.a.e., spleen
- d.n.a.e., thyroid

dog cough
dog view, scottie
Doherty sphere implant
Doherty's implant
Döhle
- D. disease
- D. disease, Heller-
- D. -Heller aortitis
- D. inclusion bodies

Dohlman implant, Brown-
Do-Jee (heroin)
doldrums, summer
dolens
- d., phlegmasia alba
- d., phlegmasia cerulea
- d. puerperarum, phlegmasia alba

Doléris' operation
Doléris' operation, Gilliam-
dolichoectatic aneurysm
dolichopellic pelvis
doll('s)
    d. eye maneuver
    d. eye reflex
    d. eye sign
    d. fetus, paper-
dolore, angina sine
dolorosa
    d., adiposis
    d., alveolitis sicca
    d., hallux
    d., nephritis
domain
    d. analysis ▸ frequency
    d. analysis ▸ time
    d. imaging ▸ frequency
    d. signal averaged
        electrocardiogram (ECG) ▸ time
dome(s) (Domes)
    D. (LSD)
    d. -and-dart configuration
    d. cells
    d., choc en
    d. complex, spike-and-
    d. configuration ▸ spike-and-
    d. cyst, blue
    d., dart and
    d. excursion
    d., injection
    d. of bladder
    d. of diaphragm
    d., patellar
    d. pulse ▸ spike-and-
    d. shaped
    d. sign, air
    d., surgical
Domeboro powder (Pwd)
domestic
    d. abuse
    d. enhancement
    d. medicine
    d. violence
    d. violence victim
domestica
    d., Musca
    d. nebulo, Musca
    d. vicina, Musca
Domiciliary Fetal Monitor, Huntleigh
dominance, hemispheric
dominant
    d. artery
    d. character

    d. characteristics
    d. complement
    d. coronary circulation ▸ left
    d. factor
    d. frequency
    d. frequency component
    d. frequency (MDF) ▸ mean
    d. gene
    d. hemisphere
    d. inheritance
    d. line
    d. pattern
    d. pattern ▸ autosomal
    d. polycystic kidney disease (PKD)
    d. side of brain
    d. transmission ▸ autosomal
dominated personality, control-
dominated personality ▸ impulse
dominating center
doming
    d., diastolic
    d. of leaflets
    d., systolic
    d. ▸ tricuspid valve
domination response (CDR) ▸ control
domino
    d. procedure
    d. reflex
    d. transplant
Donald-Fothergill operation
Donald's operation
donated
    d. blood, test
    d., body
    d., bones
    d. cornea
    d., eyes
    d. for corneal transplants ▸ eyes
    d. for kidney transplants ▸ kidneys
    d. for scientific research ▸
        authorization for body to be
    d. for scientific research ▸ consent
        form for body to be
    d., heart
    d. human organs
    d. human plasma
    d., kidney
    d., liver
    d. organ ▸ procure and allocate
    d., organs
    d. organs and tissues, surgical
        recovery of
    d. organs, surgical removal of
    d. pancreas
    d., tissue

    d. to _____ ▸ patient's body
donation
    d., altruistic
    d., autologous bland
    d., autologous predeposit
    d., blood
    d., cadaver organ
    d., consent for organ
    d., criteria for organ
    d., directed blood
    d., directed donor
    d., directed organ
    d., eye
    d. of body
    d. of bones
    d. of eyes
    d. of heart
    d. of kidney
    d. of liver
    d., organ
    d. ▸ random homologous
    d., replacement
    d., Samaritan
    d., solid organ
    d. study ▸ tissue
    d., tissue
    d., vital organ
Donders' glaucoma
Donders' law
D1-D12 ▸ T1-T12 (thoracic vertebrae)
    or
done, frozen section
D₁ syndrome, trisomy
Donne's corpuscle
donor(s) (Donor)
    d. and recipient lymphocytes
    d. and recipient ▸ transient contact
        between
    d., artificial insemination
    d. authorization form to use eyes
    d., autologous patient
    D. Awareness Program ▸ Organ
    d. bacterium
    d. bank, skin
    d., blood
    d. blood, contaminated
    d. bone, freezing
    d., bone graft
    d., cadaver
    d. candidate, vital organ
    d. card
    d. card, organ
    D. Card, Uniform
    d. cell
    d. cell ▸ phage particle maturing in

donor(s)—*continued*
- d. chromosome
- d. chromosome transferred to recipient
- d., compatible
- d., consanguineous
- d. criteria
- d. dearth
- d., deceased organ
- d. defect
- d., designated
- d., directed
- d., directed blood
- d. donation, directed
- d. duodenum
- d., egg
- d. ▸ emotionally related
- d. exchange ▸ living
- d. exchange ▸ paired
- d., eye
- d. ▸ genetically unrelated
- d. heart
- d. heart, damaged
- d. heart retrieved
- d. hospital
- d. ▸ identify potential organ
- d., infected blood
- d., infected organ
- d. infection risk
- d. insemination (TDI) ▸ therapeutic
- d., kidney
- d., living
- d., living related organ
- d. (LURD) ▸ living, unrelated
- d. maintenance
- d. maintenance ▸ principles of
- d. management
- d. match, bone marrow
- d., matched
- d., matching
- d., multiple organ
- d. organ
- d. organ ischemic time
- d. organs and tissues, distribution of
- d. organs and tissues, preservation of
- d. organs and tissues, procurement of
- d. organs readily available
- d. organs ▸ shortage of
- d., parental
- d., plasma
- d. pledge card
- d., potential

- d., potential blood
- d., potential organ
- d., potentially suitable
- d. procurement
- d. program, egg
- d., red blood cells returned to
- d., red cells transfused back into
- d., related living
- d. relative ▸ nonmatching
- d. screening
- d. screening ▸ blood
- d., sibling
- d. site
- d. site of bone graft
- d. site, skin graft
- d., skin
- d., skin graft
- d. source
- d. specific transfusion (DST)
- d. stem cells
- d. stickers
- d., stranger
- d. testing potential
- d. tissue
- d. tissue, replica of
- d. transfusion, directed
- d. transplant ▸ live
- d. transplant, unrelated
- d. transplantation, cadaveric
- d., unrelated living
- d., unsuitable
- d., volunteer blood
- d. white blood cells

Donovan bodies
Donovan bodies ▸ Leishman-donovani, Leishmania
donut, vaginal pessary
doobie (marijuana) cigarette
doom
- d., feeling of impending
- d., impending
- d., patient has sense of
- d. ▸ sense of impending

dopa, alpha methyl◇
dopamine
- d. agonist
- d. -boosting drugs
- d. deficiency
- d. deficit, chronic
- d. hypothesis
- d. infusion, saline and
- d. molecules
- d., norepinephrine and
- d. -producing nerve cells, degeneration of

- D. production, brain's natural
- d. production in brain, stimulatic
- d. receptor agonist properties
- d. receptors
- d. -releasing drugs
- d. transmission ▸ irregular
- d. transmission ▸ stimulated

dopaminergic
- d. agent
- d. and serotinergic nerve terminal ▸ central
- d. function, central
- d. neurons
- d. state induced, hyper-

dope dealers
Doppler
- D. analysis
- D. assessment
- D. auto-correlation technique
- D. blood profusion ▸ Laser
- D. cardiography
- D. cardiography, echo
- D., carotid
- D., color flow
- D. color flow mapping
- D., color flow ultrasound
- D. color jet
- D. continuity equation
- D. E:A ratio ▸ transmitral
- D., echo
- D. echocardiogram, continuous wave
- D. echocardiography
- D. echocardiography, color
- D. echocardiography, continuous wave
- D. echocardiography ▸ pulsed
- D. echocardiography ▸ pulsed wave
- D. effect
- D. energy, color
- D. examination, cardiac
- D. flow detector
- D. flow meter (FM)
- D. flowmetry ▸ pulsed
- D. imaging, continuous wave
- D. imaging ▸ tissue
- D. interrogation
- D. mapping ▸ pulsed wave
- D. measurement
- D. monitoring of fetus
- D. pressure gradient
- D. probe ▸ transcranial
- D., quantitative
- D. recording

D. scanner, Corometrics
D. Series
D. shift
D. signal
D. sound device
D. spectral analysis
D. study ▸ venous
D. test ▸ transcranial
D. tissue imaging
D. transesophageal color flow imaging
D. ultrasonography
D. ultrasonography ▸ duplex pulsed
D. ultrasound
D. ultrasound, continuous wave
D. ultrasound imaging
D. ultrasound ▸ power
D. ultrasound scan
D. velocity interrogation, deep
D. velocity probe
D. wave form analysis
Doptone, FHT (fetal heart tones) obtained with
Doptone monitoring of fetal heart tones (FHT)
d'orange
d. appearance ▸ peau
d. in breast carcinoma, peau
d., peau
Dorello's canal
Dorema ammoniacum
Dorendorf sign
Döring panencephalitis, Pette-dormant
d. cells
d. organisms
d. tuberculosis
d. tumor
dormescent jerks
Dorno's rays
dorsades de pointes
dorsal
d. aorta
d. arterial arch of foot
d. artery
d. aspect
d. aspect spinal cord
d. branch of ulnar nerve
d. column stimulator (DCS)
d. cornu
d. cutaneous nerve ▸ intermediate
d. cutaneous nerve of foot ▸ intermediate
d. cutaneous nerve of foot ▸ lateral
d. cutaneous nerve of foot ▸ medial

d. cutaneous nerve of forearm
d. decubitus position
d. digital nerves of foot
d. digital nerves of lateral surface of great toe
d. digital nerves of medial surface of second toe
d. digital nerves of radial nerve
d. digital nerves of ulnar nerve
d. digital vein of foot
d. elevated position
d. exostoses
d. flap
d. flexure
d. horn
d. horns of spinal cord
d. hump
d. interosseous metacarpal vein
d. interosseous muscles of foot
d. interosseous muscles of hand
d. interosseous vein of foot
d. kyphosis
d. lingual vein
d. lip region
d. lithotomy position
d. mediastinotomy
d. mesentery
d. metacarpal vein
d. metatarsal vein
d. nerve of clitoris
d. nerve of penis
d. nerve of scapula
d. nerve root
d. nerve root rhizotomy
d. osteophyte formation
d. pancreas
d. position
d. recumbent position
d. reflex
d. reflex of foot, Mendel's
d. regions of fingers
d. regions of toes
d. rigid position
d. root
d. root entry zone (DREZ) lesion
d. root ganglion
d. sacrococcygeal muscle
d. sclerosis
d. slit
d. spine
d. surface
d. surface of brain stem
d. sympathectomy
d. tilt
d. vein of clitoris, deep

d. vein of clitoris ▸ superficial
d. vein of penis, deep
d. vein of penis ▸ superficial
d. vein of tongue
d. venous arch of foot
d. vertebra
d. vertebrae bone
d. view
dorsalis
d., chorda
d. pedis arteries
d. pedis (DP) pulsation
d. pedis (DP) pulse
d., tabes
dorsi
d., elastofibroma
d. flap technique ▸ latissimus
d., latissimus
d. muscle, latissimus
d. procedure ▸ latissimus
dorsiflexion
d., active
d., ankle
d. sign
dorsiflexor, weakness of
dorsispinal vein
dorsoanterior, left
dorsoanterior, right
dorsocervical fat pad enlargement
dorsocuboidal reflex
dorsolateral prefrontal cortex
dorsolateral surface of knee
dorsolithotomy position
dorsomedial thalamotomy
dorsoplantar projection
dorsoposterior, left
dorsoposterior, right
dorsorecumbent position
dorsosacral position
dorsosupine position
dorsum
d. of hand, squamous cell carcinoma
d. nasi
d. sella
dosage (Dosage)
d., adjust
d., adjusting
d. adjustment
d., adult
d., biological
d., boost
d. chart
d., drug
d. effectiveness

dosage—*continued*

d., excessive drug
d. for children
d. formulation
d., high
d., increased
d., initial
d., insulin
d., Kienböck's unit of x-ray
d. levels
d., low
d., maintenance
d. ▸ maternal methadone
d., maximum
d., maximum total
d., medication
d., medium
d. (MED) ▸ minimum effective
d. of medication, regular
d., oral
d., original
d., radiation
d. range
d., recommended
d. regimen
d., roentgen
d., safe and effective
d. schedule
D. Schedule, Gradual
d., titrate
d., unit of roentgen ray;
d., x-ray

dose(s) (Doses)

d. (LSD)
d., absorbed
d., achieve high
d., air
d. and beams
d. aspirin therapy, high
d. aspirin therapy, low
d., attenuated
d., average target absorbed
d. beams of x-rays ▸ high
d., biological
d., biological surface
d., biological tumor
d. breast x-rays ▸ low-
d. calculated as given dose
d. calculated as mid-depth dose
d. calculated in a tangential plane
d. calculation
d. calculation, computer
d. calculation, irregular field
   technique for

d. calculation, isocentric technique
   for
d. calculation, rotation technique for
d., chemotherapy
d. chemotherapy, high
d. chemotherapy ▸ intense cycle of
   high
d., computation of radiatic
d. computation system, commercial
d., cumulative
d., curative
d. curves, comparative depth
d., daily supplemental
d. -dependent
d., depth
d. differential, depth
d. distribution
d. distribution and heterogeneity of
   patient
d. distribution, depth
d. distribution, Paterson and Parker
d. distribution, spatial
d. distribution system, Manchester
d. distribution system, Paris
d. distribution system, Quimby
d. distribution systems, three-
d. ▸ dose calculated as given
d. ▸ dose calculated as mid-depth
d., doubling
d., effective
d. equivalent
d., erythema
d. estimate
d., exit
d. external irradiation, high
d. fall-off, sharp
d., fatal
d. fractionation
d. fractionation, biologic factors in
d., fractionation, cell cycle
   redistribution and
d., fractionation (TDF) factor ▸ time,
d. fractionation, modification
   patterns of
d. fractionation, normal tissue
   effects of
d. fractionation radiation therapy ▸
   high
d. fractionation, reoxygenation and
d. fractionation, split course
d. fractionation, tumor control with
d. (GSD), genetically significant
d., given
d. heparin, mini-
d., high

d. hyperfractionation
d. hyperfractionation, cell cycle
   redistribution and
d. hyperfractionation,
   reoxygenation and
d., identical midplane
d. in scanning, depth
d., infective
d. infusion, total
d. inhaler (MDI) ▸ metered
d., initial
d., integral
d. intensity analysis
d., internal mammary
d., intravenous (IV)
d. intravenous (IV) insulin therapy,
   low
d., intravenous loading
d., iso◇
d., IV (intravenous)
d., lethal
d. level
d. ▸ life-threatening
d. limiting structures
d. limiting tissues
d., loading
d., localized
d., long-acting
d., maintenance
d. (MPD) ▸ maximum permissible
d., maximum target absorbed
d. (MTD) ▸ maximum tolerated
d. (MDD) ▸ mean daily
d. (MHD) ▸ mean hemolytic
d. (MLD or LD$_{50}$), median lethal
d., median curative
d., median effective
d., median fatal
d., median infective
d., median lethal
d., median tissue culture
d., median tissue culture infective
d., medical internal radiation
d. methotrexate and cisplatin, high
d., minimal effective
d., minimal erythema
d., minimal fatal
d., minimal tolerance
d., minimize normal brain
d., minimum target absorbed
d. (MHD) minimum hemolytic
d. (MID) ▸ minimum infective
d. (MLD) ▸ minimum lethal
d. (MMD) ▸ minimum morbidostatic
d. (MRD) ▸ minimum reacting

d. modification factor
d., nominal single
d. (NSD), nominal standard
d., nonpressor
d. of aspirin, liberal
d. of boluses
d. of chemotherapy, massive
d. of chemotherapy, optimal
d. of depressants, psychoactive
d. of electron beam therapy, central axis
d. of hallucinogens, psychoactive
d. of inhalants, psychoactive
d. of opioids, psychoactive
d. of phencyclidine, psychoactive
d. of rad in fractions, mid-sagittal plane
d. of rad in fractions, total
d. of rad, planned
d. of radiation, small boost
d. of steroids ▸ massive
d. of stimulants, psychoactive
d., oral
d. (OTD), organ tolerance
d., percentage depth
d. period, initial
d., precision high
d., prescribed
d. prescription
d. prescription methods, point-
d., pressor
d. priming
d. profile
d. prophylactic
d., radiatic
d., radiation
d. radiation absorbed
d. radiation, high
d. radiation, low
d. radiation therapy, high
d. radiation to tumor mass ▸ high
d. rate
d. rate, constant
d. rate, fractionated high
d. rate, hourly
d. rate irradiation, low
d. ▸ ratio of median lethal
d. reciprocity theorem
d., recommended protocol
d., rectovaginal
d. reduction factor
d. -related
d. response

d., route and method of administering medication ▸ action,
d. selection, optimal
d. size per fraction, increased
d., skin
d., skin erythema
d. (STD) ▸ skin test
d. spray ▸ metered-
d., sublethal
d., supplemental
d. survival, linear quadratic formula for
d. technique, double
d. technique, massive
d., tentative
d., therapeutic
d. therapy, biological tumor
d. therapy, high
d. therapy, low
d., thermal
d. (TED), threshold erythema
d. ▸ time interval between
d., tissue
d., tissue culture
d., tissue culture infective
d. (TTD), tissue tolerance
d., titrated initial
d. to contralateral breast
d., tolerated
d., total
d., toxic over◇
d., treatment volume and
d., tumor
d., tumor control
d. (TLD), tumor lethal
d., unit
d., vaginal
d. x-ray examination, low
d. x-ray technique, low
dosimeter
d., pencil
d., pocket
d. (TLD), thermoluminescent
d., ultraviolet fluorescent
d., Victoreen
dosimetric medicine
dosimetry
d., adjacent field x-ray beam
d. and techniques
d., classical
d. ▸ cold spots and hot spots with electron beam
d. ▸ dual x-ray beam
d., electron beam

d., external radiation
d., film
d., four field x-ray beam
d., Fricke's
d. in radiation therapy
d., internal radiation
d., large field electron beam
d., large field x-ray beam
d., pion
d., quality assurance in
d., rotational electron beam
d., rotational x-ray beam
d., single electron beam
d., single x-ray beam
dot(s)
d. blot analysis
c. cataract, blue
d., Gunn's
d. hemorrhage
d. hemorrhagic
d., Mittendorf's
d. pattern test
d. scan
d., Trantas'
dotted line
dotted tongue
dottering effect
double (Double)
d. aortic arch
d. aortic stenosis
d. apical impulse
d. -armed mattress suture
d. autograft
d. -balloon valvotomy
d. -balloon valvuloplasty
d. -barrel aorta
d. -barreled colostomy
d. -blind clinical trial
d. -blind comparison ▸ randomized
d. -blind controlled study
d. -blind experiment
d. -blind fashion
d. -blind food challenge
d. -blind placebo control prophylactic study
d. -blind placebo control study
d. -blind placebo trial
d. -blind procedure
d. -blind studies
d. -blind techniques, controlled
d. -blinded placebo controlled trial ▸ randomized
d. -blinded trial
d. -bubble appearance

double—*continued*
- d. -bubble flushing reservoir
- d. -button suture
- d. concave
- d. -contrast arthrogram
- d. -contrast barium enema
- d. -contrast enema
- d. -contrast examination
- d. -contrast roentgenography
- d. -contrast study
- d. -contrast visualization
- d. convex
- d. counting of pacer spike
- D. Cross (amphetamines)
- d. cuffed tube
- d. discharges
- d. disharmonic hearing
- d. -disk occluder prosthesis ▸ Rashkind
- d. distance
- d. dose technique
- d. -dummy technique
- d. -end flap
- d. -end graft
- d. extra stimulus
- d. -flap amputation
- d. focus, lens with
- d. footling delivery
- d. fracture
- d. harelip
- d. helix
- d. inlet left ventricle
- d. inlet ventricle
- d. inlet ventricle anomaly
- d. innervation
- d. jointed
- d. kidney
- d. lumen breast implant
- d. -lumen endobronchial tube
- d. lumen subclavian
- d. lung reduction surgery
- d. lung transplant
- d. major curve
- d. mastectomy ▸ prophylactic
- d. needle operation on cataract
- d. oscillation
- d. -outlet left ventricle (LV)
- d. -outlet left ventricle (LV) malposition
- d. -outlet right ventricle
- d. -outlet right ventricle (RV) malposition
- d. pedicle flap
- d. personality
- d. pleurisy

- d. pneumonia
- d. product
- d. puncture laparoscopy
- d. refraction
- d. scale
- d. seal
- d. -sheath bronchial brushings
- d. -shock sound
- d. spica
- d. staining
- d. -step gait
- d. -step gait, intermittent
- d. tachycardia
- d. tone, Traube's
- d. tongue
- d. triangular test
- d. -trisomy, mongolism
- d. umbrella
- d. umbrella closure
- d. umbrella device
- d. umbrella ▸ Rashkind
- d. velour graft ▸ Microvel
- d. ventricular extra stimulus
- d. vibration
- d. vision
- d. vision ▸ disabling
- d. vision ▸ dizziness with
- d. vision from myasthenia gravis
- d. vision in one eye
- d. vision, intermittent
- d. vision with eye redness
- d. vision with headache
- d. voice

doubling
- d. dose
- d. time
- d. time in lung carcinoma, tumor
- d. time, tumor

doubly
- d. clamped
- d. clamped and divided
- d. clamped, transsected and stump ligated
- d. ligated
- d. ligated and sectioned
- d. ligated, proximal stump
- d. ligated with transfixion suture

doubt or disgust ▸ fear,
doubting insanity
doubting mania
doubts, pathological
douche
- d., air
- d., alternating
- d. and gel, Betadine

- d. electromagnetic
- d., fan
- d., jet
- d. massage
- d., nasal
- d., Scotch
- d. solution, Nylmerate
- d., Tivoli
- d., transition
- d., vaginal
- d., vinegar
- d., Weber's

doughnut
- d. configuration
- d. headrest
- d. kidney
- d. pessary
- d. sign

doughy consistency
Douglas'
- D. cul-de-sac
- D. fold
- D. graft
- D. line
- D. mechanism
- D. method
- D. pouch

douloureux
- d. ▸ dizziness from tic
- d., feigned tic
- d., tic

doute, folie du
Dow
- D. Corning implant
- D. Corning shunt
- D. hollow fiber dialyzer
- D. Corning silicone

dowager hump
dowel [*towel*]
dowel crown
down (Down's)
- d. ▸ bone constantly breaks
- d., bound
- d., break◊
- d. cancer growth ▸ slow
- d. _____ cm ▸ liver
- d., complete break◊
- d., emotional break◊
- d. exercise, pull
- D. disease
- d. exercising, cool-
- d., eye rotated
- d., fallopian tube bound
- d. flap, ▸ Gillies' up-and-
- d., hernia protrudes

d. leg, pain radiating
d. legs ▸ back pain extends
d. legs, pain
d., milk let◇
d. reflex, milk let◇
d. of motor skills ▸ slowing
d. over cotton, sutures tied
d. pain, bearing-
d., patient calmed
d. ▸ patient feels
d. period, cool-
d. position, brow-
d. position, face-
d. position ▸ head
d. presentation, head
d. projection, cone-
d. reflex, let◇
d. reflex, milk let◇
d. region, build-
d. region of irradiated medium, build-
d. relaxation exercise, cool
d., run◇
d. sensation, bearing-
d. shoulder, knocked-
d. site, cut
d. slope
d. stomach, upside
D. syndrome
D. syndrome cells
D. syndrome, translocation
d. therapy ▸ step-
d. tilt test ▸ head
d. time
d. to fracture site ▸ incision carried
d. transformer, step-
d. -turned mouth corners
d. view, coned-
d. ▸ warm up and cool
downcast stare ▸ blank or
Downers (barbiturates)
downfall, emotional
downgoing bilaterally, Babinski
downgoing, toes
downhill
d. course
d. course ▸ patient had steady
d. course ▸ patient pursued rapid
d. course, progressively
d. deterioration
d. esophageal varices
d., progressive
d. running
d. ST segment depression
downsizing of hearing aid

downsloping activity
downsloping ST segment
    depression
downstairs heart ▸ upstairs-
downstream venous pressure
downward
d. compression
d. displacement
d. eye slant
d., incision curved
d. movement
d. pen deflection
d. squint, upward and
d. tilting
d., upward and
Doyen's operation
Doyen's vaginal hysterectomy
Doyne's choroiditis
Doyne's iritis
DP
DP (diastolic pressure)
DP (distopulpal)
DP (dorsalis pedis)
DPL (distopulpolingual)
dpm (disintegrations per minute)
DPT (diphtheria, pertussis and
    tetanus) immunization
dr (dram/drachm)
Dracunculus medinensis
drag(s)
d. forces
d. left lower extremity, patient
d. right lower extremity, patient
d. -to gait
Drager syndrome ▸ Shy-
Dragon (dragon)
D. (LSD), Blue
D. (LSD), Green
d. pyelogram
D. (LSD), Red
d. worm
Dragstedt's graft
drain(s) [grain]
d., brain
d. brought out through stab wound
d., cigarette
d., controlled
d. fluid build-up
d., incise and
d. inserted
d., intercostal
d., packs or
d., Penrose
d., pigtail nephrostomy
d. placed into wound

d., polyvinyl
d., rubber
d., rubber dam
d., Shiley
d. site
d., stab wound
d., tear
d. tears from eyes
d., thyroid
d., transnasal
d. trapped blood
d., umbilical tape
d., whistle-tip
drainage (dr'ge)
d., abdominal
d. about shunt site
d. and percussion ▸ postural
d. at incision site
d. bag, Hofmeister
d. bag, Hollister
d. bag with drip chamber ▸ closed urinary
d., basal
d., bladder
d. bottle, waterseal
d., bronchial
d., bronchoscopy with
d., button
d., capillary
d., cardiotomy reservoir chest
d., catheter
d. catheter, biliary
d., chest
d., chest tube
d., closed
d., closed chest water seal
d., closed pleural
d., closed tube
d., closed womb
d., continuous
d., continuous suction
d., copious
d., ear
d. from wound
d., gravity
d. (I and D) ▸ incision and
d., indwelling catheter
d. ▸ interrupted lymphatic
d., lymphatic
d. ▸ middle ear effusion and
d., Monaldi's
d., mucus
d., nasal
d., nodal
d., nonsurgical biliary

drainage—continued
- d. of abdominal cavity ▸ direct
- d. (I and D) of abscess ▸ incision and
- d. (I and D) of blister ▸ incision and
- d. of cerebral epidural space
- d. of cranial sinus
- d. of cyst, incision and
- d. of dye
- d. of esophagus, lymphatic
- d. (I and D) of fistulous tract ▸ incision and
- d. of hematoma
- d. (I and D) of ischiorectal abscess ▸ incision and
- d. of lacrimal gland
- d. of lacrimal sac
- d. of lateral sinus
- d. (I and D) of left buttock ▸ incision and
- d. of meninges
- d. of purulent material
- d. of pus
- d. (I and D) of right buttock ▸ incision and
- d. of sigmoid sinus
- d. of spinal cord
- d. of subarachnoid space
- d. of subdural space
- d. of tears, deficient
- d., open
- d., orthostatic
- d. ▸ partial anomalous pulmonary venous
- d., patent opening for bile
- d., pelvic
- d., pelvic lymph node
- d. ▸ percussion and postural
- d., percutaneous antegrade biliary
- d. ▸ percutaneous transhepatic
- d., peritoneal
- d. ▸ portal blood
- d. (PND) ▸ postnasal
- d., postural
- d. ▸ prolonged ear
- d., pulmonary
- d., pulmonary venous
- d., purulent
- d. (PND) ▸ purulent nasal
- d., sclerotomy with
- d., sinus
- d. structure
- d., suction
- d., surgical
- d. system

- d. system, closed water seal
- d. system, continuous
- d. system, continuous suction
- d. system, Glover's
- d. system, Monaldi's
- d. system, postural
- d. system, sump
- d. system, Surgivac suction
- d. system ▸ tear
- d. system, three-bottle
- d. system, tidal
- d. system tumors, lacrimal
- d. system, two-bottle
- d. system, vacuum
- d. system, waterseal
- d., tear
- d. technique
- d., Thoracoseal
- d., thoracotomy with closed
- d., thoracotomy with open
- d., through
- d., tidal
- d., total anomalous pulmonary venous
- d. tube
- d. tube in place
- d. tube, Shea polyethylene
- d. tube, thoracic
- d., underwater
- d., underwater seal
- d. unit ▸ intrapleural sealed
- d. unit, thermotic
- d., venous
- d., Wangensteen
- d., waterseal
- d., wound
- d., wound closed in layers without

drained
- d. abscess
- d. and preserved ▸ amniotic fluid
- d., emotionally
- d., fistulous tract
- d. from chest, fluid
- d. off, excess fluid
- d., physically
- d., rectal abscess
- d., rectal fistula

draining
- d. abscess
- d. atmosphere, emotionally
- d., incisional site
- d. lesion
- d. sores ▸ gaping,
- d. wound

dram [*gram*]

dram (fl dr) ▸ fluid
dramatic
- d. cluster disorder
- d. gestures ▸ exhibits

dramatizes ▸ patient self-
Drapanas mesocaval shunt
drape(s)
- d. applied, sterile
- d., Blair head
- d., foot
- d., gowns and instruments ▸ complete change of
- d., perineal prep and
- d., sterile
- d., surgical
- d., Vi-

drapeau, bruit de
draped
- d. ▸ abdomen scrubbed, prepped and
- d., area prepped and
- d. free, area
- d. in routine manner ▸ area prepped and
- d. in routine manner ▸ patient prepped and
- d., operative field prepared and
- d., patient prepared and
- d. ▸ prepped, positioned and
- d., skin
- d., skin prepped and
- d., sterilely prepped and

draping
- d. of field, sterile
- d. of field ▸ sterile preparation and
- d. of lid
- d. preparation and

drawal, with◊
Draw-a-Man Test
Draw-a-Person Test
drawer
- d. sign
- d. test, anterior
- d. test, posterior

drawing (Drawing)
- d. analysis
- d. of blood samples
- d. test, clock-
- D. Test, Projective Human Figure

drawn
- d. back, scope
- d., blood cultures
- d. blood specimen ▸ routinely
- d., interval blood count

dread
- d. of night ▸ morbid
- d. of school-related activities ▸ abnormal
- d., sensation of intense

dream(s)
- d., abnormal
- d. anxiety attacks
- d. anxiety disorder (Nightmare Disorder)
- d. associations
- d., bizarre
- d., clairvoyant
- d., day◇
- d. deprivation
- d. elements
- d. interpretation
- d. -like images
- d. pain
- d. ▸ rapid eye movement (REM) sleep anxiety
- d. recall
- d. ▸ sleep anxiety
- d. state
- d. study, sleep-
- d., veridical
- d., vivid
- d., wet

dreaming
- d. mentation
- d., self-psychology
- d. sleep

dreamless sleep
dreamy stupor
drenching night sweats
drepanocytic anemia
Dresbach's anemia
Dresbach's syndrome
dress and eat ▸ bathe,
dressed tube
dressed, wound
dresser's disease ▸ flax
dressers' phthisis, flax
dressing(s)
- d., abdominal
- d. and stockinette applied
- d., anorectal
- d. (DSD) applied ▸ dry sterile
- d. applied, pressure
- d. applied, sterile
- d., bathing, feeding, grooming
- d., binocular eye
- d., Bioclusive transparent
- d., biological
- d., bulky

- d., bulky compression
- d., butterfly
- d. change
- d., collodion
- d., compression
- d., contaminated
- d., cross-
- d., Dri-Site
- d., dry
- d. dry and intact
- d. dry and occlusive
- d. (DSD) ▸ dry sterile
- d., eye
- d., eye patch compression
- d., Flexinet
- d., fluff
- d., gauze
- d., Gelfoam
- d., immobilizing
- d., independent lower body
- d., independent upper body
- d., jacket-type chest
- d., Jobst
- d., Jobst mammary support
- d., Kerlix
- d., Kling adhesive
- d., Kling gauze
- d., Koch-Mason
- d., light bulky compression
- d., light compression
- d., light elastic
- d., lower body
- d., many-tailed
- d., mastoid
- d., maximum assistance for lower body
- d., maximum assistance for upper body
- d., minimal assistance for lower body
- d., minimal assistance for upper body
- d., moist
- d., monocular
- d., monocular eye
- d., mustache
- d., Nu-gauze
- d., occlusive
- d., patch
- d., patient independent in lower body
- d., patient independent in upper body
- d., plaster
- d., postnasal

- d. precaution
- d., pressure
- d., protective
- d., roller
- d., scultetus
- d. self-care deficit
- d., spica
- d., stent
- d., sterile
- d., stockinette
- d., subclavian Tegaderm
- d., Tegaderm
- d., Telfa
- d., triangular
- d., upper body
- d., Vaseline
- d., Vaseline wick
- d., Velpeau
- d., Velpeau sling-
- d., wound

Dressler('s)
- D. disease
- D. infarction, Roesler-
- D. syndrome

Dreyfus' syndrome, Gilbert-
DREZ (dorsal root entry zone) lesion
DRG (diagnostic-related groups)
DRG (diagnostic-related groups) payments
dr'ge (see drainage)
dribbling
- d. at end of urination
- d. of urine ▸ involuntary
- d. of urine ▸ leakage or
- d. on urination
- d. on urination ▸ dripping or

dried
- d. blood
- d., freeze-
- d. plant material
- d., slide air-

Driffield curve, Hunter-
drift(s) [shift]
- d., antigenic
- d., arm
- d. deformity, ulnar
- d. into normal sleep
- d., leg
- d., pronator
- d., ulnar

drilled
- d. bur hole
- d. in skull, bur holes
- d., tip of coracoid process

drills, agility

drills, conditioning
drink(s)
  d., compulsion to
  d. excessively
  d. moderately
  d., occasional
drinker(s)('s)(s')
  d. cardiomyopathy, beer-
  d. cardiomyopathy ▸ Quebec beer
  d., compulsive
  d. ▸ early-stage problem
  d., heavy social
  d., moderate
  d., patient heavy
  d., problem
drinking
  d. alcohol during pregnancy
  d. behavior
  d. behavior, suppress
  d. behavior ▸ unusual water
  d., binge
  d., casual social
  d., chronic
  d. client, problem
  d., continued
  d., controlled
  d. ▸ diminished levels of
  d. during pregnancy
  d., episodic
  d., excessive
  d. habit
  d., habitual
  d., hazards of
  d., inability to control
  d., long-term heavy
  d., maintenance
  d. ▸ massive water
  d. moderately
  d., pattern of
  d., problem
  d., prolonged heavy
  d. -related aggressivity
  d., resumed
  d., teenage
  d. water, contaminated
drip
  d. chamber
  d. chamber ▸ closed urinary
    drainage (dr'ge) bag with
  d. (PND) ▸ chronic postnasal
  d., ethanol
  d., heparin
  d. infusion
  d. infusion pyelography
  d. infusion technique

  d. infusion urogram
  d. infusion valve
  d., intragastric
  d., intravenous (IV)
  d., intravenous (IV) Pitocin
  d., Lidocaine prophylactic
  d. pad, nasal
  d., Pitocin
  d. (PND) ▸ postnasal
  d. pyelography
  d. rate of infusion
  d., slow IV (intravenous)
  d., succinyl choline
dripping or dribbling on urination
drippy nose
Dri-Site dressing
drive
  d., aggressive
  d., basic
  d. cycle length
  d. cycle length, basic
  d. decreased sex
  d. from diabetes ▸ loss of sexual
  d., fundamental human
  d., heightened sexual
  d., hypoxic
  d., instinctual
  d., low sex
  d. or motivation ▸ lack of
  d., physical
  d., primitive
  d., respiratory
  d., sex
  d., sexual
  d., strong depressive
  d. test, respiratory
  d. unit, pump/
  d., ventricular
driven
  d. artificial heart, air-
  d. intervention ▸ peer-
  d. pacemaker ▸ sensor-
  d. rotatory chair, computer-
  d. treatment ▸ theory-
driver(s)
  d., drunk
  d. fatigue
  d., impaired
  d. leg
  D. Program (IDP), Intoxicated
  d. teeth ▸ screw◇
  D. (amphetamines), Truck
drives, primitive
driving (Driving)
  d., photic

  D. Drunk (SADD) ▸ Students
    Against
  D. (MADD) ▸ Mothers Against
    Drunk
  d. skills
  d. while intoxicated (DWI)
dromotropic effect
drooling from mouth
drooling, patient
droop(s)
  d. ▸ eye bulges and
  d., left facial
  d., left-sided facial
  d., nasolabial
  d., right facial
  d., right-sided facial
drooping
  d. brows
  d. eyelid
  d. mouth ▸ permanent
  d. of face
  d. of mouth
  d. of upper eyelid
  d. shoulders
  d., temporary facial weakness or
droopy
  d., baggy eyelids
  d. eyelid
  d. lids
drop(s)
  d. anesthesia, open
  d., anesthetic eye
  d., ankle
  d. attacks
  d., bilateral foot
  d. brace, toe◇
  d. culture, hanging-
  d., ear
  d. examination, hanging
  d., eye
  d. finger
  d. foot
  d. foot brace
  d. -foot procedure
  d. hand
  d. heart
  d., Hoffmann's
  d. in academic performance
  d. in blood pressure (BP) ▸ marked
  d. -in center
  d. instilled
  d., knee
  d. (morning glory seeds) ▸ licorice
  d. -lock knee ▸ long leg brace with
  d., neck

d., neurological foot
d., nose
d. -out, client
d. -out, echo
d. -out, septal
d. shoulder
d. technique, hanging
d., wrist◊

droplet(s)
d. infection
d., lipid
d. nuclei

dropped
d. beat
d. beat, periodic
d. beat pulse
d., blood pressure (BP)
d. elbow
d. foot
d. sole
d. to _____ torr ‣ pressure kept at _____ torr,
d. uterus

dropsical nephritis
dropsical nephropathy
dropsy
d., abdominal
d., cardiac
d. chest
d. of pericardium
d., peritoneal

drowned lung
drowned newborn syndrome
drowning, patient victim of
drowning victim, patient near-
drowsiness
d., behavioral
d., daytime
d., drug-induced morning
d., excessive
d., extreme
d. from alcohol
d. from antihistamine
d. from depression
d. from glomerulonephritis
d. from insect sting
d. from meningitis
d. from sleep apnea
d., increased
d., induce
d. ‣ lassitude and
d., relaxation and
d., restlessness and
d., rhythmic temporal theta burst of
d., slow waves of

d. with light sensitivity
drowsing stage
drowsing state
drowsy feeling
drowsy, patient
Drualt, bundle of
drug(s) (Drug)
d. absorption
d. abuse
d. abuse, adolescent
d. abuse, alcohol or
d. abuse, alcoholism and
d. abuse and addiction ‣ treatment of
d. abuse, antisocial behavior and
d. abuse, antisocial personality and
d. abuse ‣ autogenic training in
d. abuse, behavioral treatment
d. abuse, cardiovascular complications
d. abuse, cardiovascular problems related to
d. abuse, cause of
d. abuse, complications of
d. abuse counseling
d. abuse ‣ cutaneous signs as a screening device for
d. abuse, cutaneous signs of
d. abuse, death due to
d. abuse, dermatologic complications of
d. abuse diagnoses
d. abuse, diagnostic tests as a screening device for
d. abuse, diagnostic tests in
d. abuse drug testing ‣ alcohol and
d. abuse ‣ early intervention in
d. abuse, economic costs of
d. abuse education
d. abuse, endocrinologic complications of
d. abuse, endocrinologic problems related to
d. abuse, euphoria and
d. abuse, gastrointestinal (GI) complications of
d. abuse, genetic factors in
d. abuse, genitourinary (GU) complications of
d. abuse, genitourinary (GU) problems related to
d. abuse, GI (gastrointestinal) problems related to
d. abuse, GU (genitourinary) complications of

d. abuse, hematopoietic complications of
d. abuse, hematopoietic problems related to
d. abuse, hepatic complications of
d. abuse, hepatic problems related to
d. abuse hot line
d. abuse ‣ illicit
d. abuse in alcoholics, prevalence of
d. abuse in general patient population, prevalence of
d. abuse in physician population, prevalence of
d. abuse, incidence of
d. abuse, international trends in
d. abuse, legal restrictions in
d. abuse ‣ linking cigarette smoking and
d. abuse, medical history as screening device for
d. abuse, monitoring systems in
d. abuse, multi-
D. Abuse (NIDA) ‣ National Institute on
d. abuse, neonatal complications of
d. abuse, neuromuscular complications of
d. abuse, neuromuscular problems related to
d. abuse, obstetric complications of
d., abuse of prescribed
d. abuse, patient behavior as a screening device for
d. abuse, patient education on
d. abuse, patient had flashback reactions from
d. abuse, patient interview as a screening device for
d. abuse, patient questionnaire as a screening device for
d. abuse, physical effects of
d. abuse ‣ physical examination as a screening device for
d. abuse, physician
d. abuse, physiological factors in
d., abuse potential of multiple
d. abuse ‣ prescription
d. abuse prevention
d. abuse program
d. abuse, psychiatric complications of
d. abuse, psychological effects of
d. abuse, psychological factors in

435

drug(s)—*continued*

d. abuse, psychological history as a screening device for
d. abuse, psychological problems related to
d. abuse, pulmonary complications of
d. abuse, recreational
d. abuse, renal complications of
d. abuse, renal problems related to
d. abuse, reproductive complications of
D. Abuse Resistance Education (DARE)
d. abuse, screening for
d. abuse, septic complications of
d. abuse, septic problems related to
d. abuse, sexual complications of
d. abuse, social history as a screening device for
d. abuse, sociological factors in
d. abuse, surgical complications of
d. abuse, symptoms of
d. abuse, symptoms as a screening device for
d. abuse, systemic signs of
d. abuse threat
d. abuse treatment
d. abuse treatment, alcohol and
d. abuse treatment program ▸ publicly assisted
d. abuse, trends in
d. abuse warning
D. Abuse Warning Network (DAWN)
d. abuse ▸ warning signs of
d. abuser, demanding
d. abuser ▸ indifferent
d. abuser ▸ irresponsible
d. abuser ▸ manipulative
d. abusers, assessing needs of multi-
d. abusers, attitudes of
d. abusers, attitudes of physician
d. abusers, attitudes of society towards
d. abusers, confrontation techniques with
d. abusers, dangerous
d. abusers, hard-core
d. abusers, IV (intravenous)
d. abusers, medical problems in
d. abusers, obstetrical management of

d. abusers, physical abnormalities in
d. abusers, psychiatric disorders in
d. abusers, psychological problems of
d. abusers, risk factors for
d. abusers, sexual disorders of
d. abusers, surgical management of
d. -abusing behavior, extinction of
d. -abusing mother
d. -abusing patient, identifying
d. -abusing pregnant woman
d. action
d., acute abuse of
d., acute intoxication with multiple
d. addict
d. addict ▸ tricuspid endocarditis in
d. addiction
d. addiction, dual
d., addictive
d. ▸ addictive disease-producing
d., addictive illicit
d. addictive potential
d. addicts ▸ halfway house for
d. addicts ▸ rehabilitation center for
d. administration
D. Administration (FDA), Food and
d. administration ▸ intraperitoneal
d., adulterated
D. Advisory Committee ▸ Fertility Maternal Health
d. -affected baby
d. -affected kids
d. affinity
d. allergy
d., analgesic
d. analysis, specific
d. and alcohol abuse death
d. and alcohol dependence
d. and radiation modality, combined
d., anti-alcohol
d., antianginal
d., antianxiety
d., antiarrhythmic
d., anticancer
d., anticholinergic
d., anticoagulant
d., anticonvulsant
d., antidepressant
d., antiemetic
d., antiepileptic
d., antifungal
d., antigout
d., antihypertensive

d. ▸ anti-infective
d., anti-inflammatory
d., antileukemic
d., antimalarial
d., antimanic
d., antiobesity
d., anti-Parkinson
d., antiplatelet
d., antipsychotic
d., antireflux
d., antirejection
d., antiseizure
d., antispasmodic
d., antitremor
d., antituberculous
d., antiviral
d. -associated fatality
d. -associated pericarditis
d. -associated primary acute pancreatitis
d. awareness
D. Awareness Resistance Education (DARE) Program
d., bacteria resistant to
d., beta agonist
d., beta blocker
d. biotransformation
d., blood pressure lowering
d., blood thinning
d. box, emergency
d., brand name
d., calcium channel blocking
d., cancer fighting
d., cardiac arrest
d., cardiotonic
d., cell wall active
d., chemotherapeutic
d., chemotherapy
d. chemotherapy, multiple
d. chemotherapy, triple
d., cholesterol lowering
d., chronic abuse of
d. classes
d. clearance
d., clot busting
d., clot dissolving
d., clot dissolving thrombolytic
d. coated stent
d. coated tube
d. complication
d. consumption
d., contraband
d., controlled
d. controlling patient
d., convulsant

d., corticosteroid
d. counseling
d. counseling, alcohol and
d. counselor
d. courier
d., curare-like
d. ▸ curb intravenous use of
d., cytotoxic
d., dangerous
d. ▸ dangerous build-up of
d. dealer
d. dealer, crack house
d. dealer, major
d. dealing
d. delivery systems
d. dependence
d. dependence, behavioral treatment for
d. dependence, estimating degree of
d. dependence, physical
d. dependence, psychological
d. dependency
d. dependency with Crohn's disease
d. -dependent client
d. -dependent illness
d. dependent ▸ multiple
d. -dependent, patient
d. -dependent person, alcoholic
d. -dependent pregnant woman
d., depressant
d. ▸ depressant effect of
d., designer
d. detoxification
d., detoxification from multiple
d. development
d. (DMARD) ▸ disease modifying antirheumatic
d. disorders
d., dispensing
d., diuretic
d., diversion of
d., dopamine-boosting
d., dopamine-releasing
d. dosage
d. dosage, excessive
d. -drug interaction
d. duration, effective
d. education, alcohol and
d. education and prevention program
d. education program
d. effect
d. effect, indirect

d. effect ▸ intense psychoactive
d. effect, paradoxical
d., effective anticancer
d. effects ▸ duration of
D. Enforcement Agency (DEA)
d. eruption
d. eruption dermatitis
d. eruption, fixed
d. evaluation, final
d. evaluation program, clinical
d. excretion, decreased
d. experimental
d. experimentation
d., experiments
d. exposed baby
d. exposed kids
d. -exposed offspring
d. exposure ▸ intrauterine
d. -fast
d., fat soluble
d., fertility
d., fever reducing
d., flashback reactions with multiple
d. -food interaction
d. free
d. -free environment
d. -free environment ▸ structure
d. -free, patient is
d. -free program ▸ outpatient
d. -free program ▸ residential
d. -free protocol ▸ Westminster
d. -free treatment
d. -free treatment, outpatient
d. -free treatment program
D. -Free Workplace Act
d. from licit medical channels, diversion
d., fungus-suppressing
d., general anesthetic
d., generic
d. habit
d., habit-forming
d. habit, kicking
d. habituation
d. ▸ hallucinatory state induced by
d., hallucinogenic
d., hard
d., hazardous
d. hazards
d. ▸ heart rhythm
d. history, patient's
d., homeopathic
d. hustlers
d. hypersensitivity
d., hypnotic

d. idiosyncrasy
d. ▸ idiosyncratic reaction to
d., illegal
d., illicit
d. ▸ immune suppressing
d., immunosuppressant
d., immunosuppressive
d. -impaired baby
d. -impaired child
d. ▸ inactive dummy
d. index, emergency
d. -induced abortion
d. -induced activity
d. -induced alopecia
d. -induced alterations of cardiovascular function
d. -induced amnestic syndrome
d. -induced cancer
d. -induced cardiomyopathy
d. -induced cell destruction
d. -induced death
d. -induced delirium
d. -induced dementia
d. -induced diabetes
d. -induced fever
d. -induced gastrointestinal disorder
d. -induced hallucinations
d. -induced hallucinosis
d. -induced heartburn
d. -induced hepatic injury
d. -induced hepatitis
d. -induced hyperplasia
d. -induced immune hemolytic anemia
d. -induced high
d. -induced liver toxicity
d. -induced lupus
d. -induced lupus erythematosus
d. -induced lupus syndrome
d. -induced mental disorder
d. -induced morning drowsiness
d. -induced neuropathy
d. -induced organic affective syndrome
d. -induced organic delusional syndrome
d. -induced parkinsonism
d. -induced pericarditis
d. -induced postanesthetic depression
d. -induced postanesthetic respiratory depression
d. -induced psychiatric effects
d. -induced psychosis

drug(s)—*continued*

d. -induced relaxation
d. -induced sleep
d. -induced thrombocytopenia
d. -induced tremors
d. industry, generic
d. information
d. infusion
d. infusion pump, implantable
d., ingestion of
d. ▸ ingestion of toxic
d. ingestion ▸ psychedelic
d., inotropic
d. interaction
d. interaction, hallucinogenic
d. interaction ▸ herb
d. interaction ▸ life threatening
d. interaction ▸ potential
d. interaction, toxicity or
d. interaction with alcohol
d. interactions ▸ food-
d. interdiction program
d. intervention program
d. intolerance
d., intolerance to specific
d. intoxication
d. intoxication, acute treatment for acute
d. intoxication, differential diagnosis in acute
d. intoxication, clinical manifestations of acute
d. intoxication ▸ hallucinogenic
d. intoxication, pathologic
d. intoxication, psychological state in acute
d. intoxication, subacute treatment of acute
d. intoxication, symptoms of acute
d., intra-arterial injection of
d., investigational
d. involvement
d. label
d., lethal
d. level, antiepileptic
d. level ▸ therapeutic
d. ▸ life-saving antiviral
d., light-sensitive
d., medical overuse of
d. metabolism ▸ hepatic
d. metabolizing enzymes ▸ microsomal
d. ▸ migraine aborting
d. ▸ mind-altering
d., misuse of

d. ▸ misuse of nonprescription
d. ▸ misuse of prescription
d. misuse ▸ psychotherapeutic
d. misuser
d. ▸ mood-altering
d., mood-elevating
d. ▸ mood-enhancing
d., mood-modifying
d. ▸ mood-stabilizing
d., multiple
d. ▸ muscle-building
d. ▸ muscle-relaxing
d., narcotic
d., nausea-producing
d. needles, contaminated
d. needles, infected IV (intravenous)
d. needles, sharing
d. needles ▸ sharing infected intravenous
d., nephrotoxic
d., nerve-numbing
d., neuroleptic
d., neurotoxic
d. ▸ nondependent abuse of
d. (NSAID), nonsteroidal anti-inflammatory
d., nontherapeutic
d. ▸ off label use of
d. offenders, repeat
d., OKT3
d., on-trial
d., opiate
d., oral diabetes
d. ▸ oral steroid
d., organic brain syndrome with multiple
d., organotropic
d., orphan
d., OTC (over the counter)
d. overdose
d., overuse of
d., pain suppressing
d., painkilling
d., palliative
d., panic reactions with multiple
d., paralytic
d. ▸ paranoid state induced by
d. ▸ patient craving
d., patient OD (overdosed) with multiple
d., physical dependence on
d., potent
d. -precipitated psychosis
d., prenatal

d. ▸ prenatal abuse of illicit
d., preparation of
d., prescribed
d., prescription
d., pressor
d. problem
d. products
d. profile
d. program, multiple
D. Program, Orphan
d. program, patient on multiple
d. program, traditional
d., project, coronary
d., prophylactic antimicrobial
d., prostate treatment
d. protocol, experimental
d. protocol, multiple
d. protocol, three
d., psychedelic
d., psychoactive
d., psychoactive properties of abused
d. psychosis
d., psychotic reactions with multiple
d., psychotropic
d., quack
d., radioprotective
d., radiosensitizing
d. raid
d. reaction
d. reaction, acute
d. reaction, adverse
d. reaction, antiemetic
d. reaction, clinical manifestations of
d. reaction withdrawal, treatment of acute
d. reactions, diagnosis of acute
d. reactions in organic brain syndrome
d. reactions in violent patients, treatment of acute
d. reactions, psychological manifestations of acute
d. reactions to cannabinoids, treatment of acute
d. reactions to depressants, treatment of acute
d. reactions to hallucinogens, treatment of acute
d. reactions to inhalants, treatment of acute
d. reactions to multiple drugs, treatment of acute

d. reactions to opioids, treatment of acute
d. reactions to phencyclidine, treatment of acute
d. reactions to stimulants, treatment of acute
d. reactions, symptoms of acute
d. reactions, treatment of acute
d., recreational
d. -refractory tachycardia
d. regimen
d. regimens, patient compliance with
d. regulation
D. Rehabilitation Center
d. -related crisis
d. -related death
d. -related fatal poisoning
d. -related impairment
d. -related infection
d. -related involuntary movement
d. -related homicide
d. -related medical complications
d. -related offenses
d. -related violence
d. research
d. resistance
d. resistance, genetic
d. -resistant
d. -resistant bacteria
d. -resistant disease
d. -resistant genes
d. -resistant infection
d. resistant, multi-
d. -resistant organisms
d. -resistant organisms aspirated into lungs
d. -resistant schizophrenia
d. -resistant strains
d. -resistant Streptococcus pneumoniae
d. -resistant tuberculosis
d. -resistant virus
d., restorative
d. safety profile
d. screen
d. screen ▸ positive urine
d. screen test
d. screen, urine
d. screening
d. screening panel
d. screening program
d. screening test ▸ initial
d., sedative action of
d. ▸ sedative hypnotic

d. -seeking
d. -seeking environment
d., selection of abused
d. self-administered
d. sensitivity
d., severe addiction to
d. ▸ slowly metabolize certain
d. sniffing
d. snorting, swallowing or smoking
d., social
d., soft
d., soporific
d., special effects of
d., sterile
d., stimulant
d., street
d., street names for
d. ▸ suppressive or disease-modifying
d., sympathomimetic
d., synthetic
d., tainted
d. taking behavior
d. tampering
d., tapering off
d. testing, alcohol and drug abuse
d. ▸ testing positive for
D. Testing Program ▸ Forensic Urine
d. testing, random
d., therapeutic
d. therapies, combination
d. therapies, multiple
d. therapy
d. therapy, antibiotic
d. therapy, cardiac
d. therapy, cholesterol-lowering
d. therapy, discontinuing
d. therapy, immunosuppressive
d. therapy ▸ long-term
d. therapy, new
d. therapy, oral
d. therapy, prescription
d. therapy, prolonged
d. therapy ▸ re-evaluation of existing
d. therapy ▸ three
d., thrombolytic
d. to ward off infection
d. tolerance
d., toxic
d., toxic levels of
d. toxicity
d. toxicity ▸ newborn
d., toxicity of multiple

d. traces ▸ residual
d. traffic, illegal
d. traffickers
d. treatment
d. treatment, antiviral
D. Treatment Center
d. treatment clinic, free
d. treatment group
d. treatment issues ▸ impaired employees alcohol and
d. treatment ▸ long-term
d., treatment of acute drug reactions to multiple
d., treatment of physicians who abuse
d. treatment program
d. treatment specialist
d. treatment system ▸ outpatient
d. trials
d. ▸ triangulation of
d., under the table
d. usage, hard
d. use, abstention vs. moderation of
d. use, adolescent
d. use, alcohol and
d. use, blood screen for
d. use, encouragement of
d. use, experimental
d. use, intravenous (IV)
d. use, illegal
d. use, illegal IV (intravenous)
d. use, illicit
d. use ▸ multigenerational
d. use, occasional
d., use of
d. use, patterns of
d. use ▸ post-treatment
d. use ▸ recent alcohol or
d. use ▸ recovery of alcohol or
d. use, regular
d. use, resume
d. use ▸ screening for
d. user
d. user, active
d. user, casual
d. user, chronic
d. user, dependent
d. user, intravenous (IV)
d. user, patient occasional
d. -using peer groups
d., vasoactive
d., vasodilator
d., vasospastic
d. victim

drug(s)—*continued*
d., war on
d. withdrawal
d. withdrawal, features associated
with
d., withdrawal from multiple
d. withdrawal insomnia
d. withdrawal syndrome
d., wonder
drugged, feeling
drum(s) [*gum*]
d., bowed
d., canals and
d., ear◇
d., inflated ear◇
d., injected ear◇
d., intact
d. membrane
d. perforation
d. perforation, ear
d., vacuum formed
Drummond's sign
drumstick finger
drunk (Drunk)
d. driver
D. Driving (MADD) ▸ Mothers
Against
D. (SADD), Students Against
Driving
drunken behavior
dry
d. adhesions
d. age-related macular
degeneration
d. and gritty ▸ eye
d. and intact, dressings
d. and itchy ▸ skin
d. and occlusive, dressing
d. and scaly ▸ skin
d. beriberi
d., blot
d. bronchiectasis
d. bronchitis
d. compress
d. cough
d., cracked skin
d., cracked skin on heel
d. crackling sounds
d., dead cells ▸ flush away dulling
d. dressing
d. eczema
d. eye symptoms
d. eye syndrome
d. eyes
d. eyes, chronic

d. field
d., fissured lips ▸ reddened,
d. gangrene
d. hacking cough
d. hands
d. heat
d. heaves
d. hernia
d. -house ▸ hot-
d., incision clean and
d., irritated eyes
d. itching skin
d., itchy, flaking skin
d. joint
d. labor
d. macular degeneration
d., mottled skin
d. mouth
d. mouth from antihistamine
d. mouth, patient has
d. mouth ▸ permanent
d. objective
d. pericarditis
d. pleurisy
d. rale
d., red, cracked and itchy hands
d. serosal peritoneal surfaces
d. -shelled cataract
d. skin
d. skin and hair
d. slide technology
d. socket
d. socket ▸ tooth extraction
d. sterile dressing (DSD)
d. sterile dressing (DSD) applied
d. swallow
d. throat
d. vomiting
d. weight
d. weight, fat-free
d. wrinkled skin
drying
d. and wrinkling of skin
d., freeze-
d. of eye
d., open-air
d. out ▸ patient
dryness
d. and itching of skin
d. and itching ▸ redness,
d., estrogen-dependent vaginal
d. from dermatitis ▸ eye
d. from eczema ▸ eye
d. of cornea
d. of eye

d. of eyes and mouth
d. of mouth
d. of mouth ▸ extreme
d. of mucous membranes
d. ▸ severe eye
d. ▸ severe mouth
d., vaginal
Drysdale corpuscles
DS (degenerative spinal disease)
**DSA (digital subtraction
angiography)**
DSD (dry sterile dressing)
**DSPS (delayed sleep phase
syndrome)**
DST (Daya Syphilis Test)
**DST (dexamethasone suppression
test)**
DST (donor specific transfusion)
**DTIC/DIC (dimethyl triazenoimidazole
carboxamide)**
DTP (distal tingling on percussion)
DTR (deep tendon reflexes)
DTR equal and active bilaterally
DTR hypoactive
DTR ▸ increased
DTR ▸ monitoring of
DTR symmetrical
DTs (delirium tremens)
du
d. doute, folie
d. pourquoi, folie
d. reveil, cataplexie
dual
d. affinity
d. approach to treatment
d. atrioventricular nodal pathways
d. chamber atrioventricular (AV)
pacemaker
d. chamber cardiac pacemaker
d. chamber pacemaker
d. chamber pacemaker, Aurora
d. chamber pacemaker, Autima II
d. chamber pacing
d. chamber rate responsive
d. demand pacemaker
d. contrast study
d. diagnosis
D. Diagnosis Groups
d. diagnosis patient
d. disorders
d. drug addiction
d. echophonocardiography
d. -electrode lead
d. energy linear accelerator

d. energy x-ray absorptiometry
(DEXA)

d. energy x-ray absorptiometry
(DEXA) bone density test

d. inlay bone graft

d. lock total hip replacement

d. mode, dual pacing, dual sensing
(DDD)

d. onlay graft

d. pacemaker ▸ reprogram

d. pacing, dual sensing (DDD) ▸
dual mode,

d. pass pacemaker

d. photon energy accelerator

d. photon linear accelerator

d. personality

d. reaction

d. sensing (DDD) ▸ dual mode,
dual pacing,

d. -site atrial pacing

d. use water cooler

d. x-ray beam dosimetry

dually addicted

dually diagnosed

Duane

D. classification of convergence
insufficiency

D. retraction syndrome

D. syndrome

D. syndrome, Stilling-Türk-

DUB (dysfunctional uterine bleeding)

Dubin-Johnson syndrome

Dubini's chorea

Dubini's disease

Dubois'

D. abscess

D. disease

D. method

duboisii, Histoplasma

Dubovitz's syndrome

Dubowitz developmental examination

Duchenne('s)

D. -Aran muscular atrophy

D. disease

D. dystrophy

D. -Erb paralysis

D. muscular atrophy ▸ Aran-

D. muscular disease ▸ Aran-

D. muscular dystrophy (DMD)

D. paralysis

D. sign

duckbill voice prosthesis

duck-billed speculum

duckling stage, ugly

ducreyi, Haemophilus/ Hemophilus

Ducrey's bacillus

Ducrey's disease

duct(s)

d., aberrant

d., alveolar

d., ampulla of lacrimal

d. anomaly ▸ müllerian

d., anterior lacrimal

d., arch of thoracic

d., atresia of lacrimonasal

d., Bellini's

d., bile

d., biliary

d., blocked sperm

d., blocked tear

d., Botallo's

d. cancer

d. cancer, bile

d. cancer, villous

d. carcinoma

d. carcinoma, bile

c. carcinoma, periurethral

d., catheterization of

d., catheterization of lacrimonasal

d. cell adenocarcinoma

d. cell carcinoma

d. cell carcinoma, infiltrating

d. cell carcinoma, multifocal ▸
infiltrated

d. cholangiogram, cystic

d., cicatricial stenosis of
lacrimonasal

d., cochlear

d., collecting

d., common

d., common bile

d., common hepatic

d., cupular cecum of cochlear

d. cyst, Bartholin

d. cyst, thyroglossal

d. cyst, vitelline

d., cystic

d., deferent

d., dilatation of bile

d., dilate narrowed

d., dilated

d., dilated bile

d. disease, small

d. ▸ disruption of pancreatic

d. ▸ distention of biliary

d., eccrine

d. ectasia, focal

d. ectasia, mammary

d., efferent

d., ejaculatory

d., elongated cystic

d. emphysema, alveolar

d., endolymphatic

d., excretory

d. exploration, bile

d. exploration, common

d., extrahepatic bile

d. fistula of lacrimonasal

d. fistula, thoracic

d. flow, thoracic

d. ▸ flush milk

d., functional

d., Gartner's

d., hepatic

d., Hoffmann's

d., hyperplasia of

d. hyperplasia, pancreatic

d., infection in milk

d. injection, transduodenal
fiberscopic

d., interstitial

d., lacrimal

d., lacrimonasal

d., lactiferous

d. lymph, thoracic

d., lymphatic

d., mammary

d. ▸ medullary collecting

d., mesonephric

d., milk

d., müllerian

d. ▸ narrowing of common

d., nasal

d., nasolacrimal

d., nipple

d., obstructed bile

d., obstructed common

d. obstruction, bile

d. ▸ obstruction of pancreatic

d. of Botallo

d. of Cuvier

d. of eye, excretory

d. of Rivinus

d. of sweat gland

d., omphalomesenteric

d. opening, bile

d., ovarian

d., pancreatic

d., papillary

d. papillomatosis ▸ subareolar

d., paramesonephric

d., paraurethral

d., parotid

d., patent

d. patent, pancreatic

duct(s)—*continued*
d., patent vitelline
d., plug tear
d. pressure (TDP) ▸ thoracic
d., probing of lacrimonasal
d., proliferation, bile
d., prostatic
d., Reichel's cloacal
d., salivary
d., semicircular
d., seminal
d., Skene's
d., sphincter muscle of bile
d., spiral fold of cystic
d., stenosis of lacrimonasal
d., Stensen's
d. stent, occluded common bile
d. stone, bile
d. stone, common bile
d. stone, dissolve common bile
d. ▸ stones present in pancreatic
d., stricture of bile
d., stump cystic
d., sublingual
d., submandibular
d., submaxillary
d., supernumerary lacrimonasal
d., surgical anastomosis of
   pancreatic
d. system, biliary
d., tear
d., thoracic
d., thyroglossal
d. tolerance, biliary
d. tumor, bile
d. tumor, craniopharyngeal
d. tumor, distal common
d., vestibular cecum of cochlear
d., vitelline
d., Walther's
d., Wharton's
d., wolffian

ductal
d. abnormality
d. adenoma
d. anatomy
d. cancer ▸ invasive
d. cannulation
d. carcinoma
d. carcinoma in situ (DCIS)
d. carcinoma, infiltrative
d. carcinoma of breast ▸ infiltrating
d. carcinoma ▸ poorly differentiated
d. cell carcinoma
d. cell carcinoma, infiltrating

d. dilatation
d. hyperplasia
d. hyperplasia ▸ atypical
d. lavage
d. morphology
d. papilloma
d. pattern

ductile hyperplasia
duction eye test
ductless gland
ductogram procedure
ductography, peroral retrograde
   pancreaticobiliary
ductus
d. arch
d. arteriosus
d. arteriosus, calcific
d. arteriosus, closed
d. arteriosus murmur ▸ patent
d. arteriosus, patent
d. arteriosus ▸ persistent
d. arteriosus ▸ railroad track
d. arteriosus ▸ reversed
d. arteriosus umbrella ▸ patent
d. bump
d. choledochus
d. cochlearis ▸ vas prominens
d. deferens
d. deferentis, ampulla
d. lacrimalis
d. lacrimalis, ampulla
d., patent
d. perilymphatici
d. renal agenesis with associated
   stigmata ▸ patent
d. venosus

Dudley's operation
due to
d.t. aging ▸ white matter loss
d.t. alcohol abuse ▸ sudden death
d.t. cocaine ingestion ▸ sudden
   death
d.t. drug abuse, death
d.t. embolism ▸ infarction of lung
d.t. Enterococci ▸ peritonitis
d.t. natural causes ▸ patient expired
d.t. obstruction ▸ shock
d.t. pressure ▸ exophthalmos
d.t. radiation ▸ spinal deterioration
d.t. thrombosis ▸ infraction of lung
d.t. tower skull ▸ exophthalmos
d.t. uremia, eclampsia

Dugas' test
Duguet siphon
Duhamel procedure

Duhring's disease
Dührssen's
D. incision
D. operation
D. tampon
Duke('s) (s')
D. C classification of right
   ascending colon
D. C colon cancer
D. carcinoma
D. carcinoma of colon
D. classification of carcinoma
D. -Elder Lamp
D. lesion
D. scale
D. treadmill prognostic score
dull
d. abdominal pain
d. aching pain
d., aching pressure discomfort ▸
   diffuse,
d. and lethargic
d. and lethargic ▸ patient
d. chest pain
d. curettage
d. epigastric pain
d., eyes
d. on questioning
d. pain
d., patient's affect
d. psychopath
dulled
d. emotions
d., memory
d. or lessened ▸ blunted,
d., sense of pain
dulling
d. dry, dead cells ▸ flush away
d., mental
d. of mental function
dullness
d. (ACD) ▸ absolute cardiac
d. and decreased breath sounds
d. and not caring ▸ feeling of
d., area of cardiac
d. (CD) ▸ border of cardiac
d. (CD) ▸ cardiac
d., cardiac border of
d. (CD) ▸ left border of cardiac
d., mental
d. on percussion
d. over left lung
d. over right lung
d. (RCD) ▸ relative cardiac
d., relative hepatic

d., shifting
d. to percussion
d., total
dumb ague
dumbbell form ▸ **myocardial**
infarction in
Dumdum fever
dummy (Dummy)
d. drug ▸ inactive
D. Dust (phencyclidine)
d. (placebo) medication
d. technique, double
dumoffi, Legionella
dumping
d. of barium meal
d., patient
d. stomach
d. syndrome
d. syndrome ▸ postgastrectomy
dumps, chemical waste
Duncan('s)
D. folds
D. mechanism
D. ventricle
Dunfermline scale
Dunlop traction
Dunn-Brittain operation
duodenal
d. artery
d. aspirate
d. atresia
d. brake
d. bulb
d. bulb and sweep
d. bulb, coarsening of
d. bulb, deformity of
d. bulb, irritable
d. bulb scarring
d. bulbar ulcer
d. bypass ▸ total
d. cap
d. carcinoma
d. deformity
d. diverticula
d. diverticulum
d. fluid analysis
d. fold, inferior
d. fold, superior
d. intubation ▸ endoscopically
assisted
d. irritability
d. loop
d. mucosa
d. opening
d. opening narrow

d. papilla
d. peptone infusion
d. string test
d. sweep
d. tube
d. ulcer
d. ulcer, acute
d. ulcer, healing
d. ulcer patient
d. veins
d. wall ▸ microscopic invasion of
duodenale, Ancylostoma
duodenectomy, pancreatico◊
duodenitis, superficial
duodenocolic reflex
duodenography, hypotonic
duodenojejunal
d. flexure
d. fold
d. hernia
duodenomesocolic fold
duodenopyloric constriction
duodenostomy
d., cholecysto◊
d., choledocho◊
d., esophago◊
d., gastro◊
duodenum
d., adenocarcinoma of
d., carcinoma of
d., closure of open ends of stomach
and
d. ▸ clotted blood in
d., donor
d., duplication of
d. free of ulcers
d. ▸ gallbladder anastomosed to
d., inferior flexure of
d., inflammation of
d., longitudinal fold of
d. ▸ mucosal surfaces of
d., pancreas and
d., prompt spill into
d., proximal
d., scope advanced directly into
d., second portion of
d., superior flexure of
d., suspensory muscle of
d., traumatic transection of proximal
Duografin contrast medium
Duo-Lock hip prosthesis, Mueller
Duplay('s)
D. bursitis
D. disease
D. urethroplasty, Thiersch-

duplex
d., Ferribacterium
d., Haemophilus/Hemophilus
d. imaging
d. placenta
d. pulsed Doppler ultrasonography
d., pulsus
d. scan, carotid
d. scanning
d., Siderobacter
d., Sideromonas
d. ultrasonography
d. ultrasound
d., uterus
duplication
d. anomaly
d. of colon
d. of duodenum
d. of esophagus
d. of left collecting system
d. of left kidney
d. of right collecting system
d. of right kidney
duplicitous thoughts
dupp, lubb-
Dupuy-Dutemps operation
Dupuytren's
D. amputation
D. contracture
D. contraction, false
D. fracture
D. hydrocele
D. sign
dura, cadaveric
dura, lamia
dura mater
d.m. encephali
d.m. of brain
d.m. of spinal cord
d.m. spinalis
durable power of attorney decision
durae matris, sinus
dural
d. artery
d. covering of cerebrum
d. cul-de-sac
d. defect
d. endothelioma
d. membrane
d. plate
d. sac
Duran annuloplasty ring
Durand-Nicolas-Favre disease
durans, Streptococcus
Durapulse pacemaker

duration
    d., action potential
    d., anodal
    d., cathodal
    d. contraction, anodal
    d. curve ▸ strength
    d., deep sleep of short
    d., effective drug
    d., fever of brief
    d., frequency of
    d. ▸ half amplitude pulse
    d., increased overall treatment
    d. ▸ insufficient severity of
    d., intensity and
    d., modality and
    d. ▸ monophasic action potential
    d. of cycle
    d. of drug effects
    d. of effects of opioids
    d. of epoch
    d. of expiration
    d. of inspiration
    d. of labor, abnormal
    d. of sleep interruption
    d. of symptoms
    d. of wave
    d., pulse
    d., QRS
    d., seizure
    d. ▸ symptoms fluctuate in
    d. ▸ syndrome, severity and
    d. tetanus, anodal
    d. tetanus, cathodal
    d. tetany
durazzo, Salmonelia
Dürck's granuloma
Dürck's nodes
Durham decision
during
    d. cardiac arrest, heart shocked
    d. dialysis, medications
    d. exercise ▸ sudden death
    d. expiration ▸ prolongation of air flow
    d. jogging ▸ sudden death
    d. labor ▸ emotional support
    d. massage, basic kneading maneuver
    d. massage, cat stroking maneuver
    d. massage, circular pressure maneuver
    d. massage ▸ fan stroking maneuver
    d. massage ▸ holding maneuver
    d. massage ▸ knuckling maneuver

    d. massage ▸ smooth and repetitive stroke
    d. massage ▸ thumb stroking maneuver
    d. pregnancy, bleeding
    d. pregnancy ▸ care and treatment
    d. pregnancy ▸ drinking alcohol
    d. pregnancy ▸ maternal smoking
    d. pregnancy ▸ substance abuse
    d. pregnancy ▸ uterine bleeding
    d. sleep, K complexes
    d. urination, pain
    d. withdrawal, psychological state
Durman's operation
Duroziez's
    D. disease
    D. murmur
    D. sign
Durr's operation
durum, carcinoma
dusky discoloration
dust (Dust)
    d. allergy, house
    D. (hallucinogen), Angel
    D. (phencyclidine), Angel
    d. asthma
    d. asthma, cotton
    d., background nuclear
    d. cell
    d. disease
    d. disease ▸ inorganic
    D. (phencyclidine), Dummy
    d., dysnuclear
    d. emphysema, focal
    d. exposure, minimal
    d. exposure, organic
    d., grain
    D. (cocaine), Heaven
    d. mites
    D. (phencyclidine), Monkey
    d., mushroom
    D. of Angels (phencyclidine)
    d. pneumoconiosis ▸ organic
    d. ▸ spore containing
dustborne infection
dutch cap
Dutemps operation ▸ Dupuy-
duttonii, Borrelia
duty care, private
duty factor
Duval bacillus ▸ Sonne-
Duval procedure
Duverger and Velter's operation
Duvernay operation ▸ Graber-
Duverney's fracture

DuVries hammer toe repair
dux, Sarcophaga
DVA (distance visual acuity)
DVD (dissociated vertical divergence)
DVI (Digital Vascular Imager)
DVI (Digital Vascular Imager) multicenter
DVIU (direct vision internal urethrotomy)
DVT (deep venous thrombosis)
D/W (dextrose in water)
dwarf(s)
    d., achondroplastic
    d., adult
    d., Amsterdam
    d., asexual
    d., ateliotic
    d., bird-headed
    d., Brissaud's
    d. (D.) colony
    d., cretin
    d., diastrophic
    d., geleophysic
    d., hypophyseal
    d., hypopituitary
    d., hypothyroid
    d., infantile
    d., Levi-Lorain
    d., micromelic
    d., nanocephalic
    d., normal
    d. of Seckel, bird-headed
    d., organism
    d., Paltauf's
    d., phocomelic
    d., physiologic
    d., pituitary
    d., primordial
    d., pure
    d., rachitic
    d., renal
    d., Russell
    d., sexual
    d., Silver
    d., thanatophoric
    d., thyroid deficient
    d., true
dwarfed enamel
dwarfism
    d., Kniest
    d., pituitary
    d., short limb
DWB (disordered water balance) ▸ syndrome of
DWI (driving while intoxicated)

Dx (diagnosis)
D-xylose absorption test
D-xylose tolerance test
dye(s)
    d., allergic reaction to
    d. appears promptly
    d. binding capacity
    d., bolus of
    d., brilliant green
    d., cancer-killing
    d., cardiogram
    d., concentration of
    d., contrast
    d. curve ▸ green
    d. curves
    d., delayed concentration of
    d., drainage (dr'ge) of
    d. exclusion assay
    d., excretion of
    d., faint concentration of
    d., fluorescein
    d., indigo carmine
    d. ▸ indocyanine green
    d. injected negative
    d., injection of
    d. laser
    d. laser, coumarin pulsed
    d. laser, pulsed
    d. laser treatment, tuneable
    d. laser ▸ tuneable
    d., neutral
    d., prompt appearance of
    d., prompt excretion of
    d., radiocontrast
    d., radiopaque
    d., residual
    d., rose bengal
    d. test
    d. test, methylene blue
    d. test, Sabin
    d., water soluble
    d. workers' cancer
dying
    d., aid in
    d. ▸ fear of
    d. ▸ lower risk of
    d. process
    d. process, prolong
    d., sick and
    d. ▸ thoughts of
dynamic(s)
    d. aorta
    d. block
    d. cardiomyoplasty

    d. computer tomography, atrial
        bolus
    d. computerized tomography
    d. condenser electrometer
    d. derangements, human
    d. equilibrium
    d. exercise
    d. facial line
    d., family
    d. finger exerciser
    d., fluid
    d. frequency response
    d., funnel
    d. ▸ left ventricular (LV) left atrial
        (LA) crossover
    d. left ventriculogram
    d., marital
    d. murmur
    d. of human behavior
    d. polarity
    d. pressure
    d. psychiatry
    d. psychology
    d. psychotherapy
    d., radionuclear
    d. range
    d. range ▸ logarithmic
    d. rays
    d. refraction
    d., relationship
    d. relaxation
    d. splinting
    d. stiffness, active
    d. therapist
    d. therapy
    d. venous plethysmography
    d. viscosity
dynamism, mental
dynamite headache
dynamite heart
dynamometer, sphygmo◇
dynamometer, squeeze
dyne seconds
DyoVac suction punch
dypnoidic state
dysarthria literalis
dysarthria syllabaris spasmodica
dysarthric, patient
dysautonomia, familial
dysautonomia ▸ mitral valve
dysautonomic mitochondrial
    myopathy
dysbasia [*dysphagia, dysphasia,*
    ***dysplasia*]**
    d. angiosclerotica

    d. angiospastica
    d. intermittens angiosclerotica
    d. lordotica progressiva
    d. neurasthenica intermittens
dysbulia/dysboulia
dyschondroplasia, Ollier's
dyschromicum, erythema
dysconjugate, eyes
dysconjugate gaze
dyscontrol
    d., dissociation
    d., impulse
    d. in eating disorder ▸ impulse
    d. ▸ serious affective
    d. ▸ serious impulsive
    d., trauma
dyscrasia
    d., blood
    d., food
    d., lymphatic
dyscrasic fracture
dyscrinic rhinitis
dysenteriae
    d., Bacillus
    d., Bacterium
    d., Shigella
dysenteric diarrhea
dysenteric gastroenteritis
dysentery
    d., amebic
    d., asylum
    d., bacillary
    d., balantidial
    d., bilharzial
    d., catarrhal
    d., ciliary
    d., ciliate
    d., epidemic
    d., flagellate
    d., Flexner's
    d., fulminant
    d. group, colon—typhoid
    d., institutional
    d., Japanese
    d., malarial
    d., malignant
    d. outbreak
    d., protozoal
    d., schistosomal
    d., scorbutic
    d., Shigella
    d., Sonne
    d., spirillar
    d., sporadic
    d., swine

dysentery—*continued*
d., viral
d., winter
dyserythropoietic anemia
dyserythropoietic anemia, congenital
dysesthetic sensation
dysfluency ▸ period of
dysfunction
d., acute psychiatric
d., adrenal
d., advanced left ventricular (LV)
d. after heart attack ▸ sexual
d. and stress ▸ personality
d., asymptomatic left ventricular (LV)
d., asymptomatic ventricular
d., autonomic
d., autonomic nervous system
d., benign inner ear
d., binocular
d., bladder
d., bladder and bowel
d. ▸ bladder involvement, infection or
d., blood
d., bowel and bladder
d., brain
d., cardiac
d., cell
d., central audiovestibular
d., central nervous system (CNS)
d., cognitive
d., constitutional hepatic
d., cortical
d., diastolic
d., diffuse cerebral
d. ▸ diffuse subcortical
d. disorder, childhood neurodevelopmental
d., endothelial
d. ▸ enhanced muscle
d., erectile
d., esophageal
d. ▸ esophageal motility
d., eustachian tube
d. ▸ generalized neurologic
d. ▸ glutamate receptor
d., heart
d., hepatic
d., hypertonic uterine
d., immune
d. ▸ immune system
d. ▸ inhibited sexual desire psychosexual
d., intellectual

d., intimacy
d., kidney
d., labyrinthine
d., language
d., leukocyte
d., liver
d. ▸ localized occipital
d. ▸ lower motor neuron (MN)
d., lung
d. ▸ male sexual
d., marital
d., membrane
d., memory
d., mental
d., microwave
d. (MBD) ▸ minimal brain
d., motor
d., muscle
d., muscular
d., myocardial
d. ▸ myofascial pain and
d., neurologic
d. ▸ ocular and cerebellar
d. of brain
d. of cervical spine
d. of liver, constitutional
d. of peripheral nerves
d. of sleep stages
d. of uterus
d., organic
d., ovarian
d. ▸ overt left ventricular
d., pain
d., paleocerebellar
d., papillary muscle
d., parathyroid
d., parietal
d., phagocytic
d., placental
d., platelet
d., posterior tibial
d., postoperative bladder
d. ▸ postpartum voiding
d. problem ▸ immune
d., progressive
d., psychic
d., psychological
d., psychosexual
d., psychosocial
d., psychostimulant
d., renal
d. ▸ renal tubular
d., respiratory
d. ▸ respiratory muscle
d., reversible myocardial

d. ▸ right frontal
d. ▸ right parietal
d. ▸ salivary gland
d., sensory
d. ▸ severe family
d., sexual
d. ▸ significant focal
d. ▸ sinus nodal
d., sinus node
d., social
d., sphincter
d. ▸ superimposed upper motor neuron
d. syndrome (MPD) ▸ myofacial pain
d. syndrome, placental
d. syndrome ▸ platelet
d., systolic
d., temporomandibular joint (TMJ)
d., thyroid
d., transient spinal cord
d. ▸ underlying immune
d., urinary tract
d., valvular
d., ventricular
d., vestibular
d. ▸ vocal cord
d., voiding
dysfunctional
d. attitude
d. behavior
d. client
d. cognition
d. episode, heart
d. family
d. family, adult children of
d. family systems
d. grieving
d. group
d. heart valve
d. immune system
d. labor
d. labor, primary
d. lifestyle
d. marriage
d. meibomian glands
d. myocardium
d. parenting style
d., patient disoriented and
d. pigment epithelium
d. portion of colon
d. process
d. relationship
d. staff behavior
d. thermoregulatory system

d. uterine bleeding (DUB)
d. vaginal bleeding
dysgenesis, gonadal
dysgerminoma, ovarian
dysglandular syndrome
dysgonic colony
dyshidrosis, blister from
dyshidrotic dermatitis
dyshormonogenesis, thyroid
dysjunctive motor activity
dyskeratosis syndrome, hereditary benign intraepithelial
dyskinesia
    d. algera
    d. ▸ antipsychotic-induced tardive
    d., apical
    d., biliary
    d., detrusor
    d. intermittens
    d., occupational
    d., orofacial
    d., severe
    d. tarda
    d., tardive
    d. ▸ tremor and
    d., uterine
dyskinesis
    d., anterior wall
    d., anteroapical
    d. ▸ left ventricular (LV)
    d., posteroinferior
dyskinetic
    d. and dystonic reactions
    d. labor
    d. movements ▸ persistent
dyslexia
    d., developmental
    d., severe
    d., spatial
dyslexic children
dyslipidemia, diabetic
dysmaturity syndrome
dysmaturity syndrome ▸ pulmonary
dysmelinatus, status
dysmenorrhea
    d., acquired
    d., congestive
    d., essential
    d., inflammatory
    d. intermenstrualis
    d., mechanical
    d., membranous
    d., obstructive
    d., ovarian
    d., plethoric

d., primary
d., psychogenic
d., secondary
d., spasmodic
d., tubal
d., uterine
dysmetabolic syndrome
dysmobility rehabilitation and balance
dysmorphia, facial
dysmorphic disorder (BDD), body
dysmorphic syndrome
dysmotility disorder ▸ sphincter of Oddi
dysmotility, esophageal
dysmyelinisatus, status
dysmyelopoietic syndrome of RAEB (refractory anemia with excess blasts)
dysnuclear dust
dysopia/dysopsia
dysopia algera
dysostosis
    d., cleidocranial
    d., craniofacial
    d., mandibulofacial
    d. multiplex
    d., orodigitofacial
dyspareunia, functional
dyspepsia
    d., acid
    d., appendicular
    d., appendix
    d., atonic
    d., catarrhal
    d., chichiko
    d., cholelithic
    d., fermentative
    d., flatulent
    d., functional
    d., gastric
    d., nervous
    d., nonulcer
    d., ovarian
    d., reflex
    d., salivary
dyspeptic urine
dyspeptica, angina
dysphagia [*dysphasia, dysplasia, dysbasia*]
    d., chronic esophageal
    d., contractile ring
    d., esophageal
    d., nausea and emesis
    d. nervosa

d., oropharyngeal
d. paralytica
d., pharyngeal
d., sideropenic
d. spastica
d., tropical
d., vallecular
d. valsalviana
dysphagic, patient
dysphasia, developmental
dysphonia
    d., abductor spasmodic
    d., adductor spasmodic
    d., chronic
    d., spasmodic
dysphoria
    d. and tension
    d., chronic
    d. ▸ intense episodic
dysphoric
    d. disorder ▸ late luteal phase
    d. disorder, periluteal phase
    d. disorder, premenstrual
    d. effect
    d. mood, basic
    d., patient
dysplasia
    d., anal
    d., anhidrotic ectodermal
    d. ▸ arrhythmogenic right ventricular (RV)
    d., atriodigital
    d., bone
    d., bronchial
    d. (BPD), bronchopulmonary
    d., cells indicative of mild
    d., cells indicative of moderate
    d., cells indicative of severe
    d., cerebral
    d., cervical
    d., chondrorectodermal
    d., congenital alveolar
    d., congenital thymic
    d., craniodiaphyseal
    d., cretinoid
    d., diaphyseal
    d. (BPD) ▸ early bronchopulmonary
    d., ectodermal
    d. epiphysealis punctata
    d., facial
    d., fibromuscular
    d., fibrous
    d., focal
    d., hereditary bone
    d., hidrotic ectodermal

dysplasia—*continued*
- d., hip
- d., mammary
- d., metaphyseal
- d. ▸ multiple epiphyseal
- d., myeloradicular
- d., OAV (oculoauriculovertebral)
- d., ODD (oculodentodigital)
- d. of bone ▸ fibrous
- d. of hip (DDH) ▸ developmental
- d. of jaw ▸ familial fibrous
- d. of nervous system
- d., ophthalmomandibulomelic
- d., polyostotic fibrous
- d., postradiation
- d. ▸ right ventricular (RV)
- d., severe
- d., skeletal
- d., spondyloepiphyseal
- d. syndrome, arteriohepatic
- d. syndrome ▸ dental enamel
- d. syndrome, ectodermal
- d., thymic
- d., ventriculoradial

dysplastic
- d. changes
- d. changes in epithelium
- d. left hemisphere of brain
- d. nevi
- d. nevi ▸ nonfamilial
- d. nevus syndrome
- d. right hemisphere of brain
- d. type

dyspnea (Dyspnea)
- d., acute
- d. and anasarca
- d. and fatigue ▸ palpitations,
- d. and flushing
- d. and headache ▸ cough,
- d., cardiac
- d., chronic
- d., cough and fever
- d., cough and rigors
- d., effort
- d., episodic
- d., exertional
- d., expiratory
- d., fatigue and
- d. ▸ fever, shaking chills,
- d., functional
- d. index, baseline
- D. Index ▸ Transition
- d. ▸ insidious onset of
- d., inspiratory
- d., Monday

- d., nocturnal
- d., nonexpansional
- d. on exercise (DOE)
- d. on exertion
- d. on exertion, increased
- d., one-flight exertional
- d., orthostatic
- d., paroxysmal
- d. (PND) ▸ paroxysmal nocturnal
- d., positional
- d., psychogenic
- d., renal
- d., rest
- d. scale
- d., sighing
- d. target
- d., Traube's
- d. ▸ two-flight exertional
- d. with exertion ▸ wheezing and

dyspneic
- d. breathing
- d., patient
- d., patient confused and

dysponderal amenorrhea

dyspragia intermittens angiosclerotica intestinalis

dyspraxia, constructive

dysreflexia
- d., bout of
- d., episode of
- d. of bladder, autonomic

dysregulation ▸ hedonic homeostatic

dysrhythmia(s)
- d., atrial
- d., cardiac
- d., cerebral
- d., cortical
- d., diffuse
- d., esophageal
- d., focal
- d., life-threatening
- d., negative spiking
- d. (PCD) ▸ paroxysmal cerebral
- d., seizure
- d., spiking
- d., thalamocortical
- d., ventricular

dysrhythmic
- d. activity
- d. activity, spikey
- d. change, focal

dyssocial personality

dyssynchronous depolarization, rapid

dyssynchrony, thoracoabdominal

dyssynergia, biliary
dyssynergia, detrussor-sphincter
dyssynergic bladder
dyssynergic myocardial segment
dystaxia
- d. agitans
- d., cerebral
- d., heel-to-knee

dystaxic cerebralis infantilis
dysthymia, chronic
dysthymic disorder
dystocia
- d., cervical
- d., fetal
- d., maternal
- d., placental
- d., shoulder
- d. syndrome, dystrophy-

dystonia
- d., acute
- d. ▸ blepharospasm and oromandibular
- d., cervical
- d., focal
- d., focal golfer's
- d., generalized
- d. musculorum deformans
- d., tardive
- d., torsion

dystonic
- d., ego-
- d. illness ▸ ego-
- d. movement
- d. reaction
- d. reaction, acute
- d. reactions ▸ dyskinetic and
- d. reactions, recurrence of
- d. spasm

dystopic calcification
dystrophia myotonica
dystrophic calcification
dystrophic gingivitis
dystrophica, elastosis
dystrophy
- d., asphyxiating thoracic
- d. ▸ Becker-type tardive muscular
- d. ▸ Best's macular
- d., Bietti's
- d., Cogan's
- d., Duchenne's
- d. (DMD) ▸ Duchenne's muscular
- d. -dystocia syndrome
- d., endothelial
- d., Erb's
- d. ▸ familial asphyxiant thoracic

d., Fehr's
d., fingerprint
d., Fleischer's
d., Franceschetti's
d., Francois'
d., Fuchs'
d., Groenouw's
d., infantile neuroaxonal
d., Landouzy-Déjerine
d. lattice corner
d., limb-girdle muscular
d., Maeder-Danis
d., Meesmann's
d., muscular
d., myotonic
d. ▸ myotonic muscular
d., nail
d., ocular muscle
d. of cornea
d. of cornea, endothelial
d. of cornea, marginal
d., Pillat's
d., progressive muscular
d. ▸ pseudohypertrophic infantile
    muscular
d., pseudohypertrophic muscular
d., reflex
d. (RSD) ▸ reflux sympathetic
d., Salzmann's
d., Salzmann's nodular corneal
d., Schlichting posterior
    polymorphous
d., Schnyder's
d. (RSD) syndrome ▸ reflex
    sympathetic
d. (TAD), thoracic asphyxiant
d. ▸ thoracic-pelvic-phalangeal
d., thyroneural
dysuria
d., patient has
d., psychic
d., psychogenic
d., spastic
dysynchrony, ventricular

E

E. (Escherichia)
    E. coli
    E. coli bacteremia
    E. coli, enteropathic
    E. coli, enteropathogenic
    E. coli, gram-negative
    E. coli infection ▸ gram-positive
    E. coli organisms
    E. coli sepsis peritonitis
    E. coli septicemia
    E. communior ▸ gram-negative
e antibody (HBeAb), hepatitis B
E antigen
e Antigen (Anti-HBe), Antibody to
    Hepatitis B
e Antigen (HBeAg), Hepatitis B
E. coli diarrhea
E, hemoglobin
E immunoglobulin (IgE)
    determination ▸ gamma
E point to septal separation
E slope, D to
E syndrome, trisomy
E test
E to A changes
E to F slope
E to F slope ▸ mitral
E to I changes
E velocity ▸ peak
E virus ▸ hepatitis
E wave deceleration time ▸
    transmitral
E wave to A wave
ex anopsia, amblyopia
ex ulcere, carcinoma
E:A
E:A ratio ▸ transmitral
E:A ratio ▸ transmitral Doppler
E:A wave ratio
EAC (external auditory canal)
each
    e. ear (AU)
    e. eye (OU)
    e. eye (VOU) ▸ vision of
EAD (early after depolarization)
Eagle-Barrett syndrome
Eagle syndrome

Eales disease
EAM (external auditory meatus)
EAP (Employee Assistance Program)
ear(s)
    e. ▸ abnormal facies and
    e., active
    e., acute
    e., acute middle
    e. and nose, basal cell carcinoma
      of
    e. and nose, squamous cell
      carcinoma
    e., anvil of
    e., asylum
    e. atresia ▸ inner
    e., aviator's
    e., Aztec
    e., balance mechanism of inner
    e., bat
    e., beach
    e., bionic
    e., Blainville
    e. bleeding
    e. block
    e. ▸ bone growth in
    e. bone, middle
    e., buzzing in
    e., Cagot
    e. canal
    e. canal clear
    e. canal, external
    e. canal ▸ impacted wax in
    e. canal, inflammation of
    e. canal, inflammation of external
    e. canal inspection ▸ video
      otoscopic
    e. canal skin
    e. carcinoma
    e. cartilage
    e. cartilage ▸ upper
    e., cat's
    e., cauliflower
    e. cavity
    e. cavity, middle
    e. clavicle splint ▸ elephant-
    e., cleaning of
    e. cleft, middle

    e., contralateral
    e. cough
    e., crustiness of
    e. culture
    e., cup
    e., cyanosis of
    e. damage from noise ▸ irreversible
    e., Darwin's
    e. deafness, inner
    e. deafness, middle
    e., defective
    e., deformed
    e., diabetic
    e. ▸ discharge of pus from the
    e. disease ▸ auto-immune inner
    e. disease ▸ middle
    e. disorder, inner
    e. ▸ dizziness from infection of
    e. drainage
    e. drainage ▸ prolonged
    e. drops
    e. drum vibration
    e. dysfunction, benign inner
    e. (AU) ▸ each
    e. effusion and drainage ▸ middle
    e. effusion ▸ middle
    e. effusion ▸ persistent middle
    e. electronic implantation ▸ inner
    e. ▸ erosion of inner
    e. ▸ eustachian tube blocked by
      infection of
    e., external
    e. ▸ fever from infection of
    e. ▸ fluid-filled inner
    e., folds of
    e., foreign body (FB) in
    e. from dermatitis ▸ red
    e. from eczema ▸ red
    e. from sore throat ▸ pain in
    e. from TMJ (temporomandibular
      joint) disorder ▸ pain in
    e. from tongue problem ▸ pain in
    e. from tonsil problem ▸ pain in
    e. from tooth decay ▸ pain in
    e., frostbite of
    e., fullness in
    e., glue

ear(s)—*continued*
e., hair cell in
e. hair, cells inner
e., hairy
e. hearing aid, behind-the-
e. hearing aid ▸ in-the-
e. ▸ hearing loss from infection of
e. hearing loss ▸ inner
e., Hong Kong
e., hot weather
e. implant
e. implant, inner
e. in aging ▸ wrinkled
e. ▸ increased blood flow to
e. infected
e. infection
e. infection, childhood
e. infection, chronic
e. infection, chronic middle
e. infection ▸ inner
e. infection, middle
e. infection ▸ outer
e. infection, repeated
e. infection ▸ viral inner
e., inflammation of
e., inflammation of middle
e. injury
e., inner
e. ▸ inner structures of the
e., insane
e., internal
e., ipsilateral
e., itching of
e., large and floppy
e. lavage
e. lead
e. (AS) ▸ left
e. lobe, contralateral
e. lobe creases
e. lobes, blue
e., lop
e. ▸ low-pitched ringing in
e., low-set
e. ▸ lump in front of or behind
e., malformed middle
e., malformed outer
e., microsurgery of
e., middle
e., Morel's
e., Mozart
e., No. 1 ▸ Stahl
e., No. 2 ▸ Stahl
e., noises in
e., nose and throat (ENT)

e., nose and throat (ENT)
  emergency
e., nose and throat (HEENT) ▸
  head, eyes,
e., nose and throat (HEENT) not
  remarkable ▸ head, eyes,
e., nose and throat (ENT) trauma
e. nystagmus ▸ inner
e. ▸ object lodged in
e., obstruction of
e. occlusion test
e., otosclerosis of
e., outer
e. pain
e., pierced
e. piercing
e. piercing instruments
e. pinna prosthesis
e. piston prosthesis
e., plugged
e. pressure
e., pressure in
e., prizefighter
e. problem from cold
e., protruding
e. pulse
e., pus in
e. reconstruction, Mladick
e. reconstruction, Steffanoff's
e. (AD) ▸ right
e., ringing in
e. ▸ ringing in affected
e., ringing sound in
e. roaring
e., satyr
e., scroll
e. ▸ sensory receptors of
e. sign ▸ rabbit-
e., Singapore
e., sores on
e. sponge
e., Stahl's
e. structures, inner
e. stuffiness from allergy ▸ altitude
  change,
e., stuffiness of
e., swelling of
e., swimmer's
e., tank
e., tropical
e. unit ▸ custom fit in
e. ▸ ventilate middle
e., vestibule of
e. wax build-up
e. wax, excess

e., wax in
e., Wildermuth's
earache, chronic
eardrum
e., inflated
e., injected
e., perforated
e. perforation
e., residual scarring of
e. retraction
e., ruptured
early
e. abortion
e. adult life ▸ emancipation disorder
  of
e. afterdepolarization (EAD)
e. ambulation
e. antigen
e. asterixis noted
e. bilateral bronchopneumonia ▸
  patchy
e. bronchopulmonary dysplasia
  (BPD)
e. burn treatment
e. cancer detection
e. childhood (EC)
e. childhood psychosis
e. childhood ▸ reactive attachment
  disorder of
e. childhood ▸ reactive attachment
  disorder of infancy or
e. click
e. cystic hyperplasia
e. deceleration
e. defibrillation
e. detection
e. detection and management
e. detection, cancer prevention and
e. detection of breast cancer
e. detection of cancer
e. detection of colorectal cancer
e. detection program
e. detection test
e. detection through mammography
e. development, birth and
e. diabetic retinopathy
e. diastolic murmur
e. diastolic wave
e. disc
e. erythroblast
e. family environment
e. fetal death
e. gastric emptying
e. identification of symptoms
e. infantile autism

e. infection
e. interstitial fibrosis
e. intervention in drug abuse
e. intervention, prevention and
e. labor
e. lens opacity
e. lung cancer
e. metastatic disease, palliation in
e. metastatic pulmonary lesions
e. morning arousal
e. morning awakening
e. morning sputum
e. morning stiffness
e. neonatal death
e. normoblast
e. onset alcoholic
e. onset, Alzheimer's
e. onset Alzheimer's disease
e. onset familial Alzheimer's
  disease
e. onset of menopause
e. onset of menstruation
e. onset of senility
e. otosclerosis
e. parental loss
e. parental separation
e. peaking systolic murmur
e. phases of sleep
e. pregnancy
e. prodromal stages
e. rapid repolarization
e. repolarization, benign
e. respiratory distress syndrome
e. satiety
e. secretory endometrium
e. sign of rejection
e. signs of relapse
e. stage breast cancer
e. stage cancer
e. -stage problem drinker
e. -stage prostate cancer
e. stages of sleep
e. systolic murmur, decrescendo
e. tuberculosis
e. warning signs
earth connection
earthy tongue
ease
  e., bronchoscope inserted through
    vocal cords with
  e., catheter passed with
  e. of engagement ▸ initial
  e., scope inserted into trachea with
easily
  e. annoyed

e. annoyed ▸ agitated, irritable, and
e. bored
e. bruises
e., capsules strip
e., capsules stripped
e. distracted
e. irritated
e. overexcited
e. ▸ patient cries
e. ▸ renal capsules stripped
e. startled
Easter egg contamination
eastern
  e. equine encephalitis (EEE)
  e. equine encephalitis (EEE) virus
  e. equine encephalomyelitis (EEE)
  e. equine encephalomyelitis (EEE)
    virus
easy
  e. bruisability
  e. bruising
  e. distractibility
  e. fatigability
  e. weight gain
eat ▸ bathe, dress and
eaten raw ▸ psilocybin
eater, Anspach cement
eater, compulsive
eating
  e. and purging
  e. bacteria ▸ flesh
  e. behavior
  e., binge
  e. cell
  e. disorder
  e. disorder, binge
  e. disorder ▸ dissociation in
  e. disorder ▸ evaluation and
    treatment of
  e. disorder, fatal
  e. disorder ▸ impulse dyscontrol in
  e. disorder, prolonged
  e. disorder symptoms
  e. disorder, unspecified
  e., disordered
  e. disorders, medical management
    of
  e. disorders patient
  e. disturbance
  e. ▸ episodic pattern of binge
  e., grooming, and toileting
  e. habits
  e. habits, erratic
  e. habits, good
  e. habits, stable

e. ▸ impulse control in
e. ▸ impulse dyscontrol in
e., impulsive
e. or sleeping habits ▸ change in
e. patterns, bizarre
e. patterns, unhealthy
e. plan ▸ low fat
e. syndrome, binge
e. toxin, tissue-
Eaton agent
Eaton agent pneumonia
eave flap, Cronin-Matthews
EB (epidermolysis bullosa)
EB (Epstein-Barr)
  EB disease
  EB virus infection
  EB virus syndrome
EBCT (electron beam computed
  tomography)
EBCT (electron beam computerized
  tomography)
Eberthella
  E. typhi
  E. typhi, gram-negative
  E. typhosa
EBL (estimated blood loss)
Ebola
  E. disease
  E. fever
  E. hemorrhagic fever
  E. virus
  E. virus outbreak
Ebstein('s)
  E. anomaly
  E. diet
  E. disease
  E. lesion
  E. lesion, Armanni-
  E. malformation of tricuspid valve
  E. pyrexia ▸ Pel-
  E. sign
eburnized bone ends
EBV (Epstein-Barr virus)
EC (early childhood)
ECBO (enteric cytopathic bovine
  orphan) virus
ECC (electrical contraction coupling)
eccentric
  e. amputation
  e. atrial activation
  e. atrophy
  e., focal and
  e. hypertrophy
  e. implantation
  e. ledge

eccentric—*continued*
   e. lesion, ulcerated
   e. narrowing
   e. occlusion
   e. pantomography
   e. stenosis
   e. stenosis ▸ focal
eccentricity index
ecchymosis(-es)
   e. and bruising
   e. and hematomas ▸ widespread
   e. and swelling
   e., bilateral antecubital
   e., cadaveric
   e., multiple
   e. on skin ▸ multiple
   e., periorbital
   e., soft tissue
   e., spontaneous
   e., swelling and
ecchymotic
   e. area
   e. discoloration
   e. hemorrhages
   e. mask
eccrine
   e. duct
   e. gland
   e. sweat gland
ECG/EKG(s) (electrocardiogram)
   [*EEG*]
   E., admission
   E., baseline
   E., blip
   E., borderline
   E. changes ▸ ischemic
   E., cross sectional
   E., exercise
   E. exercise stress test
   E., fetal
   E. findings
   E., flat
   E. ▸ His bundle
   E. machine, portable
   E., monitored with
   E. ▸ orthogonal
   E. ▸ scalar
   E., serial
   E. showed normal pattern
   E. ▸ signal averaged
   E. silence
   E., 6-lead
   E. ▸ 16-lead
   E. ▸ straight-line
   E., stress

E. strip
E. study
E. synchronized digital subtraction
   angiogram
E. telemetry
E. test, fetal
E. ▸ thallium
E. ▸ three-channel
E., 3-lead
E. ▸ time domain signal averaged
E. tracing
E. tracing display
E. treadmill, stress
E. triggering unit
E., 12-lead
E. ▸ unipolar
E. ▸ vector
E. waves
ECG/EKG (electrocardiograph)
   E. (electrocardiograph),
     bioimpedance
   E. (electrocardiograph), Cambridge
   E. (electrocardiograph) changes ▸
     ischemic
   E. (electrocardiograph) ▸ Marquette
   E. (electrocardiograph) monitor ▸
     transtelephonic
ECG/EKG (electrocardiographic)
   E. (electrocardiographic) gating
   E. (electrocardiographic)
     monitoring
   E. (electrocardiographic)
     monitoring, ambulatory
   E. (electrocardiographic) score,
     Brush
   E. (electrocardiographic)
     transtelephonic monitor
ECG/EKG (electrocardiography)
   E. (electrocardiography),
     esophageal
   E. (electrocardiography) ▸
     intracardiac
   E. (electrocardiography) ▸ signal
     averaged
echelon lymph nodes ▸ first or
   second
Echidnophaga gallinacea
Echinacea angustifolia
echinata, Leptothrix
Echinochasmus perfoliatus
echinococcal cyst
echinococcosis/echinococciasis
Echinococcus (echinococcus)
   E. alveolaris
   E. granulosus

E. multilocularis
e., Taenia
Echinorhynchus gigas
Echinorhynchus hominis
Echinostoma
   E. ilocanum
   E. lindoensis
   E. perfoliatum
   E. revolutum
   E., Trematoda
echo (Echo) (ECHO)
   E. (enteric cytopathic human
     orphan)
   E. (enterocytopathogenic human
     orphan)
   e., amphoric
   e. artifact ▸ stimulated
   e., atrial
   e. beat
   E. bed ▸ Stress
   e., bright
   e., cardiac
   e. catheter
   e. contrast ▸ left atrial spontaneous
   e. contrast ▸ spontaneous
   e. delay time
   e. dense structure
   e. density
   e. Doppler
   e. -Doppler cardiography
   e. drop-out
   e. -free area
   e. -free space
   e. guidance
   e. -guided pericardiocentesis
   e. -guided ultrasound
   e. imaging sequence ▸ spin-
   e. imaging ▸ spin-
   e., metallic
   e. ▸ motion display
   e. MRI (magnetic resonance
     imaging) ▸ spin-
   e. ▸ nodus sinuatrialis
   e. pattern
   e., pericardial
   e. -planar imaging
   e. probe ▸ transesophageal
   e. reverberation
   e. scan
   e. scanning technique
   e., scattered
   e. score
   e. -signal shape
   e. -spared area

e., specular
e. speech
e. -tracking device, A-mode-
e., transcutaneous
e., ultrasonographic
E. (enteric cytopathic human orphan) virus
e. zone

echocardiogram (ECG)
e. (ECG), abnormal
e. ▸ apical five-chamber view
e. ▸ apical four-chamber view
e. ▸ apical two-chamber view
e., continuous loop exercise
e., continuous wave Doppler
e., contrast enhanced
e., cross-sectional two-dimensional
e., exercise
e., Feigenbaum
e. ▸ long-axis parasternal view
e., M-mode
e., meridian
e. ▸ Ochsner-Mahorner
e. ▸ parasternal long-axis view
e. ▸ parasternal short-axis view
e. ▸ signal-averaged
e. (SBE) ▸ supine bicycle
e., transesophageal
e., two-dimensional (2-D)

echocardiograph ▸ transesophageal dobutamine stress

echocardiographic
e. assessment
e. automated border detection
e. automated boundary detection system
e. differentiation
e. scoring system
e. study
e. transducer

echocardiography
e., A-mode
e., adenosine
e., baseline
e., color Doppler
e., continuous wave Doppler
e., contrast
e., cross-sectional
e., deductive
e., digital subtraction
e., dipyridamole
e., dobutamine
e. ▸ dobutamine-atropine stress
e., dobutamine stress
e., Doppler

e. ejection fraction
e., endoscopic
e. ▸ ergonovine
e., esophageal
e., exercise
e. ▸ exercise stress
e., fetal
e. ▸ high frequency epicardial
e., interventional
e., intraoperative
e. ▸ intrauterine
e., meridian
e. ▸ mitral valve
e. (MCE) ▸ myocardial contrast
e., paraplane
e. ▸ pharmacologic stress
e. ▸ pulmonary valve
e. ▸ pulsed Doppler
e. ▸ pulsed wave Doppler
e. ▸ quantitative two-dimensional
e. ▸ real time three-dimensional
e. ▸ sector scan
e. ▸ signal-averaged
e., stress
e. ▸ supine bicycle stress
e. ▸ three-dimensional
e. (TEE) ▸ transesophageal
e. ▸ transesophageal contrast
e., transthoracic
e., treadmill
e., two-dimensional (2-D)
e. with pacing, transesophageal

echodense mass
echodense structure
echodensity, linear
echodensity, superimposed
echogenic area
echogenic mass
echogenicity, increased
echogenicity of periventricular white matter
echoing words of others
echolalia, delayed
echolalic, speech
echolucent plaque
echophonocardiography, dual
echopraxia/echopraxis
echoviral infection
echovirus myocarditis
Ecker diluting fluid ▸ Rees and Ecker fluid
eclampsia
e. due to uremia
e. of pregnancy, pre◇
e., puerperal

e., uremic
eclamptic idiocy
eclamptic toxemia
eclectic psychotherapy
eclipse blindness
ECM (erythema chronicum migrans) lesion
ECMO (extracorporeal membrane oxygenation)
ECMO (enteric cytopathic monkey orphan) virus
ECO (Environmental Control Officer)
ecological chemistry
ecological perspective
ecology, human
economic costs of drug abuse
economic dislocation
Economo's disease
Economo's encephalitis
economy
e., animal
e. class syndrome
e., cocaine/crack
e., marijuana
e., token
ECS (electrocerebral silence)
ECS (electroconvulsive shock)
ECS (electrocerebral silence) recording
ECSO (enteric cytopathic swine orphan) virus
ECT (electroconvulsant treatment)
ECT (electroconvulsive therapy)
ECT (emission computerized tomographic)
ECT body scanner
ECT system
ECT system, radionuclide
ectasia
e., alveolar
e., annuloaortic
e., aortoannular
e., arteriosclerotic
e., artery
e. cordis
e., corneal
e., diffuse arterial
e., distal
e., focal duct
e., hypostatic
e. iridis
e., mammary duct
e. of abdominal aorta
e. of cornea
e. of sclera

ectasia—*continued*
- e. of thoracic aorta
- e., papillary
- e., scleral
- e., tubular
- e., vascular

ectatic
- e. aneurysm
- e. aortic valve
- e. artery
- e. carotid artery
- e. emphysema

ectethmoid bones

ecthyma, pustular

ectocervical cell yield

Ectocor pacemaker ▸ Cordis-

Ectocor pacemaker ▸ Omni-

ectocuneiform bone

ectoderm
- e., amniotic
- e., basal
- e., blastodermic
- e., chorionic
- e., embryonic
- e., extraembryonic
- e., neural
- e., primitive

ectodermal
- e. defect
- e. defect, congenital
- e. disc
- e. dysplasia
- e. dysplasia, anhidrotic
- e. dysplasia, hidrotic
- e. dysplasia syndrome
- e. polydysplasia, hereditary

ectodermogenic neurosyphilis

ecto/endocervical cell segregation

ectophytic parasite

ectopia
- e. cordis abdominalis
- e. lentis
- e. of lens
- e. pupillae congenita
- e., renal
- e. testis
- e. vesicae

ectopic
- e. ACTH syndrome
- e. activity
- e. activity, ventricular
- e. adenoma
- e. anus
- e. atrial foci
- e. atrial tachycardia
- e. beat
- e. beats, multiple
- e. beats, ventricular
- e. Cushing's syndrome
- e. eruption
- e. focus
- e. gestation
- e. hormone production
- e. hyperparathyroidism
- e. impulse
- e. intrauterine device
- e. kidney
- e. pacemaker
- e. parathyroid adenoma
- e. pregnancy
- e. pregnancy and abortion
- e. pregnancy ▸ ruptured tubal
- e. pregnancy, unruptured
- e. rhythm
- e. systole ▸ ventricular
- e. tachycardia
- e. tachycardia (AET), atrial
- e. tachycardia, automatic
- e. tachycardia ▸ junctional
- e. testis
- e. thyroid tissue
- e. ureter
- e. ventricular beats
- e. ventricular contractions ▸ focal

ectopy
- e., asymptomatic complex
- e., atrial
- e., cervical
- e., recurrent ventricular
- e., supraventricular
- e., ventricular

ectothrix, Trichophyton

ectozoic parasite

ectropion [*entropion*]
- e. cicatriceum
- e., cicatricial
- e., flaccid
- e. lower lid, spastic
- e. luxurians
- e. of eyelid
- e. paralyticum
- e. sarcomatosum
- e. senilis
- e. spasticum
- e. uveae

eczema
- e., allergic
- e., atopic
- e., contact
- e., dry
- e. ▸ eye dryness from
- e. ▸ flaking skin from
- e. herpeticum
- e., infantile
- e. intertrigo
- e., itching from
- e. marginatum
- e. neonatorum
- e., nummular
- e., oozing from
- e., pediatric
- e. ▸ peeling skin from
- e. ▸ red ears from
- e. rubrum
- e. ▸ scalp itching from
- e., seborrheic
- e. seborrhoeicum
- e. ▸ skin cracking from
- e. ▸ skin crusting from
- e., stasis
- e. vaccinatum
- e., weeping

eczematiform vulvitis

eczematoid dermatitis ▸ infectious

eczematosa, ophthalmia

eczematous
- e. conjunctivitis
- e. dermatitis, nummular
- e. pannus

ED (emotionally disturbed)

EDC/EDOC (estimated date of confinement)

EDC/EDOC (expected date of confinement)

EDD/EDOD (estimated date of delivery)

eddy current

eddy sounds

Edelmann's anemia

edema
- e., abdominal
- e., acute
- e. (ACPE), acute cardiogenic pulmonary
- e., acute pulmonary
- e., alimentary
- e. all extremities ▸ severe pitting
- e., alveolar
- e. and congestion ▸ pulmonary
- e., angioneurotic
- e., ankle
- e., asbestosis pulmonary
- e., Berlin's
- e., bland
- e., boggy

e., brain
e., brawny
e., brown
e., cardiac
e., cardiogenic pulmonary
e., cerebral
e., chronic pulmonary
e., circumscribed
e., congestive
e., constrictive
e., corneal
e. ▸ cyanosis, clubbing or
e., cyclic
e., deformity or
e., dependent
e., dependent peripheral
e., diabetic macular
e., facial
e. ▸ fatal acute pulmonary
e., fingerprint
e. ▸ flash pulmonary
e. ▸ florid pulmonary
e. fluid
e., focal
e., focal pulmonary
e., fulminant pulmonary
e., hereditary angioneurotic
e. (HAPE) ▸ high altitude
   pulmonary
e., Huguenin's
e. ▸ idiopathic cyclic
e., intermittent angioneurotic
e., interstitial pulmonary
e., Iwanoff's retinal
e., laryngeal
e., leg
e. ▸ long-term
e. lower extremities, pitting
e., lymphatic
e., macular
e., malignant
e., massive
e., metastatic
e., mild pulmonary
e., Milroy's
e., Milton's
e., mucosal
e., myocardial
e., myx◇
e. neonatorum
e. ▸ neurogenic pulmonary
e., neuropathic
e., noncardiac pulmonary
e., noncardiogenic pulmonary
e., nonpitting

e. of ankles ▸ pitting
e. of bronchial mucosa
e. of eyelids
e. of face
e. of feet
e. of hand
e. of iris
e. of larynx
e. of legs
e. of lower extremities
e. of lung
e. of lung ▸ vernal
e. of macula
e. of optic disc
e. of upper extremity
e. of vessels, angioneurotic
e. or swelling ▸ clubbing,
e., pancreatic
e., papill◇
e. ▸ paroxysmal pulmonary
e., passive
e., pedal
e., penile
e., pericellular
e., periodic
e., periorbital
e., peripapillary retinal
e., peripheral
e., perivascular
e., permeability pulmonary
e., persistent macular
e., Pirogoff's
e., pitting
e. ▸ postanesthesia pulmonary
e. ▸ postcardioversion pulmonary
e., postinfarct
e., postlaser
e., prehepatic
e., presacral
e., presence of
e., pretibial
e., progressive
e. (PE), pulmonary
e. ▸ pulmonary interstitial
e., Quincke's
e., refractory
e., resolving pulmonary
e., sacral
e., severe pitting
e., stasis
e., Stellwag's brawny
e. ▸ stiffness, pain and
e., subepithelial corneal
e., subpleural
e. ▸ swelling, clubbing or

e., tense
e., terminal
e., transient
e. upper and lower extremities ▸
   mild
e., uremic pulmonary
e., uvula
e., vasogenic
e., vernal
e., woody
edematous
e. and congested ▸ lungs
e. and friable, trigone
e. and swollen, tube
e., brain
e., extremities
e., firm and
e., lungs
e. ▸ lungs atelectatic and
e. ▸ lungs congested and
e. material
e., myx◇
e., parenchyma
e. reaction, erythematous-
e., sinusoid
e. stroma
Eden-Hybbinette operation
edentulous [*dentulous*]
edentulous, patient
edge(s)
e., absorption
e., approximate skin
e., approximate wound
e. approximated
e. approximated, cutaneous
e. approximated, pleural
e. artifact
e., attached to skin
e. bite, edge-to-
e., Compton
e., cut
e., cutting
e. debrided, wound
e., denture
e. detection
e. detection, automated
e. detection, computerized
e. detection ▸ manual
e. detection method
e. enhancement ▸ leading
e., fimbriated
e., gaping wound
e., incisional
e., inverted
e., leading

edge(s)—*continued*
e., liver
e. ▸ lower peritoneal
e., medial ossified
e. of cartilage trimmed
e. of incision ▸ brought out near
e. of rib, upper
e. of wound
e. of wound ▸ sutured parallel with
e. palpable, liver
e. ▸ patient on
e., peritoneal
e., phonating
e., raised
e., reapproximate skin
e. retracted, wound
e., rounded
e. smooth, liver
e. -strength
e., thin
e. -to-edge bite
e. -to-edge occlusion
e. -to-edge, sutured
e. tracing
e. tracing, computerized
e. trimmed
e. trimmed, skin
e. undercut, skin
e. undermined
e. ▸ upper peritoneal
e., wound
E-dial calibration
Edinger-Westphal nucleus
EDOC/EDC (expected date of confinement)
EDOD/EDD (expected date of delivery)
EDP (end-diastolic pressure)
EDR (effective direct radiation)
EDR (electrodermal response)
educable mentally handicapped (EMH)
educable mentally retarded
educated childbirth
education (Education)
e., AIDS (acquired immune deficiency syndrome)
e., alcohol and drug
e., alcoholism
e. and prevention program ▸ drug-
e., childbirth
e., classes, stroke
e., community
e., continuing medical
e. coordinator, patient

E. Director, Inservice
e., drug abuse
E. (DARE) ▸ Drug Abuse Resistance
e., exceptional
e., family
e., formal staff
e., general grief
e., grief
e., health
E., Inservice
e. instruction sheet ▸ patient
e., medical
E. (NAPARE) ▸ National Association for Perinatal Addiction Research
e. on drug abuse, patient
e., parenting
e., patient
E. Program (NCEP) ▸ National Cholesterol
e. programs, continuing
e. programs, drug
E. (DARE) programs ▸ Drug Awareness Resistance
E. programs, Inservice
e. programs ▸ public health
e., sex
e., special
e., stress
educational
e. activities ▸ psychotherapeutic and
e. and social therapy ▸ psychological,
e. component, strong
e. difficulty
e. evaluation
e. needs, monitor
e. process, appropriate
e. programs ▸ family day
e. psychology
e. therapy
e. training
Edwards
E. aortic valve prosthesis ▸ Carpentier-
E. aortic valve prosthesis ▸ Starr-
E. ball and cage valve ▸ Starr-
E. ball valve prosthesis ▸ Starr-
E. cardiac valve prosthesis ▸ Starr-
E. disk valve prosthesis ▸ Starr-
E. graft
E. heart valve prosthesis ▸ Starr-
E. mitral prosthesis ▸ Starr-

E. mitral valve ▸ Starr-
E. pacemaker ▸ Starr-
E. patch
E. prosthesis
E. prosthesis ▸ Starr-
E. prosthetic ball valve ▸ Starr-
E. prosthetic valve ▸ Starr-
E. seamless prosthesis
E. silastic valve ▸ Starr-
E. syndrome
E. Teflon intracardiac patch implant
E. Teflon intracardiac patch prosthesis
E. valve prosthesis ▸ Starr-
E. valve ▸ Starr-
EECP (enhanced external counterpulsation)
EECP (enhanced external counterpulsation) therapy
EEE (eastern equine encephalitis) virus
EEE (eastern equine encephalomyelitis) virus
EEG(s) (electroencephalogram) [*ECG/EKG*]
E., abnormal
E. activities, unilateral
E. activity
E. activity, abnormal
E. activity, localized
E. activity, nonrhythmic
E. activity ▸ nonsimultaneous occurrence of
E. activity, normal
E. activity, rhythmic
E. activity ▸ suppress specific seizure wave
E. activity, suppression of
E. alpha activity
E. amplifier
E. amplifier, differential
E. artifact
E. biofeedback
E. biofeedback in control of hyperactivity
E. biofeedback procedure
E. brain wave activity ▸ excessive fast
E. channel
E. channel bandwidth
E. channel ▸ reduction of sensitivity of an
E. channel, sensitivity of
E. complexes
E. complexes, regularly repeated

E. components
E., conventional
E., cortical
E. delta waves
E., depth
E. derivation
E. desynchronization
E. discharges, repetitive
E. electrode
E. electrode placement
E. electrodes, pair of
E., flat
E. frequency range
E. frequency range ▸ alpha-theta
E. frequency spectrum
E. input test, common
E., intracerebral
E., isoelectric
E., low voltage
E., low voltage fast
E. Machine ▸ Offner
E., modification of
E. nonspecific depressant effect
E., nonsurgical
E. paper ▸ velocity of movement of
E. pattern development ▸ normal resting
E. pattern, normal waking
E. patterns
E. patterns ▸ autogenic training and
E., postictal
E. record, compressed
E. recording
E. recording, all-night
E. recording instrument
E. rhythms
E. rhythms, blocking of
E. rhythms, physiologic
E., scalp
E. seizure pattern
E. ▸ serial
E. sleep patterns
E. status epilepticus
E., stereotactic depth
E., stereotaxic depth
E. study
E. theta biofeedback training
E. topogram (CET), computed
E. trace
E. tracing
E. transient
E. transients, sharp
E. waves
E. waves, amplitude of
E. waves and complexes

E. waves, distortion of
E. waves, polarity
E. waves, regularly repeated
E. waves ▸ unequal development of
eel worm
EEMRI (endoesophageal magnetic resonance imaging) coil
EENT (eyes, ears, nose and throat)
effaced cervix
effacement
    e. and dilatation
    e., dilatation and transition
    e. of calyces
    e. of cervix
    e. of mucosa
    e., self-
effect(s) [*affect*]
    e., adverse
    e., adverse psychological
    e., adverse side-
    e., anabolic
    e., analgesic
    e., anticancer
    e., anticholinergic
    e., antihypertensive
    e., antitumor
    e., antiviral
    e., attendant side-
    e., Auger
    e., band saw-
    e., behavioral
    e., beta carotene
    e., biologic
    e., blooming
    e., broad range of
    e., Brockenbrough
    e., cardiac
    e., cardiovascular
    e., cathartic
    e., cause and
    e., cholinergic
    e., chronic amphetamine
    e., cidal
    e., clinical self-
    e., cocaine prenatal
    e., cognitive
    e., combined
    e., Compton
    e., copper wire
    e., cross-modal
    e., cumulative
    e. (CRE), cumulative radiation
    e., cytopathic
    e., cytotoxic
    e., delayed after-

e., deleterious
e., depressive
e. ▸ devastating side-
e., digitalis
e., direct biologic
e., disruptive
e., Doppler
e., dottering
e., dromotropic
e., drug
e. ▸ drug-induced psychiatric
e. ▸ duration of drug
e., dysphoric
e., enhanced hypothrombinemic
e., environmental
e., erectile
e., euphoric
e., euphorigenic
e., ex vacuo
e. exercises, thermogenic
e. from medication ▸ side-
e., genetic
e., gradual
e., hallucinogenic
e., harmful side-
e., hematologic
e., hepatic
e. ▸ horse race
e., hyperthermia
e., iatrogenic
e., immediate
e., immunomodulating
e., immunoregulatory
e., immunosuppressive
e., indirect biologic
e., indirect drug
e., inhibitory
e., intense
e. ▸ intense psychoactive drug
e., interface
e., inotropic
e., irradiation
e., isotope
e., jet
e. ▸ late proarrhythmic
e. ▸ lethal side-
e., lifelong
e., long-term
e., long-term adverse
e. ▸ long-term side-
e., maternal
e., medical side
e., metabolic
e. ▸ mille feuilles
e., mind-altering

effect(s)—*continued*

e., minor side
e. ▸ mood-elevating
e. ▸ mood-enhancing
e., multiplier
e., narcotic
e., negative
e., nervous system side-
e., neurological
e., neurotoxic
e., nonhemodynamic
e., nootropic
e. of aging
e. of AIDS (acquired immune deficiency syndrome) ▸ emotional
e. of AIDS (acquired immune deficiency syndrome) ▸ physical
e. of alcohol ▸ cardiovascular
e. of alcohol, cellular
e. of alcohol ▸ prenatal
e. of alcoholism ▸ ripple
e. of asthma on lung
e. of behavior therapy ▸ iatrogenic
e. of behavioral treatment
e. of cannabinoid abuse, physical
e. of cannabinoid abuse, psychological
e. of cocaine ▸ prenatal
e. of cocaine ▸ variable
e. of copper ▸ toxic
e. of depressant abuse, physical
e. of depressants, psychological
e. of dose fractionation, normal tissue
e. of drug abuse, physical
e. of drug abuse, psychological
e. of drugs, special
e. of emotional stress on rigidity
e. of emotional stress on spasticity
e. of estrogen loss, bone thinning
e. of hallucinogen abuse, physical
e. of hallucinogens, psychological
e. of heavy ions, physical
e. of hypnotic suggestion ▸ psychological
e. of ice and snow ▸ anesthetizing
e. of inhalant abuse, physical
e. of inhalants
e. of inhalants, psychological
e. of medication ▸ therapeutic
e. of methamphetamine ▸ cardiovascular
e. of old age, debilitating
e. of opioid abuse, physical

e. of opioids
e. of opioids ▸ duration of
e. of opioids, psychological
e. of pain ▸ emotional
e. of pain on the whole person
e. of particle beams, physical
e. of phencyclidine
e. of phencyclidine abuse, physical
e. of phencyclidine, psychological
e. of relaxation ▸ psychophysiological
e. of smoking ▸ prenatal
e. of stimulant
e. of stimulant abuse, physical
e. of stimulants, psychological
e. of trauma, cumulative
e. of treatment
e. of treatment, secondary
e. of treatment, side
e. of unprotected sun exposure ▸ cumulative
e. of weight ▸ ever-present
e. on brain, alcohol
e. on liver, alcohol
e. on lungs, alcohol
e. on medication ▸ deteriorating
e., oxygen (O_2)
e., pain relieving
e., palliative
e., paradoxical drug
e. ▸ peripheral autonomic nervous system
e. ▸ peripheral somatic
e. ▸ permanent, pervasive
e., photoelectric
e., photonuclear
e., physical
e., physical and biochemical
e., physiologic
e., placebo
e., positive
e. ▸ positive therapeutic
e., potential side
e., potential toxic
e., priming
e., Prinzmetal
e., proarrhythmic
e. ▸ profile ▸ side-
e. ▸ prolonged anesthetic
e. ▸ proto-oncogenic
e., pseudotumor
e., psychic
e., psychoactive
e., psychological
e. ▸ psychological and emotional

e., psychotoxic
e., quinidine
e., radiation
e., radiational
e., radiographic
e. relation, concentration
e. relationship, cause-and-
e., renal
e., repolarization
e., residual muscle relaxant
e., rubber band
e. ▸ secondary side-
e., sedative
e., sedative-like
e., sensitizing
e., serious side
e., severe side
e., side
e. ▸ silver wire
e., sneeze
e., snowplow
e., Somogyi
e., squeeze
e., stress-reducing
e., subjective
e., substantial
e., sundown
e., synergistic
e., synergistic bactericidal
e., synergistic pressor
e., systemic
e., teratogenic
e., therapeutic
e., thermal
e., thermogenic
e., toxic
e., toxic ocular
e., toxic side-
e., training
e., tranquilizing side-
e., traumatic
e., unusual side-
e. ▸ white coat
e., Zeeman

effective

e. action taken
e. antibiotic concentration
e. arterial elastance
e. atrial contraction
e. breathing function ▸ loss of
e. capillary flow
e. carotid pulse
e. chemotherapeutic support
e. circulating blood volume
e., clinically

e. communication skills
e. compliance
e., cost
e. direct radiation (EDR)
e. dosage (MED), minimum
e. dosages, safe and
e. dose
e. dose, median
e. dose, minimal
e. drug duration
e. functioning
e. half-life
e. heartbeat
e. infection control
e. intervention
e. mental health care
e. pain control
e. painkiller
e. parenting skills
e. pressure
e. ▸ proven safe and
e. pulse rate
e., quality treatment cost-
e. refractory period
e. refractory period (APERP), accessory pathway
e. refractory period, atrial
e. refractory period ▸ ventricular
e. regurgitant orifice
e. renal blood flow
e. renal plasma flow (ERPF)
e. skills
e. sterilization
e. stroke
e. surveillance practices
e. temperature
e. therapy
e. treatment
e. treatment ▸ high-quality and
e. treatment strategy
e. wavelength
effectiveness
e., antiemetic
e., assessment of
e., borderline
e., comparative
e., dosage
e., interpersonal
e., long-term
e. of electromyographic feedback ▸ differential
e. of mammogram ▸ reduced
e. of radiation
e., relative biological
e. studies, treatment

e., therapeutic
e. training, parent
effector cell
effector molecules
efferens glomeruli, vas
efferent [*afferent, aberrant*]
e. arteriole
e. artery
e. duct
e. fibers, blocking vagal
e. glomerular arteriole
e. loop
e. nerve
e. neuron
e. vessels
efferentia
e. lymphoglandulae ▸ vasa
e. nodi lymphatici ▸ vasa
e., vasa
effervescing antacid
efficacy (Efficacy)
e. ▸ enhancing self-
e., low self-
E. of Nosocomial Infection Control (SENIC) ▸ Study on the
e. ▸ potential clinical virological
e., therapeutic
e., treatment
efficiency
e., breathing
e., cardiovascular
e., enhanced intellectual
e., enhanced metabolic
e., exercise
e. factor, local
e., geometric
e. index (PEI) ▸ physical
e., index, sleep
e., lactic acid
e., loss of contractile
e., mental
e., neural
e. of heart and lungs ▸ improve
e. of oxygenation
e. particulate air ▸ high-
e. ratio (PER), protein
e., sleep
e., splicing
e., visual
efficient means of transmission
efficient performance of tasks
Effler hiatal hernia repair
effleurage on uterus
effleurage technique
effluent gas

effluent gas from respiratory therapy devices
effluvium, telogen
effluxed clear urine
effort
e. angina
e. angina ▸ first
e., decrease in respiratory
e. dyspnea
e., first
e., frantic
e. -induced thrombosis
e. intolerance
e., mental
e., muscle
e., poor respiratory
e., respiratory
e., resuscitative
e. syndrome
e. to avoid abandonment ▸ frantic
e. thrombosis
e., visual
e., voluntary
effuse colony
effused fluid
effusion(s)
e., abdominal
e., acid
e. and drainage ▸ middle ear
e. and tamponade ▸ pericardial
e., area of
e., asbestos
e., bilateral
e. ▸ bilateral and right serosanguinous pleural
e., bilateral pleural
e., bilaterally, pleural
e., bloody
e., cardiac
e., chronic pericarditis
e., chyliform pleural
e., chylous pericardial
e. ▸ cultures of pleural
e. ▸ exudative pleural
e., iatrogenic
e. in brain stem, blood
e., joint
e. left base
e., loculated pleural
e., malignant
e. ▸ malignant pleural
e., massive pleural
e. ▸ middle ear
e. of blood
e. of fluid

effusion(s)—*continued*
- e. of joint
- e. of knee joint
- e., otitis media with
- e., parapneumonic
- e., pericardial
- e., peritoneal
- e. ▸ persistent middle ear
- e. (PE), pleural
- e., pleurisy with
- e., pleuritic
- e., pulmonary
- e., recurrent pleural
- e. right base
- e., serosanguineous pleural
- e., serous
- e., serous pleural
- e. ▸ silent pericardial
- e., suprapatellar
- e. ▸ transudative pleural

effusive-constrictive disease
effusive-constrictive pericarditis
EGF (Epidermal Growth Factor)
egg(s)
- e. albumin, crystalline
- e. crate cushion
- e. crate mattress
- e. donation
- e. donor
- e. donor program
- e. envelope
- e., fertilized
- e. follicles
- e. freezing
- e. from ovary, release of
- e., implantation of fertilized
- e. inner membrane
- e. ▸ irregular release of
- e., mature
- e., nits and pubic lice
- e. retrieval procedure
- e. -shaped heart
- e. yellow reaction
- e. yolk
- e. yolk sputum

Eggers' operation
Eggers' procedure
eggshell pattern
EGL (eosinophilic granuloma of the lung)
ego
- e. analysis
- e. -analytic approach ▸ strategic, experiential and
- e. autonomy

- e. defense
- e. defense of denial
- e. deficit psychology
- e. -dystonic
- e. -dystonic illness
- e. function, executant
- e. functioning, autonomous
- e. functions
- e. functions, adaptive
- e. ideal
- e. instinct
- e. libido
- e. process
- e. psychology
- e. strengthening
- e. strengthening technique
- e. structure
- e. -syntonic

egocentric, patient
EGOT (erythrocyte glutamic oxaloacetic transaminase)
Egyptian conjunctivitis
Egyptian ophthalmia
Ehlers-Danlos syndrome
Ehrlich
- E. anemia, Biermer-
- E. ascites carcinoma
- E. bodies, Heinz
- E. degeneration, Armanni-
- E. granules
- E. -Heinz granules
- E. reaction
- E. test
- E. -Türck line
- E. units

ehrlichiosis (HGE) ▸ human granulocytic
ehrlichiosis (HME) ▸ human monocytic
Ehrmann's alcohol test meal
EI (environmental illness)
E:I ratio
EIA (enzyme immunoassay)
EIA (exercise induced asthma)
Eicher femoral prosthetic head
Eicher hip prosthesis
Eichhorst atrophy
eicosanoid excretion
eidetic image
eidetic imagery ▸ increase in
Eiger syndrome ▸ Bakwin-
eight (8)
- e. abnormality ▸ figure-of-
- e. artificial, heart ▸ Jarvik-
- e. -ball hemorrhage

- e. bandage, figure-of-
- e. heart ▸ figure-of-
- e. (HHV-8) ▸ Human Herpes Virus
- e. to 13 hertz (Hz)

VIII
- VIII deficiency, Factor
- VIII implant Choyce Mark
- VIII inhibitor, Factor
- VIII -related antigen ▸ Factor

18, fluorine F
18 syndrome, trisomy
eighth
- e. cranial nerve
- e. nerve
- e. nerve activity
- e. nerve damage
- e. nerve degeneration
- e. nerve function ▸ monitoring of
- e. nerve toxicity

#80, Arcing spring
82 imaging ▸ rubidium-
Eimeria stiedae
Eimeria tenella
Einhorn regimen of chemotherapy
Einthoven's triangle
eisenbergii, Pseudomonas
Eisenmenger's
- E. complex
- E. disease
- E. reaction
- E. syndrome
- E. tetralogy

ejaculated, fluid
ejaculation
- e. center
- e., premature
- e., retrograde

ejaculatory duct
ejectile vomiting
ejectile vomitus
ejection
- e. click
- e. click, systolic
- e. force, atrial
- e. fraction
- e. fraction, cineangiography and densitometric
- e. fraction, densitometric
- e. fraction ▸ depressed
- e. fraction, echocardiography
- e. fraction image
- e. fraction, left ventricular (LV)
- e. fraction ▸ light pen-determined
- e. fraction, normal
- e. fraction ▸ rest

e. fraction, right ventricular (RV)
e. fraction, spurious
e. fraction, Teicholz
e. murmur (EM)
e. murmur, diamond
e. murmur (SEM) ▸ systolic
e. period
e. period, systolic
e. phase
e. phase index
e., rapid
e. rate
e. rate (MER) ▸ mean
e. rate ▸ mean normalized systolic
e. rate (MSER) ▸ mean systolic
e. rate ▸ stroke
e. rate (SER) ▸ systolic
e., reduced
e. shell image
e. sound
e. systolic murmur (ESM)
e. systolic murmur ▸ blowing
e. time
e. time, carotid
e. time (LVET) ▸ left ventricular
e. time (RVET) ▸ right ventricular
e. time, systolic
e. velocity
e., ventricular
e., volumic
EKG (*see* **ECG**)
Ekbom syndrome
EKY (electrokymogram) study
EKY (electrokymography) study
El Tor vibrio
ELAM (endothelial leukocyte adhesion molecule)
elastance
e. ▸ effective arterial
e. ▸ end-systolic
e. ▸ maximum ventricular
elastase
e., leukocyte
e., neutrophil
e., pseudomonas
elastic
e. bandage
e. collision
e. component
e. compression stockings
e. connective tissue
e. dressing, light
e. element ▸ series
e. fibers
e. fibers in sputum

e. fibers stain
e. gauze, Kling
e. hose, Linton
e., intermaxillary
e., intramaxillary
e. lamina
e. lamina ▸ internal
e. ligature
e. ligature, thread-
e. line
e. membrane, external
e. membrane ▸ Henle
e. membrane, internal
e. nodule, antihelix
e. pulse
e. recall of lung
e. recoil
e. recoil of arterial wall
e. recoil tendency
e. resistance
e. skin
e. skin ▸ firm
e. soft tissue
e. stains
e. stiffness
e. support hose
e. tissue
e. tissue, thick
e. tissue, yellow
e. traction
e., vertical
elastica, cutis
elastica, helminthiasis
elasticity
e. ▸ bladder volume and
e., blood vessel
e., blood vessels with reduced
e. ▸ flexibility and
e. ▸ impaired blood vessel
e., loss of lung
e., lung
e. of air sacs
e. of aorta
e. of arteries
e. of lungs
e. of muscle ▸ physical
e. of muscle ▸ physiologic
e. of muscle ▸ total
e. of skin
e. ▸ sputum viscosity and
e., vascular tone and
elasticum, pseudoxanthoma
elasticum syndrome ▸ pseudoxanthoma
elasticus laryngis ▸ conus

elastofibroma dorsi
elastolysis, perifollicular
elastoma, juvenile
elastoma, Miescher's
Elastoplast bandage
elation
e., exaggerated
e., extreme
e., inappropriate
e. or depression
elbow(s)
e. (AE) ▸ above
e. (AE) amputation ▸ above
e. (BE) amputation ▸ below
e. arthroplasty, Schlein-type
e., articular muscle of
e., baseball pitcher's
e. (BE) ▸ below
e. capped
e., decubitus
e., dislocated
e., dropped
e. extension exercise
e. fibromyalgia
e. flexed
e. flexion
e. full range of motion (ROM) ▸ left
e. full range of motion (ROM) ▸ right
e., golfer's
e., Heelbo used on patient's
e. injury, lateral
e. injury, medial
e. jerk
e. joint replacement
e., Little Leaguer's
e., median vein of
e., miner's
e., nursemaid's
e. pronation exercise
e. protector
e. protector, disposable
e., pulled
e. reflex
e. replacement
e. ▸ silvery scales on
e., sore
e. supination exercise
e., tennis
ELCA (excimer laser coronary angioplasty)
elder (Elder)
e. abuse
E. lamp ▸ Duke-
e. misuse of medication

elderly
- e. abuse
- e. aerobics
- e. alcohol use
- e. cadaver
- e. care crisis
- e. ► depression and anxiety in
- e. ► innocent murmur of
- e. patient ► frail
- e., psychosis in the
- e. suicide
- e. ► systolic hypertension in the

Eldridge-Green lamp
Elecath pacemaker
elected palliative care
election line
elective
- e. abdominal surgery
- e. affinity
- e. cardioversion
- e. correction
- e. excision
- e. induction
- e. irradiation
- e. mastectomy
- e. medical admission
- e. mutism
- e. myocardial revascularization
- e. neck irradiation
- e. procedure
- e. repair
- e. replacement
- e. replacement indicators
- e. replacement pulse generator
- e. surgery
- e. /urgent admissions

Electra complex
electric (Electric)
- E. and Musical Industries (EMI) brain scanner
- e. approach
- e. arm
- e. baker
- e. bed
- e. cardiac pacemaker
- e. cataract
- e. cautery
- e. charge
- e. chorea
- e. chromatography
- e. current
- e. extremity
- e. field
- e. field, conductive radio frequency

- e. field hyperthermia, radio frequency
- e. field, inductive radio frequency
- e. field ► intensity of
- e. field, interstitial radio frequency
- e. field, resistive radio frequency
- e. infusion regulator
- e. leg
- e. -like pain
- e. loop
- e. ophthalmia
- E. pacemaker, General
- e. pain ► sharp, jabbing or
- e. patient lift
- e. potential
- e. pulses
- E. Response Audiometry (ERA)
- e. shock
- e. signals or messages ► transmission of
- e. sleep
- e. stimulation
- e. stimulus
- e. tension

electrical
- e. activation abnormality
- e. activity
- e. activity, abnormal
- e. activity, absence of
- e. activity between electrodes
- e. activity, brain
- e. activity, chaotic
- e. activity, identifiable
- e. activity in brain, abnormal
- e. activity in nerve and muscle
- e. activity ► increase in amplitude of
- e. activity of brain
- e. activity of cochlea
- e. activity of heart
- e. activity of retina
- e. activity ► pulseless
- e. activity ► rapidly pulsing
- e. activity, recording of
- e. activity, recruitment pattern of
- e. activity ► shift in direction and pattern of brain
- e. activity toward sleep activity ► shifting
- e. activity ► variations in
- e. alternans
- e. alternation of heart
- e. aversion
- e. aversive therapy
- e. axis

- e. axis ► instantaneous
- e. axis ► joule point
- e. axis ► mean
- e. axis ► normal
- e. bioimpedance ► thoracic
- e. brain activity ► recorded
- e. burn
- e. capacity
- e. cardiac activity
- e. cardioversion
- e. cardioversion, defibrillation and
- e. catheter ablation
- e. charge
- e. charge to heart
- e. circuit
- e. code
- e. conduction in heart
- e. conductor
- e. contraction coupling (ECC)
- e. conversion
- e. conversion of atrial fibrillation
- e. counter conditional procedures
- e. countershock
- e. current
- e. current block
- e. defibrillation
- e. diastole
- e. discharges, abnormal
- e. disease
- e. energy
- e. event
- e. events in heart, abnormal
- e. factor
- e. failure
- e. field
- e. firings of brain
- e. fulguration
- e. function of heart
- e. heart position
- e. impedance
- e. implant
- e. impulse
- e. impulse, abnormal
- e. impulse to heart
- e. injury
- e. instability of heart
- e. insulator
- e. interference
- e. interference, external
- e. interference ► extraneous scalp muscle
- e. intervention
- e. lead
- e. lead patches
- e. mechanical dissociation

e. muscle stimulation (EMS)
e. nerve stimulation
e. nerve stimulation (TENS), transcutaneous
e. potential
e. potential ▸ cell membrane
e. potential difference
e. reactivity of brain
e. resistance
e. response of skin
e. rhythm, heart's
e. shock
e. signals
e. silence
e. spinal cord stimulation
e. stimulation
e. stimulation device
e. stimulation (FES), functional
e. stimulation, neuromuscular
e. stimulation of atria
e. stimulation of auditory nerve
e. stimulation of brain
e. stimulation of hand
e. stimulation of heart
e. stimulation of leg
e. stimulation of spinal cord
e. stimulation of ventricles
e. stimulation ▸ paired
e. stimulation, repeated
e. stimulation, repetitive
e. stimulation, response of brain to
e. stimulation ▸ slaved programmed
e. stimulation to brain
e. stimulation to brain ▸ periodic
e. stimulation to nerve
e. stimulation (TES), transcutaneous
e. stimulator for pain relief
e. stimulus
e. stimulus, abnormal
e. system, myocardium
e. systole
e. therapy
e. wave, complex
electrically
e. charged body
e. generated shock waves
e. unstable, heart
electricity-induced anesthesia
electrocardiogram(s) (ECG/EKG)
e., abnormal
e., admission
e., baseline
e. blip
e., borderline

e. changes ▸ ischemic
e., cross sectional
e., exercise
e. exercise stress test
e., fetal
e. findings
e., flat
e. ▸ His bundle
e. machine, portable
e., monitored with
e. ▸ orthogonal
e. ▸ scalar
e., serial
e. showed normal pattern
e. ▸ signal averaged
e. silence
e., 6-lead
e. ▸ 16-lead
e., stress
e. ▸ stress multiple gated acquisition (MUGA)
e. strip
e. study
e. synchronized digital subtraction angiogram
e. telemetry
e. test, fetal
e. ▸ thallium
e. ▸ three-channel
e., 3-lead
e. ▸ time domain signal averaged
e. tracing
e. tracing display
e. treadmill, stress
e. triggering unit
e., 12-lead
e. ▸ unipolar
e. ▸ vector
e. waves
electrocardiograph (ECG)
e., bioimpedance
e., Cambridge
e. changes ▸ ischemic
e. ▸ Marquette
e. monitor▸ transtelephonic
electrocardiographic (ECG)
e. gating
e. leads
e. monitoring
e. monitoring (AEM), ambulatory
e. monitoring ▸ electrophysiologic vs
e. score, Brush
e. transtelephonic monitor
electrocardiography (ECG)
e. (AECG), ambulatory

e., esophageal
e., fetal
e. ▸ intracardiac
e. (AECG) monitoring, ambulatory
e. ▸ signal averaged
electrocardioscope, phono◊
electrocautery
e., Bovie
e. conization
e., cystoscopic
e., needlepoint
e. unit
electrocerebral
e. inactivity
e. inactivity, record of
e. inactivity, tracings of
e. silence (ECS)
e. silence (ECS), record of
e. silence (ECS) recording
electrochemical
e. cell
e. messages to brain ▸ transmitting
e. polarization
electrocoagulated, bleeders
electrocoagulated, bleeding points
electrocoagulation of hemorrhoids, bipolar
electroconvulsant treatment (ECT)
electroconvulsive
e. shock (ECS)
e. therapy (ECT)
e. treatment
electrocorticogram study
electrocorticography study
electrode(s)
e., active
e., adjacent
e. and brain ▸ interface between
e. and scalp ▸ interface between
e., anterior temporal
e. application
e. application, facial
e. applied
e. applied over cerebral cortex
e., array of
e. attachment
e. attachment, scalp
e. attachment, skin
e., average potential
e., ball tip
e., basal
e., bayonet tip
e., bipolar
e., bipolar depth

electrode(s)—*continued*

e., bipolar myocardial
e., bipolar needle
e., bipolar placement of
e. board
e., Bugbe
e., button
e., calomel
e. catheter
e., central terminal
e. closely spaced
e., coil
e., Collings'
e., common average reference
e., concentric needle
e., conical tip
e. connected in parallel
e. connections
e. contact
e., corneal
e., cortical
e., cutaneous thoracic patch
e., depolarizing
e., depth
e., disk
e., dispersing
e., distal
e. distance, inter-
e. distances, large inter-
e. distances, long inter-
e. distances, short inter-
e. distances, small inter-
e., EEG (electroencephalogram)
e., electrical activity between
e., electroencephalogram (EEG)
e., epicardial
e., epidural
e. equipotential
e., exciting
e., exploring
e., external
e., external canthus
e., fine wire
e. gel
e., Gradle's
e., Hamm's
e. ▸ His bundle
e., hydrogen
e. impedance
e. ▸ implantable cardioverter
e. ▸ implantable unipolar
endocardial
e., implantation subcutaneous
e., implanted
e. implanted in cerebral cortex

e. implanted within brain substance
e., implanting brain
e., impregnated
e., inactive
e., indifferent
e., inferior frontal
e. inserted in cerebral cortex
e., internal
e., intracerebral
e. ▸ intravascular catheter
e. ▸ ion selective
e., jelly
e., Kronfeld's
e. lead, dual-
e. lead, multi-
e., left arm
e., left leg
e., lens
e., localizing
e., low midoccipital
e. manipulated
e. mark, scalp
e., McCarthy's
e., measured between pairs of
e., metal
e., monopolar needle
e. ▸ monopolar temporary
e., multilead
e., multiple point
e. ▸ multipolar catheter
e., nasopharyngeal
e., needle
e., Neil-Moore
e., neutral
e., pacemaker
e., pad
e. paddles
e., pair of
e., pair of electroencephalogram
(EEG)
e. pair, stimulating
e., parietal
e. paste
e. patch
e., periacqueductal gray
e., Pischel's
e. placed in position
e. placed on scalp
e. placed on surface of head
e. placement
e. placement, biofeedback
e. placement ▸
electroencephalogram (EEG)
e. placement on forehead
e. placement, site of

e. placement, standard
e., point
e. polarization
e. polarization ▸ varying degrees of
e. potential, extraneous
e., proximal
e., recording
e. recording, nasopharyngeal
e., reference
e. reimplanted in old pocket
e., resistance
e. resistance, measurement of
e., right arm
e., right leg
e., ring
e., rod
e., scalp
e., scalp recording
e. selectors
e., silent
e. ▸ silver bead
e., single reference
e. site
e. skin interface
e., spacing between pairs of
e., special
e., sphenoidal
e. ▸ stab-in epicardial
e. stability
e., sternospinal reference
e., stick-on
e., stigmatic
e., stimulating
e. ▸ Stockert cardiac pacing
e., subdural
e., surface
e. ▸ surgically implanted
e. system
e. system, magnetic induction
coaxial
e. system ▸ 10-20 (ten-twenty)
e. technique, micro◊
e., temporary atrial pacing
e., temporary epicardial pacing
e., therapeutic
e., transvenous
e., true anterior temporal
e., ultrasonic
e., unipolar depth
e., ureteral meatotomy
e., VPL (ventroposterolateral)
thalamic
e., Weve's
e., wire
e. wire, pacing

e., crossover
e., disc
e., gel
e. ▸ gradient gel
e., hemoglobin
e., high voltage
e., lipoprotein
e., moving boundary
e., paper
e., protein
e. ▸ pulsed-field gel
e. scanning
e., thin layer
e., zone

electrophoretic
e. analysis
e. hemoglobin
e. mobility
e. pattern
e. profile
e. protein

electrophrenic respiration
electrophrenic respiration ▸
   radiofrequency
electrophysiologic
e. function
e. mapping
e. study (EPS)
e. study ▸ intracardiac
e. testing
e. testing and mapping
e. testing ▸ invasive
e. testing ▸ serial
e. vs electrocardiographic
   monitoring

electrophysiological study, chronic
electrophysiological test
electrophysiology
e. diagnostic program
e., intracardiac
e. ▸ pacemaker cell
e. study
e. test
e. testing

electroretinogram study
electroshock therapy (EST)
electrostatic
e. capacity
e. generator
e. imaging
e. unit

electrosurgery pencil
electrosurgical
e. cauterization
e. excision procedure ▸ loop

e. gingivectomies
e. pencil, Handtrol
electrotherapeutic sleep
electrothermal therapy (IDET),
   intradiskal
electrovibratory massage
element(s)
e., base
e., bony
e., causative
e., cell
e., cellular
e., contractile
e., daughter
e., dream
e., genetic
e., glandular
e., hematopoietic
e., Kollmorgen
e., magnetically traceable
e., nuclear
e. of risk
e. of the retina ▸ neuroepithelial
e., parent
e. (pixel), picture
e., radioactive
e., scattered hematopoietic
e. ▸ series elastic
e., structural
e., structured
e., toxic
e., trace
e. transfer factor, blood
e. (voxel), volume

elemental diet in nutrition
elementary [*alimentary*]
e. body
e. body ▸ Gordon
e. granules
e. particles

elephant
e. (elephantiasis) disease
e. -on-the-chest sensation
e. tranquilizer (phencyclidine)

elephantiasis (elephant) disease
elephantiasis of vulva
elevate feet above heart level
elevated
e., annulus
e. anxiety level
e. arm stress test
e. bilirubin
e., bladder flap
e. blood pressure (BP)
e. blood sugar

e. blood urea nitrogen (BUN)
e. cholesterol
e. diaphragm
e. enzymes
e. eye pressure
e. flap
e. heart rate
e. higher than heart, legs
e., kidney rest
e. lesion
e. levels of endothelin
e. mood
e. position, dorsal
e. pressure in eyeball
e. pulmonary artery pressure
e. rolled border
e. scapula
e. sed (sedimentation) rate
e. surface of brain
e. temperature of limb
e. temperature, patient had
e., triglycerides
e., venous blood pressure (BP)

elevating
e. drug, mood
e. effect ▸ mood-
e. lens
e. substances, temperature

elevation
e., blood pressure (BP)
e., bracing and rehabilitation
e., diaphragmatic
e., disc
e. exercise
e. exercises, shoulder
e., Gilles
e., heel
e. ▸ liver enzyme
e. of blood pressure (BP) ▸
   intermittent
e. of blood pressure (BP) persistent
e. of body temperature
e. of body weight
e. of BP (blood pressure) ▸
   persistent
e. of diaphragm
e. of eyelid ▸ sling
e. of head of bed
e. of injured limb
e. of mood ▸ persistent
e. of skull fracture
e., persistent S-T segment
e., prominent
e. (PRICE) ▸ protection, rest, ice,
   compression and

elevation—*continued*
- e. (RICE) ▸ rest, ice, compression,
- e., serum amylase
- e., ST segment
- e., temperature
- e. torque technique ▸ George Winter

elevator disease
elevatum, erythema
eleventh cranial nerve
eleventh nerve
elfin facies
elfin facies syndrome
Elgiloy frame
elicited, tenderness
eliciting nurturance
eliciting stimulus
eligibility criteria
eligibility, determination of
eligible, Medicare
eliminate
- e. alcohol abuse
- e. gravity
- e. smoking
- e. source of contamination

elimination
- e., alteration in
- e., alteration in bladder
- e., alteration in pattern of urinary
- e., altered patterns of urinary
- e. diet
- e., half-life
- e., immune
- e. of pancreatic digestive juices
- e. of waste
- e., urinary

ELISA (enzyme-linked immunosorbent assay) test
Elite II pacemaker ▸ Medtronic
elixir terpin hydrate
Ellestad
- E. exercise stress test
- E. protocol
- E. protocol ▸ modified

Elliot's operation
Elliott's treatment
ellipsoid joint
ellipsoid of spleen
ellipsoidal articulation
ellipsoidal cell
ellipsoideus, Saccharomyces
elliptic amputation
elliptica, Naumanniella
elliptica, Taenia
elliptical loop

elliptically, lesion excised
elliptocytotic anemia
Ellis' sign
Ellis-Jones operation
Ellison syndrome ▸ Zollinger-
Ellis-van Creveld syndrome
Ellsworth classification, Reese-
Elmslie-Cholmeley operation
Eloesser flap
Eloesser's operation
elongata, Trichomonas
elongate, stretch and
elongated
- e. aorta
- e. contractile fiber cell
- e. cystic duct
- e. cytoplasmic tail
- e. formation
- e. glands
- e. limb
- e., linear cell
- e. ovoid cells
- e. papillary muscle
- e. uvula

elongation
- e. and torsion
- e. of thoracic aorta
- e. of thoracic aorta ▸ arteriosclerotic
- e. stretch exercise

Elschnig('s)
- E. bodies
- E. conjunctivitis
- E. operation
- E. pearls
- E. spot
- E. syndrome
- E. syndrome ▸ Koerber-Salus-

Elsner's asthma
elusion (*same as* illusion)
elusive symptoms
eluting pacemaker lead ▸ steroid
eluting stent
elution, cord blood
elution, membrane
Ely's operation
Ely's test
EM (ejection murmur)
Em. (emmetropia)
EM ▸ definitive diagnosis by (electron microscopy)
emaciated
- e. and dehydrated
- e. condition ▸ weak
- e. face

- e., patient

emanation(s)
- e., actinium
- e., radium
- e., spike-like
- e., thorium

emancipation disorder of adolescence
emancipation disorder of early adult life
embalmed, body
embalming fluid (phencyclidine)
embarras gastrique
embarrassed respiration
embarrassment
- e., circulatory
- e., coronary circulation
- e., fear of
- e., respiratory

embedded (*same as* imbedded)
- e. debris
- e. ▸ foreign matter
- e. in tumor mass
- e. object
- e. tissue in paraffin block

embolectomy
- e., brachial
- e. catheter
- e. catheter, arterial
- e., femoral
- e. of aorta
- e., pulmonary

emboli
- e., acute aortic
- e., aortic occlusive
- e., atheromatous
- e., bone marrow
- e., cholesterol
- e. -induced lung injury, air
- e., multiple cholesterol
- e., multiple pulmonary
- e. ▸ occult pulmonary
- e., peripheral pulmonary
- e., pulmonary
- e., pulmonary vasculature free of
- e., recurrent
- e., retinal
- e., septic
- e. syndrome ▸ fat
- e. with small infarct

embolic
- e. abscess
- e. agent ▸ fluid
- e. aneurysm
- e. event

e. gangrene
e. infarct
e. occlusion
e. pattern
e. phenomena, peripheral
e. phenomenon
e. pneumonia
e. shower
e. stroke
e. thrombosis
embolism(s)
  e., acute arterial
  e., acute pulmonary
  e., air
  e., air pulmonary
  e., amniotic fluid
  e., aortic
  e., arterial
  e., artery
  e., bacillary
  e., bland
  e., bone marrow
  e., capillary
  e., catheter
  e., cellular
  e., cerebral
  e., cerebral air
  e., coronary
  e., crossed
  e., direct
  e. ▸ diving air
  e., fat
  e., gas
  e., hematogenous
  e. in atrial fibrillation
  e. infarction of lung due to
  e., infective
  e., lung
  e., lymph
  e., lymphogenous
  e., miliary
  e., multiple
  e. ▸ myxomatous pulmonary
  e. of artery
  e. of retinal artery
  e., oil
  e., pantaloon
  e., paradoxical
  e. ▸ paradoxical cerebral
  e., plasmodium
  e. (PE), pulmonary
  e., pyemic
  e., recurrent
  e., retinal
  e., retrograde

e., saddle
e., spinal
e., straddling
e. ▸ submassive pulmonary
e. syndrome, fat
e., trichinous
e., tumor
e., venous
embolization
  e., air
  e., bronchial artery
  e., coil
  e., fat
  e. of arteries ▸ cholesterol
  e., paradoxical
  e., pulmonary
  e., research cholesterol
  e., septic
  e., Silastic bead
  e. therapy
  e., transcatheter
  e. ▸ transcatheter arterial
  e. (THE), transhepatic
  e. treatment
  e. ▸ uterine artery
  e. ▸ uterine fibroid
embolized
  e. atheroma
  e. foreign material
  e. small arteries
embolomycotic aneurysm
embolus (emboli)
  e., air
  e., aortic saddle
  e., atheromatous
  e., bone marrow
  e., cancer
  e., catheter
  e., cellular
  e., cerebral
  e., cholesterol
  e., fat
  e., femoral
  e., foam
  e., massive pulmonary
  e., multiple cholesterol
  e., multiple pulmonary
  e., obturating
  e. ▸ patient threw an
  e., peripheral pulmonary
  e., polyurethane foam
  e., pulmonary
  e. ▸ pulmonary vasculature free of
  e., recurrent pulmonary
  e., retinal

e., riding
e., saddle
e., septic
e., straddling
e. with small infarct ▸ pulmonary
embosser, braille
embrace reflex
embrace reflex, Moro
embrasure
  e., buccal
  e., labial
  e., lingual
  e., occlusal
embryo
  e., atrial appendages in
  e., autolyzed
  e. bronchial tree
  e. development
  e., frozen
  e., hexacanth
  e., Janosik's
  e. kidney, human
  e. -lethal orphan (CELO) ▸ chicken-
  e., presomite
  e., previllous
  e., somite
  e., Spee's
  e. transfer
embryocardia, jugular
embryocardia rhythm
embryolethality study
embryology
  e., comparative
  e., descriptive
  e., experimental
  e. ▸ tracheoesophageal fistula
embryoma of kidney
embryonal
  e. adenoma
  e. carcinoma
  e. carcinoma, infantile
  e. carcinosarcoma
  e. cataract, anterior axial
  e. cataract, posterior axial
  e. cell tumor
  e. cells
  e. connective tissue cells
  e. cyst
  e. leukemia
  e. nephroma
  e. nevoblasts
  e. nuclear cataract
  e. rhabdomyosarcoma
  e. sarcoma
  e. tumor

embryonic
　e. axis
　e. cardiac monocytes
　e. cardiac muscle
　e. cell
　e. circulation
　e. development
　e. development, hindgut
　e. development ▸ mouth
　e. disc
　e. ectoderm
　e. heart
　e. membranes
　e. myocardium
　e. neural tube
　e. outpocketing
　e. period
　e. structures ▸ minute
　e. vitreous
embryonum, smegma
embryoplastic odontoma
EMC (encephalomyocarditis)
EMC (encephalomyocarditis) virus
EMC (essential mixed
　　cryoglobulinemia)
EMDR (eye movement
　　desensitization and
　　reprocessing)
emergency (Emergency)
　e. admission
　e., admitted as
　e. airway
　e. alert device
　e., altitude-related
　e., behavioral
　e., behavioral psychological
　e., breathing
　e., cardiac
　e. cardiac care
　e. cardiac care ▸ history and
　　symptoms of
　e. cardioresuscitation team
　E. Care Center (ECC)
　e. care center (ECC) ▸ admission
　　to
　e. care, enhance
　e. care of patient
　e. care, prehospital
　e. care, 24-hour
　e. cesarean (C-) section
　e. clinician
　e., dental
　E. Department
　e. department, hospital
　e., dermatologic

　e. detention
　e., diabetic
　e. drug box
　e. drug index
　e., endocrine
　e. endoscopy
　e. ▸ ENT (ear, nose and throat)
　e., environmental
　e., environmental medical
　e., gastrointestinal (GI)
　e. hospital
　e., hypertensive
　e., hysterectomy
　e., infectious disease
　e. insect-sting treatment
　e. laparotomy
　e., laryngeal
　e., life-threatening
　e. light reflex
　e. measures
　e. measures instituted
　e., medical
　e. medical care
　e. medical service (EMS)
　E. Medical Technician (EMT)
　e. medicine
　E. Medicine Clinic
　e. medicine physician
　e. medicine specialist ▸ pediatric
　e., medicolegal
　e., metabolic
　e. mouth-to-mouth resuscitation
　e. muscles
　e., neurological
　e., ocular
　e., orthopedic
　e. pain treatment
　e., pediatric orthopedic
　e. personnel
　e., procedure
　e., psychiatric
　e. radiation therapy
　e. reperfusion
　e., respiratory
　e. response system (PERS) ▸
　　personal
　e. resuscitation
　e. room care
　e. room episodes ▸ heroin-related
　E. Scale, Kent
　e. service
　e. service, psychiatric
　e. setting
　e. skin transplants feasible
　e. subtotal esophagectomy

　e. surgery
　e. therapy
　e. thoracentesis
　e. thoracotomy
　e. tracheotomy
　e., traumatic
　e. treatment
　e. treatment, anaphylaxis
　e. ventriculoperitoneal shunt
emergent liver injury
emergent psychiatric admission
emerging sobriety
emerging tumors
emersion field, oil
Emerson cuirass respirator
Emerson respirator
emery disc
emesis
　e. ▸ anorexia, pain, nausea and
　e. basin
　e., coffee ground
　e., coma, and death
　e., cycle of
　e. ▸ dysphagia, nausea and
　e., frequent
　e. gravidarum
　e., ipecac-induced
　e. of fecal material
　e. ▸ post-tussive
　e. postprandially, nausea and
　e. reaction, chemotherapy nausea-
emetic
　e., central
　e., direct
　e., indirect
　e., mechanical
　e., systemic
　e., tartar
EMF (electromotive force)
EMF (erythrocyte maturation factor)
EMG (electromyogram)
　EMG activity, decreased tonic
　EMG activity, increased tonic
　EMG biofeedback
　EMG biofeedback ▸ hyperkinesis
　　response to
　EMG biofeedback relaxation in
　　asthma
　EMG, integrated
　EMG pattern resemblance,
　　biofeedback
　EMG study
　EMG, submental
EMH (educable mentally
　　handicapped)

EMI (Electric and Musical Industries)
    brain scanner
emigrated cell
eminence
    e., arytenoid
    e., canine
    e., hyperthenar
    e., hypothenar
    e., iliopectineal
    e., intercondylar
    e., intercondyloid
    e., malar
    e., medial
    e., nasal
    e. of face, malar
    e., pyramidal
    e., thenar
eminent [*imminent*]
emissary vein
    e.v., condylar
    e.v., mastoid
    e.v., occipital
    e.v., parietal
emission
    e. computed tomography (ECT)
    e. computed tomography (SPECT)
        scan ▸ single photon
    e. computed tomography (SPECT),
        single photon
    e. computerized tomographic
        (ECT) body scanner
    e. computerized tomographic
        (ECT) system
    e. computerized tomographic
        (ECT) system, radionuclide
    e., electron
    e., negation
    e., nocturnal
    e. of radiation (laser) ▸ light
        amplification by stimulated
    e. of radiation (maser) ▸ microwave
        amplification by stimulated
    e. of radiation, stimulated
    e., otoacoustic
    e., partial
    e., photoelectric
    e., radiation
    e. scintiphoto, ▸ combined
        transmission-
    e. ▸ single photon
    e. spectroscopy ▸ flame
    e., thermonic
    e. tomographic scanning ▸
        fluorodopamine positron

e. tomography (SPET) imaging ▸
    single photon
e. tomography (PET), positron
e. transaxial tomography (PETT),
    positron
e. transverse tomography (PETT),
    positron
emitted radiation
emitter, beta
Emko Foam
Emma (narcotic), Miss
Emmert-Gellhorn pessary
emmetropia (Em.)
Emmet-Studdiford perineorrhaphy
Emmet's operation
emollient cream
emotion(s)
    e., affect and
    e., altered
    e. and behavior ▸ attitude,
    e. and conduct ▸ adjustment
        disorder with mixed disturbance
        of
    e. and conduct ▸ mixed disturbance
        of
    e. awareness
    e., brain wave activity and
    e., conflicting
    e., dulled
    e., exaggerated
    e. ▸ exaggerated expression of
    e., expressed
    e., family expressed
    e., fearful
    e. ▸ frequent changes in
    e., handling
    e. ▸ mixed disturbance of conduct
        and
    e., muscle behavior and
    e., negative
    e. ▸ predominant disturbance of
    e. ▸ rapidly shifting
    e. regulation
    e. -related itching
    e., repressed
    e. ▸ repression of
    e. ▸ restricted expression of
    e., reversed
    e. ▸ roller coaster
    e. ▸ shallow expression of
    e. specific to adolescence ▸
        disturbance of
    e. specific to childhood ▸
        disturbance of
    e., stressful

e. ▸ suppression of
e., toxic
e., unexpressed
e., unpredictable
emotional
    e. abuse
    e. activity
    e. activity, skin
    e. adjustment
    e. amalgam
    e. amnesia
    e. and behavioral disorders in
        adolescents
    e. and behavioral disorders in
        adults
    e. and behavioral disorders in
        children
    e. and conduct ▸ adjustment
        disorder with mixed disturbance
    e. and medical support
    e. and psychological aspect of pain
    e. and psychological battery
    e. anguish, severe
    e. arousal, increased
    e. arousal, internal
    e. aspects
    e. aspects of cancer
    e. aspects of cancer ▸ physical and
    e. aspects of supportive care
    e. attitude
    e. background
    e. barrier
    e. behavior
    e. behavior, erratic
    e. behavior, normal
    e. bleeding
    e. breakdown
    e. burdens
    e. burnout
    e. capability
    e. care, physical/
    e. challenge
    e. changes ▸ physical and
    e. cleansing
    e. coldness
    e. conflict
    e. considerations in palliation
    e. content flat
    e. context, negative
    e. control
    e. control in childbirth
    e. control, lack of
    e. control ▸ loss of
    e. control, weakened
    e. coping

emotional—*continued*
- e. crisis
- e. cues of stress
- e. cycle
- e. deception
- e. decision
- e. decompensation
- e. deficiency
- e. dependence, increased
- e. depression
- e. deprivation
- e. desperation
- e. deterioration
- e. devastation
- e. development
- e. development of children
- e. development ▸ social and
- e. disability
- e. disorder
- e. display ▸ lack of
- e. distance ▸ keeping
- e. distress
- e. distress, transient
- e. disturbance
- e. disturbances of adolescence ▸ mixed
- e. disturbances of childhood ▸ mixed
- e. downfall
- e. effects of pain
- e. effects ▸ psychological and
- e. etiology
- e. exhaustion
- e. experiences, hallucinatory
- e. explosiveness
- e. expression
- e. expression ▸ loss of
- e. expression ▸ positive
- e. factors
- e. factors ▸ physical or
- e. features ▸ adjustment disorder with mixed
- e. features ▸ adjustment reaction with mixed
- e. features, exaggerated
- e. features, mixed
- e. feeling tone
- e. first-aid
- e. freedom technique
- e. functioning
- e. gratification
- e. growth ▸ interference with intellectual and
- e. health
- e. illness

- e. imprinting
- e. insanity
- e. insecurity
- e. instability
- e. instability and impulsivity
- e. instability, episodic
- e. intimacy
- e. irritability
- e. lability
- e. lability, and irritability ▸ euphoria,
- e. lability, organic
- e. leveling
- e. maladaptation
- e. manipulator
- e. maturation
- e. maturity
- e. needs
- e. neglect
- e. numbing
- e. numbing and amnesia
- e. numbness
- e. -object amalgam
- e. or mixed origin ▸ organic,
- e. origin
- e. origin, illness of
- e. outbursts
- e. outbursts, patient experiences
- e. overactivity
- e. overinvolvement
- e. overlay
- e. pain
- e. paralysis
- e. perception
- e. phenomena
- e. pressure
- e. problem
- e. problems, exhibit
- e. process
- e. profile
- e. reaction
- e. reaction to crisis
- e. reactions ▸ modulate
- e. reactivity
- e. release
- e. release psychotherapy
- e. repression
- e. response
- e. response, appropriate
- e. responses ▸ suppress
- e. rigidity
- e. scars
- e. security
- e. serenity
- e. setback
- e. shift, mental-

- e. shock
- e. situation
- e. skills
- e., somatic support ▸ psychologic,
- e. speech difficulties
- e. stand-off
- e. state
- e. status, patient's
- e. stinginess
- e. strain
- e. stress
- e. stress and fatigue
- e. stress, intolerable
- e. stress on rigidity ▸ effect of
- e. stress on spasticity ▸ effect of
- e. stress, prolonged
- e. stress, severe
- e. stress, work-related
- e. suffering
- e. suffering, chronic
- e. support
- e. support during labor
- e. support ▸ physical and
- e. support to family
- e. support to patient
- e. swings
- e. symptoms
- e. tension
- e. trauma
- e. turmoil
- e. unresponsiveness
- e. upheaval
- e. upset
- e. vulnerability
- e. well-being
- e. withdrawal

emotionality, excessive
emotionally
- e. apathetic
- e. crippled
- e. deprived
- e. devastating
- e. disturbed (ED)
- e. drained
- e. -draining atmosphere
- e. exhausted
- e. ill, patient
- e. isolated
- e. maladjusted
- e. ▸ patient regresses
- e. related donor
- e. satisfied
- e. stable, patient
- e. stressful ▸ physically and
- e. unresponsive

e. unstable
e. unstable, patient
e. upset
e. vulnerable
emotive imagery
empathetic listening
empathic and attentive
empathy, biofeedback and
empathy ▸ lack of
emphysema
e., advanced
e., alveolar
e., alveolar duct
e., atrophic
e., bilateral
e., bilateral centrilobular
e., bullous
e., central acinar
e., centrilobular
e., cervical
e., chronic
e., chronic bronchitis with
e., chronic hypertrophic
e., chronic lobular
e. (COPE), chronic obstructive
   pulmonary
e., chronic pulmonary
e., compensatory
e., congenital
e., cystic
e., debilitating
e., diffuse
e., distal
e., ectatic
e. ▸ end-stage
e., false
e., focal
e. ▸ focal areas of
e., focal dust
e., gangrenous
e., generalized
e., glass blower's
e., hypertrophic
e., hypoplastic
e., idiopathic unilobar
e., infantile lobar
e., interlobular
e., interstitial
e., Jenner's
e., lobar
e., localized
e. ▸ localized obstructive
e., loculated
e. ▸ massive fibrinous pleuritis and
e., mediastinal

e. ▸ mild centri-acinar
e., obstructive
e., obstructive pulmonary
e. of conjunctiva
e. of lungs
e. of orbit
e., panacinar
e., panlobular
e., paracicatricial
e., paraseptal
e., predominant
e., pulmonary
e. (PIE), pulmonary interstitial
e., scar
e. secondary to heavy smoking
e., senile
e., small-lunged
e., subcutaneous
e., subfascial
e., subpleural
e., surgical
e., terminal
e., traumatic
e., unilateral
e., vesicular
emphysematosa
e., cervicocolpitis
e., cholecystitis
e., colpitis
emphysematous
e. alveoli
e., apex
e. asthma
e. bleb
e. blobs
e. bulla
e. changes
e. chest
e. cholecystitis
e. colpitis
e. cystitis
e. gallbladder
e. gangrene
e., lungs
e. vaginitis
empiric
e. antibiotic therapy
e. constant
e. therapy
e. therapy ▸ alternative
e. trial
empirical [*imperial*]
e. approach
e. basis
e. clinical placement ▸ rational/

e. studies
e. treatment
empirically, treat
empirically treated, patient
employed, patient gainfully
employee (Employee)
e. alcohol and drug treatment
   issues ▸ impaired
E. Assistance Program (EAP)
e. evaluation, initial
e. health coordinator
E. Health Department
e. health program
e. mental illness
employment
e. evaluation, pre-
e. examination
e. examination, pre-
e. physical, pre-
empowerment sessions ▸ family-
origin
emptied on voiding, bladder
emptied satisfactorily, colon
empties
e. normally, bladder
e. promptly, stomach
e. reflexively, bladder
emptiness
e. and boredom, chronic
e., chronic feelings of
e., chronic feelings of deep
emptive immunity, pre-
empty
e., feeling
e. ▸ feels hollow and
e. nest syndrome
e. ▸ patient feels
e. scrotal sac
e. sella syndrome
emptying
e., bladder
e. bladder, completely
e. cecum
e., early gastric
e., gastric
e. half-time, gastric
e., incomplete bladder
e. index ▸ left atrial
e., normal
e. of bladder, complete
e. of bladder, incomplete
e. of right atrium
e. of solids ▸ gastric
e. of stomach, partial
e., prompt

emptying—*continued*
  e. rate ▸ peak
  e. time
  e. time, gastric
empyema
  e., anaerobic
  e., benignum
  e., encapsulated
  e. fluid
  e., interlobar
  e., latent
  e., loculated
  e., metapneumonic
  e. necessitatis
  e. of chest
  e. of pericardium
  e., pleural
  e., pneumococcal
  e. ▸ postpneumonectomy
    tuberculous
  e., pulsating
  e., putrid
  e., sacculated
  e., streptococcal
  e., synpneumonic
  e., thoracic
  e. tube
  e., tuberculous
empyematic scoliosis
empyesis, tuberculous
EMS (electrical muscle stimulation)
EMS (emergency medical service)
EMS (eosinophilia myalgia syndrome)
EMT (Emergency Medical Technician)
emulgent vein
emulsification, fat
emulsion
  e. autoradiography, two-
  e., bacillary
  e., Bütschli's
  e., chylomicron
  e., fat
  e., hexachlorophene cleansing
  e. ▸ intravascular per fluoro-
    chemical
  e., kerosene
  e., liquid petrolatum
  e., mineral oil
  e., nuclear
  e., photographic
  e. proteinuria
  e., Pusey's

en
  en arceau, rhythm
  en bloc bilateral lung transplant
  en bloc dissection
  en bloc esophagectomy
  en bloc no touch technique
  en bloc resection
  en bloc vulvectomy
  en coin fracture
  en crochet, main
  en cuirasse, cancer
  en cuirasse, carcinoma
  en cuirasse, cor
  en dome, choc
  en face
  en face irradiation field
  en griffe, main
  en masse
  en rave, fracture
  en sabot, Coeur
  en salves ▸ tachycardia
ENA (extractable nuclear antibodies)
enable sobriety
enabling ideology
enamel
  e., curled
  e. cuticle
  e., defective
  e., dwarfed
  e. dysplasia syndrome ▸ dental
  e. germ
  e., gnarled
  e., hereditary brown
  e. hypocalcification
  e. hypoplasia
  e., hypoplasia, hereditary
  e., hypoplastic
  e., mottled
  e. rod sheath
  e., straight
  e. strand, lateral
enanthem (*same as* exanthem)
enarthrodial joint
encapsulated
  e. bacteria
  e. empyema
  e. gram-negative rods
  e. nodule
  e. organisms
  e. pleural fluid
  e. tumor
encased heart
encased in plaster
encasement, bony
encasing cell

encephali
  e., arachnoidea
  e., dura mater
  e., pia mater
encephalic
  e. angioma
  e. infant
  e. region
  e. vertigo
encephalitic behavior disorder ▸ post-
encephalitis
  e., acute disseminated
  e., acute necrotizing
  e., bacterial
  e., benign myalgic
  e., California
  e. ▸ chronic focal
  e., chronic subcortical
  e., clinical
  e., cortical
  e., Dawson's
  e. (EEE) ▸ eastern equine
  e., Economo's
  e., epidemic
  e. from coma
  e., hemorrhagic
  e., herpes simplex
  e. ▸ herpesvirus
  e., infantile
  e., influenzal
  e., Japanese B
  e., lethargic
  e., lethargica
  e., luetic
  e., measles
  e., meningo◊
  e., Murray Valley
  e. neonatorum
  e., polio◊
  e., postinfection
  e., postvaccinal
  e., postvaccination
  e., progressive
  e., purulent
  e., pyogenic
  e., Rasmussen's
  e., Rasmuten's
  e., Russian spring-summer
  e., Schilder's
  e., secondary
  e. siderans
  e., St. Louis
  e., Strümpell-Leichtenstern
  e., suppurative

e. ▸ tick-borne
e. (VEE) ▸ Venezuelan equine
e., viral
e. virus, California
e. (EEE) virus ▸ eastern equine
e. virus, Japanese B
e. virus, Murray Valley
e. virus, St. Louis
e. virus ▸ tick-borne
e. (WEE) virus ▸ western equine
e., West Nile
e. ▸ West Nile-like viral
e. (WEE) ▸ western equine
encephalitogenic factor
Encephalitozoon cuniculi
Encephalitozoon rabiei
encephaloarteriogram study
encephalogram, air
encephalogram (EEG), electro◊
encephalography, echo◊
encephaloid cancer
encephaloid carcinoma
encephalomalacia, avian
encephalomyelitis
e., acute disseminated
e., avian
e., benign myalgic
e. (EEE) ▸ eastern equine
e., equine
e., experimental allergic
e., granulomatous
e., infectious porcine
e., Mengo
e., mouse
e., murine
e., porcine
e., postinfectious
e., postvaccinal
e., sporadic bovine
e., Theiler's mouse
e., toxoplasmic
e. (VEE) ▸ Venezuelan equine
e., viral
e., virus
e. (EEE) virus ▸ eastern equine
e. virus, equine
e. virus ▸ murine
e. (VEE) virus ▸ Venezuelan equine
e. (WEE) ▸ western equine
encephalomyelopathy
e., infant necrotizing
e., postinfection
e., postvaccinal
e. with kernicterus
encephalomyocarditis (EMC) virus

encephalon
e., di◊
e., mes◊
e., ne◊
e., neo◊
e., pale◊
e., paleo◊
e., pros◊
e., rhin◊
e., rhomb◊
encephalopathy
e., alcoholic
e., biliary
e., bilirubin
e., bovine spongiform
e., corticostriatal
e., demyelinating
e., dialysis
e., diffuse
e., hemorrhagic
e., hepatic
e., hypercalcemic
e., hypernatremic
e., hypertensive
e., hypoglycemic
e. ▸ hypoxic ischemic
e., infantile myoclonus
e., lead
e., metabolic
e., mink
e. of childhood, myoclonic
e., portal-systemic
e., portasystemic
e., progressive dialysis
e., progressive subcortical
e., severe anoxic
e., spongiform
e., subacute spongiform
e., subcortical
e. symptoms, Wernicke's
e., toxic metabolic
e., transmissible spongiform virus
e., traumatic
e., Wernicke's
encephalorrhagia, pericapillary
encephalotrigeminal angiomatosis
enchondral bone formation ▸ inadequate
encircling
e. band
e. endocardial ventriculotomy
e. endocardial ventriculotomy ▸ partial
e. silicone tube

encoded cine-magnetic resonance imaging ▸ velocity
encoded velocity image ▸ phase
encoding ▸ respiratory ordered phase
encopresis, functional
encounter, therapeutic
encountered
e., considerable difficulty
e., excessive bleeding
e., resistance
encourage
e. communication
e. sense of responsibility
e. ventilation of feelings
encouragement of drug use
encouragement, verbal
encroachment
e., hypertrophic
e., luminal
e. of pterygium
e. on canal
e., tumor
encrustation theory of atherosclerosis
encrusted pyelitis
encrusted tongue
encysted
e. calculus
e. hernia
e. hydrocele
e. pleurisy
end(s) (End) [*and*]
e. airway pressure (PEAP), positive
e. anastomosis, end-to-
e. anastomosis, side-to-
e. bite, end-to-
e. -diastole
e. -diastolic area
e. -diastolic count
e. -diastolic diameter ▸ total
e. -diastolic dimension
e. -diastolic dimension ▸ left ventricular (LV)
e. -diastolic left ventricular (LV) pressure
e. -diastolic murmur
e. -diastolic pressure (EDP)
e. -diastolic pressure (LVEDP) ▸ left ventricular
e. -diastolic pressure (RVEDP) ▸ right ventricular
e. -diastolic velocity
e. -diastolic volume
e. -diastolic volume index

end(s)—*continued*
- e. -diastolic volume (LVEDV) ‣ left ventricular
- e. -diastolic volume (RVEDV) ‣ right ventricular
- e. -diastolic volume ‣ ventricular
- e., distal
- e. divided and separated
- e., eburnized bone
- e. -expiratory disease, positive
- e. -expiratory pause
- e. -expiratory pressure ‣ negative
- e. -expiratory pressure (PEEP), positive
- e. -expiratory pressure ‣ zero-
- e., fimbriated
- e. flap, double-
- e., fundal to cervical
- e. graft, double-
- e. ‣ hair-on-
- e. inspiratory crackles
- e. inspiratory pressure ‣ zero-
- e. occlusion ‣ end-to-
- e. of bone covered with flap
- e. of bone, cut
- e. -of-life care
- e. -of-life pacemaker
- e. of oviduct, fimbriated
- e. of stomach, anastomosis
- e. of stomach and duodenum ‣ closure open
- e. of stump, lower
- e. of tendon identified ‣ proximal
- e. of urination ‣ dribbling at
- e. -organ
- e. -organ damage
- e. -over-end running technique
- e. -plate
- e. -plate potential, miniature
- e. point
- e. -position nystagmus
- e. -pressure artifact
- e. product
- e. running technique ‣ end-over-
- e., severed nerve
- e. -stage
- e. -stage cancer
- e. -stage cardiac disease
- e. -stage cardiomyopathy
- e. -stage cardiopulmonary disease
- e. -stage emphysema
- e. -stage failure
- e. -stage heart and liver disease
- e. -stage heart failure
- e. -stage liver disease

- e. -stage liver failure
- e. -stage of disease
- e. -stage organ disease
- e. -stage renal disease (ESRD)
- E. -Stage Renal Disease (ESRD) Program
- e. -systole
- e. -systolic count
- e. -systolic diameter ‣ total
- e. -systolic dimension
- e. -systolic dimension ‣ left ventricular (LV)
- e. -systolic elastance
- e. -systolic force velocity indices
- e. -systolic ‣ left ventricular (LV)
- e. -systolic murmur
- e. -systolic pressure
- e. -systolic pressure volume relation
- e. -systolic pressure volume relation ‣ ventricular
- e. -systolic stress dimension relation
- e. -systolic stress ‣ left ventricular
- e. -systolic volume
- e. -systolic volume index
- e. -systolic volume, ventricular
- e. -tidal
- e. -tidal carbon dioxide (ETCO$_2$)
- e. -to-end anastomosis
- e. -to-end bite
- e. -to-end ileal colostomy ‣ resected
- e. -to-end occlusion
- e. -to-side
- e. -to-side anastomosis
- e. -to-side colostomy
- e. -to-side ileotransverse colostomy
- e. -to-side suture
- e. -to-side vein bypass
- e. tube
- e. vena caval shunt ‣ Marion-Clatworthy side-to-

Endamoeba blattae
endangerment ‣ physical self-
endaortitis, bacterial
endarterectomy
- e. and coronary artery bypass grafting
- e., blunt eversion carotid
- e., carotid artery
- e., coronary
- e., femoral
- e., gas◊
- e., iliac

- e. in peripheral vessels
- e., left carotid
- e. loop, Cannon's
- e. ‣ perforation in
- e., right carotid
- e. shunt ‣ Sundt carotid
- e. ‣ transluminal extraction

endarteritis
- e., cerebrospinal
- e. deformans
- e., Heubner's specific
- e. obliterans
- e. proliferans
- e., syphilitic

endarteropathy, digital
endaural incision, Shambaugh
ended amplifier, single-
ended support group, open
endemic
- e. fluorosis, chronic
- e. fungal infection
- e. goiter
- e. hematuria
- e. hemoptysis
- e. hospital organisms
- e. influenza

endemica, urticaria multiformis
endemicum, granuloma
endemicus, Clonorchis
ending(s)
- e. life ‣ patient thinks about
- e. life ‣ thinks about
- e., motor
- e., nerve
- e., peripheral nerve
- e., sensory nerve
- e., severed nerve
- e., skin nerve
- e. ‣ stimulation of nerve
- e., truncated nerve

endless
- e. alters ‣ endless memories
- e. loop tachycardia
- e. memories ‣ endless alters
- e. ruminations

endoaneurysmorrhaphy ‣ ventricular
endobronchial
- e. anesthesia
- e. brush biopsy
- e. malignancy
- e. round cell accumulation
- e. tree
- e. tree, distortion
- e. tree, left
- e. tree, right

e. tube
e. tube, double lumen
e. tumor

endocardial
e. balloon lead
e. bipolar pacemaker
e. cushion defects
e. cushion formation
e. electrode ▸ implantable unipolar
e. fibroelastosis
e. fibrosis
e. flow
e. lead system ▸ Medtronic Transvene
e. lesion ▸ nonbacterial thrombotic
e. mapping
e. murmur
e. plaques
e. pressure
e. resection
e. sclerosis
e. stain
e. thickening
e. tube
e. tumor
e. vegetation
e. ventriculotomy ▸ encircling
e. ventriculotomy ▸ partial encircling

endocarditis
e., abacterial thrombotic
e., acute
e. (ABE) ▸ acute bacterial
e. (AIE), acute infective
e. and flossing
e., atypical verrucous
e., bacteria-free stage of bacterial
e. (BE), bacterial
e. benigna
e., cachectic
e. chordalis
e., chronic
e., constrictive
e., culture negative
e., enterococcal
e. ▸ experimental enterococcal
e., fungal
e., gonococcal
e. ▸ green strep
e., Haemophilus
e. in drug addict ▸ tricuspid
e., infectious
e., infective
e. ▸ isolated parietal
e. lenta

e., Libman-Sacks
e., Löffler's parietal fibroplastic
e., malignant
e., marantic
e. ▸ mitral valve
e., mural
e., mycotic
e., nonbacterial thrombotic
e., nonbacterial verrucous
e., nosocomial
e., parietal
e. parietalis fibroplastica
e., plastic
e., polypous
e. prophylaxis
e. (SBE) prophylaxis ▸ subacute bacterial
e., prosthetic valve
e., pulmonic
e., pustulous
e., rheumatic
e., rickettsial
e., right-sided
e., septic
e., staphylococcal
e., streptococcal
e. (SBE) ▸ subacute bacterial
e. ▸ subacute infective
e., syphilitic
e., terminal
e., thrombotic
e., tuberculous
e., ulcerative
e., valvular
e., vegetative
e., verrucous
e., viridans

endocardium
e., infection of
e., mural
e., overlying mural
e. smooth, mural

endocavitary radiation therapy
endocellular complement
endocervical
e. canal
e. canal cautery
e. canal, secondary puncture wounds
e. carcinoma
e. cell
e. cell segregation, ecto/
e. cell yield
e. columnar mucosa
e. culture

e. curettage
e. glands
e. mucosa
e. Pap (Papanicolaou) smears ▸ Richart and VCE—vaginal, cervical and
e. (VCE) Pap (Papanicolaou) smears ▸ vaginal, cervical and
e. (VCE) Papanicolaou (Pap) smears ▸ Richart and vaginal, cervical,
e. polyp
e. polypectomy
e. (VCE) smear ▸ vaginal, cervical,

endocervicitis, chronic
endochondral bone
endochondral bone deposits
endochondroma, tibia
endocrine
e. abnormalities (MEA), multiple
e. abnormality
e. adenomatosis (MEA), multiple
e. adenopathies (MEA), multiple
e. atrophy
e. cardiopathy
e. cells ▸ pulmonary
e. disease, diabetes mellitus (DM) secondary to
e. disorder
e. emergency
e. failure
e. fracture
e. function
e. function, alteration in
e. gland
e. hormone
e. imbalance
e. inactive pituitary tumor
e. neoplasia (MEN), multiple
e. neoplasia syndrome
e. neoplasia syndromes, multiple
e. organ, atrophy of
e. organs
e. process
e. symptoms
e. system
e. therapy

endocrinologic complications of drug abuse
endocrinologic problems related to drug abuse
endocrinologist, pediatric
endocrinologist, reproductive
endocrinology, reproductive

endodermal
- e. cyst
- e. sinus tumor
- e. sinus tumor, ovarian

endodontic implant

endodontic treatment

endoergic reaction

endoesophageal magnetic resonance imaging (EEMRI) coil

endogenous
- e. anastomosis
- e. antigen
- e. anxiety
- e. bacteria
- e. biotin activity
- e. creatinine
- e. cycle
- e. depression
- e. estrogen
- e. factors
- e. fecal calcium
- e. flora
- e. group
- e. hyperlipidemia
- e. hypothermia
- e. infection
- e. interferon
- e. lipid
- e. obesity
- e. pathogens, activation of
- e. peroxidase activity
- e. retrovirus (PERV) ▸ porcine
- e. sporulation
- e. toxins

endograft exclusion of aneurysm

endolaryngeal brachytherapy mold

endolaryngeal lesion

Endolimax nana

endolumen enlargement

endoluminal
- e. graft, Cragg
- e. paving stent ▸ polymeric
- e. prosthesis
- e. radiation therapy
- e. stenting

endolymph filtration and excretion

endolymph fluid

endolymphatic
- e. duct
- e. hydrops
- e. pressure
- e. sac
- e. shunt tube, Teflon
- e. -subarachnoid shunt

endolymphaticus, aquaeductus

endometrial
- e. ablation
- e. ablation ▸ hysteroscopy and
- e. adenocarcinoma
- e. apoplexy
- e. atrophy
- e. biopsy
- e. biopsy, positive
- e. cancer
- e. carcinoma
- e. carcinoma, hormonal therapy in
- e. carcinoma, metastatic
- e. carcinoma, myometrial invasion in
- e. carcinoma, peritoneal seeding in
- e. cavity
- e. cavity sounded
- e. cell
- e. cells, atypical
- e. curettage
- e. cycle
- e. cyst
- e. glands
- e. hyperplasia
- e. hyperplasia, benign cystic
- e. implant
- e. islands
- e. lining
- e. polypi
- e. polyps
- e. secretory adenocarcinoma
- e. sloughing
- e. stromal sarcoma, metastatic
- e. tissue
- e. tissue ▸ aberrant
- e. tissue, eosinophilic
- e. tissue, fragments of
- e. tissue ▸ vagrant
- e. tumor

endometrioides ovarii, adenoma

endometriosis
- e. associated infertility
- e., chronic
- e. externa
- e. interna
- e. of colon
- e., ovarian
- e. ovarii
- e., pelvic
- e. syndrome ▸ thoracic
- e., undiagnosed
- e. uterina
- e. vesicae

endometriotic implant

endometritis
- e., bacteriotoxic
- e., decidual
- e. dissecans
- e., exfoliative
- e., glandular
- e., hyperplastic
- e., membranous
- e., nosocomial postpartum
- e., postpartum
- e., postradiation
- e., puerperal
- e., secretory
- e., syncytial
- e., tuberculous
- e. tuberosa papulosa

endometrium
- e., carcinoma of
- e., early secretory
- e., hyperplastic
- e., proliferative
- e., proliferative phase
- e., secretory phase
- e., Swiss-cheese

Endomyces
- E. albicans
- E. capsulatus
- E. epidermatidis
- E. epidermidis

endomyocardial
- e. biopsy
- e. disease, eosinophilic
- e. fibroelastosis
- e. fibrosis
- e. fibrosis, African
- e. fibrosis, biventricular
- e. fibrosis, Davies
- e. fibrosis ▸ tropical

endonuclease, restriction

endoperoxide steal

endophlebitis of retinal veins

endophlebitis, proliferative

endophytic parasite

endophytum, glioma

endoplasmic
- e. reticulum
- e. reticulum, rough
- e. reticulum, smooth

endoprosthesis plugged

endoprosthetic arthroplasty ▸ Austin-Moore

endoprosthetic femoral head replacement

endorphin
- e. activity, beta

e., beta
e. level
endoscope ▸ lung imaging fluorescence
endoscopic
e. approach ▸ retrograde
e. biliary decompression
e. biopsy
e. cholangiogram
e. coronary artery bypass (TECAB) ▸ total
e. diagnosis
e. echocardiography
e. examination
e. examination of bronchus
e. gastrostomy (PEG) ▸ percutaneous
e. intubation
e. intubation, catheter-guided
e. manipulation
e. palliation
e. papillotomy
e. plastic surgery
e. procedure
e. procedure, therapeutic
e. retrograde cholangiogram
e. retrograde cholangiopancreatography (ERCP)
e. retrograde pancreatography
e. sclerosis
e. sclerosis of bleeding esophageal varices
e. sclerotherapy, acute
e. sinus surgery
e. sinus surgery (FESS) ▸ functional
e. sphincterotomy
e. study
e. surgery
e. technique, therapeutic
e. ultrasonography
e. ultrasound (EUS)
e. vein harvesting
e. vein surgery
endoscopically assisted duodenal intubation
endoscopy
e. capsule, wireless
e., carpal tunnel
e., emergency
e. examination
e. for blood in feces
e., gastrointestinal
e. instrumentation

e., nasal
e., pelvic
e., sinus
e., therapeutic
endosmotic equivalent
endospores, bacterial
endosseous implant
endosteal implant
endosurgery procedure
endothelial
e. barrier
e. cancer
e. cells
e. cells, atrioventricular (AV)
e. cells, cardiac
e. cells ▸ human aortic
e. cells ▸ immature
e. cells ▸ inner layer of
e. denudation
e. dysfunction
e. dystrophy
e. dystrophy of comea
e. growth factor (VEGF) therapy▸ vascular
e. growth factor (VEGF) ▸ vascular
e. injury ▸ neutrophil-mediated
e. layer ▸ cornea's
e. leukocyte adhesion molecule (ELAM)
e. lining
e. localization of antigen
e. tissue
e. transformation process
endothelin concentration ▸ plasma
endothelin ▸ elevated levels of
endothelioblastoma, lymphangio◊
endotheliochorial placenta
endothelioid habit
endothelioma
e., dural
e., hemangio◊
e., lymphangio◊
e., reticulo◊
e., Sidler-Huguenin's
endothelium
e., corneal
e. -derived hyperpolarizing factor
e. -derived relaxing factor
e. -mediated relaxation
e., pulmonary
e., venous
endothrix, Trichophyton
endotoxic shock

endotracheal
e. anesthesia
e. aspirate
e. -bronchial suctioning
e. general anesthesia
e. insufflation
e. intubation
e. suctioning
e. tube
e. tube, cuffed
e. tube in place
e. tube malplacement
e. tumor
endovaginal sonography
endovaginal ultrasound
endovascular
e. repair
e. surgery
e. treatment
e. ultrasonography ▸ intracaval
endoventricular circular patch plasty
endowment, genetic
endplate abnormality ▸ vertebral
endplates, vertebral
endpoint, therapeutic
endurance
e. activities
e., anaerobic
e. and flexibility ▸ strength,
e., cardiorespiratory
e., cardiovascular
e. deteriorated, patient's
e. exercises
e. exercises ▸ muscular
e. exercises ▸ power and
e. fitness
e., muscle
e. muscle strength and
e., muscular
e., patient's tolerance and
e. ▸ physical strength and
e., stamina and
e., strength, balance and flexibility
e. training
enduring bitterness ▸ displays
enema
e., analeptic
e. (BE), barium
e., blind
e., cleansing
e., contrast
e., double contrast
e. ▸ double contrast barium
e. examination, barium
e., flatus

enema—*continued*
- e., Fleet
- e., inject
- e., normal saline (N/S)
- e., nutrient
- e., nutritive
- e., opaque
- e., pancreatic
- e., patient given
- e., preoperative
- e. prior to delivery ▸ patient given
- e. prior to examination ▸ patient given
- e. prior to surgery ▸ patient given
- e. prior to x-ray ▸ patient given
- e., rectal
- e. set, disposable cleansing
- e. (SSE), soapsuds
- e., thirst
- e., turpentine

energizer, psychic

energy (Energy) [*anergy*]
- e. absorption ▸ laser
- e. accelerator, high
- e. accelerators ▸ dual photon
- e. /alertness, increased
- e., anaerobic derived
- e., atomic
- e., atomic binding
- e. behavior ▸ high
- e. bent beam linear accelerator, high
- e., binding
- e., biologic
- e., biotic
- e. ▸ burst of boundless
- e. cardioversion, high
- e. cardioversion, low
- e., chemical
- e., color Doppler
- E. Commission (AEC), Atomic
- e. conservation
- e., continuous flow of
- e. converter
- e., decreased
- e., decreased appetite and increased
- e., depleted
- e. direct current ▸ low
- e., electrical
- e., electromagnetic
- e. electrons, high
- e. equivalence, mass
- e. ▸ fatigue or loss of
- e. ▸ fatigue, weakness, and decreased
- e. field, electromagnetic
- e. for muscle activity
- e., free
- e. frequency
- e., high quantum
- e., improved
- e., kinetic
- e., lack of
- e., laser
- e., laser ▸ low
- e., level
- e. level, decrease in
- e. level, low
- e. level ▸ markedly increased
- e. level ▸ psychic
- e. linear accelerator ▸ dual
- e. linear accelerator ▸ low
- e. ▸ loss of
- e., magnetic
- e., mean incident
- e., mental
- e. metabolism ▸ abnormal
- e., mood changes, apathy, loss of
- e., nervous
- e., nuclear
- e. of position
- e. or fatigue ▸ decrease in
- e. pathways
- e., patient has low
- e., photon
- e., physical
- e., potential
- e. production
- e. production ▸ depress cellular
- e. pulsed ruby laser ▸ high
- e., radiant
- e. radiation, high
- e., radiofrequency
- e. radiopharmaceutical, high
- e., release of
- e. resolution
- e., resting
- e., spiritual
- e. straight beam linear accelerator, low
- e. supply
- e. swings, mood and
- e. synchronized cardioversion ▸ low
- e., thermal
- e., threshold
- e. transfer (LET), linear
- e. transfer radiation, high linear
- e. transthoracic shock ▸ high
- e. ▸ units of magnetic
- e. use in brain
- e. value of food
- e., vital
- e. wave-length
- e. x-ray absorptiometry (DEXA) bone density test, dual
- e. x-ray absorptiometry (DEXA) ▸ dual
- e. x-ray therapy, combination high and low
- e. x-rays ▸ high

enforced inactivity ▸ period of

Enforcement Agency, Drug (DEA)

enforcement, alcohol

ENG (electronystagmograph)

ENG (electronystagmographic) recording

engaged in antisocial behavior

engaged in mental activity ▸ subject

engagement at term

engagement ▸ initial ease of

Engel-Lysholm maneuver

Engelmann syndrome ▸ Camurati-Engelmann's disc

engine
- e., dental
- e., high-speed
- e., surgical
- e., ultraspeed

engineered
- e. proteins ▸ genetically
- e. tissues ▸ biologically
- e. vaccine ▸ genetically
- e. virus ▸ genetically

engineering (Engineering)
- E. and Maintenance
- e., genetic
- e. ▸ stem cell
- e. techniques, genetic

English cane

English rhinoplasty

engorged blood vessels

engorged, vasculature

engorgement
- e., breast
- e., capillary
- e., liver
- e., neck vein
- e. of pulmonary vessels
- e. of veins
- e. of vessels
- e., retinal vein
- e., vascular
- e., venous

e., venule

engrafting, marrow

enhance
- e. aerobic fitness
- e. breast size
- e. contraction
- e. emergency care
- e. health and fitness
- e. lesions
- e. memory ▸ repetition
- e. muscle tone
- e. quality of life
- e. self-esteem
- e. sound
- e. sperm production
- e. treatment

enhanced
- e. accuracy
- e. automaticity
- e. care
- e. carotid magnetic resonance angiography (carotid MRA) ▸ contrast
- e. CAT (computerized axial tomography) scan
- e. computed tomography ▸ xenon
- e. echocardiogram, contrast
- e. external counterpulsation (EECP)
- e. external counterpulsation (EECP) therapy
- e. external counterpulsation (EECP) unit
- e. hypothrombinemic effect
- e. intellectual efficiency
- e. interest and concentration
- e. metabolic efficiency
- e. MRI (magnetic resonance imaging) scan
- e. muscle dysfunction
- e. quality of life
- e. recall
- e. scan
- e. sensitivity
- e. sensitivity to stress
- e. sensory awareness
- e. sociability
- e. somatosensory perceptions
- e. view, color
- e. vision

enhancement
- e., allograft survival
- e., areas of
- e., breast
- E. (CSE), Coping Strategy

- e., cosmetic
- e., domestic
- e. (RE) family therapy ▸ relationship
- e., labor
- e. ▸ leading edge
- e. ▸ mean contrast
- e. of MRI (magnetic resonance imaging)
- e., performance
- e. ▸ permanent lip
- e. ratio, oxygen (O_2)
- e. ratio, sensitizer
- e. scan ▸ computer
- e. surgery, breast
- e. therapy (MET) ▸ motivational
- e. (RE) therapy ▸ relationship

enhancer(s)
- e., absorption
- e. molecules
- e., taste

enhancing
- e. activity ▸ mast cell
- e. and pain relieving ▸ sleep-
- e. drug ▸ mood-
- e. effect ▸ mood-
- e. lesion
- e. normal breathing
- e. poor vision
- e. self-efficacy
- e. self-esteem
- e. social skills ▸ group exercises for
- e. traits ▸ health
- e. weight loss

enlarged
- e., adenoids appear
- e., adenoids do not appear
- e. air sacs
- e. and congested ▸ spleen
- e. atypical histiocyte
- e. bronchial tubes
- e. fatty liver
- e., fibroid of uterus does not appear
- e. fontanelles
- e., heart
- e., heart does appear
- e., heart does not appear
- e. heart muscle
- e., incision
- e., inflamed prostate gland
- e. left ventricle (LV)
- e., liver
- e., liver does appear
- e., liver does not appear
- e., liver not

- e., liver not palpably
- e., lump in left breast does appear
- e., lump in left breast does not appear
- e., lump in right breast does appear
- e., lump in right breast does not appear
- e. lymph glands
- e. lymph node
- e., markedly
- e. mass
- e. periaortic nodes
- e., prostate
- e. prostate gland
- e. prostate gland ▸ shrink
- e. retromandibular node
- e. Schwann cells
- e. septum
- e., spleen does appear
- e., spleen does not appear
- e., spleen not palpably
- e. subarachnoid space
- e., tender liver
- e. thyroid
- e. thyroid ▸ diffusely
- e., thyroid does appear
- e., thyroid does not appear
- e. tonsils
- e., tonsils appear
- e., tonsils do not appear
- e. turbinate
- e., uterus
- e., uterus does appear
- e., uterus does not appear

enlargement
- e., abnormal arterial
- e. ▸ acute spleen
- e., adenoidal
- e., atrial
- e., augmentation or
- e., biatrial
- e., bony
- e., breast
- e. (CE), cardiac
- e., chamber
- e., compensatory vessel
- e., congestive
- e., cosmetic
- e., cystic
- e., diffuse
- e., diffuse symmetrical uterine
- e. ▸ dorsocervical fat pad
- e., endolumen
- e., fingertip
- e., gingival

enlargement—*continued*
- e., glandular
- e., heart
- e. ▸ hereditary hypertrophic
- e., hypertrophic
- e. (LAE), left atrial
- e. (LVE) ▸ left ventricular
- e., liver
- e., lobe
- e., lymph node
- e. ▸ male breast
- e. (CE) ▸ massive cardiac
- e., mitochondrial
- e. of aorta
- e. of ascending aorta, patch
- e. of cardiac chamber
- e. of head, excessive
- e. of heart
- e. of kidney, cystiform
- e. of lens
- e. of liver
- e. of lymphadenoid tissue
- e. of periaortic lymph nodes
- e. of prostate gland ▸ noncancerous
- e. of sella turcica
- e., panchamber
- e., parotid
- e., progressive
- e., prostate
- e., prostatic
- e., relax prostate
- e., residual
- e., residual axillary lymph node
- e. (RAE), right atrial
- e. (RVE) ▸ right ventricular
- e., spleen
- e., symptomatic
- e., thrill or murmur
- e., tonsillar
- e., uterine
- e., venous
- e., ventricular

enlightenment, neurophysiology of
enophthalmos/enophthalmus
enough, biopsy not deep
enraged patient
enriched marrow
enrichment, spiritual
Enriquez operation ▸ Lopez-
ensheathing callus
ensiform appendix
ensiform cartilage
ensure proper flow of blood

ENT
- ENT (ears, nose and throat)
- ENT (ear, nose and throat) emergency
- ENT (ear, nose and throat) trauma

Entamoeba
- E. buccalis
- E. bütschlii
- E. coli
- E. gingivalis
- E. hartmanni
- E. histolytica
- E. kartulisi
- E. nana
- E. nipponica
- E. tetragena
- E. tropicalis
- E. undulans

entangling technique
entendu, déjà
enteral
- e. diarrhea
- e. feeding
- e. nutrition

entered
- e., abdomen
- e. and explored, abdomen
- e. peritoneum
- e., pleural cavity
- e., retroperitoneal space
- e. with cutting bur ▸ cortex
- e. with keratome ▸ anterior chamber

enteric (Enteric)
- e. anastomosis
- e. anastomosis, biliary
- e. bacilli, gram-negative
- e. bacilli ▸ gram's stain negative
- e. bacteria
- e. -coated
- e. -coated aspirin
- e. -coated tablet
- e. cyst
- e. cytopathic bovine orphan (ECBO) virus
- e. cytopathic human orphan (ECHO) virus
- e. cytopathic monkey orphan (ECMO) virus
- e. cytopathic swine orphan (ECSO) virus
- e. fever
- e. fistula
- e. gram-negative bacilli
- e., human

- e. infection
- e. infectious precaution
- E. Isolation
- e. nervous system
- e. orphan viruses
- e. pathogen
- e. plexus
- e. precautions
- e. secretions
- e. type of isolation
- e. virus

entering chest cavity
enteritidis
- e., Bacillus
- e., gram-negative Salmonella
- e. group, paratyphoid-
- e., Salmonella

enteritis
- e., bacterial
- e., Campylobacter
- e. choleriform
- e., cicatrizing
- e. cystica chronica
- e., granulomatous
- e. gravis
- e., myxomembranous
- e. necroticans
- e. nodularis
- e., pellicular
- e., phlegmonous
- e. polyposa
- e., protozoan
- e., pseudomembranous
- e., regional
- e., segmental
- e., shigella
- e., staphylococcal
- e., streptococcus
- e., typhlo◊
- e., viral

enteroanastomosis, gastro◊
Enterobacter
- E. aerogenes
- E. agglomerans
- E. alvei
- E. bacteremia
- E. cloacae
- E. erwinieae
- E. gergoviae
- E. glomerans
- E. hafniae
- E. infection
- E., Klebsiella-
- E. liquefaciens
- E. sakazakii

E. species
Enterobius vermicularis
enterococcal
   e. endocarditis
   e. endocarditis ▸ experimental
   e. food poisoning
   e. infection
   E. infection of heart
   e. urinary tract infection
enterococci, peritonitis due to
Enterococcus (enterococcus)
   E. faecalis
   E. faecalis strains
   e. microorganism
enterocolic fistula
enterocolic, gastro◊
enterocolitica colitis ▸ Yersinia
enterocolitica, Yersinia
enterocolitis
   e., antibiotic-associated
   e., gastro◊
   e., hemorrhagic
   e., necrotizing
   e., pseudomembranous
   e., radiation
   e., regional
   e., staphylococcal
enterocolostomy, gastro◊
enterocutaneous fistula
enterocytopathogenic human orphan
   (ECHO)
enteroenteric fistula
enterogastric reflex
enterogenic albumosuria
enterogenic proteinuria
enterohepatic circulation
enteromesenteric occlusion
Enteromonas hominis
enteromycosis bacteriacea
enteronitis, polytropous
enteropathic E. (Escherichia) coli
enteropathica, acrodermatitis
enteropathogenic Escherichia (E.)
   coli
enteropathy
   e., exudative
   e., gluten
   e., gluten sensitivity
   e., protein-losing
enteroplasty, gastro◊
enteroptosis, gastro◊
enterorrhaphy, circular
enterostomal therapist
enterostomal therapy

enterostomy
   e., cholangio◊
   e., choledocho◊
   e., electro◊
   e., entero◊
   e., esophago◊
   e., gun-barrel
   e., percutaneous
enterotome, Dupuytren's
enterotomy, gastro◊
enteroviral disease
enteroviral meningitis
enterovirus, atypical
enterovirus, nonpolio
entire limb anesthetized
entire lower limb, amputation
entitlement ▸ problem derived from
entity(-ies)
   e., clinical
   e., diagnostic
   e., histopathologic
   e., noninfectious
entocuneiform bone
entoderm, primitive
entoderm, yolk-sac
entodermal lining
Entomophthora coronata
Entomophthora muscae
entomophthorae, phycomycosis
entoptic pulse
entorbital fissure
entozoic parasite
entrained air
entrained air and particulates
entrainment
   e., concealed
   e., epicardial
   e. of tachycardia
   e. with concealed fusion
entrance
   e. block
   e. complaint
   e. diagnosis
   e. of fetal head into superior pelvic
     strait
   e. physical examination
   e., wound
entrant mechanism, re-
entrapment
   e., median nerve
   e., nerve
   e., ulnar nerve
entrapped
   e. anterior pituitary cells
   e. cells

   e. nerve
entropion [*ectropion*]
entropion/entropium
entropion, spastic
entropy wheel
entry
   e. access ▸ side-
   e., air
   e., port of
   e. site
   e. site, arterial
   e., vein
   e. zone (DREZ) lesion, dorsal root
enucleated [*nucleated*]
enucleated, follicular membranes
enucleation
   e. of cyst
   e. of eye
   e. of eyeball
   e. of subaortic stenosis
   e., radical
   e. scissors
enuresis [*anuresis*]
   e., childhood
   e., diurnal
   e., functional
   e., maturational
   e., nocturnal
   e., persistent
   e., primary nocturnal
enuretic [*anuretic*]
enuretic, patient
envelope
   e., aortic
   e., cell
   e., egg
   e. flap
   e., flow
   e., nuclear
   e. of tissue
   e., spectral
environment
   e., adaptation to
   e., adjustment
   e., adoptive family
   e. and lifestyle
   e., bacteria-free
   e., barrier against
   e., caring
   e., challenges of
   e., cognitive
   e., cold
   e., daily living
   e., drug-free
   e., drug-seeking

environment—*continued*
- e., early family
- e., electromagnetic
- e., extrauterine
- e., germ-free
- e., home
- e., home care support
- e., hospital
- e., hot
- e., impoverished
- e., intellectual
- e., intrauterine
- e., living
- e., locked
- e., loss of contact with
- e., low-stimulus
- e., medical
- e. ▸ medication and modification of behavior and
- e., microchemical
- e., natural
- e., nonthreatening
- e., normal stimulus
- e. of coercive control
- e., patient's home
- e., patient's social
- e., peer
- e. ▸ perception of
- e., physical work
- e. ▸ post-treatment
- e., rehabilitation
- e., restrictive
- e., semi-structured
- e. ▸ severely contaminated
- e., sheltered
- e., sleep
- e., smoke-free
- e., social
- e., sociocultural
- e., sterile
- e., stimulating
- e., strange
- e. ▸ stress-free
- e., stressful
- e. ▸ structure drug free
- e., structured
- e., supportive
- e. ▸ supportive care
- e., therapeutic
- e., thermoneutral
- e., toxic
- e., toxin-filled
- e., uterine
- e., ward

environmental (Environmental)
- e. allergen
- e. allergies
- e. barriers
- e. change
- e. cigarette smoke
- e. circumstances ▸ sensitive to
- e. conditions
- e. control
- E. Control Officer (ECO)
- E. Control Unit (ECU)
- e. culture
- e. culturing
- e. decontamination
- e. effects
- e. emergency
- e. estrogens
- e. factor
- e. habituation
- e. hazards
- e. health
- e. heat injury
- e. illness (EI)
- e. influence
- e. irritants
- e. irritation
- e. lung disease
- e. management
- e. manipulation
- e. medical emergency
- e. medicine
- e. modification
- e. monitoring
- e. noise
- E. Officer (EO)
- e. pollution
- e. risks
- e. staphylococcal contamination
- e. stimulation, restricted
- E. Stimulation Therapy (REST) ▸ Reduced
- e. stimuli
- e. stress
- e. surface, culturing of
- e. surface, nonsterile
- e. surveillance
- E. Surveillance Nurse (ESN)
- E. Surveillance Officer (ESO)
- e. survey
- e. technique, restricted
- e. therapy
- e. tobacco smoke (ETS)
- e. toxin
- e. triggers
- e. vector transmission

- e. waste disposal

envy, admiration and
envy, chronic intense
en-Y
- e. bypass ▸ Roux-
- e. cystojejunostomy ▸ Roux-
- e. ▸ Roux-

enzymatic
- e. abnormality of adrenal gland
- e. abnormality of ovaries
- e. activity
- e. debridement
- e. debridement technique
- e. decortication
- e. deficiency
- e. imbalance
- e. organ damage
- e. reaction
- e. synthesis
- e. zonulolysis

enzyme(s)
- e., abnormal liver
- e., acetylating
- e. activity
- e., adaptive
- e., adenylylating
- e., altered metabolizing
- e. (ACE), angiotensin converting
- e., antibiotic destroying
- e. aromatase
- e., artificial
- e. assays, erythrocyte
- e. balance
- e., cancer-dependent
- e., carbohydrase
- e., cardiac
- e., cardial
- e. changes
- e., coagulase
- e., critical
- e., cross-linking
- e. deficiencies
- e. deficiency anemia
- e., digestive
- e., elevated
- e. elevations ▸ liver
- e. glaucoma
- e., glycolytic
- e., hepatic
- e., hepatocellular
- e. imbalance of
- e. immunoassay (EIA)
- e. immunoassay ▸ nifedipine
- e., inactivating by substitution
- e. inhibitor

e. (ACE) inhibitor ▸ angiotensin converting
e. inhibitor, converting
e., initial cardiac
e. insensitive to inhibitor ▸ target
e., lactase
e., leakage
e. level
e. level ▸ cardiac
e. level, serum
e. linked immunosorbent assay (ELISA) ▸ sandwich
e. linked immunosorbent assay (ELISA) test
e., liver
e. measurements, traditional
e. ▸ microsomal drug metabolizing
e., missing
e., mitochondrial
e., modification of target
e. ▸ natural digestive
e. neutralization
e., normal substrate of
e. ointment
e., oral
e., pancreas
e., pancreatic
e., phosphorylating
e. profile, chemical
e., proteolytic
e. reactions
e., receptor destroying
e. replacement
e., restriction
e. rise
e. -secreting capacity
e. solution
e., stomach
e. studies, hepatic
e. study
e. study ▸ serum
e. supplement
e. synthesis, inducible
e. system
e., target
e. test, serum
e., testosterone synthesizing
e., thrombolytic
e., transaminase
e. units
e. values ▸ liver
enzymicum, Corynebacterium
EOB (explanation of benefits)
EOG (electro-oculogram)
EOG (electro-oculogram) apparatus

EOM (extraocular movements)
EOMI (extraocular movements intact)
eosin
e., hematoxylin and
e. methylene blue
e. methylene blue agar
eosinophil(s) (eosinophile)
e. cationic protein
e., chemotactic activity of
e., degranulation of
eosinophilia
e., Löffler's
e. myalgia syndrome (EMS)
e., peripheral
e. ▸ peripheral blood
e. (PIE), pulmonary infiltration and
e. ▸ tropical pulmonary
eosinophilic
e. adenoma
e. chemotaxis
e. cytoplasm
e. cytoplasm, granular
e. cytoplasm ▸ neurons with
e. dense cytoplasm
e. endometrial tissue
e. endomyocardial disease
e. erythroblast
e. esophagitis
e. gastroenteritis
e. granuloma
e. granuloma, Mignon's
e. granuloma of lung (EGL)
e. granulomatous vasculitis
e. hyperpituitarism
e. infiltrates ▸ perivascular
e. leukemia
e. leukocyte
e. leukocytosis
e. lung
e. material, granular
e. meningitis
e. myalgia
e. myelocyte
e. normoblast
e. pneumonia
e. pneumonia, chronic
e. pneumonia ▸ idiopathic acute
e. pneumonia ▸ primary
e. pneumonitis
e. pneumonopathy
e. pulmonary syndrome
EP (evoked potential)
epactal bones
EPCA (external pressure circulatory assist)

ependymal cells
ependymal glioma
ependymitis granularis
Ephedra
E. equisetina
E. sinica
E. vulgaris
ephemeral fever
ephemeral pneumonia
epiarterial bronchus
epibronchial right pulmonary artery syndrome
epibulbar carcinoma
epic microscope
epicanthal fold
epicanthic fold
epicanthus with telecanthus deformity
epicardial
e. activation
e. coronary artery
e. defibrillator patch
e. echocardiography ▸ high frequency
e. electrode
e. electrode ▸ stab-in
e. entrainment
e. fat
e. fat tag
e. flow
e. lead
e. lead ▸ three-turn
e. lead ▸ two-turn
e. pacemaker
e. pacing electrode, temporary
e. pacing lead, barbed
e. poudrage, Beck
e. surface
e. vessel patency
epicardium ▸ petechial hemorrhages of
Epicauta
E. cinerea
E. pennsylvanica
E. sapphirina
E. tormentosa
E. vittata
epicondyle, lateral
epicondyle, medial
epicondylitis
e., external human
e., lateral
e., medial
epicranial muscle
epicritic sensibility

epidemic
- e., acquired immune deficiency syndrome (AIDS)
- e. capillary bronchitis
- e. catarrhal fever
- e. cerebrospinal meningitis
- e. cholera
- e. chorea
- e. clusters
- e., cocaine
- e. conjunctivitis
- e., crack cocaine
- e. diarrhea of newborn
- e. disease
- e. dysentery
- e. encephalitis
- e. gangrenous proctitis
- e. hemorrhagic fever
- e. hepatitis
- e., heroin
- e., hospital
- e. hysteria
- e. infectious adenitis, acute
- e. influenza
- e. keratoconjunctivitis
- e. keratoconjunctivitis virus
- e. myalgia
- e. myositis
- e. neuromyasthenia
- e. of use and abuse, cyclic
- e. pleurodynia
- e., regional
- e., silent
- e. stage, pre-
- e. stomatitis
- e. strain
- e. threshold
- e. tremor

epidemica, panneuritis
epidemicus, genius
epidemiologic data
epidemiologic studies
epidemiological
- e. analysis
- e. history
- e. survey
- e. variations

Epidemiologist
- E., Field
- E., Hospital
- E. (NE) ▸ Nurse

epidemiology and etiology
epidemiology, hospital
epidermal (Epidermal)
- e. cancer

E. Growth Factor (EGF)
- e. inclusion cyst
- e. junction, dermal
- e. necrolysis, toxic

epidermatidis, Endomyces
epidermic graft
epidermica, Saccharomyces
epidermidis
- e., Cryptococcus
- e., Endomyces
- e., Leptomitus
- e., Staph
- e., Staphylococcus

epidermis, germinative layer of
epidermodysplasia verruciformis
epidermoid
- e. cancer
- e. carcinoma
- e. carcinoma bronchus
- e. carcinoma conjunctiva
- e. carcinoma cornea
- e. carcinoma esophagus
- e. carcinoma lung
- e. carcinoma trachea
- e. carcinoma, undifferentiated
- e. cyst
- e. cyst, degenerative
- e. tumor

epidermolysis bullosa (EB)
Epidermophyton
- E. floccosum
- E. inguinale
- E. rubrum

epidermosis bullosa
epididymidis
- e., globus major
- e., globus minor
- e., sinus
- e., vas

epididymis
- e., appendage of
- e., lobules of
- e., sinus of

epididymitis, acute
epididymitis, spermatogenic
epidural
- e. abscess
- e. abscess ▸ spinal
- e. abscess ▸ ventral
- e. aerocele
- e. analgesia
- e. anesthesia
- e. anesthetic
- e. angiolipoma
- e. angiolipoma ▸ spinal

- e. block
- e. cavity
- e. electrode
- e. hematoma
- e. hemorrhage
- e. hemorrhage ▸ surgical treatment for
- e. lipoma
- e. metastases, spinal
- e. pain control system ▸ SKY
- e. protrusion, interior
- e. space
- e. space ▸ drainage (dr'ge) of cerebral

epidurale, cavum
epiesophageal cancer
epigastric
- e. area
- e. artery
- e. artery, inferior
- e. aura
- e. bruit
- e. discomfort
- e. distress
- e. distress and burning
- e. fold
- e. hernia
- e. lymph nodes
- e. pain
- e. pain, dull
- e. pain, persistent
- e. puncture
- e. reflex
- e. region
- e. region of abdomen
- e. sensation
- e. shock
- e. tenderness
- e. vein, inferior
- e. vein, superficial
- e. vein, superior

epigenetic factor in cardiovascular development
epiglottic cartilage
epiglottica, vallecula
epiglottis
- e., cushion of the
- e., hyperplasia of
- e., hypoplasia of

epiglottitis, acute
epilans, Trichophyton
epilepsia partialis continua
epilepsy
- e., abdominal
- e., acquired

e., activated
e., adverse
e., akinetic
e. and ragged red fiber disease (MERRF) ▸ myoclonic
e. and seizure disorders
e., atonic
e., aura of
e., automatic
e., autonomic
e., biofeedback and
e., Bravais-jacksonian
e., central
e., centrencephalic
e., childhood
e., chronic focal
e., confusion from
e., continuous
e., cortical
e., cryptogenic
e., cursive
e., decerebrate
e., diurnal
e., dizziness from
e., essential
e., focal
e. from brain
e., gelastic
e., generalized
e., generalized flexion
e., grand mal
e., gustatory
e., haut mal
e., hypothalamic
e., hysterical
e., idiopathic
e., intractable
e., jacksonian
e., Jackson's
e., larval
e., laryngeal
e. laser treatment
e., latent
e., localized
e., major
e., matutinal
e., menstrual
e., minor
e., minor focal
e., mixed type
e., musicogenic
e., myoclonic
e., myoclonic petit mal
e., myoclonus
e., nocturnal

e., organic
e., petit mal
e., photic
e., photogenic
e., photosensitive
e., physiologic
e., post-traumatic
e., procursive
e., progressive familial myoclonic
e., psychic
e., psychomotor
e., questionable
e., reflex
e. research, alpha-
e., rolandic
e., sensory
e., serial
e., sleep
e., spinal
e., subclinical
e. ▸ support groups for
e., surgery
e. ▸ surgical treatment for
e., symptomatic
e. (HHE) syndrome ▸ hemiconvulsion, hemiplegia
e., tardy
e., temporal lobe
e., thalamic
e., tonic
e., tonic postural
e., toxemic
e., traumatic
e. ▸ trigger factors for
e., true
e., uncinate
e., untreatable
e., vasomotor
e., visceral
e. work-up

epileptic
e. attack
e. automatism
e. dementia
e. discharge
e. disorder
e. disorder, clinical
e. disorder, severe
e. equivalent
e. fugue
e. idiocy
e. mania
e. manifestations
e. manifestations, clinical
e., patient

e. pattern
e. process, highly active
e. psychosis
e., psychotic
e. seizure
e. seizures, continuous
e. seizures ▸ partial
e. state
e. stupor
e. tendency
e. vertigo
epileptica, absentia
epileptica, myoclonia
epilepticus
e. electroencephalogram (EEG) ▸ status
e., furor
e., ictus
e., status
epileptiform
e. abnormality
e. activity
e. convulsion
e. discharge
e. discharges, focal
e. discharges (PLED), periodic lateralized
e. pattern
epileptogenic foci
epileptogenic focus
epileptoid
e. attack
e. personality disorder
e. tremor
epimeric muscle
epinephrine, racemic
epinosic gain
epiotic center
epiphenomena of dissection
epiphrenic diverticulum
epiphyseal/epiphysial [*apophyseal*]
e. arch
e. arrest
e. center
e. center, metacarpal
e. center, phalangeal
e. chondroblastic growth and maturation
e. closure
e. dysplasia ▸ multiple
e. eye
e. fracture
e. fusion, diaphyseal-
e., juxta-
e. line

epiphyseal—*continued*
- e. plate
- e. separation
- e. syndrome

epiphysealis punctata ▸ dysplasia
epiphyses, distal radial
epiphyses, stippled
epiphysis [*apophysis*]
- e., avulsion of
- e., capital
- e., capital femoral
- e. cerebri
- e., distal femoral
- e., distal radial
- e., radial head
- e., slipped
- e., slipped upper femoral

epiphysitis, juvenile
epiphysitis, vertebral
epiphytica, Leptothrix
epiploic appendages
epiploic foramen
epiploicae, appendices
epiretinal membrane
episcleral
- e. bleeders
- e. lamina
- e. tissue
- e. veins

episcleritis, gouty
episiotomy
- e., left mediolateral
- e., Matsner
- e., midline
- e., right mediolateral
- e. stitches

episode(s)
- e., acute disabling vertiginous
- e., acute hypertensive
- e., acute schizophrenic
- e., anxiety
- e., apneic
- e., assaultive
- e., clinical
- e., crying
- e., daytime sleep
- e., depressive
- e., fainting
- e., febrile
- e., flailing
- e., heart dysfunctional
- e. ▸ heroin-related emergency room
- e., hypertensive
- e., hypoglycemic
- e. in full remission ▸ major depression, single
- e. in partial remission ▸ major depression, single
- e. ▸ induced manic
- e., intermittent
- e., isolated
- e. ▸ major depression, single
- e., major depressive
- e. ▸ major depressive disorder, recurrent
- e. ▸ major depressive disorder, single
- e., manic
- e. ▸ manic disorder, single
- e., mild ▸ major depression, single
- e., moderate ▸ major depression, single
- e. of acute abdominal pain ▸ intermittent
- e. of blurred vision
- e. of chest pain ▸ prolonged
- e. of dizziness
- e. of dysreflexia
- e. of numbness
- e. of pain, intermittent
- e. of severe depression
- e. of somnolence
- e. of terror ▸ overwhelming
- e. of vertigo
- e., panic
- e., presyncopal
- e., psycholeptic
- e., psychotic
- e., recurrent
- e., rejection
- e., seizure
- e., severe without psychotic features ▸ major depression, single
- e. ▸ silence of apneic
- e. ▸ superimposed acute inflammatory
- e., syncopal
- e., syndromal
- e., transient cerebral ischemic
- e., transient ischemic
- e., twitching
- e., unspecified ▸ major depression, single
- e., vasovagal
- e., with psychotic features ▸ major depression, single

episodic
- e. amnesia
- e. coughing spells
- e. disturbance of mental function
- e. drinking
- e. dysphoria ▸ intense
- e. dyspnea
- e. emotional instability
- e. fatigue
- e. hypertension
- e. incontinence
- e. loss of motor power
- e. memory
- e. pain
- e. pattern of binge eating
- e. positioning vertigo
- e. review
- e. sleep disturbance
- e. sweating
- e. symptom
- e. vertigo
- e. weight gain

episodica hereditaria, adynamia
episomes and plasmids
epispadias
- e., balanitic
- e., penile
- e., penopubic

epistaxis
- e., brisk
- e., frequent
- e., Gull's renal

epistenocardiaca, pericarditis
episternal impulse
epistropheus axis
epithelial
- e. attachment, Gottlieb's
- e. cancer
- e. cancer ▸ ovarian
- e. carcinoma
- e. cast
- e. cells
- e. cells, bronchial
- e. cells, ciliated
- e. cells, columnar
- e. cells, degenerated
- e. cells, desquamated renal
- e. cells, flattened
- e. cells, nucleated
- e. cells, polyhedral
- e. cells, pulmonary
- e. cells, sensory
- e. cells, squamous
- e. cells ▸ surface of
- e. cells, transitional
- e. dystrophy of cornea
- e. fragments, squamous

e. grafting, Mangoldt's
e. hyperplasia
e. hyperplasia ▸ focal
e. ingrowth
e. inlay
e. lining
e. lining fluid
e. lining of stomach
e. malignancy
e. membrane antigen
e. regeneration ▸ renal tubular
e. sloughing
e. spread
e. surface denuded
e. tissue
e. tissue ▸ functioning of normal

epitheliale adenoides, carcinoma
epithelialization deep
epitheliochorial placenta
epithelioid angiomatosis
epithelioid cell
epithelioma
e., basal cell
e., benign calcifying
e., calcified
e., calcifying
e., calcifying cell
e., chorio◊
e., chorionic
e., columnar
e., Contino's
e., cylindrical
e., diffuse
e., glandular
e., lympho◊
e., Malherbe's
e., multiple benign cystic
e., suprarenal

epithelium
e., alveolar
e., Barrett's
e., basal
e., basal layer of bronchial
e., capsular
e., ciliary
e., ciliated bronchial
e., circumoral area of columnar
e., columnar
e., corneal
e., cuboidal
e., desquamated
e., dysfunctional pigment
e. ▸ dysplastic changes in
e., free
e., germinal layer of bronchial

e., glandular
e., infantile
e., intestinal
e., low cuboidal
e., mesenchymal
e., nonkeratinizing stratified
    squamous
e. of cervix
e., pigment
e., placental
e., punctation, and mosaicism ▸
    white
e., regeneration of cervical
e., respiratory
e., retinal pigment
e., senile atrophy of pigmented
e. ▸ sloughed bronchial
e., squamous
e., stratified squamous
e., white

epithermal neutron
epitrochleoanconeus muscle
epitympanic recess
epitympanicum, os
epivaginal connective tissue
epizootic
e. abortion
e. keratoconjunctivitis
e. stomatitis

Epley maneuver
EPO ▸ genetically engineered
    (erythropoietin)
epoch, duration of
epoetin beta
eponychial fold
epoophoron cyst
EPR (electrophrenic respiration)
éprouvé, déjà
EPS (electrophysiologic study)
EPS (extrapyramidal symptoms)
EPSA (evoked potential signal
    averaging)
epsilon granules
epsilon staphylolysin
Epsom salt solution
EPSP (excitatory postsynaptic
    potential)
Epstein-Barr (EB)
E. (EB) chorioretinal disease
E. (CEBV) ▸ chronic
E. (EB) disease
E. (EB) syndrome
E. virus (EBV)
E. (EB) virus infection
E. (EB) virus syndrome

Epstein's nephrosis
Epstein's pearls
equal
e. and active bilaterally ▸ deep
    tendon reflexes (DTR)
e. and active bilaterally ▸ reflexes
e. and brisk, reflexes
e. and symmetrical, extremities
e. bilaterally, chest expansion
e. bilaterally ▸ peripheral pulses full
    and
e. bilaterally, reflexes
e. bilaterally ▸ reflexes strong and
e. bites of tissue
e., carotid pulses
e. concentration
e., excursions free and
e., extremities symmetrical and
e. in length
e. parts, divide in
e. parts (P. ae.) ▸ in
e. pulses
e., pupils
e., react to light and
    accommodation (PERLA) ▸
    pupils
e., react to light (PERL) ▸ pupils
e., reflexes
e., reflexes bilaterally
e., round, react to light and
    accommodation (PERRLA) ▸
    pupils
e. (RRE) ▸ round, regular and
e., round, regular, react to light and
    accommodation (PERRRLA) ▸
    pupils
e. thickness (CET), coefficient of

equalize air pressure
equalizer, stress
equalizing (PE) tube ▸ pressure
equally bilaterally, chest expands
equation
e., Bohr
e., continuity
e., Doppler continuity
e. ▸ Fick's diffusion
e., Gorlin
e., regression
e., Starling

equational division
equator of eye
equatorial staphyloma
equi
e., Ascaris
e., Babesia

equi—*continued*
- e., Clostridium parabotulinum
- e., Corynebacterium
- e., Nuttallia
- e., Psoroptes
- e., Salmonella abortus
- e., Streptococcus
- e., Trichodectes

equilateral hemianopia
equilibrating operation
equilibration
- e., mandibular
- e., occlusal
- e. time, helium

equilibratory ataxia
equilibratory coordination, disturbance of
equilibrium
- e., decrease in coordination or
- e., disturbance of body
- e., disturbance of mental
- e., dynamic
- e. -gated blood pool study
- e. image
- e. image ▸ supine test gated
- e., inability to maintain
- e., mental
- e. multigated radionuclide ventriculography
- e., radioactive
- e. radionuclide angiography (ERNA)
- e. radionuclide ventriculography ▸ rest-exercise
- e., secular
- e. sense
- e. syndrome, dialysis
- e., transient

equina
- e., adhesions of cauda
- e., cauda
- e. compression, cauda
- e., Setaria
- e. syndrome, cauda

equinal tumor, cauda
equine
- e. encephalitis (EEE) ▸ eastern
- e. encephalitis (VEE) ▸ Venezuelan
- e. encephalitis (EEE) virus ▸ eastern
- e. encephalitis (WEE) virus ▸ western
- e. encephalitis (WEE) ▸ western
- e. encephalomyelitis

- e. encephalomyelitis (EEE) ▸ eastern
- e. encephalomyelitis (VEE) ▸ Venezuelan
- e. encephalomyelitis virus
- e. encephalomyelitis (EEE) virus ▸ eastern
- e. encephalomyelitis (WEE) virus ▸ western
- e. gait
- e. sarcoid

equinovalgus, talipes
equinovarus, talipes
equinum, Trypanosoma
equinus
- e., pes
- e., Rhizopus
- e., talipes

equiphasic complex
equipment
- e., adaptive
- e. artifact
- e., computerized scanning
- e., contaminated
- e., contamination from anesthesia
- e., diagnostic
- e., disposable
- e., electronic scanning
- e., exercise
- e. malfunction
- e., medical
- e., monitoring respiratory
- e., nuclear cardiology
- e., nursing
- e. or tubing ▸ medical
- e., patient care
- e., rental
- e., Schoenander
- e., specialized
- e., Zimmer

equipotential electrodes
equipotential lines
equisetina, Ephedra
equisimilis, Streptococcus
equivalence, mass energy
equivalency ▸ left main
equivalent
- e., age
- e., aluminum
- e., anginal
- e., bursa-
- e., chemical
- e., combustion
- e., concrete
- e. detector, tissue-

- e., dose
- e., endosmotic
- e., epileptic
- e., generic
- e., gold
- e., gram
- e. in man (REM) ▸ radiation
- e., isodynamic
- e., Joule's
- e., lead
- e., lethal
- e., living skin
- e. -man period (REMP) ▸ roentgen-
- e. -man (REM), roentgen
- e. material
- e., migraine
- e., neutralization
- e. of task ▸ metabolic
- e. physical (REP) ▸ roentgen
- e., psychic
- e. ▸ right anterior oblique (RAO)
- e., roentgen
- e. score, age-
- e., spherical
- e., starch
- e., therapeutic
- e. therapy (RET), rad
- e. thickness (AET), absorption
- e., tissue
- e. tissue, bursal
- e., toxic
- e., ventilation
- e., ventilatory
- e., water
- e. wavelength

equivocal diagnosis
equivocal response
equorum, Ascaris
equuli, Actinobacillus
ER (Emergency Room)
ER (estrogen receptors)
ER (evoked response)
ER (estrogen receptor) assay test
ERA (Electric Response Audiometry)
era, preantibiotic
era vet counseling, Vietnam
eradicate infection
eradicate refluxing veins
eradication
- e., disease
- e. of abnormal veins
- e. rate
- e., total

erase, background
eraser, vein

erasing, ligation and stripping
erasing of veins
erasion of joint
Erb('s)
    E. area
    E. atrophy
    E. -Charcot disease
    E. disease
    E. -Duchenne paralysis
    E. dystrophy
    E. -Goldflam disease
    E. -Landouzy disease
    E. palsy
    E. paralysis
    E. paralysis ▸ Duchenne-
    E. point
    E. sclerosis
    E. sign
    E. syndrome
    E. waves
Erben's reflex
ERBF (effective renal blood flow)
ERCP (endoscopic retrograde
    cholangiopancreatography)
erect
    e. fluoro spot projection
    e. position
    e. spine
erectile
    e. carcinoma
    e. disorder, male
    e. dysfunction
    e. effect
    e. impotence
    e. tissue
erection
    e. center
    e., flexible
    e., pilo◊
    e., pilomotor
erector
    e. muscle of penis
    e. muscle of spine
    e. spinae reflex
erethismic (erethistic)
    e. idiocy
    e. idiot
    e. shock
ERG (electroretinogram)
ergograph, Mosso's
ergometer
    e. exercise stress test
    e. exercise stress test, bicycle
    e. ▸ Gauthier bicycle
    e. ▸ pedal mode

ergometric bike
ergometry treadmill, arm
ergonomic interventions
ergonovine
    e. challenge
    e. echocardiography (ECG)
    e. -induced spasm
    e. -induced vasospasm, refractory
    e. maleate provocation angina
    e. provocation test
ergophore group
ergosterol, activated
ergosterol, irradiated
ergotamine derivatives
ergotamine tartrate
ergotica, tabes
Erhard's test
Erichsen's
    E. disease
    E. ligature
    E. sign
eriksonii, Actinomyces
Eristalis tenax
Erlacher-Blount syndrome
Erlanger model of reentry ▸ Schmitt-
ERNA (equilibrium radionuclide
    angiography)
Ernst
    E. applicator
    E. granules ▸ Babès-
    E. radium applicator
    E. radium capsule
    E. radium tandem
Ernstein sedimentation rate (SR) ▸
    Rourke-
eroded
    e. by cholesteatoma, bone
    e. cartilage
    e. cervix
    e. mucosa
eroding gum tissue
erogenous zone
erosion
    e., antral
    e., area of
    e., bone
    e., cervical
    e., circumferential
    e., corneal
    e., dental
    e., Dieulafoy's
    e., esophageal
    e., gastric
    e., gastric mucosal
    e. in stomach

    e. ▸ intramucosal hemorrhages and
    e., neoplastic
    e. of cartilage
    e. of inner ear
    e. of mainstem bronchus
    e. of skin ▸ shallow
    e. ▸ pulse generator pocket
    e., spark
    e., superficial
    e. ▸ tracheotomy with tracheal
erosive
    e. anastomosis
    e. esophagitis
    e. gastritis
    e. gastritis with ulceration
    e. reflux
    e. reflux esophagitis
    e. tracheitis
eroticism (erotism)
eroticism, anal
erotism (eroticism)
erotism, muscle
erotism, oral
erotogenic zone
erotomanic delusions
ERP (exposure and response
    prevention)
ERPF (effective renal plasma flow)
erratic
    e. appetite
    e. behavior
    e. blood glucose levels
    e. cell growth
    e. eating habits
    e. emotional behavior
    e. heart rhythm
    e. heartbeat
    e. menstrual periods
    e. mood
    e. parenting ▸ unstable or
    e. sleep-wake patterns
    e. weight gain
error
    e. artifact, data spike detection
    e., correct optical
    e., diagnostic
    e., genetic
    e. of metabolism, inborn
    e. of the mean (SEM) ▸ standard
    e., operational
    e. -prone virus
    e. rate
    e., refractive
    e., statistical
ERT (estrogen replacement therapy)

eructation, nervous
erupted incisors
erupted teeth
eruption(s)
　　e., acneform
　　e., acneiform
　　e., blemishes or pigmentations
　　e., creeping
　　e., cutaneous
　　e. dermatitis, drug
　　e., drug
　　e., ectopic
　　e., fixed drug
　　e., Kaposi's varicelliform
　　e. of tooth
　　e. ▸ sea swimmer's
　　e., skin
　　e., varicelliform
eruptive
　　e. dermatitis
　　e. fever
　　e. gingivitis
　　e. stage
　　e. xanthoma
eruptivum, xanthoma
ERV (expiratory reserve volume)
erwinieae, Enterobacter
erysipeloid reaction
Erysipelothrix
　　E. insidiosa
　　E. muriseptica, gram-positive
　　E. rhusiopathiae
erythema
　　e. chronicum migrans
　　e. chronicum migrans (ECM) lesion
　　e. dose
　　e. dose, minimal
　　e. dose, skin
　　e. dose (TED), threshold
　　e. dyschromicum
　　e. elevatum
　　e. fugax
　　e., gluteal
　　e. induratum
　　e. infectiosum
　　e., Jacquet's
　　e. marginatum
　　e. migrans
　　e., mucosal
　　e. multiforme
　　e., napkin
　　e. neonatorum
　　e. neonatorum toxicum
　　e. nodosum
　　e. nodosum leprosum

　　e. nodosum syphiliticum
　　e. of extremities
　　e., palmar
　　e., paranasal
　　e., perianal
　　e. pernio
　　e., plantar
　　e. -producing rays
　　e., simple
　　e. streptogenes
　　e., surrounding
　　e., symptomatic
　　e., toxic
　　e. toxicum
　　e. toxicum neonatorum
　　e. traumaticum
　　e. venenatum
erythematopultaceous stomatitis
erythematosus
　　e., discoid lupus
　　e. discoides, lupus
　　e. disseminatus (LED), lupus
　　e. ▸ drug-induced lupus
　　e. (LE) ▸ lupus
　　e., pemphigus
　　e. vulgaris, lupus
erythematous
　　e. and inflamed ▸ bronchi
　　e., bronchi
　　e., bronchi looked
　　e. (LE) cell test, lupus
　　e. changes
　　e. -edematous reaction
　　e. macules
　　e. macules of palms and soles
　　e., maculopapular rash
　　e. mucosa
　　e. nodule
　　e. skin
　　e. (SLE), systemic lupus
　　e. tonsillitis
erythermalgia (*see* erythromelalgia)
erythredema polyneuropathy
erythremic myelosis
erythroblast
　　e., acidophilic
　　e., basophilic
　　e., definitive
　　e., early
　　e., eosinophilic
　　e., intermediate
　　e., late
　　e., orthochromatic
　　e., oxyphilic
　　e., polychromatic

　　e., primitive
erythroblastic
　　e. anemia
　　e. anemia, familial
　　e. anemia of childhood
erythroblastosis, ABO
erythroblastosis fetalis
erythroblastosis neonatorum
erythrocyte(s)
　　e., achromic
　　e. agglutination test, human
　　e., basophilic
　　e., burr
　　e. coproporphyria, free
　　e. coproporphyrin, free
　　e., crenated
　　e. enzyme assays
　　e. fragility
　　e. glutamic-oxaloacetic
　　　　transaminase (EGOT)
　　e. glutathione peroxidase
　　　　deficiency
　　e., hypochromic
　　e., immature
　　e. mass
　　e. maturation factor (EMF)
　　e., "Mexican hat"
　　e., normochromic
　　e., nucleated
　　e., orthochromatic
　　e., packed
　　e., polychromatic
　　e., polychromatophilic
　　e. protoporphyrin
　　e. protoporphyrin, free
　　e. sedimentation
　　e. sedimentation rate (ESR) test
　　e. sedimentation reaction (ESR)
　　e. sensitizing substance
　　e. survival time
　　e., target
erythrocytic ratio, myelocytic
erythrocytic ratio ▸ normal
　　myelocytic
erythrocytosis
　　e., leukemic
　　e. megalosplenica
　　e., stress
erythroderma
　　e., atopic
　　e. desquamativum
　　e., exfoliative
erythrodermic cutaneous T-cell
　　lymphoma
erythrogenesis imperfecta

erythrohepatic protoporphyria
erythroid
  e. activity
  e. cells
  e. precursors
  e. ratio, granulocyte-
  e. ratio, myeloid-
erythrokinetic studies
erythromelalgia (*same as* erythermalgia*)
erythromelalgia of the head
erythronormoblastic anemia
erythroplasia, Queyrat's
erythroplasia, Zoon's
erythropoiesis, defective
erythropoietic
  e. factor, renal
  e. porphyria (CEP), congenital
  e. protoporphyria
  e. stimulating factor
erythropoietin
  e. assay
  e. bioassay
  e. (EPO) ▸ genetically engineered
  e., plasma
erythropsia/erythropia
Erythroxylon coca
erythyroid precursors
escape
  e. and avoidance conditioning in human subjects
  e. beat ▸ junctional
  e. beats
  e. -capture bigeminy
  e. complex, AV junctional
  e. impulse
  e. interval
  e. interval, atrial
  e. interval ▸ pacemaker
  e., junctional
  e. mechanism
  e., nodal
  e. of air
  e. of gastroduodenal contents ▸ intra-abdominal
  e. ovulation
  e. pacemaker
  e. reality
  e. rhythm
  e. rhythm, atrial
  e. rhythm, atrioventricular (AV)
  e. rhythm ▸ junctional
  e. rhythm ▸ nodal
  e. rhythm ▸ slow
  e., vagal

  e., ventricular
  e. ventricular contraction
escaped ventricular contraction
escargot curve
eschar [*scar*]
eschar, neuropathic
escharotomy procedure
Escherichia (E.)
  E. aerogenes
  E. alkalescens
  E. aurescens
  E. coli
  E. coli bacteremia
  E. coli, enteropathic
  E. coli, enteropathogenic
  E. coli, gram-negative
  E. coli infection ▸ gram-positive
  E. coli organisms
  E. coli sepsis peritonitis
  E. communior, gram-negative
  E. dispar
  E. dispar var. ceylonensis
  E. dispar var. madampensis
Escherichial sepsis
Escherich's
  E. bacillus
  E. reflex
  E. test
escomili, Trypanosoma
escort patient
esculenta, Collocalia
ESD (esophagus, stomach and duodenum)
ESM (ejection systolic murmur)
Esmarch maneuver, Heiberg-
ESO (Environmental Surveillance Officer)
esodic nerve
esophageal
  e. abscess
  e. achalasia
  e., adventitia
  e. airway
  e. angina
  e. A-ring
  e. artery
  e. atresia
  e. atresia ▸ prenatal diagnosis of
  e. atresia ▸ pulmonary aspects in
  e. balloon
  e. biopsy
  e. bleeding
  e. body
  e. body function
  e. bougienage

  e. B-ring
  e. bronchus
  e. brushing, blind
  e. canal of diaphragm
  e. cancer
  e. cancer ▸ intrathoracic
  e. cancer ▸ lymphadenectomy of intrathoracic
  e. cancer ▸ proliferation of
  e. cancer ▸ thoracic
  e. candidiasis
  e. carcinoma
  e. carcinoma ▸ inoperable
  e. carcinoma ▸ intrathoracic
  e. carcinoma with respiratory tract fistula
  e. cardiogram
  e. contraction
  e. contraction ring
  e. detection device
  e. dilatation
  e. disease, colon interposition for
  e. disease, complex benign
  e. disorder
  e. diverticulectomy ▸ Harrington
  e. diverticulum
  e. dysfunction
  e. dysmotility
  e. dysphagia
  e. dysphagia, chronic
  e. dysrhythmia
  e. electrocardiography (ECG)
  e. electrogram
  e. erosions
  e. fibrous stricture formation
  e. fistula
  e., gastro◊
  e. hemorrhage, peri-
  e. hernia
  e. hiatal hernia
  e. hiatal hernia, sliding
  e. hiatus
  e. hiatus hernia
  e. introitus
  e. intubation detection
  e. lead
  e. lesion
  e. lesion ▸ brushing of
  e. lesion, constricting
  e. lesion, distal
  e. lining
  e. lumen
  e. lung
  e. lye stricture
  e. malfunction

esophageal—*continued*
- e. manometry
- e. motility
- e. motility disorder
- e. motility dysfunction
- e. motility ▸ irregular
- e. motility study
- e. motility test
- e. mucosa
- e. mucus
- e. narrowing
- e. obstruction
- e. obturator airway
- e. perforation
- e. perforation ▸ reconstruction, of
- e. peristalsis
- e. peristalsis ▸ uncoordinated
- e. plexus
- e. pressure
- e. pressure study
- e. prosthesis
- e. prosthesis placement
- e. reconstruction
- e. recording, bipolar
- e. reflux
- e. reflux, extra◊
- e. reflux, free
- e. regurgitation
- e. ring ▸ Schatzki
- e. rupture
- e. sclerosis, chronic
- e. sling procedure
- e. sound
- e. spasm
- e. spasm, diffuse
- e. spasm ▸ irregular
- e. speculum, Robert's
- e. speech
- e. sphincter
- e. sphincter disorder
- e. sphincter disorder ▸ upper
- e. sphincter, incompetent
- e. sphincter ▸ lower
- e. sphincter pressure, lower
- e. sphincter ▸ relaxed lower
- e. squamous atypia
- e. stenosis
- e. stenosis ▸ malignant
- e. stenosis ▸ palliation of malignant
- e. stricture
- e. stricture ▸ reflux-induced
- e. stricture ▸ Wickwitz
- e. tamponade
- e. tear
- e. temperature probe

- e. thrush
- e. transit study ▸ radionuclide
- e. transit time
- e. tube
- e. tumor
- e. ulcer
- e. ulceration
- e. variceal bleed
- e. variceal sclerosis
- e. varices
- e. varices, bleeding
- e. varices, downhill
- e. varices ▸ endoscopic sclerosis of bleeding
- e. varices, sclerosing of
- e. varix
- e. veins
- e. voice
- e. wall
- e. walls ▸ barium adherent to
- e. web

esophagectomy
- e., emergency subtotal
- e. ▸ en bloc
- e. for carcinoma
- e. in benign disease ▸ one stage

esophagism, hiatal
esophagitis
- e., chronic
- e. ▸ chronic reflux
- e., corrosive
- e. dissecans superficialis
- e., eosinophilic
- e., erosive
- e. ▸ erosive reflux
- e., gastro◊
- e., hemorrhagic
- e., infectious
- e., monilial
- e., peptic
- e., reflux
- e., regurgitant
- e., residual
- e., severe underlying
- e., ulcerative
- e., underlying

esophagobronchial fistula
esophagogastric
- e. anastomosis ▸ stenotic
- e. junction
- e. sphincter
- e. tamponade

esophagogastricitis, hemorrhagic
esophagogastrostomy ▸ two-stage
esophagojejunal anastomosis

esophagosalivary reflex
esophagosalivary symptom
esophagoscope tube, Mosher's
esophagoscopy
- e. examination
- e., fiberoptic
- e., motility
- e. with biopsy
- e. with dilatation

esophagostomy, gastro◊
esophagram, barium
esophagus
- e., achalasia of
- e., atresia of
- e. ▸ backwash of stomach acid into
- e., barium filled
- e., Barrett's
- e., border of
- e., brusque dilatation of
- e., carcinoma of
- e., carcinoma upper third of
- e., caustic strictures of cervical
- e., cervical
- e., cervical thoracic
- e., congenital atresia of
- e., congenital malformed
- e., constricted
- e. deviated anteriorly
- e., dilated
- e. dilated distally
- e., dilating
- e. disorder
- e., dissection of
- e., distal
- e., diverticulum of
- e., duplication of
- e., epidermoid carcinoma
- e. exposed
- e. ▸ extension denudation of distal
- e. ▸ flexible tube in
- e., foreign body (FB)
- e. ▸ histologic sections of
- e. into stomach ▸ barium passed through
- e. junction, cardio-
- e., lesions in
- e., lower
- e., lymphatic drainage of
- e. ▸ major obstruction of
- e., mega-
- e., midthoracic
- e. ▸ mucosal surfaces of
- e. ▸ multiple ulcers of
- e. ▸ muscle contractions of
- e., nutcracker

e. ▸ pneumatic dilatation of
e., proximal
e., pulsations in
e. replacement
e. replacement with colon in children
e. ▸ scarring and narrowing of
e., short
e. ▸ slight obstruction of
e., spasm of
e., spontaneous rupture of
e., stomach and duodenum
e., stretching
e. ▸ stricture of
e., stump of
e. ▸ superficial hemorrhage distal
e., tertiary contractions of
e., thoracic
e. ▸ Torek resection of thoracic
e., traumatic perforation of
e., upper
e. without varices

esophoria, alternating
esotropia [*exotropia*]
e., alternating
e., constant
e., left
e., periodic
e., right

ESP (extrasensory perception)
ESR (erythrocyte sedimentation rate)
ESR (erythrocyte sedimentation reaction)
ESRD (End Stage Renal Disease) Program
ess (essentially)
essential
e. asthma
e. atrophy of iris
e. blepharospasm (BEB) ▸ benign
e. bradycardia
e. convulsion
e. detail discrimination
e. distinctions, blurred
e. dysmenorrhea
e. epilepsy
e. fatty acids
e. fever
e. hematuria
e. hemorrhage
e. hypercholesterolemia
e. hypertension (HTN)
e. hypertension (HTN) ▸ low renin
e. hypertensive patient
e. medium (MEM) ▸ minimum

e. mixed cryoglobulinemia (EMC)
e. polyangiitis
e. pulmonary hemosiderosis
e. resistance
e. tachycardia
e. thrombocytopenia
e. thrombopenia
e. treatment
e. tremor
e. tremor, benign
e. tremor, disabling
e. tremor, hereditary
e. tumor ▸ benign
e. uterine hemorrhage
e. vertigo

essentially (ess)
e. negative
e. negative examination
e. negative, findings

Esser graft
Esser island flap, Monks-
Essex-Lopresti
E. fracture
E. method
E. reduction technique

EST (electroshock therapy)
establish treatment objectives
established
e., airway
e., satisfying relationships
e. therapy
e. treatment

establishing normative base rates
esteem
e., building self-
e. child ▸ low self-
e., chronic low self-
e., diminished self-
e. disturbance ▸ self-
e. ▸ enhance self-
e., enhancing self-
e. ▸ improve health self-
e., inflated self-
e. is fragile ▸ patient self-
e. ▸ loss of self-
e., low self-
e. of patient ▸ self-
e. or guilt ▸ low self-
e. ▸ poor self-
e., self-
e., shame and self-
e. ▸ situational low self-
e. skills ▸ self-
e. ▸ vulnerability in self-

ester
e., acetyltyrosine ethyl
e., cholesterol
e. ▸ fatty acid ethyl
e. storage disease, cholesterol
e., tyrosine ethyl

Estes' operation
esthesia (*same as* aesthesia)
esthesioneurocytoma, olfactory
esthetic massage
esthetics (*see* aesthetics)
estimate(s)
e., dose
e., platelet
e., risk-benefit

estimated
e. blood loss (EBL)
e. date of confinement (EDC/EDOC)
e. date of delivery (EDD/EDOD)
e. fluid sequestration
e. hepatic blood flow
e. MVV (maximum voluntary ventilation)
e. thyroid ratio (ETR)
e. time of arrival (ETA)
e. tissue resected

estimating degree of drug dependence
Estlander flap
Estlander's operation
estradiol
e. benzoate
e. concentration
e., ethinyl
e. production rate
e. receptor, tumor

estranged ▸ patient feels
estriol
e. irregularity
e., urinary
e. values, urinary

estrogen
e. and progestin, synthetic
e., cells respond to
e., conjugated
e. cream
e. cycle
e. deficiency
e. -dependent neoplasia
e. -dependent vaginal dryness
e., endogenous
e., environmental
e. excretion, total
e., exogenous

estrogen—*continued*
- e. hormone ▸ stimulate production female sex
- e. hypothesis
- e. -induced pancreatitis
- e., lack of
- e. level
- e. loss, bone thinning effects of
- e., ovarian
- e. patch
- e. potency
- e. /progestin interventions (PEPI) ▸ postmenopausal
- e. receptor (ER)
- e. receptor (ER), anti-
- e. receptor assay
- e. receptor (ER) assay test
- e. receptor (ER) gene
- e. receptor modulators (SERM) ▸ selective
- e. receptor negative
- e. receptor ▸ positive
- e. receptor study
- e. receptors (ER) in cancer cells ▸ suppress
- e. replacement
- e. replacement for osteoporosis
- e. replacement ▸ postmenopausal
- e. replacement therapy (ERT)
- e. -secreting granulosa cells
- e. sensitive tumor
- e. tablet
- e. therapy
- e. therapy for men
- e. therapy, oral
- e. therapy ▸ postmenopausal
- e. therapy, transdermal
- e., topical
- e. withdrawal bleeding

estrogenic stimulation
estrogenic substances
estrus cycle
Estuffa (heroin)
ESWL ▸ extracorporeal shock wave lithotripsy
et tardus pulse ▸ parvus
ETA (estimated time of arrival)
etched
- e. circled slides
- e., freeze-
- e. porcelain veneers

etching, freeze-
ETCO₂ (end-tidal carbon dioxide)
ETF (eustachian tube function)
E-thalassemia disease, hemoglobin

ethambutol hydrochloride
ethane hydroxydiphosphate
ethanol
- e. ablation
- e. ablation ▸ percutaneous
- e. abuse
- e. drip
- e. ingestion
- e. sensitivity

ethanolamine oleate
ether
- e. anesthesia
- e. bronchitis
- e., ethinylestradiol methyl
- e. gas, oxygen and
- e. (MTBE) ▸ methyl test-butyl
- e., petroleum
- e. pneumonia
- e. reflex
- e. test
- e., Vinethene and

ethical
- e. abuse
- e. code
- e. deterioration
- e. individuation
- e. issues
- e. judgment
- e. responsibility
- e. standards
- e. theory
- e. validity of assisted suicide

ethically extraordinary treatment
Ethicon [*Ethilon*]
Ethicon silk suture
ethics
- e., Golden Rule
- e., medical
- e., "outdated" medical
- e., research
- e., Western medical

ethinyl estradiol
ethinylestradiol methyl ether
Ethiodane contrast medium
Ethiodol contrast medium
ethmoid(s)
- e. air cells
- e. antrum
- e. bone
- e. bone ▸ lateral masses of
- e. bulla
- e. cells
- e., clouding of
- e. cornu
- e., cribriform plate of

- e. fissure
- e. infundibulum
- e., perpendicular plate of
- e. sinus cancer

ethmoidal
- e. artery
- e. cells, bony
- e. concha
- e. infundibulum
- e. nerve
- e. nerve, anterior
- e. nerve, posterior
- e. notch of frontal bone
- e. paranasal sinus
- e. sinus
- e. veins

ethmoidal, antrum
ethmoidal, os
ethmoidomaxillary suture
ethnic
- e. background, cultural-
- e. susceptibility
- e. susceptibility to alcohol

ethnographic research
ethnographic studies
ethnomedical therapy
ethyl
- e. alcohol
- e. ester, acetyltyrosine
- e. ester ▸ fatty acid
- e. ester, tyrosine

ethylene oxide
ethynodiol diacetate
etidronate sodium kit, Tc (technetium) 99m
etiennei, Octomyces
etiocholanolone fever
etiologic
- e. agent
- e. agent ▸ presumptive diagnosis of
- e. diagnosis
- e. diagnosis, presumptive
- e. diagnosis, specific
- e. diagnosis, tentative
- e. factor
- e. organism
- e. thesis

etiological
- e. agent
- e. conclusion
- e. diagnosis

etiology (*same as* aetiology, aitiology)
etiology [*etymology*]
- e., alcoholism

e. ▸ anemia of questionable
e., bacterial
e., disease and
e., emotional
e., epidemiology and
e., fever of obscure
e., infectious
e., nonpancreatic
e., nonspecific
e. of chronic pancreatitis
e. of headache, ocular
e., pancreatic
e., pyrexia of unknown
e. radiographically not determined
e., syncope undetermined
e., toxic metabolic
e. unknown (E.U.)
e., viral
etiopathic [*idiopathic*]
etousae, Shigella
ETR (estimated thyroid ratio)
ETS (environmental tobacco smoke)
ETT (exercise tolerance test)
etymology [*etiology*]
E.U. (etiology unknown)
EUA (examination under anesthesia)
eugenic(s)
e., negative
e., positive
e. sterilization
Euglena gracilis
Euglena viridis
euglobulin clot lysis time
euglobulin lysis time
Euler's number
eunuchism, pituitary
eunuchoid gigantism
eunuchoid voice
euphoria
e. and drug abuse
e., emotional lability, and irritability
e. ▸ feeling of
e., increased
e., initial feeling of
e., intense
e. ▸ level of
e., sense of
e. ▸ temporary mild
euphoric
e. effect
e. feeling
e. mood
e., patient
e. rush
e. sense of well-being

e. state
euphorigenic effect
eupraxic center
Euproctis chrysorrhoea
europaea, Larix
Eurotium malignum
Eurotium repens
eurystrepta, Spirochaeta
eurytrophic parasite
EUS (endoscopic ultrasound)
eusphaera, Siderocapsa
Eustace Smith's murmur
eustachian
e. canal
e. cartilage
e. muscle
e. probe
e. tonsil
e. tube
e. tube blocked by infection of ear
e. tube, catheterization of
e. tube dysfunction
e. tube function (ETF)
e. tube inflation
e. tube obstruction
e. tube pressure
e. valve
euthanasia
e., active
e. and disabilities
e., condemnation of active
e., involuntary active
e., legalize
e., nonvoluntary active
e., open practice of
e., passive
e., psychological cost of
e., voluntary
e., voluntary active
euthyroid (*same as* thyroid)
Eutrichomastix cuniculi
Eutrombicula
E. alfreddugesi
E. irritans
E. splendens
eV (electron volt)
evacuant, rectal
evacuate [*evaluate*]
evacuated
e., blood clots
e. bottle
e., bowel
e., bowel adequately
e., clot
e., tissue

evacuates satisfactorily ▸ bowel fills and
evacuates satisfactorily ▸ colon fills and
evacuation
e. ▸ bloating and disruption of
e., bowel
e., controllable
e., dilation and
e. film, pre-
e., hospital
e., normal
e. of barium, normal
e. of blood clots
e. of bowel
e. of clots
e. of trauma patient, air
e. ▸ strengthen muscles of
e., uterine
evaluate [*evacuate*]
e. abilities and limitations
e. extent of injury or illness
e. implant
e. orientation, attention and recent recall
e. protocol
e. safety and stability at home
e. treatment
evaluated, patient
evaluated, spicules
evaluation
e. (ASE) ▸ abstinence symptom
e., accessibility
e. and correction ▸ self-
e. and treatment
e. and treatment, initial
e. and treatment of eating disorders
e. and workup ▸ patient admitted for
e., annual health
e., anthropometric
e., arteriographic
e., assessment
e., audiologic
e. ▸ auditory and medical
e., baseline
e., biochemical
e., bladder
e., bronchoscopic
e., cardiac
e., cardiovascular
e., clinical
e., cognitive
e., colonoscopic
e., complete physical

evaluation—*continued*
- e., compulsory psychological
- e., computerized muscle-joint
- e., criminal
- e., custody
- e., diagnosis and
- e., diagnostic
- e., diagnostic hearing
- e., disability
- e., educational
- e., executive physical
- e., fertility
- e., final drug
- e., follow-up
- e., forensic
- e., foster home
- e. ▸ functional capacity
- e., further
- e., gastrointestinal (GI)
- e., geriatric
- e., global
- e., histologic
- e., Holter monitor
- e., home
- e., immunologic
- e., independent
- e., infertility
- e., initial
- e., initial employee
- e., intellectual
- e. ▸ intracranial vascular
- e., invasive diagnostic
- e., laboratory
- e. ▸ legally mandated
- e., medical
- e. ▸ mental status
- e., microscopic
- e., multidisciplinary
- e., musculoskeletal
- e., negative
- e., neurologic
- e., neurological
- e., neuropsychological
- e., neurosurgical
- e., noninvasive
- e. ▸ noninvasive cardiac
- e., occupational therapy
- e. of behavioral methods
- e. of coronary artery disease (CAD)
- e. of data
- e. of denervated heart at rest
- e. of pain
- e. of patient
- e. of psychomotor skills

- e. of radial keratotomy (PERK) protocol, prospective
- e. of resting activity
- e., otorhinolaryngological
- e., outpatient
- e., overnight sleep
- e. ▸ parent-child interaction
- e., patient
- e., patient admitted for medical
- e., personality
- e., physical
- e., physical disability
- e., post-therapy
- e., preemployment
- e., prehospital
- e., preoperative
- e., pretreatment
- e. prior to discharge, home
- e., proctosigmoidoscopic
- e., product
- e., prognostic
- e. program, clinical drug
- e., psychiatric
- e., psychoanalytic
- e., psychodynamic
- e., psychological
- e., psychometric
- e., psychosocial
- e., pulmonary
- e., radiological
- e., reflex
- e., renal
- e., repeat
- e., respiratory
- e., self-
- e. ▸ sequential quantitative
- e. services
- e., skin
- e., speech
- e., sperm count
- E. (D and E) Staffing ▸ Diagnosis and
- e., standardized psychiatric
- e., sterilization procedures
- e., stool
- e. studies, naturalistic
- e., suicide
- e., tumor
- e., urological
- e., urological medical
- e., vocational
- e., wound
- e., x-ray
- e., x-ray diagnostic

evaluative services

evaluative staging, surgical
Evans' operation
evansi, Trypanosoma
evaporated milk
evaporation, loss of fluids through
evaporation, moisture
evaporative water loss
evasive, patient
event(s) (Event)
- E. activated monitor
- e., adverse clinical
- e. (ALTE) ▸ apparent life-threatening
- e., behavioral
- e., cardiac
- e., cardiovascular
- e., catastrophic
- e., cerebral
- e., cerebrovascular
- e., cognitive distortions of actual
- e., coronary
- e., crisis
- e. diary
- e., electrical
- e., embolic
- e., external
- e., high-frequency
- e., impaired memory for recent
- e. in heart, abnormal electrical
- e., inability to recall
- e., internal
- e., intracardiac
- e., isolated
- e., life-threatening
- e., loss of memory for
- e., loss of memory for distant
- e. ▸ major stress evoking
- E. Master ▸ SpaceLabs
- e., memory for past
- e., memory for recent
- e. monitor
- e., phasic
- e., recalling past
- e., recalling recent
- E. recorder
- E. recorder, circadian
- e. -related brain potential
- e. -related potentials
- e. scanning ▸ rupture
- e., soft
- e., terminal
- e. transmitter

eventration
- e., diaphragmatic
- e. of leaf of diaphragm

e., umbilical
ever-present effects of weight
Eversbusch's operation
eversion [*inversion*]
    e. carotid endarterectomy, blunt
    e., cusp
    e. of organ, congenital
    e. of punctum
    e. of punctum, senile
    e. position
    e. tape strapping
everted, lid
everted, nipples
everting
    e. interrupted
    e. mattress suture
    e. suture
every (q)
evidence
    e., clinical
    e., demonstrable
    e., gross
    e., medical
    e., objective
    e. of active disease ▸ no
    e. of clearing
    e. of disease (NED), no
    e. of invasion
    e. of metastatic disease, clinical
    e. of pathology
    e. of pathology, no
    e. of recurrence (NER), no
    e. of recurrent disease (NERD), no
    e. of show ▸ patient had
    e. of trauma ▸ physical
    e. of weight loss ▸ abdomen
        showed
    e., periprocedural
    e., radiographic
    e., subjective
evisceration
    e. left eye
    e. of eyeball
    e. right eye
    e., wound
evocative mode
evocative play
evoked
    e. action potential
    e. potential (EP)
    e. potential, auditory
    e. potential (AEP), average
    e. potential (BAEP), brain stem
        auditory
    e. potential (MEP), multimodality

e. potential, pattern
e. potential, sensory
e. potential signal averaging
    (EPSA)
e. potential (SEP or SSEP),
    somatosensory
e. potential, transient
e. potential (VEP), visual
e. response (ER)
e. response audiometer
e. response audiometry
e. response (AER), auditory
e. response, average
e. response (BSER), brain stem
e. response (BAER), brain stem
    auditory
e. response, cortical
e. response, neurological
e. response ▸ paced ventricular
e. response (SER), short latency
    somatosensory
e. response (SER), somatosensory
e. response test
e. response, visual
evoking event ▸ major stress
evoking stimuli ▸ autonomic
    response to anxiety-
evolution of disease
evolutionary biology
evolutionary psychology
evolutus, Peptostreptococcus
evolving [*involving*]
    e. behavior
    e. myocardial infarction
    e. neurological lesion
    e. right parietal stroke
evulsion [*avulsion*]
Ewald's node
Ewald's test meal
Ewart's sign
EWI (Experiential World Inventory)
Ewing's
    E. sarcoma
    E. sign
    E. tumor
ex
    e. anopsia, amaurosis
    e. pleomorphic adenoma,
        carcinoma
    e. vacuo change ▸ hydrocephalus
    e. vivo
    e. vivo gene transfer
exacerbate
    e. depression
    e. the pain

e. trauma
exacerbated, headache
exacerbating factor
exacerbation(s)
    e., acute
    e. ▸ acute bacterial
    e. and hemorrhage
    e. and remission
    e. and remissions, acute
    e. of chronic bronchitis ▸ acute
    e. of disease
    e. of illness
    e. of pain
    e. of pain ▸ patient experiences
        remissions and
    e. of preexisting disorder
    e. of preexisting psychiatric illness
    e. of sinusitis ▸ acute
    e. of symptoms
    e. of tonsillitis ▸ acute
    e. ▸ schizophrenia, catatonic type,
        chronic with acute
    e. ▸ schizophrenia, catatonic type,
        subchronic with acute
    e. ▸ schizophrenia, disorganized
        type, chronic with acute
    e. ▸ schizophrenia, disorganized
        type, subchronic with acute
    e. ▸ schizophrenia, paranoid type,
        chronic with acute
    e. ▸ schizophrenia, paranoid type,
        subchronic with acute
    e. ▸ schizophrenia, residual type,
        chronic with acute
    e. ▸ schizophrenia, residual type,
        subchronic with acute
    e. ▸ schizophrenia, undifferentiated
        type, chronic with acute
    e. ▸ schizophrenia, undifferentiated
        type, subchronic with acute
exact nature unknown
exaggerated
    e. blink reflex
    e. distress
    e. elation
    e., emotional features
    e. emotions
    e. expression of emotions
    e. lows
    e. motions
    e. positive wave
    e. reflexes
    e. sense of self importance
examination(s) (Examination)
    e., abdominal ultrasound

examination(s)—*continued*

e., admission physical
e. ▸ air contrast colon
e., angiographic
e., annual
e., annual digitorectal
e., annual dilated eye
e., annual physical
e. annually ▸ complete gynecologic
e., anoscopic
e. anxiety, reduction
e. as a screening device for drug
   abuse ▸ physical
e., audiology
e., autopsy external
e., autopsy gross
e., autopsy internal
e., autopsy microscopic
e., ballistocardiogram
e., barium enema
e., barium roentgenographic
e., bimanual pelvic
e., bone marrow
e., breast
e. (BSE), breast self-
e., brief
E. (BNMSE), Brief
   Neuropsychological Mental
   Status
e., bronchographic
e., bronchoscopy
e., cardiac
e., cardiac Doppler
e., cell
e., cineradiographic
e., clinical
e. ▸ clinical breast
e., complete physical
e., comprehensive
e., concentric circle pattern on
   breast self-
e., cornea
e., cystoscopic
e., cytologic
e., dark-field
e., diaphanography
e., diascopic
e., digital
e., digital rectal
e., digitorectal
e., dilated eye
e., direct visual
e., double contrast
e., Dubowitz developmental
e., duodenoscopy

e., electron microscopic
e., employment
e., endoscopic
e., entrance physical
e., esophagoscopy
e. essentially negative
e., executive physical
e., extended
e., extensive medical
e., external
e., fluoroscopic
e., follow-up
e., frozen section
e., full blood
e., fundus
e., funduscopic
e., gastroscopy
e. glove
e. gown, disposable
e., gross
e. ▸ group medical
e., gynecological
e., hanging drop
e., histologic
e. (HPE), history and physical
e. inconclusive, pelvic
e., initial
e., initial physical
e. ▸ initial screening
e., insurance
e., intermediate
e., joint
e., laboratory
e., laminogram
e., laparoscopy
e., limited
e., low dose x-ray
e., mammography
e., manual internal
e., medical
e., mental status
e., microscopic
e., microsection
e., multiple washings taken for
e., mycology
e., neurological
e. ▸ neuro-ophthalmic
e., noninvasive
e., observation and
e. of abdomen ▸ in situ
e. of anterior chest ▸ pectus
e. of anus
e. of breast ▸ self-
e. of bronchus, endoscopic
e. of cells ▸ microscopic

e. of extremities, neurological
e. of eye, Wood's light
e. of pelvic ▸ manual
e. of prostate, digital
e. of testicle, self-
e., on-the-field
e., ophthalmoscopic
e., otoscopic
e., palpation
e., panendoscopic
e., parasternal
e., pathologic
e., pathological tissue
e., patient given enema prior to
e., pelvic
e., periodic
e., periodic health
e., peritoneoscopy
e., phlebogram
e., photofluorographic
e. (PE), physical
e., planographic
e., postmortem
e., postpartum
e., preemployment
e., preoperative (preop)
e., preoperative screening physical
e., proctoscopic
e., proctosigmoidoscopic
e. ▸ psychiatric mental status
e., psychometric
e., radiologic
e., rectal
e., rectovaginal
e., refractive
e., regional
e., repeat
e., retina
e. revealed microaneurysm ▸
   funduscopic
e., roentgen kymographic
e., roentgenographic
e., routine
e., routine gynecological
e., routine pelvic
e., routine physical
e., school
e., screen colposcopic
e., screening physical
e., self-limited
e., sensory
e., serial
e. sheet, disposable
e., sideline
e. ▸ skin self-

e., slide
e., slit-lamp
e., speculum
e., spinal
e., sputum
e., sterile pelvic
e., sterile vaginal
e., supraclavicular
e., suprasternal
e. (TSE) ▸ testicular self-
e., tissue
e., tissue removed for pathological
e., tomographic
e., topographic
e., ultrasonography
e., ultrasound
e. under anesthesia (EUA)
e. under anesthesia, pelvic
e., urethroscopic
e., vaginorectal
e., vascular
e. ▸ vertical pattern on breast self-
e., visual field
e. ▸ wedge section pattern on breast self-

examined
e., bronchial trees
e. for hemostasis, wound
e. hormone levels
e., patient

examiner, chief medical
exanthem [*enanthem*]
e., febrile
e. subitum
e., viral

exanthema subitum
exanthematica, stomatitis
exanthematous
e. disease
e. disease virus
e. fever
e. infections

excavated, interior of tumor
excavated lesion
excavation
e., atrophic
e., dental
e., pulpal

excavatum
e., pectus
e., pes
e. repair ▸ pericardioplasty in pectus

exceedingly fast activity

exceedingly slow activity ▸ generalized
exceptional child
exceptional education
excess
e., base
e. bile pigment ▸ produce
e. blasts (RAEB) ▸ syndrome of refractory anemia with
e. earwax
e. facial hair
e. fat
e. fatty acids
e. fluid
e. fluid consumption
e. fluid drained off
e. fluid in tissue
e. fluid retention
e. ▸ fluid volume
e. hemorrhoidal tissue
e. motion in spine ▸ restricted
e. mucus secretions
e. overjet
e. production of adrenalin
e. prostate tissue
e. saliva
e. salt
e. skin
e. skin and muscle
e. stress
e. tearing
e. tissue, laser
e. tissue regrowth
e. uric acid
e. weight
e. weight loss

excessive [*extensive*]
e. accommodation
e. accumulation of glycogen
e. activity
e. activity level
e. activity of thyroid gland
e. alcohol consumption
e. alcohol use
e. alcoholic intake
e. anger
e. arguing
e. artificial respiration
e. bleeding
e. bleeding encountered
e. body rocking
e. bone loss
e. brain activity
e. breast firmness
e. breast firmness and discomfort

e. breathing
e. breathlessness
e. callus formation
e. cerumen
e. clotting
e. consumption of alcohol
e. crying
e. curvature of spine
e. daytime sleepiness
e. daytime somnolence
e. devotion to work
e. discharge of urine
e. drinking
e. drowsiness
e. drug dosage
e. emotionality
e. enlargement of head
e. exercise
e. exposure to cold
e. exposure to sun
e. facial hair growth
e. fast activity
e. fast EEG brain wave activity
e. fatigability
e. feeling of inappropriate guilt
e. flow
e. flow of saliva
e. fluid
e. fluid intake
e. fluid loss
e. foot perspiration
e. functional activity
e. gambling
e. gas formation
e. grief
e. guilt
e. hair growth
e. hair shedding
e. heat production
e. hypersynchronous discharge
e. ingestion
e. intestinal gas
e. lacrimation
e. loss of body heat
e. menstrual bleeding
e. menstruation
e. mental activity
e. movement
e. mucus
e. neuronal discharge ▸ recurring
e. or inappropriate guilt
e. orbital fat
e. perspiration
e. physical activity
e. pronation

excessive—*continued*
- e. radiation exposure
- e. rage
- e. reactivity to tendon reflexes
- e. repetitive motion on muscles
- e. scars
- e. secretion
- e. sensitivity to painful stimuli
- e. sleepiness
- e. sleeping
- e. sputum production
- e. stair climbing
- e. stress and fatigue
- e. stress and tension
- e. stretching of ventricular muscle
- e. sun exposure
- e. swayback
- e. sweating
- e. tearing
- e. tearing of eyes
- e. tears
- e. thirst
- e. tiredness
- e. urination
- e. urination at night
- e. use
- e. use of involved muscle
- e. use of sick leave
- e. voltage
- e. watering of eyes
- e. wax build-up
- e. weakness
- e. weight gain
- e. weight loss
- e. worrying

excessively
- e. conscientious
- e., drinks
- e. impressionistic ▸ speech
- e. opinionated
- e. rapid heart rate
- e. self-centered
- e. thirsty, patient

exchange
- e., abnormalities in gas
- e., air
- e., bilateral air
- e. blood transfusion
- e., bread
- e., cadaver
- e., catheter
- e. column ▸ plasma
- e., daily
- e. diet
- e., disturbance in air

- e., fat
- e., fruit
- e., gas
- e., half-time of
- e. hypothermia ▸ extracorporeal
- e., impaired gas
- e. in lung ▸ oxygen (O_2)
- e., ion
- e. ▸ living donor
- e., meat
- e., milk
- e., natural air
- e., needle
- e. ▸ needle and syringe
- e., optional
- e. ▸ paired donor
- e., plasma
- e., poor air
- e. ▸ poor pulmonary air
- e., pulmonary gas
- e. ratio, expiratory
- e. ratio, respiratory
- e. resin, anion
- e., respiratory
- e. ▸ sex for crack
- e. ▸ sodium potassium
- e. technique
- e. therapy ▸ plasma
- e. transfusion
- e., vegetable

exchanger, heat
exchanger ▸ heat/moisture
excimer
- e. cool laser
- e. gas laser
- e. laser
- e. laser angioplasty
- e. laser coronary angioplasty (ELCA)
- e. laser coronary angioplasty (PELCA) ▸ percutaneous
- e. laser recanalization
- e. laser surgery
- e. laser technique

excised
- e., adenoids
- e. cornea stored
- e. elliptically, lesion
- e., old incision
- e., skin triangle

excision(s)
- e. and wedge biopsy of breast
- e. assay
- e. benign lesion
- e. benign wart

- e., bladder
- e., elective
- e., electro◊
- e., elliptical
- e. frontal lobe of brain
- e. fulguration
- e. ganglionic cyst
- e. ▸ heel spur
- e. ischemic portion of ventricle
- e., laser
- e. lesion of spinal cord
- e., local
- e., local tumor
- e. mastectomy ▸ wide
- e., maxillary
- e., mediastinal tumor
- e. Morton's neuroma
- e. mucous membrane of cervix uteri ▸ partial
- e., multiple surgical
- e. occipital lobe of brain
- e. of adenoids
- e. of apex of tooth root
- e. of arytenoid cartilage
- e. of chalazion
- e. of choroid plexus
- e. of head of pancreas
- e. of joint
- e. of lacrimal gland
- e. of lacrimal sac
- e. of neuroma
- e. of organ ▸ surgical
- e. of portion of blood vessel
- e. of tumor, radical
- e. parietal lobe of brain
- e., partial
- e. portion chest wall
- e. procedure ▸ loop electrosurgical
- e., radical
- e., radical toenail
- e., regional
- e., scar
- e. segment of artery
- e., shave
- e., simple
- e. surgery ▸ re-
- e., surgical
- e. temporal lobe of brain
- e. ▸ tissue ablation, incision and
- e., tracheoscopy with
- e., tracheotomy with
- e., tumor
- e. tumor of brain
- e., wedge
- e., Weir

e., wide
e., wide local
e. with irradiation, local tumor
e., wound
excisional
  e. biopsy
  e. biopsy of tumor mass
  e. biopsy perianal wart
  e. biopsy, wedge
  e. breast biopsy
  e. cardiac surgery
  e. conization biopsy, laser
  e. conization, laser vaporization and
  e. conization of cervix
  e. scars
  e. scars, well healed previous
  e. surgery
  e. surgical biopsy
  e. thoracoscopy
excitability, subnormal
excitability, supranormal
excitation
  e., anomalous atrioventricular
  e., atomic
  e. contraction-coupling
  e., direct
  e., levels of brain
  e. pattern, abnormal
  e., premature
  e., supranormal
  e. ▸ ventricular pre-
  e. wave
  e. wave, pre-
excitative type psychosis
excitatory
  e. cells, cardiovascular
  e. postsynaptic potential (EPSP)
  e. state ▸ central
  e. state ▸ local
  e. synapse
  e. transmitter
excited state
excitement
  e., cerebral
  e., feelings of
  e., inhibited sexual
  e., psychomotor
  e., seeking
exciter nerve
exciting
  e. cause
  e. electrode
  e. eye
excitoreflex nerve

exclamation point hair
exclusion
  e. assay ▸ dye
  e. criteria
  e., diagnosis of
  e. of aneurysm ▸ endograft
  e. principle, Pauli's
  e. rate and clinical trials
excoriating of skin, picking and
excoriation, extremity
excoriation, neurotic
excoriativa infantum, dermatitis
excorie de jeune, acne
excrements, secreta and
excrescence
  e., bony
  e., cauliflower
  e., fungating
  e., fungous
  e., Lambl's
  e., morbid
excreta precaution
excreted through urination ▸ salt
excretes waste products
excretion(s)
  e. and secretions
  e., biliary
  e., decrease in urine
  e., decreased
  e., decreased drug
  e., demonstrable
  e. ▸ disorder of urinary
  e., eicosanoid
  e. ▸ endolymph filtration and
  e., fecal
  e., fecal fat
  e., increasing urinary
  e. index (PEI) ▸ phosphate
  e. nitrogen
  e. of contrast material
  e. of contrast material ▸ prompt
  e. of contrast media ▸ poor
  e. of dye
  e. of dye, prompt
  e. of protein, increased
  e. of sodium in urine, over-
  e., pulmonary
  e. pyelography
  e. rate, aldosterone
  e. ratio, urea
  e., renal
  e., Schilling test for urine
  e. ▸ significant variation in pattern of
  e. test, breath
  e., total estrogen

e., urinary
e., urinary amylase
e., urinary sodium
e., vicarious
excretory [*expiratory, respiratory*]
  e. capacity, maximal tubular
  e. cystogram (XC)
  e. duct
  e. duct of eye
  e. function of body, loss of
  e. pyelogram
  e. system
  e. urethrogram
  e. urogram (XU)
  e. urogram, constant infusion
  e. urography
  e. urography ▸ rapid sequence
excrucians, Aedes
excruciating
  e. chest pain
  e. headache ▸ recurrent
  e. pain
excursion(s)
  e., chest
  e., costal
  e., diaphragmatic
  e., diminished, chest
  e., diminished contractile
  e., dome
  e., expansion and
  e. free and equal
  e. ▸ lateral protrusive
  e., left ventricular posterior wall
  e. of ataxic gait ▸ diminish
  e. of diaphragm
  e. of joint
  e., posterior wall
  e., protrusive
  e., respiratory
  e., retrusive
excurvatum, pectus
excuses ▸ patient provides
executant ego function
executive
  e. function test
  e. physical evaluation
  e. physical examination
exemptions, civil liability
exenteration
  e., anterior pelvic
  e. of orbital contents
  e. of sinus
  e., pelvic organ
  e., posterior pelvic
  e., total pelvic

exercise(s)
- e., abdominal
- e., abdominal crunch/curl-up
- e., abduction
- e., active
- e., active assisted
- e., active bending
- e., active quad strengthening
- e., active resistive
- e., advanced
- e., adverse
- e., aerobic
- e., aerobic aquatic
- e., aggressive
- e., anaerobic
- e. and diet
- e. and fitness
- e. and meditating ► stretching
- e. and weight reduction
- e., ankle
- e. ► ankle alphabet
- e., appetite and
- e., aquatic
- e., arm
- e., arm curl
- e., arm lift
- e. ► arm raise
- e., autogenic training relaxation
- e. ► avoid strain in
- e., back and chest
- e., back strengthening
- e., balance
- e. balance ► rest and
- e. -based rehabilitation program
- e., bench press
- e., bent leg crunch
- e., biceps curl
- e., body-building
- e., bouncing
- e., brainstorming
- e., breathing
- e. ► breathing and relaxation
- e. bulimia
- e., calf-heel stretch
- e., calf stretch
- e. capacity
- e. cardiogram
- e., cardiovascular
- e., cardiovascular aerobic
- e., chair sit-up
- e. ► chair stand
- e., chest press
- e., chest stretch
- e., Codman
- e. ► condition muscles with aerobic

- e., conditioning
- e., convergent
- e., cool down relaxation
- e. ► coordinate breathing with
- e., corrective
- e., coughing
- e. craze
- e. cycle
- e., daily moderate
- e., daily relaxation
- e., deep breathing
- e. deficiency
- e. ► desensitizing movement
- e. digital subtraction ventriculography
- e., diminished
- e., dynamic
- e. (DOE), dyspnea on
- e. echocardiogram
- e. echocardiogram, continuous loop
- e. echocardiography
- e. efficiency
- e., elbow extension
- e., elbow pronation
- e., elbow supination
- e. electrocardiogram (EKG/ECG)
- e., elevation
- e. ► elongation stretch
- e., endurance
- e. equilibrium radionuclide ventriculography ► rest-
- e. equipment
- e., excessive
- e., extension
- e., eye
- e. facility
- e. factor
- e., finger
- e., finger extension
- e., finger flexion
- e., finger opposition
- e., flexibility
- e. flexibility stretches ► post-
- e., flexion
- e. for enhancing social skills ► group
- e. for heart patient
- e. for patient in home
- e. for reminiscence ► therapeutic
- e. for remotivation ► therapeutic
- e. for validation ► therapeutic
- e., forward bending
- e., free
- e., full

- e., full weight bearing
- e. -gated nuclear angiography ► rest and
- e., gentle
- e. ► gentle range of motion
- e. ► gentle stretching
- e. ► golf ball roll foot
- e. ► hamstring stretch
- e., hand
- e. ► hatha yoga
- e., heart helping
- e., heart rate
- e. heart scan ► Thallium
- e. ► heel squat
- e. ► high impact
- e. ► high impact aerobic
- e., high intensity
- e., hip adductor stretch
- e., hydrotherapeutic
- e. hyperemia blood flow
- e., hyperextension
- e. imaging
- e., improper
- e. ► inability to
- e. index
- e. -induced amenorrhea
- e. -induced angina
- e. -induced arrhythmia
- e. -induced asthma (EIA)
- e. -induced bronchospasm
- e. -induced heart attack
- e. -induced hives
- e. -induced shortness of breath (SOB)
- e. -induced silent myocardial ischemia
- e. -induced sterility
- e. -induced urticaria
- e. -induced ventricular tachycardia
- e. -induced weight loss
- e., intensive
- e., interactive
- e. intolerance
- e., isokinetic
- e., isometric
- e. ► isometric handgrip
- e., isometric quad strengthening
- e., isotonic
- e., Kegel
- e. ► knee bend
- e. ► knee lift squat
- e., lack of
- e., lack of physical
- e., land-based
- e., lateral bending

e., leg
e., leg curl
e., leg press
e. level
e. load
e. ▸ long-term
e. ▸ low back flattener
e. ▸ low back stretch
e., low impact
e., low intensity
e., low risk
e., low stress
e., lower back extension
e. ▸ lower back stretch
e. ▸ marble pickup toe
e., maximal
e., memory
e., mental
e., minimal
e., moderate
e. ▸ moderate intensity
e. monitor ▸ transtelephonic
e., motion
e. ▸ muscle relaxation
e., muscle-setting
e. ▸ muscle strengthening
e., muscular
e., muscular control
e. ▸ muscular endurance
e. ▸ neck strengthening
e., neck stretching
e., neuromuscular control
e., obsessive
e. of function
e. of will
e. oxygen (O₂) consumption ▸ peak
e., passive
e., patient dieting with
e., patient taught leg
e., peak
e. ▸ pelvic floor muscle
e., pelvic muscle
e., pelvic tilt
e., pendulum
e. performance ▸ impairing
e. perfusion scanning
e., perineal
e., physical
e. physiologist
e. physiology
e., postsurgery
e. ▸ power and endurance
e., prenatal
e., prescribed
e. prescription

e. program
e. program, balanced
e. program ▸ diet-and-
e. program, home
e. program, moderate
e. program, specialized
e. program ▸ supervised
e. program ▸ vigorous
e. program ▸ vigorous in-flight
e. program, written home
e. progression, gradual
e., progressive
e., progressive resistant quadriceps
e. ▸ prolonged vigorous
e. ▸ proper nutrition and
e. protocol, Cornell
e., pull down
e., pulmonary
e. ▸ push-out
e., quad
e., quad strengthening
e., quadriceps
e., quadriceps extension
e., quadriceps stretch
e. radionuclide angiocardiography
e. ▸ range-of-motion
e., rapid
e., Regen's flexion
e. regime
e. regimen, regular
e., regular
e., regular aerobic
e. ▸ regular physical
e. ▸ regular weight bearing
e., rehabilitative
e. ▸ rehydrate after
e., relaxation
e. ▸ relaxation therapy
e., repetitive
e., resistance
e., resistive
e. (R and E), rest and
e. ▸ rest and rehabilitation
e., rhythmic
e. risk
e. room
e., rotation
e., rotational
e., routine
e., routine, strict
e. ▸ sand walking foot
e. schedule
e. ▸ seated rowing
e. shoes
e. ▸ shoulder abduction

e. ▸ shoulder adduction
e., shoulder elevation
e. ▸ shoulder external rotation
e. ▸ shoulder flexion
e. ▸ shoulder internal rotation
e., shoulder press
e. ▸ shoulder shrug
e. ▸ shoulder squeeze
e., shoulder stretch
e. ▸ side bend
e. ▸ side leg raise
e., simple
e. ▸ sit up
e. ▸ slow stretching
e. specialist
e. ▸ squat and lunge
e., squatting
e., static
e. ▸ stop-and-start
e. ▸ strength training
e., strengthening
e. ▸ strengthening and flexibility
e., strenuous
e. stress echocardiography
e. stress test
e. stress test, aerobic
e. stress test, arm
e. stress test ▸ Astrand bicycle
e. stress test, Balke
e. stress test, bicycle ergometer
e. stress test, Blake
e. stress test, Bruce
e. stress test, EKG
  (electrocardiogram)
e. stress test ▸ Ellestad
e. stress test ▸ Gradational Step
e. stress test ▸ Kattus
e. stress test ▸ Physical Work
  Capacity
e. stress test ▸ Sheffield
e. stress test ▸ single-stage
e. stress test ▸ treadmill
e., stressful
e., stretching
e. ▸ stretching and breathing
e. ▸ stretching and releasing
e. study
e. study, normal
e. study ▸ rest and
e. ▸ sudden death during
e., supine
e. ▸ tension relieving
e. test ▸ baseline
e. test, Bruce protocol

exercise(s)—*continued*
- e. test, cardiopulmonary
- e. test, Davidson protocol
- e. test, graded
- e. test ▸ Master "2-step"
- e. test ▸ Master two-step
- e. test ▸ negative
- e. test ▸ radioactive thallium
- e. test ▸ symptom-limited treadmill
- e. test ▸ two-step
- e. testing
- e. therapy
- e. thallium scintigraphy
- e. thallium test
- e. thallium 201 scintigraphy
- e., therapeutic
- e., thermogenic effect
- e. ▸ thigh stretch
- e. time
- e. to rehabilitate injured area
- e. ▸ toe curl
- e. ▸ toe heel raise
- e. ▸ toe point
- e. ▸ toe pull
- e. ▸ toe raise
- e. ▸ toe squeeze
- e. ▸ toe strengthening
- e. ▸ toe touch
- e. tolerance
- e. tolerance test (ETT)
- e. ▸ towel curl toe
- e. training ▸ supervised
- e., treadmill
- e. treadmill test
- e. treadmill time
- e. treatment
- e., triceps extension
- e. ▸ trunk curls
- e. ▸ tummy crunch
- e. ultrasound ▸ pre-
- e., underwater
- e., upper body
- e. ▸ upper thigh stretch
- e. ventriculography
- e., vestibular
- e., vigorous
- e. ▸ vigorous maternal
- e., visual
- e. ▸ visual imagery
- e. walking
- e. walking technique, proper
- e. ▸ wall push-up
- e., warm-up
- e., water
- e., weight-bearing

- e. ▸ weight loss and
- e. ▸ weight training
- e. ▸ weighted squat
- e., whirlpool
- e., Williams'
- e., Williams' flexion
- e., winter
- e. ▸ Yoga derived

exercised, flexibility
exerciser, cardiovascular
exerciser, dynamic finger
exercising
- e., cool-down
- e., patient
- e. regularly

exert force
exertion (Exertion)
- e., chest pain on
- e., dyspnea on
- e., heavy
- e., increased
- e., increased dyspnea on
- e., intellectual
- e. ▸ level of
- e. level ▸ peak
- e., minimal
- e., muscle
- e. ▸ pain and
- e., pain related to
- e., perceived
- e., physical
- e., precipitated by
- e. (RPE) ▸ ratings of perceived
- E. Scale (BPES), Borg Perceived
- E. Scale (BTES), Borg Treadmill
- E. Scale (PES) ▸ Perceived
- e., selective
- e., shortness of breath on
- e. test, perceived
- e., wheezing and dyspnea with

exertional
- e. activity
- e. activity, heavy
- e. angina
- e. asthma
- e. chest discomfort
- e. chest pain
- e. defibrillation
- e. dyspnea
- e. dyspnea, one-flight
- e. dyspnea ▸ two-flight
- e. fatigue
- e. headache
- e. in nature, chest pain
- e. rhabdomyolysis

- e. syncope
- e. weakness

exfoliation
- e. of lens capsule
- e. of newborn ▸ lamellar
- e. process

exfoliativa, cheilitis
exfoliativa infantum, dermatitis
exfoliative
- e. cytology
- e. dermatitis
- e. endometritis
- e. erythroderma
- e. gastritis
- e. skin
- e. skin disease

exhalation, forced
exhaled air
exhausted
- e., chronically
- e. consciousness
- e., emotionally
- e., patient
- e., physically
- e., weak and debilitated

exhausting, mentally
exhaustion
- e., adaptive
- e., anhidrotic heat
- e. ▸ anxiety from heat
- e. atrophy
- e., burnout and heart disease
- e., chronic nervous
- e., combat
- e., complete
- e. ▸ dehydration and
- e. delirium
- e., emotional
- e., extreme
- e., fatigue leading to
- e., heat
- e., mental
- e., nervous
- e., overwhelming
- e., physical
- e. psychosis
- e. psychosis, infection
- e., reaction of
- e., strain or
- e., total
- e., type II heat

exhibited muscle guarding ▸ patient
exhibitionism, narcissistic
exhibitionist, patient
exhibitionist type ▸ voyeur

exhibitionistic tendencies
exhibits
- e. constant movement
- e. dramatic gestures
- e. emotional problems
- e. hunger behavior, infant
- e. irritable negativism
- e. nonsensical speech
- e. overt hostility ▸ patient
- e. road rage
- e. spasticity, patient

exiguus, Saccharomyces
existential
- e. anxiety
- e. dilemma
- e. neurosis
- e. psychiatry

existing
- e. bipolar disorder ▸ pre-
- e. condition ▸ pre-
- e. coronary disease ▸ pre-
- e. drug therapy ▸ re-evaluation of
- e. hepatic disease ▸ pre-
- e. illness, pre-
- e. infection ▸ control
- e. psychiatric illness ▸ exacerbation of pre-
- e. psychosis
- e. renal damage ▸ pre-
- e. temporal bone fracture ▸ pre-

exit
- e. block murmur
- e. block ▸ sinoatrial (SA)
- e. block, sinus
- e. dose
- e. pause ▸ sinus
- e. point
- e. point of radiation beam
- e. wound

exitable gap
exocardial murmur
exoccipital bone
exochorial pregnancy
exocrine
- e. function, pancreatic
- e. function test ▸ pancreatic
- e. functional reserves
- e. gland
- e. insufficiency
- e. insufficiency ▸ mild chronic pancreatic
- e. insufficiency ▸ moderate chronic pancreatic
- e. insufficiency, pancreatic
- e. pancreatic insufficiency

- e. secretion, pancreatic
- e. secretion tests ▸ pancreatic
- e. tissue

exodic nerve
exoergic reaction
exoerythrocytic plasmodium
exogenous
- e. aneurysm
- e. antigen
- e. contamination
- e. cycle
- e. estrogen
- e. flora
- e. group of microorganisms
- e. hyperthyroidism
- e. infection
- e. interferon
- e. lipid
- e. obesity
- e. ochronosis
- e. sources, contamination of
- e. sources of infection
- e. sporulation
- e. steroid administration
- e. toxic agent

exophoria, alternating
exophoria, constant
exophthalmic goiter
exophthalmic ophthalmoplegia
exophthalmica, cachexia
exophthalmica ▸ tachycardia strumosa
exophthalmometer, Hertel's
exophthalmometer, Luedde's
exophthalmos
- e. due to pressure
- e. due to tower skull
- e. hyperthyroid factor
- e. producing factor
- e. producing substance

exophytic carcinoma
exophytic-type growth
exophytum, glioma
exopolysaccharide, mucoid
exore, fetor
exostosis(-es)
- e., bone
- e. bursata
- e. cartilaginea
- e., dental
- e., dorsal
- e. formation
- e., hereditary multiple
- e., ivory
- e., multiple

- e., multiple cartilaginous
- e., osteocartilaginous
- e., osteochondral

exotoxin, Pseudomonas
exotropia [*esotropia*]
- e., alternating
- e., Krimsky measurements for
- e., left
- e., periodic
- e., right

expand internal components of knee
expand narrowed valve
expandable
- e. breast implant
- e. intravascular stent, balloon
- e. stent ▸ heat

expanded
- e. cell production
- e. lungs
- e., lungs adequately
- e., lungs poorly

expander(s)
- e., blood
- e., breast tissue
- e. ▸ Hespan plasma volume
- e. ▸ hetastarch plasma
- e., plasma
- e., plasma volume
- e., tissue
- e., volume

expanding
- e. blood vessel
- e. cellular systems
- e. stent ▸ self-

expands
- e. adequately bilaterally ▸ chest
- e. equally bilaterally ▸ chest
- e., left hemithorax
- e., right hemithorax

expansile lytic lesion
expansile pulsation
expansion
- e. adequate bilaterally ▸ chest
- e. adequate, lung
- e. and excursion
- e., chest
- e. equal bilaterally ▸ chest
- e., good chest
- e., infarct
- e., intravascular volume
- e., lung
- e. ▸ lungs revealed decreased
- e. of blood vessels ▸ abnormal
- e. of chest ▸ diminished
- e. of chest ▸ restricted

expansion—*continued*
- e. of lung
- e. of lung ▸ active
- e. of lungs ▸ full
- e. of lungs ▸ limited
- e. ▸ restricted chest
- e., stent
- e., systolic
- e., tissue
- e., vein

expansive delusion

expansive, paraphrenia

expectancy
- e., alcohol
- e., extended life
- e. factor
- e., life
- e., limit life
- e. ▸ remissions, relapses and
- e. wave

expectant parents

expectant parents class

expectation (Expectation)
- e. ▸ high self-
- e. neurosis
- e. of others ▸ unreasonable
- e., pain determined by
- E. Score

expected
- e. date of confinement (EDC/EDOC)
- e. intervention strategy
- e. life span
- e. peak heart rate

expectorant [*expectorate*]
- e., cough
- e., liquefying
- e., stimulant
- e., Stokes'

expectorated sputum

expectorated sputum studies

expectoration
- e., bloody
- e., cough and
- e., mucoid
- e. of blood
- e., productive coughing and

expelled
- e., afterbirth
- e., fetus
- e. flatus, patient
- e., infant
- e., placenta
- e. ▸ total ventricular blood

expelling function

expenditure, total calorie

experience(s)
- e. ▸ aerobic and strength-building
- e., clinical
- e., clinical adverse
- e. criteria ▸ previous treatment
- e., dissociated
- e., dissociative
- e. ▸ distressing psychedelic
- e. emotional outbursts ▸ patient
- e. flashbacks ▸ patient
- e., hallucinatory
- e., hallucinatory emotional
- e., insightful
- e., latency
- e., learning
- e. (NDE) ▸ near-death
- e. of, cumulative
- e. (OBE) ▸ out-of-body
- e., patient care
- e., previous treatment
- e., psychedelic
- e. ▸ recall of traumatic
- e. remissions and exacerbations of pain ▸ patient
- e., self-object
- e., sexual
- e., sexually abusive
- e., stressful
- e., subjective
- e. symptoms
- e., traumatic
- e. ▸ traumatic childhood
- e., unrecognized past
- e. weakness, patient

experienced facilitator

experiencing
- e. problems
- e. withdrawal symptoms
- e. withdrawal symptoms ▸ patient

experiential (Experiential)
- e. and ego analytic approach ▸ strategic,
- e. resilience
- e. understanding
- E. World Inventory (EWI)

experiment(s)
- e., clinical
- e., controlled
- e., double-blind
- e., drug
- e., placebo controlled
- e., Valsalva's

experimental
- e. allergic encephalomyelitis

- e. anxiety
- e. basis
- e. breast cancer treatment
- e. cancer therapy
- e. cancer vaccine
- e. chemotherapeutic agent
- e. conditions
- e. data
- e. designs
- e. drug
- e. drug protocol
- e. drug use
- e. embryology
- e. enterococcal endocarditis
- e. laser surgery
- e. medicine
- e. pharmacology
- e. procedure
- e. psychology
- e. social psychology
- e. stage
- e. studies
- e. surgery
- e. therapeutics
- e. therapy
- e. therapy, best-chance
- e. therapy, last-chance
- e. treatment
- e. treatment program
- e. vaccine
- e. validation

experimentation, drug

expert, medical

expertise, clinical

expertise, medical

expiration [*exploration, extirpation*]
- e., agonal
- e. and inspiration
- e. ▸ duration of
- e., forced
- e., inhalation and
- e. -inspiration ratio
- e. of air ▸ alternate inspiration and
- e. ▸ prolongation of
- e., prolongation of air flow during
- e., prolonged
- e., strongest

expiratory [*excretory, respiratory*]
- e. capacity ▸ forced
- e. curve
- e. disease, positive end
- e. dyspnea
- e. exchange ratio
- e. flow
- e. flow (FEF) ▸ forced

e. flow (MEF) ▸ maximal
e. flow (MFEF) ▸ maximal forced
e. flow (MMEF) ▸ maximum mid-
e. flow (PEF) ▸ peak
e. flow rate
e. flow rate (MEFR) ▸ maximal
e. flow rate (MMEFR) ▸ maximal mid-
e. flow rate (MEFR) ▸ maximum
e. flow rate (MMEFR) ▸ maximum mid-
e. flow rate (PEFR) ▸ peak
e. flow volume (MEFV) ▸ maximal
e. grunting
e. murmur
e. pause, end-
e. positive airway pressure
e. pressure management
e. pressure ▸ negative end-
e. pressure plateau (PEPP) ▸ positive
e. pressure ▸ positive-
e. pressure (PEEP), positive end
e. pressure ▸ zero-end
e. (I/E) ratio ▸ inspiratory-
e. reserve volume (ERV)
e. retard
e. rhonchi
e. sounds
e. spirogram, forced
e. standstill
e. time (FET) ▸ forced
e. trapping of air
e. volume (FEV) ▸ forced
e. volume in one second ▸ forced
e. wheezes
e. wheezing

expired
e. air collection
e. carbon dioxide (FECO$_2$) ▸ fraction of
e. due to natural causes ▸ patient
e. following resuscitation attempt ▸ baby
e. in sleep ▸ patient
e., patient
e. quietly, patient
e. suddenly, patient
e., time patient
e. unexpectedly, patient

expirography, Godart
explanation of benefits (EOB)
explanation, psychodynamic
explanted heart
exploding, patient

exploitation of others, conscious
exploitation of others ▸ unwitting
exploitative ▸ irresponsible and
exploitative, patient
exploitativeness, interpersonal
exploited children, missing and
exploits others
exploration [*expiration, extirpation*]
e., abdominal
e., and feedback ▸ discussion
e., arteriotomy with
e., bile duct
e., bladder
e., common duct
e., liver
e., manual
e. of abdomen ▸ manual
e. of brain
e. of meninges
e. of nerve
e. of traumatic scenes
e., sclerotomy with
e., spinal cord
e., surgical
e., thoracotomy with
e., uterine
e., visual
e., wound

exploratory
e. biopsy
e., deep wound
e. incision
e. laparotomy
e. meatoantrotomy
e. puncture
e. surgery
e. surgical management
e. thoracotomy
e. treatment
e. tympanotomy
e. volume (FEV) ▸ forced

explored
e., abdomen
e., abdomen entered and
e., wound superficially

exploring electrode
explosion-proof suction unit
explosive
e. decompression
e. disorder, intermittent
e. disorder, isolated
e. personality
e. personality disorder

e. personality disorder ▸ intermittent
e. speech
e. stool
e. temper

explosiveness, emotional
exponential decay
exposed
e. baby, drug
e., bone
e. by blunt dissection ▸ kidney freed and
e., capsule
e., esophagus
e., hilar vessels
e. human infants, cocaine-
e., kidney
e. kids, drug
e., mediastinal pleura
e. offspring, drug-
e. surface
e. to asbestos, patient
e. to HIV
e. to tuberculosis ▸ patient
e., trachea
e., ureter

exposing peritoneum
exposing plaque to cutting mechanism
exposure .
e., accidental
e. and response prevention (ERP)
e., asbestos
e., automated
e., chronic alcohol
e., chronic sun
e., chronic ultraviolet
e., cocaine
e., cold
e., cue
e. ▸ cumulative effects of unprotected sun
e., electromagnetic field
e., excessive radiation
e., extreme prolonged
e. ▸ eye mucosal
e., film
e., imaginal
e., in vivo
e., incidental
e. ▸ intrauterine drug
e., lead
e., long-term
e. ▸ long-term alcohol

exposure—*continued*
- e. ▸ long-term ultraviolet
- e., low level
- e., malpractice liability
- e., minimal dust
- e., mucous membrane
- e., needle stick
- e., nursery
- e. obtained, good
- e. obtained, limited
- e., occupational
- e., organic dust
- e., passive smoke
- e., patient at high risk of
- e., percutaneous
- e., prenatal alcohol
- e. ▸ prenatal cocaine
- e., prolonged or repeated
- e., radiation
- e. rate constant
- e. rate constant, filtered
- e., recent
- e. relationship of film, density-
- e., risk of
- e., seasonal
- e. standards
- e., sun
- e., sunlight
- e. system, automatic
- e. technique, heavy
- e. therapy
- e. ▸ threshold amount of asbestos
- e. to allergens
- e. to asbestos
- e. to asbestos ▸ extensive
- e. to blood or body fluid
- e. to chemicals
- e. to chemicals ▸ occupational
- e. to cold ▸ excessive
- e. to germ ▸ initial
- e. to heat stress, brief
- e. to industrial substances
- e. to irritants
- e. to passive smoke
- e. to radiation
- e. to radium
- e. to sun, excessive
- e. to sunlight
- e. to toxic substance
- e. to toxins
- e. to ultraviolet light
- e. to virus
- e. transfusion (MET) ▸ minimal
- e. ▸ ultraviolet (UV)
- e., x-ray

express fluid buildup
expressed
- e. emotion
- e. emotion, family
- e. from breast ▸ colostrum
- e. from ventricle, air
- e. from wounds, clots
- e. guilt feelings ▸ patient
- e. in kilohms
- e. in megohms
- e. in ohms
- e., lens material
- e. sequence tags
- e. skull fracture

expression
- e., activates facial
- e., affective
- e. and reception
- e., blocking oncogene
- e., cardiac gene
- e. cystourethrography
- e., early
- e., emotional
- e., facial
- e., fixed facial
- e. ▸ fixed staring
- e. folds line
- e., gene
- e., involuntary facial
- e., Kristeller
- e. ▸ lack of facial
- e. ▸ loss of emotional
- e. ▸ loss of facial
- e., manual
- e. ▸ mask-like
- e. of anger
- e. of anger ▸ permitting safe
- e. of emotions ▸ exaggerated
- e. of emotions ▸ restricted
- e. of emotions ▸ shallow
- e. of language, verbal
- e. ▸ positive emotional
- e., ruminative
- e., verbal
- e., written

expressionless face ▸ blank
expressive
- e. ability
- e. aphasia
- e. aphasia, motor
- e. apraxia
- e. disorder
- e. language disorder ▸ developmental
- e. language function

- e. mode
- e. -receptive aphasia
- e. therapy
- e. therapy ▸ supportive
- e. writing disorder ▸ developmental

expulsion
- e. breathing
- e. contraction
- e., transition and

expulsive
- e. coughing
- e. hemorrhage
- e. pains
- e. stage

exquisite pain
exsanguinated of blood, extremity
exsanguinating hemorrhage
exsanguinating intraperitoneal hemorrhage
exsanguination protocol
exstrophy of bladder
extended
- e. anteriorly, arm
- e. care facility
- e. dissection
- e. dissection for thoracic cancer
- e. examination
- e. family
- e., head
- e., knee
- e. legs rigidly
- e. life expectancy
- e. medical treatment
- e. position, head and neck in
- e. -spectrum penicillin
- e. wear contact lens
- e. wear soft lens

extender, life
extenders, tissue
extends down legs ▸ back pain
extends knee completely
extensibility line, minimum
extension(s)
- e., abnormal
- e., active finger
- e. and flexion
- e., angle of greatest
- e., Bardenheuer's
- e., basilar
- e. bridge
- e., Buck's
- e., Codivilla's
- e., degrees of
- e. exercise
- e. exercise, elbow

e. exercise, finger
e. exercise, lower back
e. exercise, quadriceps
e., extranodal
e., flexion and
e., forceful
e., full
e. ▸ full range of flexion and
e., glottic
e., hand held in position of
e., head
e., hip
e. in stroke patients ▸ increase active
e., infarct
e., knee
e., lateral
e., leg
e., limitation of
e. limited to ___
e., maximum
e., nail
e. of cerebral infarct
e. of great toe
e. of myocardial infarction (MI)
e. of neck
e. of toes
e. of tumor cells
e. of tumor ▸ direct
e. per contiguitatem
e. per continuitatem
e. per saltam
e. position
e. projection flexion-
e., ridge
e., Steinmann's
e. study, lumbar flexion and
e. test, fabere
e. traction, Buck's
e., triceps

extensive [*excessive*]
e. acute necrosis
e. aspiration pneumonia
e. bilateral sloughing infiltrates
e. bile stasis
e. bone mass
e. comminution
e. debridement
e. denudation of distal esophagus
e. disease
e. exposure to asbestos
e. fecal impaction
e. fibrosis of portal tracts
e. hearing assessment
e. hemorrhage bronchial mucosa

e. hyaline membrane disease
e. infiltrations
e. inflammatory bowel disease
e. inoperable carcinoma
e. interstitial fibrosis
e. intra-abdominal metastases
e. manipulation of joint
e. medical examination
e. metastatic disease
e. metastatic involvement
e. new bone formation
e. penetration
e. pleural involvement
e. radiotherapy
e. resection
e. residual tumor
e. scarring
e. skin loss
e. tests
e. treatment programs
e. tumor deposits

extensively mottled, myocardium
extensor
e. carpi radialis brevis muscle
e. carpi radialis longus muscle
e. carpi ulnaris muscle
e. digiti minimi muscle
e. digiti quinti proprius muscle
e. digitorum brevis muscle
e. digitorum communis muscle
e. digitorum longus muscle
e. hallucis brevis muscle
e. hallucis longus muscle
e. indicis muscle
e. indicis proprius
e. muscle of digits ▸ common
e. muscle of fifth digit ▸ proper
e. muscle of fingers
e. muscle of great toe ▸ long
e. muscle of great toe ▸ short
e. muscle of index finger
e. muscle of little finger
e. muscle of thumb ▸ long
e. muscle of thumb ▸ short
e. muscle of toes ▸ long
e. muscle of toes ▸ short
e. plantar response
e. pollicis brevis muscle
e. pollicis brevis, musculus
e. pollicis brevis tendon
e. pollicis longus muscle
e. pollicis longus, musculus
e. reflex, quadrupedal
e. responses, plantar
e. synergy

e. tendon
e. tendon, short
e., toe
extent
e. of injury or illness ▸ evaluate
e., tumor
e., tumor border
exterior gestation
exterior pelvic device
exteriorization ▸ extra-abdominal uterine
exteriorizing uterus
externa
e., auris
e., endometriosis
e. et interna, pericarditis
e., lamina
e., mastoiditis
e., ophthalmoplegia
external
e. abdominal region
e. abnormalities
e. acoustic meatus
e. acoustic meatus ▸ nerve of
e. acute medical care facility
e. angle of mandible
e. arcuate fibers ▸ anterior
e. aspect
e. asynchronous pacemaker
e. auditory canal (EAC)
e. auditory meatus (EAM)
e. beam, definitive
e. beam irradiation
e. beam radiation
e. beam therapy
e. canal
e. canthus
e. canthus electrode
e. canthus, left-right
e. cardiac compression maneuvers
e. cardiac massage
e. cardioverter
e. cardioverter defibrillator
e. cardioverter defibrillator ▸ Medtronic
e. carotid artery
e. carotid nerves
e. carotid vein
e. chest compression
e. clock time
e. cobalt irradiation
e. compression
e. confusion
e. conjugate diameter
e. connection

external—*continued*
- e. controls, dependence on
- e. counterpressure
- e. counterpulsation
- e. counterpulsation (EECP) ▸ enhanced
- e. counterpulsation (EECP) therapy ▸ enhanced
- e. counterpulsation unit ▸ enhanced
- e. defibrillator
- e. defibrillator (AED), automated
- e. defibrillator (AED), automatic
- e. defibrillator (AED) ▸ SurVivaLink automated
- e. demand pacemaker
- e. description
- e. description, autopsy
- e. ear
- e. ear canal
- e. ear canal, inflammation of
- e. elastic membrane
- e. electrical interference
- e. electrode
- e. electronic stimulator
- e. events
- e. examination
- e. examination, autopsy
- e. factor
- e. factors ▸ patient's condition precipitated by
- e. fixation
- e. fixation of fracture
- e. genitalia
- e. grid
- e. hemorrhage
- e. hemorrhoid
- e. hemorrhoidectomy
- e. hernia
- e. humeral epicondylitis
- e. iliac artery
- e. iliac lymph nodes
- e. iliac vein
- e. impulsive form
- e. inguinal ring
- e. injuries
- e. insulin pump
- e. intercostal muscles
- e. interference
- e. -internal pacemaker
- e. irradiation
- e. irradiation, high dose
- e. irradiation therapy
- e. irradiation, volume treated in
- e. jugular vein
- e. landmarks

- e. ligament of malleus
- e. lobation
- e. loop recorder
- e. malleolus
- e. mammary artery
- e. mammary veins
- e. mastoid process
- e. meatus
- e. meningitis
- e. musculature
- e. naris
- e. nasal splint
- e. nasal veins
- e. nose deformity
- e. oblique
- e. oblique fascia
- e. oblique muscle
- e. oblique muscle of abdomen
- e. obturator muscle
- e. occipital protuberance
- e. ophthalmoplegia, chronic
- e. ophthalmoplegia, progressive
- e. orifice
- e. os
- e. os, blood exuding from
- e. otitis
- e. otitis ▸ invasive
- e. otitis ▸ malignant
- e. pacemaker
- e. palatine vein
- e. popliteal nerve
- e. pressure circulatory assist (EPCA)
- e. pterygoid muscle
- e. pterygoid nerve
- e. pudendal vein
- e. radial vein of Soemmering
- e. radiation
- e. radiation dosimetry
- e. radiation therapy
- e. rectus muscle ▸ advancement
- e. resistance
- e. respiration
- e. rotation
- e. rotation, abduction, stress test
- e. rotation exercise ▸ shoulder
- e. rotation test, fabere
- e. secretion of pancreas
- e. secretory activity of pancreas
- e. sensation
- e. sensory stimulation
- e. situation
- e. skull
- e. spermatic fascia
- e. spermatic nerve

- e. sphincter contraction
- e. sphincter muscle
- e. sphincter muscle of anus
- e. sphincter ▸ spasm of
- e. stimulation
- e. stimuli
- e. stimuli ▸ responsiveness to
- e. stimuli ▸ threatening
- e. stimulus, remote
- e. strabismus
- e. strangulation
- e. structure ▸ loss of
- e. substance of suprarenal gland
- e. therapy
- e. tokodynamometer
- e. transducer
- e. ultrasonic liposuction
- e. urethral orifice
- e. urethral resistance
- e. urethral sphincterotomy
- e. version

externally rotated
externi, urethritis orificii
externo incision ▸ ab-
externum, pericardium
externus, ab
extinction
- e. of drug-abusing behavior
- e., rapid
- e. techniques

extirpation [*exploration, expiration*]
extirpation of uterus and cervix
extra
- e. abdominal uterine exteriorization
- e. -alveolar crown
- e. -alveolar vessels
- e. -anatomic bypass
- e. digit
- e. heart sound
- e. -psychic conflict
- e. sounds
- e. stimulus, double
- e. stimulus ▸ double ventricular

extrabuccal feeding
extracanthic diameter
extracapsular
- e. cataract extraction
- e. fracture
- e. surgery

extracardiac murmur
extracardiac shunt
extracellular
- e. bean-shaped diplococci ▸ gram-negative
- e. cholestasis of liver

e. collagen matrix
e. fluid
e. fluid volume
e. fluid volume ▸ functional
e. kidney-shaped diplococci ▸ gram-negative
e. lipid
e. material
e. matrix
e. organisms
e. penicillinase
e. proteins
e. space
e. tissue
e. virus, free
e. volume
e. water

extracerebral
e. cavernous angioma
e. factors
e. potential
e. source

extrachromosomal material
extracorporeal
e. circulation
e. exchange hypothermia
e. heart
e. irradiation of blood
e. irradiation of lymph
e. life support
e. membrane oxygenation (ECMO)
e. membrane oxygenator
e. perfusion
e. pump
e. renal surgery
e. shock wave
e. shock wave lithotripsy (ESWL)

extracorticalis congenita ▸ aplasia axialis
extracostal bundles
extracostal muscles
extracranial
e. cardiac disease
e. carotid arterial disease
e. disease
e. -intracranial brain bypass

extract
e., adipose tissue
e., adrenocortical
e., anterior pituitary
e., charcoal yeast
e. of cannabis (SMASH), acetone
e., pancreatic
e., parathyroid
e., pituitary

e., Rauwolfia
e. surfactant, bovine lavage
e., thyroid

extractable
e. iodine (BEI), butanol-
e. nuclear antibodies (ENA)
e. nuclear antigen
e. tracer technique

extracted
e. in tumbling fashion ▸ lens
e., lens
e., placenta

extraction
e. atherectomy device
e. atherectomy ▸ transluminal
e., blind basket
e., breech
e., cataract
e., cryocataract
e., cryogenic cataract
e., dental
e., dry socket ▸ tooth
e. endarterectomy ▸ transluminal
e., extracapsular cataract
e., foreign body (FB)
e., full mouth
e., intracapsular cataract
e., lactate
e., magnetic
e., menstrual
e. of cataract
e. of cataract ▸ extracapsular
e. of cataract ▸ intracapsular
e. of teeth
e. operative delivery, vacuum
e., partial breech
e. reserve
e. residue (MER), methanol
e., serial
e., tooth
e., total breech
e., water

extradural
e. anesthesia
e. block
e. compression
e. cord compression
e. defect
e. hematoma
e. hemorrhage
e. laminectomy
e. metastatic disease

extraembryonic ectoderm
extraesophageal reflux
extrafascial hysterectomy

Extrafil breast implant
extrafusion defect
extragenital teratoma
extrahepatic
e. bile duct
e. biliary obstruction secondary to carcinoma
e. biliary system
e. obstruction
e. venous obstruction

extramammary Paget's disease
extramarital sex
extramedullary
e. hematopoiesis
e. hematopoiesis, focal
e. hematopoiesis ▸ foci of
e. hematopoiesis in the liver
e. hematopoiesis, widespread
e. hematopoietic cells ▸ sparse infiltration of
e. plasmacytoma

extraneous electrode potential
extraneous scalp muscle electrical interference
extranodal extension
extraocular
e. eye muscles
e. movement (EOM)
e. movements intact (EOMI)
e. muscles
e. tension

extra-oral appliance
extraordinary resistance
extraordinary treatment, ethically
extrapelvic disease
extrapericardial anastomosis ▸ Waterston
extraperitoneal
e. cesarean (C-) section
e. cesarean section ▸ paravesical
e. cesarean section ▸ supravesical
e. plombage

extrapleural
e. air
e. apicolysis
e. pneumothorax
e. space

extrapolar region
extrapsychic conflict
extrapulmonary
e. coccidioidomycosis ▸ primary
e. cough
e. loads
e. site
e. tuberculosis (TB)

extrapyramidal
- e. nerve disorder
- e. symptoms (EPS)
- e. syndrome
- e. system
- e. system (COEPS) ▸ cortically originating

extrarenal azotemia
extrarenal uremia
extrasaccular hernia
extrasensory perception (ESP)
extrastimulation ▸ **single premature**
extrastimulus method, atrial
extrastimulus test
extrasystolic beat
extrasystole
- e., atrial
- e., atrioventricular (AV)
- e., auricular
- e., auriculoventricular
- e., AV junctional
- e., infranodal
- e., interpolated
- e., junctional
- e. ▸ lower nodal
- e., midnodal
- e., nodal
- e., retrograde
- e., return
- e., supraventricular
- e. ▸ upper nodal
- e., ventricular

extrathoracic
- e. discomfort
- e. neoplasm
- e. rale
- e. spread pattern of lung carcinoma
- e. tumor

extrathyroidal thyroxine
extrauterine
- e. environment
- e. mass ▸ palpable
- e. pelvic mass
- e. pregnancy

extravagant spending sprees
extravasates, hemorrhagic
extravasation
- e. of blood ▸ subcutaneous
- e., urinary
- e., vascular

extravascular granulomatous features
extravascular lung water
extravert (see extrovert)

extreme(s)
- e. agitation
- e. breathlessness
- e. depression
- e. distress, patient in
- e. dizziness
- e. drowsiness
- e. dryness of mouth
- e. elation
- e. exhaustion
- e. fatigue
- e. hostility
- e. hunger
- e. impairment
- e. irritability
- e. jaw clenching
- e. lateralized reduction in amplitude
- e. mood swings
- e. narcissistic sensitivity and vulnerability
- e. nearsightedness
- e. of motion
- e. optimism
- e. pain
- e. paleness
- e. prolonged exposure
- e. reactivity to interpersonal stresses
- e. reluctance
- e. reticence in social situations
- e. sadness
- e. sarcasm ▸ displays
- e. sensitivity to sunlight
- e. sensitivity to touch
- e. skin photosensitivity
- e. spindles
- e. stress
- e. stress ▸ periods of
- e. thirst
- e. tiredness
- e. weakness

extremely
- e. congested, parenchyma
- e. degenerated, brain
- e. low voltage
- e. painful
- e. slow waves ▸ irregular,

extremis, patient in
extremity(-ies)
- e. abnormality
- e. abrasions
- e. (LLE) amputated ▸ left lower
- e. (LUE) amputated ▸ left upper
- e. (RLE) amputated ▸ right lower
- e. (RUE) amputated ▸ right upper

- e. ataxia
- e. atrophic
- e. atrophic ▸ muscles of upper
- e., atrophy of
- e. bilaterally amputated ▸ lower
- e. bilaterally amputated ▸ upper
- e. bypass graft ▸ lower
- e. cachectic
- e. cannulated, vessels of
- e., choreoathetosis of
- e. ▸ clubbing and cyanosis upper
- e., clubbing of
- e., coldness of
- e., creeping sensation in
- e., cyanosis of
- e. ▸ edema of lower
- e. ▸ edema of upper
- e. edematous
- e., electric
- e. equal and symmetrical
- e., erythema of
- e. excoriations
- e. exsanguinated of blood
- e., flaccid
- e., flail
- e. (LLE) flexed ▸ left lower
- e. (LUE) flexed ▸ left upper
- e. (RLE) flexed ▸ right lower
- e. (RUE) flexed ▸ right upper
- e. ▸ flicking twitches of
- e. full range of motion (ROM) ▸ left lower
- e. full range of motion (ROM) ▸ left upper
- e. full range of motion (ROM) ▸ right lower
- e. full range of motion (ROM) ▸ right upper
- e., function returned to
- e. functional
- e., gangrene in
- e., hyperthermia in
- e. immobilized in cast
- e. ▸ intention tremor of
- e. ▸ intramusclar arteries of lower
- e. ▸ intramuscular arteries of upper
- e. ischemia
- e., isolated heat perfusion of an
- e. ▸ jerking of
- e. (LLE) ▸ left lower
- e. (LUE) ▸ left upper
- e., limited motion of
- e. ▸ limited movement of
- e., malignant melanoma of
- e. ▸ marked atrophy of upper

e. ▸ mild edema upper and lower
e., mirroring of
e., mottling of
e., numbness of
e. ▸ pain in chest, jaw or
e. ▸ paresthesia of
e., patient drags left lower
e., patient drags right lower
e. ▸ peripheral cyanosis of all
e., pitting edema lower
e. ▸ progressive weakness of
e. pump ▸ Jobst
e. reattached
e. reattached surgically, severed
e., reimplanted
e., rhabdomyosarcoma of
e. (RLE) ▸ right lower
e. (RUE) ▸ right upper
e. ▸ sensory change in
e. ▸ severe pitting edema all
e., spasticity of
e., stiffness of
e. strength, lower
e. strength, patient lower
e. strength, patient upper
e. strength, upper
e. ▸ sudden weakness or numbness of
e., swelling of lower
e., swelling of upper
e. symmetrical and equal
e., temperature of
e. -threatening problem
e., tingling or numbness in
e. ▸ tingling sensation in
e., tortuous varicosities in lower
e., traction applied to
e. training ▸ upper
e. ▸ tremor in upper
e., unaffected
e., upper
e., varicosities of lower
e. vascular disorder ▸ upper
e., vasomotor changes in upper
e. vessels perfused with fresh blood
e. vessels washed out
e. weakness, lower

extrinsic
e. allergic alveolitis
e. alveolitis
e. alveolitis, acute allergic
e. alveolitis, chronic
e. asthma
e. colon deformity

e. compression
e. defect
e. factors
e. forces
e. laryngeal muscles ▸ tonus of
e. larynx
e. mass
e. mass pressure
e. muscle
e. obstruction
e. pressure

extrovert (*same as* extravert)
extroverted, patient
extruded disc
extruding at cervical os ▸ tissue
extrusion
e. angioplasty ▸ Kinsey rotation atherectomy
e., centripetal
e. of nucleus pulposus

extubated, patient
exuberant granulations
exudate(s)
e. and aneurysms (HEA) ▸ hemorrhages,
e. and fluids ▸ body secretions
e., bloody
e. ▸ diagnostic separation of transudate and
e., fibrinopurulent
e., fibrinous
e., gram stain of
e. ▸ hard waxy
e., inflammatory
e. ▸ intra-alveolar fibrinous
e., mucopurulent
e., mucosal
e., pleural
e., purulent
e., soft
e., tonsillar
e., watery

exudation, serous
exudativa, bronchiolitis
exudative
e. angina
e. arthritis
e. ascites
e. bronchitis
e. calcifying fasciitis
e. changes ▸ retinal
e. enteropathy
e. macular degeneration
e. nephritis
e. pleural effusion

e. pleurisy
e. retinitis
e. retinopathy
e. tonsillitis
e. tuberculosis
e. vitreoretinopathy ▸ familial

exuding from external os, blood
eye(s) (Eye)
e. ache
e. aerobics
e. alignment
e. amaurosis, cat's
e., amblyopic
e. analysis, bull's
e. and eyelids, sluggish movements of
e. and mouth ▸ dryness of
e. anesthesia, local
e., anterior chamber of
e., appendages of the
e., aqueous humor of
e. around optical axis ▸ rotation of
e., artifact ▸ glass
e., artificial
e., ash leaf spots in
e. (donor) ▸ authorization form to use
e. (next of kin) ▸ authorization form to use
e. bags, fatty
e., bags under
e. bank
E. Bank for Sight Restoration
E. Bank, Medical
e., benign lesion of
e., black
e., bleeding inside
e., blinking
e. blinks
e. blinks ▸ slow wave transients and
e., bloodshot
e., blurred vision in one
e. ▸ bone cavity around
e. (OU) ▸ both
e., Bright's
e. bulges and droops
e., bulging
e. ▸ burning sensation in
e. cancer
e. care, diabetic
e. care ▸ industrial
e. care ▸ pediatric
e. care ▸ primary
e. chamber

eye(s)—*continued*

E. chart
e. chart, Jaeger's
e., choroid coat of
e., chronic eye
e. circles, under-
e. closure ▸ forceful sustained
e., conformer for
e. (donor) ▸ consent form to use
e. (next of kin) ▸ consent form to use
e. contact
e. contact ▸ eye-to-
e. contact ▸ lack of
e. contact, maintain
e., convergence of
e. coordination ▸ hand-
e. correction ▸ mild
e., cross-
e., crossed
e., crossing of
e. damage
e., dark circles under
e. defects
e., deorsumduction of left
e., deorsumduction of right
e., dextroduction of left
e., dextroduction of right
e. ▸ dimmed vision in one
e., disabling eye
e. disease
e. disease ▸ age-related
e. disease, blinding
e. disease, diabetic
e. disease ▸ thyroid
e. disease ▸ warning signs of
e., diseased
e. disorder
e. disorder ▸ primary
e. distant and unfocused
e. donated
e. donated for corneal transplants
e. donation
e. donor
e. ▸ double vision in one
e. ▸ drain tears from
e. dressing
e. dressing, binocular
e. dressing, monocular
e. drops
e. drops, anesthetic
e. drops, mydriatic
e., dry
e. dry and gritty
e. ▸ dry, irritated

e., drying of
e. dryness from dermatitis
e. dryness from eczema
e., dryness of
e. dryness ▸ severe
e. dull
e. dysconjugate
e. (OU) ▸ each
e., ears, nose and throat (HEENT) ▸ head,
e., ears, nose and throat (HEENT) not remarkable ▸ head,
e., enucleation of
e., equator of
e. evisceration left
e., evisceration right
e. examination, annual dilated
e. examination, dilated
e. ▸ excessive tearing of
e. ▸ excessive watering of
e., excretory duct of
e. exercises
e. fatigue
e. ▸ feeling of film over
e. ▸ flapping of conjunctiva, left
e. ▸ flapping of conjunctiva, right
e. floaters
e. ▸ fluid pressure in
e. fluids
e. focus
e. ▸ foreign body in
e. ▸ frequent blinking of
e. from anemia ▸ spots before
e. from aneurysm ▸ bulging
e. from blood clot ▸ bulging
e., fundus of the
e. -gaze board
e., glazed
e., globe of the
e. ▸ gritty feeling in
e. -hand coordination
e. hemorrhage
e. ▸ herpes virus of left
e. ▸ herpes virus of right
e., host
e. implant
e. implant conformer
e. implant, conventional reform
e. implant, coral
e. implant, pyramidal
e. ▸ implantable rings in
e. ▸ inability to close
e. ▸ increased winking, blinking or squinting of
e., infected

e. infection
e., inferior
e. ▸ inflammation of
e. injury
e., irritated
e. irritation
e. itching from anxiety
e. ▸ itchy, runny nose and
e. ▸ itchy, watery
e., Klieg
e., lackluster
e., lacrimal sac of eye
e. (OS) ▸ left
e. lens, clouding of
e. lens ▸ dislocated
e. lesion
e. lesion, bull's
e., levoduction of left
e., levoduction of right
e. lift
e. lubricant
e. lubricated
e. lusterless
e. maculopathy, bull's
e. maneuver, doll's
e. medications, topical
e. mildly inflamed
e., misaligned
e., misalignment of
e. movement ▸ abnormal rhythmic
e. movement artifact
e. movement, conjugate
e. movement (NREM) cycle, nonrapid
e. movement (NREM-REM) cycle ▸ nonrapid eye movement-rapid
e. movement (REM) density, rapid
e. movement desensitization
e. movement desensitization and reprocessing (EMDR)
e. movement (NREM) intrusion, nonrapid
e. movement ▸ involuntary
e. movement (REM) latency, rapid
e. movement, lateral
e. movement (NREM), nonrapid
e. movement (REM) onset, rapid
e. movement (NREM) period, nonrapid
e. movement (REM) period, rapid
e. movement (REM) period, sleep onset rapid
e. movement (NREM) physiology, nonrapid
e. movement (REM), rapid

e. movement-rapid eye movement (NREM-REM) cycle, nonrapid
e. movement (REM) rebound, rapid
e. movement, saccadic
e. movement (REM) sleep anxiety dreams ▸ rapid
e. movement (REM) sleep ▸ increased rapid
e. movement (REM) sleep interruption insomnia, rapid
e. movement sleep (NREMS), nonrapid
e. movement (REM) sleep, rapid
e. movement (REM) sleep-related hypoxemia ▸ rapid
e. movement (SPEM) ▸ smooth pursuit
e. movement ▸ therapeutic
e. movement therapy
e. movements
e. movements, abnormal
e. movements, imprecise
e. movements, jerking
e. movements ▸ restricted
e. movements (REM) sleep ▸ rapid
e. movements (REMS), spindle rapid
e. movements, vertical
e. ▸ moving spots before
e. mucosal exposure
e. muscle, advancement of
e. muscle artifact
e. muscle imbalance
e. muscle, paralysis of
e. muscle, recession of
e. ▸ muscle spasms of
e. muscles, extraocular
e., muscles of
e., myopic
e., Nairobi
e., nearsighted
e. open spontaneously
e. open to pain
e. open to speech
e., orbicular muscle of
e. orientation ▸ mind's
e., outer canthus of
e., outer surface of
e. pad
e. pad and shield applied
e. pad, protective
e. pain
e. pain from cold
e. pain ▸ morning

e., painless increased pressure inside the
e. patch
e. patch compression dressing
e., periphery
e., pink◊
e. plaques ▸ cobalt-60 (Co⁶⁰)
e. polar coordinate mapping, bull's
e., posterior chamber of
e., postsurgical aphakia left
e., postsurgical aphakia right
e. pressure, controlling
e. pressure ▸ elevated
e., pressure in the
e. pressure ▸ inner
e. pressure ▸ internal
e. pressure, lowering
e. problem from atherosclerosis
e. procedure, closed
e. procedure, open
e., prominent
e., protective outer surface of
e., protrusion of
e. puffiness from alcohol
e. pupil, cat's
e., raccoon
e. ratings
e., recipient
e., red
e. redness ▸ double vision with
e. reflex, cat's
e. reflex, doll's
e., refraction of
e. response
e. (OD) ▸ right
e. -roll test
e. roll upward
e. rolled back
e. rotated down
e. rotated upward
e. rubbing ▸ habitual
e., rupture of
e. scratchy
e. screening and diagnosis
e. shield
e. shield, Fox
e. shield, perforated
e. shield, protective
e. shields for electron beam therapy
e. sign, doll's
e. slant, downward
e., slitting of canaliculus of
e., Snellen's
e., Snellen's reform

e. socket
e. socket inflammation
e. ▸ spots before
e., squinting
e., stabbing sensation in
e. stone
e., strabismus of
e. strain
e., subconjunctival hemorrhage of
e. sunken in appearance
e., sunset
e. surgery
e. surgery, laser
e. surgery, refractive
e., sursumduction of left
e., sursumduction of right
e., swollen
e. symptoms, dry
e. syndrome, dry
e. syndrome, lazy-
e. taped shut
e., teary
e. teeth
e. tension, increased
e. (TOS) ▸ tension of left
e. (TOD) ▸ tension of right
e. test, cover-uncover
e. test, duction
e. testing
e. tests, standard
e., tired
e. tissue
e. -to-eye contact
e. to light ▸ sensitivity of
e. tracked
e. tumor
e. tumors, heavy charged particle therapy in
e. twitch ▸ recurrent
e. twitches
e. ▸ twitching around
e. twitching artifact
e. twitching from caffeine
e., vascular layer of choroid of
e. vessel blockage
e. vessel ▸ blocked
e. vessels, arteriosclerosis of
e. (VOS) ▸ vision, left
e. (VOU) ▸ vision of each
e. (VOD) ▸ vision, right
e., visual acuity left
e., visual acuity right
e. wander aimlessly
e., wandering
e., watery

eye(s)—*continued*
- e. ▸ watery, itchy
- e., wet
- e., wood's light examination of
- e. worm
- e. ▸ yellowing of
- e. ▸ yellowing of whites of

eyeball(s)
- e., abnormal protrusion of
- e., absence of
- e., atrophy of
- e., avulsion of
- e., cavity of
- e. compression reflex
- e., continual irritation of
- e., crepitus of
- e., dimpling of
- e., elevated pressure in
- e., enucleation of
- e., evisceration of
- e., forward displacement of
- e. -heart reflex
- e., inferior oblique muscle of
- e. into orbit ▸ recession of
- e. ▸ involuntary movement of
- e., laceration of
- e. movement artifact potential ▸ asymmetric
- e. movements
- e., outer layer of
- e., plastic operation on
- e., protruded
- e. protrusion
- e., rhythmic horizontal oscillation of
- e., rhythmic vertical oscillation of
- e., shift in position of
- e., shrunken
- e., superior oblique muscle of
- e., suture of
- e., trauma to
- e., twitching
- e. under tension
- e., vertical oscillations of

eyebrow
- e. and eyelash loss in radiation therapy
- e., fatigue
- e., hairs of
- e. ▸ lift sagging
- e. piercing
- e. reconstruction, Brent's
- e., sagging
- e. ▸ sweating over

eyeglass lenses ▸ prism
eyeglasses, corrective

eyelash(es)
- e. follicles
- e. follicles ▸ infected
- e., inversion of
- e. loss in radiation therapy, eyebrow and
- e., trichiasis of
- e. turning in ▸ conjunctivitis with

eyelid(s)
- e., angular junction of
- e., apraxia of
- e., baggy
- e., basal cell carcinoma of
- e. bump
- e. cancer
- e., carcinoma of
- e. closure reflex
- e., crease ▸ upper
- e., crusting of
- e., crusty
- e., drooping
- e., drooping of
- e., drooping of upper
- e., droopy
- e. ▸ droopy, baggy
- e., ectropion of
- e., edema of
- e., flutter of
- e. function
- e., glands of the
- e. incision into
- e. ▸ infection of
- e. infiltrated, upper
- e., inflamed
- e., inflammation of
- e. ▸ infrequent blinking of
- e. injury
- e., insufficiency of
- e. ▸ involuntary forcible closure of
- e., lateral commissure of
- e., levator muscle of upper
- e. lift
- e., lower
- e. margin
- e., medial commissure of
- e. muscles, paralysis of
- e., plastic repair of
- e. plasty
- e., ptosis of
- e. ptosis operation
- e. ptosis ▸ upper
- e. ▸ puffy, swollen
- e. reconstruction, Landolt's
- e., reconstruction of
- e. ▸ red and swollen

- e. -related problem
- e., repositioning of
- e. resection of
- e., retraction
- e., sagging
- e. scaling from conjunctivitis
- e. skin cancer
- e. ▸ sling elevation of
- e., sluggish movements of eyes and
- e. sore
- e. ▸ spasm of
- e., squamous cell carcinoma
- e. surgery
- e. surgery, cosmetic
- e. surgery ▸ reconstructive
- e., suturing of
- e. swelling
- e., swollen
- e. ▸ tightening of
- e. tissue
- e. ▸ tremor of
- e., turned in
- e. twitching
- e., unilateral ptosis of
- e., upper
- e., vesiculation of
- e. wrinkles
- e., xanthelasma around

eyepiece, wide field
eyesight
- e., blurred
- e., reduced
- e., surgery

eyestrain ▸ patient has
eyewear, protective
Eyler's operation
E-zero offset

F

F (frontal)
F and R (force and rhythm)
F 18, fluorine
F factor, Mayneord
F function
F, hemoglobin
F point of cardiac apex pulse
F slope ▸ mitral E to
f wave of jugular venous pulse
F waves
Fa, Reichstein's substance
FA virus
fabere
  f. abduction test
  f. extension test
  f. external rotation test
  f. fixation test
  f. sign
  f. test
Faber's syndrome
fabricated illness
fabrication, illness
Fabry's disease
FAC (5-fluorouracil, Adriamycin,
  Cytoxan) chemotherapy
face
  f., adenoid
  f. and neck lift
  f., bird-like
  f. ▸ blank expressionless
  f., bruised and puffy
  f. crown, open-
  f., discrete jerking musculature of
  f. -down position
  f., drooping of
  f., edema of
  f., emaciated
  f., en
  f., flushing of
  f. irradiation field, en
  f. laser skin resurfacing
  f. -lift
  f. -lift, cervicofacial
  f. -lift, complete
  f. -lift ▸ nonsurgical
  f. -lift ▸ skin-tightening
  f. -lift surgery

f., malar eminence of
f. mask
f. mask, full-
f., mask-like
f. mask ▸ reservoir
f., masked
f., moon-shaped
f. movement, bilateral
f. ▸ numbness, weakness and
  paralysis of
f. ▸ pain on affected side of
f. ▸ paralysis of
f. presentation
f. ▸ puffiness of face
f. recognition
f. recognition ▸ object/
f., red butterfly-shaped rash on
f. ▸ seborrhea of
f. shield
f. shield, bronchoscopic
f., soft tissues of
f. ▸ sudden numbness one side off
f. ▸ sudden paralysis one side of
f. ▸ sudden weakness of
f. ▸ sudden weakness one side of
f. ▸ sudden weakness or numbness
  of
f., swelling of
f. ▸ swelling of lips, tongue and
f. symmetrical
f., transverse vein of
f. ▸ uncontrolled movement of limbs
  and
f. unremarkable
f., vitreous
f. ▸ weakness or numbness of
f. wrinkle removal ▸ laser
f. wrinkles
face-lift ▸ patient had
facet
  f. arthropathy
  f., articular
  f. cartilage, medial patellar
  f. joint arthritis
  f. joints
  f. joints, worn
  f. of cornea

f., superior articular
facetted stones, multiple
facial [fascial]
  f. abnormalities
  f. abrasions
  f. abscess, gram stain of
  f. acne
  f. anchorage
  f. and pubic hair, absence of
  f. anomalies
  f. appearance, altered
  f. appearance ▸ mask-like
  f. appearance ▸ pale
  f. area
  f. artery
  f. artery pressure point
  f. asymmetry
  f. atrophy
  f. atrophy, progressive
  f. atrophy, unilateral
  f. bones
  f. canal
  f. canal, prominence of
  f. capillaries, broken
  f. center
  f. characteristics ▸ altered
  f. contortions
  f. contours ▸ normal body or
  f. contractures, intermittent
  f. cosmetic surgery
  f. cues
  f. deformity
  f. diplegia, congenital
  f. disfigurement
  f. droop, left-sided
  f. droop, right-sided
  f. dysmorphia
  f. dysplasia
  f. edema
  f. electrode application
  f. expression
  f. expression, activates
  f. expression, fixed
  f. expression, involuntary
  f. expression ▸ lack of
  f. expression ▸ loss of
  f. features, characteristic

F

facial—*continued*
- f. flushing
- f. fracture, reduction
- f. fracture, transverse
- f. fullness ▸ sensation of
- f. grimacing
- f. hair
- f. hair, excess
- f. hair growth ▸ excessive
- f. hair ▸ growth of
- f. hair ▸ growth phase of
- f. hair ▸ resting phase of
- f. height, anterior
- f. height, posterior
- f. hemiatrophy
- f. hemiparesis
- f. hemiplegia
- f. hemispasm
- f. implant of cheek
- f. implant of chin
- f. implant of jaw
- f. implant surgery
- f. infections, oral-
- f. laceration
- f. line ▸ dynamic
- f. massage, scalp and
- f. muscle, affected
- f. muscles, lax
- f. muscles, paralysis of
- f. muscles ▸ weakness of
- f. musculature
- f. myoclonus
- f. nerve
- f. nerve block
- f. nerve deficit
- f. nerve ▸ disorder of
- f. nerve dissection
- f. nerve function
- f. nerve pain
- f. nerve palsy
- f. nerve signs
- f. nerve stimulator, Hilger
- f. nerve, temporal
- f. neuralgia
- f. neuroanastomosis, hypoglossal-
- f. neuroanastomosis, spinal accessory-
- f. or limb abnormalities
- f. orbit
- f. pain
- f. pain and twitching
- f. pain from arthritis
- f. pain ▸ intractable
- f. pain, involuntary
- f. pain ▸ residual

- f. pain ▸ severe, jabbing
- f. pain ▸ severe, searing
- f. palsy
- f. palsy, nuclear
- f. paralysis
- f. paralysis, acute
- f. paralysis, ▸ congenital abducens-
- f. paralysis ▸ idiopathic
- f. paralysis ▸ partial
- f. paresis
- f. plastic surgery
- f., professional
- f. psoriasis
- f. puffiness
- f. rash
- f. reconstruction
- f. refinement
- f. reflex
- f. regions
- f. rejuvenation
- f. rejuvenation cosmetic surgery
- f. rejuvenation ▸ laser
- f. resurfacing ▸ laser
- f. rhytidectomy
- f. ridge
- f. rosacea
- f. skin
- f. skin disease
- f. skin restoration ▸ laser
- f. skin ▸ sagging
- f. spasm
- f. structures
- f. surface of tooth
- f. surgery
- f. surgery, cosmetic
- f. swelling
- f. tic
- f. tics, chronic
- f. tissue
- f. trauma
- f. vein
- f. vein, common anterior
- f. vein, deep
- f. vein, posterior
- f. vein, transverse
- f. vision
- f. weakness
- f. weakness, left
- f. weakness ▸ onset of
- f. weakness or drooping, temporary
- f. weakness, right
- f. wrinkles
- f. wrinkles ▸ laser resurfacing for
- f. wrinkling

facialis, genu nervi

facialis, herpes
facies
- f., abnormal
- f., adenoid
- f. and ears ▸ abnormal
- f., anxious
- f., aortic
- f., Corvisart's
- f., cushingoid
- f., elfin
- f., flat
- f., Hutchinson's
- f., mitral
- f., moon-shaped
- f., Parkinson's
- f. syndrome, elfin

facile ▸ voluble and verbally
facilitate
- f. amebic invasion
- f. interaction
- f. transfer

facilitated angioplasty
facilitated communication (FC)
facilitation, postactivation
facilitation (PNF) ▸ proprioceptive neuromuscular
facilitators, experienced
facility(-ies)
- f., acquired immune deficiency syndrome (AIDS) residential treatment
- f., acute care
- f., alternate care nursing
- f. ▸ assisted living
- f., cardiac rehabilitation
- f., certified skilled nursing
- f. ▸ certified sleep-disorder
- F. (CBRF), Community-Based Residential
- f., exercise
- f., extended care
- f. ▸ external acute medical care
- f. ▸ free-standing private psychiatric
- f. ▸ free-standing psychiatric
- f., health care
- f., inpatient
- f. ▸ inpatient non-psychiatric medical
- f., intensive care
- f., intermediate care
- f., long-term health care
- f., medical
- f., narcotic treatment
- f., neurorehabilitation
- f., nursing

f., outpatient
f. ▸ outpatient non-psychiatric medical
f., private toilet
f., recipient
f., residential care
f., residential treatment
f., skilled
f., skilled nursing
f., tertiary care
faciobrachial hemiplegia
faciolingual hemiplegia
facioscapulohumeral artery
fact and fantasy
faction [*fraction, traction*]
factitial dermatitis
factitial lesions
factitious
f. air
f. disorder
f. disorder, adult
f. disorder with physical symptoms
f. disorder with psychological symptoms
f. fever
f. illness with physical symptoms ▸ chronic
f. illness with psychological symptoms
factor(s) (Factor) [*fracture*]
f., acidic fibroblast growth
f., adverse
f. affecting physical condition ▸ psychological
f., ambient
f., amplification
f., amplifying
f., anatomical
f., anti-angiogenesis
f. antigen ▸ Rh (Rhesus)
f. (AHF) ▸ antihemophilic
f., anti-metastatic
f., antinuclear
f., anti-oncogenic
f., antipernicious anemia
f. (ANF) ▸ atrial natriuretic
f. (AMF), autocrine motility
f., backscatter
f., basic fibroblast growth
f., behavioral
f., biochemical
f., biologic
f., biological
f., bleeding
f., blood clotting

f. (I-XIII), blood coagulation
f., blood element transfer
f., blood type
f., calculation
f., capacitance
f. ▸ cardiac risk
f., cardiovascular risk
f., causative
f., (N~gas~), cavity-gas calibration
f. (CAF), cell antiviral
f. cell loss
f. cell ▸ rheumatoid arthritis (RA)
f., chemical clotting
f., chemotactic
f., Christmas
f., circulatory
f., citrovorum
f., citrovorum rescue
f., clotting
f. (I-XIII) ▸ coagulation
f., colicinogenic
f., colonization
f., colony-stimulating
f., common sense
f. concentrate, intrinsic
f., contributing
f., controlling risk
f. ▸ coronary risk
f., corticotropin-releasing
f. counseling, risk
f., cultural
f., cytolysis prognastic
f. D
f., decapacitation
f. deficiency disease ▸ Stuart-Prower
f., demographic
f., diastolic heart
f., dietary
f., dilution
f., dominant
f., dose modification
f., dose reduction
f., duty
F. VIII deficiency
F. VIII inhibitor
F. VIII-related antigen
f., electrical
f., emotional
f., encephalitogenic
f., endogenous
f. ▸ endothelium-derived hyperpolarizing
f. ▸ endothelium-derived relaxing
f. ▸ end-stage heart

f., environmental
F. (EGF), Epidermal Growth
f. (EMF), erythrocyte maturation
f., erythropoietic-stimulating
f., etiologic
f., exacerbating
f., exercise
f., exophthalmos hyperthyroid
f., exophthalmos-producing
f., expectancy
f., external
f., extracerebral
f., extrinsic
f., faith
f., father
f., fatigue
f., fibrin-stabilizing
f. ▸ fibrin-stabilizing blood coagulation
f. ▸ florid congestive heart
f. for drug abusers, risk
f. for epilepsy ▸ trigger
f. for migraine ▸ trigger
f. 4 ▸ platelet
f., genetic
f. ▸ genetic and physiological
f., genetic risk
f., genetic transmission of risk
f., geometry
f., gravitation
f., growth
f., growth hormone-releasing
f. H
f., Hageman
f. ▸ health risk
f. ▸ heart attack risk
f. ▸ heart disease risk
f., hereditary
f., heredocongenital
f., histamine-releasing
f., histologic
f., hormonal
f. (GM-CSF), human granulocytic-macrophage colony-stimulating
f., humoral thymic
f., hyperglycemic-glycogenolytic
f. ▸ hypermobility as risk
f. ▸ hypersomnia related to a known organic
f., hypoxic gain
f., immune
f. in cardiovascular development, epigenetic
f. in dose fractionation, biologic
f. in drug abuse, genetic

523

factor(s)—*continued*
f. in drug abuse, physiological
f. in drug abuse, psychological
f. in drug abuse, sociological
f. in shock ▸ toxic
f. in treatment choices
f. influencing anxiety
f. ▸ inherited risk
f. ▸ insomnia related to a known organic
f. ▸ insulin-like growth
f., intellectual power
F. Intervention Trial (MRFIT), Multiple Risk
f., intensification
f., internal
f., intrinsic
f. IX deficiency
f., known risk
f. ▸ lack of intrinsic
f., Laki-Lorand
f., latex rheumatoid
f. ▸ leukemia inhibitory
f., leukocytosis-promoting
f., lifestyle
f., local efficiency
f., luteinizing hormone-releasing
f., lymph node permeability
f., macrophage-inhibiting
f. ▸ major risk
f., mauve
f., Mayneord F
f., medical
f. ▸ medical risk
f. (MIF) ▸ migration inhibition
f. ▸ modifiable risk
f., modification, cardiac risk
f. modification ▸ risk
f., monocytosis-inducing
f., motivating
f. ▸ multiple cardiac risk
f., multiple-risk
f., myocardial depressant
f., necrosis
f. negative, Rhesus
f. (NGF) ▸ nerve growth
f., neurohumoral
f., neurophysiologic
f., neurotrophic
f. IX antigen
f., nonuniformity
f., nutritional
f. of longevity ▸ psychological
f., off-axis
f., output

f., Ovenstone
f., pain
f., pathologic prognostic
f., patient's condition precipitated by external
f., peakscatter
f. ▸ personal risk
f., personality
f., pharmacokinetic
f. ▸ physical or emotional
f., physiological
f., platelet
f. ▸ platelet-activating
f. ▸ platelet-aggregating
f. (PDGF) ▸ platelet-derived growth
f. positive, Rhesus
f., precipitating
f., predetermined biological
f., predisposing
f. ▸ primary pulmonary hypertension risk
f. ▸ primary risk
f. ▸ proatrial natriuretic
f., prognostic
f., prolactin-inhibiting
f., provocative
f., psychic
f., psychodynamic
f., psychogenic
f., psychologic
f., psychological
f., purify blood-clotting
f., RA (rheumatoid arthritis)
f. reduction ▸ risk
f., regret
f., rejection
f., releasing
f., renal erythropoietic
f., rescue
F. (RTF) ▸ Resistance Transfer
f., Rh (Rhesus) blood
f., Rh (Rhesus) negative (Rh-)
f., Rh (Rhesus) positive (Rh+)
f., Rhesus (Rh)
f., rheumatoid
f., rheumatoid arthritis (RA)
f., risk
f. VII antigen
f., Simon's septic
f. social
f., somatotropin-releasing
f., stress
f. ▸ stress-amplifying
f. ▸ stress-attenuating
f. ▸ stress-moderating

f. ▸ stress-producing
f., stress-related
f. ▸ Stuart-Prower
f., sufficient intrinsic
f. (SPF), sun protection
f. (SPF) ▸ sunscreen protection
f., survival
f., symptomatologic
f. test, rheumatoid
f., therapeutic
f., therapy, transfer
f. (VEGF) therapy ▸ vascular endothelial growth
F. III deficiency
f., thymic humoral
f. (TRF) ▸ thyrotropin-releasing
f. ▸ time dose fractionation (TDF)
f., tissue
f., tissue-coding
f., tissue-damaging
f., toxic
f., transfer
f. ▸ transforming growth
f., transmission
f., trophic
f., tumor angiogenesis
F. (TGF), Tumor Growth
f. (TNF) ▸ tumor necrosis
f., undergraded insulin
f., unknown risk
f. (VEGF) ▸ vascular endothelial growth
f., von Willebrand's
f. X antigen
F. X deficiency
facultative
f. aerobes
f. anaerobes
f. bacteria
f. hyperopia
f. parasite
faculties
f., gradual loss of mental
f., loss of intellectual
f., mental
FAD (familial Alzheimer's disease
FAD (fetal activity determinations)
fad diet
Faden procedure
faecalis
f., Alcaligenes
f. alcaligenes, Bacillus
f. ▸ Enterococcus
f., gram-positive Streptococcus
f. strains ▸ enterococcus

f., Streptococcus (Strep)
f., Vibrio
Fahey's operation
Fahrenheit scale
Fahrenheit thermometer
failed
f. forceps delivery
f. suicide attempt
f. to respond, patient
failing
f. heart ▸ pumping ability of
f. lung sign
f. vision
fails to keep appointment
failure
f., acute
f., acute cardiorespiratory
f., acute congestive heart
f., acute fulminant liver
f., acute heart
f., acute hepatic
f., acute kidney
f., acute left ventricular heart
f., acute liver
f. (ARF), acute renal
f., acute respiratory
f., acute right ventricular heart
f. ▸ adrenal gland
f. (CHF) ▸ advanced stage of
    congestive heart
f. and cardioversion, congestive
    heart
f. artifact, calibration
f., backward heart
f. ▸ bone marrow
f., breathing
f., cardiac
f., cardiopulmonary
f., cardiorespiratory
f. cells, heart-
f., chronic cardiac
f., chronic congestive heart
f., chronic heart
f., chronic kidney
f., chronic renal
f., chronic respiratory
f., cocaine-induced respiratory
f., compensated heart
f. ▸ confusion from heart
f., congenital
f., congenital heart
f., congestive
f., congestive cardiac
f. (CHF), congestive heart
f., decompensated heart

f. ▸ deteriorating heart
f., dilatation
f., electrical
f., endocrine
f., end-stage
f., end-stage liver
f., fatal respiratory
f. ▸ florid congestive heart
f., forward heart
f. ▸ fulminant liver
f., growth hormone
f., heart
f., hemorrhagic diathesis
f., hepatic
f., hepatocellular
f., hepatorenal
f., high-output heart
f., hypoventilation
f., hypoxemic
f. ▸ impending respiratory
f. in prevention
f. in ventriclar lead ▸ insulation
f., incipient heart
f., infection
f., intractable heart
f., irreversible kidney
f., kidney
f. ▸ lasting impression of impending
f. ▸ late-stage heart
f. ▸ left heart
f., left-sided heart
f., left ventricular
f., left ventricular heart
f., liver
f. ▸ loss of appetite from heart
f. ▸ low-output
f. ▸ low-output heart
f. ▸ major-organ
f., marginal heart
f., massive hepatic
f., mental
f. ▸ mild thyroid
f. ▸ multisystem organ
f., myocardial
f. ▸ myoglobinuric renal
f. (CHF) ▸ natural history of
    congestive heart
f. ▸ neonate respiratory
f. of breast development
f. of immediate recall
f. of muscular coordination
f. of ovulation
f. of recognition
f. of ventilation

f. of vital organs, total system
f. ▸ onset of overt heart
f., organ
f., ovarian
f., overt congestive
f., overt heart
f., ovulatory
f., pacemaker
f. pattern after surgical resection
f. pattern, treatment
f. (PTARF) ▸ post-traumatic acute
    renal
f. ▸ premature reproductive
f., progressive kidney
f., progressive respiratory
f., prosthetic
f., pulmonary
f., pump
f. rate
f. rate, primary
f. rate, success and
f. (CHF), recurrent congestive heart
f., refractory heart
f., renal
f., repeated
f., respiratory
f. ▸ reverse heart
f. ▸ right heart
f., right-sided heart
f., right ventricular (RV)
f., right ventricular (RV) heart
f. ▸ stable, controlled heart
f. (CHF) ▸ sudden congestive heart
f. ▸ sudden heart
f. ▸ symptom of heart
f. syndrome, respiratory
f. ▸ systolic heart
f., testicular
f., therapeutic
f. (CHF) therapy ▸ congestive heart
f. to identify and respond
f. to plan ahead
f. to progress
f. to thrive
f. to thrive ▸ nonorganic
f., treatment
f. treatment ▸ heart
f., vascular
f., vein valve
f., ventilatory
faint
f., common
f. diastolic murmur
f. opacification
f., physiological

fainting
- f., chest discomfort with
- f. episode
- f. from anemia
- f. from diuretics
- f., hysterical
- f. reflex
- f. spell
- f. spell ▸ near-
- f. spells ▸ repeated
- f. ▸ sudden loss of strength or

faintness and unsteadiness
faintness ▸ dizziness and
fair complexion
fair-skinned, patient
fairly consistent form
fait, déjà
faith
- f. factor
- f. healer
- f. healing
- f. tradition

Fajersztajn's sign
faking illness ▸ patient
falciform
- f. body
- f. cartilage
- f. fold of fascia lata
- f. hymen
- f. ligament
- f. lobule

falciforme, Cephalosporium
falcine region
falciparum malaria
falciparum, Plasmodium
Falk-Shukuris operation
Falk's operation
fall(s)
- f. and fractures ▸ immobility,
- f., ▸ frequent staggering and
- f., Marshall
- f., sudden
- f. ▸ sudden, unexplainable
- f. ▸ unsteadiness or sudden

fallacy, Berckson's
fallax, Clostridium
fallback therapy
fallen arches
falling
- f. asleep ▸ momentary
- f., frequent
- f. palate
- f., risk of
- f. sickness
- f. spells of Tumarkin

- f. ▸ tremors, shakes, jerks and
fallopi, knee of acqueductus
fallopian
- f. aqueduct
- f. pregnancy
- f. transfer (ZIFT) ▸ zygote intra-
- f. tube
- f. tube blockage
- f. tube, blocked
- f. tube bound down
- f. tube cancer
- f. tube carcinoma
- f. tube, infundibulum of
- f. tube, isthmus of
- f. tube, obstruction of
- f. tube, scarred
- f. tubes ▸ open blocked
- f. tubes, patent
- f. tubes ▸ surgical absence of

Fallopius, aqueduct of
Fallot
- F., pentalogy of
- F. ▸ pink tetralogy of
- F. tetrad
- F., tetralogy of
- F. triad
- F., trilogy of

fallout, radioactive
Falope ring
FALS (familial amyotrophic lateral sclerosis)
false
- f. aneurysm
- f. angina
- f. aortic aneurysm
- f. belief
- f. bruit
- f. cardiomegaly
- f. cardiomyopathy
- f. colonic obstruction
- f. combined hyperlipidemia
- f. cord
- f. croup
- f. cyanosis
- f. dentures
- f. dextrocardia
- f. diverticulum
- f. Dupuytren's contraction
- f. emphysema
- f. fungi
- f. ganglion
- f. hematuria
- f. highs
- f. hypercholesterolemia
- f. hypertrophy

- f. idea ▸ idiosyncratic
- f. idea ▸ overvalued
- f. idea ▸ superstitious
- f. idea ▸ unpersuasive
- f. identity ▸ induced
- f. joint
- f. labor
- f. labor contractions
- f. labor pains
- f. ligament, lateral
- f. lumen
- f. macula
- f. membrane
- f. memory
- f. memory syndrome
- f. -negative
- f. -negative flu diagnoses
- f. -negative results
- f. -negative results in clinical trials
- f. -negative test
- f. pains
- f. pelvis
- f. perception
- f. personal belief
- f. -positive
- f. -positive, biologic
- f. -positive, chronic
- f. -positive reaction
- f. -positive reactor ▸ biologic
- f. -positive results
- f. -positive results in clinical trials
- f. -positive screening test
- f. -positive serology
- f. -positive syphilis serology
- f. -positive test
- f. pregnancy
- f. restenosis
- f. ribs
- f. security
- f. sensory perception
- f. spatial orientation
- f. stricture
- f. suture
- f. teeth
- f. tendon
- f. transmitter
- f. twins
- f. tympanites
- f. vision
- f. vocal cord
- f. vocal fold

falsification ▸ retroactive memory
falsification, retrospective
Falta's triad

falx
- f. artery
- f. cerebelli
- f. cerebri
- f. inguinalis
- f. ligamentosa
- f. of maxillary antrum

familial
- f. adenomatous polyposis (FAP)
- f. advanced sleep phase syndrome (FASPS)
- f. aggregation
- f. alobar holoprosencephaly
- f. Alzheimer's disease (FAD)
- f. Alzheimer's disease ▸ early-onset
- f. amyloidosis
- f. amyotrophic lateral sclerosis (FALS)
- f. angiomatosis, hemorrhagic
- f. asphyxiant thoracic dystrophy
- f. bilateral giant-cell tumor
- f. centrolobar sclerosis
- f. cerebral sclerosis
- f. characteristic
- f. chloride diarrhea
- f. cholemia
- f. cholestasis syndrome
- f. colon cancer
- f. colorectal cancer
- f. craniofacial anomaly
- f. diabetic history
- f. disease
- f. disease, hereditary
- f. disorder
- f. dysautonomia
- f. erythroblastic anemia
- f. exudative vitreoretinopathy
- f. fibrous dysplasia of jaw
- f. gastrointestinal polyposis
- f. hepatitis
- f. high-cholesterol
- f. high-density lipoprotein deficiency
- f. hypercholesterolemia (FH)
- f. hypercholesterolemia, heterozygous
- f. hypercholesterolemia, homozygous
- f. hypertrophic cardiomyopathy
- f. hypertrophic obstructive cardiomyopathy
- f. hypocalciuric hypercalcemia
- f. hypophosphatemia
- f. idiocy
- f. idiocy, amaurotic

- f. illness, hereditary
- f. immunity
- f. incidence
- f. influence
- f. insomnia, fatal
- f. juvenile nephrophthisis (FJN)
- f. lipidosis
- f. melanoma
- f. mutation
- f. myoclonic epilepsy ▸ progressive
- f. nephritis
- f. neuropathy
- f. nonhemolytic jaundice, chronic
- f. osteochondrodystrophy
- f. polyposis
- f. polyposis and cancer
- f. predisposition
- f. pulmonary fibrosis
- f. spinal muscular atrophy
- f. tasks ▸ difficulty performing
- f. tendency
- f. tremor
- f. xanthomatosis, primary

familiarity ▸ sense of
family(-ies) (Family)('s)
- f. adaptation
- f. adjustment to illness
- f. adjustments
- f., adult children of dysfunctional
- f. advocate, patient-
- f. alcoholic
- f. at risk
- f. ataxia
- f. awareness and change
- f. -based treatment
- f., blended
- f. -borne disease
- f. cancer-prone
- f. cancer syndrome
- f. circumstances
- f. circumstances ▸ other specified
- f. conflict
- f. conflict and violence
- f. constellation
- f. coping
- f. coping, compromised ineffective
- f. coping ▸ disabling ineffective
- f. coping ▸ ineffective
- f. counseling
- f. counselor
- f. couples, step-
- f. day educational programs
- f. discord
- f. disintegration
- f. disruption

- f. doctor
- f. dynamics
- f. dysfunction
- f. dysfunction ▸ severe
- f. education
- f., emotional support to
- f. environment, adoptive-
- f. environment, early
- f. expressed emotion
- f., extended
- f. -focused sessions
- f., friends or school activities ▸ withdrawal from
- f. functional
- f. goals
- F. Group, Al-Anon
- f. group counseling ▸ multi-
- f. group therapy
- f. history (FH)
- f. history (FH) noncontributory
- f. history (FH) not remarkable
- f. history of cancer
- f. history, positive
- f. ▸ intake interview of
- f. interaction
- f. intervention
- f. intervention program
- f. involvement
- f. issues
- F. Medicine
- f. members
- f., nuclear
- f. of organic molecules
- f. -of-origin empowerment sessions
- f. of viruses ▸ herpes
- f. -oriented activities
- f. -oriented issues
- f. outreach program
- f. outreach sessions
- f. pattern, behavioral
- f. patterns of addiction
- f. physician
- f. physician ▸ patient discharged to care of
- f. planning, natural
- f., postdivorce
- f. practice
- f. practitioner
- f. present at time of death
- f. present at time of demise
- f. pressure
- f. processes, altered
- f. program
- F. Program, Weekend
- f. psychotherapy

family(-ies)—*continued*
- f. reaction to illness
- f. recovery, adolescents in
- f. relationship
- f. roles
- f. rules
- f. services
- f. services intake process
- f. sessions
- f. sexual abuse treatment
- f. situation, current
- f., stable
- f. strain
- f. stress
- f. stressors
- f. support
- f. support groups
- f. syndrome, cancer
- f. syndrome, single
- f. system, abusive
- f. systems, alcohol
- f. systems approach
- f. systems, dysfunctional
- f. tension
- f. therapist coordinator
- f. therapy
- f. therapy, group and
- f. therapy, long-term
- f. therapy, multiple-
- f. therapy ▸ relationship enhancement (RE)
- f. therapy ▸ strategic
- f. to view body, prepare
- f. treatment agreement
- f. values ▸ redefining
- f. violence
- f., Zero

famine psychosis
fan douche
fan stroking maneuver during massage
Fañana, glia of
fanatic
- f., political
- f., racial
- f., religious

Fanconi('s)
- F. -Albertini-Zellweger syndrome
- F. anemia
- F. -Debre syndrome, ▸ de Toni
- F. disease ▸ Lignac-
- F. pancytopenia
- F. -Petrassi syndrome
- F. syndrome
- F. syndrome, Abderhalden-

- F. syndrome, Lignac-

fancy, flights of
Fannia, Anthomyiidae
Fannia canicularis
fanning of toes
fantasizer, habitual
fantastica, pseudologia
fantasy(-ies)
- f., act out
- f., age-appropriate
- f. and delusion
- f. and reality
- f. ▸ denial in
- f., fact and
- f. ▸ fragmentation of
- f. ▸ highly prone to
- f., latent
- f., manifest
- f. ▸ normal childhood
- f. of grandeur ▸ preoccupation with
- f. of loneliness ▸ universal
- f. play
- f. ▸ preoccupation with
- f. ▸ preoccupied with
- f., preoedipal
- f. proneness and absorption
- f. ▸ trauma-based mastery
- f., verbal

FAP (familial adenomatous polyposis)
FAP (fibrillating action potentials)
far
- f. advanced carcinoma
- f. advanced disease
- f. field
- f. sight
- f. suture

Farabeuf's amputation
Faraco stain ▸ Wade-Fite-
faradic
- f. current
- f. current into larynx ▸ passing
- f. response
- f. shock
- f. stimulation

faradization, galvanic
Farber's test
farciminosus, Blastomyces
farciminosus, Histoplasma
farcinica, Nocardia
farinata, cornea
farm-related deaths
farmer's lung
farmer's lung disease
Farrar prosthesis ▸ McKee-

Farrar total hip arthroplasty ▸ McKee-
Farre's line
Farre's tubercles
Farris' test
farsighted, patient
farsightedness, premature
FAS (fetal acoustic stimulation)
FAS (fetal alcohol syndrome)
Fasanella operation
Fasanella-Servat operation
fascia
- f. abdominal wall
- f. bulbi
- f., cervical
- f., cremasteric
- f., dartos
- f., dentate
- f. divided
- f., external oblique
- f., external spermatic
- f., Gerota's
- f. graft
- f. incised
- f. incised transversely
- f., inferior
- f. internal spermatic
- f. ▸ irritated plantar
- f. lata
- f. lata, falciform fold of
- f. lata femoris
- f. lata graft
- f. lata prosthesis
- f. lata, tensor of
- f. lata, tensor muscle of
- f., level, prevertebral
- f., lumbodorsal
- f., muscle
- f. of urogenital trigone
- f. opened posteriorly ▸ lumbodorsal
- f., palmar
- f., paraspinous
- f., pectoral
- f., perinephric
- f., perirenal
- f., perivaginal
- f., perivesical
- f., plantar
- f., pretracheal
- f., pubocervical
- f., pubovesicocervical
- f., rectovaginal
- f., rectovesical
- f., rectus
- f., release plantar
- f., renal

f., Scarpa's
f., subvesical
f., superficial
f., supraclavicular
f., temporalis
f., Tenon's
f., tightened
f. transversalis
f. transversalis, semilunar fold of
f., transverse
f., underlying
f., vesicovaginal
fasciae latae muscle, tensor
fascial [*facial*]
f. flap
f. graft
f. graft, underlay
f. layer
f. planes
f. sheath
fasciatus
f., Ceratophyllus
f., Nosopsyllus
f., Tabanus
fascicular
f. achromatin
f. beat
f. block
f. graft
f. heart block
f. keratitis
f. neuroglia
f. ophthalmoplegia
f. twitching
f. ventricular pathways
fasciculata, zona
fasciculated bladder
fasciculation(s) [*vesiculation*]
f., muscle
f. ► muscle wasting and
f. potential
f. ► tremors, tics and
fasciculi atrioventricularis, truncus
fasciculoventricular Mahaim fiber
fasciculus
f. aberrans of Monokow
f., anterior cerebrospinal
f. cuneatus
f., Foville's
f. gracilis
f., lateral cerebrospinal
f. lenticularis
f. of Gowers
f. of Rolando
f., uncinate

fasciitis
f., exudative calcifying
f., necrotizing
f., nodular
f., palmar
f., perirenal
f., plantar
f., proliferative
f., pseudosarcomatous
fasciogram study
Fasciola
F. cervi
F. gigantica
F. hepatica
F. heterophyes
F. magna
F., Trematoda
fasciolaris
f., Cysticercus
f., Fimbriaria
f., gyrus
Fasciolopsis
F. buski
F. fuelleborni
F. goddardi
F. rathouisi
F. spinifera
F. Trematoda
fasciotomy wound biopsy
fashion
f., appendectomy performed in routine
f., criss-cross
f., double-blind
f., homeostatic
f., incision closed in serial
f., interrupted
f., inverted T
f., lens extracted in tumbling
f., over-and-over
f., prepped in routine
f., ray-like
f., simple interrupted
f., stoichiometric
f. ► string of pearls
f., tumbling
fashioned and sutured, flap
fashioned, flap
FASPS (familial advanced sleep phase syndrome)
fast (Fast)
f., acid-
f. -acting insulin
f. activity
f. activity, abnormally

f. activity, exceedingly
f. activity excessive
f. activity, generalized
f. activity, high-voltage
f. activity, intermediate
f. activity, low-voltage
f. alpha variant rhythm
f. and slow component
f. bacilli, acid-
f. bacillus (AFB), acid-
f. bacteria, acid-
f., bed◊
f. channel
f. component
f., drug-
f. EEG brain wave activity ► excessive
f. electroencephalogram (EEG) ► low-voltage
f. growth rate
f. -growing tumor
f. heart rate
f. heartbeat
f. hemoglobins
f., low-voltage
f. mitten pattern
f. neutron
f. neutron beam therapy
f. neutrons, unit for
f. organism, acid-
f. pathway
f. pathway radiofrequency ablation
f. pathway ► retrograde
F. -Scan Computerized Tomography (CT)
f. sodium current
f. stain, acid-
f. stain of sputum ► acid-
f. tachycardia ► slow-
f. wave
f. wave sleep
fasting
f. blood sugar (FBS)
f. blood sugars (FBS) ► daily
f. glucose ► impaired
f. glucose levels
f. plasma cholesterol
f. plasma glucose
f. plasma triglyceride
f. protocol, medically supervised
f. type diet
fat(s)
f., abdominal
f., abdominal body
f. absorption

fat(s)—*continued*
f. -absorption studies
f. -absorption study ‣ triolein
f. -absorption test
f. analysis, body-
f., artery-clogging
f. atrophy ‣ focal serous
f., axillary
f., body
f., bound
f., brown
f., bulging
f., burning body
f. cast
f. cell
f. cells, alpha 2
f. cholesterol diet, low-
f., chyle
f., circulating
f. clot, chicken
f. consumption, dietary-
f. -controlled diet
f., controlling
f., corpse
f. density area
f. deposits
f. deposits, abdominal-
f. deposits, body-
f. diet, high-
f. diet, low-
f. diet, low-saturated-
f. diet, reduced-
f., dietary
f. digestion
f. disorder, blood-
f. distribution
f. distribution, gynecoid
f. eating plan ‣ low-
f. emboli syndrome
f. embolism
f. embolism syndrome
f. embolization
f. embolus
f. emulsification
f. emulsion
f., epicardial
f., excess
f. ‣ excessive orbital
f. exchange
f. excretion, fecal
f. food, high-
f. fractionation
f. -free
f. -free diet
f. -free dry weight

f. -free mass
f. -free meal
f. -free wet weight
f. ‣ gluteal body
f. graft
f. graft, autologous
f., grave
f. heart
f. hernia
f., high-cholesterol diet ‣ high-
f., hydrous wool
f. in diet
f. ‣ indentation for thymus and
        mediastinal
f. index, cholesterol saturated
f. injection
f. intake
f. intake, dietary
f. intake ‣ saturated
f. intake, total
f., interstitial
f., IV (intravenous)
f. ketogenic diet ‣ high-
f. KP (keratic precipitates), mutton
f. -laden microphages
f. -laden plaque
f. layer, subcutaneous
f. level, blood-
f. liquefaction
f., ‣ low-cholesterol diet, low-
f., low-cholesterol food ‣ low-
f., low-fiber diet ‣ high-
f. marrow
f., masked
f. mass, decreased
f. meal
f. meal response
f., metabolism of
f., milk
f. milk ‣ low-
f. -mobilizing substance
f., molecular
f., monounsaturated
f. ‣ mortality and body
f., moruloid
f., mulberry
f. necrosis
f. necrosis ‣ postinjectional
f., neutral
f., nonacidic diet ‣ low-
f., omental
f. oppression
f. pad
f. pad biopsy, scalene
f. pad enlargement ‣ dorsocervical

f. pad, pericardial
f. pad, pleural
f. pad, retropatellar
f. pad sign
f., pericolic
f., perinephric
f., perinephritic
f., perirenal
f. plug, Imlach's
f., polyunsaturated
f. profile
f. profile, blood
f., qualitative
f., reducing saturated
f., reduction of blood
f. refined wool
f. -related disease
f. replacement atrophy
f. -restricted diet
f. saturated
f. saturation
f. screening, body-
f. solubility
f. -soluble drugs
f. -soluble vitamin
f. stains
f., stored
f. stripe ‣ subepicardial
f., subcutaneous
f., subcuticular
f., subepicardial
f. suctioning
f. suctioning ‣ ultrasonic
f. tag, epicardial
f. test, fecal
f. ‣ thymus and mediastinal
f. tissue
f. tissue, brown
f., total body
f. transplant
f. transplantation
f., unsaturated
f. vegetarian diet, low-
f., visceral

fatal
f. acute pulmonary edema
f. allergic reaction
f. allergic reaction to penicillin
f. arrhythmia
f. blood disease
f. blood disorder
f. bone marrow aplasia
f. brain damage
f. burn
f. cardiac spasm

f. child abuse
f. complications
f. condition, potentially
f. disease
f. disease, potentially
f. disorder
f. dose
f. dose, median
f. dose, minimal
f. eating disorder
f. familial insomnia
f. genetic illness
f. granulomatous disease
f. heart arrhythmias
f. heart attack
f. heart attack ▸ sudden
f., heart rhythm
f. heart rhythm disturbance
f. hemorrhage
f. hemorrhagic pancreatitis
f. hepatitis
f. hereditary disorder
f. hypersensitivity reaction
f. illness
f. infection
f. injury, non-
f. liver toxicity
f. lung condition
f. medical condition
f. myoglobinuria
f. neuromuscular disease
f. nosocomial infection
f. overdose
f. poisoning ▸ drug-related
f. pulmonary hemorrhage
f. respiratory failure
f. seizure
f. stroke
f. systemic infection
f. transfusion reaction
f. virus
fatalistic attitude
fatality(-ies)
f. alcohol-related
f., drug-associated
f., huffing
f. rate, breast cancer
f. rate, cancer
fate map
father
f., diabetic
f. factor
f. figure
f., foster
fatigability, easy

fatigability, excessive
fatigans, Culex
fatigue
f. and agitation
f. and breathlessness ▸
   unexplained
f. and depression
f. and dyspnea
f. and insomnia
f., and insomnia ▸ pain,
f. and lethargy
f. and loss of appetite
f. and malaise
f. and/or nausea
f. and pallor
f. and shortness of breath (SOB) ▸
   weakness,
f. and sleeplessness
f. and tension
f. and weakness ▸ progressive
f., anemia and
f. ▸ anger, tension and
f. ▸ breathlessness and
f., chronic
f., combat
f., compassion
f., constant
f. damage
f. ▸ decrease in energy or
f., depression and impotence
f. ▸ depression, insomnia and
f. ▸ detrimental impact of
f., driver
f., episodic
f. ▸ excessive stress and
f., exertional
f., extreme
f., eye
f., eyebrow
f. factor
f. fever
f., fluctuating
f., foot
f. fracture
f. from antihistamine
f. from anxiety
f. from birth control pill
f. from depression
f., general
f., generalized
f. ▸ generalized,
   debilitating,longstanding
f. ▸ generalized weakness and
f. in leg muscles ▸ sense of
f. ▸ inactivity, lethargy and

f., inappropriate
f., increased
f., increasing
f. leading to exhaustion
f. ▸ loss of appetite with
f., marked
f., mental
f., muscle
f., muscle aches, and pains
f. ▸ muscular pain and
f., neurosis
f., neurotic
f. of muscles and tendons
f. or loss of energy
f., overwhelming
f. ▸ palpitations, dyspnea, and
f., persistent
f., physiopathology of
f., progressive
f., prolonged generalized
f., pupillary
f., reaction
f., relentless
f., retina
f., severe
f. ▸ severe joint pain and
f. syndrome (CFS) ▸ chronic
f., tremendous
f., unrelieved
f. weakness and
f., weakness, and decreased energy
f. ▸ withdrawal, isolation, depression
   and
fatigued
f. and stressed
f., patient awakes
f., patient is
f., patient routinely
fatness, intense fear of
fatty
f. acid
f. acid crystals
f. acid, essential
f. acid ethyl ester
f. acid, excess
f. acid, free
f. acid, long-chain
f. acid, medium-chain
f. acid, polyunsaturated
f. acid production, free
f. acid, radioiodinated
f. acid, synthesize
f. acid, total
f. acid, trans-
f. acid, triglyceride

fatty—*continued*
f. acid, unesterified
f. ascites
f. atrophy
f. bags
f. capsule of kidney
f. cardiopathy
f. cell membranes
f. change ▸ hyaline
f. cholesterol deposits
f. cirrhosis
f. degeneration of heart
f. deposits
f. diarrhea ▸ pancreatogenous
f. diet, high
f. diet, low
f. eye bags
f. food intolerance
f. foods
f. granule cell
f. heart
f. heart, Quain's
f. infiltration
f. infiltration, bulging
f. infiltration of liver
f. layer
f. liver
f. liver, acute
f. liver ▸ alcoholic
f. liver disease
f. liver, enlarged
f. lobules
f. material
f. meal
f. meal, after
f. metamorphosis
f. metamorphosis, mild
f. metamorphosis of liver
f. molecules ▸ oxidized
f. necrosis, Balser's
f. liver ▸ nonalcoholic
f. panniculus
f. plaque
f. plaque build-up
f. plaque in arteries
f. plaque in blood vessels
f. plaque in vessel walls
f. sheath
f. stool
f. streak
f. substance
f. thickened
f. tissue
f. tissue, abnormal
f. tissue ▸ underlying

f. tissues, mediastinal
f. tumor
f. tumor, cortical
f. vacuoles
f. vacuolization
fauces [*fossae*]
f., muscles of
f., muscles of palate and
f., pillar of
Fauchard's disease
faucial
f. arch
f. arch carcinoma
f. area
f. reflex
f. tonsil
faucium, Mycoplasma
faulty
f. airways
f. bone growth
f. coordination
f. gene
f. heart rhythm
f. heart's normal rhythm ▸ reboot
f. memories ▸ confused or
f. memory
f. prescriptions
f. valve action
f. vision
f. warning system
Fauvel's granules
faviform, Trichophyton
favorite supplements
favosa, mycosis
favosa, trichomycosis
Favre
F. disease
F. disease ▸ Durand Nicolas-
F. disease ▸ Nicolas-
favus circinatus
favus herpeticus
Fazio-Londe atrophy
FB (fingerbreadth)
FB (foreign body)
FB, electromagnetic removal of
FB esophagus
FB extraction
FB from cornea, removal of
FB giant cell
FB granuloma
FB impacted
FB in air passage
FB in anterior chamber
FB in bronchus
FB in ciliary body

FB in cornea
FB in ear
FB in iris
FB in lacrimal sac
FB in lens
FB in lung
FB in nose
FB in optic nerve
FB in trachea
FB, inhalation of
FB, intraocular
FB, intrauterine
FB, metallic
FB, nostril obstructed by
FB obstructing airway
FB, opaque
FB papule
FB passed
FB, removal of
FB removed
FB retained
FB, sclerotomy with removal of
FB seen on x-ray
FB, soft-tissue
FB, tracheal
FBP (femoral blood pressure)
FBS (fasting blood sugar)
FBS (fasting blood sugars) ▸ daily
FC (facilitated communication)
FC (5-fluorocytosine) ▸ 5-
fc (foot-candles)
FCC (fracture compound, comminuted)
fcm (foot-candle meter)
FDA (Food and Drug Administration)
FDA ▸ advisory committee of
fear(s)
f., abandonment of
f., age-related
f. and anxiety
f. and confusion
f. and hopelessness
f. and rage
f. and rejection
f. and tension
f., anger and depression
f., attack of intense
f. conditioning
f. ▸ disabling irrational
f., doubt or disgust
f. ▸ hopelessness and
f., housebound by
f. ▸ intense abandonment
f. ▸ level of
f. of aloneness

f. of anxiety
f. of being alone
f. of being attacked
f. of being demeaned
f. of being influenced
f. of being manipulated
f. of dark
f. of doctors, patient has
f. of dying
f. of embarrassment
f. of fatness, intense
f. of future
f. of going crazy
f. of hospitals, patient has
f. of imminent death
f. of impending loss
f. of losing control
f. of panic attack
f. of personal harm
f. of social situations
f. of suffocation
f. of the future
f., phobias and anxieties
f. response, conditioned
f. -tension-pain cycle

fearful
f., anxious and
f. emotions
f., patient

feasible ▸ emergency skin transplants
feather analysis
feathering or redness ▸ light
feature(s)
f. ▸ adjustment disorder with mixed emotional
f. ▸ adjustment reaction with mixed emotional
f. and disorders, associated
f. ▸ arteriosclerotic dementia depressive
f. ▸ arteriosclerotic dementia with delusional
f. ▸ bipolar disorder, depressed, severe, without psychotic
f. ▸ bipolar disorder, depressed, with psychotic
f. ▸ bipolar disorder, manic, severe, without psychotic
f. ▸ bipolar disorder, manic, with psychotic
f. ▸ bipolar disorder, mixed, severe, without psychotic
f. ▸ bipolar disorder, mixed, with psychotic

f., characteristic
f., characteristic facial
f., exaggerated emotional
f. ▸ extravascular granulomatous
f. ▸ major depression, recurrent, severe, without psychotic
f. ▸ major depression, recurrent, with psychotic
f. ▸ major depression, severe, without psychotic
f. ▸ major depression, single-episode, severe, with psychotic
f. ▸ major depression, single-episode, with psychotic
f. ▸ major depression, with psychotic
f., mixed emotional
f., mongoloid
f., personality
f., salient
f., squamoid

febrile [*afebrile*]
f. agglutinin
f. convulsion
f. convulsion, benign
f. delirium
f. delirium, specific
f. disease
f. episode
f. exanthem
f. illness
f. morbidity
f. morbidity ▸ maternal
f. morbidity ▸ puerperal
f. neutropenia
f. neutropenic patient
f. paroxysm
f., patient
f. polyneuritis, acute
f. proteinuria
f. psychosis
f. pulse
f. reaction, acute
f. respiratory disease
f. seizures
f. state
f. syndrome, acute
f. transfusion reaction
f. tropical splenomegaly
f. urine

febrilis
f., calor
f., herpes
f., placenta

fecal [*fetal*]
f. anaerobes
f. analysis
f. blood
f. calcium, endogenous
f. carcinoembryonic antigen
f. contamination, direct
f. contents
f. continence
f. control ▸ loss of
f. discharge
f. excretion
f. excretion, maximal
f. fat excretion
f. fat test
f. fistula
f. flora
f. frequency
f. impaction
f. impaction, constipation and
f. impaction, extensive
f. incontinence
f. leukocytes
f. mass
f. material
f. material, emesis of
f. material, impacted
f. material, passing
f. material, retained
f. occult blood testing (FOBT)
f. -oral route
f. -oral route of infection
f. particle, retained
f. residue
f. shedding, chronic
f. smears
f. soilage
f. urobilinogen
f. vomiting
f. vomitus

fecalith, appendiceal
fecalith obstruction
fecally contaminated vehicle
feces
f. and gas
f. and colonic cancer
f., bacteria in
f., blood in
f. defecation
f., discharge of
f. ▸ endoscopy blood in
f., gas and
f. in the colon
f. incontinence
f., incontinence of the

feces—*continued*
f. ▸ involuntary discharge of
f., normal
f., patient incontinent of
f., pooled rat
f., retained
f., scybalous
FECG (fetal electrocardiogram)
FECO₂ (fraction of expired carbon dioxide)
fed infant ▸ bottle-
fed, infant breast-
federal immunization program
Federov's implant
fee scale, sliding-
feeble pulse
feebleminded, patient
feedback
f., accurate
f., analogue
f. and cognition, temperature
f., anticipatory bogus heart rate
f. as relaxation technique ▸ electromyograph
f., auditory
f., binary
f., delayed auditory
f., discrete post-trial
f. ▸ discussion, exploration, and
f., group
f. groups, tension in
f., haptic
f. heart rate
f. -induced muscle relaxation
f. mechanisms of hormonal control
f., mechanoelectrical
f. monitoring
f. monitoring, anesthesia
f. negative
f. of myoelectric output ▸ visual
f. of speech muscle activity
f., positive
f., respiratory
f., sensory
f. session
f. signals, artificial
f. technique for deep relaxation
f. therapy, sensory
f. training, autogenic
f. training, neuromuscular
f. training of parts of buccinator muscle
f., visual
feeder channels
feeder vessel

feeding(s)
f. and grooming ▸ dressing, bathing
f., artificial
f., blenderized tube
f., breast-
f., casein-based tube
f. center ▸ hypothalamic
f. difficulties
f., enteral
f., extrabuccal
f., Finkelstein's
f., forced
f. ▸ forced tube
f., forcible
f., formula
f. gastrostomy
f., gavage
f., glucose
f., glucose and water
f., hyperalimentation
f., intravenous (IV)
f., jejunostomy
f., long-term breast
f., milk-based tube
f., nasal
f., nipple
f., NJ (nasojejunal)
f., oral
f., Osmolite
f., parenteral
f., patient breast-
f., patient independent in
f. self-care deficit
f., sham
f., Similac
f. tube
f. tube, infant
f. tube, intraesophageal
f. tube, nasoesophageal
f. tube, nasogastric
f. tube ▸ surgically implanted
f. tube ▸ withdrawal
f. tube ▸ withholding

feel(s) [*seal*]
f. abandoned, patient
f. blue ▸ patient
f. damaged ▸ patient
f. degraded
f. demoralized ▸ patient
f. down ▸ patient
f. empty ▸ patient
f. estranged ▸ patient
f. giddy, patient
f. guilty ▸ patient
f. hollow and empty

f. isolated ▸ patient
f. pleasure ▸ inability to
f. rejected or ridiculed, patient
feelei, Legionella
feeling(s)
f., absence of
f., aggressive
f., ambivalent
f. and actions, addictive
f., and perceptions ▸ memories,
f. anxious
f., bloated
f., burning, tingling, prickly
f., crisis-related
f., depressed
f., depressive
f., drowsy
f. drugged
f., empty
f. ▸ encourage ventilation of
f., euphoric
f. ▸ fidgeting, aching, pulling, or itching
f. hostile, patient
f. in eye ▸ gritty
f. in head ▸ tight
f. in leg ▸ crampy, achy
f., inferiority
f., intense
f., internal
f., lethargic
f., listless and tired
f., loss of
f., mixed
f., negative
f. numb
f., Oedipal
f. of abandonment
f. of anger
f. of anxiety ▸ persistent
f. of choking
f. of confidence
f. of deep emptiness, chronic
f. of depersonalization
f. of depression
f. of derealization
f. of despair
f. of despondency
f. of detachment
f. of dissociation
f. of dullness and not caring
f. of emptiness, chronic
f. of euphoria, initial
f. of excessive feeling of inappropriate guilt

f. of excitement
f. of film over eyes
f. of futility
f. of guilt
f. of guilt ▸ persistent
f. of guilt, worthlessness, and helplessness
f. of hopelessness
f. of hopelessness ▸ persistent
f. of humiliation ▸ sustained
f. of immobilization
f. of impending disaster
f. of impending doom
f. of inadequacy
f. of inappropriate guilt
f. of inner tension
f. of intellectual and physical power
f. of isolation
f. of isolation and being misunderstood
f. of malaise, generalized
f. of melancholy
f. of mistrust
f. of others ▸ indifferent to
f. of pins and needles
f. of pressure
f. of resentment
f. of restlessness
f. of sadness and grief ▸ overwhelming
f. of sadness ▸ persistent
f. of shame ▸ sustained
f. of social inadequacy
f. of terror, sudden unexplainable
f. of tightness in chest
f. of tingling or stiffness
f. of uneasiness
f. of unreality
f. of weakness
f. of well-being
f. of worthlessness
f. off-balance
f. out-of-control
f. overwhelmed
f., paresthetic
f., patient expressed guilt
f., patient has floating
f., pent-up
f. ▸ perception of
f., persistent
f., positive
f. pressure
f. rejected
f. removed from reality
f. sad

f. sick to stomach
f. spaced out
f., stabilization of
f. stressed, patient
f. ▸ stuffed-up
f., stunned
f., subjective
f. ▸ suicidal or homicidal
f. tone
f. tone, emotional
f., tranquilize
f. uncoordinated
f., unexplained
f., unsteady
f., ventilate
f., verbalization of
f. washed out

feet

f. above heart level, elevate
f., aching
f., bacterial growth on
f., bony changes of
f., bromhidrosis of
f., burning
f., callus on
f., cavus
f., cold
f., digits of
f. ▸ flaking and chafing of
f., flat
f. from atherosclerosis ▸ burning
f., neuropathy of
f. ▸ numbness of
f. ▸ painful burning of
f., paresthesias of
f., peeling of hands and
f. ▸ persistent swelling of
f. ▸ physical complications of problem
f., planovalgus
f., poor circulation to the
f. ▸ puffiness of
f., scaly
f. ▸ spring-loaded
f., sweaty
f., swelling of
f. ▸ swelling of hands or
f., swollen
f. ▸ tender blisters on
f. tingle
f. ▸ tingling and numbness in
f. ▸ tingling in hands and
f., tingling sensations in
f., tired, aching

FEF (forced expiratory flow)

Fehleisen's streptococcus
Fehr's dystrophy
Feigenbaum echocardiogram
feigned
f. psychological problems
f. renal colic
f. tic douloureux
f. toothache
feigning symptoms
Feil syndrome ▸ Klippel-
Feingold diet
Feist-Mankin position
Feldman adaptometer
Feldman test, Sabin-
Feldstein syndrome ▸ Klippel-
félé, bruit de pot
Felig insulin pump
feline ataxia virus
feline leukemia
felineum, Microsporum
felineus, Opisthorchis
felis, Miyagawanella
Felix reaction ▸ Weil-
Felix-Weil reaction
fell, blood pressure (BP)
felo-de-se
felt
f. gauze pad
f. patch
f. pledget ▸ Meadox Teflon
f., Teflon
Felty's syndrome
female
f. adult genitalia, normal
f. breast reduction
f. breasts
f. condom
f. fertility
f. gender
f. genital tract
f. genitalia, infantile
f. genitalia, normal
f. gonadotropins ▸ level of
f. hormones
f. hypospadias
f. infant, viable
f. infertility
f. intersex
f., multiparous
f. neonate, term AGA (appropriate for gestational age)
f. orgasm, inhibited
f. (b/fe) ▸ patient black
f., patient Caucasian
f., patient Indian

female—*continued*
  f. patient, menopausal
  f., patient Oriental
  f. (wh/fe) ▸ patient white
  f. pattern baldness
  f. -pattern hair loss
  f. pelvic floor
  f., prepubescent
  f. rat brain
  f. reproductive cycle
  f. reproductive tract
  f. sex estrogen hormone ▸
    stimulate production of
  f. sex hormone
  f. sexual arousal disorder
  f. sterility
  f. textured breast augmentation
  f. urethra, cervical colliculus of
  f. urethral lesions
feminae, hydrocele
feminina, urethra
femininae, crista urethralis
femininum, pudendum
feminization, testicular
feminizing syndrome, testicular
femora
  f., lower
  f., proximal
  f., upper
femoral
  f. approach
  f. approach ▸ retrograde
  f. arteriogram
  f. arteriography
  f. artery
  f. artery approach
  f. artery cannulated
  f. artery, common
  f. artery contusion ▸ superficial
  f. artery, deep
  f. artery, left
  f. artery occlusion
  f. artery pressure point
  f. artery repair
  f. artery, right
  f. artery, stenotic
  f. artery ▸ superficial
  f. artery thrombosis
  f. arthritis, patellar
  f. blood pressure (FBP)
  f. bone
  f. bypass, cross femoral-
  f. bypass, descending thoracic
    aortofemoral-
  f. bypass ▸ femoral-

  f. canal
  f. condyle
  f. condyle, medial
  f. cortices
  f. cutaneous nerve ▸ lateral
  f. Dacron graft ▸ aorto◊
  f. embolectomy
  f. embolus
  f. endarterectomy
  f. epiphysis, capital
  f. epiphysis, distal
  f. epiphysis, slipped upper
  f. -femoral bypass
  f. -femoral bypass, cross
  f. graft
  f. head
  f. head prosthesis ▸ Zimaloy
  f. head replacement ▸
    endoprosthetic
  f. head replacement ▸ Matchett-
    Brown
  f. head, Thompson
  f. hernia
  f. herniorrhaphy
  f. (SAF) hip replacement, self-
    articulating
  f. lymphadenopathy, palpable
  f. muscle
  f. neck
  f. neck fracture ▸ displaced
  f. neck fracture site
  f. nerve
  f. nerve block
  f. nodes
  f. perfusion cannula
  f. popliteal bypass surgery
  f. popliteal occlusive disease
  f. prosthesis, Xenophor
  f. prosthetic head ▸ Eicher
  f. prosthetic head ▸ Judet-type
  f. prosthetic head ▸ Naden-Rieth
  f. pulse
  f. pulse, palpable
  f. reflex
  f. route
  f. runoff angiography
  f. runoff arteriography
  f. shaft
  f. shortening osteotomy
  f. sound ▸ pistol-shot
  f. tibial bypass
  f. -tibial-peroneal bypass
  f. triangle
  f. vascular injury
  f. vein

  f. vein, common
  f. vein, deep
  f. vein, lateral circumflex
  f. vein ligation
  f. vein, medial circumflex
  f. vein occlusion
  f. venous thrombosis
  f. vessel
femorale, calcar
femoris
  f. artery ▸ profunda
  f., biceps
  f., fascia lata
  f., ligamentum teres
  f., linea aspera
  f. muscle, biceps
  f., rectus
  f. tendon, rectus
  f. vein ▸ profunda
femoroaxillary bypass
femorocerebral catheter angiography
femorofemoral crossover bypass
femoroiliac disease
femoropopliteal
  f. artery occlusion
  f. bypass graft
  f. vein
femorotibial bypass
femur
  f., anteversion neck of
  f., bone graft
  f. dislocation
  f. displaced
  f. fractured
  f. full range of motion (ROM) ▸ left
  f. full range of motion (ROM) ▸ right
  f., head of
  f., intercondylar notch of
  f., left
  f., nail inserted into neck and head
    of
  f., neck of
  f. ▸ osteonecrosis of
  f. osteotomized
  f. pinned
  f. (UPF) prosthesis, Bateman
    universal proximal
  f., proximal metaphysis of
  f. repaired with prosthesis
  f., right
  f., shaft of
  f., supracondylar fracture of
  f., torque of
fence, Kirklin
fender fracture, bumper-

Fendt sarcoid ▸ Spiegler-
fenestra
    f. cochlea
    f. ovalis
    f. rotunda
    f. vestibuli
fenestrata, placenta
fenestrated
    f. catheter
    f. compress
    f. hymen
    f. membrane
    f. membrane ▸ Henle
    f. septum
    f. valve
fenestration
    f., aortopulmonary
    f., baffle
    f. bur, Lempert's
    f. cavity
    f., cusp
    f. of semicircular canal
    f. operation
fensor, noci◊
Féréol's nodes
Ferguson's method
Fergusson and Critchley's ataxia
Fergusson's incision
ferment fever
fermental diarrhea
fermentans, Lactobacillus
fermentation
    f., mannitol
    f., self-
    f. tube
fermentative diarrhea
fermenti, Lactobacillus
fermenting, nonmannite
fern
    f. leaf tongue
    f. phenomenon
    f. test
Fernwald sign, Braun-
Fernwald's sign, Von
ferox, Psorophora
Ferrata's cells
Ferraton disease ▸ Perrin-
Ferree-Rand perimeter
Ferrein's canal
Ferribacterium duplex
ferritin conjugated antibodies
Ferrobacillus ferrooxidans
ferrokinetic data
ferromagnetic artifact
ferrooxidans, Ferrobacillus

ferrous
    f. carbonate mass
    f. fumarate
    f. gluconate
    f. hydroxide, macroaggregated
ferrugineum, Trichophyton
ferruginous bodies
fertile, patient
fertile period
fertility (Fertility) [*virility*]
    F. and Maternal Health Drugs
       Advisory Committee
    f. awareness
    f. clinic
    f. drugs
    f. evaluation
    f., female
    f. from chemotherapy ▸ loss of
    f. from radiation ▸ loss of
    f. ▸ impairment of
    f. problem
    f. specialist
    f. test
fertilization
    f. (IVF), in vitro
    f., self-
    f. services, in vitro
fertilize ovum
fertilized
    f. egg
    f. egg, implantation of
    f. ovum, implantation of
fervens, calor
fervescence, stage of
FES (functional electrical
    stimulation)
feseri, Clostridium
FESS (functional endoscopic sinus
    surgery)
festering skin sores
festinating gait
FET (forced expiratory time)
fetal (Fetal) [*fecal*]
    f. abnormality
    f. acoustic stimulation (FAS)
    f. activity
    f. activity determinations (FAD)
    f. adenoma
    f. age
    f. AIDS (acquired immune
       deficiency syndrome)
    f. air sign ▸ intravascular
    f. alcohol baby
    f. alcohol retardation
    f. alcohol syndrome (FAS)

    f. anomalies ▸ pneumococcus in
       vitro
    f. anomaly
    f. appendages
    f. arrhythmia
    f. ascites
    f. asphyxia
    f. back
    f. basiotripsy
    f. bladder ▸ malformation of
    f. bleed, large
    f. blood analysis
    f. blood cells, Rh positive
    f. blood, Rh positive
    f. bradycardia
    f. brain cells
    f. brain formation
    f. cardiac anomaly
    f. cell transplant
    f. cells
    f. cells ▸ human
    f. cells ▸ purified
    f. cells, transplanted
    f. chamber communication
    f. chest anomaly
    f. circulation
    f. circulation, inhibit
    f. circulation ▸ persistent
    f. cleidotomy
    f. congenital diaphragmatic hernia
       (CDH)
    f. cord
    f. cranial diameters
    f. cranioclasis
    f. craniotomy
    f. death
    f. death, antepartum
    f. death, early
    f. death, intermediate
    f. death ▸ intrauterine
    f. death, late
    f. decelerations
    f. demise
    f. development
    f. disposition
    f. distress
    f. distress, impending
    f. distress, severe
    f. dystocia
    f. echocardiography
    f. electrocardiogram (ECG/EKG)
       test
    f. electrocardiography
    f. gastrointestinal (GI) anomaly
    f. gastroschisis

fetal—*continued*
f. genetic disorder
f. gestation
f. gigantism
f. growth
f. growth and development
f. growth, normal
f. growth ▸ retard
f. growth, slow
f. head
f. head into superior pelvic strait ▸ entrance
f. head ▸ rotate
f. head ▸ wedged
f. heart
f. heart monitor
f. heart monitor, electronic
f. heart monitor tracing
f. heart monitoring
f. heart rate
f. heart rate, baseline variability of
f. heart rate monitoring ▸ internal
f. heart rate reading
f. heart sound (FHS)
f. heart tones (FHT)
f. heart tones (FHT), Doptone monitoring of
f. heart tones (FHT) obtained with Doptone
f. heart tones (FHT) ▸ stable
f. heartbeat
f. hemoglobin
f. hemoglobin test
f. hemorrhage ▸ maternal
f. hydrops
f. hypertensive crisis ▸ potential
f. inclusion
f. infection
f. intervention
f. karyotyping
f. kidney development
f. life
f. lobulation
f. lobulations, normal
f. lung liquid production
f. lung maturity
f. lung tumor
f. lungs, immature
f. macrosomia
f. malformation
f. maternal bleed
f. maternal hemoglobin
f. maturity
f. maturity ▸ premature
f. medicine

f. medicine, maternal-
f. membrane
f. membranes, prolonged rupture of
f. metabolism
f. monitor
F. Monitor (CFM) ▸ Corometrics
F. Monitor, Huntleigh Domiciliary
f. monitoring
f. monitoring, advanced
f. monitoring system
f. morbidity and mortality
f. motion
f. movement
f. nerve cell transplant
f. nuchal fluid
f. nuchal translucency
f. oophoritis
f. outcomes, adverse
f. ovary
f. pancreas transplant ▸ human
f. parasite
f. part ▸ protrusion of
f. pelvic disproportion
f. pig cell transplant
f. placenta
f. placental membrane
f. position
f. position ▸ patient in
f. protein test, alpha
f. quickening
f. renal hamartoma
f. respiration
f. rhythm
f. scalp
f. scalp sampling
f. skeleton
f. souffle
f. spine
f. stage
f. suprarenal gland
f. surgery
f. tachycardia
f. therapist
f. tissue
f. tissue transplant
f. tissue ▸ transplanting human
f. tolerance, normal
f. ultrasound
f. urine
f. uterus
f. wastage
Fetaldex test
fetalis
f. calcificans, chondrodystrophia
f., chondromalacia

f., erythroblastosis
f., hydrops
f., opisthotonos
f., placentae, pars
fetally malnourished ▸ intrauterine
fetid odor
fetid sweat
fetishism, transvestic
fetogram study
fetomaternal hemorrhage
fetomaternal incompatibility
fetopelvic disproportion
fetoprotein, alpha-
fetoprotein test, alpha
fetor
f. ex ore
f., hepaticus
f. oris
fetu, fetus in
fetus
f., abnormal
f., aborted
f., aborted human
f. acardiacus
f., amniotic adhesions of
f. amorphus
f., anemic
f., calcified
f., Campylobacter
f. compressus
f. continuously monitored
f., crushing procedure skull of
f., dead
f., developing
f., Doppler monitoring of
f. expelled
f., full-term
f., harlequin
f., ichthyosis
f., impact on
f., imperfect
f. in fetu
f. in utero
f. in utero ▸ dead
f. into activity ▸ stimulating
f., intrauterine
f., length of
f., macerated
f., malformed
f., mummified
f., no abnormality of
f., nonviable
f., paper-doll
f., papyraceous
f. papyraceus

f., parasitic
f., patient delivered macerated
f. rotated
f. sanguinolentis
f. sireniform
f. ▸ spontaneously aborted human
f. stem cell transplant ▸ fetus-to-
f. -to-fetus stem cell transplant
f., viable
f., Vibrio
f. with hydrocephalus

feuilles effect ▸ mille
Feulgen strain
FEV (forced expiratory volume)
fever(s)

f., absorption
f., acute rheumatic
f., adynamic
f., American mountain
f. and chills
f. and cough ▸ chills,
f. and disorientation
f. and nausea
f., and night sweats ▸ chills,
f., aphthous
f., Argentinian hemorrhagic
f., artificial
f., aseptic
f., Assam
f., asthenic
f., Australian Q
f., bilious
f., black
f. blister
f., blue
f., Bolivian hemorrhagic
f., bouquet
f., brain
f., Brazilian spotted
f., breakbone
f., cabin
f., cachectic
f., cachexial
f., camp
f., carbuncular
f., catarrhal
f., cat-bite
f., cat-scratch
f. caused by infection
f., cerebrospinal
f., Charcot's
f., childbed
f., chills and
f., chronic
f., Colombian tick

f., Colorado tick
f., continued
f., continuous
f., convulsion accompanying
f., cough, and disorientation
f., cough, confusion, or weakness
f., coughing with
f., Crimean Congo hemorrhagic
f., dandy
f., dehydration
f., delirium of
f., delirium with high
f., dengue
f., desert
f. ▸ diarrhea, abdominal pain, and
f., digestive
f., discomfort and
f., drug-induced
f., Dumdum
f. ▸ dyspnea, cough and
f., Ebola
f. ▸ Ebola hemorrhagic
f., enteric
f., ephemeral
f., epidemic catarrhal
f., epidemic hemorrhagic
f., eruptive
f., essential
f., etiocholanolone
f., exanthematous
f., factitious
f., fatigue
f., ferment
f., field
f., food
f., Fort Bragg
f. from arthritis
f. from cold
f. from infection of ear
f., glandular
f., Haverhill
f., hay
f., hectic
f., hemorrhagic
f. ▸ hemorrhagic dengue
f., hepatic
f., herpetic
f., hospital
f., humidifier
f., hyperpyrexial
f., hysterical
f. immunization, yellow
f., inanition
f., induced
f. -induced dehydration

f., inhalation
f., intermenstrual
f., intermittent
f., intermittent chills and
f., intermittent hepatic
f., irritation
f. ▸ Jaccoud dissociated
f. ▸ jaundice, chills, and
f. ▸ jaundice, lethargy, and
f., jungle
f., jungle yellow
f., Korean hemorrhagic
f., land
f., Lassa
f., low-grade
f., lung
f., macular
f., malarial
f., Malta
f. ▸ Marburg hemorrhagic
f., Mediterranean
f., milk
f., Monday
f., night sweats, cough, foul sputum
f., nonseasonal hay
f. of brief duration
f. of obscure etiology
f. of undetermined origin (FUO)
f. of unknown origin (FUO)
f. ▸ Omsk hemorrhagic
f., onset of chills and
f., Oroya
f. ▸ pain in abdomen with
f., Panama
f., paratyphoid
f., parrot
f., patient spiked
f., perennial hay
f., periodic
f., persistent
f., petechial
f., pharyngoconjunctival
f., phlebotomus
f., pneumonic
f., postoperative
f., pretibial
f., psittacosis, cocci triad ▸ Q
f., puerperal
f., pulmonary
f., pulmonary infiltrate
f., Q (query)
f., quartan
f., query (Q)
f., quinine
f., quintana

fever(s)—*continued*
- f., quotidian
- f., rabbit
- f., rat-bite
- f., recurrent
- f., reduce
- f. -reducing drugs
- f., relapsing
- f., remittent
- f., rheumatic
- f., Rift Valley
- f., Rocky Mountain spotted
- f., San Joaquin
- f., scarlet
- f., septic
- f., shaking chills
- f., shaking chills, dyspnea
- f., shoddy
- f., South American hemorrhagic
- f., Southeast Asian mosquito-borne hemorrhagic
- f. spike
- f., spiking
- f., splenic
- f., spotted
- f., sthenic
- f., stiffneck
- f., streptobacillary
- f. subsided spontaneously
- f., sudden onset of
- f., swelling and tenderness of transplant
- f., swelling and tissue destruction
- f. symptoms, hay
- f. therapy ▸ malaria
- f., thermic
- f., threshing
- f., tick
- f., transitory
- f., traumatic
- f., treatment of rheumatic
- f., trench
- f., tsutsugamushi
- f., typhoid
- f. undetermined origin (FUO)
- f., undulant
- f. unknown origin (FUO)
- f. unresponsive to antibiotic therapy
- f., urethral
- f., urinary
- f., vaccinal
- f., valley
- f. ▸ Venezuelan hemorrhagic
- f. ▸ viral hemorrhagic
- f. virus, Colorado tick

- f. virus, pappataci
- f. virus, pharyngoconjunctival
- f. virus, Rift Valley
- f. virus ▸ yellow
- f., West Nile
- f. ▸ West Nile-like
- f. with renal syndrome ▸ hemorrhagic
- f., wound
- f., yellow

feverish, patient
F-F (finger-to-finger) testing
FFA-labelled scintigraphy
FFDR (full florid diabetic retinopathy)
FH (familial hypercholesterolemia)
FH (family history)
FHS (fetal heart sound)
FHT (fetal heart tones)
FHT (fetal heart tones) obtained with Doptone
fiber(s)
- f., accessory nodoventricular
- f., activating inhibitory
- f., afferent
- f., afferent nerve
- f., afferent spinal nerve
- f. and bowel movement
- f. and colonic cancer
- f. and diverticulitis
- f. and hemorrhoids
- f. and sheaths ▸ medullated
- f., annular
- f., anterior external arcuate
- f., asbestos
- f., association
- f., atrial muscle
- f., atrio-Hisian
- f., atrophic muscle
- f., Berneheimer's
- f., beta
- f., blocking vagal efferent
- f., brain nerve
- f., Brücke's
- f., bundle of nerve
- f. bundles, myocardial
- f., bundles of nonmyelinated nerve
- f., C-
- f., capsule
- f., cardiac muscle
- f. catheter ▸ optical
- f. cell
- f. cell, elongated contractile
- f. cell, nucleated contractile
- f., circular
- f. ▸ clumps of tangled

- f., collagen
- f., collagenous
- f., corticopontine
- f., cotton
- f., crude
- f., damage to nerve
- f., Darkschweitsch's
- f., deep transverse
- f., demyelinated nerve
- f., deterioration of nerve
- f. dialyzer, Dow hollow
- f. dialyzer, hollow
- f. diameter
- f. diet, high-
- f. diet ▸ high-fat, low-
- f. diet, low-
- f., dietary
- f. dietary requirements
- f. (MERRF) disease ▸ myoclonic epilepsy and ragged red
- f. ▸ disorganized muscle
- f., elastic
- f. ▸ fasciculoventricular Mahaim
- f., fermentation of
- f., flexible glass
- f. friction, cross
- f., frontopontile
- f., fusiform
- f., gamma
- f., glial
- f., heart muscle
- f., Herxheimer's
- f. ▸ His-Purkinje
- f., hyperplastic muscle
- f. in sputum, elastic
- f., inhibitory
- f., interstitial
- f., intrafusal
- f. ▸ ischemic muscle
- f., large nerve
- f., light-conducting
- f. ▸ loss of muscle
- f., Mahaim
- f., medullated nerve
- f., motor
- f., motor nerve
- f., Müller's
- f., muscle
- f., muscles split in line of
- f., myelinated nerve
- f., myocardial
- f., natural food
- f., nerve
- f., nodoventricular
- f. of connective tissue ▸ reticular

f. of Kent
f. of Mahaim
f. of Remak
f., optical
f., pain
f., pain-bearing nerve
f., parasympathetic
f. ▸ parasympathetic nerve
f., peripheral nerve
f., Prussak's
f., Purkinje's
f., regeneration after damage to nerve
f., Sappey's
f., sensory nerve
f., Sharpey's
f. shortening, circumferential
f. shortening ▸ myocardial
f. shortening ▸ velocity of circumferential
f., small nerve
f. ▸ soluble dietary
f. stain, elastic
f., Stilling's
f., striated muscle
f. ▸ striations of myocardial
f. supplement, daily high-
f., surrounding myocardial
f. suture, polyester
f. ▸ terminal Purkinje
f. traction
f., unmyelinated nerve
f., von Monakow's
f., wavy
f., zonular
f., zonule
fiberglass-cancer link
fiberglass casting tape
fiberoptic
f. bronchoscope
f. bronchoscope ▸ flexible
f. bronchoscopy
f. bronchoscopy ▸ flexible
f. camera
f. catheter delivery system
f. cold light source
f. colonoscope
f. esophagoscopy
f. gastroscope
f. headlight
f. light source
f. system, flexible
f. telescope
f. thermometers
f. tube

f. viewing
fiberscopic bronchoscopy
fiberscopic duct injection, trans-duodenal
fibrillar mass of Flemming
fibrillar twitching
fibrillary
f. astrocytoma
f. chorea
f. collagen network
f. contractions
f. glia
f. tremor
f. twitching of tongue
f. waves
fibrillating
f. action potentials (FAP)
f. arrest ▸ hypothermic
f. atria
fibrillation
f. ▸ acute onset of atrial
f., atrial
f. ▸ atrial fibrillation
f., auricular
f., cardiac
f. ▸ chaotic activity of ventricular
f., continuous atrial
f., control atrial
f., controlled atrial
f., controlled auricular
f. detection
f. ▸ electrical conversion of atrial
f. ▸ embolism in atrial
f., flutter-
f. flutter, atrial
f. ▸ idiopathic ventricular
f., induced
f. ▸ lone atrial
f., paroxysmal atrial
f. ▸ postoperative atrial
f. potential
f. potentials, repetitive
f., primary ventricular
f. rhythm
f., risk of ventricular
f. therapy
f. threshold
f., uncontrolled atrial
f. (VF) ▸ ventricular
f. waves ▸ flutter-
fibrillatory tremors
fibrillatory wave
fibrils, amyloid
fibrils, collagen

fibrin
f. balls ▸ pleural
f. bodies
f. bodies of pleura
f. calculus
f. clot
f. conversion syndrome ▸ fibrinogen
f. degradation product
f. degradation product ▸ fibrinogen
f. deposition
f. film
f. foam
f. glue
f. in urine
f., interalveolar
f. lytic activity
f. plug
f., split products of
f. sponge
f. -stabilizing blood coagulation factor
f. stabilizing factor
f. thrombi
f. thrombus
Fibrindex test
fibrinogen
f. breakdown products
f. deficiency
f. degradation product
f. fibrin conversion syndrome
f. fibrin degradation product
f., iodinated I-125
f. level
f., radiolabeled
f. -split products
f. test
f. uptake test, radioactive
fibrinohematic material
fibrinoid
f. arteritis
f. changes
f. degeneration
f. necrosis
fibrinolysin, seminal
fibrinolysis, secondary
fibrinolytic
f. activity of mesothelial surface
f. activity ▸ peritoneal
f. hemorrhage
f. reaction
f. -split products
f. system
f. therapy
f. therapy, anti-
fibrinoplatelet aggregate

fibrinopurulent exudate
fibrinopurulent peritonitis
fibrinosa, chorditis
fibrinous
    f. acute lobar pneumonia
    f. acute pleuritis
    f. adhesions
    f. adhesions, multiple
    f. adhesions, pericardial
    f. bronchitis
    f. exudate
    f. exudate ▸ intra-alveolar
    f. intraseptal pleural adhesions
    f. material
    f. material, intra-alveolar
    f. pericarditis
    f. pericarditis, acute
    f. peritonitis, focal
    f. pleural adhesions
    f. pleurisy
    f. pleuritis and emphysema ▸
      massive
    f. pleuritis ▸ fibrous and
    f. pleuritis, marked
    f. pleuritis, severe
    f. pneumonia
    f. polyp
    f. rhinitis
    f. tissue
fibrinsplint products
fibroadenoma, microscopic
fibroadenoma of breast ▸ giant
fibroadenomatous hyperplasia of
    prostate gland
fibroadenosis, breast
fibroadipose tissue
fibroblast(s)
    f., active
    f. cell
    f. growth factor, acidic
    f. growth factor, basic
    f., human
    f., proliferation of
fibroblastic activity ▸ areas of
fibroblastoma, meningeal
fibrocalcareous disease
fibrocalcareous scarring
fibrocalcific lesion
fibrocartilages, intervertebral
fibrocartilaginous joint
fibrocartilaginous material
fibrochondrosarcoma
fibrocollagenous tissue
fibrocystic
    f. breast

f. breast change
f. breast condition
f. breast disease
f. changes in breast
f. cytoma
f. disease
f. disease from caffeine
f. disease of breasts, bilateral
f. nodules
f. sarcoidosis
fibroelastoma ▸ papillary
fibroelastosis, endomyocardial
fibroelastosis, subendocardial
fibroepithelial polyp
fibroepithelial polypoid anorectal
    lesion
fibrofatty plaque
fibrofatty tissue
fibrofibrinous adhesions
fibrogenic pneumoconiosis
fibroglandular densities ▸ scattered
fibroglandular proliferation
fibrohyaline tissue
fibroid [*thyroid*]
    f. adenoma
    f., calcified uterine
    f. cataract
    f. embolization ▸ uterine
    f. heart
    f. induration
    f., intramural
    f. lung
    f. mass, degenerating
    f. of uterus does appear enlarged
    f., palpable
    f., pedunculated
    f. phthisis
    f., prolapsed
    f., serosal
    f., submucosal
    f., subserosal
    f., symptomatic
    f. treatment
    f. tumor of uterus
    f. tumor, vaporize
    f., uterine
    f., uterus
fibrointimal hyperplasia
fibrolipomatous nephritis
fibrolipomatous tissue
fibroma [*lipoma*]
    f., cardiac
    f., chondromyxoid
    f., histiocytic
    f., lymphangio◊

f., neuro◊
f. of conjunctive
f. of lung
f. of orbit
f. of sclera
f., osteo◊
f., plantar
f., uterine
f. virus, rabbit
fibromata, leiomyoma
fibromata, non-osteogenic
fibromatosis gingivae
fibromatosis, mucoperiosteal
fibromuscular
    f. dysplasia
    f. hyperplasia
    f. walls
fibromusculoelastic lesion
fibromyalgia
    f., elbow
    f., linked to
    f., pain of
    f. ▸ patient has
    f., shoulder
    f. symptoms, relieve
    f. syndrome
    f. victim
fibromyelinic plaques
fibromyoadenomatous hyperplasia
fibromyomata uteri
fibromyomatous stroma ▸ loose
fibroplasia (RLF) ▸ retrolental
fibroplastic
    f. cardiomyopathy
    f. diathesis
    f. endocarditis, Löffler's parietal
fibroplastica, gastritis granulomatosa
fibrosa
    f. cystica, osteitis
    f., myositis
    f. obliterans, bronchiolitis
    f., pseudophakia
    f. renis, capsula
fibrosarcoma
    f., myxo◊
    f., odontogenic
    f. of orbit
    f. of soft tissue
    f. of uterus ▸ recurrent
    f., recurrent
fibrosing alveolitis ▸ mural
fibrosis
    f., African endomyocardial
    f., apical pleural
    f., arteriocapillary

f., biventricular endomyocardial
f., bundle branch
f. choroideae corrugans
f., chronic interstitial pulmonary
f. ▸ chronic pulmonary interstitial
f., conglomerate
f. (CF), cystic
f., Davies endomyocardial
f., Davies myocardial
f., debilitating pulmonary
f., dense
f., diffuse
f., diffuse interstitial pulmonary
f., diffuse patchy
f., early interstitial
f., endocardial
f., endomyocardial
f., extensive interstitial
f., familial pulmonary
f., focal
f. ▸ focal areas of minimal
f., focal interstitial
f., focal myocardial
f., focal pleural
f. ▸ focal subpleural interstitial
f. gene, cystic
f., idiopathic
f. (IPF) ▸ idiopathic pulmonary
f., interstitial
f. ▸ interstitial left ventricular
   myocardial
f., interstitial pulmonary
f., intimal
f., liver
f., lung
f., marrow
f., matchline
f., mediastinal
f., multifocal
f., myocardial
f. of anteroseptal wall
f. of liver ▸ portal
f. of pancreas ▸ cystic
f. of placenta
f. of portal tracts ▸ extensive
f. of ventricular myocardium ▸
   patchy
f., pancreatic
f., papillary muscle
f., parenchymal
f. ▸ partial intermixed
f., patchy
f. ▸ patchy area of old
f., patchy interstitial
f., patchy myocardial

f., peribronchial
f., pericardial
f., perielectrode
f., periportal
f., perivascular
f., pleural
f. ▸ primary pulmonary
f. ▸ progressive interstitial
   pulmonary
f., progressive massive
f., pulmonary
f., pulmonary interstitial
f., radiation
f. regulator, cystic
f. ▸ rejection-associated pulmonary
f., retroperitoneal
f., silicotuberculosis
f., subendocardial
f., subendocardial focal
f. ▸ tropical endomyocardial
f. without pigmentation ▸ scattered

fibrosum, carcinoma
fibrosum, pericardium
fibrosus, annulus
fibrotic
  f. areas
  f. changes
  f. changes, interstitial
  f. infiltration
  f. lung
  f. markings
  f. mass, black
  f., pancreas
  f. pattern, pulmonary
  f. scarring
  f. scarring, pulmonary
  f. serosa
  f. strands
  f. tissue, hyalin

fibrous
  f. adhesion
  f. adhesion, focal
  f. adhesions, dense
  f. adhesions, multiple
  f. adhesions ▸ multiple apical
  f. adhesions, old
  f. and fibrinous pleuritis
  f. ankylosis
  f. appendage of liver
  f. body
  f. body, central
  f. cap
  f. cap ▸ thin
  f. capsule
  f. capsule of corpora

f. cell mass
f. connective tissue
f. dysplasia
f. dysplasia of bone
f. dysplasia of jaw ▸ familial
f. dysplasia, polyostotic
f. goiter
f. histiocytoma, malignant
f. joint
f. layers
f., liver capsule
f. mass
f. mediastinitis
f. membrane
f. mesothelioma, benign
f. mesothelioma ▸ benign pleural
f. mesothelioma, malignant
f. myocarditis
f. nephritis
f. nodule
f. odontoma
f. or scar tissue ▸ formation of
f. papule
f. pericarditis
f. pericardium
f. plaque
f. pleural adhesions
f. pleural adhesions ▸ bilateral
   apical
f. pleuritis
f. pneumonia
f. pneumonia, chronic
f. process
f. replacement
f. sac
f. scar tissue
f. sheath
f. skeleton
f. strands
f. strands, cut
f. streaking
f. stricture formation, esophageal
f. subaortic stenosis
f. thickening ▸ indistinct semicircumferential
f. thickening mitral valve
f. thickening of chordae
f. tissue
f. tissue, dense
f. tissue formation
f. tissue, hyalinized
f. tissue ▸ interfascicular
f. tissue, white
f. tumor proliferation

fibrous—*continued*
    f. tunic
    f. union
fibrovascular stroma ▸ loose
fibroxanthoma, atypical
fibula, distal
fibula, shaft of
fibular
    f. bone
    f. malleolus
    f. muscle, long
    f. muscle, short
    f. muscle, third
    f. nerve, common
    f. nerve, deep
    f. nerve, superficial
    f. notch
    f. shaft
    f. shaft, distal
    f. vein
Fick's
    F. bacillus
    F. diffusion equation
    F. halo
    F. law
    F. position
    F. technique
FICO$_2$ (fraction of inspired carbon dioxide)
fictitious occurrence
fidgeting, aching, pulling, or itching feeling
fidgets, patient
fidgety-leg syndrome
Fiedler's myocarditis
field(s)
    f. ▸ abnormal visual
    f., alcoholism treatment
    f. anesthetized, operative
    f., beam overlap in orthogonal
    f. block
    f. block anesthesia
    f. block, local
    f., bloodless
    f. cautery, wet
    f., central
    f., clear lung
    f., clear pulmonary
    f. cobalt, large
    f., conductive radiofrequency electric
    f., confrontation of visual
    f. created, bloodless
    f. cut, visual
    f. defect, temporal

f. defect, visual
f. deficit, visual
f. dependence
f., direct
f., dry
f., electric
f., electrical
f., electromagnetic
f., electromagnetic energy
f. electron beam dosimetry, large
f., en face irradiation
f., epidemiologist
f. examination, dark-
f. examination ▸ on-the-
f. examination, visual
f. exposure, electromagnetic
f. eyepiece, wide-
f., far
f. fever
f. for radiation therapy, lumbosacral
f., Forel's
f. gel electrophoresis ▸ pulsed-
f. (hpf) ▸ high-power
f. hospital
f. in radiation therapy, mantle
f. in radiation therapy, subdiaphragmatic
f., inductive radiofrequency electric
f., inferior lung
f. inhomogeneity artifact ▸ main magnetic
f. ▸ intensity of electric
f., interstitial radiofrequency electric
f. isocentric technique ▸ four-
f., Krönig's
f. laryngectomy, wide-
f. lesion, wide-
f., limited radiation
f. localization, therapy
f. loss, temporal
f. (lpf) ▸ low-power
f., lower margin of
f., lung
f. machine, computerized visual
f., magnetic
f., matching supraclavicular and tangential
f., matching tangential field with internal mammary
f., maximal potential
f. method electromagnetic
f., midlung
f., minimal potential
f. modification, radiation
f., narrowing of visual

f., nasal
f., near
f. of radiation
f. of radiotherapy
f. of view
f. of vision
f. of vision, center of
f. of vision, central
f. of vision ▸ narrowed
f. of vision, nasal
f. of vision, temporal
f., oil emersion
f., operative
f., opposing lateral
f. (organisms/hpf) ▸ organisms per high-power
f., parallel opposing tangential
f., peripheral
f., peripheral lung
f. (PMN/LPF), polymorphonuclears per low-powered
f. ▸ poor aeration both lungs
f., potential
f. prepared and draped ▸ operative
f. procedure in cardiac arrest
f. protocol
f., pulmonary
f. (PEMF), pulsing electromagnetic
f., quadrant
f., radiation
f., resistive radiofrequency electric
f. simulated
f. size
f. size in half body irradiation
f., sterile
f., sterile draping of
f., sterile operative
f., sterile preparation and draping of
f. stimulation, full
f. ▸ substance abuse treatment
f., surgical
f. team
f. technique for dose calculation, irregular
f. technique, four-
f. technique, shrinking-
f., temporal
f. test, visual
f. therapy ▸ thought
f., treatment
f. treatment, rib
f., tubular visual
f. uniformity determination
f. verified
f. verified with beam films

f. ▸ virtual radiation
f. (VF), visual
f., visual half-
f. (WBC/hpf) ▸ white blood cells per high-power
f. with internal mammary field, matching tangential
f. x-ray beam dosimetry, adjacent-
f. x-ray beam dosimetry, large-
f. x-ray dosimetry, four-

FIF (forced inspiratory flow)
fifth
f. cranial nerve
f. digit ▸ proper extensor muscle of
f. digits of foot ▸ first through
f. digits of hand ▸ first through
f. disease
f. disease virus
f. intercostal space (ICS)
f. intercostal space (PMI 5th ICS) ▸ point of maximum impulse
f. nerve
f. shock count ▸ second through
f. toe
f. trigeminal nerve

50%, hypaque
fight(s)
f. -or-flight mode
f. -or-flight reaction
f. -or-flight response
f. -or-flight syndrome
f. ▸ repeated physical

fighting
f. cells, cancer-
f. cells, infection-
f. drug, cancer-
f. immune system ▸ body's infection-
f. lymphocytes, tumor-
f. molecules, disease-
f. T cells, disease-
f. T cells ▸ infection-
f. white cells ▸ infection-

figure(s)
f., authority
F. Drawing Test, Projective Human
f., father
f., fortification
f., mitotic
f., mother
f. -of-eight abnormality
f. -of-eight bandage
f. -of-eight heart
f. -of-eight suture
f., parent authority

f., parental
f., predominant

fil d'Arion silicone tube
filament(s)
f. ▸ abnormal tangles of
f., beaded
f. in cells
f., nerve
f. of spinal nerves
f. polymorphonuclear
f., protein
f. proteins, abnormal
f. theory ▸ sliding
f. transformer

filamented forms
filamentosa, keratitis
filamentous
f. actin and myosis molecule
f. adhesion
f. appendage
f. component
f. forms
f. prosthesis ▸ Sauvage

Filaria
F. bancrofti
F. conjunctivae
F. hominis oris
F. immitis
F. juncea
F. labialis
F. lentis
F. lymphatica
F. palpebralis
F. philippinensis

filariasis
f., Bancroft's
f. of orbit
f., Ozzard's

Filatov-Marzinkowsky operation
Filatov's operation
filial
f. generation ▸ first
f. generation ▸ second
f. maturity

filiform
f. catheter
f. followers
f. implantation
f. Jackson bougie
f. papillae
f. pulse

filled
f. abdomen, fluid-
f. alveoli, fluid-
f. atherosclerotic plaques ▸ lipid-

f. blister ▸ fluid
f. blisters ▸ pus-
f. breast implant ▸ gel-
f. breast implant, saline-
f. breast implant, silicone-
f. bursa ▸ fluid-
f. canal, fluid-
f. cavities, air-
f. chamber ▸ fluid
f. cyst, fluid-
f. cystic mass, fluid-
f. cysts in breast, fluid-
f. environment, toxin-
f. esophagus, barium-
f. follicles, colloid-
f. ganglion ▸ fluid
f. implant ▸ gel-
f. implant, silicone-
f. implants, silicone gel-
f. inner ear ▸ fluid
f. loop of bowel ▸ fluid-
f. nodule ▸ fluid-
f. plaque ▸ cholesterol
f. sac, fluid-
f. sacs in breast, fluid-
f., stomach
f. teeth
f. tub, air-
f. ventricle, fluid-
f. vitreous, blood-
f. with contrast material ▸ vein
f. with self-pity ▸ patient

filler(s)('s)
f. disease, silo
f. graft
f. in plastic surgery ▸ injectable
f. lung ▸ silo-

filling
f., amalgam
f., collateral
f., complete
f., coronary
f. defect
f. defect in bladder ▸ negative
f. defect, intraluminal
f. defect, luminal
f., dental
f., diastolic
f. disease ▸ diffuse alveolar
f. fraction
f. fraction ▸ first-third
f., fragmentary
f., gallop
f., incomplete
f., mercury amalgam

filling—*continued*
f. of bladder
f. of right atrium
f. pattern, alveolar
f. period, diastolic
f. pressure, atrial
f. pressure, diastolic
f. pressure ▸ left ventricular (LV)
f. pressures, right-sided
f. pressures, ventricular
f., rapid ventricular
f. rate (PFR) ▸ peak
f. rate ▸ peak diastolic
f., reduced ventricular
f., reflux
f., retrograde
f., root canal
f. rumble
f., silicate
f., ventricular
f. wave, occasional late
f. wave, rapid
fills and evacuates satisfactorily ▸ bowel
fills and evacuates satisfactorily ▸ colon
film(s)
f., additional
f., AP (anteroposterior)
f. badge
f., beam
f., Bucky
f., chest
f., comparison
f. density calibration
f. ▸ density-exposure relationship of
f. device, spot
f., dirty
f. dosimetry
f. exposure
f., fibrin
f., fields verified with beam
f. fluorography ▸ spot
f., follow-up
f., gallbladder (GB)
f., gastrointestinal (GI)
f. ▸ kidneys, ureters and bladder (KUB)
f., lateral decubitus
f., localization
f. localization, suitable beam
f., neurosensory
f., oblique
f. of abdomen ▸ portable
f. of abdomen ▸ preliminary

f. of abdomen ▸ upright
f. of ankles ▸ forced inversion
f. of chest, portable semi-upright
f. of liquid ▸ surface
f. over eyes ▸ feeling of
f. oxygenation
f., PA (posteroanterior)
f. packs
f., plain
f., portable
f., portable recumbent
f., portable recumbent AP (anteroposterior) and lateral
f., postevacuation
f., postreduction
f., post-thoracentesis chest
f., postvoiding
f., preevacuation
f., preliminary
f., prereduction
f. pressure spot
f., progress
f., prone
f., rapid processing
f. radiography, spot
f., repeat
f., retention
f. roentgenography ▸ spot-
f., scout
f. screen mammography
f., sequential
f., serial
f., serial cut
f., skull
f., spine spot
f., spot
f., stereoscopic chest
f., strain
f., stress
f. -stripping autoradiography
f. study
f. study, spot
f., subtraction
f., supine
f., tear
f. test, malaria
f., translateral
f., upright
f. (VCF) ▸ vaginal contraceptive
f., verification
f., wet
filming, rapid sequence
filming, serialographic
filmy
f. adhesions

f. tongue
Filoviridae virus
filter
f., anti-glare
f., arterial
f., bandpass
f., caval
f., clot-trapping
f. control, high-frequency
f. control, low-frequency
f. controls, operation of
f. ▸ Greenfield vena cava
f. ▸ heparin arterial
f., high-frequency
f., high-pass
f., low-frequency
f. media, hydrophilic
f. media, hydrophobic
f. ▸ mediastinal sump
f., notch
f., oxygen
f. paper chromatography
f. paper microscopic test
f., platinum
f. ▸ triple bandpass
f., umbrella
f., variable
filterable virus
filtered
f. and cultured ▸ sample
f. by dialysis, blood
f. exposure rate constant
f. fluid
f. hot air
f. tap water
f., volume
filtering cicatrix
filtering toxins from blood
filtrable virus
filtrate, tuberculin
filtration
f. and excretion ▸ endolymph
f. coefficient, capillary
f. fraction
f., glomerular
f. of lung fluid
f. pressure, screen
f. rate (GFR), glomerular
f. slit
f. technique, dilution-
f. ▸ x-ray beam
filum terminale
fimbria ovarica
fimbria, ovarian
fimbriae of uterine tube

fimbriae, taenia
Fimbriaria fasciolaris
fimbriated
    f. end
    f. end of oviduct
    f. fold
fimbrioplasty, bilateral
fin deformity, seal-
final [*spinal*]
    f. closure
    f. common pathway
    f. diagnosis
    f. drug evaluation
    f. impression
    f. pathological diagnosis
    f. rapid repolarization
    f. stage of labor
financial
    f. abuse
    f. assessment
    f. counseling
    f. irresponsibility
    f. obligations ▸ honor
    f. problems
    f. services (PFS), patient
    f. status, stable
    f. stress
    f. stressors
    f. support
finding(s)
    f. and diagnosis, postcannulation
    f., audiometric
    f., clinical
    f. compatible
    f., concurrent
    f. consistent
    f., cystoscopic
    f., ECG (electrocardiogram)
    f. essentially negative
    f., focal
    f., incidental
    f., laboratory
    f. limited, x-ray
    f., mammographic
    f., microscopic
    f., negative
    f., negative microscopic
    f., negative x-ray
    f., operative
    f., paucity of
    f., pelvic
    f., personality assessment
    f., pertinent laboratory
    f., pertinent physical
    f., positive

f., positive microscopic
f., positive x-ray
f., postmortem
f., preliminary
f., prominent
f., psychophysical
f., pure tone audiometric
f., radiographic physical
f., reporting positive
f., sonographic
f., specific
f., suggestive
f., urinary
f., x-ray
fine [*line*]
    f. -angled curette
    f. crepitant rale
    f. hair
    f. -hair movement
    f. -hand dexterity
    f. -mesh gauze
    f. moist rales
    f. -motor behavior
    f. -motor coordination
    f. -motor coordination ▸ gross and
    f. -motor movements, bilateral
    f. -needle aspiration (FNA)
    f. -needle aspiration (FNA) biopsy
    f. -needle aspiration (FNA) biopsy, thoracic
    f. -needle biopsy
    f. -needle biopsy investigation
    f. -needle transhepatic cholangiography (FNTC)
    f. plain catgut
    f. rales
    f. root canal
    f. -silk sutures
    f. -silk sutures ▸ interrupted
    f. structure
    f. tremor
    f. -type nystagmus
    f. -wire electrodes
finger(s)
    f., abductor muscle of little
    f. agnosia
    f. and/or toes ▸ numbness in
    f., baseball
    f. blood pressure (BP) monitor ▸ electronic
    f., bolster
    f., Brodie's
    f., clubbing of
    f., contracted
    f., count

f. (CF) ▸ counting
f. counting test of vision
f. cuff
f., dead
f., deep flexor muscle of
f. dilation
f. dissection
f., dorsal regions of
f., drop
f., drumstick
f. exerciser, dynamic
f. exercises
f. extension, active
f. extension exercise
f., extensor muscle of
f., extensor muscle of index
f., extensor muscle of little
f., first
f. flap, cross-
f. flexed
f. flexion exercise
f. flexion reflex
f., fore◊
f. fracture
f. fracture, baseball
f., frostbite
f., giant
f., hammer
f., hippocratic
f., index
f. infected
f. -in-glove appearance
f. injury
f., insane
f. jerk
f. joint
f. joint implant, Swanson
f. joint ▸ knobby growth on
f., little
f., lock
f., Madonna
f., mallet
f., middle
f. mobility, restore
f. motion
f. muscles
f. -nose (F-N) test
f., numb
f. ▸ numbness and tingling in
f., numbness of
f., opposing muscle of little
f. opposition exercises
f. oximetry
f., palpating
f. percussion

finger(s)—*continued*
- f. plethysmograph
- f. prick test
- f. probing
- f. prosthesis, two-prong stem
- f. replacement
- f. ring
- f., short flexor muscle of little
- f., snapping
- f., spider
- f., spring
- f. -stick medicine
- f. -sucking
- f., superficial flexor muscle of
- f., swelling of
- f., swollen
- f. syndrome, blue
- f. tamponade
- f. (F-F) test ▸ finger-to-
- f., thumb
- f. -thumb reflex
- f., tingling of
- f. -to-finger (F-F) test
- f. -to-nose (F-N) test
- f., trigger
- f., tulip
- f. ▸ vasospasm in
- f. vision
- f., volar regions of
- f., waxy
- f., webbed
- f., webs of

fingerbreadth (FB)
fingernail(s)
- f. ▸ blood clot under
- f., bluish
- f., brittle
- f., cyanosis of
- f., deformed
- f. deformity
- f., gnarled
- f., horizontally ridged
- f. onychomycosis
- f., splitting
- f., vertically ridged

fingerprint(s)
- f. analysis
- f., DNA (deoxyribonucleic acid)
- f. dystrophy
- f. edema
- f., genetic

fingerstick test
fingertip(s)
- f. amputation
- f. ▸ change of color in

- f., cyanosis of
- f. enlargement
- f., frostbite of
- f. ▸ injury and reimplantation
- f., postmortem
- f., tingling of
- f., tingling sensations in

Finkelstein's feeding
Finkelstein's test
finkleri, Vibrio
finned pacemaker lead
Finney's pyloroplasty
Finochietto's stirrup
Finsen
- F. lamp
- F. rays
- F. -Reya lamp

FIO₂ (fraction of inspired oxygen)
FIRDA (frontal irregular rhythmic delta activity)
fire
- f. electronically
- f. in synchrony ▸ thalamus and cortex
- f. -related injury
- f. -setting potential
- f. treatment, cross-

firemen's lift
firing(s)
- f. area
- f., high-voltage
- f. in normal subjects ▸ neuromuscular
- f. in spastic subjects ▸ neuromuscular
- f., laser
- f. of brain ▸ electrical

firm
- f. and ateletatic
- f. and edematous
- f. cell mass
- f. circumscribed nodule ▸ small
- f. consistency
- f. elastic skin
- f., irregular, nodular liver
- f. lenses
- f., liver
- f., red, nodular, or flat growth
- f., tan parenchyma ▸ lobulated,
- f. tissue
- f., uterus

firmness and discomfort, excessive breast
firmness, excessive breast

first (First)
- f. aid
- f. aid ▸ emotional
- f. aid, perform
- f. aid techniques
- f. cartilaginous ring
- f. circulation
- f. course of chemotherapy (second, third, etc.)
- f. cranial nerve
- f. -degree atrioventricular block with intraventricular conduction delay
- f. -degree AV (arteriovenous) block
- f. -degree burn
- f. -degree burns ▸ patient sustained
- f. -degree heart block
- f. -degree uterine prolapse
- f. digit of foot
- f. digit of hand
- f. -echelon or second-echelon lymph nodes
- f. effort
- f. -effort angina
- f. filial generation
- f. finger
- f. heart attack ▸ risk of
- f. heart sound
- f. impression
- f. incisor
- f. intention, healing by
- f. intention, wound healed by
- F. Line (Dilaudid)
- F. Line (Morphine)
- f. metacarpal of wrist
- f. (M1), mitral
- f. nerves
- f. obtuse marginal
- f. obtuse marginal artery
- f. -order kinetics
- f. -pass radionuclide angiocardiography (ACG)
- f. -pass technique
- f. pregnancy
- f. pregnancy, delayed
- f. renal transplant
- F. Response manual resuscitator
- f. rib
- f. -rib thoracic syndrome, anomalous
- f., second- or third-degree sprain
- f. shock count
- f. sound (M1) ▸ mitral
- f. stage of labor
- f. -station or second-station lymph nodes

f. strength
f. -strength tuberculin test
f. -third filling fraction
f. through fifth digits of foot
f. through fifth digits of hand
f. toe
f. transplant, removal of
f. trimester of pregnancy
f. -trimester spotting
f. ventricle of cerebrum
Fischer sign
Fischer's test meal
fish
f. -hook injury
f. insulin, bonito
f. meal lung
f. meal lung disease
f. -mouth cusp
f. -mouth incision
f. -mouth mitral stenosis
f. -mouthed cervix
f. oil supplements
Fishberg's concentration test
Fisher miliary plaques ▸ Redlich-
Fisher's murmur
fishhook lead
fishnet pattern
fission fungus
fissura prima
fissuratum, granuloma
fissure(s)
f., ambient
f., anal
f., anterior median
f., arteriovenous (AV)
f. bleeding, anal
f., Broc's
f., bulging of minor
f., calcarine
f., corneal
f., dentate
f., entorbital
f., ethmoid
f. fracture
f. from childbirth ▸ anal
f., glaserian
f., Henle's
f., horizontal
f., inferior accessory
f., interlobar
f., intrahemispheric
f., intralobular
f., lateral
f., lateral cerebral
f. lips ▸ reddened, dry,

f., longitudinal cerebral
f., minor
f., oblique
f. of anus
f. of cerebrum ▸ longitudinal
f. of lung
f. of Sylvius
f. on brain surface
f., palpebral
f., Pansch's
f., petrotympanic
f., posterior median
f., primary
f., rectal
f., Schwalbe's
f., sylvian
f. tongue
fissuring
f., blister
f., fragmentation and
f., plaque
fist(s)
f. clenched
f., patient makes
f. percussion
f. sign, clenched
f. technique ▸ gloved
fistula
f., anal
f., anorectal
f., antro-aural
f., aortocaval
f., atriovenous (AV)
f., atrioventricular
f., brachioaxillary bridge graft
f., Brescio-Cimino arteriovenous
f., bronchocutaneous
f., bronchopleural
f., bronchopulmonary
f., carotid cavernous
f., chronic anal
f., Cimino
f., circulation in
f., closure of tracheal
f., colocutaneous
f., colovesical
f., congenital coronary
f., congenital tracheoesophageal
f., coronary artery
f., coronary artery right ventricular
 (RV)
f. drained, rectal
f., Eck's
f. embryology ▸ tracheoesophageal
f., enteric

f., enterocolic
f., enterocutaneous
f., enteroenteric
f., esophageal
f. ▸ esophageal carcinoma with
 respiratory tract
f., esophagobronchial
f., fecal
f., gastric
f., gastrojejunocolic
f. ▸ gross tracheoesophageal
f. hook
f., internal
f., jejunal
f., jejunocolic
f., labyrinthine
f., Latzko repair for vesicovaginal
f. ▸ malignant tracheoesophageal
f., mucus
f. of bronchus
f. of carotid cavernous sinus
f. of cornea
f. of lacrimal gland
f. of lacrimal sac
f. of lacrimonasal duct
f. of orbit
f. of sclera
f., oozing
f., open
f. operation, scleral
f., oroantral
f., oronasal
f., pancreatic
f., penoscrotal
f., perilymph
f. (PLF), perilymphatic
f., pleuroesophageal
f., pulmonary arteriovenous (AV)
f., rectal
f., rectocutaneous
f., rectolabial
f., rectovaginal
f., renal
f. ▸ respiratory tract
f. site
f. site occluded
f. ▸ solitary pulmonary
 arteriovenous
f. ▸ subclavian arteriovenous
f., symptomatic
f., thoracic duct
f., tracheal
f., tracheoesophageal
f., traumatic
f. ▸ trifurcation tracheoesophageal

fistula—*continued*
f., urinary
f., uterovaginal
f., vaginoperineal
f., vesicocervical
f., vesicocolic
f., vesicocutaneous
f., vesicouterine
f., vesicovaginal
f., vulvorectal
f. with good bruits, arteriovenous (AV)
fistulization, perilymphatic
fistulous
f. tract
f. tract drained
f. tract, incision and drainage (I and D) of
fisturata, lingua
fit(s)
f. in ear unit ▸ custom
f., nicotine
f. of dentures ▸ improper
f., patient had
f., running
Fite-Faraco stain ▸ Wade-
fitness
f. activity
f. addict
f. aerobic
f. assessment
f., biological
f., cardiorespiratory
f., cardiovascular
f., endurance
f., enhance aerobic
f. ▸ enhance health and
f., exercise and
f., health and
f. ▸ lack of physical
f. level
f. level, current
f., mental
f., muscular
f., overall
f., physical
f. pole striding
f. pole walking
f. program, physical
f. program, total
f., prolapsed
f. test
f. -walking
f., walking for
fitters' asthma, steam-

fitting
f., appliance
f., breast prosthesis
f. dentures, ill-
f. dentures, poorly
f., shoes ill-
Fitz('s)
F. -Hugh-Curtis syndrome
F. -Hugh's syndrome
F. law
F. syndrome
FIVC (forced inspiratory vital capacity)
five
5 -azacytidine
f. -chamber view
f. -chamber view echocardiogram ▸ apical
5 -FC (5-fluorocytosine)
#5 floating catheter
5 -fluorouracil, Adriamycin, Cytoxan (FAC) chemotherapy
5 -fluorouracil, combined radiation and
5 -fluorouracil combined with radiotherapy
5 -fluorouracil (CMF) ▸ cytoxan, methotrexate,
5 -fluorouracil ▸ high-dose methotrexate and
5 -FU, infusion of
5 -HIAA (5-hydroxy-indoleacetic acid)
5 -hydroxy-indoleacetic acid (5-HIAA)
5 % dextrose in water (D-5-W/D_5W)
f. senses
5, Transderm-Nitro
f. -year survival rate
fix diets, quick-
fixation
f. and dissection
f. and sectioning of the brain
f., binocular
f., bizarre
f., cardiolipin complement
f., cleanliness
f. (CF) ▸ complement
f. device, insertion of
f. device, intramedullary
f. device, metallic
f., external
f., Freudian
f. graft

f., hip
f. hysteria
f. in vivo
f., intermaxillary
f., internal
f., intramaxillary
f., intramedullary
f., intramural
f., latex
f. muscles
f. neurosis
f. of calcaneus ▸ axial
f. of carina
f. of fracture ▸ external
f. of fracture ▸ internal
f. on a single object
f. (ORIF), open reduction and internal
f., otosclerotic
f., parent
f. point
f. reaction, complement
f., sexual
f., stapes
f., surgical
f. suture
f. test, complement
f. test, fabere
f. test, latex
f. test ▸ RA (rheumatoid arthritis) latex
f. test, Reiter protein complement
f. titers, complement
f., visual
f. with osteogenesis
fixative, Zenker's
fixator muscle of base of stapes
fixator muscles
fixe, idée
fixé, virus
fixed
f. -action pattern
f. airflow obstruction
f. and dilated ▸ pupils
f. antibody, cell-
f. appliance
f. -arch bar
f. bridge
f. bridgework
f. coupling
f. delusions
f. drug eruption
f. facial expression
f. footplate
f. idea

f. joint
f. lingual arch
f. macrophage
f. perfusion defect
f. P-R interval
f. pupil
f. -rate mode
f. -rate pacemaker
f. -rate pacemaker, Cordis'
f. -rate pulse generator
f., slide heat
f. spasm
f. specimen, formalin
f., stapes
f. stare
f. staring expression
f. stenotic area
f. -tissue cells
f. value
f. virus
fixing
f. antibody, complement
f. antibody, kidney-
f., complement
f. fluid, Flemming's
f. time
fixture titanium
FJN (familial juvenile nephrophthisis)
fl dr (fluid dram)
fl. oz. (fluid ounce)
flabby airway
flabby flesh
flaccid
f. and blue
f. ectropion
f. extremity
f. glottis
f. hemiparalysis
f. hemiplegia
f. paralysis
f. paralysis (AFP), acute
f. paraplegia
f., patient
f. skin
flaccida, pars
Flack node ▸ Keith-
Flack's node
flagellar agglutinin
flail [frail]
f. chest
f. chordae
f. extremity
f. joint
f. leaflet
f. mitral valve

f. segments
f. wildly, arms
f. wildly ▸ legs
flailing episode
flailing, legs
flair valve
Flajani's disease
Flajani's operation
Flake (flake)
F. (cocaine)
F. (cocaine), Peruvian
f. fracture
flaked out, patient
flakiness from athlete's foot ▸ redness and
flaking
f. and chafing of feet
f. skin
f. skin ▸ dry, itchy,
f. skin from dermatitis
f. skin from eczema
flamboyant, patient
flame
f., alcohol lamp
f. cells
f. emission spectroscopy
f. ionization detector
f. -retardant gowns
f. -retardant linens
f. -retardant material
f. -shaped hemorrhage
f. spots
flammeus, nevus
flange [phalanges]
f., buccal
f., dental
f., labial
f., lingual
flank [frank]
f. area
f. bone
f. incision
f. incision, lateral
f. incision, subcostal
f. pain
f. pain, acute
f. stripe
f. tenderness
f. wound, lateral
flap [flat]
f., Abbe
f., abdominal jump
f., abdominothoracic
f. advancement procedure
f. amputation

f. amputation ▸ double-
f. and zap surgery
f., Argamaso-Lewin composite
f. artery island
f., Bakamjian
f., bilobed
f., bipedicle
f., bladder
f. bleeding uterine
f., bone
f., Bunnell's
f., caudal
f., Charretera's
f. chest wall
f., circular
f., compound
f., conchal
f., conjunctival
f., corneal
f., Crane's
f., craniotomy
f., Cronin-Matthews eave
f., cross-arm
f., cross-finger
f., cross-leg
f. deflected, skin
f., delayed
f., delayed transfer
f. developed
f. developed, adequate
f., direct transfer
f., distant
f., dorsal
f., double-end
f., double-pedicle
f. elevated
f. elevated, bladder
f., Eloesser's
f. end of bone covered with
f., envelope
f., Estlander
F. fascial
f. fashioned
f. fashioned and sutured
f., fornix-based conjunctival
f., French
f., French sliding
f., Frickle's
f., gauntlet
f., Gillies'
f., Gillies' up-and-down
f., Gunderson conjunctival
f., Hodgson-Tuksu tumble
f., horseshoe-shaped skin
f., Hueston spiral

flap—*continued*
f., immediate transfer
f. incision ▸ Z-
f., Indian
f., Indian rotation
f. injury, avulsion
f., interpolated
f., intimal
f., inverted horseshoe
f., island
f., island leg
f., Italian
f., Italian distant
f., jump
f., Limberg
f., lingual tongue
f., liver
f., local
f., localized advancement
f., long rectangular
f. ▸ lower abdominal
f. ▸ lower peritoneal
f., MacFee neck
f., marsupial
f., McGregor's forehead
f., medial
f. ▸ microvascular free
f., Millard's island
f., Monks-Esser island
f., Moore and Chong sandwich
f., mucoperiosteal
f., muscle
f., musculocutaneous
f., New's sickle
f. of abdominal tissue
f. of conjunctiva
f. of periosteum reflected
f. of tissue
f. of tissue, crescent-shaped
f. operation, cataract
f., osteoplastic
f. otoplasty
f., over-and-out cheek
f., pedicle
f., pericardial
f., pericoronal
f., posterolateral
f. procedure ▸ four-
f. procedure ▸ gluteal-free
f. raised, periosteal
f. raised, skin
f. reflected, skin
f. repair of lip ▸ Abbe
f. repair, pharyngeal
f., rope

f., rotation
f., rotation advancement
f., rotation of
f., scalp
f., scleral
f., Sewell-Boyden
f., short rectangular
f., skin
f., sliding
f., Stein-Abbé lip
f., Stein-Kazanjian lower lip
f., Stenstrom foot
f. surgery
f. surgery ▸ scalp
f., surgical
f., synovial
f., Tagliacozzi's
f., tailoring of
f. technique ▸ latissimus dorsi
f. technique, Waldhausen
   subclavian
f., Thom
f. tracheostomy
f. transplant technique
f. transplanted, tissue
f. trimming, mucoperiosteal
f., tube
f., tubed pedicle
f., tumbler
f., tunnel
f., turn a
f., tympanomeatal
f., tympanotomy
f. -type laceration
f. ▸ upper abdominal
f. ▸ upper peritoneal
f., Van Lint conjunctival
f., viable
f., volar
f., von Langenbeck's bipedicle
   mucoperiosteal
f., V-Y
f. ▸ V-Y advancement
f., Wookey's neck
f., Z-
f., Zimany's bilobed
f., Zovickian's
flapless amputation
flapping
f., hand
f. of conjunctiva, left eye
f. of conjunctiva, right eye
f. sound
f. tremor
f. valve syndrome

flare
f., aqueous
f., asthma
f. reaction, wheal-
f. shoes, out-
f. -up of Crohn's
f. -up of _____ ▸ patient had
f. ▸ wheal and
flared nostrils
flaring
f., alar
f., nasal
f. of nostrils
flash(es)
f. and retinal detachment ▸ floaters,
f. burn
f. burn cases
f. conjunctivitis, arc-
f., hot
f., hot or cold
f. keratoconjunctivitis
f., menopausal
f. of light ▸ diffused
f. of light ▸ intermittent
f. of light ▸ isolated
f. ophthalmia
f. pulmonary edema
f. stimulation
f. triggers ▸ hot
flashback(s)
f. and anxiety disorder
f., nightmares and
f. ▸ patient experiences
f., patient has
f. ▸ post-traumatic
f. reactions, acute treatment for
f. reactions, clinical manifestations
   of
f. reactions from drug abuse,
   patient had
f. reactions, psychological state in
f. reactions, subacute treatment of
f. reactions, treatment of
f. reactions with cannabinoids
f. reactions with depressants
f. reactions with hallucinogens
f. reactions with inhalants
f. reactions with multiple drugs
f. reactions with opioids
f. reactions with phencyclidines
f. reactions with stimulants
f., re-enactments/
flashes and floaters ▸ recent onset of
flashing lights
flashing patterns of light ▸ irregular,

flashlight test, swinging-
flask culture
flask-shaped heart
flat [*flap*]
    f., abdomen
    f. affect
    f. affect, blunted or
    f. affect, patient has
    f. cells
    f. chamber
    f. chest
    f. curve
    f. electrocardiogram (ECG/EKG)
    f. electroencephalogram (EEG)
    f., emotional content
    f. facies
    f. feet
    f., fontanelle
    f. growth ▸ firm, red, nodular, or
    f. hand
    f., jugular veins
    f. pelvis
    f. plate of abdomen
    f. polyp
    f. suture
    f. tongue
    f., white patches on mucosa of
        stomach ▸ small,
    f. worm
Flatau's law
flatfoot, spastic
flattened
    f. affect
    f. diaphragm
    f. epithelial cells
    f. nipple
    f. nose
    f. nuclei
    f. tissue cells
flattener exercise ▸ low back
flattening
    f., affective
    f., curvilinear
    f., focal
    f. of affect
    f. of lordosis
    f. of lumbar curve
    f. of lumbosacral curve
    f. of normal lumbar curvature
    f., T wave
flatulence, coughing with
flatulence from dairy products
flatulent dyspepsia
flatuous melancholia

flatus
    f. enema
    f. material, passing
    f., passage of
    f., patient expelled
    f., patient passing
flatworm, nervous system
flava, Neisseria
flaval ligament
flavescens, Aedes
flavescens, Cellvibrio
flavin mononucleotide
Flavobacterium meningosepticum
flavum, ligamentum
flavus, Aspergillus
flax dresser's disease
flax dressers' phthisis
flea-bitten kidney
Flechsig's area
fleck of barium
flecked retinopathy
fledged disease, full-
fleece, Stilling's
Fleet enema
fleeting
    f. chest pain
    f. illusions
    f. pain
    f. pain, nagging
Fleischer's dystrophy
Fleischmann's hygroma
Fleischner syndrome
Fleming's operation
Flemming
    F. center
    F., fibrillar mass of
    F. fixing fluid
    F. ▸ interfibrillar substance of
flesh
    f., flabby
    f. -eating bacteria
    f. trabeculae of heart
fleshy growths
fleshy lesion, soft
Fletcher
    F. after-loading colpostat
    F. after-loading tandem
    F. loading applicator
    F. -Suit applicator
Flex diaphragm, All-
flexa, coxa
flexed
    f., ankle
    f. at wrist, hand
    f., elbow

    f., fingers
    f., hip
    f., knee
    f., left lower extremity (LLE)
    f., left upper extremity (LUE)
    f., LLE (left lower extremity)
    f., LUE (left upper extremity)
    f. muscles
    f., neck passively
    f. position ▸ spine in
    f. posture, forward
    f., right lower extremity (RLE)
    f., right upper extremity (RUE)
    f., RLE (right lower extremity)
    f., RUE (right upper extremity)
    f., shoulder
    f., toes
    f. lower back ▸ patient
    f. upper back ▸ patient
    f., wrist
flexibilitas cerea
flexibility
    f. and elasticity
    f., decrease in
    f. drills
    f. ▸ endurance, strength, balance
        and
    f. exercise
    f. exercises ▸ strengthening and
    f., improved
    f., increased
    f., joint
    f., loss of
    f., maintain muscle
    f., mental
    f., muscle
    f. ▸ muscle strength and
    f., normal
    f. of bronchial tree
    f. of hip
    f., parental
    f. ▸ regain muscle strength and
    f., shoulder
    f. ▸ spontaneity, creativity, and
    f. ▸ strength and
    f. ▸ strength, endurance and
    f. ▸ strength, stamina and
    f. stretches ▸ post-exercise
    f. test
    f. ▸ trunk and hip
    f., waxy
flexible
    f., arms
    f. collodion
    f. erection

flexible—*continued*
f. fiberoptic bronchoscope
f. fiberoptic bronchoscopy
f. fiberoptic system
f. glass fiber
f. joint
f. lens
f., lighted tube
f. pencil
f. plastic gel
f. proctoscopy
f. round silicone rod
f. rubber endoscopic tube
f. scar tissue
f. sigmoidoscopy
f. sigmoidoscopy ‣ postradiation
f. tube in esophagus
f. tubing
Flexicair Low Airloss Therapy
Flexicair Therapy
Flexinet dressing
Flexing, joint
flexing, lifting, straining
flexion
f., abnormal
f., active knee
f. and extension
f. and extension ‣ full range of
f. and extension study, lumbar
f., angle of greatest
f. contracture
f. contracture deformity
f. contracture of hip
f. contracture of knee
f. contractures, digital
f. contractures of digits
f. crease
f., degrees of
f., elbow
f. epilepsy, generalized
f. exercise
f. exercise, finger
f. exercise, Regen's
f. exercise ‣ shoulder
f. exercise, Williams'
f., extension and
f. -extension projection
f., forceful
f., forward
f., full
f., gentle active
f., hand splinted in
f., hip
f., knee
f., limitation of

f. line
f., loss of
f., neck
f. of great toe ‣ normal
f. of leg, passive
f. of spine
f. of thigh
f. of thigh on abdomen
f. of toes
f. of trunk, forward
f., palmar
f., passive
f., plantar
f. position
f. reflex, finger
f. reflex of leg
f. ‣ shoulder horizontal
f. ‣ trunk forward
Flexner('s)
F. bacillus
F. dysentery
F. serum
F. -Strong bacilli
F. -Strong bacillus
flexneri, Shigella
flexor(s) [*flexure*]
f. carpi radialis muscle
f. carpi radialis tendon
f. carpi ulnaris muscle
f. digitorum brevis muscle
f. digitorum longus muscle
f. digitorum profundus muscle
f. digitorum profundus tendon
f. digitorum sublimis muscle
f. digitorum sublimis ‣ tendinous chiasm of musculus
f. digitorum sublimis tendon
f. digitorum superficialis muscle
f. hallucis brevis muscle
f. hallucis longus muscle
f. muscle, accessory
f. muscle of fingers ‣ deep
f. muscle of fingers ‣ superficial
f. muscle of great toe ‣ long
f. muscle of great toe ‣ short
f. muscle of little finger ‣ short
f. muscle of little toe ‣ short
f. muscle of thumb ‣ long
f. muscle of thumb ‣ short
f. muscles of toes ‣ long
f. muscles of toes ‣ short
f., neck
f., plantar reflexes
f. plantar response
f. pollicis brevis muscle

f. pollicis brevis, musculus
f. pollicis longus muscle
f. pollicis longus, musculus
f. profundus tendon
f. reflex, paradoxical
f. retinaculum
f. spasticity, inhibit
f. sublimis, tendinous chiasm of
f. surface
f. synergy
f., toe
f. tone
f. tone, increased
f. weakness of plantar
flexorplasty, Steindler's
flexure [*flexor*]
f., basicranial
f., carcinoma splenic
f., caudal
f., cephalic
f., cerebral
f., cervical
f., cranial
f., dorsal
f., duodenojejunal
f., hepatic
f. line
f., lumbar
f., mesencephalic
f., nuchal
f. of colon, hepatic
f. of colon, iliac
f. of colon, left
f. of colon, right
f. of colon, sigmoid
f. of colon, splenic
f. of duodenum, inferior
f. of duodenum, superior
f. of rectum, perineal
f. of rectum, sacral
f., pontine
f., sacral
f., splenic
f. syndrome ‣ splenic
flicker
f. frequency, critical
f. fusion, critical
f. fusion test, critical
f. fusion threshold
f. phenomenon
f. test
flickering pulse
flicking twitches of extremities
Flieringa operation, Bonaccolto-
Flieringa scleral ring

flight(s)
- f. angiography ▸ time-of-
- f. blindness
- f. exertional dyspnea ▸ one-
- f. exertional dyspnea ▸ two
- F. for Life
- f. mode ▸ fight or
- f. of fancy
- f. of ideas
- f. of stairs claudication ▸ two
- f. phobia
- f. radiation, airline
- f. reaction ▸ fight-or-
- f. response ▸ fight-or-

flint (Flint)('s)
- f. disease
- F. murmur
- F. respiration, Austin
- F. rumble, Austin

flip angle
flip angle ▸ pulse
flipped T wave
flittering scotoma
Flo carotid shunt ▸ Vascu-
float supinely
float to top of container ▸ red cells
floater(s)
- f., dark
- f., eye
- f., flashes and retinal detachment
- f. in vision
- f. ▸ recent onset of flashes and
- f., stringy vitreous
- f., visual
- f., visual field
- f., vitreous

floating
- f. anxiety, free-
- f. bone chip ▸ free-
- f. cartilage
- f. feeling, patient has
- f. fragment, free-
- f. kidney
- f. kidney, free-
- f. otoconia ▸ free-
- f. patella
- f. ribs
- f., vertex
- f. wall motion study

FLOC (cephalin flocculation) ▸ CEPH
floccosum, Acrothesium
floccosum, Epidermophyton
flocculate [loculate, lobulate]
flocculation
- f. (CEPH FLOC) ▸ cephalin

- f., cephalin-cholesterol
- f., cholesterol
- f., limit
- f., Ramon
- f. reaction
- f. test
- f. test, bentonite
- f. test, cephalin
- f. test, cephalin-cholesterol
- f. test, Kline
- f. test, latex
- f. test, zinc
- f., thymol

floccule, toxoid-antitoxin
flocculonodular lobe
flocculus, peduncle of
flooding
- f., alveolar
- f., manage memory floor
- f. therapy

floor
- f., antral
- f. cells
- f. electromyography ▸ pelvic
- f., female pelvic
- f., jugular
- f., laceration of pelvic
- f. muscle exercise ▸ pelvic
- f. muscles ▸ pelvic
- f. of bladder
- f. of inguinal canal
- f. of mouth
- f. of mouth, carcinoma of
- f. of orbit
- f. of orifice
- f. of third ventricle
- f., orbital
- f., pelvic
- f., peritoneal
- f. pressure, pelvic
- f. prosthesis, orbital
- f., relaxed pelvic
- f. weakness ▸ pelvic

floppy
- f. disk
- f. ears ▸ large and
- f. infant
- f. infant syndrome
- f. mitral valve
- f. valve
- f. valve syndrome

flora
- f., bacterial
- f., balance of bacterial
- f., endogenous

- f., exogenous
- f., fecal
- f., gastrointestinal
- f., hospital
- f., intestinal
- f., mixed bacterial
- f., mixed common
- f., natural bacterial
- f., normal
- f. ▸ normal bacterial
- f., normal oropharyngeal
- f., normal vaginal
- f., oral
- f., respiratory
- f., skin
- f., sputum showed mixed
- f., stools showed normal
- f., throat
- f., vaginal

Florentine iris
florid
- f. congestive heart factor
- f. congestive heart failure
- f. diabetic retinopathy (FFDR) ▸ full
- f. pulmonary edema

floriform cataract
floriformis, cataract
flossing
- f. ▸ endocarditis and
- f. of teeth
- f. teeth, brushing and
- f., tooth brushing and

flotation
- f. center
- f. cushion
- f., direct centrifugal
- f. tank
- f. units, Svedberg

Flourens' law
flow(s) [slow]
- f. ▸ abnormal myocardial blood
- f., acceleration of blood
- f., acid
- f. across orifice
- f., adequate blood
- f. ▸ alterations in blood
- f. and dilution ▸ back
- f., anterograde
- f., aortic
- f., aortic blood
- f., arterial blood
- f. artifact
- f. -assisted, short-term
- f. ▸ atherosclerosis and blood
- f., axoplasmic

flow(s)—*continued*
f. backward into bladder ▸ semen
f., bile
f., block air
f., blocked blood
f., blood
f., brain
f. brain scan, rapid
f. capacity, heart
f., cerebral blood
f., choroidal blood
f., collateral
f., coronary
f., coronary blood
F. coronary graft ▸ Perma-
f., coronary sinus blood
f. culture, continuous
f., current
f. cytometric analysis
f., decreased blood
f. detector, Doppler
f. detector, ultrasound blood
f., diminished blood
f., diminution of blood
f. -directed pulmonary artery
　catheter
f. ▸ disruption of blood
f. Doppler, color
f. during expiration ▸ prolongation
　of air
f., effective capillary
f., effective renal blood
f. (ERPF) ▸ effective renal plasma
f., electron
f. endocardial
f. envelope
f., epicardial
f., estimated hepatic blood
f., excessive
f., exercise hyperemia blood
f., expiratory
f. (FEF) ▸ forced expiratory
f. (FIF) ▸ forced inspiratory
f. ▸ forced midexpiratory
f., forearm
f., free
f., fresh gas
f. from artery ▸ blood
f. from capillary ▸ blood
f. from constipation ▸ change in
　urine
f. gradient (PFG) ▸ pressure
f. headaches, vascular
f., heavy
f., heavy menstrual

f. hemostatic catheter, return
f., hepatic blood
f., hepatofugal
f., hepatopetal
f., high
f. imaging ▸ Doppler
　transesophageal color
f. ▸ impair blood
f. ▸ impaired blood
f., impairment of air
f. ▸ impairment of subendocardial
　blood
f. ▸ impede blood
f., improved blood
f. in heart, blood
f., inadequate blood
f. incentive spirometry ▸ Tri-
f., increase of blood
f., increased calcium
f., increased cutaneous blood
f. ▸ increased urinary
f. injector
f. ▸ insufficient blood
f., interrupted urine
f., intracranial blood
f. (LAF) isolation room ▸ laminar air
f. (LAF) ▸ laminar air
f. ▸ laminar blood
f. limiting stenosis
f., lymph
f. mapping
f. mapping, color
f. mapping, color-coded
f. mapping ▸ Doppler color
f. mapping technique
f. (MEF) ▸ maximal expiratory
f. (MFEF) ▸ maximal forced
　expiratory
f. (MMEF) ▸ maximal midexpiratory
f. (MTF) ▸ maximum terminal
f. ▸ mean forced midexpiratory
f., measure blood
f. ▸ measure rate of blood
f. measurement, blood
f. measurement, coronary blood
f. measurement ▸ venous
f., menstrual
f. (MRF), mitral regurgitant
f. mode
f., moderate menstrual
f. murmurs
f., myocardial blood
f., normal
f., normal blood
f., normal urine

f. ▸ obstructed blood
f., obstruction of
f. of air, obstruct
f. of alternating current (AC) ▸
　opposition of
f. of aqueous humor
f. of barium ▸ retrograde
f. of blood and oxygen to heart
f. of blood ▸ augment
f. of blood ▸ backward
f. of blood ▸ ensure proper
f. of blood ▸ preventing adequate
f. of blood, turbulence of
f. of blood ▸ vaginal
f. of direct current (DC) ▸ opposition
　of
f. of energy, continuous
f. of lungs ▸ blood
f. of saliva
f. of saliva, decreased
f. of saliva ▸ excessive
f. of saliva ▸ reduced
f. of sperm
f. of tears, decreased
f. of tears, diminished
f. of thought
f. of urinary bladder, peak
f. of urinary stream
f. of urination, interruption of
f. of urine
f. ▸ ovulation and menstrual
f., palmar arch
f., pansystolic
f. (PEF) ▸ peak expiratory
f. (PIF) ▸ peak inspiratory
f. ▸ peak tidal inspiratory
f. ▸ petal fugal
f. (PVF) ▸ portal venous
f. probe, blood
f., prolongation of air
f., pulmonary
f. (PBF) ▸ pulmonary blood
f., pulsatile
f. rate
f. rate, arterial blood
f. rate (BFR) ▸ blood
f. rate, coil
f. rate, expiratory
f. rate, increased
f. rate (IFR) ▸ inspiratory
f. rate ▸ low
f. rate (MIFR) ▸ maximal inspiratory
f. rate (MMEFR) ▸ maximal mid-
　expiratory
f. rate ▸ maximum

f. rate (MEFR) ▸ maximum expiratory
f. rate (MIFR) ▸ maximum inspiratory
f. rate (MMEFR) ▸ maximum mid-expiratory
f. rate ▸ mean mid-expiratory
f. rate (MFR) ▸ mucus
f. rate (PFR) ▸ peak
f. rate (PEFR) ▸ peak expiratory
f. rate (PIFR) ▸ peak inspiratory
f. rate ▸ peak jet
f. rate, varying
f. ratio
f. ratio ▸ pulmonary systemic blood
f., reactive hyperemia blood
f., reduce blood
f., reduced cerebral blood
f. ▸ reduced urinary
f. ▸ regional myocardial blood
f. regulator clamp
f. relationship ▸ pressure
f. (RBF) ▸ renal blood
f. (RPF) ▸ renal plasma
f. ▸ rerouting of blood
f. reserve, coronary
f. reserve technique, coronary
f. ▸ respirator on maximum
f. ▸ restore blood
f. restricted, air
f., return
f., reverse
f., ▸ revision of in-
f., ▸ revision of out-
f. room (LAFR) ▸ laminar air
f. rumbling murmur, atrioventricular (AV)
f., scanty menstrual
f., sequential
f. sheet
f. sheet, medication
f. sheet, treatment
f., sluggish blood
f. ▸ small-vessel inadequate blood
f., splanchnic blood
f., stimulating blood
f. studies, cerebral blood
f. study, blood
f. study, cerebral blood
f. study, pulmonary blood
f. study ▸ salivary
f., systemic
f., systemic blood
f. test ▸ urinary
f., thoracic duct

f. to brain, blood
f. to brain, collateral arterial
f. to brain ▸ reduced blood
f. to ear ▸ increased blood
f. to heart ▸ insufficient blood
f. to heart muscle, increased blood
f. to scalp ▸ blood
f. to the brain ▸ tracking blood
f. to transplanted organ ▸ blood
f. to tumor, oxygen
f. (TF) ▸ total
f. (TCF) ▸ total coronary
f. (TPBF) ▸ total pulmonary blood
f. (TRBF) ▸ total renal blood
f. tract, left
f. tract, right
f., transvalvular
f. ▸ tricuspid valve
f., tumor blood
f. unimpeded, blood
f. unit (LAFU) ▸ laminar air
f., urinary
f., uterine blood
f. velocity
f. velocity, coronary blood
f., velocity of blood
f. velocity ▸ translesional spectral
f. ventilation, continuous
f. ventilation ▸ volume cycled decelerating
f. volume curve
f. volume loop
f. volume (MEFV) ▸ maximal expiratory
f. wire

flowmeter (FM)
f., blood
f. (FM) ▸ Doppler
f., electromagnetic
f., Gould electromagnetic
f., peak
f., Statham electromagnetic
flowmetry (MRF) ▸ magnetic resonance
flowmetry ▸ pulsed Doppler
floxuridine (FUDR)
flu
f., Asian
f., chills with
f. diagnoses ▸ false-negative
f. inoculation
f., intestinal
f. -like syndrome
f. ▸ loss of appetite from

f. mortality
f. shot
f., Spanish
f. stomach
f. strain
f. vaccine ▸ nasal spray
f. vaccine ▸ swine
f. virus
f. virus, deadly
f., yuppie
fluctuant mass
fluctuant nodular lesions ▸ soft
fluctuate in duration ▸ symptoms
fluctuated
f., blood pressure (BP)
f., hemoglobin (Hgb)
f., serum cholesterol
f., weight
fluctuating
f., blood pressure
f. fatigue
f. hearing loss
f. hormone levels
f. level of consciousness
f. mental status
f. periods of remission and relapse
f. sensorineural hearing loss
fluctuation(s)
f., blood pressure (BP)
f., blood urea nitrogen (BUN)
f. ▸ diurnal weight
f., hormonal
f., mental
f., mood
f. of temperature
f., response
f., symptom
f., weight
fluence, radiation
fluency ▸ period of
fluency, verbal
fluent aphasia
fluff dressing
fluff, vitreous
fluffy
f. alveolar infiltrate
f. bibasilar infiltrate
f. cuffed tube
fluid(s) (Fluid)
f. ▸ abdominal cavity free of
f., abnormal accumulation of
f., abnormal sac containing
f. (CSF), absorption of cerebrospinal

fluid(s)—*continued*

f. access, controlled
f., accumulating
f. accumulation
f. accumulation and inflammation
f. accumulation and swelling
f. accumulation in arm
f. accumulation in leg
f. accumulation in lung
f., accumulation of
f., acidic
f., allantoic
f., Altmann's
f., amniotic
f. analysis, duodenal
f. analysis, joint
f. and electrolyte imbalance
f. and electrolyte replacement
f. and electrolyte therapy in trauma
f. and humidity, increased
f. and secretions, body
f., ascites
f., ascitic
f. aspirated
f. aspirated from abdomen
f. aspirated from chest
f. aspirated from joint
f. aspirated from knee
f. aspiration, amniotic
f., aspiration of
f., aspiration of food or
f. aspiration ▸ pleural
f. at term, amniotic
f. balance
f. balance, body's
f. balance in neonatal lung
f. balance, maintaining
f., Bamberger's
f. barrier, blood cerebrospinal
f., bleaching
f. (CSF) ▸ blocking of passage of cerebrospinal
f. (CSF) ▸ blood in cerebrospinal
f., blood in seminal
f., blood-tinged
f., bloody
f., bloody peritoneal
f., bodily
f., body
f. ▸ body secretions, exudates and
f., Bouin's
f. (CSF) brain barrier, cerebrospinal
f., bronchoalveolar lavage
f. buildup
f. buildup ▸ drain

f. buildup ▸ express
f., Burnett's disinfecting
f., Callison's
f., Carrel-Dakin
f. cataract
f. cavity, air
f. cell count ▸ spinal
f. (CSF) ▸ cerebrospinal
f. changes, pleural
f., chlorpalladium
f., circulatory
f., clear
f., clear, spinal
f., cloudy
f., Coley's
f. collection
f., Condy's
f. congestion
f. consumption
f. consumption, excess
f., contaminated with bodily
f. content
f. content blood-tinged
f., controlled access to
f., crystalline
f., cul-de-sac
f. culture, amniotic
f. cultured and analyzed ▸ amniotic
f. (CSF) cytology ▸ cerebrospinal
f., Dalkin's
f., dark blood-stained
f., decalcifying
f. deficit
f. deficit, hypernatremia and
f., Delafield's
f. density
f. density in left/right base
f., dialysis
f. drained and preserved ▸ amniotic
f. drained from chest
f. drained off ▸ excess
f. dram (fl. dr.)
f. dynamics
f., Ecker's
f., edema
f., effused
f., effusion of
f. ejaculated
F. (phencyclidine), Embalming
f., embolic agent
f. embolism, amniotic
f., empyema
f., encapsulated pleural
f., endolymph
f., epithelial lining

f., excess
f., excessive
f., exposure to blood or body
f., extracellular
f., eye
f., fetal nuchal
f. -filled abdomen
f. -filled alveoli
f. -filled blister
f. -filled bursa
f. -filled canal
f. -filled chamber
f. -filled cystic mass
f. -filled cysts
f. -filled cysts in breast
f. -filled ganglion
f. -filled inner ear
f. -filled loop of bowel
f. -filled nodule
f. -filled sac
f. -filled sacs in breast
f. -filled ventricle
f., filtered
f. ▸ filtration of lung
f., Flemming's fixing
f., follicular
f., force
f. formation
f. formation, controlling
f. formation ▸ reduce
f., formol-Müller
f., foul-smelling amniotic
f., free
f., gastric
f., Gauvain's
f., glandular
f. (CSF) glucose ▸ cerebrospinal
f. gradient
f., gram stain of body
f., gram stain of peritoneal
f. gram stains ▸ spinal
f., grossly cloudy
f. ▸ hazardous spills of
f., Helly's
f., hemorrhagic
f. ▸ human spinal
f., hyperalimentation
f. imbalance
f. in abdomen
f. in abdomen ▸ ascitic
f. in body tissue
f. in cul-de-sac ▸ free
f. in heart sac
f. in knee
f. in lungs

f. in peritoneal cavity ▸ blood
f. in pleural cavity
f. in pleural cavity ▸ watery
f. in scrotal area
f. in tissues, excess
f. ▸ inadequate intake of
f., infectious
f., infectious body
f. inflow ▸ gradient of
f., ingested food and
f. intake
f. intake, excessive
f. intake, insufficient
f. intake ▸ manage
f. intake/output
f. intelligence
f., interarterial
f., interstitial
f., intestinal
f. intoxication
f. intoxicator
f., intracellular
f., intravascular
f., intravenous (IV)
f. ▸ jelly-like
f., joint
f., Kaiserling's
f., labyrinthine
f., Lang's
f., leakage of
f. left base
f. level
f. level, air
f. level ▸ spinal
f. levels ▸ multiple air
f., loculated
f., loculation of
f. loss
f. loss ▸ excessive
f. loss, immeasurable
f. losses, replace
f., lymph
f., lymphatic
f. maintenance
f. mechanics
f., meconium
f., meconium-stained
f., meconium-stained amniotic
f., meniscus
f., Mitchell's
f. movement
f., Morton's
f. mucinous cyst
f., mucous
f., Müller's

f., nipple
f., normal spinal
f. ▸ odorous amniotic
f., oncotic
f., oozing
f., organ preservation
f. ounce (fl. oz.)
f. outflow ▸ net gradient of
f. output
f. output, insensible
f. overload
f., parenteral
f., Parker's
f., Pasteur's
f., patient to push
f., patient treated initially with
    intravenous (IV)
f., pericardial
f., perilymph
f., peritoneal
f., Piazza's
f., piggy-backing IV (intravenous)
f., Pitfield's
f., pleural
f. ▸ pleural sac free of
f., potentially infective bodily
f. precautions, body
f., preserved vitreous
f. pressure
f. pressure (CSFP) ▸ cerebrospinal
f. pressure in eye
f. pressure ▸ increased
f. pressure, ocular
f. pressure (SFP) ▸ spinal
f. pressure (VFP) ▸ ventricular
f. production
f., proteinaceous
f., purulent
f., push
f. reaccumulation
f., red hemorrhagic
f., Rees and Ecker diluting
f., release of biological
f. released from anterior chamber
f. replacement
f. replacement, adequate
f. (CSF) ▸ replacement of cerebro-
    spinal
f. replacement therapy
f. repletion
f. repletion of shock patients
f. reservoir
f. (RTF), respiratory tract
f. restriction
f. restriction ▸ patient on

f. resuscitation
f. ▸ retained lung
f. retention
f. retention and swelling
f. retention, excess
f. retention, minimize
f. rhinorrhea, spinal
f. right base
f. ▸ sac of
f., Scarpa's
f., Schaudinn's
f., secrete
f. secretion, blood and body
f. -seeking behavior ▸ unrecognized
f., seminal
f. sequestration, estimated
f., serosanguineous
f., serosanguineous turbid
f., serous
f. ▸ serous straw-colored
f. ▸ shrinkage of vitreous
f. sobriety
f. spilling into upper abdomen
f., spinal
f. started ▸ intravenous (IV)
f., sterile
f., stomach
f., stomach distended with
f. ▸ stopping or never starting food
    and
f., straw-colored
f. ▸ straw-colored pericardial
f. ▸ straw-colored serous
f. streaked with blood ▸ mucous
f., subdural
f., subretinal
f. ▸ sub-zero cryogenic
f., swell with
f. syndrome, amniotic
f., synovial
f. tap, spinal
f. tapped daily ▸ ascitic
f., tapping of chest for
f., Tellyesniczky's
f. therapy
f., Thoma's
f. through evaporation, loss of
f., tissue
f., Toison's
f., transcellular
f., transudation of
f., tubular
f., tumescent
f., turbid
f., turbid milky

fluid(s)—*continued*
f. ▸ umbilical cord
f. vascular occluding agent
f., ventricular
f., vesicle
f., vitreous
f. volume
f. volume deficit
f. volume excess
f. volume, extracellular
f. volume, functional extracellular
f. volume, intracellular
f., volume of
f. volume overload
f., von Behring's
f., Waldeyer's
f., watery
f. wave
f., Wickersheimer's
f. withdrawn
f., withholding food and
f., xanthochromic
f., yellow serous
f., Zenker's
fluidization, membrane
fluke(s)
f., intestinal
f., lung
f. worm
flu-like symptoms
fluoranthene carcinogens
fluorescein
f. angiography
f. dye
f. material
f. uptake
fluorescence
f. endoscope ▸ lung imaging
f. ▸ laser-induced arterial
f. microscope
f. microscopy
f., relative
f. spectroscopy
fluorescens, Azotomonas
fluorescens, Pseudomonas
fluorescent
f. antibody
f. antibody darkfield
f. antibody, direct
f. antibody, indirect
f. antibody stain
f. antibody test
f. antinuclear antibody
f. cytoprint assay
f. dosimeter, ultraviolet

f. in situ hybridization (FISH)
f. ray
f. scan
f. screen
f. staining
f. thyroid imaging
f. treponemal, absorption
f. treponemal antibody
f. treponemal antibody absorption
test
fluoric cachexia
fluoridated water
fluoridation, water
fluoride(s)
f., hydrogen
f. pills
f., topical
fluorine F 18
fluorite objective
fluoro spot projection, erect
fluorocarbon poisoning
fluorocytosine (5-FC) ▸ 5-
**fluorodopamine positron emission
tomographic scanning**
fluorography, cine◊
fluorography ▸ spot film
**fluorometric technique,
chromatographic-**
fluorophotometry, vitreous
fluoroscope, biplane
fluoroscopic
f. examination
f. guidance
f. study
f. unit, digital
f. visualization
fluoroscopy
f., biplane
f., cardiac
f., electro-
f., kV
fluorosis, chronic endemic
fluorosis, dental
fluorouracil (5-FU)
f., Adriamycin, Cytoxan (FAC)
chemotherapy ▸ 5
f., combined radiation and 5-
f. combined with radiotherapy, 5-
f. (CMF) ▸ Cytoxan, methotrexate, 5-
f. ▸ high-dose methotrexate, 5-
f., infusion of
f. ribo side
Fluosol artificial blood

flush(es)
f. and bathe technique
f. aortogram
f. aortography
f. away dulling dry, dead cells
f., carcinoid
f., hectic
f. heparin lock
f., hot
f., hot and cold
f., mahogany
f., malar
f. milk ducts
f. out kidneys
f. out plaque
f. percutaneous catheter ▸ straight
f. syndrome ▸ Asian
flushed
f., aspirated and
f. cheeks
f. complexion
f. countenance
f. skin
f. skin ▸ reddened,
f. with saline
f. with saline ▸ catheter aspirated
and
flushing
f., alcohol skin
f. and heat
f., cutaneous
f. ▸ dyspnea and
f., facial
f. from alcohol
f. from caffeine
f. of artery
f. of face
f. of skin
f. of upper body
f. reaction
f. reservoir, double-bubble
f. sensation of heaviness
f. time
flutter
f., atrial
f., atrial fibrillation
f., auricular
f. cycle length
f., diaphragmatic
f. -fibrillation
f. -fibrillation waves
f., heart
f., impure
f., mediastinal
f. of eyelids

f., pure
f. R interval
f., recurrent atrial
f., ventricular
f. with 4:1 conduction, atrial
f. with 3:1 conduction, atrial

fluttering
f. aortic valve, diastolic
f. heart
f. heartbeat
f. sensation in chest

flux
f., bilious
f., celiac
f., hepatic
f., menstrual
f., soldering
f. ▸ transmembrane calcium

fluxionary hyperemia
fly, Hessian wheat
fly, tsetse
Flying Saucers (morning glory seeds)
FM (flowmeter)
FM., blood
FM., Doppler
FM., electromagnetic

fMRI (functional magnetic resonance imaging)
fMRI (functional magnetic resonance imaging) brain scan
F-N (finger-to-nose) test
FNA (fine-needle aspiration)
FNTC (fine-needle transhepatic cholangiography)
foam
f. cell
f., Dalkon
f., Delfen
f. embolus
f. embolus, polyurethane
f., fibrin
f., polyurethane
f. rubber
f. rubber vaginal graft
f. rubber vaginal stent
f. stability test

foamy
f. histiocytes and lymphocytes
f. interstitial plaque
f. macrophage
f. myocardial cell
f. plaques, intimal
f. urine

FOBT (fecal occult blood test)

focal [*vocal, local*]
f. abnormality
f. abscess
f. abscess formation
f. accumulation
f. acute bronchopneumonia
f. acute pericarditis
f. acute pneumonia
f. adenocarcinoma
f. aggregation of cells
f. and eccentric
f. and lateralizing neurologic signs
f. anterior temporal spikes
f. antrum
f. area
f. area of bronchiectasis
f. area of emphysema
f. area of hemorrhage
f. area of hyperemia
f. area of infarction
f. area of intrapulmonary hemorrhage
f. area of lymphoid infiltrate
f. area of minimal fibrosis
f. area of squamous metaplasia
f. atelectasis
f. atherosclerosis
f. atrophy
f. atypical changes
f. bile stasis
f. block
f. brain disease
f. brain lesion
f. bronchopneumonia
f. calcified granulomata ▸ multiple
f. cardiomyopathy
f. cerebral seizure
f. chronic inflammatory infiltrate ▸ mild
f. colloid nodules
f. convulsive seizure
f. cortical nodular hyperplasia ▸ mild
f. cortical process
f. defects
f. delta waves
f. dermal hypoplasia syndrome
f. disorders of brain and spinal cord
f. distance
f. disturbance
f. duct ectasia
f. dust emphysema
f. dysfunction ▸ significant
f. dysplasia
f. dysrhythmia

f. dysrhythmic change
f. dystonia
f. dystonia, golfer's
f. eccentric stenosis
f. ectopic ventricular contractions
f. edema
f. emphysema
f. encephalitis ▸ chronic
f. epilepsy
f. epilepsy, chronic
f. epilepsy, minor
f. epileptiform discharges
f. epithelial hyperplasia
f. extramedullary hematopoiesis
f. fibrinous peritonitis
f. fibrosis
f. fibrous adhesion
f. finding
f. flattening
f. hemorrhage
f. hemorrhage, small
f. hemorrhages ▸ superficial subendocardial
f. hemorrhagic cystitis
f. hemorrhagic infarct
f. hemorrhagic, necrotizing cystitis
f. hepatic hemorrhages
f. herpes of vulva
f. hyalinization
f. illumination
f. infarct of liver
f. infarction
f. infection
f. infiltrating tumor metastases
f. infiltration
f. inflammatory change
f. inflammatory mucosal changes
f. interstitial fibrosis
f. interstitial hemorrhage
f. interstitial scarring
f. interstitial scarring ▸ mild
f. intrapulmonary hemorrhage
f. invasion
f. involvement
f. keratinization
f. length
f. lesions
f. limb abnormality
f. lymphocytic aggregates
f. metastases to spleen
f. metastasis left adrenal gland
f. moderately slow activity
f. motor signs
f. mucin
f. mucosal autolysis

focal—*continued*
- f. mucosal ulcerations
- f. muscle weakness
- f. myocardial fibrosis
- f. nephritis
- f. neurologic signs
- f. neurological deficit
- f. nodular hyperplasia
- f. nodularity
- f. nodules of residual tumor
- f. occult blood test
- f. onset
- f. pancreatitis
- f. petechiae
- f. petechial hemorrhages
- f. plane tomography
- f. pleural fibrosis
- f. pleural thickening
- f. point
- f. pulmonary edema
- f. radiation therapy
- f. reaction
- f. retinal detachment
- f. scarring
- f. scarring ‣ areas of
- f. scarring of interstitium
- f. sclerosis
- f. seizure
- f. seizures, continuous
- f. serosal abscess formation
- f. serous fat atrophy
- f. shallow subpleural hemorrhage
- f. slow activity
- f. slow waves
- f. slowing
- f. spikes
- f. spot
- f. subendocardial
- f. subendocardial fibrosis
- f. subendocardial hemorrhages
- f. subpleural interstitial fibrosis
- f. temporal slowing
- f. tenderness
- f. thickening of alveolar septum
- f. ulceration, superficial
- f. ulcerations
- f. zone (FZ)

focally cystic gray medulla

foci
- f., arrhythmia
- f., calcified
- f., ectopic atrial
- f., epileptogenic
- f., hyaline scarred
- f., low-voltage

- f. multiple
- f., multiple-spike
- f., occipital slow-wave
- f. of extramedullary hematopoiesis
- f. of infarcts
- f. of infection
- f. of infection, abdominal
- f. of inflammatory cells
- f. of mucosal ulceration
- f., Simon
- f., slow-wave

focus
- f., adenomatous
- f., anterior temporal slow-wave
- f., anterior temporal spike
- f., Assmann's
- f. attention ‣ inability to
- f., bilateral
- f., calcified
- f., central slow-wave
- f., central spike
- f., ectopic
- f., epileptogenic
- f., eye
- f., frontal slow-wave
- f., frontal spike
- f., Ghon
- f. ‣ inability to
- f., known metastatic
- f. lens ‣ single-
- f., lens with double-
- f., microscopic
- f., midtemporal
- f., midtemporal slow-wave
- f., midtemporal spike
- f., minimal
- f., obsessive
- f., occipital slow-wave
- f., occipital spike
- f. of aggression discharge
- f. of atelectasis
- f. of attention
- f. of carcinoma
- f. of cells ‣ microscopic
- f. of clinical attention
- f. of hepatic necrosis ‣ small
- f. of infection
- f. of slow activity
- f. of slow activity ‣ mid-temporal
- f. of tuberculosis, calcified
- f. on self
- f., parietal slow-wave
- f., parietal spike
- f. ‣ poor intellectual
- f., primary

- f., primary seizure
- f., right temporal lobe
- f., seizure
- f., slow-wave
- f., solitary
- f., spike
- f. ‣ strengthen reality
- f. to skin distance

focused
- f. approach to psychotherapy ‣ trauma-
- f. beams
- f. care ‣ patient
- f. concentration
- f. cryosurgery
- f. grid
- f. group therapy ‣ solution
- f. imagery
- f. psychotherapy
- f. relaxation
- f. sessions, family-

focusing collimator
focusing ‣ shock wave
Foegella method, Sommer-
foetalis, placenta
foetus, Trichomonas
fogginess, mental
fogging system of refraction
foggy thinking
foggy vision
foils in electron beam therapy, scattering
Foix sign, Marie-
Foix's syndrome
folate
- f. antagonist
- f. deficiency
- f. preventable birth defect

fold(s)
- f., alar
- f., amniotic
- f. and groove, conoventricular
- f., antral
- f. artifact ‣ skin
- f., aryepiglottic
- f., axillary
- f., bulboventricular
- f., caval
- f., cecal
- f., ciliary
- f., circular
- f., coarse
- f., congested rugal
- f., conjunctival
- f., costocolic

f., Douglas'
f., Duncan's
f., duodenojejunal
f., duodenomesocolic
f., epicanthal
f., epicanthic
f., epigastric
f., eponychial
f., false vocal
f., fimbriated
f., gastric
f., gastric rugal
f., gastropancreatic
f., genital
f., glossoepiglottic
f., gluteal
f., Guérin's
f., Hasner's
f., head
f., Heister's
f., Hensing's
f., ileocecal
f., ileocolic
f. incision, skin
f., incudal
f., inferior duodenal
f., inframammary
f., infrapatellar synovial
f., infraumbilical
f., interureteric
f., iridial
f., Kerckring's
f., Kohlrausch's
f., labial
f., lacrimal
f. line, expression
f., malleolar
f., mammary
f., Marshall
f., medial umbilical
f., median umbilical
f., medullary
f., mesolateral
f., mesonephric
f., mesouterine
f., middle umbilical
f., mucobuccal
f., mucolabial
f., mucosobuccal
f., mucous
f., nasolabial
f., nasopharyngeal
f., Nélaton's
f., neural
f. of colon, semilunar

f. of colon, sigmoid
f. of conjunctiva, semilunar
f. of cystic duct ▸ spiral
f. of duodenum, longitudinal
f. of ear
f. of fascia lata ▸ falciform
f. of fascia transversalis, semi-lunar
f. of hip, synovial
f. of large intestine
f. of mucous membrane of
   tympanum ▸ anterior mallear
f. of peritoneum
f. of rectum, horizontal
f. of rectum, mucous
f. of rectum, transverse
f. of skin
f. of stomach, rugal
f. of stomach, villous
f. of tympanic membrane ▸ anterior
   mallear
f. of tympanic membrane ▸
   posterior mallear
f. of uterine tube ▸ tubal
f., opercular
f., palatine
f., palmate
f., palpebral
f., palpebronasal
f., pancreaticogastric
f., paraduodenal
f., parietocolic
f., parietoperitoneal
f., patellar synovial
f. pattern, coarsened mucosal
f. pattern, mucosal
f., Pawlik's
f., pharyngoepiglottic
f., pituitary
f., primitive
f., proximal nail
f., Rathke's
f., rectal
f., rectouterine
f., rectovaginal
f., rectovesical
f., retrotarsal
f., Rindfleisch's
f., rugal
f., sacrogenital
f., salpingopalatine
f., salpingopharyngeal
f., Schultze's
f., semilunar
f., serosal
f., serous

f., skin
f., soft
f., stapedial
f., sublingual
f., superior duodenal
f., synovial
f., tail
f., thickened
f., transverse palatine
f., transverse vesical
f., Treves'
f., triangular
f., urogenital
f., uterovesical
f., vaginal
f., vascular cecal
f., ventricular
f., Veraguth's
f., vestibular
f., vestigial
f., vocal
f. ▸ wrinkled skin
foldable
   f. artificial lens, soft
   f. intraocular lenses
   f. silicone intraocular lens (IOL)
Foley Y-type ureteropelvicoplasty
foliacée, lame
foliaceus, pemphigus
foliate lamina
foliate papillae
folic acid (FA)
   FA anemia
   FA antagonist
   FA deficiency
   FA synthesis
folie
   f. à deux
   f. circulaire
   f. du doute
   f. du pourquoi
   f. gemellaire
   f. musculaire
   f. raisonnante
foliforme, paracolon
Folius' muscle
folk medicine
follicle(s)
   f., colloid-filled
   f., eff
   f., eyelash
   f. formation ▸ secondary
   f., graafian
   f., hair
   f. ▸ infected eyelash

follicle(s)—*continued*
  f. ▸ infected hair
  f., Lieberkühn's
  f., lymph
  f., lymphoid
  f. ▸ lymphoid depletion of
  f., malpighian
  f., nabothian
  f., Naboth's
  f., ovarian
  f., primary
  f., primordial
  f., ruptured
  f. ▸ segmental analysis of hair
  f. -stimulating hormone (FSH)
  f. ▸ unencapsulated, colloid
  f., vesicular
follicular
  f. adenoma
  f. adenomata
  f. bronchiectasis
  f. bronchiolitis
  f. cells
  f. cholecystitis
  f. conjunctivitis
  f. cyst
  f. fluid
  f. gait
  f. gastritis
  f. germinal centers
  f. goiter
  f. hyperplasia, giant
  f. iritis
  f. lupus
  f. lutein cells
  f. lymphadenopathy, giant
  f. lymphoblastoma, giant
  f. lymphoma, giant
  f. lymphosarcoma
  f. membranes
  f. membranes enucleated
  f. pattern
  f. pharyngitis
  f. phase
  f. stigma
  f. thyroiditis, giant
  f. tonsillitis
  f. unit grafts
  f. vulvitis
  f. xeroderma
follicularis, hydrosalpinx
follicularis, keratosis
folliculi
  f., hydrops
  f., liquor

  f., theca
folliculitis, pseudomonas
folliculorum, Demodex
Follmann's balanitis
followed
  f. as outpatient, patient
  f. in office, patient
  f. on outpatient basis ▸ patient
followers, filiform
following
  f. abdominal surgery, ileus
  f. defibrillation, arrhythmias
  f. infarction ▸ rupture of
    myocardium
  f. ingestion
  f. response, frequency
  f. resuscitation attempt ▸ baby
    expired
  f. trauma, cardiac arrest
follow-through, clinical
follow-through (SBFT), small-bowel
follow-up
  f., bereavement
  f. biopsy
  f., cardiac
  f. care
  f. chest x-ray
  f., discharged to
  f., discharged to office
  f. evaluation
  f. examination
  f. film
  f., high-risk
  f. instructions understood
  f., lab
  f., office
  f., outpatient
  f., pastoral
  f., patient discharged to
  f., patient discharged to office
  f., patient referred to
  f. period
  f., postnatal
  f., postoperative
  f., postpartum
  f., postradiation
  f., postsurgical
  f. procedures ▸ systematic
  f., radiation therapy
  f., short-term
  f. studies
  f. treatment
  f. urine cultures
  f. visit, office
  f. wound care

  f., x-ray
Foltz's valve
fond, bas-
fond formation, bas-
Fonsecaea compactum
Fonsecaea pedrosoi
Fontan
  F. atriopulmonary anastomosis
  F. procedure
  F. repair
Fontana's spaces
fontanelle/fontanel
  f., anterior
  f., anterolateral
  f., bregmatic
  f., bulging
  f., bulging anterior
  f., Casser's
  f., enlarged
  f. flat
  f., frontal
  f., Gerdy's
  f., mastoid
  f., occipital
  f. open
  f., posterior
  f., posterolateral
  f. reflex
  f., sagittal
  f., sphenoid
food(s) (Food)
  f., acidic
  f. allergens
  f. allergies
  f. allergy, acute
  F. and Drug Administration (FDA)
  f. and fluid, ingested
  f. and fluid ▸ stopping or never
    starting
  f. and fluids, withholding
  f. angina
  f., artery-clogging
  f. asthma
  f., bolus of
  f. -borne
  f. -borne bacteria
  f. -borne disease
  f. -borne illness
  f. -borne illness, bacterial
  f. -borne illness outbreak
  f. -borne infection
  f. -borne transmission of viral
    hepatitis
  f., carbohydrate
  f. challenge ▸ double-blind

f., cholesterol-laden
f., comfort
f. consumption
f., contaminated
f. craving
f. diary
f. diet, junk
f., digested
f. digestion
f. /drug interactions
f. dyscrasia
f., energy value of
f., fatty
f. fever
f. fiber, natural
f. /fluids, time of last
f. -free diet ▸ caffeine, alcohol, pepper, spicy (CAPS)
f., gas-forming
f. group, negative calorie
f., health
f., high-fat
f. in pharynx, regurgitated
f. intake
f. intake ▸ restricting
f. interaction, drug-
f. intolerance
f. intolerance, fatty
f., intolerance to certain
f., intolerance to specific
f., irradiated
f. irradiation ▸ partial
f., junk
f. labels
f. lodged in trachea
f. ▸ low-fat, low-cholesterol
f. obstructing airway
f., obstructing bolus of
f. or fluid, aspiration of
f. particle
f. particles, aspiration of
f. particles, ingested
f. particles, patient vomited undigested
f. particles, regurgitated
f. particles, undigested
f. poisoning
f. poisoning, Bacillus cereus
f. poisoning, clostridial
f. poisoning ▸ diarrhea from
f. poisoning, enterococcal
f. poisoning ▸ pain in abdomen from
f. preference
f., preoccupation with

f. preparation
f., rapid ingestion of large amounts of
f., regurgitated
f. -related headache ▸ cold
f. service
f. substance, accessory
f. supplement
f., tainted restaurant
f. trapped in trachea
f. trigger
f., undigested
f. vacuole

food-borne outbreak
Foolpills (barbiturates)
foot

f., abscess of
f., adductor reflex of
f. alignment ▸ improper
f. and mouth disease ▸ hand,
f. at ankle ▸ amputation of
f., athlete's
f. bacteria
f., ball of
f. ▸ blister from athlete's
f. bone
f. brace, drop
f., bursitis of
f. -candle meter (fcm)
f. -candles (fc)
f. care
f. care, diabetic
f. care, improper
f. care ▸ routine
f. cells
f., cellulitis of
f., Charcot's
f., claw◊
f., cleft
f., club
f., common digital vein of
f. control of corrective orthotics
f. cradle
f., cross◊
f. deformity, congenital vertical talus
f. disorder
f., dorsal arterial arch of
f., dorsal digital nerves of
f., dorsal digital veins of
f., dorsal interosseous muscles of
f., dorsal interosseous veins of
f., dorsal venous arch of
f. drape
f. drop, bilateral

f., dropped
f. exercise ▸ golf ball roll
f. exercise ▸ sand walking
f. fatigue
f., fifth digit of
f., first digit of
f. flap, Stenstrom
f., fore◊
f., fourth digit of
f. fracture
f. freedom
f., frostbite
f. fungus
f. hazard ▸ indirect
f. hygiene, regular
f. ▸ improper functioning of
f. in neutral position
f. infection
f. infection, diabetic
f., intercapitular veins of
f., intermediate dorsal cutaneous nerve of
f. ▸ itching from athlete's
f., lateral aspect of
f., lateral dorsal cutaneous nerve of
f. ▸ longitudinal arch of
f., lumbrical muscles of
f., Madura
f., march
f. massage
f., medial dorsal cutaneous nerve of
f., Mendel's dorsal reflex of
f. muscles ▸ weakness of
f., musculocutaneous nerve of
f. ▸ nail breaking from athlete's
f. neuroma
f. odor
f. orthotic
f. orthotic ▸ custom-designed
f. pain
f., pain in ball of
f. pain, incapability
f., perspiration, excessive
f., plantar aspect of
f. problem from arthritis
f. problem from circulatory problem
f. problem from diabetes
f. procedure ▸ drop-
f. ▸ redness and flakiness from athlete's
f. rest, padded
f., rocker-bottom
f. rot
f., sag
f. scab

foot—*continued*
f. screening
f., second digit of
f. sensation, burning
f., sensory nerves in
f. shuffling
f. ▸ skin cracking from athlete's
f. ▸ skin peeling from athlete's
f. sprained
f. syndrome, burning
f., tabetic
f., taut
f., third digit of
f., trash
f., trench
f. ulcer
f. ulcer ▸ persistent
f., weak
Football (amphetamine)
football knee
footdrop
f. after stroke
f. after stroke ▸ biofeedback treatment of
f., neurological
footed gait ▸ glue-
footling
f. breech presentation
f. delivery, double-
f. delivery, single-
f., double
f. presentation
footplate
f., fixed
f. fragments
f. of stapes, congenital defect in
f., stapes
footprint
f. identification
f. taken of infant in delivery room
f. taken of newborn in delivery room
footprinted in delivery room ▸ infant
footprinted in delivery room ▸ newborn
foramen
f., apical
f., Bochdalek
f., bulboventricular
f. cecum
f., closed oval
f., epiploic
f., Galen's
f., Huschke's
f. incisivum
f., infraorbital
f., interventricular
f. lacerum
f., Luschka's
f., Magendie's
f. magnum
f., mandibular
f. mastoideum
f., meibomian
f. mental
f., Morgagni's
f., neural
f., obturator
f., occipital
f. occipitale magnum
f. of Bochdalek hernia
f. of Monro
f. of Morgagni hernia
f. of sclera, optic
f. of Winslow
f. of Winslow ▸ epiploic
f., optic
f. ovale
f. ovale basis cranii
f. ovale closed
f. ovale cordis
f. ovale ossis sphenoidalis
f. ovale, patent
f., pacchionian
f. primam
f., rivinian
f. rotundum ossis sphenoidalis
f., Scarpa's
f., Schwalbe's
f. secundum
f. sphenopalatinum
f. spinosum
f., Stensen's
f. stylomastoideum
f. syndrome, jugular
f. venae cavae
f., vertebral
foramina
f., intervertebral
f., neural
f., Scarpa's
f., thebesian
foraminal bone ▸ supratrochlear
foraminal hernia
foraminotomy operation
foraminotomy procedure
Forbes-Albright syndrome
Forbe's amputation
forcé, accouchement

force(s) (Forces)
f. and rhythm (F and R)
f., atrial ejection
f., brisement
f., chemical
f., contractile
f., coulomb
f., drag
f. (EMF), electromotive
f., exert
f., extrinsic
f. fluids
f. frequency relation
f., generate
f., inspiratory
F. Institute of Pathology (AFIP) ▸ Armed
f. ▸ left ventricular (LV)
f. length relation
f. ▸ level of
f. line
f., maximum inspiratory
f. microscope, atomic
f. (NIF) ▸ negative inspiratory
f. of contraction, rate and
f. of muscle contraction
f. on spine ▸ compressive
f. on spine ▸ twisting
f. on urethra, closing
f. on uterus and upper vagina
f. ▸ P terminal
f. ▸ peak twitch
f., physical
f., relative centrifugal
f., repetitive
f., rotational
f., shear
f., Starling
F. (LSD), The
f. trauma ▸ blunt
f., twisting
f. velocity indices ▸ end-systolic
f. velocity length relation
f. velocity relation
f. velocity volume relation
f., vertical
f., vital
forced
f. air
f. awakening
f. beat
f. blowing out ▸ shallow breathing with
f. breathing
f. cycle

f. exhalation
f. expiration
f. expiratory capacity
f. expiratory flow (FEF)
f. expiratory flow (MFEF) ▸ maximal
f. expiratory spirogram (FES)
f. expiratory time (FET)
f. expiratory volume (FEV)
f. expiratory volume in one second
f. feeding
f. inspiratory flow (FIF)
f. inspiratory vital capacity (FIVC)
f. inversion
f. inversion film of ankles
f. ischemia-reperfusion transition
f. mandatory intermittent ventilation
f. midexpiratory flow
f. midexpiratory flow ▸ mean
f. movement
f. oscillation technique
f. respiration
f. tremor
f. tube feeding
f. ventilation
f. vital capacity (FVC)
f. vital capacity analysis
f. vital capacity ratio

forceful
f. contraction, synchronous
f. extension
f. flexion
f. heart contractions
f. sustained eye closure
f. vomiting

forceps
f. delivery
f. delivery, failed
f. delivery, high
f. delivery, low
f. delivery, outlet

forcible
f. closure of eyelids ▸ involuntary
f. feeding
f. sexual activity

Fordyce disease ▸ Fox-Fordyce's granules

forearm
f. and wrist, immobilize
f., anterior interosseous nerve of
f. crutch
f., dorsal cutaneous nerve of
f. flow
f. fracture
f., immobilize wrist and
f., lateral cutaneous nerve of

f., lower
f., medial cutaneous nerve of
f., median vein of
f. obstruction
f., posterior cutaneous nerve of
f., posterior interosseous nerve of
f., rotating

forebrain
f., basal
f. cells, basal
f. stimulation

forefoot
f., amputated
f. hyperpronation
f., swelling of

forego life supports
foreground program
foreground system
**foregut malformation,
    bronchopulmonary**
forehead
f., armpits, palms ▸ sweating
f., bruised
f., electrode placement on
f. flap, McGregor's
f. lift
f., prominence of
f., prominent

foreign
f. accent syndrome
f. cancer cells
f. material artifact
f. material, aspirated
f. material deposit
f. material ▸ embolized
f. material, inhalation of
f. matter embedded
f. object
f. object in wound
f. object, patient ▸ swallowed
f. organ
f. particles
f. pigmentation
f. substance
f. substance, inhalation of
f. substance ▸ invasion of
f. tissue

foreign body (FB)
FB ▸ accidentally swallowed
FB airway obstruction
FB, aspiration of
FB, contamination
FB, electromagnetic removal of
FB esophagus
FB extraction

FB from cornea, removal
FB giant cell
FB granuloma
FB granulomatous reaction
FB impacted
FB in air passage
FB in anterior chamber
FB in bronchus
FB in ciliary body
FB in cornea
FB in ear
FB in eye
FB in iris
FB in lacrimal sac
FB in lens
FB in lung
FB in nose
FB in optic nerve
FB in stomach
FB in trachea
FB, inhalation of
FB, intraocular
FB, intrauterine
FB ▸ intravascular
FB (MFB), metallic
FB, nostril obstructed by
FB obstructing airway
FB obstruction
FB, opaque
FB papule
FB passed
FB reaction
FB, removal of
FB removed
FB, retained
FB retrieval ▸ intravascular
FB, sclerotomy with removal of
FB seen on x-ray
FB, soft-tissue
FB, tracheal

Forel('s)
F. commissure
F. decussation
F. field
F., fornix longus of
F. space

forensic (Forensic)(s)
f. assessment
f. chemistry
f. evaluation
f. mapping
f. medicine
f. neuropsychology
f. psychology
f. stomatology

forensic—*continued*
- f. toxicologist
- F. Urine Drug Testing Program

forequarter amputation

foreskin
- f., bifurcation of
- f., redundant
- f. ▸ removal of

Forest disease virus ▸ Kyasanur

Forest virus, Semliki

Forestier's disease

forgetful and confused ▸ patient

forgetful, patient

forgetfulness
- f. from aging
- f. from alcohol
- f. from antidepressant
- f. from anxiety
- f., irritability and confusion ▸ patient has
- f. of old age ▸ benign
- f., poor concentration/

forgetting, directed

forgetting, traumatic

fork
- f. deformity, silver-
- f. fracture, silver-
- f., Hartmann tuning
- f. -like stump
- f. test, tuning
- f., tuning

Forlanini's method

Forlanini's treatment

form(s) (Form)
- f., abnormal wave
- f., abstract
- f., accident
- f., accident-related
- f., alteration in wave
- f. analysis, Doppler wave
- f. analysis ▸ wave-
- f. and pattern, perception of
- f. and topography ▸ frequency,
- f., anesthetic authorization
- f., anesthetic consent
- f., autopsy authorization
- f., autopsy consent
- f., background
- f., blood transfusion refusal
- f., complex wave
- f., consent
- f., cosmetic surgery authorization
- f., cosmetic surgery consent
- f. ▸ Diagnostic, Social, and Addiction History

- f., diphtheroidal
- f., discrete delta
- f., disseminated
- f., external impulsive
- f., fairly consistent
- f., filamented
- f., filamentous
- f. for operation and grafting of tissue ▸ authorization
- f. for operation and grafting of tissue ▸ consent
- f. for operation ▸ authorization
- f. for operation ▸ consent
- f. for recipient of organ transplant ▸ authorization
- f. for recipient of organ transplant ▸ consent
- f. for refusal to submit to treatment
- f. for removal of organ for transplant ▸ authorization
- f. for removal of organ for transplant ▸ consent
- f. for removal of tissue for grafting ▸ authorization
- f. for removal of tissue for grafting ▸ consent
- f. for ritual circumcision ▸ release
- f. for taking and publication of photographs ▸ authorization
- f. for taking and publication of photographs ▸ consent
- f. for taking of motion pictures of operation ▸ authorization
- f. for taking of motion pictures of operation ▸ consent
- f. for televising of operation ▸ authorization
- f. for televising of operation ▸ consent
- f., free-base
- f. gradually
- f. granulocyte, band-
- f., informed consent
- f., instrumental elevation in wave
- f., mesenchymal
- f., mutated
- f. ▸ myocardial infarction in dumbbell
- f. ▸ myocardial infarction in H-
- f., nonfilamented
- f. of amplitude ▸ frequency and
- f. of cancer ▸ localized
- f. of cerebral palsy ▸ hemiplegic
- f. of cerebral palsy ▸ paraplegic
- f. of methamphetamine ▸ smokable

- f. of occlusion, spherical
- f. of penicillin ▸ repository
- f. of preexcitation, combined
- f., operation consent
- f., patient release
- f., polyhedral-shaped
- f., pressure wave
- f., pulmonary
- f., pulmonary pressure wave
- f., recrystallized
- f., rectangular wave
- f. refusing permission for blood transfusion
- f., release
- f., request
- f., rod-like
- f., rod-shaped
- f., sarcomatoid
- f. ▸ seclusion/restraint observation
- f., segmented
- f. sense
- f., sharp transient wave
- f. signed ▸ against medical advice (AMA)
- f., smokable
- F. Sorting Test ▸ Color-
- f., spectral wave
- f., spherical-shaped
- f., stab
- f., stimulus wave
- f., subclinical
- f., tablet
- f. to admit observers ▸ authorization
- f. to delivery by alternate physician ▸ consent
- f. to use eyes (donor) ▸ authorization
- f. to use eyes (next of kin) ▸ authorization
- f. to use eyes (donor) ▸ consent
- f. to use eyes (next of kin) ▸ consent
- f. to use kidneys (donor) ▸ authorization
- f. to use kidneys (next of kin) ▸ authorization
- f. to use kidneys (donor) ▸ consent
- f. to use kidneys (next of kin) ▸ consent
- f., wave
- f., W wave

Formad's kidney

formal

f. developmental history
f. monitoring of patient
f. protocol
f. staff education
formalin fixed specimen
formant gene
format
  f. ▸ quad-screen
  f., scanning
  f., treatment-planning
formation
  f. ability, verbal concept
  f., abscess
  f., adhesion
  f. and increase mass in bone ▸ stimulate
  f. and release of hormone
  f. and resportion ▸ bone
  f., aspergilloma
  f., bas-fond
  f., blast
  f., bone
  f., bone cell
  f., callous
  f., callus
  f., cancellous
  f., cancer
  f., cellule
  f., cervical rib
  f., clot
  f., coagulum
  f., contracture
  f., controlling fluid
  f., crust
  f., cyst
  f., cystocele
  f., desmoplastic
  f., dorsal osteophyte
  f., elongated
  f. ▸ endocardial cushion
  f., esophageal fibrous stricture
  f., excessive callus
  f., excessive gas
  f., exostosis
  f. ▸ extensive new bone
  f. ▸ fetal brain
  f. ▸ fibrous tissue
  f., fluid
  f., focal abscess
  f., focal serosal abscess
  f., gallstone
  f., granular
  f., impulse
  f. in cornea, hyaline
  f. ▸ inadequate enchondral bone

f. ▸ increased risk of clot
f., inhibiting clot
f. ▸ intraperitoneal adhesion
f., keloid
f., larval
f., liver
f., localized plaque
f., median bar
f., mesencephalic reticular
f., mesoderm
f., new bone
f. ▸ new lesion
f., nodule
f. of brain stem ▸ reticular
f. of corpus luteum
f. of fibrous or scar tissue
f. of scar tissue
f. of stoma
f., osteoarthritic hypertrophic spur
f., osteophyte
f., pancreatic abscess
f., paravertebral mass
f., pearl
f., plaque
f., platelet plug
f., pneumothorax
f., polymorphous wave
f. postcesarean section, abscess
f., pseudocyst
f., pseudojoint
f. rate, bone
f., reaction
f. ▸ reduce fluid
f., reducing clot
f., rouleaux
f., sac-like
f., scar
f., scar tissue
f., secondary adhesions
f. ▸ secondary follicle
f., sequestrum
f., sparsity of bone
f., spike-like
f., spore
f., spur
f. ▸ stimulate bone
f., stomach
f., stone
f., stricture
f., symptom
f., syncytial knot
f., thrombus
f., tumor
formative cell
formative yolk

forme fruste
forme tardive
formed drum, vacuum
formicant pulse
formiminoglutamic acid
forming
  f. cells, burst-
  f. cells, cancer-
  f. cells, plaque-
  f. drugs, habit-
  f. foods, gas-
  f., habit-
  f. laxative, bulk-
  f. sarcoma, bone-
  f. substances, organ-
  f. tissues, blood-
  f. units, colony-
  f. units (PFU) ▸ plaque-
  f. units, spleen colony-
formol-gel test
formol Müller fluid
formosanum, Stamnosoma
formula
  f., autotransformer
  f. feeding
  f. for dose survival, linear quadratic
  f. ▸ geometric cube
  f. ▸ Gorlin hydraulic
  f., isoeffect
  f., liquid diet
  f., Poisson-Pearson
  f., Poisson statistical
  f., projection
  f. ▸ tension-relieving
formulation
  f., clinical case
  f., dosage
  f., therapeutic
fornicatus, gyrus
forniceal invasion
fornicis
  f., carina
  f., crus
  f., taenia
fornix
  f., anterior
  f., anterior pillar of
  f. -based conjunctival flap
  f. cerebri
  f., commissure of
  f., conjunctival
  f., inferior
  f., lateral
  f. longus of Forel

fornix—_continued_
  f., posterior
  f., posterior pillar of
  f., vaginal
Foroblique lens
Forrester-type head halter
Förster('s)
  F. choroiditis
  F. -Fuchs' black spot
  F. operation
  F. -Penfield operation
  F. syndrome
  F. uveitis
Fort Bragg fever
fortification figure
fortified vitamin D milk
fortress mentality
fortuitum, Mycobacterium
40 (SV 40) ▸ simian virus
48 hours incubation ▸ growth after
49er knee brace
46 chromosomes
forward
  f. bending
  f. -bending exercise
  f. -bending maneuver
  f. conduction
  f. displacement of eyeball
  f. -flexed posture
  f. flexion
  f. flexion of trunk
  f. heart failure
  f. movement
  f. subluxation
  f. triangle technique
fossa
  f. abscess ▸ iliac
  f., antecubital
  f., anterior
  f., axillary
  f., canine
  f. carcinoma, tonsillar
  f., cerebellar
  f., cerebral
  f. cerebri lateralis
  f., chondrosarcoma posterior
  f., Claudius'
  f., coronoid
  f., cranial
  f. cranii anterior
  f. cranii media
  f. cranii posterior
  f., fusiform
  f., glenoid
  f., hypophyseal

f., interpeduncular
f., kidney replaced in renal
f., lateral cerebral
f., left antecubital
f., left iliac
f. mandibularis, glenoid
f. metastasis syndrome ▸ parasellar
  and middle
f., middle
f. ▸ middle cranial
f., Morgagni's
f., nasal
f., navicular
f. navicularis
f. navicularis urethrae
f., obturator
f. of cerebrum ▸ cistern of lateral
f. of male urethra, navicular
f. of Sylvius ▸ cistern of
f. of Trietz
f. of vestibule of vagina
f., olecranon
f. ovalis
f. ovalis cordis
f., ovarian
f. ovarica
f., paravesical
f., pelvic
f., piriform
f., pituitary
f., popliteal
f., posterior
f., posterior cranial
f., prostatic
f., radial
f., radical
f., renal
f., right antecubital
f. (RIF) ▸ right iliac
f., scaphoid
f., supraclavicular
f., sylvian
f., temporal
f., tonsil
f., tonsillar
f., triangular
f., tumor, posterior
f., vein of sylvian
f., vestibuli vaginae
fossae [_fauces_]
fossae, antecubital
fossae, condylar
foster (Foster)
  f. care
  f. confidence

f. father
f. home
f. home care
f. home evaluation
f. home placement
F. Kennedy syndrome
f. mother
f. parent
f. placement
Fothergill('s)
  F. neuralgia
  F. operation
  F. operation ▸ Donald-
foul
  f. -smelling amniotic fluid
  f. -smelling phlegm
  f. -smelling sputum
  f. -smelling ▸ sputum purulent and
  f. -smelling urine
  f. sputum ▸ fever, night sweats,
    cough,
  f. sputum ▸ malnourished multiple
    caries
  f. -tasting discharge around tooth
Foundation
  F. (AHAF) ▸ American Health
    Assistance
  F., Arthritis
  F. support garment ▸ Frederick
founders' ague, brass-
fountain decussation of Meynert
four (4) (Four)
  f. -A Magovern valve prosthesis
  4 antireflex procedure, Belsey Mark
  f. -chambered human heart
  f. -chamber view
  f. -chamber view echocardiogram ▸
    apical
  F., Code
  f. field isocentric technique
  f. field x-ray beam dosimetry
  f. -flap procedure
  f. hour delayed lymph nodal stage
    radiograph ▸ twenty-
  f. hour urines ▸ twenty-
  4 ▸ platelet factor
  f. -point assay
  f. -point biopsy
  f. -point gait
  f. -point leather restraints
  f. -portal technique
  f. -poster cervical brace
  f. -pronged cane
  f. -quadrant biopsy
  f. quick breaths

f. -site GC (gonococcus) cultures
f. times a day (q.i.d.)
f. -vessel angiogram
f. -vessel angiography, total absence of circulation on
f. -vessel arteriogram
F. -Way (LSD)

400, Conray-
400 resin ▸ IRA-
fourché, main
Fourier transformation imaging, direct
Fourier two-dimensional imaging
Fournier's disease
Fournier teeth
14
14 and six hertz (Hz) positive bursts
14 and six hertz (HZ) positive spikes
14 and six per second positive spikes
14 positive spikes ▸ six and
14 spike rhythm, six and

fourth
f. circulation
f. cranial nerve
f. -degree burn
f. digit of foot
f. digit of hand
f. heart sound
f. nerve
f. stage of labor
f. toe
f. ventricle ▸ glial membrane of
f. ventricle of brain
f. ventricle of cerebrum

4:1 conduction, atrial flutter with
fovea
f., anterior
f., central
f. centralis retinae
f., inferior
f., posterior
f., superior

foveal blindness, complete
foveal vision
foveated chest
foveolar reflex
Foville('s)
F. fasciculus
F. syndrome
F. tract
F. -Wilson syndrome

Fowler('s)
F. angular incision
F. loudness balance test
F. maneuver
F. operation
F. position
F. single-breath test
F. solution

Fox('s)
F. eye shield
F. -Fordyce disease
F. implant
F. operation

fps (frames per second)
fraction(s) [*traction, faction*]
f., absorbed
f., blood
f., branching
f., cineangiography and densitometric ejection
f., CK/MB
f., densitometric ejection
f. ▸ depressed ejection
f. ▸ echocardiography ejection
f., ejection
f., filling
f., filtration
f. ▸ first-third filling
f. ▸ global left ventricular (LV) rejection
f., growth
f., heparin precipitable
f. image, ejection
f., increased dose size per
f., indirect
f., (LDH) lactic dehydrogenase
f., left ventricular (LV) ejection
f. ▸ light pen-determined ejection
f., low
f., mid-sagittal plane dose of rad in
f., normal ejection
f. of expired carbon dioxide (FECO$_2$)
f. of inspired carbon dioxide (FICO$_2$)
f. of inspired oxygen (FIO$_2$)
f., packing
f., penetration
f., plasma
f., prostatic
f., regurgitant
f. ▸ rest ejection
f., right ventricular (RV) ejection
f., scatter
f., shortening

f., spurious ejection
f., Teicholz ejection
f., total dose of rad in
f., Weber

fractional
f. biopsy
f. culture
f. curettage
f. D and C
f. myocardial shortening
f. retrograde amnesia
f. sterilization

fractionated high-dose rate
fractionated radiotherapy
fractionation
f., accelerated
f., biologic factors in dose
f., cell cycle redistribution and dose
f., dose
f. (TDF) factor ▸ time, dose,
f., fat
f., modification patterns of dose
f., normal tissue effects of dose
f. radiation therapy ▸ high-dose
f. rate of rad ▸ daily
f., reoxygenation and dose
f., split-course dose
f., tumor control with dose
f. with chemotherapy
f. without chemotherapy

fracture(s) [*factor*]
f., advancing union of
f., agenetic
f., alignment of
f. and/or subluxation
f., apposition
f., articular
f., atrophic
f., aviator's
f., avulsion chip
f., backfire
f. bar
f., Barton's
f., basal neck
f., basal skull
f., baseball finger
f., basilar
f., basilar skull
f. bed
f., bedpan
f., bending
f., Bennett
f., bent
f. bilaterally in a horizontal plane

fracture(s)—*continued*

f., bimalleolar
f., blow-in
f., blow-out
f., bone
f., bony vertebral
f., bowing of
f., boxer's
f., bucket-handle
f., bumper
f., bumper-fender
f., bursting
f., butterfly
f., buttonhole
f. by contrecoup
f., capillary
f., carpal
f., carpal scaphoid
f. caused by disease
f. caused by malignancy
f., cementum
f., chance
f., chauffeur's
f., chip
f., chisel
f., Chopart's
f., circumferential
f., clay-shoveler
f., cleavage
f., closed
f., closed reduction of
f., closed segmental
f., closed skull
f., Colles'
f., comminuted
f., comminuted femoral
f., comminuted tibial
f., complete
f., complex
f., complex simple
f., complicated
f., composite
f., compound
f., compound comminuted
f., compound skull
f., compression
f., condylar
f., congenital
f., cortical
f., Cotton
f., cough
f., crack
f., crushing
f., dashboard
f., debridement of compound skull

f., deferred
f., delayed healing of
f., delayed union of
f., dentate
f., depressed
f., depressed skull
f., Desault's
f., diacondylar
f., diastatic skull
f. diet, high
f., direct
f., dish-pan
f. -dislocation
f., displaced
f., displaced femoral neck
f., displacement of
f., double
f., Dupuytren's
f., Duverney's
f., dyscrasic
f., elevation of skull
f. en coin
f. en rave
f., endocrine
f., epiphyseal
f., Essex-Lopresti
f., expressed skull
f. ▸ external fixation of
f., extracapsular
f., fatigue
f., finger
f., fissure
f., flake
f., foot
f., forearm
f. fragments
f. fragments, clavicular
f. fragments, displacement of
f. fragments, manipulation of
f. fragments, pushed inward
f. fragments, realignment of
f. fragments wired
f. frame
f. frame, head
f. ▸ frequency of vertebral
f. fusi
f., Galeazzi's
f., gamekeeper's thumb
f., Gosselin's
f., greenstick
f., grenade-thrower
f., growing
f., Guérin's
f., gutter
f., hairline

f., hangman's
f., healed
f., healing
f., hickory-stick
f., hip
f., humeral
f., iatrogenic
f. ▸ immobility, falls and
f., impacted
f. in vertebra ▸ compression
f., incomplete
f., indirect
f., inflammatory
f., intercondylar
f., internal fixation of
f., interperiosteal
f., intertrochanteric
f. ▸ intertrochanteric region
f., intra-articular
f., intracapsular
f., intraperiosteal
f., intrauterine
f., Jefferson's
f., joint
f., Kocher's
f., lead pipe
f., LeFort's
f., leg
f., leverage
f. line
f., linear
f., linear skull
f., Lisfranc's
f., long bone
f., longitudinal
f., loose
f., lunate
f., Maisonneuve's
f., major
f., Malgaigne's
f., malleolar
f., malunited
f., mandible
f. manipulated
f., march
f., marginal
f., metacarpal
f., metatarsal
f., Monteggia's
f., Moore's
f., multiple
f., multiple old nasal
f., multiple pathologic
f., multiple rib
f. nail

f., nasal
f., nasomaxillary
f., navicular
f. neck of radius
f., neoplastic
f., neurogenic
f., nightstick
f., nondisplaced
f., nondisplaced crack
f. ▸ nondisplaced zygomati arch
f., nonunion of
f. ▸ nonvertebral osteoporotic
f., numerous compression
f., oblique
f., occipital
f., occult
f. of ankle
f. of ankle, bimalleolar
f. of ankle, trimalleolar
f. of bone, incomplete
f. of calcaneus
f. of femur
f. of femur, supracondylar
f. of hip, intercondylar
f. of maxilla, LeFort's
f. of patella
f. of patella, tripartite
f. of radius at wrist
f. of radius, Galeazzi's
f. of rib ▸ hairline
f. of spine, compression
f. of Tillaux
f. of ulnar shaft
f. of zygoma
f., old
f., old healed
f., old nasal
f., open
f., open reduction of
f., open reduction of skull
f., orbital
f., osteoporosis-related spine
f., osteoporotic
f., osteoporotic compression
f., out
f. ▸ outlet strut
f. ▸ pacemaker lead
f., paratrooper
f., parry
f., partial union of
f., pathologic
f., pathologic compression
f., Pauwel
f., pelvic
f. ▸ pelvic stress

f., perforating
f., periarticular
f., perilunate
f., pertrochanteric
f., phalangeal
f., Piedmont
f., pillion
f., ping-pong
f., plaque
f. plaque obstructing artery
f., pond
f., position and alignment of
f., postmortem
f., postmortem induced
f., Pott's
f. ▸ pre-existing temporal bone
f., pressure
f., proper alignment and apposition of
f., puncture
f., pyramidal
f., Quervain's
f. rate
f., recent
f. reduced
f. reduced, nasal
f., reduction facial
f., reduction of
f., resecting
f., rotation and reduction of
f. running length of bone
f., Salter's
f., secondary
f., segmental
f., segmented
f., Segond's
f., septal
f., Shepherd's
f., shin bone
f., Shoveller's
f., sideswipe
f., silver-fork
f., simple
f. ▸ simple, comminuted
f., simple skull
f. site
f. site, base of
f. site, comminuted tibial
f. site, crepitus at
f. site, femoral neck
f. site, incision carried down to
f. site, motion at
f. site, radial
f. site, remottling
f. site, separation at

f. site, tibial
f., Skillern's
f., skull
f., Smith's
f., spinal compression
f., spiral
f. splint, Clayton greenstick
f., splintered
f., spontaneous
f., sprain
f., sprinter's
f., stabilization of
f. stabilized
f., stabilizing
f., stable
f., stellate
f., Stieda's
f., strain
f., stress
f., strut
f., subcapital
f., subcutaneous
f., subluxation and/or
f., subperiosteal
f., subtrochanteric
f., supracondylar
f., susceptible to
f., synthesis of continuity of
f. table
f. table, Albee
f. table, Bell
f., teardrop
f. ▸ temporal bone
f., terminal tuft
f. threshold
f., thumb
f., tibial plateau
f., Tillax's
f., tonus
f., torsion
f., torus
f., total transverse
f., tracheal
f., transcervical
f., transcondylar
f., transverse
f., transverse facial
f., transverse maxillary
f., trimalleolar
f., tripod
f., trophic
f., T-shaped
f., tuft
f. /ultrasound study
f., undisplaced

fracture(s)—*continued*
  f., union of
  f. united
  f., ununited
  f. vertebrae of spine
  f., vertebral
  f. ▸ vertebral compression
  f. ▸ volar plate
  f., wagon wheel
  f., Wagstaffe's
  f., willow
  f. with cross union
  f. with delayed union
  f. with malunion
  f. with nonunion
  f., zygomaticomaxillary
fractured
  f., crura
  f. jaw
  f. rib
  f. trachea
  f. valve
  f. windpipe
fracturing, freeze-
fracturing the stricture
Fraenkel's nodules
Fraentzel's murmur
fragi, Pseudomonas
fragile (Fragile)
  f. child syndrome
  f. ▸ patient self-esteem is
  F. X syndrome
fragilis
  f., Bacillus
  f., Bacteroides
  f., Dientamoeba
  f. infection ▸ Bacteroides
  f. isle, Bacteroides
fragilitas ossium
fragilitas sanguinis
fragility [*frigidity*]
  f., bone
  f., erythrocyte
  f. of blood
  f. of nails
  f., osmotic
  f., red cell
  f., Rumpel-Leede's capillary
  f. test
  f. test, capillary
  f. test of blood
fragmatic buttress
fragment(s)
  f., acetabular
  f., antibody

  f. antigen binding
  f., avulsed
  f., bone
  f., bony
  f., butterfly
  f., clavicular fracture
  f., cortical
  f., displacement of fracture
  f., displacement of lower
  f., endometrial tissue
  f., footplate
  f., fracture
  f., free-floating
  f., glistening
  f., irregular osseous
  f. length polymorphism (RFLPs) ▸
    restriction
  f., manipulation fracture
  f., media
  f., metallic
  f., nasal bone
  f. of adventitia
  f. of bone
  f. of medial tissue
  f. of placenta
  f., ovarian
  f. pared with motor saw
  f., placental
  f., realignment of fracture
  f., retention of decidual
  f., retention of placental
  f., separation of
  f., shell
  f., shrapnel
  f. splintered to pieces
  f., squamous epithelial
  f. stones
  f. wired, fractured
  f. wound
  f. wounds, multiple
fragmentary
  f. filling
  f. images
  f. sensory memories
fragmentation
  f. and fissuring
  f., continued
  f. ▸ kidney stone
  f., multiple
  f. myocarditis
  f. of fantasy
  f. of myocardium
  f. of thought
  f. process
  f. ▸ renal stone

  f., transverse
fragmented plaque
**fragmented psychological sense of
  self**
fragmenter, ultrasonic
frail [*flail*]
frail elderly patient
frame(s)
  f., arc-shaped stereotactic
  f., B-scan
  f., Balkan
  f., Bradford
  f., Deiters' terminal
  f., Elgiloy
  f., Foster
  f., fracture
  f., head fracture
  f., Hibbs'
  f., Leksell's stereotactic
  F., Mobile Standing
  f., occluding
  f. of death, Kübler-Ross time
  f. per second (fps)
  f., Putti
  f., quadriplegic standing
  f., stereotactic
  f., Stryker
  f., trial
  f., Whitman's
framework, basic trauma
Framingham Heart Study
Franceschetti's
  F. disease
  F. dystrophy
  F. operation
  F. syndrome
Francisella tularensis
francisi, Thrassis
Francke's strae
Francois' dystrophy
Franconi's anemia
**Frangenheim-Goebell-Stoeckel
  operation**
frank (Frank) [*flank*]
  f. breech presentation
  F. gastrostomy ▸ Ssabanejew-
  f. prolapse
  f. rales
  F. -Starling curve
  F. -Starling mechanism
  F. -Starling reserve
  F. -Straub-Wiggers-Starling
    principle
  f. vaginal breech

Fränkel('s)
- F. appliance
- F. sign
- F. treatment

Frankl-Hochwart's disease

Franklin('s)
- F. disease
- F. glasses
- F. unit (RFU) ▸ Reitland-

frantic effort

frantic effort to avoid abandonment

fraternal twins

fraud, health

Frazier-Spiller operation

Frazier suction tube

Frederick Foundation support garment

free
- f. abdominal air
- f. accessibility, barrier-
- f., adhesions dissected
- f. air
- f. air in diaphragm
- f. -air ionization chamber
- f. and equal, excursions
- f. ankle, long leg brace with
- f., area draped
- f. area ▸ echo
- f. association
- f. -base (cocaine sulphate)
- f. -base abusers ▸ cocaine
- f. -base cocaine ▸ long-term use of
- f. -base cocaine ▸ smoking
- f. -base crystal
- f. -base form
- f. -base heroin
- f. -based cocaine
- f. -basing cocaine
- f. beam laser
- f. bland diet, milk-
- f. blood pressure (BP) screening
- f. blood sugar screening
- f. bodies, opaque
- f. body, calcified
- f., cancer-
- f., carrier-
- f. clinic
- f. communication, chemically
- f. diet ▸ caffeine, alcohol, pepper, spicy (CAPS) foods-
- f. diet, fat-
- f. diet, gluten-
- f. diet, lactose-
- f. diet, purine-
- f. diet, salt-

- f., disease-
- f., dissected
- f., drug-
- f. drug treatment clinic
- f. dry weight, fat-
- f. electrons
- f. energy
- f. environment, bacteria-
- f. environment, drug-
- f. environment, germ-
- f. environment, smoke-
- f. environment ▸ stress-
- f. environment ▸ structure drug-
- f. epithelium
- f. erythrocyte coproporphyria
- f. erythrocyte coproporphyrin
- f. erythrocyte protoporphyrin
- f. esophageal reflux
- f. exercise
- f. extracellular virus
- f., fat-
- f. fatty acid production
- f. fatty acids
- f. flap ▸ microvascular-
- f. flap procedure ▸ gluteal
- f. -floating anxiety
- f. -floating bone chip
- f. -floating fragment
- f. -floating kidney
- f. -floating otoconia
- f. flow
- f. fluid
- f. fluid in cul-de-sac
- f., germ-
- f. gingival
- f. gingival groove
- f. glaucoma screening
- f., gluten-
- f. graft
- f. health screening
- f. hemoglobin ▸ pyridoxilated stroma
- f. hemoglobin solution, stroma-
- f. hydrochloric acid
- f., inferior rectus muscle dissected
- f. interval ▸ symptom-
- f. intraperitoneal air
- f. iris scraped
- f., irritation
- f. isolation units, germ-
- f. life, cancer-
- f. lifestyle, chemically
- f. lifestyle, smoke-
- f. living, chemical-
- f. macrophage

- f. magnesium ▸ low intracellular-
- f. mass, fat-
- f. meal, fat-
- f. medical screening
- f. motion, pain-
- f. nipple transplants
- f. nuclei
- f. of chemical dependency
- f. of disease
- f. of emboli ▸ pulmonary vasculature
- f. of fluid ▸ abdominal cavity
- f. of fluid ▸ pleural sac
- f. of obstruction, tube
- f. of significant risks
- f. of ulcers ▸ duodenum
- f., pain-
- f. passage of urine
- f. path, mean
- f., patient is drug-
- f., patient pain-
- f. period, disease-
- f. period, pain-
- f. peritoneal air
- f. position, gravity
- f. posture screening
- f. program ▸ outpatient drug-
- f. program ▸ residential drug-
- f. program, smoke-
- f. protocol ▸ Westminster drug-
- f. radical
- f. radical damage
- f. radical molecules
- f. radical oxidants (FRO)
- f. radical poisoning
- f. radical theory
- f. radicals ▸ oxygen (O_2)
- f. radicals ▸ oxygen (O_2) derived
- f. radioisotope, carrier-
- f. ratio, bound-
- f., seizure-
- f. space ▸ echo-
- f. space, retrosternal
- f. (SPF) ▸ specific pathogen
- f. stage of bacterial endocarditis, bacteria-
- f. -standing clinic
- f. -standing detoxification
- f. -standing private psychiatric facility
- f. state ▸ pain-
- f. surgery, pain-
- f. surgery, risk-
- f. survival rate, disease-
- f., symptom

free—*continued*

    f. thyrotoxin index
    f. thyroxine
    f. thyroxine index (FTI)
    f. treatment, drug-
    f. treatment, out-patient drug-
    f. treatment program, drug-
    f. tuberculin, albumose-
    f. walking time ▸ pain-
    f. wet weight ▸ fat-
    f. work site, smoke-
    F. Workplace Act ▸ Drug-
    f. zone, pain-

freed

    f. and exposed by blunt dissection
        ▸ kidney
    f. by blunt dissection
    f. by sharp dissection
    f., kidney
    f. up
    f. up, appendix
    f., ureter

freedom

    f., chemical
    f., degree of
    f., foot
    f., sexual
    f. technique ▸ emotional
    f., total chemical

freely

    f. mobile, uterus
    f. movable
    f. movable, carina
    f. movable joint
    f. movable, uterus

freestyle stroke injury

freeze

    f. -cleaving
    f. -dried
    f. -drying
    f. -etched
    f. -etching
    f. -fracturing
    f. -slow thaw treatment ▸ rapid
    f. -substitution
    f. technique ▸ freeze-thaw-
    f. thaw cryotherapy
    f. -thaw-freeze technique

freezing

    f. donor bone
    f., egg
    f., gastric
    f. microtome
    f. pain, burning or
    f. point

    f. with liquid nitrogen

Fregoli delusion
Freiberg's disease
Freiberg's infraction
Freiburg method
Frei's test
fremitus

    f., auditory
    f., bronchial
    f., friction
    f., hydatid
    f., pectoral
    f., pericardial
    f., peripheral
    f., pleural
    f., rhonchial
    f., subjective
    f., tactile
    f., tussive
    f., vocal

frenata, lingua
French

    F. (SKF) culture ▸ Smith, Klein and
    F. flap
    F. paradox
    F. scale
    F. sliding flap

frenetic [*phrenetic, phonetic*]
frenoplasty procedure
frenulum

    f. labiorum pudendi
    f. of clitoris
    f. of prepuce of penis
    f. veli

frenum, labial
frenum, lingual
Freon 12
frequency(-ies)

    f. AC (alternating current) signals,
        low
    f. activity, alpha
    f. activity, high
    f., alpha
    f., amplifier input
    f., amplifier output
    f. analysis
    f. analysis, narrow band
    f. and form of amplitude
    f. and intensity ▸ running
    f. and urgency of urination
    f., attack
    f., attenuated
    f., audio
    f. band
    f. band, narrow

    f. bands, selected
    f., basic rhythmic
    f., beta
    f. blood group, high
    f. blood group, low
    f., burst of theta
    f., ciliary beat
    f. component, dominant
    f. components, low
    f., controlled variable
    f., critical flicker
    f., critical fusion
    f. current, high
    f., decrease in
    f., delta
    f. dependent
    f. domain analysis
    f. domain imaging
    f., dominant
    f., energy
    f. epicardial echocardiography ▸
        high
    f. event, high
    f., fecal
    f. filter control, high
    f. filter control, low
    f. filter, high
    f. filter, low
    f. following response (FFR)
    f., form and topography
    f., fundamental
    f., fusion
    f., gene
    f., headache
    f., hearing
    f. hearing loss, high
    f., high
    f., infrasonic
    f., intermediate
    f. jet ventilation ▸ high
    f. jet ventilator ▸ high
    f., low
    f. (MDF) ▸ mean dominant
    f., medium
    f. modulation
    f. murmur ▸ high
    f. murmur ▸ low
    f., natural
    f. of contractions
    f. of diarrhea ▸ volume and
    f. of duration
    f. of infection
    f. of medication
    f. of recording, high
    f. of rhythm

f. of seizures ► reducing
f. of sound waves, shifts in
f. of testing
f. of undetermined etiology ► urinary
f. of urination ► increased
f. of urination, patient has
f. of vertebral fractures
f. of waves
f. oscillation ► high
f. oscillation ventilator ► high
f. pacemaker, radio-
f. positive pressure ventilation ► high
f. potentials, bizarre high
f. pulsations, low
f. ► pulse repetition
f. range ► alpha-theta EEG (electroencephalogram)
f. range, brain wave
f. range, electroencephalogram (EEG)
f., range of
f., recombination
f., reduce tension headache
f. ► reduced hearing at high
f. relation ► force
f., resonant
f., response
f. response curve
f. response, dynamic
f. response, high
f. response, low
f., rhythm of alpha
f., rhythmic wave
f. sensorineural hearing loss ► high
f. sensorineural hearing loss ► low
f. shifter
f., slow brain wave
f. sound waves, high
f. spectrum
f. spectrum, electroencephalogram (EEG)
f., speech
f., spurious
f., square waves of high
f. stimulation ► high
f., stimulus
f., subsonic
f., supersonic
f., theta
f. thrombolysis ► high
f. tracer
f., ultrasonic
f., uniform

f., unit of
f., urgency and
f., urinary
f. ► urinary urgency and
f. ventilation ► high
f. ventilation ► ultra high
f. vibrations, low
f. voltage, zero
f., wave
f., waves of alpha
f., zero

frequens, Ixodes
frequent
f. assessment
f. attacks of disabling vertigo
f. blinking of eyes
f. blowing respirations
f. bowel movements
f. change in body position
f. changes in emotion
f. colds
f. contractions
f. depression
f. emesis
f. epistaxis
f. falling
f., headache
f. heartburn
f. individual bursts of alpha
f. infections
f. intoxication
f. mastalgia
f. monitoring
f. mood changes
f. mood swings
f. nausea and diarrhea
f. night-time urination
f. pulse
f. seizures
f. spasms
f. staggering and falls
f. stools
f. urinary incontinence
f. urination
f. urination ► burning and
f. vaginal bleeding
f. vaginal yeast infections
f. visits to physician

fresh
f. bleeding
f. blood, extremity vessels perfused with
f. corneal tissue
f. cut on hand
f. frozen allograft

f. frozen plasma
f. frozen plasma infusion
f. frozen plasma ► patient admitted and transfused with
f. frozen plasma, transfusion of
f. gas flow
f. granulation tissue
f. hemorrhage
f. traumatic wounds ► open

freshening peel
freshly clotted blood
freshly clotted blood in stomach
Fresnel zone plate
Freudian censor
Freudian fixation
Freud's
F. catharsis
F. cathartic method
F. theory
Freund('s)
F. adjuvant
F. adjuvant, complete
F. adjuvant ► incomplete
F. anomaly
F. law
F. operation
freundii, Citrobacter
freundii urinary tract infection ► Citrobacter
Frey's hairs
Frey's implant
friability, patchy
friable [viable]
f. cervix
f. necrotic tissue
f., trigone edematous and
f. tumor mass
Fricke's dosimetry
Fricke's operation
Frickle's flap
friction
f. blisters
f. burn
f., cross fiber
f. fremitus
f. murmur
f. of pericardial surfaces
f. rub
f. rub, absence of
f. rub, pericardial
f. rub, pleural
f. rub, saddle leather
f. rub ► systolic pericardial
f. rub, thrills and/or
f. ► skin subjected to

friction—*continued*
- f. sound
- f. sound, Beatty-Bright
- f. sound ▸ pericardial
- f. sound, to-and-fro
- f., systematic therapeutic

Friderichsen syndrome, Waterhouse-
Friedenwald's operation
Friedenwald's syndrome
Friede's operation
friedländeri, Klebsiella
Friedländer's
- F. bacillus
- F. bacillus pneumonia
- F. disease
- F. pneumobacillus
- F. pneumonia

Friedman('s)
- F. -Lapham test
- F. position
- F. test

Friedmann's vasomotor syndrome
Friedreich's
- F. ataxia
- F. disease
- F. operation
- F. sign
- F. tabes

friend, bereaved
friendly, patient
friends, or school activities ▸
    withdrawal from family,
fright reaction
frigidity [*fragility*]
fringe joint
fringent viral
Fritsch-Asherman syndrome
Fritsch's operation
Fritz-Asherman syndrome
Fritz-Lang operation
FRO (free radical oxidants)
fro
- f. friction sounds ▸ to-and-
- f. murmur ▸ to-and-
- f. sound ▸ to-and-

frog
- f. breathing
- f. -leg projections
- f. -leg view
- f. -legged position
- f. test

Fröhlich's syndrome
Froin's syndrome
froissement, bruit de
frolement, bruit de

Froment's sign
Frommel syndrome, Chiari-
Frommel's operation
frondosum, chorion
fronds of connective tissue ▸ long
fronds, sea
frons cranii
front
- f. kicks
- f. of or behind ear ▸ lump in
- f. punches, straight
- f. -tap reflex
- f. teeth

frontal (F) [*fundal*]
- f. abscess
- f. activity, abnormal
- f. alopecia
- f. antrotomy, radical
- f. antrum
- f. area
- f. artery
- f. ataxia
- f. balding
- f. bone
- f. bone, ethmoidal notch of
- f. bone, inner table
- f. bone, outer table
- f. cells
- f. cortex
- f. cortex watershed
- f. diploic vein
- f. dysfunction ▸ right
- f. electrode, inferior
- f. fontanelle
- f. gyrus, ascending
- f. gyrus, inferior
- f. gyrus, middle
- f. gyrus, superior
- f. headache
- f. hematoma, left
- f. hematoma, right
- f., inferior
- f. intermittent rhythmic delta activity
- f. irregular rhythmic delta activity
- f. leads
- f. lobe
- f. lobe, inferior
- f. lobe of brain
- f. lobe of brain ▸ excision
- f. lobe syndrome
- f. lobes of cerebral cortex
- f. lobotomy
- f. nerve
- f. notch
- f. paranasal sinus

- f. plane
- f. process of maxilla
- f. projection
- f. region
- f. segment
- f. sinus
- f. sinus, aperture of
- f. sinus, subperiosteal abscess of
- f. sinusectomy
- f. slow activity
- f. slow wave focus
- f. slowing spikes, right
- f. spike focus
- f. spindle
- f. spindle, slow
- f. suture
- f. vein
- f. zygomatic suture line

frontale, os
frontalis
- f. inferior, gyrus
- f. interna, hyperostosis
- f. medialis, gyrus
- f. medius, gyrus
- f. muscle
- f. muscle tension
- f., pars
- f., sulcus
- f. superior, gyrus
- f., torus

frontoanterior
- f., left
- f. position
- f., right

frontocentral
- f. beta rhythm
- f. beta rhythm ▸ variable
- f. region

frontocortical aphasia
frontocortical damage
frontodextra posterior
frontodextra transversa
frontoethmoid sphenoidectomy
frontoethmoidal suture
frontolacrimal suture
frontolaeva
- f. anterior
- f. posterior
- f. transverse

frontolenticular aphasia
frontomalar suture
frontomaxillary suture
frontomental diameter
frontonasal process
frontonasal suture

fronto-occipital diameter
frontoparietal
  f. area
  f. spike-and-wave discharge
  f. suture
frontopolar artery
frontopontile fibers
frontoposterior
  f., left
  f. position
  f., right
frontosphenoid suture
frontotemporal dementia
frontotransverse
  f., left
  f., position
  f., right
frontozygomatic suture
Froriep's induration
frost (Frost)
  F. -Lang operation
  F. suture
  f., uremic
frostbite
  f. cocktail
  f., deep
  f. ears
  f. finger
  f. fingertips
  f. foot
  f. hand
  f. injury
  f. lungs
  f. nose
  f., preventing
  f., superficial
  f. toe
  f., victim of
frosted heart
frosting heart
froth
  f., blood-tinged
  f. in upper airway
  f., meibomian
frothing at mouth
frothy sputum
frottement, bruit de
frown furrows
frozen
  f. allograft ▸ fresh
  f. angioplasty
  f. cells
  f. corneal tissue
  f. embryo
  f. hand

  f. joint
  f. pelvis
  f. plasma
  f. plasma, fresh
  f. plasma infusion ▸ fresh
  f. plasma ▸ patient admitted and
    transfused with fresh
  f. plasma, transfusion of fresh
  f. red cells
  f. saline
  f. section
  f. section, biopsy submitted for
  f. section done
  f. section examination
  f. section, specimen submitted for
  f. section, tissue submitted for
  f. shoulder
  f. skin sloughs off
  f. sleep
  f. thorax
fructose intolerance
fructose intolerance, hereditary
fruit exchange
fruit sugar
fruste, forme
frustrate systole
frustrated, patient
frustration
  f. and belligerency ▸ rage,
  f., anger and
  f. ▸ depression, anxiety, and
  f. ▸ pent-up
  f. tolerance
  f. tolerance ▸ low
FSC (fracture simple, comminuted)
FSH (follicle-stimulating hormone)
FSR (fusiform skin revision)
FTI (free thyroxine index)
FTLB (full-term living birth)
FTND (full-term normal delivery)
FU (fluorouracil)
FU (fluorouracil) ▸ infusion of 5-
Fuchs(')
  F. atrophy
  F. black spot ▸ Förster-
  F. coloboma
  F. dimples
  F. dystrophy
  F. heterochromia
  F. iritis
  F. keratitis
  F. -Kraupa syndrome
  F. nodules, Dalen-
  F. operation
  F. spot

  F. syndrome
fuchsin ▸ trypsin, aldehyde-
fuchsinophil granules
FUDR (floxuridine)
Fuel (phencyclidine analog), Rocket
fuelleborni, Fasciolopsis
Fueth operation, Mayo-
fugal flow ▸ petal-
fugax
  f., amaurosis
  f., amaurosis partialis
  f., amblyopia
  f., coxitis
  f., erythema
  f., hemianopia bitemporalis
  f., proctalgia
fugitive swelling
Fukala's operation
Fukuda test
fulcrum height adjustment ▸
  automatic
fulfilling prophesies, self-
fulfillment, personal
fulgurant pains
fulgurating migraine
fulguration
  f., cystoscopic
  f., direct
  f., electrical
  f., excision
  f., indirect
  f. of recurring bladder tumors
  f., tubal
fulica, Achatina
full
  f. activity
  f. alcohol syndrome
  f. and equal bilaterally ▸ peripheral
    pulses
  f. arousal
  f. artificial airway
  f. blood examination
  f. blood workup
  f. -blown addiction
  f. -blown AIDS
  f. -blown compulsion
  f. -blown convulsion
  f. -blown dementia
  f. -blown infection
  f. -blown manic depressive illness
  f. -blown panic disorder
  f. -blown psychosis
  f. -blown stroke
  f. -blown symptoms
  f. -blown ulcer

full—*continued*
- f. body CT (computerized) scan
- f. body immersion
- f. body massage
- f. body radiation
- f. body weight
- f. brain radiation therapy
- f. breech presentation
- f. cardiac arrest
- f. contact lens
- f. course of radiation
- f. course of radiation ▸ patient tolerated
- f. course radiation therapy
- f. course, radiation therapy resumed in
- f. criteria
- f. crown
- f. denture
- f. exercise
- f. expansion of lungs
- f. extension
- f. -face mask
- f. field stimulation
- f. fist, patient makes
- f. -fledged disease
- f. flexion
- f. florid diabetic retinopathy (FFDR)
- f. function
- f. head of hair
- f. inspiration
- f. leather restraints
- f. leathers, patient in
- f. liquid diet
- f. monitoring
- f. mouth dentures
- f. mouth extraction
- f. mouth series
- f. mouth x-rays
- f. of blood ▸ abdomen
- f. of self-pity
- f. pulse
- f. range of flexion and extension
- f. range of motion (ROM)
- f. range of motion (ROM) ▸ left ankle
- f. range of motion (ROM) ▸ left elbow
- f. range of motion (ROM) ▸ left femur
- f. range of motion (ROM) ▸ left knee
- f. range of motion (ROM) ▸ left lower extremity (LLE)
- f. range of motion (ROM) ▸ left shoulder
- f. range of motion (ROM) ▸ left upper extremity (LUE)
- f. range of motion (ROM) ▸ left wrist
- f. range of motion (ROM) ▸ neck
- f. range of motion (ROM) ▸ right ankle
- f. range of motion (ROM) ▸ right elbow
- f. range of motion (ROM) ▸ right femur
- f. range of motion (ROM) ▸ right knee
- f. range of motion (ROM) ▸ right lower extremity (RLE)
- f. range of motion (ROM) ▸ right shoulder
- f. range of motion (ROM) ▸ right upper extremity (RUE)
- f. range of motion (ROM) ▸ right wrist
- f. range of symptoms
- f. remission ▸ bipolar disorder, depressed, in
- f. remission ▸ bipolar disorder, manic, in
- f. remission ▸ bipolar disorder, mixed, in
- f. remission ▸ major depression, in
- f. remission ▸ major depression, recurrent, in
- f. remission ▸ major depression, single episode, in
- f. respiratory failure
- f. ROM (range of motion)
- f. scale
- f. -scale delusion
- f. -scale IQ (intelligence quotient) test
- f. set of dentures
- f. strong pulse
- f. term
- f. -term delivery, normal
- f. -term fetus
- f. -term infant
- f. -term living birth (FTLB)
- f. -term normal delivery (FTND)
- f. term, patient went
- f. -term pregnancy
- f. -thickness graft
- f. -thickness postauricular graft
- f. -thickness skin graft
- f. -thickness transplant

- f. veneer crown
- f. voluntary contraction of muscle
- f. wakefulness
- f. weight bearing
- f. weight-bearing exercises
- f. width at half maximum (FWHM)

Fuller shield
fullness
- f., abdominal
- f., aural
- f., borderline left ventricular
- f., borderline right ventricular
- f., chest
- f., hilar
- f. in abdomen
- f. in chest ▸ sensation of
- f. in ear
- f. of breasts
- f. of cul de sac
- f. ▸ sensation of facial

fully
- f. automatic pacemaker
- f. dilated cervix
- f. roused, patient

fulminans, purpura
fulminant
- f. dysentery
- f. glaucoma
- f. hepatitis
- f. liver disease
- f. liver failure
- f. liver failure, acute
- f. pulmonary edema
- f. recurrence

fulminating
- f. apoplexy
- f. appendicitis
- f. colitis
- f. disease
- f. meningococcemia, acute

fulvum, Microsporum
fulvus, Cellvibrio
fumarate, ferrous
fume(s)
- f., cadmium
- f., soldering
- f., toxic

fumigatus, Aspergillus
function(s) [*junction*]
- f. ▸ abnormal brain
- f., abnormal brain wave
- f., abnormal cardiac
- f., abnormal heart valve
- f., abnormal liver
- f., abnormal primary

f., abnormal pulmonary
f. abnormality ▸ immune
f. activity, brain
f., adaptive ego
f., adenoid
f., airway
f. ▸ alcohol impairs cardiac
f., alter gastric
f., alteration in endocrine
f., alteration in respiratory
f., alteration of mental
f., altered brain
f., altering brain
f. analysis ▸ transfer
f. and cineangiography ▸ ventricular
f. antigen ▸ lymphocyte
f., artificially maintained ▸ vital
f., assessing ventricular
f., assessment
f. assessment ▸ myocardial
f., atrial transport
f., auditory
f., auditory recovery
f., autocorrelation
f., automatic
f., autonomic
f. autonomously
f., barrier
f., basic human
f., basic life-preserving
f., behavioral
f., bilateral renal
f., biliary
f., biofeedback hypnotic control of
    autonomic
f., biofeedback voluntary control of
    autonomic
f., biological
f., bladder
f., blood
f., blood vessel
f. blood work ▸ liver
f., bodily
f., body
f., bowel
f., bowel and bladder
f., brain
f., brain stem
f., breathing
f. ▸ caloric testing of vestibular
f., capacity to
f., cardiac
f. ▸ cardiac size and
f., cardiovascular
f., ceased to

f., cell
f. cell growth, division and
f., cellular
f., central dopaminergic
f., cerebellar
f., cerebral
f., cerebral metabolic
f. ▸ chronic loss of
f., circulatory system
f., cognitive
f. ▸ common cognitive
f., compromised renal
f., contractile
f., cortical
f. curve
f. curve ▸ ventricular
f., cyclical
f. ▸ decline in mental
f., decline in sexual
f., decrease of
f., decreased ability to
f., decreased bowel
f., decreased immune
f., decreased kidney
f., decreased renal
f., depressed
f. ▸ deterioration in renal
f., detrusor
f., diastolic
f. ▸ diminished heart, kidney and
    brain
f., diminished motor
f., discriminant
f. ▸ disintegration of cognitive brain
f. disorder ▸ motor
f., disordered mind
f., disorganization of neuronal
f., disruption of bladder
f., disruption of motor
f., disturbance of visual
f. ▸ drug-induced alterations of
    cardiovascular
f. dulling of mental
f., ego
f., electrophysiologic
f., endocrine
f. ▸ episodic disturbance of mental
f. ▸ esophageal body
f. (ETF), eustachian tube
f., executant ego
f. exercise of
f., expelling
f., expressive language
f., eyelid
f., F

f., facial nerve
f., full
f., gallbladder
f., gene
f. ▸ general deterioration of brain
f., global assessment of
f., heart
f. ▸ heart, kidney, and brain
f. ▸ heart valve
f., hemispheric
f., hepatic
f. ▸ high level of
f., higher mental
f., Hipputope renal
f., host's leukotactic
f., immune
f., immune system
f. ▸ impair immune
f., impair nerve
f., impair receptor
f., impaired
f., impaired cardiac
f., impaired hepatic
f., impaired kidney
f., impaired left ventricular
f., impaired liver
f., impaired motor
f., impaired neurological
f., impaired renal
f., impaired systolic
f., impaired ventricular
f., impairment of kidney
f., impairment of liver
f., impairment of social
f., improved immune
f. in cells of myocardium ▸
    contractile
f., inability to
f., inadequate sexual
f., increased kidney
f. independently, ability to
f. independently ▸ decreased ability
    to
f. ▸ ineffective valve
f., intellectual
f., involuntary
f., involuntary body
f., irregular brain
f., irreversible cessation of
    circulatory and respiratory
f., kidney
f., knee
f. laboratory, pulmonary
f., labyrinthine
f. ▸ left ventricular (LV)

function(s)—*continued*
f., leukotactic
f. ▸ level of cognitive
f. ▸ level of independent
f., liver
f. ▸ long-term memory
f., loss of
f. ▸ loss of control of bladder
f. ▸ loss of effective breathing
f. ▸ loss of language
f. ▸ loss of motor
f. ▸ loss of sensation or
f. ▸ loss of sphincter
f. ▸ loss of valvular
f. ▸ loss of vestibular
f. ▸ low memory
f. ▸ low thyroid
f., lung
f. lung test ▸ split
f. ▸ luteal cell
f., marginal cardiac
f., meaningful brain
f., measuring heart
f., membrane
f., memory
f., menstrual
f., mental
f., metabolic
f., mind-brain
f., mitochondrial
f., mode of
f. (MTF), modulation transfer
f., monitor
f. monitor (CFM), cerebral
f., monitor liver
f., monitor vital
f., monitoring of eighth nerve
f., monitoring of renal
f., motor
f., motor and sensory
f., muscle
f., musculoskeletal
f., myoneuronal
f. ▸ nerve cell
f., neurohormonal
f., neurologic
f., neurological
f., neuropsychological
f. ▸ nondistorting memory
f., normal
f., normal bowel
f., normal cell
f., normal heart
f. ▸ normal immune system
f., normal jaw

f., normal organ
f., normal physical
f., normal physiologic
f., normal pulmonary
f., normal renal
f. ▸ normal stomach and bowel
f., normal urinary
f. of body ▸ loss of excretory
f. of brain stem ▸ impairment of
f. of cell ▸ physiological
f. of heart
f. of heart ▸ electrical
f. of heart, pumping
f. of joint
f. of mitochondria ▸ abnormalities
    of structure and
f. of neurofilaments
f. of ovaries
f. of ▸ sympathetic nervous system,
f. of thalamus
f. of valve ▸ structure and
f., ophthalmologic
f. or memory ▸ intellectual
f., organ
f., organically impaired brain
f., organized mental
f., ovarian
f., overall level of mental
f., pacemaker
f., pacing
f., pancreatic exocrine
f., parasympathetic
f. ▸ parathyroid gland
f., parotid
f., partial
f., partial loss of motor
f. partially suspended ▸ bodily
f., perceptual
f. ▸ permanent decline in intellectual
f., personality
f. ▸ perturbed autonomic nervous
    system
f., phagocytic
f., physiologic
f., platelet
f. ▸ poor liver
f., position of
f. ▸ postoperative pulmonary
f. ▸ probability density
f. profile ▸ thyroid
f., profundus
f. ▸ progressive decline in
f. ▸ progressive decline in intellec-
    tual
f., progressive loss of cerebral

f., pulmonary
f., pump
f., pyramidal
f., radial nerve
f. reaction, thyroid
f., receptive language
f. ▸ receptor sites lose
f., recurrent laryngeal nerve
f. ▸ reduced cognitive
f. ▸ reduced kidney
f., reduced renal
f. ▸ regenerative metabolic
f., renal
f., reproductive
f., respiratory
f., restoration of oral
f. ▸ return of sensation and
f. returned to extremity
f. ▸ right ventricular (RV)
f. ▸ salivary gland
f. screen ▸ normal pulmonary
f. screening, pulmonary
f. ▸ self-care
f. ▸ sensation and motor
f., sensing
f., sensory
f. ▸ sensory aspect of neurologic
f. ▸ sensory neurologic
f., sexual
f., shunt
f., sigh
f. ▸ sinus node
f., slowed intellectual
f., specific
f., spinal cord
f. ▸ stabilize heart
f. ▸ stimulate mental
f. study ▸ nuclear ventricular
f. study, pulmonary
f. study, quantitative regional
f. study, renal
f. study, split
f. study, split renal
f. study, thyroid
f., sustained adrenal
f., swallowing
f., systolic
f. test, airway
f. test, biliary
f. test ▸ gallbladder
f. test, kidney
f. test (LFT), liver
f. test, pancreatic
f. test ▸ pancreatic exocrine
f. test ▸ pancreatic secretory

f. test ▸ pretransplant pulmonary
f. test (PFT), pulmonary
f. test, thyroid
f. testing, cortical
f. testing, pulmonary
f., thymus gland
f., thyroid
f., tonsil
f., total loss of motor
f., transient loss of
f., unimpaired
f., various body
f. ventilation studies ▸ pulmonary
f., ventricular
f., vestibular
f., vision
f., visual
f., visual-motor
f., vital
f. ▸ vital body
f. waxed and waned ▸ left motor
f. waxed and waned ▸ right motor

functional
f. ability ▸ independent
f. ability, patient's
f. activation
f. activity
f. activity, excessive
f. adjustment
f. amenorrhea
f. analysis
f. aphasia
f. appliance
f. aspects of heart
f. asplenia
f. assessment
f. attitude
f. bleeding
f. block
f. bowel disease
f. bowel problems ▸ intermittent
f. bowel syndrome
f. capacity, cardiac
f. capacity classification
f. capacity evaluation
f. cardiac murmur
f. cardiovascular disease
f. change
f. changes, irreversible
f. class
f. colitis, intestinal control in
f. command, concrete
f. communication system
f. congestion
f. constipation

f. deafness
f. death
f. decline
f. decortication from hypoglycemia
f. decortication from hypoxia
f. decortication from trauma
f. deficiency
f. delusion
f. depression
f. diarrhea
f. disability
f. disorder
f. duct
f. dyspareunia
f. dyspepsia
f. dyspnea
f. electrical stimulation (FES)
f. encopresis
f. endoscopic sinus surgery
    (FESS)
f. enuresis
f. extracellular fluid volume
f., extremity
f. family
f. gastrointestinal (GI) disorder
f. headache
f. hearing test
f., heart
f. heart murmur
f. hypertrophy
f. hypoglycemia
f. illness
f. image
f. imaging
f. impairment
f. impairment ▸ alcohol-induced
f. impairment, major
f. impairment ▸ restrictive
f. improvement
f. incontinence
f. independence
f. indigestion
f. inquiry
f. insufficiency, severe
f. kidney
f. level, stabilized
f. limb
f. limitations
f. limits, movement within
f. limits, within
f. losses, permanent
f. magnetic resonance imaging
    (fMRI)
f. magnetic resonance imaging
    (fMRI) brain scan

f. medicine
f. megacolon, acquired
f. memory
f. memory skills
f. memory test
f. menstrual pain
f. murmur
f. neglect
f. nursing
f. occlusal harmony
f. occlusion
f. overlay
f. overlay, significant
f. pain
f. position
f. prognosis
f. progress, overall
f. protoplasm
f. psychomotor retardation
f. psychosis
f. purpose ▸ cosmetic and
f. range of motion (ROM)
f. recovery
f. refractory period
f. reserve capacity
f. reserves, exocrine
f. residual capacity
f. spasm
f. status
f. status ▸ poor
f. stenosis
f. stricture
f. studies
f. subtraction
f. subunit
f. subunit of hair
f. subunit tissue
f. symptom
f. system
f. tendon nerve deficit
f. test, severe
f. validation
f. viability of human islets
f. vision ▸ residual
f. vital capacity (FVC)
functionally
f. blind ▸ patient
f. illiterate, patient
f. independent
functioning
f., abstract
f., adaptive
f., affective
f. after treatment
f. alcoholic ▸ patient

functioning—*continued*
f. at normal ability level ‣ difficulty
f. at _____% normal capacity
f., autonomous ego
f., bilaterally
f., borderline intellectual
f. change, prohealthy
f., CNS (central nervous system)
f., cognitive
f. colostomy
f., daily
f., degree of physical
f., difficulty
f., disordered
f. effective
f. emotional
f. gallbladder
f., graphomotor
f. ileal transverse colostomy ‣ normal,
f., impaired cognitive
f., impaired mental
f. ‣ impairment in occupation
f. impeded
f., improved overall
f., intellectual
f. level
f. level, highest
f. ‣ level of present
f. lymphocytes
f., mental
f. ‣ modes of ineffective
f. normally, kidney
f. of GI tract ‣ normal
f. of normal epithelial tissue
f. of foot ‣ improper
f. of heart ‣ abnormal
f. of heart ‣ assess
f., optimal levels of
f., optimal physiological
f. optimally, shunt
f., overall
f., perceptual
f., physical
f., physiological
f., psychological
f., psychosocial
f. ‣ retardation of normal psycho-motor
f., social
f. ‣ social role
f., sufficient cognitive
f. test, lung
f., vocational

fundal [*frontal, fungal***]**
f. height
f. placenta
f. plication
f. portion of uterus
f. to cervical end
fundamental
f. bundles
f. cause
f. frequency
f. human drive
funded programs, state-
fundi
f. intact
f. negative
f., ocular
f., optic
fundiforme penis, ligamentum
funding
f. base
f., indigent care
f., subsidized
fundoplasty ‣ modified Thal
fundoplication
f., Nissen
f. procedure
f. ‣ Rossetti modification of Nissen
funduliformis, Bacteroides
fundus [*fungus***]**
f., albinotic
f., bladder
f. examination
f., gastric
f. microscopy
f., ocular
f. oculi
f. of eyes
f. of gallbladder
f. of stomach
f. of urinary bladder
f. of uterus
f. of vagina
f. photography, retinal
f., pigmentation of
f., tessellated
f. tigre
f., tigroid
f. tympani
f. uteri
f., uterine
f. vaginae
funduscopic examination
funduscopic examination revealed
microaneurysms

funeral
f. director contacted
f. home arrangements
f. home notification
fungal [*fundal, frontal***]**
f. abscess
f. dermatitis
f. disease
f. disease, cutaneous
f. drug, anti-
f. endocarditis
f. growth
f. hyphae
f. infection
f. infection, aspergillus
f. infection ‣ clinically undetected
f. infection, disseminating
f. infection ‣ endemic
f. infection in mouth
f. infection, mixed
f. infection, nosocomial
f. infection of cornea
f. infection of nail unit
f. infection of nervous system
f. intracellular pathogen
f. invasion
f. nail disease
f. nail infection
f. organisms
f. scalp infection
f. sepsis
f. septicemia
f. serology
f. sinusitis, allergic
f. toenail
fungating
f. brain
f. excrescence
f. lesion
f. mass
f. masses, necrotic
f. mucosal masses ‣ small
f. tumor
f. wound
fungi
f., Achorion
f. and protozoal organisms
f., ascomycetous
f., bacteria and
f., basidiomycetous
f., Coccidioidomyces
f., false
f., kefir
f., Madurella
f., nonpathogenic

f., parasitic
f., pathogenic
f., phycomycetous
f., Rhinocladium
f. smear
f. spores
fungiform, papillae
fungoides
    f. dermatitis ▸ mycosis
    f., granuloma
    f., mycosis
fungosa gastrosia
fungosa, gastroxynsis
fungous
    f. cancer
    f. excrescence
    f. gonitis
fungus
    f., algae-like
    f., alpha
    f. ball
    f. ball ▸ renal
    f., beta
    f., cerebral
    f. cerebri
    f., chignon
    f. ▸ chronic toenail
    f., club
    f. culture
    f., cutaneous
    f., fission
    f. foot
    f., gamma
    f. ▸ generalized infection involving
    f. haematodes
    f., imperfect
    f. infected nail
    f. infection
    f. infection of skin
    f., kefir
    f., mold
    f., mosaic
    f., mycelial
    f. nail
    f. of the brain
    f. organisms, skin test for
    f., perfect
    f., proper
    f., ray
    f., sac
    f., slime
    f. -suppressing drug
    f. testis
    f., thread
    f., toenail

f., Trichosporon
f., true
f., umbilical
f., yeast
f., yeast-like
funic pulse
funic souffle
funicola, Siphunculina
funicular
    f. hernia
    f. hydrocele
    f. souffle
funis presentation
funnel
    f. chest
    f. deformity
    f. dynamics
    f., mitral
    f. -shaped pelvis
    f., vascular
FUO (fever of undetermined origin)
FUO (fever of unknown origin)
FUR (fluorouracil riboside)
Furacin gauze
furcal nerve
furcate placenta
furfur
    f., Malassezia
    f., Microspora
    f., Microsporum
furfuracea, impetigo
Furman Type II electrogram
Furniss' anastomosis
furor epilepticus
furosemide therapy
furred tongue
furrier's
    f. lung
    f. lung disease
    f. suture
furrow(s)
    f., atrioventricular
    f., dental
    f., frown
    f., palpebral
    f., Schmorl's
furrowed tongue
Fürstner's disease
further evaluation
further outbreak, prevent
furuncular otitis
fury ▸ panic or
fusca, Cellfalcicula
fuscicauda, Sarcophaga

fused
    f. commissure
    f. kidney
    f. teeth
    f. vertebrae
    f. vulva
fuser pump
fusi, cortical
fusi, fracture
fusidic acid
fusiform
    f. aneurysm
    f. aneurysmal widening
    f. aortic aneurysm
    f. bronchiectasis
    f. cataract
    f. cells
    f. cells, nucleated
    f. deformity
    f. dilatation
    f. fibers
    f. fossa
    f. gyrus
    f. lobule
    f. muscle
    f. narrowing
    f., papillae
    f. skin revision (FSR)
    f. widening of abdominal aorta
fusiforme, Fusobacterium
fusiformis (Fusiformis)
    f., Bacteroides
    f., gyrus
    F. necrophorus
fusing of personalities
fusion
    f., abnormal
    f., Albee spinal
    f., amplitude of
    f., ankle
    f. beat
    f., binocular
    f., bony
    f., cervical
    f., Charnley compression
    f., commissural
    f. complex
    f., critical flicker
    f. data
    f. defect
    f., diaphyseal-epiphyseal
    f. ▸ entrainment with concealed
    f. frequency
    f. frequency, critical
    f., Hibbs' spinal

fusion—*continued*
  f., joint
  f., knee
  f., magnetic
  f., multilevel spinal
  f., nerve
  f., nuclear
  f. of teeth
  f. of vertebrae
  f., pericardial
  f. procedure
  f. reflex
  f., Rogers' type spinal
  f., Schneider's hip
  f., slow
  f., spinal
  f. surgery, spinal
  f. test, critical flicker
  f. threshold, flicker
  f. tubes
  f., ventricular couplet with
  f., wrist
Fusobacterium
  F. fusiforme
  F. plautivincenti
  F. varium
fusospirochetal
  f. angina
  f. disease
  f. gingivitis
  f. stomatitis
fussy about details ▸ patient
futility, feeling of
future ▸ fear of
future problems, studies to serve as
    baseline for
fuzzy, distant objects
fuzzy vision ▸ blurred or
FVC (functional vital capacity)
FWHM (full width at half maximum)
FZ (focal zone)

G

g (gram)
G banding technique
G benzathine, penicillin
G immunoglobulin (IgG) determin-
   ation ▸ gamma
G, potassium penicillin
G, procaine penicillin
G suit, anti-
G virus ▸ hepatitis
Ga (gallium)
   Ga, radioactive
   Ga scanning
   Ga 67 scan
GA (Gamblers Anonymous)
GA (gastric analysis)
GA (gingivoaxial)
GABA (gamma aminobutyric acid)
Gabarro's graft
Gabastou's hydraulic method
Gabriel-Tucker tube
Gad's hypothesis
Gaenslen's sign
Gaffky scale
Gaffkya tetragena
gag(s)
   g. gene
   g. junction
   g. reflex
   g. reflex, hair-trigger
   g. reflexively, patient
Gaillard-Arlt suture
gain [pain, stain]
   g., abnormal diurnal weight
   g. and bloating ▸ weight
   g., body weight
   g. control
   g. control switch
   g. control ▸ time-
   g. control ▸ time-varied
   g., desire for personal
   g. diet, weight
   g. ▸ easy weight
   g., epinosic
   g., episodic weight
   g., erratic weight
   g., excessive weight
   g., factor, hypoxic

g., gradual weight
g. in aging ▸ weight
g. in weight, significant
g., infant weight
g., maternal weight
g., near
g. nurturance ▸ manipulates to
g., paranosic
g. perspective
g. ▸ postmenopause weight
g. power ▸ manipulates to
g., primary
g. profit ▸ manipulates to
g., rapid weight
g. ratio, modified
g., secondary
g., significant weight
g., subsequent weight
g., sudden weight
g. ▸ time compensation
g., voltage
g., weight
gainfully employed, patient
Gaisböck's syndrome
gait
   g., abnormal
   g. abnormalities
   g. analysis
   g. and balance disorder
   g. and posture, change in
   g. and speech ▸ deterioration of
      coordination,
   g. and stance
   g. and stance ▸ disturbance of
   g. and station
   g. and station, abnormal
   g. and station adequate
   g. and tremor ▸ slowed
   g., antalgic
   g. apraxia
   g. assessment
   g., ataxic
   g., balance and coordination
   g., cerebellar
   g., change in
   g., Charcot's
   g. ▸ diminish excursion of ataxic

g., disturbances in
g., double-step
g., drag-to
g., equine
g., festinating
g., follicular
g., four-point
g. ▸ glue-footed
g., gluteal
g., heel-toe
g., hemiplegic
g. imbalance
g. imbalance and oscillopsia
g. imbalance ▸ progressive
g., intermittent double-step
g., lilting
g., listing
g., magnetic
g., Oppenheim's
g., osteoarthritis
g. ▸ patient unsteady in
g. pattern
g. pattern, bizarre
g. ▸ reeling, staggering
g., scissor
g., shambling
g., shuffling
g., slapping
g., spastic
g., staggering
g., standard
g., steppage
g., swaying
g., swing-through
g., swing-to
g., tabetic
g., tandem
g., three-point
g., toppling
g. training
g. trait
g., Trendelenburg
g., two-point
g., unsteady
g., waddling
g. ▸ wide-based
gaiter brace

G

galacticolus, Saccharomyces
galactokinase deficiency
galactose
    g. in diet ▸ utilize
    g. phosphate uridyl transferase
    g. tolerance test
galactosemia
    g. diet
    g. ▸ lactose intolerance and
    g. ▸ testing of newborn for
galactosidase deficiency
Galassi reflex, Gifford-
galaxioides, Sisyrinchium
galea aponeurotica
galea, tendinous
Galeati's glands
Galeazzi's fracture of radius
Galeazzi's sign
Galen aneurysm ▸ vein of
galenic medicine
Galen's
    G. anastomosis
    G. foramen
    G. vein
    G. ventricle
gall, knee
gall sickness (gallsickness)
gallbladder (GB)
    g., ampulla of
    g. anastomosed to duodenum
    g. and liver scan
    g. bed
    g. bed, gallbladder shelled out from
    g., calcified
    g., calcified wall of
    g. calculus
    g. cancer
    g., chronically inflamed
    g. contraction
    g. disease
    g. disease, symptomatic
    g., emphysematous
    g. films (GB films)
    g. function
    g. function test
    g., functioning
    g., fundus of
    g., hydrops of
    g., inflamed
    g. ▸ inflammation of
    g. meridian
    g., nonfunctioning
    g., nonvisualization of
    g., notch of
    g., perforated

    g., poorly visualizing
    g., porcelain
    g., primary adenocarcinoma of
    g., sac-like
    g. (GB) series
    g. (GB) shadow
    g. shelled out from gallbladder bed
    g., sluggish
    g. surgery, laparoscopic
    g. ultrasound
    g. visualized
    g. wall
    g. with stones ▸ chronically
        inflamed
Galli-Mainini test
gallinacea, Echidnophaga
gallinae
    g., Ceratophyllus
    g., Dermanyssus avium et
    g., Trichomonas
    g., Trichophyton
gallinarum, Salmonella
gallinarum, Trichomonas
gallinatum, pectus
gallium (Ga)
    g., radioactive
    g. scan
    g. scanning
    g. -67 imaging
    g. -67 scan
    g. -67 scintigraphy
gallop
    g., atrial
    g., diastolic
    g., filling
    g., presystolic
    g., protodiastolic
    g. rhythm
    g. rhythm, systolic
    g. sound
    g. summation
    g., systolic
    g., ventricular
    g. (VDG), ventricular diastolic
galloping consumption
galloping paresis
gallstone(s)
    g. colic
    g. detection
    g. detection, ultrasound
    g. disease
    g., dissolve
    g. formation
    g. ileus
    g. imaging

    g., multiple
    g. ▸ pain in abdomen from
    g. ▸ palpable stones in
    g. pancreatitis
    g. ▸ pancreatitis secondary to
    g. ▸ prone to developing pigment
    g. removal
    g., silent
    g. surgery
    g., symptomatic
galop, bruit de
GALT (gut-associated lymphoid
    tissue) maturation
Galt's trephine
galvanic
    g. cautery
    g. contractility
    g. current
    g. faradization
    g. response
    g. skin reflex
    g. skin resistance
    g. skin response
    g. stimulation
galvanization, gastro◊
galvanocaustic amputation
galvanometer, pen
galvanotonic contractions
Galveston Orientation and Amnesia
    Test (GOAT)
GAM injection, Rho◊
GAM test, Rho◊
gambiense, Trypanosoma
Gamble syndrome, Darrow-
Gamblers Anonymous (GA)
gamblers, compulsive
gambling
    g. addiction
    g., compulsive
    g., excessive
    g., pathologic
    g., pathological
    g., video
gamekeeper's thumb fracture
gamete intrafallopian transfer (GIFT)
Gamgee tissue
gamma
    g. A globulin (IgA) deficiency
    g. A immunoglobulin (IgA)
        deficiency
    g. A immunoglobulin (IgA)
        determination
    g. aminobutyric acid (GABA)
    g. camera
    g. camera ▸ multicrystal

g. camera ▸ single-crystal
g. decay
g. fibers
g. fungus
g. globules
g. globulin
g. globulin, human
g. globulin injection
g. globulin M (IgM) deficiency
g. globulin, prophylactic
g. globulin, synthesize
g. glutamine peptidase (GGP)
g. -glutamyl transpeptidase
g. hydroxybutyrate
g. hydroxybutyrate (GHB) Liquid X
g. immunoglobulin D (IgD)
    determination
g. immunoglobulin E (IgE)
    determination
g. immunoglobulin G (IgG)
    determination
g. immunoglobulin M (IgM)
    deficiency
g. immunoglobulin M (IgM)
    determination
g. interferon
g. knife, neurosurgical
g. knife procedure
g. knife stereotactic radiosurgery
G. Med II
g. motoneurons
g. probe localization ▸ introperative
g. radiation
g. ray, capture
g. ray constant, specific
g. ray, detection of
g. ray spectra
g. ray spectrometer
g. ray surgery
g. ray therapy
g. rays
g. rhythm
g. roentgen
g. scintigraphy ▸ single-photon
g. scintillation camera
g. secretase
g. staphylolysin
g. streptococcus
g. unit, Leksell
g. well counter
gammaglobulinemia, hyper◊
gammopathy
g., IgA monoclonal
g., monoclonal
g., polyclonal

Gamna('s)
G. disease
G. -Gandy bodies
G. nodules
G. nodules, Gandy-
G. spleen, Gandy-
Gandhi strategy
Gandy bodies ▸ Gamna
gangles, stringy
ganglia
g., accessory
g., basal
g. calcification, basal
g., cardiac
g. cardiaca
g., celiac
g., cerebrospinal
g., diaphragmatic
g. ▸ histologic sections of basal
g., intermediate
g., lumbar
g. of sympathetic plexuses
g. of sympathetic trunk
g., pelvic
g., prevertebral
g., renal
g., sacral
g., sympathetic
g., thoracic
g., Wrisberg's
gangliated nerve
ganglioma, para◊
ganglion
g., auditory
g., Auerbach's
g., auricular
g., azygous
g., basal
g. block, stellate
g., Bock
g., carotid
g. cells
g. cells, giant
g., cephalic
g., cervicothoracic
g., cervicouterine
g., ciliary
g., Cloquet's
g., coccygeal
g., compound
g., Corti's
g. cyst
g., diffuse
g. disease, basal
g., dorsal root

g., false
g. ▸ fluid-filled
g., Ganser's
g., gasserian
g., geniculate
g., hepatic
g., hypogastric
g., hypoglossal
g., inferior carotid
g., inferior cervical
g., inferior jugular
g., inferior mesenteric
g., inferior petrosal
g., inferior vagal
g., infiltration
g., inhibitory
g., intercarotid
g., interpeduncular
g., lingual
g., Lobstein's
g., Loetwig's
g., Ludwig's
g., Luschka's
g., maxillary
g., Meckel's
g., Meissner's
g., middle cervical
g., nephrolumbar
g. nerve block ▸ stellate
g. nodosum
g. of cochlea ▸ spiral
g. of cochlear nerve ▸ spiral
g. of glossopharyngeal nerve ▸
    inferior
g. of glossopharyngeal nerve ▸
    jugular
g. of glossopharyngeal nerve ▸
    lower
g. of glossopharyngeal nerve ▸
    superior
g. of head ▸ posterior intervertebral
g. of Meckel, lesser
g. of uterus, cervical
g. of vagus nerve, inferior
g. of vagus nerve, jugular
g. of vagus nerve, lower
g. of vagus nerve, superior
g., olfactory
g., ophthalmic
g., optic
g., orbital
g., otic
g., periosteal
g., petrosal
g., petrous

ganglion—*continued*
- g., phrenic
- g., primary
- g., prostatic
- g., pterygopalatine
- g., Remak's
- g. retinae
- g., Ribes'
- g., Scarpa's
- g., Schmiedel's
- g., semilunar
- g., sensory
- g., simple
- g., sinoatrial
- g., sinus
- g., sphenomaxillary
- g., sphenopalatine
- g., spinal
- g., spiral
- g., splanchnic
- g., stellate
- g. stimulation, stellate
- g., submandibular
- g., submaxillary
- g., superior carotid
- g., superior cervical
- g., superior mesenteric
- g., superior vagal
- g., suprarenal
- g., synovial
- g., terminal
- g., trigeminal
- g., Troisier's
- g., tympanic
- g., upper
- g., ventricular
- g., vertebral
- g., vestibular
- g., Walther's
- g., Wrisberg's
- g., wrist

ganglionated chain

ganglionectomy
- g., cerebral nerve
- g., gasserian
- g., Meckel's
- g., sphenopalatine

ganglionic
- g. blocking agent
- g. center
- g. cyst
- g. cyst ▸ excision
- g. glioma
- g. saliva
- g. synapse, autonomic

gangraenescens, granuloma

gangraenosa, balanitis

gangrene
- g., angiosclerotic
- g., clostridial gas
- g., cold
- g., diabetic
- g., digital
- g., dry
- g., embolic
- g., emphysematous
- g. from atherosclerosis
- g. from diabetes
- g., gas
- g., hot
- g. in extremity
- g., incipient
- g. -like infection
- g., moist
- g. of bowel
- g. of lung
- g. of lung, diabetic
- g., Potts
- g., Raynaud's
- g. stomatitis
- g. tissue, necrotic
- g. wound, gas

gangrenosa
- g., angina
- g. infantum, dermatitis
- g., vaccinia
- g., varicella

gangrenosum, pyoderma

gangrenous
- g. appendicitis
- g. appendix
- g. balanitis
- g. emphysema
- g. pharyngitis
- g. pneumonia
- g. proctitis, epidemic
- g. rhinitis
- g. skin
- g. small bowel

Ganja (marijuana)

gannister disease

Ganong-Levine syndrome ▸ Long-

Ganong-Levine syndrome ▸ Lown-

Ganser's
- G. ganglion
- G. symptom
- G. syndrome

Gantry angle

Gant's operation

gap(s)
- g., air-bone
- g., anion
- g., auscultatory
- g. conduction phenomenon
- g. correction, air
- g. correction, isodose shift method for air
- g., exitable
- g., gender
- g. junction
- g. junction protein, cardiac
- g., low anion
- g., memory
- g. metabolic acidosis, anion
- g., silent

gaping, draining sores

gaping sores

garbled speech

Garcinia mangostana

Garcin's syndrome

Garden procedure

Gardner's
- G. chair
- G. operation
- G. syndrome

gargantuan mastitis

Gariel's pessary

Garland-White syndrome, Bland-

garlic ▸ medical benefits of

garlic therapy

garment
- g., antishock
- g. ▸ Jobst pressure
- g. ▸ pneumatic antishock

garnet (Nd:YAG) laser ▸ neo-dymium: yttrium-aluminum-

Garrés osteomyelitis

Garrison rongeur

GART (genotypic antiretroviral resistance testing)

gartnerian cyst

Gärtner('s)
- G. bacillus
- G. duct
- G. method
- G. tonometer
- G. vein phenomenon

gas(es)
- g., abdominal
- g., abnormal sac containing
- g. abnormality, arterial blood
- g. alterations, blood
- g. amplification
- g. analysis, arterial blood

g. analyzer
g. and feces
g. (ABG), arterial blood
g. artifact, bowel
g. at room air, capillary blood
g. barrier, blood
g., bloating and
g., bloating and abdominal
  tenderness
g., bloating and/or diarrhea ▸
  cramps
g., blood
g. ▸ burns to respiratory tract from
g. calibration factor (N_{gas}) ▸ cavity-
g. (CBG), capillary blood
g. cautery
g. chromatography
g. clearance
g. clearance measurement
g. clearance method
g., colorless
g. constant
g. (ABG) ▸ deteriorating arterial
  blood
g., deteriorating blood
g. distribution
g., effluent
g. embolism
g., excessive intestinal
g. exchange
g. exchange ▸ abnormalities in
g. exchange, impaired
g. exchange, pulmonary
g., feces and
g. flow, fresh
g. formation, excessive
g. -forming foods
g. from respiratory therapy devices
  ▸ effluent
g. gangrene
g. gangrene, clostridial
g. gangrene wound
g. (HPVG) ▸ hepatic portal venous
g. in stomach
g. insufflation, retroperitoneal
g., intestinal
g., intestinal tract
g., intraluminal
g. laser
g. laser ▸ (CO_2) carbon dioxide
g. laser ▸ excimer
g., laughing
g. level
g. -liquid chromatography
g. measurement, blood

g. mixture, anaerobic
g., nerve
g., overlying intestinal
g., oxygen and ether
g. pack
g. partition coefficient, blood
g., passing
g. pattern
g. pattern, bowel
g. pattern, intestinal
g. permeable (RGP) contact lenses
  ▸ rigid
g. permeable lens
g. poisoning ▸ nerve
g., poisonous
g. samplings, arterial
g. shadows, overlying
g. -solid chromatography
g. sterilization
g. sterilized instruments
g. sticks, blood
g. studies, blood
g., superimposed bowel
g., toxic
g. transfer
g. tube
g. values, Astrup blood
g. volume, intrathoracic
g. volume, thoracic
g. volume ▸ trapped

gaseous
g. cholecystitis
g. dilatation, gastric
g. distention
g. pericholecystitis
g. pulse

gasiness and cramping
gasless abdomen
gasp reflex
gasping
g., agonal
g. and cyanotic, patient
g. for air
g. for breath
g. respirations

gasserian ganglion
gasserian ganglionectomy
Gasser's syndrome
Gastaut syndrome
Gastaut syndrome, Lennox-
Gasterophilus genus
Gasteva seizure ▸ Laennec's
gastralgia, appendicular
gastrectomy
g., bilateral

g., esophago◊
g., Hofmeister type
g., partial
g., subtotal
g. total

gastric
g. acid
g. acid inhibitor
g. acid secretion
g. acidity
g. adenocarcinoma, distal
g. air bubble
g. anacidity
g. analysis
g. antrum
g. antrum ▸ retained
g. artery
g. aspirant ▸ vomitus or
g. aspirate
g. aspiration
g. aspiration ▸ preoperative
g. atony
g. atrophy
g. band operation
g. band procedure
g. bleeding
g. bubble
g. bypass
g. bypass operation
g. bypass procedure
g. bypass ▸ substernal
g. bypass surgery
g. cancer
g. carcinoma
g. carcinoma, inoperable
g. cardia
g. chromoscopy
g. component of reflex barrier
g. contents
g. contents, aspiration of
g. contents, reflux of
g. contents ▸ terminal aspiration of
g. culture
g. cycle
g. cytology
g. decompression
g. dilatation
g. dilatation, acute
g. disorder
g. distention
g. distress
g. diverticula
g. dyspepsia
g. emptying
g. emptying, early

gastric—*continued*
- g. emptying half-time
- g. emptying of solids
- g. emptying time
- g. erosion
- g. fistula
- g. fluid
- g. folds
- g. freezing
- g. function, alter
- g. fundus
- g. gaseous dilatation
- g. glands
- g. hypersecretion
- g. indigestion
- g. insufficiency
- g. irritation
- g. juice
- g. juice, secretes
- g. lavage
- g. lung
- g. lymph nodes ▸ left
- g. lymph nodes ▸ right
- g. lymphoma
- g. mucosa (GM)
- g. mucosal atrophy
- g. mucosal erosions
- g. mucosal hemorrhages
- g. nerves
- g. neurectomy
- g. notch
- g. outlet
- g. outlet, deformity of
- g. outlet irritability
- g. outlet, narrowing of
- g. outlet obstruction
- g. pacemaker
- g. parietography
- g. pars media
- g. pits
- g. pressure
- g. pylorus
- g. resection
- g. resection, Balfour
- g. rugal folds
- g. rugal prominence
- g. sclerosis
- g. secretion, basal
- g. secretion ▸ caustic
- g. secretion, control
- g. secretory testing
- g. -stapling procedure
- g. stimulator ▸ implantable
- g. stoma
- g. suction

- g. torsion
- g. tract disorder
- g. tumor
- g. ulcer (GU)
- g. ulcer, benign
- g. ulcer, chronic
- g. ulcer, superficial
- g. varices
- g. vein, left
- g. vein, right
- g. vein, short
- g. volvulus
- g. washings

gastrica
- g., adenasthenia
- g., adenohypersthenia
- g. haemorrhagica, achylia
- g., myasthenia
- g., zymosis

gastricus nervosus, singultus
gastricus, status
gastrin, synthetic human
gastritis
- g., acute
- g., alcoholic
- g., antral
- g., aspirin
- g., atrophic
- g., catarrhal
- g., chemical
- g., chronic
- g., chronic active
- g., chronic atrophic
- g., chronic cystic
- g., cirrhotic
- g., erosive
- g., exfoliative
- g., follicular
- g. from alcohol
- g. from aspirin
- g., giant hypertrophic
- g. granulomatosa fibroplastica
- g., hemorrhagic
- g., hyperpeptic
- g., hypertrophic
- g., interstitial
- g. ▸ loss of appetite from
- g., mycotic
- g. ▸ pain in abdomen from
- g., phlegmonous
- g., polypous
- g., pseudomembranous
- g., purulent
- g., radiation
- g., superficial

- g., suppurating
- g. ▸ tenderness in abdomen from
- g., toxic
- g. with ulceration ▸ erosive

gastroanastomosis, esophago◊
gastrocardiac syndrome
gastrocnemius
- g. muscle
- g. muscle, lateral
- g. muscle, medial
- g. reflex

gastrocolic omentum
gastrocolic reflex
gastrocystostomy, patient had
gastrocystostomy, pseudocyst
Gastrodiscoides hominis
Gastrodiscoides, Trematoda
gastroduodenal
- g. artery
- g. contents, intra-abdominal escape of
- g. mucosa
- g. ulcer, acute

gastroenteritis
- g., acute
- g., acute infantile
- g., acute infectious
- g., bloating from
- g., Campylobacter
- g., dehydration from
- g., diarrhea from
- g., dysenteric
- g., eosinophilic
- g. from alcohol
- g. from anxiety
- g., infantile
- g. of swine (TGS) ▸ transmissible
- g. paratyphosa B
- g., rotavirus
- g. treatment
- g. typhosa
- g., viral

gastroenterogenous cyst
gastroenterostomy
- g., Balfour's
- g., Hofmeister's
- g. I, Billroth's
- g. stoma
- g. II, Billroth's

gastroepiploic
- g. artery
- g. lymph nodes
- g. vein, left
- g. vein, right
- g. vessels

gastroesophageal
g. angle
g. disorder
g. hernia
g. incompetence
g. junction
g. reflux
g. reflux disease (GERD)
g. -related chest pain
g. sphincter
gastrogenic diarrhea
Gastrografin contrast medium
gastrogram, electro◊
gastrography, electro◊
gastrography study, electro◊
gastrohepatic ligament
gastrohepatic omentum
gastroileal reflex
gastrointestinal (GI)
g. anomaly ▸ fetal
g. anthrax
g. biofeedback
g. biopsy
g. bleed
g. bleed, massive upper
g. bleeding
g. blood loss test
g. cancer
g. complications of drug abuse
g. decontamination
g. derangement
g. diet, liberal
g. disease
g. disorder
g. disorder, chronic
g. disorder ▸ drug-induced
g. (GI) disorder ▸ functional
g. distress
g. disturbances
g. emergency
g. endoscopy
g. (GI) endoscopy ▸ upper
g. evaluation
g. film
g. flora
g. hemorrhage
g. hemorrhage, acute
g. hemorrhage ▸ massive
g. hypermotility
g. infection
g. infection, nosocomial
g. intubation
g. irritation
g. irritation and ulceration
g. lesion

g. lesion ▸ chronic blood loss of
g. lesion, coagulation of bleeding
g. malignancy
g. motility ▸ postoperative
g. organisms ▸ aspiration of
g. perforation
g. polyposis, familial
g. problems related to drug abuse
g. procedure, lower
g. protein loss test
g. reaction, psychogenic
g. reaction, psychophysiological
g. series
g. series, upper
g. spasm
g. stromal tumor (GIST)
g. symptom
g. symptomatology
g. system
g. therapeutic system
g. toxicity
g. tract
g. tract adenocarcinoma
g. tract carcinoma
g. tract tissue repair
g. ulcer
g. ulcers, bleeding
g. (UGI) ▸ upper
g. viral infection
g. workup
gastrointestinalis, pseudoleu-
kemia
gastrojejunal anastomosis
gastrojejunal constipation
gastrojejunocolic fistula
gastrojejunostomy
g., palliative
g., patent
g., posterior
g., Roux-en-Y
gastromotor insufficiency
gastromyotomy, esophago◊
gastronomical distress
gastropancreatic folds
gastropancreatic reflex
gastroparesis, diabetic
gastroplasty
g., esophago◊
g., Mason vertical banded
g., vertical banded
gastrorrhea continua chronica
gastroschisis, fetal
gastroscope, fiberoptic
gastrosia fungosa
gastrosplenic omentum

gastrostomy
g., Billroth I
g., Billroth II
g., cholangio◊
g., cholecysto◊
g., choledocho◊
g., Depage-Janeway
g., esophago◊
g., feeding
g., gastro◊
g. (PEG) ▸ percutaneous endoscopic
g., Ssabanejew-Frank
g., Stamm's
gastrosuccorrhea, digestive
gastrosuccorrhea mucosa
gastroxynsis fungosa
Gatch bed
gate(s)
g., acquisition
g., M
G. (morning glory seeds) ▸ Pearly
gated
g. acquisition (MUGA) electrogram
   ▸ stress, multiple
g. acquisition (MUGA) ▸ multiple
g. angiography (MUGA) scan ▸
   multiple-
g. blood pool angiography
g. blood pool imaging
g. blood pool scanning
g. blood pool scintigraphy
g. blood pool study
g. blood pool study ▸ equilibrium-
g. cardiac scan
g. computed tomography
g. equilibrium image ▸ supine rest
g. list mode
g. nuclear angiogram
g. nuclear angiography ▸ rest and
   exercise
g. radionuclide angiocardiography
g. radionuclide angiography
g. sweep magnetic resonance
   imaging
g. system
g. techique
Gatellier's operation
gating
g., cardiac
g., electrocardiographic (ECG)
g. ▸ in-memory
g. mechanism
g. ▸ R wave
g. signal

Gaucher's
 G. cell
 G. disease
 G. splenomegaly
gauge(s)
 g., autoclave
 g., catheter
 g., Magna-Helic
 g. plethysmography, strain
 g., pressure
 g., Statham strain
 g., strain
Gaule's spots
Gault's cochleopalpebral reflex
Gault's test
gauntlet flap
gauntlet graft
Gauss' sign
gaussian distribution
Gauthier bicycle ergometer
Gauthier syndrome, de Morsier-
Gauvain's fluid
gauze [*pause*]
 g., absorbent
 g., Adaptic
 g., Aquaflo
 g., Aureomycin
 g. bandage
 g., cellulose
 g., cotton
 g. dressing
 g. dressing, Kling
 g. dressing ▸ Nu-
 g., fine-mesh
 g., Furacin
 g., Gelfoam
 g. implant placement ▸ Surgicel
 g., impregnated
 g., iodoform
 g., Kling elastic
 g. packing, cotton
 g. pad, felt
 g., rayon
 g. roll, Kerlix
 g., strip of
 g., surgical
 g., Surgicel
 g., uterus packed with
 g., Vaseline
 g. wick
 g., Xeroform
gavage [*lavage*]
 g. feeding
 g., gastro◊
 g., gastrosto◊

 g., nasal
 g. tube
Gavard's muscle
gay
 g. bashing
 g. bowel syndrome
 g. disease
 g. immunocompromise syndrome
 g. -related immune deficiency
 (GRID)
Gayet's operation
Gaylor punch
Gaynor-Hart position
gaze [*phase*]
 g. board ▸ eye
 g., conjugate
 g., disconjugate
 g., dysconjugate
 g. palsy
 g. palsy ▸ vertical
 g., paralysis of upward
 g. ▸ slight nystagmus on upward
 g. to right ▸ moderate nystagmus
 on
 g., upward
GB (gallbladder)
 GB films
 GB series
 GB shadow
GC
 GC (gas chromatography)
 GC (gastrointestinal catastrophe)
 GC (glucocorticoid)
 GC (gonococcus)
G-cal (gram-calorie)
GCM (geriatric care manager)
g-cm (gram-centimeter)
GDM (gestational diabetes mellitus)
GDS (Gradual Dosage Schedule)
GE (General Electric) pacemaker
Gehrig disease, Lou
Gehrung pessary
Geigel's reflex
Geiger counter
Geiger Müller counter
Geist operation, Henry-
gel
 g., aluminum hydroxide
 g. barrier
 g. ▸ Betadine douche and
 g. breast implant, silicone
 g. cushioning, air or
 g., electrode
 g. electrophoresis
 g. electrophoresis ▸ gradient

 g. electrophoresis ▸ pulsed-field
 g. -filled breast implant ▸ silicone
 g. -filled implant
 g. -filled implants, silicone
 g., flexible plastic
 g. implant, silicone
 g. ▸ leakage or seepage of
 g., leaking silicone
 g. patch
 g. test, formol-
 g., vaginal
 g., viscous, silicone
 g., vitreous
gelastic epilepsy
gelatiginous tissue
gelatin
 g. capsule
 g. compression boot
 g. disc
 g. sponge
 g. sponge, absorbable
 g. sugar
 g., Wharton's
 g., zinc
gelatiniform carcinoma
gelatinous
 g. acute pneumonia
 g. ascites
 g. carcinoma
 g. marrow
 g. material
 g. silicone
 g. substance
 g. substance of gray substance
 g. substance of spinal cord
 g. substance, Rolando's
 g. tissue
geleophysic dwarf
gel-filled implant
Gelfoam
 G. cookie
 G. dressing
 G. gauze
 G. pack
 G. packing
 G. powder
 G. sponge
 G. strips
 G. ▸ thrombin-soaked
 G., Topical
Gelidium cartilagineum
Gélineau's syndrome
Gellé's test
Gellhorn pessary, Emmert-
gémellaire, folie

gemellary pregnancy
gemellus muscle, inferior
gemellus muscle, superior
geminata, Solenopsis
geminate teeth
gemistocytic astrocytoma
gender
    g. assignment
    g., biological
    g., female
    g. gap
    g. identity disorder
    g. identity disorder of adolescence
    g. identity disorder of adolescence
       or adulthood, nontranssexual
       type
    g. identity disorder of adult life
    g. identity disorder of childhood
    g., male
    g., psychological
    g. selection, baby
    g. -specific treatment programs
gene(s)
    g., abnormal
    g. ▸ abnormal cholesterol related
    g., alcoholism
    g. alterations, inherited
    g., altered
    g. -altered cells ▸ TNF (tumor
       necrosis factor)
    g. amplification
    g., angiotensinogen
    g., anti-aging
    g., anticancer
    g., antiviral
    g., bacterial
    g. bank
    g. -based disease
    g., behavioral
    g., beta myosin heavy chain
    g. bomb
    g., breast cancer
    g., cancer
    g., cancer-causing
    g. carrier
    g., cell growth
    g., chromosomal
    g. cloning
    g. ▸ colon cancer
    g. copying
    g., cystic fibrosis
    g. defect
    g., defective
    g., defective recessive
    g. deletion

g., disease-causing
g. disease ▸ single-
g., diseased
g. disorder ▸ single-
g., dominant
g., drug-resistant
g., estrogen receptor
g. expression
g. expression, cardiac
g., faulty
g., format
g. frequency
g. function
g., gag
g., hemochromatosis
g. ▸ human preproendothelin-1
g., Huntington's
g., identical
g., identification
g., individual
g. inheritance, single-
g., insulin
g. malfunction
g. mapping
g., medical
g. microbe
g., mitochondrial
g., multiple
g., mutant chromosomal
g., mutant mitochondrial
g., mutated
g. mutation
g., nonmutated
g., normal
g., nucleotide sequence of
g., obesity
g., predisposing
g. problem, defective
g. profile
g. regulation of cardiovascular
    development
g., reproductive
g., RTF (Resistance Transfer
    Factor)
g. screening ▸ colon cancer
g., sequencing
g. ▸ sickle cell
g., silent
g. ▸ single causative
g. splicing
g. ▸ superoxide dimutase
g., suppress abnormal
g., suppressor
g., susceptibility
g., thalassemia

g. therapy
g. therapy, abnormal
g. therapy ▸ cardiac
g. therapy, coronary
g. therapy contamination
g. therapy ▸ development of
g. therapy for heart
g. therapy injection
g. therapy procedure
g. therapy program ▸ coronary
g. therapy research
g. therapy technique
g. therapy trials
g. transcription
g. transfer
g. transfer, adenovirus mediated
g. transfer ▸ ex vivo
g. transfer ▸ in vivo
g. transfer transcription assay
g. transfer ▸ vascular
g. transplants
g., tumor suppression
g., tumor suppressor
g. variant
g., viral
**Genentech biosynthetic human
  growth hormone**
genera, bacterial
general (General)
    g. aches and pains
    g. achiness
    g. adaptation syndrome
    g. alcohol cleansing
    g. anatomy
    g. anesthesia
    g. anesthesia, endotracheal
    g. anesthesia, satisfactory
    g. anesthetic
    g. anesthetic drug
    g. anxiety
    g. anxiety disorder
    g. body pain
    g. care
    g. cataract
    G. Classification Test (AGCT) ▸
      Army
    g. clinical service
    g. cognitive impairment ▸ normal
    g. deterioration of brain function
    g. diet
    g. disability
    g. discoloration
    g. disease
    G. Electric (GE) pacemaker
    g. fatigue

general—continued

g. gonadotropic activity
g. grief education
g. health
g. health problem
g. hepatic circulation
g. inhalational anesthesia
g. joint pain
g. malaise
g. medical
g. medical and surgical
g. medicine
g. mental health
g. metastatic disease
g. muscle pain
g. muscle weakness
g. nursing assistance (GNA)
g. nursing care (GNC)
g. nursing supervision
g. paralysis
g. paresis
g. paroxysm, involuntary
g. patient population, prevalence of drug abuse in
g. peritoneal cavity
g. population
g. posture
g. practice
g. practitioner
g. practitioner care ▸ routine
g. pseudoparalysis, arthritic
g. purpose lens
g. reconstructive surgery
g. relaxation training technique
g. sensation
g. slowing of movements
g. stimulant
g. supportive measures
g. surgery
g. tonic
g. well-being
g. well-being index

generalisata ossium, xanthomatosis
generalisata, osteitis condensans
generalisatus, herpes
generalized

g. abdominal pain
g. aches and pains
g. aching
g. activity
g. anxiety
g. anxiety, comorbid
g. arteriosclerosis
g. arthritis
g. atrophy ▸ moderately prominent

g. atrophy of brain
g. bisynchronous delta activity
g. blood infection
g. body radiation
g. body weakness
g. candidiasis
g. coldness
g., debilitating, longstanding fatigue
g. degenerative tic
g. disc bulging
g. distribution, pains of
g. dystonia
g. emphysema
g. epilepsy
g. exceedingly slow activity
g. fast activity
g. fatigue
g. fatigue, prolonged
g. feeling of malaise
g. flexion epilepsy
g. grand mal seizures ▸ uncontrolled
g. headache
g. infection involving fungus
g. irradiation of body
g. itching
g. low voltage
g. lymph node swelling
g. lymphadenopathy
g. macrodontia
g. malignancy
g. metastasis
g. muscle ache
g. muscle weakness
g. neurologic dysfunction
g. osteoarthritis
g. osteoporosis
g. pain
g. peritonitis
g. personality deterioration
g. plane xanthoma
g. pruritus
g. reduced voltage
g. seizure
g. seizure disorder ▸ primary
g. seizure ▸ secondary
g. Shwartzman's reaction
g. slightly slow activity
g. slow activity
g. spikes
g. tenderness
g. tonic clonic seizures ▸ uncontrolled
g. transduction
g. weakness

g. weakness and fatigue
g. weakness, unexplained
g. xanthelasma

generate force
generated

g. artifact, computer-
g. images, computer-
g. neutrophils recruitment ▸ host

generating thesis ▸ stress-
generation

g., affect self-
g., crack
g., first filial
g. of breast, heat
g., sandwich
g., second filial
g. test, Hicks-Pitney thromboplastin
g., thrombin
g. time
g. time, thromboplastin

generational problems, cross-
generator(s)

g., asynchronous pulse
g., atrial synchronous pulse
g., atrial triggered pulse
g., Aurora pulse
g., cardiac
g., change of cardiac
G. Chardack-Greatbatch Implantable Cardiac Pulse
g., defective
g., demand pulse
g. ▸ elective replacement pulse
g., electrostatic
g. ▸ fixed-rate pulse
g., medical pion
g. ▸ Medtronic pulse
g. ▸ Microlith pacemaker pulse
g. ▸ Minilith pacemaker pulse
g. ▸ NeuroCybernetic Prosthesis (NCP)
g. pocket erosion ▸ pulse
g. pocket infection ▸ pulse
g., polyphase
g. pouch ▸ Parsonnet pulse
g. ▸ Programalith III pulse
g., pulse
g., replacement of
g., resonance
g., slow-wave
g. ▸ standby pulse
g., supervoltage
g., Tc (technetium) 99m
g., three-phase
g., unipolar pacemaker

g., Van de Graaff
g. ▸ ventricular inhibited pulse
g. ▸ ventricular synchronous pulse
g. ▸ x-ray
generic
g. drug
g. drug industry
g. equivalent
g. name
g. screening criteria, medical
generosity of time
generous in size, liver
genes, defective
genes, recessive
genesial cycle
genetic(s)
g. abnormality
g. abnormality ▸ inherited
g. activity
g. alcoholism
g. alterations
g. analysis
g. analysis ▸ molecular
g. and physiological factors
g. approach
g. aspects of alcoholism
g. aspects of criminality
g., bacterial
g. basis
g., behavioral
g., biochemical
g. birth defect
g. bone disease
g., cancer
g. characteristics
g., clinical
g. code
g. code ▸ human
g. component
g. component to alcoholism
g. condition
g. conjugation
g. connective tissue disorder
g. continuity
g. control
g. counseling
g. counselor
g. damage
g. death
g. defect
g. defect, inherited
g. defect ▸ sex-linked
g. defect ▸ X-linked
g. determinants
g. digestive disorder

g. disease
g. disorder
g. disorder, degenerative
g. disorder, disabling
g. disorder, fetal
g. disorder, human
g. disorder ▸ terminal
g. effects
g. element
g. endowment
g. engineering
g. engineering techniques
g. error
g. factor
g. factors in drug abuse
g. fingerprint
g. heritage
g. heterogeneity
g., human
g. ▸ human molecular
g. hypertrophic cardiomyopathy
g. illness, fatal
g. illness ▸ terminal
g. immunity
g. impairment
g. imprinting
g. induction
g. influence
g. information
g. inheritance
g. intervention
g. level
g. link
g. linkage map
g. locus
g. makeup
g. manipulation
g. map
g. mapping
g. markers
g. match
g. material
g. material, human
g. material ▸ microinjection of
g., medical
g. medicine
g. message
g. metabolic abnormality
g., mitochondrial
g., molecular
g. mother and father
g. mutation
g. neurological disease
g. of drug resistance
g. origin

g. pattern
g. predisposition
g. predisposition testing
g. predisposition to alcohol
g. predisposition to psychiatric
   illness
g. process
g. profile
g. prognosis
g. psychology
g. relationship
g. repertoire ▸ identical
g. replication
g., reproductive
g. research
g. research center
g. revascularization
g. risk
g. risk factor
g. risk, high
g. screening study
g. sequence
g. strand
g. structures
g. studies, behavioral
g. study
g. susceptibility
g. technology
g. tendency
g. termination
g. testing
g. testing ▸ preembryotic
g. therapy
g. trait
g. transduction
g. transformation
g. transmission
g. transmission of risk factors
g. transplant
g. treatment
g. underlying lipid abnormality
g. variations, bacterial
g. vulnerability
genetically
g. altered cells
g. altered tumor cells
g. altered tumor infiltrating
   lymphocytes (TIL)
g. at risk
g. determined, disease
g. engineered cells
g. engineered erythropoietin
g. engineered proteins
g. engineered vaccine
g. engineered virus

genetically—*continued*
- g. heterogeneous
- g. manipulated cells
- g. matched marrow
- g. predisposed
- g. programmed yeast
- g. prone to diabetes
- g. significant dose (GSD)
- g. unrelated donor
- g. vulnerable

geneticist, medical
genetotrophic disease
genetous idiocy
Gengou, Bordet-
genial apophysis
genic balance
genicular artery
genicular veins
geniculata, Trypanosoma
geniculate
- g. bodies
- g. body, lateral
- g. body, medial
- g. ganglion
- g. neuralgia

geniculatus, Panstrongylus
geniculi, gyrus
geniculocalcarine tract
genioglossus muscle
geniohyoid muscle
geniohyoideus muscle
genital
- g. anomaly
- g. area
- g. cancer
- g. candidiasis
- g. center
- g. dermatoses
- g. fold
- g. herpes
- g. herpes infection
- g. herpes ▸ recurrent
- g. herpes virus
- g. mycoplasma
- g. neoplasia
- g. pain in males ▸ chills with
- g. papillomavirus infection
- g. reflex
- g. secretion
- g. sores
- g. sores, open
- g. stage
- g. stimulant
- g. swelling
- g. teratoma

- g. tract
- g. tract, female
- g. tract lesions
- g. ulcer
- g. warts

genitalia
- g., external
- g., indifferent
- g., infantile female
- g., infantile male
- g., normal female
- g., normal female adult
- g., normal male
- g., normal male adult
- g., premature male
- g., swelling of

genitalis, herpes
genitalis, Treponema
genitofemoral nerve
genitospinal center
genitourinary (GU)
- g. anomaly
- g. cancer
- g. complications of drug abuse
- g. (GU) infection, Chlamydia
- g. malfunction, psychogenic
- g. problems related to drug abuse
- g. region
- g. system
- g. tract

genius
- g. epidemicus
- g. loci
- g. morbi

genome
- g., bacterial
- g., human
- g. ▸ mapping and sequencing the
- g., mitochondrial
- g., plant
- g., viral

genomics research
genotypic antiretroviral resistance testing (GART)
Gensini index
gentian
- g. violet
- g. violet, aniline
- g. violet, area painted with
- g. violet, area swabbed with
- g. violet treatment

gentle
- g. active flexion
- g. active mobilization
- g. exercise

- g. physiotherapy
- g. pressure bandage applied
- g. range of motion exercises
- g. resistance training
- g. resistance ▸ water provides
- g. rocking motion
- g. stimulation
- g. stretching exercises
- g. traction

gently brought into view
genu
- g. corporis callosi
- g. impressum
- g. nervi facialis
- g. recurvatum
- g. valgum
- g. varum

Genupak tampon
genus
- g., Diplococcus
- g., Dirofilaria
- g., Gasterophilus
- g., Gnathostoma
- g., Shigella
- g., Spirillum
- g., Spirochaeta
- g., Staphylococcus
- g., Streptococcus
- g., Streptothrix
- g., Trichomonas

geodesic sensor net
geographic landmarks
geographic tongue
geographica, lingua
geometric
- g. cube formula
- g. efficiency
- g. knee prosthesis
- g. mean (GM)
- g. mean titer (GMT)

geometry
- g. factor
- g., normal
- g. of stenosis
- g., ventricular

Georgariou's operation
George
- G. Lewis technique
- G. position, Leonard-
- G. Washington strut
- G. Winter elevation torque technique

Geotrichum candidum
Geraghty's test, Rowntree and
Gerbode defect

GERD (gastroesophageal reflux disease)
Gerdy's
  G. fontanelle
  G. interauricular loop
  G. tubercle in knee
gergoviae, Enterobacter
Gerhardt's change of sound
Gerhardt's test
geriatric
  g. acute care
  g. alcoholism
  g. assessment, comprehensive
  g. care
  g. care manager (GCM)
  g. chair pad
  g. clinic
  G. Depression Scale
  g. evaluation
  g. medicine
  g. patient
  g. psychiatry
  g. service
Gerlach's tonsil
Gerlier's disease
germ(s)
  g. agglutinin ▸ wheat
  g., airborne
  g. -cell determinant
  g. cell mediastinal tumor, malignant
  g. cell tumor
  g. cells
  g. cells, primordial
  g., dental
  g., enamel
  g. -free
  g. -free environment
  g. -free flexible plastic bubble
  g. -free isolation units
  g., hair
  g. ▸ initial exposure to
  g. -laden air
  g. obsession
  g. plasm
  g. warfare
  g., wheat
German measles
germicides, quaternary
germinal
  g. aplasia
  g. cell
  g. centers
  g. centers, follicular
  g. centers ▸ hyalinized burned out
  g. disc

g. infection
g. layer
g. layer of bronchial epithelium
g. plate hemorrhages ▸ subependymal
g. rod
g. streak
germinative layer of epidermis
germine diacetate
germline band
germline mutations
geroderma osteodysplastica
geromorphism, cutaneous
gerontology, clinical
Gerontology Service
Gerota's capsule
Gerota's fascia
Gerson diet ▸ Sauerbruch-Herr-mannsdorfer
Gerson-Herrmannsdorfer diet
gerstaeckeri, Trypansoma
Gerstmann's syndrome
gestalt
  g. designs
  g. psychology
  g. test, Bender
  g. theory
gestation
  g., ectopic
  g., exterior
  g., fetal
  g., interior
  g., intrauterine
  g., near-term
  g., pulmonary
  g., twin
gestational
  g. age
  g. age (AGA), appropriate for
  g. age assessment
  g. age (AGA) female neonate, term appropriate for
  g. age (LGA), large for
  g. age (AGA) male neonate, term appropriate for
  g. age neonate ▸ large for
  g. age neonate ▸ small for
  g. age (SGA), small for
  g. diabetes
  g. diabetes mellitus (GDM)
  g. diabetic
  g. months
  g. mother
  g. period
  g. psychosis

g. sac, intrauterine
g. size
g. trophoblastic disease
g. weeks
gestationis, herpes
gesticulatory tic
gestures
  g. ▸ exhibits dramatic
  g. ▸ makes obscene
  g. ▸ patient displays obscene
  g., suicidal
GET (gastric emptying time)
GET½ (gastric emptying half-time)
getting behavior, attention-
GFR (glomerular filtration rate)
gft (graft)
GGP (gamma glutamine peptidase)
GHB (gamma hydroxybutyrate) Liquid X
ghinda, Vibrio
Ghon('s)
  G. complex
  G. focus
  G. lesion
  G. primary lesion
  G. -Sachs bacillus
  G. tubercle
Ghormley's operation
ghost
  g. cell
  g. vessel
  g. vessel in cornea
ghoul hand
GI (gastrointestinal)
  GI biofeedback
  GI biopsy
  GI bleed, massive upper
  GI bleed with anemia
  GI bleeding
  GI blood loss test
  GI cancer
  GI complications of drug abuse
  GI decontamination
  GI derangement
  GI disease
  GI disorder ▸ functional
  GI distress
  GI disturbances
  GI endoscopy ▸ upper
  GI evaluation
  GI film
  GI hemorrhage
  GI hemorrhage, acute
  GI hemorrhage ▸ massive
  GI infection, nosocomial

GI—*continued*
- GI intubation
- GI irritation
- GI lesions
- GI malignancy
- GI perforation
- GI problems related to drug abuse
- GI procedure, lower
- GI protein loss test
- GI reaction, psychogenic
- GI reaction, psychophysiological
- GI series
- GI series, upper
- GI spasm
- GI symptomatology
- GI system
- GI tract
- GI tract ▸ normal functioning of
- GI ulcer
- GI ulcers, bleeding
- GI upper

Gianotti-Crosti syndrome

giant
- g. a wave
- g. aneurysm
- g. cell
- g. cell aortitis
- g. cell arteries
- g. cell arteritis
- g. cell astrocytoma
- g. cell astrocytoma ▸ subependymal
- g. cell carcinoma
- g. cell, foreign body (FB)
- g. cell hepatitis
- g. cell hepatitis, neonatal
- g. cell, Langhans'
- g. cell ▸ multinucleated
- g. cell myeloma
- g. cell myocarditis
- g. cell pneumonia
- g. cell pneumonitis ▸ marked
- g. cell reaction
- g. cell reparative granuloma
- g. cell reparative granuloma ▸ central
- g. cell reparative granuloma ▸ peripheral
- g. cell thyroiditis
- g. cell, Touton
- g. cell tumor
- g. cell tumor ▸ familial bilateral
- g. cell ▸ histiocyte
- g. fibroadenoma of breast

- g. finger
- g. follicular hyperplasia
- g. follicular lymphadenopathy
- g. follicular lymphoblastoma
- g. follicular thyroiditis
- g. ganglion cells
- g. hives
- g. hypertrophic gastritis
- g. papillary conjunctivitis (GPC)
- g. plasma cells ▸ bizarre
- g. swelling
- g. urticaria
- g. v wave
- g. vertebral artery aneurysm ▸ thrombosed
- g. vulvar condylomata

Gianturco method, Camp-
Giardia lamblia
Giardia parasite diarrhea
giardiasis, intestinalis
gibberish aphasia
Gibbon('s)
- G. hernia
- G. hydrocele
- G. -Landis test

gibbus deformity
Gibney's bandage
Gibney's perispondylitis
Gibson('s)
- G. approach
- G. bandage
- G. circularity index
- G. murmur
- G. operation
- G. operation, Potts-Smith-
- G. rule
- G. vestibule

gibsoni, Babesia
gibsoni, Nuttallia
gibsoni, Onchocerca
giddy laughter
giddy, patient feels
Giemsa('s)
- G. stain
- G. stain, Jenner-
- G. stain, May-Grunwald-

Gierke's disease, von
Gies' joint, von
Gieson stain, van
Gifford('s)
- G. -Galassie reflex
- G. operation
- G. operation, Machek-
- G. reflex
- C. sign

gift(s) (GIFT) (Gift)
- G. (gamete intrafallopian transfer)
- G. Act, Uniform Anatomical
- g., anatomical
- g. and creativity ▸ strengths,
- g. card, uniform anatomical
- G. of Life
- g. statement, anatomical

gifted child, specially
gifted children
giganteum, Trichosporon
giganteus, Aspergillus
gigantica, Fasciola
gigantism
- g., acromegalic
- g., cerebral
- g., eunuchoid
- g., fetal
- g., hyperpituitary
- g., normal
- g., pituitary

gigantocellulare, carcinoma
gigas, Echinorhynchus
Gigli's operation
Gilbert('s)
- G. cholemia
- G. disease
- G. -Dreyfus' syndrome
- G. -Lereboullet syndrome
- G. syndrome

gilchristi, Cryptococcus
Gilchrist's disease
Gilchrist's mycosis
Gilford syndrome, Hutchinson-
gill slit
Gilles
- G. de la Tourette's disease
- G. de la Tourette's disorder
- G. de la Tourette's syndrome
- G. elevation

Gillespie's operation
Gilliam('s)
- G. -Doleris' operation
- G. operation
- G. suspension, Abell-
- G. suspension of uterus

Gillies'
- G. approach
- G. flap
- G. graft
- G. operation
- G. up-and-down flap

Gill's operation
gin and tonic purpura

gingiva
g., alveolar
g., areolar
g., attached
g., buccal
g., cemented
g., free
g., interdental
g., labial
g., lingual
g., marginal
g., septal
g., squamous cell carcinoma
g., treatment of
gingivae, fibromatosis
gingival
g. and oral mucosa pigmentation
g. cartilage
g. crevice
g. enlargement
g. groove ▸ free
g. hyperplasia
g. lancet
g. line
g. margin
g. pocket
g. sulci
g. sulcus
g. surface of tooth
g. trough
g. wall
gingivalis
g., Bacteroides
g., Entamoeba
g., porphyromonas
gingivarum, stomatorrhagia
gingivectomies, electrosurgical
gingivectomy/gingivoectomy
gingivectomy, Ochsenbein's
gingivitis
g., bismuth
g., catarrhal
g., cotton-roll
g., desquamative
g., dystrophic
g., eruptive
g., fusospirochetal
g. gravidarum
g., hemorrhagic
g., herpetic
g., hormonal
g., hyperplastic
g., marginal
g., necrotizing ulcerative
g., phagedenic

g., scorbutic
g., senile atrophic
g., simple marginal
g., streptococcal
g., suppurative marginal
g., ulceromembranous
g., Vincent's
gingivolabial sulci
gingivostomatitis
g., herpes simplex
g., herpetic
g., necrotizing ulcerative
Giordano-Giovannetti diet
Giordano's operation
Giraldés, organ of
Girard's operation
Giraud-Teulon law
girdle(s)
g., hip
g. muscular dystrophy ▸ limb-
g. pain
g., pectoral
g. pelvic
g. sensation
g., shoulder
Girdlestone
G. arthroplasty
G. joint resection
G. operation
G. -Taylor procedure
Girout's method
girth, abdominal
girth, increased abdominal
GIST (gastrointestinal stromal tumor)
gitter [*glitter*]
Giuffrida-Ruggieri stigma
given
g. dose
g. dose ▸ dose calculated as
g. enema prior to examination ▸ patient
g. enema prior to surgery ▸ patient
g. enema prior to x-ray ▸ patient
giver
g., care-
g., designated care-
g., in-home care-
g., primary care-
giving up response
GLA (gingivolinguoaxial)
glabelloalveolar line
glabrata
g., Candida
g. pneumonia, Torulopsis
g., Torulopsis

gladiatorum, herpes
gladiolus bone
gladius, Xiphias
gland(s) [*glans*]
g. activity, thyroid
g. adenocarcinoma of lacrimal
g. adenoma, sebaceous
g. adenoma, sweat
g., adrenal
g., Albarran's
g., anterior lobe of pituitary
g., anterior lobule of pituitary
g., anterior pituitary
g., apocrine
g., apocrine sweat
g., areola of mammary
g. ▸ atrophy of salivary
g. ▸ atrophy of tear-producing
g., autolysis of mucosal
g., Bartholin's
g., Bartholin's, urethral and Skene's (BUS)
g. biopsy, adrenal
g., bulbourethral
g., calcification, pineal
g., calculus of lacrimal
g., cancer of prostate
g., cancerous
g. carcinoma, meibomian
g. carcinoma, salivary
g. carcinoma, sebaceous
g. carcinoma, sweat
g., cardiac
g., carotid
g., central vein of suprarenal
g., chronic infection in prostate
g. ▸ cortical substance of suprarenal
g., Cowper's
g. cyst, marsupialization Bartholin
g., cystically dilated
g., digestive
g. disease ▸ salivary
g., dislocation of lacrimal
g. disorder ▸ salivary
g. drainage (dr'ge) of lacrimal
g., duct of sweat
g., ductless
g. dysfunction ▸ salivary
g. ▸ dysfunctional meibomian
g., eccrine
g., elongated
g., endocervical
g., endocrine
g., endometrial

gland(s)—*continued*

g. ▸ enlarged, inflamed prostate
g., enlarged lymph
g., enlarged prostate
g. ▸ enzymatic abnormality of adrenal
g. ▸ excessive activity of thyroid
g., excision of lacrimal
g., exocrine
g. ▸ external substance of suprarenal
g. failure ▸ adrenal
g., fetal suprarenal
g., fibroadenomatous hyperplasia of prostate
g., fistula of lacrimal
g. ▸ focal metastasis left adrenal
g. function ▸ parathyroid
g. function ▸ salivary
g., function, thymus
g., Galeati's
g., gastric
g., goiter or stiffness of
g. ▸ hemorrhagic infarcts of adrenal
g., hilus of suprarenal
g., hormone output of pituitary
g., hormones, adrenal
g., hypertrophy ▸ submucosal
g., hypothalamus
g. ▸ infected lymph
g., inferior thyroid
g., insufficiency, adrenal
g., intermediate lobe of pituitary
g. ▸ intermediate substance of suprarenal
g. ▸ internal secretion
g. ▸ internal substance of suprarenal
g., interstitial
g., intestinal
g., Krause's
g., labial
g., lacrimal
g. lesions, salivary
g., levator muscle of thyroid
g., Lieberkühn's
g., Littre's
g., lobules of mammary
g., lobules of thyroid
g., luxation of lacrimal
g., lymph
g., lymphosarcoma of lacrimal
g., mammary
g., Manz
g., medulla of adrenal

g. ▸ medullary substance of suprarenal
g., meibomian
g., milk
g. ▸ milk-secreting
g., mixed tumor of lacrimal
g., Moll's
g., mucous
g. multinodular, thyroid
g., nabothian
g., Naboth's
g. neoplasm, sebaceous
g. ▸ nodular hyperplasia of prostate
g. ▸ noncancerous enlargement of prostate
g. of eyelid
g. of Moll
g. of skin
g. of trigeminal nerve
g. of Zeis
g. ▸ overactive parathyroid
g., overactive thyroid
g., overstimulation of salivary
g., pacchionian
g. ▸ painful swollen
g. ▸ painfully swollen
g., parathyroid
g., paraurethral
g., parotid
g., Philip's
g., pineal
g., pituitary
g., posterior lobe of pituitary
g., preputial
g., prostate
g., removal of thymus
g., retention cyst lacrimal
g. ▸ right submaxillary salivary
g., Rivinus
g., Rosenmüller's
g., salivary
g., sebaceous
g. ▸ shrink enlarged prostate
g., Skene's
g., stimulate pituitary
g., sublingual
g., submandibular salivary
g., submaxillary
g., submental
g., superior lacrimal
g., superior thyroid
g., supernumerary lacrimal
g., suprarenal
g., sweat
g., swollen

g. ▸ swollen lymph
g., swollen lymphoma
g., syphilis of lacrimal
g., tarsal
g., TB (tuberculosis) of lacrimal
g., Theile's
g., thymus
g., thyroid
g. tissue transplant, adrenal
g., tortuosity of
g., trigeminal
g., tuberculosis (TB) of lacrimal
g. tumor, adrenal
g. tumor, ceruminous
g. tumor, lacrimal
g. tumor, salivary
g. tumor, submaxillary
g., underactive thyroid
g. urethral
g., vestibular
g. virus, salivary
g., Wolfring's
g., zeisian

glanders bacillus
glanders of lung
glandis clitoridis, crus
glandis penis, septum
glandulae suprarenalis, hilus
glandular [*granular*]

g. abnormality
g. atrophy
g. cancer
g. carcinoma
g. cells
g. cells, bronchial
g. disorder
g. elements
g. endometritis
g. enlargement
g. epithelioma
g. epithelium
g. fever
g. fluid
g. hyperplasia
g. involvement
g. mastitis
g. pharyngitis
g. secretion
g. structure
g. swelling
g. therapy
g. tissue
g. tissue, atrophy of
g. tissue, intracranial calcification benign

g. tissue, radiation treatment of
g. vaginitis
glandularis
   g. apostematosa, cheilitis
   g. proliferans, cholecystitis
   g., pyelitis
   g., urethritis
glandulosum, corpus
glans
   g. clitoridis
   g. of clitoris
   g. penis, septum of
Glantz derivative method ▸ Raff-
Glanzmann's disease
Glanzmann's syndrome
glare
   g. around lights
   g. filter, anti-
   g. ▸ sensitivity to light and
   g. ▸ video display terminal (VDT)
glaserian fissure
Glasgow Coma Scale
Glasgow's sign
glass (Glass)
   G. (crystal methamphetamine)
   g. appearance ▸ ground-
   g. eye artifact
   g. fiber, flexible
   g. graft, fiber
   g. hand, opera-
   g. murmur, hour-
   g. opacification ▸ ground-
   g. pathway ▸ ground-
   g. pipe
   g. rays
   g. screen, nonreflective
   G. sphere implant
   g. test, red
   g. thermometer
   g. vials
glassblower's cataract
glassblower's emphysema
glasses
   g., bifocal
   g., cataract
   g., crutch
   g., distance
   g., Franklin
   g., Hallauer's
   g., hyperbolic
   g., microscopic
   g., polarized
   g., prism
   g., single-vision
   g., snow

g., sun
g., telescopic
g., trifocal
glassing, hour-
glassy degeneration
glassy swelling
glauca, Magnolia
glaucoma
   g., absolute
   g., acute
   g. ▸ acute angle closure
   g., acute congestive
   g., air block
   g., angle-closure
   g., angle-recession
   g., aphakic
   g., apoplectic
   g., auricular
   g., capsular
   g. check
   g., chronic
   g., chronic narrow-angle
   g., chronic open-angle
   g., chronic simple
   g., closed-angle
   g., congenital
   g., congestive
   g., Contino's
   g., Donder's
   g., enzyme
   g., fulminant
   g., hemorrhagic
   g. imminens
   g., incipient
   g., infantile
   g., inflammatory
   g., juvenile
   g., lenticular
   g., malignant
   g., narrow-angle
   g., neovascular
   g., noncongestive
   g., obstructive
   g., open-angle
   g., painful hemorrhagic
   g., phakogenic
   g., phakolytic
   g., pigmentary
   g., primary
   g. ▸ primary open-angle
   g. screening
   g. screening, free
   g., secondary
   g., simple
   g. simplex

g. surgery ▸ laser
g., suspect
g. therapy
g., traumatic
g. treatment
g., vitreous-block
g., wide-angle
glaucomatous
   g. cataract
   g. cup
   g. habit
   g. halo
glaucum, Penicillium
glaucus, Aspergillus
glazed eyes
Gleason grading system
Gleason score
Glénard's syndrome
Glenn
   G. anastomosis
   G. operation
   G. shunt
glenohumeral joint
glenohumeral joint ▸ prosthetic
glenoid
   g. cavity
   g. fossa
   g. fossa mandibularis
   g. labrum
   g. process
glia
   g., ameboid
   g. cell
   g., cytoplasmic
   g., fibrillary
   g. membrane
   g. membrane of fourth ventricle
   g. of Fañana
   g., proliferation of
   g. sheath
glial
   g. cells
   g. fibers
   g. matrix, subependymal
   g. membrane
   g. membrane of fourth ventricle
   g. sheath
glib, patient
glide
   g., mandibular
   g., occlusal
   g., reach and sway ▸ sweep and
gliding joint
gliding motion
glioblastoma multiforme

gliocladium, Aspergillus
glioma
  g., astrocytic
  g., brain stem
  g. endophytum
  g., ependymal
  g. exophytum
  g., ganglio◊
  g., ganglionic
  g., infiltrating
  g., mixed
  g. multiforme
  g., nasal
  g., oligodendro◊
  g., optic nerve
  g., peripheral
  g., primary
  g. retinae
  g. sarcomatosum
  g. telangiectatic
gliosis
  g., basilar
  g., cerebellar
  g., diffuse
  g., hemispheric
  g., hypertrophic nodular
  g. in brain ▸ inflammation and
  g., isomorphic
  g., lobar
  g. of anterior column
  g. of cerebral aqueduct
  g. of lateral column
  g., perivascular
  g. spinal
  g., unilateral
glissement, hernia par
Glisson's
  G. capsule
  G. cirrhosis
  G. sling
glistening
  g., brain
  g. ▸ capsular surface smooth and
  g. fragments
  g. ▸ peritoneal surfaces smooth and
  g. ▸ peritoneum smooth and
  g. serosa ▸ smooth,
  g. transparent meninges
glitter [*gitter*]
glitter cells
global
  g. amnesia
  g. amnesia ▸ temporary
  g. amnesia (TGA) ▸ transient
  g. anoxia

  g. aphasia
  g. assessment index
  g. assessment of function
  g. distribution
  g. evaluation
  g. hypokinesis
  g. left ventricular (LV) ejection
    fraction
globe
  g. -cell anemia
  g., disorganized
  g., luxation of
  g., ocular
  g. of the eye
  g., ulceration of the
globin insulin
globoid cell leukodystrophy
globoid heart
globosa
  g., cornea
  g. albuminuria
  g. proteinuria
  g. sputum
globular heart
globular thrombus
globule [*lobule, nodule*]
  g., dentin
  g., Dobie's
  g., Marchi's
  g., milk
  g., Morgagni's
  g., myelin
  g., polar
globuliferum, Sideronema
globulin(s)
  g., AC (accelerator)
  g., accelerator
  g., alpha
  g. antibodies, alpha
  g., antidiphtheritic
  g. (AHG) ▸ antihemophilic
  g., antihuman
  g., antilymphocyte
  g., antimacrophage
  g. (ATG), antithymocyte
  g., antithymocytic
  g., antitoxic
  g., A-1
  g., A-2
  g., Bence Jones
  g., beta
  g. (CBG) ▸ corticosteroid-binding
  g., cortisol-binding
  g. (IgA) deficiency, gamma A
  g. (IgM) deficiency, gamma M

  g., gamma
  g., hepatitis B immune
  g., human gamma
  g., human rabies immune
  g., immune
  g., immune serum
  g. injection, gamma
  g. ▸ lymphocyte immune
  g., measles immune
  g. (human) ▸ measles immune
  g., pertussis immune
  g. (human) ▸ pertussis immune
  g., prophylactic gamma
  g. ▸ rabbit antihymocyte
  g. (A/G) ratio ▸ albumin-
  g. ▸ respiratory syncytial virus IV
    immune
  g., Rh immune
  g., Rh$_o$ (D antigen) immune
  g., serum
  g., synthesize gamma
  g., tetanus immune
  g., thyroxine-binding
  g., unbound thyroxine-binding
  g. (VZIG), varicella-zoster
    immune
  g. X
  g., zoster immune
globus
  g. abdominalis
  g. hystericus
  g. major epididymidis
  g. minor epididymidis
  g. of the heel
  g. palatum
  g. pallidus
  g. pharyngis
glomera aortica
glomerans, Enterobacter
glomeratus, Halogeton
glomerular
  g. arteriole
  g. arteriole, afferent
  g. arteriole, efferent
  g. basement membrane
  g. capsule
  g. capsule of kidney
  g. disorder
  g. filtration
  g. filtration rate (GFR)
  g. hyalinization
  g. kidney disease
  g. membrane antibodies
  g. nephritis
  g. sclerosis

g. -stimulating hormone
glomerule infiltration
glomeruli
  g., capsula
  g., cellularity of
  g., congestion of
  g., hyalinization of
  g., immature
  g., sclerosed
  g., sclerotic
  g., vas afferens
  g., vas efferens
glomerulocapsular nephritis
glomerulonephritis
  g., acute
  g., chronic
  g., chronic membranous
  g., drowsiness from
  g., membranoproliferative
  g., membranous
  g., poststreptococcal
  g., rapidly progressive
glomerulosclerosis
  g. and arteriosclerosis, widespread
  g., diabetic
  g., intercapillary
glomerulus, capsule of
glomerulus, malpighian
glomus jugulare
glomus tumor
Glory
  G. seeds injected ▸ Morning
  G. seeds (Flying Saucers) ▸ Morning
  G. seeds (Heavenly Blue) ▸ Morning
  G. seeds (Licorice Drops) ▸ Morning
  G. seeds (Pearly Gates) ▸ Morning
glossodynia ▸ burning tongue syndrome of
glossoepiglottic folds
glossokinesthetic center
glossopalatine, arcus
glossopalatine muscle
glossopalatinus, arcus
glossopharyngeal
  g. breathing
  g. muscle
  g. nerve
  g. nerve, inferior ganglion of
  g. nerve, jugular ganglion of
  g. nerve, lower ganglion of
  g. nerve signs
  g. nerve, superior ganglion of

g. neuralgia
g. neurotomy
glossoptosis syndrome, micrognathia-
glottic
  g. atresia
  g. carcinoma
  g. chink
  g. extension
  g. spasm
glottidis, atrium
glottidis, vestibulum
glottis
  g. atrium of
  g., flaccid
  g. focal
  g. patent
glove(s)
  g. appearance ▸ finger-in-
  g., compression
  g., disposable
  g. distribution ▸ stocking
  g., examination
  g., medical
  g., protective
  g. type hypesthesia ▸ stocking-and-
  g. -wearing
gloved-fist technique
Glover's drainage system
glovers' suture
glow modular tube
glucagon, immunoreactive
glucagon test
glucocorticoid therapy, adjunctive
glucogen, intravenous (IV)
gluconate
  g., calcium
  g., ferrous
  g., magnesium
  g., potassium
  g., quinidine
gluconic acid
glucophore group
glucose
  g. absorption test
  g. and saline
  g. assimilation
  g., blood
  g., cerebral metabolic rate of
  g., cerebrospinal fluid (CSF)
  g. concentration
  g. control
  g., CSF (cerebrospinal fluid)
  g. determinations, blood

g. determinations, interim
g. disappearance rate, plasma
g., fasting plasma
g. feeding
g. ▸ impaired fasting
g., insulin and potassium
g. intolerance
g. level
g. level, blood
g. level control
g. levels ▸ erratic blood
g. levels, fasting
g. levels, maintain blood
g. medium, Brun's
g. metabolism
g. metabolism in brain
g. meter ▸ home blood
g. monitor
g. monitor, blood
g. monitor, electronic
g. monitor ▸ noninvasive
g. monitoring
g. monitoring, home
g. -nitrogen (G-N) ratio
g. oxygen quotient ▸ cerebral
g. phosphate dehydrogenase
g. phosphate isomerase
g., postprandial
g. ▸ postprandial plasma
g. radioactive
g. self-monitoring
g. sensor, implantable
g. -6-phosphate dehydrogenase deficiency
g. -6-phosphate dehydrogenase deficiency anemia
g. strip
g. test
g. tolerance (IGT) ▸ impaired
g. tolerance test
g. tolerance test, abnormal
g. tolerance test, borderline
g. tolerance test, cortisone-
g. tolerance test, intravenous (IV)
g. tolerance test, oral
g. tolerance test, plasma
g., tubular reabsorption of
g. uptake
g., urine
g. water feedings
glucosidase deficiency ▸ a-1, 3-
glucosides, cardiac
glucuronic acid
glucosuria (*same as* glycosuria)

glue(s)
- g. ear
- g., fibrin
- g., Histoacryl
- g., methyl methacrylate

glum and moody ▸ **patient**

glutamate
- g., monosodium
- g., neurotransmitter
- g. receptor dysfunction

glutamic
- g. -oxalic transaminase (SGOT), serum
- g. -oxaloacetic transaminase (GOT)
- g. -oxaloacetic transaminase (EGOT) ▸ erythrocyte
- g. -oxaloacetic transaminase (SGOT) ▸ serum
- g. -pyruvic transaminase (GPT)
- g. -pyruvic transaminase (SGPT) ▸ serum

glutamine peptidase (GGP) ▸ **gamma-glutamyl transpeptidase**

glutamyl transpeptidase ▸ **gamma-glutaraldehyde, activated**

glutaric aciduria

glutaric aciduria ▸ **test for**

glutathione
- g., oxidized
- g. peroxidase deficiency ▸ erythrocyte
- g., reduced
- g. reductase

glutea, linea

gluteal
- g. artery
- g. body fat
- g. bonnet
- g. bursitis
- g. erythema
- g. fold
- g. free-flap procedure
- g. gait
- g. hernia
- g., left
- g. limp
- g. line
- g. muscle
- g. muscle, least
- g. nerve, inferior
- g. nerve, middle
- g. nerve, superior
- g. reflex
- g. region

- g., right
- g. vein, inferior
- g. vein, superior

gluteale infantum, granuloma

gluten
- g. enteropathy
- g. -free
- g. -free diet
- g. intolerance
- g. -restricted diet
- g. sensitivity enteropathy

gluteus
- g. maximus muscle
- g. medius muscle
- g. minimus muscle

glutinis, Rhodotorula

glutinis, Saccharomyces

glycated hemoglobin

glycemia/glycohemia

glycemic control

glycemic index

glyceraldehyde phosphate dehydrogenase

glycerin suppository

glycerin suppository inserted

glycerol kinase

glycerophosphate dehydrogenase

glycerophosphatide, choline

glycerophosphatide, serine

glyceryl
- g. guaiacolate
- g. methacrylate
- g. trinitrate

glycogen
- g. cardiomegaly
- g. depletion
- g. ▸ excessive accumulation of
- g. loading
- g. nephrosis
- g. storage disease
- g. storage test
- g. synthetase
- g. vacuolization

glycogenic cardiomegaly

glycogenolytic factor, hyperglycemic

glycogenosis, cardiac

glycol methacrylate

glycolysis, anaerobic

glycolytic enzymes

glycoprotein ▸ **platelet receptor**

glycoproteins, viral

glycoside
- g., cardiac
- g., cardioactive
- g., digitalis

glycosphingolipid disorder

glycosuria (*same as* glucosuria)

glycosuria, renal

glycosylated hemoglobin

glycosylated hemoglobin level

GM (gastric mucosa)

GM (geometric mean)

GM (grand mal)

GMA (glyceryl methacrylate)

GM-CSF (granulocytic-macrophage colony-stimulating factor), human

Gmelin's test

gm-m (gram-meter)

GMT (geometric mean titer)

GMW (gram-molecular weight)

GN (gram-negative)

G/N (glucose-nitrogen) ratio

GNA (general nursing assistance)

gnarled
- g. enamel
- g. fingernails
- g. joints, deformed
- g. knuckles ▸ thickly

gnashing and clenching of teeth

gnashing of teeth

Gnathostoma genus

Gnawing discomfort

gnawing sensation

GNC (general nursing care)

gnostic sensation

Gn-RH (gonadotropin-releasing hormone)

goal(s)
- g., abstinence
- g. ambulation
- g., appropriate
- g. attainment method
- g. attainment scaling
- g. ▸ apathy and lack of interest in personal
- g. attitudinal
- g. behavior
- g., family
- g. -gradient
- g., inaccessible
- g. ▸ long-term
- g., nursing
- g. -oriented behavior
- g. -oriented psychotherapy
- g. -oriented tasks
- g., overall therapeutic
- g., patient
- g., personal
- g. pursuit

g., primary
g., realistic
g., rehabilitation team
g., safety technique
g., shifting
g. ▸ short-term
g., treatment
g. weight
g., ultimate
GOAT (Galveston Orientation and Amnesia Test)
goat lice
goat louse
goblet cell
goblet cell degranulation
goblet cell metaplasia
Gocht osteoclast, Phelps-
God, patient angry at
Godart expirography
goddardi, Fasciolopsis
GOE (gas, oxygen and ether)
Goebell-Stoeckel operation
Goebell-Stoeckel operation ▸ Frangenheim-
Goffe's operation
goggle, pinhole
goggles, translucent
going crazy ▸ fear of
going rectification ▸ inward-
goiter
g., aberrant
g., adenomatous
g., Basedow's
g., benign multinodular
g., colloid
g., congenital
g., cystic
g., diffuse
g., diffuse colloid
g., diving
g., endemic
g., exophthalmic
g., fibrous
g., follicular
g., intrathoracic
g., multinodular
g., nodular
g., nontoxic
g., or stiffness of glands
g., papillomatous
g., parenchymatous
g., plunging
g., simple
g., substernal
g., suffocative

g., thyrotoxic
g., toxic
g., vascular
g., wandering
Golaski graft
gold (Gold)
G. (marijuana)
G. (grade of marijuana), Acapulco
g., colloidal
g. curve
g. curve, colloidal
g. equivalent
g. grain implant
g. grains, radioactive
g. implant
g. implant material
g. injection
g. inlay
g. marker
g. 198 (Au^{198})
g. 195m radionuclide
g., radioactive
g. salts
G. sphere implant
g. test, colloidal
Goldblatt's hypertension
Goldblatt's kidney
Golden Rule ethics
Golden's sign
Goldflam's disease
Goldflam disease, Erb-
Goldman cardiac risk index score
Goldmann's applanation tonometer
Goldmann's goniolens
Goldstein('s)
G. hematemesis
G. hemoptysis
G. rays
Goldthwait('s)
G. operation
G. operation, Roux-
G. sign
golf ball roll foot exercise
golfer's elbow
golfer's focal dystonia
Golgi('s)
G. body
G. cells
G. complex
Goll's tract
Goltz syndrome
Goltz-Gorlin syndrome
Goma (Numorphan)
Goma de Mota (hashish)

Gomco suction
Gomez-Marquez's operation
Gompertzian tumor growth
gonad shield, lead
gonadal
g. agenesis
g. aplasia
g. artery
g. disease
g. dysgenesis
g. hormone
gonadotropic (same as gonadotrophic)
g. activity, general
g. cycle
g. hormone
g. hormone assay
gonadotropin(s)
g. (CG), chorionic
g. (HCG) ▸ human chorionic
g. (HMG), human menopausal
g., human pituitary
g. -inhibitory material
g. ▸ level of female
g. -releasing agent
g. -releasing hormone (Gn-RH)
g. test, chorionic
g. titer
g. (TUG) ▸ total urinary
g., urinary chorionic
gondii, Toxoplasma
gondii, toxoplasmosis
G1 (grid 1)
gonecystic calculus
Gongylonema
G. ingluvicola
G. neoplasticum
G. pulchrum
G. scutatum
gonidial colony
Gonin's operation
Goniobasis silicula
goniolens
g., Allen-Thorpe
g., Barkan
g., Goldmann's
g,. Koeppe
goniometer, Conzett's
goniometer, electro◊
goniophotography study
goniopuncture operation
goniopuncture procedure
gonitis, fungous
gonitis tuberculosa
Gonnin-Amsler marker

gonococcal
- g. arthritis
- g. conjunctivitis
- g. dermatitis
- g. endocarditis
- g. meningitis
- g. ophthalmia
- g. stomatitis
- g. urethritis

gonococcus (GC) cultures, four-site
gonococcus (GC) microorganism
gonorrhea (GC)
- g., arthritis from
- g., insomnia from
- g. (VDG), venereal disease—

gonorrheal
- g. arthritis
- g. bubo
- g. conjunctivitis
- g. heel
- g. ophthalmia
- g. urethritis

gonorrhoeae, Diplococcus
gonorrhoeae, gram-negative
  Neisseria
gonorrhoeica, macula
gonotrophic cycle
Gonzales blood group
good
- g. appetite
- g. breath sounds
- g. bruits, arteriovenous (AV) fistula
  with
- g. chest expansion
- g., color and cry
- g. concentration
- g. condition, patient discharged in
- g. contact with skin
- g. cosmetic result
- g. dental condition ▸ teeth in
- g. dental repair ▸ teeth in
- g. eating habits
- g. exposure obtained
- g. hemostasis
- g. nutrition
- g. patient's appetite
- g. pelvic support
- g. peripheral circulation
- g. prenatal care
- g. rapport with others ▸ patient has
- g. response
- g. self-image
- g. self-talk
- g. support, introitus with
- g. support, uterus has

- g. tissue turgor

Goodall-Power operation
Goodell's law
Goodell's sign
Goodenough test
Goodpasture's syndrome
Goofballs (barbiturates)
Goon (phencyclidine)
goose bumps ▸ skin
goose-honk murmur
gooseneck deformity
Gordan-Overstreet syndrome
Gorder operation, Van
Gordon elementary body
gordonae, Mycobacterium
Gordon's reflex
Gore-Tex (GT)
- GT baffle
- GT cardiovascular patch
- GT jump graft
- GT surgical patch
- GT vascular graft

Gorlin
- G. constant
- G. equation
- G. hydraulic formula
- G. syndrome, Goltz-

gormanii, Legionella
Goslee tooth
Gosselin's fracture
Gothic arch tracing
Gott('s)
- G. and Daggett valve prosthesis
- G. low-profile prosthesis
- G. prosthesis
- G. shunt

Gottlieb's epithelial attachment
Gottschalk's operation
gouge [gauge]
Gougerot's syndrome
Goulain mastopexy
Gould electromagnetic flowmeter
gout
- g., abarticular
- g., acute
- g., articular
- g., attack
- g., calcium
- g., chalky
- g., from alcohol
- g., latent
- g., lead
- g., misplaced
- g., oxalic
- g., polyarticular

- g., retrocedent
- g., rheumatic
- g., saturnine
- g., tophaceous

gouty
- g. arthritis
- g. arthritis, acute
- g. arthropathy
- g. diabetes
- g. diathesis
- g. diet
- g. episcleritis
- g. iritis
- g. nephropathy
- g. node
- g. phlebitis
- g. proteinuria
- g. urethritis
- g. urine

governed behavior, rule-
government-mandated guidelines
Gower(s')
- G. contractions
- G. disease
- G., fasciculus of
- G. hemoglobin
- G. maneuver
- G. sign
- G. syndrome

gown(s)
- g. and bootees, cover
- g. and instruments ▸ complete
  change of drapes,
- g., disposable examination
- g., disposable mortuary
- g., flame-retardant
- g., steam-sterilized masks and

Goyrand's hernia
GPC (giant papillary conjunctivitis)
GPMAL (gravida, para, multiple
  births, abortion, live births)
GPT (glutamic-pyruvic transaminase)
gr (grain)
Graaff generator, Van de
graafian
- g. follicle
- g. ovules
- g. vesicle

grab bar
grabbing technique
Graber-Duvernay operation
Gracilaria confervoides
gracilis
- g., Euglena
- g., fasciculus

g. muscle
g., nucleus
g., Siderobacter
Gradational Step exercise stress test
grade [*grate, great*]
  g. disease ‣ low-
  g. fever, low-
  g. lesion, high-
  g., low
  g. of marijuana (Acapulco Gold)
  g. of marijuana (Berkeley Boo)
  g. of marijuana (Panama Red)
  g. I-IV astrocytoma
  G. 1 through 6 murmur
  g. point average
  g. stenosis ‣ high-
  g. temperature, low-
  g., thrombus
  g., tumor
graded exercise test
Gradenigo's syndrome
gradient(s)
  g. acquisition
  g., alveoloarterial oxygen (O_2) tension
  g., alveolocapillary partial pressure
  g. amplitude
  g., aortic pressure
  g., aortic valve
  g. ‣ aortic valve peak
  g., arm-leg
  g., atrioventricular (AV)
  g., axial
  g. bandwidth
  g. ‣ colloid hydrostatic pressure
  g., density
  g., diastolic
  g., Doppler pressure
  g., fluid
  g. gel electrophoresis
  g., goal-
  g., hemodynamic
  g. ‣ intracavitary pressure
  g., mean
  g. measurement ‣ transstenotic pressure
  g., mitral
  g. (MVG) ‣ mitral valve
  g. of approach
  g. of avoidance
  g. of fluid inflow
  g. of fluid outflow ‣ net
  g. ‣ peak instantaneous
  g. (PSG) ‣ peak systolic
  g. ‣ peak transaortic valve

g., peak-to-peak systolic
g., potential
g., pressure
g. pressure ‣ peak systolic
g. ‣ pulmonary valve
g. (PVC) ‣ pulmonic valve
g. reduction
g., residual
g. support stockings ‣ venous pressure
g., systolic
g. ‣ transaortic valve
g., transplacental
g. ‣ transvalvular aortic
g., tricuspid valve
g., ventricular
g. ‣ vertical pleural pressure
grading system ‣ Gleason
Gradle's electrode
Gradle's operation
gradual (Gradual)
  g. ambulation
  g. blurring of vision
  g. desensitization
  g. deterioration
  g. distortion of sound
  G. Dosage Schedule
  g. effect
  g. exercise progression
  g. increase
  g. lifestyle modification
  g. loss of alertness
  g. loss of auditory discrimination
  g. loss of bone tissue
  g. loss of mental faculties
  g. memory loss
  g. mental deterioration
  g. onset
  g. relaxation
  g. weight bearing
  g. weight gain
  g. withdrawal
gradually, form
graduated
  g. compress
  g. compression stockings
  g. stairs
  g. tenotomy
graduation, volumetric
Graefe's
  G. disease
  G. disease, von
  G. incision
  G. operation, von
  G. sign

G. sign, von
G. syndrome
Graenslen test
Graffi virus
graft (gft) (Graft) [*graph*]
  g., accordion
  g., activated
  g., albumin-coated vascular
  g., allo◊
  g., allogeneic
  g. anastomosis
  g. angiography ‣ internal mammary artery
  g. angiography ‣ saphenous vein bypass
  g. angioplasty ‣ patch
  g., aortic aneurysm
  g., aortic tube
  g., aortocoronary bypass
  g. (AFBG), aortofemoral bypass
  g., aortofemoral Dacron
  g., aortoiliac bypass
  g., aortovein bypass
  g. area rejected (TGAR) ‣ total
  g., arrow-shaped
  g., arterial
  g., artery bypass
  g., atherosclerosis
  g., autochthonous
  g., autodermic
  g., autoepidermic
  g., autogenic
  g., autogenous
  g., autogenous bone
  g. (VG) ‣ autogenous vein
  g., autologous
  g., autologous fat
  g., autoplastic
  g., avascular
  G. Bank, Bone
  g., B-B
  g., bifurcation
  g., Blair-Brown skin
  g., blood vessel
  g., bolus tie-over
  g., bone
  g., Bonfiglio bone
  g., bovine
  g., Braun
  g., Braun-Wangensteen
  g., brephoplastic
  g., Brett bone
  g., B's
  g., B-W
  g., bypass

graft—*continued*
g., bypass vein
g., cable
g., cadaveric
g., cancellous
g., cancellous-cortical bone
g., cardiac bypass
g., cartilage
g. ▸ catheter placed
g., chessboard
g., chorioallantoic
g., clogged bypass
g., composite
g., compressed Ivalon patch
g., Cooley
g., Cooley woven Dacron
g., corneal
g. (CABG), coronary artery bypass
g., coronary bypass
g., cortical
g., Cragg endoluminal
g., Creech aortoiliac
g., cross-leg
g., Cryolife valve
g., cutis
g., Dacron
g., Dacron arterial
g., Dacron sleeve
g., Dacron tube
g., Davis
g., DeBakey's
g. defatted, skin
g., delayed
g., dermal
g., dermic
g., diamond inlay
g., diamond inlay bone
g., diced cartilage
g., donor, bone
g., donor site of bone
g. donor site, skin
g., donor, skin
g., double-end
g., Douglas'
g., Dragstedt's
g., dual-inlay bone
g., dual-onlay
g., Edwards
g., epidermic
g., Esser
g., fascia
g., fascia lata
g., fascial
g., fascicular
g., fat

g., femoral
g., femoropopliteal bypass
g., fiber glass
g., filler
g. fistula, brachioaxillary bridge
g., fixation
g., foam rubber vaginal
g. ▸ follicular unit
g. for vascular reconstruction ▸
    bifurcated vein
g., free
g., full-thickness
g., full-thickness postauricular
g., full-thickness skin
g., Gabarro's
g., gauntlet
g., Gillies'
g., Golaski
g., Gore-Tex
g. ▸ Gore-Tex jump
g. ▸ Gore-Tex vascular
g., H-
g., hair
g., hair-bearing
g. ▸ Hancock pericardial valve
g. ▸ Hancock vascular
g., hemicylindrical
g., hemicylindrical bone
g., hetero◇
g., heterodermic
g., heterogenous
g., heterologous
g., heteroplastic
g., homo◇
g., homogenous
g., homogenous bone
g., homologous
g., homoplastic
g., hyperplastic
g., iliac
g., implantation
g., Impra vein
g. inclusion technique, Crawford
g. infection
g. infection ▸ vascular
g., inlay
g., inlay bone
g., intermediate skin
g., intermediate split-thickness skin
g. ▸ internal mammary
g., interposition
g., interracial
g., intramedullary and spongiosa
g., intramedullary bone
g. ▸ Ionescu-Shiley vascular

g., island
g., iso◇
g., isogeneic
g., isologous
g., isoplastic
g., Ivalon
g., jump
g., Kebab's
g., Kiel
g. ▸ kimura cartilage
g., Konig's
g., Krause-Wolfe
g., lamellar
g., lay-on
g. ▸ lower extremity bypass
g. ▸ mammary artery
g., Marlex
g., massive sliding
g. material ▸ MycroMesh
g., material, polytetrafluoroethylene
    (PTFE) arterial
g. material, surrounding
g. material, synthetic
g., Meadox Microvel Dacron
g., medullary
g., medullary bone
g., Mersilene
g. ▸ mesenteric bypass
g. ▸ Microknit patch
g. ▸ microsurgically implanted
g. ▸ Microvel double velour
g., Milliknit vascular
g., mucosal
g., mucous membrane
g., muscle
g., myringoplasty (VGM) ▸ vein
g., nerve
g. occlusion
g. of pigskin, split-thickness
g., Ollier-Thiersch
g., omental
g., onlay
g., onlay bone
g., ooze
g., organ
g., osseous
g., osteoperiosteal
g., osteoperiosteal bone
g., osteoperiosteal iliac bone
g., outer table
g., Padgett's
g., partial-thickness skin
g., patch
g., pedicle
g., peg

g., peg bone
g., penetrating
g., perichondrial
g., periosteal
g. ▸ peripheral nerve
g. ▸ Perma-Flow coronary
g., Phemister
g., pinch
g. ▸ popliteal tibial bypass vein
g., porcine
g. ▸ portacaval H
g., preclotted
g. procedure, Damian
g., prop
g. prosthesis ▸ Milliknit vascular
g. prosthesis ▸ vascular
g., PTFE (polytetrafluoroethylene) Gore-Tex
g., PTFE (polytetrafluoroethylene) Impra
g., reaction, white-
g. rejection
g. rejection, immediate
g. rejection, late
g. ▸ renal artery bypass
g., replacement
g. replacement ▸ aortic
g. restenosis
g., Reverdin
g. ▸ reversed saphenous vein
g., ring
g. ring marker ▸ vein
g., rope
g., Russe's bone
g., saphenous
g. ▸ saphenous vein
g., saphenous vein bypass
g., Sauvage Dacron
g., seamless arterial
g., Seddon's nerve
g., seed
g. ▸ Shiley Tetraflex vascular
g., sieve
g., single-onlay cortical
g. site, bone
g. sizer ▸ Meadox
g., skin
g., sleeve
g., slice
g., sliding inlay bone
g., slough, skin
g., snake
g. ▸ solid-organ
g., Solvang
g., split

g., split-skin
g., split-thickness
g., split-thickness skin
g., sponge
g. stenosis ▸ saphenous vein
g., Stent
g. ▸ subclavian artery bypass
g., surgery, brain
g. ▸ surgically placed
g., sutured in place
g., syngeneic
g., synthetic
g., Tanner-Vanderput
g., tantalum mesh
g. technique, Braun pinch
g., Teflon
g., temporofacial
g. tendon,
g., thick-split
g., Thiersch's
g., thin-split
g., three-vein
g. thrombosis
g., tibial
g., tissue
g., to femur, bone
g., tube
g., tubular
g., tunnel
g., umbilical
g., underlay fascial
g., valise handle
g., Van Millingen's
g. vascular prosthesis ▸ Medi-
g. ▸ vascularized bone
g. vasculopathy
g., (VG) ▸ vein
g. ▸ vein bypass
g. ▸ Velex woven Dacron vascular
g. ▸ velour collar
g., venous
g. -versus-host (GVH)
g. -versus-host disease (GVHD)
g. -versus-host disease (GVHD) ▸ life-threatening
g. -versus-host reaction (GVHR)
g. ▸ vertebral artery bypass
g. ▸ Vitagraft vascular
g., Weavenit patch
g., white
g. whole-bone transplant
g., Wolfe
g., Wolfe-Krause
g. ▸ woven Dacron tube

g., xeno◊
g., Y
grafted
g. blood vessel
g. cells
g. kidney rejection
g. skin
g. skin vulnerable to injury
grafting
g., authorization form for removal of tissue for
g. ▸ autologous cultured skin
g., bone
g., bypass
g., consent form for removal of tissue for
g. ▸ endarterectomy and coronary artery bypass
g., Mangoldt's epithelial
g. of tissue ▸ authorization form for operation and
g. of tissue ▸ consent form for operation and
g., orthopedic
g., periodontal
g. ▸ port-access coronary artery bypass
g., repeated skin
g., skin
g. surgery, coronary artery bypass
g., vascular
Graham Steell murmur of heart
Grahamella peromysci
Grahamella talpae
grahami, Culicoides
grain [*drain*]
g. cayenne pepper
g. dust
g. implant, gold
g., radioactive gold
g. stool, sago-
gram (g) [*dram*]
g. -amphophilic
g. -calorie (G-cal)
g. -centimeter (g-cm)
g., cholangio◊
g., cholecysto◊
g., entero◊
g. equivalent
g., lymphangio◊
g. -meter (gm-m)
g. -molecular weight (GMW)
g. -negative (GN)
g. -negative Aerobacter aerogenes
g. -negative aerobes

gram—*continued*

g. -negative aerobic bacilli
g. -negative bacilli
g. -negative bacilli ▸ enteric
g. -negative bacilli infection
g. -negative bacteria
g. -negative bean-shaped diplococci
g. -negative Brucella abortus
g. -negative Brucella melitensis
g. -negative Brucella suis
g. -negative cigar-shaped rods
g. -negative cocci
g. -negative coccobacilli Acinetobacter
g. -negative coccobacilli ▸ lightly staining
g. -negative coccobacilli ▸ pleomorphic
g. -negative coccobacilli, small
g. -negative E. (Escherichia) coli
g. -negative Eberthella typhi
g. -negative endocarditis
g. -negative enteric bacilli
g. -negative enterococcus
g. -negative Escherichia (E.) coli
g. -negative Escherichia (E.) communior
g. -negative extracellular bean-shaped diplococci
g. -negative extracellular kidney-shaped diplococci
g. -negative Hemophilus influenzae
g. -negative Hemophilus pertussis
g. -negative infection
g. -negative intracellular bean-shaped diplococci
g. -negative intracellular diplococci
g. -negative intracellular kidney-shaped diplococci
g. -negative kidney-shaped diplococci
g. -negative Klebsiella ozogenes
g. -negative Klebsiella pneumoniae
g. -negative Malleomyces mallei
g. -negative Neisseria gonorrhoeae
g. -negative Neisseria intracellularis
g. -negative organisms
g. -negative organisms ▸ nosocomial
g. -negative organisms ▸ proteolytic
g. -negative Pasteurella lepiseptica
g. -negative Pasteurella pestis
g. -negative Pasteurella tularensis
g. -negative pericarditis
g. -negative pneumonia
g. -negative Proteus vulgaris
g. -negative Pseudomonas aeruginosa
g. -negative rods
g. -negative rods, anaerobic
g. -negative rods and cocci
g. -negative rods ▸ cluster of short
g. -negative rods ▸ encapsulated
g. -negative rods ▸ pleomorphic
g. -negative Salmonella aertrycke
g. -negative Salmonella enteritidis
g. -negative Salmonella schottmülleri
g. -negative Salmonella suipestifer
g. -negative sepsis
g. -negative septicemia
g. -negative Shigella paradysenteriae
g. -negative species
g. -negative spirilla
g. -negative surgical pathogens
g. -negative Vibrio comma
g. -positive
g. -positive Actinomyces bovis
g. -positive Bacillus anthracis
g. -positive bacteria
g. -positive Clostridium butyricum
g. -positive Clostridium septicum
g. -positive Clostridium sordellii
g. -positive Clostridium tetani
g. -positive Clostridium welchii
g. -positive cocci
g. -positive cocci ▸ aerobic
g. -positive cocci ▸ clusters of
g. -positive cocci in pairs and chains
g. -positive cocci ▸ short-chain
g. -positive Corynebacterium diphtheriae
g. -positive diplococci ▸ helmet-shaped
g. -positive diplococci ▸ lancet-shaped
g. -positive Diplococcus pneumonias
g. -positive E. (Escherichia) coli infection
g. -positive Erysipelothrix muriseptica
g. -positive Mycobacterium tuberculosis
g. -positive nosocomial infection
g. -positive organisms
g. -positive organisms ▸ nosocomial
g. -positive penicillin-sensitive coccus
g. -positive rods
g. -positive rods and cocci
g. -positive rods ▸ large darkly staining
g. -positive species
g. -positive Staphylococcus aureus
g. -positive Streptococcus faecalis
g. -positive Streptococcus hemolyticus
g. -positive Streptococcus lactis
g. -positive Streptococcus salivarius
g. -positive Streptococcus viridans
g. -positive surgical pathogens
g. reaction
g., sphygmo◊
g. stain
g. stain method
g. stain negative bacteremias
g. stain negative enteric bacilli
g. stain of body fluid
g. stain of cervix
g. stain of exudate
g. stain of facial abscess
g. stain of pelvic abscess
g. stain of peritoneal fluid
g. stain of purulent discharge
g. stain of skin lesion
g. stain of stool specimen
g. stain of throat
g. stain of unspun urine
g. stain of urethra
g. stain procedure
g. stain, spinal fluid
g. stain, sputum
g. -staining technique
g. stains
g., veno◊

gramicidin, Soviet
grammatical complexity
grand mal (GM)
g.m., compatible with
g.m. convulsion
g.m. epilepsy
g.m. seizure
g.m. seizures, isolated
g.m. seizures ▸ uncontrolled generalized
g.m. status
grand multiparity

grandeur
g., delusions of
g., ideas of
g. ▸ preoccupation with fantasies of
grandiose
g. ideas
g. mania
g. notions
g. sense of self-importance
g. thoughts
grandiosity ▸ sustained periods of
grandis, Diplogonoporus
Grandmont's operation, de
Granger x-ray view
Granger's sign
Grant-Ward operation
granted, permission for autopsy
granola, Amoebobacter
granular [*glandular*]
g. atrophy of kidney
g., breasts ropy or
g. casts
g. cell
g. cell layer
g. cell tumor
g. cell tumor ▸ microscopic
g. cells ▸ cyanophilic,
g., cervix
g. component
g. conjunctivitis
g. eosinophilic cytoplasm
g. eosinophilic material
g. formation
g. induration
g. inflammation
g. inflammatory nodules
g. lesion
g. leukocytes, basophil
g., lungs coarsely
g. lymphocyte antigen ▸ large
g. masses, Schultze's
g. material
g. ophthalmia
g. pharyngitis
g. pneumonocyte
g. precipitate
g. protoplasm
g. respiration
g. stricture of urethra
g. surface
g. urethritis
g. vaginitis
granularis, ependymitis
granulata, Amoeba urinae
granulated tissue

granulating
g. in
g. in and healing
g. in, incision
g. in, wound
g. wound, chronic
granulation(s)
g., arachnoidal
g., Bayle's
g., Bright's
g., cell
g., cellular
g., exuberant
g., healing by
g. index (JGI) ▸ juxtaglomerular
g., pacchionian
g., pyroninophilic
g., Reilly
g. stenosis
g. tissue
g. tissue, fresh
g. tissue, tuberculosis
g. tissue, vascular
g. tube
g., Virchow's
granule(s)
g., acidophil
g., acrosomal
g., albuminous
g., aleuronoid
g., alpha
g., Altmann's
g., amphophil
g., argentaffine
g., azur
g., azurophil
g., Babès-Ernst
g., Balfour infective
g., basal
g., basophil
g., beta
g., Bettelheim's
g., Bollinger's
g., Bütschli's
g., carbohydrate
g. cell, fatty
g., cellular
g., chromatic
g., chromophilic
g., cone
g., cortical
g., cytoplasmic
g., delta
g., Dioscorides'
g., Ehrlich

g., Ehrlich-Heinz
g., elementary
g., epsilon
g., Fauvel's
g., Fordyce's
g., fuchsinophil
g., gamma
g., Grawitz's
g., Heinz
g., hyperchromatin
g., iodophil
g., Isaac's
g., juxtaglomerular
g., kappa
g., keratohyaline
g., Kölliker's interstitial
g., Kretz's
g., Langley's
g., melanin
g., meningeal
g., metachromatic
g., Mezei
g., Much's
g., Neusser's
g., neutrophil
g., Nissl's
g., oxyphil
g., pale transparent
g., Paschen's
g., pigment
g., polar
g., proacrosomal
g., protein
g., rod
g., Schridde's
g., Schrön-Much
g., Schrön's
g., Schüffner's
g., secretary
g., seminal
g., sphere
g., sulfur
g., thread
g., toxic
g., volutin
g., zymogen
granulocyte(s)
g., band-form
g. -erythroid ratio
g., mature
g. pool, circulating
g. pool, marginal
g. pool, total blood
g. specific activity ▸ blood
g. transfusion

granulocytic
- g. ehrlichiosis (HGE) ‣ human
- g. leukemia
- g. leukemia, acute
- g. leukemia, chronic
- g. -macrophage colony-stimulating factor (CM-CSF) ‣ human
- g. sarcoma

granuloma(s)
- g., actinic
- g., amebic
- g. annulare
- g., apical
- g., balnei
- g., beryllium
- g., calcified
- g., calcified benign
- g., candida
- g., candidal
- g., central giant-cell reparative
- g., cholesterol
- g., cocci
- g., coccidioidal
- g., dental
- g., Durck's
- g. endemicum
- g., eosinophilic
- g., FB (foreign body)
- g. fissuratum
- g. fungoides
- g. gangraenescens
- g., giant-cell reparative
- g. gluteale infantum
- g., Hodgkin's
- g. in canaliculus
- g., infectious
- g., infective
- g. inguinale
- g. iridis
- g., laryngeal
- g., lipoid
- g., lipophagic
- g., lycopodium
- g., lympho◊
- g., Majocchi's
- g., malarial
- g., midline
- g., Mignon's eosinophilic
- g., monilial
- g., multiforme
- g., noncaseating
- g. of lung
- g. of lung, eosinophilic
- g. of orbit
- g. of sinus

- g. of the lung (EGL), eosinophilic
- g. of the pudenda ‣ ulcerating
- g. of thyroid, benign
- g., para◊
- g., paracoccidioidal
- g., peripheral giant-cell reparative
- g., plasma cell
- g. pudendi
- g. pudente tropicum
- g., pyogenic
- g., reticulohistiocytic
- g., rheumatic
- g., sarcoid
- g. sarcomatodes
- g., septic
- g., silicotic
- g. swimming pool
- g. telangiectaticum
- g., trichophytic
- g. tropicum
- g., umbilical
- g., venereal
- g. venereum
- g., xanthomatous
- g., zirconium

granulomata, caseating
granulomata ‣ multiple focal calcified
granulomatis, Cephalosporium
granulomatosa, cheilitis
granulomatosa fibroplastica, gastritis
granulomatosis
- g., allergic
- g., bronchocentric
- g., lipophagia
- g., lipophagic intestinal
- g., lympho◊
- g., lymphomatoid
- g., malignant
- g., necrotizing respiratory
- g., pulmonary
- g. ‣ pulmonary Wegener's
- g. siderotica
- g., Wegener's

granulomatosus, Saccharomyces
granulomatous
- g. abscess
- g. angiitis, allergic
- g. arteritis
- g. arteritis, cranial
- g. arteritis ‣ temporal
- g. cervicitis
- g. colitis
- g. disease
- g. disease, chronic

- g. disease, fatal
- g. disease ‣ infectious
- g. disease of childhood
- g. encephalomyelitis
- g. enteritis
- g. features ‣ extravascular
- g. ileojejunitis
- g. inflammation
- g. iridocyclitis
- g. lesion
- g. lining
- g. lung disease
- g. lymphoma
- g. orchitis, spermatogenic
- g. pneumonitis
- g. process, chronic inflammatory
- g. prostatitis
- g. thyroiditis
- g. vasculitis, eosinophilic

granulosa
- g. cell carcinoma
- g. cell tumor
- g. cells ‣ estrogen-secreting
- g., colpitis
- g. lutein cyst
- g., pyelitis
- g. theca cell carcinoma
- g., urethritis

granulosis virus
granulosum, stratum
granulosus, Echinococcus
granulovacuolar degeneration
grape(s)
- g. appearance, cluster of
- g., Carswell's
- g. cell
- g. sugar

graph(s) [*graft*]
- g., basal metabolic temperature
- g., entero◊
- g., isoeffect
- g., (SCG) ‣ serum chemistry
- g., temperature

graphic(s)
- g., computer
- g. recording
- g., 3-D computer

graphica, asemia
graphii, Verticillium
graphomotor aphasia
graphomotor functioning
graphy, veno◊
Graseby pump
Grashey's aphasia
Grashey's position

grasp [*rasp, clasp*]
g., hand
g., Moro's
g. reflex
g. reflex, palmar
g. response
g. strength
grasped
g., cecum
g., cervix
g., tonsil
g. with single-tooth tenaculum ▸ cervix
grasping reflex
Grass (grass)
G. (marijuana)
g., scurvy
G. Ten-Channel Instrument
grate [*great, grade*]
gratification
g., delay of
g., emotional
g., material
grating
g. pain
g. sensation
g. sensation under kneecap
g. sound
Gratiolet, convolutions of
gratissima, Persea
gratus, Tabanus
Graves' (grave)
G. disease
g. fat
G. ophthalmopathy
g. prognosis
G. scapula
gravid uterus
Gravida (gravida)
g. I (II, III, etc.)
G., para, multiple births, abortions, live births (GPMAL)
g., primi◊
gravidarum
g., chloasma
g., chorea
g., colostrum
g., emesis
g., gingivitis
g., hydrorrhea
g., hyperemesis
g., melasma
g., nephritis
g., pyelitis
g., retinitis

g., striae
gravidic retinitis
Gravindex test
gravis
g. and mediastinal tumors, myasthenia
g., colitis
g. ▸ double vision from myasthenia
g., enteritis
g. hypophyseogenea, asthenia
g., icterus
g., icterus castrensis
g. (MG) ▸ muscle-weakening myasthenia
g., myalgia
g., myasthenia
g. neonatorum, icterus
g. pseudoparalytica, myasthenia
g., Tensilon test for myasthenia
gravitate to bottom of container ▸ red cells
gravitating hemorrhage
gravitation factor
gravitational line
gravitational movement
gravity
g., decreased specific
g. -dependent movement of cupula
g. drainage (dr'ge)
g., eliminate
g. free position
g. -settling culture
g., specific
g. stimulation, anti-
g. test, specific
Grawitz's globules
Grawitz's tumor
Gray's (gray) (*same as* grey)
G. Anatomy
g. area, neutral or
g. atrophy
g. baby syndrome
g. cataract
g. columns of spinal cord ▸ ventral
g. commissure, anterior
g. commissure, posterior
g. electrode, periacqueductal
g. induration
g. line
g. masses, central
g. matter
g. matter of brain
g. matter of spinal cord
g. medulla ▸ focally cystic
g. patches

g. scale
g. -scale imaging
g. -scale ultrasonography
g. -scale ultrasound
g. scale ▸ voxel
g. softening
g. substance
g. substance ▸ gelatinous substance of
g. substance of cerebrum, central
g. substance of spinal cord
g. substance, periventricular
g. substance, Soemmering's
g., tympanic membrane
graying hair from aging
grayish tissue
Grayson's ligament
Grease (hashish)
grease, silicone
great [*grate, grade*]
g. adductor muscle
g. alveolar cells
g. anterior radicular artery
g. arteries, complete transposition of
g. arteries, corrected transposition of
g. arteries ▸ malposition of
g. arteries ▸ transposition of
g. artery
g. auricular nerve
g. cardiac vein
g. cerebral vein
g. cistern
g. distress, patient in
g. saphenous vein
g. toe
g. toe, abductor muscle of
g. toe, adductor muscle of
g. toe, dorsal digital nerve of lateral surface of
g. toe, extension of
g. toe implant, Swanson
g. toe, lateral surface of
g. toe, long extensor muscle of
g. toe, long flexor muscle of
g. toe, normal flexion of
g. toe, short extensor muscle of
g. toe, short flexor muscle of
g. toe sign
g. toe, weakness of
g. transverse commissure
g. vessels
g. vessels, corrected transposition of

great—*continued*
- g. vessels, heart and
- g. vessels, penetrating wounds of
- g. vessels, transposition of

Greatbatch Implantable Cardiac Pulse Generator ▸ Chardack-
Greatbatch pacemaker, Chardack-
greater
- g. circulation
- g. curvature
- g. curvature aspect
- g. curvature of antrum
- g. curvature of stomach
- g. curvature site
- g. ischiatic notch
- g. multangular bone
- g. occipital nerve
- g. omentum
- g. oval center
- g. palatine nerve
- g. pectoral muscle
- g. pelvis
- g. petrosal nerve
- g. psoas muscle
- g. sacrosciatic notch
- g. saphenous vein
- g. sciatic notch
- g. splanchnic nerve
- g. superficial nerve
- g. than air conduction (BC > AC) ▸ bone conduction
- g. trochanter muscle
- g. tubercle
- g. zygomatic muscle

greatest
- g. extension, angle of
- g. flexion, angle of
- g. strength
- g. weakness

greedy bowel
Greeff bodies, Prowazek-
green (Green)('s)
- g. algae, blue-
- g. angiography ▸ indocyanine
- g. argon laser
- g. bile ▸ viscid dark
- g., brilliant
- g. cancer
- G., Cardio-
- g. cataract
- g. color perception deficiency ▸ red-
- G. Dragon (barbiturate)
- G. Dragon (LSD)
- g. dye, brilliant
- g. dye curve
- g. dye ▸ indocyanine
- g. indicator dilution technique ▸ indocyanine
- G., Indocyanine
- G. lamp, Eldridge
- g. method ▸ indocyanine
- G. operation, Grice-
- g., outlined with brilliant
- G. replacer
- g. sickness
- g. softening
- g. sputum
- g. strep endocarditis
- g. sweat
- g. tea leaves (hallucinogens)
- G. technique, Indocyanine
- g. test for diplopia ▸ Lancaster's red-
- g. tobacco sickness
- g. urine from antidepressant
- g. viscous bile ▸ dark

Greene sign
Greenfield vena cava filter
Greenough microscope
greenstick fracture
gregarium, Myconostoc
Gregory Pell sectioning technique
Greig syndrome
grelot, bruit de
grenade-thrower fracture
grenz ray
grenz ray treatment
Greulich and Pyle ▸ bone age according to
grew organisms, culture
grey (*see*** gray)**
- g. code
- g. column, anterior
- g. column, posterior
- g. column, ventral

greyhound therapy
Grice stabilization
Grice-Green operation
grid (Grid)
- g., Amsler
- g., baby
- g., Bucky
- g. cassette
- g. cassette, camp
- g., external
- g., focused
- g., moving
- g. 1
- g., oscillating
- g., parallel

- g., Potter-Bucky
- g. ratio
- g., stationary
- g. technique
- G. Test, Amsler
- g. 2
- g., Wetzel

grief
- g., actual
- g., acute
- g. and loss counseling
- g. and mourning
- g. and mourning ▸ children's
- g. and separation
- g., anticipatory
- g. assessment
- g., attention span in
- g., chronic
- g. counseling
- g. counselor
- g. cycle, adult
- g. education
- g. education, general
- g., excessive
- g., impacted
- g., maladaptive
- g., normal
- g. ▸ overwhelming feelings of sadness and
- g., physical symptoms in
- g. process
- g., prolonged
- g., prophetic dimension of
- g. reaction
- g. reaction with depression
- g. recovery
- g., resolution of
- g., spiritual dimension of
- g. support group
- g. therapist
- g. therapy
- g., traumatic
- g., unresolved
- g. worker

grievance procedure
grieving
- g., dysfunctional
- g. process
- g. process ▸ normal
- g. process, therapeutic

Griffa (marijuana)
griffe, main en
grimacing
- g., and spasm ▸ twitching,
- g., facial

g. in pain
g., patient
grinders'
    g. asthma
    g. disease
    g. phthisis
grinding
g. disorder, teeth
g., jaw
g. ‣ nocturnal teeth
g. of teeth
g. of teeth ‣ clenching and
g. of teeth, night
g. pain
grinds teeth, patient
grip
g., devil's
g., loss of
g., Pawlik's
g. strength
g. strength ‣ hand
grippe, la
grippotyphosa, Leptospira
grisea, Madurella
Gritti amputation
Gritti-Stokes amputation
gritty ‣ eye dry and
gritty feeling in eye
groaning murmur
Groenouw's dystrophy
groin, bubonic lymphadenopathy of
groin complications
grooming
g. and hygiene
g., and toileting ‣ eating,
g., decline in personal
g. ‣ dressing, bathing, feeding,
g. ‣ loss of interest in personal
g. self-care deficit
groove(s)
g., arterial
g. artery ‣ left atrioventricular (LAV)
g., atrioventricular
g., auriculoventricular
g., bulboventricular
g., conoventricular fold and
g. created
g., deltopectoral
g. depression
g. ‣ free gingival
g., Harrison
g., interatrial
g., intercondylar
g., intercostal
g., limbal

g., linear
g. meningioma, olfactory
g., pectoral
g., peroneal
g., sinus
g. stitched together ‣ tongue-and-
g. suture ‣ tongue-and-
g., terminal
g., vascular
g., venous
g., Verga's lacrimal
g., vertical
g., vomerine
grooved nails, brittle
grooved tongue
gross (Gross)
g. adenopathy
g. alteration
g. anatomy
g. and fine-motor coordination
g. anomalies
g. appearance, normal
g. bleeding or perforation
g. blood
g. changes, abnormal
g. continuity broken
g. continuity not broken
g. defects
g. deformity
g. description
g. distortion
g. evidence
g. examination
g. examination, autopsy
g. hematuria
g. hemorrhage
g. lesion
g. morphology
g. neurological parameters
g. pathological process
g. pyuria
g. stress reaction
g. testing
G. tracheoesophageal atresia
G. tracheoesophageal fistula
g. tumor
G. virus
G. virus antigen
grossly
g. cloudy, fluid
g. congested, spleen
g. disorganized behavior
g. intact, cranial nerves
g. normal
g. preserved

g. purulent material
g. purulent, sputum
g. symmetrical, brain
g. unremarkable
Grossman('s)
G. operation
G. scale
G. sign
ground(s)
g. bundles
g. connection
g. emesis, coffee
g. for arrest
g. -glass appearance
g. -glass opacification
g. -glass pathway
g. illumination, dark-
g. itch anemia
g. state
g. substance
g. water contamination
group(s) (Group) [*loop*]
g. A, B, AB, O ‣ blood
G. A beta hemolytic streptococci
G. A beta streptococcal pharyngitis
g. A Streptococcus ‣ autopsy-
    acquired
g. activities
g. agglutinin
G., Al-Anon
G., Al-Anon Family
G., Alateen
g., alcohol
G. Alert
g. and family therapy
g. anorexia support
g. antigens, blood
g. average, age-
g. bereavement recovery
g., bereavement support
g., blood
g. care
g., cognitive therapy
g., coli-aerogenes
g., colon-typhoid dysentery
g., combined-treatment
G., Community Self-Help
g., community support
g., complementophil
g., control
g., conventional therapy
g., correctional
g. counseling
g. counseling ‣ multi-family
g. cytophil

group(s)—*continued*

g. desensitization and relaxation
G. (DRG) ▸ Diagnosis-Related
g. (DRG), diagnostic-related
g., divorce support
g., drug treatment
g., drug-using peer
G., Dual Diagnosis
g., dysfunctional
g., endogenous
g., ergophore
g. exercises for enhancing social skills
g., family support
g. feedback
g. for Alzheimer's disease ▸ support
g. for epilepsy ▸ support
g. for infections, risk
g. for paraplegics ▸ support
g. for quadriplegics ▸ support
g., glucophore
g., Gonzales blood
g., grief support
g., haptophore
g., heboid-paranoid
g., hemorrhagic-septicemia
g., high-frequency blood
g., high-risk
g. home
g., hog cholera
g. ▸ inability to play in
g. ▸ intensive therapy
g. interaction
g. ▸ interactive process-oriented
g., isoxazolyl
g. junkie, support
g. ▸ long-term support
g., low-frequency blood
g. ▸ low-stress treatment
g., major motor
g. medical examination
g. medicine
g. meeting, peer
g. methods
g., methyl
g. modalities
g., multidisciplinary
g. ▸ multiple skills
g., multispecialty medical
g., muscle
g. ▸ mutual aid
g., negative-calorie food
g. of microorganisms ▸ exogenous
g., open-ended support

g., osmophore
g. ▸ pacemaker support
g., pain support
g., paratyphoid-enteritidis
g., patient sub-
g. (DRG) payments, diagnostic-related
g., peer
g., peptide
g., placebo control
g. play therapy ▸ directive
g., prosthetic
g., proteus
g., pseudomallei
g. psychotherapy
g. reaction
g., recovery
g., referral to support
g., relapsed
g. resistant, isoxazolyl
g., Rhesus (Rh) blood
g., saccharide
g., salmonella
g., sapophore
g., self-help
g. ▸ self-help support
g., self-improvement
g. services, support
g. session
g., sexual abuse
g. situation
g. -specific
g. -specific component
g. ▸ strengthen and tone muscle
g. ▸ structured adolescent psychotherapy
g. substances, blood
g., sulfonic
g. support
g. support sessions
g., susceptible
g. system, blood
g., tension in feedback
g. ▸ thematic process
g. therapy
g. therapy, daily
g. therapy, family
g. therapy, psychoeducational
g. therapy sessions
g. therapy, small
g. therapy ▸ solution-focused
g. ▸ topic-oriented process
G. ▸ Tough Love Parents Support
g., toxophore
g. -transfer

g. treatment for children
g. treatment of insomnia
g. type ▸ conduct disorder,
g. ▸ youth/parent support

grouping

g., antigenic structural
g., haptenic
g., histopathologic
g. specific substances ▸ blood

Grover's disease

grow ▸ villus hairs to thicken and

growing

g. acoustic neuroma ▸ slow-
g. brain tumor ▸ rapidly
g. cortical neoplasm, slow
g. fracture
g. in bone ▸ lump
g. invasive adenocarcinoma ▸ slowly
g. lesion, rapidly
g. neoplasm, rapidly
g. pains
g. tumor
g. tumor ▸ fast
g. tumor, rapidly
g. tumor, slowly
g. virus, slow

growling, intestinal

growling stomach

growth(s)

g., abnormal bone
g. ▸ abnormal brain
g., abnormal hair
g., abnormal mass of tissue
g. abnormality
g., adaptive
g. after 48 hours incubation
g. and breakdown, bone
g. and development, altered
g. and development ▸ fetal
g. and development, normal
g. and maturation ▸ epiphyseal chondroblastic
g. and maturation of new skin
g. and preserved ▸ generic skin
g. and transformation
g., anorectal
g. arrest
g., axonal
g., bacterial
g., benign
g. ▸ blood vessel
g., bone
g., bony
g., cancer

g., cancerous
g., cartilaginous
g., cell
g., cellular
g., circumscribed new
g., constitutional delayed
g., culture negative for
g. cycle
g. deficiency
g. deficiency ▸ postnatal
g., disordered bone
g., disproportionate
g., distorted cell
g., division and function cell
g., erratic cell
g. ▸ excessive facial hair
g. ▸ excessive hair
g., exophytic-type
g. factor
g. factor, acidic fibroblast
g. factor, basic fibroblast
G. Factor (EGF), Epidermal
g. factor ▸ insulin-like
g. factor (NGF), nerve
g. factor (PDGF) ▸ platelet-derived
g. factor (VEGF) therapy ▸ vascular endothelial
g. factor ▸ transforming
G. Factor (TGF), Tumor
g. factor (VEGF) ▸ vascular endothelial
g. factors (NGF) ▸ nerve
g. ▸ faulty bone
g., fetal
g. ▸ firm, red, nodular, or flat
g., fleshy
g. fraction
g., fungal
g. genes, cell
g., Gompertzian tumor
g., hair
g., head
g., Hodgkin's-like
g. hormone
g. hormone, artificial
g. hormone, biosynthetic human
g. hormone deficiency
g. hormone deficiency ▸ human
g. hormone failure
g. hormone, Genentech biosynthetic human
g. hormone (HGH), human
g. hormone, immunoreactive human
g. hormone, natural

g. hormone, pituitary
g. hormone, placental
g. hormone prolactin ▸ chorionic
g. hormone releasing factor
g. hormone, synthetic human
g. hormone therapy, supplemental
g., impaired
g. in ear ▸ bone
g. ▸ increased hair
g. ▸ inhibit nerve cell
g., inhibit tumor
g. inhibition
g. inhibitor, nerve
g. ▸ interference with intellectual and emotional
g. interval
g., malignant
g., neoplastic
g., noncancerous
g. ▸ noncancerous skin
g., normal fetal
g. of blood cells ▸ cancerous
g. of blood vessels ▸ invasive
g. of cancer ▸ uncontrolled cell
g. of cells, progressive
g. of facial hair
g. of neuronal connections, abnormal
g. of prostate ▸ stimulate
g. of spine ▸ abnormal bone
g. of tissue ▸ nodular
g. of tissues, progressive
g. of tumor, inhibit
g. on feet, bacterial
g. on finger joint ▸ knobby
g., osteocartilaginous
g. pattern
g., pedunculated
g., personal
g. phase of facial hair
g., physical
g., pigmented
g. plate, epiphyseal
g. plates ▸ bone
g., precancerous
g., precancerous cervical
g., primary
g. process, abnormal
g. process, psychophysiological
g. ▸ prostate cell
g., protein stimulate
g., protruding
g., psychological
g., rapid muscle
g. rate

g. rate, fast
g. rate, intrauterine
g. rate, slow
g. ▸ retard fetal
g. retardation
g. retardation in children
g. retardation (IUGR), intrauterine
g., retarded
g., revitalize hair
g., scar-like
g., secondary
g., skin
g., slow
g. ▸ slow down cancer
g., slow fetal
g., small
g., social
g., spurts
g., stimulate new vessel
g., stimulates bone
g. -stimulating hormones
g. stimulator, implantable bone
g., stunted
g., suppression of tumor
g., testicular
g., tissue
g. tumor
g. ▸ uncontrolled cell division
g., wart-like
Gruber('s)
  G. hernia
  G., petrospheno-occipital suture of
  G. -Widal reaction
grumose (*same as* grumous)
grumous debris
grumous material
Grünfelder's reflex
Grüning's magnet
grunt(s)
  g. and squeals
  g. and squeals ▸ patient
  g., audible
  g., diastolic
grunting
  g. and retractions
  g., expiratory
  g. ▸ infant retracting and
  g. or retraction
  g. respirations
  g., retraction or
Grunwald-Giemsa stain ▸ May-Grynfeltt hernia
GSD (genetically significant dose)
GSR (galvanic skin reflex)
GSR (galvanic skin response)

gt (drop)
GTT (glucose tolerance test)
gtt (drops)
G2 (grid 2)
GU
    GU (gastric ulcer)
    GU (genitourinary) cancer
    GU (genitourinary) infection,
        Chlamydia
    GU (genitourinary) problems
        related to drug abuse
    GU (genitourinary) tract
guaiac
    g., bicolor
    g. -negative stool
    g. -positive stool
    g. test of stool
Guaiacolate, glyceryl
guajava, Psidium
Guama virus
Guanarito virus
guanidinoacetic acid
guanine cytosine
guanine phosphoribosyl transferase
    ▸ hypoxanthine
guanosine triphosphate
guar gum
guard [*hard*]
guard, Sachs'
guarded postoperative period
guarded, prognosis
guardian, court-appointed
guardian, patient's legal
guarding
    g., abdominal muscle
    g. and/or rebound
    g. and/or rigidity
    g., muscle
    g. or rigidity ▸ rebound,
    g., patient exhibited muscle
    g., rebound and/or
    g., rigidity and/or
    g., voluntary
Guarnieri's inclusions
Guaroa virus
Guatamahri's nodules
gubernaculum
    g., chorda
    g. dentis
    g., Hunter's
    g. testis
Gubler('s)
    G. hemiplegia
    G. icterus
    G. syndrome, Millard-

Gudden('s)
    G. atrophy
    G. commissure
    G., nucleus of
    G. tract
Guepar hinge knee prosthesis
Guérin('s)
    G. (BCG) ▸ bacille Calmette-
    G. fold
    G. fracture
    G. (BCG) immunization ▸ bacille
        Calmette-
    G. (BCG) vaccine ▸ bacille
        Calmette-
Guerry cataract implant lens, Lieb
    and
guidance
    g., career
    g., echo
    g., fluoroscopic
    g., vocational
guide
    g., adjustable anterior
    g., anterior
    g. catheter
    g., incisal
    g. inclination, condylar
    g. pin
    g. suture
guided
    g. biopsy, catheter-
    g. biopsy ▸ image-
    g. bronchoscopy ▸ ultrasound-
    g. endoscopic intubation, catheter-
    g. imagery
    g. imagery ▸ biofeedback and
    g. imagery therapist
    g. injection therapy ▸ ultrasound-
    g. into bladder, sound
    g. laser beam ▸ computer-
    g. laser-induced prostatectomy
        (TULIP) ▸ transurethral
        ultrasound-
    g. laser beam, computer-
    g. lasik (laser-assisted in situ
        keratomileusis) surgery ▸
        wavefront-
    g. medial therapy ▸ ischemia
    g. open biopsy ▸ imaging-
    g. pericardiocentesis, echo-
    g. procedure ▸ image-
    g. relaxation
    g. surgical resection, activation
        map-
    g. surgical technique, image-

    g. therapy, angina-
    g. ultrasound ▸ echo-
guideline(s)
    g., clasp
    g., dietary
    g., government-mandated
    g., income poverty
guidewire perforation
guiding catheter, angioplasty
Guiffrida-Ruggieri stigma
Guilford stapedectomy technique
Guilford-Zimmerman personality test
Guillain-Barré
    G. polyneuritis
    G. syndrome
    G. syndrome, Landry-
Guilland's sign
guilliermondi, Candida
guillotine amputation
guillotine technique
guilt
    g. and shame
    g. and survival ▸ surviving
    g. complex
    g., deep-seated
    g., delusions of
    g., excessive
    g. ▸ excessive or inappropriate
    g. feelings
    g. ▸ feelings of excessive feeling of
        inappropriate
    g. feelings, patient expressed
    g., inappropriate
    g., increased
    g. ▸ low self-esteem or
    g., or depression ▸ anxiety-
    g. over disloyalty
    g. ▸ persistent feelings of
    g. reaction
    g. ▸ sense of
    g., shame and
    g., survivor
    g., worthlessness and helplessness
        ▸ feeling of
guilty
    g., ashamed and intimidated
    g. ▸ patient feels
    g. ruminations
guinea (Guinea)
    G. Pig ABS
    g. pig inoculation
    g. wing
    g. worm
Guinon, tic de
Guist sphere implant

Guleke-Stookey operation
Gulf War syndrome
gull murmur, sea◊
Gull's renal epistaxis
Gullstrand's law
Gullstrand's slit lamp
gum(s) [*drum*]
- g. acacia
- g., bleeding
- g. care ▸ periodontal
- g., discoloration of
- g. disease
- g. disease, advanced
- g. disease, serious
- g. from dentures ▸ red
- g., guar
- g. infected
- g. infection
- g. infection ▸ chronic
- g., inflamed
- g. inflammation
- g. lancet
- g. line
- g., nicotine
- g. ▸ physical dependence on nicotine
- g., prescription
- g. problems from aging
- g., receded
- g. recession
- g., red and puffy
- g. ▸ red, swollen, tender
- g. shrinkage
- g., shrinking
- g., swelling of
- g. ▸ swollen and tender
- g. tissue
- g. tissue breakdown
- g. tissue ▸ eroding

gumma
- g., miliary
- g., rib
- g., scrofulous
- g., tuberculous

gummatous meningitis
gummifer, Bursera
gummosa, periarteritis
gummy clots
gun (Gun)
- g. approach, shot-
- g. -barrel enterostomy
- g. cough, minute
- G. Hill, hemoglobin
- g. injury, pressure
- g., skin

Gunderson conjunctival flap
Gunn('s)
- G. crossing sign
- G. dot
- G. phenomenon, Marcus
- G. syndrome
- G. syndrome, Marcus

gunshot wound
Günther's disease
Günther's syndrome
Gupta bodies
Gurd operation, Mumford-
gurgle test ▸ water
gurgling rales
gurney (*same as* guerney)
gurney, patient transported on
GUS (genitourinary system)
gustatoria, anosmia
gustatory
- g. anesthesia
- g. audition
- g. cells
- g. center
- g. epilepsy
- g. hallucination
- g. stimuli

gustolacrimal reflex
gut [*cut*]
- g. -associated
- g. -associated lymphoid tissue (GALT)
- g., blind
- g., development of
- g. intestinal cells
- g., lumen of the
- g. peptide, brain
- g., plain
- g., postanal
- g., preoral
- g., primitive
- g., ribbon
- g., silkworm
- g. suture, chromic
- g. suture, plain
- g. suture, silkworm
- g. syndrome ▸ short
- g. syndrome, slick-
- g., tail
- g., upper

Guthrie's muscle
gutless organisms
Gutman unit
gutta-percha
gutta-percha, baseplate
guttata, cornea

guttata senilis, choroiditis
guttate hypomelanosis ▸ idiopathic
gutter(s)
- g. fracture
- g. ▸ packing of paracolic
- g., paracolic
- g., pelvic

guttulatus, Saccharomyces
guttulatus, Saccharomycopsis
guttural
- g. pulse
- g. rales
- g. sound

Gutzeit's operation
Guyon's amputation
Guyon's canal
Guyton-Friedenwald suture
Guyton's suture
GVH (graft-versus-host)
GVHD (graft-versus-host disease)
GVHD ▸ life-threatening (graft-versus-host disease)
GVHR (graft-versus-host reaction)
gymnastics injury
Gymneman sylvestre
GYN (gynecology)
gynecoid
- g. fat distribution
- g. pelvis
- g. pelvis, adequate

gynecologic
- g. applicators, intracavitary
- g. cryosurgery
- g. examination
- g. examination annually ▸ complete
- g. infection
- g. lesions
- g. malignancy
- g. oncology
- g. urology

gynecological
- g. care
- g. disease, benign
- g. examination
- g. examination, routine
- g. history
- g. infection, nosocomial
- g. malignancy
- g. oncologist

gynecology and obstetrics
gynecomastia
- g., irradiation for
- g., male
- g. surgery

gynefold pessary

gypseum, Microsporum
gypseum, Trichophyton
gyri
- g. and/or sulci
- g., annectant
- g. breves insulae
- g. cerebri
- g. insulae
- g., lateral occipital
- g. of cerebrum
- g. of insula, short
- g. operti
- g., orbital
- g. orbitales
- g., preinsular
- g. profundi cerebri
- g. temporales transverse
- g. transitivi cerebri
- g., transverse temporal

gyriform carcinoma
gyrous area
gyrus
- g., angular
- g. angularis
- g., anterior central
- g., anterior transverse temporal
- g., ascending frontal
- g., Broca's
- g., callosal
- g. callosus
- g. centralis anterior
- g. centralis posterior
- g. cerebelli
- g., cingulate
- g. cinguli
- g., dentate
- g. dentatus
- g. fasciolaris
- g. fornicatus
- g. frontalis inferior
- g. frontalis medialis
- g. frontalis medius
- g. frontalis superior
- g., fusiform
- g. fusiformis
- g. geniculi
- g. herniation
- g., Heschl's
- g., hippocampal
- g. hippocampi
- g., inferior frontal
- g., inferior occipital
- g., inferior temporal
- g., infracalcarine
- g., infracalcarinus

- g., lateral occipitotemporal
- g. limbicus
- g., lingual
- g. lingualis
- g. longus insulae
- g., marginal
- g. marginalis
- g., medial occipitotemporal
- g., middle frontal
- g., middle temporal
- g. occipitotemporalis lateralis
- g. occipitotemporalis medialis
- g. of brain ▸ superior insular
- g. of insula, long
- g. of Turner, marginal
- g. olfactorius lateralis of Retzius
- g. olfactorius medialis
- g. olfactorius medialis of Retzius
- g., paracentral
- g. paracentralis
- g., parahippocampal
- g. parahippocampalis
- g., paraterminal
- g. paraterminalis
- g., parietal
- g. postcentralis
- g., posterior central
- g., precentral
- g. precentralis
- g., quadrate
- g. rectus
- g., subcallosal
- g. subcallosus
- g., subcollateral
- g., superior frontal
- g., superior occipital
- g., superior temporal
- g., supracallosal
- g. supracallosus
- g., supramarginal
- g. supramarginalis
- g., temporal
- g. temporalis inferior
- g. temporalis medius
- g. temporalis superior
- g., uncinate
- g. uncinatus

H

H
- H (heroin)
- H (heroin) abuser, Big
- H (heroin) addict, Big
- H (heroin) addiction, Big
- H (heroin), Big
- H (heroin) dependency, Big
- H (heroin) habit, Big
- H (heroin) substance
- H (heroin) user, Big
- H (heroin) withdrawal
- H (hypo)
- H incision, lazy

H agglutination
H agglutinin
H and P (history and physical)
H. (Hauch) colony
H factor
H graft ▸ portacaval
H, hemoglobin
H, influenza
h plateau
H rays
H space
H wave
- h. arteriolar nephrosclerosis
- H. arteriosclerosis
- h. carcinoma
- h. cartilage
- h. cast
- h. degeneration
- h. formation in cornea
- h. membrane
- h. membrane disease (HMD)
- h. scarred foci

HA lines
Haab('s)
- H. -Dimmer degeneration ▸ Biber-
- H. magnet
- H. reflex

Haag-Streit slit lamp
HAART (highly active antiretroviral therapy)
Haas' operation
Haas position
Haase's rule
habenular commissure
habit(s)

- h., alcohol
- h., altered bowel
- h., apoplectic
- h., asthenic
- h., bad dietary
- h., Big H (heroin)
- h., bladder
- h., bowel
- h., change in bladder
- h., change in bowel
- h. ▸ change in eating or sleeping
- h., change in sexual
- h., changing
- h. chorea
- h., chronic
- h., clamping
- h., dietary
- h. disorder, stereotype
- h., drinking
- h., drug
- h., eating
- h., endothelioid
- h., erratic eating
- h. forming
- h. -forming drugs
- h., glaucomatous
- h., good eating
- h., health
- h., healthy dietary
- h., healthy lifestyle
- h., heroin (Big H)
- h., kicking drug
- h., kicking smoking
- h. ▸ kicking the
- h., leptosomatic
- h., leukocytoid
- h., LSD (lysergic acid diethylamide)
- h., modify stressful living
- h. of blame ▸ parental
- h. of praise ▸ parental
- h., opium
- h., oral
- h., physiologic
- h., poor dietary
- h., pycnic
- h. reversal
- h., revising sleep

- h., sedentary
- h. ▸ self-injurious
- h. ▸ severe nail-biting
- h., smoking
- h., stable eating
- h., visual

habitation, sexual co-
habitual
- h. abortion
- h. behavior
- h. cocaine smokers
- h. dislocation
- h. drinking
- h. eye rubbing
- h. fantasizer
- h. labor
- h. occlusion
- h. patterns

habituation
- h., alcohol
- h. and balance rehabilitation
- h. and overdose
- h., drug
- h., environmental
- h., impaired
- h., poor

habitus (LBBH) ▸ limited by body
habitus ▸ patient's body
hack, smoker's
hacing
- h. cough
- h. cough, dry
- h. cough ▸ persistent

had
- h. elevated temperature ▸ patient
- h. evidence of show ▸ patient
- h. face lift ▸ patient
- h. fit ▸ patient
- h. flashback reactions from drug abuse ▸ patient
- h. gastrocystostomy ▸ patient
- h. mini-peel ▸ patient
- h. previous workup ▸ patient
- h. relapse of disease ▸ patient
- h. respiratory arrest ▸ patient
- h. sclerotherapy ▸ patient

had—*continued*
  h. seizure ‣ patient
  h. steady downhill course ‣ patient
  h. stillbirth ‣ patient
  h. stormy course ‣ patient
  h. uneventful postoperative course
    ‣ patient
Hadefield syndrome, Clarke-
Haemadipsa
  H. ceylonica
  H. chiliani
  H. japonica
  H. zeylandica
Haemaphysalis
  H. concinna
  H. humerosa
  H. leachi
  H. leporispalustris
  H. punctata
  H. spinigera
Haematobia irritans
haematobium, Schistosoma
haematodes, fungus
Haematosiphon indorus
Haementeria officinalis
Haemobartonella canis
Haemobartonella muris
Haemodipsus ventricosus
haemolyticum, Clostridium
haemolyticum, Corynebacterium
haemolyticus, Staphylococcus
Haemonchus contortus
Haemonchus placei
Haemophilus (haemophilus) [*same*
  ***as* Hemophilus]**
  H. aegyptius
  H. aphrophilus
  H. bovis
  H. bronchisepticus
  H. ducreyi
  H. duplex
  H. endocarditis
  H. hemoglobinophilus
  H. hemolyticus
  H. influenzae, gram-negative
  H. influenzae infection
  H. influenzae meningitis
  H. influenzae pneumonia
  h., Koch-Weeks
  h., Morax-Axenfeld
  H. parahemolyticus
  H. parainfluenzae
  H. parapertussis
  H. pertussis
  H. pertussis, gram-negative

  H. pertussis vaccine
  H. suis
  H. vaginalis
Haemopis paludum
Haemopis sanguisuga
Haemoproteus
  H. columbae
  H. danielewskyi
  H. noctuae
  H. passeris
haemorrhagica
  h., achylia gastrica
  h., otitis
  h., purpura
  h., retinitis
haemorrhoidalis, Sarcophaga
Haemosporidia, Sporozoa
Haenel's symptom
Hafnia alvei
hafniae, Enterobacter
hag teeth
Hageman factor
hageni, Otomyces
Hagie hip pin
Haglund's deformity
Haidinger's brushes
Haik's implant
hair(s)
  h., absence of facial and pubic
  h. analysis test
  h. and blood ‣ semen,
  h., arm
  h., arrector muscles of
  h., auditory
  h., bamboo
  h., beaded
  h. bearing area
  h. bearing graft
  h., body
  h. bulb
  h., burrowing
  h. cell
  h. cell, acoustic
  h. cell in ear
  h. cell, inner
  h. cell, outer
  h. cell receptors ‣ damaged
  h. cells, inner ear
  h. cells, sensory
  h., chest
  h., club
  h., coarse scalp
  h. cycle
  h. decreased, body
  h. ‣ dermatophyte infections of

  h. disease ‣ kinky
  h. distribution, body
  h., dry skin and
  h., excess facial
  h., exclamation point
  h., facial
  h., fine
  h. follicle
  h. follicle ‣ infected
  h. follicles ‣ segmental analysis
  h., Frey's
  h. from aging ‣ graying
  h. from anemia ‣ limp
  h., functional subunit
  h. germ
  h. graft
  h. growth
  h. growth, abnormal
  h. growth ‣ excessive
  h. growth ‣ excessive facial
  h. growth ‣ increased
  h. ‣ growth of facial
  h. ‣ growth phase of facial
  h. growth, revitalize
  h., ingrown
  h., knotted
  h., lanugo
  h. -like cell
  h. loss
  h. loss and nausea
  h. loss ‣ female-pattern
  h. loss from antidepressant
  h. loss from birth control pill
  h. loss from childbirth
  h. loss, minoxidil and
  h. loss, temporary
  h. loss treatment
  h. loss ‣ treatment for
  h., masculine pubic
  h. matrix
  h. -matrix carcinoma
  h., micrografting
  h., mole
  h., moniliform
  h. movement, fine
  h., nasal
  h., normal distribution of
  h. normal texture
  h. of eyebrow
  h. of nose
  h. of pubis
  h. on end
  h. on head
  h. papilla
  h. papilla, capillary loop in

h. ▸ patient pulls
h. pigment, regenerate
h. -producing region
h., pubic
h. pulling, compulsive
h. pulling ▸ pathological
h. (RIAH) ▸ radioimmunoassay of
h., regrow
h. removal
h. removal ▸ laser
h. removal treatment
h. removal treatment ▸ laser
h. replacement
h. replacement surgery
h., resting
h. ▸ resting phase of facial
h. restoration surgery
h. ▸ restore lost or thinning
h., sensory
h. shaft
h. shedding, excessive
h., stellate
h., superfluous
h., tactile
h., taste
h. teeth
h., terminal
h. testing
h., thigh
h., thinning
h. to thicken and grow ▸ villus
h. transplant
h. transplanting
h. transplantation
h. -trigger gag reflex
h., twisted
h. unit
h., vellus
h., woolly

hairline
h. fracture
h. fracture of rib
h., low
h. of brow
h., receding

hairpin loop

hairy
h. cell leukemia
h. ears
h. heart
h. leukoplakia
h. leukoplakia, oral-
h. nevus
h. tongue
h. tongue, black

Hakim shunt, Cordis-
Hakim-Cordis pump
HAL (hemorrhoidal artery ligation)
Halban's disease
Halban's sign
Halbeisen syndrome, Stryker-
Halberstaedter bodies, Prowazek-
Halbrecht's syndrome
half
h. amplitude pulse duration
h. -axial projection
h. body irradiation, field size in
h. -cap crown
h. -field, visual
h. -hour interval
h. -life
h. -life, biological
h. -life, effective
h. -life, elimination
h. -life, physical
h. -life, serum
h. -life ▸ short
h. maximum (FWHM), full width at
h. -power distance
h. -retinal
h. sit-ups
h. -thickness
h. -thickness, narrow-beam
h. -time, gastric-emptying
h. -time method
h. -time of exchange
h. -time ▸ pressure
h. -time technique ▸ pressure
h., upper
h. -value
h. -value layer (HVL)
h. -value thickness
h. vision

halfway house
h.h. for alcoholics
h.h. for drug addicts
h.h. for mentally retarded
h.h. for penal rehabilitation
h.h. for physically handicapped
h.h. for runaways
h.h. placement

halitosis, chronic
Hall
H. device ▸ Medtronic-
H. heart valve prosthesis ▸
    Medtronic-
H. -Kaster mitral valve prosthesis
H. sign, Soto-
H. tilting disk valve prosthesis ▸
    Medtronic-

Hallauer's glasses
Hallermann-Streiff syndrome
Haller's layer
Hallervorden-Spatz syndrome
Hallopeau's acrodermatitis
Hallpike
H. caloric stimulation response
H. caloric stimulation test
H. maneuver
H. maneuver ▸ Dix-

hallucinating, patient
hallucinating, patient actively
hallucination(s)
h., active
h. and delusions
h. and delusions ▸ schizophrenic
h. and incoherent thinking
h. and loss of reality
h., auditory
h., command
h., delusions and paranoia
h. ▸ delusions or
h., depressive
h., derogatory
h. ▸ distorted visual images and
h., drug-induced
h. from alcohol
h. from brain
h., gustatory
h., haptic
h., hypnagogic
h., hypnopompic
h. ▸ inhalant-induced
h., kinesthetic
h., lilliputian
h., minor
h. ▸ occasional auditory
h. ▸ occasional tactile
h., olfactory
h., patient has disorientation and
h., possible
h., prominent
h., recurring
h., reflex
h., religious
h., schizophrenic
h., stump
h., tactile
h., transitory
h., visual
h., vivid
h. ▸ vivid visual, auditory and
    olfactory

hallucinatory
h. emotional experiences

hallucinatory—*continued*
- h. experience
- h. mania, acute
- h. neuralgia
- h. odor
- h. paranoia
- h. paranoia, acute
- h. state induced by drugs
- h. visions
- h. voices

hallucinogen(s)
- h. (Cogentin)
- h. (Magic Mushroom)
- h. (Mappine)
- h. (moon)
- h. (Morning Glory seeds)
- h. (PCP)
- h. (PCP/PeaCe Pill)
- h. (Sacred Mushroom)
- h. (Silly Putty)
- h. (Supergrass)
- h. (Superjoint)
- h. (Surfer)
- h. (T)
- h. (Tic Tac)
- h. (Tranq)
- h. abuse
- h. abuse, pattern of
- h. abuse, physical effects of
- h., abuse potential of
- h. abuse, prevalence of
- h. abusers, assessing needs of
- h., acute intoxication with
- h. delusional disorder
- h., dependence on
- h., flashback reactions with
- h. hallucinosis
- h., mode of administration with
- h. mood disorder
- h., organic brain syndrome with
- h., overdose with
- h., panic reactions with
- h., patient OD (overdosed) with
- h. persisting perception disorder
- h., potential tolerance to
- h., psychoactive doses of
- h., psychoactive properties of
- h., psychological effects of
- h., short-acting
- h., tolerance to
- h., toxicity of
- h., treatment of acute drug reactions to
- h., (LSD) user
- h., withdrawal from

hallucinogenic
- h. amphetamine
- h. drug interactions
- h. drug intoxication
- h. effects
- h. mushrooms

hallucinosis
- h., acute
- h., alcohol withdrawal
- h., alcoholic
- h., drug-induced
- h., hallucinogen
- h., organic
- h. syndrome, organic

hallucis
- h. brevis muscle, extensor
- h. brevis muscle, flexor
- h. longus muscle, extensor
- h. longus muscle, flexor
- h. muscle, adductor

hallux
- h. dolorosa
- h. malleus
- h. rigidus
- h. valgus
- h. valgus deformity
- h. varus

halo(s)
- h. around lights
- h. cast
- h. cast, supportive
- h., Crutchfield tongs or
- h., Fick's
- h. glaucomatosus
- h. nevus
- h. -pelvic traction
- h. saturninus
- h., senile
- h. traction
- h. vision

Halobacterium
- H. cutirubrum
- H. halobium
- H. marismortui
- H. salinarium
- H. trapanicum

halobium, Halobacterium
halogenated hydrocarbon
Halogeton glomeratus
halothane anesthesia
Halpin's operation
Halstead
- H. Category Test
- H. maneuver

- H. Neuropsychological Test Battery for Adults or Children
- H. -Reitan test
- H. -Wepman Aphasia Screening Test

Halsted('s)
- H. incision
- H. operation
- H. radical mastectomy
- H. suture

halter
- h., Forrester-type head
- h., head
- h. traction, Forrester-Brown head
- h. traction, head
- h. traction, Zimfoam head

halting nystagmus
halves, cerebral
Hamamelis virginiana
hamartoma
- h., fetal-renal
- h. (HH) ▸ hypothalamic
- h., intrapulmonary
- h., myocardial
- h. of lung
- h., pulmonary

hamartomatosis, systemic
hamate bone
hamate, capitate and
hamatometacarpal ligament
Hamburger's test
Hamilton('s)
- H. method
- H. Rating Scale
- H. test

Hamman('s)
- H. click
- H. crunch
- H. disease
- H. murmur
- H. Rich syndrome
- H. sign

hammer
- h. bone
- h. finger
- h. ▸ labyrinth area
- h., Mayor's
- h., Neef's
- h. nose
- h. pulse, trip-
- h. pulse, water-
- h. syndrome ▸ hypothenar
- h. toe
- h. toe correction
- h. toe defect

h. toe repair, DuVries
h., Wagner's
hammering head pain
hammocking of posterior mitral leaflet
Hammond's disease
Hammond's operation
Hamm's electrode
Hampton's hump
hamstring(s)
h. curls
h., inner
h. muscles
h., outer
h. stretch exercise
h. ▸ stretching calves, thighs, and
h. tightness
hamular process
Hancock('s)
H. mitral valve prosthesis
H. pericardial valve graft
H. vascular graft
hand(s) (Hand)
h., accoucheur's
h. and feet, peeling of
h. and feet ▸ tingling in
h., ape
h. arthroplasty
h., benediction
h., blanching of
h. -breath coordination
h., callus on
h., carcinoma of
h., carcinomatous arthritis in
h., chiasm of digits of
h. circulation, decreased
h. clapping
h., claw
h., cleft
h. -clenched
h., club
h., cold
h. contracture
h. controls
h. coordination, eye-
h., dead
h. deficit
h. deformity
h., dermatomyositis in
h. dexterity, fine
h., digits of
h. disorder
h., dorsal interosseous muscles of
h., drop
h., dry

h. dry, red, cracked and itchy
h., edema of
h. ▸ electrical stimulation of
h. exercise
h. -eye coordination
h., first through fifth digits of
h. flapping
h., flat
h. flexed at wrist
h., foot and mouth disease
h., fresh cut on
h., frostbite
h., frozen
h., ghoul
h. grasp
h. grip exercise ▸ isometric
h. grip strength
h. grip test ▸ isometric
h. -held defibrillator
h. -held in position of extension
h. -held mammotome
h. injury
h., intercapitular vein of
h., intercostal veins of
h., in tetany ▸ contraction of
h., Krukenberg's
h. ▸ laying on of
h., left major
h., lobster-claw
h., lumbrical muscle of
h., Marinesco's succulent
h., mirror
h., mitten
h., monkey
h. motion ▸ repetitive
h. movements
h., myoelectric
h., numb
h., obstetrician's
h. -off violence
h. -on-care
h., opera-glass
h. or feet ▸ swelling of
h. or tongue, outstretched
h., palm of
h., paw-like
h., phantom
h., poor circulation in
h., preacher's
h. pronated
h. ▸ puffiness of
h., ratio
h., right major
H. -Schüller-Christian disease
H. -Schüller-Christian syndrome

h. scrubs, surgical
h., skeleton
h. smoke, second-
h. smoking, second-
h., spade
h. splinted in flexion
h. splinting
h., split
h. squamous cell carcinoma dorsum of
h. steadiness
h. strength test
h. surgery
H. suture, Perma-
h., swelling of
h. syndrome, heart-
h. syndrome, shoulder-
h. synkinesis, mouth-and-
h., tingling sensations in
h. -to-hand transmission
h. -to-mouth movement
h. transmission, hand-to-
h. transplant
h., transplanted
h., trembling of
h., tremor of
h. tremors, coarse
h., trench
h. trident
h., volar region of
h. washing in critical care areas
h. washing in nursery
h. -washing technique
h. ▸ weakness in
h. /wrist joint replacement
h., writing
handed
h. individual, left-
h. individual, right-
h., left-
h., patient left-
h., patient right-
h., right-
handedness
h., left-
h. ▸ pathological, left-
h., right-
handicap(s)
h., multiple
h., neurologic
h., physical
h., residual
h. ▸ severe disabling
h., social
h., special

handicapped
- h. accessibility
- h. (EMH), educable mentally
- h., halfway house for physically
- h., mentally
- h., neuromuscularly
- h., parking for
- h., patient
- h., physically
- h. (P/MH), physically/multiple
- h., rehabilitation center for physically
- h. (TMH) ▸ trainable mentally
- h., visually

handle
- h. cane, curved-
- h. fracture, bucket-
- h. graft, valise
- h., malleus
- h. tear, bucket-
- h. tear of meniscus ▸ bucket-
- h. traction

handling emotions
Handtrol electrosurgical pencil
handwashing compulsion
handwriting progressively shaky
handwriting, small
Hanger-Rose skin test
Hanger's test
hanging
- h. -block culture
- h. cast
- h. -drop culture
- h. -drop examination
- h. -drop technique
- h. heart
- h. skin

hangman's
- h. break
- h. fracture
- h. injury
- h. surgery

hangout interval
hangover headache
Hanhart's syndrome
Hanlen operation, Blalock-
Hanlen procedure, Blalock-
Hanot('s)
- H. -Chauffard syndrome ▸ Troisier-
- H. cirrhosis
- H. disease
- H. -Rössle syndrome

Hansen('s)
- H. bacillus
- H. disease

H. -Street intramedullary nail
H. -Street pin
hansenii, Debaryomyces
hansenii, Saccharomyces
Hantaan virus
Hantavirus outbreak
Hantavirus pulmonary syndrome
HA1 (type 1 hemadsorption virus)
haptic feedback
HAPE (high-altitude pulmonary edema)
haploscopic vision
happy puppet syndrome
haptenic grouping
haptens loops
haptic hallucination
haptics loops
haptoglobin serum
haptophore group
haptosporus, Basidiobolus
Harada's disease
Harada's syndrome
harboring deep rage
hard [*guard*]
- h. abdomen
- h. alcoholic user
- h. and soft palates
- h. cancer
- h. cataract
- h. core alcoholics
- h. core drug abuser
- h. cyst
- h. drug
- h. drug usage
- h. indurated colon mass
- h. lens
- h. metal disease
- h. -nose strategy
- h. palate
- h. palate, bony
- h. palate, carcinoma of
- h. pulse
- h. rays
- h. stool passage
- h. subcutaneous nodule
- h. ticks
- h. tumor
- h., waxy exudate

hardened tissue
hardening
- h. artifact, beam
- h. artifact, bone
- h. from dermatitis ▸ skin
- h. of aorta
- h. of arteries

- h. of breast tissue
- h. of coronary arteries
- h. of walls of arteries
- h. program, work
- h. tissue

hardness, permanent
hardness, temporary
Hardy sign, Béhier-
Hare test, Hickey-
harelip
- h., acquired
- h., complete
- h., double
- h., incomplete
- h., median
- h., single
- h. suture

Harkins valve prosthesis
Hark's operation
harlequin fetus
harm
- h. ▸ fear of personal
- h. or violence ▸ physical
- h. ▸ potential for self-
- h. reduction
- h. reduction psychotherapy
- h., self
- h. ▸ threats of physical

harmful
- h. antibiotic-resistant bacteria
- h. behavior
- h. side-effects

harming behavior ▸ self-
harmonic component
harmonic content
harmonious movement
harmonious retinal correspondence
Harmon's operation
harmony, functional occlusal
harmony, occlusal
harness, head
harness, Pavlik
Harrington('s)
- H. esophageal diverticulectomy
- H. operation
- H. solution
- H. spinal instrumentation

Harris(')
- H. -Beath operation
- H. broach
- H. HD hip prosthesis
- H. migrainous neuralgia
- H. staining method
- H. syndrome
- H. tube

Harrison('s)
- H. groove
- H. interlocked mesh prosthesis
- H. method

harsh
- h. murmur
- h. pain ▸ constant,
- h. respiration
- h. systolic murmur

Hart position, Gaynor-

Hartel's
- H. method
- H. technique
- H. treatment

Hartford Test, Shipley-

Hartley implant

Hartmann's point pouch

Hartmannella hyalina

hartmanni, Entamoeba

Hartnup's disease

Hartnup's syndrome

Hart's syndrome

Harvard
- H. infusion pump
- H. P.B. test
- H. Spondee Word test

harvest
- h. bone marrow
- h., marrow
- h. mites
- h. organ
- h. tissue

harvested stem cells

harvester's lung

harvesting
- h. ▸ endoscopic vein
- h., organ

has
- h. agoraphobia ▸ patient
- h. brain mets (metastases) ▸ patient
- h. chills ▸ patient
- h. diarrhea ▸ patient
- h. difficulty swallowing ▸ patient
- h. disequilibrium ▸ patient
- h. dry mouth ▸ patient
- h. dysuria ▸ patient
- h. endotracheal tube in place ▸ patient
- h. fear of doctors ▸ patient
- h. fear of hospitals ▸ patient
- h. fibromyalgia ▸ patient
- h. flashbacks ▸ patient
- h. flat affect ▸ patient
- h. floating feeling ▸ patient

- h. forgetfulness, irritability and confusion ▸ patient
- h. frequency of urination ▸ patient
- h. generalized weakness ▸ patient
- h. good rapport with others ▸ patient
- h. headache ▸ patient
- h. heartburn ▸ patient
- h. indigestion ▸ patient
- h. insomnia ▸ patient
- h. interest in surroundings ▸ patient
- h. labored breathing ▸ patient
- h. lack of concentration ▸ patient
- h. leathery skin ▸ patient
- h. lipedema ▸ patient
- h. lockjaw ▸ patient
- h. low energy ▸ patient
- h. lump in throat ▸ patient
- h. lymphedema ▸ patient
- h. mastalgia, patient
- h. memory loss ▸ patient
- h. multiple trauma ▸ patient
- h. natural immunity to hepatitis B virus ▸ patient
- h. needle tracks ▸ patient
- h. neuropathy ▸ patient
- h. nightmares ▸ patient
- h. no interest in surroundings ▸ patient
- h. no purposeful movement ▸ patient
- h. nocturia ▸ patient
- h. occasional palpitations ▸ patient
- h. persistent pain ▸ patient
- h. phobias ▸ patient
- h. polydipsia ▸ patient
- h. polyuria ▸ patient
- h. poor concentration ▸ patient
- h. poor insight ▸ patient
- h. poor memory ▸ patient
- h. potential for violence ▸ patient
- h. progeria ▸ patient
- h. quinsy ▸ patient
- h. rash ▸ patient
- h. religious values ▸ patient
- h. scanning speech ▸ patient
- h. sense of doom, patient
- h. stretchmarks ▸ patient
- h. suicidal tendencies ▸ patient
- h. swelling of upper arm ▸ patient
- h. tachycardia ▸ patient
- h. tantrums ▸ patient
- h. the shakes ▸ patient
- h. toothache ▸ patient

- h. tremors ▸ patient
- h. urinary retention ▸ patient
- h. urostomy ▸ patient
- h. vertigo and unsteadiness ▸ patient
- h. vertigo ▸ patient
- h. whiplash injury ▸ patient

hash (marijuana) (*same as* hashish)
- h. (Goma de Mota)
- h. (hashish)
- h. (Soles)
- h. brownies (hashish)
- h. oil (hashish oil)

Hashimoto's
- H. disease
- H. struma
- H. thyroiditis

hashish
- h. (Black)
- h. (Goma de Mota)
- h. (Grease)
- h. (Hash)
- h. (Honey Oil)
- h. (Smoke)
- h. (Soles)
- h. (Solids)
- h. (Tea)
- h. (Weed Juice)
- h. (Weed Oil)
- h. brownies
- h. oil (Hash Oil)
- h. smoked

Hasner's fold

Hasner's operation

Hassall-Henle warts

Hassall's corpuscles

hata yoga exercise

Hatafuku fundus onlay patch esophageal repair

Hatcher's operation

Hatcher's pin

hate crimes

HA2 (type 2 hemadsorption virus)

Hauch (H.) colony

Hauch (O.) colony ▸ ohne

haughty behavior ▸ arrogant,

Haultaim's operation

haunch bone

haunted womb syndrome

haupt agglutinin

hauptganglion of Küttner

Hauser('s)
- H. operation
- H. procedure
- H. transplant

haustra of colon
haustral
  h. markings
  h. pattern
  h. segmentation
haustrum coli
haut mal epilepsy
HAV (hepatitis A virus)
Haverhill fever
Haverhillia multiformis
haversian canal
Hawaiian (marijuana)
hawaiiensis, Xenopsylla
Hawley appliance
Hay (hay)
  H. (marijuana)
  h. fever
  h. fever, nonseasonal
  h. fever, perennial
  h. fever symptoms
  H. (marijuana) ▸ Indian
Hayem's icterus
Hayem-Widal syndrome
Haygarth's nodes
Haynes' operation
hazard(s)
  h. ▸ alcohol-related health
  h. awareness
  h., environmental
  h. from microwave radiation
  h., health
  h. ▸ indirect foot
  h., infection
  h., occupational
  h. of drinking
  h. of drugs
  h. of smoking
  h. of surgery
  h. of yo-yo dieting
  h., public health
  h., radiation
  h., relapse
hazardous
  h. activity
  h. blood
  h. drugs
  h. spills of fluid
  h. stress
  h. substance ▸ potentially
  h. to health ▸ job
  h. waste
haze (Haze)
  H. (LSD)
  h., hilar
  h. of cornea

H. (LSD), Purple
hazing ritual
hazy
  h. appearance
  h. infiltrate
  h., urine
  h. vision
HB (heart block)
Hb (hemoglobin)
HBc IgM (Antibody "IgM class" to
  Hepatitis B Core Antigen) ▸ Anti-
HBcAb (Hepatitis B core Antibody)
HBe (Antibody to Hepatitis B "e"
  Antigen) ▸ Anti-
HBeAb (Hepatitis B "e" Antibody)
HBeAg (Hepatitis B "e" Antigen)
HBO (hyperbaric oxygen) chamber
HBP (high blood pressure)
HBs (Antibody to Hepatitis B Surface
  Antigen) ▸ Anti-
HBsAb (Hepatitis B surface
  Antibody)
HBsAg (Hepatitis B surface Antigen)
HBsAg (Hepatitis B surface Antigen)
  reactivity
HBV (Hepatitis B virus)
HC (hospital course)
HCG (human chorionic
  gonadotropin) antibody ▸ anti-
HCG (human chorionic
  gonadotropin) molecule
HCT (hematocrit)
HCT ▸ mean circulatory hematocrit
Hct (hematocrit), repeat venous
HCVD (hypertensive cardiovascular
  disease)
HCW (health care workers)
HD
  HD (hearing distance)
  HD (heart disease)
  HD (Hodgkin's disease)
  HD hip prosthesis, Harris
  HD (heart disease), restrictive
  HD II total hip prosthesis
HDD (humor deficit disorder)
HDH (heart disease history)
HDL (high-density lipoprotein)
HDN (hemolytic disease of the
  newborn)
HDPE ▸ (high-density polyethylene)
HDV (hepatitis D virus)
HEA (hemorrhages, exudates and
  aneurysms)
head (Head)
  h. analysis ▸ optic nerve

h. anastomosis, cobra-
h. and neck, clenched muscles in
h. and neck in extended position
h. and neck normal
h. and neck, rhabdomyosarcoma of
h. and trunk ▸ rhythmic instability of
h. assessment ▸ initial
h. birth
h., blow to
h., bone
h. brace
h. cancer
h. cap
h. cap, anterior
h., choking of optic nerve
h. circumference
h. cold
h. compression
h. control
h., contusion of
h., crowning of infant's
h. dependent position
h. dermatitis
h. -down position
h. -down presentation
h. -down tilt test
h. drape, Blair
h., Eicher femoral prosthetic
h., electrodes placed on surface of
h. epiphysis, radial
h. ▸ erythromelalgia of the
h., excessive enlargement of
h. extended
h. extension
h., eyes, ears, nose and throat
  (HEENT)
h., eyes, ears, nose and throat
  (HEENT) not remarkable
h., femoral
h., fetal
h. fold
h., fore◊
h. fracture frame
h. growth
h., hair on
h. halter
h. halter, Forrester-type
h. halter traction
h. halter traction ▸ Forrester-Brown
h. halter traction, Zimfoam
h. harness
h. higher than heart
h. implant, Swanson radial
h. implant, Swanson ulnar
h. injury

h. injury, closed
h. injury ▸ confusion with
h. injury, severe
h. into superior pelvic strait ▸ entrance of fetal
h. jerking
h., Judet-type femoral prosthetic
h., left side of
h. lice
h., longissimus muscle of
h. louse
h. maneuver
h., metacarpal
h., metatarsal
h., molding of
h. motion
h. motion, active
h. movement
h. movement ▸ control
h. movement ▸ rapid
h., Naden-Rieth femoral prosthetic
h., nodding of
h. normocephalic
H. Nurse
h., occipital regions of
h. of bed, elevation of
h. of caudate nucleus
h. of femur
h. of femur ▸ nail inserted into neck and
h. of hair, full
h. of humerus
h. of malleus
h. of pancreas
h. of pancreas ▸ adenocarcinoma in
h. of pancreas, excision
h. of pancreas, carcinoma
h. of pancreas, resection
h. of pterygium
h. of radius
h. of radius, dislocation
h. of radius, resection
h. of talus
h., opposite sides of
h., optic nerve
h. pain
h. pain, blinding
h. pain ▸ hammering
h. pain ▸ intractable
h. pain, unilateral
h. ▸ pointless side-to-side swinging of
h. position

h., posterior intervertebral ganglion of
h., posterior region of
h. prosthesis, Zimaloy femoral
h., radial
h. replacement, endoprosthetic femoral
h. replacement, Matchett-Brown femoral
h. rest, Light-Veley
h. rest, Veley
h., right side of
h. rolling, rocking and crying
h. ▸ rotate fetal
h. scab
h., semispinal muscle of
h. size, small
h., splenius muscle of
h., stuffy
h. subluxation ▸ radial
h., surface of
h., Thompson femoral
h. ▸ throbbing pain in
h. ▸ tight feeling in
h. tilt
h. tilt and chin lift maneuver
h. tilt method
h. tilt test
h. tilt with chin tilt
h. tilt with neck lift
h. tilting
h. to rump length
h., tomographic images of the
h. traction, Crile
h. trauma
h. trauma, coma secondary to
h. trauma, severe
h. tremor
h. unengaged
h. unremarkable
h. up ▸ loss of ability to hold
h. -up tilt table test
h. -up tilt test
h. vein, primary
h. ▸ wedged fetal

headache(s)
h. activity
h. activity and desensitization
h. after spinal tap
h., alcohol-related
h. ameliorated
h. and dizziness
h. and tension
h., anemic
h. ▸ anxiety, tension and

h., autogenic training for
h., autogenic training for migraine
h., bicarb
h., bicranial vascular
h., bifrontal
h., bilious
h., bioccipital
h., biofeedback and
h., biparietal
h., bitemporal
h., blind
h., childhood migraine
h., chronic
h., chronic migraine
h., chronic progressive
h. clinic
h., cluster
h. ▸ cocaine-related vascular
h. ▸ cold food-related
h. ▸ confusion from migraine
h., congestive
h., cough
h. ▸ cough, dyspnea and
h., crippling
h., debilitating
h. disorder ▸ primary
h. ▸ double vision with
h., dynamite
h. exacerbated
h., exertional
h. frequency
h. frequency, reduce tension
h. from alcohol
h. from birth control pill ▸ migraine
h. from caffeine
h. from cold ▸ sinus
h., frontal
h., functional
h., generalized
h., hangover
h., helmet
h., hemicranial vascular
h., histamine
h., histaminic
h., hormone
h., Horton's
h., hunger
h., hyperemic
h., ice cream
h., incapacitating
h., inflammatory
h., intensity of
h., intracranial neoplasm
h., lateralized
h., localized

headache(s)—*continued*
h., lumbar puncture
h. medication
h., migraine
h., miners'
h., Monday morning
h., morning
h., muscle contraction
h., muscle tension
h., nervous tension
h., occipital
h., ocular etiology of
h., one-sided
h., organic
h., pain
h., pain, chronic
h., pain, intense
h. pain ▸ temporary relief of
h., parietal
h. ▸ patient has
h. pattern
h., persistent
h., postcoital
h., postconcussive
h., postdelivery
h., postlumbar puncture
h., postspinal
h. ▸ post-traumatic
h. preceded by aura, classic
h., primary
h., puncture
h., pyrexial
h., rebound
h. ▸ recurrent excruciating
h., recurring
h. reduction
h., reflex
h., rhinogenous
h. secondary to cervical spine
  disease
h., severe
h. ▸ severe throbbing
h., sex
h., sick
h., sinus
h., soda
h., spinal
h., stress
h., stress-related
h., sudden
h. ▸ sudden, severe
h., symptomatic
h. ▸ syncopal migraine
h. syndrome, vascular
h., temporal

h., tension
h. therapy
h. therapy, relaxation response in
h., throbbing
h., thunderclap
h., toxic
h., traction
h., traumatic
h. triggers
h. ▸ tumor-caused
h. ▸ unilateral throbbing
h., vacuum
h., vascular
h., vascular flow
h., vasomotor
h., vertex
h., voluntary control of tension
h., vomiting and
h., vomiting or confusion ▸
  persistent
h. ▸ weather-related migraine
h., withdrawal
headed
h. dwarf, bird-
h. dwarf of Seckel, bird-
h. worm, thorny-
headgear, Kloehn's
headhunter angiography catheter
headlight, fiberoptic
headrest
h., doughnut
h,. Light-Veley
h., Mayfield-Kees
h., Multipoise
h., neurosurgical
headwall system
Heaf test
heal [*heel*]
heal slowly
heal spontaneously
healed
h. blister
h. by first intention ▸ wound
h. by second intention ▸ wound
h. cutdown site
h. fracture
h. fracture, old
h. incision site
h. myocardial infarct
h. myocardial infarction
h. myocardial infarction ▸ old
h., operative wounds clean and
h. per primam ▸ incision
h. per primam ▸ wound
h. perforation

h. previous excisional scars ▸
  well
h. rheumatic valvulitis
h. scar, well
h. stump
h. superficial laceration
h. surgical incision
h., well
h. wound clean and
h. yellow atrophy
healer, faith
healing
h. ability ▸ body's natural
h. biopsy incision
h., bony
h. by first intention
h. by granulation
h. by second intention
h. by third intention
h. capability, wound
h., consolidation and
h., crystal
h., delayed
h. duodenal ulcer
h., faith
h. fracture
h., granulating in and
h., holistic
h. incision site
h. injury
h. labyrinth
h., mental
h. method, bone
h. method, natural
h. myocardial infarction
h. of fracture, delayed
h., per primam
h., per secundum
h. personality ▸ self-
h. ▸ poor wound
h., postabortion
h., postsurgical
h. power of warm baths
h., primary
h. process
h. process ▸ stall the
h., radiographic
h. ▸ rate of
h. satisfactorily, wound
h. sores ▸ slow
h., spiritual
h. surgical incision
h. the sick
h. touch
h. well, wound

h. with approximation
h. wound
health (Health)
  h. aide, home
  h., analyze tissue
  h. and fitness
  h. and fitness ▸ enhance
  h. and well-being
  h. assessment
  H. Assistance Foundation (AHAF)
    ▸ American
  h. awareness
  h., behavioral
  h. benefits, mental
  h. benefits of walking
  h. care
  h. care agency
  h. care agency ▸ home
  h. care agent
  h. care alternative
  h. care, ancillary
  h. care ▸ availability of
  h. care consultant
  h. care cost reduction
  h. care costs
  h. care costs, rising
  h. care coverage
  H. Care Coverage Act, Catastrophic
  h. care decision
  h. care decision, informed
  h. care decision-making
  h. care declaration
  h. care document ▸ Power of
    Attorney (POA)
  h. care documents
  h. care ▸ effective mental
  h. care facilities
  h. care facilities ▸ long-term
  h. care, home
  h. care industry
  h. care institution
  h. care institution ▸ comprehensive
  h. care, medical
  h. care, mental
  h. care personnel
  h. care ▸ prepaid
  h. care products
  h. care professional
  h. care provider
  h. care, quality
  h. care questionnaire
  h. care rationing plan
  h. care resources
  h. care services
  h. care specialist

h. care system
h. care team
h. care technology
h. care, total
h. care utilization
h. care workers (HCW)
h. center
h. center, community mental
h. claims, unproven
h. club
h., comprehensive mental
h. -conscious
h. coordinator, employee
h. coverage ▸ mandated mental
h. decisions
h. delivery system ▸ mental
H. Department, Employee
H. Department of Mental
H. Discharge Survey (NHDS) ▸
  National
H. Drugs Advisory Committee ▸
  Fertility Maternal
h. education
h. education programs ▸ public
h., emotional
h. enhancing traits
h., environmental
h. evaluation, annual
h. examination, periodic
h. food
h. fraud
h., general
h., general mental
h. habits
h. hazard
h. hazard ▸ alcohol-related
h. hazard, public
h., heart
h. history
h. information, vital
h. insurance
h. insurance, catastrophic
h. insurance, national
h. ▸ job hazardous to
h. literacy ▸ marginal
H. Locus of Control Scale
h. maintenance, altered
h. maintenance organization
  (HMO)
h., managed mental
h., mental
H. Nurse
H. Nurse (PHN) ▸ Public
h., occupational
H. Organization (WHO), World

h. patients, mental
h. patients ▸ public mental
h. perception
h., physical
h. plan, comprehensive
h. plans ▸ managed behavioral
h. practitioner, mental
h., preservation of
h. problem, chronic
h. problem, general
h. problems ▸ nature of mental
h. problems, public-
h. problems ▸ stress caused
h. problems ▸ weight-related
h. professional, mental
h. professionals, allied
h. program, employee
h. program, mental
h. program, personnel
h. program, public
h. provider, mental
h., public
h. records analyst
h. -related legislation
h. responsibility
h. risk
h. risk appraisal
h. risk, maternal
h. risk, occupational
h., psychological
h. risk factor
h. risk, serious
h. screening
h. screening, free
h. self-esteem ▸ improve
H. Service (PHS) ▸ Public
h. services ▸ home
h. services, mental
h. services ▸ outpatient mental
h. spa ▸ holistic
h. spiritual aspect of
h. status
h. status, assessment of
h. status, mental
h. status, stable
h. threat, major
h. treatment, behavioral
h. treatment, mental
h. visits, home
h. wellness
h. workers, paraprofessional
healthy
  h. appearing organ
  h. conflict management
  h. coping strategies

healthy—*continued*
- h. diet
- h. dietary habits
- h. lifestyle
- h. lifestyle habits
- h. lifestyle ▸ heart
- h. motile sperm
- h. nerve cells
- h. pregnant women
- h. reaction
- h. self-assertion
- h. tissue
- h. tissue, burn
- h. tissue ▸ damage to
- h. tissue, destroy
- h. tissue stained

Healy position, Blackett-Heaney's vaginal hysterectomy
hear [*here*]
heard at hip joint, click
hearing
- h. acuity
- h. acuity screening
- h. aid
- h. aid ▸ analog
- h. aid, behind-the-ear
- h. aid, binaural
- h. aid, body worn
- h. aid, completely in the canal
- h. aid, digital
- h. aid ▸ downsizing of
- h. aid ▸ in-the-canal
- h. aid ▸ in-the-ear
- h. aid ▸ traditional
- h. and balance
- h. and sight ▸ diminished
- h. assessment, extensive
- h. at high frequency ▸ reduced
- h. center, brain's
- h. damage
- h., decreased
- h. defect
- h., diminished
- h. disorder
- h. distance (HD)
- h. disturbance
- h., double disharmonic
- h. evaluation, diagnostic
- h. frequencies
- h., hypersensitive
- h. impaired
- h. impairment
- h. impairment ▸ speech and
- h. level
- h. loss

- h. loss, age-related
- h. loss, bilateral progressive
- h. loss, conductive
- h. loss, delayed
- h. loss ▸ fluctuating
- h. loss ▸ fluctuating sensorineural
- h. loss from aging
- h. loss from antibiotic
- h. loss from aspirin
- h. loss from diuretics
- h. loss from infection of ear
- h. loss, high frequency
- h. loss ▸ high frequency sensorineural
- h. loss, high tone
- h. loss, impaired
- h. loss ▸ inner ear
- h. loss ▸ low frequency sensorineural
- h. loss ▸ minor
- h. loss, monaural
- h. loss, noise-induced
- h. loss, partial
- h. loss, permanent
- h. loss profile ▸ personal
- h. loss ▸ profound
- h. loss, progressive
- h. loss ▸ progressive unilateral
- h. loss ▸ rapidly progressing bilateral
- h. loss, retrocochlear
- h. loss (SHL) ▸ selective
- h. loss, sensorineural
- h. loss ▸ sensory neural
- h. loss ▸ severe
- h. loss studies
- h. loss, sudden
- h. loss, symptomatic
- h. loss ▸ temporary
- h. loss ▸ unilateral
- h. loss, visual
- h. loss ▸ warning signs of
- h., monaural
- h. nerve
- h., normal
- h. normalized
- h., organ of
- h. patterns, modify
- h. problems
- h., receptor cells of
- h., receptor organ of
- h. screening
- h., sense of
- h., sensory nerve of
- h. ▸ severe impairment of

- h., sharper
- h. system
- h. test
- h. test, decibel (DB)
- h. test, functional
- h., visual
- h. voices

hears voices ▸ patient
heart(s) Heart('s)
- H. (amphetamines)
- h., abdominal
- h., abnormal electrical events in
- h. ▸ abnormal functioning of
- h., above level of
- h. action
- h. action ▸ ineffective
- h. action ▸ irregular
- h. action, rapid
- h. activity
- h. activity, abnormal
- h. activity, normal
- h., adhesions of pericardium around
- h. affliction
- h. ailment
- h. ailment, advanced
- h., air-driven artificial
- h., alternans of the
- h. amyloidosis of
- h. and breathing rate ▸ increase
- h. and great vessels
- h. and liver damage
- h. and liver disease, end stage
- h. and lung function
- h. and lungs
- h. and lungs ▸ autopsy limited to
- h. and lungs ▸ improve efficiency of
- h. anomaly
- h. anomaly, congenital
- h. antigen, beef
- h., aortic ventricle of
- h., apex of
- h., armored
- h., armour
- h. arrhythmia
- h. arrhythmias, fatal
- h. arrhythmias ▸ life-threatening
- h. arrest
- h. artery, blocked
- h., artificial
- h. ▸ assess functioning of
- h. assessment
- h. -assist pump
- H. Association (NYHA) classification ▸ New York

H. Association (AHA) diet, American
h. at rest, evaluation of denervated
h., athlete's
h., athletic
h. attack
h. attack, acute
h. attack apoptosis ▸ post-
h. attack ▸ aspirin and
h. attack, asymptomatic
h. attack, atypical
h. attack, cocaine
h. attack death, sudden
h. attack ▸ dizziness from
h. attack, exercise induced
h. attack, fatal
h. attack from aspirin
h. attack from blood clot
h. attack, initial
h. attack, massive
h. attack ▸ Monday morning
h. attack ▸ nonfatal
h. attack, pain of
h. attack pain ▸ pre-
h. attack patient
h. attack patient, depressed
h. attack ▸ recurrent
h. attack rehabilitation
h. attack ▸ repeat
h. attack risk
h. attack risk factor
h. attack ▸ risk of first
h. attack ▸ sexual dysfunction after
h. attack, silent
h. attack ▸ sudden fatal
h. attack survivor
h. attack survivor, depressed
h. attack ▸ suspected
h. attack symptoms
h. attack trigger
h. attack victim
h. attack victim, cocaine-related
h. attack ▸ warning signs of
h., atrium of
h., auscultation of
h., baggy
h., balloon-shaped
h., Baylor total artificial
h. beat ▸ chaotic
h., beating
h., beer
h., beriberi
h., Berlin total artificial
h. biopsy
h. block (HB)

h. block, arborization
h. block, atrioventricular (AV)
h. block, atrioventricular (AV) junctional
h. block, bifascicular
h., block, bundle branch
h. block (CHB), complete
h. block, congenital
h. block, diversional
h. block, divisional
h. block fascicular
h. block, first degree
h. block ▸ His bundle
h. block, incomplete
h. block, interventricular
h. block, intraventricular
h. block, Mobitz
h. block, partial
h. block, second degree
h. block, sinoatrial
h. block, sinoauricular
h. block, subjunctional
h. block, third degree
h. block, 3:1
h. block, 3:2
h. block ▸ transient
h. block ▸ trifascicular
h. block, Wenckebach
h., blood flow in
h., blood supply to
h., blunt injury
h., boat-shaped
h., boot-shaped
h., bony
h., booster
h. border
h., bovine
h. bypass, left
h. bypass ▸ percutaneous left
h. bypass, right
h. bypass surgery
h. cannulated
h. cardiac bypass ▸ beating
h., CardioWest total artificial
h. catheterization
h. catheterization, combined
h. catheterization ▸ left
h. catheterization, right
h. catheterization stylet
h. catheterization ▸ transseptal left
h. cell death
h. cells
h., cervical
h. chamber
h. changes ▸ radiation-induced

h., chaotic
h. circulates blood
h., compliance of
h. condition
h. condition ▸ stress-related
h. configuration
h., congenital defect interventricular septum of
h., congenital displacement of
h., conjoined
h., contour of
h. contracted
h. ▸ contraction and relaxation of
h., contraction cycle of
h. contraction ▸ physiology of
h. contractions
h. contractions, abnormal
h. contractions ▸ forceful
h., contusion of
h., crisscross
h., crux of
h. damage
h. damage, irreparable
h. damage ▸ irreversible
h. damage ▸ silent
h., damaged donor
h., decompression of
h., decortication of
h., decreased venous return to
h. defect
h. defect, congenital
h. defect, cyanotic
h. defect ▸ hereditary
h. defect ▸ structural
h. defibrillated
h. defibrillated with single shock of _____ joules
h., dextroposition of
h., dextroversion of
h., digitalization of
h. dilated
h., dilation of the
h. disease
h. disease, acromegalic
h. disease, acute ischemic
h. disease, acyanotic
h. disease, advanced
h. disease, amyloid
h. disease (ASHD) ▸ arteriosclerotic
h. disease, asymptomatic
h. disease, atherosclerotic
h. disease, beriberi
h. disease, carcinoid
h. disease, causes of

heart(s)—*continued*

h. disease cells
h. disease, chronic
h. disease, clinical
h. disease (CHD), congenital
h. disease (CHD) ▸ congestive
h. disease (CHD), coronary
h. disease, coronary atherosclerotic
h. disease, cyanotic
h. disease ▸ decreased risk of
h. disease (DHD), degenerative
h. disease, diastolic
h. disease ▸ exhaustion, burnout and
h. disease history (HDH)
h. disease (HHD), hypertensive
h. disease, hypertensive arteriosclerotic
h. disease (IHD), ischemic
h. disease ▸ lower risk of
h. disease, organic
h. disease, overt symptom of
h. disease ▸ postmenopausal
h. disease, premature
h. disease, prevent
h. disease, rehabilitation of
h. disease (HD), restrictive
h. disease ▸ reverse
h. disease, rheumatic
h. disease risk factor
h. disease, risk of
h. disease screening
h. disease ▸ silent ischemic
h. disease ▸ stress of
h. disease therapy
h. disease, thyrotoxic
h. disease ▸ traumatic
h. disease, treatment of
h. disease, valvular
h. disease ▸ vascular
h., diseased
h., diseased human
h., disembodied
h. disorder
h. (DAH) ▸ disordered action of
h. disorders, alcohol-related
h. disorders, related
h. ▸ dissection of
h. disturbance
h. does appear enlarged
h. does not appear enlarged
h. donated
h., donation of
h., donor
h., drop

h., dynamite
h. dysfunction
h. dysfunctional episode
h. ▸ egg-shaped
h., electrical activity of
h. ▸ electrical alternation of
h., electrical charge to
h. ▸ electrical conduction in
h. ▸ electrical function of
h., electrical impulse to
h. ▸ electrical instability of
h. electrical rhythm
h. ▸ electrical stimulation of
h. electrically unstable
h. ▸ electromechanical artificial
h., embryonic
h., encased
h., enlarged
h., enlargement of
h. ▸ Enterococcal infection of
h., explanted
h., extracorporeal
h. factor, diastolic
h. factor ▸ end-stage
h. factor ▸ florid congestive
h. failure
h. failure, acute
h. failure, acute congestive
h. failure, acute left ventricular
h. failure, acute right ventricular
h. failure (CHF) ▸ advanced stage of congestive
h. failure and cardioversion, congestive
h. failure, backward
h. failure cells
h. failure, chronic
h. failure, chronic congestive
h. failure, compensated
h. failure ▸ confusion from
h. failure, congenital
h. failure (CHF), congestive
h. failure, decompensated
h. failure ▸ deteriorating
h. failure ▸ florid congestive
h. failure, forward
h. failure, high output
h. failure, incipient
h. failure, intractable
h. failure ▸ late-stage
h. failure ▸ left
h. failure, left-sided
h. failure, left ventricular
h. failure ▸ loss of appetite from
h. failure ▸ low-output

h. failure, marginal
h. failure (CHF) ▸ natural history of congestive
h. failure ▸ onset of overt
h. failure, overt
h. failure (CHF), recurrent congestive
h. failure, refractory
h. failure ▸ reverse
h. failure ▸ right
h. failure, right-sided
h. failure, right ventricular
h. failure ▸ stable, controlled
h. failure ▸ sudden
h. failure (CHF) ▸ sudden congestive
h. failure ▸ symptoms of
h. failure ▸ systolic
h. failure (CHF) therapy ▸ congestive
h. failure treatment
h., fat
h., fatty
h., fatty degeneration of
h., fetal
h., fibroid
h. ▸ figure-of-eight
h., flask-shaped
h., flesh trabeculae of
h. flow capacity
h., flow of blood and oxygen to
h. flutter
h., fluttering
h., four-chambered human
h., frosted
h., frosting
h. function
h. function, measuring
h. function, normal
h. function ▸ stabilize
h., functional
h., functional aspects of
h. ▸ gene therapy for
h., globoid
h., globular
h., Graham-Steell murmur of
h. -hand syndrome
h., hairy
h., hanging
h., head higher than
h. health
h. -healthy lifestyle
h. -helping exercise
h. ▸ Hershey total artificial
h., Holmes

h., horizontal
h. hormone
h., hyperthyroid
h. hypertrophied and dilated
h., hypertrophy of
h., hypoplastic
h., icing
h., imaging
h., immune rejection of transplanted
h. implant, artificial
h., implantable artificial
h. in diastole
h. infection
h., inflammation of
h., inflammation of lining of
h., infundibulum of
h. infusion, brain-
h. ▸ insufficient blood flow to
h., interventricular sulcus of
h. into normal rhythm, shock
h. intracorporeal
h. irregular
h., irritable
h. ▸ ischemic damage to
h. ▸ Jarvik-8 artificial
h., Jarvik-7 artificial
h. ▸ Jarvik 7-70 artificial
h. ▸ Jarvik 2000 artificial
h. ▸ jump-start
h. jump-started
h., kidney, and brain function
h., kidney, and brain function ▸ diminished
h. ▸ Kolff-Jarvik artificial
h., laceration of
h. laser revascularization
h. ▸ law of the
h., left
h., left atrium of
h. left pump, artificial
h., left ventricle (LV) of
h., legs elevated higher than
h. lesion cells
h. level, elevate feet above
h. level, tonic
h. lining
h. lining, inflammation of
h. ▸ Liotta total artificial
h. living, prudent
h., longitudinal sulcus of
h. loop
h., lower chamber of
h. -lung bloc
h., -lung bypass
h. -lung machine

h. -lung resuscitation
h. -lung resuscitator
h. -lung transplant
h., luxus
h., lymph
h. malformation
h. malposition, crisscross
h. map
h., markedly dilated
h. massage
h., mechanical
h. ▸ mechanical alternation of
h. meridian
h. ▸ metabolic balance of
h. monitor
h. monitor, fetal
H. Monitor ▸ King of
h. monitor tracing, fetal
h. ▸ monocytolysis of
h., movable
h., movement of
h. ▸ multiple thrombi in vessels of
h. murmur
h. murmur ▸ apical mid-diastolic
h. murmur, apical systolic
h. murmur ▸ benign
h. murmur, continuous
h. murmur, functional
h. murmur ▸ innocent
h. muscle
h. muscle abnormality
h. muscle activity ▸ chaotic
h. muscle, beating
h. muscle, blood diffuses into
h. muscle cell
h. muscle cells, autorhythmic
h. muscle ▸ compensatory hypertrophy of
h. muscle ▸ contractility of
h. muscle, contraction of
h. muscle cramps
h. muscle damage
h. muscle, dead area of
h. muscle death
h. muscle degeneration ▸ acute
h. muscle, deterioration of
h. muscle disease
h. muscle disease ▸ alcoholic
h. muscle disease ▸ chronic alcoholic
h. muscle disease ▸ preclinical
h. muscle disease ▸ symptomatic alcohol
h. muscle distress, silent
h. muscle, enlarged

h. muscle fibers
h. muscle, increased blood flow to
h. muscle ▸ inflammation of
h. muscle ▸ injured
h. muscle ▸ ischemic
h. muscle ▸ oxygen (O_2)-starved
h. muscle ▸ reconstruct
h. muscle, relaxation of
h. muscle removed ▸ slice of
h. muscle ▸ revascularize
h. muscle, scarring of
h. muscle, stimulate
h. muscle, thickened
h. muscle tissue
h. muscle tissue, blood-starved
h. muscle tissue, death of
h. muscle to digitalis toxicity ▸ sensitize
h. muscle ▸ weakened
h. muscle weakness
h. myocytes
h. ▸ myocytolysis of
h., myxedema
h., normal contour of
h. ▸ normal rhythm of
h. normal rhythm ▸ reboot faulty
h. normal size
h. observed
h. ▸ one-ventricle
h. or heart valve ▸ malformed
h. ▸ orthotopic biventricular artificial
h. ▸ orthotopic univentricular artificial
h., overburdened
h., ox
h. pacemaker of
h. pain, intermittent
h. palpitations
h., paracorporeal
h., parchment
h. patient
h. patient, exercises for
h., pear-shaped
h., pectoral
h., pendulous
h., penetrating wound of
h., Penn State total artificial
h., perfusion of
h., Phoenix total artificial
h. port surgery
h. position
h. position ▸ electrical
h. positioner ▸ starfish
h., postischemic
h., pounding of

heart(s)—*continued*

h., precontractile
h. preparation ▸ Langendorff
h. probe ▸ Norwood univentricular
h. problem
h. problem, activity-related
h. problem ▸ chest pain from
h. production, increase
h., prosthesis
h. prosthesis, Cartright
h., pulmonary
h. pump
h. pump, mechanical
h. pumping
h. ▸ pumping ability of failing
h. ▸ pumping ability of weakened
h. pumping action
h. pumping chamber
h., pumping function of
H. (barbiturates), Purple
h., Quain's fatty
h., racing
h., rapid beating of
h. rate
h. rate, abnormality in
h. rate, abnormally rapid
h. rate, accelerating
h. rate, apneic infant with decreased
h. rate, arousal
h. rate, baseline variability of fetal
h. rate, change in
h. rate changes ▸ large magnitude voluntary
h. rate conditionability
h. rate conditioning ▸ human operant
h. rate control
h. rate control learning and awareness
h. rate control, voluntary
h. rate, decreased
h. rate disorder
h. rate during oxygen deprivation ▸ control of
h. rate ▸ elevated
h. rate, exercise
h. rate ▸ excessively rapid
h. rate ▸ expected peak
h. rate ▸ fast
h. rate feedback
h. rate feedback ▸ anticipatory bogus
h. rate, fetal
h. rate, increased

h. rate, increasing
h. rate, intrinsic
h. rate, maximal
h. rate, maximum
h. rate (MPHR), maximum predicted
h. rate monitor
h. rate monitored
h. rate monitoring ▸ internal fetal
h. rate, operant acceleration of
h. rate, operant deceleration of
h. rate ▸ peak
h. rate perception
h. rate, precordial
h. rate ▸ QT corrected for
h. rate rapid
h. rate reading, fetal
h. rate recovery
h. rate, reduced
h. rate regular
h. rate reserve
h. rate responses
h. rate responses ▸ instrumental
h. rate ▸ resting
h. rate ▸ rising
h. rate, self-control of
h. rate, slow
h. rate ▸ standing
h. rate, target
h. rate ▸ training
h. rate variability
h. rate zone (THRZ) ▸ target
h. recipient
h. recipient, artificial
h., reconditioned
h. ▸ reduced blood supply to
h. reduced to normal size
h. reduction surgery
h. reflex
h. reflex, Abrams'
h. reflex, eyeball-
h. rehabilitation program
h. rejected
h. ▸ rejuvenate damaged
h. relaxed phase
h. relaxes
h. remodeling
h. reshaping
h. response to stress
h. resting
h. resuscitated
h. retrieved, donor
h. ▸ revascularization of blood vessels of
h. ▸ rheumatism of

h. rhythm
h. rhythm, abnormal
h. rhythm abnormality
h. rhythm abnormality ▸ life-threatening
h. rhythm, change in
h. rhythm ▸ chaotic
h. rhythm disorder
h. rhythm disturbance
h. rhythm disturbance ▸ controlled
h. rhythm disturbance ▸ fatal
h. rhythm drug
h. rhythm, erratic
h. rhythm, fatal
h. rhythm ▸ faulty
h. rhythm, irregular
h. rhythm ▸ lethal
h. rhythm ▸ life-threatening
h. rhythm ▸ normal
h. rhythm ▸ normal sinus
h. rhythm problems
h. rhythm, racing
h. rhythm ▸ rapid
h. rhythm, regular
h. rhythm regulation
h. rhythm ▸ slow
h., right
h., right atrium of
h., right ventricle (RV) of
h. risk
h. risk assessment
h., round
h. ▸ RTV total artificial
h., rupture of
h., sabot
h. sac
h. sac ▸ fluid in
h. scan
h. scan, nuclear
h. scan ▸ Thallium exercise
h., scarred
h. screening
h. ▸ secondary morphogenesis of
h., semihorizontal
h., semivertical
h., senescent
h. sensible diet
h. ▸ septation of
h. ▸ septum of
h. ▸ severely weakened
h. shadow
h. shock
h. shocked during cardiac arrest
h., silhouette of
h. size

h. size and outline
h. size and shape
h. size, increased
h. size, normal
h., skin
h. slows
h., small vein of
h., smoker's
h., snowman
h., soldier's
h. ▸ sonogram of
h. sound, first
h. sound (atrial gallop) ▸ fourth
h. sound ▸ physiologic third
h. sound ▸ rubbing
h. sound (A₂) ▸ second
h. sound, splitting of
h. sound, third
h. sounds
h. sounds, distant
h. sounds, extra
h. sounds (FHS), fetal
h. sounds ▸ muffled
h. sounds ▸ quiet
h. sounds (S1, S2, S3, S4)
h., Starling's law of the
h., stiff
h. stimulant
h. ▸ stimulate calcium receptors in
h., stone
h. stoppage
h. strain, right
h. stroke
h. ▸ stroke volume of
h., structural change in
h. study
H. Study ▸ Framingham
H. Study ▸ Helsinki
h. sugar
h., superoinferior
h. surgery
h. surgery ▸ beating
h. surgery, closed
h. surgery ▸ laser
h. surgery, open
h. surgery, triple bypass
h., suspended
h., swinging
h. syndrome ▸ athletic
h. syndrome ▸ holiday
h. syndrome, hyperkinetic
h. syndrome ▸ hypoblastic right and left
h. syndrome, hypoplastic, left
h. syndrome ▸ pediatric

h. syndrome ▸ suspended
h. syndrome, stiff-
h., systemic
h., tabby cat
h. table ▸ Siemens open
h. tamponade
h. ▸ Taussig-Bing
h., teardrop
h. ▸ tendinous zones of
h. therapy ▸ regenerative
h. -threatening hypertension
h., three-chambered
h., thrust breast
h., thrust of apex of
h., tiger
h., tiger lily
h. tissue
h. tissue ▸ recreating
h. to lungs, blood from
h., tobacco
h. tones (HT)
h. tones (FHT), Doptone monitoring of fetal
h. tones (FHT) ▸ fetal
h. tones (FHT) obtained with Doptone, fetal
h. tones regular
h. tones, stable fetal
h., total artificial
h. transplant
h. transplant, long-term survivor of
h. transplant ▸ orthotopic
h. transplant patient
h. transplant recipient
h. transplant, temporary
h. transplantation
h., transverse diameter of
h. ▸ transverse section of
h., transverse sulcus of
h., Traube's
h., triatrial
h., trilocular
h. trimming procedure
h., univentricular
h. ▸ University of Akron artificial
h., unstressed
h., upper chamber of
h. ▸ upstairs-downstairs
h. ▸ Utah total artificial
h. valve
h. valve abnormality
h. valve allograft, cryopreserved
h. valve, artificial
h. valve, biological
h. valve, bioprosthetic

h. valve, bovine
h. valve, broken
h. valve, calcium deposits on
h. valve damage
h. valve defect
h. valve, defective
h. valve, defective artificial
h. valve disease
h. valve disorder
h. valve disorder ▸ pulmonary
h. valve ▸ dysfunctional
h. valve function
h. valve function, abnormal
h. valve ▸ Heimlich
h. valve infection
h. valve infection ▸ bacterial
h. valve ▸ leaking
h. valve ▸ leaky
h. valve ▸ malformed heart or
h. valve ▸ mechanical
h. valve ▸ metal
h. valve ▸ myxomatous degeneration of
h. valve, narrowed
h. valve, narrowing of
h. valve narrowing, severe
h. valve ▸ plastic
h. valve ▸ porcine
h. valve prosthesis
h. valve prosthesis ▸ Hufnagel low profile
h. valve prosthesis ▸ Medtronic-Hall
h. valve prosthesis ▸ SCDT
h. valve prosthesis ▸ St. Jude
h. valve prosthesis ▸ Starr-Edwards
h. valve prosthesis ▸ Wada hingeless
h. valve ▸ prosthetic
h. valve replacement
h. valve, scarring of
h. valve ▸ Shiley
h. valve ▸ Shiley convexoconcave
h. valve ▸ Smeloff
h. valve ▸ staphylococcal infection of
h. valve surgery
h. valve surgery ▸ prosthetic
h. valve ▸ synthetic
h. valve, tricuspid
h. (VDH), valvular disease of
h. ▸ vascular disease in diabetic
h., venous
h. ▸ venous return to
h., vertical

heart(s)—*continued*
- h., viable
- h. ▸ Vienna total artificial
- h. ▸ waist of
- h. wall, ischemic
- h. wall thickening
- h., wandering
- h. ▸ water-bottle
- h., weakened
- h. ▸ weakly pumping
- h. with pericardium
- h., wooden-shoe
- h. worm

heartbeat
- h., abnormal
- h. absent
- h., accentuated
- h., arrest of
- h., depressed breathing and
- h. disorder, rhythm of
- h., effective
- h., fast
- h., fetal
- h., fluttering
- h., initiate
- h., irregular
- h., irregularities
- h., life-threatening abnormal
- h., monitoring
- h., multifocal
- h., nocturnal
- h., normal
- h., racing
- h., rapid
- h. ▸ rapid pounding
- h. rhythm ▸ irregular
- h., skipped
- h., slow
- h., symptoms of
- h., synchronous with

heartburn
- h., acid
- h., disabling
- h., drug-induced
- h., frequent
- h. from antibiotic
- h., nighttime
- h. ▸ patient has
- h., persistent
- h., severe

heartworm disease
heartworm larvae
HEAT (human erythrocyte agglutination test)

heat
- h. and massage therapy
- h. and work, acclimation to
- h., atomic
- h., body
- h. capacity
- h. capacity, unit of
- h. coagulation (IRC) ▸ infrared
- h., conductive
- h., convective
- h., conversive
- h. cramp
- h., delayed
- h. detection test
- h. device ▸ radiant
- h., dry
- h. ▸ excessive loss of body
- h. exchanger
- h. exhaustion
- h. exhaustion, anhidrotic
- h. exhaustion ▸ anxiety from
- h. exhaustion, type II
- h. expandable stent
- h. fixed, slide
- h., flushing and
- h. generation of breast
- h., humidify and
- h. illness syndrome
- h., increased local
- h. -induced illness
- h., initial
- h. injury
- h. injury, environmental
- h., internal body
- h. intolerance
- h. intolerance from alcohol
- h. intolerance from chlorpromazine
- h. intolerance from diuretics
- h. -killed cells
- h., latent
- h. lesion
- h. load
- h. loss
- h. loss by radiation
- h., moist
- h. /moisture exchanger
- h. mold
- h., molecular
- h. ▸ overexposure to
- h. packs ▸ microwaveable
- h. pattern, abnormal
- h. pattern thermography
- h. perfusion ▸ isolated

- h. perfusion of an extremity, isolated
- h., prickly
- h. production, excessive
- h. production ▸ increase metabolic
- h. prostration
- h., radiant
- h. radiated by breast
- h., radiating
- h. radiation
- h. rash
- h. rash, prickly
- h. -ray cataract
- h. rays
- h., recovery
- h. -regulating centers
- h. -related disorders
- h. -related illness
- h. -related injury
- h. sensation
- h., sensible
- h. sensitivity
- h. shock protein
- h., specific
- h. stable
- h. stable alkaline phosphates
- h. sterilization
- h. stress
- h. stress, brief exposure to
- h. stress, tolerate
- h. stroke
- h. stroke, dizziness from
- h. stroke in aging
- h. stroke, life-threatening
- h. syncope
- h. therapy
- h. tolerance
- h. transfer
- h. transfer agent
- h. treatment, moist
- h., ultrasonic
- h., warm moist
- h. wheel

heated bed cradle
heater probe cauterization
Heath's
- H. curette
- H. dilator
- H. expressor
- H. forceps

heating
- h. cancer cells
- h. devices
- h., ohmic

h., regional deep
h., resistive
heave(s)
  h., dry
  h., parasternal
  h., precordial
  h. ▸ right ventricular (RV)
  h., systolic
  h., ventricular
Heaven Dust (cocaine)
Heavenly Blue (morning glory seeds)
Heavens (barbiturates), Blue
heaviness
  h., chest
  h. ▸ flushing sensation of
  h. in legs
  h. of limbs
  h. of limbs ▸ stiffness or
  h., sensation of
heavy
  h. alcohol consumption
  h. alcohol usage
  h. alcohol user
  h. chain gene, beta myosin
  h. chain ▸ myosin
  h. charged particle beam therapy
  h. charged particle therapy in eye tumors
  h. clamps applied
  h. consumption of alcohol
  h. drinker, patient
  h. drinking, long-term
  h. drinking, prolonged
  h. exertion
  h. exertional activity
  h. exposure technique
  h. flow
  h. infection
  h. ion irradiation
  h. ions, physical effects of
  h. menstrual flow
  h. menstrual period from anemia
  h. menstrual periods
  h. metal
  h. metal poisoning
  h. metal stain
  h. particle therapy
  h. periods
  h. retention suture
  h. scaling of skin
  h. sedation
  h. smoker, patient
  h. smoking, emphysema secondary to

h. social drinkers
h. vaginal discharge
hebdomidis, Leptospira
hebephrenic-type schizophrenia
Heberden('s)
  H. anomaly
  H. asthma
  H. disease
  H. nodes
  H. rheumatism
  H. signs
hebetomy/hebotomy
heboid paranoia
heboid-paranoid group
hebotomy/hebetomy
hebraeum, Amblyomma
Hecht's pneumonia
heckle cell
hectic fever
hectic flush
hedger's cataract
hedonic homeostatic dysregulation
heel [*heal*]
  h., abscess of
  h. and sole ▸ hyperpigmented macules on
  h., anterior
  h., basketball
  h., big
  h. bone
  h. bone density scan
  h. bowl
  h., Bush walking
  h., cellulitis of
  h., contracted
  h. cord
  h. cord, contracted
  h. cord lengthening
  h., cracked
  h., crown-to-
  h., decubitus
  h. elevation
  h., globus of the
  h., gonorrheal
  h., Heelbo used on patient's
  h. -knee test
  h. length (RHL), rump
  h. pad
  h. pain
  h., painful
  h., policeman's
  h., prominent
  h. protector
  h. protector, disposable
  h. raise exercise ▸ toe-

h., SACH
h. (WACH) shoe, wedge adjustable cushioned
h. spur
h. spur excision
h. spur ▸ painful
h. spur syndrome
h. squat exercise
h. stick pain
h. stretch exercise, calf-
h. strike
h. strike, palm-
h., Stryker walking
h. syndrome, painful
h. -tap reflex
h., Telson hinged walking
h. test, knee-
h., Thomas
h. -to-crown
h. -to-knee
h. -to-knee dystaxia
h. -to-shin test
h. -to-toe gait
h. -to-toe walking
h. -toe motion
h. ulcer
h., walking
h., wedge
Heelbo used on patient's elbow
Heelbo used on patient's heel
HEENT (head, eyes, ears, nose and throat)
HEENT (head, eyes, ears, nose and throat) not remarkable
Heerfordt's disease
Heerfordt's syndrome
Heerman incision
Hefke-Turner sign
Hegar's
  H. dilators
  H. operation
  H. sign
Hegglin's anomaly
Hegglin's anomaly, May-
Heiberg-Esmarch maneuver
Heidenhain's
  H. cells
  H. iron hematoxylin stain
  H. law
  H. rods
  H. stain
Heifitz's operation
height
  h. adjustment, automatic fulcrum
  h. age

height—*continued*
- h. analyzer ▸ pulse
- h., anterior facial
- h., apex
- h., cusp
- h., fundal
- h., mid-parental
- h. of contour
- h., posterior facial
- h., sitting
- h., sitting suprasternal
- h., sitting vertex
- h. spectrometry, pulse
- h. spectrum, pulse-
- h., standing
- h., vertebral body

heighten sexual response
heightened
- h. awareness of touch or taste
- h. irritability ▸ lapse into
- h. perception of colors
- h. sense of awareness
- h. sensitivity to odors
- h. sensitivity to sounds
- h. sexual drive
- h. startle reactions
- h. stress

Heimlich
- H. heart valve
- H. maneuver
- H. sign

Heineke-Mikulicz pyloroplasty
Heine's operation
Heinz
- H. bodies
- H. body anemia
- H. body hemolytic anemia
- H. -Ehrlich bodies
- H. granules
- H. granules, Ehrlich-
- H. stain

Heisler diet, Moro-
Heister's
- H. diverticulum
- H. fold
- H. valve

Helanca seamless tube prosthesis
helicine artery
held
- h. defibrillator ▸ hand-
- h. in position of extension ▸ hand
- h. mammotome ▸ hand-

Helic gauge, Magna-
helical CAT (computerized axial tomography) scanner

helical rim
helicis
- h., crus
- h. major, musculus
- h. minor, musculus

Helicobacter
- H. pylori
- H. pylori bacterium
- H. pylori infection

heliotrope infraorbital discoloration
helium
- h. cadmium diagnostic laser
- h. equilibration time
- h. neon laser
- h. washout

helix
- h., amphipathic
- h., caudal
- h., crus of
- h., double

Heller('s)
- H. aortitis, Döhle-
- H. -Döhle disease
- H. myotomy

Helly's fluid
helmet
- h. headache
- h. -shaped gram-positive diplococci
- h. sign ▸ Prussian

Helmholtz theory, Young-
helminthiasis
- h., cutaneous
- h. elastica
- h. wuchereri

helminthic disease
help
- h. abortion, self-
- h. course, mutual self-
- h. course, self-
- H. Groups, Community Self-
- h. groups, self-
- h., medical self-
- h. patient achieve independence
- h., professional
- h. program, self-
- h. -seeking behavior
- h., self-
- h. -skill ▸ self
- h. support group ▸ self-
- h. techniques, self-

helper T cell
helper virus
helping exercise, heart

helplessness
- h. ▸ feeling of guilt, worthlessness and
- h. ▸ sense of
- h. ▸ sense of increasing

Helsinki Heart Study
Helweg's bundle
Helweg's tract
hemachromatosis (*see*** hemochromatosis)**
hemachromatosis (see hemochromatosis) gene
hemachromatosis (see hemochromatosis) in wrist
hemadsorption
- h., mixed
- h. virus (HA1) ▸ type 1
- h. virus (HA2) ▸ type 2

hemagglutinating
- h. antibody
- h. antipenicillin antibody
- h. unit

hemagglutination
- h., indirect
- h. inhibition
- h. -inhibition antibody
- h. -inhibition reaction
- h. -inhibition test
- h. titer

hemagglutinin inhibition
hemagglutinin spike
hemal arch
hemal nodes
hemangioblastoma
- h., capillary
- h., cerebellar
- h., inoperable

hemangioma
- h., ameloblastic
- h., calcified
- h., capillary
- h., cavernous
- h., choroidal
- h., mixed capillary cavernous
- h. of choroid
- h. of conjunctiva
- h. of iris
- h. of meningeal vessels
- h. of orbit
- h. of retina
- h. of skin, cavernous
- h., papillary
- h., pericardial
- h., port wine
- h., sclerosing

h. simplex
h., strawberry
h. thrombocytopenia syndrome
h., vertebral
hemangiomatosis of meningeal vessels
Hemantigen screening
hemapheresis
h. methodology
h. technology
h. therapeutic
hemarthrosis, acute
hemarthrosis knee
hemate, ammonia
hematemesis
h. and/or melena
h., Goldstein's
h. ▸ melena, hematochezia, or
hematidrosis/hematohidrosis
hematin (*see* heme)
hematin albumin
hematinic, oral
hematocele
h., parametric
h., pudendal
h., retrouterine
h., scrotal
h., vaginal
hematochezia, or hematemesis ▸ melena,
hematocrit (HCT)
h., large vessel
h. (HCT), mean circulatory
h. ratio ▸ body hematocrit/venous
h. (HCT), repeat venous
h., venous
h., whole blood
h., whole body
hematodepressive disease, viral
hematogenic shock
hematogenous
h. contamination
h. dissemination
h. embolism
h. jaundice
h. metastases
h. osteomyelitis, acute
h. pigmentation
h. proteinuria
h. pyelitis
h. siderosis
h. tuberculosis
hematoid cancer
hematoid carcinoma
hematoidin crystals

hematologic
h. disease
h. disorder
h. effects
h. malignancy
h. parameters
h. toxicity
hematological disease
hematological disorder
hematology rocker
hematology within normal limits (WNL)
hematoma(s)
h., aneurysmal
h., aortic intramural
h. auris
h., chronic subdural
h., dissection
h., epidural
h., extradural
h., intracerebral
h., left frontal
h. ▸ liquefaction of subdural
h. of chest wall
h. of liver ▸ subscapular
h. of orbit
h. of placenta
h. of scalp
h., pelvic
h. ▸ pelvic viscera surrounded by
h., perianal
h. periorbital
h., pulsatile
h., residual
h., retrosternal
h., retrouterine
h., right frontal
h., scalp
h., soft tissue
h. ▸ sonography of subfascial
h., subcapsular
h., subdural
h., sublingual
h., submental
h., subungual
h. ▸ widespread ecchymoses and
hematopneic index
hematopoiesis
h., extramedullary
h., focal extramedullary
h., foci of extramedullary
h. in the liver ▸ extramedullary
h., widespread extramedullary
hematopoietic
h. cells

h. cells ▸ sparse infiltration of extramedullary
h. complications of drug abuse
h. elements
h. elements, scattered
h. problems related to drug abuse
h. stem cell
h. system
h. tissue
hematoporphyrin derivative
hematoxylin
h., alum
h. and eosin
h., Delafield's
h., iron
h. method, iron
h. stain, Heidenhain's iron
h. stain, Weigert's
hematozoic parasite
hematuria
h., angioneurotic
h., endemic
h., essential
h., false
h., gross
h., intermittent
h., microscopic
h., painless
h., painless intermittent
h., pyuria and
h., renal
h., urethral
h., vesical
heme (*same as* hematin)
heme iron
hemelytrometra lateralis
Hemerocampa leukostigma
hemianesthesia
h., alternate
h., cerebral
h., crossed
h. cruciata
h., mesocephalic
h., pontile
h., spinal
hemianopia/hemianopsia
h., absolute
h., altitudinal
h., bilateral
h., binasal
h., binocular
h., bitemporal
h. bitemporalis fugax
h., complete
h., congruous

hemianopia—*continued*
   h., crossed
   h., equilateral
   h., heteronymous
   h., homonymous
   h., horizontal
   h. in intracranial neoplasms
   h., incomplete
   h., incongruous
   h., lateral
   h., lower
   h., nasal
   h., quadrant
   h., quadratic
   h., relative
   h., temporal
   h., true
   h., unilateral
   h., uniocular
   h., upper
   h., vertical
hemi-arthroplasty procedure
hemiatrophy, facial
hemiatrophy, progressive lingual
hemiaxial view
hemiaxial view, caudocranial
hemiazygos vein
hemiazygos vein, accessory
hemiblock
   h. ▸ left middle
   h. ▸ left posterior
   h. ▸ left septal
hemibody irradiation
hemibody radiation therapy
hemic
   h. distomiasis
   h. murmur
   h. systole
hemicolectomy, left
hemicolectomy, right
hemiconvulsion, hemiplegia,
   epilepsy (HHE) syndrome
hemicranial vascular headache
hemicylindrical bone graft
hemicylindrical graft
hemidiaphragm, tenting of
hemifacial atrophy
   h. atrophy
   h. hypertrophy
   h. spasm
hemigastrectomy and vagotomy
hemihypoplasia, cerebral
hemilaminectomy for cervical disc
hemilateral chorea
hemilingual atrophy

hemiopic pupillary reaction
hemiparalysis, flaccid
hemiparesis
   h. and aphasia ▸ right
   h., facial
   h. left arm
   h. right arm
hemiplegia
   h., acute
   h., alternate
   h., alternating oculomotor
   h., ascending
   h., capsular
   h., cerebral
   h., contralateral
   h., crossed
   h., dense
   h., epilepsy (HHE) syndrome ▸
     hemiconvulsion,
   h., facial
   h., faciobrachial
   h., faciolingual
   h., flaccid
   h., Gubler's
   h., infantile
   h., puerperal
   h., spastic
   h., spinal
   h., Wernicke-Mann
hemiplegic
   h. form of cerebral palsy
   h. gait
   h. idiocy
   h. migraine, basilar
   h., neuromuscular re-education of
     the
   h., patient
   h., rigidity
hemipterus, Cimex
hemisection
   h., mandibular
   h. of kidneys
   h. of spinal cord
hemispasm, facial
hemisphere(s)
   h., activity of both
   h., animal
   h., brain
   h., cerebellar
   h., cerebral
   h. deficit, left
   h. deficit, right
   h., dominant
   h., implant
   h., lateral

   h., left cerebral
   h., medial surface of cerebral
   h. of brain
   h. of brain ▸ dysplastic left
   h. of brain ▸ dysplastic right
   h. of brain, left
   h. of brain, right
   h., right cerebral
   h. spikes
   h., two cerebral
   h., vegetal
hemispherectomy procedure
hemispheric
   h. activities
   h. alpha synchrony biofeedback
   h. attack ▸ transient
   h. derivation, intero◊
   h. dominance
   h. functions
   h. gliosis
   h. parietal damage ▸ right
   h. synchrony, biofeedback
hemisphincter, pharyngeal
Hemispora stellata
hemisuccinate, prednisolone sodium
hemithorax [*hemothorax*]
hemithorax expands, left
hemitransfixion incision
hemoblastic leukemia
hemochorial placenta
hemochromatosis
   h. (*same as* hemachromatosis)
     gene
   h. (*same as* hemachromatosis) in
     wrist
   h., neonatal
hemoclastic reaction
hemoclastic shock
hemocult (Hemocult)
   h. positive stools
   H., screening
   h. screening
hemoculture negative
hemocytoblastic leukemia
hemodialysis
   h. arthropathy
   h., chronic
   h. ▸ joint swelling in
   h. maintenance
   h. transmission of viral hepatitis
   H. Unit
   h., vascular access in
hemodialyzer, ultrafiltration
hemodynamic(s)
   h. abnormalities

h. abnormalities ▸ left ventricular
h. angiographic study
h. assessment
h. calculation
h. collapse
h. data, derived
h. derangements
h. gradient
h. instability
h., intraoperative
h. maneuver
h. measurement
h. monitoring
h. monitoring, cardiac
h. parameters
h. parameters ▸ systemic
h., postanesthesia
h. principle
h. study
h. support
h., systemic
h. tolerance
h. vise
hemodynamically significant
  stenosis
hemoendothelial placenta
hemofiltration, continuous
  arteriovenous
hemofiltration, continuous
  venovenous
hemofuscin pigment
hemoglobin (Hgb)
  h. A
  h., admission
  h., Bart's
  h. C
  h. C disease, sickle cell-
  h. carbamate
  h. Chesapeake
  h. concentration (MCC/MCHC) ▸
    mean corpuscular
  h. C-thalassemia disease
  h. D
  h. D disease, sickle cell-
  h. E
  h. electrophoresis
  h. E-thalassemia disease
  h. F
  h., fast
  h., fetal
  h., fetal-maternal
  h. fluctuated
  h., glycated
  h., glycosylated
  h., Gower

h. Gun Hill
h. H
h. I
h. imbibition
h. Lepore
h. level, glycosylated
h. M
h. (MCH) ▸ mean corpuscular
h., muscle
h., nitric oxide
h., oxidized
h. oxygen (O_2) dissociation curve
h., oxygenated
h., peripheral ring of
h. production
h. ▸ pyridoxilated stroma-free
h. Rainier
h., reduced
h. S
h. Seattle
h., sickling
h., slow
h. solution, stroma-free
h., synthetic
h. test, fetal
h., total circulating
h., un-ionized
h. Yakima
hemoglobinophilus, Haemophilus
hemoglobinuria
  h., paroxysmal
  h., paroxysmal cold
  h. (PNH) ▸ paroxysmal nocturnal
hemologic parameters
hemolymph nodes
hemolysin test, ox cell
hemolytic
  h., alpha
  h. anemia
  h. anemia, acquired
  h. anemia, autoimmune
  h. anemia, chronic
  h. anemia, congenital
  h. anemia, congenital
    nonspherocytic
  h. anemia ▸ drug induced immune
  h. anemia ▸ Heinz body
  h. anemia, hereditary
  h. anemia ▸ idiopathic
  h. anemia ▸ immune
  h. anemia, microangiopathic
  h. anemia (HHA) test ▸ hereditary
  h. aureus
  h., beta
  h. blood transfusion disease

h. ▸ incompatible
h. complement assay
h. complement (C'H₅₀), total
h. disease
h. disease of the newborn (HDN)
h. dose, mean
h. dose (MHD) ▸ minimum
h. icterus
h. icterus, acholuric
h. index
h. jaundice
h. plaque assay
h. process
h. reaction, delayed
h. resistance
h. splenomegaly
h. staph aureus
h. strains, beta
h. strep, beta
h. streptococci
h. streptococci, beta
h. streptococci ▸ Group A beta
h. streptococcus
h. streptococcus, alpha
h. streptococcus, beta
h. substance
h. uremic syndrome (HUS)
hemolyticus
  h., gram-positive Streptococcus
  h., Haemophilus
  h., Hemophilus
  h. icterus
  h., Streptococcus
hemolyzed serum
hemopericardium
  h., cardiac lacerations and
  h., clotted
  h., minor
  h., resultant
  h., traumatic
hemophil/hemophile
hemophilia
  h., mild
  h., para
  h., severe
hemophilic arthropathy
Hemophilus (*see* Haemophilus)
  H. influenza type B (HIB)
  H. influenza type B (HIB) vaccine
  H. influenzae
  H. pertussis
  H. vaginalis
hemopleuropneumonic syndrome
hemoptysis
  h., cardiac

hemoptysis—*continued*
- h., cough and/or
- h., endemic
- h., Goldstein's
- h., intermittent
- h., Manson's
- h., oriental
- h., parasitic
- h., persistent cough with
- h., vicarious

Hemopure blood substitute
hemorrhage(s)
- h., acute gastrointestinal (GI)
- h., acute intraventricular
- h., acute pulmonary
- h., acute rectal
- h. ▸ agonal spinal cord
- h., alveolar
- h. and clotted blood
- h. and erosions ▸ intramucosal
- h. and necrosis ▸ areas of
- h. and stroke
- h., aneurysmal
- h., antepartum
- h. ▸ area of recent
- h., arterial
- h., atrial subendocardial
- h., bladder mucosal
- h., bowel wall
- h., brain
- h., brain damage from cerebral
- h., brain stem
- h., brisk
- h. bronchial mucosa ▸ extensive
- h., capillary
- h., capsuloganglionic
- h., cerebral
- h., concealed
- h., conjunctival
- h., cranial
- h., diffuse alveolar
- h., diffuse petechial
- h. ▸ diffuse pulmonary alveolar
- h. distal esophagus ▸ superficial
- h., dot
- h., Duret
- h., ecchymotic
- h., eight-ball
- h., epidural
- h., essential
- h., essential uterine
- h., exacerbation and
- h., expulsive
- h., exsanguinating
- h., exsanguinating intraperitoneal

- h., external
- h., extradural
- h., exudates and aneurysms (HEA)
- h., eye
- h., fatal
- h., fatal pulmonary
- h., fetomaternal
- h., fibrinolytic
- h., flame-shaped
- h., focal
- h., focal area of
- h. ▸ focal areas of intrapulmonary
- h., focal hepatic
- h., focal interstitial
- h., focal intrapulmonary
- h., focal petechial
- h. ▸ focal shallow subpleural
- h., focal subendocardial
- h., fresh
- h. from aneurysm ▸ recurrent
- h., gastric mucosal
- h., gastrointestinal (GI)
- h., gravitating
- h., gross
- h., hypertensive
- h. in brain
- h. in brainstem ▸ Duret's
- h. in cranium ▸ subarachnoid
- h. in cranium ▸ subdural
- h. in medulla
- h. in orbit
- h. in retina
- h. in vitreous
- h., infiltration by
- h., intermediary
- h., intermediate
- h., internal
- h., interstitial
- h., intestinal
- h. into mesentery ▸ soft tissue
- h. into submucosa
- h. into wall of bladder
- h., intra-abdominal
- h., intra-alveolar
- h., intracerebral
- h. ▸ intracerebral and subarachnoid
- h., intracranial
- h. ▸ intractable postpartum
- h., intramedullary
- h., intramucosal
- h., intraocular
- h., intrapartum
- h., intratesticular
- h., intraventricular
- h., laceration or

- h. ▸ linear-shaped
- h., lung
- h., massive
- h. ▸ massive gastrointestinal (GI)
- h., massive intracerebral
- h., massive midbrain
- h. ▸ maternal fetal
- h., meningeal
- h., mucosal
- h. ▸ multiple interstitial pulmonary
- h., multiple punctate
- h., nasal
- h. of bowel ▸ petechial
- h. of epicardium ▸ petechial
- h. of eye ▸ subconjunctival
- h. of iris
- h. of kidneys ▸ petechial
- h. of midbrain ▸ dissecting
- h. of pericardium ▸ petechial
- h. of peritoneum ▸ petechial
- h. of skin ▸ petechial
- h. or laceration
- h., parenchymal
- h., parenchymatous
- h., patchy purpuric
- h. per rhexis
- h., peri-adrenal
- h., peri-esophageal
- h., periventricular
- h., petechial
- h., plasma
- h., postcesarean
- h., postpartum
- h., post-tonsillectomy
- h., primary
- h., profuse
- h., pulmonary
- h. ▸ pulmonary alveolar
- h., punctate
- h., recent soft tissue
- h. ▸ recurrent variceal
- h., recurring
- h., renal
- h., renopelvic
- h. ▸ reperfusion-induced
- h., retroperitoneal
- h., scleral
- h., secondary
- h., serosal
- h. ▸ shaped retinal
- h. ▸ small brain
- h., small focal
- h., soft tissue
- h., splinter
- h., spontaneous

h., sternocleidomastoid
h., stroke due to cerebral
h., subarachnoid
h., subchorionic
h., subconjunctival
h., subdural
h., subendocardial
h., subendocardial petechial
h. ▸ subependymal germinal plate
h., subhyaloid
h., submucosal
h., subpleural
h., superficial cortical
h. ▸ superficial subendocardial focal
h., surface infiltration by
h. ▸ surgical procedure for
    subarachnoid
h. ▸ surgical treatment for epidural
h., transmural
h., transplacental
h., traumatic
h., traumatic multiple
h., unavoidable
h., urinary
h., uterine
h., vaginal
h., venous
h., vicarious
h., vitreous
hemorrhagic
h. adrenals
h. appearance, mottled
h. area, mottled
h. ascites
h. bronchitis
h. bronchopneumonia
h. bronchopneumonia, acute
h. bursitis, traumatic
h. colitis
h. corpus luteum
h. cyst
h. cyst, organizing
h. cystitis
h. cystitis, focal
h. diathesis
h. diathesis secondary to hepatic
    failure
h. discoloration
h. disease of the newborn
h. dot
h. encephalitis
h. encephalopathy
h. enterocolitis
h. esophagitis
h. esophagogastricitis

h. extravasation
h. familial angiomatosis
h. fever
h. fever, Argentinian
h. fever, Bolivian
h. fever, Crimean Congo
h. fever ▸ dengue
h. fever ▸ Ebola
h. fever, epidemic
h. fever, Korean
h. fever ▸ Marburg
h. fever ▸ Omsk
h. fever, South American
h. fever, Southeast Asian
    mosquito-borne
h. fever ▸ Venezuelan
h. fever ▸ viral
h. fever with renal syndrome
h. fluid
h. fluid, red
h. gastritis
h. gingivitis
h. glaucoma
h. glaucoma, painful
h. infarct, focal
h. infarcts of adrenal glands
h. infarctions
h. infiltration
h. lesion
h. leukoencephalitis, acute
h. manifestations
h. material
h. measles
h. metastasis
h. mucosa
h. necrosis, pulmonary
h., necrotizing cystitis ▸ focal
h. nephritis
h. nephrosonephritis
h. nephrosonephritis, Korean
h. omental lymph nodes
h. pancreatitis
h. pancreatitis, acute
h. pancreatitis ▸ fatal
h. pancreatitis, severe
h. pericarditis
h. peritonitis
h. petechiae
h. pleurisy
h. polioencephalitis, superior
h. purpura
h. pyelitis
h. salpingitis
h. scurvy
h. -septicemia group

h. shock
h. softening
h. spots on skin ▸ purplish
h. sputum
h. stools
h. stroke
h. telangiectasia, hereditary
h. telangiectasis
h. tumor metastasis
h. virus
hemorrhagica
h., aleukia
h., purpura
h., urticaria
hemorrhagicum, corpus
hemorrhaging
h., catastrophic
h., petechial
h., uncontrollable
hemorrhoidal artery ligation (HAL)
hemorrhoidal tissue, excess
hemorrhoidal tissue ▸ vaporized
hemorrhoid(s)
h., bipolar electrocoagulation of
h. ▸ chronic constipation or
h., combined
h., external
h., fiber and
h. ▸ infrared coagulation of
h., internal
h., lingual
h. ▸ laser therapy of
h., mixed
h., mucocutaneous
h., nonsymptomatic
h. of rectum ▸ internal
h. pain
h., prelapsed
h., prolapsing
h., rectal
h., rectal bleeding secondary to
h., rosette of
h. ▸ rubber band ligation of
h., shrinkage of
h., strangulated
h., thrombosed
hemorrhoidal
h. disease
h. nerves, inferior
h. skin tags
h. vein, inferior
h. vein, middle
h. vein, superior
h. vessels
hemorrhoidectomy, external

647

hemorrhoidectomy, internal
hemosiderin deposit
hemosiderin-laden macrophages
hemosiderosis
  h. ▸ essential pulmonary
  h., hepatic
  h., idiopathic pulmonary
  h., pulmonary
  h., secondary pulmonary
  h., transfusional
hemostasis
  h. accomplished
  h., adequate
  h. assured
  h. complete
  h., electrofulguration
  h. good
  h. maintained, adequate
  h. obtained
  h. secured
  h. secured with ties
  h. valve
  h., wound examined for
hemostatic
  h. bag, Pilcher's
  h., capillary
  h. catheter, return flow
  h. clamps, bleeding controlled with
  h. material
  h. processes, natural
  h. suture
  h. suture, continuous
hemothorax [*hemithorax*]
  h., left
  h., right
  h., spontaneous left
  h., spontaneous right
  h., traumatic
hemovac
  h. suction
  h. tube
  H. unit
Hemp (hemp)
  H. (marijuana)
  h. plant, Indian
  h. seed calculus
Henderson operation
Hendry's operation
Henle('s)
  H. ampulla
  H., ascending loop of
  H. cells
  H. elastic membrane
  H. fenestrated membrane
  H. fissures

H. loop
H. membrane
H. reaction
H. sphincter
H. spine
H. warts, Hassall-
Henoch's
  H. chorea
  H. disease
  H. purpura
  H. purpura ▸ Schönlein-
  H. -Schönlein purpura
  H. -Schönlein syndrome
  H. -Schönlein vasculitis
Henry-Geist operation
henselae, Rochalimaea
henselae topical bacteria ▸ Bartonella
Hensen's disc
Hensen's node
Hensing's fold
HEP (hepatoerythropoietic porphyria)
hepar
  h. adiposum
  h. lobatum
  h. siccatum
  h. sulfuris
heparin
  h. arterial filter
  h. block
  h. drip
  h. flush
  h. lock
  h. lock, flush
  h., mini-dose
  h. precipitable fraction
  h. therapy
  h. thrombocytopenia
heparinized
  h. blood
  h., patient
  h. saline
  h. solution infusion
hepatic [*herpetic*]
  h. abscess
  h. adenoma
  h. amebiasis
  h. angiography
  h. angiosarcoma
  h. angle
  h. artery
  h. artery aneurysm
  h. artery, common
  h. biliary system ▸ extra-
  h. blood flow
  h. blood flow, estimated

h. calculus
h. capsule
h. carcinoma
h. catalase
h. catheterization
h. catheterization, intra-arterial
h. cecum
h. cells
h. circulation, general
h. cirrhosis
h. colic
h. coma
h. coma, deep
h. complications of drug abuse
h. congestion
h. disease
h. disease ▸ pre-existing
h. disease, primary
h. disease ▸ protein loss in
h. distention
h. distomiasis
h. diverticulum
h. drug metabolism
h. duct
h. duct, common
h. dullness, relative
h. dysfunction
h. dysfunction ▸ constitutional
h. effects
h. encephalopathy
h. enzyme studies
h. enzymes
h. failure
h. failure, acute
h. failure ▸ hemorrhagic diathesis
  secondary to
h. failure, massive
h. fever
h. fever, intermittent
h. flexure
h. flexure of colon
h. flux
h. function
h. function ▸ impaired
h. ganglion
h. hemorrhages, focal
h. hydrothorax
h. impairment
h. infarct
h. infusion, intra-arterial
h. injury ▸ drug-induced
h. insufficiency
h. lipase
h. lobe, left
h. lobe, right

h. lobules
h. lobules, central vein of
h. lymph nodes
h. metabolism
h. metastases
h. necrosis
h. necrosis, massive
h. necrosis ▸ small focus of
h. obstruction
h. parenchyma
h. portal
h. portal vein (HPV)
h. portal venous gas (HPVG)
h. problems related to drug abuse
h. pulse
h. radicals
h. scan
h. schistosomiasis
h. segments
h. siderosis
h. softening, diffuse
h. stimulant
h. transplant, orthotopic
h. triad
h. tumor
h. vein
h. vein catheterization

hepatica
h., adiposis
h., Fasciola
h., pseudohemophilia

hepaticolenticular degeneration
hepaticum, coma
hepaticus, fetor
hepatis
h., hilus
h., lues
h., Myrtophyllum
h., pons
h., porta
h. ▸ vasa aberrantis

hepatitis
h. A virus (HAV)
h. ▸ acute, alcoholic
h., acute toxic
h., acute viral
h., alcohol-related
h., alcoholic
h., Allopurinol-induced
h., amebic
h. and acetaminophen
h. and alcoholism
h., anicteric
h., antigen ▸ serum
h. -associated antigen(s)

h., autopsy-acquired
h. B antibody
h. B carrier
h. B core antibody (HBcAb)
h. B core antigen (Anti-HBc IgM),
    antibody IgM class to
h. B core antigen (Anti-HBc), total
    antibody to
h. B immune globulin
h. B infection
h. B infection, patient immune to
h. B surface antibody (HBsAb)
h. B surface antigen (HBsAg)
h. B surface antigen (Anti-HBs),
    antibody to
h. B surface antigen (HBsAg)
    reactivity
h. B vaccine
h. B virus (HBV)
h. B virus infection ▸ chronic
h. B virus, patient has natural
    immunity to
h. B'e' antibody (HBeAb)
H. B'e' antigen (HBeAg)
H. B'e' antigen (Anti-HBe), antibody
    to
h. C, acute
h. C infection, chronic
h. C screening
h. C virus
h., cholangiolitic
h., cholestatic
h., chronic active
h., chronic aggressive
h., chronic interstitial
h., chronic persisting
h., cirrhosis from
h., clinical
h., clinical alcoholic
h. ▸ confirmed transmission of viral
h. D virus (HDV)
h. ▸ drug-induced
h. E virus
h., epidemic
h., familial
h., fatal
h. ▸ food-borne transmission of viral
h. from birth control pill
h., fulminant
h. G virus
h., gastro◊
h., giant cell
h. ▸ hemodialysis transmission of
    viral
h., homologous serum

h., hospital-acquired viral
h., icteric
h. icteric serum
h. -induced liver cancer
h. infection
h., infectious
h., inoculation
h. ▸ inoculation transmission of viral
h. ▸ intrafamily transmission of viral
h. ▸ intrainstitutional transmission of
    viral
h., lingering
h., lupoid
h. ▸ maternal-neonatal transmission
    of viral
h., neonatal
h., neonatal giant cell
h. ▸ non-A, non-B
h., nonicteric
h., nonviral
h. ▸ oral transmission of viral
h. ▸ pain in abdomen from
h. panel, viral
h. patients ▸ secretion spills from
h., plasma cell
h., post-transfusion
h. profile
h. sequestrans
h., serodiagnosis
h., serum
h. ▸ sexual transmission of viral
h., suppurative
h. surface antigen studies
h. -tainted blood
h. ▸ tenderness in abdomen
h., toxic
h., toxipathic
h., transfusion
h. ▸ transfusion transmission of viral
h., transient clinical
h., transmission
h., trophopathic
h., undiagnosed
h. vaccine
h., viral
h. viremia
h. virus
h. virus A
h. virus B
h. virus IH
h. virus SH
h. ▸ waterborne transmission of
    viral
h. with infection

hepatobiliary
- h. cholangiography, percutaneous
- h. scan
- h. tract disease

hepatocellular
- h. abnormality, nonspecific
- h. adenoma
- h. carcinoma
- h. carcinoma ▸ well-differentiated
- h. injury
- h. degeneration, diffuse
- h. disease
- h. enzymes
- h. failure
- h. liver disease
- h. necrosis, acute

hepatodiaphragmatic adhesions
hepatoerythropoietic porphyria (HEP)
hepatofugal flow
hepatofugal venous collateral circulation
hepatoid adenocarcinoma
hepato-iminodiacetic acid (HIDA) scan
hepatojejunal anastomosis
hepatojugular reflex
hepatojugular reflex test
hepatolenticular degeneration
hepatolenticular disease
hepatoma, human
hepatomegaly/hepatomegalia
hepatopancreatic ampulla ▸ sphincter muscle of
hepatopancreatica, ampulla
hepatopetal flow
hepatorenal
- h. disease
- h. failure
- h. syndrome

hepatosplenomegaly with liver metastases
hepatostomy, choledocho◊
hepatotoxicity, serious
herald patch
Herb (marijuana)
herb-drug interaction
herbal
- h. medicine
- h. remedy
- h. supplement
- h. therapy
- h. treatment

herbalism, medicinal
herbarum, Cladosporium
Herbert's operation

Herculon suture
herd immunity
herd instinct
here [hear]
hereditaria, adynamia episodica
hereditaria, anemia hypochromica siderochrestica
hereditary
- h. angioneurotic edema
- h. ataxia
- h. atrophy optic nerve
- h. benign intraepithelial dyskeratosis syndrome
- h. bleeding disorder
- h. bone disease
- h. bone dysplasia
- h. breast cancer
- h. breast-ovarian cancer syndrome
- h. brown enamel
- h. cancer
- h. cerebellar ataxia
- h. cerebral leukodystrophy
- h. chorea
- h. chorea, chronic progressive
- h. colon cancer
- h. coproporphyria
- h. defect
- h. disease
- h. disease ▸ irreversible
- h. disease of nervous system
- h. disorder
- h. disorder ▸ slowly progressive
- h. ectodermal polydysplasia
- h. enamel hypoplasia
- h. essential tremor
- h. factors
- h. familial disease
- h. familial illness
- h. fructose intolerance
- h. heart defect
- h. hemolytic anemia (HHA) test
- h. hemorrhagic telangiectasia
- h. hypertrophic enlargement
- h. insanity
- h. methemoglobinemic cyanosis
- h. motor neuron disease, juvenile
- h. multiple exostosis
- h. nephritis
- h. nonpolyposis colon cancer (HNPCC)
- h. nonpolyposis colorectal cancer
- h. nonspherocytic
- h. optic atrophy
- h. optic neuropathy ▸ Leber's
- h. osteo-onychodysplasia

- h. pancreatitis
- h. predisposition
- h. prostate cancer
- h. progressive ataxia
- h. psychoses
- h. respiratory disease
- h. sclerosis
- h. spherocytosis
- h. tabes
- h. tendencies
- h. traits
- h. tremor ▸ benign

heredity
- h., autosomal
- h., sex-linked
- h., X-linked

heredocongenital factors
heredocongenital nucleus of personality
heredoconstitutional disease
heredodegenerative disease
heredofamilial tremor
Hérelle phenomenon ▸ Twort-d'
Herellea vaginicola
Hering('s)
- H. -Breuer reflex
- H. inflation reflex, Breuer-
- H. law
- H. nerve
- H. phenomenon
- H. test
- H. theory
- H. waves, Traube-

heritage, genetic
hermanni, Argas
Hermetia illucens
hermetic medicine
hermsi, Damalinia
hermsi, Trichodectes
hermsii, Borrelia
hernia
- h., abdominal
- h., acquired
- h. adiposa
- h., amniotic
- h. and constipation ▸ hiatal
- h., Barth's
- h., Béclard's
- h., Birkett's
- h., bladder
- h., Bochdalek
- h., cecal
- h. celomic
- h., cerebri
- h., Cloquet's

h., complete
h., concealed
h., congenital
h., congenital diaphragmatic
h., Cooper's
h., crural
h., cystic
h., diaphragmatic
h., direct
h., direct inguinal
h., diverticular
h., dry
h., duodenojejunal
h., encysted
h., epigastric
h., esophageal hiatal
h., esophageal hiatus
h., external
h., extrasaccular
h., fat
h., femoral
h. (CDH) ► fetal congenital diaphragmatic
h., foremen of Bochdalek
h., foremen of Morgagni
h., foraminal
h., funicular
h., gastroesophageal
h., Gibbon's
h., gluteal
h., Goyrand's
h., Gruber's
h., Grynfeltt's
h., Hesselbach's
h., Hey's
h., hiatal
h., hiatus
h., Holthouse's
h. in recto
h., incarcerated
h. ► incarcerated inguinal
h., incisional
h., incomplete
h., indirect
h., indirect inguinal
h., infantile
h., inguinal
h., inguinocrural
h., inguinofemoral
h., inguinoproperitoneal
h., inguinosuperficial
h., intermuscular
h., internal
h., interparietal
h., intersigmoid

h., interstitial
h., intestinal
h., iris
h., irreducible
h., ischiatic
h., ischiorectal
h., Krönlein's
h., labial
h., Laugier's
h., levator
h., linea alba
h., Littre-Richter
h., Littre's
h., lumbar
h., Maydi's
h., McVay repair of
h., mesenteric
h., mesocolic
h., Morgagni
h., mucosal
h., oblique
h., obturator
h. of bladder
h. of diaphragm
h. of esophagus
h. of lung
h., omental
h., ovarian
h. ► pain in abdomen from
h., pantaloon inguinal
h. par glissement
h., paraduodenal
h., paraesophageal
h., paraperitoneal
h., parasaccular
h., parietal
h., parumbilical
h., pectineal
h., pectineal crural
h., perineal
h., peritoneopericardial
h., Petit's
h., pleuroperitoneal
h., posterior labial
h., posterior vaginal
h., properitoneal
h. protrudes down
h., pudendal
h., pulp
h., pulsion
h., rectal
h., rectovaginal
h., recurrent
h., reducible
h. repair

h. repair, Allison hiatal
h. repair, Bassini inguinal
h. repair, Bassini-type
h. repair, Boerema
h. repair ► Effler hiatal
h. repair ► laparoscopic
h. repair ► pants-over-vest
h., retrocecal
h., retrograde
h., retroperitoneal
h., retrosternal
h., Richter's
h., Rieux's
h., Rokitansky's
h., rolling
h., root
h. sac ► large inguinal
h., sciatic
h., scrotal
h., Serafini
h., sliding
h., sliding esophageal hiatal
h., sliding hiatal
h., slip
h., slipped
h., spigelian
h., strangulated
h., subdiaphragmatic
h., subpubic
h. ► supportive device to restrain
h., synovial
h., thyroidal
h., tonsillar
h., transmesenteric
h., Treitz's
h., tunicary
h., umbilical
h., uterine
h., vaginal
h., vaginolabial
h., Velpeau's
h., ventral
h., vesical
h., voluminous
h., Von Bergmann's
h., w

hernial
h. aneurysm
h. protrusion
h. sac

herniated
h. disc
h. disc syndrome
h. disk, vaporize water in
h. intervertebral disc

herniated—*continued*
   h. nucleus pulposus (HNP)
herniation
   h., bilateral uncal
   h., cardiac
   h., cingulate gyrus
   h., disc
   h., gyrus
   h., intervertebral disc
   h., intestinal
   h., massive
   h. of disc
   h. of muscle
   h. of nucleus pulposus (HNP)
   h. of the brain
   h., sacular
   h., tentorial
   h., tonsillar
   h., transtentorial
   h. ▸ traumatic transtentorial
   h., uncal
   h., vitreous
hernioplasty, diaphragmatic
herniorrhaphy
   h., bilateral
   h., femoral
   h. incision, LaRoque
   h., inguinal
heroic measures
heroin
   h. (Big H)
   h. (Boy)
   h. (Brown)
   h. (Brown Sugar)
   h. (Caballo)
   h. (Chiva)
   h. (Crap)
   h. (Do-Jee)
   h. (Estuffa)
   h. (H)
   h. (Heroina)
   h. (Hombre)
   h. (Horse)
   h. (Jive)
   h. (Junk)
   h. (Material)
   h. (Mexican Med)
   h. (Mud)
   h. (Polvo)
   h. (Product)
   h. (Scag)
   h. (Skag)
   h. (Smack)
   h. (Stofa)
   h. (Stuff)

   h. (Thing)
   h. (Big H) abuser
   h. (Big H) addict
   h. addict, detoxification of
   h. (Big H) addiction
   h. addicts ▸ long-term
   h. chasers
   h. (Big H) dependency
   h. detoxification
   h. epidemic
   h., free-base
   h. (Big H) habit
   h. intoxication
   h. (Dava), Iranian
   h. (Persian), Iranian
   h. (Persian Brown), Iranian
   h. (Rufus), Iranian
   h., Persian
   h. plague
   h. -related emergency room
      episodes
   h. smoking
   h., snorting
   h. substitute (Ts and Blues)
   h. (Big H) user
   h. -using population
   h. (Big H) withdrawal
Heroina (heroin)
herpangina pharyngitis
herpangina virus
herpes (Herpes)
   h. catarrhalis
   h. corneae
   h., dermal or oral
   h. facialis
   h. family of viruses
   h. febrilis
   h. generalisatus
   h., genital
   h. genitalis
   h. gestationis
   h. gladiatorum
   h. infection
   h. infection, genital
   h. infection, ocular
   h. keratitis
   h. labialis
   h. -like lesions
   h. -like virus
   h. meningoencephalitis
   h. menstrualis
   h. of vulva, focal
   h. ophthalmicus
   h. oticus
   h. pain

   h., penile
   h. pneumonia
   h. praeputialis
   h. progenitalis
   h. recurrens
   h. ▸ recurrent genital
   h. retinitis
   h. simplex
   h. simplex antibody titers
   h. simplex encephalitis
   h. simplex infection
   h. simplex gingivostomatitis
   h. simplex pneumonitis
   h. simplex Type 1
   h. simplex Type 2
   h. simplex virus
   h. simplex, visceral
   h. -type virus
   h. virus
   h. virus, genital
   h. virus (KSHV) ▸ Kaposi's
      sarcoma
   h. virus of right eye
   h. virus vesicles
   H. Virus-8 (HHV 8) ▸ Human
   H. Virus-7 (HHV 7) ▸ Human
   h. vulvitis
   h. zoster (shingles)
   h. zoster infection ▸ disseminated
   h. zoster of cornea
   h. zoster of iris
   h. zoster virus
herpesvirus
   h. encephalitis
   h. hominus
   h. infection
   h., Marek's disease
herpetic [*hepatic*]
   h. fever
   h. gingivitis
   h. gingivostomatitis
   h. keratitis
   h. keratitis, stromal
   h. lesions
   h. neuralgia (PHN) ▸ post-
   h. ocular disease
   h. stomatitis
   h. tonsillitis
   h. ulcerations
   h. whitlow
herpetica, pharyngitis
herpetica, stomatitis
herpeticum, eczema
herpeticus, favus
herpetiform lesion

herpetiform lesion of Cole
herpetiformis, dermatitis
herpetiformis, impetigo
Herrick's anemia
herring, red
herring sperm
Herrmannsdorfer diet, Gerson-
Herrmannsdorfer Gerson diet ▸
    Sauerbruch-
Hers' disease
Hershey total artificial heart
Hertel's exophthalmometer
Hertwig-Magendie syndrome
hertz (Hz)
    h. (Hz) ▸ eight to 13
    h. positive bursts ▸ 14 and six
    h. positive spikes ▸ 14 and six
    h. spike-and-slow waves ▸ three
    H. (Hz) unit
hertzian rays
Herxheimer's
    H. fibers
    H. reaction
    H. spirals
Heschl's convolution
Heschl's gyrus
hesitancy, urinary
hesitant urinary stream ▸ slow,
hesitation and retreat ▸ symptoms of
Hespan plasma volume expander
Hess diplopia screen
Hess operation
Hessburg trephine
Hesselbach's
    H. hernia
    H. ligament
    H. triangle
Hessian wheat fly
hetastarch plasma expander
heterochromia, Fuchs'
heterochromia iridis
heterochromic
    h. cataract
    h. cyclitis
    h. uveitis
heterochronicus, pulsus
heterocladic anastomosis
heterodermic graft
heteroduplex analysis
heterogeneic antigen
heterogeneities, patient
heterogeneity(-ies)
    h., genetic
    h. of patient ▸ dose
    h. of patient ▸ dose distribution

    h. of psychiatric disorder
    h. of viral lode
    h., patient
heterogeneous
    h. attenuation
    h., genetically
    h. graft
    h. noises
heterogenetic antibody
heterograft
    h., bovine
    h., porcine
    h. valve ▸ stent-mounted
heterologous
    h. antigen
    h. blood transfusion
    h. cardiac transplant
    h. chimera
    h. graft
    h. insemination
    h. stimulus
    h. strain
    h. tissue
heterometric autoregulation
heteronymous
    h. diplopia
    h. hemianopia
    h. hemianopsia
    h. motoneurons
    h. parallax
hetero-osteoplasty
heterophil/heterophile
    h. agglutination
    h. antibody
    h. antibody reaction
    h. antibody test
    h. antibody titer
    h. antigen
    h. negative mononucleosis
heterophilic agglutinin
heterophyes (Heterophyes)
    h., Fasciola
    H. heterophyes
    H., Trematoda
heteroplastic graft
heterosexual
    h. contact
    h. contact with male carriers of
      AIDS (acquired immune
      deficiency syndrome)
    h. intercourse
    h. men
    h. transmission
    h. women
heterosomal aberration

heterotaxia, cardiac
heterotaxy
    h. syndrome
    h. syndrome ▸ visceroatrial
    h., visceral
heterotopia cerebralis
heterotopia cerebrum
heterotopic
    h. cardiac transplant
    h. pain
    h. pregnancy
    h. stimulus
    h. tissue
heterotrema, Paragonimus
heterotropia
    h., alternating
    h., left
    h., periodic
    h., right
heterozygous achondroplasia
heterozygous familial
    hypercholesterolemia
Heublein's method
Heubner's specific endarteritis
Heuter's operation
hexacanth embryo
hexachlorophene
    h. cleansing emulsion
    h. scrub
    h. soap
hexagonus, Ixodes
hexamibi ▸ technetium-99m
hexaxial reference system
hexokinase reaction
hexosaminidase deficiency
hexose monophosphate shunt
Hey('s)
    H. amputation
    H. hernia
    H. internal derangement
    H. ligament
    H. operation
Heyer-Schulte breast implant
Heyman operation
Heyns' decompression
H-form ▸ myocardial infarction in
Hg 197, chlormerodrin
Hg 203, chlormerodrin
Hgb (hemoglobin)
HGE (human granulocytic
    ehrlichiosis)
HGF (hyperglycemic-glycogenolytic
    factor)
HGH (human growth hormone)
H-graft

HHA (hereditary hemolytic anemia) test
HHD (hypertensive heart disease)
HHE (hemiconvulsion, hemiplegia, epilepsy) syndrome
HHV-7 (Human Herpes Virus-7)
HIAA (5-hydroxyindoleacetic acid) ▸ 5-
hiatal
   h. esophagism
   h. hernia
   h. hernia and constipation
   h. hernia, esophageal
   h. hernia repair, Allison
   h. hernia repair ▸ Effler
   h. hernia, sliding
   h. hernia, sliding esophageal
   h. hernia, sliding-type
   h. insufficiency
hiatus
   h., aortic
   h., esophageal
   h. hernia
   h. hernia, esophageal
   h. semilunaris
HIB (Hemophilus influenza type B)
HIB (Hemophilus influenza type B) vaccine
Hibbs(')
   H. frame
   H. operation
   H. spinal fusion
   H. technique, modified
hibernating myocardium
hibernation, myocardial
hiccoughing, patient
hiccups, prolonged
Hickey('s)
   H. -Hare test
   H. position
   H. projection ▸ Lauenstein and
hickory-stick fracture
Hicks'
   H. contraction
   H. contraction, Braxton-
   H. -Pitney thromboplastin generation test
   H. sign
   H. sign, Braxton-
   H. version
   H. version, Braxton-
HIDA (hepatoiminodiacetic acid) scan
hidden
   h. determinant
   h. sensitivity

h. suicidal tendencies
h. trauma
hidradenitis (*same as* hydradenitis)
hidradenitis, axillary
hidradenitis suppurativa
hidrosadenitis axillaris
hidrosadenitis destruens suppurativa
hidrotic ectodermal dysplasia
hiemalis, arthritis
hiemis, hyperemesis
Higashi syndrome ▸ Arakawa-
Higashi syndrome ▸ Chédiak-
high
   h. acid level in blood
   h. affinity antibody
   h. altitude pulmonary edema (HAPE)
   h. altitude related disorders
   h. altitude related illnesses
   h. altitude sickness
   h. altitude simulation test
   h. and low energy x-ray therapy, combination
   h. anxiety
   h. arch deformity
   h. arched palate
   h. antiembolilc stockings ▸ thigh-
   h. anxiety sensitivity
   h. beam intensity
   h. birth weight
   h. blood alcohol level
   h. blood cholesterol
   h. blood pressure (BP)
   h. blood pressure (BP), borderline
   h. blood pressure (BP), chronic
   h. blood pressure (BP), controlled
   h. blood pressure (BP) from birth control pill
   h. blood pressure (BP) ▸ primary
   h. blood pressure (BP) ▸ secondary
   h. blood pressure (BP), uncontrolled
   h. bulk diet
   h. calorie diet
   h. carbohydrate diet
   h. ceiling diuretic
   h. cholesterol diet ▸ high fat,
   h. cholesterol ▸ familial
   h. cholesterol ▸ inherited
   h. cholesterol level
   h. clotting risk
   h., cocaine
   h. concentration
   h. concentration of urine ▸ abnormally

h. content, abnormally
h. cure rate
h. death rate
h. degree atrioventricular block ▸ atrial tachycardia with
h. degree of risk
h. density bile
h. density lipoprotein (HDL)
h. density lipoprotein deficiency ▸ familial
h. density polyethylene (HDPE)
h. dosage
h. dose
h. dose, achieve
h. dose aspirin therapy
h. dose beams of X-rays
h. dose chemotherapy
h. dose chemotherapy ▸ intense cycle of
h. dose external irradiation
h. dose fractionation radiation therapy
h. dose methotrexate and cistoplatin
h. dose methotrexate and 5-fluorouracil
h. dose, precision
h. dose radiation
h. dose radiation therapy
h. dose radiation to tumor mass
h. dose rate
h. dose rate, fractionated
h. dose therapy
h. ▸ drug-induced
h. -efficiency particulate air
h. energy accelerator
h. energy behavior
h. energy bent beam linear accelerator
h. energy cardioversion
h. energy electrons
h. energy pulsed ruby laser
h. energy radiation
h. energy radiopharmaceuticals
h. energy transthoracic shock
h. energy x-rays
h., false
h. fat diet
h. fat food
h. fat, high cholesterol diet
h. fat ketogenic diet
h. fat, low fiber diet
h. fever, delirium with
h. fiber diet
h. fiber supplement, daily

h. flow
h. forceps delivery
h. fracture risk
h. frequencies of recording
h. frequency
h. frequency activity
h. frequency blood group
h. frequency current
h. frequency epicardial echocardiography
h. frequency filter
h. frequency filter control
h. frequency hearing loss
h. frequency jet ventilation
h. frequency jet ventilator
h. frequency murmur
h. frequency oscillation
h. frequency oscillation ventilator
h. frequency oscillatory ventilation
h. frequency positive pressure ventilation
h. frequency potentials, bizarre
h. frequency ▸ reduced hearing at
h. frequency response
h. frequency sensorineural hearing loss
h. frequency sound waves
h. frequency ▸ square waves of
h. frequency stimulation
h. frequency thrombolysis
h. frequency ventilation
h. genetic risk
h. grade lesion
h. grade stenosis
h. impact activity
h. impact aerobic exercise
h. impact exercise
h. impact trauma
h. impulsiveness
h. in fiber, diet
h. incision
h. input impedance
h., intense
h. intensity exercise
h. intensity light source
h. intracranial pressure
h. -jumper's strain
h. level of anxiety
h. level of function
h. levels of arousal
h. levels of care
h. levels of kidney protein renin
h. ligation and stripping
h. linear energy transfer radiation
h. lung volume

h. membranous interventricular septum
h. molecular weight
h. occlusion
h. output heart failure
h. oxygen
h. oxygen concentration
h. oxygen pressure (HOP)
h. pass filter
h. ▸ patient on a
h. peak powered
h. -pitched
h. -pitched murmur
h. -pitched noises ▸ loud,
h. -pitched sounds
h. position
h. potassium diet ▸ low sodium,
h. potency vitamin
h. power field (hpf)
h. power field (hpf) ▸ organisms per
h. power field (WBC/hpf) ▸ white blood cells per
h. -powered magnification
h. pressure chamber
h. pressure chamber ▸ walk-in
h. pressure oxygen
h. pressure, oxygen under
h. pressure treatment
h. probability of survival
h. profile research
h. protein
h. protein diet
h. -quality and effective treatment
h. -quality care
h. -quality medical care
h. quantum energy
h., rapid
h. rate
h. residue diet
h. resolution B mode ultrasonography
h. resolution computed tomography
h. resolution computed tomography (HRCT) scan
h. right atrium
h. -risk
h. -risk adolescent population
h. -risk angioplasty
h. -risk baby
h. -risk behavior
h. -risk candidate
h. -risk category
h. -risk follow-up
h. -risk for breast cancer
h. -risk group

h. -risk infant
h. -risk lifestyle
h. -risk mother
h. -risk mother, infant of
h. risk of developing cervical cancer
h. risk of exposure, patient at
h. risk of HIV infection
h. risk of suicide
h. -risk patient
h. -risk population
h. -risk potential victims
h. -risk pregnancy
h. -risk procedure
h. -risk sexual activity
h. -risk sexual behavior
h. -risk situation
h. -risk systolic pressure
h., runner's
h. saphenous vein ligation
h. self-expectation
h. sensitivity C-reactive protein (hs-CRP)
h. serum-bound iron
h., short-lived
h. socks, knee
h. socks, thigh
h. -speed drill
h. -speed engine
h. -speed rotational atherectomy
h. -speed volumetric imaging
h. -stress job
h. -stress workout
h. -strung, patient
h. -tension pulse
h. thoracic cord lesion
h. tone
h. tone hearing loss
h. toxicity
h. tracheotomy
h. -velocity electron beams
h. -viscosity barium and air
h. voltage
h. voltage activity
h. voltage arrhythmic slow waves
h. voltage brain waves
h. voltage bursts
h. voltage diphasic slow wave
h. voltage discharge ▸ paroxysmal
h. voltage electrophoresis
h. voltage fast activity
h. voltage firing
h. voltage pattern
h. voltage ▸ periodic bursts of
h. voltage slow wave activity

high—*continued*
- h. voltage slow waves ▸ paroxysmal
- h. voltage transformer
- h. voltage waves, slow

higher
- h. air pressure
- h. mental functions
- h. than heart, head
- h. than heart, legs elevated

highest
- h. functioning level
- h. intercostal vein
- h. level of activity
- h. risk for disease

highly
- h. active antiretroviral therapy (HAART)
- h. active epileptic process
- h. addictive
- h. addictive and isolated
- h. compulsive, patient
- h. motivated
- h. prone to fantasy
- h. reactive oxygen (O_2) molecules

Highmore, antrum of
highmori, antrum
hilar
- h. adenopathy
- h. cell
- h. clouding
- h. dance
- h. fullness
- h. haze
- h. infiltrate
- h. infiltrates, bilateral
- h. lesion
- h. lymph node, left
- h. lymph node, right
- h. lymph nodes
- h. lymphadenopathy
- h. mass
- h. node
- h. node metastasis
- h. nodes, anthracotic
- h. nodes, calcified
- h. prominence
- h. region
- h. scarring
- h. shadow
- h. structures
- h. substance of lung
- h. vasculature
- h. vessels exposed

Hildreth('s)
- H. cautery
- H. cautery ▸ Rommel-
- H. mercury lamp

Hilgenreiner line
Hilger facial nerve stimulator
hili of lungs
hill (Hill)
- h. diarrhea
- H., hemoglobin Gun
- H. -Sachs lesion

Hillis maneuver, Müller-
Hillis obstetric stethoscope ▸ DeLee-
hillock, axon
Hilton sac
Hilton's muscle
hilum
- h. convergence sign
- h., left
- h. overlay sign
- h., prominence of left
- h., prominence of right
- h., pruned
- h., right

hilus
- h. glandulae suprarenalis
- h. hepatis
- h., kidney
- h. lienis
- h., lung
- h., lymph node
- h. nodi lymphatici
- h. nuclei dentati
- h. of ovary
- h. olivary nucleus
- h. ovarii
- h., pulmonary
- h. renalis
- h., suprarenal gland
- h. tuberculosis

him/her, world around
Himmelsbach rating scale
Himmelstein's valvulotome
hind kidney
hindgut embryonic development
hinge
- h. joint
- h. knee prosthesis, Guepar
- h. knee prosthesis, Kinematic rotating

hinged articulation
hingeless heart valve prosthesis ▸ Wada
hip(s)
- h., abduction contracture of
- h., adduction contracture of
- h., adductor spasticity of
- h. adductor stretch exercise
- h. and pelvis
- h., arthrodesis of
- h. arthroplasty, Crawford-Adams
- h. arthroplasty, McKee-Farrar total
- h. arthroplasty, total
- h. -associated bursitis
- h. bone
- h., ceramic total
- h. clicks
- h., congenital dislocation
- h. contracture
- h. cup prosthesis ▸ Smith-Petersen
- h. (DDH) developmental dysplasia of
- h., dislocated
- h. dislocation, congenital
- h. displacement, congenital
- h. dysplasia
- h. extension
- h. fixation
- h. flexed
- h. flexibility ▸ trunk and
- h. flexion
- h., flexion contracture of
- h. fracture
- h. fusion, Schneider's
- h. girdle
- h., intercondylar fracture of
- h., internal rotation contracture of
- h. joint
- h. joint, click heard at
- h. lipectomy
- h. locking prosthesis ▸ modified Moore
- h., marked degenerative change of
- h. motion
- h. musculature
- h. nailing
- h., orbicular zone of
- h., osteoarthritis of
- h. pain
- h., pelvis and
- h. pin, Hagie
- h. pinning
- h. pointer
- h. prosthesis, Austin-Moore
- h. prosthesis, DePalma
- h. prosthesis, Eicher
- h. prosthesis, Harris HD
- h. prosthesis, HD II total
- h. prosthesis, left
- h. prosthesis, Lippman
- h. prosthesis, Moore

h. prosthesis, Mueller Duo-Lock
h. prosthesis, right
h. prosthesis, Vitallium
h. ratio (WHR) ▸ waist-
h. replacement
h. replacement ▸ dual lock total
h. replacement ▸ metal-on-metal
h. replacement ▸ metal-on-plastic
h. replacement operation ▸ total
h. replacement procedure ▸ total
h. replacement, self-articulating femoral
h. replacement surgery
h. replacement surgery ▸ primary
h. replacement surgery ▸ repeat
h. replacement surgery ▸ revision
h. replacement, total
h., snapping
h. spica
h. spica cast
h. stiffness
h. surgery, reconstructive
h., synovial fold of

Hippel('s)
H. disease
H. disease, Lindau-von
H. -Lindau disease, von
H. -Lindau syndrome ▸ von
H. operation

hippicum, Trypanosoma
hippocampal
h. atrophy
h. cell loss
h. degeneration
h. gyrus
h. neurons, degeneration of
h., right

hippocampi
h., gyrus
h., sulcus
h., taenia

hippocampus ▸ histologic sections of
Hippocrates manipulation
hippocratic (Hippocratic)
h. angina
h. fingers
H. Oath
h., sound
h. succession

Hippuran contrast medium
Hippuran (RAH) test ▸ radioactive
hippuric acid
hippuric acid test
Hipputope renal function
Hirano body

Hirschberg('s)
H. magnet
H. method
H. reflex
H. sign

Hirschfield disease
Hirschfield lamp, Birch-
Hirschsprung's disease
Hirst's operation
hirsutism, amenorrhea and
hirsutum, cor
Hirtz's rale
hirudinaceus, Macracanthorhynchus
hirudinis, Oeciacus
Hirudo
H. aegyptiaca
H. japonica
H. javanica
H. medicinalis
H. quinquestriata
H. sanguisorba
H. troctina

His(')
H. bundle ablation
H. bundle activity
H. bundle branch block
H. bundle deflection
H. bundle depolarization
H. bundle electrocardiogram (ECG)
H. bundle electrode
H. bundle electrogram
H. bundle heart block
H., bundle of
H. bundle recording
H. canal
H. pathway, atrio-
H. perivascular space
H. -Purkinje conduction
H. -Purkinje fibers
H. -Purkinje system
H. -Purkinje tissue
H. rule
H. ▸ space of
H. spindle
H. -Tawara node

Hisian
H. block ▸ supra-
H. bypass tract, atrio-
H. bypass tract ▸ nodo-
H. connection, atrio-
H. fiber, atrio-
H. interval, atrio-

hispanica, Borrelia
histamine
h. antagonist

h., blood
h. cephalalgia
h. challenge
h. dihydrochloride
h. headache
h. phosphate
h. phosphate acid
h. releasing factor
h. shock
h. stimulation test
h. test
h. test, augmented
h. toxicity

histaminic headache
histidine
h. decarboxylase
h. production
h., tissue

histiocyte(s) (*same as* histocyte)
h. and giant cells
h. and lymphocytes ▸ foamy
h., cardiac
h., enlarged atypical
h., pallisading
h., scattered
h., sea-blue
h., wandering

histiocytic
h. fibroma
h. hyperplasia of lymph nodes
h. leukemia
h. lymphocyte depleted type ▸ Hodgkins disease of diffuse,
h. lymphoma
h. lymphoma (DHL), diffuse
h. lymphoma, malignant
h. lymphoma of stomach ▸ diffuse
h. type ▸ abdominal lymphoma, diffuse
h. type lymphoma ▸ non◊

histiocytoma
h., malignant
h., malignant fibrous
h. of soft tissue

histiocytosis
h., infantile malignant
h., lipid
h., sinus
h. X
h. X ▸ primary pulmonary

Histoacryl glue
histocompatibility
h. agent B27
h. antigen
h. complex antigen ▸ major

histocompatibility—*continued*
  h. locus
histocyte (*see* **histiocyte**)
histogram mode
histologic
  h. analysis
  h. anatomy
  h. appearance of liver
  h. architecture
  h. confirmation
  h. diagnosis
  h. evaluation
  h. examination
  h. factors
  h. lesion
  h. morphology
  h. pattern, nonspecific
  h. pattern, normal
  h. sections
  h. sections of basal ganglia
  h. sections of bladder
  h. sections of brain
  h. sections of cerebellum
  h. sections of cortex
  h. sections of esophagus
  h. sections of hippocampus
  h. sections of kidney
  h. sections of liver
  h. sections of lungs
  h. sections of pancreas
  h. sections of pons
  h. sections of prostate
  h. sections of spleen
histological diagnosis
histological spectrum
histologically benign
histologically malignant
histology, normal
histology, pathologic
histolytica
  h., Amoeba
  h., Entamoeba
  h., Torula
histolyticum, Clostridium
histolyticus, Cryptococcus
Histomonas meleagridis
histopathologic
  h. abnormality
  h. data
  h. entity
  h. grouping
histopathology, surgical
Histoplasma
  H. capsulatum
  H. duboisii

H. farciminosus
H. myocarditis
histoplasmic pericarditis
histoplasmin skin test
histoplasmosis
  h., acute
  h., African
  h., bronchopulmonary
  h. of lung
  h., pulmonary
  h. syndrome ▸ ocular
historical retrospect
history(-ies)
  h. and physical (H and P)
  h. and physical examination (HPE)
  h. and symptoms of emergency
    cardiac care
  h. as screening device for drug
    abuse, medical
  h. as screening device for drug
    abuse, psychological
  h. as screening device for drug
    abuse, social
  h. as screening device,
    psychological
  h. (BH), birth
  h., case
  h., chemical
  h., childhood
  h., clinical
  h., complete psychosocial
  h., comprehensive medical
  h., congenital
  h., detailed medical
  h., developmental
  h., diet
  h., epidemiological
  h., familial diabetic
  h. (FH), family
  H. form ▸ Diagnostic, Social, and
    Addiction
  h., formal developmental
  h., gynecological
  h., health
  h. (HDH), heart disease
  h., long smoking
  h. (MH), marital
  h. (MH), medical
  h., natural
  h. (FH) noncontributory ▸ family
  h. (PH) noncontributory ▸ past
  h. (FH) not remarkable ▸ family
  h. (PH) not remarkable ▸ past
  h., obstetrical (OB)
  h., occupational

h. of blackouts
h. of cancer, family
h. of congestive heart failure (CHF)
  ▸ natural
h. of heart disease
h. of interpersonal difficulty
h. of maladjustment
h. of needle sharing
h. of opioid addiction
h. of panic disorder ▸ agoraphobia
  without
h. of pathological use
h. of present illness (HPI)
h. of research
h. of stroke
h. (PH) ▸ past
h. (PMH) ▸ past medical
h. (PSH) ▸ past surgical
h., patient's chemical
h., patient's drug
h., patient's medical
h., positive family
h., self-reported
h., sleep
h., smoking
h., social
h., surgical
histrionic
  h. personality
  h. personality disorder
  h. personality traits
hitch, clove
Hits (LSD)
hitting bottom
Hitzig's test
HIV (human immunodeficiency
  virus)
  HIV antibodies
  HIV ▸ antibodies to
  HIV -associated cognitive disorder
  HIV -associated dementia
  HIV ▸ carriers of
  HIV encephalopathy
  HIV ▸ high risk of
  HIV -infected blood
  HIV ▸ infected with
  HIV infection ▸ high risk of
  HIV infection ▸ symptomatic
  HIV positive
  HIV prevention and control
  HIV seroconversion
  HIV -tainted blood
  HIV -2
hives
  h., cold

h., exercise-induced
h., giant
HLA (human leukocyte antigens)
HLA (human lymphocyte antigen)
HMD (hyaline membrane disease)
HME (human monocytic ehrlichiosis)
HMG (human menopausal
  gonadotropin)
HMO (health maintenance
  organization)
HNP (herniated nucleus pulposus)
HNPCC (hereditary nonpolyposis
  colon cancer)
hoarse voice
hoarseness
h. ▸ chest pain with
h. ▸ nagging cough or
h., persistent
h., progressive
hobbies, stimulating
Hoboken's nodules
hoc analysis, post
Hochwart disease ▸ Frankl-
hockey
h. -stick deformity
h. -stick incision
h. -stick incision ▸ Meyer's
Hocus (morphine)
Hodge('s)
H. maneuver
H. pessary
H. pessary, Smith-
Hodgkin('s)
H. cells
H. cycle
H. disease (HD)
H. disease in relapse
H. disease, mixed nodular type
H. disease of diffuse, histiocytic
  lymphocyte depleted type
H. disease, recurrent
H. granuloma
H. -like growth
H. lymphoma, diffuse non-
H. lymphoma, nodular non-
H. lymphoma, non-
H. lymphoma, null-type non-
H. sarcoma
Hodgson-Tuksu tumble flap
Hoehne's sign
Hoen's skull plate
Hoffa-Lorenz operation
Hoffa's operation
Hoffmann('s)
H. anodyne

H. atrophy
H. disease ▸ Werdnig-
H. drops
H. duct
H. phenomenon
H. reflex
H. sign
H. syndrome ▸ Charcot-Marie-
  Tooth-
H. syndrome, Werdnig-
hofmannii, Corynebacterium
Hofmann's bacillus
Hofmeister('s)
H. drainage (dr'ge) bag
H. gastrectomy
H. gastroenterostomy
H. test
Hog (phencyclidine)
hog cholera group
Hogan operation
Hogben's test
Hoguet's maneuver
Hohmann operation
hold
h. -back carrier
h., director's
h. head up ▸ loss of ability to
holdaway ration
holder, chart
Holder deformity ▸ Ilfeld-
holding maneuver during massage
holding test, breath
hole(s) [*whole*]
h. angiographic catheter ▸ one
h., burr
h. collimator, parallel-
h. collimator, pin-
h. collimator, single-
h. drilled in skull ▸ bur
h. in brain ▸ sponge-like
h. in retina
h., retinal
h. tomography ▸ slant-
holiday
h. anxiety
h. depression
h., dobutamine
h. heart
h. heart syndrome
Holinger tube
holistic
h. approach
h. healing
h. health spa
h. medicine

h. nursing
h. perspective
h. technique ▸ natural
h. therapy
Hollander's solution
Hollenberg treadmill score
Hollenhorst plaques
Hollister drainage (dr'ge) bag
hollow
h. and empty ▸ feels
h. fiber analyzer ▸ Dow
h. fiber dialyzer
h. fiber dialyzer, Dow
h. organs
H. organs, T categories in
h. sphere implant
h. sphere implant material
h. sphere prosthesis
h. viscus organs
Holme('s)(s')
H. degeneration
H. heart
H. operation
H. -Rahe Scale
H. sign
Holmgren's test
Holmgren's wool skein test
holmium laser
Holocaine anesthesia
holocaust survivors ▸
  psychopathology of
holocyclus, Ixodes
holodiastolic murmur
hologram of skull
hologram-assisted surgery
holographic CAT (computerized axial
  tomography) scan ▸ digital
holographic contact lens
holoprosencephaly, familial alobar
holosystolic murmur
Holothyrus coccinella
holster, shoulder
Holter
H. diary
H. monitor
H. monitor, ambulatory
H. monitor evaluation
H. monitor ▸ SpaceLabs
H. monitor, three channel
H. monitoring (AHM), ambulatory
H. shunt
H. technology
H. tube
H. valve

Holthouse's hernia
Holth's operation
Holt-Oram syndrome
Holzknecht's
    H. chromoradiometer
    H. scale
    H. space
    H. stomach
    H. unit
Homans' sign
homatropine
    h. dilatation
    h. ▸ hydrocodone and
    h. refraction
Hombre (heroin)
home (Home)
    h. arrangements, funeral
    h. assessment
    h. bacteriuria ▸ nursing
    h. blood glucose meter
    h. blood pressure (BP) measurement
    h. blood pressure (BP) monitoring
    h. blood sugar monitoring
    h. care
    h. care assistance
    h. care bereavement
    h. care, continuous
    H. Care Coordinator
    h. care, foster
    h. care givers, in-
    h. care, palliative
    h. care ▸ patient discharged to
    H. Care Program
    H. Care Program, Coordinated
    H. Care Program, Hospice
    H. Care Program ▸ patient discharged to Coordinated
    h. care program ▸ specialized AIDS (acquired immune deficiency syndrome)
    H. care, routine
    h. care support
    h. care support environment
    h. care, supportive
    H. Care Team
    h. care, traditional
    h. chemotherapy, in
    h. delivered meals
    h. dialysis
    h. environment
    h. environment, patient's
    h. ▸ evaluate safety and stability at
    h. evaluation

    h. evaluation, foster
    h. evaluation prior to discharge
    h. exercise program
    h. exercise program, written
    h., exercises for patient in
    h., foster
    h. glucose monitoring
    h., group
    h. health aide
    h. health care
    h. health care agency
    h. health services
    h. health visits
    h. maintenance management ▸ impaired
    h. management
    h. medical test kits
    h. modification
    h. monitoring
    h. nebulizer
    h. notification, funeral
    h., nursing
    h. nursing care
    h. O₂ (oxygen)
    h. oxygen (O₂) therapy
    h. pass ▸ therapeutic
    h., patient discharged to
    h., patient discharged to nursing
    h., patient transferred to nursing
    h. placement, foster
    h. placement, nursing
    h. ▸ rebellion in
    h. recovery period ▸ at-
    h. -related activities
    h. therapist
    h., transfer to nursing
homebound
    h. individual
    h. needs
    h. patient
    h. person
homeless children
homeless population
homemaker companion
homemaker service
Homén's syndrome
homeometric autoregulation
homeopathic
    h. drug
    h. medicine
    h. remedy
    h. therapy
    h. treatment
homeostasis, developmental
homeostasis, magnesium

homeostatic
    h. dysregulation ▸ hedonic
    h. fashion
    h. mechanisms, calcium
    h. reflex mechanism
    h. system
homicidal
    h. feeling ▸ suicidal or
    h. ideation
    h. insanity
    h. risk
    h. tendencies
    h. thoughts
homicide, drug-related
hominis
    h., Actinobacillus
    h., Amphistoma
    h., Cardiobacterium
    h., Cercomonas
    h., Coccidium
    h., Cryptococcus
    h., Dermatobia
    h., Echinorhynchus
    h., Enteromonas
    h., Gastrodiscoides
    h., herpesvirus
    h., Isospora
    h., Mycoplasma
    h., Octomitus
    h., Oestrus
    h. oris, Filaria
    h., Pentatrichomonas
    h., Saccharomyces
    h., Staphylococcus
    h. streptothrica, pseudotuberculosis
    h., Trichomonas
hominivorax, Cochliomyia
homme rouge
homochronous insanity
homocladic anastomosis
homocollateral reconstitution
homocysteine level
homocysteine test
homocystinuria syndrome
homodimer, alpha-alpha
homodimer, beta-beta
homogeneity, coefficient
homogenized milk
homogeneous [*homogenous*]
    h. antibody
    h. clouding
    h. component
    h. density
    h. immersion
    h., musculature

h. nature
h. sound
h. strain
homogenous [*homogeneous*]
  h. bone graft
  h. graft
  h. transplant
homogentisic acid
homogentisic acid test
homograft
  h., aortic
  h. cadaver
  h., denatured
  h. implant
  h. implant material
  h. reaction
  h. rejection
  h., skin
  h. valve, cryopreserved
homologous
  h. antigen
  h. areas
  h. areas of cortex
  h. artificial insemination
  h. cardiac transplant
  h. chimera
  h. donation ▸ random
  h. graft
  h. insemination
  h. regions
  h. serum hepatitis
  h. serum jaundice
  h. stimulus
  h. tissue
  h. transfusions
homonymous
  h. diplopia
  h. hemianopia
  h. hemianopsia
  h. motoneurons
  h. parallax
homoplastic graft
homosexual
  h. activity
  h. anal intercourse
  h. contact, male
  h. men, sexually active
  h. neurosis
  h. panic
  h. panic, acute
  h. patient
  h. transmission
homosexuality, latent
homosexuality, overt
homostatic reflex mechanism

homostatic transplants
homotopic pain
homotransplantation, renal
homovanillic acid
homovital transplants
homozygous achondroplasia
homozygous familial
  hypercholesterolemia
Honan manometer
Honan pressure reducer
Honey Oil (hashish)
honey-colored plasma
honeycomb
  h. lesion
  h. lung
  h. pattern
honeycombed appearance
honeycombed bones
honeymoon cystitis
Hong Kong ear
Hong Kong influenza
honk
  h. murmur ▸ goose
  h., precordial
  h., systolic
honking murmur
honor financial obligations
hood (Hood)
  h. Braun-Jardine DeLee
  H. chemistry profile
  H., OXY-
hooked acromion
hookworm
  h. anemia
  h., anemia from
  h. disease
  h. larvae
hooped knee
hooping compression, barrel
hoops, cartilage
Hoorn's maneuver, Van
HOP (high oxygen pressure)
hope (Hope)('s)
  h. ▸ level of
  H. resuscitator
  H. sign
hopeana, Brunfelsia
hopelessness
  h. and fear
  h., displays
  h., feelings of
  h. ▸ persistent feelings of
  h., sense of
  h. ▸ stress, anger and
Hoplopsyllus anomalus

Hopmann's polyp
Horay operation
Horgan operation, Lyon-
horizontal
  h. beam study
  h. canal
  h. cells
  h. fissure
  h. flexion ▸ shoulder
  h. folds of rectum
  h. heart
  h. hemianopia
  h. incision across lower abdomen
  h. jugular vein, anterior
  h. long axis view
  h. mattress suture
  h. nystagmus
  h. nystagmus, sustained
  h. oscillation of eyeballs, rhythmic
  h. overlap
  h. plane
  h. plane ▸ fracture bilaterally in a
  h. position
  h. ridging of nails
  h. sternotomy
  h. strabismus
  h. tube
  h. uterine incision
horizontally ridged fingernail
hormic psychology
Hormodendrum
  H. carrionii
  H. compactum
  H. pedrosoi
hormonal
  h. activity
  h. agent
  h. assay
  h. balance
  h. balance ▸ normal
  h. cancer treatment
  h. changes
  h. components
  h. control
  h. control, feedback mechanisms of
  h. cycles
  h. deficiency
  h. deficiency ▸ parathyroid
  h. disorder
  h. disturbance
  h. factor
  h. fluctuation
  h. gingivitis
  h. imbalances
  h. influences

hormonal—*continued*
- h. manipulation
- h. or chemotherapy treatment ▸ adjuvant
- h. reactions
- h. receptors
- h. status, postmenopausal
- h. stimulation
- h. system, control of
- h. therapy
- h. therapy, ablative
- h. therapy, additive
- h. therapy in endometrial carcinoma
- h. treatment

hormone(s)
- h., adrenal
- h., adrenal gland
- h., adrenal steroid
- h., adrenocortical
- h. (ACTH) ▸ adrenocorticotropic
- h. analysis
- h., androgen
- h. angiotensin II ▸ potent
- h., anterior lobe
- h. (ADH), antidiuretic
- h., antitumor
- h., artificial growth
- h. assay, gonadotropic
- h. binding studies
- h., biosynthetic human growth
- h. changes ▸ postovulation
- h., circulating pituitary
- h., corticosteroid
- h. (CRH), corticotropin-releasing
- h. deficient children
- h. deficiency, antidiuretic
- h. deficiency, growth
- h. deficiency ▸ human growth
- h. disorder
- h., endocrine
- h. failure, growth
- h., female
- h., female sex
- h. (FSH) ▸ follicle-stimulating
- h. ▸ formation and release of
- h., Genentech biosynthetic human growth
- h., glomerular-stimulating
- h., gonadal
- h., gonadotropic
- h. (Gn-RH), gonadotropin-releasing
- h., growth
- h., growth stimulating
- h. headaches

- h., heart
- h. (HGH), human growth
- h., human luteinizing
- h. hypercalcemia
- h., hypothalamic
- h., imbalance of
- h., immunoreactive human growth
- h. (IPTH), immunoreactive parathyroid
- h. implant
- h., inactive
- h. (IADH), inappropriate antidiuretic
- h., interstitial cell stimulating
- h., lactogenic
- h. levels
- h. levels, examined
- h. levels, fluctuating
- h., long-acting thyroid-stimulating (LATS)
- h. (LH), luteinizing
- h. (LTH), luteotropic
- h., male
- h., male sex
- h., mammotropic
- h. manipulation
- h. (MSH) ▸ melanocyte-stimulating
- h. (MSH) ▸ melanophore-stimulating
- h., messenger
- h. migraine
- h., mineralocorticoid
- h., natriuretic
- h., natural growth
- h., natural or synthetic
- h. output of pituitary gland
- h., ovine lactogenic
- h. (PTH), parathyroid
- h., peptide
- h., pituitary
- h., pituitary growth
- h. ▸ pituitary reproductive
- h., placental growth
- h., posterior pituitary
- h. production
- h. production, ectopic
- h. production, male
- h., production of sex
- h. production ▸ thyroid
- h., progestational
- h. prolactin, chorionic growth
- h. receptor negative tumor
- h. receptor positive tumor
- h. receptor test
- h. receptors
- h., releases of

- h. releasing factor, growth
- h. releasing factor, luteinizing
- h. replacement
- h. replacement medication
- h. replacement therapy (HRT)
- h. replacement (THR) ▸ thyroid
- h., reproductive
- h. resistance, thyroid
- h. response ▸ thyrotropin-releasing
- h. secretion of
- h. secretion rate, parathyroid
- h. (SIADH) secretion ▸ syndrome of inappropriate anti-diuretic
- h., sex
- h. ▸ slow release of
- h., somatotropic
- h., steroid
- h. ▸ stimulate production female sex estrogen
- h., stress
- h., stress-related
- h., stress-released
- h. supplement
- h., synthetic
- h., synthetic human growth
- h., synthetic male
- h., synthetic thyroid
- h. testosterone, male
- h. therapy
- h. therapy ▸ postmenopausal
- h. therapy ▸ prostate
- h. therapy, supplemental growth
- h., thyroid
- h. (TSH), thyroid stimulating
- h., thyrotropic
- h., thyrotropin releasing
- h. titer
- h. treatment
- h. treatment ▸ thyroid
- h. trigger ovulation ▸ pituitary

horn(s)
- h., Ammon's
- h. calculus, stag-
- h. cell, anterior
- h. cell, ventral
- h. cells
- h., dorsal
- h. of clitoris
- h. of lateral ventricle
- h. of lateral ventricle, interior
- h. of lateral ventricle, temporal
- h. of medial meniscus ▸ posterior
- h. of spinal cord
- h. of spinal cord ▸ anterior
- h. of spinal cord, dorsal

h. of spinal cord, lateral
h. of spinal cord, ventral
h. of uterus
h., pulp
h., temporal
h., ventricular
Horner('s)
H. -Bernard syndrome
H. law
H. muscle
H. ptosis
H. pupil
H. syndrome
H. teeth
H. -Trantas spots
horny cell layer
Horse (horse)
H. (Heroin)
h. asthma
h., charley
h. lice
h. -race effect
h. tranquilizer (phencyclidine)
horsehair worm
horseshoe
h. configuration
h. flap, inverted
h. lung
h. placenta
h. -shaped skin flap
h. -type kidney
Horsley's bone wax
Horsley's operation
hortae, Piedraia
Hortega's cell
Horton's
H. arteritis
H. disease
H. headache
H. syndrome
Horvath's operation
Horwitz-Adams operation
hose
h., compression
h. ► elastic support
h., Juzo
h., Linton elastic
h., TED (thromboembolic disease)
hosiery, special
Hoskins distribution law, Doerner-
hospice
h. approach
h. care
h. coordinator
H. Home Care Program

h. inquiry
h. nurse
H. Organization (NHO), National
h. philosophy
h. program
h. support
h. team
h. volunteer
hospital (Hospital)
h., accredited psychiatric
h. -acquired infection
h. -acquired organism
h. -acquired organism infection
h. -acquired pneumonia
h. -acquired urinary tract infection
h. -acquired viral hepatitis
h., acute care
h. addiction medicine service
h. admission
h. air, ambient
h. air ► contamination from ambient
h. air, normal
H. ► American Association of
Private Psychiatric
h. -associated infections
h. -associated infections ► reduce
risk of
h. -associated respiratory tract
infection
h., base
h. -based blood bank
h. -based physician
h. -based stress management
h. bed
h. benefit (MHB) ► maximum
h. benefit ► patient reached
maximum
h. birth certificate
h. camp
h. cardiac catheterization
laboratory
h. care, acute
h. care cost
h. care ► prolonged
h., certified
h., closed
h. (CSH), combat support
h. course
h. course benign
h. course turbulent ► patient's
h. day
h., donor
h., emergency
h. emergency department
h. environment

h. epidemic
H. Epidemiologist
h. epidemiology
h., evacuation
h. fever
h., field
h. flora
h. infection control
h. infections, prevention of
h. inservice program
h., isolation
H. Laundry
h., lying-in
h. medical staff
h., mobile
h., night
h., open
h. operation
h. organisms, endemic
h., orientation to
h. origin
h., patient discharged from
h., patient has fear of
h., patient treated in
H. Pharmacy
h. policy
h., private
h., private psychiatric
H. Program, Night
h. protocol
h., psychiatric
h., recipient
h., rehabilitation
h. -related infection
h., remote
h. residency program
h. resources
h. setting
h. ship
h., specialty
h. stay
h. stay, length of
h. stay unremarkable
h. study
h. systems
h. team
h. treatment assistant (SHTA) ►
security
h. treatment program ► partial
h. treatment, standard
h. -wide practice
Hospitalization
(Hospitalization)(s)
H. ► American Association for
Partial

hospitalization—*continued*
- h., intensive structured
- h., long-term
- h., multiple
- h. programs, partial
- h., prolonged
- h., psychiatric
- h. ▸ psychological stress of

hospitalized
- h. for workup, patient
- h., patient
- h., patient previously
- h. patients on bail

host
- h. body
- h. cell
- h. cell, living
- h. cell, new
- h. cell, original
- h. cell ▸ phage particle infects new
- h. cell vacuole
- h. chromosome
- h., classification of
- h., colonization of
- h., compromised
- h. defense
- h. disease (GVHD) ▸ graft-versus-
- h. disease (GVHD) ▸ life-
  threatening graft vs.
- h. eye
- h. generated neutrophils
  recruitment
- h. (GVH) ▸ graft-versus-
- h., human
- h., humoral
- h., immune compromised
- h., immunocompetent
- h., immunocompromised
- h., immunological
- h., impaired
- h., intermediate
- h. leukotactic function
- h., nonimmunocompromised
- h., normal
- h. reaction (GVHR) ▸ graft-versus-
- h. resistance
- h. susceptibility
- h., susceptible
- h., transmission of microbe to
- h., weakened

hostile
- h. and anxious
- h. and depressed
- h. conflict
- h. dependence

- h. dependency
- h. or aggressive behavior ▸
  unusually
- h., patient
- h., patient abusive and
- h., patient feeling
- h. personality
- h. relationship

hostility
- h. and anger ▸ diffusing
- h. and depression
- h., extreme
- h., patient exhibits overt
- h., pent-up
- h. scale ▸ overcontrolled
- h., thoughtless

**HOT Hypertension Optimal
Treatment**

hot
- h. air, filtered
- h. and cold flushes
- h. and cold sensation
- h. appendix
- h. balloon ▸ radiofrequency
- h. biopsy
- h. biopsy technique
- h. -cathode tube
- h. -cold lysis
- h. -cold system
- h. compress
- h. cone
- h. -dry-house
- h. environment
- h. flash triggers
- h. flashes
- h. flashes, menopausal
- h. flush
- h. gangrene
- h. knife
- h. lesion
- h. moist compresses
- h. moist packs
- h. moist poultice
- h. or cold flashes
- h. packs and bed rest
- h. reactor syndrome
- h. spot
- h. spot imaging
- h. spot scintigraphy ▸ infarct avid
- h. spots on scan
- h. spots with electron beam
  dosimetry ▸ cold spots and
- h. stage
- h. stupes
- h., swollen and tender

- h. tip laser probe
- h. tub dermatitis
- h. tub lumg
- h. vs. cold breast tumor
- h. water
- h. weather ear

hotline
- h., antisuicide
- h., crisis
- h., drug abuse
- h., suicide

Hotz's operation

Hough hole

Hough stapedectomy technique

Hounsfield units

hour(s)
- h. at one meter (rhm) ▸ roentgens
  per
- h. emergency care, 24
- h. incubation ▸ growth after 48
- h. interval, half-
- h. (Kw-hr), kilowatt
- h. (mah), milliampere
- h. (mch), millicurie-
- h. (mgh), milligram-
- h. monitoring, 24-
- h. of sleep (h.s.) ▸ at bedtime or
- h., organism isolated after 72
- h. period of observation and
  hydration ▸ 24-
- h. postprandial, two
- h. sleep-wake cycle ▸ phase-shift
  disruption of 24-
- h. urine, 24-
- h., visiting
- h., waking

hourglass
- h. chest
- h. contractions
- h. murmur
- h. pathway
- h. stenosis
- h. stomach

hourglassing

hourly dose rate

house (House)
- h. drug dealer, crack
- h. dust allergy
- h. dust mite
- h. for alcoholics, halfway
- h. for drug addicts, halfway
- h. for mentally retarded ▸ halfway
- h. for penal rehabilitation ▸ halfway
- h. for physically handicapped ▸
  halfway

h. for runaways, halfway
h., halfway
h., hot-dry-
H. incus replacement prosthesis ▸ Sheehy-
h. kicks, round-
h. mouse, patient is
h. murmur, mill-
h. physician
h. placement, halfway
h. programs, in-
h. resident
h. staff member
H. stainless steel mesh prosthesis
H. stapedectomy
H. stapedectomy technique
H. Test ▸ Draw Person, Tree,
h. -tree-person (HTP)
housebound by fear
housebound, patient
Housekeeping Department
housemaid's knee
housing, congregate
housing, sheltered
Houston's muscle
Houston's operation
Houttuynia californica
Howard test
Howell('s) bodies
Howell-Jolly bodies
Howmedica prosthesis
Howorth operation
Hoyer anastomosis, Sucquet-
Hoyer lift
HPA (hypothalamic-pituitary-adrenal) axis
HPAA (hypothalamic pituitary adrenocortical axis)
HPE (history and physical examination)
hpf (high power field)
hpf (per high power field) ▸ organisms
HPI (history of present illness)
HPL (human placental lactogen) and plasma
HPV (hepatic portal vein)
HPV (human papilloma virus)
HPV (human papillomavirus) infection
HPVG (hepatic portal venous gas)
HRCT (high resolution computed tomography) scan
H-reflex
HRS (Hamilton Rating Scale)

HRT (hormone replacement therapy)
Hruby lens
h.s. (at bedtime or hour of sleep)
HSA (human serum albumin)
Hs-CRP (high sensitivity C-reactive protein)
HSG (hysterosalpingogram)
HT (heart tones)
HTLV (Human T cell Lymphotropic Virus)
HTN (hypertension)
HTN, Essential
HTN evaluation ▸ initial
HTN low renin essential
HTP (house-tree-person)
Hubbard
H. tank
H. tank massage
H. tank therapy
H. tub
Huchard's disease
Hudson's brace
Hudson's line
Hueston spiral flap
Huet
H. anomaly, Pelger-
H. cells, Pelger-
H. nuclear anomaly, Pelger-
Hueter's maneuver
Hueter's sign
huffing fatality
huffing inhalant
Hufnagel('s)
H. low profile heart valve prosthesis
H. operation
H. valve prosthesis
hug therapy
Hugh Syndrome ▸ Fitz
Hugh-Curtis Syndrome ▸ Fitz
Hughes
H. implant
H. operation
H. reflex
Hughston, jerk test of
Huguenin's edema
Huguenin's endothelioma ▸ Sidler-
Huguier's sinus
Huhner test
Huhner test ▸ Sims-
hum, cervical venous
hum, venous
human
h. ability
h. aortic allograft, cryopreserved
h. aortic endothelial cells

h. atrial natriuretic peptide
h. behavior
h. behavior, dynamics of
h. betterment ▸ potential for
h. bites
h. blood cells, packed
h. blood substitute ▸ recycled
h. body
h. bonding
h. brain
h. brain disease
h. breast milk
h. carriers of infection
h. cell nucleus
h. chorionic gonadotropic
h. chorionic gonadotropin
h. chorionic somatomammotropin
h. chromosomes
h. condition
h. development
h. development, normal
h. drive, fundamental
h. dynamic derangements
h. ecology
h. embryo kidney
h. enteric
h. erythrocyte agglutination test
h. fetal cells
h. fetal pancreas transplant
h. fetal tissue ▸ transplanting
h. fetus, aborted
h. fetus ▸ spontaneously aborted
h. fibroblast
H. Figure Drawing Test, Projective
h. functions, basic
h. gamma globulin
h. gastrin, synthetic
h. genetic code
h. genetic disorder
h. genetic material
h. genetics
h. genome
h. GM-CSF (granulocytic-macrophage colony stimulating factor)
h. granulocytic ehrlichiosis (HGE)
h. growth hormone
h. growth hormone, biosynthetic
h. growth hormone deficiency
h. growth hormone, Genentech biosynthetic
h. growth hormone, immunoreactive
h. growth hormone, synthetic
h. heart, diseased

human—*continued*
- h. heart, four-chambered
- h. hepatoma
- H. Herpes Virus-8 (HHV 8)
- H. Herpes Virus-7 (HHV 7)
- h. immune cells
- h. immunodeficiency virus (HIV)
- h. immunodeficiency virus (HIV-2)
- h. immunodeficiency virus (HIV) antibodies
- h. immunodeficiency virus (HIV) ▸ antibodies to
- h. immunodeficiency virus (HIV) encephalopathy
- h. immunodeficiency virus (HIV) infected blood
- h. immunodeficiency virus (HIV) infection ▸ high risk of
- h. immunodeficiency virus (HIV) seroconversion
- h. immunodeficiency virus (HIV)-associated dementia
- h. immunodeficiency virus (HIV)-associated motor cognitive disorder
- h. infants, cocaine-exposed
- h. infection
- h. insulin
- h. insulin antibodies
- h. intelligence
- h. interaction
- h. interferon
- h. intracisternal A type retroviral particle
- h. iodinated I 131 serum albumin
- h. islets ▸ functional viability of
- h. leukocyte antigen (HLA)
- h. leukocyte antigen (HLA) system
- h. leukocyte interferon
- h. luteinizing hormone
- h. lymphocyte antigen (HLA)
- h. lymphocyte antigen typing
- h. lymphocyte transformation
- h. menopausal gonadotropin (HMG)
- h. milk
- h. milk lysozyme
- h. molecular genetics
- h. monocytic ehrlichiosis (HME)
- h. myoglobulin ▸ radioimmunoassay
- h. needs
- h. nutrition
- h. oncology
- h. operant heart rate conditioning

- h. organ transplantation
- h. organs
- h. organs, donated
- h. orphan (ECHO) ▸ enterocytopathogenic
- h. orphan (ECHO) 28 virus ▸ enteric cytopathic
- h. orphan (ECHO) virus ▸ enteric cytopathic
- h. pancreatic cancer
- h. papilloma virus (HPV)
- h. papillomavirus (HPV) infection
- h. pharmacology
- h. pituitary
- h. pituitary gonadotropin
- h. placental lactogen
- h. placental lactogen (HPL) and plasma
- h. plague
- h. plasma, antipseudomonas
- h. plasma ▸ donated
- h. plasma level
- h. pregnancy
- h. preproendothelin-1 gene
- h. psychopathology
- h. rabies immune globulin
- h. relations
- h. retrovirus
- h. serum albumin (HSA)
- h. serum albumin, iodinated
- h. serum albumin, normal
- h. serum albumin ▸ radioactive iodinated
- h. serum, normal
- h. ▸ sexual maturation in
- h. sexuality
- h. skin
- h. somatomammotropin
- h. spinal fluid
- h. spiritual concerns
- h. subject
- h. subjects ▸ escape and avoidance conditioning in
- H. T cell Lymphotropic Virus (HTLV)
- h. tau
- h. testing
- h. therapeutics
- h. therapy
- h. thymus antiserum
- h. tissue
- h. touch
- h. traits
- h. transmission
- h. tumor xenograft

- h. uniparental disomy
- h. umbilical vein
- h. umbilical vein (HUV) bypass graft
- h. variation
- h. violence

humane individuals ▸ caring,
humanistic psychology
humanized antibody
humanized monoclonal antibody
humanus
- h. capitis, Pediculus
- h., Pediculus
- h. var. capitis, Pediculus
- h. var. corporis, Pediculus
- h. var. vestimentorum, Pediculus

humeral [*humoral*]
- h. block in radiation therapy
- h. bone
- h. epicondylitis, external
- h. fracture
- h. shaft

humeri, capitulum
humeri, proximal
humeroperoneal neuromuscular disease
humeroradial articulation
humerosa, Haemaphysalis
humeroulnar articulation
humerus
- h., anatomical neck of
- h., head of
- h., open reduction of
- h., shaft of
- h. splint, Magnuson abductor
- h., surgical neck of

humid asthma
humidifier
- h. and oxygen (O_2)
- h., bubble
- h., cold mist
- h. fever
- h., jet
- h. lung
- h., passover
- h., ultrasonic
- h., warm mist

humidify and heat
humidity
- h. and oxygen
- h., increased fluids and
- h., relative

humiliated, patient
humiliation ▸ sustained feelings of
humming murmur

humming-top murmur
humor
  h., aqueous
  h., crystalline
  h. deficit disorder (HDD)
  h. ▸ flow of aqueous
  h. movement ▸ therapeutic
  h., ocular
  h. of eye, aqueous
  h., therapeutic
  h. ▸ therapeutic benefits of
  h. therapist
  h., vitreous
humoral [*humeral*]
  h. antibody
  h. antibody response
  h. factor, thymic
  h. host
  h. immune defect
  h. immune response
  h. immunity
  h. immunologic reactivity
  h. response
  h. system
  h. thymic factor
hump [*lump*]
  h., biparietal
  h., bony
  h., dorsal
  h., dowager's
  h., Hampton's
  h. in upper back
  h., parietal
  h., widow's
humped back
humped pressure pulse ▸ triple-
hunched back
hundredth-normal solution
hunger
  h., air
  h. behavior, infant exhibits
  h., extreme
  h. headache
  h. pain
  h. pangs
  h. respiration
  h., stimulus
  h., stimulus-action
  h. swelling
Hunner's stricture
Hunt('s)
  H. atrophy
  H. disease
  H. method
  H. neuralgia

  H. paradoxical phenomenon
  H. phenomenon
  H. reaction
  H. striatal syndrome
  H. syndrome
  H. syndrome ▸ Ramsay
  H. syndrome ▸ Tolosa-
  H. test
  H. tremor
Hunter('s)
  H. canal
  H. Driffield curve
  H. gubernaculum
  H. ligament
  H. syndrome
hunting reaction
Huntington's
  H. chorea
  H. disease
  H. gene
  H. operation
Huntleigh Domiciliary Fetal Monitor
Hurler('s)
  H. disease
  H. polydystrophy ▸ pseudo-
  H. syndrome
Hürthle
  H. cell
  H. cell adenoma
  H. cell carcinoma
  H. cell tumor
Hurting (MASH) ▸ Make Arthritis Stop
HUS (hemolytic uremic syndrome)
husband
  h., battered
  h. syndrome, battered
  h. /wife, bereaved
Huschke('s)
  H. auditory teeth
  H. canal
  H. foramen
  H. valve
husky voice
hustlers, drug
hustlers, patient
Hutchinson('s)
  H. disease
  H. facies
  H. -Gilford syndrome
  H. incisors
  H. mask
  H. pupil
  H. syndrome
  H. syndrome ▸ Siegrist-
  H. teeth

  H. triad
Hutinel's disease
HUV (human umbilical vein) bypass
graft
HV (hyperventilation)
  HV build-up
  HV, deliberate
  HV interval
HVD (hypertensive vascular
disease)
HVL (half-value layer)
HVS (hyperventilation syndrome),
chronic
hyacinthi, Xanthomonas
hyalin fibrotic tissue
hyalina, Hartmannella
hyaline
  h. acellular areas
  h. arterionecrosis
  h. cytoplasmic inclusion
  h. deposition, marked
  h. fatty change
  h. inclusion bodies ▸ alcoholic
  h. inclusions, intracytoplasmic
  h. membrane
  h. membrane disease
  h. membrane disease ▸ extensive
  h. membranes lining alveolar
    spaces
  h. membranes, pulmonary
  h. sclerosis
  h. thrombi
  h. thrombus
hyalinization
  h., focal
  h., glomerular
  h. of alveolar walls
  h. of glomeruli
hyalinized burned out germinal
centers
hyalinized fibrous tissue
hyalinizing vasculitis ▸ segmented
hyalinosis, arteriolar
hyalitis
  h., asteroid
  h. punctata
  h. suppurativa
hyaloid
  h. artery
  h. canal
  h. corpuscle
  h. membrane
  h. vessel
hyaloserositis
    ▸ **progressive multiple**

Hyam's operation
Hybbinette operation ▸ **Eden-**
hybrid cells
hybrid unit
hybridization analysis ▸ **slot blot**
hybridization ▸ **in situ**
hybridum, Trifolium
hydatid
    h. cyst
    h. cyst disease
    h. disease
    h. disease, alveolar
    h. of Morgagni
    h. pregnancy
    h., sessile
    h., stalked
hydatidiform/hydatiform
hydatidiform mole
Hydatigena infantis
hydatigena, Taenia
hydradenitis (see hidradenitis)
hydragogue diuretic
hydralizine lupus syndrome
hydramnios, oligo◊
Hydrastis canadensis
hydrate, chloral
hydrate elixir, terpin
hydrated
    h., inadequately
    h., patient well-
    h. pyelogram
hydration
    h., adequate
    h. and turgor
    h. intake, alteration in
    h., intravenous (IV)
    h., normal
    h. of mucous membranes
    h. oral
    h., skin
    h., 24-hour period of observation
       and
hydraulic formula ▸ **Gorlin**
hydraulic method, Gabastou's
hydrazide, isonicotinic acid
hydremic ascites
hydremic nephritis
hydrocarbon
    h., halogenated
    h., polycyclic aromatic
    h. toxicity
hydrocele
    h., chylous
    h. colli
    h., communicating

h., Dupuytren's
h., encysted
h. feminae
h. funicular
h., Gibbon's
H., Maunoir's
h. muliebris
h., noncommunicating
h. of Nuck
h., scrotal
hydrocephalic idiocy
hydrocephaloid disease
hydrocephalus
    h., acquired
    h., acute
    h., chronic
    h., communicating
    h., congenital
    h. ex vacuo
    h. ex vacuo change
    h., fetus with
    h., internal
    h., noncommunicating
    h. (NPH), normal pressure
    h., normopressure
    h., normotensive
    h., obstructive
    h., otitic
    h., primary
    h., secondary
    h. shunt
    h., undiagnosed
    h., unsuspected
hydrochloric acid
hydrochloric acid, free
hydrochloride, cocaine
hydrochloride, ritodrine
hydrocodone and homatropine
hydrocollator pack
hydrocollator pads
hydrocortisone acetate
hydrocortisone injection
Hydrocurve contact lenses
hydrogen
    h. breath test
    h. density
    h. electrodes
    h. fluoride
    h. ion
    h. ion concentration
    h. isotopes, nonradioactive
    h. isotopes, radioactive
    h. peroxide
hydrolysis of surfactant
hydroma [hygroma]

hydrometer scale
hydronephrosis
    h., caliceal sign of
    h., crescent sign of
    h., left
    h., right
hydrophila, Aeromonas
hydrophilic filter media
hydrophilus, Proteus
hydrophobic filter media
hydropic nephrosis
hydropigenous nephritis
hydropneumatic massage
hydrops
    h. abdominis
    h., endolymphatic
    h., fetal
    h. fetalis
    h. folliculi
    h., hypertensive meningeal
    h., meningeal
    h. of gallbladder
    h. of pleura
    h. pericardii
    h. spurius
hydrorrhea gravidarum
hydrorrhea, nasal
hydrosalpinx
    h., bilateral
    h., both tubes
    h. follicularis
    h., intermittent
    h. simplex
hydrostatic
    h. pressure
    h. pressure, capillary
    h. pressure gradient ▸ colloid
    h. pressure ▸ intravascular
Hydrotaea, Anthomyiidae
hydrotherapeutic exercise
hydrotherapy (Hydrotherapy)
    h., colonic
    h., scientific
    h., tank suit
    H. Treatment
hydrothermal ablation
hydrothorax, chylous
hydrothorax, hepatic
hydrotubation, chromo◊
hydroureteral nephrosis
hydrous wool fat
hydroxide
    h., aluminum
    h. gel, aluminum
    h., iron

h., macroaggregated ferrous
hydroxyapatite spheres
hydroxyapatite (THA) ▸ **total**
hydroxybutyrate
  h. dehydrogenase, serum
  h., gamma
  h. (GHB) Liquid X ▸ gamma
hydroxybutyric dehydrogenase
hydroxycorticosteroid test ▸ **17-**
hydroxydiphosphate, ethane
hydroxyindoleacetic acid
hydroxyindoleacetic acid (5-HI-AA)
  ▸ **5-**
hydroxyl
  h. aminobutyric acid
  h. concentration
  h. radical
hydroxylase deficiency syndrome
  ▸ **17-**
hydroxyproline, total
hydroxyurea radiotherapy (PH-RT)
  ▸ **procarbazine**
hydruria, oligo
hygiene
  h., basic
  h., daily oral
  h., dental
  h., grooming and
  h., mental
  h., oral
  h., personal
  h., poor dental
  h., regular foot
  h. self-care deficit
  h., sleep
hygienic practices, standard
hygienist, dental
hygroma
  h., cystic
  h., Fleishmann's
  h., subdural
Hyland method
Hylemyia, Anthomyiidae
hylic tissue
hymen
  h., annular
  h. bifenestratus
  h. biforis
  h., circular
  h., cribriform
  h., denticular
  h., falciform
  h., fenestrated
  h., imperforate
  h., infundibuliform

h., intact
h., lunar
h., rigid
h., septate
h. subseptus
hymenal
  h. band
  h. caruncles
  h. cyst
  h. orifice
  h. ring
  h. syndrome
Hymenolepis
  H. diminuta
  H. nana
  H. nurina
hyoepiglottic ligament
hyoglossal muscle
hyoglossus muscle
hyoid
  h. arch
  h. bone
  h. bone, central
  h. bone, cornu of
  h. bone, muscles of
  h. region
hyoideum, os
hyos, Leptospira
hyoscine chorea
hyothyroid ligament
hyothyroid membrane
hypacusia/hypacusis (*see***
  hypoacusis)**
Hypaque (hypaque)
  H. contrast medium
  H. -Cysto contrast medium
  h. 50%
  H. M contrast medium
  h. -M 75%
  h. -M 90%
  H. Meglumine contrast medium
  H. sodium contrast medium
  h. sodium powder and liquid
  h. 20%
hyparterial bronchi
hyparterial bronchus
hypaxial muscles
hypazoturic nephropathy
hyperabduction maneuver
hyperabduction syndrome
hyperactive
  h. and risky behavior
  h. and violent
  h. asthma
  h. behavior

h. bowel sounds
h. bowel tones
h. carotid sinus reflex
h. child
h. children
h. immune system
h., patient
h. reflex
h. thyroid
hyperactivity
  h. and decreased appetite ▸
    insomnia
  h. and irritability anxiety
  h. ▸ attention deficit disorder with
  h. ▸ attention deficit disorder without
  h., autonomic
  h. disorder (ADHD), attention
    deficit
  h. ▸ electroencephalogram (EEG)
    biofeedback in control of
  h. from anxiety
  h. ▸ peripheral nerve
  h. ▸ pharmacotherapy for
  h., physical
  h., progressive relaxation under
  h. ▸ relaxation therapy for
hyperacusis/hyperacusia
hyperacute phase
hyperacute xenograft rejection
hyperadrenergic state
hyperaerated chest
hyperalbuminosa, polyemia
hyperalimentation
  h. catheter
  h. feeding
  h. fluid
  h. line ▸ infected
  h. management
  h. solution
  h. therapy
  h. tubing
hyperapolipoprotein B syndrome
hyperarousal and intrusive
  memories
hyperbaric
  h. bed
  h. chamber
  h. medicine
  h. oxygen (O_2)
  h. oxygen (HBO) chamber
  h. oxygen (O_2) therapy
  h. oxygen (O_2) treatment
  h. oxygenation
  h. pressure
  h. tank

hyperbilirubinemia, prolonged unexplained
hyperbolic glasses
hypercalcemia
- h., familial hypocalcuric
- h., hormone
- h., idiopathic
- h. stenosis, infantile
- h. syndrome ▸ supravalvular aortic

hypercalcemic
- h. crisis
- h. encephalopathy
- h. nephropathy

hypercalciuria, idiopathic
hypercapnia, permissive
hypercapnic acidosis
hyperchloremic acidosis
hyperchloremic renal acidosis
hypercholesterolemia
- h., essential
- h., false
- h. (FH), familial
- h., homozygous familial
- h., polygenic

hypercholesterolemic splenomegaly
hypercholesterolemic xanthomatosis, biliary
hyperchromatic
- h. cell
- h. macrocythemia
- h. nuclei
- h. nuclei, pleomorphic
- h. ovoid nuclei

hyperchromatin granule
hyperchromatism ▸ loss of polarity and
hyperchromatism, macrocytic
hyperchromic microcytic
hypercoagulable state
hypercontractility, detrusor
hypercorbia pulmonary hypertension
hypercyanotic angina
hyperdicrotic pulse
hyper-dopaminergic state induced
hyperdynamic state
hyperdynamic ventricle
hyperelastics, cutis
hyperemesis gravidarum
hyperemesis hiemis
hyperemia
- h., active
- h., arterial
- h. blood flow, exercise
- h. blood flow, reactive
- h., collateral

- h., conjunctival
- h., fluxionary
- h., focal area of
- h. of arytenoids
- h. of iris
- h. of retina
- h. of retina, active
- h. of retina, passive
- h., passive
- h. peristaltic
- h., pulp
- h., reactive
- h., unit
- h., venous

hyperemic
- h. headache
- h. laryngeal mucosa
- h. membranes
- h. mucosa
- h. mucosal pattern
- h. nasal mucosa

hypereosinophilia syndrome
hypereosinophilic syndrome ▸ idiopathic
hyperesthesia, cutaneous
hyperexcitability, neuronal
hyperextension
- h. brace
- h. exercise
- h. of spine
- h. postures and maneuvers

hyperflexed wire
hyperfractionation
- h., biologic basis of
- h., cell cycle redistribution and dose
- h., dose
- h., reoxygenation and dose

hyperfunction, pituitary
hyperfunctional occlusion
hyperfunctional pituitary tumor
hypergammaglobulinemia, polyclonal
hyperglobulinemica, purpura
hyperglycemic
- h. glycogenolytic factor
- h. hyperosmolar syndrome
- h. nonketotic coma
- h., patient

hypergranulation tissue
hyperhidrosis ▸ patient has
hyperhidrosis unilateralis
hyperinflated lungs
hyperinsulinar obesity
hyperinsulinemic level
hyperinterrenal obesity

hyperirritability of labyrinth
hyperkalemia [*hypercalcemia*]
hyperkalemia, spurious
hyperkalemic cardioplegia
hyperkeratosis
- h. lacunaris
- h. linguae
- h., mucosal
- h. of soles

hyperkeratotic
- h. area
- h. lesion
- h. verrucoid surfaced lesion

hyperkinesis
- h. response to electromyogram (EMG) biofeedback
- h. sign, Claude's
- h. with developmental delay

hyperkinetic
- h. conduct disorder
- h. heart syndrome
- h. pulse
- h. reaction of childhood
- h. state
- h. syndrome
- h. syndrome of childhood

hyperlipidemia, endogenous
hyperlipidemia, false combined
hyperlobulated nuclei
hyperlucency of lung ▸ unilateral
hyperlucent lung
hyperlucent lung syndrome
hypermature cataract
hypermetabolic syndrome
hypermetabolism of bone cells
hypermetropia, latent
hypermetropia, total
hypermetropic astigmatism (As.H.)
hypermetropic astigmatism, compound
hypermobile kidney
hypermobility as risk factor
hypermotility, gastrointestinal
hypermotility, intestinal
hypernatremia and fluid deficit
hypernatremic dehydration
hypernatremic encephalopathy
hypernephroid carcinoma
hypernephroid tumor
hypernephroma, primary
hyperopia, facultative
hyperopia, manifest
hyperopic [*hypertrophic*]
- h. astigmatism

h. astigmatism, compound
h., patient
hyperosmolality, iatrogenic
hyperosmolar
 h. coma
 h. nonketotic coma
 h. syndrome
 h. syndrome ▸ diabetic
 h. syndrome, hyperglycemic
hyperosmotic, nonketotic
hyperostosis
 h., ankylosing
 h. cranii
 h. frontalis interna
 h. ▸ idiopathic skeletal
 h., infantile cortical
 h., Morgagni's
 h. totalis
hyperoxaluria, primary
hyperparathyroidism
 h., adenomatous
 h., ectopic
 h., primary
 h., secondary
hyperpeptic gastritis
hyperphoria
 h., alternating sursumduction
 h., left
 h., right
hyperpigmented macules on heel
 and sole
hyperpituitarism, basophilic
hyperpituitarism, eosinophilic
hyperpituitary gigantism
hyperplasia
 h., adenomatous
 h., adrenal
 h., adrenocortical
 h., alveolar cell
 h., angiolymphoid
 h., atypical
 h. ▸ atypical ductal
 h., benign cystic endometrial
 h., benign prostatic
 h., cementum
 h., chronic inflammatory
 h., congenital adrenal
 h., congenital virilizing adrenal
 h., cortical stromal
 h., cystic
 h., drug-induced
 h., ductal
 h., early cystic
 h., endometrial
 h., epithelial

h., fibrointimal
h., fibromuscular
h., fibromyoadenomatous
h. ▸ focal epithelial
h., focal nodular
h., giant follicular
h., gingival
h., glandular
h., inflammatory
h., intimal
h., juxtaglomerular cell
h., lipoid
h., lobar
h. ▸ lymph node
h., lymphoid
h., mesothelial
h. ▸ mild focal cortical nodular
h., mucosal inflammatory
h., neoplastic
h., nodular
h., nodular cortical adrenal
h., nonpapillary
h. of ducts
h. of epiglottis
h. of lymph nodes ▸ histocytic
h. of ovary ▸ nodular
h. of prostate gland,
 fibroadenomatous
h. of prostate gland ▸ nodular
h. of pulp ▸ chronic perforating
h., ovarian stromal
h., pancreatic duct
h., polar
h., postmenopausal
h., proliferative
h., prostate
h., prostatic
h., pseudoepitheliomatous
h., pulmonary vascular
h., quantitative
h., reactive
h., renal
h., sebaceous
h., simple
h., stromal
h., Swiss-cheese
h., trilobar
h., true
h., unilateral
h., uterine
h., verrucose
h., vicarious
hyperplasmic obesity
hyperplastic(s)
 h. achondroplasia

h. arteriolar nephrosclerosis
h. arteriolosclerosis
h., arteritis
h. bone marrow ▸ mildly
h. cholecystosis
h. endometritis
h. endometrium
h. gingivitis
h. graft
h. membrane
h. muscle fibers
h. nodules
h. nodules, cortical
h. primary vitreous (PHPV),
 persistent
h. rectal polyp
h. sclerosis
h. tissue
h. vitreous, primary persistent
hyperpnea, isocapneic
hyperpnea, voluntary
hyperpolarizing factor ▸ endothelium-
 derived
hyperpronation, forefoot
hyperpyrexia, malignant
hyperpyrexial fever
hyperpyrexial insolation
hyperreactive airway
hyperreactive bronchial tubes
hyperreactivity, bronchial
hyperreactivity to stimuli
hyperreflexia, autonomic
hyperreflexia, detrusor
hyperreflexic bladder
hyperresonance to percussion ▸
 lungs revealed
hypersalivating, patient
hypersecretion, gastric
hypersecretion, mucus
hypersecretory activity
hypersensitive
 h. carotid sinus syndrome
 h. dentin
 h. hearing
 h., patient
 h. skin
 h. to aspirin ▸ patient
hypersensitivity
 h. angiitis
 h., bee sting
 h., brain
 h., carotid sinus
 h., delayed
 h. disorder
 h., drug

hypersensitivity—*continued*
- h. myocarditis
- h. pneumonia
- h. pneumonitis
- h. pneumonitis, interstitial
- h. reaction
- h. reaction, delayed-type
- h. reaction ▸ fatal
- h. reaction, immunologic
- h. to aspirin
- h., tuberculin-delayed
- h. vasculitis

hyperserotonemia ▸ vasculocardiac syndrome of

hypersomnia
- h., chronic
- h., primary
- h. related to a known organic factor
- h. related to another mental disorder (nonorganic)
- h. related to mental disorder (nonorganic)
- h., semichronic

hypersplenic anemia

hypersplenism/hypersplenia

hypersynchronous cerebral discharge

hypersynchronous discharge, excessive

hypertelorism, ocular

hypertelorism, orbital

hypertension [*hypotension*]
- h., accelerated
- h., adolescent
- h., adrenal
- h., alveolar
- h. and tachycardia
- h., arterial
- h., autogenic training for
- h., benign
- h., benign intracranial
- h., borderline
- h., borderline systolic
- h. ▸ chronic thromboembolic pulmonary
- h., curable
- h., decreasing
- h., diabetic
- h., episodic
- h. (HTN), essential
- h. (HTN) evaluation ▸ initial
- h., Goldblatt's
- h. ▸ heart-threatening
- h., hypercorbia pulmonary
- h. ▸ hypoxic pulmonary

- h., idiopathic
- h. ▸ idiopathic hypertrophic subaortic
- h., inherited
- h. in pregnancy
- h. in the elderly ▸ systolic
- h., intracranial
- h., intrahepatic portal
- h. ▸ isolated systolic
- h., labile
- h. ▸ left atrial
- h. (HTN) ▸ low renin essential
- h., malignant
- h., mild
- h. murmur ▸ primary pulmonary
- h., neurogenic
- h., neuromuscular
- h., ocular
- h. of newborn ▸ persistent pulmonary
- h. of the liver ▸ portal
- h., office
- H. Optimal Treatment (HOT)
- h. optimal treatment study
- h. ▸ oral contraceptive-induced
- h., orthostatic
- h., pale
- h., paroxysmal
- h., pediatric
- h., portal
- h., postpartum
- h., postural
- h., pregnancy-induced
- h. pressure ▸ pulmonary
- h., primary
- h., primary pulmonary
- h., pulmonary
- h. (PAH), pulmonary artery
- h., recalcitrant
- h., red
- h., Regitine test for
- h., renal
- h., renoprival
- h., renovascular
- h., resistant
- h. risk factor ▸ primary pulmonary
- h. screening program
- h., secondary
- h., secondary pulmonary
- h., severe
- h., splenoportal
- h. ▸ Stage 1
- h. ▸ stress-related
- h., sustained
- h., symptomatic

- h., systemic
- h. ▸ systemic vascular
- h. ▸ systemic venous
- h., systolic
- h., transitory
- h. treatment
- h., treatment for
- h., uncontrolled
- h., unspecified
- h., vascular
- h., venous
- h., white coat
- h. with ascites ▸ portal

hypertensive(s)
- h. agent
- h., arteriopathy
- h., arteriosclerosis
- h. arteriosclerotic heart disease
- h., biofeedback for
- h. cardiomyopathy
- h. cardiopathy
- h. cardiovascular disease (HCVD)
- h. choroidopathy
- h. crisis
- h. crisis ▸ potential
- h. crisis ▸ potential fetal
- h. disease, choroidal
- h. disease, chronic
- h. emergency
- h. encephalopathy
- h. episode
- h. episode, acute
- h. heart disease (HHD)
- h. hemorrhage
- h. hypertrophic cardiomyopathy
- h. meningeal hydrops
- h. nephropathy
- h. neuroretinopathy
- h. ocular disease
- h. optic neuropathy
- h. patient
- h. patient, essential
- h. patient, stress in
- h. personality
- h. pulmonary vascular disease
- h. retinitis
- h. retinopathy
- h. smoker
- h., stressed
- h. therapy
- h. therapy, rational
- h. urgency
- h. vascular crisis
- h. vascular disease (HVD)
- h. vasculopathy

hyperthermia
h., adjuvant
h. and radiation treatment ▸ combined
h., cooling blanket for
h. effect
h., malignant
h., microwave
h. in breast
h. in extremities
h. in pelvis
h., interstitial
h., radiofrequency electric field
h., sensitivity to
h., thermometer monitoring in
h., ultrasound
h. whole body
hyperthermic limb perfusion ▸ isolated
hyperthyroid factor, exophthalmos
hyperthyroid heart
hyperthyroidism
h., amiodarone-induced
h., apathetic
h., exogenous
hypertonic
h. bladder
h. solution
h. sphincter
h. uterine dysfunction
hypertonica, polycythemia
hypertriglyceridemia, diabetic
hypertrophic [*hyperopic*]
h. adenoids
h. arthritis
h. arthropathy, secondary
h. burn scar
h. cardiomyopathy
h. cardiomyopathy, concentric
h. cardiomyopathy, familial
h. cardiomyopathy ▸ genetic
h. cardiomyopathy ▸ hypertensive
h. catarrh
h. change
h. changes, normal
h. cirrhosis
h. emphysema
h. emphysema, chronic
h. encroachment
h. enlargement
h. enlargement ▸ hereditary
h. gastritis
h. gastritis, giant
h. infiltrative tendinitis

h. interstitial neuropathy ▸ progressive
h. lipping
h. muscular subaortic stenosis
h. myopathy
h. nodular gliosis
h. obstructive cardiomyopathy
h. obstructive cardiomyopathy, familial
h. osteoarthropathy, idiopathic
h. osteoarthropathy ▸ pulmonary
h. osteoarthropathy, secondary
h. pharyngitis
h. pulmonary osteoarthropathy
h. pyloric stenosis
h. rhinitis
h. salpingitis
h. scar
h. smooth muscle layer
h. spondylitis
h. spur
h. spur formation ▸ osteoarthritic
h. spurring
h. subaortic hypetension ▸ idiopathic
h. subaortic stenosis (IHSS), idiopathic
h. synovitis
hypertrophied
h. adenoids
h. and dilated ▸ heart
h. muscle
h. muscle ▸ impaired contactibility of
h. papilla
h. scar
h. tonsil
h. ▸ ventricles dilated and
hypertrophy
h., adaptive
h., adenoid
h., apical
h. (ASH), asymmetrical septal
h., atrial
h., basal septal
h., benign
h. (BPH) ▸ benign prostatic
h., biatrial
h., Billroth's
h., biventricular
h. ▸ biventricular dilatation and
h. ▸ borderline septal
h., breast
h., cardiac
h., combined ventricular

h., compensatory
h., complementary
h., concentric
h., concentric left ventricular (LV)
h., eccentric
h., false
h., functional
h., hemifacial
h. (IMH), idiopathic myocardial
h. ▸ isolated septal
h. (LAH), left atrial
h. (LVH), left ventricular
h., lipomatous
h., lymphoid
h., Marie's
h. ▸ marked left ventricular
h. ▸ mild biventricular dilatation
h., muscle
h., muscular
h., myocardial
h., myocardial idiopathic
h., myocyte
h., nodular prostatic
h., numeric
h. of adenoids
h. of cardiomegaly
h. of heart
h. of heart muscle ▸ compensa- tory
h. of prostate ▸ benign
h. of pulmonary vessels ▸ medial
h. of tonsils and adenoids
h. of trigone
h., papillary
h., physiologic
h., prostatic
h., pseudomuscular
h. (RAH), right atrial
h. (RVH), right ventricular
h., septal
h., stromal
h. ▸ submucosal gland
h., trabecular
h., true
h., unilateral
h., ventricular
h., vicarious
h. ▸ volume load
h., work
hypertropia
h., alternating
h., constant
h., left
h., right
hyperuricemic nephropathy

hyperventilating, patient
hyperventilating, sweating and
   shaking
hyperventilation (HV)
   h., alveolar
   h. build-up
   h., deliberate
   h. from anxiety
   h. maneuver
   h. procedure
   h., prolonged intensive
   h. syndrome
   h. syndrome (HVS), chronic
   h. tetany
hyperviscosity
   h. retinopathy
   h., serum
   h. syndrome
hypesthesia (*same as* hypoesthesia)
   h. and paralysis
   h., median nerve
   h., numbness and
   h. of left leg
   h. of right leg
   h., stocking-and-glove type
hyphae
   h., broad septate
   h., fungal
   h., yeast and
hyphema, total
hypnagogic
   h. hallucination
   h. imagery
   h. perceptions
   h. phenomena
   h. startle
   h. starts
   h. state
hypnic jerks
hypnociastic shock
hypnoidal state
hypnoleptic state
hypnopompic hallucinations
hypnopompic state
hypnosis
   h., behavioral
   h., clinical
   h., memory, and distortion
   h. ▸ patient under self-
   h., self-
   h. study
   h., technique
hypnotherapy and medication
hypnotherapy, clinical
hypnotic (Hypnotic)

   h. abuse
   h. -alpha procedure
   h. amnestic disorder
   h. control of autonomic functions ▸
     biofeedback
   h. drug
   h. drug ▸ sedative
   h. imagery
   h. induction
   H. Induction Profile
   h., or anxiolytic abuse ▸ sedative,
   h., or anxiolytic dependence ▸
     sedative,
   h., or anxiolytic intoxication ▸
     sedative,
   h. relaxation for insomnia
   h. similarly acting dependence
   h. state
   h. suggestions
   h. suggestions, post-
   h. suggestions, psychological
     effects of
   h. susceptibility
   h. training
   h. trance
   h. treatment
   h., undesirable
   h. withdrawal delirium
hypnotically suggested relaxation
hypnotized, patient
hypo (H)
hypoactive
   h. bowel sounds
   h. bowel tones
   h. deep tendon reflexes (DTR)
   h. movements
   h. reflex
   h. sexual desire disorder
hypoacusis (*same as*
   hypacusia/hypacusis)
hypoaldosteronism, hyporeninemic
hypobaric hypoxia
hypoblastic right and left heart
   syndrome
hypocalcemia [*hypokalemia*]
hypocalcemia [*hypokalemia*] -
   induced arrhythmia
hypocalcemia [*hypokalemia*] ▸ renal
   tubule
hypocalcification, enamel
hypocalcuric hypercalcemia, familial
hypocellular bone marrow
hypochloraemicum, coma
hypochloremic azotemia
hypochloruric nephropathy

hypochondriac
   h. region
   h. region of abdomen ▸ left
   h. region of abdomen ▸ right
hypochondriaca, melancholia
hypochondriacal
   h. delusions
   h. neurosis
   h., patient
   h. personality
   h. reflex
hypochondriasis, severe
hypochordal arch
hypochromemia, idiopathic
hypochromic
   h. anemia
   h. anemia ▸ idiopathic
   h. erythrocyte
hypochromica siderochrestica
   hereditaria, anemia
hypocratic medicine, neo-
Hypoderma bovis
Hypoderma lineatum
hypodermic
   h. implantation
   h. microscope
   h. needle
   h. tablet
hypodynamia cordis
hypoesthesia (*see* hypesthesia)
hypoexemia, circulatory
hypofunction, vestibular
hypogammaglobulinemia
   h., acquired
   h., congenital
   h., physiologic
   h., transient
hypogastric
   h. artery
   h. ganglion
   h. ligation
   h. nerve
   h. occlusion
   h. plexus
   h. pressure
   h. region
   h. region of abdomen
   h. vein
hypogenetic nephritis
hypoglossal
   h. artery ▸ primitive
   h. -facial neuroanastomosis
   h. ganglion
   h. nerve
   h. nerve, accompanying vein of

h. nerve, loop of
h. nerve signs
h. neuroanastomosis, spinal
   accessory-
hypoglycemia
h., alimentary
h. ▸ functional decortication from
h., chronic
h., functional
h., metabolic
h., spontaneous
hypoglycemic
h. agent
h. coma
h. encephalopathy
h. episode
h., patient
h. shock
h. syncope
hypogonad obesity
hypohomycetica, stomatitis
hypokalemia [*hypocalcemia*]
h. -induced arrhythmia
h. ▸ renal tubule
hypokalemic nephrosis
hypokalemic rhabdomyolysis
hypokinesia of left ventricle
hypokinesis
h., anteromesial
h., cardiac wall
h., diffuse
h., global
hypokinetic
h. movement
h. pulse
h. septum
hypomaniac
h. mood
h. personality
h. personality disorder, chronic
hypomastia with ptosis
hypomelanosis ▸ idiopathic guttate
hypomeric muscle
hyponatremia ▸ disorder of
hyponatremic, patient
hypo-osmolarity of blood and urine
hypoparathyroidism, pseudo◊
hypoperfusion, cerebral
hypopharyngeal carcinoma
hypopharyngeal diverticulum
hypopharynx, caustic strictures of
hypophosphatemia, familial
hypophyseal/hypophysial
h. cachexia
h. dwarf

h. fossa
h. infantilism
h. -pituitary adrenal axis
h. stalk
hypophyseogenea, asthenia gravis
hypophyseoportal veins
hypophysiopriva cachexia
hypophysis
h. cerebri
h., peduncle of
h. sicca
h. tentorium of
hypopiesis, orthostatic
hypopigmented macules on legs
hypopituitarism, congenital
hypopituitary dwarfs
hypoplasia
h., congenital idiopathic adrenal
h., enamel
h., hereditary enamel
h. membrane disease ▸ pulmonary
h. ▸ mitral valve
h. of epiglottis
h. of right ventricle (RV)
h. of zonule
h., pulmonary
h. ▸ right ventricular (RV)
h., secondary pulmonary
h. syndrome, focal dermal
hypoplasmic obesity
hypoplastic
h. anemia
h. anemia, congenital
h. emphysema
h. enamel
h. heart
h. kidney
h. left heart syndrome
h. lung syndrome
hypopnea index (AHI), apnea
hypopnea syndrome ▸ sleep apnea/
hypopyon keratitis
hyporeflexia, detrusor
hyporeflexic bladder
hyporeninemic hypoaldosteronism
hypospadias, female
hypostatic
h. bronchopneumonia
h. congestion
h. ectasia
h. pneumonia
h. splenization
hypotelorism, orbital
hypotension [*hypertension*]
h., acute severe

h. and coma
h. and tachycardia
h., arterial
h., chronic idiopathic orthostatic
h., chronic orthostatic
h. ▸ idiopathic orthostatic
h. ▸ increased peripheral
   vasodilation and
h. (NMH) ▸ neurally mediated
h., orthostatic
h., postexercise
h., postprandial
h., postural
h., prolonged
h., systolic
h., vasovagal
h. ▸ vertigo, syncope and
hypotensive
h. agent
h. and unresponsive ▸ patient
   weak,
h. and ventilatory support
h., bradycardia
h. hamartoma (HH)
h., patient
h. period
h. syndrome, supine
hypothalamic
h. amenorrhea
h. epilepsy
h. feeding center
h. hormones
h. lesions
h. pituitary adrenocortical axis
   (HPAA)
h. -pituitary-adrenal (HPA) axis
h. stimulation ▸ pulmonary
hypothalamicus, sulcus
hypothalamus
h., anterior
h. gland
h., inferior aspect of
h. (INAH), interstitial nuclei of
   anterior
hypothenar eminence
hypothenar hammer syndrome
hypothermia
h., accidental
h. and alcoholism
h. blanket
h., chills with
h. circulatory arrest, deep
h., dilated pupils and
h., endogenous
h. ▸ extracorporeal exchange

hypothermia—*continued*
- h. in aging
- h., limited
- h., local
- h., topical

hypothermic
- h. blanket
- h. cardiac arrest surgery
- h. cardioplegic arrest
- h. fibrillating arrest
- h. mattress
- h. procedure
- h. surgery
- h. technique

hypothesis [*apophysis*]
- h., attenuation
- h., beta amyloid
- h., dopamine
- h., estrogen
- h., Gad's
- h. ▸ leading circle
- h., lipid
- h., Lyon
- h., modification
- h., monoclonal
- h., null
- h. of atherogenesis ▸ response-to-injury
- h. ▸ premature ventricular complex trigger
- h. ▸ response-to-injury

hypothrombinemic effect, enhanced
hypothyroid dwarf
hypothyroid obesity
hypothyroidism, congenital
hypothyroidism, depression from
hypotonia/hypotonus/hypotony
hypotonia oculi
hypotonia of muscles
hypotonic
- h. bladder
- h. colon
- h. duodenography

hypotropia, alternating
hypotropia, constant
hypoventilating patient
hypoventilation
- h. failure
- h. syndrome, congenital central
- h. syndrome ▸ obesity

hypovolemic sequelae
hypovolemic shock
hypoxanthine guanine phosphoribosyl transferase

hypoxemia
- h., arterial
- h. ▸ rapid eye movement (REM) sleep-related
- h. rest
- h. test

hypoxemic failure
hypoxia
- h., altitude
- h., alveolar
- h. and anoxia
- h., anemic
- h., cerebral
- h., chronic
- h., circulatory
- h., diffusion
- h., functional decortication from
- h., hypobaric
- h., hypoxic
- h., ischemic
- h., sleep
- h., stagnant
- h., tumor cell

hypoxic
- h. cells
- h. change in brain
- h. drive
- h. gain factor
- h. hypoxia
- h. ▸ infant acidotic and
- h. -ischemic encephalopathy
- h. lap swimming
- h. neuronal changes ▸ mild
- h. pulmonary hypertension
- h. pulmonary vasoconstriction
- h. response study
- h. syncope

hypsarrhythmia, compatible with
hypsarrhythmia pattern
Hyrtl's
- H. anastomosis
- H. nerve
- H. sphincter

hysterectomy
- h., abdominal (ab hys/abd. hyst.)
- h., Bonney's
- h., celio◊
- h., cesarean
- h., chemical
- h., complete
- h., cunei◊
- h. Doyen's vaginal
- h., emergency
- h., etro◊
- h., extrafascial

- h., Heaney's vaginal
- h., laparo◊
- h. (LAVH) ▸ laparoscopically assisted vaginal
- h., Latzko's radical
- h., Mayo-Ward vaginal
- h., modified radical
- h., ovario◊
- h., pan◊
- h., paravaginal
- h., partial
- h., Porro's
- h., prophylactic
- h., radical
- h., radical abdominal
- h., Ries-Wertheim
- h., subtotal
- h. support
- h., supracervical
- h., supravaginal
- h., total
- h., total abdominal
- h. (TVH) ▸ total vaginal
- h., vaginal
- h., Ward-Mayo vaginal
- h., Wertheim's radical

hysteresis
- h., pacemaker
- h., pacing
- h., rate

hysteria
- h., anxiety
- h., canine
- h., conversion
- h., epidemic
- h., fixation
- h. libidinosa
- h. major
- h. minor
- h., monosymptomatic
- h., psychosomatic

hysteric
- h. amaurosis
- h, amblyopia
- h. angina
- h. aphonia
- h. ataxia
- h. insanity
- h. joint
- h. lethargy
- h. pregnancy
- h. stigma

hysterical
- h. chorea
- h. conversion disorder

h. convulsion
h. deafness
h. disorder
h. epilepsy
h. fainting
h. fever
h. laughter
h. mania
h. mutism
h. neurosis
h. paralysis
h. paralysis ▸ trauma-induced
h., patient
h. personality
h. reaction
h. state
h. stricture
h. syncope
h. tremor
h. vertigo
h. vomiting
hystericus, globus
hysterogram, electro◊
hysterogram study
hysteroid convulsion
hysterosalpingogram (HSG)
hysterosalpingogram study
**hysterosalpingo-oophorectomy,
    laparo◊**
**hysteroscopy and endometrial
    ablation**
hystrix, icthyosis
Hz (hertz)

Hz, eight to 13
Hz positive bursts ▸ 14 and six
Hz positive spikes ▸ 14 and six
Hz spike-and-slow waves ▸ three
Hz unit

I

I (iodine)
I and D (incision and drainage)
    I and D of abscess
    I and D of blister
    I and D of fistulous tract
    I and D of ischiorectal abscess
    I and D of left buttock
    I and D of right buttock
I and O (in and out)
I and O (intake and output)
I changes ▸ E to
I disorder, bipolar
I, hemoglobin
I, Mobitz
I substance
IA
    IA (internal auditory)
    IA (intra-aortic)
    IA (intra-arterial)
IABP (intra-aortic balloon pumping)
IAC (internal auditory canal)
IAC (interposed abdominal compression)
IADH (inappropriate antidiuretic hormone)
ialo photocoagulation
IAM (integrated anger management)
IAS (interatrial septum)
IASD (interatrial septal defect)
iatrogenic
    i. anemia
    i. atrial septal defect
    i. disorder
    i. effects
    i. effects of behavior therapy
    i. effusion
    i. fracture
    i. hyperosmolality
    i. illness
    i. infection
    i. injury
    i. pneumothorax
    i. trauma
    i. ureteral injury
IB (instrument birth)
IBC (iron-binding capacity)
I-beam, Jergesen

I-beam nail
IBS (irritable bowel syndrome)
IBU (international benzoate unit)
IC
    IC (inspiratory capacity)
    IC (intermediate care)
    IC (irritable colon)
ICA (internal carotid artery)
ICAO (internal carotid artery occlusion)
ICC (Infection Control Coordinator)
ICCU (Intensive Coronary Care Unit)
ice (Ice) (ICE)
    I. (cocaine)
    I. (crystal methamphetamine)
    i. and snow ▸ anesthetizing effect of
    i. bag
    i. chips
    i., compression and elevation (PRICE) ▸ protection, rest,
    i., compression, elevation (RICE) ▸ rest,
    i. cream headache
    i. mapping
    i. massage
    i. pack
    i. -pick view
    i. ▸ therapeutic qualities of
    i. therapy
    i. victim
    i. whirlpool treatment ▸ cold or
iced saline
Icelandic disease
ichorous pleurisy
ichthyosis
    i. congenital
    i. fetalis
    i. fetus
    i. hystrix
    i., lamellar
    i. linguae
icing compression
icing heart
ICL (intraocular contact lens)
ICM (intercostal margin)
ICM Tele-Sensor, Cosman

ICN (Infection Control Nurse)
ICN (Intermediate Care Nursery)
ICO (Infection Control Officer)
Icon molecule
ICP (Infection Control Practitioner)
ICP (intracranial pressure) catheter
ICS
    ICS (intercostal space)
    ICS (intercostal space) ▸ fifth
    ICS (intercostal space) ▸ PMI (point of maximum impulse) fifth
ICT (insulin coma therapy)
ICT (integrative couple therapy)
ict ind (icteric index)
ictal paroxysmal activity ▸ inter◊
ictal slowing, post-
icteric
    i., conjunctivae
    i. hepatitis
    i. index (ict ind)
    i., infant mildly
    i. necrosis
    i. sclerae
    i., sclerae markedly
    i. serum hepatitis
    i. sputum
icterohaemorrhagiae, Leptospira
icterohemolytic anemia
icterohemorrhagica, leptospirosis
icterus
    i., acholuric hemolytic
    i., bilirubin
    i. castrensis gravis
    i. castrensis levis
    i. catarrhalis
    i., cythemolytic
    i. gravis
    i. gravis neonatorum
    i., Gubler's
    i., Hayem's
    i., hemolytic
    i. hemolyticus
    i. index
    i. index test
    i. infectiosus
    i., Liouvilles
    i., marked

icterus—*continued*
- i. melas
- i. neonatorum
- i. praecox
- i., scleral
- i. simplex
- i., spirochetal
- i., urobilin
- i. viridans

ictus
- i. cordis
- i. epilepticus
- i. paralyticus
- i. sanguinis
- i. solis

ICU (Intensive Care Unit)
- ICU ‣ Neonatal
- ICU psychosis
- ICU syndrome

ID (identification) bracelet, patient
ID (identification) number, laboratory
id reaction
idahoensis, Ceratophyllus
idahoensis, Oropsylla
IDD (iodine deficiency disorder)
IDDM (insulin-dependent diabetes mellitus)
idea(s)
- i., confusion of
- i. density
- i., fixed
- i., flight of
- i., grandiose
- i. ‣ idiosyncratic false
- i. of grandeur
- i. of reference
- i. of reference ‣ delusion or
- i. of reference ‣ transient
- i., overvalued
- i. ‣ overvalued false
- i. ‣ overvalued obsessional
- i., poverty of
- i. ‣ senseless thoughts and
- i., sphere of
- i. ‣ superstitious false
- i. ‣ unpersuasive false

ideal
- i. arch wire
- i. body weight
- i., ego
- i. occlusion

idealize potential caregivers
idealized ‣ nurturing qualities
ideation
- i., aggressive

- i., homicidal
- i., incoherent
- i., paranoid
- i., suicidal
- i., suicide

ideational agnosia
ideational apraxia
idée fixe
identical
- i. genes
- i. genetic repertoire
- i. midplane doses
- i. patterns
- i. stimuli
- i. twin transplants
- i. twins

identifiable electrical activity
identifiable psychiatric syndrome
identification
- i., body
- i. bracelet
- i. (ID) bracelet, patient
- i., footprint
- i., isolation and
- i., medical information
- i. of genes
- i. of symptoms ‣ early
- i., organism
- i., warning sign

identified
- i. and ligated
- i. at-risk
- i., bleeders
- i., capsule
- i., causative organism
- i. criteria
- i. high-risk mother
- i. needs, patient's
- i. proximal ends of tendon
- i., tumor

identify
- i. and respond ‣ failure to
- i. infection
- i. patient at-risk
- i. potential organ donor

identifying a drug-abusing patient
identifying resources
identity
- i. and role counseling
- i. ‣ assumption of new
- i. disorder
- i. disorder ‣ dissociative
- i. disorder, gender
- i. disorder of adolescence ‣ gender

- i. disorder of adolescence or adulthood, nontranssexual type ‣ gender
- i. disorder of adult life ‣ gender
- i. disorder of childhood ‣ gender
- i. ‣ disorders of psychosexual
- i. disturbance
- i. disturbance, persistent
- i. disturbance ‣ personal
- i. ‣ induced false
- i. problem
- i., reaction of
- i., sexual

ideokinetic apraxia
ideology, controlling
ideology, enabling
ideomotor apraxia
ideo-obsessional constitution
IDET (intradiskal electrothermal therapy)
idiocy
- i., absolute
- i., amaurotic familial
- i., athetosic
- i., axonal
- i., Aztec
- i., cretinoid
- i., developmental
- i., diplegic
- i., eclamptic
- i., epileptic
- i., erethistic
- i., familial
- i., genetous
- i., hemiplegic
- i., hydrocephalic
- i., intrasocial
- i., Kalmuk
- i., microcephalic
- i., mongolian
- i., paralytic
- i., paraplegic
- i., plagiocephalic
- i., profound
- i., scaphocephalic
- i., sensorial
- i., spastic amaurotic axonal
- i., torpid
- i., traumatic
- i., xerodermic

idiogenous pain
idiojunctional rhythm
idiomuscular contractility
idiomuscular contractions
idionodal rhythm

idionodal rhythm, accelerated
idiopathic
- i. acute eosinophilic pneumonia
- i. adrenal hypoplasia, congenital
- i. anemia
- i. angioedema
- i. arteritis of Takayasu
- i. bradycardia
- i. brown induration
- i. cardiomegaly
- i. cardiomyopathy
- i. cardiomyopathy, degenerative
- i. CNS (central nervous system) hypersomnolence
- i. cyclic edema
- i. dilatation
- i. dilated cardiomyopathy
- i. disorder
- i. epilepsy
- i. facial paralysis
- i. fibrosis
- i. guttate hypomelanosis
- i. hemolytic anemia
- i. hypercalcemia
- i. hypercalcinuria
- i. hyperchromemia
- i. hypereosinophilic syndrome
- i. hypertension
- i. hypertrophic osteoarthropathy
- i. hypertrophic subaortic hypertension
- i. hypertrophic subaortic stenosis (IHSS)
- i. hypochromic anemia
- i. interstitial pneumonia
- i. isosexual puberty
- i. long Q-T interval syndrome
- i. megacolon
- i. megakaryocytic aplasia
- i. mental deficiency
- i. muscular atrophy
- i. myocardial hypertrophy (IMH)
- i. myocardiopathy
- i. myocarditis
- i. myoglobinuria
- i. nephralgia
- i. nephritis
- i. nephrotic syndrome
- i. neuromuscular disease ▸ progressive
- i. orthostatic hypotension
- i. orthostatic hypotension, chronic
- i. osteoporosis
- i. pericarditis
- i. polyneuritis, acute

- i. polyserositis
- i. pulmonary fibrosis (IPF)
- i. pulmonary hemosiderosis
- i. purpura
- i. Raynaud's disease
- i. restrictive cardiomyopathy
- i. respiratory distress of newborn
- i. respiratory distress syndrome (IRDS)
- i. scoliosis ▸ juvenile
- i. seizure disorder
- i. skeletal hyperostosis
- i. steatorrhea
- i. subaortic stenosis
- i. thrombocytopenia
- i. thrombocytopenic purpura (ITP)
- i. unilobar emphysema
- i. ventricular fibrillation
- i. ventricular tachycardia
- i. vertigo
- i. xanthomatosis, chronic

idiophrenic insanity
idiophrenic psychosis
idiosyncrasy, drug
idiosyncratic
- i. alcohol intoxication
- i. false idea
- i. food preference
- i. intoxication
- i. intoxication, alcohol
- i. obsessions and rituals
- i. reaction
- i. reaction to drug

idiot
- i., erethistic
- i., mongolian
- i., pithecoid
- i., profound
- i. -savant
- i., superficial
- i., torpid

idiotype antibody
idiotypic antigen
idioventricular
- i. bradycardia
- i. kick
- i. rhythm
- i. rhythm, accelerated
- i. rhythm ▸ pulsed
- i. rhythm ▸ pulseless
- i. tachycardia
- i. tachycardia, accelerated

IDM (infant of diabetic mother)
IDP (Intoxicated Driver Program)

IDSA (intraoperative digital subtraction angiography)
IDT (interdisciplinary team) meeting
I/E (inspiratory-expiratory ratio)
I:E ratio
IFR (inspiratory flow rate)
Ig (immunoglobulin)
IgA
- IgA (gamma A globulin) deficiency
- IgA (gamma A immuno-globulin) deficiency
- IgA (gamma A immuno-globulin) determination
- IgA monoclonal gammopathy

IgD (gamma D immuno-globulin) determination
IgE (gamma E immuno-globulin)
- IgE determination
- IgE sensitized cell
- IgE ▸ serum

IgG (gamma G immuno-globulin) determination
Iglesias bridge
IgM
- IgM (Antibody IgM class to Hepatitis B Core Antigen), Anti-HBc
- IgM class to Hepatitis B Core Antigen (Anti-HBc IgM), Antibody
- IgM (gamma M globulin) deficiency
- IgM (gamma M immuno-globulin) deficiency
- IgM (gamma M immuno-globulin) determination

IH, hepatitis virus
IHD (ischemic heart disease)
IHSS (idiopathic hypertrophic subaortic stenosis)
I-IDDM (insulin dependent diabetes mellitus) ▸ Type
IJP (internal jugular pressure)
Ilazarov operation
Ilazarov procedure
ileac [iliac]
ileal
- i. atresia
- i. bypass ▸ partial
- i. colostomy, resected end-to-end
- i. conduit
- i. loop stoma
- i. loop, terminal
- i. stasis
- i. transverse colostomy ▸ normal functioning
- i. vein

ileitis
 i., distal
 i., regional
 i., terminal
ileoanal anastomosis
ileoanal pouch
ileocecal
 i. bladder
 i. incompetence
 i. insufficiency
 i. intussusception
 i. junction
 i. region
 i. valve
ileocolic
 i. artery
 i. fold
 i. intussusception
 i. lymph nodes
 i. vein
ileogastric reflex
ileojejunitis, granulomatous
ileojejunitis, nongranulomatous
ileorectal anastomosis
ileostomy
 i. bag
 i., cholecysto◊
 i., choledocho◊
 i., gastro◊
 i., permanent
 i. pouch
 i. procedure
 i. sac
 i., uretero◊
ileotransverse colostomy
ileotransverse colostomy, end-to-side
ileum [*ilium*]
 i. adhesed ▸ jejunum and
 i., distal
 i. ▸ inflammation of
 i. normal ▸ reflux into terminal
 i., terminal
ileus
 i., adynamic
 i. following abdominal surgery
 i., gallstone
 i., meconium
 i., paralytic
 i., postoperative
 i., reflex
 i., reflexive
 i., reflex-type
 i., spastic
Ilfeld-Holder deformity

Ilheus virus
iliac [*ileac*]
 i. adenopathy, internal
 i. aneurysm, ruptured
 i. artery
 i. artery aneurysm
 i. artery, common
 i. artery, external
 i. artery, internal
 i. artery occlusion
 i. augmentation
 i. autograft
 i. bifurcation
 i. bone
 i. bone, crest of
 i. bone graft ▸ osteoperiosteal
 i. bypass, aortobi-
 i. cancellous bone
 i. chain
 i. colon
 i., common
 i. crest
 i. crest biopsy
 i. endarterectomy
 i., external
 i. flexure of colon
 i. fossa abscess
 i. fossa, left
 i. fossa, right
 i. graft
 i. joint, sacro◊
 i. lymph nodes
 i. lymph nodes ▸ common
 i. lymph nodes ▸ external
 i. lymph nodes ▸ internal
 i. muscle
 i. pulse
 i. region
 i. region of abdomen ▸ left
 i. region of abdomen ▸ right
 i., sacro
 i. spine
 i. spine (ASIS), anterior superior
 i. steal
 i. vein
 i. vein, common
 i. vein, deep circumflex
 i. vein, external
 i. vein, internal
 i. vein, superficial circumflex
 i. vein thrombosis
iliacus, muscle
ilii, osteitis condensans
iliocana, Fascioletta
iliococcygeal muscle

iliocostal muscles
iliocostalis
 i. cervicis muscle
 i. lumborum muscle
 i. thoracis muscle
iliofemoral artery
iliofemoral deep vein thrombosis
iliohypogastric nerve
ilioinguinal artery
ilioinguinal nerve
iliolumbar vein
iliopectineal eminence
iliopectineal line
iliopopliteal bypass
iliopsoas muscle
iliosacral articulation
iliotibial
 i. band
 i. band (ITB) tendinitis
 i. tract
iliotrochanteric ligament
ilium [*ileum*]
 i., ala
 i. bone
 i., crest of
 i., posterior crest of
ill
 i., acutely
 i. children, terminally
 i., chronically
 i. critically
 i. -defined
 i. -defined density
 i. -fitting dentures
 i. -fitting shoes
 i., patient acutely
 i., patient chronically
 i., patient emotionally
 i., patient incurably
 i., patient mentally
 i., patient seriously
 i., patient terminally
 i. (SI), seriously
 i., terminally
 i. virus, louping
illegal
 i. chemicals
 i. controlled substances
 i. drug traffic
 i. drug use
 i. drugs
 i. intravenous drug
 i. intravenous (IV) drug use
illegible prescriptions

illicit
- i. drug
- i. drug, addictive-
- i. drug ▸ prenatal abuse of
- i. drug use
- i. substance use

illinii, Miyagawanella
illiterate, functionally
illiterate, patient functionally
illness (Illness)
- i., accepting
- i., acute
- i., acute clinical
- i., acute medical
- i., addictive
- i., affective
- i., AIDS (acquired immune deficiency syndrome)
- i., alcohol-related
- i., asbestos-related
- i., bacterial food-borne
- i., biphasic
- i., bipolar
- i., catastrophic
- i., catastrophic life-threatening
- i., chronic
- i., chronic and progressive
- i., chronic long term
- i., chronic medical
- i., clinical
- i., co-morbid
- i., course of
- i., debilitating
- i. ▸ delusional mental
- i., dementing
- i., depression triggered by physical
- i., depressive
- i., destructive
- i., devastating
- i., disabling
- i. ▸ disabling mental
- i., drug-dependent
- i. ▸ ego-dystonic
- i., emotional
- i., employee mental
- i. (EI), environmental
- i. ▸ evaluate extent of injury or
- i., exacerbation of
- i. ▸ exacerbation of pre-existing psychiatric
- i., fabricated
- i. fabrication
- i., family adjustment to
- i., family reaction to
- i., fatal

- i., fatal genetic
- i., febrile
- i., food-borne
- i. ▸ full-blown manic depressive
- i., functional
- i. ▸ genetic predisposition to psychiatric
- i. ▸ heat-induced
- i. ▸ heat-related
- i., hereditary familial
- i., high altitude related
- i. (HPI) ▸ history of present
- i., iatrogenic
- i., immune
- i. ▸ increased risk for
- i., incurable
- i. index, definable
- i., infectious
- i. ▸ influenza-related
- i., insight into
- i., length of awareness of
- i., level and degree of mental
- i., life-threatening
- i., long-term
- i. ▸ major mental
- i., manic depressive
- i., mass psychogenic
- i., medical
- i., mental
- i., mild
- i., mononucleosis-like
- i., neurotic
- i. (PI) ▸ noncontributory to present
- i. of emotional origin
- i. outbreak, food-borne
- i. outbreak, waterborne
- i. ▸ patient concealed
- i. ▸ patient faking
- i., persistent
- i., persistent mental
- i. ▸ pervasive mental
- i. ▸ pet-borne
- i., phantom
- i. ▸ potentially life-threatening
- i., predisposition toward
- i., preexisting
- i., present
- i., prevalent
- i. ▸ prevention of mental
- i. ▸ previously unrecognized mental
- i., prolonged
- i., prolonged symptomatic
- i., psychiatric
- i., psychological
- i., psychosomatic

- I. ▸ Psychosocial Adjustment to
- i., psychotic
- i., recurrent
- i. (RI), respiratory
- i., salmonella
- I. Scale ▸ Psychosocial Adjustment to
- i., self-awareness in
- i. ▸ self-induced
- i., self-limiting
- i., severe
- i. ▸ severe and persistent mental
- i. ▸ severe depressive
- i. ▸ severe mental
- i. ▸ severe paralytic
- i., site of
- i., sudden
- i. ▸ swimming-related
- i. syndrome, heat
- i., systemic
- i., terminal
- i. ▸ terminal genetic
- i. ▸ terminal stage of
- i. ▸ tick-borne
- i., treatable
- i., treatment of mental
- i., underlying
- i. ▸ underlying physical
- i., viral
- i. ▸ warning signs of serious
- i. with physical symptoms ▸ chronic factitious
- i. with psychological symptoms ▸ factitious

illucens, Hermetia
illumination
- i., axial
- i., central
- i., contact
- i., critical
- i., darkfield
- i., dark-ground
- i., direct
- i., focal
- i., lateral
- i., oblique
- i. ▸ red laser
- i., through

illusion(s) [*elusion*]
- i., auditory
- i., fleeting
- i., Kuhnt's
- i. of control
- i., optical
- i. or perceptual distortions

illusion(s)—*continued*
- i. of transparency
- i., pain blocking
- i., passive
- i., perception
- i., visual

illusional seizure
illusory child abuse
ilocanum, Echinostoma
IM (intramuscular)
- IM (intramuscular) administration
- IM (intramuscular) cocktail
- IM (intramuscular) injection

IM (intermenstrual) spotting
IMA (inferior mesenteric artery)
image(s)
- i., accidental
- i. agnosia, body-image aliasing
- i. -amplified fluoroscopy
- i. amplifier
- i., amplitude
- i. analysis
- i. analysis, digital
- i. analysis ► phase
- i. and hallucinations ► distorted visual
- i. artifact ► split
- i., body
- i. bundle
- i. changes, body
- i., cognitive change of body
- i., comfortable self-
- i., computer generated
- i., computerized
- i. converter
- i. -converter infrared
- i. dextrocardia, mirror-images, digital mammography
- i. display and analysis
- i., dissection quality
- i., distorted body
- i. distortions, body
- i. disturbance, body
- i., disturbance in self-
- i., dream-like
- i., eidetic
- i. ► ejection fraction
- i. ► ejection shell
- i., equilibrium
- i., fragmentary
- i., functional
- i. ► good-self
- i. -guided biopsy
- i. -guided procedure
- i. -guided surgical technique

- i. ► improve self-
- i. intensifier
- i. laryngoscopy ► mirror
- i. lung syndrome ► mirror
- i., magnetic resonance
- i. management
- i., mental
- i. modulation
- i., negative
- i., negative self-
- i. of body organs
- i. of body, tomographic
- i. of brain, delayed
- i. of head, tomographic
- i. of mines
- i. on screen, detailed
- i. -oriented
- i., paradox
- i., parametric
- i. ► patient self-
- i. patterns of anxiety
- i. ► persistently unstable self-
- i., phase
- i. ► phase encoded velocity
- i., photo
- i. ► poor body
- i. ► poor self-
- i., positive self-
- i. processor
- i. produced by computerized tomography
- i. ► profound change in self-
- i., Purkinje
- i., Purkinje-Sanson
- i., Purkinje-Sanson mirror
- i. puzzle, body
- i., readable
- i., self-
- i. slices
- i. ► stability of self-
- i. ► stress washout myocardial perfusion
- i. ► supine rest gated equilibrium
- i., three-dimensional
- i. ► three-dimensional x-ray
- i. ► T1-T2 weighted
- i. ► T2 weighted
- i., ultrasound
- i. ► unstable self-
- i., video
- i., visual
- i., x-ray

Imager (imager)
- I. (DVI), Digital Vascular

- I. (DVI) Multicenter ► Digital Vascular
- i., ultrasonic

imagery
- i. and relaxation techniques ► biofeedback,
- i. and visualization
- i., aversive
- i. ► biofeedback and guided
- i. device
- i., emotive
- i. exercise ► visual
- i., focused
- i., guided
- i., hypnagogic
- i., hypnotic
- i. ► increase in eidetic
- i., mastery
- i. ► meditation, visualization and
- i., mental
- i., negative
- i. ► relaxation, distraction, and
- i., reverie
- i. ► stress management and
- i., stressful
- i. therapist, guided
- i., visual
- i. ► vivid visual
- i., x-ray

imaginal exposure
imaginary line
imagination and reality
imaginative play ► pretend/
imagined
- i. abandonment
- i. ugliness
- i. ugliness ► irrational obsession

imaging
- i., acoustic
- i., adenosine radionuclide perfusion
- i., advanced
- i. agent
- i., anatomical
- i. and localization ► stone
- i., antifibrin antibody
- i., antimyosin antibody
- i., biliary
- i., biplane
- i., blood pool
- i., bone
- i., brain
- i. (fMRI) brain scan ► functional magnetic resonance
- i., breast
- i., cardiac

i., cardiac blood pool
i. chain
i., coded-aperture
i. (EEMRI) coil ▸ endoesophageal magnetic resonance
i. ▸ computer
i. ▸ computer based digital
i., continuous wave Doppler
i. (MRI), conventional magnetic resonance
i., coronary
i. device
i. (DI), diagnostic
i. (MRI) ▸ diffusion weighted magnetic resonance
i., digital
i., digital subtraction
i., digital vascular
i. ▸ dipyridamole thallium
i. ▸ direct Fourier transformation
i., Doppler tissue
i. ▸ Doppler transesophageal color flow
i., Doppler ultrasound
i., duplex
i. ▸ echo planar
i., electrostatic
i. (MRI) ▸ enhancement of magnetic resonance
i., exercise
i. fluorescence endoscope ▸ lung
i., fluorescent thyroid
i. ▸ Fourier two-dimensional
i. ▸ frequency domain
i., functional
i. (fMRI) ▸ functional magnetic resonance
i., gallium (Ga) 67
i., gallstone
i. ▸ gated blood pool
i. ▸ gated sweep magnetic resonance
i., gray-scale
i. -guided open biopsy
i., heart
i. ▸ hot spot
i. infarct avid
i. live x-ray
i. machine ▸ magnetic resonance
i. (MRI), magnetic resonance
i. (MRSI) ▸ magnetic resonance spectroscopy
i. (MSI) ▸ magnetic source
i. ▸ mask-mode cardiac
i., multislice

i., myocardial
i. ▸ myocardial perfusion
i., nuclear
i. (MRI) ▸ nuclear magnetic resonance
i. of arteries
i., parametric
i. ▸ pharmacologic stress perfusion
i., phase
i. ▸ planar myocardial
i., platelet
i. procedures
i., pyrophosphate
i., radioisotope
i., radionuclide
i., radionuclide thyroid
i., redistribution
i. ▸ rest redistribution thallium 201
i. ▸ rubidium-82
i. scan ▸ advanced
i. scan ▸ brain
i. (MRI) scan, enhanced magnetic resonator
i. (MRI) scan ▸ magnetic resonance
i. (MRI) scan, side-view magnetic resonance
i. (MRI) scanner, magnetic resonance
i. screen ▸ viewer self-
i. sequence ▸ spin-echo
i., sestamibi
i. ▸ single photon emission tomography (SPET)
i. (MRI) spectrometer, magnetic resonance
i. ▸ spin-echo
i. (MRI) ▸ spin-echo magnetic resonance
i., staging process and
i. ▸ stress thallium-201 myocardial perfusion
i. studies
i. studies ▸ arteriographical
i. studies ▸ pelvic radiation
i. study, brain
i. system
i. system, computer-
i. system, digital cardiac
i. system, radial subtraction
i., teboroxime
i. ▸ technetium-99m
i. ▸ technetium-99m MIBI
i. technique
i. technique, brain
i. technique, cardiac

i. technique, neuro-
i. techniques, computerized
i. techniques, sonic
i. technology
i. technology, breast
i. ▸ thallium perfusion
i. ▸ tissue Doppler
i. ▸ transient response
i., ultrasound
i., vascular
i. ▸ velocity encoded cine-magnetic resonance
i. ▸ ventilation/perfusion
i., video
i. window
i. ▸ xenon lung ventilation
i., x-ray
Imatron Ultrafast CT scanner
imbalance(s)
i., acid/base
i. and oscillopsia ▸ gait,
i., chemical
i., electrolyte
i., endocrine
i., enzymatic
i. ▸ eye muscle
i., fluid
i., fluid and electrolyte
i., gait
i., hormonal
i. in neurotransmitter level
i., liver
i., metabolic
i., mineral
i., muscle
i., muscular
i., nutritional
i. of enzymes
i. of hormones
i. of neurochemicals
i. of oxygen
i. ▸ progressive gait
i. ▸ protease-antiprotease
i., salt and water
i., sympathovagal
i. ▸ vertigo and
IMBC (indirect maximum breathing capacity)
imbecile, moral
imbecility, moral
imbedded (*see* embedded)
imbibes, patient
imbibition, hemoglobin
imbricating layer
imbricating stitch

IMCU (Intermediate Medical Care Unit)
IMH (idiopathic myocardial hypertrophy)
imidazole carboxamide (DTIC/DIC) ▸ dimethyl triazine
iminodiacetic acid (HIDA) scan ▸ hepato-
imitating movements of others
imitative chorea
imitative synkinesis
Imlach's fat plug
immature
   i. blood cells
   i. bone
   i. brain, microscopically
   i. brain tissue ▸ normal
   i. cataract
   i. cells
   i. endothelial cells
   i. erythrocytes
   i. fetal lungs
   i. glomeruli
   i. infant
   i., kidneys
   i. labor
   i. lung ▸ oxygen (O_2) toxicity in
   i. lungs
   i., microscopically
   i. muscle cells ▸ transferring
   i. ovarian teratoma
   i., patient
   i. phage
   i. phenomenon
   i. prostate
   i. teratoma
immaturity
   i. and atelectasis ▸ pulmonary
   i. of lungs
   i. of lung ▸ interstitial
   i., physical
immeasurable fluid loss
immediate
   i. allergy
   i. amputation
   i. and delayed recall
   i. and delayed recognition
   i. auditory memory
   i. auditory recall
   i. auscultation
   i. cause
   i. contact
   i. contagion
   i. diagnosis
   i. discharge

   i. effect
   i. graft rejection
   i., intense need to void
   i. interpretation
   i. memory
   i. patient care
   i. reaction
   i. recall
   i. recall, failure of
   i. response
   i. sensory trace recall
   i. transfer flap
   i. transfusion
   i. transfusion reaction
   i. transport
immersion
   i., cold
   i., full body
   i., homogenous
   i. lens
   i. objective
   i., oil
   i., silicone
   i., water
imminens, glaucoma
imminent
   i. abortion
   i. death
   i. death ▸ fear of
immite, Mycoderma
immitis
   i., Blastomycoides
   i., Coccidioides
   i., Dirofilaria
   i., Filaria
immobile, patient
immobile tissues
immobility
   i., falls and fractures
   i. ▸ stiffness, tremors and
   i., total
immobilization
   i., ankle
   i. ▸ feeling of
   i. of back injury
   i. of injured arm
   i. of injured leg
   i. of joint ▸ surgical
   i. of neck injury
   i. of spinal injury
   i., spinal
   i. (TPI) ▸ Treponema pallidum
immobilize forearm and wrist
immobilized
   i. and unconscious

   i. in cast, extremity
   i. in plaster cast
   i., knee
   i., patient
immobilizing
   i. and splinting leg
   i. bandage
   i. dressing
immotile cilia syndrome
immovable joint
immune
   i. agglutinin
   i. augmentative therapy (IAT)
   i. booster
   i. capability
   i. cells
   i. cells, human
   i. complex disease
   i. complex precipitation
   i. complex reaction
   i. complexes
   i. compromised host
   i. defect ▸ humoral
   i. defense
   i. defense system
   i. deficiency
   i. deficiency, congenital
   i. deficiency disease ▸ combined
   i. deficiency (GRID) ▸ gay-related
   i. deficiency syndrome (AIDS), acquired
   i. deficiency syndrome (AVIDS), acquired violence
   i. deficiency syndrome (AIDS) antibodies, acquired
   i. deficiency syndrome (AIDS) antibody test, acquired
   i. deficiency syndrome (AIDS) associated transfusion, acquired
   i. deficiency syndrome (AIDS) carrier, patient acquired
   i. deficiency syndrome (AIDS) carrier, patient unknown acquired
   i. deficiency syndrome (AIDS) crisis, acquired
   i. deficiency syndrome (AIDS) dementia complex ▸ acquired
   i. deficiency syndrome (AIDS) ▸ emotional effects of acquired
   i. deficiency syndrome (AIDS) epidemic ▸ acquired
   i. deficiency syndrome (AIDS) ▸ fetal acquired

i. deficiency syndrome (AIDS) ▸ heterosexual contact with male carriers of acquired
i. deficiency syndrome (AIDS) illness ▸ acquired
i. deficiency syndrome (AIDS) infected child ▸ acquired
i. deficiency syndrome (AIDS) mandatory testing ▸ acquired
i. deficiency syndrome (AIDS) ▸ mother infected with acquired
i. deficiency syndrome (AIDS) patient ▸ acquired
i. deficiency syndrome (AIDS) ▸ patient at risk for acquired
i. deficiency syndrome (AIDS) ▸ prevention, acquired
i. deficiency syndrome (AIDS) primary pathogen ▸ acquired
i. deficiency syndrome (AIDS) related complex (ARC) ▸ acquired
i. deficiency syndrome (AIDS) related dementia
i. deficiency syndrome (AIDS) related dementia acquired
i. deficiency syndrome (AIDS) related macular degeneration
i. deficiency syndrome (AIDS) related pneumonia, acquired
i. deficiency syndrome (AIDS) residential treatment facility, acquired
i. deficiency syndrome ▸ severe combined
i. deficiency syndrome (AIDS) tainted-transfusion acquired
i. deficiency syndrome (AIDS) testing, acquired
i. deficiency syndrome (AIDS) testing, mandatory acquired
i. deficiency syndrome (AIDS) transfusion-transmitted ▸ acquired
i. deficiency syndrome (AIDS) transmission ▸ acquired
i. deficiency syndrome (AIDS) treatment ▸ acquired
i. deficiency syndrome (AIDS) treatment trials ▸ federal acquired
i. deficiency syndrome (AIDS) vaccine, anti-acquired
i. deficiency syndrome (AIDS) victim, acquired

i. deficiency syndrome (AIDS) virus infection, acquired
i. deficiency syndrome (AIDS) virus testing, acquired
i. depressed patient
i. destructive process
i. deviation
i. disease, autoimmune disorder
i. disorder, chronic
i. disorder ▸ inherited
i. dysfunction
i. dysfunction problem
i. dysfunction ▸ underlying
i. electron microscopy
i. elimination
i. factor
i. function
i. function abnormality
i. function, decreased
i. function ▸ impair
i. function ▸ improved
i. globulin
i. globulin, hepatitis B
i. globulin, human rabies
i. globulin ▸ lymphocyte
i. globulin, measles
i. globulin (human) ▸ measles
i. globulin, pertussis
i. globulin (human) ▸ pertussis
i. globulin ▸ respiratory syncytial virus
i. globulin, Rh
i. globulin ▸ Rho (D antigen)
i. globulin, tetanus
i. globulin (VZIG), varicella-zoster
i. globulin, zoster
i. hemolytic anemia
i. hemolytic anemia ▸ drug-induced
i. illness
i. injury ▸ mesangial
i. inner ear disease ▸ auto-
i. interferon
i. kidney disease
i. -mediated disease
i. -mediated membranous nephritis
i. modulation procedure
i. modulator
i. platelet (ZIP), zoster
i. potential
i. reaction
i. reaction, auto◊
i. reaction, localized
i. reaction ▸ suppress
i. reactions, cell mediated
i. rejection of transplanted heart

i. response
i. response ▸ active
i. response and combined modality therapy
i. response, antibody
i. response, body's
i. response, cellular
i. response, cellular mediated
i. response, defective
i. response, initial
i. response, patient's
i. response, secondary
i. response, slow
i. response, suppressed
i. serum
i. serum globulin
i. state, tolerate
i. substance, anti-
i. suppressing drugs
i. suppression
i. -suppressive medication
i. system
i. system, activate
i. system, allergy/
i. system anatomy
i. system, body's infection-fighting
i. system cancer
i. system cells
i. system, cellular
i. system damage
i. system disorder
i. system dysfunction
i. system, dysfunctional
i. system function
i. system function ▸ normal
i. system ▸ hyperactive
i. system ▸ impair the
i. system, inhibit
i. system, malfunctioning
i. system of body
i. system of cancer patient
i. system ▸ overactive
i. system proteins
i. system, stimulate the
i. system ▸ suppression of
i. system ▸ underactive
i. system ▸ vaccine stimulates
i. system ▸ weakened
i. systems, overactive
i. therapy
i. to hepatitis B infection, patient
i. to rejection
immunity
i., acquired
i., active

immunity—*continued*
- i., actual
- i., adoptive
- i., antibacterial
- i., antiblastic
- i., antitoxic
- i., artificial
- i., athreptic
- i., bacteriolytic
- i., cell
- i., cell mediated
- i., cellular
- i., chemotherapy
- i., community
- i., congenital
- i., cross
- i., deficiency state
- i. deficiency syndrome ▸ cellular
- i., familial
- i., genetic
- i., herd
- i., humoral
- i., impair
- i., impaired
- i., inborn
- i., infection
- i., inherited
- i., innate
- i., intrauterine
- i., local
- i., maternal
- i., maturation
- i., mixed
- i., native
- i., natural
- i., nonspecific
- i., nutritional
- i., opsonic
- i., passive
- i., phagocytic
- i., placental
- i., postoncolytic
- i., preemptive
- i., Profeta's
- i., radial
- i., reaction
- i., residual
- i., response
- i., rubella
- i., species
- i., specific
- i., sterile
- i., tissue
- i. to hepatitis B virus, patient has natural
- i., toxin-antitoxin
- i., transplanted
- i. ▸ vaccine-induced
- i., varicella
- i., weakened

immunization
- i., active
- i., adenovirus
- i., bacille Calmette-Guérin (BCG)
- i., basic
- i., childhood
- i., collateral
- i., DPT (diphtheria, pertussis and tetanus)
- i., influenza
- i., isopathic
- i., mandatory
- i., occult
- i., oral polio
- i., passive
- i., poliomyelitis
- i. program, federal
- i., Rh (rhesus)
- i., rubella
- i., side-to-side
- i., tetanus
- i., tetanus and diphtheria toxoid
- i., tetanus toxoid
- i. therapy
- i., yellow fever

immunizing agents
immunizing unit
immunoassay
- i. (EIA), enzyme
- i. ▸ nifedipine enzyme
- i., optical

immunoblastic lymphoma
immunochemical abnormalities
immunochemical abnormality
immunocompetent
- i. cells
- i. host
- i. patient

immunocompromise syndrome, gay
immunocompromised
- i. cancer patient
- i. host
- i. patient
- i. person

immunocytochemical
- i. analysis
- i. assay
- i. study ▸ muscle

immunodeficiency
- i., combined
- i., common
- i., congenital
- i. disease
- i. ▸ primary-acquired
- i., severe combined
- i., variable
- i. virus (HIV) antibodies, human
- i. virus (HIV) associated dementia ▸ human
- i. virus (HIV) associated motor cognitive disorder ▸ human
- i. virus (HIV) encephalopathy ▸ human
- i. virus (HIV), human
- i. virus (HIV-2), human
- i. virus (HIV) infected blood ▸ human
- i. virus (HIV) seroconversion ▸ human
- i. virus (SIV), simian

immunodeficient disorder
immunodeficient syndrome (SCIDS) ▸ severe combined
immunodepressed patient
immunoelectron microscopy
immunoelectro-osmophoresis
immunoelectrophoresis, protein
immunoenhancement, radiation induced
immunofiltration, analytical
immunofiltration, preparative
immunofluorescence
- i. analysis
- i. analysis, direct
- i. assay test
- i., cytometric indirect
- i., indirect
- i., mixed

immunofluorescent microscopy
immunofluorescent technique
immunogenic infection
immunogenotypic analysis
immunoglobulin(s) (Ig)
- i. deficiency
- i. (IgA) deficiency, gamma A
- i. (IgM) deficiency, gamma M
- i. (IgA) determination ▸ gamma A
- i. (IgA) determination ▸ gamma D
- i. (IgE) determination ▸ gamma E
- i. (IgG) determination ▸ gamma G
- i. (IgM) determination ▸ gamma M
- i., gamma A
- i., gamma D
- i. gamma E
- i., gamma G

i., gamma M
i. M syndrome ▸ X-linked
i., synthesis of
i. (VZIG) ▸ varicella zoster
immunohematologic diagnostic procedure
immunohematologic disorder
immunohistochemical analysis
immunologic
  i. abnormalities
  i. amnesia
  i. competence, alteration
  i. deficiencies
  i. deficiency disorder
  i. disorder
  i. evaluation
  i. hypersensitivity reaction
  i. potency
  i. reactivity, cellular
  i. reactivity, humoral
  i. response, abnormal
  i. test
  i. tumor suppression
  i. workup
immunological
  i. barrier to skin transplantation
  i. defenses
  i. disease
  i. evaluation
  i. host
  i. suppression
  i. theory
  i. therapy
immunology
  i., allergies and
  i., radiation
  i., reproductive
  i., research design for
immunomagnetic bead
immunomodular therapy
immunomodulating effect
immunomodulators, noninterferon
immunonephelometry, rate
immunophenotypic analysis
immunopotentiating agents
immunoproliferative lesion, angiocentric
immunoradiometric assay
immunoreactive
  i. glucagon
  i. human growth hormone
  i. insulin
  i. parathyroid hormone (IPTH)
immunoregulatory effect

immunosorbent assay (ELISA) test ▸ enzyme-linked
immunosorbent assay ▸ sandwich enzyme linked
immunosuppressant drug
immunosuppressant therapy
immunosuppressed patient
immunosuppressed person
immunosuppression
  i. lack
  i. therapy
  i. ▸ tumor-derived
immunosuppressive
  i. agents
  i. drug therapy
  i. drugs
  i. effect
  i. measures, x-ray
  i. medication
  i. therapy
immunotherapy
  i., adaptive
  i. ▸ BCG (bacille Clamette Guërin)
  i., cancer
  i. treatment
impact(s) [*intact*]
  i. activity ▸ high
  i. activity ▸ low
  i. aerobic exercise ▸ high
  i. aerobic workout ▸ low
  i. aerobics
  i. aerobics, low
  i. exercise ▸ high
  i. exercise, low
  i. movement, low
  i. of depression
  i. of fatigue, detrimental
  i. of trauma, destabilizing
  i. on fetus
  i., psychological
  i., therapeutic
  i. trauma ▸ high
  i. trauma ▸ low
impacted
  i. cerumen
  i. fecal material
  i. foreign body (FB)
  i. fracture
  i. grief
  i. molar
  i. molar teeth
  i., patient
  i. stone
  i. stool

i. teeth
i. tooth
i. twins
i. wax in ear canals
impaction
  i., bowel
  i., ceruminal
  i. ▸ constipation and fecal
  i., dental
  i., extensive fecal
  i., fecal
  i. lesion
  i., mucoid
  i., posterior
  i., septal
impactor, electromechanical
impactor, spondylophyte
impair(s)
  i. blood flow
  i. cardiac function ▸ alcohol
  i. immune function
  i. immunity
  i. nerve function
  i. protein synthesis
  i. receptor function
  i. the immune system
impaired
  i. ability to smell
  i. ability to swallow
  i. abstract thinking
  i. adjustment
  i. alertness
  i. assisted living ▸ memory
  i. attention
  i. baby, drug-
  i. balance
  i. behavior
  i. blood flow
  i. blood vessel elasticity
  i. brain activity
  i. brain function, organically
  i. breaking and swallowing
  i. cardiac function
  i. cartilage
  i. child, drug-
  i. child ▸ learning
  i., child speech
  i. circulation
  i. cognitive functioning
  i. cognitive performance
  i., cognitively
  i. communication
  i. comprehension
  i. concentration
  i. consciousness

impaired—*continued*
i. contractility of hypertrophied muscle
i. coordination
i. coronary artery
i. coronary vascular reserve
i. dark adaptation
i. dexterity
i. difficult speech
i. discriminatory, vibratory and position sensation
i. drivers
i. employees' alcohol and drug treatment issues
i. fasting glucose
i. function
i. gas exchange
i. glucose tolerance (IGT)
i. growth
i. habituation
i. hearing
i. hearing loss
i. hepatic function
i. home maintenance management
i. host
i. immunity
i. individual, speech
i. intelligence
i. interpersonal relations
i. judgment
i. kidney function
i. Kupffer's cell phagocytosis
i. language ability
i. left discrimination
i. left ventricular function
i. liver function
i. memory
i. memory for recent events
i. memory of unknown cause
i. mental functioning
i., mentally
i. ▸ mild to moderately
i. mobility
i. motor coordination
i. motor function
i. movement
i. muscular activity
i. neurological function
i., neurologically
i. normal activities
i. parent
i., patient physically
i. patient ▸ renal
i., perception
i. physical mobility

i., physically
i. posture and balance
i., psychiatrically
i., psychologically
i. pumping ability
i. reality testing
i. renal function
i. respirations
i. reticuloendothelial system
i. right discrimination
i. sensation
i. sexual development
i. short term memory
i. side
i. skin integrity
i. social interaction
i. speech
i. ▸ speech and language
i. speech, delayed or
i. support ▸ sensory
i. swallowing
i. systolic function
i. thinking
i. thinking or concentration
i. tissue integrity
i. ventilation
i. ventricular function
i. verbal communication
i. (VI), vision
i., visually

impairing exercise performance
Impairment (impairment)
I. (AAMI), Age-Associated Memory
i., age-related visual
i., alcohol
i. ▸ alcohol-induced functional
i. and confabulation ▸ recent memory
i., autonomic
i., biochemical
i., brain
i., cardiac
i., cerebellar
i., chronic orthopedic
i., cognitive
i., cranial nerve
i., disability
i., drug-related
i., extreme
i. from disorder
i., functional
i., genetic
i., hearing
i., hepatic
i. in alcoholism, cognitive

i. in interpretation of reality ▸ severe
i. in judgment
i. in liver function
i. in occupation functioning
i. in thinking ▸ severe
i., intellectual
i., kidney
i., language
i. ▸ low vision
i., major
i., major functional
i., memory
i., mental
i. ▸ mental ability
i. ▸ mild cognitive
i., minor
i., motivational
i., neurobehavioral
i., neurological
i., neuropsychological
i. ▸ normal general cognitive
i. ▸ occupational and social
i. of air flow
i. of conduction, complete
i. of conduction, partial
i. of consciousness
i. of diffusion
i. of fertility
i. of functions of brain stem
i. of hearing ▸ severe
i. of judgment
i. of kidney function
i. of liver function
i. of memory
i. of power of voluntary movement
i. of skin integrity
i. of social function
i. of subendocardial blood flow
i. of systolic and diastolic performance
i. of ventricle ▸ severe
i. of vision, progressive
i., permanent
i. ▸ permanent visual
i., psychomotor
i., pulmonary ventilation
i., respiratory
i. ▸ restrictive functional
i., sensory
i., severe neurological
i., sexual
i. ▸ sexual/reproductive system
i., speech
i. ▸ speech and hearing

i., sufficient
i., temporary
i., transient
i., vision
i., visual
impassable scar tissue
impassable stricture
impasses ▸ negotiate therapeutic
impatient, patient
impedance(s)
i., acoustic
i. aggregometry
i. angle
i., aortic
i., arterial
i., atrial lead
i. catheter
i., electrical
i., electrode
i., high input
i., input
i., lead
i., low output
i., measure
i. meter
i. of meninges
i., pacemaker
i. plethysmography (IPG)
i., skin
i., thoracic
i., transthoracic
i. variables
i., vascular
impede blood flow
impeded, functioning
impediment, speech
impediment, stressor or
impending
i. cord compression
i. disaster ▸ feeling of
i. doom
i. doom, feeling of
i. doom ▸ sense of
i. failure ▸ lasting impression of
i. fetal distress
i. infarction
i. loss ▸ fear of
i. myocardial infarction (MI)
i. psychosis
i. respiratory failure
i. retinal detachment
i. seizure
i. separation ▸ perception of
i. stroke
imperative pain

imperceptible, pulse
imperfect
i. closure
i. fetus
i. fungus
imperfecta
i., amelogenesis
i. cystica, osteogenesis
i., dentinogenesis
i., erythrogenesis
i., osteogenesis
imperforate anus
imperforate hymen
imperial [*empirical*]
impermeable stricture
impetiginous cheilitis
impetigo
i. bullosa
i., bullous
i. contagiosa
i. furfuracea
i. herpetiformis
i. neonatorum
i. simplex
i. staphylogenes
i. streptogenes
i. vulgaris
impingement
i., disc
i., nerve
i. on spinal cord
i. on spinal nerve
i. syndrome
impinging on cortex, tumor
implant(s)
i., acorn-shaped
i., acrylic
i., adhesive silicone
i., adjustable breast
i., Allen's
i., Alpar's
i., Arruga's
i., artificial
i., artificial heart
i., artificial joint
i., artificial lens
i. ▸ artificial sphincter
i., augmentation with
i., Berens
i., Berens conical
i., Berens pyramidal
i., Berens sphere
i., Berens-Rosa scleral
i., Binkhorst's
i., Biocell RTV

i., biodegradable
i., Biomatrix ocular
i., bioresorbable
i., bone
i., Boyd's
i., brain tissue
i., breast
i., Brown-Dohlman
i., build-up
i., Bunker's
i., cartilage
i. cataract lens, Anis Staple
i. cataract lens, Appolionio
i. cataract lens, Azar Tripod
i. cataract lens, Baron
i. cataract lens, Bietti
i. cataract lens, Binkhorst
   iridiocapsular
i. cataract lens, Choyce
i. cataract lens, Krasnov
i. cataract lens, Pearce Tripod
i. cataract lens, Platina Clip
i. cataract lens, Ridley
i. cataract lens, Schachar's
i. cataract lens, Scharf's
i. cataract lens, Strampelli
i., cataract surgery with
i., celluloid
i., cheek
i., chin
i., Choyce Mark VIII
i., Choyce's
i., cochlear
i., collagen
i. conformer, eye
i., conical
i., conventional reform eye
i., conventional shell type
i., Copeland's
i., coral eye
i., Core-Vent
i., corneal
i., corrected cosmetic contact shell
i., cosmetic
i., Cronin
i., Custodis'
i., Cutler's
i., DeBakey
i., defective
i., defibrillator
i., dental
i., disulfiram
i., Doherty
i., Doherty sphere
i., double lumen breast

implant(s)—*continued*
i., Dow Corning
i., ear
i., Edwards Teflon intracardiac
    patch
i., electrical
i., electronic
i., endodontic
i., endometrial
i., endometriotic
i., endosseous
i., endosteal
i., evaluate
i., expandable breast
i., Extrafil breast
i., eye
i., Federov's
i. ▸ finger joint
i. fork
i., Fox's
i., Frey's
i., gel-filled
i. ▸ gel-filled breast
i., Glass sphere
i., gold
i., gold grain
i., Gold sphere
i., Guist sphere
i., Haik's
i., Hartley
i., hemisphere
i., Heyer-Schulte breast
i., hollow sphere
i., homograft
i., hormone
i., Hughes'
i. infection ▸ orthopedic
i., initial
i., inner ear
i., insert radioactive
i., insertion of polyethylene
i., intact
i., interstitial
i. ▸ intraocular lens (IOL)
i., intraperitoneal
i., iridium wire
i., Ivalon sponge
i., Kratz
i., Lash-Löffler
i. ▸ leaking breast
i., leaky saline
i., Leiske #10 lens
i., lens
i. lens, Lieb and Guerry cataract
i., Levitt's

i., Lincoff's
i., lucite
i., lymphoma
i., magnetic
i., Marlex mesh
i. material, acrylic ball
i. material, adhesive silicone
i. material, artificial joint
i. material, augmentation with
i. material, Berens
i. material, bone
i. material, celluloid
i. material, gold
i. material, hollow sphere
i. material, homograft
i. material, Ivalon sponge
i. material, Marlex mesh
i. material, paraffin
i. material, plastic
i. material, polyethylene
i. material, Silastic
i. material, Silastic corneal
i. material, Silastic Cronin
i. material, Silastic subdermal
i., material, silicone
i. material, subdermal
i. material, subperiosteal
i. material, Supramid
i. material, tantalum
i. material, tantalum mesh
i. material, Teflon
i. material, Teflon mesh
i. material, Tensilon
i. material, ureteral
i. material, Usher's Marlex mesh
i. material, Vitallium
i. material, Vivosil
i. material, Wheeler's
i. material, wire mesh
i. McGhan's
i., medical
i., meshed ball
i., metallic
i., metastatic
i., Mules
i., multichannel
i. ▸ multifocal lens
i., multiple channel
i., nerve
i. of cheek ▸ facial
i. of chin ▸ facial
i. of jaw ▸ facial
i., open bladder brachytherapy
i., orbital
i., osseointegrated

i., pacemaker
i., paraffin
i., patient
i., penile
i., permanent
i. ▸ pig cell
i., pin
i. placement
i. placement, mucoperiosteal
i. placement, Surgicel
i. placement, Surgicel gauze
i., plastic
i., plastic sphere
i., Plexiglas
i., polyethylene
i., polyethylene metal
i., polyurethane
i., polyvinyl sponge
i., porous
i., primary
i. ▸ pump-operated penile
i., pyramidal eye
i., radiation
i., radioactive
i. ▸ radioactive seed
i., radioisotope
i. radiotherapy
i., radium
i., radon seed
i., Rayner-Choyce
i., removable
i., reverse-shape
i., rupture of
i., saline
i., saline-filled breast
i., salt water
i., scalp
i., scleral
i., scleral buckler
i., self-sealing breast
i., semishell
i., shelf-type
i., shell
i., Silastic
i., Silastic corneal
i., Silastic Cronin
i., Silastic medical adhesive silicone
i., Silastic scleral buckler
i., Silastic subdermal
i., Silastic trapezoid
i., silicone
i., silicone breast
i., silicone-filled
i., silicone-filled breast
i., silicone gel

i., silicone gel breast
i., silicone gel-filled
i., silicone gel-filled breast
i., silicone rod
i., silicone sponge
i. site
i., Snellen conventional reform
i., sphere
i., spherical
i., sponge
i., stainless steel
i., Stone's
i., subdermal
i., submucosal
i., subperiosteal
i. ▸ subthalamic nucleus
i., superficial
i. support device ▸ Medtronic defibrillator
i. supported denture
i., Supramid
i., surface
i. surgery, brain
i. surgery ▸ facial
i., surgical
i., Surgite mammary
i., Swanson
i., Swanson carpal lunate
i., Swanson carpal scaphoid
i., Swanson finger joint
i., Swanson great toe
i., Swanson radial head
i., Swanson radiocarpal
i., Swanson trapezium
i., Swanson ulnar head
i., Swanson wrist joint
i. System, Nobelpharma
i., tantalum
i., tantalum mesh
i. techniques
i. technology, dental
i., Teflon
i., Teflon mesh
i., temporary breast
i. ▸ temporary pacemaker
i., tendon
i., Tensilon
i., testicular
i. therapy
i. therapy, permanent
i., tire
i., titanium
i., transmandibular
i., transosteal
i., trapezoid

i., Troutman's
i., tumor
i., tunneled
i., two plane needle
i., two plane radium
i., ureteral
i., Usher's Madex mesh
i., Vitallium
i., Vivosil
i., Weber
i., Wheeler's
i., wire mesh

implantable
i. atrial defibrillator
i. artificial heart
i. bone growth stimulator
i. cardiac defibrillator (ICD)
i. cardiac defibrillator insertion
i. cardiac pacemaker ▸ Maestro
i. Cardiac Pulse Generator, Chardack-Greatbatch
i. cardioverter
i. cardioverter defibrillator (ICD)
i. cardioverter defibrillator (AICD) ▸ automatic
i. cardioverter defibrillator ▸ Medtronic PCD
i. cardioverter defibrillator ▸ nonthoracotomy
i. cardioverter defibrillator ▸ nonthoracotomy lead
i. cardioverter defibrillator ▸ Telectronics ATP
i. cardioverter defibrillator ▸ Transvene nonthoracotomy
i. cardioverter defibrillator ▸ Ventritex Cadence
i. cardioverter electrodes
i. defibrillator
i. defibrillator (AID), automatic
i. defibrillator in cardioversion
i. defibrillator (AID) malfunction ▸ automatic
i. device
i. drug infusion pump
i. gastric stimulator
i. glucose sensor
i. insulin infusion pump
i. left ventricular (LV) assist system
i. lens
i. medication system (PIMS) ▸ programmable
i. pacemaker
i. pacing device
i. pump

i. rings in eyes
i. unipolar endocardial electrode
implantation
i., artificial lens
i., autologous chondrocyte
i., Bergenhem
i. bleeding
i., cataract lens
i., central
i., circumferential
i., cornual
i., coronary stent
i. cyst
i. cyst of iris
i. ▸ dual chamber pacemaker
i., eccentric
i., filigree
i., graft
i., hypodermic
i. ▸ inner ear electronic
i., interstitial
i. ▸ intraocular lens
i. left ventricular assist device
i., lens
i. loop recorder
i. memory
i. metastasis
i., nerve
i. of cardioverter defibrillator ▸ subpectoral
i. of cardioverter defibrillator ▸ transvenous
i. of fertilized egg
i. of fertilized ovum
i. of pacemaker
i. of radioactive isotopes, interstitial
i. of radium
i. of ureter into rectum
i., Oreton pellets for subcutaneous
i., periosteal
i. ▸ permanent pacemaker
i., pigment
i., radon seed
i. response
i., silk
i., stent
i., steroid
i., subcutaneous electrode
i., superficial
i. surgical
i., Surgicel
i. techniques
i., teratic
i. test
i., ureteral

implanted
- i. battery
- i. cancer cells
- i. cells
- i., chemo wafers
- i. device
- i. device ▸ surgically
- i. device tether
- i. diagnostic device
- i. electrode
- i. electrode ▸ surgically
- i. feeding tube ▸ surgically
- i. graft ▸ microsurgically
- i. in cerebral cortex ▸ electrodes
- i. medication tube ▸ surgically
- i. neurostimulator, surgically
- i. pacemaker
- i. pumps, surgically
- i. radioactive pellets
- i. receiver
- i. secondary transformer coil
- i. surgically ▸ metal sieve
- i. sutures
- i. tube, surgically
- i. under skin ▸ pacemaker
- i. ventricular assist device (VAD), permanently
- i. within brain substance ▸ electrode

implanting
- i. brain electrodes
- i., dental
- i. radioactive sources
- i. stent
- i. teeth

implantology, dental
implantology, oral
implementation of advance directives
implementation ▸ prevention, diagnosis and
implications
- i., cardiovascular
- i., clinical
- i., community
- i. for treatment
- i., legal
- i., moral
- i., peripheral vascular
- i., treatment

implicit memory
implied consent
implosive therapy
importance
- i. ▸ exaggerated sense of self-
- i. ▸ grandiose sense of self-

- i. of touch

important warning sign
imposed
- i. abstinence
- i. abstinence ▸ self-
- i. starvation ▸ self-

impotence
- i. after childbirth ▸ male
- i., atonic
- i., chronic
- i., erectile
- i. from antidepressant
- i. from diabetes
- i., paretic
- i., psychic
- i., psychogenic
- i., psychological
- i. rage
- i., sexual
- i., symptomatic
- i., temporary
- i., vasculogenic

impotent, patient
impoverished
- i. environment
- i. thought
- i. thought and speech, confused or

impoverishment, spousal
Impra graft, PTFE (polytetrafluoroethylene)
Impra vein graft
imprecise eye movements
imprecisely aimed laser
impregnated electrode
impregnated gauze
impression(s)
- i., anatomic
- i., basilar
- i., bridge
- i., cardiac
- i., clinical
- i., complete denture
- i. cup
- i., defective
- i., dental
- i., final
- i., first
- i., initial
- i., lasting
- i., lower
- i., mandibular
- i. material
- i., maxillary
- i. of impending failure ▸ lasting
- i., partial denture

- i., preliminary
- i., primary
- i., sectional
- i., sensory
- i. tonometer
- i., upper

impressionistic speech, excessively
impressionistic speech, overly
impressive aphasia
impressum, genu
imprinting, emotional
imprinting, genetic
improper
- i. bite
- i. exercise
- i. fit of dentures
- i. foot alignment
- i. foot care
- i. functioning of foot
- i. management
- i. nail trimming
- i. use of prescription

improve
- i. circulation
- i. efficiency of heart and lungs
- i. healthy self-esteem
- i. muscle contraction
- i. muscle tone
- i. quality of life
- i. self-image

improved
- i. blood flow
- i. condition
- i. energy
- i. flexibility
- i. immune function
- i. muscle tone
- i. overall functioning
- i., patient
- i., patient discharged
- i., patient partially
- i., patient symptomatically
- i. performance and tolerance
- i. psychological adjustment
- i. self-concept
- i. stamina
- i. symptom relief
- i. thought process

improvement
- i., cosmetic
- i., diabetic neuropathy
- i., functional
- i. groups, self-
- i., interval
- i., objective

i., patient showed subjective
i. program, self-
i., progressive
i., short-term
i. skills, self-
i., subjective
i. technique, balance
i., treatment

improving lenses ▸ vision
improving skin texture
impulse(s)
i., abnormal electrical
i., afferent
i., apex
i., apical
i., atrial
i., auditory
i., block pain
i., brain
i., cardiac
i., chemical
i., conduction of
i., conduction of nerve
i. control
i. control difficulty
i. control disorder
i. control disorder, compulsive
i. control in eating
i. control, poor
i. control skills
i., cough
i. disorder control
i. -dominated personality
i., double apical
i. dyscontrol
i. dyscontrol in eating disorder
i., ectopic
i., electrical
i., episternal
i., escape
i. fifth intercostal space (PMI 5th
   ICS) ▸ point of maximum
i. formation
i. in brain ▸ activate chemical
i., inguinal
i., intensity of
i. ▸ interrupting conduction of nerve
i., irresistible
i., left parasternal
i., loss of nerve
i., motor
i., nerve
i., nervous
i., neural
i., neurochemical

i., neuronal
i. on coughing
i., pacing
i., pain
i. ▸ paradoxical rocking
i. (PMI) ▸ point of maximum
i. propagation
i., right parasternal
i., seizure
i., sinus node
i., stimulate nerve
i. stimulator
i., sudden
i., suicidal
i. summation
i., sustained apical
i. ▸ systolic apical
i. test, irresistible
i. to heart, electrical
i. transmission
i., transmission of nerve
i. transmitted pain
i. ▸ uncoordinated atrial
i. violence
i., visual

impulsion, wandering
impulsive
i. acting out
i. actions
i. activity ▸ reckless and
i. aggression
i. behavior
i. child
i. dyscontrol ▸ serious
i. eating
i. form, external
i. insanity
i., patient

impulsiveness
i. and inattention
i., high
i., sexual

impulsivity
i., aggression and deceit
i. and inattentiveness
i. ▸ emotional instability and
i., marked
i. ▸ pattern of
i. to plan ahead

impurities, street
Imre
i. operation
i. operation, Knapp-
i., treatment

IMS (irritable male syndrome)

imvic characters
in fracture, blow-
inability
i. to arrange words
i. to arrange words properly
i. to chew or swallow
i. to close eye
i. to communicate
i. to concentrate
i. to control anger
i. to control appetite
i. to control blood pressure (BP)
i. to control drinking
i. to control stool
i. to control urine
i. to control weight
i. to cope
i. to defecate
i. to digest lactose
i. to exercise
i. to feel pleasure
i. to focus
i. to focus attention
i. to function
i. to interpret written word
i. to maintain attention
i. to maintain equilibrium
i. to make decisions
i. to move a joint
i. to move tongue
i. to pass urine
i. to perform purposeful movements
i. to play in groups
i. to recall
i. to recall events
i. to recognize objects
i. to relate to people
i. to relax
i. to remember spoken words
i. to sleep
i. to speak
i. to speak ▸ difficulty or
i. to stand
i. to straighten back
i. to suckle
i. to sustain consistent work
   behavior
i. to swallow
i. to talk
i. to tolerate boredom
i. to urinate ▸ partial
i. to urinate ▸ total
i. to walk
i. to walk ▸ progressive
inaccessibility, psychological

inaccessible goals
inaction, passivity and
inactivate the molecule
inactivated
 i. influenza vaccine
 i. polio vaccine (IPV)
 i. poliovirus vaccine
 i. vaccine
inactivating agent, virus
inactivating by substitution,
 enzymes
inactive
 i., biologically
 i. colon
 i. dummy drug
 i. electrode
 i. hormone
 i. lifestyle
 i. lifestyle ▸ physically
 i. medication
 i. muscles
 i., optically
 i., physically
 i. pituitary tumor ▸ endocrine
 i. placebo
 i. placebo, medically
 i. tuberculosis
 i. vaccines and toxoids
inactivity
 i. ▸ cycle of pain and
 i., electrocerebral
 i., lethargy and fatigue
 i., mental
 i. ▸ obesity and
 i. ▸ period of enforced
 i., physical
 i., prolonged
 i., record of electrocerebral
 i., tracings of electrocerebral
inadequacy
 i., feelings of
 i., feelings of social
 i. of systemic circulation
 i., sexual
inadequate
 i. blood flow
 i. blood flow ▸ small vessel
 i. blood supply
 i. cardiac output
 i. circulation
 i. coping
 i. enchondral bone formation
 i. intake of fluids
 i. literacy skills
 i. pelvis

 i. personality
 i. sexual function
 i. tissue maintenance
 i. tissue repair
 i. ventilation
inadequately
 i. cleaned x-ray tables
 i. hydrated
 i. sterilized instruments
 i. sterilized needles
 i. sterilized syringes
INAH (interstitial nuclei of anterior
 hypothalamus)
Inahara carotid shunt, Pruitt-
inanimate possession
inanition fever
inappropriate
 i. actions
 i. admission
 i. affect
 i. anger
 i. antidiuretic hormone
 i. antidiuretic hormone (SIADH)
  secretion ▸ syndrome of
 i. attachments to objects
 i. behavior
 i. behavior ▸ socially
 i. child behavior
 i. dangerous behavior
 i. elation
 i. fatigue
 i. guilt
 i. guilt ▸ excessive or
 i. guilt ▸ excessive feeling of
 i., intense anger
 i. irritability
 i. overt anger
 i., patient
 i. polycythemia
 i. sexual behavior
 i. sexually provocative behavior
 i. social behavior
 i. suspicion
 i. thinking, inconsistent and
 i. verbalization
 i. vocalization
 i. words ▸ patient uses
inappropriately, patient acting
inappropriately, patient laughs
inarticularis, pars
inarticulate, patient
inattention ▸ impulsiveness and
inattentive, child
inattentiveness ▸ impulsivity and
inaudible sound waves

inborn
 i. error of metabolism
 i. immunity
 i. personality differences
 i. reflex
incapability foot pain
incapable
 i. of caring for self ▸ patient
 i. of caring for self ▸ totally
 i. of making decisions
incapacitance, input shunt
incapacitated
 i. by alcohol
 i., mentally
 i., patient
 i., severely
incapacitating
 i. ailment
 i. chest pain
 i. depression
 i. disease
 i. fatigue
 i. headaches
 i. insulin reaction
 i. nerve damage
 i. pain
 i. tremor
 i. vertigo, severe
incapacity, bowel
incapacity, physical
incarcerated
 i. hernia
 i. inguinal hernia
 i. parents, children of
 i. placenta
incarceration, in lieu of
incarceration of iris
incarial bone
incarnatus, unguis
incasing cells
incentive spirometry
incentive spirometry ▸ Tri-flow
incessant
 i. coughing
 i. movements
 i. tachycardia
incest
 i., childhood
 i. ▸ memories of
 i. ▸ unverifiable memories of
incestuous abuse
I$_n$ chelate
inch (psi) ▸ pounds per square
incidence [*incidents*]
 i., angle of

i., cancer
i., disease
i., familial
i. of drug abuse
i. of infection, rate
i. of maternal mortality
i. of peptic ulcers, low
i., peak
i., point of
i., risk, and prognosis
i. surveys

incident [*incidence*]
i. ▸ distressing recollection of
i. energy, mean
i. ▸ preoccupation with
i. ray
i. reduction ▸ trauma
i. review, critical
i. stress management, critical
i., vascular

incidental
i. appendectomy
i. exposure
i. finding
i. murmur
i. parasite

incipient [*incipid*]
i. cataract
i. degenerative brain disease
i. gangrene
i. glaucoma
i. heart failure
i. respiratory infection

incisal surface of tooth
incise and drain
incise peritoneum
incised
i., abscess
i. and retracted, periosteum
i., cartilaginous rings
i., central suture
i., fascia
i., mediastinal pleura
i., periosteum
i., peritoneum
i. perpendicular
i., platysma
i. renal parenchyma
i., trachea
i. transversely, fascia
i., visceral pleura
i. wound

incision(s)
i., abdominal
i., ab-externo

i. across lower abdomen ▸
    horizontal
i. and drainage (I and D)
i. and drainage (I and D) of
    abscess
i. and drainage (I and D) of blister
i. and drainage (I and D) of cyst
i. and drainage (I and D) of
    fistulous tract
i. and drainage (I and D) of
    ischiorectal abscess
i. and drainage (I and D) of left
    buttock
i. and drainage (I and D) of
    paronychia
i. and drainage (I and D) of right
    buttock
i., and excision ▸ tissue ablation,
i., angle of
i., apex of
i., appendix brought into surgical
i., Auvray
i., Bar's
i., Battle
i., Battle-Jalaguier-Kammerer
i., Bergmann's
i., Bevan's
i., bikini
i., bimastoid coronal
i., Boyd's
i., Boyd's posterior
i., brought out near edge of
i., Bruser's
i., buttonhole
i. carried down to fracture site
i. cataract surgery ▸ small
i., celiotomy
i., cervical
i., Cherney
i., Chernez
i., chevron
i., circular
i., circumareolar
i., circumcorneal
i., circumferential
i., circumoral
i., circumscribing
i., classic
i., classical
i. clean and dry
i. closed anatomically
i. closed in layers
i. closed in serial fashion
i. closed musculofascially
i. closed, skin

i., collar
i., confirmatory
i., conjunctival
i., corneoscleral
i., corollary
i., coronal
i. ▸ coronary mastoid-to-mastoid
i., counter
i., crescent
i., crescent-shaped
i., cross-shaped
i., crucial
i., cruciate
i., Cubbins
i., culdotomy
i., curved
i. curved downward
i., curved periscapular
i., curvilinear
i., curvilinear skin
i., Deaver's
i. deepened
i., deltopectoral
i., Dührssen's
i., elliptical
i., endaural
i. enlarged
i. excised, old
i., exploratory
i. extended bilaterally
i., Fergusson's
i. ▸ fish mouth
i., flank
i., forceps passed up through
i., Fowler's angular
i., Graefe's
i. granulating in
i., Halsted's
i. healed per primam
i., healing biopsy
i., healing surgical
i., Heerman
i., hemitransfixion
i., high
i., hockey stick
i. ▸ horizontal uterine
i. ▸ induration along skin
i., infected
i., infraorbital
i., infraumbilical
i., inguinal
i., intercartilaginous
i. into an artery
i. into aorta
i. into bladder

incision(s)—*continued*
- i. into blood vessel
- i. into eyelid
- i. into intestine
- i. into joint
- i., intracapsular
- i., inverted T
- i., Kehr's
- i., keratome
- i., keyhole
- i., Kocher
- i., Kocher collar
- i., Küstner's
- i., ladder
- i., Langenbeck's
- i., LaRoque herniorrhaphy
- i., lateral flank
- i., lateral portion of
- i., lateral rectus
- i., lateral to the
- i., lazy H
- i., lazy S
- i., lazy Z
- i., Lempert's
- i., limbal
- i. line
- i., linear
- i., longitudinal
- i., Longuet's
- i., loosely closed
- i., low
- i., lower pole of
- i., lower transverse abdominal
- i., Lynch
- i., Maylard
- i., McArthur's
- i., McBurney's
- i., median
- i. ▸ median sternotomy
- i., Meyer's hockey stick
- i., midline
- i., midline skin
- i., midsternal
- i., Morison's
- i., muscle splitting
- i., Nagamatsu
- i., oblique
- i. of coccyx
- i. of pancreas
- i. of prostate (TUIP) ▸ transurethral
- i., operative
- i., original
- i., paracostal
- i., parallel
- i., paramedian
- i., paramuscular
- i., pararectus
- i., paravaginal
- i., perilimbal
- i., peripatellar
- i., periscapular
- i., peritoneal
- i., Perthes'
- i., Pfannenstiel's
- i., postauricular
- i., pyelotomy
- i., racquet
- i., radial
- i., recovery
- i., rectus muscle splitting
- i., relaxing
- i., relief
- i., Rocky-Davis
- i., Schuchardt's
- i., scratch-type
- i., semilunar
- i., semishelving
- i., serpentine
- i., Shambaugh endaural
- i., shelving
- i., shoulder-strap
- i. site
- i. site, drainage at
- i. site, healed
- i. site, healing
- i. site, infected
- i. site, irritation of
- i. site ▸ pain at
- i. site, pus at the
- i. site, redness along
- i. site ▸ redness at
- i. site ▸ swelling at
- i. site ▸ warmth at
- i., skin
- i., skin fold
- i., skinline
- i. ▸ smaller rib
- i., smile
- i., spiral
- i., S-shaped
- i., stab
- i., stab wound
- i., standard "Y"
- i., stellate
- i., sternal splitting
- i. ▸ stocking seam
- i., subcostal
- i., subcostal flank
- i., suboccipital
- i., superficial
- i., supracervical
- i., suprapubic
- i., surgical
- i., tenderness at site of
- i., thoracotomy
- i. through wall of cavity
- i., tracheal
- i., transverse
- i., transverse linear
- i., T-shaped
- i., upper pole of uterine
- i., U-shaped
- i., uterine
- i., vermis
- i., vertical
- i., vertical uterine
- i., Vischer's lumboiliac
- i., V-shaped
- i., Warren's
- i., wide skin
- i. widened
- i., Wilde's
- i., W-shaped
- i., Yorke-Mason
- i., Y-type
- i., Z
- i., Z-flap
- i., Z-plasty
- i., Z-shaped

incisional
- i. biopsy
- i. care
- i. discomfort
- i. edge
- i. hernia
- i. pain
- i. site draining

incisive
- i. muscles of inferior lip
- i. muscles of lower lip
- i. muscles of superior lip
- i. muscles of upper lip
- i. suture

incisivum, foramen

incisor(s)
- i., central
- i., erupted
- i., first
- i., Hutchinson's
- i., lateral
- i., medial
- i., permanent
- i., second
- i., shovel-shaped
- i. teeth

i., temporary
i., winged
incisura
  i. angularis
  i., Anthomyia
  i. apicis cordis
  i., cardiac
  i. intertragica
  i. pulse
  i. Rivini
  i. tympanica
incisure, thoracic
inclination, condylar guide
inclusion
  i. blennorrhea
  i. bodies
  i. bodies ▸ alcoholic hyaline
  i. bodies, cytomegalic
  i. bodies, cytoplasmic
  i. body encephalitis, subacute
  i. cell
  i. conjunctivitis
  i. conjunctivitis (TRIC) ▸ trachoma
  i. conjunctivitis virus
  i. criteria, patient
  i. cyst
  i. cyst, epidermal
  i. cyst, vaginal
  i., dental
  i. disease (CMID) ▸ cytomegalic
  i. disease (CMID) of newborn b-
    cytomegalic
  i. disease (CMID) virus ▸
    cytomegalic
  i., fetal
  i., Guarnieri's
  i., hyaline cytoplasmic
  i., intracytoplasmic hyaline
  i., intranuclear
  i., leukocyte
  i. ▸ Rocha-Lima
  i. technique, Bentall
  i. technique, Crawford graft
  i., Walthard's
inclusum, Chiracanthium
incognita, Oxyuris
incognitus, Mycoplasma
incoherence, restlessness and
incoherent
  i. ideation
  i., patient
  i. speech
  i. thinking
  i. thinking, bizarre
  i. thinking ▸ hallucinations and

  i. thoughts
income poverty guidelines
incoming pain signals
incoming signal
incomitant strabismus
incompatibility
  i., ABO
  i., blood
  i., chemical
  i., fetomaternal
  i. medication
  i. ▸ parental Rh (Rhesus)
  i., physiologic
  i., Rh
  i., therapeutic
incompatible
  i. blood transfusion
  i. bone marrow
  i. hemolytic blood transfusion
    disease
incompetence
  i., aortic
  i., cervical
  i., chronotropic
  i., gastroesophageal
  i., ileocecal
  i. (MI) ▸ mitral
  i., muscular
  i. of the cardiac valves
  i. (PI), pulmonary
  i., pulmonic
  i., pyloric
  i., relative
  i. (TI), tricuspid
  i., urethral
  i., valvular
  i., venous
incompetent [*incontinent*]
  i. atrioventricular valve
  i., cardia
  i. cervical os
  i. cervix
  i. esophageal sphincter
  i. individual ▸ direct killing of
  i. murmur, aortic
  i., patient
  i. patient, legally
  i. perforating vein
  i., socially
  i. valve
  i. vein
incomplete
  i. abortion
  i. angiography
  i. antigens

  i. atrioventricular (AV) block
  i. atrioventricular (AV) dissociation
  i. bladder emptying
  i. breech position
  i. bundle branch block (BBB)
  i. development of autonomic
    nervous system
  i. dislocation
  i. emptying of bladder
  i. filling
  i. fracture of bone
  i. Freund adjuvant
  i. harelip
  i. heart block
  i. hemianopia
  i. hernia
  i. left bundle branch block (LBBB)
  i. miscarriage
  i. Moro reflex
  i. opening
  i. paralysis
  i. pregnancy
  i. right bundle branch block (RBBB)
  i. Sentence Blank, Rotter
  i. separation
  i. situs inversus
  i. thrombosis
incompletely treated pain
incomprehensible speech
inconclusive
  i. pattern
  i., pelvic exam
  i. results
incongruous hemianopia
inconsistency, Zinsser
inconsistent and inappropriate
thinking
inconsistent parental discipline
inconsolable crying
inconsolable screaming
inconstans, Proteus
inconstant period
inconstant period ▸ sequence of
waves of
incontinence
  i., active
  i., after childbirth
  i., anal
  i., and constipation
  i., bladder
  i., bowel
  i., chronic
  i., episodic
  i., fecal
  i., feces

incontinence—*continued*
  i. ▸ frequent urinary
  i., from diabetes
  i., functional
  i., increased stress
  i. ▸ minimize or delay urinary
  i. of stool
  i. of the feces
  i. of urine
  i., overflow
  i., paradoxical
  i., paralytic
  i., passive
  i., persistent
  i., postoperative
  i., postprostatectomy
  i. products
  i., rectal
  i., reflex
  i. stress
  i., total
  i. urge
  i. urinary
  i. urinary stress

incontinent [*incompetent*]
  i. of feces, patient
  i. of stool, patient
  i. of urine, patient

incoordination
  i., cerebellar
  i., motor
  i., muscle
  i., muscular
  i. of all voluntary movement
  i. of limbs
  i., weakness and

increase
  i. active extension in stroke
    patients
  i. awareness
  i. awareness and decrease
    discomfort
  i. cardiac output ▸ vasodilators
  i., gradual
  i. heart and breathing rate
  i. heart production
  i. heart rate
  i. in amplitude of electrical activity
  i. in compliance ▸ abnormal
  i. in eidetic imagery
  i. in motor activity ▸ mild
  i. in muscle size
  i. in occupational activity
  i. in pancreatic density ▸ diffuse
  i. in polymorphonuclear leukocytes

  i. in sexual activity
  i. in social activity
  i. in social, occupational, sexual
    activity
  i. in temperature, sudden
  i. in voltage, progressive
  i. mass in bone ▸ stimulate
    formation and
  i. metabolic heat production
  i. of blood flow
  i. sexual activity

increased
  i. abdominal girth
  i. action of reflexes
  i. activity
  i. activity, area of
  i. activity, bone scan reveals
  i. activity level
  i. alertness
  i. amplitude
  i. and labored breathing
  i. anxiety
  i. appetite
  i. attention span
  i. attenuation
  i. blood flow to ear
  i. blood flow to heart muscle
  i. blood pressure
  i. blood sugar
  i. bone density
  i. bone mass
  i. calcium flow
  i. cellularity
  i. central venous pressure
  i. clotting
  i. compliance with medications
  i. confusion
  i. convexity of lens
  i. correlation
  i. craving for sweets
  i. cutaneous blood flow
  i. deep tendon reflexes (DTR)
  i. density
  i. density, linear
  i. density ▸ vague
  i. depression
  i. dosage
  i. dose size per fraction
  i. drowsiness
  i. dyspnea on exertion
  i. echogenicity
  i. emotional arousal
  i. emotional dependence
  i. energy/alertness
  i. energy, decreased appetite

  i. energy level ▸ markedly
  i. euphoria
  i. excretion of protein
  i. exertion
  i. eye tension
  i. fatigue
  i. flexibility
  i. flexor tone
  i. flow rates
  i. fluid pressure
  i. fluids and humidity
  i. frequency of urination
  i. guilt
  i. hair growth
  i. heart rate
  i. heart size
  i. in severity, symptoms
  i. in size, tumor
  i. intake
  i. intracranial pressure
  i. intraocular pressure
  i. kidney function
  i. knee jerks
  i. lacrimation
  i. level of blood sugar
  i. libido
  i. local heat
  i. lumbar curve
  i. lung permeability
  i. medical risk
  i. memory
  i. mental tension
  i. metabolism
  i. muscle mass
  i., muscle strength
  i. muscle tone
  i. obtundation
  i. overall treatment duration
  i. pain threshold
  i. pain tolerance
  i. painless
  i. penile inflow
  i. peripheral vasodilation and
    hypotension
  i. personality disintegration
  i. phlegm
  i. physical activity
  i. pigmentation, area of
  i. platelets
  i. prenatal care
  i. pressure
  i. pressure inside the eye
  i. pressure of blood
  i. pressure on nerves
  i. psychomotor activity

i. pulmonary artery pressure
i. pulse
i. pulse rate
i. rapid eye movement (REM) sleep
i. recoil
i. reflex activity
i. reflexes
i. respiratory rate
i. rhythm disturbances
i. rigidity
i. risk for illness
i. risk of breast cancer
i. risk of clot formation
i. risk of miscarriage
i. risk of stroke
i. sadness
i. secretion of parathyroid
i. self-confidence
i. sensitivity
i. sexual appetite
i. sexual desire
i. shortness of breath
i. skin temperature
i. stereotypical behavior
i. stress incontinence
i. stresses
i. susceptibility to infection
i. sweating
i. talking
i. tension
i. tension line
i. thirst
i. thyroid activity
i. tolerance of pain
i. tonic EMG (electromyogram) activity
i. toxicity
i. uptake, areas of
i. uptake of isotope
i. urinary flow
i. urinary output
i. urination
i. urine osmolality
i. venous pressure
i. wandering
i. weight
i. winking, blinking or squinting of eyes

increasing
i. abdominal discomfort
i. airway resistance
i. amplitude, waves of
i. capillary permeability
i. confusion
i. congestion

i. debility
i. debility and weakness
i. demands
i. fatigue
i. heart rate
i. helplessness ▸ sense of
i. in severity, pain
i. insomnia
i. jaundice
i. oncotic pressure
i. respiratory acidosis
i. stress incontinence
i. symptomatology
i. urinary excretion
i. weakness, debility and dyspnea

increasingly irritable
Increment Sensitivity Index (SISI) Test, Short
incremental
i. atrial pacing
i. decline
i. lines, Salter's
i. ventricular pacing

incrementing response
increta, placenta
incrustation of cornea, lead
incubate [*intubate*]
incubated sperm
incubating syphilis
incubation
i., growth after 48 hours
i. period
i. period (MIP) ▸ mean

incubative stage
incubative stage of infection
incubator, infant placed in
incudal fold
incudal joint, malleo-
incudiformis, uterus
incudis, crus breve
incudomalleal joint
incudomalleolar joint
incudostapedial joint
incurable
i., affliction
i. autoimmune disease
i. brain disease
i. brain disease ▸ progressive, debilitating,
i. brain disorder
i. cancer
i. chronic dementia
i. chronic mania
i. condition
i. condition ▸ progressive and

i. disease
i. disease, chronic or
i. disorder
i. illness
i. mental disorder
i., progressive disease
incurably ill, patient
incus
i. bone
i., lenticular process of the
i., modified
i., posterior ligament of the
i. replacement prosthesis ▸ Sheehy-House
i. repositioning
i., short crus of the
i., superior ligament of the
ind (icteric index)
indecisive, patient
indentation for thymus and mediastinal fat
independence
i., architectural barriers to
i., cohesion
i., functional
i. ▸ help patient achieve
i., maximum level of
i. of living, maximum
i., optimal level of
independent
i. ambulation
i. antigen ▸ thymus
i., bilaterally
i. evaluation
i. function ▸ level of
i. functional ability
i., functionally
i. in ADL (activities of daily living)
i. in ambulation, patient
i. in bathing with cueing, patient
i. in bedmatic activities, patient
i. in boosting and rolling, patient
i. in feeding, patient
i. in lower body dressing, patient
i. in transfers, patient
i. in upper body dressing, patient
i., insulin
i. lifestyle
i. living
i. living, capable of
i. living needs
i. living skills
i. lower body dressing
i. metabolism
i. mobility ▸ maximum level of

independent—*continued*
- i. practice
- i. psychiatrist
- i. self-care
- i. slow waves
- i. toxicity in combined modality therapy
- i. transfer, patient completes
- i. upper body dressing
- i. with small based quad cane, patient

independently
- i., ability to function
- i. ► decreased ability to function
- i., patient rolls

in-depth
- i. perspective
- i. shoes
- i. study

index(es) (Index)
- i., acidophilic
- i. (ASI), addiction severity
- i. (AVI) ► air velocity
- i. (ARI) ► airway reactivity
- i., alpha
- i. ametropia
- i., ankle arm
- i. (ABI), ankle brachial
- i. (AHI), apnea hypopnea
- i., asynchrony
- i., atherectomy
- i., atherogenicity
- i., bacteriological
- i., baseline dyspnea
- i. (BMI) ► body mass
- i., brachial-ankle
- i., brain wave
- i., Broders'
- i., burn
- i. (CMI) ► carbohydrate metabolism
- i. (CI) ► cardiac
- i., cardiac output
- i., cardiac risk
- i. (CWI), cardiac work
- i., cephalic
- i., Charlson comorbidity
- i., chemotherapeutic
- i., cholesterol saturated fat
- i., cicatrization
- i. (CI) ► color
- i., contractile work
- i. (CPI) ► coronary prognostic
- i., definable illness
- i. (DBI) ► development-at-birth
- i. ► diastolic pressure time
- i., eccentricity
- i., ejection phase
- i., emergency drug
- i. ► end-diastolic volume
- i. ► end-systolic volume
- i., exercise
- i. finger
- i. finger, extensor muscle of
- i. ► free thyrotoxin
- i. (FTI) ► free thyroxine
- i. ► general well-being
- i., Gensini
- i. ► Gibson circularity
- i., global assessment
- i., glycemic
- i., hematopneic
- i., hemolytic
- i. (ict ind) ► icteric
- i. ► isovolumetric phase
- i., isovolumic
- i. (JGI) ► juxtaglomerular granulation
- i., Krebs' leukocyte
- i. ► left atrial (LA) emptying
- i. ► left ventricular (LV) diastolic phase
- i. (LVWI) ► left ventricular stroke work
- i., Lewis
- i., maturation
- i. (MCI) ► mean cardiac
- i. measurement ► Reid
- I. (MPI) ► Medical Phrase
- i., Mengert's
- i., mitotic
- i. ► mitral valve closure
- i. ► myocardial jeopardy
- i. (NPI) ► nucleoplasmic
- i. of cardiac risk ► modified multifactorial
- i. of refraction
- i. of refraction, relative
- i. of response (IR)
- i. ► oxygen (O_2) consumption
- i., patient psychologic
- i. ► penile-brachial pressure
- i., performance
- i., phagocytic
- i. (PEI) ► phosphate excretion
- i. (PEI) ► physical efficiency
- i., ponderal
- i. ► pulmonary vascular resistance
- i., pyknotic
- I. ► Quality of Well Being
- i. (RI) ► refractive
- i., Reid
- i. (RVI) ► relative value
- i. ► relaxation time
- i. ► respiratory disturbance
- i., risk
- i. (SI) ► saturation
- i., Schneider
- i. score ► Goldman cardiac risk
- i., sedimentation
- i. ► segmental pressure
- i., shock
- i. (SISI) ► short increment sensitivity
- i., sleep efficiency
- i., sphericity
- i. (SLI) ► splenic localization
- i. (SPAI) ► steroid protein activity
- i., stiffness
- i. (SI), stroke
- i. (SVI) ► stroke volume
- i. (SWI) ► stroke work
- i. , systemic vascular resistance
- i. ► systolic pressure time
- i. ► tension-time
- i. test, icterus
- i. (SISI) Test, Short Increment Sensitivity
- i. test, thyroxine binding
- i., thoracic
- i. (TBI) ► thyroid binding
- i. (TBI) ► thyroxine binding
- i. (TTI) ► time-tension
- i. ► total peripheral resistance
- I. Transition Dyspnea
- i., trauma
- i. ► vascular resistance
- i. (VI) ► volume
- i. ► volume thickness
- i. ► wall motion score

indiam scan

Indian
- I. childhood cirrhosis
- I. female, patient
- I. flap
- I. hay (marijuana)
- I. hemp plant
- I. male, patient
- I. medicine
- I. rhinoplasty
- I. rotation flap
- I. tick typhus

Indiana aphasic screening test, Reitan-indica, Serratia

indica, trichosporosis

indican test

indicated, treatment as
indication(s)
i. for long-term treatment
i. for therapy
i., medical
i., serological
indicative
i. of brain metastases ▸ seizure activity
i. of carcinoma in situ
i. of infection, amniocentesis
i. of mild dysplasia, cells
i. of moderate dysplasia, cells
i. of severe dysplasia, cells
indicator(s)
i., clinical
i., diagnostic and prognostic
i. dilution technique ▸ indocyanine green
i. ▸ elective replacement
i., intervention
i. of ischemia, chemical
i., surgical discharge
i. (MBTI) test ▸ Myers-Briggs Type
i., xylol pulse
indices
i., arm-ankle
i. ▸ end-systolic force velocity
i., normal blood
i. of death
i. predicting response
i., red cell
i., wall shortening
i., Wintrobe
indicial myopia
indicis
i. artery, radialis
i. muscle, extensor
i. proprius, extensor
indicus, Azotobacter
indifference
i., depraved
i., personal
i. to pain
indifférence, la belle
indifferent
i. cell
i. drug abuser
i. electrode
i. genitalia
i., patient
i. tissue
i. to feelings of others
indigent
i. care funding

i. patient
i. population
indigestion
i., acid
i., belching and
i., bloating and
i. from appendicitis
i. from cirrhosis
i. from constipation
i., functional
i., gastric
i. ▸ loss of appetite with
i., nervous
i. ▸ pain in abdomen from
i., patient has
i., persistent
i., prolonged
indignation, bitterness and
indigo
i. calculus
i. carmine dye
i. carmine test
indirect
i. ballottement
i. bilirubin
i. bilirubin test
i. biologic effects
i. cell division
i. contact
i. contact with contaminated instruments
i. contact with contaminated laboratory apparatus
i. Coombs' test
i. diuretic
i. drug effect
i. emetic
i. fecal contamination
i. fluorescent antibody
i. foot hazard
i. fraction
i. fracture
i. fulguration
i. hemagglutination
i. hernia
i. immunofluorescence
i. immunofluorescence, cytometric
i. infection
i. inguinal hernia
i. lead
i. maximum breathing capacity (IMBC)
i. murmur
i. ophthalmoscopy

i. ophthalmoscopy, binocular
i. personal contact
i. platelet count
i. rays
i. reflex
i. sequelae
i. transfusion
i. vision
indiscretion, dietary
indiscriminate lesion
indiscriminate socializing
indistinct
i. blur
i. borders
i. cell borders
i. margin
i. semicircumferential fibrous thickening
i. speech ▸ slurred,
indium 111 scintigraphy
individual(s)
i. adult children of alcoholics counseling
i., alcoholic
i. beamlets
i. bursts of alpha ▸ frequent
i. caring humane
i. cells
i. codependent counseling
i. complex
i. components
i. coping ▸ ineffective
i. counseling
i. counseling, long-term
i. counseling sessions
i. couple's counseling
i. defense mechanisms
i. dependent counseling
i., depressed
i. differences
i. ▸ direct killing of incompetent
i., emotionally disturbed
i. genes
i., homebound
i. layers
i., left-handed
i., leukemic
i., mentally disturbed
i., motivated
i. motor unit action potentials
i. organisms, morphology of
i., paranoid
i. preference
i. psychodynamic psychotherapy

individual(s)—*continued*
- i. psychology
- i. psychotherapy
- i., psychotic
- i., resistant
- i., right-handed
- i., sedentary
- i. seeking information
- i. sense of self-worth, augment
- i. sensory modality
- i., severely affected
- i., severely debilitated
- i. solution-based therapy
- i., speech impaired
- i. stress
- i. subject
- i. therapy
- i., totally dependent
- i. treatment plan
- i. voluntary control
- i. vulnerability
- i. wave
- i. well-being

individualized
- i. behavior therapy
- i. care
- i. transfusion therapy
- i. treatment plan

individually clamped and coagulated ► muscle bleeding points

individually ligated

individuation, ethical

indoctrination, cultural

indocyanine
- i. dilution curve
- i. green angiography
- i. green dye
- i. green indicator dilution technique
- i. green method

Indoklon therapy

indoleacetic acid (5-HIAA) ► 5-hydroxy-

indole-negative

indole-positive

indorus, Haematosiphon

induce
- i. drowsiness
- i. labor
- i. nausea

induced
- i. ablation, catheter-
- i. abortion
- i. abortion, drug-
- i. activity, drug-
- i. affect ► marijuana-

- i. aggression ► stress-
- i. allergy
- i. alopecia, drug-
- i. alterations of cardiovascular function ► drug-
- i. amnestic disorder ► alcohol-
- i. amnestic syndrome ► drug-
- i. anesthesia, electricity-
- i. angina, cold-
- i. angina, exercise-
- i. angina ► pacing-
- i. angina ► smoking-
- i. angina ► treadmill-
- i. anxiety, cocaine-
- i. arrhythmia ► exercise-
- i. arrhythmia ► hypokalemia-
- i. arterial fluorescence ► laser-
- i. asthma, allergen-
- i. asthma (EIA), exercise-
- i. bacterial antagonism
- i. birth defects ► thalidomide-
- i. blackouts, alcohol-
- i. bronchospasm ► exercise-
- i. by alcohol, delirium
- i. by alcohol, dementia
- i. by cocaine ► psychosis
- i. by drugs ► hallucinatory state
- i. by drugs ► paranoid state
- i. by medication, condition
- i. cancer, drug-
- i. cancer ► radiation-
- i. carcinogenesis, radiation-
- i. cardiomyopathy, alcohol-
- i. cardiomyopathy, drug-
- i. cardiomyopathy ► tachycardia-
- i. cell destruction, drug-
- i. change
- i. changes, tumor-
- i., chemotherapy
- i. chest pain ► stress-
- i., cocaine-
- i. convulsion, anesthetic-
- i. damage, alcohol-
- i. damage, light-
- i. deafness, noise-
- i. death, cocaine-
- i. death, drug-
- i. dehydration, fever-
- i. dementia, alcohol-
- i. delirium, drug-
- i. delivery
- i. dementia, drug-
- i. depression, cocaine-
- i. diabetes, drug-
- i. diarrhea, antibiotic-

- i. disease, radiation-
- i. disorder, alcohol-
- i. disorder, methamphetamine-
- i. disorder, nonsubstance-
- i. disorder ► substance-
- i. emesis, ipecac-
- i. esophageal stricture ► reflux-
- i. false identity
- i. fever
- i. fever, drug-
- i. fibrillation
- i. fractures, postmortem
- i. functional impairment ► alcohol-
- i. gastrointestinal disorder ► drug-
- i. hallucinations, drug-
- i. hallucinations ► inhalant-
- i. hallucinosis, drug-
- i. hearing loss, noise-
- i. heart attack, exercise-
- i. heart changes ► radiation-
- i. heartburn, drug-
- i. hemorrhage ► reperfusion-
- i. hepatic injury ► drug
- i. hepatitis, Allopurinol
- i. hepatitis ► drug-
- i. high ► drug-
- i. hives, exercise
- i., hyperdopaminergic state
- i. hyperplasia, drug-
- i. hypertension ► oral contraceptive-
- i. hypertension, pregnancy
- i. hyperthyroidism, amiodarone-
- i. hysterical paralysis ► trauma-
- i. illness ► heat-
- i. illness ► self-
- i. immune hemolytic anemia ► drug-
- i. immunity ► vaccine-
- i. immunoenhancement, radiation-
- i. injury, alcohol-
- i. keratosis ► noncancerous sun-
- i. labor
- i. lethargy
- i. liver cancer, hepatitis-
- i. liver disease ► alcohol-
- i. liver toxicity ► drug-
- i. lung disease ► cigarette
- i. lung disease ► irradiation-
- i. lung injury, air emboli-
- i. lung injury ► oxidant-
- i. lung injury ► smoke-
- i. lupus, drug-
- i. lupus erythematosus ► drug-
- i. lupus syndrome ► drug-
- i. malignancy ► radiation-
- i. manic episode

i. mediator release, allergen-
i. memory
i. mental disorder ▸ drug-
i. metabolic acidosis, cannulation-
i. morning drowsiness, drug-
i. movement therapy ▸ constraint-
i. muscle relaxation
i. muscle relaxation, feedback-
i. nausea, chemotherapy-
i. neuropathy ▸ drug-
i. nystagmus ▸ thermally
i. obstructive lung disease ▸
   cigarette-
i. organic affective syndrome ▸
   drug-
i. organic delusional syndrome ▸
   drug-
i. organic mental disorder ▸
   methamphetamine-
i. organic mental disorder ▸
   psychoactive substance-
i. organic mental disorder ▸
   substance-
i. osteoporosis ▸ steroid-
i. pain, anxiety
i. pain, disease-
i. pain, stimulus-
i. pancreatitis, alcohol-
i. pancreatitis, estrogen-
i. panic attack, cannabis-
i. paranoid psychotic state ▸
   amphetamine-
i. parkinsonism, drug-
i. Parkinson's syndrome, drug-
i. pericarditis, drug-
i. pericarditis ▸ radiation-
i. pneumopericardium ▸ ventilator-
i. pneumothorax
i. pneumothorax ▸ ventilator-
i. postanesthetic depression ▸ drug-
i. postanesthetic respiratory
   depression ▸ drug-
i. prostatectomy (TULIP) ▸
   transurethral ultrasound-guided
   laser-
i. psychiatric effects ▸ drug-
i. psychosis, drug-
i. psychosis ▸ lysergic acid
   diethylamide (LSD)-
i. psychotic disorder
i. purging, self-
i. reaction, stress-
i. reflex voiding
i. relaxation, drug-
i. respiratory depression, narcotic-

i. respiratory failure, cocaine-
i. shortness of breath (SOB) ▸
   exercise
i. silent myocardial ischemia ▸
   exercise-
i. situation, stress-
i. sleep
i. sleep, drug-
i. spasm, catheter
i. spasm ▸ ergonovine-
i. state of relaxation
i. sterility, exercise-
i. stress ▸ medication-
i. tardive dyskinesia ▸
   antipsychotic-
i. tattoos, self-
i. thrombocytopenia, drug-
i. thrombosis ▸ effort-
i. thrombosis ▸ laser-
i. tremors, drug-
i. urticaria ▸ cold-
i. urticaria, exercise-
i. vasoconstriction, cold-
i. vasospasm, refractory
   ergonovine-
i. ventricular tachycardia ▸
   exercise
i., virus-
i. vomiting, chemotherapy-
i. vomiting, self-
i. weight loss ▸ exercise-

inducer
i., inducible
i., interferon
i., menses
i., stress

inducible
i. arrhythmias
i. enzyme synthesis
i. inducers
i. polymorphic ventricular
   tachycardia

inducing
i. adverse influences ▸ relapse-
i. cravings
i. factor, monocytosis
i. sleep
i. suppression
i. virus ▸ cancer-

inductance, self-
induction (Induction)
i. anesthesia
i., autonomous
i. chemotherapy

i. coaxial electrode system,
   magnetic
i., coefficient of
i., complementary
i., coronary spasm
i., elective
i., electromagnetic
i., genetic
i., hypnotic
i., medical
i. of anesthesia
i. of coma
i. of convulsion
i. of labor
i. of sleep
i. (RSI) orotracheal intubation ▸
   rapid sequence
I. Profile, Hypnotic
i. (RSI) ▸ rapid sequence
i., seizure
i., somatic
i., Spemann's
i., spinal
i., sputum

inductive
i. radiofrequency
i. radiofrequency electric field
i. reasoning
i. resistance

indurata, acne
indurated
i. cellulitis
i. colon mass ▸ hard,
i. mass

induration
i. along skin incision
i. and swelling
i., black
i., brawny
i., brown
i., cyanotic
i., fibroid
i., Froriep's
i., granular
i., gray
i. ▸ idiopathic brown
i., laminate
i. of lung, brown
i. of tissue
i. or tenderness ▸ masses,
i., parchment
i., penile
i., phlebitic
i., plastic
i., red

indurative
- i. myocarditis
- i. nephritis
- i. pleurisy
- i. pneumonia

induratum, erythema

industrial
- i. accident
- i. anthrax
- i. chemistry
- i. clinic
- i. disease
- i. eye care
- i. injury
- i. medicine
- i. monitoring
- i. psychiatry
- i. psychology
- i. substances, exposure to
- i. toxicity

Industries (EMI) brain scanner ▸ Electric and Musical

industry
- i., alcohol
- i., generic
- i., health care

indux, rale

indwelling
- i. bladder catheter
- i. catheter
- i. catheter drainage (dr'ge)
- i. catheter ▸ prolonged
- i. Foley catheter
- i. line
- i. prosthetic joint
- i. prosthetic medical device
- i. urethral catheter
- i. urinary catheter
- i. vascular catheter
- i. venous catheter

ineffective
- i. airway clearance
- i. breastfeeding
- i. breathing pattern
- i. coping mechanism
- i. denial
- i. family coping
- i. family coping, compromised
- i. family coping ▸ disabling
- i. functioning ▸ modes of
- i. heart action
- i. individual coping
- i. intervention
- i. thermoregulation
- i. treatment

- i. valve function

inefficiency, chronic pump

inefficient pumping of blood

inelastic collision

inept , socially

inertia
- i., colonic
- i., law of
- i., sedentary
- i., sleep
- i. uteri
- i., uterine

inertial confinement

inevitable abortion

inevitable miscarriage

infancy
- i. or early childhood ▸ reactive attachment disorder of
- i. ▸ reactive attachment disorder of
- i. ▸ rumination disorder of

infant (Infant) ('s)
- i. abnormal position of
- i. acidotic and hypoxic
- i. Ambu resuscitator
- i., anencephalic
- i. bonding, mother-
- i. bonding, parent-
- i. born with congenital anomalies
- i., bottle-fed
- i. breast-fed
- i. burns
- i. car seat
- i. care, newborn
- i. caretaking
- i., cocaine-exposed human
- i., colicky
- i., cord about neck of
- i. course
- i. CPR (cardiopulmonary resuscitation) techniques ▸ child and
- i. crowning
- i., cyanotic
- i. death
- I. Death Syndrome (SIDS), Sudden
- i. delivered
- i. development
- i. exhibits hunger behavior
- i. expelled
- i. feeding tube
- i., floppy
- i. footprinted in delivery room
- i., full-term
- i. had weak cry
- i. head, crowning of

- i., high risk
- i., immature
- i. in acute respiratory distress
- i. in delivery room ▸ footprint taken of
- i. in respiratory distress
- I. Intelligence Scale, Cattell
- i. interaction ▸ mother-
- i. intubated
- i. jaundice
- i., liveborn
- i. (LBWI), low birth weight
- i., macerated
- i. massage
- i., mature
- i. mildly icteric
- i. minimally active
- i. morbidity and mortality
- i. mortality
- i. mortality rate
- i. neck, cord around
- i. necrotizing encephalomyelopathy
- i. newborn
- i. nutrition
- i. of diabetic mother (IDM)
- i. of high risk mother
- i. of infected mother
- i. omphalitis
- i., patient delivered congenitally deformed
- i., patient delivered normal
- i. placed in incubator
- i. placed in isolette
- i. placed in warmer
- i. placed under bili-lites
- i., postmature
- i., post-term
- i., premature
- i., pre-term
- i. psychotherapist
- i. pyoderma
- i. respiratory distress syndrome
- i. rooming-in
- i. rotated
- i. ▸ sexual arousal in
- I. Special Care Unit (ISCU)
- i. stillborn
- i. stimulation program
- i. suck is poor
- i. syndrome, floppy
- i., Tay-Sachs
- i., term
- i. tracks movement
- i., transmission from infected mother to

i. ventilator, Bourns
i., viable
i., viable female
i., viable male
i. vision
i. weight gain
i. weight loss
i. with decreased heart rate, apneic
i. with oxygen (O₂)
i. with seizures
i. with sepsis
i. with umbilical catheter

infantile
i. agranulocytosis, Kostmann's
i. amnesia
i. arteriosclerosis
i. arteritis
i. atrophy
i. autism
i. autism, early
i. beriberi
i. cataract
i. celiac disease
i. cortical hyperostosis
i. diarrhea
i. diarrhea, acute
i. diplegia
i. dwarf
i. eczema
i. embryonal carcinoma
i. encephalitis
i. epithelium
i. female genitalia
i. gastroenteritis
i. gastroenteritis, acute
i. glaucoma
i. hemiplegia
i. hernia
i. hypercalcemia syndrome ▸
   supravalvular aortic stenosis
i. kala-azar
i. lichenoid acrodermatitis
i. liver
i. lobar emphysema
i. male genitalia
i. malignant histiocytosis
i. motor neuron disease
i. muscular dystrophy ▸
   pseudohypertrophic
i. myoclonus encephalopathy
i. myxedema
i. neuroaxonal dystrophy
i. panmyelopathy, constitutional
i. papular acrodermatitis
i. paralysis

i. pelvis
i. periarteritis nodosum
i. period
i. polycystic disease
i. pseudoleukemia
i. psychosis
i. scurvy
i. skeleton
i. spasms
i. state
i. tantrum
infantilis ▸ dystaxic cerebralis
infantilis, roseola
infantilism, hypophyseal
infantis, Hydatigena
infantum
i., acrodermatitis papulosa
i., anemia pseudoleukemica
i., cholera
i., dermatitis excodativa
i., dermatitis exfoliativa
i., dermatitis gangrenosa
i., granuloma gluteale
i., Leishmania
i., roseola
i., tabes
infarct
i., acute
i. ▸ acute subendocardial
   myocardial
i., anterior lateral myocardial
i., anteroposteroseptal
i., anteroseptal
i. (ASMI), anteroseptal myocardial
i. avid hot spot scintigraphy
i. avid imaging
i. avid myocardial scintigraphy
i. avid scintigraphy
i. avid scintigraphy, antimyosin
i., bilateral occipital lobe
i., bile
i., bilirubin
i., brain
i., Brewer's
i. bulging
i., cerebellar
i., cerebral
i., chronic
i., chronic cystic
i., cystic
i. dementia, multi-
i. dementia, uncomplicated ▸ multi-
i. dementia, with delirium ▸ multi-
i. dementia, with delusions ▸ multi-

i. dementia, with depression ▸
   multi-
i., diaphragmatic pulmonary
i. disease ▸ multi-
i., embolic
i. expansion
i. extension
i. ▸ extension of cerebral
i., focal hemorrhagic
i., foci of
i., healed myocardial
i., hemorrhagic
i., hepatic
i., lacunar
i., lung
i., medullary
i., multiple
i., multiple pulmonary
i., myocardial
i., myocardial subendocardial
i. of adrenal glands ▸ hemorrhagic
i. of brain stem, massive
i. of liver ▸ focal
i. of myocardium
i., old
i., old cystic
i. patient, post-
i., posterior wall
i., pulmonary
i. ▸ pulmonary emboli with small
i., recent
i., recent myocardial
i., red
i. -related vessel
i., renal
i. scar
i. scintigraphy, acute
i., size of
i., small cystic
i., splenic
i. thinning
i., triangular
i., undetected
i., uric acid
i., watershed
i. zone, ischemia in peri-
infarcted transverse colon
infarction [*infraction*]
i., acute anterolateral myocardial
i. ▸ acute anteroseptal myocardial
i. (AMI) ▸ acute myocardial
i., age-undetermined myocardial
i., anterior
i. (AMI) ▸ anterior myocardial
i. (AWI) ▸ anterior wall

infarction—*continued*
- i. (AWMI) ▸ anterior wall myocardial
- i., anteroinferior myocardial
- i., anterolateral
- i., anterolateral myocardial
- i., anteroposterior
- i., anteroseptal
- i., anteroseptal myocardial
- i., apical
- i., atrial
- i. (MI), atrial myocardial
- i. block, peri-
- i., cardiac
- i., cerebral
- i. (MI) ▸ chills from myocardial
- i., chronic cystic
- i., complete myocardial
- i., complicated myocardial
- i., conduction defects in acute myocardial
- i., cystic
- i., diaphragmatic
- i. ▸ diaphragmatic myocardial
- i. ▸ evolving myocardial
- i. (MI), extension of myocardial
- i., focal
- i. ▸ focal areas of
- i., healed myocardial
- i., healing myocardial
- i., hemorrhagic
- i., impending
- i. (MI) ▸ impending myocardial
- i. in dumbbell form ▸ myocardial
- i. in H-form ▸ myocardial
- i. (IWMI) ▸ inferior wall myocardial
- i. ▸ inferolateral, myocardial
- i., intestinal
- i. ▸ ischemic cerebral
- i., kidney
- i., lacunar
- i., large necrotic
- i., lateral
- i. ▸ lateral myocardial
- i., macular
- i., massive
- i., massive recent
- i., mesenteric
- i., multiple previous
- i. (MI) ▸ myocardial
- i. ▸ nontransmural myocardial
- i. of choroid
- i. of lung
- i. of lung due to embolism
- i. of lung due to thrombosis
- i. of placenta

- i. of retina
- i. (MI) ▸ old healed myocardial
- i. (MI), old inferior wall myocardial
- i. (MI) ▸ old myocardial
- i. ▸ old subcortical
- i., pathogenesis of acute myocardial
- i. (MI) ▸ patient candidate for myocardial
- i., posterior
- i. (MI) ▸ posterior myocardial
- i., posterior wall
- i., posterolateral
- i., postmyocardial
- i. (MI) ▸ previous posterior myocardial
- i. ▸ primary angioplasty in myocardial
- i. (PI), pulmonary
- i. ▸ Q wave myocardial
- i., recurrent myocardial
- i., renal
- i. (MI) research unit ▸ myocardial
- i., right ventricular
- i., Roesler-Dressler
- i. ▸ rule out myocardial
- i. ▸ rupture of myocardium following
- i., septal
- i. ▸ silent myocardial
- i. ▸ stuttering myocardial
- i. ▸ subacute myocardial
- i., subendocardial
- i. ▸ subendocardial myocardial
- i. syndrome ▸ postmyocardial
- i. syndrome ▸ pulmonary
- i. therapy ▸ myocardial
- i. ▸ through-and-through myocardial
- i., transmural
- i. ▸ transmural myocardial
- i., watershed

infarctional disturbance ▸ peri-
infarctional ventricular arrhythmias ▸ peri-
infarctoid cardiopathy
infected [*inspected*]
- i. adenoids
- i. aneurysm
- i. area
- i. blood donor
- i. blood, HIV (human immunodeficiency virus)
- i. cartilage
- i. callus
- i. cells
- i. cells, nonvirus

- i. child, acquired immune deficiency syndrome (AIDS)
- i. decubitus ulcer
- i. ear
- i. eyes
- i. eyelash follicles
- i. finger
- i. gums
- i. hair follicle
- i. hyperalimentation line
- i. incision site
- i. intravenous (IV) drug needles
- i. intravenous (IV) drug needles ▸ sharing
- i. joint
- i. joint lining
- i. lung tissue
- i. lymph gland
- i. membrane
- i. mother, infant of
- i. mother to infant, transmission from
- i. mucous membranes
- i. myxoma
- i. nail ▸ fungus
- i. organ donor
- i. parturient women
- i., perinatally
- i. personnel
- i. pilonidal cyst
- i. pseudocysts
- i. sebaceous cyst
- i. skin, debridement
- i. tissue
- i. tissue cultures
- i. toe
- i. tonsils
- i. tonsils, chronically
- i. tooth
- i. tumor cells ▸ virus
- i. with AIDS (acquired immune deficiency syndrome) virus, mother
- i. with HIV (human immunodeficiency virus)
- i. wound

infecting organism
infection(s) (Infection)
- i., abdominal
- i., abdominal foci of
- i., absence of
- i., acquired immune deficiency syndrome (AIDS) virus
- i., active
- i., acute

i., acute respiratory
i., acute respiratory tract
i., acute throat
i., acute toxoplasmosis
i., acute viral
i., adenovirus
i., aerial
i., aerobic
i., agents of
i., airborne
i., amebic
i., amniocentesis indicative of
i., anaerobic
i., anaerobic respiratory
i. and care, nail
i. and inflammation
i., anthrax
i. ▸ anthrax cutaneous
i., apical
i., aspergillus fungal
i., asymptomatic
i., asymptomatic urinary tract
i., atypical mycobacteria
i., auto-
i., bacterial
i., bacterial blood
i. ▸ bacterial heart valve
i., bacterial pathogenesis of
i., bacterial skin
i. ▸ Bacteroides fragilis
i., baseline
i., benign pulmonary
i., benign viral
i., bladder
i., bleeding and
i., blister without
i., blood-borne
i. (BSI) ▸ bloodstream
i., bone
i., bone and joint
i., bone marrow
i., brain
i., burn
i., Campylobacter jejuni
i., cancer-linked microbial
i., Candida bloodstream
i., Candida urinary tract
i. ▸ Candida yeast
i., candidal
i., cardiac
i., catheter-related
i., catheter-related urinary tract
i., central venous catheter
i., cerebral
i., cervical

i., chickenpox virus
i., childhood ear
i., Chlamydia
i., Chlamydia genitourinary (GU)
i., Chlamydia pneumoniae
i., chronic
i. ▸ chronic gum
i. ▸ chronic hepatitis B virus
i., chronic hepatitis C
i. ▸ chronic irritation or
i., chronic lid
i., chronic middle ear
i., chronic minor
i. ▸ chronic periodontal
i., chronic pulmonary
i. ▸ chronic sinus
i. ▸ chronic skin
i., chronic syphilitic
i., chronic urinary
i. ▸ chronic yeast
i. ▸ Citrobacter freundii urinary tract
i. cleared, urinary tract
i. ▸ clinically undetected fungal
i., cluster of
i., CNS (central nervous system) nosocomial
i., community-acquired
i., community-acquired bladder
i., compiling surveillance data on
i. complications
i., concurrent upper respiratory tract
i., congenital
i. (UTI), congenital urinary tract
i., congenital viral
i., conjunctival
i., contact
i. ▸ contact lens
i. contained
I. Control Committee
I. Control Coordinator (ICC)
i. control, effective
i., control existing
i. control, hospital
i. control, neonatal
I. Control Nurse (ICN)
i., control of nosocomial bacterial
I. Control Officer (ICO)
i. control policy
I. Control Practitioner (ICP)
i. control procedure
i. control program
i. control program, nosocomial
I. Control (SENIC) ▸ Study on the Efficacy of Nosocomial
i. control surveillance

I. Control Team
i., counter current
i., Coxsackie viral
i., Coxsackie virus
i., cross
i., cryptococcal
i., cryptosporidiosis
i., cutaneous
i., cytomegalovirus (CMV)
i., data
i., dermatophyte
i., determine source of
i. ▸ device-related
i., diabetic foot
i., direct
i., disguised
i., disseminated
i., disseminated herpes zoster
i., disseminating fungal
i., droplet
i., drug-related
i., drug-resistant Cyclospora
i. ▸ drugs to ward off
i., dustborne
i., ear
i., early
i., echoviral
i. ▸ endemic fungal
i., endogenous
i., enteric
i., Enterobacter
i., enterococcal
i. ▸ enterococcal urinary tract
i. eradicated
i., exanthematous
i. exhaustion psychosis
i., exogenous
i., exogenous sources of
i., eye
i. failure
i., fatal
i., fatal nosocomial
i., fecal-oral route of
i., fetal
i., fever caused by
i. -fighting T cells
i. -fighting immune system, body's
i. -fighting white cells
i., focal
i., foci of
i., focus of
i., food-borne
i., foot
i., frequency of
i., full-blown

infection(s)—*continued*

i., fungal
i. ▸ fungal nail
i., fungal scalp
i., fungus
i., gangrene-like
i., gastrointestinal (GI)
i., gastrointestinal (GI) nosocomial
i., gastrointestinal (GI) viral
i., generalized blood
i., genital herpes
i. ▸ genital papillomavirus
i., germinal
i., graft
i. ▸ gram-negative bacilli
i., gram-positive E. (Escherichia) coli
i., gram-positive nosocomial
i., gum
i., gynecologic (GYN)
i. ▸ Haemophilus influenzae
i. hazard
i., heart
i. ▸ heart valve
i., heavy
i. ▸ Helicobacter pylori
i., hepatitis
i., hepatitis B
i. ▸ hepatitis with
i., herpes
i., herpes simplex
i. ▸ high risk of HIV (human immunodeficiency virus)
i., hospital-acquired
i., hospital-acquired bloodstream
i., hospital-acquired urinary tract
i., hospital-associated
i., hospital-associated respiratory tract
i. ▸ hospital-related
i. ▸ human
i., human carriers of
i. ▸ human papillomavirus (HPV)
i., iatrogenic
i. immunity
i., immunogenic
i. in children, urinary
i. in leg tissue
i. in milk ducts
i. in mouth, fungal
i. in pregnancy ▸ parasitic
i. in prostate gland, chronic
i., incipient respiratory
i. ▸ increased susceptibility to
i. ▸ incubative stage of

i., indirect
i., influenza
i. ▸ inner ear
i., initial
i., insect-home
i., interamniotic
i., intestinal
i. ▸ intra-abdominal
i., intrauterine viral
i., intravascular
i. ▸ intravascular device
i. ▸ intravenous (IV) line
i., invasive
i. involving fungus ▸ generalized
i., IV (intravenous) associated
i., IV (intravenous) site
i., joint
i., kidney
i. ▸ Klebsiella urinary tract
i., laryngeal
i., latent
i., life-threatening
i., local
i., localized
i. ▸ lower respiratory
i. ▸ lowered resistance to
i., lung
i., lymphogranuloma venereum psittacosis
i., marine
i., mass
i., massive
i., meningococcal
i., middle ear
i., mixed
i. ▸ mixed aerobic-anaerobic
i., mixed bacterial
i., mixed fungal
i., mode of spread of
i., monilial
i., mouth
i., musculoskeletal
i. ▸ Mycobacterium avium complex (MAC)
i. ▸ Mycobacterium avium intracellulare (MAI)
i. ▸ Mycobacterium pneumonia
i., Mycoplasma
i., mycotic
i., nailbed
i., nasal
i., natural defense against
i., nematode
i. no rejection (NI NR) ▸ no
i. ▸ non-Q-wave myocardial

i., nosocomial
i., nosocomial central nervous system (CNS)
i., nosocomial cutaneous
i., nosocomial fungal
i., nosocomial gastrointestinal (GI)
i., nosocomial gynecological (GYN)
i., nosocomial respiratory tract
i., nosocomial vascular
i. ▸ nosocomial wound
i., obstetrical
i., occult
i., ocular
i., ocular herpes
i., odontogenic
i. of bloodstream, bacterial
i. of brain
i. of cornea, bacterial
i. of cornea, fungal
i. of ear
i. of ear ▸ dizziness from
i. of ear ▸ eustachian tube blocked by
i. of ear ▸ fever from
i. of ear ▸ hearing loss from
i. of endocardium
i. of eyelid
i. of hair ▸ dermatophyte
i. of heart ▸ Enterococcal
i. of heart valve ▸ staphylococcal
i. of liver
i. of lung, bacterial
i. of meninges, bacterial
i. of mouth and throat
i. of nail unit ▸ fungal
i. of nails ▸ dermatophyte
i. of nerve pathways
i. of nervous system ▸ fungal
i. of scalp ▸ dermatophyte
i. of skin, bacterial
i. of skin ▸ dermatophyte
i. of skin ▸ fungus
i. of the bones
i. of the cervix
i. of the uterus
i., operative site
i. (OI), opportunistic
i. or dysfunction ▸ bladder involvement,
i., oral
i. ▸ oral yeast
i., oral-facial
i., originating
i. ▸ orthopedic implant
i. outbreak, nosocomial

i. ▸ outer ear
i., overwhelming
i., pacemaker
i., parasitic
i., paratyphoid
i., parvovirus
i., pathogenesis of
i., patient admitted with active
i., patient admitted with disguised
i., patient immune to hepatitis B
i., pelvic
i. penetrated bone
i., periodic yeast
i., persistent tolerant
i., pilonidal
i., pin tract
i., pinworm
i., pneumococcal
i. ▸ pneumococcal bloodstream
i., polymicrobial
i., postabortal
i., postoperative
i., postoperative wound
i., postpartum
i., postsurgical
i. ▸ potential for
i., potential source of
i., presence of
i., prevent spread of
i., preventable nosocomial
i. prevention
i. prevention and control
i. prevention in crush injury
i., prevention of
i., prevention of hospital
i., prevention of nosocomial
    bacterial
i. prevention ▸ opportunistic
i. prevention, surgical
i., primary
i., primary cytomegalovirus (CMV)
i., prostatic
i. ▸ prosthetic device
i. ▸ prosthetic joint
i., protozoal
i., Pseudomonas
i., Pseudomonas aeruginosa
i., pulmonary
i. ▸ pulse generator pocket
i., pyogenic
i. rate
i., rate of incidence of
i., recent acute
i., recurrent
i., recurrent upper respiratory tract

i., recurrent urinary tract
i. ▸ recurrent vaginal yeast
i. ▸ recurrent kidney
i., recurring
i., recurring bladder
i., red
i., reduce risk of hospital-associated
i., re-emerging
i. -related crisis
i., repeated ear
i. ▸ reproductive tract
i., resistance to
i., respiratory
i., respiratory tract
i., retrograde
i., retroviral
i. ▸ rhinocerebral
i. ▸ rhinoviral respiratory
i., rickettsial
i. risk
i. risk, donor
i., risk groups for
i., risk of
i., route of
i., scabetic
i., secondary
i., secondary bacterial
i., self-
i., Serratia marcescens
i., severe
i., severe intestinal
i., severe skin
i. ▸ sexually transmitted
i., shingles
i., shunt
i., silent
i., sinus
i. site
i., site of nosocomial
i., site of primary
i., skin
i. ▸ skin structure
i., soft tissue
i., source of
i., source of bacterial
i., spirochetal
i., spread bacterial
i., spread of
i. ▸ spread of skin
i., staph
i. ▸ staph (Staphylococcus) aureus
    prosthetic joint
i., staphylococcal
i., sternal
i. ▸ sternal wound

i. stones
i., Streptococcus pyogenes
i., streptococcal
I. Study (NNIS) ▸ National
    Nosocomial
i., subclinical
i., superficial
i., suppurative
i., surgical
i. (SSI) ▸ surgical site
i., surgical wound
i., surveillance of
i., symptomatic
i., symptomatic HIV (human
    immunodeficiency virus)
i. ▸ symptomatic urinary tract
i. syndrome, amniotic
i. syndromes, clinical
i., systemic
i. ▸ systemic body
i. ▸ systemic Candida
i., systemic mycotic
i. ▸ systemic yeast
i., terminal
i., throat
i., transfusion-associated
i., transfusion-related
i., transmissible
i., transmission of
i., transmitting
i. ▸ treatment of pericular
i., Trichomonas
i., umbilical
i., uncomplicated skin
i. (URI) ▸ upper respiratory
i., urinary
i. (UTI) ▸ urinary tract
i., vaginal
i., vaginal yeast
i., valve
i., valvular
i. ▸ varicella virus
i. ▸ vascular graft
i., venereal
i., vibrio
i., Vincent's
i., viral
i. ▸ viral inner ear
i., viral respiratory
i., viral-like
i. vs. total admissions ▸ total
i., water-borne
i., wound
i., yeast
infectiosa, dermatitis

infectiosa, spondylitis
infectiosum, erythema
infectiosus, conjunctivitis necroticans
infectiosus, icterus
infectious (Infectious)
i. abortion
i. adenitis, acute epidemic
i. agent
i. agent, blood-borne
i. agent, life-threatening
i. arthritis
i. asthmatic bronchitis
i. blood plasma
i. blood specimen, potentially
i. body fluid
i. bulbar paralysis
i. carcinoma
i. cardiomyopathy
i. cause
i. colitis
i. conjunctivitis
i. diarrhea
i. disease
i. disease, acute
i. disease, associated
i. disease control
i. disease, diagnosed
i. disease emergency
i. disease of lungs
i. disease ▸ risk of
I. Disease Service
i. disease, suspected
i. disorder
i. eczematous dermatitis
i. endocarditis
i. esophagitis
i. etiology
i. fluid
i. gastroenteritis, acute
i. granuloma
i. granulomatous disease
i. hepatitis
i. illness
i. material, potentially
i. mononucleosis
i. mononucleosis ▸ acute
i. morbidity
i. morbidity, maternal
i. myxomatosis
i. organism
i. patient
i., patient currently
i., patient potentially
i. polyneuritis

i. porcine encephalomyelitis
i., potentially
i. precaution, enteric
i. process
i. process ▸ active invasive
i. process, acute
i. stomatitis
i. wart virus
infective
i. asthma
i. bodily fluids, potentially
i. disorder
i. dose
i. dose, median
i. dose ▸ median tissue culture
i. dose (MID) ▸ minimum
i. dose, tissue culture
i. drug ▸ anti-
i. embolism
i. endocarditis
i. endocarditis (AIE), acute
i. endocarditis ▸ subacute
i. granule, Balfour
i. granuloma
i. morbidity
i. pericarditis
i. polyneuritis, acute
i., potentially
i. silicosis
i. thrombosis
i. thrombus
infectivity rate
infects new host cell ▸ phage particle
inferior [*interior*]
i. accessory fissure
i. alveolar nerve
i. ampullar nerve
i. anastomotic vein
i., arcus palpebralis
i. aspect
i. aspect of hypothalamus
i. border of wound
i. cardiac nerve
i. carotid ganglion
i. cerebellar artery (PICA) aneurysm, posterior
i. cerebellar artery (PICA), posterior
i. cerebellar peduncle
i. cerebellar vein
i. cerebral veins
i. cervical cardiac nerve
i. cervical ganglion
i. clunial nerves
i. colliculi

i. communicating artery (AICA), anterior
i. communicating artery (PICA), posterior cornu
i. constrictor muscle
i. defect, posterior
i. dental nerve
i. displacement
i. duodenal fold
i. epigastric artery
i. epigastric vein
i. eye
i. fascia
i. flexure of duodenum
i. fornix
i. fovea
i. frontal
i. frontal electrode
i. frontal gyrus
i. frontal lobe
i. ganglion of glossopharyngeal nerve
i. ganglion of vagus nerve
i. gemellus muscle
i. gluteal nerve
i. gluteal vein
i., gyrus frontalis
i., gyrus temporalis
i. hemorrhoidal nerve
i. hemorrhoidal vein
i. horn of lateral ventricle
i. jugular ganglion
i. labial region
i. labial vein
i. lacrimal gland
i. lamina of sphenoid bone
i. laryngeal nerve
i. laryngeal vein
i. lateral cutaneous nerve of arm
i. lip ▸ incisive muscles of
i. lobe
i. longitudinal diameter
i. longitudinal muscle of tongue
i. lung field
i. margin
i. margin of left lung
i. margin of right lung
i. meatus
i. mesenteric angiogram
i. mesenteric artery (IMA)
i. mesenteric ganglion
i. mesenteric lymph nodes
i. mesenteric vascular occlusion
i. mesenteric vein
i. muscle, obliquus

i. muscle, rectus
i. myocardial infarction (MI)
i. oblique muscle
i. oblique muscle ▸ advancement of
i. oblique muscle of eyeball
i. occipital gyrus
i. ophthalmic vein
i. organ
i. ossea, concha nasalis
i. palpebrae, tarsus
i. palpebral region
i. palpebral veins
i. parietal lobule
i. pedicle
i. peduncle of thalamus
i. petrosal ganglion
i. phrenic vein
i. polioencephalitis
i. posterior serratus muscle
i. pulmonary vein, left
i. pulmonary vein, right
i. ramus
i. rectal nerve
i. rectal vein
i. rectus muscle
i. rectus muscle, advancement of
i. rectus muscle dissected free
i. semilunar lobule
i., sinus sagittalis
i. splanchnic nerve
i. -superior projection
i. -superior tangential projection
i. tarsal muscle
i. temporal gyrus
i. temporal venule of retina
i. thyroid gland
i. thyroid notch
i. thyroid vein
i. tracheobronchial lymph nodes
i. turbinate
i. vagal ganglion
i. vena cava (IVC)
i. vena cava pressure (IVCP)
i. vena cava (TIVC) ▸ thoracic
i. vena cava (IVC) obstruction
i. vena cava occlusion
i. venacavography
i., venula macularis
i., venula nasalis retinas
i., venula temporalis retinas
i. vertebral notch
i. wall
i. wall ischemia
i. wall myocardial infarction (IWMI)

i. wall myocardial infarction (MI) ▸ old

inferiority
i. complex
i., constitutional psychopathic
i. feelings
inferiorly, viscera packed
inferobasal wall
inferolateral aspect
inferolateral myocardial infarction
inferosuperior axial projection
infertile couple
infertility
i. acupuncture
i., endometriosis associated
i. evaluation
i., female
i. from alcohol
i. from chemical
i. from diabetes
i. in women
i., male
i., primary
i. problem, male
i., secondary
i. studies
i. tests
i. treatment
i., tubal
i. workup
infestans, Triatoma
infestans, Trypanosoma
infestation
i., Armillifer
i., cestode
i., lice
i., louse
i., nematode
i., parasitic
i., skin
i., Trichomonas
infested, insect-
infiltrate(s)
i., abundant leukemic
i., active
i., Assmann tuberculous
i., Assmann's
i., basilar
i., bibasilar pulmonary
i. ▸ bilateral alveolar pulmonary
i., bilateral hilar
i. ▸ bilateral lower lobe
i., bronchopneumonic
i., chronic inflammatory
i. ▸ chronic interstitial inflammatory

i., clearing of
i., corneal
i., dense lobar
i. ▸ deteriorating kidney
i., diffuse leukemic
i., diffuse lymphomatous
i. ▸ extensive bilateral sloughing
i. fever, pulmonary
i. ▸ fluffy alveolar
i., fluffy bibasilar
i. ▸ focal areas of lymphoid
i., hazy
i., hilar
i., interstitial
i. ▸ interstitial polymorphonuclear
   leukocyte
i., left lower lobe (LLL)
i. left lung base
i., leukemic
i., lymphocytic
i., lymphocytic peribronchial
i., lymphoid
i., marked plasmocytic
i. ▸ migratory pulmonary
i. ▸ mild focal chronic inflammatory
i., mixed bacterial
i., moderate
i., multilobe
i. of adrenals ▸ leukemic
i. of colon ▸ leukemic
i. of kidneys ▸ leukemic
i. of liver ▸ leukemic
i. of lymphocytes ▸ perivascular
i., parenchymal
i., patchy
i. ▸ patchy chronic inflammatory
i., patchy pneumonic
i. ▸ peribronchial chronic
   inflammatory
i. ▸ perivascular eosinophilic
i., plasma cell
i., pneumonic
i., pulmonary
i., residual
i., right lower lobe (RLL)
i., right lung base
i. ▸ scattered chronic inflammatory
i., scattered lymphocytic
i., strandy
i., streaky
i. ▸ Wasserman-positive pulmonary
infiltrated
i., diffusely
i. duct cell carcinoma ▸ multifocal
i., upper eyelid

infiltrated—*continued*
i. ▸ washed, prepped and
i. with Xylocaine
infiltrating
i. carcinoma
i. ductal carcinoma of the breast
i. ductal cell carcinoma
i. glioma
i. irregular tumor mass
i. lobular cancer
i. lymphocytes (TIL) ▸ genetically altered tumor
i. lymphocytes (TIL) technique, tumor
i. lymphocytes, tumor
i. single cells ▸ anaplastic
i. squamous cell carcinoma
i. tumor metastases ▸ focal
infiltration
i., active
i., amyloid
i. and eosinophilia (PIE), pulmonary
i. anesthesia
i. anesthetics
i., bulging fatty
i. by hemorrhage, surface
i. by tumor cells
i., chronic inflammatory
i., chronic inflammatory cell
i., diffuse lymphoid
i. ductal carcinoma
i., extensive
i., fatty
i., fibrotic
i., focal
i., glomeruli
i., hemorrhagic
i., leukemic
i., local
i., lymphocytic cell
i., malignant
i., massive
i., mottled
i. of extramedullary hematopoietic cells ▸ sparse
i. of ganglion
i. of liver ▸ acute inflammatory
i. of liver, fatty
i. of liver ▸ leukemic
i. of spleen ▸ leukemic
i. of urinary tract
i., parenchymal
i., patchy
i., perilymphatic
i., perineural

i., perivascular
i., pneumonic
i., polymorphonuclear
i., pulmonary
i., scant
i., stringy
i., tumor
infiltrative
i. cardiomyopathy
i. change
i. disease ▸ lymphocytic
i. disorder ▸ lymphocytic
i. ductal carcinoma
i. lung disease, diffuse
i. process
i. process, active
i. process, patchy
i. tendinitis, hypertrophic
inflamed
i., air passages become
i. airway, chronically
i. airway tissue
i. appendix
i. appendix, acutely
i. arch
i. area
i. area ▸ painful,
i. artery
i. ▸ bronchi erythematous and
i. cartilage
i. cyst, chronically
i. diverticulum
i. diverticulum rupture
i. ▸ eye mildly
i. eyelid
i. gallbladder
i. gallbladder, chronically
i. gallbladder with stones ▸ chronically
i. gums
i. intestines
i. joint
i. joints ▸ swollen, stiff
i. ligament
i., mucosa appeared
i. muscle fibers
i. nerve
i. nipple
i. ovary
i. pharynx
i., placenta
i. pleura mildly
i. prostate gland ▸ enlarged,
i. socket
i. spinal nerve

i. surfaces
i. swollen joint
i. synovial tissue
i. tendon
i. ▸ thumb joint swollen and
i. tissue
i., tonsils
i., trachea markedly
i. veins
inflammation
i., acute
i. ▸ acute and chronic
i., acute catarrhal
i., acute kidney
i., acute portal
i. and gliosis in brain
i. and/or swelling
i., aortic
i., atherosclerotic
i., blood vessel
i., bowel
i., cardiac
i., chronic
i., chronic bladder
i., chronic kidney
i., colonic mucosal
i., development of
i. ▸ diseased joint with
i. ▸ eye socket
i. ▸ fluid accumulation and
i. from pernicious anemia ▸ tongue
i., granular
i., granulomatous
i., gum
i. in tooth socket
i. ▸ infection and
i. ▸ ischemic ocular
i., interstitial
i., intestinal
i., jaundice without
i., joint
i., local
i., localized
i. ▸ lower respiratory tract
i., meningeal
i. ▸ nasal passage
i., nonlocalized
i. of arterial lining
i. of biopsy tissue
i. of bladder
i. of bladder and urethra
i. of bladder wall
i. of brain
i. of brain, chronic
i. of breastbone and ribs

i. of bronchial tubes
i. of cartilage of rib cage
i. of cerebral sinus
i. of colon
i. of conjunctiva
i. of connective tissue
i. of cornea
i. of coronary arteries
i. of diaphragm
i. of diverticular
i. of duodenum
i. of ear
i. of ear canal
i. of external ear canal
i. of eye
i. of eyelid
i. of gallbladder
i. of heart
i. of heart lining
i. of heart muscle
i. of ileum
i. of intestine
i. of joint
i. of joints, chronic
i. of joints, painful
i. of kidney
i. of lamina propria ▸ chronic
i. of lid margins
i. of lining of abdominal cavity
i. of lining of heart
i. of lining of organ
i. of liver
i. of lungs
i. of meninges
i. of middle ear
i. of mucous membrane of nose
i. of muscles
i. of nerve
i. of nerves, viral
i. of optic nerve
i. of oral mucosa
i. of pancreas
i. of pancreas, purulent
i. of pericardium
i. of pleura
i. of portal tracts ▸ acute
i. of prostate
i. of retina
i. of semicircular canal
i. of seminal vesicle
i. of skin
i. of spinal cord
i. of spinal cord ▸ acute
i. of stomach
i. of stomach ▸ persistent

i. of synovial membrane
i. of synovium
i. of tendons
i. of tooth socket
i. of urethra
i. of urinary bladder
i. of uvea
i. of vaginal tissues
i. of vein
i. of vessel
i. of voice box
i., painful
i., pancreatic
i., persistent
i., persistent tissue
i., postoperative
i., progressive
i. ▸ redness and
i., respiratory
i. ▸ respiratory tract
i., septic
i., severe
i., sinus
i., sterile
i., synovial
i., systemic
i., throat
i. ▸ tympanic membrane
i., vaginal
i., vascular
i., viral
i. with alveolar sloughing ▸ chronic
i. within affected area
i. within joint

inflammatory
i. activity
i. adhesions
i. agent, ▸ nonsteroidal anti-
i. aneurysm
i. aortic aneurysm
i. arthritis
i. atrophy
i. bowel disease
i. bowel disease ▸ extensive
i. bowel disorder
i. breast carcinoma, locally
   advanced and
i. breast cancer
i. carcinoma
i. carcinoma of breast
i. cell
i. cell infiltration, chronic
i. cells, acute
i. cells, chronic
i. cells ▸ foci of

i. cells ▸ interstitial acute
i. cells, necrotic
i. change
i. change, focal
i. change, pleural
i. condition
i. cyst
i. diarrhea
i. disease
i. disease, chronic
i. disease (chr. PID) ▸ chronic
   pelvic
i. disease from Chlamydia ▸ pelvic
i. disease of bowel
i. disease of pancreas ▸ chronic
i. disease (PID) ▸ pelvic
i. disease, peptic
i. disease process
i. disease (PID) residues, pelvic
i. disease (PID) ▸ sexually
   transmitted pelvic
i. disorder
i. drug, anti-
i. drug (NSAID), nonsteroidal anti-
i. dysmenorrhea
i. episodes ▸ superimposed acute
i. exudate
i. fracture
i. glaucoma
i. granulomatous process, chronic
i. headache
i. hyperplasia
i. hyperplasia, chronic
i. hyperplasia, mucosal
i. infiltrate, chronic
i. infiltrate ▸ chronic interstitial
i. infiltrate ▸ mild focal chronic
i. infiltrate ▸ patchy chronic
i. infiltrate ▸ peribronchial chronic
i. infiltrate ▸ scattered chronic
i. infiltration, chronic
i. infiltration of liver ▸ acute
i. intestinal disorder
i. joint disorder
i. lesion
i. macrophage
i. malignant fibrous histiocytoma
i. mass
i. medication, anti-
i. mucosal changes, focal
i. myopathy
i. nodules, granular
i., nonsteroidal anti-
i. pelvic disease
i. pericarditis

inflammatory—*continued*
- i. polyp
- i. polyradiculoneuropathy, acute
- i. process
- i. protein
- i. protein, anti-
- i. reaction
- i. reaction, characteristic
- i. reaction, peritoneal
- i. response
- i. response syndrome ▸ systemic
- i. rheumatoid arthritis
- i. softening
- i. spine arthritis
- i. steroid, anti-
- i. stimulation ▸ persistent
- i. suppression
- i. tissue

inflatable
- i. balloon, small
- i. comfort ring
- i. cuff
- i. limb splint

inflated
- i., balloon
- i. eardrum
- i. judgment of accomplishments
- i., lungs
- i. self-appraisal
- i. self-esteem
- i., tourniquet

inflates accomplishments

inflation
- i., automatic
- i., balloon
- i., eustachian tube
- i., intra-aortic balloon
- i., manual
- i. reflex
- i. reflex, Breuer-Hering
- i., tubal
- i. with oxygen (IPPO) ▸ intermittent positive pressure

inflexible
- i. antisocial personality traits
- i. insistence
- i. spine
- i. trait

inflicted
- i. abuse behavior ▸ self-
- i. injury, self-
- i. wound, self-

inflight exercise program ▸ vigorous

inflow
- i. conduit

- i. ▸ gradient of fluid
- i., increased penile
- i. obstruction ▸ right ventricular (RV)
- i. of arterial blood
- i., revision of
- i. tract
- i. tract obstruction ▸ left ventricular (LV)
- i. ▸ turbulent diastolic mitral

influence(s)
- i., cognitive
- i., constitutional
- i., controlling
- i., cultural
- i., environmental
- i., familial
- i., genetic
- i., hormonal
- i., interpersonal
- i., media
- i. of trauma
- i., parental
- i., peer
- i., prenatal
- i., proprioceptive
- i., psychic
- i., psychosocial
- i. ▸ relapse-inducing adverse
- i., ruling
- i., sensory
- i., traumatic
- i. ▸ working under the

influenced character, sex-
influenced ▸ fear of being
influencing anxiety, factors
influenza
- i. A, B, C
- i., Asian
- i., Avian
- i. bacilli
- i., Bacillus
- i., epidemic
- i., endemic
- i. H
- i. ▸ Hong Kong
- i. immunization
- i. infection
- i. inoculation
- i. lymphatica
- i. nostras
- i., pandemic
- i. -related illness
- i., Russian
- i. strain, swine

- i., swine
- i., Texas
- i. type B (HIB), Hemophilus
- i. type B (HIB) vaccine ▸ Hemophilus
- i. vaccination
- i. vaccine
- i. vaccine, bivalent
- i. vaccine ▸ inactivated
- i. vaccine ▸ intranasal
- i. vaccine, monovalent
- i. vaccine ▸ swine
- i. virus
- i. virus pneumonia
- i. virus vaccine
- i., yuppie

influenzae
- i., Bacillus
- i., gram-negative Haemophilus
- i., Haemophilus/Hemophilus
- i. infection ▸ Haemophilus
- i. meningitis, Haemophilus
- i. pneumonia, Haemophilus

influenzal encephalitis
influenzal pneumonia
informal support
information
- i., accurate
- i., clinical
- i., cognitive
- i., confidentiality of
- i., critical
- i., demographic
- i., didactic
- i., disclosure of
- i., drug
- i., genetic
- i. identification, medical
- i., individual seeking
- i., medical
- i. monitoring system ▸ quality
- i., parse
- i. ▸ perception, thought and recognition of
- i., pre-admission
- i. processing
- i., release of
- i., retaining new
- i. system, medical
- i., toxicity
- i., visual
- i., vital health

informed
- i. consent
- i. consent form

i. decision
i. health care decision
i. waiver and consent
infracalcarine gyrus
infracalcarinus, gyrus
infraclavicular
i. area
i. triangle
infracted turbinate
infraction [*infarction*]
infraction, Freiberg's
infracubital bypass
infradian rhythm
infradiaphragmatic portion
infrahepatic arteriography
infrahepatic arteriography and
infusion
infrahilar area
infrahyoid muscles
inframammary
i. crease
i. fold
i. region
infranodal block
infranodal extrasystole
infraoccipital nerve
infraorbital
i. block
i. discoloration, heliotrope
i. foramen
i. incision
i. line
i. nerve
i. region
i. suture
infraorbitomeatal line
infrapatellar synovial fold
infrapopliteal angioplasty
infrapopliteal transluminal
angioplasty
infrared
i. coagulation
i. coagulation of hemorrhoids
i. heat coagulation (IRC)
i. image-converter
i. light therapy
i. microscope
i. photocoagulation
i. pulsed laser
i. pulsed laser ▸ mid-
i. radiation
i. rays
i. spectrophotometry
i. spectroscopy ▸ near-
i. thermography

infrarenal
i. abdominal aorta
i. abdominal aortic aneurysm
i. aortic thrombosis
i. node, periaortic
infraroentgen rays
infrascapular region
infrasonic frequency
infraspinatus reflex
infraspinous muscle
infrasternal retraction
infratemporal region
infratentorial parts of central nervous
system (CNS)
infratrochlear nerve
infraumbilical fold
infraumbilical incision
infrequent
i. blinking
i. blinking of eyelids
i. menstruation
i. pulse
infundibula of kidney
infundibular
i. obstruction
i. septal defect
i. stalk
i. stenosis ▸ myocardial
i. wedge resection
infundibulectomy, Brock
infundibuliform hymen
infundibuloarterial inversion
infundibuloarterial inversion ▸
isolated
infundibulopelvic ligament
infundibulum
i., Choanotaenia
i., dilatation of
i., ethmoidal
i. of fallopian tube
i. of heart
i. of urinary bladder
i. of uterine tube
i. tubae uterinae
infuse
i. antibiotics
i. -a-port
i. marrow
Infuser, Button
Infuser, Pen Pump
infusing solutions
infusing solutions, priming of
infusion(s)
i., bone
i., bone marrow

i., brain-heart
i. chemotherapy, continuous
i., continuous insulin
i. ▸ continuous wound
i. device, positive pressure
i. device, pressure
i., dextrose
i., drip
i., drip rate of
i., drug
i. ▸ duodenal peptone
i. excretory urogram, constant
i. ▸ fresh frozen plasma
i., heparinized solution
i., infrahepatic arteriography and
i., intra-amniotic saline
i., intra-arterial hepatic
i., intracoronary streptokinase
i. ▸ intraduodenal peptone
i., intravenous (IV)
i., isolated
i. needle, intraosseous
i., nephrotomography
i., nitroprusside
i. of chemotherapeutic agent
i. of 5-FU (fluorouracil)
i. of magnesium ▸ intravenous
i. period, total
i., peripheral
i. phlebitis
i. phlebitis, IV (intravenous)
i., plasma
i. pump
i. pump, Abbott
i. pump, Acupressure
i. pump, Harvard
i. pump, implantable drug
i. pump ▸ implantable insulin
i. pump, IVAC volumetric
i. pyelogram
i. pyelographic study
i. pyelography
i. pyelography, drip
i. rate
i., regular insulin
i. regulator, electric
i., saline and dopamine
i. site
i. site discomfort
i., slow
i., slow intravenous (IV)
i. suction cutter (VISC), vitreous
i. system ▸ portable insulin
i. technique, drip
i. therapy

infusion(s)—*continued*
  i. therapy, arterial
  i. ▸ tissue plasminogen activator
    (TPA)
  i., total
  i., total dose
  i. urogram, drip-
  i. valve, drip
Inge procedure
ingested [*injected*]
  i., amphetamines
  i. (amphetamines), Speed
  i., barbiturates
  i., cocaine
  i. contrast medium, patient
  i. food and fluid
  i. food particles
  i., Ketamine
  i., lysergic acid diethylamide
    (LSD)
  i., marijuana
  i. material
  i., mescaline
  i. ▸ nutmeg (trimethoxy-
    amphetamine)
  i., orally
  i. orally ▸ peyote
  i., PCP (phencyclidine)
  i. poison
  i., psilocybin
  i. ▸ trimethoxy-amphetamine
    (nutmeg)
ingestion [*injection*]
  i. ▸ acute or chronic alcohol
  i., aspirin
  i. ▸ crack cocaine
  i., drug
  i., ethanol
  i., excessive
  i., following
  i. of barium
  i. of drugs
  i. of large amounts of food, rapid
  i. of poisonous substance
  i. of potentially poisonous
    substance
  i. of toxic agents
  i. of toxic drug
  i., oral
  i. ▸ psychedelic drug
  i., rapid
  i. ▸ sudden death due to cocaine
ingluvicola, Gongylonema
ingravescent apoplexy
ingredients, active painkilling

ingrown
  i. hair
  i. nail
  i. positive strains
  i. toenails
ingrowth
  i., endothelial
  i., epithelial
  i. prosthesis, bone
inguinal
  i. arch
  i. area
  i. artery, ilio◊
  i. canal
  i. canal, floor of
  i. hernia
  i. hernia, direct
  i. hernia ▸ incarcerated
  i. hernia, indirect
  i. hernia, pantaloon
  i. hernia repair, Bassini
  i. hernia sac ▸ large
  i. herniorrhaphy
  i. ilio
  i. impulse
  i. incision
  i. ligament
  i. ligament, shelving border of
  i. lymph nodes
  i. lymph nodes, deep
  i. lymph nodes, superficial
  i. lymphadenopathy, palpable
  i. nerve, ilio◊
  i. node dissection, radical
  i. nodes
  i. orchiectomy
  i. reflex
  i. region
  i. region of abdomen, left
  i. region of abdomen, right
  i. ring
  i. ring, external
  i. ring, internal
  i. sphincter
inguinale
  i., Epidermophyton
  i., granuloma
  i., lymphogranuloma
inguinalis
  i., falx
  i., pediculosis
  i., Pediculus
  i., phthiriasis
inguinocrural hernia
inguinofemoral hernia

inguinoproperitoneal hernia
inguinosuperficial hernia
INH (isoniazid)
INH (isonicotine hydrazine)
inhalable poison
inhalant(s)
  i. abuse
  i. abuse, chronic
  i. abuse, pattern of
  i., abuse, physical effects of
  i. abuse potential of
  i. abuse, prevalence of
  i. abusers, assessing needs of
  i., acute intoxication with
  i., antifoaming
  i. antigen
  i., dependence on
  i., effects of
  i., flashback reactions with
  i., huffing
  i. -induced hallucinations
  i. intoxication
  i., mode of administration with
  i., organic brain syndrome with
  i., panic reactions with
  i., patient OD (overdosed) with
  i., potent
  i., potential tolerance to
  i., psychoactive doses of
  i., psychoactive properties of
  i., psychological effects of
  i., psychotic reactions with
  i., toxicity of
  i., treatment of acute drug reactions
    to
  i., withdrawal from
inhalation
  i. accidental
  i. agent
  i. and expiration
  i. anesthesia
  i. anesthetic ▸ respiratory
    depression
  i. bronchography
  i. challenge
  i. challenge apparatus, quantitative
  i. chemotherapy treatment
  i., chronic antibiotic
  i. fever
  i. injury
  i., long-term
  i. of FB (foreign body)
  i. of foreign material
  i. of foreign substance
  i., marijuana

i. ‣ oxygen (O₂)
i., patient treated for smoke
i. pneumonia
i., smoke
i. solution
i., steam
i. test
i. therapy
i. therapy ‣ steam
i. tuberculosis

inhalational
i. anesthesia
i. anesthesia ‣ general
i. anesthetic, alveolar partial pressure of
i. anthrax
i. lung disease

inhale cocaine
inhaleable insulin
inhaled
i. bronchodilator
i., LSD
i., Mescaline
i. steroids

inhaler(s)
i., beta agonist
i., insulin
i., (MDI) metered dose
i., nicotine
i., steam spray

inhaling spores
inherent
i. capabilities
i. density
i. filter
i. mechanism
i. risk
i. strength of myocardial contraction
i. weakness in arterial wall

inheritable brain disease
inheritance
i., dominant
i., genetic
i. pattern ‣ recessive
i., recessive
i., single gene
i. ‣ X-linked

inherited
i. abnormality in brain
i. anemia
i. bleeding disorder
i. blood disease
i. blood disorder
i. brain disorder

i. cancer syndrome
i. colon cancer
i. color deficiency
i. defect
i. disease
i. disorder
i. disorder, severe
i. gene alterations
i. genetic abnormality
i. genetic defect
i. high cholesterol
i. hypertension
i. immune disorder
i. immunity
i. iron storage disease
i. metabolic disorder
i. motor neuron (MN) disease
i. mutations
i. nerve disorder
i. neuromuscular disorder
i. predisposition ‣ multifactorially
i. procoagulant deficiency
i. risk factor
i. tendencies
i. trait
i. vulnerability

inhibit
i. blood clots
i. bone resorption
i. fetal circulation
i. flexor spasticity
i. growth of tumor
i. immune system
i. labor
i. nerve cell growth
i. tumor growth

inhibited
i. behavior
i. female orgasm
i. male orgasm
i. pacemaker, atrial demand
i. pacemaker ‣ atrial synchronous ventricular
i. pacemaker ‣ atrial triggered ventricular
i. pacemaker ‣ ventricular demand
i. pacing
i. pulse generator ‣ ventricular
i. sexual desire psychosexual dysfunction
i. sexual excitement

inhibiting
i. behavioral injury device (SIBID), self-

i. clot formation
i. dilution (MID) ‣ maximum
i. factor (MIF) ‣ macrophage
i. factor, prolactin
i. stress response

inhibition
i. ‣ academic or work
i. ‣ adjustment disorder with academic
i. antibody, hemagglutination-
i. assay, agglutination
i., behavioral
i., chemical
i., contact
i., diminished
i. factor (MIF) ‣ migration-
i., growth
i., hemagglutination
i., hemagglutinin
i., leukotriene
i. of action
i. of activity
i. of shivering
i., potassium
i., protein synthesis
i., psychomotor
i. reaction, hemagglutination-
i., reduced
i., relaxed
i., relieve
i., suppress
i. test, adrenocortical
i. test, agglutination
i. test, hemagglutination
i. test, latex agglutination
i., tetrazolium-reduction
i. titer, agglutination
i., zone of

inhibitor(s)
i., ace
i., angiogenesis
i. ‣ angiotensin-converting enzyme (ACE)
i., beta lactamase
i., bronchial mucus
i., cholinesterase
i. coagulant complex, anti-
i., converting enzyme
i., culture
i., cyclooxygenase
i. diet ‣ restricted tyramine and MAO (monoamine oxidase)
i., enzyme
i., Factor VIII
i., gastric acid

inhibitor(s)—*continued*
- i. ▸ lipoprotein-associated coagulation
- i. ▸ longer acting ACE
- i. ▸ mast cell
- i., monoamine oxidase (MAO)
- i., mucus
- i., nerve growth
- i. ▸ nucleoside reverse transcriptase
- i., plaque
- i. ▸ plasminogen activator
- i., platelet
- i. protein ▸ secretory leukoprotease
- i. ▸ proton pump
- i., renin
- i., rhinovirus
- i., secretase
- i., sympathetic
- i., target enzyme insensitive to
- i. therapy ▸ protease
- i., viral

inhibitory
- i. capacity, trypsin-
- i. cells, cardiovascular
- i. center
- i. concentration (MIC) ▸ minimum
- i. effect
- i. factor ▸ leukemia
- i. fibers
- i. fibers, activating
- i. ganglion
- i. material, gonadotropin-
- i. nerve
- i. neurotransmitter action
- i. postsynaptic potential (IPSP)
- i. state, central
- i. transmitter

in-home care givers

in-home care, respite and

inhomogeneity(-ies)
- i. artifact ▸ main magnetic field
- i., correct for
- i. in electron beam therapy

inhumane, slow and

initial
- i. Apgar score
- i. apnea
- i. assessment
- i. assessment phase
- i. attack
- i. attack of vertigo
- i. autopsy
- i. baseline level
- i. bleed
- i. breathing difficulty

- i. cardiac enzymes
- i. case assessment
- i. cells
- i. cocaine abstinence
- i. complaint
- i. consultation
- i. contact
- i. crisis
- i. cryotherapy
- i. diagnosis and treatment
- i. dosage
- i. dose
- i. dose period
- i. dose, titrated
- i. drug screening test
- i. ease of engagement
- i. employee evaluation
- i. evaluation
- i. evaluation and treatment
- i. examination
- i. exposure to germ
- i. feeling of euphoria
- i. head assessment
- i. heart attack
- i. heat
- i. hypertension (HTN) evaluation
- i. immune response
- i. implant
- i. impression
- i. infection
- i. insomnia
- i. interview
- i. investigation
- i. levels of alcohol intake
- i. linear survival curve
- i. management
- i. manifestation
- i. paralysis
- i. physical examination
- i. prognostic score
- i. psychiatric treatment plan
- i. reaction
- i. resuscitation
- i. screening
- i. screening examination
- i. site
- i. stabilization phase of treatment
- i. stroke
- i. study
- i. symptom
- i. syphilitic lesion
- i. target volume
- i. therapy
- i. trauma
- i. treatment

- i. treatment plan
- i. tumor
- i. urinalysis
- i. urine specimen
- i. vector
- i. venous shunt
- i. visit

initialization, parameter

initially, patient treated

initially with intravenous (IV) fluids ▸ patient treated

initiate
- i. cardiopulmonary resuscitation (CPR)
- i. heartbeat
- i. pulmonary ventilation
- i. treatment

initiating
- i. abstinence
- i. sleep
- i. sleep ▸ persistent disorder
- i. sleep ▸ transient disorder of
- i. therapy
- i. urination ▸ difficulty in
- i. wakefulness ▸ persistent disorder of
- i. wakefulness ▸ transient disorder of

initiation
- i. and management ▸ chemotherapy
- i. of medication
- i., treatment

initiative
- i. and spontaneity, lack of
- i. ▸ lack of
- i., loss of
- i., nutrition screening
- i. ▸ reduced spontaneity, curiosity and

inject sterile liquid cement

injectable diuretic

injectable fillers in plastic surgery

injected [*ingested*]
- i., amphetamines
- i., barbiturates
- i., cocaine
- i., conjunctivae
- i., eardrum
- i. into uterus ▸ Pituitrin
- i., Ketamine
- i., LSD
- i., Mescaline
- i. ▸ morning glory seeds
- i. negative ▸ dye-

i., PCP (phencyclidine)
i., pharynx
i., pharynx not
i., psilocybin
i., posterior pharynx (posteropharynx) not
i. radiation
i. radioactive isotopes
i. Speed (amphetamines)
i. steroids
i. tendon sheath
i. therapy ‣ virus
i., throat
i., tympanic membranes
i. under conjunctiva, medication
i. with lethal substance ‣ patient
i. with liposomes ‣ patient

injecting bone cement
injecting contrast media
injection(s) [*ingestion*]
i., bleeding at site of
i., blood patch
i., bolus
i. ‣ Botulinum Toxin (Bo-Tox)
i., cocaine
i., collagen
i., conjunctival
i., conjunctival vascular
i., corticosteroid
i., cortisone
i., daily
i., desensitization
i. ‣ direct killing by lethal
i. dome
i., fat
i., gamma globulin
i. ‣ gene therapy
i., gold
i., hydrocortisone
i., insulin
i., intra-arterial
i., intracardiac
i., intramuscular (IM)
i., intrathecal
i., intravenous (IV)
i., left ventricular
i., lethal
i. ‣ lump at site of
i., marrow
i., mass
i., microlips
i. ‣ monthly/bimonthly contraceptive
i., nasal
i., nasopalatine
i., nerve

i. of air
i. of bursae, aspiration and
i. of contrast media
i. of contrast medium, intravenous (IV) bolus
i. of contrast substance
i. of drugs, intra-arterial
i. of dye
i. of joints, aspiration and
i. of radiopaque contrast medium
i. of radiopaque material
i. of radiopaque substance
i. of silicone into breast ‣ direct
i. of tendons, aspiration and
i. ‣ pain-relieving
i., parenteral
i., perinephric air
i., pharyngeal
i., placebo
i. port
i., radioactive
i., recumbivax
i., RhoGAM
i., right ventricular
i., root
i. sclerotherapy ‣ long-term
i., self-administered
i., Silastic
i., silicone
i. site
i. site ‣ original
i. site reaction
i., steroid
i., subconjunctival
i., subcutaneous (SC)
i., systemic
i., Tensilon
i. therapy
i. therapy ‣ ultrasound-guided
i., transduodenal fiberscopic duct
i. treatment
i. ‣ trigger point

injector
i. ‣ air-jet insulin
i., flow
i. ‣ insulin pen
i., power

injured
i. area ‣ exercise to rehabilitate
i. arm ‣ immobilization of
i. heart muscle
i. joint
i. knees ‣ protect and stabilize
i. leg ‣ immobilization of
i. limb

i. limb, elevation of
i. patient, head-
i. rotator cuff
i. tissue

injuring behaviors, self-
injurious habits ‣ self-
injurious motor vehicle crash
injury(-ies)
i., abdominal
i., abdominal muscle
i., accidental
i., acute
i., acute knee
i., acute lung
i., advanced
i., air emboli-induced lung
i., alcohol-induced
i., alcohol-related
i. and reimplantation fingertip
i. and repair ‣ peritoneal
i., animal bite
i., anoxic brain
i., aortic
i., avulsion
i., avulsion flap
i., backstroke
i., birth
i., bladder
i., blast
i., blunt
i., blunt renal
i., bony
i., brain
i., brain damage
i., breaststroke
i., broken
i., burn
i., butterfly stroke
i. by chronic alcoholism ‣ persistent
i., cardiac
i., cervical cord
i., cervical spine
i., chemical
i., childbirth
i., closed
i., closed head
i. ‣ confusion with head
i., contrecoup
i., corneal
i., craniocerebral
i., crush
i., crushed chest
i., crushing
i., current
i., debilitating

injury(-ies)—*continued*
 i., deceleration
 i., deglove
 i., dental
 i., destructive
 i. device (SIBID), self-inhibiting
   behavioral
 i., diaphragmatic
 i. ▸ diastolic current of
 i., diffuse lung
 i., diving
 i. ▸ drug-induced hepatic
 i., ear
 i., electrical
 i. ▸ emergent liver
 i., environmental heat
 i., external
 i., eye
 i., eyelid
 i. ▸ femoral vascular
 i., finger
 i., fire-related
 i., fishhook
 i., freestyle stroke
 i. from Addison's disease ▸
   bleeding
 i. from ozone ▸ lung
 i., frostbite
 i. ▸ grafted skin vulnerable to
 i., gymnastics
 i., hand
 i., hangman's
 i., head
 i., healing the
 i., heat
 i. ▸ heat-related
 i., hepatocellular
 i. hypothesis of atherogenesis ▸
   response-to-
 i. hypothesis ▸ response-to-
 i., iatrogenic
 i., iatrogenic ureteral
 i. ▸ immobilization of back
 i. ▸ immobilization of neck
 i. ▸ immobilization of spinal
 i., industrial
 i. ▸ infection prevention in crush
 i., inhalation
 i., internal
 i., intimal
 i., intracranial
 i., irradiation
 i. ▸ irreversible brain
 i., irreversible catastrophic brain
 i. ▸ ischemic reperfusion

 i., job-related
 i., joint
 i., kidney
 i., knee
 i., knee ligament
 i., lateral elbow
 i., lethal
 i., life-threatening
 i., life-threatening brain
 i., ligament
 i., limb
 i., lip
 i., liver
 i., local defense against
 i. ▸ localized brain
 i., localized cold
 i., lung
 i., maxillofacial
 i., mechanisms of testicular
 i., medial elbow
 i. ▸ median nerve
 i. ▸ mesangial immune
 i., microvascular
 i., motor vehicle
 i., movement
 i., multihit
 i. ▸ muscle relaxation in patients
   with neck
 i., myocardial
 i. ▸ myocardial reperfusion
 i., nail
 i., neck
 i., needle stick
 i., nerve
 i. ▸ neutrophil-mediated endothelial
 i. ▸ neutrophil-mediated lung
 i. ▸ nipple discharge from breast
 i., non-fatal
 i., obstetrical
 i. of major airway, blunt
 i. of major airway, penetrating
 i. of target cells, radiation
 i. of vascular system, radiation
 i. open
 i. or illness ▸ evaluate extent of
 i., orbital
 i., overuse
 i. ▸ overuse strain
 i. ▸ oxidant-induced lung
 i. ▸ oxygen (O_2)-mediated lung
 i. ▸ pain in back from whiplash
 i. paralysis, post-
 i. paralysis ▸ spinal cord
 i., paralyzing

 i., patient has whiplash
 i., penetrating
 i., penetrating renal
 i., penile
 i., perinatal
 i., peripheral nerve
 i., personal
 i., physical
 i. (PIRI) ▸ postischemic reperfusion
 i. ▸ postischemic skeletal muscle
   reperfusion
 i., potential
 i., prenatal
 i., pressure gun
 i., radial nerve
 i., reality of
 i., receptor stimulated by
 i., recreational
 i. renal problem, crush
 i., reperfusion
 i., repetitive motion
 i. (RSI), repetitive strain
 i. (RSI) ▸ repetitive stress
 i., retinal
 i., rotator cuff
 i., running
 i. score ▸ lung
 i., self-inflicted
 i., severe head
 i., severity of
 i. ▸ side splash lightning
 i. site
 i., skin
 i. ▸ smoke-induced lung
 i., soft structure
 i., soft tissue
 i., soft tissue compression
 i., spinal
 i., spinal cord
 i., spleen
 i., sports
 i., sports-related
 i. stages, stress
 i., steering wheel
 i. strain, myocardial
 i., subendocardial
 i., subepicardial
 i., swimming
 i. syndrome, crush
 i. ▸ systolic current of
 i., tampon
 i., tendon
 i., testicular
 i. theory ▸ response to
 i., thermal

i., thigh
i., thoracic
i., throat
i., through-and-through avulsion
i., tissue
i. to brain ▸ acute
i. to heart, blunt
i. to joint, twisting
i. to lid margins
i. to meningeal vessel
i. to neck, whiplash
i., toe
i., toxic
i., traumatic
i. ▸ traumatic brain
i., traumatic ureteral
i. treatment ▸ sports
i. untreatable
i., ureteric
i., urinary tract
i., vascular
i., vertebral
i., vesicovaginal
i., volar plate
i., whiplash
i., work-related
i., wrist

ink blot test
ink blot test, Rorschach
inlay(s)
i. bone graft
i. bone graft, diamond
i. bone graft ▸ dual
i. bone graft, sliding
i., cast
i., crowns or
i., epithelial
i., gold
i. graft
i. graft, diamond
i. graft, sliding
i., porcelain

inlet
i., conjugate diameter of pelvic
i. left ventricle (LV), double
i., pelvic
i. position
i., thoracic
i. ventricle anomaly, double
i. ventricle, double

Inman's disease
innate immunity
innatus, calor
inner
i. artery walls

i. aspect
i. canthus
i. canthus, left
i. canthus, right
i. cell mass
i. child issues
i. dimension
i. ear
i. ear atresia
i. ear, balance mechanism of
i. ear deafness
i. ear disease ▸ auto-immune
i. ear disorder
i. ear dysfunction, benign
i. ear electronic implantation
i. ear ▸ fluid-filled
i. ear hair cells
i. ear hearing loss
i. ear implant
i. ear inflammation
i. ear infection
i. ear infection ▸ viral
i. ear ▸ erosion of
i. ear nystagmus
i. ear structures
i. eye pressure
i. hair cell
i. hamstring
i. layer of aorta
i. layer of cornea
i. layer of endothelial cells
i. lining of bladder
i. malleolus
i. membrane, egg's
i. mucous membrane
i. phalangeal cells
i. pillar cells
i. pillars
i. quadrant, lower
i. quadrant, upper
i. rods
i. structures of the ear
i. surface of abdominal wall
i. surface of ribs
i. table frontal bone
i. table of skull
i. tension, feeling of
i. world

innermost intercostal muscles
innermost membrane of
meninges
innervated, muscles
innervation
i., aberrant peripheral
i. apraxia

i., autonomic sensory
i., disruption of normal
i., double
i. of bladder ▸ normal motor
i. of lung, autonomic
i. of lung, cholinergic
i. of lung ▸ parasympathetic
i. of lung ▸ sympathetic
i., reciprocal

innocent
i. appearing tissue
i. heart murmur
i. murmur
i. murmur of elderly

innocuous lumps
innocuous tumor
innominate
i. aneurysm
i. artery
i. artery, right
i. bone
i. osteotomy
i. vein

innovation, scientific
innovative
i. psychiatric nursing intervention
strategies
i. therapy
i. treatment

INO (intranuclear ophthalmo-
plegia)
inoculate, varicella
inoculated virus, auto-
inoculation
i., curative
i., cutaneous
i., direct
i., flu
i., guinea pig
i. hepatitis
i., influenza
i., intracerebral
i., parenteral
i., periodic
i., physical
i., pneumonia
i., protective
i., stress
i. training ▸ stress
i. transmission of viral hepatitis

inopectic diathesis
inoperable
i. bladder malignancy
i. brain tumor
i. cancer

inoperable—_continued_
  i. carcinoma, extensive
  i. esophageal carcinoma
  i. gastric carcinoma
  i. hemangioblastoma
  i. malignancy
  i. metastatic lung cancer
  i. ovarian cancer
  i. pancreatic cancer
  i., patient totally
  i., tumor
  i. tumor, shrink
inorganic
  i. chemistry
  i. dust disease
  i. iodine, plasma
  i. iron
  i. murmur
inorata, Culiseta
inotrope, negative
inotropic
  i. agent ‣ nonglycoside
  i. agents
  i. arrhythmia
  i. drugs
  i. effect
  i. medication
  i. state
  i. support
inotropy, negative
inpatient
  i. admission, potential
  i. care
  i. care, standard
  i. care, surgical
  i. counselor
  i. days
  i. detoxification
  i. facility
  i. non-psychiatric medical
    facilities
  i. psychiatric care
  i. psychiatric consultation
  i. psychiatric treatment
  i. rehabilitation
  i. service, specialty
  i. setting
  i. status
  i. surgery
  i. to outpatient transfer
  i. treatment
  i. treatment protocols
  i. unit
in-phase discrimination
in-phase signals

input
  i. circuit
  i. device
  i. frequency, amplified
  i. from spinal cord ‣ sensory
  i. impedance
  i. impedance, high
  i. ‣ lowered levels of
  i. resistance
  i. shunt in capacitance
  i. signal, isolate
  i. signal voltage, ratio of
  i. stage
  i. terminal
  i. terminal 1
  i. terminal 2
  i. terminals, respective
  i. terminals, two
  i. test ‣ common
    electroencephalogram (EEG)
  i. voltage
**INPAV (intermittent negative-
  pressure assisted ventilation)**
inquiry
  i., functional
  i., hospice
  i., judicial
INR (international normalized ratio)
insane
  i., criminally
  i. ear
  i. finger
insaniens, chorea
insanity
  i., adolescent
  i., affective
  i., alcoholic
  i., alternating
  i., anticipatory
  i., bordering on
  i., choreic
  i., circular
  i., climacteric
  i., communicated
  i., compound
  i., compulsive
  i., confusional
  i., consecutive
  i., cyclic
  i., doubting
  i., emotional
  i., hereditary
  i., homicidal
  i., homochronous
  i., hysteric

  i., idiophrenic
  i., impulsive
  i., manic-depressive
  i., moral
  i., perceptional
  i., periodic
  i., polyneuritic
  i., primary
  i., puerperal
  i., recurrent
  i., senile
  i., simultaneous
  i., toxic
insatiable appetite from depression
insatiable appetite from diabetes
insect
  i. bite, stinging
  i. bites
  i. -borne infection
  i. -infested
  i. ring ‣ drowsiness from
  i. sting allergy
  i. sting anaphylaxis
  i. sting ‣ blister from
  i. sting ‣ dizziness from
  i. sting ‣ pain in abdomen from
  i. sting treatment
  i. sting treatment ‣ emergency
  i. venom ‣ allergic to
  i. venom ‣ allergy to
  i. viruses
insecticide poisoning
insecure, patient
insecurity
  i., emotional
  i., lifelong
  i., ligamentous
  i. ‣ manifestation of latent
insemination
  i., artificial
  i. donor, artificial
  i., heterologous
  i., homologous
  i., homologous artificial
  i. (TDI) ‣ therapeutic donor
insensible fluid output
insensible thirst
insensitive
  i. current ‣ toxin
  i. limbs
  i. to inhibitor, target enzyme
  i. to others
  i. to pain
insensitivity, carotid
insensitivity to pain

insert
- i., intramucosal
- i. mattress sutures
- i. of shunt, peritoneal
- i. radioactive implant
- i., shoe
- i. teeth, metal

inserted
- i. and positioned, monitoring lines
- i., cardiac catheter with balloon
- i., catheter
- i., Copper 7 intrauterine device (IUD)
- i., drain
- i., glycerin suppository
- i. in cerebral cortex ▸ electrodes
- i. into neck and head of femur ▸ nail
- i. into trachea with ease ▸ scope
- i., rib spreader
- i., speculum
- i., suction tubes
- i. through vocal cords with ease ▸ bronchoscope
- i., tracheostomy tube
- i., tube
- i. under shoulder, pillow

insertion
- i. activity
- i., arterial line
- i., bony
- i., cesium
- i., cystoradium
- i. ▸ implantable cardiac defibrillator
- i., medial transplantation of patellar tendon
- i., muscle reflected from
- i. of arterial pressure (AP) line
- i. of fixation device
- i. of intraocular lens
- i. of placenta, low
- i. of prosthesis
- i. of radium, cervical
- i. of stent
- i. of synthetic tube
- i. of vascular prosthesis
- i., pacemaker
- i., patellar tendon
- i., permanent pacemaker
- i. plastic ball
- i. polyethylene implant
- i., radium
- i. ▸ route of
- i., Rush rod
- i., scleral

- i. site
- i. site, catheter
- i. site ▸ selected
- i., tandem
- i. technique, direct
- i. ▸ tympanostomy tube
- i., vasopacemaker

Inservice
- I. Education
- I. Education Director
- I. Education programs
- I. Program, Hospital
- I., Staff

inside
- i. diameter
- i. eye, bleeding
- i. neurons
- i. out, suturing cyst
- i. skull, bleeding
- i. the eye, painless increased pressure

insidiosa, Erysipelothrix
insidiosus, Triphleps
insidious onset of dyspnea
insight
- i. and self-care ▸ understanding,
- i. into illness
- i., lack of
- i. oriented psychotherapy, intensive
- i. -oriented therapy
- i., patient has poor
- i., psychoanalytic
- i. psychotherapy
- i. skills
- i., sudden

insightful experience
insipid
insipidus (DI), diabetes
insipidus, nephrogenic diabetes
insipient gangrene
insistence, inflexible
insistence on sameness
insolation, asphyxial
insolation, hyperpyrexial
insolita, Azotomonas
insoluble amidine
insomnia
- i. and fatigue ▸ depression,
- i. and nightmares
- i. and orthopnea ▸ breathlessness,
- i. and paranoia
- i., autogenic training for
- i., chronic
- i., conditioned
- i., drug withdrawal

- i., fatal familial
- i., fatigue and
- i. from alcohol
- i. from anxiety
- i. from caffeine
- i. from depression
- i. from gonorrhea
- i., group treatment of
- i., hyperactivity and decreased appetite
- i., hypnotic relaxation for
- i., increasing
- i., intermittent
- i., internal arousal
- i., initial
- i., management of
- i. ▸ pain, fatigue, and
- i. ▸ patient has
- i., primary
- i., progressive relaxation for
- i., psychic
- i., psychophysiological
- i. ▸ rapid eye movement (REM) sleep interruption
- i. related to a known organic factor
- i. related to mental disorder (nonorganic)
- i., severe
- i., short-term
- i., sleep maintenance
- i., sleep onset
- i., transient

insomniac
- i., chronic
- i., paranoid
- i., patient
- i., sleep patterns of

inspected [*infected*]
inspected, larynx
inspected, pelvis
inspection(s)
- i., cataract
- i., direct
- i., regular self-
- i. ▸ video otoscopic ear canal
- i., visual

inspirated, volume of air
inspiration
- i. and expiration
- i. and expiration of air ▸ alternate
- i., deep
- i. ▸ duration of
- i., full
- i., jerky
- i. ▸ prolonged deep

inspiration—*continued*
- i. ratio, expiration-
- i., wheezing on

inspiratory
- i. capacity (IC)
- i. crackles ▸ end-
- i. dyspnea
- i. expiratory (I/E) ratio
- i. flow (FIF) ▸ forced
- i. flow (PIF) ▸ peak
- i. flow rate (IFR)
- i. flow rate (MIFR) ▸ maximal
- i. flow rate (PIFR) ▸ peak
- i. force
- i. force, maximum
- i. force (NIF) ▸ negative
- i. murmur
- i. muscles
- i. positive airway pressure
- i. pressure (MIP) ▸ maximum
- i. pressure ▸ positive
- i. pressure ▸ zero-end
- i. rales
- i. reserve capacity
- i. reserve volume (IRV)
- i. respiration
- i. rhonchi
- i. sounds
- i. spasm
- i. standstill
- i. stridor
- i. vital capacity (FIVC) ▸ forced
- i. wheezing

inspired oxygen (F/0₂) ▸ fraction of
inspired oxygen (O₂), supplemental
inspissated cerumen
inspissated milk syndrome
instabilis, Trichostrongylus
instability
- i., affective
- i. and impulsivity ▸ emotional
- i. artifact ▸ temporal
- i., atlantoaxial
- i., cardiac
- i., cardiovascular
- i., catheter
- i., chronic
- i., cruciate
- i., emotional
- i., episodic emotional
- i., hemodynamic
- i., inversion
- i., joint
- i., lateral
- i., ligamentous

- i., lumbosacral
- i., mood
- i., nervous
- i., neurologic
- i. of head and trunk ▸ rhythmic
- i. of heart ▸ electrical
- i. of knee
- i. of lumbosacral joint
- i. ▸ pervasive pattern of
- i., postural
- i., psychiatric
- i. to straighten ▸ pain in back with
- i., truncal
- i., vascular
- i., vasomotor

installation [*instillation*]
instant delivery
instant thin layer chromatography
instantaneous
- i. electrical axis
- i. gradient ▸ peak
- i. pressure (IP)
- i. spectral peak velocity
- i. vector

instillation [*installation*]
- i., intratracheal
- i., lavage
- i., local
- i. of diagnostic media
- i. of x-ray contrast media

instilled
- i., carbon dioxide (CO₂)
- i., drops
- i. in anterior chamber ▸ air bubble
- i., x-ray contrast media

instinct(s)
- i., death
- i., ego
- i., herd
- i., mother
- i., sexual

instinctual decision
instinctual drive
Institute
- I. (NCI) ▸ National Cancer
- I. of Pathology (AFIP) ▸ Armed Forces
- I. on Drug Abuse (NIDA) ▸ National

instituted, emergency measures
institution
- i. ▸ comprehensive health care
- i., health care
- i. of therapy
- i., recipient

institutional
- i. activities
- i. care
- i. clinical trials, multi-
- i. communication
- i. dysentery
- i. respite care, short-term
- I. Review Board (IRB)
- i. units

institutionalized adult patient
instructing nursing students
instructing students, nursing
instruction(s)
- i., binary
- i. in self-management
- i., intratreatment therapeutic
- i., mnemonic
- i., postdischarge
- i., pretreatment therapeutic
- i. sheet, discharge
- i. sheet ▸ patient education
- i. understood ▸ follow-up

instrument(s) (Instrument)
- i., acupuncture
- i., attempted passage of
- i., binocular
- i., biofeedback
- i. birth (IB)
- i. ▸ complete change of drapes, gowns and
- i., contamination from
- i. ▸ ear piercing
- i., electroencephalogram (EEG) recording
- i., gas sterilized
- I., Grass Ten Channel
- i., inadequately sterilized
- i., indirect contact with contaminated
- i., microsurgical
- i., or syringes ▸ used needles,
- i., pachometer
- i. passed with ease
- i. passed without difficulty
- i. performance
- i., puncturing of skin by contaminated
- i., successful passage of
- i., tattooing
- i., telescope-like
- i., viewing

instrumental
- i. alteration in wave form
- i. compression
- i. conditioning

i. conditioning of diastolic blood
   pressure (BP)
i. distortion
i. heart rate responses
i. labor
i. malfunction
i. means
i. percussion
i. phase reversal
i. sensitivities

instrumentation
i., advanced
i. (AB-BI) ▸ advanced breast biopsy
i., angiographic
i., biofeedback
i., endoscopy
i., Harrington spinal
i., urethral

insufferable pain

insufficiency
i., active
i., acute cardiac
i., adrenal
i., adrenal gland
i., adrenocortical
i. (AI) ▸ aortic
i., aortic valvular
i., arterial
i., atrioventricular (AV) valve
i., autonomic
i., basilar
i., capsular
i. (CI) ▸ cardiac
i., cerebrovascular
i. ▸ chronic adrenocortical
i., chronic venous
i. (CI), coronary
i., deep venous
i., dietary
i., divergence
i. ▸ Duane classification of
   convergence
i., exocrine
i. ▸ exocrine pancreatic
i., gastric
i., gastromotor
i., hepatic
i., hiatal
i., ileocecal
i. ▸ mild chronic pancreatic exocrine
i. (MI) ▸ mitral
i. ▸ mitral valve
i. ▸ moderate chronic pancreatic
   exocrine
i., multivalve

i., muscular
i., myocardial
i., myovascular
i. of aorta
i. of eyelids
i. of prematurity, chronic pulmonary
i. of thyroid secretion
i., oxygen (O_2)
i., pancreatic
i., pancreatic exocrine
i., parathyroid
i. ▸ permanent adrenocortical
i., placental
i. ▸ primary adrenocortical
i., pseudoaortic
i., pulmonary
i., pulmonic
i., renal
i., respiratory
i. revascularization syndrome ▸
   pulmonary
i. ▸ rheumatic mitral
i. ▸ secondary adrenocortical
i., severe autonomic
i., severe functional
i., severe pancreatic
i., severe respiratory
i. ▸ Sternberg myocardial
i. syndrome, coronary
i. syndrome, pancreatic
i., thyroid
i. (TI), tricuspid
i., uterine
i., uteroplacental
i., valvular
i., vascular
i., velopharyngeal
i., venous
i. ▸ venous valvular
i., vertebrobasilar
i. ▸ vertebrobasilar arterial
i. with malabsorption, pancreatic

insufficient
i. blood flow
i. blood flow to heart
i. blood supply
i. coronary artery circulation
i. fluid intake
i. government reimbursements
i. severity of duration

insufflated, peritoneal cavity

insufflation
i., air
i. anesthesia
i., cranial

i., endotracheal
i., methylene blue
i. of carbon dioxide (CO_2)
i. of the lungs
i., perirenal
i., presacral
i., retroperitoneal gas
i., thoracoscopic
i. ▸ thoracoscopic talc
i., tubal
i., tubo-

insufflator, tube

insula
i., limen of
i., long gyrus of
i., short gyri of

insulae
i., gyri
i., gyri breves
i., gyrus longus
i., limen

insular
i. gyrus of brain ▸ superior
i. sclerosis
i. scotoma

insulated leads

**insulation failure in ventricular
   lead**

insulator, electrical

insulin [*inulin*]
i. activity, plasma
i., allergy to
i. and potassium ▸ glucose,
i. antibodies ▸ human
i., artificial
i., beef
i., bonito fish
i. clearance
i. clearance test
i. coma therapy
i. coma treatment
i., crystalline
i. deficiency
i. delivery system ▸
   preprogrammed
i. -dependent
i. -dependent, diabetes
i. dependent diabetes mellitus
   (IDDM), Type I
i. dosage
i. factor, undergraded
i., fast-acting
i. gene
i., globin
i., human

insulin—*continued*
- i., immunoreactive
- i. independent
- i. infusion, continuous
- i. infusion pump ▸ implantable
- i. infusion, regular
- i. infusion system ▸ portable
- i., inhaleable
- i. inhaler
- i. injection
- i. injector ▸ air-jet
- i. iodine
- i., Lente
- i. level
- i. -like activity
- i. -like growth factor
- i., long-acting
- i. molecule
- i., nasal
- i. nasal spray
- i., oral
- i., pancreas secretes
- i. pen injector
- i. pen pump
- i., pig
- i., pork
- i., premixed
- i. preparation
- i. producing cells
- i. production
- i., protamine
- i. pump, Autosyringe
- i. pump ▸ closed loop
- i. pump, external
- i. pump, Felig
- i. pump, internal
- i. pump, mechanical
- i. rainbow, regular
- i. reaction
- i. reaction ▸ incapacitating
- i. receptor
- i. receptor cells ▸ malfunctioning
- i. ▸ regular purified pork
- i. regulation
- i. release ▸ stimulating
- i. resistance
- i. resistance ▸ severe
- i. resistance syndrome
- i. -resistant diabetes
- i., secreted
- i. secretion
- i. sensitivity
- i. sensitivity test
- i. shock
- i. shock ▸ confusion from
- i. shock therapy
- i. shock treatment
- i., short-acting
- i., soluble
- i. stimulation
- i., synthetic
- i. therapy
- i. therapy, intensive
- i. therapy, low
- i. therapy, low dose intravenous (IV)
- i. therapy, sliding scale
- i. tolerance test
- i. tolerance test ▸ glucose-
- i. treatment
- i. treatment, subcoma
- i. treatment, subshock
- i., Ultralente

insult
- i., cardiac
- i., pathologic
- i., vascular

insurance
- i., catastrophic health
- i. claim
- i. coordinator
- i. examination
- i., health
- i., national health
- i. policy
- i., private medical
- i., supplemental

intact [*impact*]
- i. anastomosis
- i. auditory nerve
- i. blister ▸ painless, small,
- i. bone structure
- i. breast, radiation therapy for
- i. chest muscles
- i., cognitively
- i., cranial nerves
- i., cranial nerves grossly
- i., dressings dry and
- i. drum
- i. ▸ extraocular movements (EOM)
- i. (EOMI), extraocular movements
- i., fundi
- i. hymen
- i. implants
- i. motor skills
- i. motor tract
- i., neurologically
- i. neurons
- i. outer rim
- i. pedicles

- i., peripheral pulses
- i., placenta
- i., placenta delivered
- i. rib cage
- i. round window
- i., sensory tract
- i., septum
- i., skin sutures
- i. spinal cord
- i., tendons
- i. tissues
- i., tonsils
- i. vision

intake
- i., adequate calories
- i., alcohol
- i., alteration in hydration
- i., alteration in nutrition
- i. and output
- i. and output ▸ monitor fluid
- I. Assessment
- i. assessment staff
- i., caffeine
- i., calcium
- i., caloric
- i., calorie
- i., daily caloric
- i. data
- i., dietary
- i., dietary cholesterol
- i., dietary fat
- i., diminished salt
- i., excessive alcoholic
- i., excessive fluid
- i., fat
- i. fluid
- i., increased
- i. ▸ initial levels of alcohol
- i., insufficient fluid
- i. interview
- i. interview of family
- i. interview, pre-
- i., limit salt
- i., limiting alcohol
- i., low sodium
- i. ▸ manage fluid
- i., nutrient
- i. of fluids ▸ inadequate
- i. of food
- i. of liquid
- i. ▸ optimum calorie
- i., oral
- i., output and
- i. /output, fluid
- i., poor dietary

i., poor oral
i., potassium
i. process ▸ family services
i., protein
i., reduce
i., reduce salt
i., reduce sodium
i. ▸ reduction of salt
i. ▸ restricting food
i., salt
i. ▸ saturated fat
i., saturated for
i., sodium
i., sugar
i., therapeutic nutritional
i., total fat
i., water
i. withdrawal, alcohol

integral
i. dose
i., secant
i., sievert

integrated
i. anger management (IAM)
i. approach
i. bipolar sensing
i. electromyogram
i. lead system
i. medicine
i. psychotherapy
i. therapy
i. treatment

integrating microscope
integration
i., biological
i., internal
i., neuromuscular
i., primary
i., secondary
i., sensory
i. training ▸ sensory

integrative
i. couple therapy (ICT)
i. neurobehavioral approach
i. problem ▸ sensory

integrity
i., arterial wall
i., cell
i., impaired skin
i. ▸ impaired tissue
i. ▸ impairment of skin
i., skin

integrum, restitutio
integument, common
integumentary barrier

integumenti communis ▸ vasa sanguinea
intellectual
i. abilities ▸ decline in
i. ability
i. activity ▸ continuous
i. and emotional growth ▸ interference with
i. and motor skills
i. and physical power ▸ feeling of
i. decline
i. deficiencies
i. deficit
i. deterioration
i. deterioration ▸ progressive
i. development
i. dysfunction
i. efficiency, enhanced
i. environment
i. evaluation
i. exertion
i. faculties, loss of
i. focus ▸ poor
i. function
i. function or memory
i. function ▸ permanent decline in
i. function ▸ progressive decline in
i. function, slowed
i. functioning
i. functioning, borderline
i. impairment
i. level
i. life
i. potential
i. power factor
i. stimulation
i. stimuli

intellectualization, philosophical
intellectually
i. conscious
i. stimulated
i. stimulating activities

intelligence (Intelligence)
i., borderline
i., crystallized
i., decreased
i., fluid
i., human
i., impaired
i., limited
i., memory, perception and sensation
i. quotient (IQ)
i. quotient (IQ), performance
i. quotient (IQ) test

I. Quotient Test, full scale (IQ)
i. quotient (IQ), verbal
I. Scale, Cattell Infant
I. Scale for Children (WISC) Test, Wechsler
I. Scale (WAIS) Test, Wechsler Adult
I. Scale (WAIS) ▸ Wechsler Adult

intelligible speech
intended overdose
intense [*intent*]
i. abandonment fears
i. anger ▸ inappropriate,
i. back pain
i. burning pain
i. concentration
i. confrontations
i. coughing
i. course, short
i. cramping
i. craving ▸ irritability, restlessness, and
i. cycle of high dose chemotherapy
i. dread, sensation of
i. effects
i. envy, chronic
i. episodic dysphoria
i. euphoria
i. fear, attack of
i. fear of fatness
i. feelings
i. headache pain
i. high
i. interpersonal relationship
i. itching
i. levels
i. motor agitation
i. need to void ▸ immediate
i. outpatient programs
i. outpatient treatment program
i. pain
i., patient
i., prolonged chest pain
i. psychoactive drug effect
i. relationship
i. relationships ▸ unstable and
i., short-term anxiety
i., short-term irritability
i., short-term moodiness
i. stabbing pain
i. sweating
i. tantrums
i. terror, attack of
i. therapy ▸ aggressive
i. throbbing pain

intensification factor
intensifier, image
intensifying screen
intensity (Intensity)
    i., absolute
    i. analysis, dose
    i. and duration
    i., echo
    i. exercise, high
    i. exercise, low
    i. exercise ▸ moderate
    i., high beam
    i. ▸ levels of shock
    i. light source, high
    i., luminous
    i., maximal
    i., medical
    I. Modulated Radiation Therapy
      (IMRT)
    i. of contractions
    i. of electric field
    i. of headache
    i. of impulse
    i. of labor contractions
    i. of magnetism
    i. of movement ▸ diminished
    i. of pain
    i. of roentgen rays
    i. of service
    i., optimal
    i., performance
    i. (PMI) ▸ point of maximum
    i. ▸ running frequency and
    i., spatial
    i. stimulation, low
    i., stimulus
intensive (Intensive)
    i. addiction treatment unit ▸
      medically managed
    i. antimicrobial therapy
    i. care
    i. care facility
    I. Care (NIC) ▸ Neonatal
    I. Care Unit (ICU)
    I. Care Unit (CICU) ▸ Cardiology
    I. Care Unit (CICU) ▸ Coronary
    I. Care Unit (MICU) ▸ Medical
    I. Care Unit (MICU) ▸ Mobile
    I. Care Unit (NICU) ▸ Neonatal
    I. Care Unit (PICU), Prenatal
    I. Care Unit (PICU) ▸ Pulmonary
    i. care unit (ICU) psychosis
    I. Care Unit (SICU) ▸ Surgical
    i. care unit (ICU) syndrome
    i. chemotherapy

i. chemotherapy treatment
I. Cocaine Program
i. colposcopy
i. combination chemotherapy
i. coronary care
I. Coronary Care Unit (ICCU)
i. dietary therapy
i. exercise
i. hyperventilation, prolonged
i. insight-oriented psychotherapy
i. insulin therapy
i. nursing care
i. outpatient program
I. Outpatient Program ▸ Day
i. outpatient treatment program
i. postnatal intervention
i. prenatal care
i. scientific investigation
i. stimulation of senses
i. structured hospitalization
i. supportive programs
i. therapy
i. therapy group
i. therapy observation unit (ITOU)
i. therapy unit (ITU)
i. topical antibiotic therapy
i. treatment
i. use
intent [*intense*]
intent to control
intent, volitional
intention
    i. healing by first, second or third
    i. spasm
    i. tremor
    i. tremor, ataxia and
    i. tremor of extremities
    i. tremor, slight
    i. ▸ wound healed by first, second or
      third
intentional
    i. overdose
    i. recall
    i. replantation
    i. vomiting
intentionally causing death
intentionem, per primam
intentionem, per secundum
interabdominal pressure
inter-acinar connective tissue,
    overgrowth of
interact with others
interacting determinants of pain
interacting massive particle (WIMP) ▸
    weakly

interaction(s)
    i., alcohol
    i. and detoxification, clinical
    i., antagonistic
    i., aspirin
    i. between anxiety and pain ▸
      circular
    i., biomaterial
    i., chemical
    i., child-centered
    i., clinical and pharmacological
    i., complex
    i., drug
    i., drug-drug
    i., drug-food
    i. evaluation ▸ parent-child
    i., facilitate
    i., family
    i., group
    i., hallucinogenic drug
    i. ▸ herb drug
    i., human
    i. ▸ impaired social
    i., interpersonal
    i. ▸ laser tissue
    i. ▸ life-threatening drug
    i., medical
    i., medical-legal
    i., mind body
    i. ▸ mother-infant
    i., parent-child
    i., photoelectric
    i. ▸ potential drug
    i. ▸ protein-protein
    i., radiative
    i., social
    i. ▸ staff patient
    i. ▸ staff training and
    i. surgical navigation (ISN)
    i., synergistic
    i., toxicity or drug
    i. with alcohol, drug
    i. with peers
interactive exercise
interactive process-oriented
    group
interalveolar fibrin
interalveolaria maxillae, septa
interamniotic infection
interannular segment
interaortic balloon pump
interarterial
    i. communication
    i. fluid
    i. septum

i. shunt
i. volume
interarticular cartilage
interarticular disc
interarticularis, pars
interarytenoid muscle
interarytenoid notch
interatrial
i. groove
i. septal defect
i. septal defect closure
i. septum (IAS)
interauditory canal tomogram
interauricular loop, Gerdy's
interauricular septum
intercalary cell
intercalary staphyloma
intercalated disc
intercalatum, Schistosoma
intercanthic diameter
intercapillary glomerulosclerosis
intercapillary nephrosclerosis
intercapital vein
intercapitular vein of foot
intercapitular vein of hand
intercarotid ganglion
intercarpal joint
intercartilaginous incision
intercartilaginous rim
intercellular
i. bridges
i. coupling
i. junction
i. organisms, obligate
i. parasites
i. spaces
i. tissue space
intercept angle
interclavicular
i. notch
i. notch of occipital bone
i. notch of temporal bone
intercondylar
i. eminence
i. fracture
i. fracture of hip
i. groove
i. notch
i. notch of femur
i. process
interconnection, neuronal
intercostal
i. anesthesia
i. artery
i. block

i. brachial nerve
i. catheter
i. drain
i. groove
i. lymph nodes
i. margin
i. muscle
i. muscles, external
i. muscles, innermost
i. muscles, internal
i. myalgia
i. nerve
i. nerve block
i. nerve cut
i. nerve resected
i. retraction
i. retraction, sternal
i. space (ICS)
i. space (ICS) ▸ fifth
i. space (PMI 5th ICS) ▸ point of
   maximum impulse fifth
i. tenderness
i. tenderness, parasternal
i. tube
i. vein
i. vein, anterior
i. vein, highest
i. vein, left superior
i. vein of hand
i. vein (IV-XI) ▸ posterior
i. vein, right superior
i. vessels
i. vessels ligated
i. zoster
intercostobrachial nerve
intercourse
i., anal
i., heterosexual
i., homosexual anal
i. ▸ involuntary deviate sexual
i., painful
i., sexual
i., vaginal
intercristal diameter
intercurrent diagnosis
interdental gingiva
interdermal buried suture
interdiction program, drug
interdigital neuroma
interdisciplinary
i. approach
i. care, physician directed
i. team
i. team approach
i. team (IDT) meeting

interectopic interval
interelectrode
i. distance
i. distances, large
i. distances, long
i. distances, short
i. distances, small
interest(s)
i. and aptitude, activity
i. and concentration ▸ enhanced
i., appetite and concentration ▸ loss
   of
i., decreased sexual
i. in activities ▸ loss of
i. in others ▸ lack of
i. in peer social activities ▸ loss of
i. in personal goals ▸ apathy and
   lack of
i. in personal grooming ▸ loss of
i. in society ▸ apathy and lack of
i. in surroundings, patient has no
i. in usual activities ▸ loss of
i. ▸ lack of reciprocal
i. ▸ loss of sexual
i. of opposite sex, decline in
i., sexual
interesting sociological phenomenon
(ISP)
interface
i. arterial blood filter
i. between electrode and brain
i. between electrode and scalp
i. effects
i., electrode skin
interfacial surface tension
interfascicular fibrous tissue
interference
i. beat
i., blood crossmatching
i. device (SQUID) ▸
   superconducting quantum
i. ▸ dissociation by
i., electrical
i., electromagnetic
i., external
i., external electrical
i., extraneous scalp muscle
   electrical
i., isorhythmic atrioventricular (AV)
   dissociation with
i. microscope
i. microscopy (RIM) ▸ reflection
i. movement
i. pattern
i. pattern, reduced

interference—*continued*
- i. phenomenon
- i. (RFI), radiofrequency
- I. with circulation, localized
- i. with intellectual and emotional growth
- i. with judgment and decision making

interfering artifacts
interfering thoughts
interferon
- i., alpha
- i. alpha ▸ recombinant
- i. alpha therapy
- i., Alpha II
- i., autologous
- i., endogenous
- i., exogenous
- i., gamma
- i., human
- i., human leukocyte
- i., immune
- i. inducers
- i., mouse
- i., murine
- i., recombinant
- i. therapy
- i. treatment

interfibrillar substance of Flemming
interfilar substance
interfoveolar muscle
interhemispheric derivation
interictal paroxysmal activity
interim
- i. analysis
- i. glucose determinations
- i. period

interior [*inferior*]
- i. chest wall
- i. epidural protrusion
- i. gestation
- i. of tumor excavated
- i. resources

interlaced scanning
interlacing blood vessels
interlacing ligature
interleukin-1 beta
interleukin-2 treatment
interlobar
- i. artery
- i. empyema
- i. fissures
- i. notch
- i. pleurisy
- i. vein
- i. vein of kidney

interlobular
- i. artery
- i. emphysema
- i. pleurisy
- i. septa
- i. septum
- i. vein of kidney
- i. vein of liver

interlobularis purulenta, pneumonia
interlocked mesh prosthesis, Harrison
interlocking ligature
interlocking sutures
intermaxillary
- i. bone
- i. elastic
- i. fixation
- i. suture

intermedia, beta thalassemia
intermedia, pars
intermediary
- i. hemorrhage
- i. nerve
- i. sleep stage
- i. tissue, Kuhnt's
- i. vesicle

intermediate (Intermediate)
- i. abutment
- i. acting barbiturate
- i. age-related macular degeneration (AMD)
- i. bronchus
- i. callus
- i. care
- i. care facility
- I. Care Nursery (ICN)
- i. cell mass
- i. density lipoprotein
- i. disc
- i. dorsal cutaneous nerve
- i. dorsal cutaneous nerve of foot
- i. erythroblast
- i. examination
- i. fast activity
- i. fetal death
- i. frequencies
- i. ganglia
- i. hemorrhage
- i. host
- i. lobe of pituitary gland
- i. malignant teratoma
- i. mass
- I. Medical Care Unit (IMCU)
- i. membrane

- i. nerve
- i. neutron
- i. normoblast
- i. nursing care
- i. operation
- i., Purified Protein Derivative (PPD)
- i. rays
- i. skin graft
- i. split-thickness skin graft
- i. storage
- i. substance of spinal cord, central
- i. substance of spinal cord, lateral
- i. substance of suprarenal gland
- i. sulcus, postero-
- i. supraclavicular nerves
- i. syndrome
- i. thickness skin graft
- i. tissue ▸ vascular

Intermedics pacemaker
intermedium, Paracolobactrum
intermedium, paracolon
intermedius
- i. artery ▸ ramus
- i., Bacteroides
- i., bronchus
- i. muscle, vastus
- i. nerve
- i., Phlebotomus
- i., Prevotella
- i., sulcus

intermenstrual
- i. bleeding
- i. fever
- i. pain
- i. (IM) spotting

intermenstrualis, dysmenorrhea
intermetacarpal articulations
intermetatarsal articulations
interminable affliction
intermittens
- i. angiosclerotica ▸ dysbasia
- i. angiosclerotica intestinalis ▸ dyspragia
- i. ▸ dysbasia neurasthenica
- i., dyskinesia
- i., ischemia cordis
- i., otalgia
- i. ▸ pulsus respiration

intermittent
- i. affective disorder
- i. angina
- i. angioneurotic edema
- i. asthma
- i. atrial fibrillation
- i. attacks of severe vertigo

i. bleeding
i. catheterization
i. catheterization of bladder
i. cervical traction
i. cessation
i. chills and fever
i. claudication
i. confusion
i. contraction
i. contracture
i. coronary sinus occlusion
i. cramps
i. diarrhea
i. diplopia
i. diuretic therapy
i. double-step gait
i. double vision
i. elevation of blood pressure (BP)
i. episodes
i. episodes of acute abdominal pain
i. episodes of pain
i. explosive disorder
i. explosive personality disorder
i. facial contractures
i. fever
i. flashes of light
i. functional bowel problems
i. heart pain
i. hematuria
i. hematuria, painless
i. hemoptysis
i. hepatic fever
i. hydrosalpinx
i. insomnia
i. low back pain, chronic
i. mandatory ventilation
i. mandatory ventilation ▸ synchronized
i. menorrhagia
i. negative-pressure assisted ventilation (INPAV)
i. or continuous spasms
i. otorrhea
i. pain
i. parasite
i. periods of depression
i. photic stimulation
i. pneumatic compression
i. pneumatic compression boots
i. porphyria (AIP), acute
i. positive pressure (IPP)
i. positive pressure breathing (IPPB)
i. positive pressure inflation with oxygen (IPPO)

i. positive pressure respiration (IPPR)
i. positive pressure ventilation (IPPV)
i. pulse
i. radiation
i. reflux
i. reinforcement
i. rhythmic delta activity ▸ frontal
i. rhythmical delta activity (OIRDA), occipital
i. self-catheterization
i. skilled nursing care
i. small bowel obstruction
i. spotting
i. spotting and cramping
i. sterilization
i. steroid therapy
i. strabismus
i. therapy
i. tonic muscular contractions
i. traction
i. tremor
i. ventilation ▸ forced mandatory
i. vomiting
intermittently anxious
intermixed fibrosis ▸ partial
intermixed with alpha rhythm
intermuscular hernia
intern (*same as* interne)
interna
 i., auris
 i., endometriosis
 i., hyperostosis frontalis
 i., lamina
 i., leptomeningitis
 i., mastoiditis
 i., ophthalmoplegia
 i., pericarditis externa et
internae, vasa auris
internal
 i. acoustic meatus
 i. adhesive pericarditis
 i. anatomy
 i. antifungal therapy
 i. arousal insomnia
 i. auditory (IA)
 i. auditory canal (IAC)
 i. auditory meatus (IAM)
 i. auditory veins
 i. auricular nerve
 i. auris
 i. awareness
 i. bladder, artificial
 i. bleeding

i. body clock
i. body heat
i. body temperature
i. canthal ligament
i. capsule, knee of
i. cardiac massage
i. cardioverter defibrillator
i. cardioverter defibrillator (AICD), automatic
i. carotid artery (ICA)
i. carotid artery, cavernous
i. carotid artery occlusion (ICAO)
i. carotid nerve
i. cerebral veins
i. cervical os
i. changes
i. clock
i. components of knee ▸ expand
i. conflicts
i. conjugate diameter
i. conversion
i. derangement
i. derangement, Hey's
i. derangement of joint
i. derangement of knee
i. diameter
i. diastolic diameter ▸ left ventricular (LV)
i. diastolic dimension ▸ left ventricular
i. dimension—diastole
i. dimension—left lateral
i. dimension—supine
i. dimension—systole
i. disconnection
i. disorder
i. ear
i. elastic lamina
i. elastic membrane
i. electrode
i. emotional arousal
i. events
i. examination, autopsy
i. examination, manual
i. eye pressure
i. factor
i. feelings
i. fetal heart rate monitoring
i. fistula
i. fixation
i. fixation of fracture
i. fixation (ORIF), open reduction and
i. hemorrhage
i. hemorrhoid

internal—*continued*
- i. hemorrhoidectomy
- i. hemorrhoids of rectum
- i. hernia
- i. hydrocephalus
- i. iliac adenopathy
- i. iliac artery
- i. iliac lymph nodes
- i. iliac vein
- i. inguinal ring
- i. injuries
- i. injury
- i. insulin pump
- i. integration
- i. intercostal muscles
- i. jugular chain lymph nodes
- i. jugular pressure (IJP)
- i. jugular vein
- i. jugular vein cannulation
- i. jugular vein, left
- i. jugular vein, right
- i. laryngeal nerve, superior
- i. learning process
- i. malleolus
- i. mammary artery
- i. mammary artery bypass
- i. mammary artery catheter
- i. mammary artery graft angiography
- i. mammary artery (LIMA) ‣ left
- i. mammary artery ‣ right
- i. mammary chain
- i. mammary dose
- i. mammary field, matching tangential field with
- i. mammary graft
- i. mammary involvement
- i. mammary lymph nodes
- i. mammary lymphoscintigraphy
- i. mammary vein
- i. medicine
- i. meningitis
- i. nares
- i. node involvement
- i. oblique
- i. oblique approximated
- i. oblique muscle
- i. oblique muscle of abdomen
- i. obstruction
- i. obturator muscle
- i. occipital nerve
- i. orifice
- i. os
- i. pacemaker
- i. pacemaker, external-

- i. popliteal nerve
- i. psychological conflict
- i. pterygoid muscle
- i. pterygoid nerve
- i. pudendal vein
- i. radiation
- i. radiation dose, medical
- i. radiation dosimetry
- i. radiation therapy
- i. rectus muscle, advancement of
- i. resistance
- i. respiration
- i. rotation
- i. rotation contracture of hip
- i. rotation exercise ‣ shoulder
- i. scalp stimulation test
- i. scar tissue
- i. secretion
- i. secretion gland
- i. secretions of body
- i. sensation
- i. sense
- i. shock
- i. spermatic fascia
- i. spermatic vessel
- i. sphincter
- i. sphincter muscle
- i. sphincter muscle of anus
- i. sphincter ‣ relaxation
- i. sphincterotomy ‣ lateral
- i. states, voluntary control of
- i. strabismus
- i. structures, differentiated
- i. substance of suprarenal gland
- i. tarsorrhaphy
- i. thoracic artery
- i. thoracic veins
- i. thyroarytenoid muscle
- i. transmission
- i. urethral orifice
- i. urethrotomy (DVIU), direct vision
- i. version

internasal suture
international (International)
- I. Association of Laryngectomees
- i. benzoate unit (IBU)
- I. Montage
- i. normalized ratio (INR)
- i. system, standard
- i. trends in drug abuse
- i. trials
- I. Unit (IU)
- i. units (MIU) ‣ million

interne (*see* intern)

internodal
- i. conduction
- i. pathway
- i. pathway, antegrade
- i. pathway, anterior
- i. tracts
- i. tracts, atrial

intern-on-call
internum, pericardium
internus, calor
interobserver variability
interorbital line
interosseous
- i. artery
- i. cartilage
- i. metacarpal vein ‣ dorsal
- i. muscle
- i. muscles of foot ‣ dorsal
- i. muscles of hand ‣ dorsal
- i. muscles, palmar
- i. muscles, planter
- i. muscles, volar
- i. nerve of forearm ‣ anterior
- i. nerve of forearm ‣ posterior
- i. nerve of leg
- i. vein of foot ‣ dorsal

interparietal
- i. bone
- i. hernia
- i. sulcus
- i. suture

interparietale, os
interpeak latency
interpedicular joint spaces
interpedicular spaces
interpeduncular
- i. cistern
- i. fossa
- i. ganglion

interperiosteal fracture
interpersonal
- i. conflict
- i. contact
- i. difficulty ‣ history of
- i. effectiveness
- i. exploitativeness
- i. influences
- i. interaction
- i. issues
- i. problem
- i. problem, other
- i. psychotherapy
- i. relations ‣ impaired
- i. relationship
- i. relationship ‣ intense

i. relationship ▸ unstable
i. situation, social or
i. skills
i. skills ▸ limited
i. skills, social
i. stresses ▸ extreme reactivity to
i. therapy
interpersonally objective
interphalangeal
  i. articulations
  i. (DIP) ▸ distal
  i. joint
  i. joint (DIPJ), distal
  i. joint (PIPJ), proximal
interpleural space
interpolated
  i. beat
  i. extrasystole
  i. flap
interposed abdominal compression (IAC)
interposed abdominal counterpulsation
interposition
  i. for esophageal disease, colon
  i., graft
  i., jejunal
  i. of colon
  i. operation
interpret written word ▸ inability to
interpretation
  i. and suggestion ▸ undisciplined
  i., auditory
  i., clinical
  i., dream
  i., immediate
  i. of reality
  i. of reality ▸ severe impairment in
  i., primary
  i., scan
  i., secondary
  i., visual
interpreter, language
interprismatic substance
interproximal space
interpubic disc
interpupillary distance (PD)
interpupillary line
interquartile range
interracial grafts
interradiculare, septum
interrogans, Leptospira
interrogation
  i., deep Doppler velocity
  i., Doppler

i. of telemetry
i., stereoscopic
interrupted
  i. aortic arch
  i. black silk sutures
  i. chromic sutures
  i. cotton sutures
  i. fashion
  i. fashion, simple
  i. fine silk sutures
  i. lymphatic drainage
  i. mattress sutures
  i. mattress sutures, silk
  i. plain catgut
  i. pledgeted suture
  i. respiration
  i. silk, skin closed with
  i. sleep
  i. suture
  i. suture, evening
  i. urine flow
  i. urine stream ▸ weak or
interrupting conduction of nerve impulses
interruption(s)
  i., aortic arch
  i., azygoportal
  i. ▸ duration of sleep
  i. in continuity of bone
  i. insomnia ▸ rapid eye movement (REM) sleep
  i. of blood supply
  i. of flow of urination
  i., response
  i., sleep
  i. (STI) structured treatment
interscalene nerve block
interscapular reflex
interscapular region
intersection point ▸ beam
interseizure period
Intersept cardiotomy
intersex
  i., female
  i., male
  i., true
intersigmoid hernia
interspace
  i., junctional
  i., lumbar
  i., narrowing of
  i., second left
  i., vertebral
  i., widening of
interspinal muscles

interspinal muscles of thorax
interspongioplastic substance
interstimulus interval (ISI)
interstitial
  i. acute inflammatory cells
  i. and perivascular collagen network
  i. atrophy
  i. brachytherapy
  i. cell stimulating hormone
  i. cell tumor
  i. cells
  i. clefts
  i. congestion
  i. cystitis
  i. disease
  i. disorder ▸ pulmonary
  i. ducts
  i. edema ▸ pulmonary
  i. emphysema
  i. emphysema (PIE), pulmonary
  i. fat
  i. fibers
  i. fibrosis
  i. fibrosis ▸ chronic pulmonary
  i. fibrosis, early
  i. fibrosis, extensive
  i. fibrosis, focal
  i. fibrosis ▸ focal subpleural
  i. fibrosis, patchy
  i. fibrosis, pulmonary
  i. fibrotic changes
  i. fluid
  i. gastritis
  i. glands
  i. granules, Kölliker's
  i. hemorrhage
  i. hemorrhage, focal
  i. hepatitis, chronic
  i. hernia
  i. hypersensitivity pneumonitis
  i. hyperthermia
  i. immaturity of lung
  i. implantation
  i. implantation of radioactive isotopes
  i. implants
  i. infiltrates
  i. inflammation
  i. inflammatory infiltrate ▸ chronic
  i. irradiation
  i. keratitis
  i. left ventricular myocardial fibrosis
  i. lung disease
  i. lung disease, chronic

interstitial—*continued*
- i. lung disease ▸ diffuse
- i. markings
- i. mastitis
- i. myocarditis
- i. nephritis
- i. neuropathy, progressive hypertrophic
- i. nuclei
- i. nuclei of anterior hypothalamus (INAH)
- i. organizing pneumonia
- i. pancreatitis
- i. pattern
- i. plaque, foamy
- i. plasma cell pneumonia
- i. pneumonia
- i. pneumonia, acute
- i. pneumonia, desquamative
- i. pneumonia ▸ idiopathic
- i. pneumonia ▸ lymphoid
- i. pneumonia oxygen (O₂) therapy ▸ organizing
- i. pneumonitis
- i. pneumonitis, acute
- i. pneumonitis (DIP), desquamative
- i. pneumonitis ▸ lymphocytic
- i. polymorphonuclear leukocyte infiltrate
- i. polymorphonuclear leukocytes
- i. pregnancy
- i. pulmonary edema
- i. pulmonary fibrosis
- i. pulmonary fibrosis, chronic
- i. pulmonary fibrosis, diffuse
- i. pulmonary fibrosis ▸ progressive
- i. pulmonary hemorrhages ▸ multiple
- i. radiation
- i. radiofrequency
- i. radiofrequency electric field
- i. radiotherapy
- i. restrictive lung disease
- i. salpingitis, chronic
- i. scarring
- i. scarring, focal
- i. scarring ▸ mild focal
- i. spaces
- i. substances
- i. tabes
- i. therapy
- i. tissue
- i. vessels, vascular congestion of
- i. water

interstitialis, calcinosis

interstitium
- i.. cardiac
- i. ▸ focal scarring of
- i. of lung
- i. ▸ subcapsular scarring in

intersystolic period
Intertach II pacer
intertarsal joints
interthalamic commissure
intertragic notch
intertragica, incisura
intertransverse muscles
- i.m., anterior
- i.m. of neck, anterior
- i.m. of neck, posterior
- i.m. of thorax

intertriginous vulvitis
intertrigo
- i., areas of
- i., eczema
- i. labialis

intertrochanteric
- i. fracture
- i. line
- i. plate
- i. region
- i. region fracture

intertropica, psilosis stomatitis
intertropica, stomatitis
intertuberal diameter
intertubular substance of tooth
intertubular tissue
intertypic recombinant
iterureteric fold
interureteric ridge
intervaginal [*intravaginal*]
interval(s)
- i., A-H
- i., anxiety
- i., atrial escape
- i., atriocarotid
- i., atrio-Hisian
- i., atrioventricular
- i., auriculocarotid
- i., auriculoventricular
- i., automatic
- i., A-V delay
- i. between doses ▸ time
- i. blood count
- i. blood count drawn
- i., cardioarterial
- i. CBC (complete blood count)
- i. chemotherapy
- i. clearing
- i., coupling

- i., critical coupling
- i., electromechanical
- i., escape
- i., fixed P-R
- i. ▸ flutter R
- i. growth
- i., half-hour
- i., hangout
- i., H-V
- i. improvement
- i., interectopic
- i. (ISI), interstimulus
- i., irregular
- i., isoelectric
- i., isometric
- i., isovolumic
- i., JT
- i. ▸ magnet pacing
- i. (MTI) ▸ minimum time
- i., monthly
- i. of time, predetermined
- i., P-A
- i. ▸ pacemaker escape
- i., passive
- i., P-H
- i., P-J
- i. platelet count
- i. postsphygmic
- i., P-P
- i., P-Q
- i., P-R
- i., presphygmic
- i., prolonged Q-T
- i., Q-H
- i., Q-M
- i., Q-R
- i., Q-RB
- i., QRS
- i., QRST
- i., Q-S2
- i., Q-T
- i., Q-Tc
- i., QU
- i. ▸ right ventricular (RV) systolic time
- i., R-P
- i., R-R
- i. ▸ R-R prime
- i., RS-T
- i. sensing pacemaker ▸ Q-T
- i., short P-R
- i., sphygmic
- i., S-QRS
- i., S-R
- i., ST

i. strength relation
i. ▸ symptom-free
i. syndrome ▸ idiopathic long Q-T
i. syndrome ▸ prolonged Q-T
i. syndrome ▸ Q-TU
i. systolic time
i., 30-minute
i., time
i., T-P
i., ventriculoatrial
i., wave
i., weekly
intervene with patient-at-risk
intervener survival
intervening period
intervening tissues
intervention(s)
i., abuse
i., active
i., acute medical management/
i., alcohol
i., behavioral
i., cardiac
i., clergy
i., clinical
i., cognitive behavioral
i., conflict
i., consent to
i., crisis
i., delayed
i., directional vascular
i. ▸ disaster crisis
i., effective
i., electrical
i., ergonomic
i., family
i., fetal
i., genetic
i. in drug abuse ▸ early
i., indicator
i., ineffective
i., intensive postnatal
i., lifestyle
i., medical
i. ▸ milieu management
i., neurosurgical
i., nonpharmacological
i., nursing
i., on-site
i. ▸ peer-driven
i., percutaneous
i., pharmacological
i., physical
i. ▸ physician-based
i. ▸ point of

i. (PEPI) ▸ postmenopausal
estrogen/progestin
i., prevention and early
i. ▸ primary care
i., program, drug
i., program, family
i., psychiatric
i. ▸ psychiatric nursing assessment
and
i., psychosocial
i., psychotherapeutic
i., rape
i., right to refuse
i. ▸ school-based
i., secondary
i., service, crisis
i., skills, crisis
i., social
i., social service
i., strategies
i., strategies ▸ innovative psychiatric
nursing
i. strategy ▸ expected
i., supportive
i., surgical
i., therapeutic
i., treatment
i. trial (MRFIT), multiple risk factor
i., vagomimetic
interventional
i. angiography
i. cardiac catheterization
i. echocardiography
i. radiologic technique
i. radiological technique
i. radiology
i. study
i. therapy
i. vascular stent ▸ Medtronic
interventricular
i. artery
i. conduction delay
i. foramen
i. heart block
i. septal amplitude ▸ apical
i. septal defect (IVSD)
i. septal motion
i. septal rupture
i. septum
i. septum aneurysm
i. septum, high membranous
i. septum of heart, congenital
defect
i. septum ▸ Swiss cheese
i. sulcus of heart

i. veins
intervertebral
i. body
i. cartilage
i. cartilage, calcification
i. cartilage, chondritis
i. disc
i. disc calcification
i. disc, crushing of
i. disc disease
i. disc, herniated
i. disc herniation
i. disc protrusion
i. disc, rupture of
i. disc space
i. disc space, narrowing of
i. fibrocartilages
i. foramina
i. ganglion of head, posterior
i. notch
i. spaces, wide
i. vein
interview
i. as a screening device for drug
abuse, patient
i. as a screening device, patient
i., clinical
i., collateral
i., initial
i., intake
i. of family ▸ intake
i., police
i., pre-intake
i. psychiatric diagnostic
i., risk assessment
interviewing, motivational
intervillous circulation
intervillous lacuna
interwoven bundle
intestinal
i. abscess
i. absorption
i. adhesions
i. amebiasis
i. anastomosis
i. angina
i. angiodysplasia
i. anthrax
i. atony
i. atresia
i. atresia, congenital
i. bacteria
i. biopsy
i. bleeding
i. bleeding, massive

intestinal—*continued*
i. bleeding ▸ painless
i. blockage
i. brush border
i. bypass
i. bypass surgery
i. candidiasis
i. cells, gut
i. claudication
i. complaint
i. contents
i. contraction ▸ painful
i. control in functional colitis
i. descending colon ▸ large
i. disease
i. disorder
i. disorder ▸ inflammatory
i. disorder ▸ upper
i. distomiasis
i. disturbance
i. dyspepsia
i., entero▸
i. epithelium
i. flora
i. flu
i. fluid
i. flukes
i. gas
i. gas, excessive
i. gas, overlying
i. gas pattern
i., gastro◊
i. glands
i. granulomatosis, lipophagic
i. growling
i. hemorrhage
i. hernia
i. herniation
i. hypermotility
i. infarction
i. infection
i. infection, severe
i. inflammation
i. intoxication
i. ischemia
i. lining
i. lipodystrophy
i. loop
i. lymphoma
i. malabsorption
i. malfunction
i. malrotation
i. metaplasia
i. movement
i. mucosa

i. myoneurosis
i. myxoneurosis
i. neuropathy
i. neurosis
i. obstruction
i. obstruction ▸ constipated from
i. obstruction ▸ diarrhea from
i. obstruction, partial
i. obstruction syndrome ▸ distal
i. parasites
i. parasites ▸ microscopic
i. peptidase
i. peptide (VIP) ▸ vasoactive
i. perforation
i. peristalsis
i. peritoneum
i. polyp
i. pouch
i. problems
i. protozoa
i. pseudo-obstruction
i. queasiness
i. secretions
i. serosa
i. spasm
i. spasticity
i. stasis
i. stimulant
i. strangulation
i. submucosa ▸ porcine small
i. submucosa ▸ small
i. sutures
i. tissue
i. tonic
i. tonsil
i. tract
i. tract carcinoid
i. tract gas
i. transplantation
i. tuberculosis
i. upsets
i. villi
i. wall
i. wall perforation
i. wall, small
i. wall ▸ spasm of
intestinalis
i., Campylobacter
i. ▸ dyspragia intermittens angiosclerotica
i. giardiasis
i., Lamblia
i., mycosis
i., Trichomonas

intestine(s)
i. absorption, small
i. as a defense barrier ▸ small
i., benign polyps of large
i. cancer ▸ small
i., carcinoid tumor of
i., carcinoma of large
i., demucosation of
i., distal portion of small
i., folds of large
i., incision into
i., inflamed
i., inflammation of
i., kinking of
i., large
i. meridian ▸ large
i. meridian ▸ small
i. ▸ mucosal surfaces of large
i. ▸ mucosal surfaces of small
i., rent of
i., resection of
i., small
i., solitary lymphatic nodules of large
i. solitary lymphatic nodules of small
i. ▸ spasms in walls of
i. transplant, small
intestinitenuis, vasa
intestinointestinal reflex
intima
i., aortic aortic
i. -pia
i., thickening of tunica
i., tunica
intimacy dysfunction
intimacy, emotional
intimal
i. arteriosclerosis
i. cell ▸ mesenchymal
i. deformity
i. fibrosis
i. flap
i. foamy plaques
i. hyperplasia
i. injury
i. layer
i. medial thickness
i. tear
i. thickening
i. thickening, diffuse
intimectomy for Leriche syndrome
intimidated ▸ guilty, ashamed, and
intimidated, patient

intolerable
  i. emotional stress
  i. pain
  i. situation
intolerance
  i., activity
  i., alcoholic
  i. and galactosemia ▸ lactose
  i. ▸ bloating from lactose
  i., carbohydrate
  i., cold
  i. ▸ diarrhea from lactose
  i., drug
  i., effort
  i., exercise
  i., fatty food
  i., food
  i. from alcohol ▸ heat
  i. from antibiotic ▸ lactose
  i. from chlorpromazine ▸ heat
  i. from diuretics ▸ heat
  i., fructose
  i., glucose
  i., gluten
  i., heat
  i., hereditary fructose
  i., lactose
  i., milk
  i. of being alone
  i. of criticism
  i. of defeat
  i. ▸ pain in abdomen from lactose
  i., sucrose
  i. to certain foods
  i. to cold
  i. to light, abnormal
  i. to specific drugs
  i. to specific foods
  i. with Crohn's disease ▸ lactose
intolerant to aspirin therapy ▸ patient
intoxicated (Intoxicated)
  i. behavior
  I. Driver Program (IDP)
  i. (DWI), driving while
  i. minors
  i., patient
intoxication
  i., acid
  i., acute
  i., acute alcoholic
  i., acute cocaine
  i., acute treatment for acute drug
  i., alcohol
  i., alcohol idiosyncratic
  i., alkaline

  i. amaurosis
  i., amphetamine
  i. ▸ amphetamine or similarly acting
     sympathomimetic
  i., anaphylactic
  i., bongkrek
  i., bromide
  i., caffeine
  i., cannabis
  i., chronic methamphetamine
  i., chronic methedrine
  i., clinical manifestations of acute
     drug
  i., cocaine
  i., continued
  i., differential diagnosis in acute
     drug
  i., digitalis
  i., drug
  i., fluid
  i., frequent
  i. ▸ hallucinogenic drug
  i., heroin
  i. idiosyncratic
  i., idiosyncratic alcohol
  i., inhalant
  i., intestinal
  i. ▸ lysergic acid diethylamide (LSD)
  i., marijuana
  i., opiate
  i., opioid
  i. ▸ other or unspecified
     psychoactive substance
  i., pathologic drug
  i., peyote
  i. ▸ Phencyclidine (PCP)
  i., point of
  i., psychological state in acute drug
  i., radiation
  i., roentgen
  i. ▸ sedative, hypnotic, or anxiolytic
  i., serum
  i., subacute treatment of acute
     drug
  i., symptoms of acute drug
  i., thyroid
  i., treatment of acute
  i., water
  i. with cannabinoids, acute
  i. with depressants, acute
  i. with hallucinations, acute
  i. with inhalants, acute
  i. with multiple drugs, acute
  i. with opioids, acute
  i. with phencyclidines, acute

  i. with stimulants, acute
intoxicator, fluid
intra-
  i. -abdominal abscess
  i. -abdominal bleeding ▸ massive
  i. -abdominal carcinoma
  i. -abdominal escape of
     gastroduodenal contents
  i. -abdominal hemorrhage
  i. -abdominal infection
  i. -abdominal laser procedure
  i. -abdominal masses
  i. -abdominal metastases
  i. -abdominal metastases ▸
     extensive
  i. -abdominal pain
  i. -abdominal pressure
  i. -abdominal procedure
  i. -abdominal surgery ▸ major
  i. -abdominal tumor debulking
  i. -abdominal varices
  i. -alveolar debris
  i. -alveolar fibrinous exudate
  i. -alveolar fibrinous material
  i. -alveolar hemorrhage
  i. -alveolar neutrophils
  i. -amniotic saline infusion
  i. -aortic (IA)
  i. -aortic balloon
  i. -aortic balloon counterpulsation
  i. -aortic balloon deflation
  i. -aortic balloon inflation
  i. -aortic balloon pump
  i. -aortic balloon pumping
     (IABP)
  i. -arterial (IA)
  i. -arterial chemotherapy
  i. -arterial counterpulsation
  i. -arterial digital subtraction
     angiography
  i. -arterial hepatic catheterization
  i. -arterial hepatic infusion
  i. -arterial infusion
  i. -arterial injection
  i. -arterial injection of drugs
  i. -arterial line
  i. -arterial measurement of blood
     pressure
  i. -articular component
  i. -articular disc
  i. -articular fracture
  i. -articular osteophytosis
  i. -articular status
  i. -atrial activation sequence
  i. -atrial baffle

intra- —*continued*
- i. -atrial baffle, Senning-type
- i. -atrial block
- i. -atrial conduction
- i. -atrial conduction time
- i. -atrial mass
- i. -atrial reentrant tachycardia
- i. -atrial site
- i. -aural distance
- i. -aural plane
- i. -auricular muscles

intrabronchial vegetable matter
intracapsular
- i. cataract extraction
- i. fracture
- i. incision

intracapsularly, lens delivered
intracardiac
- i. atrial activation sequence
- i. catheter
- i. defibrillator, automatic
- i. electrocardiography (ECG)
- i. electrophysiologic study
- i. electrophysiology
- i. event
- i. injection
- i. lead
- i. malformation
- i. mapping
- i. mass
- i. medication
- i. pacing
- i. patch
- i. patch, Dacron
- i. patch implant, Edwards Teflon
- i. patch ▸ polypropylene
- i. patch prosthesis, Edwards Teflon
- i. patch ▸ Teflon
- i. phonocardiography
- i. phonocatheterization
- i. pressure
- i. pressure curve
- i. shunt
- i. thrombus

intracath catheter
intracaval device
intracaval endovascular
ultrasonography
intracavernous carotid aneurysm
intracavitary
- i. application
- i. cesium
- i. cesium therapy
- i. container placement
- i. gynecologic applicators

- i. irradiation
- i. pressure electrogram dissociation
- i. pressure gradient
- i. radiation
- i. radiation sources
- i. radiation therapy
- i. radiotherapy
- i. therapy

intracellular
- i. activation
- i. antigen
- i. bacteria
- i. bean-shaped diplococci ▸ gram-negative
- i. bridges
- i. calcium concentration
- i. diplococci, gram-negative
- i. fluid
- i. fluid volume
- i. -free magnesium ▸ low
- i. kidney-shaped diplococci ▸ gram-negative
- i. level of magnesium
- i. lipid
- i. magnesium deficiency
- i. magnesium test
- i. organisms
- i. pathogen, fungal
- i. water

intracellulare (MAI) infection ▸
Mycobacterium avium
intracellulare (MAI), Mycobacterium
avium
intracellularis
- i., gram-negative Neisseria
- i., Mycobacterium
- i., Neisseria

intracerebral
- i. and subarachnoid hemorrhage
- i. bleed, massive
- i. bleeding
- i. electrode
- i. electroencephalogram (EEG)
- i. hematoma
- i. hemorrhage
- i. hemorrhage, massive
- i. inoculation
- i. vessels ▸ atherosclerosis of
- i. vessels ▸ basilar of
- i. vessels ▸ vertebral arteries of

intracerebrovascular accident
intracholestasis of liver
intrachondrial bone
intracisternal A-type retroviral
partical, human

intraclavicular triangle
intracoronary
- i. thrombolysis balloon valvuloplasty
- i. thrombolysis ▸ selective
- i. ultrasound

intracorporeal heart
intracranial
- i. abnormality
- i. aerocele
- i. aneurysm
- i. aneurysm clipped
- i. arterial aneurysm
- i. arterial stenosis ▸ symptomatic
- i. bleeding
- i. blood flow
- i. blood pressure (BP)
- i. brain bypass ▸ extracranial-
- i. bruit
- i. calcification
- i. calcification benign glandular tissue
- i. cavity
- i. disease
- i. hemorrhage
- i. hypertension
- i. hypertension, benign
- i. injury
- i. lesion
- i. lesion, severe
- i. mass lesion
- i. metastases
- i. monitor
- i. MR (magnetic resonance) angiography
- i. neoplasm
- i. neoplasm headache
- i. neoplasm, hemianopsia in
- i. neoplasm, primary
- i. neoplasm, seizures in nervous system
- i. part of central nervous system (CNS)
- i. pressure
- i. pressure (ICP) catheter
- i. pressure, high
- i. pressure, increased
- i. pressure monitor in skull
- i. pressure monitoring
- i. pressure, relief of
- i. sinus thrombosis
- i. surgery
- i. thrombosis
- i. tumor
- i. vascular abnormality

i. vascular evaluation
i. vascular malformation
i. vasospasm
intractable
  i. bone pain
  i. diarrhea
  i. epilepsy
  i. facial pain
  i. head pain
  i. heart failure
  i. junctional tachycardia
  i. pain
  i. pain treatment
  i. pelvic pain
  i. postpartum hemorrhage
  i. seizures
  i. shock
  i. skin rash
intracutaneous reaction
intracuticular nylon suture
intracytoplasmic hyalin inclusions
intracytoplasmic mucin
intradermal
  i. mattress suture
  i. nevus
  i. reaction
  i. salt solution test
  i. test
  i. test, Casoni's
intradermic suture
intradiskal electrothermal therapy (IDET)
intraductal
  i. carcinoma, noninfiltrating
  i. carcinoma of breast
  i. papillary mucinous neoplasm (IPMN)
  i. papilloma, benign
  i. papilloma of breast
  i. papillomatosis
intraduodenal peptone infusion
intraepidermal carcinoma
intraepidermal neoplasia
intraepithelial
  i. carcinoma
  i. dyskeratosis syndrome, hereditary benign
  i. neoplasia (CIN), cervical
  i. neoplasia, laser destruction of
  i. neoplasia, vaginal
  i. neoplasia, vulvar
  i. plexus
  i. vesicles
intraesophageal feeding tube

intrafallopian
  i. transfer
  i. transfer (GIFT), gamete
  i. transfer (ZIFT), zygote
intrafamily transmission of viral hepatitis
intrafusal fibers
intragastric drip
intrahemispheric fissure
intrahepatic portosystemic shunt ▸ transjugular
intrainstitutional transmission of viral hepatitis
intraligamentous pregnancy
intralobular fissures
intralocular (*same as* intraocular)
intraluminal
  i. adenocarcinoma
  i. filling defects
  i. gas
  i. mass
  i. palliation
  i. plaque
  i. pressure
  i. pressure, abnormal
  i. radiation therapy
  i. stripper
  i. tube prosthesis, Mackler
  i. ultrasound
intralymphatic radioactivity administration
intramaxillary elastic
intramaxillary fixation
intramedullary
  i. and spongiosa graft
  i. bone graft
  i. canal
  i. device
  i. fixation
  i. fixation device
  i. hemorrhage
  i. nail
  i. nail, Hansen-Street
  i. nail, Rush
  i. nail, Schneider
  i. nailing
  i. pin, Rush
  i. rod
intramucosal
  i. hemorrhage
  i. hemorrhages and erosions
  i. insert
intramural
  i. air in colon
  i. air in large bowel

  i. aneurysm
  i. coronary arteries
  i. fibroid
  i. fixation
  i. hematoma, aortic
  i. pregnancy
  i. thrombi
  i. thrombosis
intramuscular
  i. (IM) administration
  i. arteries ▸ occlusion of
  i. arteries of lower extremities
  i. arteries of upper extremities
  i. (IM) bleeding
  i. (IM) cocktail
  i. (IM) injection
  i. (IM) medications
intramyocardial prearteriolar vessel
intranasal
  i. anesthesia
  i. application
  i. block
  i. influenza vaccine
intranuclear
  i. cycle
  i. inclusions
  i. ophthalmoplegia (INO)
intraocular [*intralocular*]
  i. biopsy
  i. contact lens (ICL)
  i. disorder
  i. foreign body (FB)
  i. hemorrhage
  i. leaking wound
  i. lens (IOL)
  i. lens (IOL), Cilco
  i. lens (IOL), Coburn
  i. lens (IOL) ▸ foldable silicone
  i. lens (IOL) implant
  i. lens (IOL) implantation
  i. lens (IOL), insertion of
  i. lens (IOL), Iolab
  i. lens (IOL), Liteflex
  i. lens (IOL) McGhan
  i. lens (IOL), Optiflex
  i. lens (IOL), Sinskey/Sinskey modified blue loop
  i. lens (IOL), Surgidev
  i. lenses (IOL) ▸ foldable
  i. light
  i. lymphoma
  i. metastasis
  i. muscles
  i. node, subcutaneous
  i. pressure (IOP)

intraocular—*continued*
- i. pressure monitoring
- i. site
- i. tension
- i. tension, normal
- i. toxicity
- i. tumor

intraoperative
- i. angiography
- i. arrhythmias
- i. atrial ischemia
- i. bleeding
- i. care
- i. cholangiogram
- i. cholangiography
- i. conduction disturbance
- i. digital subtraction
- i. digital subtraction angiography (IDSA)
- i. echocardiography
- i. gamma probe localization
- i. hemodynamics
- i. mapping
- i. radiation surgery
- i. radiation therapy
- i. radiotherapy
- i. recanalization
- i. salvage
- i. vascular angiography (IVA)

intraoral
- i. anesthesia
- i. cancer
- i. cone for electron beam therapy
- i. dental molds
- i. device
- i. lesion
- i. projection
- i. stent
- i. wire

intraosseous infusion needle
intraparenchymal air spaces
intraparietal sulcus
intraparietal sulcus of Turner
intrapartum
- i. blood loss
- i. death ▸ term delivery
- i. hemorrhage
- i. period

intrapelvic kidney pelvis
intrapelvic protrusion
intrapericardial anastomosis, Cooley
intraperiosteal fracture
intraperitoneal
- i. abscess
- i. adhesion formation

- i. air
- i. air, free
- i. bleeding
- i. bleeding ▸ source of
- i. chemotherapy
- i. drug administration
- i. hemorrhage, exsanguinating
- i. implant
- i. pregnancy
- i. rupture
- i. transfusion

intrapersonal determinants of relapse ▸ potential
intrapleural
- i. chemotherapy
- i. pressure
- i. rupture
- i. sealed drainage unit

intrapsychic
- i. ataxia
- i. conflict
- i. coping

intrapulmonary
- i. hamartoma
- i. hemorrhage, focal
- i. hemorrhage ▸ focal areas of
- i. metastases
- i. nodal metastases
- i. shunting

intraracial grafts
intrarenal vein
intraretinal microangiopathy (IRMA)
intraretinal microvascular abnormalities (IRMA)
intrascrotal abscess
intrascrotal pain, acute
intraseptal pleural adhesions ▸ fibrinous
intrasocial idiocy
Intrasound pain reliever ▸ Medtronic Pulsor
intraspinal
- i. administration
- i. anesthesia
- i. block

intrastent recurrent disease
intrastent restenosis
intratesticular band
intratesticular hemorrhage
intrathecal
- i. contrast material
- i. injection
- i. space
- i. therapy

intrathecal pump

intrathecally, Methotrexate
intrathoracic
- i. blood volume ▸ augmentation of
- i. esophageal cancer
- i. esophageal cancer ▸ lymphadenectomy of
- i. esophageal carcinoma
- i. gas volume
- i. goiter
- i. pressure
- i. pressure variations
- i. stomach
- i. thyroid

intrathyroid cartilage
intratracheal
- i. instillation
- i. medication
- i. oxygen (O_2) catheter
- i. tube

intratreatment therapeutic instructions
intrauterine
- i. clotting (DIC), disseminated
- i. contraceptive
- i. contraceptive device
- i. contraction
- i. death
- i. device (IUD)
- i. device (IUD), bow
- i. device (IUD), coil
- i. device (IUD) dislodged
- i. device (IUD), ectopic
- i. device (IUD) inserted, Copper 7
- i. device (IUD), Lippes loop
- i. device (IUD) string
- i. dislocation
- i. distress
- i. drug exposure
- i. echocardiography
- i. environment
- i. FB (foreign body)
- i. fetal death
- i. fetally malnourished
- i. fetus
- i. fracture
- i. gestation
- i. gestational sac
- i. growth rate
- i. growth retardation (IUGR)
- i. immunity
- i. isodose
- i. life
- i. pneumonia
- i. polyp
- i. pregnancy (IUP)

i. pregnancy at term
i. pregnancy, multiple
i. pregnancy, single
i. pregnancy, twin
i. pressure
i. pressure catheter
i. respiration
i. transfusion
i. viral infection

intravaginal [*intervaginal*]
intravaginal therapy
intravasation, venous
intravascular
i. agent
i. agglutination
i. catheter culture
i. catheter electrode
i. coagulation (DIC), diffuse
i. coagulation (DIC) ▸ disseminated
i. coagulopathy
i. coagulopathy (DIC), diffuse
i. coagulopathy, disseminated
i. consumption coagulopathy
i. device infection
i. fetal air sign
i. fluid
i. foreign body
i. foreign body retrieval
i. hydrostatic pressure
i. infection
i. mass
i. oxygenator
i. perfluorochemical emulsion
i. pressure (AIP) ▸ average
i. pressure ▸ normal
i. space
i. stent
i. stent, balloon expandable
i. stent ▸ Schatz-Palmaz
i. thrombus
i. ultrasound
i. ultrasound catheter
i. volume
i. volume ▸ adequacy of
i. volume expansion

intravenous (IV)
i. administration of medication
i. administration, peripheral
i. alimentation
i. ammonium chloride
i. anesthesia
i. anesthetic agents
i. angiocardiography
i. angiography
i. antibiotic

i. anticoagulant therapy
i. antioxidant therapy
i. -associated infections
i. barbiturate
i. bolus injection of contrast medium
i. catheter
i. chemotherapy
i. cholangiogram (IVC)
i. cholangiography
i. cholecystography
i. cocktail
i. contrast material
i. digital angiography
i. digital subtraction angiography (IVDSA)
i. discontinued
i. diuretic
i. dose
i. drip
i. drip, slow
i. drug abuser
i. drug needles, infected
i. drug needles ▸ sharing infected
i. drug use
i. drug use, illegal
i. drug user
i. fats
i. feeding
i. fluid
i. fluids, patient treated initially with
i. fluids, piggy-backing
i. fluids started
i. glucose
i. glucose tolerance test
i. hydration
i. infection site
i. infusion
i. infusion of magnesium
i. infusion phlebitis
i. infusion, slow
i. injection
i. insulin therapy, low dose
i. intubation
i. line
i. (IV) line infection
i. (IV) line, subclavian
i. loading dose
i. magnesium
i. needle sharing
i. needle site care
i. needle stick
i. nitroprusside
i. nutritional therapy
i. Pitocin (DIVP) ▸ dilute

i. Pitocin drip
i. pump
i. pyelogram (IVP)
i. pyelogram (IVP) ▸ rapid sequence
i. pyelography (IVP)
i. sedation
i. sedative
i. site of infection
i. system ▸ self-controlled
i. tension
i. therapy
i. tolbutamide tolerance test
i. transfusion
i. urogram
i. urography
i. usage
i. use of drugs ▸ curb

intraventricular
i. aberration
i. block
i. catheter
i. conduction
i. conduction block
i. conduction defect (IVCD)
i. conduction defect (IVCD), nonspecific
i. conduction delay
i. conduction delay ▸ first degree atrioventricular block with
i. conduction pattern
i. delay
i. heart block
i. hemorrhage
i. hemorrhage, acute
i. pressure
i. rhythm, accelerated
i. site
i. tunnel ▸ Kawashima

intravesical
i. chemotherapy
i. prostatic tissue
i. space

intravital staining
intra vitam
intrinsic
i. asthma
i. bronchial lesions
i. colon abnormality
i. defect
i. deflection
i. factor
i. factor concentrate
i. factor ▸ lack of
i. factor, sufficient

intrinsic—*continued*
- i. heart rate
- i. larynx
- i. lesions
- i. mass
- i. muscle
- i. obstruction
- i. pressure
- i. proteinuria
- i. refractory period
- i. religiosity
- i. resistance to antibiotic
- i. sympathomimetic activity

intrinsicoid deflection
introduced
- i., catheter
- i., scope
- i., speculum

introducer, Carter's
introitus
- i., esophageal
- i., marital
- i., nonmarital
- i., nulliparous
- i., parous
- i., patulous
- i., relaxed
- i., vaginae
- i., virginal
- i. with good support

Intropaque contrast medium
introspection, positive self-
introvert-type schizophrenia
introverted
- i. behavior in adolescent
- i. disorder of childhood
- i., patient
- i. personality
- i. tendencies

intrusion(s)
- i., alpha
- i., NREM (nonrapid eye movement)
- i. of sleep ▸ repetitive

intrusive
- i. memories ▸ hyperarousal and
- i. memories ▸ involuntary
- i. reliving ▸ uncontrolled
- i. surgery
- i. thoughts
- i. thoughts and compulsions ▸
  persistent,

intubate [*incubate*]
intubate patient
intubated
- i., baby

- i., infant
- i. patient
- i., patient rapidly
- i. with bronchoscope, patient

intubation
- i. and suction
- i. anesthesia
- i. anesthesia, nasotracheal
- i., catheter-guided endoscopic
- i. detection ▸ esophageal
- i., endoscopic
- i. ▸ endoscopically assisted
  duodenal
- i., endotracheal
- i., gastrointestinal (GI)
- i., intravenous (IV)
- i., nasal
- i., nasoendotracheal
- i., nasogastric
- i., nasotracheal
- i. of airway
- i., oral
- i., orotracheal
- i. ▸ rapid sequence induction (RSI)
  orotracheal
- i., tracheal
- i. tube

intuitive skills
intumescent cataract
intussusception
- i., cecolic
- i., colocolic
- i., ileocolic
- i., ileoileal
- i., postmortem

inulin [*insulin*]
inulin clearance
invading
- i. bacteria
- i. mucosa and submucosa,
  carcinoma
- i. muscularis, carcinoma
- i. viruses

invaginated nipple
invalidate memory
invasion
- i., adenocarcinoma with myometrial
- i., blood vessel
- i., bone marrow
- i. by foreign substance
- i. by tumor, bone marrow
- i. depth ▸ radiography
- i., evidence of
- i., facilitate amebic
- i., focal

- i., fungal
- i. in endometrial carcinoma,
  myometrial
- i., myometrial
- i. of duodenal wall ▸ microscopic
- i. of lymphatics
- i., parametrial
- i. ▸ soft tissue
- i., tissue
- i., tumor
- i., vascular

invasive
- i. activity test
- i. adenocarcinoma
- i. adenocarcinoma ▸ slowly growing
- i. aspergillosis ▸ semi-
- i. assessment
- i. bacteremia
- i. biopsy technique ▸ minimally
- i. brain surgery
- i. brain surgery, minimally
- i. breast biopsy procedure ▸
  minimally
- i. breast cancer
- i. breast tissue cells
- i. cancer
- i. carcinoma
- i. carcinoma, cells consistent with
- i. carcinoma, circumferential
- i. carcinoma of breast
- i. cervical cancer
- i. cervical carcinoma
- i. diagnostic evaluation
- i. diagnostic procedure
- i. direct coronary artery bypass
  (MIDCAB) ▸ minimally
- i. disease
- i. ductal cancer
- i. electrophysiologic testing
- i. external otitis
- i. growth of blood vessels
- i. infection
- i. infectious process ▸ active
- i. laparoscopy surgery ▸ minimally
- i. lesion
- i. lobular cancer
- i. management strategy
- i. medical procedure
- i. method
- i. monitoring, continuous
- i. person, abusive
- i. pneumococcal disease
- i. pressure measurement
- i. procedure
- i. procedure (CIP), cardiac

i. procedure ▸ minimally
i. pulmonary aspergillosis
i. spinal surgery
i. surgery
i. surgical technique
i. technique
i. technique ▸ minimally
i. technique, vascular
i. tendency
i. test
i. therapy
i. thymoma
i. thyroiditis
i. treatment
i. tumor
i. valve replacement surgery ▸ minimally
i. vascular study ▸ mini-
i. vulvar carcinoma

Inventory (inventory)
I. (AUI), Alcohol Use
i., assertiveness
I. (BSRI), Bem Sex Role
I. by systems
I. (EWI), Experiential World
I., (MMPI) ▸ Minnesota Multiphasic Personality
I., State Trait Anxiety
I. (MMPI) Test, Minnesota Multiphasic Personality

inversa, angina
inverse
i. comma appearance
i. ratio ventilation
i. ratio ventilation ▸ pressure controlled
i. square law
i. symmetry

inversion [*aversion*]
i. deformity
i. film of ankles, forced
i., forced
i., infundibuloarterial
i. instability
i. ▸ isolated conotruncal
i. ▸ isolated infundibuloarterial
i. of eyelashes
i. of uterus
i. position
i. range
i., sexual
i. sprain
i. strain
i. strain x-ray
i. stress

i. stress test
i., T wave
i., temperature
i. ▸ U wave
i., ventricular

inversional trend
inversus
i., complete situs
i. ▸ dextrocardia with situs
i., incomplete situs
i. ▸ levocardia with situs
i., situs
i. viscerum, situs

invert sugar
inverted
i., cardiac stump
i. edge
i. horseshoe flap
i. nipple
i. radial reflex
i. reflex
i., stump
i., stump phenolized and
i. -T appearance
i. T fashion
i. T incision
i. T wave
i. testis
i. waves
i. Y and spleen pedicle

inverting
i. appendiceal stump
i. stitches
i. suture
i. suture, continuous
i. suture, continuous circular

Investigate Memory and Aging (OPTIMA) ▸ Oxford Project to
investigation
i., clinical
i., controlled
i., fine needle biopsy
i., intensive scientific
i., limited
i. of brain
i., outbreak
i. terminated
i., ultrasonographic

investigational drug
investigational therapy
invisible main pulmonary artery
invisible radiation
involuntary
i. active euthanasia
i. admission

i. body function
i. body movements
i. commitment
i. contraction
i. contraction of muscle ▸ sudden,
i. contraction of voluntary muscles ▸ violent
i. deviate sexual intercourse
i. discharge of feces
i. discharge of urine
i. dribbling of urine
i. eye movement
i. facial expression
i. facial pain
i. forcible closure of eyelids
i. function
i. general paroxysm
i. intrusive memories
i. jerking movements of legs
i. jerks
i. motor movement
i. motor tics
i. movement
i. movement disorder
i. movement ▸ drug-related
i. movement, irregular
i. movement irregular, spas-modic
i. movement of chorea
i. movement of eyeball
i. movements ▸ twitches and
i. muscle
i. muscle contraction
i. muscle spasm
i. muscular contraction
i. muscular movements
i. nervous system
i. rapid movement
i. repetitive movement
i. response
i. rhythmic oscillation
i. sinuous movements ▸ slow, repeated,
i. smoking
i. spasm of diaphragm
i. spasmodic blinking or squint-ing
i. sterilization
i. trembling
i. trembling of body
i. trembling of limbs
i. tremors
i. twitching
i. verbal tics

involution
- i. cyst
- i. ▸ moderate degree of
- i. of uterus

involutional
- i. changes of ovaries
- i. depression
- i. melancholia
- i. psychosis

involved muscle ▸ excessive use of
involved site
involvement
- i., active
- i., artery
- i., axillary lymph node
- i., brachial plexus
- i., ciliary body
- i., cranial nerve
- i., dermal lymphatic
- i., drug
- i., extensive metastatic
- i., extensive pleural
- i., focal
- i., glandular
- i. in breast carcinoma, survival relative to nodal
- i. in reckless activities
- i., infection or dysfunction ▸ bladder
- i., internal mammary
- i., internal node
- i., leptomeningeal
- i., liver
- i., local
- i., lymphatic
- i., massive
- i., massive retroperitoneal
- i., metastatic
- i., microscopic cervical
- i., motor
- i., nerve
- i., nodal
- i., node
- i., periaortic lymph
- i., pneumonic
- i., primary node
- i., regional
- i., regional lymph
- i., regional lymph node
- i., regional node
- i., religious cult
- i., rib
- i., sensory
- i., serial lymph node
- i., soft tissue
- i., subdiaphragmatic

- i., tumor
- i., vascular

involving [*evolving*]
involving fungus ▸ **generalized infection**
involving pulmonary valve ▸ **carcinoid**
inward
- i. aggression
- i. current ▸ transient
- i. -going rectification
- i. movement
- i. rotation

Iodamoeba bütschlii
Iodamoeba williamsi
iodide
- i., calcium
- i. (SSKI), saturated solution of potassium
- i. (I^{123}, I^{125}, I^{131}) ▸ sodium

iodinated
- i. contrast media
- i. human serum albumin
- i. human serum albumin ▸ radioactive
- i. I^{131} aggregated albumin (human)
- i. I^{131} serum albumin (human)
- i. I^{125} fibrinogen
- i. I^{125} serum albumin
- i. macroaggregated albumin
- i. serum albumin
- i. serum albumin (RISA) study, radioactive
- i. serum, radio◊

iodination of antibodies
iodine (I)
- i. allergy
- i. -azide test
- i. (BEI), butanol-extractable
- i. deficiency
- i. deficiency disorder (IDD)
- i., insulin-
- i. -medicated bath
- i. (mcl) ▸ millicuries
- i. 131 MIBG scintigraphy
- i. 131 with triiodothyronine (I^{131}-T3)
- i., plasma inorganic
- i. (PBI) ▸ protein-bound
- i. PVP (polyvinylpyrrolidone)
- i. (I^{131}) ▸ radioactive
- i., radiolabeled
- i. sensitivity
- i. (SPBI) ▸ serum protein-bound
- i., serum-bound
- i., serum-precipitable

- i. solution povidone-iodine treatment ▸ radioactive
- i. uptake (AIU) ▸ absolute
- i. (RAI) uptake ▸ radioactive
- i. (I^{131}) uptake test ▸ radioactive

iodipamide
- i. contrast medium
- i. contrast medium, meglumine
- i. contrast medium, sodium
- i., sodium

iodized oil, residual
iodized oil study
iodo prep
iodoalphionic acid contrast medium
iodoform gauze
iodoform gauze packing
iodohippurate contrast medium, sodium
iodohippurate I^{131} sodium
iodomethmate
- i. contrast medium
- i. contrast medium, sodium
- i., sodium

iodophil granules
iodophor solution
iodophthalein sodium contrast medium
iodopyracet contrast medium
IOL (intraocular lens)
- IOL (intraocular lens), Coburn
- IOL (intraocular lens) implant
- IOL (intraocular lens), Liteflex
- IOL (intraocular lens), McGhan
- IOL (intraocular lens), Optiflex
- IOL (intraocular lens), Sinskey/ Sinskey modified blue loop lens
- IOL (intraocular lens), Surgidev

Iolab intraocular lenses
ion(s)
- i., amphoteric dipolar
- i., calcium
- i. channel
- i., chloride
- i. concentration, hydrogen
- i. exchange
- i. irradiation, heavy
- i. laser
- i. laser, argon
- i. microscope
- i., physical effects of heavy
- i., potassium
- i. pump
- i. selective electrode
- i., sodium

i. therapy, carbon
i. therapy ▸ negative
i. therapy, neon
i. therapy, silicon
Ionescu
  I. method
  I. -Shiley aortic valve prosthesis
  I. -Shiley pericardial patch
  I. -Shiley pericardial xenograft
  I. -Shiley prosthesis
  I. -Shiley valve
  I. -Shiley vascular graft
I^{131} (radioactive iodine)
  I^{131} aggregated albumin (human), ionated
  I^{131} (sodium iodide) ▸ I^{123}, I^{125},
  I^{131} serum albumin (human), iodinated
  I^{131}, sodium iodohippurate
  I^{131}, sodium rose bengal
  I^{131}, triolein
  I^{131} (radioactive iodine) uptake test
I^{125}
  I^{125} fibrinogen, iodinated
  I^{121}, I^{131} (sodium iodide) ▸ I^{123},
  I^{125} serum albumin, iodinated
  I^{125}, sodium iothalamate
  I^{123}, I^{125}, I^{131} (sodium iodide)
ionic contrast material, non-ionic medicine
ionization
  i. chamber
  i. chamber, free-air
  i. density
  i. detector, flame
ionized hemoglobin, un-
ionized serum calcium, low
ionizing radiation
ionizing radiation ▸ therapeutic
ionometric studies
ionotropic effect
iontophoresis procedure
iontophoresis sweat test ▸
  quantitative pilocarpine
IOP (intraocular pressure)
iopanoic acid contrast medium
iopax contrast medium, Neo-
iophdone contrast medium
iophendylate contrast medium
iophenoxic acid contrast medium
iopydol contrast medium
iothalamate
  i. contrast medium
  i. contrast medium, meglumine

i. contrast medium, sodium
i. I^{125}, sodium
Iowa Test
IP (instantaneous pressure)
IPCO/Partridge defibrillator
IPD (inflammatory pelvic disease)
ipecac-induced emesis
ipecac, syrup of
ipecacuanha, Cephaelis
IPF (idiopathic pulmonary fibrosis)
IPG (impedance plethysmography)
IPJ (interphalangeal joint)
IPMN (intraductal papillary mucinous neoplasm)
ipodate
  i. calcium contrast medium
  i. contrast medium, sodium
  i., sodium
IPP (intermittent positive pressure)
IPPB (intermittent positive pressure breathing)
IPPO (intermittent positive pressure inflation with oxygen)
IPPR (intermittent positive pressure respiration)
IPPV (intermittent positive pressure ventilation)
ipsilateral
  i. antegrade arteriography
  i. aspect
  i. breast tumor recurrence
  i. contraction
  i. ear
  i. mentalis muscle
  i. rhinorrhea
  i. stroke
IPSP (inhibitory postsynaptic potential)
IPTH (immunoreactive parathyroid hormone)
IPV (inactivated polio vaccine)
IQ (intelligence quotient)
  IQ (intelligence quotient), performance
  IQ (intelligence quotient) test, full scale
  IQ (intelligence quotient), verbal
IR (index of response)
IRA-400 resin
Iranian
  I. heroin (Dava)
  I. heroin (Persian)
  I. heroin (Persian Brown)
  I. heroin (Rufus)
IRB (Institutional Review Board)

IRC ▸ (infrared heat coagulation)
IRDS (idiopathic respiratory distress syndrome)
iridectomy
  i., basal
  i., optic
  i., optical
  i., peripheral
  i., preliminary
  i., preparatory
  i., sclerecto◊
  i., sector
  i., stenopeic
  i., surgical
  i., therapeutic
iridencleisis procedure
iridescent vision
iridesis/iridodesis
iridial folds
iridial tent
iridic muscles
iridocapsular implant cataract lens, Binkhorst
iridis
  i., atresia
  i., coloboma
  i., ectasia
  i., granuloma
  i., heterochromia
  i. major, anulus
  i. minor, anulus
  i., plicae
  i., rubeosis
  i., sphincter
  i., stroma
  i., xanthomatosis
iridium
  i. capsule, platinum
  i. 192 (Ir^{192})
  i. seeds
  i. strand
  i. wire implant
iridocapsular fixation lens
iridocorneal angle
iridocyclitis, granulomatous
iridodialysis, sclerecto◊
iridomedialysis/iridomesodialysis
iridotomy (*same as* iritomy)
iris
  i., atrophy of
  i. bombé
  i. ciliary body
  i. cloudy
  i., coloboma of
  i. contraction reflex

iris—_continued_
- i., cyst of
- i. dehiscence
- i. diaphragm
- i. diastasis
- i., edema of
- i., essential atrophy of
- i., FB (foreign body) in
- i. fixation lens
- i., Florentine
- i. forceps, closed
- i., foreign body (FB) in
- i., hemangioma of
- i., hemorrhage of
- i. hernia
- i., herpes zoster of
- i., hyperemia of
- i., implantation cyst of
- i., incarceration of
- i., late prolapse of
- i., leiomyoma of
- i. metastasis
- i. pillars
- i. pillars replaced
- i. plane lens
- i., plane of
- i., postoperative coloboma left
- i., postoperative coloboma right
- i., prolapse of
- i., protrusion of
- i. replaced with spatula ▸ pillars of
- i. reposited
- i. scraped free
- i. stretching operation
- i., stroma of
- i., suture of
- i., syphilis of
- i., transfixation of
- i., tremulous
- i., umbrella

iritis
- i. catamenialis
- i., diabetic
- i., Doyne's
- i., follicular
- i., Fuchs'
- i., gouty
- i. papulosa
- i., plastic
- i., purulent
- i., serous
- i., spongy
- i., sympathetic
- i., tuberculous
- i., uratic

iritomy (_see_ **iridotomy**)
IRMA (intraretinal microangio-pathy)
IRMA (intraretinal microvascular abnormalities)
iron
- i. absorption
- i. binding
- i. -binding capacity
- i. -binding capacity, latent
- i. -binding capacity test
- i. -binding capacity (TIBC) ▸ total
- i. -binding capacity (UIBC) ▸ unsaturated
- i. chelator
- i., colloidal
- i. complex ▸ polysaccharide
- i. damage ▸ toxic
- i. deficiency
- i. deficiency anemia
- i. deposits
- i. dextran complex
- i. disappearance, plasma
- i. hematoxylin
- i. hematoxylin method
- i. hematoxylin stain, Heidenhain's
- i., heme
- i., high serum-bound
- i. hydroxide
- i., inorganic
- i. level
- i. low serum-bound
- i. lung
- i. metabolism disease
- i. overload disease
- i. -poor blood
- i., radioactive
- i. saturation level
- i., serum
- i., serum-bound
- i. stain
- i., stainable
- i. storage disease
- i. storage disease ▸ inherited
- i. supplement
- i. turnover (PIT), plasma
- i. turnover rate, plasma

irradiated
- i. cells
- i. ergosterol
- i. food
- i. medium
- i. medium, build-down region of
- i. medium, build-up region of
- i. surgical defects

- i. victim
- i. volume

irradiation
- i., adjuvant
- i., adjuvant pulmonary
- i. and chemotherapy
- i. and phytohemagglutinin, lymphocyte
- i. and surgery
- i., axillary lymph node
- i., biopsy after
- i. cataract
- i., cesium
- i., chest
- i., conservative surgery and
- i., cranial sanctuary
- i., craniospinal
- i. cystitis
- i., definitive
- i. effect
- i., elective
- i., electron beam scalp
- i., external
- i., external beam
- i., external cobalt
- i. field, en face
- i., field size in half body
- i. for allograft survival, total lymphoid
- i. for gynecomastia
- i., generalized body
- i., heavy ion
- i., hemibody
- i., high dose external
- i. in arthritis, total lymphoid
- i. in organ transplantation, total lymphoid
- i. in radiation therapy neuraxis
- i. in rheumatoid arthritis, total lymphoid
- i. -induced lung damage
- i. injury
- i., interstitial
- i., intracavitary
- i., local
- i., local tumor excision with
- i., long wave
- i., low dose rate
- i., lymphoid
- i. neck, elective
- i., neuraxis
- i. of blood, extracorporeal
- i. of lymph, extracorporeal
- i. of raw meat
- i. of transplant, local

i. ▸ partial food
i., pelvic
i., periaortic
i., postoperative
i., preoperative
i., preoperative pelvic
i. process
i., prophylactic cranial
i. sterilization
i. technique in radiation therapy, photon
i. therapy
i. therapy, external
i. therapy, supervoltage rotational
i. ▸ total axial node
i., total body
i., total lymphoid
i. (TNI) ▸ total nodal
i., ultraviolet
i., ultraviolet blood
i., volume treated in external
i., whole body
i., whole brain
i., whole skull

irrational
i. anxiety
i. behavior
i. beliefs
i. fear ▸ disabling
i. obsession with imagined ugliness
i., patient
i. phobia
i. rationality
i. thinking
i. thoughts
i. violence

irrationality and disorientation ▸ irritability,

irreducible hernia

irregular
i. astigmatism
i. astigmatism, corneal
i. astigmatism, lenticular
i. bleeding
i. bone
i. bowel movements
i. brain function
i. breathing
i. breathing pattern
i. calcification
i. cervix
i. changes in cervical cells
i. contractions
i. defects
i. disfigured cells

i. dopamine transmission
i. esophageal motility
i. esophageal spasm
i., extremely slow waves
i. field technique for dose calculation
i., firm, nodular liver
i., flashing patterns of light
i., heart
i. heart action
i. heart rhythm
i. heartbeat
i. heartbeat rhythm
i. intervals
i. involuntary movement
i. jerking motions ▸ violent and
i., jerky movements
i., low voltage
i. menses
i. menstrual cycles
i. menstrual periods
i., nodular liver ▸ firm,
i. nuclei, large
i. osseous fragments
i. ovulation
i. periods
i. pulse
i. pulse ▸ irregularly
i. rate
i. release of egg
i. respirations
i. rhythm
i. rhythm ▸ irregularly
i. rhythm ▸ regularly
i. rhythmic delta activity ▸ frontal
i. septum
i., spasmodic, involuntary movements
i. tumor mass ▸ infiltrating
i. twitching
i. uterine bleeding
i. vaginal bleeding
i. wandering cells
i. with nodulation

irregularity(-ies)
i., border
i., cardiac
i., cyclic
i., estriol
i., heartbeat
i. in brain chemistry
i. ▸ lethal rhythmic
i., luminal
i., menstrual
i., mucosal

i., neurological
i. of pulse
i. of teeth
i., periosteal
i., vascular

irregularly
i. irregular pulse
i. irregular rhythm
i. shaped body
i. shaped bone
i. shaped nuclei ▸ basophilic pleomorphic

irreparable heart damage
irreparable tissue damage
irrepressible sleep attacks
irresistible impulse
irresistible impulse test
irresponsibility, consistent
irresponsibility, financial
irresponsible
i. and exploitative
i. behavior
i. drug abuser
i. work behavior

irreversible
i. blindness
i. bone loss
i. brain damage
i. brain death
i. brain injury
i. catastrophic brain damage
i. catastrophic brain injury
i. cessation of circulatory and respiratory functions
i. coma
i. coma, prolonged
i. damage
i. damage to brain cells
i. dementia
i. depression
i. disability
i. disorder
i. disorder, progressive
i. ear damage from noise
i. functional changes
i. heart damage
i. hereditary disease
i. kidney failure
i. laser surgery
i. legal blindness
i. medical condition
i. mental or physical condition
i. motor deterioration
i. neurological damage
i. pain

irreversible—*continued*
    i. psychosis, potentially
    i. shock
    i. structural changes
    i. weakness
irrevocable blindness
irrigate [*irritate*]
irrigated
    i., bladder
    i., operative site
    i., pelvis
    i., retroperitoneum
    i., stoma
    i. with normal saline ▸ wound
    i. with saline
    i. with saline ▸ anterior chamber
    i. with saline ▸ operative site
    i. with saline solution ▸ wound
    i., wound
irrigating
    i. catheter, three-way
    i. solution, contamination from
    i. solution, prepackaged
irrigation [*irritation*]
    i. and curettage
    i., bronchoscopy with
    i., cold caloric
    i., colonic
    i., colostomy
    i., continuous
    i., copious
    i., curettage and
    i., daily
    i., debridement and
    i., local
    i. of bladder
    i. of nose
    i. of urinary bladder
    i., postoperative
    i., preoperative
    i. smear, vaginal
    i., sterile
    i. techniques
    i. techniques, nonsterile
    i., tracheoscopy with
    i. tubes, salvarsan throat
    i., Zephiran
irrigator
    i., Buie
    i., DeVilbiss
    i., Dougherty's
    i., Fox's
    i., Gibson's
    i., Rollet's
    i., Sylva's

irritability
    i., agitation and
    i., agitation and restlessness
    i. and aggressiveness
    i. and confusion ▸ patient has
        forgetfulness,
    i. and depression
    i. and mood swings
    i. and tremor
    i. and/or anxiety
    i. ▸ apathy and
    i., depression and personality
        changes
    i., disorientation and
    i., duodenal
    i., emotional
    i. ▸ euphoria, emotional lability,
    i., extreme
    i., gastric outlet
    i., hyperactivity, and anxiety
    i., inappropriate
    i. ▸ intense, short-term
    i., irrationality and disorientation
    i. ▸ lapse into heightened
    i., nervousness and
    i. or anxiety
    i. or nervousness
    i., persistent
    i., reflex
    i. ▸ restlessness, anorexia and
    i., restlessness and intense craving
    i. ▸ sadness and
    i., sleeplessness and
    i., tension
    i., uterine
irritable
    i. and aggressive ▸ moody,
    i. and easily annoyed ▸ agitated,
    i. and jumpy, patient
    i. and lightheaded
    i. and tense, patient
    i. bladder
    i. bowel
    i. bowel syndrome
    i. bowel syndrome ▸ bloating and
    i. bowel syndrome ▸ pain in
        abdomen from
    i. bowel syndrome with constipation
    i., clinical pharmacology patient
    i. colon (IC)
    i. colon syndrome
    i. duodenal bulb
    i. heart
    i., increasingly
    i. joint

    i. male syndrome (IMS)
    i. mood
    i. mood, depressed or
    i. negativism ▸ exhibits
    i., patient
    i. stomach
    i. stricture
    i. testis, Cooper's
irritans
    i., Eutrombicula
    i., Haematobia
    i., Leptus
    i., Lyperosia
    i., Pulex
    i., Siphona
    i., Trombicula
irritant(s)
    i., blood-borne
    i., chemical
    i. cosmetic reactions
    i. in airway ▸ nonspecific
    i., lung tissue
    i., menopausal
    i., mucosal
    i. receptor
irritate [*irrigate*]
irritate nasal passages
irritated
    i. area, persistent
    i., easily
    i. eyes
    i. eyes, dry,
    i. plantar fascia
    i., red, and swollen
    i. ▸ tired and
irritates stomach lining, aspirin
irritating spurs on vertebral bodies
irritating toxin
irritation [*irrigation*]
    i., acute throat
    i., anal
    i. and anger ▸ bursts of
    i. and rubbing, constant skin
    i. and ulceration ▸ gastrointestinal
    i., bronchial
    i., cerebral
    i., chronic
    i., environmental
    i., eye
    i. fever
    i. free
    i. from Benadryl ▸ skin
    i., gastric
    i., gastrointestinal (GI)
    i. ▸ itching and

i., local
i., localized
i., localized tissue
i., meningeal
i., mild skin
i., nasal
i., nerve
i., nerve root
i. of bladder
i. of conjunctiva
i. of cornea
i. of cortex
i. of eyeball, continual
i. of incision site
i. of sciatic nerve
i. of stomach lining
i. of urethra
i. or infection ▸ chronic
i., perianal
i., peritoneal
i., rectal
i., respiratory
i., skin
i., spinal
i., stomach
i., superficial
i., total body
i., trigeminal nerve
i., vaginal
i., vulvar

irritative
i. diarrhea
i. lesion
i. miosis
i. radiation
i. reaction
i. reaction, localized
i. response

IRV (inspiratory reserve volume)
Irving's operation
Irving-type tubal ligation
IS (inventory by system)
Isaac's differential distortion divergent method
Isaac's granules
Isaacs-Ludwig arteriole
ischemia
i., acute
i. ▸ acute mesenteric
i., acute myocardial
i., anterior wall
i., asymptomatic
i. (ACI), asymptomatic cardiac
i., brachiocephalic
i., cardiac

i., cerebral
i., cerebrobasilar
i., chemical indicators of
i., chronic
i. ▸ chronic mesenteric
i., clandestine myocardial
i., colonic
i. cordis intermittens
i., cystic
i., daily
i., digital
i., distal
i., documented silent
i. ▸ exercise-induced silent myocardial
i., extremity
i. -guided medial therapy
i. in peri-infarct zone
i., inferior wall
i., intestinal
i. ▸ intraoperative atrial
i., lateral wall
i. ▸ life-threatening
i., limb
i., manifest
i., mesenteric
i., midgut
i. monitoring, ambulatory
i., muscle
i., myocardial
i. of myocardium
i. of retina
i., persistent
i., plantar
i. ▸ recurrent mesenteric
i. reperfusion transition ▸ forced
i. retinae
i., reversible
i., silent
i. ▸ silent myocardial
i. ▸ skeletal muscle
i. ▸ small bowel
i., spontaneous
i., ST-T wave changes compatible with
i., subendocardial
i., temporary
i. test ▸ plantar
i., tourniquet
i., transient
i., transient cerebral
i. ▸ transient mesenteric

ischemic
i. arrhythmia
i. attack and aging ▸ transient

i. attack (TIA), transient
i. attack (TIA) ▸ warning signs of transient
i. burden
i. cardiomyopathy
i. cerebral infarction
i. change
i. claudication
i. colitis
i. contracture
i. contracture of the left ventricle (LV)
i. damage of heart
i. disease, myocardial
i. ECG (electrocardiogram) changes
i. ECG (electrocardiograph) changes
i. encephalopathy ▸ hypoxic
i. episode, transient
i. episode, transient cerebral
i. heart disease (IHD)
i. heart disease, acute
i. heart disease ▸ silent
i. heart muscles
i. heart wall
i. hypoxia
i. left ventricle (LV)
i. leg disease
i. limb disease
i. lumbago
i. mitral regurgitation
i. muscle
i. muscle contracture
i. muscle fibers
i. muscle necrosis
i. muscular atrophy
i. myocardial disease
i. myocardium
i. myopathy
i. necrosis
i. neurologic defect ▸ reversible
i. neuropathy
i. ▸ nonocclusive mesenteric
i. ocular inflammation
i. optic neuropathy
i. optic neuropathy, anterior
i. paralysis
i. paralysis and contracture
i. paralysis ▸ Volkmann
i. pattern
i. pericarditis
i. portion of ventricle ▸ excision
i. pressure necrosis
i. reflex

ischemic—*continued*
- i. reperfusion injury
- i. rest angina
- i. skeletal muscle
- i. stroke
- i. stroke risk
- i. sudden death
- i. sylvian waves
- i. syndrome ▸ myocardial
- i. syndrome ▸ ocular
- i. threshold
- i. time
- i. time ▸ donor organ
- i. tissue
- i. tissue reperfusion
- i. ulcer
- i. vascular disease

ischiadic nerve

ischial
- i. bone
- i. brace
- i. bursitis
- i. ramus
- i. spine
- i. tuberosity
- i. weight bearing leg brace

ischiatic
- i. hernia
- i. notch, greater
- i. notch, lesser
- i. scoliosis

ischiocavernous muscle

ischiopubic ramus

ischiopubica, osteochondritis

ischiorectal
- i. abscess
- i. abscess ▸ incision and drainage (I and D)
- i. hernia

ISCU (Infant Special Care Unit)

iseikonic lens

Isherwood's position

Ishihara's plate

Ishihara's test

ISI (interstimulus interval)

island(s) (Islands)
- i., bone
- i., endometrial
- i. flap
- i. flap, artery
- i. flap, Millard's
- i. flap, Monks-Esser
- i. graft
- i. leg flap
- I., Life
- i. of Langerhans
- i. of Reil

islandica, Cetraria

isle, Bacteroides fragilis

islet(s)
- i. cell
- i. cell adenoma
- i. cell ▸ pancreatic
- i. cell transplant procedure
- i. cell transplantation
- i. cell transplants
- i. cell tumor
- i., digestive
- i. ▸ functional viability of human
- i. isolation process
- i. of Langerhans
- i. of Langerhans ▸ sclerosis of
- i. structures
- i., transplanted

ISN (interaction surgical navigation)

isoactin switch

isoamylase levels, pancreatic

isobaric transition

isocapneic condition

isocapneic hyperpnea

isocenter system

isocentric
- i. oblique
- i. technique for dose calculation
- i. technique, four field

isochronal rhythm

isocitric dehydrogenase

isocitric dehydrogenase, serum

isodense with surrounding tissues

isodiphasic complex

isodose
- i. chart
- i. curve
- i. distribution
- i., intrauterine
- i. line
- i. shift method
- i. shift method for air gap correction

isodynamic equivalent

isoeffect
- i. curve
- i. formula
- i. graphs

isoelectric
- i. electroencephalogram (EEG)
- i. interval
- i. level
- i. line
- i. period
- i. point
- i. T waves

isoenzyme, CPK

isoenzyme, LDH (lactic dehydrogenase)

isogeneic antigen

isogeneic graft

isohydric cycle

isoimmunization, Rh

Isoiodeikon test

isokinetic exercise

isolate input signal

isolate of bacteria, clinical

isolated
- i. after 72 hours, organism
- i. and tagged, muscles
- i. arbovirus
- i., artery
- i. brain
- i. bursts
- i. conotruncal inversion
- i. dextrocardia
- i., emotionally
- i. episode
- i. events
- i. explosive disorder
- i. flashes of light
- i. from patients, viruses
- i. grand mal seizures
- i. heat perfusion
- i. heat perfusion of an extremity
- i. ▸ highly addictive and
- i. hyperthermic limb perfusion
- i. in urine, diphtheroids
- i. infundibuloarterial inversion
- i. infusion
- i. myocarditis, acute
- i., organ
- i. pancreatitis
- i. parietal endocarditis
- i., patient
- i. ▸ patient feels
- i. perfusion
- i. phobias
- i. premature beats
- i. renal cyst
- i. septal hypertrophy
- i. Shigella
- i., socially
- i. spike transients
- i. spikes
- i., superior pulmonary vein
- i. systolic hypertension
- i. units

isolates, cluster of

isolating mesoappendix
isolation (Isolation)
- i. and asepsis
- i. and being misunderstood ▸ feeling of
- i. and demoralization
- i. and identification
- i. and withdrawal
- I., Blood
- i., cell
- i., denial and
- i., depression and fatigue ▸ withdrawal
- I., Enteric
- i., enteric type of
- i., feeling of
- i. hospital
- i., local
- i., loneliness and
- i., maximum
- i. measures
- i., minimum
- i. of patient
- i., partial
- i., patient placed in
- i. policies
- i. ▸ post-transplant
- i., potential
- i. precautions
- i. precautions, specific
- i. procedure ▸ left atrial
- i. process ▸ islet
- I., Protective
- I., Respiratory
- i., reverse
- i. room, laminar air flow (LAF)
- i., sensory
- i., social
- i., stimulus
- I., Strict
- i. technique
- i. techniques, develop
- i. techniques, standard
- i. techniques, update
- i. trash
- I. Unit (SIU), Stimulus
- i. units, germ-free
- i., viral
- i., wound
- I., Wound and Skin

isolator, plastic tent
isolator, surgical
isolette, infant placed in
isologous chimera
isologous graft

isomerase
- i., glucose phosphate
- i., phosphoribose
- i., triosephosphate
- i., uroporphyrin

isomeric decay
isometric(s)
- i. contraction
- i. contraction period
- i. exercise
- i. hand grip
- i. hand grip exercise
- i. hand grip test
- i. interval
- i., neck
- i. period of cardiac cycle
- i. pressure
- i. program
- i. quad strengthening exercises
- i. relaxation period
- i. ▸ stretching and neck
- i. transition

isomorphic gliosis
isomyosin switch
isonicotinic acid hydrazide
Isopaque contrast medium
Isoparorchis trisimilitubis
isopathic immunization
isoperistaltic anastomosis
isophil antigen
isoplastic graft
isopotential axis, zero
isopropyl alcohol
isopropyl chlorophenol
isoproterenol stress test
isoproterenol tilt table test
isorhythmic AV (atrioventricular) dissociation
isorhythmic AV (atrioventricular) dissociation with interference
isosensitization, Rh (Rhesus)
isosexual puberty ▸ idiopathic
Isospora bigemina
Isospora hominis
isotonic contraction
isotonic exercise
isotope(s)
- i. bone scan
- i. calibrator, digital
- i. effect
- i., increased uptake of
- i. ▸ injected radioactive
- i., interstitial implantation of radioactive
- i., nonradioactive hydrogen

- i., radio◊
- i., radioactive
- i., radioactive hydrogen
- i., radioactive labeled
- i. renogram
- i. scanning studies
- i. scanning studies of brain
- i., stable
- i. studies
- i. therapy

isotopic linkage of antibodies
isotropic (*same as* isotopic)
isotropic disc
isovaleric acid level
isovaleric acidemia
isovelocity surface area ▸ proximal
isovolumetric
- i. contractility
- i. phase index
- i. relaxation
- i. relaxation period

isovolumic
- i. contraction time
- i. index
- i. interval
- i. relaxation
- i. relaxation period
- i. relaxation time
- i. systole

isoxazolyl
- i. group
- i. group resistant
- i. penicillin

ISP (interesting sociological phenomenon)
israelii, Actinomyces
israelii, Nocardia
issue(s)
- i., clinical
- i., clinical practice
- i., cross-cultural
- i., damaged
- i., ethical
- i., family
- i., family-oriented
- i. ▸ impaired employees alcohol and drug treatment
- i., inner child
- i., interpersonal
- i., key
- i., legal
- i., parenting
- i., patient management
- i. ▸ quality of life
- i., sexual

issue(s)—*continued*
- i., sexuality
- i., social
- i., special teaching

IST (insulin shock therapy)
isthmica nodosa
isthmica nodosa, salpingitis
isthmicae tubae uterinae, plica
isthmus
- i., aortic
- i., Krönig's
- i. of fallopian tube
- i. of uterus
- i., thyroid
- i. tubae uterinae
- i. uteri

Italian distant flap
Italian rhinoplasty
itch
- i., anal
- i. -and-scratch syndrome ▸ chronic
- i. anemia ▸ ground
- i., barber's
- i., dhobie
- i., diabolical
- i., jock
- i., mad
- i. medication, anti-
- i. mites
- i. -scratch cycle
- i., vaginal
- i., winter

itchiness of abdomen
itching
- i., anal
- i. and antibiotic ▸ anal
- i. and irritation
- i. and redness of skin ▸ burning,
- i. and sneezing, control
- i., dandruff with
- i. ▸ emotion-related
- i. feeling ▸ fidgeting, aching, pulling or
- i. from anxiety ▸ eye
- i. from athlete's foot
- i. from conjunctivitis
- i. from dermatitis
- i. from dermatitis ▸ scalp
- i. from diabetes
- i. from diabetes ▸ vaginal
- i. from eczema
- i. from eczema ▸ scalp
- i. generalized
- i. in anus
- i., intense

- i., lacrimation and
- i. of ear
- i. of jaundiced skin
- i. of skin
- i. of skin, dryness and
- i. or burning sensation
- i., perianal
- i. rash
- i., rectal
- i. ▸ redness, dryness and
- i. sensation
- i. skin ▸ dry
- i. syndromes, chronic-
- i., vaginal
- i., vulvar

itchy
- i. ▸ blister red, scaly, and
- i. crop of blisters
- i. eyes ▸ watery,
- i., flaking skin ▸ dry,
- i. hands ▸ dry, red, cracked and
- i. lesion
- i. nose ▸ runny,
- i. or chapped skin
- i. patches of skin ▸ thick, red,
- i., red, and swollen
- i., runny nose and eyes
- i., scratchy sore throat
- i. skin
- i. ▸ skin dry and
- i. skin rash
- i. swelling of tongue
- i., watery eyes
- i., whitish vaginal discharge

I:E ratio
ITOU (intensive therapy observation unit)
itself, catheter coiled upon
ITU (intensive therapy unit)
IU (International Units)
IUD (intrauterine device)
- IUD, bow
- IUD, coil
- IUD dislodged
- IUD inserted, Copper 7
- IUD, Lippes loop
- IUD spotting
- IUD string

IUGR (intrauterine growth retardation)
IUP (intrauterine pregnancy)
IV (intravenous)
- IV ▸ add-a-line
- IV administration of medication
- IV administration, peripheral

- IV anesthesia
- IV angiocardiography
- IV antibiotic
- IV antireflux procedure, Belsey Mark
- IV -associated infections
- IV barbiturate
- IV bolus injection of contrast medium
- IV catheter
- IV cholangiogram
- IV cholangiography
- IV cholecystography
- IV cocktail
- IV contrast material
- IV discontinued
- IV diuretic
- IV dose
- IV drip, slow
- IV drug abuser
- IV drug needles, infected
- IV drug use
- IV drug use, illegal
- IV drug user
- IV fats
- IV feeding
- IV fluid
- IV fluids, patient treated initially with
- IV fluids, piggy-backing
- IV fluids started
- IV glucose
- IV glucose tolerance test
- IV hydration
- IV immune globulin ▸ respiratory syncytial virus
- IV infection site
- IV infusion
- IV infusion phlebitis
- IV infusion, slow
- IV injection
- IV insulin therapy, low dose
- IV intubation
- IV line
- IV line infection
- IV needle sharing
- IV needle site care
- IV nutritional therapy
- IV, peripheral
- IV Pitocin (DIVP) ▸ dilute
- IV Pitocin drip
- IV sedation
- IV site of infection
- IV tension
- IV therapy

IV tolbutamide tolerance test
IV transfusion
IV urogram
IV urography
IV use of drugs ▸ curb

IVA (intraoperative vascular angiography)

IVAC volumetric infusion pump

Ivalon
I. graft
I. patch
I. patch graft, compressed
I. sponge
I. sponge implant
I. sponge implant material

IVC (inferior vena cava)

IVC (intravenous cholangiogram)

IVCD (intraventricular conduction defect)

IVCP (inferior vena cava pressure)

IVDSA (intravenous digital subtraction angiography)

Ivemark's syndrome

IVF (in vitro fertilization)

ivory
i. bones
i. exostosis
i. substance of tooth

IVP (intravenous pyelogram)

IVP (intravenous pyelogram) ▸ rapid sequence

IVSD (interventricular septal defect)

ivy (Ivy's)
i. blisters ▸ poison
I. loop wiring
I. method bleeding time
i., poison

Iwanoff cyst, Blessig-Iwanoff's retinal edema

IWMI (inferior wall myocardial infarction)

IX antigen, factor

Ixodes
I. bicornis
I. calvipalpus
I. canisuga
I. dammini
I. frequens
I. hexagonus
I. holocyclus
I. pacificus
I. persulcatus
I. pilosus
I. rasus
I. ricinus

I. rubicundus
I. scapularis
I. spinipalpus

J

J (marijuana) (*same as* Jay)
J curve
J junction
J point treadmill test
J pouch
J wave
jabbing
   j. facial pain ▸ severe,
   j. or electric pain ▸ sharp,
   j. pain ▸ sharp,
Jaboulay's
   J. amputation
   J. button
   J. operation
   J. pyloroplasty
Jaccoud('s)
   J. arthropathy
   J. dissociated fever
   J. phenomenon
   J. sign
jack box
jacket(s) (Jackets)
   j., Bonchek-Shiley cardiac
   j. cancer
   j., cardiac cooling
   j. cast, Minerva
   j. crown
   j., cuirass
   j., Kydex body
   j. ▸ Medtronic cardiac cooling
   j., Minerva
   j., plaster of Paris
   j., Royalite body
   j., Sayre's
   j. -type chest dressing
   J. (barbiturates), Yellow
   j. ▸ Willock respiratory
jackknife position
Jackson('s)
   J. bistoury
   J. epilepsy
   J. law
   J. rule
   J. syndrome
   J. tube
   J. veils

jacksonian
   j. attack
   j. epilepsy
   j. epilepsy, Bravais-
   j. seizure
jacobaeus operation
Jacob's membrane
Jacobson's
   J. anastomosis
   J. nerve
   J. retinitis
Jacquemier's sign
Jacquet's dermatitis
Jacquet's erythema
Jaeger's eye chart
Jaeger's test types
Jaesche-Arlt operation
Jaesche operation, Arlt-
Jaffe sign, Pfuhl-
jail bars appearance
Jako biopsy
Jakob('s)
   J. -Creutzfeldt disease
   J. -Creutzfeldt syndrome
   J. disease
   J. disease (vCJD) ▸variant
      Creuzfeldt-
   J. syndrome, Creutzfeldt-
Jaksch's anemia, von
Jalaguier-Kammerer incision ▸
   Battle-
Jamaican (marijuana)
Jamaican vomiting sickness
jamais vu
James bundle
Jameson's operation
Jane (marijuana), Mary
Janet's disease
Janet's test
Janeway('s)
   J. gastrostomy, Depage-
   J. lesions
   J. spots
jangled nerve
Janosik's embryo
Jansen's syndrome
Jansen's test

Jansky's classification
Janthinum, Chromobacterium
Japanese B encephalitis virus
Japanese dysentery
japonica, Haemadipsa
japonica, Hirudo
japonicum, Schistosoma
jargon
   j. agraphia
   j. aphasia
   j., medical
   j. speech
Jarjavay's muscle
Jarotsky's diet
jarring motion
Jarvik
   J. artificial heart ▸ Kolff-
   J. -8 artificial heart
   J. -7 artificial heart
   J. -7 mechanical pump
   J. 7-70 artificial heart
   J. 2000 artificial heart
Jatene arterial switch probe
jaundice
   j. and lethargy
   j. associated with sepsis
   j., chills and fever
   j., cholestatic
   j., chronic familial nonhemo-
      lytic
   j., decreasing
   j., diarrhea ▸ lethargy,
   j., diffuse
   j. from anemia
   j. from cancer
   j. from cirrhosis
   j., hematogenous
   j., hemolytic
   j., homologous serum
   j., infant
   j. leptospiral
   j., lethargy, and fever
   j., neonatal
   j., obstructive
   j., painless
   j., physiologic
   j., progressive

jaundice—*continued*
  j. pruritus
  j., rapid onset of
  j. without inflammation
jaundiced sclerae
jaundiced, skin
Javal's ophthalmometer
javanica, Hirudo
Javid's bypass clamp
Javid's shunt
jaw
  j. and shoulder ▸ chest pain
    radiating to
  j., broken
  j. claudication
  j., clenched
  j. clenching, extreme
  j. deformity
  j. ▸ facial implant of
  j., familial fibrous dysplasia of
  j., fractured
  j. function, normal
  j. grinding
  j. jerk
  j. jerk reflex
  j., misaligned
  j. movement
  j. muscle activity
  j. or extremities ▸ pain in chest,
  j. pain
  j., receding lower
  j. roentgenogram, lateral oblique
  j. strain
  j. support
  j. tension
  j. thrust maneuver
  j. -winking syndrome
  j. wired
jawbone
  j., denuded
  j. loss
  j., lower
  j., upper
Jay (marijuana)
jealousy
  j., alcoholic
  j. and control ▸ obsessive
  j. and persecution, delusions of
  j., delusional
  j., sibling
Jeanselme nodules, Lutz-
Jeanselme's nodules
jecoral tone
Jefferson's fracture
Jeghers syndrome, Peutz-

jejunal
  j. artery
  j. autotransplantation
  j. bypass
  j. diverticula
  j. diverticulosis
  j. feeding tube
  j. fistula
  j. interposition
  j. loop
  j. mucosa
  j. ulcer
  j. vein
  j. villi
jejuni infection, Campylobacter
jejuni, Vibrio
jejunocolic fistula
jejunocolic, gastro◊
jejunoileal bypass
jejunojejunostomy anastomosis
jejunoplasty, esophago◊
jejunostomy
  j., cholecysto◊
  j., choledocho◊
  j., esophago◊
  j. feeding
  j., gastro◊
  j., jejuno◊
  j., pancreatico◊
jejunum and ileum adhesed
Jelenko's arch bar
jelly
  j. belly appearance
  j., cardiac
  j., electrode
  j., lidocaine
  j. -like fluid
  j. -like mass, transparent
  j. nodules, apple
  j. sputum, currant
  j., vitreous
  j., Wharton's
Jendrassik's maneuver
Jenner-Giemsa stain
Jenner's emphysema
Jensen('s)
  J. classification
  J. disease
  J. retinitis
jeopardized myocardium
jeopardy index ▸ myocardial
jeopardy score
jequirity ophthalmia
Jergesen I-beam

jerk(s)
  j., Achilles
  j. and falling ▸ tremors, shakes,
  j. (AJ) ▸ ankle
  j., biceps
  j., crossed
  j. (AJ) ▸ depressed ankle
  j., dormescent
  j., elbow
  j., finger
  j., hypnic
  j., increased knee
  j., involuntary
  j., jaw
  j. (KJ) ▸ knee
  j., muscular
  j., myoclonal
  j., myoclonic
  j., quadriceps
  j. reflex, knee
  j., sudden body
  j., tendon
  j. test of Hughston
  j., triceps surae
  j. ▸ wild limb
jerking
  j. eye movements
  j., head
  j. motions ▸ violent and irregular
  j. movement
  j. movements ▸ massive
  j. movements of legs ▸ involuntary
  j. movements, rhythmic
  j. musculature of face, discrete
  j. of body
  j. of extremity
  j. of limb
jerky
  j. movements
  j. movements, irregular
  j. movements ▸ tremors and
  j. pulse
  j. respiration
  j. step-wise movement
Jervell-Lange-Nielsen syndrome
Jesionek lamp
jet
  j., anteriorly directed
  j., aortic stenosis
  j. area ▸ regurgitant
  j., Doppler color
  j. douche
  j. effect
  j. flow rate ▸ peak
  j. humidifier

j. insulin injector ▸ air-
j. lag
j. lag, occupational
j. lesion
j. ▸ mitral regurgitant
j., mosaic
j., residual
j. signals ▸ mosaic
j., turbulent
j. velocity, aortic
j. ventilation ▸ high frequency
j. ventilator ▸ high frequency
jeune, acne excorie de
Jewell pacer cardioverter
jewelry allergy
Jewett('s)
J. brace
J. classification
J. plate
JGI (juxtaglomerular granulation index)
JH virus
Jianu operation, Beck-
jitteriness ▸ shakiness and
jittery, unfocused behavior
Jive (heroin)
JMD (juvenile memory deficit)
Joaquin fever, San
Joaquin Valley disease ▸ San
job(s)
j., accidents off-the-
j. burn out
j. hazardous to health
j., high stress
j., modified
j. performance
j. performance, decline in
j. performance, diminished
j. -related
j. -related activities
j. -related ailments
j. -related disability
j. -related injury
j. -related stress
j. stress
Jobst('s)
J. bra
J. dressing
J. extremity pump
J. mammary support dressing
J. pressure garment
J. stockings
jock itch
jocked stand crutch
Joffroy's reflex

jogger's nipples
jogging
j., aqua
j. bra
j. craze
j., regular
j. shoes
j. ▸ sudden death during
j., walking and
Johansson disease, Larsen-
johimbe, Corynanthe
Johne's bacillus
Johnson('s)
J. calculation
J. position
J. syndrome, Dubin-
J. syndrome, Stevens-
J. technique
J. twin wire appliance
joint(s) (Joint) [point]
J. (marijuana cigarette)
j. abnormality
j. ▸ accumulation of blood within
j. aches
j. aching
j. (AC joint) ▸ acromioclavicular
j., affected
j., afflicted
j. alignment disorder, knee
j., amphidiarthrodial
j., amputation at
j. and bones
j. and muscle ache
j. and muscle ▸ tender
j., ankle
j. ankylosis, cricoarytenoid
j., anterior dislocation of shoulder
j., apophyseal
j., arthrodial
j. arthroplasty
j., arthritic
j. arthritis, facet
j. arthritis ▸ metatarsophalangeal
j. arthrocentesis
j., artificial knee
j., aspiration and injection of
j., ball-and-socket
j., biaxial
j., bilocular
j., bleeding into
j., bones and
j., Brodie's
j., Budin's
j., bunion
j., capsular

j. capsule
j., capsulitis
j., carpometacarpal
j. cartilage
j., cartilaginous
j., cemented
j., Charcot's
j. chondroma
j., Chopart's
j., chronic inflammation of
j., click heard at hip
j., Clutton's
j., cochlear
j., composite
j., compound
j., condyloid
j. contracture and swelling
j. contractures
j., copious lavage of
j., Cruveilhier's
j. damage
j. damage, permanent
j. debridement
j., deformed gnarled
j. deformity
j. degeneration
j. destruction
j., diarthrodial
j. disease
j. disease (DJD) ▸ degenerative
j. disease, polyradicular
j. dislocation
j. (TMJ) dislocation, temporomandibular
j. disorder
j. disorder ▸ disabling
j. disorder ▸ inflammatory
j. disorder ▸ metatarsophalangeal
j. (TMJ) disorder ▸ temporomandibular
j. (DIPJ) ▸ distal interphalangeal
j., dry
j. dysfunction, temporomandibular
j. effusion
j., effusion of knee
j., elbow
j., ellipsoid
j., enarthrodial
j., erasion of
j. evaluation, computerized muscle-
j. examination
j., excision of
j., excursion of
j. ▸ extensive manipulation of
j., facet

joint(s)—*continued*

j., false
j., fibrocartilaginous
j., fibrous
j., fixed
j., flail
j. flexibility
j. flexible
j. flexing
j. fluid
j. fluid analysis
j., fluid aspirated from
j. fracture
j., freely movable
j., fringe
j., frozen
j. function
j. fusion
j., glenohumeral
j., gliding
j., hinge
j., hip
j., hysteric
j., immovable
j. implant, artificial
j. implant ▸ finger
j. implant material, artificial
j. implant, Swanson finger
j. implant, Swanson wrist
j., incision into
j., incudomalleal
j., incudomalleolar
j., incudostapedial
j. ▸ indwelling prosthetic
j., infected
j. infection
j. infection, bone and
j. infection ▸ prosthetic
j. infection ▸ staph
   (Staphylococcus) aureus
   prosthetic
j., inflammation of
j., inflamed
j. ▸ inflamed swollen
j. injury
j., instability of lumbosacral
j., intercarpal
j., internal derangement of
j., interphalangeal
j., intertarsal
j., irritable
j., knee
j. ▸ knobby growth on finger
j. level, medial
j., ligamentous

j. line
j. line, anteromedial
j. line, medial
j. lining ▸ infected
j., Lisfranc's
j., locking of
j., loose
j., loose body in
j., loosening
j., lumbosacral
j., Luschka's
j., malleo-incudal
j., manipulation of
j., manipulation of dislocated
j., medial meniscus of knee
j., meniscus of acromioclavicular
j., meniscus of temporomaxillary
j. (MPJ), metacarpophalangeal
j., metatarsal cuneiform
j., metatarsophalangeal
j. mice
j., midcarpal
j., midcervical apophyseal
j., mixed
j. mobility
j. mobility ▸ knee
j., mortise of
j. motion
j. motion, limited
j. mouse
j. movement, limited
j. movement, loss of
j., multiaxial
j., natural
j. of Luschka
j. of thumb, basal
j., osteoarthritis of
   temporomandibular
j., osteonecrosis of
j. ▸ overuse of
j. pain
j. pain and discomfort
j. pain and fatigue ▸ severe
j. pain and stiffness
j. pain and swelling
j. pain, chronic
j. pain, general
j. ▸ pain in muscles and
j. pain ▸ peripheral
j. pain, sacroiliac
j. pain, severe
j. pain ▸ stabbing
j. pain, transient
j. pain ▸ weakness, dizziness, and
j., painful

j., painful inflammation of
j., painful swollen
j. parts ▸ wear-resistant artificial
j. pathology
j., pathology, bone or
j., pivot
j., plane
j., polyaxial
j., popliteal
j. position sensation
j. position sense (JPS)
j., pressure on toe
j. problems from arthritis
j. (TMJ) proper alignment of
   temporomandibular
j., prosthetic
j. ▸ prosthetic glenohumeral
j. protection
j. (PIPJ), proximal interphalangeal
j. range of motion
j. range of motion ▸ maintaining
j. reconstruction
j. reconstruction ▸ total
j. ▸ red swollen
j. reflex, basal
j. -related disorder
j., relaxation of
j. repair, customized
j., repair of
j. replacement, elbow
j. ▸ repetitive motion in the
j. ▸ repetitive motion of wrist
j. replacement
j. replacement, knee
j. replacement surgery
j. replacement, total
j. resection, Girdlestone
j., reshaping
j. rheumatoid arthritis (JRA)
j., rotary
j., sacrococcygeal
j., sacroiliac
j., saddle
j., scapuloclavicular
j. (TMJ) screening,
   temporomandibular
j. sensibility
j., separated acromioclavicular (AC)
j., septic
j., shoulder
j. (MPJ), silastic
   metacarpophalangeal
j. ▸ silicone-based artificial
j., simple
j. site

j., socket
j., sore
j. space
j. space, interpedicular
j. space, narrowing of
j., spheroid
j., spiral
j., sprained
j. stability
j. stabilized
j., stable
j., sternoclavicular
j., stiff
j. stiffening
j. stiffness
j. ▸ structural changes in
j. subluxation
j., subtalar
j., supple
j. surface
j. surface, lateral plateau
j., surgical immobilization of
j. swelling
j. swelling and tenderness
j. swelling in hemodialysis
j. swelling ▸ loss of appetite with
j., swollen
j. swollen and inflamed ▸ thumb
j., swollen and painful
j. ▸ swollen, stiff, inflamed
j., synarthrodial
j. syndrome, temporomandibular
j., synovial
j., synovial membrane of
j., talonavicular
j., tarsal
j., temporary opening in
j. (TMJ) ▸ temporomandibular
j., tender
j. tenderness
j., tibiofibular
j. tissues
j. toilet
j., transitional lumbosacral
j. trauma
j. treatment planning
j., trochoid
j. twisting injury to
j., uncemented
j., uniaxial
j., unilocular
j., von Gies'
j., warm
j. weight-bearing
j. with inflammation ▸ diseased

j., worn facet
j., wrist
j., zygapophyseal
jointed, double
jointedness, loose
Jolly('s)
J. bodies
J. bodies, Howell-
J. reaction
Jones(')
J., albumin of Bence
J. albumosuria, Bence
J. closure, Tom
J. cylinder
J. globulin, Bence
J. light chain type ▸ Bence
J. operation
J. operation, Blundell-
J. operation, Ellis-
J. operation, Strassman-
J. operation, Watson-
J. position
J. procedure
J. protein, Bence
J. protein method, Bence-
J. protein test, Bence
J. proteinuria, Bence
J. -Reinhard unit ▸ Shinowara-
J. suspension traction
J. tenodesis
J. tenosuspension
J. toe repair
J. urine, Bence-
J. valve prosthesis ▸ Cross-
Joplin toe prosthesis
Joplin's operation
jordanis, Legionella
Joseph's syndrome
Josephs-Diamond-Blackfan
syndrome
Jostra cardiotomy reservoir
Joule('s)
j. curve
J. equivalent
j., heart defibrillated with single
shock of _____
j. junction
j. per kilogram
j. point
j. point electrical axis
j. wave
Journal of Substance Abuse
Treatment (JSAT)
journal writing skills
jovial disposition

JPS (joint position sense)
JRA (joint rheumatoid arthritis)
JRA (juvenile rheumatoid arthritis)
JSAT (Journal of Substance Abuse
Treatment)
JT interval
Judd's pyloroplasty
Judet's prosthesis
Jude('s)
J. annuloplasty ring ▸ St.
J. heart valve prosthesis ▸ St.
J. valve ▸ St.
Judet-type femoral prosthetic head
judge memory
judgment
j., aberration of
j. and decision making ▸
interference with
j., change in
j., clinical
j., common sense
j., decreased
j., deficiency in
j. ▸ disintegration of
j., ethical
j., impaired
j., impairment of
j. ▸ loss of
j. ▸ loss of recent memory,
confusion and poor
j. ▸ mental abilities and
j., moral
j. of accomplishments ▸ inflated
j. of distance
j., poor
j., weaker
judicial inquiry
jugal suture
jugular
j. bulb anomaly
j. bulb, thrombosis of
j. chain lymph nodes, internal
j. embryocardia
j. floor
j. foramen syndrome
j. ganglion, inferior
j. ganglion of glossopharyngeal
nerve
j. ganglion of vagus nerve
j. lymph nodes
j. lymph nodes, internal
j. notch of occipital bone
j. notch of sternum
j. notch of temporal bone
j. pressure (IJP) ▸ internal

jugular—*continued*
- j. pulse
- j. test, abdominal
- j. test, aortic
- j. trunk
- j. vein (JV)
- j. vein (JV) ▸ anterior
- j. vein (JV) ▸ anterior horizontal
- j. vein cannulation, internal
- j. vein, collapsed
- j. vein distention (JVD)
- j. vein, external
- j. vein, flat
- j. vein, internal
- j. vein ▸ left internal
- j. vein, right internal
- j. vein, severed
- j. venous arch
- j. venous (JV) blocking
- j. venous catechol spillover
- j. venous distention (JVD)
- j. venous pressure
- j. venous pulse
- j. venous pulse, CV wave of
- j. venous pulse ▸ f wave of
- j. venous pulse tracing
- j. venous pulse ▸ y depression of
- j. venous pulse ▸ y descent of
- j. wall

jugulare, glomus
jugularis, bulbus venae
jugularis, paries
jugulodigastric nodes
jugulotympanic paraganglioma
juice(s)
- j. ▸ elimination of pancreatic digestive
- j., gastric
- j., pancreatic
- j., secretes gastric
- j. sputum, prune
- j. (hashish) ▸ Weed

jumbled speech
jump
- j. collaterals
- j., depth
- j. flap
- j. flap, abdominal
- j. graft
- j. graft ▸ Gore-Tex
- j. -start heart
- j. -started ▸ heart

jumper's knee
jumper's strain, high-
jumping pain

jumping thrombosis
jumpy, patient irritable and
juncea, Filaria
junction(s) [*function*]
- j., amelodentinal
- j., angular
- j. anomaly, atrioventricular (AV)
- j., atrioventricular
- j., cardioesophageal
- j., cardioesophagus
- j., cortical medullary
- j., costochondral
- j., dentinocemental
- j., dentinoenamel
- j., dermal epidermal
- j., dermal subcutaneous
- j., dermoepidermal
- j. escape rhythm, atrioventricular (AV)
- j., esophagogastric
- j., gap
- j., gastroesophageal
- j., ileocecal
- j., intercellular
- j., ischiopubic
- j., J
- j., joule
- j., loose
- j. motion, atrioventricular (AV)
- j., mucocutaneous
- j., myoneural
- j., nasolabial
- j., nerve
- j., nerve-muscle
- j., neuromuscular
- j. obstruction, ureteropelvic
- j. of distal third
- j. of eyelids, angular
- j. of middle third
- j. of optic nerve
- j. of pharynx
- j., osteochondral
- j., pontine
- j., pontine medullary
- j. protein, cardiac gap
- j., QRS-ST
- j., rectosigmoid
- j., saphenofemoral
- j., sclerocorneal
- j., sinotubular
- j., splice
- j., squamocolumnar
- j., ST
- j., sternochondral
- j., sternoclavicular

- j. tachycardia ▸ nonparoxysmal atrioventricular (AV)
- j., tear in mucosa at cardioesophageal
- j., tight
- j., tracheoesophageal
- j., triadic
- j. (UP), ureteropelvic
- j. (UVJ), ureterovesical

junctional
- j. arrhythmia
- j. axis
- j. beats, premature
- j. bigeminy
- j. bigeminy, atrioventricular (AV)
- j. bradycardia
- j. cavity
- j. complex
- j. complex ▸ premature atrioventricular (AV)
- j. contractions
- j. depression
- j. ectopic tachycardia
- j. escape
- j. escape beat
- j. escape complex, AV (atrioventricular)
- j. escape rhythm
- j. extrasystole
- j. extrasystole, AV (atrioventricular)
- j. heart block, atrioventricular (AV)
- j. interspace
- j. lymph nodes
- j. nevus
- j. pacemaker
- j. pacemaker, atrioventricular (AV)
- j. reciprocating tachycardia
- j. reciprocating tachycardia, AV (atrioventricular)
- j. reciprocating tachycardia (PJRT) ▸ permanent
- j. rhythm
- j. rhythm, accelerated
- j. rhythm, accelerated atrioventricular (AV)
- j. rhythm after cardiac surgery
- j. rhythm, arteriovenous
- j. rhythm, atrioventricular (AV)
- j. rhythm, AV (atrioventricular)
- j. systoles, premature
- j. tachycardia
- j. tachycardia, arteriovenous
- j. tachycardia, atrioventricular (AV)
- j. tachycardia, AV (atrioventricular)
- j. tachycardia ▸ intractable

j. tachycardia ▸ nonparoxysmal
j. tachycardia ▸ nonparoxysmal
  atrioventricular
j. tachycardia ▸ paroxysmal
j. tissue
junctioning reciprocating tachycardia
juncture, saphenofemoral
juncture stricture ▸ UP
  (ureteropelvic)
Jungbluth, vasa propria of
Jungian theory
jungle fever
jungle yellow fever
Jüngling's disease
Jung's method
Jung's muscle
Junin virus
Junin virus ▸ South American
Junius disease, Kuhnt-
Junk (junk)
  J. (heroin)
  j. food
  j. food diet
junkie, support group
junky aorta
Jürgens syndrome, Willebrand-
Jürgensen's sign
Juster reflex
justo major, pelvis aequabiliter
justo minor, pelvis aequabiliter
jutting mandible
juvenile
  j. acquired hypothyroidism
  j. alcoholic
  j. aldosteronism
  j. angiofibroma
  j. anxiety disorder
  j. arrhythmia
  j. cataract
  j. cell
  j. chorea
  j. chronic polyarthritis
  j. diabetes
  j. diabetic, patient
  j. elastoma
  j. epiphysitis
  j. glaucoma
  j. hereditary motor neuron disease
  j. idiopathic scoliosis
  j. macular degeneration
  j. melanoma
  j. memory deficit (JMD)
  j. muscular atrophy
  j. nephrophthisis (FJN), familial
  j. neutrophil

j. onset
j. onset diabetes mellitus (DM)
j. osteomalacia
j. pattern
j. pernicious anemia
j. pilocytic astrocytoma
j. polyp, pedunculated
j. polyps
j. reflex
j. residential care
j. rheumatoid arthritis
j. wart
j. xanthogranuloma
juvenilis
  j., acne
  j., arcus
  j., osteochondritis deformans
  j., verruca plana
juxta-articular nodules
juxtacapillary receptor
juxtacardiac pleural pressure
juxtaductal coarctation
juxtaglomerular
  j. cell hyperplasia
  j. cells
  j. granulation index (JGI)
  j. granules
juxtapapillaris, retinochoroiditis
juxtapapillary chorioretinitis, acute
juxtapapillitic choroiditis
Juzo hose
JV (jugular vein)
JV (jugular venous) blocking
JVD (jugular vein distention)
JVP (jugular venous pulse)

K

K (potassium)
K complex
    K.c. burst
    K.c. during sleep
    K.c. waves
K current
K nail
K pad, Aqua-
K (Ketamine) ▸ Special
K virus
K (Ketamine) ▸ Vitamin
Kagel exercises
Kahn's test
Kaiserling's fixative
Kaiserling's fluid
kala azar
    k., canine
    k., infantile
    k., Mediterranean
Kalischer's disease
Kallmann's syndrome
Kameruns' swelling
Kammerer incision ▸ Battle-
    Jalaguier-
Kamofsky status
Kanavel's sign
kang cancer
kangaroo ligature
kangri cancer
Kanner's syndrome
kansasii, Mycobacterium
Kanter's sign
kaolin partial thromboplastin time
Kapeller-Adler test
Kapel's operation
Kapetansky, method of
Kaposi('s)
    K. sarcoma
    K. sarcoma herpes virus (KSHV)
    K. sarcoma ▸ pseudo-
    K. varicelliform eruption
    K., xeroderma of
kappa
    k. angle
    k. angle, large
    k. granule
    k. light chains

    k. opioid
    k. rhythm
    k. wave
Kappeler's maneuver
karate chop
Kardex card, patient's
Kardex system
Karell's diet
Karell's treatment
Karmen technique
Karmen units
Karnofsky rating scale
Karnofsky status
Kartagener's
    K. disease
    K. syndrome
    K. triad
kartulisi, Entamoeba
karyoblastoma, mega◊
karyopyknotic cells
karyotype, abnormal
karyotyping, fetal
karyozoic parasite
Kasabach-Merritt syndrome
Kasai procedure
Kashin-Bek disease
Kaster
    K. cardiac valve prosthesis ▸
        Lillehei-
    K. mitral valve prosthesis ▸
        Lillehei-
    K. prosthesis ▸ Lillehei-Cruz-
Katena trephine
Kattus exercise stress test
Katz-Wachtel phenomenon
Kaufman('s)
    K. (M-K) medium, McCarey-
    K. pneumonia
    K. vitrector
Kawasaki's disease
Kawasaki's syndrome
Kawashima intraventricular tunnel
Kaycel towels
Kay-Shiley valve prosthesis
Kay-Suzuki disc valve prosthesis
Kayser-Fleischer ring
Kazanjian lower lip flap, Stein-

Kaznelson's syndrome
K-capture
kc (kilocycle)
K-cal (kilocalorie)
kcps (kilocycles per second)
Kearns-Sayre syndrome
Kebab's graft
keel, McNaught
keel stent
keeled chest
Keeler cryophake unit
Keeler polarizing ophthalmoscope
Keen's sign
keep appointment, fails to
keeping emotional distance
Kees headrest, Mayfield-
kefir fungi
Kegel exercises
Kehrer's reflex
Kehr's incision
Kehr's sign
Keith('s)
    K. bundle
    K. -Flack node
    K. node
    K. -Wagener-Barker classification
Keller
    K. bunion
    K. bunion osteotomy
    K. bunionectomy
    K. procedure
kellicotti, Paragonimus
Kellner questionnaire
Kellogg-Speed operation
Kelly('s)
    K. operation
    K. syndrome ▸ Paterson-Brown
    K. tube
Kelman phacoemulsification
keloid
    k. formation
    k. of cornea
    k. scar
Kelvin scale
Kempf's disease
Kempner's diet
Ken nail

K

Kennedy('s)
- K. classification
- K. operation
- K. syndrome
- K. syndrome ▸ Foster-

Kent('s)
- K. bundle
- K. bundle ablation
- K., bundle of Stanley-
- K. Emergency Scale
- K. ▸ fibers of
- K. -His bundle
- K. potential

Keogh feeding tube

kept at ____torr, dropped to____torr ▸ pressure

keratectomy
- k., complete
- k., partial
- k. (PRK) ▸ photorefractive
- k. (Lasek) procedure, laser-assisted subepithelial
- k., radial

keratic precipitates (KP)

keratic precipitates (KP), mutton fat

keratin ball

keratin whorls

keratinization, focal

keratinized cell

keratitis
- k., Acanthamoeba
- k., acne rosacea
- k., actinic
- k., aerosol
- k., alphabet
- k., arborescent
- k., artificial silk
- k., bacterial
- k., band
- k. bandelette
- k. bullosa
- k., dendriform
- k., dendritic
- k., Dimmers
- k. disciformis
- k., fascicular
- k. filamentosa
- k., Fuchs'
- k., herpes
- k., herpetic
- k., hypopyon
- k., interstitial
- k., lagophthalmic
- k., lattice
- k., marginal

- k., metaherpetic
- k., mycotic
- k., neuroparalytic
- k., neurotropic
- k. nummularis
- k., oyster shuckers'
- k., parenchymatous
- k. petrificans
- k., phlyctenular
- k. profunda
- k. punctata
- k. punctata subepithelialis
- k., punctate
- k. pustuliformis profunda
- k. ramificata superficialis
- k., reaper's
- k., reticular
- k., ribbon-like
- k., rosacea
- k., Schmidt's
- k., sclerosing
- k., sclerotic
- k., scrofulus
- k., serpiginous
- k. sicca
- k., striate
- k., stromal herpetic
- k., suppurative
- k., Thygeson's
- k., trachomatous
- k., trophic
- k., ulcerative
- k., vascular
- k., vasculonebulous
- k., vesicular
- k., xerotic

keratoconjunctivitis
- k., epidemic
- k., epizootic
- k., flash
- k. sicca
- k., superior limbic
- k., viral
- k. virus, epidemic
- k., welder's

keratohyaline granules

keratoma, malignant

keratome incision

keratomileusis
- k. (LASIK) correction ▸ laser-assisted in situ
- k. (LASIK) ▸ laser assisted in situ
- k. (LASIK) ▸ laser in situ
- k., myopic

- k. (LASIK) surgery ▸ laser-assisted in situ
- k. (LASIK) surgery ▸ wavefront-guided laser-assisted in situ

keratopathy, band

keratopathy, bullous

keratoplasty
- k. (ALK), automated lamellar
- k. (CK), conductive
- k., lamellar
- k. ▸ laser thermal
- k., optic
- k., partial penetrating
- k., tectonic

keratosa, pharyngitis

keratoses
- k., actinic
- k., benign lichenoid
- k., multiple
- k., multiple seborrheic
- k. ▸ pre-cancerous
- k., pruritic
- k., senile
- k., stucco

keratosis(-es)
- k. blennorrhagica
- k. follicularis
- k. ▸ noncancerous sun-induced
- k. palmaris
- k. pharyngea
- k. pilaris
- k. plantaris
- k. precancerous actinic
- k. punctata
- k., roentgen
- k., seborrheic
- k. seborrheica
- k., senile
- k. senilis
- k., solar

keratotic lesion

keratotomy
- k., astigmatic
- k., delimiting
- k. (PERK) protocol ▸ prospective evaluation of radial
- k. (RK), radial
- k. ▸ radial and astigmatic
- k. technique ▸ radial

Kerckring('s)
- K. folds
- K., nodules of
- K., valve of

Kergaradec's sign

Kerley's A line

Kerley's B line
Kerlix
  K. bandage
  K. dressing
  K. gauze roll
kerma rate constant, air
kernicterus, encephalomyelopathy
  with
Kernig's sign
Kernohan's notch
kerosene emulsion
Kerr('s)
  K. cesarean (C-) section
  K. maneuver, Munro-
  K. sign
Kerrison's technique
Kessler's operation
Kestenbach-Anderson procedure
Ketamine (K)
  K. (Ketalar)
  K. (Special K)
  K. (Vitamin K)
  K. ingested
  K. injected
  K. snorted
ketoacidosis (DKA), diabetic
ketogenic
  k. -antiketogenic ratio
  k. diet ▸ high fat
  k. steroid
ketone(s)
  k. bodies
  k. body test
  k., Ketostix test for
ketosis, starvation
ketosteroid test
Ketostix test for ketones
ketotic acidosis
kev (kilo electron volts)
Kevorkian punch biopsy
key
  k. issues
  k. kid, latch
  k. muscles, stretching
keyed up, patient
keyhole
  k. bypass surgery
  k. incision
  k. mastectomy
  k. surgery
  k. surgical technique
keying, sound
Key's operation
keystone ligament
kg (kilogram)

Kg-cal (kilogram-calorie)
kg/m² (kilogram per meter squared)
Khz (kilohertz)
kick(s)
  k., atrial
  k. counts
  k., front
  k., idioventricular
  k., knee
  k., round-house
  k., side
kicking
  k. cocaine
  k. drug habit
  k. smoking habit
  k. the habit
kid(s)
  k., crack
  k., drug affected
  k., drug exposed
  k., latch key
Kidner's operation
kidney(s)
  k., adenocarcinoma
  k. adenoma
  k., amyloid
  k. ▸ anaplastic carcinoma of
  k. anatomically normal
  k. and bladder, tuberculosis of
  k. and brain function ▸ diminished
    heart,
  k. and brain function ▸ heart,
  k. and spleen (LKS) ▸ liver,
  k. anomaly
  k., arcuate vein of
  k., arteriolonecrosis of
  k., arteriosclerotic
  k. artery
  k., artificial
  k., atrophic
  k. (donor) ▸ authorization form to
    use
  k. (next of kin) ▸ authorization form
    to use
  k., blocked
  k., cadaver
  k., cadaveric
  k., cake
  k. calcium stones
  k. cancer
  k., carcinoma of
  k. cell cultures
  k., cicatricial
  k., cirrhosis of
  k., clump

k., congenital absence of
k., congested
k. (donor) consent form to use
k. (next of kin) ▸ consent form to
  use
k., contracted
k. cortex
k., cortical lobules of
k., cortical scarring of
k. ▸ cortical substance of
k., crush
k., cyanotic
k., cystic
k., cystiform dilatation of
k., cystiform enlargement
k. cysts
k. damage
k. damage ▸ permanent
k. damage, progressive
k., decapsulation of
k. development ▸ fetal
k. dialysis
k., disc
k. disease
k. disease, active lupus
k. disease (APKD), adult polycystic
k. disease (PKD) ▸ autosomal
  dominant polycystic
k. disease, chronic
k. disease ▸ glomerular
k. disease ▸ immune
k. disease (PKD), polycystic
k. disease ▸ risk of
k. disorder
k. donated
k. donated for kidney transplant
k., donation of
k. donor
k., double
k., doughnut
k., duplication of left
k., duplication of right
k. dysfunction
k., ectopic
k., embryoma of
k. exposed
k. failure
k. failure, acute
k. failure, chronic
k. failure, irreversible
k. failure, progressive
k., fatty capsule of
k. -fixing antibody
k., flea-bitten
k., floating

kidney(s)—*continued*
k., flush out
k., Formad's
k., free floating
k. freed
k. freed and exposed by blunt dissection
k. function
k. function, decreased
k. function, impaired
k. function, impairment of
k. function, increased
k. function ▸ reduced
k. function tests
k., functional
k. functioning normally
k., fused
k., glomerular capsule of
k., Coldblatt's
k., granular atrophy of
k., hemisection of
k. hilus
k., hind
k. ▸ histologic sections of
k., horseshoe-type
k., human embryo
k., hypermobile
k., hypoplastic
k. immature
k. impairment
k. infarction
k. infection
k. infection ▸ recurrent
k. infiltrate ▸ deteriorating of
k. inflammation, acute
k. inflammation, chronic
k., inflammation of
k., infundibula of
k. injury
k., interlobar vein of
k., interlobular vein of
k., lardaceous
k., large red
k., left
k. ▸ leukemic infiltrates of
k. ▸ living unrelated
k., lobe of
k., lobulated
k., long axis of
k., lump
k. machine, artificial
k. malformation
k. malfunction
k., malignant tumor of
k., medullary sponge

k. ▸ medullary substance of
k. meridian
k. mobile
k., mortar
k., mural
k., myelin
k. ▸ Nephros bioartificial
k., nonfunctioning
k., non-visualized
k. (LSK) not palpable ▸ liver, spleen,
k. obstruction
k. pale and swollen
k. palpated
k. -pancreas transplants
k., parenchyma of
k., parental
k. pedicle clamps
k. pelvis, intrapelvic
k., pelvis of
k. perfused
k. perfused and cooled
k., ▸ petechial hemorrhages of
k., piecemeal removal of
k., polycystic
k., portable mechanical
k., priming of artificial
k., primordial
k. protein renin, high levels of
k., ptosis of
k., ptotic
k. punch
k., putty
k., pyramids of
k. recipient
k. rejection, grafted
k., renal cell carcinoma of
k. replaced in renal fossa
k. rest elevated
k. ▸ retention cyst of
k., right
k., Rokitansky's
k., Rose-Bradford
k., rotated
k., sacciform
k. scan
k., scar lower pole left
k., scar lower pole right
k., scarred
k., sclerotic
k., segments of
k. shadow
k. -shaped diplococci ▸ gram-negative

k. -shaped diplococci ▸ gram-negative extracellular
k. -shaped diplococci ▸ gram-negative intracellular
k., shrunken
k., shutdown of
k., sigmoid
k., soapy
k., sponge
k., stellate vein of
k. stimulant
k. stone
k. stone, disintegrating
k. stone, dissolve
k. stone fragmentation
k. stone, passing of
k., suitcase
k., supernumerary
k., suspension of
k. tissue
k. tissue, necrotic
k., tomography of both
k. toxicity
k. transplant
k. transplant ▸ kidney donated for
k. transplant patient
k. transplant rejection
k. transplant ▸ spousal
k. transplantation
k. tubules, dilated
k. tumor in children
k., ureters and bladder (KUB)
k., ureters and bladder (KUB) film
k., urine secreted in
k., vein of
k. ▸ venous arches of
k., wandering
k. washout
k., waxy
k. (WAK) ▸ wearable artificial
k. worm

Kiel graft
Kien respiration, Kussmaul-
Kienböck's dislocation
Kienböck's unit of x-ray dosage
Kiesselbach's
K. area
K. plexus
K. triangle
kif (tobacco and marijuana mix)
kiliense, Acremonium
kiliensis, Serratia
kill patient, directly
killed cells, heat
killed poliomyelitis vaccine

Killeen pacemaker, Amtech
killer
- k. bacteria
- k. blood cells
- k., cancer
- k. (LAK) cell, lymphokine-activated
- k. (NK) cells ▸ natural
- k., pain
- k., silent
- k. virus vaccine
- K. Weed (phencyclidine)

Killian's operation
Killian's tube
killing
- k. ability, body's tumor
- k. ability, cancer-
- k. brain tumors
- k. by lethal injection ▸ direct
- k., cell
- k. dye, cancer-
- k., mercy
- k. of incompetent individual ▸ direct

kilo electron volts (kev)
kilocycles per second (kcps)
kilogram
- k. -calorie (kg-cal)
- k., joule per
- k. per meter squared (kg/m²)

Kiloh-Nevin syndrome
kilohms, expressed in
kilovolt peak (Kvp)
kilowatt-hour (kw-hr)
Kimmelstiel-Wilson disease
Kimmelstiel-Wilson syndrome
Kimura cartilage graft
kin, next-of-
kin, permission of next-of-
kinase
- k. activity ▸ receptor
- k., bacterial
- k., creatine
- k., glycerol
- k., neurofilament
- k., phosphoglycerate
- k., protein
- k., pyruvate
- k., serum creatine
- k. test, serum creatine

Kindling phenomenon
kinematic rotating hinge knee prosthesis
kinematic viscosity
kinesiology, applied
kinesograph, gastro◊

kinesthetic
- k. aura
- k. disorder
- k. hallucinations
- k. sense

kinetic(s)
- k. abrasion
- k. analysis, cell cycle
- k. apraxia, limb-
- k. ataxia
- k., cell
- k., cellular
- k. center
- k. energy
- k. ▸ first order
- k. of adenocarcinoma, cell
- k. of tumors, cell
- k., radionuclide
- k. strabismus
- k. tremor
- k., tumor cell
- k. type, amyostatic-
- k. ▸ zero-order

kinetocardiogram study
kinetocardiography study
Kinevac contrast medium
King
- K. -Armstrong unit
- K. cervical brace
- K. of Hearts Monitor
- K. operation ▸ Reichenheim-
- K. -Richards operation
- K. Tut (LSD)

kinked aorta
kinking of bowel
kinking of intestine
kinky hair disease
Kinsey rotation atherectomy extrusion angioplasty
Kinyoun stain
Kipp's coronary arteries
Kirby's operation
Kirby's suture
Kirkaldy-Willis operation
Kirklin fence
Kirklin staging system
Kirk's amputation
Kirmisson's operation
Kirschner wire (K-wire)
Kirschner's apparatus
Kisch's reflex
kissing
- k. balloon angioplasty
- k. balloon technique
- k. ulcers

Kistner tracheal button
kit(s)
- k., catheter care
- k., colorectal cancer
- k., home medical test
- k., Medi-
- k., Tc (technetium) 99m aggregated albumin
- k., Tc (technetium) 99m albumin microspheres
- k., Tc (technetium) 99m etidronate sodium
- k., Tc (technetium) 99m medronate sodium
- k., Tc (technetium) 99m penetate sodium
- k., Tc (technetium) 99m serum albumin
- k., urinary catheter care

Kitahara disease ▸ Masuda-
k.j. (knee jerk)
Kjeldahl method, micro-
Kjeldahl technique, macro-
KK (knee kicks)
Klebs' disease
Klebs-Löffler bacillus
Klebsiella
- K. -Enterobacter
- K. friedländeri
- K. oxytoca
- K. ozaenae
- K. ozogenes, gram-negative
- K. pneumonia
- K. pneumoniae
- K. pneumoniae, gram-negative
- K. rhinoscleromatis
- K. species
- K. urinary tract infection

Kleihauer-Betke test
Kleijn neck reflex ▸ Magnus and de
Klein & French (SKF) culture ▸ Smith,
Kleine-Levin syndrome
Klein's bacillus
Kleinschmidt technique
Klieg eye
Kline flocculation test
Klinefelter's syndrome
Kling
- K. adhesive dressing
- K. bandage
- K. elastic gauze
- K. gauze dressing

Klippel-Feil sign
Klippel-Feil syndrome
Kloeckera apiculatus

Kloehn's headgear
Kloepfer's syndrome
Kluge's method
Klumpke's paralysis
Klüver-Bucy syndrome
kluyveri, Clostridium
Knapp-Imre operation
Knapp's operation
knäuel stage
kneading maneuver during massage,
   basic
kneading of body
knee(s)
   k. (AK) ▸ above
   k., acromegaly of
   k. action
   k. alignment
   k. (AK) amputation ▸ above
   k. (BK) amputation ▸ below
   k., arcuate ligament of
   k. arthroplasty, total
   k., articular muscle of
   k. artificial
   k. baby
   k., back
   k., beat
   k. bend
   k. bend exercise
   k. bends, cartilage-wearing
   k. bends, deep
   k., big
   k. bone
   k. boot
   k. brace
   k. brace, custom
   k. brace, 49er
   k. brace, preventive
   k. brace, prophylactic
   k. breech presentation
   k., Brodie's
   k., buckling and/or locking of
   k., calcification collateral ligament of
   k. cap
   k. cap splinting
   k. cap, stabilize
   k., capped
   k. cartilage
   k. cartilage, torn
   k. -chest position
   k., chondrocalcinosis of
   k., chronically painful
   k. clonus
   k. completely, extends
   k. ▸ congenital subluxation of
   k., contracture of

k. crackling
k., cyst meniscus of
k. ▸ degenerative arthritis of
k., disability in
k., dislocation of
k., dorsolateral surface of
k. drop
k. -elbow position
k. ▸ expand internal components of
k. extended
k. extension
k. flexed
k. flexion
k. flexion, active
k. flexion contracture of
k., fluid aspirated from
k., fluid in
k., football
k. full range of motion (ROM) ▸ left
k. full range of motion (ROM) ▸
   right
k. function
k. fusion
k. -gall
k., Gerdy's tubercle in
k. -heel test
k., heel-to-
k. hemarthrosis
k. -high socks
k., hooped
k., housemaid's
k. immobilized
k. in children ▸ knock-
k. injury
k. injury, acute
k., instability of
k., internal derangement of
k. jerk (KJ)
k. jerk (KJ) ▸ increased
k. jerk (KJ) reflex
k. joint
k. joint alignment disorder
k. joint, artificial
k. joint, effusion of
k. joint, medial meniscus of
k. joint mobility
k. joint replacement
k. kicks
k., knock
k., lateral surface of
k. lift squat exercise
k. ligament, artificial
k. ligament injury
k. ligament repair
k. ligament ▸ torn

k., locked
k. locks
k., long leg brace with droplock
k., medial compartment of
k., misalignment of
k., mobilize
k. monarthritis caused by
   tuberculosis
k. motion, range of
k. of acquaductus fallopi
k. of internal capsule
k. osteonecrosis
k., out
k., overflex
k. pain, chronic debilitating
k. pain in runner
k. pain ▸ osteoarthritis
k. ▸ painful osteoarthritis of
k. prosthesis, geometric
k. prosthesis, Guepar hinge
k. prosthesis, Kinematic rotating
   hinge
k. prosthesis, Shier's total
k. prosthesis ▸ unicompartmental
k. prosthesis ▸ Walldius Vitallium
   mechanical
k. ▸ protect and stabilize injured
k. ▸ pseudogout in
k., reconstruct
k. reflex
k. replacement ▸ partial
k. replacement surgery
k. replacement, total
k., robotic
k., rugby
k., runner's
k., septic
k. ▸ silvery scales on
k., sprung
k., stabilize
k. stiffness
k. stress
k. (AK) support, above
k., surgery, arthroscopic
k., swelling of
k. ▸ synovial cell sarcoma of the
k. test, heel-
k. to chest raise
k. to shoulder stretch
k., trick
k., unstable
Kniest dwarfism
knife (knives)
   k. advanced upward
   k. and scissors dissection

k. cone biopsy, cold
k. cone, cold
k. conization
k. conization biopsy, cold
k. conization, cold
k., hot
k. -like pain, burning
k., neurosurgical gamma
k. procedure ▸ gamma
k. reflex, clasp-
k. rigidity, clasp-
k., roller
k. stereotactic radiosurgery ▸ gamma
k., tympanoplastic
k. wound
Knight's brace
knitted sewing ring
knitted vascular prosthesis
knob, aortic
knobby growth on finger joint
knobs, synaptic
knock
k. -knee
k. -knee in children
k., pericardial
knocked-down shoulder
knot formation, syncytial
knot tying
knotted muscles ▸ tight,
knowing limitations
knowledge
k., accumulated
k. deficit
k. ▸ loss of self-
k., medical
k. situation
Knowles pin
known
k. asthmatic, patient
k. cardiac risk
k. cure, no
k. deficits
k. metastatic focus
k. organic factor ▸ hypersomnia related to a
k. organic factor ▸ insomnia related to a
k. risk factor
knuckle
k., aortic
k., arthritic
k., cervical aortic
k. cracking
k. sign

k. sobriety, white
knuckling maneuver during massage
Koby's cataract
Koch('s)
K. -Mason dressing
K. node
K. reservoir
Koch-Weeks
K.W. bacillus
K.W. conjunctivitis
K.W. Haemophilus
Kocher('s)
K. collar incision
K. fracture
K. incision
K. maneuver
K. -McFarland approach
K. operation
K. reflex
kochii, Borrelia
Kocks' operation
Koebner's phenomenon
Koenig-Wittek operation
Koeppe('s)
K. disease
K. goniolens
K. lens
K. nodule
Koerber-Salus-Elschnig syndrome
Koester's nodule
Kofler's operation
Köhler's bone disease
Köhler's disease
Kohlrausch's folds
Kohlrausch's veins
koinotropic type
Kolff-Jarvik artificial heart
Kölliker's interstitial granules
Kollmorgen elements
Kolmer's test
Kolomnin's operation
Kong ear, Hong
Kong influenza ▸ Hong
König's
K. graft
K. operation
K. rods
koningi, Scopulariopsis
Kono procedure
kopf tetanus
Koplik's sign
Koplik's spots
Korányi's auscultation
Korean hemorrhagic fever

Korean hemorrhagic nephroso-nephritis
Kornzweig syndrome, Bassen-
Korotkoff's sounds
Korotkoff's test
Korsakoff('s)
K. psychosis
K. syndrome
K. syndrome, Wernicke-
Koshevnikoff's disease
Kossa staining, von
Kostmann's infantile agranulocytosis
Kotex pad
Koyanagi syndrome, Vogt-
Koyter's muscle
Kozlowski's degeneration
KP (keratic precipitates)
KP (keratic precipitates), mutton fat
Krabbe('s)
K. disease
K. leukodystrophy
K. sclerosis
krabbei, Taenia
Kraepelin disease, Morel-
Kraepelin's classification
Krantz operation, Marshall-Marchetti-
Kraske procedure
Krasnov implant cataract lens
Kratz implant
Kratz scratcher
Kraupa operation
Kraupa syndrome, Fuchs-
kraurosis penis
kraurosis vulvae
Krause('s)
K. corpuscles
K. gland
K. graft, Wolfe-
K. operation
K. syndrome
K., transverse suture of
K. ventricle
K. -Wolfe graft
Krebs(')
K. cycle
K. leukocyte index
K. pentose
K. -Ringer phosphate
Kreibig's operation
Kreibig's opticomalacia
Kreiker's operation
Kreiselman unit
Kretschmer types
Kretz, paradox of
Kretz's granules

Kreuscher's operation
Krimsky measurements for exotropia
Kristeller technique
Kristeller's method
Kroener's operation
Krogh's apparatus spirometer
Kromayer's lamp
Krompecher's carcinoma
Kronecker's center
Kronfeld's electrode
Krönig's
    K. area
    K. cesarean section (CS)
    K. field
    K. isthmus
    K. percussion
    K. steps
Krönlein('s)
    K. -Berke operation
    K. hernia
    K. operation
Krukenberg's
    K. hand
    K. operation
    K. spindle
    K. tumor
    K. veins
krusei, Candida
krypton laser
Krystal (phencyclidine)
K-shell
KSHV ▸ Kaposi's sarcoma herpes virus
k-space segmentation
KTP laser
KUB (kidneys, ureters and bladder)
KUB (kidneys, ureters and bladder) film
Kübler-Ross time frame of death
kuetzingianus, Acetobacter
Kugel anastomosis
Kugel anastomotic artery
Kugelberg-Welander disease
Kugler capsule, Crosby-
Kuhlmann cervical traction
Kuhn's mask
Kuhnt('s)
    K. illusion
    K. intermediary tissue
    K. -Junius disease
    K. operation
    K. operation, Szymanowski-
    K. postcentral vein
    K. -Szymanowski operation

    K. -Szymanowski operation ▸ Smith-
    K. -Szymanowski procedure
Kulchitzky cell carcinoma
Kulmuk idiocy
Kumba virus
Kümmell('s)
    K. disease
    K. spondylitis
    K. -Verneuil disease
Kundrat's lymphosarcoma
Kunkel syndrome, Bearn-
Küntscher's nail
Kuntz ▸ nerve of
Kupffer's cell phagocytosis ▸ impaired
Kupffer's cells
Kupperman's test
Kupressoff's center
Kurtzke score
Kurzbauer's position
Kurz's syndrome
Kussmaul's
    K. aphasia
    K. breathing
    K. coma
    K. disease
    K. -Kien respiration
    K. -Maier disease
    K. paradoxical pulse
    K. pulse
    K. respirations
    K. sign
Küstner's
    K. incision
    K. law
    K. operation
    K. sign
Küttner, hauptganglion of
Kv (kilovolt)
kV fluoroscopy
Kveim
    K. antigen
    K. antigen skin test
    K. reaction
    K. -Siltzbach test
    K. test
KVO (constant verbal order)
Kvp (kilovolt peak)
kw (kilowatt)
Kwell lotion shampoo
kw-hr (kilowatt-hour)
K-wire (Kirschner wire)
Kyasanur Forest disease virus
Kydex body jacket

Kydex brace
kymograph, electro◊
kymography, electro◊
kymography study, roentgen
kyphectomy, Sharrard-type
kyphoplasty procedure
kyphoplasty treatment
kyphosis
    k., dorsal
    k. ▸ lordosis, scoliosis and
    k., postural
    k., Scheuermann's

L

L and A (light and accommodation)
L and W (living and well)
LA
    LA (left atrial)
    LA (left atrium)
    LA (linguoaxial)
la
    l. belle indifference
    l. Camp's sign, de
    l. grippe
    l. roue de moulin, bruit
    l. Tourette's disease, Gilles de
    l. Tourette's syndrome, Gilles de
La:A ratio
lab (Lab)
    l. assistant
    l., cultures sent to
    l. follow-up
    l., maximum containment
    L., Radiobiology Research
    l., sleep
    L. -Tek cryostat ▸ Ames
    l., tissue specimen sent to
    l., workup ▸ mobile mass
LABA (laser-assisted balloon
    angioplasty)
Labbé's vein
label(s)
    l., alcoholic
    l., drug
    l., food
    l. memory
    l. study ▸ open
    l. use of drugs ▸ off
    l. use of medication ▸ off
    l., warning
labeled isotopes, radioactive
labeled scintigraphy ▸ FFA
labia
    l., anterior commissure of
    l. majora
    l. majus
    l. minora
    l., posterior commissure of
labial
    l. cyst
    l. embrasure

    l. flange
    l. fold
    l. frenum
    l. gingiva
    l. gland
    l. hernia
    l. hernia, posterior
    l. nerves, anterior
    l. nerves, posterior
    l. region, inferior
    l. region, superior
    l. swelling
    l. teeth
    l. vein, anterior
    l. vein, inferior
    l. vein, posterior
    l. vein, superior
labialis
    l., Filaria
    l., herpes
    l., intertrigo
labile
    l., acid
    l. affect
    l. blood pressure (BP)
    l. diabetic
    l. hypertension
    l. mood
    l. muscle movements
    l. personality
    l. pulse
lability
    l., affective
    l., and irritability ▸ euphoria,
      emotional
    l., emotional
    l., mood
    l., organic emotional
labiochoreic stuttering
labiodental sulcus
labioglossopharyngeal nerve
labioglossopharyngeal paralysis,
    progressive
labiorum pudendi, frenulum
labioscrotal swelling
labor
    l., abnormal duration of

    l., accelerated painless
    l., active
    l. activity
    l. and delivery ▸ pregnancy,
    l., atonic
    l., augmentation of
    l., back
    l., complicated
    l. contraction
    l. contractions during
    l. contractions ▸ false
    l. contractions, intensity of
    l., deep relaxation in
    l., desultory
    l., dry
    l., dysfunctional
    l., dyskinetic
    l., early
    l. ▸ emotional support during
    l. enhancement
    l., false
    l., final stage of
    l., first stage of
    l., fourth stage of
    l., habitual
    l., immature
    l., induced
    l., induction of
    l., inhibit
    l., instrumental
    l. ▸ mandatory trial of
    l., mechanism of
    l., mimetic
    l., missed
    l. monitor
    l., obstructed
    l., onset of
    l. pains
    l. pains, false
    l. pains ▸ psychogenic aversion to
    l. pains ▸ spurious
    l., patient in
    l., pitocin augmentation of
    l., postponed
    l., precipitate
    l., precipitous
    l., premature

labor—*continued*
l., preterm
l., primary dysfunctional
l., prodromal
l. program, active management of
l. progressed
l. prolonged
l. protracted
l., second stage of
l., spontaneous
l., spontaneous onset of
l., spontaneous premature
l., term in
l. terminated
l. ▸ termination of
l. ▸ third stage of
l., threatened
l. time, total
l., trial of
l., true

laboratory(-ies) (Laboratories)
l. abnormalities
l. analysis
l. animal medicine
l. apparatus, indirect contact with
    contaminated
l. assessment ▸ noninvasive
    vascular
l., cardiac catheterization
l. computer system
l. data
l. determinations
l. diagnosis
l. evaluation
l. examination
l. findings
l. findings, pertinent
l. ▸ hospital cardiac catheterization
l. ID (identification) number
l. monitoring
L., Motion Study
l. ▸ peripheral vascular
l., pulmonary function
l. results
l., screening
l., sleep
l. studies
l. studies, precatheterization
l. technician-on-call
L. (VDRL) Test, Venereal Disease
    Research
L., Tissue Typing
l., toxicology
l., transplant tissue-typing

L. (VDRL), Venereal Disease
    Research
l. workup
l. workup ▸ preoperative
l. workup ▸ presurgical

labored
l. breathing
l. breathing ▸ increased and
l. breathing, patient has
l. respiration

labrum, acetabular
labyrinth
l., acquired defect of
l. area hammer
l., bony
l., cochlear
l., concussion of
l., congenital defect of
l., defect of
l. disease
l., healing
l., hyperirritability of
l. membrane
l., membranous
l., Minotaur's
l. of brain
l., osseous
l., veins of
l., vestibular

labyrinthectomy, transmastoid
labyrinthic ataxia
labyrinthine
l. concussion
l. deafness
l. defect
l. disease
l. disorder
l. dysfunction
l. fistula
l. fluid
l. function
l. nystagmus
l. placenta
l. sclerosis
l. sense
l. symptoms

labyrinthitis
l., acute
l., acute purulent
l., acute suppurative
l., bacterial
l., chronic
l., purulent
l., serous
l., suppurative

l., viral
labyrinthotomy, transmeatal
Lacarrere's operation
lace-like appearance
lacerated [*macerated***]**
l. cervix
l. perineum
l. tendon
l. wound

laceration(s) [*maceration***]**
l. and/or abrasions
l. and hemopericardium, cardiac
l., avulsing
l., bleeding
l., facial
l., flap-type
l., hemorrhage or
l. middle meningeal artery
l., minor
l., nasal
l. of eyeball
l. of heart
l. of liver
l. of lung
l. of pleura
l. or hemorrhage
l. pelvic floor
l., puncture
l., scar from
l., skin
l., soft tissue
l., superficial
l., superficial healed
l. sutured
l., tape closure of
l., traumatic
l. undermined
l., uterine
l., vermilion

lacerum, foramen
Lachman's test
laciniate ligament
lack(s)
l. cartilage ▸ tiny bronchioles
l., immunosuppression
l. of affection
l. of awareness and alertness
l. of balance and coordination
l. of blood to the brain
l. of communication
l. of concentration
l. of concentration, patient has
l. of consciousness
l. of coordination
l. of coordination and control

l. of drive or motivation
l. of emotional control
l. of emotional display
l. of empathy
l. of energy
l. of estrogen
l. of exercise
l. of eye contact
l. of facial expression
l. of initiative
l. of initiative and spontaneity
l. of insight
l. of interest in others
l. of interest in personal goals ▸
   apathy and
l. of interest in society ▸ apathy and
l. of intrinsic factor
l. of medical care
l. of memory
l. of mobility ▸ stiffness, pain and
l. of motivation
l. of motor control
l. of motor coordination
l. of muscle tone
l. of normal response
l. of nurturing
l. of oxygen (O_2)
l. of oxygen (O_2) to cardiac muscle
l. of oxygen (O_2) to the brain
l. of physical exercise
l. of physical fitness
l. of pleasure or motivation
l. of reciprocal interest
l. of regular exercise
l. of remorse
l. of self-destructiveness
l. of social support
l. of sufficient tears
l. of support
l. of tolerance to treatment
l. of ultraviolet protection
l. of understanding
lacking cells, myosin
lacking in detail ▸ speech
lackluster eyes
lacrimal
l. artery
l. bone
l. canals
l. caruncle
l. crest
l. drainage system tumors
l. duct
l. duct, ampulla of
l. duct, anterior

l. fold
l. gland
l. gland, adenocarcinoma of
l. gland, calculus of
l. gland, dislocation of
l. gland, drainage of
l. gland, excision of
l. gland, fistula of
l. gland, inferior
l. gland, luxation of
l. gland, lymphosarcoma of
l. gland, mixed tumor of
l. gland, retention cyst
l. gland, superior
l. gland, supernumerary
l. gland, syphilis of
l. gland, tuberculosis (TB) of
l. gland tumors
l. groove, Verga's
l. lake
l. nerve
l. notch of maxilla
l. obstruction ▸ congenital
l. papilla
l. papilla, splitting of
l. passage, atresia of
l. passage, stenosis of
l. punctum
l. reflex
l. sac
l. sac, drainage of
l. sac, excision of
l. sac ▸ FB (foreign body) in
l. sac, fistula of
l. sac of eye
l. sac, polyp in
l. sac, rhinoscleroma
l. sac, sporotrichosis of
l. sac, streptotrichosis of
l. secretions ▸ salivary and
l. sound
l. system
l. trephine, Arruga's
l. vein
lacrimale, os
lacrimalis
l., ampulla canaliculi
l., ampulla ductus
l., canaliculus
l., caruncula
l., ductus
l., lacus
l., nucleus
l., papilla
l., rivus

l., sacculus
lacrimation
l. and itching
l., increased
l. ▸ yawning, sweating and
lacrimoconchal suture
lacrimo-ethmoidal suture
lacrimomaxillary suture
lacrimonasal duct
l.d., atresia of
l.d., catheterization of
l.d., cicatricial stenosis of
l.d., fistula of
l.d., probing of
l.d., stenosis of
l.d., supernumerary
lacrimoturbinal suture
lacrymans, Merulius
lactam
l. antibiotics, beta
l., beta
l. ring, beta
lactamase, beta
lactamase inhibitor, beta
lactase
l. deficiency
l. enzyme
l. -treated milk
lactate
l., arterial blood
l. concentration
l. dehydrogenase
l. extraction
l. measurements, blood
l. -pyruvate ratio
l. solution, Ringer's
l. stain, Ringer's
l. threshold
lactated Ringer's solution
lactating
l. adenoma
l. breast
l. patient
l. women
lactation amenorrhea
lactation atrophy
lactational mastitis
lactea, macula
lacteal cataract
lactic
l. acid
l. acid efficiency
l. acid ▸ metabolic waste product
l. acid test
l. acidosis

lactic—*continued*
   l. dehydrogenase (LDH)
   l. dehydrogenase (LDH) fraction
   l. dehydrogenase (LDH) ▸ serum
   l. dehydrogenase (LDH) test
   l. dehydrogenase (LDH) virus
lactici, Bacillus acidi◊
lactiferous duct
lactis
   l., gram-positive Streptococcus
   l. R. Streptococcus
   l., Streptococcus
lactobacilli diphtheroides
Lactobacillus
   L. acidophilus
   L. arabinosus
   L. bifidus
   L. bulgaricus
   L. casei
   L. fermentans
   L. fermenti
   L. leichmannii
   L. of Boas-Oppler
   L. plantarum
lactogen
   l. (HPL) and plasma, human
     placental
   l. (HPL), human placental
   l., placental
lactogenic hormone
lactogenic hormone, ovine
lactoglobulin, beta
lacto-ovo vegetarian diet
lactose
   l. allergy, milk
   l. deficient
   l. -free diet
   l. ▸ inability to digest
   l. intolerance
   l. intolerance and galactosemia
   l. intolerance ▸ bloating from
   l. intolerance ▸ diarrhea from
   l. intolerance from antibiotic
   l. intolerance ▸ pain in abdomen
     from
   l. intolerance with Crohn's disease
   l. placebo, pure
   l. reduced diet
   l. restricted diet
   l. tolerance test
lacuna, intervillous
lacunae of Morgagni
lacunar
   l. amnesia
   l. angina

   l. cerebrovascular accidents (CVA)
   l. infarct
   l. infarction
   l. ligament
   l. skull
   l. stroke
   l. tonsillitis
lacunaris, hyperkeratosis
lacunata, Moraxella
lacus lacrimalis
lacustris, Chaoborus
lacy red rash
LAD
   LAD (left anterior descending)
   LAD (left anterior descending)
     artery
   LAD (left axis deviation) abnormal
ladder diagram
ladder incisions
laded macrophages, brown pigment
laden
   l. air, germ-
   l. food, cholesterol-
   l. macrophages, hemosiderin-
   l. microphages, fat-
   l. plaque, cholesterol-
   l. plaque, fat-
Ladies (barbiturates), Pink
Ladin's sign
Lady (cocaine)
LAE (left atrial enlargement)
Laennec's
   L. catarrh
   L. cirrhosis
   L. disease
   L. Gasteva seizure
   L. pearls
   L. serology
   L. sign
   L. thrombus
laevis test, Xenopus
LAF (laminar air flow)
LAF (laminar air flow) isolation room
Lafora body
Lafora's sign
LaForce tonsillectomy
LAFR (laminar air flow room)
LAFU (laminar air flow unit)
LAG (labiogingival)
LAG (lymphangiogram)
lag
   l., jet
   l., lid
   l., nitrogen
   l., occupational jet

   l., respiratory
   l. syndrome, jet-
   l. time
   l. time ▸ pacemaker
Lagleyze's operation
Lagochilascaris minor
lagophthalmic keratitis
Lagrange's operation
LAH (left atrial hypertrophy)
LAI (left atrial involvement)
laid back view
laidlawii, Acholeplasma
Laidlaw's clotting time ▸ Dale-
Laing's plate
lait spots ▸ café au
laiteuse, tache
LAK (lymphokine-activated killer) cell
lake (Lake's)
   l., lacrimal
   l., marginal
   L. pigment
   l., venous
Laki-Lorand factor
LaLeche method
Lam procedure
Lamaze
   L. method of childbirth
   L. technique
   L. training
lambda (Lambda)
   l. disease
   l. light chain component
   L. pacemaker
   l. wave
lambdoid
   l. suture
   l. suture lines
   l. wave
lambing sickness
lamblia, Giardia
Lamblia intestinalis
Lambl's excrescence
Lambrinudi triple arthrodesis
Lambrinudi's operation
lame foliacée
lamellar
   l. cataract
   l. exfoliation of newborn
   l. graft
   l. ichthyosis
   l. keratoplasty
   l. keratoplasty (ALK), automated
   l. transplant ▸ deep
   l. transplant ▸ surface
   l. zonular perinuclear cataract

lamina
- l. dura
- l., elastic
- l., episcleral
- l. externa
- l., foliate
- l. interna
- l. ▸ internal elastic
- l. of sphenoid bone ▸ inferior
- l., orbital
- l. propria
- l. propria ▸ chronic inflammation of
- l., suprachoroid

laminar
- l. air flow (LAF)
- l. air flow (LAF) isolation room
- l. air flow room (LAFR)
- l. air flow unit (LAFU)
- l. blood flow

Laminaria tent
laminate induration
laminate, porcelain
laminated
- l. clot
- l. thrombus
- l., yellowish-brown cortex

laminectomy
- l., decompression
- l., decompressive lumbar
- l., extradural
- l., lumbar
- l., thoracic

laminogram examination
laminotomy procedure
lamp
- l., annealing
- l., arc
- l., Birch-Hirschfeld
- l., carbon arc
- l., cold quartz mercury vapor
- l., diagnostic
- l., Duke-Elder
- l., Eldridge-Green
- l. examination, slit-
- l., Finsen
- l., Finsen-Reya
- l. flame, alcohol
- l., Gullstrand's slit
- l., Haag-Streit slit
- l., Hildreth mercury
- l., Jesionek
- l., Kromayer's
- l., Lortet
- l. microscope, slit-
- l., mignon

- l., quartz
- l., Simpson
- l., slit
- l., tungsten arc
- l., ultraviolet
- l., Wood's

Lamprocystis roseopersicina
Lamy syndrome, Maroteaux-
Lanager's axillary arch
lanata, Digitalis
Lancaster's magnet
Lancaster's red-green test for diplopia
lance, Rolf's
Lancefield classification
lanceolatus, Streptococcus
Lancereaux's diabetes
Lancereaux's nephritis
lancet (Lancet)
- l., abscess
- l., acne
- L. coefficient
- l., gingival
- l., gum
- l., laryngeal
- l. -shaped gram-positive diplococci
- l., spring

lancinating pain
Lancisi, longitudinal nerves of
Lancisi, nerves of
land
- l. -based exercises
- l. fever
- l. mine amputees

Landau reflex
Landau test
Landis test, Gibbon-
landmarks
- l., anatomical
- l., bony
- l. check
- l., external
- l., geographic
- l. preserved

Landolt's
- L. bodies
- L. broken ring
- L. eyelid reconstruction
- L. operation

Landou's sign
Landouzy('s)
- L. -Déjerine atrophy
- L. -Déjerine dystrophy
- L. -Déjerine syndrome
- L. disease, Erb-

- L. purpura

Landry-Guillain-Barré syndrome
Landry's paralysis
Landström's muscle
Lane's plate
Lang operation, Frost-
Lange('s)
- L. -Nielsen syndrome ▸ Jervell
- L. operation
- L. operation, Fritz-
- L. position
- L. syndrome, Brachmann-de
- L. syndrome, Cornelia de
- L. syndrome, de

Langenbeck('s)
- L. amputation
- L. bipedicle mucoperiosteal flap ▸ von
- L. incision
- L. operation

Langendorff heart preparation
Langerhans(')
- L. cell
- L., islands of
- L., islets of
- L. ▸ sclerosis of islets
- L. stellate corpuscles

langerhansian adenoma
langeroni, Arthrographis
Langer's muscle
Langhans'
- L. cell
- L. giant cell
- L. layer
- L. stria
- L. type

Langley's granules
Langley's nerves
Langoria's sign
Lang's fluid
language
- l. ability
- l. ability ▸ impaired
- l. acquisition
- l. (ALGOL), ALGOrithmic
- l. alphabet, sign
- l. assembly
- l., auditory comprehension of
- l. barrier
- l. -based learning disability
- l. -based learning problem
- l., body
- l. center in brain
- l. comprehension
- l. control

language—*continued*
l. deficit
l. deficits, auditory verbal
l. -delayed (LD) children
l. development
l. disability
l. disability, child has
l. disorder
l. disorder, developmental
l. disorder ▸ developmental expressive
l. disorder ▸ developmental receptive
l. disorders ▸ speech and
l., disturbed
l. dysfunction
l. function, expressive
l. function ▸ loss of
l. function, receptive
l. impaired ▸ speech and
l. impairment
l. interpreter
l. loss ▸ disorientation, confusion, and
l., moral
l. nonfunctional, written
l., normal comprehension of spoken
l. of body posture ▸ nonverbal
l. pathologist, speech and
l. pathology service
l., positive body
l., preferred
l. referral
l. (signing), sign
l. skill ▸ oral
l. skills
l. skills and perception ▸ attention, orientation
l. skills, loss of
l. spoken
l. test
l. therapy
l. ▸ unable to understand
l., verbal expression of
l. within normal limits, speech and
Lankesterella ranarum
Lankesteria culicis
lanosum, Microsporum
Lansing virus
lansingensis, Legionella
lantern test
lanthanic patient
lanugo hair
LAO (left anterior oblique)
LAO (left anterior oblique) position

lap [*flap, flat*]
l. count, sponge and
l. packs
l. packs, moist
l. sponge
l. swimming ▸ hypoxic
LAP (left atrial pressure)
LAP (leukocyte alkaline phosphatase) test
laparohysterosalpingo-oophorectomy
laparoscope, laser surgery via
laparoscopic
l. cholecystectomy
l. gallbladder surgery
l. hernia repair
l. myomectomy
l. radical prostatectomy
l. salpingo-oophorectomy
l. sterilization
l. surgery
l. technique
l. tubal ligation
laparoscopically assisted vaginal hysterectomy (LAVH)
laparoscopy
l., diagnostic
l., double puncture
l. examination
l., laser
l., pelvic
l. surgery ▸ minimally invasive
laparotomy
l., abdominal
l., diagnostic
l., emergency
l., exploratory
l., hystero◊
l., negative
l., pelvic
l., staging
Lapham test, Friedman-
lapillosum, scrotum
Lapiné maneuver, Chassard-
Lapiné projection, Chassard-
Laplace relationship
lapping murmur
lapse
l. in normal breathing ▸ momentary
l. in short term memory
l. into heightened irritability
l. of awareness ▸ momentary
l. of consciousness
l. of memory
l., time

lapsed into coma, patient
lapsing into coma
lapsus linguae
lapsus memoriae
Laquerrière-Pierquin position
larabensis, Cricetulus
larch sugar
lardaceous
l. kidney
l. liver
l. spleen
l. tissue
large
l. amounts of food, rapid ingestion of
l. and floppy ▸ ears
l. artery thrombosis
l. base quad cane
l. blood vessel
l. bowel
l. bowel distended
l. bowel ▸ intramural air in
l. bowel obstruction
l. cell carcinoma
l. cell carcinoma ▸ poorly differentiated
l. cell carcinoma ▸ underlying undifferentiated
l. cell carcinoma ▸ undifferentiated
l. cell undifferentiated carcinoma
l. cell undifferentiated carcinoma ▸ metastatic
l. colon
l. column of Bertin
l. core breast biopsy, automated
l. darkly staining gram-positive rods
l. fetal bleed
l. field cobalt
l. field electron beam dosimetry
l. field x-ray beam dosimetry
l. for gestational age neonate
l. granular lymphocyte antigen
l. inguinal hernial sac
l. inter-electrode distances
l. intestinal descending colon
l. intestine
l. intestine, benign polyps of
l. intestine, carcinoma of
l. intestine, folds of
l. intestine meridian
l. intestine ▸ mucosal surfaces
l. intestine, solitary lymphatic nodules of
l. irregular nuclei
l. kappa angle

l. lipid core
l. magnitude voluntary heart rate changes
l. necrotic infarction
l. nerve fibers
l. oval nucleus
l. pelvis
l. physiologic cup
l. polyp
l. quantities of blood ▸ patient vomited
l. red kidney
l. sacral decubitus ulcer
l. scale screening
l. scale testing
l. septum of Bertin
l. stones, crush
l. tibial cuff ▸ long leg brace with
l. tongue
l. veins on abdomen
l. vessel disease
l. vessel hematocrit
l. voltage waves
Larix europaea
Lark riser ▸ morning
Larkin's position
LaRocca's tube
LaRoque herniorrhaphy incision
Larrey spaces
Larrey's amputation
Larsen-Johansson disease
Larsen's syndrome
larva
l. currens
l. migrans
l. migrans ▸ ocular
l. migrans, visceral
l., rat-tailed
larvae
l., Anopheles
l., Bacillus
l., heartworm
l., hookworm
l., nematode
l. ▸ Taenia solium
larval
l. conjunctivitis
l. discharge
l. epilepsy
l. formations
l. migration
l. nephrosis
l. seizures
l. spike-and-slow waves
larvicide, Panama

laryngeal [*pharyngeal*]
l. adhesions
l. applicator
l. atresia
l. block in radiation therapy
l. cancer
l. carcinoma
l. cartilage of Luschka
l. catheterization
l. chorea
l. commissure
l. crisis
l. diphtheria
l. edema
l. emergency
l. epilepsy
l. granuloma
l. infection
l. lancet
l. mirror
l. mucosa
l. mucosa, hyperemic
l. muscles, tonus of extrinsic
l. nerve
l. nerve function, recurrent
l. nerve, inferior
l. nerve paralysis
l. nerve, recurrent
l. nerve, superior
l. nerve, superior internal
l. papillomatosis
l. plexus
l. pouch
l. prominence
l. prosthesis
l. protuberance
l. punch
l. rale
l. reconstruction
l. reflex
l. reflexes, protective
l. region
l. respiratory murmur
l. saccules
l. sinus
l. spasm, terminal
l. stridor
l. stridor, congenital
l. swabs
l. syncope
l. syringe
l. tic
l. tracheitis, acute
l. tube
l. tumor

l. vein, inferior
l. vein, superior
l. vertigo
l. web
Laryngectomees, International
laryngectomy [*pharyngectomy*]
l., partial
l., total
l., wide-field
laryngei, plica nervi
laryngis
l., aditus
l., atrium
l., conus elasticus
l., corniculum
l., myasthenia
l., phlebectasia
l., vestibulum
laryngismus paralyticus
laryngitis
l. and alcoholism
l., atrophic
l., catarrhal
l., chronic
l., chronic catarrhal
l., croupous
l. from breathing
l. from chemical
l., diphtheritic
l., membranous
l., phlegmonous
l., progressive
l. sicca
l. stridulosa
l., subglottic
l., syphilitic
l., tuberculous
l., vestibular
laryngography, contrast
laryngopharyngeal reflexes
laryngoscopic visualization
laryngoscopy
l., direct
l. ▸ mirror image
l., suspension
laryngotomy, subhyoid
laryngotomy, thyroid
laryngotracheal bronchitis, acute
laryngotracheal trauma
laryngotracheobronchitis, acute
laryngotracheobronchitis virus ▸ acute
larynx [*pharynx*]
l. and trachea anesthetized ▸ pharynx,

larynx—*continued*
- l., aperture of
- l., artificial
- l., arytenoid cartilage of
- l., atrium of
- l. backward and upward, displacement of
- l., cancer of
- l., carcinoma of
- l., dilatation of
- l., edema of
- l., electronic
- l., extrinsic
- l. inspected
- l., intrinsic
- l., passing faradic current into
- l., pneumatic
- l., polyps of
- l., saccules of
- l., tuberculosis of
- l., ventricle of
- l., vestibule of
- l. with vocal cords

Larzel's anemia

LAS (lymphadenopathy syndrome)

Lasegue's
- L. disease
- L. maneuver
- L. sign

LASEK (laser-assisted subepithelial keratectomy) procedure

Laseque test

LASER (light amplification by stimulated emission of radiation)
- l. ablation
- l. ablation, continuous wave
- l. ablation ▸ pulsed
- l., ablative
- l. acupuncture
- l., alexandrite
- l. alignment system
- l. angiography, absorption in coronary
- l. angioplasty
- l. angioplasty, ablative
- l. angioplasty, balloon
- l. angioplasty, coronary
- l. angioplasty, coronary artery
- l. angioplasty, excimer
- l. angioplasty (PLA) ▸ peripheral
- l., argon
- l., argon ion
- l. -assisted balloon angioplasty (LABA)
- l. -assisted in situ keratomileusis (LASIK)
- l. -assisted in situ keratomileusis (LASIK) correction
- l. -assisted in situ keratomileusis (LASIK) surgery
- l. -assisted in situ keratomileusis (LASIK) surgery ▸ wavefront-guided
- l. -assisted subepithelial keratectomy (LASEK) procedure
- l. -assisted uvula palatoplasty (LAUP)
- l. -assisted vascular anastomosis
- l., atheroblation
- l. balloon
- l., balloon centered argon
- l. beam
- l. beam ▸ computer guided
- l. beam machine
- l. beam surgery
- l. burst
- l. ▸ carbon dioxide (CO_2) gas
- l., cardiac
- l. catheter
- l. clinic, walk-in
- l., computer controlled
- l., computerized
- l. conization
- l., continuous wave
- l., cool tip
- l. coronary angioplasty (ELCA) ▸ excimer
- l. coronary angioplasty (PELCA) ▸ percutaneous excimer
- l., cosmetic
- l., coumarin pulsed dye
- l. destroyed tissue
- l. destruction of intraepithelial neoplasia
- l. disk decompression, percutaneous
- l. Doppler blood profusion
- l., dye
- l. energy
- l. energy absorption
- l. excess tissue
- l., excimer
- l. ▸ excimer cool
- l. ▸ excimer gas
- l. excision
- l. excisional conization biopsy
- l. eye surgery
- l. face wrinkle removal
- l. facial rejuvenation
- l. facial resurfacing
- l. facial skin restoration
- l. firing
- l. ▸ free beam
- l., gas
- l. glaucoma surgery
- l., green argon
- l. hair removal
- l. hair removal treatment
- l. heart surgery
- l. ▸ helium cadmium diagnostic
- l., helium neon
- l., high energy pulsed ruby
- l., holmium
- l. illumination ▸ red
- l., imprecisely aimed
- l. in situ keratomileusis (LASIK)
- l. -induced arterial fluorescence
- l. -induced prostatectomy (TULIP) ▸ transurethral ultrasound-guided
- l. -induced thrombosis
- l. ▸ infrared pulsed
- l., ion
- l. keratectomy
- l., krypton
- l., KTP
- l. laparoscopy
- l. light
- l. light ray
- l. ▸ low energy
- l. mammoplasty
- l., manganese
- L. Medicine and Surgery (ASLMS) ▸ American Society of
- l. ▸ Metalase copper vapor
- l. microdiscectomy, arthroscopic
- l. microscope
- l. microsurgery, computer assisted stereotactic
- l. ▸ mid-infrared pulsed
- l., Nd:YAG (neodymium: yttrium-aluminum-garnet)
- l., nonablative
- l., nonthermal
- l., ophthalmic
- l. ophthalmologist's
- l. ophthalmoscope (SLO) ▸ scanning
- l. peel
- l. photocoagulator
- l., photodisruptive
- l. ▸ potassium titanyl phosphate
- l. probe ▸ hot tip
- l. procedure, intra-abdominal
- l. pulsed dye

l. radiation
l. recanalization ▸ excimer
l. refractive surgery
l. resurfacing
l. resurfacing for facial wrinkles
l. revascularization
l. revascularization ▸ heart
l. revascularization (TMLR) ▸ transmyocardial
l. ▸ rotational ablation
l., ruby
l. scanner
l. scanning
l., Sharplan 733 carbon dioxide (CO_2)
l., short pulsed
l. skin rejuvenation
l. skin resurfacing, carbon dioxide (CO_2)
l. skin resurfacing ▸ face
l. skin surgery
l. skin treatment
l. speckle
l. ▸ spectroscopy-directed
l. spots
l. surgery
l. surgery, argon
l. surgery, computer assisted
l. surgery ▸ cosmetic
l. surgery, excimer
l. surgery, experimental
l. surgery ▸ irreversible
l. surgery treatment
l. surgery via laparoscope
l., surgical
l. technique
l. technique ▸ excimer
l. technique ▸ nonablative
l. therapy
l. therapy, cryosurgery and
l. therapy of diabetic retinopathy
l. therapy of hemorrhoids
l., thermal
l. thermal keratoplasty
l. tip
l. tissue interaction
l. tomograph ▸ scanning
l. trabeculoplasty (LTP)
l. treatment
l. treatment, aggressive
l. treatment, diabetic
l. treatment, epilepsy
l. treatment of cervical neoplasia
l. treatment of vaginal neoplasia
l. treatment ▸ stand-alone

L. Treatment, Tuneable Dye
l. ▸ tunable dye
l. ▸ ultraviolet (UV)
l. utilizing ruby ▸ solid state
l. vaporization
l. vaporization and excisional conization
l. vaporization, carbon dioxide (CO_2)
l. vaporization of lesion
l. vaporized plaques
l. vaporized tissue
l. vision correction
l. xenon (Xe) arc
laseroscopy, video
Lash('s)
L. -Löffler implant
L. operation
l. reflex
L. technique
LASIK (laser-assisted in situ keratomileusis)
L. correction
L. surgery
L. surgery ▸ wavefront-guided
Lassa fever
Lassa virus
Lassar's paste
Lassar's plain zinc paste
lassitude
l. and drowsiness
l., prolonged
l., sudden
last
l. -chance experimental therapy
l. food/fluids, time of
l. menstrual period (LMP)
l. normal menstrual period (LNMP)
lasting impression
lasting impression of impending failure
lata
l., fascia
l. femoris, fascia
l. graft, fascia
l. prosthesis, fascia
l., tensor muscle of fascia
l., tensor of fascia
latae muscle, tensor fasciae
latch key kid
late
l. abortion
l. antigen
l. apical systolic murmur

l. apnea
l. bone marrow depression
l. convalescence
l. cyanosis
l. death
l. deceleration
l. diastole
l. diastolic murmur
l. erythroblast
l. fetal death
l. filling wave, occasional
l. graft rejection
l. -life
l. -life anxiety
l. -life depression
l. -life disability
l. luteal phase dysphoric disorder
l. menopause
l. menstrual period
l. onset alcoholic
l. onset asthma
l. onset crack dependence
l. paraphrenia
l. passage of meconium
l. peaking systolic murmur
l. period
l. phase reaction
l. positive component
l. proarrhythmic effect
l. prolapse of iris
l. reactions to radiation therapy
l. reperfusion
l. responding tissue, acute responding versus
l. responding tumor
l. -stage heart failure
l. systole
l. systolic murmur (LSM)
l. tuberculosis
latency(-ies) [*patency*]
l. age development
l. age period
l. and adult sublimation
l. -based cognitive skills
l., distal
l. experience
l., interpeak
l. of conduction
l. of response
l. period
l., rapid eye movement (REM)
l., sleep
l. somatosensory evoked response (SER), short
l., stage of

latency(-ies)—*continued*
   L. Test, Multiple Sleep
   l. theory
latent [*patent*]
   l. cancer
   l. content
   l. diabetes
   l. diabetic, patient
   l. empyema
   l. epilepsy
   l. fantasy
   l. gout
   l. heat
   l. homosexuality
   l. hypermetropia
   l. infection
   l. insecurity ▸ manifestation of
   l. iron-binding capacity
   l. paroxysmal activity
   l. period
   l. phase
   l. pleurisy
   l. schizophrenia
   l. squint
   l. strabismus
   l. syphilis
   l. tetany
   l. virus
lateral [*collateral*]
   l. abdominal region
   l. ampullar nerve
   l. anconeus muscle
   l. aneurysm
   l. angle
   l. ankle sprain
   l., anteroposterior and
   l. aperture
   l. arch
   l. aspect
   l. aspect of foot
   l. basal
   l. bending
   l. bending exercise
   l. bending, left
   l. bending, right
   l. border
   l. canal
   l. cerebral fissure
   l. cerebral fossa
   l. cerebrospinal fasciculus
   l. chest wall, left
   l. chromatic aberration
   l. circumflex femoral veins
   l. collateral ligament
   l. column

   l. column ▸ gliosis of
   l. commissure of eyelids
   l. compartment
   l. condyle bone
   l. constriction phenomenon
   l. conus
   l. cortical margin
   l. cricoarytenoid muscle
   l. crus
   l. curvature of spine
   l. cutaneous nerve of arm ▸ inferior
   l. cutaneous nerve of arm ▸
      superior
   l. cutaneous nerve of calf
   l. cutaneous nerve of forearm
   l. cutaneous nerve of thigh
   l. decubitus film
   l. decubitus position
   l. displacement
   l. dorsal cutaneous nerve of foot
   l. elbow injury
   l. enamel strand
   l. epicondyle
   l. epicondylitis
   l. epileptiform discharges ▸ periodic
   l. extension
   l. eye movement
   l. false ligament
   l. femoral cutaneous nerve
   l. fields, opposing
   l. films, portable recumbent AP
      (anteroposterior) and
   l. fissure
   l. flank incision
   l. flank wound
   l. fornix
   l. fossa of cerebrum, cistern of
   l. gastrocnemius muscle
   l. geniculate body
   l. hemianopia
   l. hemispheres
   l. horns of spinal cord
   l. illumination
   l. incisor
   l. infarction
   l. instability
   l. ▸ intermediate substance of spinal
      cord,
   l., internal dimension—left
   l. internal sphincterotomy
   l., left
   l. ligament
   l. ligament of the malleus
   l. ligature
   l. lobe

   l. malleolus
   l. malleolus muscle
   l. mammillary nucleus of Rose
   l. mass of atlas
   l. mass of sacrum
   l. mass of vertebrae
   l. masses of ethmoid bone
   l. membranous wall
   l. meniscectomy
   l. menisci ▸ medical and
   l. meniscus
   l. meniscus bone
   l. meniscus, torn
   l. movement
   l. myocardial infarct ▸ anterior
   l. myocardial infarction
   l. nystagmus
   l. oblique axial projection
   l. oblique jaw roentgenogram
   l. occipital gyri
   l. occipitotemporal gyrus
   l. occlusion
   l. orbital rim
   l. pectoral nerve
   l. planter nerve
   l. planter nerve ▸ common planter
      digital nerves of
   l. planter nerve ▸ proper plantar
      digital nerves of
   l. plateau joint surface
   l. popliteal nerve
   l. portion of incision
   l. position, cross-table
   l. position, left
   l. position, pivot shift test in
   l. position, right
   l. positioning, quick
   l. pressure
   l. process of the malleus
   l. projection
   l. projection ▸ left
   l. projection, oblique
   l. projection, recumbent
   l. projection, stereo left
   l. projection, stereo right
   l. projections ▸ PA (posteroanterior)
      and
   l. protrusive excursion
   l. pterygoid muscle
   l. pterygoid nerve
   l. puboprostatic ligament
   l. ramus roentgenogram
   l. rectus incision
   l. rectus muscle
   l. rectus muscle, advancement of

l. recumbent position
l. region of abdomen, left
l. region of abdomen, right
l. region of spinal cord
l., right
l. sac
l. sacral vein
l. sclerosis
l. sclerosis (ALS) ▸ amyotrophic
l. sclerosis (FALS), familial amyotrophic
l. sclerosis, primary
l. sinus
l. sinus, drainage (dr'ge) of
l. sinus, phlebitis of
l. sinus, thrombosis of
l. skull roentgenogram
l. spurring, degenerative
l. subluxation
l. sulcus
l. supraclavicular nerves
l. surface
l. surface of great toe
l. surface of great toe ▸ dorsal digital nerves of
l. surface of knee
l. tangential breast, medial and
l. thalamus
l. thoracic vein
l. thorax, left
l. thorax, right
l. thrombus
l. tibial plateau
l. tilt
l. to the incision
l. transcranial projection
l. transfacial projection
l. umbilical fold
l. ventricle
l. ventricle cholesteatoma
l. ventricle, horn of
l. ventricle, inferior horn of
l. ventricle of cerebrum
l. ventricle, temporal horn of
l. view
l. views ▸ AP (anteroposterior) and
l. wall
l. wall ischemia

lateralis
l., fossa cerebri
l., hemelytrometra
l., hyperhidrosis
l. medullae oblongatae, nucleus
l. muscle, rectus
l. muscle, vastus

l., musculus rectus
l., musculus vastus
l. of LeGros Clark, nucleus
l. of Retzius, gyrus olfactorius

lateralization, cerebral
lateralization, paradoxical
lateralized
l. epileptiform discharges (PLED), periodic
l. headache
l. reduction in amplitude ▸ extreme
l. reduction of voltage

lateralizing neurologic signs, focal and
laterally reflected
laterocollateral ligament
lateromedial oblique projection
latex
l. agglutination
l. agglutination inhibition test
l. allergy, severe
l. balloon
l. catheter
l. fixation
l. fixation test
l. fixation test ▸ RA (rheumatoid arthritis)
l. flocculation test
l. microspheres ▸ polystyrene
l. protein allergy
l. rheumatoid factor
l. sensitivity, potential
l. slide agglutination test

latissimus
l. dorsi flap technique
l. dorsi muscle
l. dorsi procedure

La:A ratio
LATS (long-acting thyroid-stimulating) hormone
lattice
l. corner dystrophy
l. degeneration
l. keratitis
l. time ▸ spin-

latum, condyloma
latum, Diphyllobothrium
latus, metatarsus
latus, Siderobacter
Latzko's
L. cesarean section (CS)
L. closure
L. operation
L. radical hysterectomy
L. repair for vesicovaginal fistula

Lauber's disease
Lauenstein and Hickey projection
laugh and squint lines
laughing gas
laughing sickness
laughs inappropriately, patient
laughter
l., giddy
l., hysterical
l., reflex
l., senseless
l., weeping or rage ▸ senseless

Laugier's hernia
Laugier's sign
Laundry, Hospital
Launois syndrome
LAUP (laser-assisted uvulopalatoplasty)
Laurence-Moon-Biedl syndrome
Laurens-Alcatel pacemaker, Medtronic-
Laurentii, Streptococcus
Lautier's test
lavage [*gavage*]
l., bronchial
l., bronchoalveolar
l., bronchoscopic
l., continuous pericardial
l., ductal
l., ear
l. extract surfactant, bovine
l. fluid, bronchoalveolar
l., gastric
l., gastrosto◊
l. instillation
l. of bronchi
l. of joint, copious
l. of sinus
l. performed, copious
l., pericardial
l., peritoneal
l., pleural
l., tracheal
l., tracheobronchial

lavaged with sterile saline ▸ area
LAVH (laparoscopically assisted vaginal hysterectomy)
law(s) (Law)
l., all or none
l., Babinski
l., Bell-Magendie
l., Bell's
l., Cushing's
l., Descartes'
l., Desmarres'

law(s)—*continued*
- l., Diday's
- l., Doerner-Hoskins distribution
- l., Donders'
- l., Fick's
- l., Fitz's
- l., Flatau's
- l., Flourens'
- l., Freund's
- l., Giraud-Teulon
- l., Goodell's
- l., Gullstrand's
- l., Heidenhain's
- l., Hering's
- l., Homer's
- l., inverse-square
- l., Jackson's
- l., Küstner's
- l., Leopold's
- l., Levret's
- l., Listing's
- l., Louis'
- l., Magendie's
- l. of inertia
- l. of reciprocity
- l. of the heart
- l. of the heart, Starling's
- l. of thermodynamics
- l., Ohm's
- l., Ollier's
- l. or principle, Talion
- l., Pajot's
- L. position
- l., Rayleigh scattering
- L., Required Request
- l., Sherrington's
- l., Snell's
- l., Starling's
- L. x-ray view
- l., wallerian

lawful behavior
Lawman's sling procedure
Lawrence's position
Lawson-Thornton plate
lax anal sphincter
lax facial muscles
laxa syndrome, cutis
laxative(s)
- l. abuse
- l., bulk forming
- l. dependency
- l., diarrhea from
- l., natural vegetable
- l., osmotic
- l., psyllium-based

- l., water-retaining

layer(s)
- l., abdomen closed in
- l., adventitial
- l. autoradiography, thick-
- l., basal
- l., basal cell
- l., Buffy
- l., capsid
- l., chest closed in anatomic
- l., choroid
- l. chromatography, instant thin
- l. chromatography, thin
- l., closed in anatomic
- l. closure
- l. ▸ compacted dead skin cell
- l. ▸ cornea's endothelial
- l. damage, ozone
- l., deep
- l., desquamating
- l. electrophoresis, thin
- l., fascial
- l., fatty
- l., fibrous
- l., germinal
- l. ▸ granular cell
- l. (HVL), half-value
- l., Haller's
- l. ▸ horny cell
- l. ▸ hypertrophic smooth muscle
- l., imbricating
- l., incision closed in
- l., individual
- l., intimal
- l., Langhans'
- l., malpighian
- l., molecular
- l., mucosal
- l., muscle
- l., muscular
- l. of alveolar wall, outer
- l. of aorta ▸ inner
- l. of bone marrow, Buffy
- l. of bowel
- l. of brain, protective
- l. of bronchial epithelium ▸ basal
- l. of bronchial epithelium ▸ germinal
- l. of cervix ▸ superficial
- l. of cervix ▸ surface
- l. of choroid of eye, vascular
- l. of connective tissue
- l. of cornea ▸ inner
- l. of cornea, superficial
- l. of cortex, deep
- l. of endothelial cells ▸ inner

- l. of epidermis, germinative
- l. of eyeball, outer
- l. of muscle
- l. of scalp, subdermal
- l. of skin ▸ outer
- l. of skin, outermost
- l. of spinal cord ▸ protective
- l. of valve ▸ mucinous
- l., Ollier's
- l., papyraceous
- l. phlebotomy
- l., polymorphic
- l., seromuscular
- l., serosal
- l., skin
- l., soft tissue
- l. ▸ spinous cell
- l., subcutaneous fat
- l., subendocardial
- l. ▸ superficial myocardial
- l., tenth value
- l. upon layer
- l., visceral pleural
- l. without drainage (dr'ge) wound closed in
- l., wound closed in
- l., wound closed in anatomic

laying on of hands
layoff survivor sickness
lay-on graft
laziness, mental
lazy
- l. bowel
- l. eye
- l. -eye syndrome
- l. H incision
- l. leukocyte syndrome (LLS)
- l. S incision
- l. tongue
- l. Z incision

LBBB (left bundle branch block)
LBBH (limited by body habitus)
LBJ (LSD)
LBNP (lower-body negative pressure)
LBP (low blood pressure)
LBW (low birth weight)
LBWI (low birth weight infant)
LCA
- LCA (left circumflex coronary artery)
- LCA (left coronary angiogram)
- LCA (left coronary artery)

LCD (liquor carbonis detergens)
L-chain concentration (TLC) ▸ total
LCM (left costal margin)

LCM (lymphocytic choriomeningitis) virus
LCT (liquid crystal thermogram)
LCU (life change units)
LD
    LD (language delayed) children
    LD (learning disability)
    LD (linguodistal)
LD$_{50}$ or MDL (median lethal dose)
LDH
    LDH (lactic dehydrogenase)
    LDH (lactic dehydrogenase) fraction
    LDH (lactic dehydrogenase) isoenzyme
LDL (low density lipoprotein)
LE (lupus erythematosus)
LE (lupus erythematosus) cell test
leachi, Haemaphysalis
lead(s) (Lead)
    l. artifact
    l., atrial
    L. AVF
    L. AVL
    L. AVR
    l., barb-tip
    l., barbed epicardial pacing
    l. beads for radiation beam
    l., bipolar
    l., black
    l., capped
    l., chest
    l. cutout
    l., direct
    l. dislodgement, atrial
    l., dual-electrode
    l., ear
    l., ECG/EKG (electrocardiogram)
    l., electrical
    l. electrocardiogram (ECG), 6-
    l. electrocardiogram (ECG) ▸ 16
    l. electrocardiogram (ECG), 3-
    l., electrocardiographic
    l. encephalopathy
    l. ▸ endocardial balloon
    l., epicardial
    l. equivalent
    l., esophageal
    l. exposure
    l. ▸ finned pacemaker
    l., fishhook
    l. fracture ▸ pacemaker
    l., frontal
    l. gonad shield
    l. gout
    l. impedance

l. impedance, atrial
l. implantable cardioverter defibrillator ▸ nonthoracotomy
l. in blood, level of
l. incrustation of cornea
l., indirect
l., insulated
l. ▸ insulation failure in ventricular
l., intracardiac
l., Leo's
l. letter marker
l., Lewis
l., limb
l., Medtronic
l., monitor
l., multi-electrode
l., myocardial
l., nasal
l., noncephalic
l. ▸ nonintegrated transvenous defibrillation
l. ▸ nonintegrated tripolar
L. I (one)
l., 1 thru 6
l. pace ▸ ventricular
l., pacemaker
l., parietal
l. patches, electrical
l. per deciliter
l. ▸ permanent cardiac pacing
l., pharyngeal
l. pipe colon
l. pipe fracture
l. pipe rigidity
l. placement
l. placement, nonthoracotomy
l. poisoning
l. pollution risk
l., precordial
l. reversal
l. ▸ reversed arm
l., scalar
l. ▸ segmented ring tripolar
l., semidirect
l. shielding in radiation
l. ▸ single pass
l. ▸ standard limb
l., sternal
l. ▸ steroid eluting pacemaker
l. strip
l., sugar of
l. syndrome ▸ nonthoracotomy defibrillation
l. system
l. system ▸ integrated

l. system ▸ Medtronic transvene endocardial
l. system ▸ orthogonal
l., tetramethyl
L. III
l. ▸ three-turn epicardial
l. threshold
l. ▸ transvenous defibrillator
l., tripolar
L. II (two)
l. ▸ two-turn epicardial
l., tympanic
l., unipolar
l. ▸ unipolar limb
l. ▸ unipolar precordial
l., ventricular
L. V-1 through V-6
l., white
l., Wilson's
leader ▸ treatment team
leading
    l. cause of death
    l. circle concept
    l. circle hypothesis
    l. edge
    l. edge enhancement
    l. to exhaustion, fatigue
leaf
    l., digitalis
    l. of diaphragm
    l. of diaphragm, eventration of
    l. spots in eye, ash
    l. tongue, fern
leaflet(s)
    l., anterior
    l., aortic
    l. aortic prosthesis ▸ tri-
    l., aortic valve
    l., bowing of mitral valve
    l., calcified mitral
    l., cardiac valve
    l. cardiac valve prosthesis ▸ Omniscience single
    l., cleft anterior
    l., delayed closing of
    l., doming of
    l., flail
    l. ▸ hammocking of posterior mitral
    l. ▸ mitral valve
    l. ▸ mitral valve anterior
    l. ▸ mitral valve posterior
    l. motion, posterior
    l., mural
    l., posterior
    l. ▸ posterior mitral

leaflet(s)—*continued*
- l. prolapse, aortic valve
- l. prosthesis, Teflon tri-
- l. thickening
- l. ‣ tricuspid valvular
- l., valve
- l. ‣ valve rings and
- l. vegetation

leaguer's elbow, little

leak(s)
- l., air
- l., alveolar
- l., anastomotic
- l., baffle
- l., peripheral air
- l., perivalvular
- l. syndrome, capillary
- l. technique ‣ minimal
- l. technique ‣ no-
- l., transient capillary

leakage
- l., blood
- l. current
- l. of air
- l. of blood into brain
- l. of enzymes
- l. of fluid
- l. or dribbling of urine
- l. or seepage of gel
- l. ‣ replacement valve
- l., spectral

leaking
- l. about shunt site
- l. aortic valve
- l., arteriovenous (AV)
- l. breast implant
- l. heart valve
- l. of aortic valve ‣ mild
- l. of aortic valve ‣ moderate
- l. of mitral valve ‣ moderate
- l., pseudocyst
- l. pulmonary capillaries
- l. retinal vessels
- l. silicone gel
- l. valve
- l. wound, intraocular

leaky
- l. artery
- l. capillaries
- l. heart valve
- l. mitral valve
- l. saline implant
- l. valve

lean body mass

lean muscle mass

leaping atrophy

learned
- l. behavior
- l. control
- l. relaxation

learner, auditory

learner, slow

learning (Learning)
- l. ability
- l. and awareness ‣ heart rate control
- l. and behavior problems
- l. and motivation
- l., behavior role
- l. change
- l., cognition and communication
- l., cognitive
- l. difficulties
- l. disabilities
- l. disability (LD)
- l. disability ‣ language-based
- l. disabled
- l. disabled child
- l. disorder, childhood
- l. experience
- l. impaired child
- l., nonverbal
- l., observational
- l. problem ‣ language-based
- l. process
- l. process, internal
- l. process, self-actuated
- l., rate of
- l. skills
- l., social
- l. support
- l. tasks
- L. Test, Rey Auditory Verbal
- l. theories of anxiety
- l. theorist
- l., verbal

least
- l. gluteal muscle
- l. occipital nerve
- l. squares analysis
- l. squares regression

leather(s)
- l. bottle stomach
- l. friction rub, saddle
- l., patient in full
- l. restraints
- l. restraints, four-point
- l. restraints ‣ full
- l. sound ‣ squeaky

leathery skin, patient has

leave(s)
- l. ‣ excessive use of sick
- l. (hallucinogens), green tea
- l. leave, maternity
- l. of broad ligament
- l. of diaphragm
- l. of mesentery
- l., separation of

Leber's
- L. amaurosis
- L. disease
- L. hereditary optic neuropathy
- L. neuropathy
- L. optic atrophy

Leboyer method of delivery

lecithin
- l., cardiolipin natural
- l., cardiolipin synthetic
- l. sphingomyelin (LS) ratio

lectin agglutination

lectularius, Cimex

LED (lupus erythematosus disseminatus)

Ledbetter maneuver

Lederer's anemia

ledge
- l., dental
- l., eccentric
- l., limbic

Ledgeriana, Cinchona

Lee-White clotting time method

Lee-White method

leech saliva

Leede('s)
- L. capillary fragility ‣ Rumpel-
- L. phenomenon, Rumpel-
- L. sign, Rumpel-

LeFort('s)
- L. amputation
- L. fracture
- L. fracture of maxilla
- L. I apertognathia repair
- L. operation
- L. suture
- L. uterine prolapse repair

left
- l. acetabular region
- l. adrenal gland ‣ focal metastasis
- l. ankle full range of motion (ROM)
- l. antecubital fossa
- l. anterior descending (LAD) artery
- l. anterior descending (LAD) lumen
- l. anterior hemiblock
- l. anterior oblique (LAO)
- l. anterior oblique (LAO) projection

l. aortic angiography
l. arm
l. arm electrode
l. arm ▸ hemiparesis
l. arm recumbent
l. atrial (LA)
l. atrial (LA) abnormality
l. atrial (LA) angiography
l. atrial (LA) aortic bypass ▸ Litwak
l. atrial (LA) appendage
l. atrial (LA) crossover dynamics ▸ left ventricular (LV)-
l. atrial (LA) dilation
l. atrial (LA) dimension
l. atrial (LA) emptying index
l. atrial enlargement (LAE)
l. atrial (LA) hypertension
l. atrial hypertrophy (LAH)
l. atrial (LA) isolation procedure
l. atrial (LA) Maze procedure ▸ modified
l. atrial (LA) myxoma
l. atrial (LA) partitioning
l. atrial pressure (LAP)
l. atrial pressure (MLAP) ▸ mean
l. atrial (LA) spontaneous echo contrast
l. atrial (LA) to aortic
l. atrioventricular (LAV) groove artery
l. atrium (LA)
l. atrium (LA), oblique vein of
l. atrium (LA) of heart
l. atrium (LA) ratio, aorta
l. axis deviation (LAD)
l. axis deviation (ALAD) ▸ abnormal
l. azygos vein
l. base, effusion
l. base, fluid density in
l. border of cardiac dullness
l. brachiocephalic vein
l. branch ▸ block in anterosuperior division of
l. branch ▸ block in posteroinferior division of
l. breast does appear enlarged ▸ lump in
l. breast does not appear enlarged ▸ lump in
l. bronchial tree
l. bronchus
l. bronchus, occlusion of
l. bundle branch
l. bundle branch block (LBBB)

l. bundle branch block (LBBB) ▸ complete
l. bundle branch block (LBBB) ▸ incomplete
l. buttock ▸ incision and drainage (I & D) of
l. calyces, blunting of
l. cardiac catheterization
l. carotid artery ▸ occlusion of
l. carotid endarterectomy
l. cataract surgery
l. central cortical area
l. cerebral hemisphere
l. chest opacity
l. circumflex artery
l. colic lymph node
l. colic vein
l. collecting system ▸ duplication of
l. colon syndrome, small
l. common carotid artery
l. coronary angiogram (LCA)
l. coronary artery (LCA)
l. coronary artery (LCA) angiography
l. coronary artery (LCA) ▸ calcification of
l. coronary artery (LCA) ▸ severe stenosis
l. coronary cineangiography
l. coronary vein
l. costal margin (LCM)
l. decubitus position
l. deltoid
l., deviation to the
l. diaphragm
l. discrimination, impaired
l. dominant coronary circulation
l. dorsoanterior
l. dorsoposterior
l. ear (AS)
l. endobronchial tree
l. esotropia
l. exotropia
l. eye (OS)
l. eye, deorsumduction of
l. eye, dextroduction of
l. eye, evisceration
l. eye ▸ flapping of conjunctiva,
l. eye, levoduction of
l. eye, postsurgical aphakia
l. eye, sursumduction of
l. eye (TOS) ▸ tension of
l. eye (VOS) ▸ vision
l. eye, visual acuity

l. facial droop
l. facial weakness
l. femoral artery
l. femur
l. femur full range of motion (ROM)
l. flexure of colon
l. flow tract
l. frontal hematoma
l. frontoanterior
l. frontoposterior
l. frontotransverse
l. gastric lymph nodes
l. gastric vein
l. gastroepiploic vein
l. gluteal
l. -handed
l. -handed individual
l. -handed, patient
l. -handedness
l. -handedness, pathological
l. heart
l. heart bypass
l. heart bypass ▸ percutaneous
l. heart catheterization
l. heart catheterization ▸ transseptal
l. heart failure
l. heart syndrome ▸ hypoblastic right and
l. heart syndrome, hypoplastic
l. hemicolectomy
l. hemisphere
l. hemisphere deficit
l. hemisphere of brain
l. hemisphere of brain ▸ dysplastic
l. hemithorax expands
l. hemothorax
l. hemothorax, spontaneous
l. hepatic lobe
l. heterotropia
l. hilar lymph node
l. hilum
l. hilum, prominence of
l. hip prosthesis
l. hydronephrosis
l. hyperphoria
l. hypertropia
l. hypochondriac region of abdomen
l. iliac fossa
l. iliac region of abdomen
l. inferior pulmonary vein
l. infundibulum, dilatation of
l. inguinal region of abdomen
l. inner canthus

left—*continued*

l. internal jugular vein
l. internal mammary artery (LIMA)
l. interspace, second
l. iris, postoperative coloboma
l. kidney
l. kidney, duplication of
l. kidney, scar lower pole
l. knee full range of motion (ROM)
l. lateral
l. lateral bending
l. lateral chest wall
l. lateral, internal dimension—
l. lateral position
l. lateral projection
l. lateral projection, stereo
l. lateral region of abdomen
l. lateral thorax
l. leg
l. leg electrode
l. leg, hypesthesia of
l. lower extremity (LLE)
l. lower extremity (LLE) amputated
l. lower extremity (LLE) flexed
l. lower extremity (LLE) full range of
   motion (ROM)
l. lower extremity (LLE), patient
   drags
l. lower lobe (LLL)
l. lower lobe (LLL) bronchial orifice
l. lower lobe (LLL) infiltrate
l. lower lobe (LLL) lesion
l. lower lobe (LLL) of lung
l. lower lobectomy
l. lower quadrant (LLQ)
l. lower quadrant (LLQ) of abdomen
l. lumbar region of abdomen
l. lung
l. lung, adenocarcinoma
l. lung ▸ apex of
l. lung base
l. lung base, atelectasis
l. lung base, infiltrate
l. lung, cardiac notch of
l. lung ▸ diaphragmatic surface of
l. lung ▸ dullness over
l. lung ▸ inferior margin of
l. lung ▸ lower lobe of
l. lung ▸ sternal margin of
l. lung ▸ upper lobe of
l. main bronchus
l. main coronary artery
l. main coronary artery (ALMCA),
   anomalous
l. main coronary artery disease

l. main coronary stenosis
l. main disease
l. main equivalency
l. main stem bronchus ▸ distortion
l. major hand
l., maternal
l., mediastinal shift to the
l. mediolateral episiotomy
l. mentoanterior
l. mentoposterior
l. mentotransverse
l. middle hemiblock
l. middle lobe (LML) of lung
l., moderate shift to
l. motor function waxed and waned
l. occipitoanterior
l. occipitoposterior
l. occipitotransverse
l. outer canthus
l. ovarian vein
l. ovary atrophic
l. parasternal impulses
l. pleural sac
l. pneumothorax
l. posterior cerebral artery
l. posterior hemiblock
l. posterior oblique (LPO)
l. prefrontal cortex
l. pubic ramus
l. pulmonary apex
l. pulmonary artery
l. pulmonary veins
l. pump, artificial heart
l. radical mastectomy
l. radical pneumonectomy
l. renal pelvis
l. -right external canthus
l., rotated to
l. sacroanterior
l. sacroposterior
l. sacrotransverse
l. scapuloanterior
l. scapuloposterior
l. sciatic radiation
l., scoliosis with concavity to
l., scoliosis with convexity to
l. septal hemiblock
l., shift to
l. shoulder full range of motion
   (ROM)
l. shunt, right-to-
l. side
l. side of body
l. side of brain
l. side of head

l. -sided
l. -sided appendicitis
l. -sided facial droop
l. -sided heart failure
l. -sided weakness
l. stem bronchus
l. sternal border (LSB)
l. subclavian artery
l. subclavian vein (LSV)
l. subcostal area
l. superior intercostal vein
l. superior pulmonary vein
l. suprarenal vein
l. testicular vein
l. thalamus
l. thigh
l. thoracostomy
l. thoracotomy
l. -to-right shunt
l. umbilical vein
l. upper extremity (LUE)
l. upper extremity (LUE) amputated
l. upper extremity (LUE) flexed
l. upper extremity (LUE) full range
   of motion (ROM)
l. upper lobe (LUL)
l. upper lobe (LUL) bronchial orifice
l. upper lobe (LUL) lesion
l. upper lobe (LUL) of lung
l. upper lobe (LUL) pneumonia
l. upper quadrant (LUQ)
l. upper quadrant (LUQ) of
   abdomen
l. ureter
l. ureteral calculus
l. ventricle (LV)
l. ventricle ▸ anterior papillary
   muscle of
l. ventricle ▸ apical thickening of
l. ventricle, damaged
l. ventricle (LV), double inlet
l. ventricle (LV), double outlet
l. ventricle (LV), enlarged
l. ventricle, hypokinesia of
l. ventricle (LV) ▸ ischemic
l. ventricle (LV) ▸ ischemic
   contracture of
l. ventricle (LV) malposition ▸
   double outlet
l. ventricle (LV) of heart
l. ventricle ▸ papillary muscle of the
l. ventricle ▸ posterior papillary
   muscle of
l. ventricle ▸ posterior vein of
l. ventricular (LV) aneurysm

l. ventricular (LV) aneurysm, congenital
l. ventricular angiography
l. ventricular (LV) apex
l. ventricular assist device (LVAD)
l. ventricular assist device (ALVAD), abdominal
l. ventricular assist system (LVAS)
l. ventricular (LV) assist system ▸ implantable
l. ventricular (LV) bypass pump
l. ventricular (LV) chamber compliance
l. ventricular compliance ▸ diminished
l. ventricular (LV) contractility
l. ventricular decompensation
l. ventricular (LV) diameter
l. ventricular (LV) diastolic phase index
l. ventricular diastolic pressure (LVDP)
l. ventricular (LV) diastolic relaxation
l. ventricular disease
l. ventricular (LV) dysfunction
l. ventricular (LV) dysfunction, advanced
l. ventricular (LV) dysfunction ▸ asymptomatic
l. ventricular (LV) dysfunction ▸ overt
l. ventricular (LV) dyskinesis
l. ventricular ejection fraction
l. ventricular (LV) ejection fraction ▸ global
l. ventricular ejection time (LVET)
l. ventricular end-diastolic pressure (LVEDP)
l. ventricular end-diastolic volume (LVEDV)
l. ventricular (LV) end-systolic stress
l. ventricular enlargement (LVE)
l. ventricular failure
l. ventricular (LV) failure ▸ acute
l. ventricular (LV) filling pressure
l. ventricular (LV) forces
l. ventricular fullness, borderline
l. ventricular (LV) function
l. ventricular (LV) function ▸ impaired
l. ventricular heart failure
l. ventricular heart failure, acute

l. ventricular (LV) hemodynamic abnormalities
l. ventricular hypertrophy (LVH)
l. ventricular (LV) hypertrophy, concentric
l. ventricular (LV) hypertrophy ▸ marked
l. ventricular (LV) inflow tract obstruction
l. ventricular injection
l. ventricular (LV) internal diastolic diameter
l. ventricular internal diastolic dimension
l. ventricular (LV) left atrial (LA) crossover dynamics
l. ventricular (LV) mass
l. ventricular mean (LVM)
l. ventricular (LV) muscle compliance
l. ventricular (LV) muscle disease
l. ventricular (LV) myocardial fibrosis ▸ interstitial
l. ventricular (LV) myocardium
l. ventricular (LV) myxoma
l. ventricular (LV) outflow tract
l. ventricular (LV) outflow tract obstruction
l. ventricular (LV) outflow tract velocity
l. ventricular (LV) output
l. ventricular posterior wall exclusion
l. ventricular posterior wall thickness
l. ventricular (LV) power
l. ventricular pressure (LVP)
l. ventricular (LV) pressure ▸ end-diastolic
l. ventricular (LV) pressure ▸ mean diastolic
l. ventricular (LV) pressure ▸ mean systolic
l. ventricular (LV) pressure ▸ systolic
l. ventricular (LV) pressure volume
l. ventricular (LV) pressure volume curve
l. ventricular (LV) puncture
l. ventricular (LV) puncture ▸ apical
l. ventricular (LV) reduction
l. ventricular (LV) reduction surgery
l. ventricular (LV) rejection
l. ventricular (LV) rejection fraction ▸ global

l. ventricular (LV)-right atrial communication murmur
l. ventricular strain
l. ventricular stroke volume (LVSV)
l. ventricular stroke work (LVSW)
l. ventricular stroke work index (LVSWI)
l. ventricular study
l. ventricular (LV) systolic performance
l. ventricular systolic pressure (LVSP)
l. ventricular (LV) tension
l. ventricular (LV) tunnel murmur, aortic
l. ventricular wall
l. ventricular wall motion
l. ventricular (LV) wall motion abnormality
l. ventricular (LV) wall stress
l. ventricular (LV) weakness
l. ventricular work (LVW)
l. ventricular work index (LVWI)
l. ventriculectomy (LV) ▸ partial
l. ventriculogram, dynamic
l. ventriculography
l. ventriculography ▸ quantitative
l. wave-spike ▸ parietal area
l. wrist full range of motion (ROM)

leg(s)
l., angina in
l., artificial
l., atrophy of
l., back pain extends down to
l., baker's
l., blood pools in
l. bone
l., bowed
l. brace, long
l. brace, short
l. brace with drop-lock knee ▸ long
l. brace with free ankle ▸ long
l. brace with large tibial cuff ▸ long
l. cast, long
l. cast, short
l. circulation
l. circulation, decreased
l. ▸ claudication in the
l., coarse tremors of
l., congenital pseudarthrosis of
l. cramp
l. cramping
l. cramps ▸ nighttime
l. cramps, nocturnal
l. cramps ▸ painful

leg(s)—*continued*
- l. cramps, potassium
- l., crampy, achy feeling in
- l., creepy-crawly syndrome of
- l. crunch exercise, bent
- l. curl exercise
- l. drift
- l., driver's
- l. edema
- l., electric
- l. ► electrical stimulation of
- l. electrode, left
- l. electrode, right
- l. elevated higher than heart
- l. exercises
- l. exercises, patient taught
- l. extensions
- l. flail wildly
- l. flailing
- l. flap, cross-
- l. flap, island
- l., flexion of
- l., flexion reflex of
- l. ► fluid accumulation in
- l. fracture
- l. from caffeine ► restless
- l. gradient, arm-
- l. graft, cross-
- l. ► heaviness in
- l., hypesthesia of fight
- l. ► hypopigmented macules on
- l. ► immobilizing and splinting
- l., interosseous nerve of
- l. ► involuntary jerking movements of
- l., left
- l. lift
- l. list
- l., milk
- l. motion
- l. movement ► uncoordinated
- l. movements, periodic
- l. muscles, anesthesia of
- l. muscles, atrophy of
- l. muscles ► oxygen (O₂)-deprived
- l. muscles ► sense of fatigue in
- l., musculocutaneous nerve of
- l. ► numbness of lower
- l. ► numbness, weakness and paralysis of
- l. pain
- l., pain and swelling of
- l. pain, chronic
- l., pain down
- l., pain radiating down

- l. ► painful claudication of
- l. ► paralysis of
- l., passive flexion of
- l. positioned in stirrups
- l. press exercise
- l. prosthesis ► sea
- l. raise exercise ► side
- l. raising
- l. raising (SLR) limited ► straight
- l. raising (SLR) negative straight
- l. raising, straight
- l. raising tenderness (SLRT), straight
- l. raising test (SLRT), straight
- l. ► reduce swelling in
- l., restless
- l., right
- l. rigidly extended
- l. ► silvery scales on
- l. sit-ups ► straight
- l. sparing stress test
- l. spasm
- l. ► spasticity of
- l. ► stiffening and deformity of
- l. stiffness
- l. strength
- l. ► sudden numbness of
- l. ► sudden paralysis of
- l. ► sudden weakness of
- l. swelling
- l., swollen
- l. syndrome, fidgety
- l. syndrome, restless
- l. tissue ► infection in
- l. type
- l. ulcer
- l. ► uncontrollable shakiness in
- l., varicosities of
- l., vascular disease of
- l. vein
- l. vein clotting
- l. vein treatment
- l. view, frog-
- l. walking cast, short
- l. weakness, bilateral
- l., weakness of
- l. ► weakness or numbness of

legal
- l. advice
- l. aspects of resuscitation
- l. blindness
- l. blindness ► irreversible
- l. complications
- l. conceptions
- l. document

- l. guardian, patient's
- l. implications
- l. interaction, medical-
- l. issue
- l. medicine
- l. requirements
- l. responsibility
- l. restrictions in drug abuse
- l. stressors

legalize euthanasia

legally
- l. competent patient
- l. mandated evaluation
- l. sane patient

Legendre's nodes

legends, urban

Legg-Calvé-Waldenstrom disease

Legg-Perthes syndrome ► Calvé-

legged, patient is bow-

legged position, frog-

Legionella
- L. anisa
- L. birminghamensis
- L. bozemanii
- L. cincinnatiensis
- L. dumoffi
- L. feelei
- L. gormanii
- L. jordanis
- L. lansingensis
- L. longbeachae
- L. micdadei
- L. oakridgensis
- L. pneumonia
- L. pneumophila

Legionnaires'
- L. disease
- L. pneumonia
- L. titer

legislation, health-related

legitimate therapeutic activity

LeGros Clark, nucleus lateralis of

Legroux's remission

leichmannii, Lactobacillus

Leichtenstern encephalitis, Strümpell-

Leichtenstern's sign

Leinbach's prosthesis

Leiner's disease

leiomyoma(s)
- l., fibro◊
- l. fibromata
- l. ► multiple small calcified
- l. of iris
- l. of orbit

l. of uterus, calcified
l., pericardial
l., sclerosed
l., sclerotic
l., submucous
l. uteri
leiomyomata, multiple
leiomyomata uteri
leiomyosarcoma
l. of orbit
l. of soft tissue
l., uterine
Leipmann's apraxia
Leishe #10 lens implant
Leishman('s)
L. anemia
L. -Donovan bodies
L. nodules
L. stain
Leishmania
L. braziliensis
L. braziliensis pifanoi
L. donovani
L. infantum
L. tropica
leishmaniasis
l., cutaneous
l., mucocutaneous
l., naso-oral
l., nasopharyngeal
l., visceral
leisure
l. activity
l. skills ▸ sober
l. skills ▸ social and
l. social time activities
Leitner's syndrome
Leitz microscope
Leksell's
L. gamma unit
L. stereotactic device
L. stereotactic frame
Lembert suture
Lembert suture, Czerny-
LeMesurier's method
Lemli-Opitz syndrome ▸ Smith-
lemniscus, medial
lemonnieri, Saccharomyces
Lempert('s)
L. fenestration
L. incision
L. instruments
L. procedure
Lenard rays
Lenegre's disease

length
l. active tension curve
l. alternans, cycle
l. alternation, cycle
l., antegrade block cycle
l., atrial-paced cycle
l., basic cycle
l., basic drive cycle
l., block cycle
l., chordal
l. (CRL) ▸ crown rump
l., cycle
l. data, wave
l., deBroglie wave
l. -dependent activation
l., drive cycle
l., equal in
l. ▸ flutter cycle
l., focal
l. (HRL) ▸ head to rump
l. method, area
l. of awareness of illness
l. of bone, fracture running
l. of fetus
l. of hospital stay
l. of rhythmic activity, wave
l. of stay
l. of stay, appropriate
l. ▸ paced cycle
l. ▸ pacing cycle
l., period
l. polymorphisms (RFLPs) ▸
  restriction fragment
l. relation ▸ force
l. relation ▸ force velocity
l. relation ▸ tension-
l. resting tension relation
l. (RHL) ▸ rump to heel
l. ▸ sinus cycle
l. speech, phrase
l. ▸ tachycardia cycle
l. tension relation
l. tension relation ▸ resting
l., tumor
l., uterus normal in
l. utterance, phrase
l. ▸ ventricular tachycardia cycle
l., wave
l. window, cycle
lengthening
l., crown
l., heel cord
l. operation ▸ limb
l. reaction
l., tendon

l. tibia
lengthy recuperation
Lennarson's tube
Lennox-Gastaut, syndrome
Lennox's syndrome
lens(es) (Lens)
l., achromatic
l., acrylic
l., adherent
l., Anis Staple implant cataract
l., aplanatic
l., apochromatic
l., Appolionio implant cataract
l., artificial
l., asymmetric refraction of
l., Azar Tripod implant cataract
l., Baron implant cataract
l., biconcave
l., biconvex
l., bicylindrical
l., Bietti implant cataract
l., bifocal
l., Binkhorst iridiocapsular cataract
l., bispherical
l., Brücke's
l. capsule
l. capsule, exfoliation of
l., cataract
l. cells
l., Choyce anterior chamber
l., Choyce implant cataract
l., Cilco intraocular
l., clouded
l., clouding of eye
l., cloudy
l. (IOL), Coburn intraocular
l., concave
l., concavoconcave
l., concavoconvex
l., conoid
l., contact
l. contact lens, T
l., contaminated contact
l., converging
l., convex
l., convexoconcave
l., Coquille plano
l., corrective
l. ▸ cortical substance of
l., cosmetic
l., Crookes'
l., crystalline
l., curvature of
l., custom contact
l., cylindrical

lens(es)—*continued*

l. ▸ daily-wear soft
l., decentered
l., decentration of
l. delivered
l. delivered by tumbling procedure
l. delivered intracapsularly
l., discission of
l. ▸ dislocated eye
l., dislocation of the
l., dispersing
l. ▸ disposable bifocal contact
l., distortion of
l., ectopia of
l. electrodes
l. elevated
l., enlargement of
l., express
l., extended wear contact
l., extended wear soft
l. extracted
l. extracted in tumbling fashion
l., fiberoptic
l., firm
l., flexible
l. ▸ foldable intraocular
l. (IOL) ▸ foldable silicone
  intraocular
l., foreign body (FB) in
l., Foroblique
l., full contact
l., gas permeable
l., general purpose
l., gonio◊
l., hard
l., Hruby
l., Hydrocurve contact
l., immersion
l. implant
l. implant, artificial
l. (IOL) implant ▸ intraocular
l. implant, Leiske #10
l., implantable
l. implantation
l. implantation, artificial
l. implantation, cataract
l. implantation ▸ intraocular
l. implants ▸ multifocal
l., increased convexity of
l. infection ▸ contact
l., insertion of intraocular
l. (IOL), intraocular
l. (ICL) ▸ intraocular contact
l., lolab intraocular
l., iridocapsular fixation

l., iris fixation
l., iris plane
l., iseikonic
l., Koeppe
l., Krasnov implant cataract
l., Lieb and Guerry cataract implant
l. (IOL), Liteflex intraocular
l., luxation of
l., magnifying
l. material expressed
l. (IOL), McGhan intraocular
l., meniscus
l., meter
l., minus
l., monofocal
l., needling of
l., omnifocal
l. opacification
l. opacity, early
l., opaque contact
l., opening through
l. (IOL), Optiflex intraocular
l., orthoscopic
l., parenchyma of
l., Pearce Tripod implant cataract
l., periscopic
l., piggyback
l., pigmentary deposits on
l., plane of contact
l., planoconcave
l., planoconvex
l. plastic
l., Platina Clip implant cataract
l. plus ultraviolet (PUVA) light
  treatment, psora-
l. ▸ prism eyeglass
l. prism, Goldmann's contact
l. ▸ progressive clouding of the
l., prosthetic
l., punktal
l., retroscopic
l., Ridley implant cataract
l., right-angle
l. ▸ rigid gas permeable (RGP)
  contact
l., Sauflon PW contact
l., Schachar's cataract
l., Schachar's implant cataract
l., Scharf's implant cataract
l., shagreen lesions of
l. ▸ single focus
l. (IOL), Sinskey/Sinskey modified
  blue loop intraocular
l., Soflens contact
l., soft

l. ▸ soft contact
l. ▸ soft disposable contact
l. ▸ soft foldable artificial
l., special purpose
l., spherical
l. spoon, Daviel's
l. stars
l., stiffening of
l., Stokes'
l., Strampelli implant cataract
l., subluxation of
l., substance of
l. (IOL), Surgidev intraocular
l., suspensory ligament of
l. system
l. system, angled-vision
l., T lens contact
l., Thorpe plastic
l., toric
l., trifocal
l. ▸ vision improving
l., Volk conoid ophthalmic
l. washed out, remnants of
l. whorl
l. with double focus
L., Worst Medallion

lenta

l., cholangitis
l., endocarditis
l., sepsis
l., tonsillitis

Lente insulin
lente insulin, Ultra◊
lenticular

l. aphasia
l. astigmatism
l. bone
l. carcinoma
l. cataract
l. degeneration, progressive
l. glaucoma
l., irregular astigmatism
l. nucleus
l. process of the incus
l. ring, Vossius'

lenticulare, carcinoma
lenticularis, fasciculus
lenticulostriate arteries
lentiform nodule
lentigines, senile
lentigines syndrome, multiple
lentiginous melanoma, sacral
lentigo

l. maligna
l. maligna melanoma

l. senilis
lentil agglutination binding
lentis
l., caligo
l., capsula
l., chalcosis
l., coloboma
l., cortex
l., ectopia
l., Filaria
l., tunica vasculosa
lentivirus, rare
Leon virus
Leonard-George position
leopard retina
leopard syndrome
Leopold's
L. law
L. maneuver
L. operation
Leo's lead
lepidic tissue
L'Episcopo's operation
lepiseptica, gram-negative
  Pasteurella
Lepore, hemoglobin
leporispalustris, Haemaphysalis
leprae
l., Bacillus
l. murium, Mycobacterium
l., Mycobacterium
leproticum, erythema nodosum
Leptocimex boueti
Leptodera pellio
leptomeningeal
l. anastomosis
l. carcinomatosis
l. disease
l. involvement
leptomeningitis
l., circumscribed
l. interna
l., nonserous
l., sarcomatous
l., serous
l., syphilitic
l., tuberculous
Leptomitus
L. epidermidis
L. urophilus
L. vaginae
Leptopsylla musculi
Leptopsylla segnis
leptosomatic habit

Leptospira
L. australis
L. autumnalis
L. bataviae
L. biflexa
L. canicola
L. grippotyphosa
L. hebdomidis
L. hyos
L. icterohaemorrhagiae/
  icterohemorrhagiae
L. interrogans
L. pomona
L. pyrogenes
leptospiral jaundice
leptospirosis
l., anicteric
l., benign
l., canine
l. icterohaemorrhagica
l. species ▸ saprophytic
Leptothrix
L. buccalis
L. echinata
L. discophora
L. epiphytica
L. lopholea
L. major
L. ochracea
L. pseudovacuolata
L. sideropous
L. skujae
L. thermalis
L. volubilis
L. winogradskii
Leptotrichia buccalis
Leptotrichia placoides
leptotrichosis conjunctivae
Leptus akamushi
Leptus irritans
Lereboullet syndrome, Gilbert-
Leredde's syndrome
Leri('s) sign
Leriche('s)
L. operation
L. syndrome
L. syndrome, intimectomy for
L. syndrome, Sudeck-
Lerman-Means scratch
Lermoyez's syndrome
Lerous method
lesbian, sexually active
Lesch-Nyhan syndrome
lesion(s) [*region*]
l., abnormal anatomical

l. accessible for biopsy
l., active
l., adrenal
l., anatomic
l., aneuploid
l., angiocentric immunoproliferative
l., annular
l., antibiotic-treated
l., aorto-ostial
l., apical
l., apparent
l., apple core
l., areatic
l., Armanni-Ebstein
l., arterial
l., arterial bend
l. artifact ▸ skin
l., asymptomatic
l., atheromatous
l., atherosclerotic
l., atrophic
l., bacterial
l., Baehr-Löhlein
l., Bankart
l., basal cell
l., benign
l., benign lymphoepithelial
l. ▸ benign skull base
l., bifurcation
l. biopsy
l. biopsy, skin
l., birds' nest
l., black sunburst
l., bladder
l., blistering
l., Blumenthal
l., blunt arterial
l., borderline malignant
l., braid-like
l., brain
l., branch
l., Brown-Sequard
l. ▸ brushing of esophageal
l., buccal
l., bulging
l., bull's eye
l., calcified
l. ▸ calvarium without palpable
l., cancerous
l., candida
l., carcinomatous
l., carious
l., cavitary
l. cells, heart
l., cellular

lesion(s)—*continued*

l., central
l., central audiovestibular
l., cerebral
l., cerebrovascular
l., cervical cord
l., cervical spinal
l., chest
l. ▸ chronic blood loss of gastrointestinal
l., circular
l., circumscribed
l., coagulation of bleeding gastrointestinal (GI)
l., coin
l., cold
l., collar button
l., colonic
l., congenital
l., constricting
l., constricting esophageal
l., coronary artery
l., cortical
l., corticospinal
l., corticospinal tract
l., Councilman's
l., culprit
l., cystic
l., de novo
l., deep-seated
l., dendritic
l. desiccated
l., dilatable
l., discrete
l. ▸ discrete coronary
l. disease ▸ retina vascular
l., distal esophageal
l., draining
l., DREZ (dorsal root entry zone)
l., Duke's III
l., Duret's
l., early metastatic pulmonary
l., Ebstein's
l., elevated
l., endolaryngeal
l., enhancing
l. ▸ erythema chronicum migraines
   (ECM)
l., esophageal
l. ▸ evolving neurological
l., excavated
l. excised elliptically
l. ▸ excision benign
l., expansile lytic
l. eye

l., factitial
l., female urethral
l., fibrocalcific
l., fibroepithelial polypoid anorectal
l. ▸ fibromusculoelastic
l., focal
l. ▸ focal brain
l. formation ▸ new
l., fungating
l., gastrointestinal (GI)
l., genital tract
l., Ghon
l., Ghon's primary
l., gram stain of skin
l., granular
l., granulomatous
l., gross
l., gynecologic
l., heat
l., hemorrhagic
l., herpes-like
l., herpetic
l., herpetiform
l., high grade
l., high thoracic cord
l., hilar
l., Hill-Sachs
l., histologic
l., honeycomb
l., hot
l., hyperkeratotic
l., hyperkeratotic verrucoid surfaced
l., hypothalamic
l., impaction
l. in Broca's area
l. in coronary arteries, asymmetric
l. in dermatomyositis
l. in esophagus
l. in the brain
l., indiscriminate
l., inflammatory
l., initial syphilitic
l., intracranial
l. ▸ intracranial mass
l., intraoral
l. intrinsic
l., intrinsic bronchial
l., invasive
l., irritative
l., itchy
l., Janeway's
l., jet
l., keratotic
l., laser vaporization of
l., left lower lobe (LLL)

l., left upper lobe (LUL)
l. ▸ Libman-Sacks
l., lichenified
l., linear skin
l., lipomatous
l., LLL (left lower lobe)
l., local
l., localized
l. ▸ Löhlein-Baehr
l., long
l., LUL (left upper lobe)
l., lytic
l., lytic bone
l., macroscopic
l. ▸ macroscopic central nervous
   system (CNS)
l. ▸ macrovascular coronary
l., maculopapular
l., malignant
l. ▸ malignant metastatic or benign
l. ▸ malignant skull base
l., marsupialization of
l., mass
l., metastatic
l., metastatic bone
l. ▸ microscopic central nervous
   system (CNS)
l. milked out
l., mixed
l., molecular
l., monmalignant chest
l., monotypic
l., mucosal
l., multiple
l. ▸ multiple punctate mucosal
l., myocardial
l., nailbed
l., neck
l., necrotic
l., neoplastic
l., nevoid
l., nodular
l. ▸ nonbacterial thrombotic
   endocardial
l., noninvasive
l., obstructing
l., obstructive
l., occlusive
l., occult
l. of bone, benign
l. of brain stem
l. of cervix
l. of Cole, herpetiform
l. of cortical center
l. of corticospinal tracts

l. of eye, benign
l. of lens, shagreen
l. of lung, coin
l. of soft tissue, benign
l. of spinal cord, excision
l. of uterus ▸ nonmalignant
l. of vagina
l. of vulva
l. on the cornea
l. ▸ onion scale
l., onionskin
l., oral
l., organic
l., organic cardiac
l., original rectal
l., osteoblastic
l., osteolytic
l., osteolytic calvarial
l., ostial
l., outcropping of
l., painful
l. ▸ painful, blister type
l. palpable
l., pancreatic
l., parasagittal
l. ▸ paring of
l., partial
l. ▸ pathogenesis of ocular
l., pearly
l., pedunculated
l. ▸ penetrating arterial
l., penile
l., periapical
l., peripheral
l., peripheral nerve
l., petechial
l., pigmented
l., pinkish
l., pituitary
l., plaque-like
l., plexiform
l., pneumatic
l., polypoid
l., polypoidal
l., pontine
l., posterior vaginal septal
l., posterior vaginal wall
l., precancerous
l., preinvasive
l., premalignant
l., primary
l. ▸ proliferative skin
l., pulmonary
l., punctiform
l., purpuric

l., pustular
l., questionable
l., radiographic
l., radiographic stability of
l., radiopaque
l., raised
l., rapidly growing
l., rectal
l., rectosigmoid polypoid
l., recurrent
l., renal vascular
l. resectable
l., restenosis
l., retinal
l., rib
l., right lower lobe (RLL)
l., right upper lobe (RUL)
l., ring-wall
l., RLL (right lower lobe)
l. ▸ rotator cuff
l., RUL (right upper lobe)
l., salivary gland
l., satellite
l. scabbing
l., scalene
l., scalp
l., scalp without palpable
l., seizure-triggering
l., sessile
l., severe intracranial
l., sharply demarcated
      circumferential
l., skin
l., skip
l., slowly developing
l., soft fleshy
l. ▸ soft fluctant nodular
l., solitary
l., sore
l., space occupying
l., spherical
l. ▸ spinal cord
l., spontaneous
l., stability of
l., stenotic
l., structural
l., surface of
l., surgical
l., suspicious
l., suspicious mammogram
l. ▸ synchronous airway
l., systemic
l., tandem
l., target
l., temporal lobe

l., tongue
l., total
l., treatable
l., trophic
l., tuberculous
l., ulcerated
l., ulcerated eccentric
l., ulcerating
l., ulcerative
l., underlying
l., undifferentiated
l., unresectable
l., variceal
l., vascular
l., vegetative
l., verrucous
l., vestibular
l., wide field
l. ▸ widespread bony osteolytic
l., wire-loop
l. with small white centers, oval
lesionectomy procedure
lesioning, stereotactic
   radiofrequency
L'Esperance's erysiphake
less
   l. restrictive diet
   l. restrictive measures
   l. than air conduction (BC < AC) ▸
      bone conduction
lessened ▸ blunted, dulled or
lessening of pain
lessening sense of taste
lesser
   l. afar cartilage
   l. circulation
   l. curvature
   l. curvature aspect
   l. curvature of stomach
   l. curvature site
   l. ganglion of Meckel
   l. ischiatic notch
   l. multangular bone
   l. occipital nerve
   l. omentum
   l. palatine nerves
   l. pancreas
   l. pelvis
   l. peritoneal cavity
   l. petrosal nerve
   l. resection
   l. rhomboid muscle
   l. sacrosciatic notch
   l. saphenous system
   l. sciatic notch

lesser—*continued*
- l. splanchnic nerve
- l. superior azygos vein
- l. trochanter
- l. tubercle
- l. zygomatic muscle

LET (linear energy transfer)

letdown
- l., milk
- l. reflex
- l. reflex, milk

lethal
- l. arrhythmia
- l. childhood tumors
- l. concentration
- l. concentration, approximate
- l. condition
- l. convulsion
- l. damage
- l. disease
- l. dose
- l. dose (MLD or LD$_{50}$), median
- l. dose (MLD) ► minimum
- l. dose ► ratio of median
- l. dose (TLD), tumor
- l. drugs
- l. equivalent
- l. heart rhythm
- l. injection
- l. injection ► direct killing by
- l. injury
- l. midline granuloma
- l. neuromuscular disease
- l. organisms
- l. orphan (CELO) ► chicken-embryo-
- l. overdose of morphine
- l. rhythmic irregularities
- l. side-effects
- l. substance
- l. substance ► patient injected with
- l. toxicity
- l. underlying disease ► non-

lethargic
- l. and dull
- l. and weak ► somnolent,
- l. encephalitis
- l. feeling
- l., patient
- l., somnolent and
- l. state
- l. stupor

lethargica, encephalitis

lethargy
- l. and fatigue ► inactivity

- l. and fever ► jaundice
- l., confusion and
- l., fatigue and
- l., hysteric
- l., induced
- l., jaundice and
- l., jaundice, diarrhea
- l., lucid
- l. ► nausea, vomiting and
- l. unexplained depression and

letter marker ► lead

Letterer-Siwe
- L. disease
- L. syndrome
- L. syndrome, Abt-

letters and punctuation, perseverated

Leuber's neuropathy

Leube's test meal

leucine
- l. aminopeptidase
- l. aminopeptidase test
- l. sensitive

leucocelaenus, Aedes

leucovorin rescue

leucurus, Ammospermophilus

Leudet's bruit

leukemia
- l., acute childhood
- l., acute granulocytic
- l. (ALL), acute lymphoblastic
- l., acute lymphocytic
- l. (AMOL), acute monoblastic
- l. (AML), acute monocytic
- l. (AML), acute myeloblastic
- l. (AML), acute myelocytic
- l. (AMMOL), acute myelomonoblastic
- l. (AMML), acute myelomonocytic
- l. (ANLL), acute nonlymphocytic
- l. (ANLL), acute nonlymphoid
- l. (APL), acute promyelocytic
- l., acute undifferentiated
- l., aleukocythemic
- l. antigen, common acute
- l. antigen, common acute lymphoblastic
- l., aplastic
- l., basophilic
- l., blast cell
- l. cell structure, basic
- l., chronic lymphatic
- l. (CLL), chronic lymphocytic
- l., chronic lymphosarcoma cell
- l. (CML), chronic myelocytic
- l. (CML), chronic myelogenous

- l., chronic myeloid
- l., chronic myelomonocytic
- l., chronic neutrophilic
- l. cutis
- l., embryonal
- l., eosinophilic
- l., erythro◊
- l., feline
- l., granulocytic
- l., hairy cell
- l., hemoblastic
- l., hemocytoblastic
- l., histiocytic
- l. inhibitory factor
- l., leukopenic
- l., lymphatic
- l., lymphoblastic
- l., lymphocytic
- l., lymphogenous
- l., lymphoid
- l., lymphoidocytic
- l., lymphosarcoma cell
- l., mast cell
- l., megakaryocytic
- l., meningeal
- l., micromyeloblastic
- l., monocytic
- l., myeloblastic
- l., myelocytic
- l., myelogenous
- l., myeloid
- l., null cell lymphoblastic
- l., plasma cell
- l., plasmacytic
- l., promyelocytic
- l. -protection, radiation-
- l., Reider cell
- l. relapse rate
- l., reticuloendothelial cell
- l., Schilling's
- l. ► Schilling-type monocytic
- l., splenomedullary
- l., splenomyelogenous
- l., stem cell
- l., subacute myelomonocytic
- l., subleukemic
- l., undifferentiated cell
- l. variant, chronic lymphocytic
- l. virus
- l. virus, murine
- l. virus, Schwartz's

leukemic
- l. adenia
- l. erythrocytosis
- l. individual

l. infiltrate, abundant
l. infiltrate, diffuse
l. infiltrates of adrenals
l. infiltrates of colon
l. infiltrates of kidneys
l. infiltrates of liver
l. infiltration
l. meningitis
l. reaction
l. reticuloendotheliosis
l. retinitis
l. retinopathy
l. transformation ▸ multiple myeloma with

leukemogenic virus, Moloney's
leukemoid reaction, stress-type
leukoagglutinin reaction
leukocyte(s)
l. adhesion molecule (ELAM) ▸ endothelial
l. agglutinin
l. alkaline phosphatase (LAP) test
l. antigen, common
l. antigens (HLA) ▸ human
l. ascorbic acid
l., basophil granular
l. chemotaxis
l. common antigen
l. count, polymorphonuclear
l. culture (MLC), mixed
l. dysfunction
l. elastase
l., eosinophilic
l., fecal
l. inclusions
l. ▸ increase in polymorphonuclear
l. index, Krebs'
l. infiltrate ▸ interstitial polymorphonuclear
l. interferon, human
l., interstitial polymorphonuclear
l. mobilization, localized
l., neutrophilic
l., neutrophilic polymorphonuclear
l., polymorphonuclear
l. reaction
l. reaction, mixed
l. response, polymorphonuclear
l. ▸ sequestration of polymorphonuclear
l. syndrome (LLS), lazy
l., transfusion of

leukocythemia, oligo◊
leukocytoblastic vasculitis
leukocytoclastic angiitis

leukocytoclastic vasculitis
leukocytoid habit
leukocytosis
l., eosinophilic
l., lymphocytic
l. -promoting factor
l., transient
leukodystrophy
l., globoid
l., globoid cell
l., hereditary cerebral
l., Krabbe's
l. (MLD) ▸ metachromatic
l., spongiform
l., sudanophilic
leukoencephalitis
l., acute hemorrhagic
l., chronic subacute
l., subacute sclerosing
leukoencephalopathy, progressive multifocal
leukoerythroblastic anemia
leukopenia
l., basophil
l., basophilic
l., congenital
l., malignant
leukopenic leukemia
leukoplakia
l. from alcohol
l. from dentures
l., hairy
l., oral
l., oral-hairy
l. penis
l. vulvae
leukoplakic changes
leukoplakic vulvitis
leukoprotease inhibitor protein ▸ secretory
leukorrhea, menstrual
leukorrhea, periodic
leukorrheal discharge
leukosis
l., acute
l., avian
l. complex, avian
l., fowl
l., lymphoid
l., myeloblastic
l., myelocytic
l., skin
leukostigma, Hemerocampa
leukotactic function
leukotactic function, host's

leukotome, Love's
leukotomy, transorbital
leukotriene inhibition
levator
l. ani
l. ani muscle
l. hernia
l. muscle
l. muscle of angle of mouth
l. muscle of palatine velum
l. muscle of prostate
l. muscle of scapula
l. muscle of thyroid gland
l. muscle of upper eyelid
l. muscle of upper lip
l. muscle of upper lip and ala of nose
l. muscle of velum palatini
l. muscle, resection
l. muscles of ribs
l. muscles of ribs ▸ long
l. muscles of ribs ▸ short
l. nerve
l. palpebrae superior muscle
l. palpebrae superioris, musculus
l. slings
l. veli palatini muscle
levatorius, torus
LeVeen
L. dialysis shunt
L. peritoneal shunt
L. peritoneovenous shunt
L. plaque cracker
level(s)
l., abnormal
l., abnormal calcium
l., abnormal magnesium
l., abnormal potassium
l., acetaldehyde
l., activity
l. ▸ age-appropriate articulation
l., air fluid
l., ammonia
l. and degree of mental illness
l., antibody
l., antimicrobial
l., antiepileptic drug
l., anxiety
l., average cholesterol
l., baseline
l., baseline cortisol
l., blood
l., blood alcohol
l., blood carbon dioxide (CO_2)
l., blood cholesterol

level(s)—*continued*

l., blood fat
l., blood oxygen (O₂)
l., blood phosphorus
l., blood sugar
l., blood triglyceride
l., bone pain at minimal
l., border
l., butyrocholinesterase
l., calcitonin
l., calcium
l., cancericidal
l. ▸ cardiac enzyme
l., carotene
l., cellular
l., centimeter (cm)
l., cholesterol
l., cholesterol blood
l., comfort
l., consumption
l., control glucose
l., creatinine
l., crisis
l., critical
l., current fitness
l., decrease in energy
l., dermatome
l. ▸ difficulty functioning at normal ability
l., digoxin
l., disruptive
l., dosage
l., dose
l., electrolyte
l., elevate feet above heart
l., elevated anxiety
l., endorphin
l., energy
l., enzyme
l. ▸ erratic blood glucose
l., estrogen
l., examined hormone
l., excessive activity
l., exercise
l. exposure, low
l., fasting glucose
l., fibrinogen
l., fitness
l., fluctuating hormone
l., fluid
l. for pain ▸ tolerance
l., functioning
l., gas
l., genetic
l., glucose

l., glycosylated hemoglobin
l., hearing
l. ▸ high blood alcohol
l., high cholesterol
l., highest functioning
l., homocysteine
l., hormone
l. ▸ human plasma
l., hyperinsulinemic
l. ▸ imbalance in neurotransmitter
l. in blood ▸ high acid
l., increased activity
l., initial baseline
l. insulin
l., intellectual
l., intense
l., iron
l. ▸ iron saturation
l., isoelectric
l., isovaleric acid
l., Lidocaine
l., lipid
l., loudness
l., loudness discomfort
l. ▸ low blood potassium
l., low energy
l., low magnesium
l., low noise
l., magnesium blood
l., maintain blood glucose
l., maintenance
l. ▸ markedly increased energy
l. ▸ maternal neonatal methadone
l., maximal comfort
l., medial joint
l., melatonin
l., microscopic
l., minimal bactericidal
l., molecular
l. ▸ multiple air fluid
l. ▸ multiple shunt
l., muscle
l., narrowing at lumbosacral
l., natural stress
l., neural thread protein
l., neurobiological
l., nicotine
l., noise
l., normal triglyceride
l., normalize thyroxin
l. ▸ noxious noise
l., occlusal
l. of achievement
l. of activity
l. of activity, highest

l. of alcohol consumption
l. of alcohol intake ▸ initial
l. of amphetamine, blood
l. of amphetamine, urine
l. of anesthesia
l. of anger
l. of annulus
l. of antibody titers
l. of anxiety ▸ high
l. of anxiety ▸ pain determined by
l. of anxiety, patient's
l. of arousal, high
l. of awareness
l. of blood alcohol
l. of blood sugar ▸ increased
l. of brain excitation
l. of calcium, blood
l. of care
l. of care, appropriate
l. of care criteria ▸ skilled
l. of care ▸ high
l. of cocaine, blood
l. of cocaine, urine
l. of cognitive function
l. of communication
l. of confidence
l. of consciousness (LOC)
l. of consciousness altered
l. of consciousness, decreased
l. of consciousness, depressed
l. of consciousness ▸ fluctuating
l. of consciousness, patient's
l. of cricoid cartilage
l. of denial
l. of dependency
l. of depressant, blood
l. of depressant, urine
l. of depression
l. of depression ▸ mild-to-moderate
l. of despair
l. of development, prepsychotic
l. of diaphragm
l. of disability, patient's
l. of disease
l. of drinking ▸ diminished
l. of drugs, toxic
l. of endothelin ▸ elevated
l. of estrogen
l. of euphoria
l. of exertion
l. of fear
l. of female gonadotropins
l. of force
l. of function ▸ high
l. of functioning, optimal

l. of heart, above
l. of hope
l. of independence, maximum
l. of independence, optimal
l. of independent function
l. of independent mobility ▸ maximum
l. of input ▸ lowered
l. of kidney protein renin, high
l. of lead in blood
l. of magnesium ▸ intracellular
l. of malignant melanoma, Clark's
l. of medication
l. of mental function, overall
l. of mobility
l. of opioids, blood
l. of opioids, urine
l. of orientation
l. of pain
l. of perceived pain ▸ significant
l. of personality development
l. of phencyclidine, blood
l. of present functioning
l. of rationalization
l. of shock intensity
l. of significance
l. of social support ▸ low
l. of spontaneous activity ▸ low
l. of stimulation
l. of urinary bladder
l., optimal
l., oxygen
l. ▸ oxygen and carbon dioxide
l. ▸ oxygen (O_2) saturation
l., pancreatic isoamylase
l., parahormone
l. ▸ peak and trough
l. ▸ peak exertion
l., peak serum
l., periosteal
l., pharynx
l., plasma
l., plasma renin
l., plasminogen
l., platelet
l., postmenopausal
l., postprandial
l., potassium
l. practitioner ▸ advanced
l., predose
l., pregnanediol
l., pretreatment
l., prevertebral fascia
l., pseudocholinesterase
l., psychic

l. ▸ psychic energy
l., radiation
l. radiation, low
l. radioactive tracer, low
l., radon
l., reflecting
l., sarcolemmal
l., semiconscious
l., sensation
l., sensory
l. (SAL) ▸ sensory acuity
l. ▸ sensory dermatome
l., serum
l., serum alcohol
l., serum antibiotic
l., serum complement
l., serum enzyme
l., serum peak
l., serum protein
l. ▸ serum renin
l., serum thyroxin
l., serum triglyceride
l., skin potential
l., somatomedin
l., soreness
l., sound
l. (SPL) ▸ sound pressure
l. ▸ spinal fluid
l., stabilized functional
l., strength
l., stress
l., subcuticular
l., sugar
l., sulfa
l. surface
l. surfaces, assistive device on
l. synaptic
l. test ▸ protein
l. (SAL) test ▸ sensory acuity
l., testosterone
l. ▸ therapeutic blood
l. ▸ therapeutic drug
l., thiocyanate
l., thromboxane
l., tissue
l., tolerable
l., tonic heart
l. ▸ total blood cholesterol
l., toxic
l., treatment
l., triglyceride
l., trough
l. ▸ trough and peak
l. 2 ultrasound
l., uric acid

l. ▸ urinary calcium
l., urine
l., visual detection
l., vitamin
l. walking
l., weight
leveling, emotional
Leventhal syndrome ▸ Stein-
lever pessary
leverage fracture
Levi-Lorain dwarf
Levin
    L. medium smear, Pagano-
    L. syndrome ▸ Keine-
    L. tube
Levine('s)
    L. operation
    L. shunt
    L. sign
    L. syndrome, Long-Ganong-
    L. syndrome, Lown-Ganong-
Levinson test
levis, icterus castrensis
Levitt's implant
levoatriocardinal vein
Levocardia
    l. malposition
    l., mixed
    l. with situs inversus
levoduction of left eye
levoduction of right eye
levotransposed position
Levret's law
Lev's disease
levulose tolerance test
Lévy
    L. disease ▸ Roussy-
    L. polyneuropathy ▸ Roussy-
    L. syndrome ▸ Roussy-
lewd affect
Lewin composite flap, Argamaso-
Lewis(')
    L. index
    L. lead
    L. lines
    L. position
    L. scoop
    L. technique, George
    L. thoracotomy
    L. tube
    L. upper limb cardiovascular disease
lewisite (BAL) ▸ British anti-
Lewy('s)
    L. body

Lewy('s)—*continued*
  L. body disease
  L. holder
Leyden crystals ▸ Charcot-
Leyden's ataxia
Leydig cell tumor, Sertoli-
Leydig's cells
LFA (left frontoanterior)
L-5 S-1 projection
LFG (large for gestational age)
LFP (left frontoposterior)
LFT (left frontotransverse)
LFT (liver function test)
LH (luteinizing hormone)
Lhermitte's sign
LI (linguoincisal)
liability
  l., criminal
  l. of nicotine, addiction
  l., vicarious
liaison psychiatry, consultation-
liaison, surgical
liar, idiopathic
liar, pathological
lib, patient up ad
liberal doses of aspirin
liberal gastrointestinal (GI) diet
libidinal response
libidinosa, hysteria
libidinous pleasure
libido
  l., bisexual
  l., decreased
  l., ego
  l., increased
  l. ▸ loss of
  l., reduced
Libman-Sacks
  LS endocarditis
  LS lesion
  LS syndrome
lice (*see* louse)
  l., biting
  l., body
  l., chicken
  l., clothes
  l., crab
  l. ▸ eggs, nits, and pubic
  l., goat
  l., head
  l., horse
  l. infestation
  l., pubic
  l., sucking
licensed consulting psychologist

Licensed Practical Nurse (LPN)
lichen
  l. acuminatus
  l. albus
  l. amyloidosus
  l. annularis
  l. myxedematosus
  l. nitidus
  l. planus
  l. planus from dentures
  l. ruber
  l. sclerosis
  l. sclerosus et atrophicus
  l. simplex chronicus
  l. spinulosus
  l. starch
  l. striatus
  l. urticatus
lichenified lesions
licheniformis, Bacillus
lichenoid acrodermatitis, infantile
lichenoid keratoses, benign
lichenoides, tuberculosis
Lichtheimia corymbifera
Lichtheim's
  L. aphasia
  L. plaques
  L. sign
licit drugs ▸ prenatal abuse of
licit medical channels, diversion of
  drugs from
licking of lips ▸ smacking and
Licorice Drops (morning glory
  seeds)
licorice powder
lid(s) [*lip*]
  l. block, Atkinson-type
  l., draping of
  l., droopy
  l. infection, chronic
  l. lag
  l., lower
  l. margin
  l. margins, inflammation of
  l. margins, injury to
  l. plate, Jaeger's
  l., previously split
  l. ptosis
  l. reflex
  l., satisfactory akinesia of
  l. skin ▸ wrinkled
  l., spastic ectropion lower
  l. surgery
  l., upper
Liddel and Sherrington reflex

lidocaine
  l. drip
  l. jelly
  L. level
  L. prophylactic drip
lie
  l., low
  l. presentation, transverse
  l., transverse
Lieb and Guerry cataract implant
  lens
Lieberkühn's
  L. crypts
  L. follicles
  L. glands
Liebermeister rule
lienis
  l., hilus
  l., porta
  l., pulpa
lienteric diarrhea
lienteric stool
Lieou-Barré syndrome
lieu of incarceration, in
Life (life)
  L. Alert
  l. and death struggle
  l. and disability rights ▸ pro-
  l., animal
  l., antenatal
  l. anxiety, late-
  l., artificial prolongation of
  l., average
  l., biological half-
  l., cancer-free
  l. care ▸ end of
  L. Care Pump
  l. ▸ cell replication
  l., cellular
  l., change of
  l. change units (LCU)
  l. -changing decisions
  l. -changing skills
  l. circumstance problem
  l. crisis
  l. cycle
  l. depression ▸ late
  l. disability, late-
  l., effective half-
  l. ▸ elimination half-
  l. ▸ emancipation disorder of early
  l., enhance quality of
  l. ▸ enhanced quality of
  l. expectancy
  l. expectancy, extended

l. expectancy, limit
l. expectancy ▸ remissions, relapses and
l. extender
l., fetal
L., Flight for
l. ▸ gender identity disorder of adult
L., Gift of
l., half-
l. ▸ improve quality of
l., in control of
l., intellectual
l., intrauterine
L. Islands
l. issues ▸ quality of
l. -long disability
l. -long medication
l. -long, relapsing disease
l., low quality of
l., mental
l. ▸ near-normal quality
L. orthopedic Shoes, Child
l. pacemaker, end-of-
l. ▸ patient thinks about ending
l. ▸ patient withdrawn from
l., physical half-
l., preservation of quality of
l. -preserving functions, basic
l. problem ▸ phase of
l., prolong
l. prolonged
l., prolonging
l. -prolonging machine
l. -prolonging measures
l. -prolonging treatment
l., psychic
l., quality of
l., quality of daily
l. ▸ quality versus quantity of
l. -saving antiviral drug
l. -saving assistance
l. -saving decision
l. -saving measures
l. -saving medical care
l. -saving medical treatment
l. -saving medical treatment ▸ denial of
l. -saving organ
l. -saving skills
l. -saving treatment
l. -saving treatment ▸ withdrawal of
l. -saving treatment ▸ withholding of
l., serum half-
l., shelf

l. ▸ short half-
l. skills support
l. span, expected
l. span (MLS) ▸ mean
l. sting, marine-
l. stressor
l. stressors, assessing
l., subconscious
L. Suit
l. support (ALS), advanced
l. support (ACLS) ▸ advanced cardiac
l. support (ATLS), advanced trauma
l. support, artificial
l. support (BLS), basic
l. support (BCLS), basic cardiac
l. support ▸ extracorporeal
l. support, forgo
l. support measures
l. support (ACLS) protocol ▸ advanced cardiac
l. support, removal of
l. -support system
l. -support system ▸ withdrawing
l. -support technology
l. -supporting treatment
l. surgery ▸ face
l. -sustaining measures
l. -sustaining procedure
l. -sustaining procedures, withdraw
l. -sustaining procedures, withhold
l. -sustaining treatment
l. -threatening abnormal heartbeat
l. -threatening allergic reaction
l. -threatening angina
l. -threatening arrhythmias
l. -threatening asthma attack
l. -threatening behavior ▸ problematic
l. -threatening bleeding
l. -threatening blood clots
l. -threatening blood clots ▸ dissolve
l. -threatening brain injury
l. -threatening circumstances
l. -threatening complications
l. -threatening conditions
l. -threatening crisis
l. -threatening disease
l. -threatening disease ▸ chronic
l. -threatening disease process
l. -threatening disorder
l. -threatening dose
l. -threatening drug interaction

l. -threatening dysrhythmias
l. -threatening effect
l. -threatening emergency
l. -threatening event
l. -threatening event (ALTE), apparent
l. -threatening graft vs. host disease (GVHD)
l. -threatening heart arrhythmias
l. -threatening heart rhythm
l. -threatening heart rhythm abnormality
l. -threatening heatstroke
l. -threatening illness
l. -threatening illness, catastrophic
l. -threatening illness ▸ potentially
l. -threatening infection
l. -threatening infectious agent
l. -threatening injury
l. -threatening ischemia
l. -threatening manifestation
l. -threatening microbial contamination
l. -threatening problems
l. -threatening reaction
l. -threatening respiratory complications
l. -threatening rhythm disorder
l. -threatening rhythm disturbance
l. -threatening situation
l. -threatening surgery
l. -threatening ventricular arrhythmia
l. -threatening ventricular tachyarrhythmias
l. transition
l., uterine
l., vegetative
l. ▸ withdrawn from
lifeless body
lifeline for medication
lifeline necklace
lifelong
l. abstinence
l. anxiety
l. carriers of virus
l. effect
l. insecurity
lifestyle
l., active
l. activity
l., alcoholic
l., alteration in
l., alternative

lifestyle—*continued*
- l. change, personal
- l. changes
- l., chemically free
- l., dangerous
- l., disease preventive
- l., dysfunctional
- l., environment and
- l. factor
- l. habits, healthy
- l., healthy
- l. ► heart healthy
- l., high-risk
- l., inactive
- l., independent
- l. intervention
- l. management
- l. modification
- l. modification ► gradual
- l., normal
- l., patient's
- l. patterns
- l. ► physically inactive
- l., radical change in
- l., resume active
- l., resume normal
- l., sedentary
- l., smoke-free
- l., stressful
- l., vigorous
- l., workaholic

lifetime
- l., average remaining
- l. reserve days
- l. risk

lift [*lisp, list*]
- l., breast
- l., brow
- l., buttock
- l., cervicofacial face
- l., chair
- l. chair, patient
- l., chin
- l., complete face
- l., electric patient
- l. exercises, arm
- l., eye
- l., eyelid
- l., face-
- l. ► face and neck
- l., firemen's
- l., forehead
- l., head tilt with neck
- l., Hoyer
- l., leg

- l. maneuver ► head tilt and chin
- l., neck
- l. ► nonsurgical face
- l. ► parasternal systolic
- l., platform
- l., porch
- l. sagging eyebrows
- l. ► skin-tightening face-
- l. squat exercise ► knee
- l., stairway
- l., straight-arm
- l. surgery ► brow
- l. surgery ► neck
- l., throat
- l., ventricular
- l., wheelchair

Lifter, portable Medi-lifting
- l. and/or straining
- l., straining ► flexing
- l. techniques

ligament(s)
- l., accessory
- l., acromioclavicular (AC)
- l., acromiocoracoid
- l., adipose
- l., annular
- l., anterior
- l., anterior cruciate
- l., arcuate
- l., Arnold's
- l., artificial knee
- l., axis
- l., Bertin's
- l., Bigelow's
- l., brachioradial
- l., broad
- l., Brodie's
- l., calcaneofibular
- l., calcaneonavicular
- l., canthal
- l., capsular
- l., cardinal
- l., carpometacarpal
- l., caudal
- l., chronic pain in
- l., ciliary
- l., Cleland's
- l., collateral
- l. contracture
- l., Cooper's
- l., coracoacromial
- l., coracoclavicular
- l., coracohumeral
- l., coronary

- l., costoclavicular
- l., Cowper's
- l., cricoarytenoid
- l., cricothyroarytenoid
- l., cricothyroid
- l., cricotracheal
- l., cruciate
- l., crural
- l., cuboideonavicular
- l., cuneiform
- l., cuneonavicular
- l., deltoid
- l., dentate
- l., denticulate
- l., detachment of
- l., falciform
- l., flaval
- l., gastrohepatic
- l., Gore-Tex
- l., Grayson's
- l., hamatometacarpal
- l., Hesselbach's
- l., Hunter's
- l., hyoepiglottic
- l., hypothyroid
- l., iliofemoral
- l., iliotrochanteric
- l., inflamed
- l., infundibulopelvic
- l., inguinal
- l. injury
- l. injury, knee
- l., internal canthal
- l., keystone
- l., laciniate
- l., lacunar
- l., lateral
- l., lateral collateral
- l., lateral false
- l., lateral puboprostatic
- l., laterocollateral
- l., leaves of broad
- l., longitudinal
- l., lucinate
- l., Mackenrodt's
- l., Marshall
- l., medial collateral
- l., medial palpebral
- l., medial puboprostatic
- l., middle umbilical
- l. of incus, posterior
- l. of incus, superior
- l. of knee, arcuate
- l. of knee ► calcification mediocollateral

l. of lens, suspensory
l. of malleus, anterior
l. of malleus, external
l. of malleus, lateral
l. of Toldt
l. of Treitz
l., olecranon
l., ovarian
l., partial tearing of
l., patellar
l., pectinate
l., pericardiosternal
l., pisohamate
l., pisometacarpal
l., planter
l., popliteal
l., posterior
l., posterior cruciate
l., Poupart's
l., pubocapsular
l., pubofemoral
l., pubovesical
l., pulmonary
l., radiocarpal
l., rectouterine
l. repair ▸ knee
l., rhomboid
l., round
l., rupture of
l., rupture of anterior and posterior
    longitudinal
l., sacrogenital
l., sacrospinous
l., sacrouterine
l., Scarpa's
l., shelving border of inguinal
l. stability test
l., sternoclavicular
l., sternocostal
l. ▸ stiffness and discomfort in
l., stretch
l., superior
l., suspensory
l., talocalcaneal
l., talofibular
l., talonavicular
l. tear, cruciate
l., tear of
l., tendinotrochanteric
l., thyroepiglottic
l., thyrohyoid
l., torn
l. ▸ torn anterior cruciate
l. ▸ torn knee
l. transplant

l., transverse
l., trapezoid
l., Treitz
l., ulnar
l., ulnocarpal
l., uterosacral
l., vesicouterine
l., volar
l., volar carpal
l., Whitnall
l., Winslow's
l., Wrisberg's
l., yellow
l., Zinn's

**ligament, Cooper's [*ligament,*
    Poupart's]**
ligamentosa, falx
ligamentous
  l. calcification
  l. insecurity
  l. instability
  l. joint
  l. relaxation
  l. strain
  l. structures
ligamentum
  l. arteriosum
  l. denticulatum
  l. flavum
  l. fundiforme penis
  l. teres cardiopexy
  l. teres femoris
  l. teres, notch of
ligand, macromolecular
ligate [*migrate, plicate*]
ligated
  l. and amputated, appendix
  l. and retracted mesially ▸ vein
  l. and sectioned, doubly
  l. and transected, vein
  l., bleeders
  l., bleeders clamped and
  l., clamped and
  l., doubly
  l., identified and
  l. ▸ mesoappendix serially clamped,
      cut and
  l. with silk
  l. with transfixion suture ▸ doubly
ligation [*plication*]
  l. and stripping
  l. and stripping, high
  l. clip
  l., femoral vein
  l. (HAL), hemorrhoidal artery

l., high saphenous vein
l., hypogastric
l., Irving type tubal
l. ▸ laparoscopic tubal
l. middle meningeal artery
l. of hemorrhoids ▸ rubber band
l. of meningeal vessels
l., proximal
l., rubber band
l., stripping and
l. and stripping ▸ erasing,
l. superior longitudinal sinus
l., suture
l., tubal
l. ▸ varicose vein stripping and

ligature(s)
  l., anchor with suture
  l. and avulsion ▸ vein
  l., chain
  l., chromic
  l., elastic
  l., Erichsen's
  l., interlacing
  l., interlocking
  l., kangaroo
  l., lateral
  l., occluding
  l., provisional
  l., proximal
  l., soluble
  l., suboccluding
  l., terminal
  l., thread-elastic
  l. wire

light(s) (Light)
  l., abnormal intolerance to
  l. absorption
  l., acute sensitivity to
  l. adaptation
  l. -adapted eye
  l. amplification
  l. amplification by stimulated
      emission of radiation (laser)
  l. amplification by stimulated
      emission of radiation (laser)
      beam
  l. and accommodation (L and A)
  l. and accommodation (PERLA) ▸
      pupils equal, react to
  l. and accommodation (PERRLA) ▸
      pupils equal, round react to
  l. and accommodation (PRLA) ▸
      pupils react to
  l. and color perception
  l. and glare ▸ sensitivity to

light(s)—*continued*
- l. and noise ▸ sensitivity to
- l. and sound ▸ sensitivity to
- l. -beam therapy
- l. bulb appearance
- l. bulky compression dressing
- l. camera, TV
- l. chain component ▸ lambda
- l. chain disease
- l. chain, kappa
- l. chain ▸ myosin
- l. chain type ▸ Bence Jones
- l. chains
- l. coagulation
- l. -colored stools
- l. compression dressing
- l. -conducting fibers
- l., constriction caused by
- l. -dark discrimination
- l. -dark ratio
- l. diet
- l. difference
- l., diffused flashes of
- l. discrimination
- l. discrimination, two-
- l., dispersion of
- l. elastic dressing
- l. examination of eye, Wood's
- l., exposure to ultraviolet
- l. feathering or redness
- l., flashing
- l., glare around
- l., halos around
- l. -induced damage
- l., intermittent flashes of
- l., intraocular
- l. ▸ irregular, flashing patterns of
- l., isolated flashes of
- l., laser
- l., Lumiwand
- l. microscope
- l. microscopy
- l. pen
- l. pen-determined ejection fraction
- l. perception (LP)
- l. perception (NLP), no
- l. perception only (LPO)
- l. (PERL) ▸ pupils equal, react to
- l. pupils sluggish to
- L., Questran
- l. ray, laser
- l. reaction, consensual
- l. reflection rheography (LRR)
- l. reflex
- l. reflex, arteriolar

- l. reflex, consensual
- l. reflex, direct
- l. reflex, emergency
- l. reflex, tapetal
- l. refraction
- l. regimen, psora-lens plus ultraviolet (PUVA)
- l. scanning
- l. sensation
- l. sense
- l. -sensing cells
- l. -sensitive cells
- l. -sensitive chemicals
- l. -sensitive drug
- l. sensitivity
- l. sensitivity ▸ confusion with
- l. sensitivity ▸ drowsiness with
- l. sensitivity from coldness
- l. sensitivity, minor
- l. ▸ sensitivity of eyes to
- l. ▸ sensitivity to
- l. ▸ sensitivity to bright
- l., Simpson
- l. sleep
- l. sleep stage
- l. source, fiberoptic
- l. source, fiberoptic cold
- l. source, high intensity
- l., starbursts of
- l. stimulation
- l. stimulation, response to
- l. stroke
- l. tactile pressure
- l. therapy
- l. therapy, infrared
- l. therapy, laser
- l. therapy ▸ pulsed
- l. therapy, red
- l. therapy, ultraviolet
- l. to dark adaptation
- l. touch sensors
- l., transillumination
- l. transmission, blockage of
- l. treatment, psora-lens plus ultraviolet (PUVA)
- l., ultraviolet
- L. -Veley head rest
- l. velocity
- l. waves
- l., xenon arc

lighted tube ▸ flexible
lightening depression
lightening pains
lighter stage of sleep
lightheaded, irritable and

lightheaded on standing
lightheadedness
- l. and weakness
- l., chest discomfort with
- l., orthostatic
- l., positional

lighting module
lightly staining coiled bacteria
lightly staining gram-negative coccobacilli
lightning (Lightning)
- l. cataract
- l. injury ▸ side splash
- l. module
- l. -related death
- l. stroke
- L. (LSD), White

lightweight cast
lightweight object
Lightwood-Albright syndrome
Lignac('s)
- L. disease
- L. -Fanconi disease
- L. -Fanconi syndrome

ligneous thyroiditis
Lignières test
lignieresii, Actinobacillus
lignocaine, M
like [*type*]
- l. angina, band-
- l. appearance, bubble-
- l. appearance ▸ lace-
- l. atelectasis ▸ plate-
- l. attack, trance-
- l. behavior ▸ schizophrenia-
- l. behavior ▸ trance-
- l. bleeding ▸ menstrual-
- l. blisters ▸ pus-
- l., board-
- l. calcification, tooth-
- l. cell, hair-
- l. cells, rod-
- l. cholesterol, lipid-
- l. complications, shock-
- l. configuration ▸ spade-
- l. consistency, clay-
- l. defect, sac-
- l. deformity, claw-
- l. dilation of artery, balloon-
- l. discharge, cottage cheese-
- l. disturbances ▸ Parkinsonian-
- l. drug, curare-
- l. effects, sedative-
- l. emanation, spike-
- l. expression ▸ mask-

l. face, bird-
l. facial appearance ▸ mask-
l. fever ▸ West Nile-
l. fluid ▸ jelly-
l. formation, sac-
l. formation, spike-
l. forms, rod-
l. fungus, algae-
l. gallbladder, sac-
l. growth factor ▸ insulin-
l. growth, scar-
l. growth, wart-
l. holes in brain ▸ sponge-
l. illness, mononucleosis-
l. images, dream-
l. infection, viral-
l. instrument, telescope-
l. lesion, braid-
l. lesions, herpes-
l. lesions, plague-
l. -mad syndrome ▸ scratch-
l. pain, burning knife-
l. pain, electric-
l. pain, vise-
l., patient zombie-
l. pelvic pain, cramp-
l. polygonal cells ▸ squamous-
l. probe, needle-
l. protrusion, sac-
l. psychosis ▸ schizophrenia-
l. psychotic state ▸ schizophrenic-
l. reaction, reflex-
l. rigidity, board-
l. secretion, wax-
l. sensation, cramp-
l. state ▸ chronic schizophrenia-
l. state, psychosis-
l. state, sleep-
l. state, trance-
l. stools ▸ soft and ribbon-
l. structures, cell-
l. symptoms, flu-
l. symptoms ▸ panic-
l. symptoms ▸ psychotic-
l. symptoms ▸ shock-
l. syndrome, flu-
l. syndrome of aphasia ▸ stroke-
l. tremor, Parkinson-
l. viral encephalitis ▸ West Nile-
l. virus ▸ West Nile-
l. vision, tunnel-

Lilienfeld's position
Liliequist, membrane of
Lillehei
 L. -Cruz-Kaster prosthesis

L. -Kaster cardiac valve prosthesis
L. -Kaster mitral valve prosthesis
lilliputian hallucination
lilting gait
lily heart, tiger
LIMA (left internal mammary artery)
Lima inclusion ▸ Rocha-
limax, Amoeba
limb(s)
 l. abnormalities ▸ facial or
 l. abnormality
 l. abnormality, focal
 l., amputation entire lower
 l., amputation of
 l. amputee ▸ patient bilateral lower
 l. amputee ▸ patient bilateral upper
 l., anacrotic
 l. and face ▸ uncontrolled
  movement of
 l. anesthetized, entire
 l., artificial
 l. ▸ bandaging and splinting
 l., cardiac
 l. cardiovascular disease ▸ Lewis
  upper
 l., contralateral
 l. deficiency
 l., deformed
 l., deformity
 l. ▸ discoloration of
 l. disease, ischemic
 l. dwarfism, short
 l. elevated, temperature of
 l., elevation of injured
 l., elongated
 l., functional
 l. -girdle muscular dystrophy
 l., heaviness of
 l., incoordination of
 l. injury
 l. ischemia
 l., insensitive
 l., involuntary trembling of
 l. ▸ jerking of
 l. jerks ▸ wild
 l. -kinetic apraxia
 l. lead
 l. lead ▸ standard
 l. leads ▸ unipolar
 l. lengthening operation
 l., missing
 l. movement
 l. movement, bilateral
 l. movement disorder (PLMD) ▸
  periodic

l. movement ▸ periodic
l. movements in sleep (PLMS) ▸
 periodic
l. movements, passive
l. movements, uncontrolled
 rhythmic
l. ▸ no spontaneous movement of
l. pain, claudication
l. pain, phantom
l., paresthesias of
l. perfusion ▸ isolated hyperthermic
l., peripheral
l., phantom
l., prosthetic
l. reanastomosis
l. reattached surgically, severed
l., reattaching severed
l., reconstructed
l. reduction abnormality
l. reduction anomaly
l. replant
l. restrained
l., rigid
l., rigidity of paralyzed
l. salvage
l. salvage technique, severed
l., severed
l., spastic
l. stance, single
l. ▸ stiffness or heaviness of
l., stump of
l. ▸ sudden weakness of
l., surgical absence of
l. swelling
l. syndrome ▸ uneven
l. temperature
l., thoracic
l. -threatening problem
l. tiredness
l. ▸ uncontrolled shaking of
l. venography
limbal
 l. groove
 l. incision
 l. stem cell transplant
 l. suture
limber up stiff back and hips
Limberg flap
limbic
 l. brain
 l. center
 l. keratoconjunctivitis, superior
 l. ledge
 l. lobe
 l. lobe of brain

limbic—*continued*
  l. region
  l. system
  l. system, brain's
limbicus, gyrus
limbus
  l., cicatrix of
  l. conjunctivae
  l. corneae
  l., cystoid cicatrix of
  l. luteus retinas
  l. of cornea
  l., surgical
  l., upper
lime, bruit de
lime, soda
limen
  l. difference
  l. insulae
  l. nasi
  l. of insula
  l. of twoness
limensis, Phaseolus
limes zero
limicola, Chlorobium
liminal [*minimal*]
liminal consciousness
liminal stimulus
limit(s)
  l., age
  l. flocculation
  l. (WNL) ▸ hematology within
    normal
  l. joint motion
  l. life expectancy
  l. milk consumption
  l., movement within functional
  l. of normal ▸ upper
  l. salt intake
  l. sodium
  l., speech and language within
    normal
  l. swelling
  l. value, threshold
  l., within functional
  l. (WNL) ▸ within normal
  l., within physiologic
limitans, sulcus
limitation(s)
  l., evaluate abilities and
  l., functional
  l., knowing
  l., medical
  l., musculoskeletal
  l., occupational

  l. of chemotherapy
  l. of delayed recall ▸ therapeutic
  l. of extension
  l. of flexion
  l. of motion (LOM)
  l. of movement
  l. of physical activity
  l. of radiation therapy
  l. of rotation
  l. of surgery
  l. on bending
  l., orthopedic
  l., physical
  l., strict
limited
  l. activity
  l. activity range
  l. attention span
  l., autopsy
  l. basis
  l. by body habitus (LBBH)
  l. character, sex-
  l. examination
  l. examination, self-
  l. expansion of lungs
  l. exposure obtained
  l. hypothermia
  l. intelligence
  l. interpersonal skills
  l. investigation
  l. joint motion
  l. joint movement
  l. mobility, pain and
  l. motion of extremity
  l. movement
  l. movement of extremity
  l. pericardiotomy ▸ subxiphoid
  l. peripheral vision
  l. physical activity
  l. prognosis
  l. radiation field
  l. range of motion (ROM)
  l., self-
  l., separation ▸ realistic time
  l., straight leg raising (SLR)
  l. surgery
  l. to abdomen, autopsy
  l. to brain, autopsy
  l. to _____ ▸ extension
  l. to heart and lungs ▸ autopsy
  l. treadmill exercise test ▸ symptom-
  l. visitation
  l., x-ray findings
limiting
  l. alcohol intake

  l. illness, self-
  l. pain, self-
  l. stenosis ▸ flow
  l. structures, dose-
  l. tissues, dose
limoniticus, Siderococcus
limp
  l. chorea
  l., gluteal
  l. hair from anemia
limpness ▸ rapid breathing and
Lincoff's implant
Lincoff's operation
lincolnensis, Streptomyces
Lindau
  L. disease ▸ von Hippel-
  L. syndrome ▸ Hippel-
  L. syndrome ▸ von Hippel-
  L. -von Hippel's disease
Lindblom's position
Linde walker
Linder's sign
Lindner's operation
lindoensis, Echinostoma
Line(s) (line) [*fine*]
  L. (cocaine)
  l., abdominal
  l., acanthomeatal
  l., Amici's
  l. angle
  l. (AAL) ▸ anterior axillary
  l., anteromedial joint
  l. appointment system ▸ on-
  l., arterial
  l., arterial mean
  l. artifact, center
  l., auricular
  l., axillary
  l. ▸ blank spots and distortion
    of
  l., blood
  l., breast
  l., Brödel's
  l., canthomeatal
  l., cell
  l., central venous
  l., cleavage
  l., contour
  l., coronal suture
  l., crease
  l., crinkle
  l., dashed
  l., dentate
  l., dependency
  l., division

l., dominant
l., dotted
l., Douglas'
l. ▸ dynamic facial
l., Ehrlich-Turck
l. EKG (electrocardiogram) ▸
   straight-
l., elastic
l., election
l., epiphyseal
l., equipotential
l., expression folds
l., Farre's
L. (morphine), First
l., flexion
l., flexure
l., force
l., fracture
l., frontal zygomatic suture
l., gingival
l., glabelloalveolar
l., gluteal
l., gravitational
l., gray
l., gum
l., HA
l., Hilgenreiner
l., Hudson's
l., iliopectineal
l., imaginary
l. in place ▸ subclavian
l., incision
l., increased tension
l., indwelling
l. ▸ infected hyperalimentation
l. infection ▸ intravenous (IV)
l., infraorbital
l., infraorbitomeatal
l. inserted and positioned ▸
   monitoring
l. insertion, arterial
l., interorbital
l., interpupillary
l., intertrochanteric
l., intra-arterial
l., intravenous (IV)
l., isodose
l., isoelectric
l. IV ▸ Add-a-
l., joint
l., Kerley's A
l., Kerley's B
l., lambdoid suture
l. ▸ laugh and squint
l., Lewis

l., lip
l., M
l., main solution
l., maximal tension
l., McGregor's
l., medial joint
l., median
l., mesenteric artery
l. (MAL) ▸ midaxillary
l. (MCL) ▸ midclavicular
l., midcostal
l., midsternal
l., minimal tension
l., minimum extensibility
l. monitor catheter placement,
   arterial
l., mylohyoid
l., natural
l., Nélaton's
l., nuchal
l., occipitomastoid suture
l. of cocaine, snorting
l. of demarcation
l. of demarcation, no
l. of fibers ▸ muscles split in
l. of occlusion
l. of skull, suture
l. of Toldt
l. of Zahn
l., Ogston's
l., orthostatic
l., parietomastoid suture
l., patient walks straight
l., pectate
l., pectinate
l., pectineal
l., peripheral
l. placement, arterial
l., posterior axillary
l., primary suture
l. protein ▸ M-
l., pubococcygeal
l., radiolucent
l. ▸ red vermilion lip
l. (RSTL), relaxed skin tension
l., relieve pressure on primary
   suture
l. sagittal suture
l., Salter's incremental
l., Schwalbe's
l., semilunar
l., Sergent's white
l., Shenton's
l. ▸ shimmering zigzag
l. sign ▸ plumb

l., skin
l., soup
l., sphenofrontal suture
l., sphenoparietal suture
l., squamous suture
l., Stähli's
l., subclavian
l., subclavian intravenous
l., suture
l., sylvian
l., temporal
l., tension
l., tentorial
l., terminal
l., total parenteral nutrition (TPN)
l., tram
l., transvenous pacemaker
l., Ullmann's
l., umbilical arterial
l. up arm ▸ red
l., visual
l., widening of suture
l., wrinkle
l., Z
l., Zahn's
l., zigzag
l., zygomaticofrontal suture
linea
l. alba
l. alba cervicalis
l. alba hernia
l. aspera femoris
l. corneas senilis
l. glutea
l. terminalis pelvis
lineage
l. antigen ▸ macrophage
l. antigen ▸ monocyte
l. antigen ▸ myeloid
l. -associated antigen
linear
l. absorption co-efficient
l. accelerator
l. accelerator, Clinic 18
l. accelerator ▸ dual energy
l. accelerator ▸ dual-photon
l. accelerator, high energy bent
   beam
l. accelerator, low energy straight
   beam
l. amplifier
l. amputation
l. array
l. array, convex
l. array, research logic

linear—*continued*
- l. atelectasis
- l. atrophy
- l. attenuation
- l. cell, elongated
- l. compartmental system
- l. density
- l. depressions
- l. displacement analysis
- l. echodensity
- l. energy transfer (LET)
- l. energy transfer radiation, high
- l. fracture
- l. groove
- l. incision
- l. increased density
- l. markings
- l. opacification, opaque
- l. opacities
- l. osteotomy
- l. phonocardiograph
- l. phonocardiography
- l. quadratic survival relationship
- l. raphe
- l. regeneration
- l. regression
- l. scarring
- l. -shaped hemorrhage
- l. skin lesion
- l. skull fracture
- l. sources
- l. strands
- l. survival curve, initial
- l. system
- l. transverse incision

linearis, Siderobacter
linearity, amplitude
lineatum, Hypoderma
linen(s)
- l., blood-contaminated
- l. change
- l., contamination from
- l., flame-retardant

liner, bedpan
lingering depression
lingering hepatitis
lingua
- l. dissecta
- l. fisturata
- l. frenata
- l. geographica
- l. nigra
- l. plicata
- l. scrotalis
- l. villosa nigra

linguae
- l., anthracosis
- l., apex
- l., hyperkeratosis
- l., ichthyosis
- l., lapsus
- l., psoriasis
- l., tremor

lingual
- l. arch
- l. arch ▸ fixed
- l. arch ▸ passive
- l. arch ▸ stationary
- l. artery
- l. braces
- l. embrasure
- l. flange
- l. frenum
- l. ganglion
- l. gingiva
- l. gyrus
- l. hemiatrophy, progressive
- l. hemorrhoid
- l. nerve
- l. occlusion
- l. papillae
- l. quinsy
- l. saliva
- l. sulcus
- l. surface of tooth
- l. thyroid
- l. titubation
- l. tongue flap
- l. tonsil
- l. tonsillitis
- l. vein
- l. vein, deep
- l. vein, dorsal

lingualis, gyrus
Linguatula rhinaria
Linguatula serrata
linguistic disability
linguistic programming, neuro-
lingula cerebelli
lingula cerebri
lingular
- l. bronchus
- l. pneumonia
- l. segment

linguoplate, palatal
lining
- l. alveolar spaces ▸ hyaline membranes
- l. anesthesia
- l., arterial

- l., aspirin irritates stomach
- l., bronchial
- l. brushed and washed
- l., cancer of chest
- l., cell
- l., cellular
- l., colonic
- l., discharge of
- l., endometrial
- l., endothelial
- l., entodermal
- l., epithelial
- l., esophageal
- l. fluid, epithelial
- l., granulomatous
- l., heart
- l. ▸ infected joint
- l. ▸ inflammation of arterial
- l., inflammation of heart
- l., intestinal
- l. ▸ irritation of stomach
- l., mucosal
- l., mucous membrane
- l. of abdominal cavity ▸ inflammation of
- l. of bladder ▸ inner
- l. of brain
- l. of cavity
- l. of heart, inflammation of
- l. of mouth ▸ mucous
- l. of mucous ▸ stomach's protective
- l. of nasal passages
- l. of organ ▸ inflammation of
- l. of spinal cord
- l. of stomach, epithelial
- l. of trachea
- l. of uterus
- l. of uterus, cauterize
- l. of vagina
- l., periosteal membranous
- l., pleural membrane
- l. ▸ precancerous overgrowth of uterine
- l. ▸ repeated stress to tissue
- l., sclerosis tubular
- l., skin-like cells
- l., stomach
- l. ▸ swollen tissue
- l. ▸ thickening of uterine
- l. tissue, uterine
- l., urethral
- l., uterine

linitis plastica
link(s)
- l., fiberglass-cancer

l., genetic
l., potential breast cancer

linkage
l. analysis
l., cellular transducer
l. map, genetic
l. of antibodies, isotopic
l. theory, cross

linked
l. antibodies, radiation-
l. agammaglobulinemia, Bruton sex-
l. agammaglobulinemia ▸ X-
l. bipolar derivations
l. character, sex-
l. defect ▸ sex-
l. dilated cardiomyopathy ▸ X-
l. disease, radiation-
l. disease ▸ sex-
l. disorder, sex-
l. disorder ▸ X-
l. genetic defect ▸ sex-
l. genetic defect ▸ X-
l. heredity, sex-
l. heredity, X-
l. immunoglobulin M syndrome ▸ X-
l. immunosorbent assay ▸ sandwich enzyme-
l. immunosorbent assay (ELISA) test ▸ enzyme-
l. inheritance ▸ X-
l. lymphoproliferative syndrome (XLP) ▸ X-
l. lymphoproliferative, X-
l. microbial infections, cancer-
l. retardation syndrome ▸ alpha thalassemia X-
l. to fibromyalgia
l. traits, sex-

linking cigarette smoking and drug abuse
linking enzyme, cross-
Lint
L. akinesia, Van
L. block, Van
L. conjunctival flap, Van
L. Pic-Ups, Surgical
L. technique, Van

Linton elastic hose
Linuche unguiculata
Liotta total artificial heart
Liouville's icterus
lip(s) [lid]
l., Abbe flap repair of

l. and ala of nose ▸ levator muscle of upper
l. and mouth care before and after chemotherapy
l. and nailbeds, bluish tinge to
l. and palate ▸ cleft
l., basal cell carcinoma of
l., blue
l. breathing ▸ pursed
l., cancer of
l. carcinoma
l., chapped
l., cleft
l., corneal
l., cracked
l., cyanosis of
l., depressor muscle of lower
l. enhancement ▸ permanent
l. flap, Stein-Abbé
l. flap, Stein-Kazanjian lower
l. from caffeine ▸ chapped
l., harre
l., incisive muscles of inferior
l., incisive muscles of lower
l., incisive muscles of superior
l., incisive muscles of upper
l. injury
l., levator muscle of upper
l. line
l. line ▸ red vermilion
l., lower
l. movements
l. mucosa, lower
l. mucosa, upper
l. ▸ numbness of
l. of cervix
l. of mouth ▸ commissure of
l. of wound
l., pink mucous membranes of
l. pursing
l., quadrate muscle of lower
l., quadrate muscle of upper
l. reading
l. ▸ reddened, dry, fissured
l. reflex
l. region, dorsal
l., scarred
l., skin cancer of
l. ▸ smacking and licking of
l., smacking movements of tongue and
l., squamous cell carcinoma
l. ▸ swelling of
l., tongue and face ▸ swelling of

l. tumors
l., upper
l., vermilion border of
l., vermilion surface of
l. wrinkles

lipase
l., diacylglycerol
l., hepatic
l., lipoprotein
l., pancreatic
l., serum
l. test
l., triglyceride

lipectomy
l., buttock
l., hip
l., submental
l., suction
l. ▸ suction-assisted

lipedema ▸ patient has
lipemia, postprandial
lipemia retinalis
lipemic serum
lipid(s)
l. abnormality
l. abnormality ▸ genetic underlying
l., adrenals slightly
l. accumulation
l., blood
l. body
l. core ▸ large
l., cytoplasmic
l. depleted, adrenals
l. depletion
l. diet, low
l. disorder
l. droplets
l., endogenous
l., exogenous
l., extracellular
l. -filled atherosclerotic plaques
l. histiocytosis
l. hypothesis
l., intracellular
l. level
l. -like cholesterol
l. management
l. metabolism
l. nephrosis
l. panel
l. peroxidation product
l. profile
l. profile ▸ serum
l. profile, total

lipid(s)—*continued*
 l., renomedullary
 l. -rich plaque
 l., sarcolemma
 l. screening
 l., skin
 l. test
 l. therapy
 l. (TL) ▸ total
lipidosis, familial
Lipiodol ascendant
Lipiodol contrast medium
lipochrome pigment
lipodystrophy, intestinal
lipofuscin pigment
lipogenesis syndrome
lipogenic theory of atherosclerosis
lipohypertrophy, localized
lipoid
 l. granuloma
 l. hyperplasia
 l. material
 l. nephrosis
 l. pneumonia
 l. stain
lipoides corneae, arcus
lipoides myringis, arcus
lipoidica diabeticorum, necrobiosis
lipoidica, necrobiosis
lipolytic activity, postheparin
lipoma [*fibroma*]
lipoma, benign
lipoma, epidural
lipomatosis, ptosis
lipomatosis, symmetrical
lipomatous
 l. carcinoma
 l. hypertrophy
 l. lesion
 l. nephritis
 l. paranephritis
lipophagia granulomatosis
lipophagic granuloma
lipophagic intestinal granulomatosis
lipophilicity ▸ properties of
lipopolysaccharide vaccine
lipoprotein(s)
 l., alpha
 l. analysis
 l. -associated coagulation inhibitor
 l., beta
 l. deficiency ▸ familial high density
 l. electrophoresis
 l. (HDL), high density
 l. ▸ intermediate density

 l. lipase
 l. (LDL), low density
 l. ▸ pre-beta
 l. (VLDL) ▸ very low density
lipoproteinemia, a-beta-
liposarcoma of soft tissue
liposomes ▸ patient injected with
liposuction
 l. cosmetic surgery
 l. ▸ external ultrasonic
 l. of body part
 l. procedure
 l. surgery
 l. tube
 l., tumescent
 l., ultrasonic
 l., ultrasound
lipothiamide pyrophosphate
Lippes loop intrauterine device (IUD)
lipping
 l., arthritic
 l., hypertrophic
 l., narrowing and
 l., osteoarthritic
 l., posterior
 l. style of breathing ▸ pursed-
Lippman hip prosthesis
lipsoideus, Saccharomyces
LIQ (lower inner quadrant)
liquefaciens
 l., Aeromonas
 l., Enterobacter
 l., Moraxella
 l., Pseudomonas non◊
 l., Serratia
 l., Streptococcus
liquefaction
 l., fat
 l. of subdural hematoma
 l. of vitreous
liquefactum, phenol
liquefying expectorant
liquid (Liquid)
 l. air
 l. anesthetic
 l. bowel preparation
 l. cement, inject sterile
 l. chromatography, gas-
 l. crystal device
 l. crystal thermogram (LCT)
 l. crystal thermography
 l. diet
 l. diet,clear
 l. diet, cold
 l. diet formula

 l. diet, full
 l. diet, nonresidue
 l. diet program
 l., hypaque sodium powder and
 l., intake of
 l. nitrogen
 l. nitrogen ▸ freezing with
 l. oxygen (O₂)
 l. petrolatum emulsion
 l. production ▸ fetal lung
 l. silicone
 l. supplement to diet
 l., surface film of
 l. tissue ▸ soft, spongy, semi-
 l. ventilation
 l. ventilation (PLV) ▸ partial
 L. X ▸ gamma hydroxybutyrate
   (GHB)
Liquipake contrast medium
liquor
 l. amnii
 l. carbonis detergens (LCD)
 l. chorii
 l. corneae
 l. folliculi
 l., Morgagni's
 l. prostaticus
 l. seminis
Lisfranc's
 L. amputation
 L. fracture
 L. joint
lisp [*list, lift*]
Lissauer's
 L. paralysis
 L. tract
 L. zone
list
 l., leg
 l. memory ▸ word-
 l. mode
 l. mode ▸ gated
 l. or scoliosis
 l., patient on waiting
 l. specific symptoms
 l., waiting
listening
 l., auditory
 l. device (ALD) ▸ personal assistive
 l. skills ▸ recall and
Listeria
 L. monocytogenes
 L. monocytogenes meningitis
 L. monocytogenes strain
listing gait

Listing's law
listless
- l. and apathetic
- l. and tired feeling
- l., weak and

lite, bili-
lite ▸ infant placed under bili-
Liteflex intraocular lens (IOL)
liter(s)
- l. (mEq/L) ▸ milliequivalent per
- l. (Mm/L) ▸ millimole per
- l. of oxygen
- l. per minute (LPM)
- l. per minute per meter squared
- l. per second (LPS)

literacy
- l. ▸ marginal health
- l. skills, adequate
- l. skills ▸ inadequate
- l. skills ▸ marginal

literal agraphia
literal paraphasia
literalis, dysarthria
Literature (literature)
- L. Analysis and Retrieval System (MEDLARS) ▸ Medical
- l., clinical
- l., treatment

lith II pacemaker, Intermedics thin
lithiasis
- l., cholecystitis
- l., choledocho◊
- l. conjunctivae
- l., entero◊
- l., gastro◊
- l., renal

lithium
- l. pacemaker
- l. pacemaker, Arco
- l. poisoning
- l. relapse
- l. therapy
- l. treatment

lithogenes, Saccharomyces
lithotomy
- l., chole◊
- l., choledocho◊
- l. position
- l. position, dorsal

lithotripsy
- l., biliary
- l., chole◊
- l., cholecysto◊
- l., choledocho◊

- l. (ESWL) ▸ extracorporeal shock wave
- l., noninvasive
- l. procedure

lithotripter machine
lithotrite, Bigelow's
litigious paranoia
litmus milk
Litten diaphragm sign
Little('s) (little)
- L. area
- l. clusters of seizures
- L. disease
- l. finger
- l. finger ▸ abductor muscle of
- l. finger ▸ extensor muscle of
- l. finger ▸ opposing muscle of
- l. finger ▸ short flexor muscle of
- l. leaguer's elbow
- l. toe
- l. toe ▸ abductor muscle of
- l. toe ▸ short flexor muscle of

Littler's operation
Littlewood's operation
Littman defibrillation pad
Littre('s)
- L. gland
- L. hernia
- L. -Richter hernia

Litwak left atrial-aortic bypass
Litzmann's obliquity
live
- l. birth
- l. births (GPMAL) ▸ Gravida, para, multiple births, abortions,
- l. cell analysis
- l. donor transplant
- l. poliomyelitis vaccine
- l. sperm
- l. vaccine
- l. virus
- l. -virus vaccine
- l. x-ray imaging

liveborn infant
lived
- l. high, short-
- l. pain, short-
- l., short-

livedo
- l. racemosa
- l. reticularis
- l. vasculitis

livedoid dermatitis
liver [*livor*]
- l. abscess

- l. abscess, amebic
- l., acute fatty
- l. ▸ acute inflammatory infiltration of
- l. ▸ acute passive congestion of
- l. agenesis
- l., alcohol effect on
- l. ▸ alcoholic fatty
- l., amyloid
- l. and lung metastasis ▸ retroperitoneal
- l. atrophic
- l. autolytic
- l. bed
- l., biliary cirrhotic
- l. biopsy
- l. biopsy ▸ percutaneous
- l. block in radiation therapy, thin
- l. breath
- l., brimstone
- l. cancer
- l. cancer cells
- l. cancer, hepatitis-induced
- l. cancer, primary
- l. capsule
- l. capsule fibrous
- l., carcinoid metastatic malignancy of
- l., carcinoma of
- l., cardiac
- l., caudate lobe of
- l. cell adenoma
- l. cell carcinoma
- l. cell cytoplasm
- l. cell nuclei
- l. cells
- l., central veins of
- l. ▸ centrilobular necrosis of
- l. cholesterol production
- l., chronic passive congestion of
- l., cirrhosis of
- l., cirrhotic
- l. concentrate
- l. congested on cross-section
- l. congested with central necrosis
- l., congestion of
- l., constitutional dysfunction of
- l. cords ▸ compression of
- l., cyanotic atrophy of
- l. damage
- l. damage, accelerated
- l. damage ▸ advanced
- l. damage, heart and
- l. death
- l. degeneration of
- l. deposition

liver—*continued*
- l. disease
- l. disease, active
- l. disease, advanced
- l. disease, alcoholic
- l. disease ► clinical alcoholic
- l. disease, chronic
- l. disease, degenerative
- l. disease ► end stage
- l. disease, end stage heart and
- l. disease, fatty
- l. disease, fulminant
- l. disease, hepatocellular
- l. disease ► severe alcoholic
- l. disorder
- l. does appear enlarged
- l. does not appear enlarged
- l. donated
- l., donation of
- l. down _____ cm
- l. dysfunction
- l. edge
- l. edge palpable
- l. edges smooth
- l. engorgement
- l. enlarged
- l., enlarged fatty
- l. ► enlarged, tender
- l. enlargement
- l. enzyme elevations
- l. enzyme values
- l. enzymes
- l. enzymes, abnormal
- l. exploration
- l. ► extracellular cholestasis of
- l. ► extramedullary hematopoiesis in the
- l. failure
- l. failure, acute
- l. failure, acute fulminant
- l. failure, end-stage
- l. failure ► fulminant
- l., fatty
- l., fatty infiltration of
- l., fatty metamorphosis of
- l. fibrosis
- l., fibrous appendage of
- l. firm
- l. ► firm, irregular, nodular
- l. flap
- l. ► focal infarct of
- l. formation
- l. function
- l. function, abnormal
- l. function blood work
- l. function, impaired
- l. function, impairment of
- l. function, monitor
- l. function ► poor
- l. function studies
- l. function test (LFT)
- l. generous in size
- l. ► histologic appearance of
- l. ► histologic sections of
- l. imbalance
- l., infantile
- l., infection of
- l., inflammation of
- l. injury
- l. injury ► emergent
- l., interlobular veins of
- l. ► intracholestasis of
- l. involvement
- l. ► irregular, firm and nodular
- l., kidneys and spleen (LKS)
- l., laceration of
- l., lardaceous
- l. ► leukemic infiltrates of
- l., lobe of
- l., lobules of
- l. malfunction
- l. meridian
- l. metastases
- l. metastases ► hepatosplenomegaly with
- l. ► metastases to the
- l., metastatic carcinoma
- l., metastatic disease of
- l. multinodular
- l., needle biopsy of
- l., nodular
- l. nodule, metastatic
- l. ► nonalcoholic fatty
- l. not enlarged
- l. not palpably enlarged
- l. palm
- l. parenchyma
- l. parenchyma congested
- l. parenchyma ► cut section of
- l. percussed
- l. pigmentation
- l. ► portal fibrosis of
- l. ► portal hypertension of the
- l. ► portal tracts of
- l. profile
- l. pulse, atrial
- l. recipient
- l. resection
- l. rupture
- l. scan
- l. scan, gallbladder and
- l. scan, pancreatic
- l. scan, rose bengal
- l. scintiphoto
- l., segments of
- l. shadow
- l. shock
- l., sinusoids of
- l., spleen, kidneys (LSK) not palpable
- l. spots
- l., stellate cells of
- l. studies with nodules
- l. ► subcapsular of
- l., submassive necrosis of
- l. sugar
- l. tender
- l. ► thin-walled cyst of
- l., thromboembolism in
- l. tissue
- l. tissue abnormality
- l. toxicity
- l. toxicity ► drug-induced
- l. toxicity, fatal
- l. transplant
- l. transplant patient
- l. ► tumor nodules on
- l. tumors

livid cyanosis

livida, asphyxia

lividity
- l. and coldness of skin
- l., mild dependent
- l., postmortem

Livierato's
- L. reflex
- L. sign
- L. test

living
- l. (ADL) ► activities of daily
- l. and well (L/W)
- l. arrangements, special
- l., assisted
- l. birth (FTLB), full term
- l. birth, term
- l. brain
- l., capable of independent
- l., chemical-free
- l. child ► premature birth,
- l. conditions, change in
- l. donor
- l. donor exchange
- l. donor, related
- l. donor, unrelated
- l. environment

l. environment, daily
l. habits, modify stressful
l. host cell
l., independent
l. (ADL), independent in activities of daily
l. mammalian tissue
l., maximum independence of
l. ▸ memory-impaired assisted
l. needs ▸ independent
l. organisms
l., prudent heart
l. quotient (TLQ) ▸ total
l. related organ donor
l. ▸ relearn skills of daily
l. residence, assisted
l. situation
l. situation, long-term
l. skills, daily
l. skills ▸ independent
l. syndrome (DLS) ▸ depressive
l. under stress
l. unrelated donor (LURD)
l. unrelated kidney
l. (ADL), verbal cueing for activities of daily
l. will
l. (ADL) with supervision, patient does activities of daily

livor [*liver*]
livor mortis
LKS (liver, kidneys and spleen)
LLE (left lower extremity) amputated
LLE (left lower extremity) flexed
LLL (left lower lobe)
    LLL bronchial orifice
    LLL infiltrate
    LLL lesion
    LLL of lung
LLQ (left lower quadrant)
LLQ (left lower quadrant) of abdomen
LLS (lazy leukocyte syndrome)
LM (linguomesial)
LMA (left mentoanterior)
LML (left middle lobe) of lung
LMO (low midoccipital) electrode
LMP (last menstrual period)
LMP (left mentoposterior)
LMT (left mentotransverse)
LNMP (last normal menstrual period)
LO (linguo-occlusal)
LOA (leave of absence)
LOA (left occipitoanterior)
Loa

load(s)
l., average daily patient
l. -bearing activity
l. ▸ electronic pacemaker
l., exercise
l., extrapulmonary
l., heat
l. hypertrophy ▸ volume
l. ▸ peak work
l. perception
l., sodium
l. test, water
loaded
l. breathing sensation
l. feet ▸ spring-
l. stent ▸ spring-
loading
l. applicator, Fletcher's
l. colpostat ▸ Fletcher after-
l. course
l. dose, intravenous
l. doses
l., glycogen
l., relaxation
l., saline
l. system, after-
l. tandem ▸ Fletcher after-
l., 2:1
l., volume
loaf cornea, sugar-
lobar
l. atelectasis
l. atrophy
l. bronchi
l. bronchus
l. emphysema
l. emphysema, infantile
l. gliosis
l. hyperplasia
l. infiltrate, dense
l. overinflation, congenital
l. pneumonia
l. pneumonia ▸ community-acquired
l. pneumonia ▸ fibrinous acute
l. sclerosis
lobation, external
lobatum, hepar
lobe(s)
l. artifact ▸ side
l., azygos
l., blue ear
l. (LLL) bronchial orifice ▸ left lower
l. (LUL) bronchial orifice ▸ left upper
l. (RLL) bronchial orifice ▸ right lower

l. (RML) bronchial orifice ▸ right middle
l. (RUL) bronchial orifice ▸ right upper
l. bronchus, lower
l. bronchus, middle
l. bronchus, upper
l., cavitation of
l. collapse ▸ lower
l. collapse ▸ middle
l., contralateral ear
l. creases, ear
l. decompression, median
l., diseased
l., ear
l. enlargement
l. epilepsy, temporal
l., flocculonodular
l. focus, right temporal
l., frontal
l. hormone, anterior
l. infarcts, bilateral occipital
l., inferior
l., inferior frontal
l. infiltrate ▸ bilateral lower
l. (LLL) infiltrate ▸ left lower
l. (RLL) infiltrate ▸ right lower
l., lateral
l., left hepatic
l. (LLL) ▸ left lower
l. (LUL) left upper
l. (LLL) lesion ▸ left lower
l. (LUL) lesion ▸ left upper
l. (RLL) lesion ▸ right lower
l. (RUL) lesion ▸ right upper
l. lesion, temporal
l., limbic
l., lower
l., medial surface occipital
l., middle
l., occipital
l. of brain
l. of brain, excision frontal
l. of brain, excision occipital
l. of brain, excision parietal
l. of brain, excision temporal
l. of brain, frontal
l. of brain, limbic
l. of brain, mesial surface of occipital
l. of brain, occipital
l. of brain, olfactory
l. of brain, parietal
l. of brain, temporal
l. of cerebral cortex ▸ frontal

lobe(s)—*continued*
l. of cerebrum
l. of kidney
l. of left lung ▸ lower
l. of left lung ▸ upper
l. of liver
l. of liver, caudate
l. of lung
l. (LLL) of lung ▸ left lower
l. (LML) of lung ▸ left middle
l. (LUL) of lung ▸ left upper
l. (RLL) of lung ▸ right lower
l. (RML) of lung ▸ right middle
l. (RUL) of lung ▸ right upper
l. of pituitary gland, anterior
l. of pituitary gland, intermediate
l. pituitary gland, posterior
l. of prostate
l. of right lung ▸ lower
l. of right lung ▸ middle
l. of right lung ▸ upper
l. of thyroid
l. orifice, middle
l., parietal
l. (RLL) partial collapse ▸ right
   lower
l. (LUL) pneumonia ▸ left upper
l. (RUL) pneumonia ▸ right upper
l., prostatic
l., Riedel's
l., right hepatic
l. (RLL) ▸ right lower
l. (RML) ▸ right middle
l. (RUL) ▸ right upper
l. segmental atelectasis ▸ lower
l. segmental bronchi, upper
l., side
l. ▸ sulci of occipital
l., superior
l. syndrome, frontal
l. syndrome, middle
l. (RML) syndrome ▸ right middle
l., temporal
l., upper
lobectomy
l., complete
l., left lower
l., partial
l., sleeve
lobed placenta
lobotomy
l., frontal
l., prefrontal
l., radical
l., transorbital

Lobstein's cancer
Lobstein's ganglion
lobster-claw deformity
lobster-claw hand
lobular
l. bronchiole
l. cancer, infiltrating
l. cancer ▸ invasive
l. carcinoma
l. carcinoma in situ
l. congestion, central
l. emphysema, chronic
l. in situ
l. necrosis, central
l. neoplasia
l. patches of atelectasis
l. pattern
l. pneumonia
lobulate [*loculate, flocculate*]
lobulated
l. atrioventricular (AV) bundle
l. contour
l., firm, tan parenchyma
l. kidney
l. mass
l. pancreas
l. tongue
l. tumor mass
lobulation, fetal
lobulation, normal fetal
lobule(s) [*globule, nodule*]
l., atelectatic
l., biventral
l., central veins of hepatic
l., crescentic
l., falciform
l., fatty
l., fusiform
l., hepatic
l., inferior parietal
l., inferior semilunar
l. of auricle
l. of cerebellum, central
l. of cerebellum, quadrangular
l. of epididymis
l. of kidney, cortical
l. of liver
l. of lung
l. of lung, primary
l. of lung, secondary
l. of mammary gland
l. of pituitary gland ▸ anterior
l. of testis
l. of thymus
l. of thyroid gland

l., paracentral
l., posteromedian
l., primary respiratory
l., pulmonary
l., superior parietal
l., superior semilunar
l., tumor
lobuli, coloboma
lobulus auriculae
lobulus biventer
lobus simplex
LOC (level of consciousness)
local [*focal, vocal*]
l. adverse reaction
l. and regional metastases ▸ painful
l. and systemic disease ▸ control of
l. anesthesia
l. anesthesia ▸ toxic reaction to
l. anesthetic
l. application
l. area network
l. asphyxia
l. brain activity
l. brain radiation therapy, whole
   brain versus
l. cancer
l. cause
l. chorea
l. contact
l. control
l. convulsion
l. death
l. defense against injury
l. diminution in blood supply
l. disease
l. disease of cortex
l. efficiency factor
l. excision
l. excision, wide
l. excitatory state
l. eye anesthesia
l. field block
l. flap
l. heat, increased
l. hypothermia
l. immunity
l. infection
l. infiltration
l. inflammation
l. instillation
l. involvement
l. irradiation
l. irradiation of transplant
l. irrigation
l. irritation

l. isolation
l. lesion
l. metastases
l. neoplasm
l. occurrence
l. prophylaxis
l. radiation therapy
l. reaction
l. recurrence
l. recurrence after radiation therapy
l. recurrence of carcinoma
l. recurrence of tumor
l. resection of rectal tumor
l. skin swelling
l. spinal reflex
l. spread in cancer, pattern of
l. spread pattern of lung carcinoma
l. stimulant
l. swelling
l. syncope
l. tenderness over scalp
l. therapy
l. thrombophlebitis
l. tic
l. treatment
l. tumor control
l. tumor excision
l. tumor excision with irradiation
l. ulcer

localization
l., anatomic
l. audiometry
l., beam
l., Comberg
l., diagnosis and
l., field
l. films
l. index (SLI) ▸ splenic
l. ▸ intraoperative gamma probe
l., needle
l. of antigen ▸ endothelial
l., portal
l. scan, tumor
l., source
l., stereotactic
l., stone
l. ▸ stone imaging and
l., suitable beam film
l., Sweet's
l., target volume
l., therapy field
l., tumor
l., wire

localized
l. absence of skin ▸ congenital

l. aching pain
l. advancement flap
l. alveolar osteitis
l. amnesia
l. aneurysmal dilation
l. bladder cancer
l. bone destruction
l. brain activity
l. brain injury
l. cancer
l. cancerous breast tumor
l. clonic seizures
l. cold injury
l. damage
l. defect
l. degenerative tic
l. depressive reaction
l. dermatitis, treatment of
l. disease
l. distribution, pains of
l. dose
l. electroencephalogram (EEG)
    activity
l. emphysema
l. epilepsy
l. form of cancer
l. headache
l. immune reaction
l. in original site ▸ cancer
l. infection
l. inflammation
l. interference with circulation
l. irritation
l. irritative reaction
l. lesion
l. leukocyte mobilization
l. lipohypertrophy
l. malignant melanoma
l. mass
l. moderate decrease in voltage
l. neurological signs
l. non-Hodgkin's lymphoma
l. numbness
l. obstructive emphysema
l. occipital dysfunction
l. pain
l. pain in breast
l., pain primarily
l. pain ▸ sharp,
l. pancreatitis
l. pericarditis
l. peritonitis
l. plaque formation
l. post-seizure stupor
l. prostate cancer

l. pyelonephritis
l. radiotherapy
l. rales
l. reduction of voltage
l. sacculation
l. scleroderma
l. sepsis
l. signs
l. signs of weakness
l. stage
l. tenderness
l. tingling or numbness
l. tissue irritation
l. trauma
l., tumor
l., unresectable disease
l. visceral arteritis

localizer cast, Risser
localizing
l. electrode
l. neurological signs
l. sign

**locally advanced and inflammatory
    breast carcinoma**
**locally advanced squamous cell
    carcinoma**
location(s)
l., anatomic
l., anatomical
l., memory storage
l., primitive
l., topographic
l., usual anatomic

lochia
l. alba
l. cruenta
l. purulenta
l. rubra
l. sanguinolenta

loci, genius
loci mnemonic
lock (Lock)('s)
l. finger
l., flush heparin
l., heparin
L. hip prosthesis, Mueller Duo-
l., knee
l. knee ▸ long leg brace with drop-
l. -stitch, running
l. -stitch suture
l. suture, continuous running
l. suture, running
l. total hip replacement ▸ dual

locker room odor of body
locker room syndrome

locking
  l. device
  l. manner, continuous
  l. of joint
  l. of knee ▸ buckling and/or
  l. prosthesis ▸ modified Moore hip
  l. prosthesis ▸ Vitallium Moore self-
  l. running suture
  l. stitch, self-
lockjaw, patient has
Lockwood's tendon
locomotion, brachial
locomotor
  l. activity
  l. ataxia
  l. stimulation
loco-regional spread
Locoweed (marijuana)
locular cyst
loculate [lobulate, flocculate]
loculated
  l. abscess
  l. cyst
  l. emphysema
  l. empyema
  l. fluid
  l. pleural effusion
locus
  l. ceruleus
  l., genetic
  l., histocompatibility
  l. of control
locustae, Malameba
lode ▸ heterogeneity of viral
lode testing ▸ viral
lodge, cholesterol
lodged in ear ▸ object
lodged in trachea, food
Loetwig's ganglion
Loewenstein tumor, Buschke-
Löffler('s)
  L. bacillus ▸ Klebs-
  L. disease
  L. endocarditis
  L. eosinophilia
  L. implant, Lash-
  L. parietal fibroplastic endocarditis
  L. pneumonia
  L. syndrome
Loft-Strand crutches
log
  l. amplifier
  l. rank test
  l. sleep

logarithmic
  l. dynamic range
  l. phonocardiograph
  l. unit
logic
  l. linear array, research
  l. signal
  l., trance
logical
  l. reasoning
  l. sequential approach
  l. thinking
Löhlein's
  L. -Baehr lesion
  L. diameter
  L. lesion, Baehr-
  L. nephritis
  L. operation
Lok catheter connection, Luer-
Lok syringe, Luer-
lollipop bite-block
lollipop, narcotic
LOM (limitation of motion)
Lombardi's sign
Lombard's test
Londe atrophy, Fazio-
Londermann's operation
lone atrial fibrillation
loneliness
  l. and isolation
  l., boredom and
  l. ▸ displays passive
  l. ▸ universal fantasies of
L1-L5 (lumbar vertebrae)
long
  l. abductor muscle of thumb
  l. abductor tendon
  l. -acting anesthetic
  l. -acting barbiturate
  l. -acting calcium blocker
  l. -acting dose
  l. -acting insulin
  l. -acting thyroid stimulant
  l. -acting thyroid-stimulating (LATS) hormone
  l. -acting thyroid stimulator
  l. adductor muscle
  l. arm cast
  l. attention span
  l. axial oblique view
  l. axis
  l. axis of kidney
  l. -axis parasternal view echo-cardiogram
  l. -axis view

  l. -axis view echocardiogram ▸ parasternal
  l. -axis view ▸ horizontal
  l. -axis view ▸ parasternal
  l. -axis view ▸ vertical
  l. bone
  l. -bone fracture
  l. -bone survey
  l., cervix
  l. -chain fatty acid
  l. -chain triglyceride
  l. chest
  l. ciliary nerves
  l. crus
  l. disability, life-
  l. -distance runner
  l. extensor muscle of great toe
  l. extensor muscle of thumb
  l. extensor muscle of toes
  l. fibular muscle
  l. flexor muscle of great toe
  l. flexor muscle of thumb
  l. flexor muscle of toes
  l. fronds of connective tissue
  L. -Ganong-Levine syndrome
  l. gyrus of insula
  l. inter-electrode distances
  l. -lasting muscular atrophy
  l. leg brace
  l. leg brace with drop-lock knee
  l. leg brace with free ankle
  l. leg brace with large tibial cuff
  l. leg cast
  l. lesion
  l. levator muscles of ribs
  l. palmar muscle
  l. peroneal muscle
  l. philtrum
  l. posterior ciliary artery
  l. posterior ciliary axis
  l. process of incus
  l. pulse
  l. Q-T interval syndrome ▸ idiopathic
  l. Q-T syndrome
  l. QT syndrome ▸ congenital
  l. Q-TU syndrome
  l. rectangular flap
  l., regular discharges
  l. relapsing disease ▸ life-
  l. rods
  l. rotator muscles
  l. -short cycle ▸ short-
  l. -short sequences
  l. sight

l. smoking history
l. -standing
l. -standing arthritic deformities
l. -standing diabetes mellitus (DM)
l. -standing symptomatology
l. term
l. -term acupuncture treatment
l. -term adjustment
l. -term adverse effects
l. -term aftercare treatment
l. -term alcohol exposure
l. -term anticoagulation therapy
l. -term aspirin therapy
l. -term behavior modification treatment
l. -term behavioral change
l. -term biofeedback relaxation therapy
l. -term breast feeding
l., -term care
l. -term care facility
l. -term care services
l. -term chronic pain
l. -term cohabitation
l. -term complications
l. -term consequences
l. -term counterconditioning treatment
l. -term damage ▸ acute and
l. -term depression
l. -term depression ▸ severe
l. -term detoxification treatment
l. -term dialysis
l. -term drug therapy
l. -term drug treatment
l. -term edema
l. -term effectiveness
l. -term effects
l. -term exercise
l. -term exposure
l. -term family therapy
l. -term goals
l. -term health care facility
l. -term heavy drinking
l. -term heroin addicts
l. -term hospitalization
l. -term illness
l. -term illness, chronic
l. -term individual counseling
l. -term inhalation
l. -term injection sclerotherapy
l. -term living situation
l. -term management
l. -term mechanical assistance
l. -term mechanical ventilation

l. -term memory (LTM)
l. -term memory function
l. -term mood disorder
l. -term morbidity and mortality
l. -term neurologic disease
l. -term outpatient treatment
l. -term oxygen (O_2) therapy
l. -term pain
l. -term pain relief
l. -term paralysis
l. -term prognosis
l. -term psychological morbidity
l. -term psychotherapy
l. -term reaction
l. -term recovery
l. -term recovery ▸ support
l. -term relief
l. -term remission
l. -term restoration of muscle strength
l. -term safety studies
l. -term self-administration of opioids
l. -term sequelae
l. -term side-effects
l. -term skilled nursing care
l. -term smoker
l. -term steroid therapy
l. -term steroids
l. -term support group
l. -term survival data
l. -term survival period
l. -term survival rate
l. -term survivor of heart transplant
l. -term tendency
l. -term toxicity
l. -term trauma
l. -term treatment
l. -term treatment, indications for
l. -term ultraviolet exposure
l. -term unit, adult
l. -term use
l. -term use of free-base cocaine
l. -term ward ▸ restrictive
l. -term weight control
l., thick and closed ▸ cervix
l. thoracic nerve
l. tract signs
l. wave irradiation

longbeachae, Legionella
longer
l. acting ACE inhibitor
l. periods of sleep
l. runs

longevity (Longevity)
l., battery
L. Center, Pritikin
l. ▸ psychological factors of
longicauda, Cercomonas
longissimus
l. muscle of back
l. muscle of head
l. muscle of neck
l. muscle of thorax
longitudinal
l. anteroposterior arrays
l. arch
l. arch of foot
l. axis
l. bipolar montage
l. bundle, posterior
l. cerebral fissure
l. chromatic aberration
l. diameter, inferior
l. dissociation
l. fissure of cerebrum
l. fold of duodenum
l. fracture
l. incision
l. ligament
l. ligaments, rupture of anterior and posterior
l. medial bundle
l. muscle
l. muscle of tongue ▸ inferior
l. muscle of tongue ▸ superior
l. nerves of Lancisi
l. pancreaticojejunostomy
l. plane
l. presentation
l. sinus, ligation superior
l. sulcus
l. sulcus of heart
l. support
l. suture
l. suture of palate
l. wave
longitudinally, muscles split
longstanding fatigue ▸ generalized, debilitating,
Longuet's incision
longus
l., adductor
l., extensor carpi radialis
l., extensor hallicus
l. insulae, gyrus
l. muscle, adductor
l. muscle avulsion ▸ peroneus
l. muscle, extensor carpi radialis

longus—*continued*
l. muscle, extensor digitorum
l. muscle, extensor hallucis
l. muscle, flexor digitorum
l. muscle, flexor hallucis
l. muscle, flexor pollicis
l. muscle, palmaris
l. muscle, peroneus
l., musculus abductor pollicis
l., musculus extensor pollicis
l., musculus flexor pollicis
l. of Forel, fornix
l., palmaris
l., peroneus
l. reflex, supinator
l. tendon, palmaris

look
l. -alike case, AIDS
l. operation ▸ second
l. surgical management, second

looked erythematous, bronchi
looking, patient pasty
loop(s) [*Toupe, group*]
l., afferent
l., archoplasmic
l., atrial vector
l., bowel
l., bulboventricular
l., Cannon's endarterectomy
l., capillary
l., cardiac
l., cine
l., closed
l. colostomy
l. colostomy, sigmoid
l., Cordonnier ureteroileal
l. delivery, closed
l. device, closed
l. diuretic
l., duodenal
l., efferent
l., electric
l. electrosurgical excision
    procedure
l., elliptical
l. exercise echocardiogram,
    continuous
l., flow volume
l., Gerdy's interauricular
l., hairpin
l., haptens
l., haptics
l., heart
l., Henle's
l. in dermal papilla ▸ capillary

l. in hair papilla ▸ capillary
l. insulin pumps ▸ closed
l. intraocular lens (LOL), Sinskey/
    Sinskey modified blue
l. intrauterine device (IUD), Lippes
l., jejunal
l., lenticular
l. lesion, wire-
l., Lippe's
l. ▸ maxi-vessel
l., memory
l., Meyer's
l. of bowel, anastomosed to
l. of bowel, dilated
l. of bowel ▸ fluid-filled
l. of Henle, ascending
l. of hypoglossal nerve
l. of roux-en-y ▸ proximal
l. of small bowel ▸ multiple
l. of spinal nerves
l. of suture material
l. of Vieussens
l., P
l., peduncular
l., platinum
l., QRS
l. recorder
l. recorder ▸ external
l. recorder ▸ implantable
l., reentrant
l. ▸ sewing ring
l., Stoerck's
l. stoma, ileal
l. strut, wire-
l., subclavian
l. suture
l. syndrome, blind
l., T
l. tachycardia ▸ endless
l., terminal ileal
l. test, wire-
l., vascular
l., vector
l., ventricular
l. ▸ ventricular pressure volume
l., video
l. wire, continuous
l. wiring, Ivy

loose
l. associations
l. black stool
l. bodies
l. body
l. body, detached
l. body in joint

l. bowel movement
l. cartilage particles
l. cheeks
l. connective tissue
l. dentures
l. fibromyomatous stroma
l. fibrovascular stroma
l. fracture
l. jointedness
l. joints
l. junction
l. peritoneum
l. rectal mucous membrane
l. shoulder
l. skin
l. stools
l. watery stools

loosely
l. approximated, wound
l. closed, incision
l., wound closed

looseness of association
loosening joints
loosening of components
Looser-Milkman syndrome
Looser's zone
LOP (left occipitoposterior)
lop ear
Lopez-Enriquez operation
lopholea, Leptothrix
Lopresti method, Essex-
Lopresti reduction technique ▸
    Essex-
LOQ (lower outer quadrant)
Lorain dwarf, Levi-
Lorand factor, Laki-
lordosis
l., flattening of
l., lumbar
l., scoliosis and kyphosis

lordotic
l. curve
l. curve, lumbar
l. projection, anteroposterior
l. projection, apical
l. projection, PA (postero-
    anterior)
l. roentgenogram, apical
l. view
l. view, apical

lordotica progressiva ▸ dysbasia
Lorenz('s)
L. operation
L. operation, Hoffa-
L. osteotomy

L. position
L. sign
Lorenzo SMO prosthesis
lorgnette, main en
Loring's ophthalmoscope
Lortet lamp
LOS (length of stay)
lose
    l. ability to swallow
    l. control
    l. excess weight
    l. function ▸ receptor sites
losing
    l. control ▸ fear of
    l. enteropathy, protein-
    l. nephritis, potassium-
    l. nephritis, salt-
loss
    l. ▸ abandonment, separation or
    l., abdomen showed evidence of weight
    l., abdominal pain associated with blood
    l., acceptance of
    l., actual or perceived
    l., age-related memory
    l. and confusion, memory
    l. and exercise ▸ weight
    l. and nausea ▸ hair
    l. anemia, blood
    l., anemia secondary to blood
    l. attempt, weight
    l., attention
    l., bilateral progressive hearing
    l., blood
    l., body weight
    l., bone
    l., bone conduction
    l., bone density
    l., bone-mineral
    l., bone-thinning effects of estrogen
    l. by radiation ▸ heat
    l., cartilage
    l., central vision
    l., cerebral cortex
    l., chronic blood
    l., conductive
    l., conductive hearing
    l., coincidence
    l. counseling, grief and
    l., delayed hearing
    l. diet, weight
    l. disorder
    l. ▸ disorientation, confusion, and language

l. ▸ dissociative memory
l. due to aging ▸ white matter
l. ▸ early parental
l., enhancing weight
l. (EBL) ▸ estimated blood
l., evaporative water
l., excessive bone
l. ▸ excessive fluid
l. ▸ excessive weight
l. ▸ exercise-induced weight
l., extensive skin
l. factor, cell
l. ▸ fear of impending
l. ▸ female-pattern hair
l. ▸ fluctuating hearing
l. ▸ fluctuating sensorineural hearing
l., fluid
l. from aging ▸ hearing
l. from an adenocarcinoma ▸ chronic blood
l. from antibiotic ▸ hearing
l. from antidepressant ▸ hair
l. from anxiety ▸ weight
l. from aspirin ▸ hearing
l. from birth control pill ▸ hair
l. from brain ▸ memory
l. from cancer ▸ appetite
l. from cancer ▸ weight
l. from depression ▸ appetite
l. from depression ▸ memory
l. from depression ▸ weight
l. from diabetes ▸ weight
l. from diuretics ▸ hearing
l. from infection of ear ▸ hearing
l. from pain in abdomen ▸ appetite
l. from pernicious anemia ▸ appetite
l. from pernicious anemia ▸ memory
l. from pernicious anemia ▸ weight
l., gradual memory
l., hair
l., hearing
l., heat
l., high-frequency hearing
l. ▸ high-frequency sensorineural hearing
l., high-tone hearing
l., hippocampal cell
l., immeasurable fluid
l., impaired hearing
l. in hepatic disease ▸ protein
l. in radiation therapy, eyebrow and eyelash
l., infant weight

l. ▸ inner ear hearing
l. ▸ intrapartum blood
l. ▸ irreversible bone
l., jawbone
l. ▸ low-frequency sensorineural hearing
l. medication ▸ weight
l., memory
l. method, weight
l., minimal blood
l. ▸ minor hearing
l., Minoxidil and hair
l., momentary
l., monaural hearing
l., muscle
l., negligible blood
l., nerve cell
l., noise-induced hearing
l. of ability to speak
l. of ability to hold head up
l. of ability to sit up
l. of ability to smile
l. of ability to walk
l. of ability to write
l. of acuity
l. of aerobic capacity
l. of alertness ▸ gradual
l. of ambition and motivation
l. of appetite
l. of appetite and weight
l. of appetite, fatigue and
l. of appetite from Addison's disease
l. of appetite from AIDS
l. of appetite from anxiety
l. of appetite from Crohn's disease
l. of appetite from flu
l. of appetite from gastritis
l. of appetite from heart failure
l. of appetite from hepatitis
l. of appetite, mild
l. of appetite with fatigue
l. of appetite with indigestion
l. of appetite with joint swelling
l. of associated movements
l. of auditory discrimination ▸ gradual
l. of automatic movement
l. of balance
l. of balance and coordination
l. of balance ▸ sudden
l. of bladder control
l. of blood supply
l. of body heat ▸ excessive

loss—*continued*

l. of bone density
l. of bone mass
l. of bone strength
l. of bone tissue ▸ gradual
l. of bowel control
l. of cartilage
l. of cerebral function ▸ progressive
l. of concentration
l. of consciousness
l. of consciousness ▸ abrupt
l. of consciousness and motor control
l. of consciouness ▸ brief
l. of consciousness ▸ periodic
l. of consciousness, specific
l. of consciousness, total
l. of consciousness, transient
l. of contact with environment
l. of contact with reality
l. of contractile efficiency
l. of control
l. of control consumption
l. of control of bladder function
l. of control of muscular coordination
l. of coordination
l. of coordination ▸ sudden
l. of coordination ▸ weakness and
l. of desire to attend religious services
l. of dexterity
l. of effective breathing function
l. of emotional control
l. of emotional expression
l. of energy
l. of energy ▸ fatigue or
l. of energy, mood changes, apathy
l. of excretory function of body
l. of external structure
l. of facial expression
l. of fecal control
l. of feeling
l. of fertility from chemotherapy
l. of fertility from radiation
l. of flexibility
l. of flexion
l. of fluids through evaporation
l. of function
l. of function ▸ chronic
l. of function, transient
l. of gastrointestinal lesion ▸ chronic blood
l. of grip
l. of initiative

l. of intellectual faculties
l. of interest
l. of interest, appetite and concentration
l. of interest in activities
l. of interest in peer social activities
l. of interest in personal grooming
l. of interest in usual activities
l. of joint movement
l. of judgment
l. of language function
l. of language skills
l. of libido
l. of lung elasticity
l. of memory
l. of memory for distant events
l. of memory for recent events
l. of memory for smell
l. of memory for words
l. of memory, pathologic
l. of memory, progressive
l. of memory, temporary
l. of mental faculties ▸ gradual
l. of mental skills ▸ progressive
l. of motion
l. of motivation
l. of motor coordination
l. of motor function
l. of motor function ▸ total
l. of motor power, episodic
l. of motor skills
l. of movement
l. of muscle ▸ age-related
l. of muscle control
l. of muscle fiber
l. of muscle mass
l. of muscle strength
l. of muscle tone
l. of muscle tone and collapse
l. of nerve cells, age-related
l. of nerve impulse
l. of normal architecture
l. of peripheral vision
l. of polarity and hyperchromatism
l. of postural sensation
l. of postural tone
l. of power of voluntary movement
l. of prestige
l. of proprioception
l. of reality ▸ hallucinations and
l. of recent memory, confusion and poor judgment
l. of respiratory reflex ▸ transient
l. of self-confidence ▸ severe
l. of self-control

l. of self-esteem
l. of self-knowledge
l. of sensation
l. of sensation, complete
l. of sensation of pain
l. of sensation or function
l. of sense of time
l. of sensitivity to scent
l. of sexual desire
l. of sexual desire from anxiety
l. of sexual drive from diabetes
l. of sexual interest
l. of sight
l. of sight, complete
l. of skeletal muscular tone, momentary
l. of skin
l. of smell from aging
l. of speech
l. of sphincter function
l. of strength
l. of strength, momentary
l. of strength or fainting ▸ sudden
l. of strength ▸ sudden
l. of substantia Nigra cells
l. of taste
l. of teeth
l. of valvular function
l. of vestibular function
l. of vision
l. of vision, complete
l. of vision ▸ dimness or
l. of vision, partial
l. of vision, permanent
l. of vision ▸ spotty
l. of vision ▸ sudden
l. of vision ▸ sudden dimness or
l. of vision, total
l. of vision, transient
l. of vitality
l. of voice
l. of weight
l. of weight, significant
l., partial hearing
l. ▸ partial or complete memory
l., patient has memory
l., perceptive
l., permanent functional
l., permanent hearing
l. ▸ permanent memory
l. ▸ permanent vision
l. profile ▸ personal hearing
l. ▸ profound hearing
l. program, weight
l., progressive hearing

l. ▸ progressive memory
l. ▸ progressive unilateral hearing
l. ▸ progressive vision
l. ▸ rapid bone
l., rapid weight
l. ▸ rapidly progressing bilateral
  hearing
l., reality of
l. ▸ recent memory
l., recurring sense of
l. ▸ red blood cell
l., replace fluid
l., retrocochlear hearing
l. (SHL) ▸ selective hearing
l., sense of
l., sensorineural hearing
l., sensory
l. ▸ sensory neural hearing
l. ▸ severe bone
l. ▸ severe hearing
l. ▸ severe memory
l. ▸ severe vision
l. ▸ severe visual
l., short-term memory
l., significant weight
l., sleep
l. ▸ slowly progressing memory
l., soft tissue
l., spinal-bone
l., sudden hearing
l. ▸ sudden vision
l., sudden weight
l. surgery ▸ weight
l., symptomatic hearing
l., temporal field
l., temporary hair
l. ▸ temporary hearing
l., temporary memory
l. ▸ temporary vision
l. test, gastrointestinal (GI) protein
l. test, GI (gastrointestinal) blood
l., tissue
l., total blood
l. ▸ total memory
l., transepidermal water
l. ▸ treatment for hair
l. treatment, hair
l., unexplained weight
l. ▸ unilateral hearing
l., vision
l. ▸ visual and perceptual
l., visual hearing
l. ▸ warning signs of hearing
l. ▸ weakness, anorexia, weight
l., weight

LOT (left occipitotransverse)
lotion
  l., bootleg
  l., moisturizing
  l. shampoo, Kwell
Lottes'
  L. nail
  L. operation
  L. pin
  L. reduction technique
Lou Gehrig disease
loud
  l., high-pitched noises
  l. intermittent snoring
  l. piping rales
  l. systolic murmur
loudness
  l. balance, alternate binaural
  l. balance, monaural bi-frequency
  l. balance test, Fowler
  l., binaural
  l. decreased
  l. discomfort level
  l. level
  l., maximum
Louis
  L. angle
  L. -Bar syndrome
  L. encephalitis virus, St.
  L. law
Louisiana pneumonia
louisianae, Miyagawanella
Lounger, Wheel-
loupe [*loop*]
loupe, corneal
loupe, magnifying
louping ill virus
louse (lice)
  l., biting
  l., body
  l., chicken
  l., clothes
  l., crab
  l., goat
  l., head
  l., horse
  l. infestation
  l., pubic
  l., sucking
love (Love)
  l. assessment
  L. nerve root retractor
  L. Parents Support Group ▸ Tough
  L. Pill (phenylisopropylamine)

Lovelace, Bulbulian (BLB) mask ▸
  Boothby,
Lovén reflex
loving care (TLC) ▸ tender
Lovset's maneuver
low (Low)
  L. Airloss Therapy, Flexicair
  l. amplitude ▸ delta activity of
  l. anion gap
  l. anterior resection
  l. anxiety
  l. aridity antibodies
  l. attention span
  l. back
  l. back discomfort
  l. back flattener exercise
  l. back pain
  l. back pain, chronic intermittent
  l. back pain ▸ postpartum
  l. back strain
  l. back strain, chronic
  l. back stretch exercise
  l. back syndrome
  l. backache, chronic
  l. bacteria diet
  l. bandwidth
  L. -Beer position
  L. -Beer projection
  L. -Beer view
  l. birth weight (LBW)
  l. birth weight infant (LBWI)
  l. blood count
  l. blood potassium level
  l. blood pressure (LBP)
  l. blood pressure ▸ postural
  l. blood sugar
  l. blood sugar, severe
  l. body temperature
  l. bone density
  l., borderline
  l. calorie diet
  l. cardiac output
  l. cervical cesarean (C-) section
  l. cesarean (C-) section
  l. cholesterol
  l. cholesterol diet
  l. cholesterol diet ▸ low fat,
  l. cholesterol food ▸ low fat,
  l. cholesterol, low fat diet
  l. concentration
  l. content, abnormally
  l. cuboidal epithelium
  l. cure rate
  l. current Bovie
  l. delirium

low—*continued*

l., demand
l. density lipoprotein (LDL)
l. density lipoprotein (VLDL) ▸ very
l. diffusing capacity
l. dosage
l. dose aspirin therapy
l. dose breast x-rays
l. dose intravenous insulin therapy
l. dose radiation
l. dose rate irradiation
l. dose therapy
l. dose x-ray examination
l. dose x-ray technique
l. energy cardioversion
l. energy direct current
l. energy laser
l. energy level
l. energy linear accelerator
l. energy, patient has
l. energy radionuclide emission computerized tomographic (ECT) system
l. energy straight beam linear accelerator
l. energy synchronized cardio-version
l. energy x-ray therapy, combination high and
l., exaggerated
l. fat cholesterol diet
l. fat diet
l. fat eating plan
l. fat, low cholesterol diet
l. fat, low cholesterol food
l. fat milk
l. fat, nonacidic diet
l. fat vegetarian diet
l. fiber diet
l. fiber diet ▸ high fat
l. flow rate
l. forceps delivery
l. fractions
l. frequency
l. frequency blood group
l. frequency components
l. frequency filter
l. frequency filter control
l. frequency murmur
l. frequency pulsations
l. frequency response
l. frequency sensorineural hearing loss
l. frequency vibrations
l. frustration tolerance

l. grade
l. grade disease
l. grade fever
l. grade temperature
l. hairline
l. impact activities
l. impact aerobic workout
l. impact aerobics
l. impact exercise
l. impact movement
l. impact trauma
l. incidence of peptic ulcers
l. incision
l. insertion of placenta
l. insulin therapy
l. intensity exercise
l. intensity stimulation
l. intracellular-free magnesium
l. ionized serum calcium
l. level exposure
l. level of social support
l. level of spontaneous activity
l. level radiation
l. level radioactive tracer
l. lie
l. lipid diet
l. lying placenta
l. magnesium concentration
l. magnesium level
l. memory function
l. methionine diet
l. midoccipital electrode
l. molecular weight
l. molecular weight dextran
l. motivation
l. noise level
l. osmolality contrast material
l. -output failure
l. -output heart failure
l. output impedance
l. oxygen conditions
l. pain threshold
l. pass filter
l. pitched murmur
l. pitched ringing in ear
l. platelet count
l. power field (lpf)
l. powered field (PMN/LPF), poly-morphonuclear per
l. pressure bleed
l. pressure tamponade
l. probability of recovery
l. profile heart valve prosthesis ▸ Hufnagel
l. profile prosthesis, Gott

l. profile ▸ ultra-
l. protein
l. protein diet
l. purine diet
l. quality of life
l. radiation
l. rate
l. Renin essential hypertension (HTN)
l. residual urine volume
l. residue diet
L. resistance voice prosthesis ▸ Ultra-
l. risk
l. risk category patient, ultra
l. risk exercise
l. salt diet
l. -salt syndrome
l. saturated fat diet
l. self-confidence
l. self-efficacy
l. self-esteem
l. self-esteem child
l. self-esteem, chronic
l. self-esteem or guilt
l. self-esteem ▸ situational
l. septal atrium
l. septal right atrial electrogram
l. serum albumin
l. serum-bound iron
l. -set ears
l. sex drive
l. sodium diet
l. sodium, high potassium diet
l. sodium intake
l. -sodium syndrome
l. -speed rotational angioplasty
l. sperm count
l. spinal anesthesia
l. stimulus environment
l. stress angioplasty ▸ percutaneous
l. stress angioplasty (PLSA) ▸ physiologic
l. stress exercise
l. stress treatment group
l. tar/nicotine (T/N) cigarette
l. -tension cycling
l. -tension pulse
l. threshold
l. thyroid function
l. tones
l. tracheotomy
l. uric acid diet
l. viscosity cement, Zimmer

l. vision aids
l. vision impairment
l. vision rehabilitation
l. vision services
l. vision therapy
l. vision training
l. voltage
l. voltage activity
l. voltage brain waves
l. voltage electroencephalogram (EEG)
l. voltage, extremely
l. voltage fast
l. voltage fast activity
l. voltage fast electroencephalogram (EEG)
l. voltage foci
l. voltage, generalized
l. voltage, irregular
l. voltage record
l. voltage waking activity
l. voltage waves
Löwenberg cuff sign
Löwenberg, scala of
Löwenstein's culture medium
Löwenstein's operation
lower
l. abdomen
l. abdomen ▸ horizontal incision across
l. abdominal flap
l. abdominal pain
l. air pressure
l. airway obstruction
l. and upper
l. angle of scapula
l. back, arched
l. back extension exercise
l. back ▸ numbness in
l. back pain
l. back, patient flexed
l. back ▸ persistent pain in
l. back stretch exercise
l. basilar aneurysm
l. body dressing
l. body dressing, independent
l. body dressing, maximum assistance for
l. body dressing, minimal assistance for
l. body dressing, patient independent in
l. -body negative pressure (LBNP)
l. body strength
l. border of pupil

l. bowel cancer
l. bowel, stimulation of
l. brain stem
l. brain tumor
l. cervical region
l. chamber of heart
l. collecting system
l. cul-de-sac
l. denture
l. denture, complete
l. denture, partial
l. end of stump
l. esophageal sphincter
l. esophageal sphincter pressure
l. esophageal sphincter ▸ relaxed
l. esophagus
l. extremities bilaterally amputated
l. extremities ▸ edema of
l. extremities ▸ intramuscular arteries of
l. extremities ▸ mild edema upper and
l. extremities, pitting edema
l. extremities, swelling of
l. extremities ▸ tortuous varicosities in
l. extremities, varicosities of
l. extremity (LLE) amputated ▸ left
l. extremity (RLE) amputated ▸ right
l. extremity bypass graft
l. extremity (LLE) flexed ▸ left
l. extremity (RLE) flexed ▸ right
l. extremity full range of motion (ROM) ▸ left
l. extremity full range of motion (ROM) ▸ right
l. extremity (LLE) ▸ left
l. extremity, patient drags left
l. extremity, patient drags right
l. extremity strength
l. extremity strength, patient
l. extremity (RLE) ▸ right
l. extremity weakness
l. eyelid
l. femora
l. forearm
l. fragment, displacement of
l. ganglion of glossopharyngeal nerve
l. ganglion of vagus nerve
l. gastrointestinal (GI) procedure
l. hemianopia
l. impression
l. inner quadrant
l. jaw, receding

l. jawbone
l. leg ▸ numbness of
l. lid
l. lid, spastic ectropion
l. limb, amputation entire
l. limb amputee ▸ patient bilateral
l. lip
l. lip ▸ depressor muscle of
l. lip flap, Stein-Kazanjian
l. lip ▸ incisive muscles of
l. lip mucosa
l. lip ▸ quadrate muscle of
l. lobe
l. lobe (LLL) bronchial orifice ▸ left
l. lobe (RLL) bronchial orifice ▸ right
l. lobe bronchus
l. lobe infiltrate ▸ bilateral
l. lobe collapse
l. lobe (LLL) infiltrate ▸ left
l. lobe (RLL) infiltrate ▸ right
l. lobe (LLL) ▸ left
l. lobe (LLL) lesion ▸ left
l. lobe (RLL) lesion ▸ right
l. lobe (LLL) of lung ▸ left
l. lobe (RLL) of lung ▸ right
l. lobe (RLL) partial collapse ▸ right
l. lobe (RLL) ▸ right
l. lobe segmental atelectasis
l. lobectomy, left
l. lumbar discomfort
l. mantle
l. margin of field
l. motoneuron/motor neuron (MN)
l. motor neuron (MN) dysfunction
l. motor neuron paralysis
l. nephron nephrosis
l. nodal extrasystole
l. nodal rhythm
l. obstructive airway disease
l. obstructive lung disease
l. outer quadrant (LOQ)
l. peritoneal edge
l. peritoneal flap
l. plate
l. pole calyx
l. pole left kidney ▸ scar
l. pole of incision
l. pole right kidney ▸ scar
l. quadrant (LLQ) ▸ left
l. quadrant (LLQ) of abdomen ▸ left
l. quadrant (RLQ) of abdomen ▸ right
l. quadrant (RLQ) ▸ right
l. respiratory infection

lower—*continued*
- l. respiratory tract
- l. respiratory tract inflammation
- l. retina
- l. risk of dying
- l. risk of heart disease
- l. segment
- l. segment cesarean (C-) section
- l. serum calcium
- l. teeth
- l. teeth, pyorrhea around
- l. transverse abdominal incision
- l., upper and
- l. uterine canal curettings
- l. uterine segment

Löwe's ring
Lowe's syndrome
lowered
- l. blood pressure (BP)
- l. in Addison's disease ▸ blood pressure
- l. levels of input
- l. resistance to infection
- l. tumor antigenicity

lowering
- l. diet, cholesterol
- l. drug, blood pressure
- l. drug, cholesterol
- l. drug therapy, cholesterol
- l. eye pressure
- l. medication, cholesterol

lowest splanchnic nerve
Löwn-Ganong-Levine syndrome
Lowry unit, Bessey-
LP
- LP (light perception)
- LP (linguopulpal)
- LP (lumbar puncture)

lpf (low power field)
L-plasty repair
lpm (liter per minute)
LPN (Licensed Practical Nurse)
LPO (left posterior oblique)
LPO (light perception only)
lps (liters per second)
LRR (light reflection rheography)
LS (lecithin sphingomyelin) ratio
LS (lumbosacral)
L/S ratio
LSA (left sacroanterior)
LSB (left sternal border)
L.Sc.A. (left scapuloanterior)
L.Sc.P. (left scapuloposterior)
LSD (lysergic acid diethylamide)
- LSD (acid)

LSD (Barrels)
LSD (Big D)
LSD (Blotter Acid)
LSD (Blue Cap)
LSD (Blue Dragon)
LSD (California Sunshine)
LSD (Camel)
LSD (Candies)
LSD (Cubes)
LSD (Cupcake)
LSD (Domes)
LSD (Doses)
LSD (Four-Way)
LSD (Green Dragon)
LSD (Haze)
LSD (Hits)
LSD (King Tut)
LSD (LBJ)
LSD (Microdots)
LSD (Mr. Natural)
LSD (Orange Sunshine)
LSD (Paper Acid)
LSD (Peace pill)
LSD (Purple Haze)
LSD (Raggedy Ann)
LSD (Red Dragon)
LSD (Sunshine)
LSD (Tabs)
LSD (The Force)
LSD (Wedges)
LSD (White Lightning)
LSD (Windowpanes)
LSD (Zig-Zag Man)
LSD addict
LSD addiction
LSD dependency
LSD habit
LSD -induced psychosis
LSD ingested
LSD inhaled
LSD injected
LSD intoxication
LSD smoked
LSD snorted
LSD (hallucinogen) user
LSD user
LSD withdrawal

LSK (liver, spleen, kidneys) not palpable
LSM (late systolic murmur)
LSP (left sacroposterior)
LST (left sacrotransverse)
LSV (left subclavian vein)
LTH (luteotropic hormone)
LTM (long-term memory)

LTP (laser trabeculoplasty)
L-type nose bridge prosthesis ▸ Rosi
lubb-dupp
lubricant, eye
lubricated, eyes
lubrication, vaginal
Luc
- L. approach ▸ Caldwell-
- L. operation ▸ Caldwell-
- L. procedure ▸ Caldwell-

Lucas
- L. -Championnierre's disease
- L. -Cottrell operation
- L. operation ▸ Abbott-

lucent calculi
lucent defect
lucid
- l. lethargy
- l., patient
- l. rage
- l. recognition

lucidity, periods of
lucidity ▸ periods of alertness and
luciflavum, Mycobacterium
lucinate ligament
lucite implant
Luck operation
Ludes (barbiturates)
luding out
Lüdloff('s)
- L. -Laewen disease, Budinger-
- L. operation
- L. sign

Ludwig('s)
- L. angina
- L. angle
- L. arteriole, Isaacs-
- L. ganglion

LUE (left upper extremity)
LUE (left upper extremity) amputated
LUE (left upper extremity) flexed
Luedde's exophthalmometer
Luedde's transparent rule
Luer-Lok catheter connection
Luer-Lok syringe
lues
- l. hepatic
- l. nervosa
- l. syphilitica
- l. tarda
- l. venerea

luetic
- l. aneurysm
- l. aortitis

l. disease
l. encephalitis
Luft's syndrome
Lugol's solution
Lugol's stain
LUL (left upper lobe)
LUL bronchial orifice
LUL lesion
LUL of lung
LUL pneumonia
lumbago, ischemic
lumbar
l. aorta
l. aortography
l. arteriogram
l. artery
l. body
l. car seat
l. corpectomy
l. curvature
l. curvature ▸ flattening of normal
l. curve
l. curve, flattening of
l. curve reversal
l. discectomy
l. discectomy, automated
percutaneous
l. discomfort, lower
l. flexion and extension study
l. flexure
l. ganglia
l. hernia
l. interspace
l. laminectomy
l. laminectomy, decompressive
l. lordosis
l. lordotic curve
l. lymph nodes
l. musculature
l. myelogram
l. myositis
l. nephrectomy
l. nephrotomy
l. nerves
l. pain
l. Pantopaque column
l. plexus
l. pseudosacralization
l. puncture (LP)
l. puncture headache
l. radiculopathy
l. reflex
l. region
l. region of abdomen ▸ left
l. region of abdomen ▸ right

l. root avulsion
l. scoliosis
l. space
l. spinal root origin
l. spinal stenosis
l. spine
l. spine motion
l. spine, spurring of
l. splanchnic nerves
l. spurring
l. spurring, degenerative
l. subarachnoid catheter
l. subarachnoid space
l. sympathectomy
l. vein, ascending
l. veins I and II
l. veins III and IV
l. vertebrae (L1-L5)
l. vertebrae bones
l. vertebrae, decalcified
lumbodorsal fascia
lumbodorsal fascia opened
posteriorly
lumboiliac incision, Vischer's
lumboinguinal nerve
lumboperitoneal shunt, Spetzler
lumborum muscle, iliocostalis
lumbosacral (LS)
l. agenesis
l. belt
l. curve, flattening of
l. disc protrusion
l. fields for radiation therapy
l. instability
l. joint
l. joint, instability of
l. joint, transitional
l. level, narrowing at
l. projection
l. radiculopathy
l. spine
l. sprain
l. strain
l. support
lumbrical muscles of foot
lumbrical muscles of hand
lumbricoides, Ascaris
lumen(s)
l., arterial
l. breast implant, double
l., bronchial
l. catheter, triple
l. endobronchial tube, double
l., esophageal
l., false

l., left anterior descending (LAD)
l., narrowing of
l. of appendix
l. of artery
l. of bowel
l. of bronchial artery
l. of gut
l. of vein
l., patent
l., single
l. subclavian, double
l., true
l. tube, multiple
l., vaginal
l., vessel
lumenal narrowing
luminal
l. diameter ▸ minimal
l. encroachment
l. filling defect
l. irregularity
l. narrowing
l. occlusion
luminous intensity
luminous rays
Lumiwand light
lump [*hump*]
l. at site of injection
l., benign breast
l., breast
l., cancerous
l. growing in bone
l. in abdomen
l. in anus
l. in front of or behind ear
l. in left breast does appear
enlarged
l. in left breast does not appear
enlarged
l. in right breast does appear
enlarged
l. in right breast does not appear
enlarged
l. in throat
l. in throat, patient has
l., innocuous
l. kidney
l. on breast
l. or swelling under chin
l., palpable breast
l. pressing, breast
l., suspicious
l. with Crohn's disease ▸ abdominal
lumpectomy and radiation
lumpectomy procedure

lumpiness, breast
lumpy breasts
Lumsden's center
lunar hymen
lunata, Curvularia
lunate
    l. bone
    l. dislocation
    l. fracture
    l. implant, Swanson carpal
lunatum, os
lunatus, sulcus
Lund's operation
Lundvall's blood crisis
lung(s)
    l. abscess
    l. abscess, anaerobic
    l. abscess, aspiration
    l., abscess of
    l. acinus
    l. ▸ active expansion of
    l., adenocarcinoma left
    l., adenocarcinoma right
    l., adenosquamous carcinoma of
    l. adequately expanded
    l., aeration of
    l. ailment, terminal
    l., alcohol effect on
    l. allograft
    l. and bone metastases
    l., angioma of
    l., anterior segment of
    l. ▸ apex of left
    l. ▸ apex of right
    l., apical segment of
    l. apices
    l., apicoposterior segment of
    l. appearance, dirty
    l., arc welder
    l. architecture
    l., arterial circulation to the
    l., artificial
    l., artificial collapse of upper portion of
    l. aspirate, direct
    l. atelectatic and edematous
    l., atrium of
    l., auscultation of
    l., autonomic innervation of
    l. ▸ autopsy limited to heart and
    l., bacterial infection of
    l. base
    l. base, atelectasis left
    l. base, atelectasis right
    l., base, infiltrate left

    l. base, infiltrate right
    l. base, left
    l. base, right
    l., basilar portion of
    l. biopsy
    l. biopsy, open
    l. biopsy ▸ surgical
    l. biopsy, transbronchial
    l., bird-breeder's
    l., black
    l., blast
    l. ▸ bleeding into
    l. ▸ bloc ▸ heart-
    l. blockage
    l. blocks in radiation therapy, thin
    l. ▸ blood clot in
    l. ▸ blood clot in brain or
    l. ▸ blood flow of
    l., blood from heart to
    l., brown induration of
    l. brushings
    l. bypass, heart-
    l., calcification of
    l. calculus
    l. cancer
    l. cancer, early
    l. cancer, inoperable metastatic
    l. cancer ▸ metachronous
    l. cancer ▸ nonsmall cell
    l. cancer, occult
    l. cancer, small cell
    l. cancer, sputum cytology in
    l. cancer, terminal
    l. ▸ cannonball metastasis to
    l. capacity
    l. capacity (RV/TLC) ratio ▸ residual volume to total
    l. capacity ▸ reduced
    l. capacity (RLC), residual
    l. capacity (TLC) ▸ total
    l. carcinoma, extrathoracic spread pattern of
    l. carcinoma, local spread pattern of
    l. carcinoma, lymphatic spread pattern of
    l. carcinoma, metastatic
    l., carcinoma of
    l. carcinoma, supraclavicular node metastasis in
    l. carcinoma, tumor doubling time in
    l., cardiac
    l., cardiac notch of left
    l., cheese worker's
    l., cholinergic innervation of

    l., chondroma of
    l., chronic passive congestion of
    l., circulation to
    l., cirrhosis of
    l. clear
    l. clear to percussion and auscultation (P and A)
    l., coal miner's
    l., coarsely granular
    l., coin lesion of
    l., collapsed
    l. complaints, chronic
    l. compliance (TLC) ▸ total
    l. complication, postoperative
    l. condition, fatal
    l. congested and edematous
    l. congestion
    l., consolidation of
    l., contusion of
    l., crackling in
    l., crackling sounds in
    l., cystic disease of
    l. damage
    l. damage ▸ irradiation-induced
    l., decortication of
    l. destruction, recurrent
    l. destruction, scarring
    l. ▸ detergent worker's
    l., developing
    l., diabetic gangrene of
    l. ▸ diaphragmatic surface of left
    l. ▸ diaphragmatic surface of right
    l., diffusing capacity of
    l., discrete nodulation of
    l. disease
    l. disease, active
    l. disease, black
    l. disease, brown
    l. disease, cheese worker's
    l. disease, chronic
    l. disease, chronic interstitial
    l. disease, chronic obstructive
    l. disease, chronic progressive
    l. disease ▸ cigarette induced
    l. disease ▸ cigarette induced obstructive
    l. disease, diffuse
    l. disease ▸ diffuse alveolar
    l. disease, diffuse infiltrative
    l. disease ▸ diffuse interstitial
    l. disease, environmental
    l. disease, farmer's
    l. disease ▸ fish meal
    l. disease ▸ furrier's
    l. disease ▸ granulomatous

l. disease, inhalational
l. disease, interstitial
l. disease ▸ interstitial restrictive
l. disease, lower obstructive
l. disease, metastatic
l. disease, obstructive
l. disease, occupational
l. disease ▸ parenchymal
l. disease, primary
l. disease ▸ radiation
l. disease, residual
l. disease, restrictive
l. disease ▸ rheumatoid
l. disorder
l. disorder, chronic
l. disorder ▸ occupational
l. disorder ▸ severe
l., drowned
l., drug-resistant organisms aspirated into
l. due to embolism ▸ infarction of
l. due to thrombosis ▸ infarction of
l. ▸ dullness over left
l. ▸ dullness over right
l. dysfunction
l., edema of
l. edematous
l. edematous and congested
l. ▸ effects of asthma on
l. ▸ elastic recall of
l. elasticity, loss of
l., elasticity of
l. embolism
l., emphysema of
l. emphysematous
l., eosinophilic
l. (EGL), eosinophilic granuloma of the
l., epidermoid carcinoma of
l., esophageal
l., expanded
l. expansion adequate
l., farmer's
l., FB (foreign body) in
l. fever
l., fibroid
l., fibroma of
l., fibrosis of
l., fibrotic
l. field
l. field, inferior
l. fields, clear
l. fields, peripheral
l. fields ▸ poor aeration both
l. ▸ fish meal

l., fissure of
l. ▸ fluid accumulation in
l. ▸ fluid balance in neonatal
l. fluid ▸ filtration of
l., fluid in
l. fluid ▸ retained
l. fluke
l., foreign body (FB) in
l., frostbite of
l., full expansion of
l. function
l. function studies
l. function study, quantitative regional
l. functioning test
l., gangrene of
l., gastric
l., glanders of
l., granuloma of
l., hamartoma of
l., harvester's
l., heart and
l. hemorrhage
l., heparin beef
l., hernia of
l. ▸ hilar substance of
l., hili of
l. hilus
l. ▸ histologic sections of
l., histoplasmosis of
l., honeycomb
l., horseshoe
l. ▸ hot tub
l., humidifier
l., hyperinflated
l., hyperlucent
l. imaging fluorescence endoscope
l., immature
l., immature fetal
l., immaturity of
l. ▸ improve efficiency of heart and
l. infarct
l., infarction of
l. infection
l., infectious disease of
l. ▸ inferior margin of left
l. ▸ inferior margin of right
l. infiltrate, right
l., inflammation of
l. inflated
l. injury
l. injury, acute
l. injury, air emboli-induced
l. injury, diffuse
l. injury from ozone

l. injury ▸ neutrophil-mediated
l. injury ▸ oxidant-induced
l. injury ▸ oxygen (O_2)-mediated
l. injury score
l. injury ▸ smoke-induced
l., insufflation of
l. ▸ interstitial immaturity of
l. ▸ interstitium of
l., iron
l., laceration of
l., left
l., left lower lobe (LLL) of
l., left middle lobe (LML) of
l., left upper lobe (LUL) of
l., limited expansion of
l. liquid production ▸ fetal
l., lobe of
l., lobules of
l. machine, heart-
l. malignancy, advanced
l. markings
l., mason's
l. maturity
l. maturity, fetal
l. mechanics
l. meridian
l. metastases
l. metastasis ▸ retroperitoneal liver and
l. ▸ metastatic disease of
l., microembolic disease of
l. ▸ middle lobe of right
l., ▸ mucus in
l. ▸ mushroom worker's
l. ▸ needle aspiration of
l. ▸ nerves of
l. ▸ neuroepithelial bodies in
l. nodules
l., nutrition of
l. ▸ oxygen (O_2) exchange in
l. ▸ oxygen (O_2) toxicity in immature
l. pap smear
l. ▸ parasympathetic innervation of
l. parenchyma
l. parenchyma, surrounding
l., passive congestion of
l., pigeon breeder's
l. pink white
l., polycystic
l. poorly expanded
l., posterior segment of
l., postperfusion
l. pressure

lung(s)—*continued*
l. ▸ pressure in blood vessel of
l., primary lobule of
l. problem, peripheral
l. ▸ pumping chamber of
l. puncture
l., punctured
l. radiation therapy
l. ▸ rattling sound in
l. reduction procedure
l. reduction ▸ stapled
l. reduction surgery
l. reduction surgery, double
l. reduction surgery ▸ single
l. reduction surgery ▸ unilateral
l. redux procedure
l., re-expansion of
l. reinflated
l. rejection, acute
l. resection
l. resection ▸ segmental
l. respirator
l. resuscitator, heart-
l. revealed decreased expansion
l. revealed diminished breath
    sounds
l. revealed hyperresonance to
    percussion
l., rheumatoid
l., right
l., right lower lobe (RLL) of
l., right middle lobe (RML) of
l. (RL), right
l., right upper lobe (RUL) of
l., root of
l. scan
l. scan ▸ ventilation defect on
l. scan, ventilation perfusion
l. scanning
l. scanning ▸ ventilation perfusion
l. scarring
l., scleroderma
l., secondary lobule of
l. secretion
l., segment of
l., senile atrophy of
l. ▸ sensory nerves of
l., shock
l. shunt ▸ vascular
l. sign, failing
l. ▸ silo filler's
l. ▸ small cell cancer of
l., small cell carcinoma of
l. sound, abnormal
l., squamous cell carcinoma of

l. ▸ sternal margin of left
l. ▸ sternal margin of right
l., stiff
l. stones
l., subclavian sulcus of
l. subcrepitant
l. substance
l., superior segment of
l. ▸ sympathetic innervation of
l. syndrome, bubbly
l. syndrome, busulfan
l. syndrome, hyperlucent
l. syndrome, hypoplastic
l. syndrome ▸ mirror image
l. syndrome, wet
l. test ▸ split function
l., thresher's
l. tissue
l. tissue atelectatic
l. tissue congested
l. tissue ▸ infected
l. tissue irritant
l. tissue ▸ necrotic
l. tissue, replacement of
l. tissue, scarring of
l. ▸ total collapse of
l. transplant
l. transplant, bilateral
l. transplant, double
l. transplant ▸ en bloc bilateral
l. transplant, heart-
l. transplant, single
l. transplantation
l., traumatic wet
l., trench
l., tuberculosis of
l. tumors, fetal
l., tumors of the
l., underdeveloped
l. ▸ unilateral hyperlucency of
l. ▸ unilateral nonfunctioning
l. ▸ upper lobe of left
l. ▸ upper lobe of right
l. uptake
l., vanishing
l. ventilation imaging ▸ xenon
l. ventilation ▸ split
l. ▸ vernal edema of
l. volume
l. volume ▸ high
l. volume reduction surgery
l. volume ▸ restriction of
l. volume ▸ total
l. ▸ volumetric aspect of
l. washings

l. water ▸ extravascular
l. well aerated
l. well aerated and crepitant
l., wet
l. ▸ wheezing in
l., white
l. with brain metastases ▸
    choriocarcinoma
l. ▸ wood pulp worker's
l. worm
lunge exercise ▸ squat and
lunged emphysema, small-
lunula(-ae)
l., nail
l. of aortic valves
l. of pulmonary trunk valves
l. of scapula
l. of semilunar valves
l. of semilunar valves of aorta
l. unguis
l. valvularum semilunarium aortae
l. valvularum semilunarium arteriae
    pulmonalis
l. vaivularum semilunarium trunci
    pulmonalis
Lunyo virus
lupoid hepatitis
lupus
l. anticoagulant
l. -associated valve disease
l., cutaneous
l. diathesis
l., drug-induced
l. erythematosus (LE)
l. erythematosus (LE) cell test
l. erythematosus (LE) ▸ discoid
l. erythematosus disseminatus
    (LED)
l. erythematosus ▸ drug-induced
l. erythematosus (SLE), systemic
l. erythematosus (LE) vulgaris
l., follicular
l. kidney disease, active
l. miliaris
l. nephritis
l. pernio
l. pleuritis
l. syndrome ▸ drug-induced
l. syndrome, hydralizine
l., systemic
l. vulgaris
LUQ (left upper quadrant)
LUQ (left upper quadrant) of
    abdomen
LURD (living, unrelated donor)

Lurid-Nebraska Test
lurida, Nocardia
Luscher-Zwislocki test
Luschka('s)
  L. crypts
  L. foramen
  L. ganglion
  L. joints
  L., laryngeal cartilage of
  L. muscles
  L., nerve of
  L. tonsil
luster, cornea
luster eyes, lack◊
lusterless, eyes
Lust's reflex
lutea retinae, macula
luteal
  l. cell function
  l. phase
  l. phase dysphoric disorder, late
lutein
  l. cells
  l. cells, follicular
  l. cells, theca-
  l. cyst
  l. cyst, granulosa
  l. cyst, theca-
  l. granulosa
luteinizing
  l. hormone (LH)
  l. hormone, human
  l. hormone releasing factor
Lutembacher's
  L. complex
  L. disease
  L. syndrome
luteola, Auchmeromyia
luteola, Musca
luteotropic hormone (LTH)
luteum
  l. cell
  l. cells ▸ progesterone-producing corpus
  l., corpus
  l. cyst, corpus
  l. ▸ formation of corpus
  l., hemorrhagic corpus
luteus retinas, limbus
Lutz
  L. -Cogan syndrome ▸ Bielschowsky-
  L. -Jeanselme nodules
  L. -Splendore-de Almeida syndrome

lutzii, Psorophora
luxans, coxa vara
luxation
  l., anterior
  l., Malgaigne's
  l. of globe
  l. of lacrimal gland
  l. of lens
luxurians, ectropion
luxus heart
Luys, nucleus of
LV (left ventricle) of heart
LV (left ventricle) study
LV (left ventricular)
  LV aneurysm
  LV assist system (LVAS)
  LV diameter
  LV diastolic pressure (LVDP)
  LV dysfunction
  LV ejection fraction ▸ global
  LV end-diastolic pressure (LVEDP)
  LV end-diastolic volume (LVEDV)
  LV enlargement (LVE)
  LV function
  LV mean (LVM)
  LV myocardium
  LV pressure (LVP)
  LV reduction surgery
  LV rejection fraction ▸ global
  LV stroke volume (LVSV)
  LV stroke work (LVSW)
  LV systolic pressure (LVSP)
  LV tunnel murmur, aortic
  LV weakness
  LV work (LVW)
  LV work index (LVWI)
LVAS (left ventricular assist system)
LVDP (left ventricular diastolic pressure)
LVE (left ventricular enlargement)
LVEDP (left ventricular end-diastolic pressure)
LVEDV (left ventricular end-diastolic volume)
LVM (left ventricular mean)
LVP (left ventricular pressure)
LVSP (left ventricular systolic pressure)
LVSV (left ventricular stroke volume)
LVSW (left ventricular stroke work)
LVW (left ventricular work)
LVWI (left ventricular work index)
L/W (living and well)
lwoffi, Acinetobacter
lycopodium granuloma

lye stricture, esophageal
Lyell's syndrome
lying placenta, low
lying, repeated
lying-in hospital
Lyle's syndrome
Lyman rays
Lyman-Smith brace
Lyme
  L. borreliosis
  L. carditis
  L. disease vaccine
  L. titer
lymph
  l. capillary
  l. cell
  l. cell lymphoma
  l. channels
  l. circulation
  l. dialysis
  l. embolism
  l., extracorporeal irradiation of
  l. flow
  l. fluid
  l. follicle
  l. gland
  l. gland ▸ infected
  l. glands, enlarged
  l. glands ▸ swollen
  l. heart
  l. involvement, periaortic
  l. involvement, regional
  l. nodal stage radiograph ▸ 24-hour delayed
  l. node swelling ▸ generalized
  l. node tenderness
  l. nodule
  l. scrotum
  l. spaces, perivascular
  l. system
  l., thoracic duct
  l. tissue appendix
  l. vessel
lymph node(s)
  l.n., abdominal
  l.n., anterior
  l.n., anterior mediastinal
  l.n., anterior tibial
  l.n., anthracotic
  l.n., aplastic
  l.n., axillary
  l.n. biopsies, selected retro-peritoneal
  l.n. biopsy
  l.n. biopsy, abdominal

lymph node(s)—*continued*
l.n. biopsy ▸ mediastinal
l.n. biopsy, scalene
l.n. biopsy ▸ supraclavicular
l.n., bronchial
l.n., bronchopulmonary
l.n., buccal
l.n., calcified
l.n., cancer of
l.n., cecal mesocolic
l.n., celiac
l.n., cervical
l.n. classification in squamous cell carcinoma, cervical
l.n., common iliac
l.n. ▸ cortical substance of
l.n., cubital
l.n., deep cervical
l.n., deep inguinal
l.n., Delphian
l.n. disease
l.n. dissection
l.n. dissection, axillary
l.n. drainage (dr'ge) ▸ pelvic
l.n., enlarged
l.n. enlargement
l.n. enlargement periaortic
l.n. enlargement ▸ residual axillary
l.n., epigastric
l.n., external iliac
l.n. ▸ first or second echelon
l.n. ▸ first or second station
l.n., gastroepiploic
l.n. ▸ hemorrhagic omental
l.n., hepatic
l.n., hilar
l.n., hilus of
l.n., histiocytic hyperplasia of
l.n. hyperplasia
l.n., ileocolic
l.n., iliac
l.n., inferior mesenteric
l.n., inferior tracheobronchial
l.n., inguinal
l.n., intercostal
l.n., internal iliac
l.n., internal jugular
l.n., internal mammary
l.n. involvement, axillary
l.n. involvement in nasopharyngeal carcinoma
l.n. involvement, regional
l.n. involvement, serial
l.n. irradiation, axillary
l.n., jugular

l.n., junctional
l.n., left colic
l.n., left gastric
l.n., left hilar
l.n., lumbar
l.n. ▸ lymphoid depletion of
l.n., mandibular
l.n., mediastinal
l.n., mesenteric
l.n. metastases, axillary
l.n. metastases, periaortic
l.n. metastasis
l.n., middle colic
l.n., neck
l.n., occipital
l.n. ▸ painless
l.n., pancreaticosplenic
l.n., pancreatoduodenal
l.n., parapharyngeal
l.n., paraportal
l.n., parasternal
l.n., paratracheal
l.n., pelvic
l.n., periaortic
l.n., perigastric
l.n. ▸ perihilar
l.n., peripancreatic
l.n. permeability factor
l.n., pharyngeal
l.n., phrenic
l.n., pleural
l.n., popliteal
l.n. ▸ positive
l.n., posterior mediastinal
l.n. ▸ pretracheal
l.n., pulmonary
l.n., pyloric
l.n., regional
l.n., regional node bearing area of
l.n., retroperitoneal
l.n. ▸ retropharyngeal
l.n., right colic
l.n., right gastric
l.n., right hilar
l.n., scalene
l.n. scintigraphy ▸ thyroidal
l.n., shotty
l.n., shotty residual
l.n. ▸ small, tender
l.n., spinal accessory chain
l.n., subdigastric
l.n., submandibular
l.n., submental
l.n., superficial and deep parotid
l.n., superficial cervical

l.n., superficial inguinal
l.n., superior mesenteric
l.n., superior tracheobronchial
l.n., supraclavicular
l.n., swollen
l.n. syndrome (MLNS), mucocutaneous
l.n. system
l.n., tracheal
l.n., tracheobronchial
l.n. ▸ underarm
lymphadenectomy
l., cervical
l. of intrathoracic esophageal cancer
l., staging
lymphadenia ossea
lymphadenitis
l., caseous
l., mesenteric
l., Mycobacterium
l., paratuberculous
lymphadenoid tissue
lymphadenoid tissue ▸ enlargement of
lymphadenoma cells
lymphadenopathy
l., angioblastic
l., angioimmunoblastic
l. -associated virus
l., axillary
l., benign
l., dermatopathic
l., generalized
l., giant follicular
l., hilar
l., mesenteric
l., neck
l. of axilla, bubonic
l. of groin, bubonic
l., palpable
l., palpable femoral
l., periaortic
l., subcarinal
l. syndrome (LAS)
lymphangiectasis, chronic pulmonary cystic
lymphangiectasis, congenital pulmonary
lymphangiogram, abdominal
lymphangiogram study
lymphangioma circumscriptum
lymphangioma cysticum
lymphangitic
l. carcinoma

l. carcinomatosis
l. metastases
l. pattern of cancer spread
l. spread
l. spread of prostatic adenocarcinoma
lymphatic(s)
l. cachexia
l. cancer
l. capillaries
l. chain
l. channel
l. channel ▸ dilated
l. channels, para-aortic
l. choriomeningitis (LCM)
l. disorder
l. drainage (dr'ge)
l. drainage ▸ interrupted
l. drainage of esophagus
l. duct
l. dyscrasia
l. edema
l. fluid
l., invasion of
l. involvement
l. involvement, dermal
l. leukemia
l. leukemia, chronic
l. mapping
l. metastases
l. metastases, cervical
l. nodules
l. nodules ▸ minute,
l. nodules of large intestine ▸ solitary
l. nodules of small intestine ▸ solitary
l. nodules of stomach
l. obstruction
l. ▸ obtuse marginal
l. sinuses
l. spread
l. spread of nasopharyngeal carcinoma
l. spread pattern of lung carcinoma
l., subclavian
l. system
l. system ▸ malignancy of
l. tissue
l. tuberculosis
l. vessels
lymphatica
l., Filaria
l., influenza

l., pseudoleukemia
l., vasa
lymphatici, hilus nodi
lymphatici ▸ vasa afferentia nodi
lymphatici ▸ vasa efferentia nodi
lymphaticum profundum ▸ vas
lymphaticum superficiale ▸ vas
lymphaticus, status
lymphedema
l. ▸ patient has
l. praecox
l. therapy
lymphoblast mutation assay
lymphoblastic
l. leukemia
l. leukemia (ALL), acute
l. leukemia antigen, common acute
l. leukemia, null cell
l. lymphoma
l. lymphosarcoma
l. transformation
lymphoblastoma, giant follicular
lymphocapillare, vas
lymphocyte(s)
l. activator
l. antigen, cutaneous
l. antigen (HLA), human
l. antigen ▸ large granular
l. antigen ▸ thymic
l. antigen typing ▸ human
l., atypical
l. binding ▸ T-
l. count, decreased peripheral
l. count, peripheral
l. culture, mixed
l. depleted type ▸ Hodgkin's disease of diffuse, histiocytic
l. depletion
l., donor and recipient
l. ▸ foamy histiocytes and
l. function antigen
l., functioning
l., (TIL) ▸ genetically altered tumor infiltrating
l. immune globulin
l. irradiation and phytohemagglutinin
l., mature
l., mitogenic stimulation of
l., neoplastic
l. (NPDL), nodular poorly differentiated
l. ▸ perivascular infiltrate of
l., plasmacytoid

l. proliferation assay
l. ratio (M:L) ▸ monocyte-
l., reticular
l. serum, antihuman-
l., suppressor
l., T
l. (TIL) technique, tumor infiltrating
l. test ▸ primed
l., T-4
l. transfer test
l. transfer test, normal
l. transformation ▸ antigen specific
l. transformation, human
l. trapping
l., tumor fighting
l. (TIL), tumor infiltrating
lymphocytic
l. aggregates, focal
l. cell infiltration
l. cells
l. choriomeningitis (LCM)
l. choriomeningitis (LCM) virus
l. depletion, severe
l. disease, chronic
l. infiltrate
l. infiltrates, scattered
l. infiltrative disease
l. infiltrative disorder
l. interstitial pneumonitis
l. leukemia
l. leukemia, acute
l. leukemia, Burkitt-type acute
l. leukemia (CLL), chronic
l. leukemia variant, chronic
l. leukocytosis
l. lymphoma
l. lymphoma, diffuse
l. lymphoma, poorly differentiated
l. lymphosarcoma
l. meningitis
l. meningitis, benign
l. nodules, scattered
l. peribronchial infiltrate
l. thyroiditis
l. thyroiditis, chronic
l. thyroiditis ▸ nonspecific chronic
lymphocytoma cutis
lymphocytosis, neutrophilic
lymphoepithelial carcinoma
lymphoepithelial lesion, benign
lymphoepithelioma
l., nasopharyngeal
l. of nasopharynx
l. of thymus
lymphogenous embolism

lymphogenous leukemia
lymphoglandulae ▸ vasa afferentia
lymphoglandulae ▸ vasa efferentia
lymphogranuloma
- l. benignum
- l. inguinale
- l., Schaumann's benign
- l., venereal
- l. venereum
- l. venereum antigen
- l. venereum psittacosis infection
- l. venereum virus

lymphogranulomatosis, Miyagawanella
lymphoid
- l. aggregate
- l. alveolitis
- l. depletion
- l. depletion of follicles
- l. depletion of lymph nodes
- l. follicles
- l. hyperplasia
- l. hypertrophy
- l. infiltrate
- l. infiltrate ▸ focal areas of
- l. infiltration, diffuse
- l. interstitial pneumonia
- l. irradiation
- l. irradiation for allograft survival, total
- l. irradiation in arthritis, total
- l. irradiation in organ transplantation, total
- l. irradiation in rheumatoid arthritis, total
- l. irradiation, total
- l. leukemia
- l. leukosis
- l. masses
- l. plasma
- l. polyps
- l. thyroiditis
- l. tissue
- l. tissue (GALT) ▸ gut-associated
- l. tissue, residual

lymphoidocytic leukemia
lymphokine-activated killer (LAK) cell
lymphoma
- l. ▸ African Burkitt's
- l., B cell
- l., Burkitt's
- l., clasmocytic
- l., cutaneous T-cell
- l. (DHL), diffuse histiocytic

- l. ▸ diffuse histiocytic type abdominal
- l., diffuse lymphocytic
- l., diffuse non-Hodgkin's
- l., disseminated malignant
- l. ▸ erythrodermic cutaneous T-cell
- l., gastric
- l., giant follicular
- l. glands, swollen
- l., granulomatous
- l., histiocytic
- l., histiocytic malignant
- l., immunoblastic
- l. implant
- l., intestinal
- l., intraocular
- l., lymph cell
- l., lymphoblastic
- l., lymphocytic
- l., malignant
- l., malignant histiocytic
- l. ▸ mantle cell
- l., nodular
- l., nodular non-Hodgkin's
- l. ▸ noncleaved cell
- l., nonhistiocytic type
- l., non-Hodgkin's
- l., null-type non-Hodgkin's
- l. of ocular adnexa
- l. of orbit
- l. of retina, malignant
- l. of stomach ▸ diffuse histiocytic
- l. of stomach ▸ non-Hodgkin's
- l., poorly differentiated lymphocytic
- l., primary central nervous system (CNS)
- l., pulmonary
- l., stem cell
- l. ▸ T-cell
- l., testicular
- l. treatment
- l., undifferentiated
- l., undifferentiated malignant

lymphomatoid granuloma
lymphomatosa, struma
lymphomatosum, papillary adenocystoma
lymphomatous infiltrate, diffuse
lymphonodular pharyngitis
lymphopathia venereum
lymphoproliferative
- l. disease
- l. disorder
- l. syndrome
- l. (XLP) syndrome ▸ X-linked

- l., X-linked

lymphosarcoma
- l. cell leukemia
- l. cell leukemia, chronic
- l., follicular
- l., Kundrat's
- l., lymphoblastic
- l., lymphocytic
- l., malignant
- l. of lacrimal gland
- l. reticulum cell sarcoma

lymphosarcomatous nodules
lymphoscintigraphy, internal mammary
lymphoscintigraphy, nuclear
Lymphotropic Virus (HTLV), Human T-Cell
lymphotropic virus type ▸ simian T-cell
Lynch syndrome
Lynchia maura
Lyon hypothesis
Lyon-Horgan operation
Lyperosia irritans
lyra
- l. uteri
- l. uterina
- l. vaginae

lyre of uterus
lyre of vagina
lysed, adhesions
lysed, clot
lysergic acid diethylamide (LSD)
- l. acid diethylamide (LSD) addict
- l. acid diethylamide (LSD) addiction
- l. acid diethylamide (LSD) dependency
- l. acid diethylamide (LSD) habit
- l. acid diethylamide (LSD)-induced psychosis
- l. acid diethylamide (LSD) ingested
- l. acid diethylamide (LSD) intoxication
- l. acid diethylamide (LSD) user
- l. acid diethylamide (LSD) withdrawal

Lysholm maneuver, Engel-lysine pitressin spray
lysing system ▸ transluminal
lysis
- l., clot
- l., dilute blood clot
- l., hot-cold
- l. of adhesions
- l. of bacteria, transmissible

    l. of cell
    l. pelvic adhesions
    l. time
    l. time, blood clot
    l. time, clot
    l. time, euglobulin
    l. time, euglobulin clot
    l. time ▸ streptokinase clot
lysodeikticus, Micrococcus
lysozyme, human milk
Lyssa body
lytic
    l. activity, fibrin
    l. area
    l. blastic changes
    l. bone lesions
    l. cocktail
    l. defect
    l. disease
    l. lesion
    l. lesion, expansile
    l., osteo◊
    l. state
    l. virus

M

M (megohm)
m (meter)
m (minim)
M cell
M. (mucoid) colony
M component
M contrast medium, Hypaque
M gate
M protein
MA (ma)
    MA (mental age)
    ma (meter-angle)
    ma (milliampere)
MAA (macroaggregated albumin)
MABP (mean arterial blood pressure)
MAC (maximum allowable
    concentration)
MAC (minimum alveolar
    concentration)
MAC (Mycobacterium avium
    complex) infection
Macaca
    M. cynomulgus
    M. mulatta
    M. speciosa
MacAusland's operation
macedonicum, Phlebotomus
macellaria, Chrysomyia
macerated [*lacerated*]
    m. fetus
    m. infant
    m. stillborn
maceration [*laceration*]
maceration, perianal
maceration, skin
Macewen's
    M. operation
    M. osteotomy
    M. sign
macfadyani, Malassezia
MacFee neck flap
Mache unit
Machek('s)
    M. -Blaskovics operation
    M. Gifford operation
    M. operation
machination [*maturation*]

machine(s)
    m., artificial kidney
    m., bypass
    m., cardiopulmonary bypass
    m., cesium 137 teletherapy
    m., cobalt-60 teletherapy
    m., computerized visual field
    m., dialysis
    m. for cleansing ▸ patient's blood
        circulated to
    m., heart-lung
    m., laser beam
    m., life-prolonging
    m., lithotripter
    m. ▸ magnetic resonance imaging
    m., MediPort
    m., MixEvac
    m., Offner electroencephalogram
        (EEG)
    m., polygraph
    m. ▸ polymerase chain reaction
        (PCR)
    m., portable analyzing
    m., portable electrocardiogram
        (ECG/EKG)
    m., portable x-ray
    m., quality assurance in treatment
    m., rowing
    m., suction
    m. units (mu)
    m., Van de Graaff
machinery murmur
MacIntosh
    M., pivot shift test
    M. prosthesis
    M. tibial plateau prosthesis
Mackay-Marg tonometer
Mackenrodt's ligament
Mackenrodt's operation
MacKenty('s)
    M. choanal plug
    M. nasal pack
    M. tube
MacKenzie's amputation
Mackler intraluminal tube prosthesis
MacLeod's capsular rheumatism
Macracanthorhynchus hirudinaceus

macro [*micro*]
macroaggregated
    m. albumin (MAA)
    m. albumin, iodinated
    m. ferrous hydroxide
macroangiopathy, coronary
Macrobdella decora
macrobiotic diet
macrobiotic therapy
macrocheilia/macrochilia
macrocythemia, hyperchromatic
macrocystic
    m. adenoma
    m. pilocytic astrocytoma
    m. pilocytic cerebellar astro-
        cytoma
macrocytic
    m. anemia
    m. anemia ▸ tropical
    m. hyperchromatism
macrodentium, Treponema
macrodontia, generalized
macrofollicular adenoma
macrofolliculoid, carcinoma
macroglobulinemia, Waldenstrom's
macro-Kjeldahl technique
macrolide antimicrobial agent
macromaniacal delirium
macromastia, severe
macromelia paresthetica
macromolecular ligand
Macromonas bipunctata
Macromonas mobilis
macrophage(s)
    m., alveolar
    m., brown pigment laden
    m. cells
    m. colony stimulating factor (GM-
        CSF), human granulocytic-
    m. defects
    m., fixed
    m., foamy
    m., free
    m., hemosiderin laden
    m., inflammatory
    m. inhibiting factor
    m. lineage antigen

macrophage(s)—*continued*
- m. -mediated cytotoxicity
- m., tissue

macroreentrant atrial tachycardia
macroreentrant circuit
macroreentry orthodromic
   tachycardia ▸ reciprocating
macroscopic [*microscopic*]
- m. agglutination
- m. anatomy
- m. central nervous system (CNS) lesion
- m. lesion

macrosomatia adiposa congenital
macrosomia, fetal
Macrostoma mesnili
Macrotherapy dermagraphic
macrovascular
- m. complication
- m. coronary lesion
- m. disease, accelerated

macula
- m. acustica sacculi
- m. acustica utriculi
- m. albida
- m. corneae
- m. ▸ deterioration of
- m., edema of
- m., false
- m. gonorrhoeica
- m. lactea
- m. lutea retinae
- m. retinae
- m. sacculi
- m., Saenger's
- m. tendinea
- m. utriculi

macular
- m. atrophy
- m. change
- m. degeneration
- m. degeneration (ARMD) ▸ advanced age-related
- m. degeneration (AMD), age-related
- m. degeneration ▸ atrophic
- m. degeneration, congenital
- m. degeneration, dry
- m. degeneration (ARMD) ▸ dry, age-related
- m. degeneration ▸ exudative
- m. degeneration (ARMD) ▸ intermediate age-related
- m. degeneration ▸ juvenile
- m. degeneration, senile

- m. degeneration, vitelliform
- m. degeneration ▸ wet
- m. degeneration (ARMD) ▸ wet age-related
- m. depression
- m. deterioration of retina
- m. displacement
- m. dystrophy ▸ Best's
- m. edema
- m. edema, diabetic
- m. edema, persistent
- m. fever
- m. infarction
- m. ischemia
- m. motion
- m. neuroretinopathy, acute
- m. rash
- m. rash, polymorphous
- m. seborrhea

macularis inferior, venula
macularis superior, venula
maculata, Cicuta
maculation, pernicious
maculatum, Amblyomma
macules
- m., erythematous
- m. of palms and soles, erythematous
- m. on heel and sole ▸ hyperpigmented
- m. on legs ▸ hypopigmented
- m., reddish
- m., violaceous

maculipennis, Anopheles
maculopapular
- m. lesion
- m. rash
- m. rash ▸ erythematous

maculopathy, bull's eye
maculopathy, Valsalva
maculosa, purpura
maculosa, urticaria
mad
- m. cow disease
- m. itch
- m. syndrome ▸ scratch like

madagascariensis, Raillietina
madagascariensis, Taenia
madampensis ▸ Escherichia dispar var.
madampensis, Shigella
Maddox
- M. prism
- M. rod test
- M. rods

made arch bar ▸ custom-
made chorea ▸ school-
Madlener operation
Madelung's deformity
Madonna fingers
Madox
Madura foot
madurae
- m., Actinomadura
- m., Nocardia
- m., Streptomyces

Madurella
- M. fungi
- M. grisea
- M. mycetomi

Maeder-Danis dystrophy
Maestro implantable cardiac pacemaker
Maffucci's syndrome
magalhaesi, Dirofilaria
Magee syndrome ▸ Shy-
Magendie('s)
- M. foramen
- M. law
- M. law, Bell-
- M. phenomenon
- M. solution
- M. space
- M. syndrome, Hertwig-

magenta, basic
magenta tongue
magic (MAGIC)
- m. angle
- m. mushrooms (psilocybin)
- M. (Magnesium in Coronaries) trial

magical thinking
Magitot's operation
magna (Magna)
- m., cisterna
- m., coxa
- m., Fasciola
- M. -Helic gauge

magnesia, milk of
magnesium (Magnesium)
- m. blood levels
- m. carbonate
- m., chelated
- m. chloride
- m. concentration, low
- m. deficiency
- m. deficiency ▸ intracellular
- m. deficiency, symptomatic
- m. ▸ depletion of potassium
- m. gluconate
- m. homeostasis

M. in Coronaries (MAGIC) trial
m. ▸ intracellular level of
m., intravenous
m. ▸ intravenous infusion of
m. level, abnormal
m. level, low
m. ▸ low intracellular-free
m. oxide
m., patient's serum
m. poisoning
m. ribonuclease
m. test
m. test, intracellular
m. therapy

magnet
m., beam-bending
m., bronchoscopic
m., Grüning's
m., Haab's
m., Hirschberg's
m., Lancaster's
m. mode
m. operation
m. pacing interval
m. rate
m., Storz
m. testing
m. therapy
m. wire

magnetic (Magnetic)
m. bead
m. circuit
m. energy
m. energy ▸ units of
m. extraction
m. field
m. field inhomogeneity artifact ▸ main
m. fusion
m. gait
m. implant
m. induction coaxial electrode system
m. moment
m. relaxation time
m. removal
m. resonance angiography (MRA)
m. resonance angiography (carotid MRA) ▸ contrast enhanced carotid
m. resonance angiography (MRA) ▸ intracranial
m. resonance angiography (MRA) ▸ selective arterial

m. resonance angiography (MRA) ▸ selective venous
m. resonance (MR) brain scan
m. resonance flowmetry (MRF)
m. resonance image (MRI)
m. resonance imaging (MRI)
m. resonance imaging (fMRI) brain scan ▸ functional
m. resonance imaging (EEMRI) coil ▸ endoesophageal
m. resonance imaging (MRI), conventional
m. resonance imaging (MRI) ▸ diffusion weighted
m. resonance imaging (MRI) ▸ enhancement of
m. resonance imaging (fMRI/MRI) ▸ functional
m. resonance imaging (MRI) ▸ gated sweep
m. resonance imaging (MRI) machine
m. resonance imaging (NMRI) ▸ nuclear
m. resonance imaging (MRI) scan
m. resonance imaging (MRI) scan, side-view
m. resonance imaging (MRI) scanner
m. resonance imaging (MRI) spectrometer
m. resonance imaging (MRI) ▸ spin-echo
m. resonance imaging (MRI) ▸ velocity encoded cine-
m. resonance (NMR), nuclear
m. resonance scanner
M. Resonance Scanner (NMRS), Nuclear
m. resonance (MR) signal
m. resonance spectography (MRS)
m. resonance spectroscopy (MRS)
m. resonance spectroscopy imaging (MRSI)
m. resonance (NMR) spectroscopy ▸ nuclear
m. resonator imaging (MRI) scan, enhanced
m. source imaging (MSI)
m. stimulation ▸ transcranial
m. susceptibility artifact
magnetically confined plasma
magnetically traceable element
magnetism, intensity of

magnetization precession angle
magnetoencephalography (MEG) technique
magnification
m. angiography
m., cardiologic
m., high-powered
m. ▸ x-ray
magnifying lens
magnifying loupe
magnitude
m., average pulse
m. of QRS ▸ maximum
m. of risk
m., peak
m., sensation
m. shunt
m., stimulus
m. voluntary heart rate changes ▸ large
Magnolia
M. acuminata
M. glauca
M. tripetala
magnum
m., foramen
m., foramen occipitale
m., os
magnus (Magnus)
M. and de Kleijn neck reflex
m., Diplococcus
m. muscle, adductor
Magnuson('s)
M. abductor humerus splint
M. modified arthroplasty
M. operation
M. reduction technique
M. -Stack operation
M. -Stack shoulder arthroplasty
M. -Cromie prosthesis
M. -Cromie valve prosthesis
M. valve prosthesis ▸ 4-A
mah (milliampere hours)
Mahaim bundle
Mahaim fiber ▸ fasciculoventricular
Maher's disease
mahogany flush
Mahorner echocardiogram ▸ Ochsner-
MAI (Mycobacterium avium intracellulare) complex
MAI (Mycobacterium avium intracellulare) infection
Maier disease ▸ Kussmaul-
maieutic, Horrocks'

mailed in prior to admission
- ▸ orders

Mailith pacemaker, CPI

main
- m. bronchi
- m. bronchus, left
- m. bronchus, partial occlusion
- m. bronchus, right
- m. bundle
- m. circumflex, distal portion
- m. coronary artery (ALMCA), anomalous left
- m. coronary artery disease ▸ left
- m. coronary artery ▸ right
- m. coronary stenosis ▸ left
- m. en crochet
- m. en griffe
- m. en lorgnette
- m. en pince
- m. equivalency ▸ left
- m. fourché
- m. magnetic field inhomogeneity artifact
- m. pulmonary artery ▸ invisible
- m. pulmonary artery, right
- m. renal vein
- m. sensory pathways
- m. solution line
- m. stem
- m. stem bronchus
- m. stem bronchus ▸ distortion left
- m. stem bronchus, right

Mainini test, Galli-

mainliner and/or skin popper

mainstem bronchus ▸ occlusion of

mainstream smoke

maintain
- m. abstinence
- m. attention ▸ inability to
- m. balance and coordination
- m. blood glucose levels
- m. equilibrium ▸ inability to
- m. eye contact
- m. mobility of patient
- m. muscle flexibility
- m. muscle strength
- m. sobriety and abstinence
- m. stable weight
- m. systolic pressure

maintained
- m., adequate hemostasis
- m. pressure
- m., vital functions artificially

maintaining
- m. fluid balance

- m. joint range of motion
- m. sleep
- m. sleep (DIMS), disturbance in
- m. sleep ▸ persistent disorder of
- m. sleep ▸ transient disorder of
- m. sobriety
- m. wakefulness ▸ persistent disorder of
- m. wakefulness ▸ transient disorder of

maintenance (Maintenance)
- m., airway
- m., altered health
- m. chemotherapy
- m. chemotherapy, continuing
- m., cognitive
- m. depth
- m. dialysis
- m. dialysis, chronic
- m. diet
- m. disorder, sleep
- m., donor
- m. dosage
- m. dose
- m. drinking
- M., Engineering and
- m., fluid
- m. hemodialysis
- m. ▸ inadequate tissue
- m. infection
- m. insomnia, sleep
- m. level
- m. management ▸ impaired home
- m., medical
- m., methadone
- m. of nervous system
- m., opioid
- m. organization (HMO), health
- m., preventive
- m. ▸ principles of donor
- m. program
- m. skills
- m. therapy
- m. therapy, chronic
- m. treatment program ▸ methadone
- m., weight

Maisonneuve's
- M. amputation
- M. fracture
- M. sign

maitre, tour de

Maixner's cirrhosis

Masjewsky's operation

Majocchi's granuloma

major
- m. affective disorder
- m. affective disorder, predominance of
- m. airway, blunt injury of
- m. airway, penetrating injury of
- m. amputation
- m. anemia, thalassemia
- m., anulus iridis
- m. arterial thrombosis
- m., beta thalassemia
- m. blockage
- m. blockage carotid vessels
- m. blood vessel
- m. body movements
- m. calyces
- m., chorea
- m. contraindication to surgery
- m. convulsions
- m. curve, double
- m. depression
- m. depression, in full remission
- m. depression, in partial remission
- m. depression, mild
- m. depression, moderate
- m. depression, recurrent
- m. depression, recurrent, in full remission
- m. depression, recurrent, in partial remission
- m. depression, recurrent, mild
- m. depression, recurrent, moderate
- m. depression, recurrent, severe, without psychotic features
- m. depression, recurrent, unspecified
- m. depression, recurrent, with psychotic features
- m. depression, severe, without psychotic features
- m. depression, single episode
- m. depression, single episode, in full remission
- m. depression, single episode, in partial remission
- m. depression, single episode, mild
- m. depression, single episode, moderate
- m. depression, single episode, severe without psychotic features
- m. depression, single episode, unspecified
- m. depression, single episode, with psychotic features

m. depression, with psychotic features
m. depressive disorder (MDD)
m. depressive disorder, recurrent episode
m. depressive disorder, single episode
m. depressive episode
m. drug dealer
m. epididymidis, globus
m. epilepsy
m. fracture
m. functional impairment
m. hand, left
m. hand, right
m. health threat
m. histocompatibility antigen
m. histocompatibility complex antigen
m. impairment
m. intra-abdominal surgery
m., Leptothrix
m. mental disorder
m. mental illness
m. mood disorder
m. motivator
m. motor group
m. muscle, pectoralis
m., musculus pectoralis
m., musculus teres
m., musculus helicis
m. obstruction carotid vessels
m. obstruction of esophagus
m. organ failure
m. organ replacement
m. organ system malfunctions
m. organs, obstruction of
m. overload
m., pectoralis
m. pelvis aequabiliter justo
m. physical trauma
m. risk factor
m., Siderocapsa
m., Sideromonas
m. spinal nerves
m. stress evoking event
m. stroke
m. surgery, risk of
m., thalassemia
m. thoracic surgery
m. tranquilizers
m. trauma
m. treatment modality
m. vessel, venous-
m. viral strains

majora, labia
Majorner-Mead operation
majus
  m., Ammi
  m., labia
  m., omentum
Make-A-Picture-Story Test
make(s) (Make)
  m. abuse statements
  m. arthritis stop hurting (MASH)
  m. deliberate actions ▸ patient
  m. decisions ▸ inability to
  m. decisions ▸ unwilling to
  m. full fist, patient
  m. obscene gestures
  m. obscene statements
maker(s) Maker('s)
  m. disease, barometer
  m., DNA (deoxyribonucleic acid)
  m., surrogate decision
makeup, genetic
makeup, psychological
making
  m., clinical decision-
  m., decision
  m. decisions ▸ incapable of
  m. ▸ difficulty in decision
  m., health care decision-
  m. ▸ interference with judgment and decision
  m., personal decision-
  m. process, decision-
  m. skills, decision-
Makin's murmur
MAL (midaxillary line)
mal
  m., compatible with grand
  m., compatible with petit
  m. convulsion ▸ petit
  m. de mer
  m. discharge, miniature petit
  m. discharge, petit
  m. discharge, pseudo petit
  m. epilepsy, grand
  m. epilepsy, haut
  m. epilepsy, myoclonic petit
  m. epilepsy, petit
  m. (GM) ▸ grand
  m., petit
  m., pseudo petit
  m. seizure, grand
  m. seizures, isolated grand
  m. seizures ▸ uncontrolled generalized grand
  m. status, grand

m. status, petit
m. substances, antipetit
m., true petit
m. variant ▸ compatible with petit
m. variant discharge, petit
m. variant, petit
malabsorption
  m., intestinal
  m., nutrient
  m. of vitamins and minerals
  m., pancreatic insufficiency with
  m., small bowel
  m. syndrome
  m. syndrome ▸ bloating from
  m. syndrome, methionine
malacia, chondrodystrophy
malacoplakia/malakoplakia
malacotic teeth
maladaptation, emotional
maladaptive
  m. antisocial personality traits
  m. behavior, continued
  m. consequences
  m. grief
  m. pattern
  m. technique
  m. traits
maladie-de-Roger disease
maladjusted, emotionally
maladjusted, sexually
maladjustment
  m., adult
  m., history of
  m., psychological
  m., social
maladroit, socially
malady, crippling
malady, physical
malaise
  m. and weakness
  m., fatigue and
  m., general
  m., generalized feeling of
malaligned teeth
Malameba locustae
malar
  m. arch
  m. area
  m. bone
  m. eminence
  m. eminence of face
  m. flush
malaria
  m., benign tertian
  m., cerebral

malaria—*continued*
- m., falciparum
- m. fever therapy
- m. film test
- m. prophylaxis

malariae, Plasmodium

malarial
- m. cachexia
- m. cirrhosis
- m. dysentery
- m. fever
- m. granuloma
- m. parasite
- m. pneumonitis
- m. stippling

Malassezia
- M. furfur
- M. macfadyani
- M. tropica

malayi, Brugia

malayi, Wuchereria

maldeveloped nervous system

maldevelopment, cardiovascular

male
- m. adult genitalia, normal
- m. alopecia
- m. baldness
- m. breast enlargement
- m. breast reduction
- m. carriers of AIDS (acquired immune deficiency syndrome), heterosexual contact with
- m. ▸ chills with genital pain in
- m. erectile disorder
- m. gender
- m. genitalia, infantile
- m. genitalia, normal
- m. genitalia, premature
- m. gynecomastia
- m. homosexual contact
- m. hormone
- m. hormone production
- m. hormones, synthetic
- m. hormone testosterone
- m. impotence after childbirth
- m. infant, viable
- m. infertility
- m. infertility problem
- m. intersex
- m. menopause
- m. neonate, term AGA (appropriate for gestational age)
- m. orgasm, inhibited
- m. (b/m) ▸ patient black
- m., patient Caucasian

- m., patient Indian
- m., patient Oriental
- m. (wh/m) ▸ patient white
- m. pattern baldness
- m. pattern obesity
- m., prepubescent
- m. rat brain
- m. reproductive tract, cancer of
- m. sex hormone
- m. sexual dysfunction
- m. sterility
- m. syndrome (IMS) ▸ irritable
- m., uncircumcised
- m. urethra, navicular fossa of
- m. urethra, orifice of

maleate provocation angina ▸ ergonovine

malformation
- m., aneurysm or vascular
- m., Arnold-Chiari
- m., arteriovascular
- m. (AVM), arteriovenous
- m. (AVM), atrioventricular
- m. at birth
- m., brain
- m., bronchopulmonary foregut
- m., cardiovascular
- m., cerebellar
- m., congenital
- m., congenital cardiovascular
- m., fetal
- m., heart
- m., intracardiac
- m. ▸ intracranial vascular
- m., kidney
- m., Mondini
- m. ▸ Mondini pulmonary arteriovenous
- m. ▸ neural crest
- m. of blood vessel
- m. of brain, arteriovenous
- m. of brain vessels
- m. of chest wall
- m. of fetal bladder
- m. of pinna
- m. of tricuspid valve ▸ Ebstein's
- m., organ
- m. ▸ pulmonary arteriovenous
- m., tooth
- m., vascular

malformed
- m. esophagus, congenital
- m. fetus
- m. heart or heart valve
- m. maxilla

- m. middle ear
- m. nails
- m. outer ear
- m. reproductive systems

malfunction
- m. ▸ age-related muscle
- m. ▸ automatic implantable defibrillator (AID)
- m. ▸ bone marrow
- m., brain
- m. ▸ brain cell
- m., cardiac
- m., cognitive
- m., equipment
- m., esophageal
- m., gene
- m., instrumental
- m., intestinal
- m., kidney
- m., liver
- m. ▸ major organ system
- m., nerve
- m. of permanent demand ventricular pacing system
- m. of valve
- m., organ
- m., pacemaker
- m., peripheral nerve
- m., physiological
- m. ▸ protein calorie
- m., psychogenic genitourinary
- m., psychophysiological
- m., thyroid
- m., valve
- m., vein-valve

malfunctioning
- m. cells
- m. immune system
- m. insulin-receptor cells
- m., mental
- m., sexual
- m., sphincter
- m. valve, clicking of

Malgaigne's fracture

Malgaigne's luxation

Malherbe's epithelioma

malic dehydrogenase

maligna, lentigo

maligna melanoma, lentigo

malignancy
- m., advanced
- m., advanced lung
- m. -associated changes
- m., bone marrow
- m., bowel

m., brain
m., breast
m., carcinoid
m., cytology brushings for
m., dermal
m. endobronchial
m., epithelial
m., fracture caused by
m., gastrointestinal (GI)
m., generalized
m., gynecologic
m., gynecological
m., hematologic
m., inoperable
m., inoperable bladder
m., ocular adnexal
m. of liver, carcinoid metastatic
m. of lymphatic system
m., pelvic
m., progressive
m. ▸ radiation-induced
m., renal
m., reticuloendothelial
m., tissue negative for
m., underlying

malignant

m. alopecia
m. angioendotheliomatosis
m. anthrax
m. astrocytoma
m. beat
m. blood disorder
m. brain tumor
m. calcifications of breast
m. carcinoid syndrome
m. cardiac tumor, primary
m. cells
m. cell change
m. diagnosis
m. disease
m. disease of blood
m. disease of pleura
m. disorder ▸ pre-
m. dysentery
m. edema
m. effusion
m. endocarditis
m. esophageal stenosis
m. esophageal stenosis ▸ palliation of
m. external otitis
m. fibrous histiocytoma
m. fibrous mesothelioma
m. germ cell mediastinal tumor
m. glaucoma

m. granulomatosis
m. growth
m. histiocytic lymphoma
m. histiocytoma
m. histiocytosis, infantile
m., histologically
m. hyperpyrexia
m. hypertension
m. hyperthermia
m. infiltration
m. keratoma
m. lesion
m. lesion, borderline
m. leukopenia
m. lymphoma
m. lymphoma, disseminated
m. lymphoma, histiocytic
m. lymphoma of retina
m. lymphoma, undifferentiated
m. lymphosarcoma
m. mediastinal tumor
m. melanoma
m. melanoma, Clark's level of
m. melanoma, cutaneous
m. melanoma, localized
m. melanoma, metastatic
m. melanoma of extremity
m. melanoma, unpigmented
m. meningitis, metastatic
m. mesothelioma
m. mesothelioma of peritoneum
m., metastatic or benign lesion
m. myeloma
m. neoplasm
m. nephrosclerosis
m. neuroleptic syndrome
m. ovarian cyst
m. parotid tumor
m. pleural effusion
m. polymorphic reticulosis, midline
m. polyp
m. polyp ▸ pre-
m. process
m. renal tumor
m. reticulopathy
m. schwannoma
m. skull base lesion
m. stricture
m. teratoma
m. teratoma, intermediate
m. teratoma, trophoblastic
m. thrombocytopenia
m. thyroid nodule
m. tissue
m. tracheoesophageal fistula

m. transformation of cell
m. trophoblastic tumor
m. tumor
m. tumor of kidney
m. tumor of urinary bladder
m. tumors, classification of
m. uterine cancer
m. vascular tumor
m. ventricular arrhythmia
m. ventricular tachycardia

maligni No. II ▸ Bacillus oedematis
malignum

m., chorioepithelioma
m., Eurotium
m., syncytioma

malignus, pemphigus
mali-mali
malingering and deception
malingering, patient
mall walk
mall walking program
malleability, memory
mallear

m. fold of mucous membrane of tympanum
m. fold of tympanic membrane ▸ anterior
m. fold of tympanic membrane ▸ posterior

malleatory chorea
mallei

m., Actinobacillus
m., Bacillus
m., gram-negative Malleomyces
m., Malleomyces
m., Pseudomonas

mallein test
malleo-incudal joint
malleolar fold
malleolar fracture
malleolus [*malleus*]

m., external
m., fibular
m., inner
m., internal
m., lateral
m., medial
m. muscle, medial
m. of tibia ▸ medial
m., outer
m., radial
m., tibial
m., ulnar

Malleomyces

M. mallei

Malleomyces—*continued*
- M. mallei, gram-negative
- M. pseudomallei
- M. whitmori

mallet finger

mallet toe

malleus [*malleolus*]
- m., anterior ligament of
- m. bone
- m., cog-tooth of
- m., external ligament of
- m., hallux
- m. handle
- m., head of
- m., lateral ligament of
- m., lateral process of
- m., manubrium of
- m., spur of

Mallinckrodt radioimmunoassay

Mallory
- M. bodies
- M. pacemaker
- M. stain
- M. -Weiss syndrome
- M. -Weiss tear

Mallotus philippinensis

malnourished
- m., intrauterine fetally
- m., multiple caries, foul sputum
- m. patient
- m. patient with chronic disease
- m., severely

malnourishment, severe

malnutrition
- m., alcoholic
- m., marked
- m., myocardial
- m. of child
- m., patient suffering from
- m., protein calorie

malocclusion, closed-bite

malocclusion, open-bite

malodorous
- m. breath
- m. discharge, purulent
- m. stools ▸ pale and
- m. sweat
- m. vaginal discharge

malomaxillary suture

Malpighamoeba mellifcae

Malpighia punicifolia

malpighian
- m. bodies
- m. capsule
- m. cells
- m. corpuscle
- m. follicles
- m. glomerulus
- m. layer
- m. rete
- m. stigma
- m. tuft

Malpighi's vesicles

malplacement ▸ endotracheal tube

malposed tooth

malposition
- m., crisscross heart
- m. ▸ double outlet left ventricle (LV)
- m. ▸ double outlet right ventricle (RV)
- m., levocardia
- m., mesocardia
- m. of great arteries
- m. ▸ single ventricle

malpractice
- m. crisis
- m. defense
- m. liability exposure
- m., medical

malrotation, intestinal

malsensing, atrial

malt sugar

Malta fever

maltophilia
- m., Pseudallescheria
- m., Pseudomonas
- m., Xanthomonas

maltreatment, medical

malum
- m. articulorum senilis
- m. cordis
- m. coxae senilis

malunion, fracture with

malunited fracture

MAM (milliampere minute)

mamillary suture

mamillary system

mammae, areola

mammae, cirrhosis

mammalian cells

mammalian tissue, living

mammaplasty (mammoplasty)

mammaplasty, Aries-Pitanguy

mammaplasty, augmentation

mammary
- m. artery
- m. artery bypass, internal
- m. artery catheter ▸ internal
- m. artery, external
- m. artery graft

- m. artery graft angiography ▸ internal
- m. artery, internal
- m. artery (LIMA) ▸ left internal
- m. artery ▸ right internal
- m. artery transplant
- m. cancer, metastatic
- m. chain, internal
- m. cycle
- m. dose, internal
- m. duct
- m. duct ectasia
- m. dysplasia
- m. field, matching tangential field with internal
- m. fold
- m. gland
- m. gland, areola of
- m. gland, lobules of
- m. graft ▸ internal
- m. implant, Surgitek
- m. involvement, internal
- m. lymphoscintigraphy, internal
- m. lymph nodes, internal
- m. prosthesis
- m. ptosis procedure, Aries-Pitanguy
- m. region
- m. serum antigen
- m. souffle murmur
- m. souffle sound
- m. support dressing, Jobst
- m. tumor virus
- m. vein, external
- m. vein, internal
- m. vessels

mammillary bodies

mammillary nucleus of Rose, lateral

mammogram(s)
- m., annual
- m., baseline
- m. checkup
- m., digital
- m. lesion, suspicious
- m. ▸ reduced effectiveness of
- m., regular
- m., routine
- m. screening
- m., suspicious

mammographic findings

mammography
- m. center
- m., computerized digital
- m., early detection through
- m. examination

m., film screen
m. images, digital
m. radiation
m., routine
m., screening
m. unit, mobile
m. (XEM) ▸ xonics electron
m., x-ray

mammoplasty/mammiplasty
m. augmentation
m., laser
m., McKissock
m., poststatus augmentation
m., reduction

mammotome biopsy
mammotome procedure
mammotropic hormone
man (Man)
m. period (REMP), roentgen equivalent-
m. (REM) ▸ radiation equivalent in
m. (REM), roentgen equivalent-
M. Test, Draw-A-
M. (LSD), Zig-Zag

manage [*damage*]
m. abreactions
m. behavior
m., child difficult to
m. fluid intake
m. memory flooding
m. patient at-risk

manageable disease
managed
m. behavioral health plans
m. care
m. care-based psychiatry
m. care system
m. intensive addiction treatment unit ▸ medically
m. medically, patient
m. mental health
m. symptomatically

management
m., acute symptom
m., advanced
m., advanced medical pain
m., aggressive
m. ▸ aggressive medical
m., airway
m. and imagery ▸ stress
m. and prognosis
m. and survival
m., anger
m., anxiety
m., behavior

m., behavioral
m., cancer
m., cancer pain
m., case
m. ▸ chemotherapy initiation and
m., choking
m., clinical
m., combination therapy inpatient
m., conservative
m., contingency
m., contractual
m. control (PMC) ▸ pain
m., conventional
m., crisis
m., critical incident stress
m., current medical
m., cytoreductive surgical
m., data base
m., decision trees in patient
m., diabetes
m. ▸ diabetes self-
m., dietetic
m., disease
m., donor
m. ▸ early detection and
m., environmental
m., expiratory pressure
m., exploratory surgical
m., healthy conflict
m., home
m. ▸ hospital-based stress
m., hyperalimentation
m., image
m. ▸ impaired home maintenance
m., improper
m., initial
m., instruction in self
m. (IAM) ▸ integrated anger
m. interventions ▸ milieu
m. issues, patient
m. /intervention ▸ acute medical
m. lifestyle
m., lipid
m. ▸ long-term
m., medical
m., medication
m., milieu
m., multidisciplinary approach to pain
m. ▸ noninvasive pain
m., nursing
m. of acute pancreatitis
m. of bacterial shock
m. of cardiac arrhythmias
m. of chronic pain

m. of chronic pain ▸ psychological
m. of chronic pancreatitis
m. of drug abuser, obstetrical
m. of drug abusers, surgical
m. of eating disorders, medical
m. of insomnia
m. of labor program, active
m. of metastatic disease, surgical
m. of pain
m. of patient, conservative
m. of patient, medical
m. of psychiatric services
m. operative
m., optimal
m., osteoporosis
m., pain
m., pain and symptom
m., pain causation and
m., palliative
m., permanent pacemaker
m., perioperative
m., personal stress
m., pharmaceutical
m., pharmacologic
m., postexposure
m., postoperative pain
m., postprocedural
m., prehospital
m. program
m. program ▸ bowel
m. program, pain
m. program ▸ psychiatric case
m. program, stress
m. protocol
m. protocol ▸ milieu
m. relapse prevention, anger
m. relaxation training ▸ stress
m., risk
m. ▸ routine aggressive
m., second look surgical
m., self-
m. ▸ self-care
m. services, utilization
m. skills, anger
m. skills, anxiety
m. skills ▸ depression
m. skills ▸ poor
m. skills ▸ self-
m. skills ▸ sleep
m. skills ▸ stress
m. skills ▸ time
m., skin
m. specialist, pain
m., stone
m. strategy ▸ invasive

management—continued
- m. strategy ▸ pain
- m. strategy ▸ therapeutic milieu
- m., stress
- m., surgical
- m., symptom
- m., symptomatic
- m. technique, behavioral
- m. techniques, stress
- m., temporary pacemaker
- m. therapy ▸ stress
- m. training, stress
- m., trauma
- m., ventilator
- m., warning sign
- m., weight
- m., wound

manager
- m., clinical nurse
- m. (GCM) ▸ geriatric care
- m., nurse
- m., therapy

managing
- m. anger
- m. anxiety
- m. arthritis ▸ self-
- m. detoxification
- m. pain
- m. satanic alters
- m. stress

Manchester
- M. bacillus, Newcastle-
- M. dose distribution system
- M. operation
- M. ovoid

manchouricus, Parafossarulus

Manchurian symptoms

mandated
- m. choice
- m. evaluation ▸ legally
- m. guidelines, government
- m. metabolic screening

mandatory
- m. AIDS (acquired immune deficiency syndrome) testing
- m. blood testing
- m. contact tracing ▸ complete,
- m. immunization
- m. intermittent ventilation ▸ forced
- m. minute volume
- m. testing, acquired immune deficiency syndrome (AIDS)
- m. trial of labor
- m. vaccination program
- m. ventilation, continuous

- m. ventilation ▸ intermittent
- m. ventilation ▸ synchronized intermittent

Mandel Social Adjustment Scale (MSAS)

mandelic acid

mandible
- m., alveolar yokes of
- m., condyle of
- m., external angle of
- m., fractured
- m., jutting
- m., prognathic
- m., protruding
- m., sagittal splitting of
- m., semilunar notch of

mandibulae, alveoli dentales

mandibular
- m. anchorage
- m. arch
- m. arch bar
- m. bone
- m. deformities
- m. dentitional odontectomies
- m. equilibration
- m. foramen
- m. glide
- m. hemisection
- m. impression
- m. lymph nodes
- m. movement
- m. nerve
- m. notch
- m. port
- m. protraction
- m. recontouring alveolectomy
- m. reflex
- m. ridge
- m. teeth
- m. torus

mandibularis, glenoid fossa

mandibularis, torus

mandibulofacial dysostosis

maneuver(s)
- m., Adson
- m., Allen
- m., Bracht's
- m., Brandt-Andrews
- m., cervioprecordial
- m., Chassard-Lapine
- m., cold pressor testing
- m., Crede's
- m., clinical
- m., DeLee's
- m., doll's eye

- m. during massage, basic kneading
- m. during massage, cat stroking
- m. during massage, circular pressure
- m. during massage ▸ fan stroking
- m. during massage ▸ holding
- m. during massage ▸ knuckling
- m. during massage ▸ thumb stroking
- m. ▸ Dix-Hallpike
- m., Engel-Lysholm
- m., Epley
- m., external cardiac compression
- m., forward bending
- m., Fowler
- m., Gowers'
- m., Hallpike
- m., Halstead
- m., head
- m. ▸ head tilt and chin lift
- m., Heiberg-Esmarch
- m., Heimlich
- m., hemodynamic
- m., Hodge's
- m., Hoguet's
- m., Hueter's
- m., hyperabduction
- m. ▸ hyperextension postures and
- m., hyperventilation
- m. ▸ jaw thrust
- m., Jendrassik's
- m., Kappeler's
- m., Lasegue's
- m., Ledbetter
- m., Leopold
- m., Lovset's
- m., Massini's
- m., Mauriceau-Smellie
- m., Mauriceau-Smellie-Veit
- m., Mauriceau's
- m., McDonald's
- m., McMurray
- m., Müller-Hillis
- m., Müller's
- m., Munro-Kerr
- m., Nägeli's
- m., Nylen-Barany
- m., Pajot's
- m., Patrick's
- m., Phalen
- m., Phaneuf's
- m., physical
- m., Pinard's
- m., positives
- m., Prague

m., provocative
m., Queckenstedt's
m., Ritgen
m., Saxtorph's
m., Scanzoni's
m., Schatz's
m., Schreiber's
m., Sellick
m., Shobert's
m., therapeutic
m., Toynbee
m., Valsalva's
m., Van Hoom's
m., Wigand's

manganese laser

mange
m., demodectic
m., psoroptic
m., sarcoptic
m., Texas

Mangoldt's epithelial grafting
mangostana, Garcinia
Manheim
mania
m., acute
m., acute hallucinatory
m., akinetic
m., apotu
m., Bell's
m., dancing
m. ▸ depression and
m., doubting
m., epileptic
m., grandiose
m., hysterical
m. ▸ incurable chronic
m., mitis
m., periodical
m., puerperal
m., Ray's
m., reasoning
m., religious
m., secandi
m. ▸ symptoms of severe
m., transitory
m., unproductive
m., untreated

maniacal chorea
maniacal movements
manic [*panic*]
m. behavior, uncontrollable
m. ▸ bipolar affective disorder,
m. depression
m. -depressive disease, bipolar
m. -depressive disorder

m. -depressive illness
m. -depressive illness ▸ full-blown
m. -depressive insanity
m. -depressive, patient
m. -depressive personality
m. -depressive psychosis
m. disorder, atypical
m. disorder, recurrent episode
m. disorder, single episode
m. episode
m. episode ▸ induced
m., in full remission ▸ bipolar
disorder,
m., in partial remission ▸ bipolar
disorder,
m., mild ▸ bipolar disorder,
m., moderate ▸ bipolar disorder,
m. period
m. phase
m. phase of bipolar disorder
m. psychosis
m., severe, without psychotic
features ▸ bipolar disorder,
m. symptoms
m., unspecified ▸ bipolar disorder,
m., with psychotic features ▸ bipolar
disorder,

manicata, Anthomyia
manifest(s)
m. behavior
m. content
m. deviation
m. fantasy
m. hyperopia
m. ischemia
m. refraction
m. strabismus
m. suicidal tendencies ▸ patient
m. vector
m. vector ▸ mean

manifesta ▸ spina bifida
manifestation(s)
m., clinical
m., clinical epileptic
m., clinicopathologic
m., dermatologic
m., epileptic
m., hemorrhagic
m., initial
m. ▸ life-threatening
m. of acute drug intoxication,
clinical
m. of acute drug reactions,
psychological
m. of anxiety, behavioral

m. of disease, physical
m. of drug reaction, clinical
m. of flashback reactions, clinical
m. of latent insecurity
m. of organic brain syndrome,
clinical
m. of overdosing, clinical
m. of panic reactions, clinical
m. of physical disease ▸
psychological
m. of psychotic reactions, clinical
m. of withdrawal, clinical
m., predominant
m., psychiatric
m., psychological
m., psychotoxic
m., sympathetic
m., symptom
m., visceromotor

manipulated
m. cells ▸ genetically
m., electrodes
m. ▸ fear of being

manipulates
m. to gain nurturance
m. to gain power
m. to gain profit

manipulation
m., artificial
m., chest wall
m., chiropractic
m., chirospinal
m., conjoined
m., dietary
m., endoscopic
m., environmental
m., genetic
m., Hippocrates
m., hormonal
m., hormone
m., manual
m. of body, treatment by
m. of dislocated joint
m. of fracture
m. of fracture fragments
m. of joint
m. of joint ▸ extensive
m. of prosthetic device
m., osteopathic
m., percutaneous stone
m., physical
m., spinal
m. technique
m. techniques, body
m., uterine

manipulation—*continued*
   m., vertebral
   m., visceral
manipulative
   m. behavior
   m. behavior, attention-seeking
   m. drug abuser
   m. patient
   m. personality
   m. therapy
   m. therapy ▸ naturopathic
manipulator, emotional
manner
   m., area prepped and draped in
      routine
   m., continuous locking
   m., detached
   m., McLean's
   m., patient prepared and draped in
      routine
   m., patient prepped and draped in
      routine
   m., Pomeroy's
   m., self-assured
mannitol fermentation
mannitol pretreatment
manometer, aneroid
manometer, Honan
manometric cicatrix
manometric pressure
manometry
   m., anal
   m., anorectal
   m., esophageal
   m., sphincter of Oddi
   m. study
Mansonella ozzardi
mansoni, Cladosporium
mansoni, Schistosoma
Mansonioides annulifera
Manson's hemoptysis
mantle
   m. block
   m., brain
   m. cell lymphoma
   m. field in radiation therapy
   m. in radiation therapy,
      supramediastinal
   m., lower
   m. radiation therapy ▸ post◊
   m. radiation treatment ▸ modified
      upper
   m. radiation, upper
   m. technique
   m. technique in radiation therapy

   m. technique, radiation
   m. therapy
   m. therapy, upper
mantled rads, modified
Mantoux
   M. conversion
   M. diameter
   M. skin test
manual
   m. activity
   m. chest compression
   m. delivery of placenta
   m. dexterity
   m. edge detection
   m. examination of pelvis
   m. exploration
   m. exploration of abdomen
   m. expression
   m. inflation
   m. internal examination
   m. manipulation
   m. means
   m. movements
   m. muscle test
   m. muscle testing
   m. palpation
   m. percussion of suprapubic area
   m. positioning, rapid
   m. reduction
   m. removal of placenta
   m. resuscitator ▸ BagEasy
      disposable
   m. resuscitator ▸ First Response
   m. resuscitator ▸ Safe Response
   m. traction
manually
   m., placenta delivered
   m., placenta removed
manubrium bone
manubrium of the malleus
manus, chiasma tendinum digitorum
many-tailed bandage
many-tailed dressing
Manz glands
MAO (monoamine oxidase) inhibitor
   diet ▸ restricted tyramine and
MAOI (monoamine oxidase inhibitor)
MAP (mean aortic pressure)
MAP (mean arterial pressure)
map
   m., fate
   m., genetic
   m., genetic linkage
   m. -guided surgical resection,
      activation

   m., heart
   m., linkage
   m. ▸ polar coordinate
maple
   m. bark disease
   m. sugar
   m. syrup urine disease (MSUD)
mapper, brain
Mappine (hallucinogen)
mapping
   m. activation, sequence
   m. and sequencing the genome
   m., atrial activation
   m., brain
   m., bull's eye polar coordinate
   m., cardiac
   m., catheter
   m., color-coded flow
   m., color flow
   m. ▸ Doppler color flow
   m., electrophysiologic
   m. ▸ electrophysiologic testing and
   m., endocardial
   m., flow
   m., forensic
   m., gene
   m., genetic
   m., ice
   m., intracardiac
   m., intraoperative
   m., lymphatic
   m., pace
   m. ▸ pulsed wave Doppler
   m. ▸ retrograde activation
   m. ▸ retrograde atrial activation
   m. sequence, direct
   m. ▸ spectral temporal
   m. ▸ spectral turbulence
   m. ▸ tachycardia pathway
   m. technique ▸ flow
   m., ventricular
mappy tongue
Maquet technique
Maragliano body
marantic
   m. endocarditis
   m. thrombosis
   m. thrombus
marasmic thrombosis
marasmic thrombus
marathon runner
marathon training
marble pickup toe exercise
marble state
Marburg hemorrhagic fever

Marburg virus
marcescens infection, Serratia
marcescens, Serratia
march foot
march fracture
Marchand's adrenals
Marchesani syndrome, Weill-Marchetti
    M. operation, Marshall-
    M. procedure, Marshall-
    M. -Krantz operation, Marshall-
    M. test
Marchiafava
    M. -Bignami disease
    M. -Bignami syndrome
    M. -Micheli syndrome
Marchi's globule
Marckwald's operation
Marcus Gunn phenomenon
Marcus Gunn syndrome
mare, night◊
Marek's disease
Marek's disease herpesvirus
Marfan syndrome, Dennie-
Marfan's syndrome
Marg tonometer, Mackay-
Margaropus annulatus
Margaropus winthemi
margin(s)
    m., anterior
    m., apposition of cutaneous
    m., cord
    m., corneal
    m., costal
    m., costochondral
    m., distinct
    m., eyelid
    m., first obtuse
    m., gingival
    m., indistinct
    m., inferior
    m., inflammation of lid
    m., injury to lid
    m. (ICM) ▸ intercostal
    m., lateral cortical
    m., left costal
    m., lid
    m. of field, lower
    m. of left lung ▸ inferior
    m. of left lung ▸ sternal
    m. of right lung ▸ inferior
    m. of right lung ▸ sternal
    m. of wound brought into apposition
    m., opposing

    m., orbital
    m., peripheral
    m., psoas
    m., rectal
    m. revised, wound
    m., rib
    m., right costal
    m., second obtuse
    m., sharp
    m., skin
    m., smooth
    m., ulcer
    m. undermined, wound
    m., vermilion
    m., well-defined
    m., well-demarcated
    m., wound
marginal
    m. abruptio placentae
    m. artery
    m. artery ▸ first obtuse
    m. artery ▸ obtuse
    m. artery of colon
    m. artery ▸ second obtuse
    m. benefits
    m. branch, callosal
    m. branch ▸ obtuse
    m. cardiac function
    m. cardiac output
    m. cells
    m. circumflex artery
    m. degenerative changes
    m. dystrophy of cornea
    m. fracture
    m. gingiva
    m. gingivitis
    m. gingivitis, simple
    m. gingivitis, suppurative
    m. granulocyte pool
    m. gyrus
    m. gyrus of Turner
    m. health literacy
    m. heart failure
    m. keratitis
    m. lakes
    m. literacy skills
    m. lymphatic ▸ obtuse
    m. (OM), obtuse
    m. placenta praevia
    m. portion
    m. rales
    m. ridge
    m. separation
    m. ulcer
marginale, Anaplasma

marginalis
    m., abruptio placentae
    m., blepharitis
    m., gyrus
    m., para
    m., placenta
    m., placenta previa
marginata
    m., Ascaris
    m., placenta
    m., Taenia
marginatum, eczema
marginatum, erythema
Margulles' coil
Marie('s)
    M. ataxia
    M. disease, Bamberger-
    M. Foix sign
    M. hypertrophy
    M. Sainton syndrome, Scheuthauer-
    M. sclerosis
    M. sign
    M. -Strümpell arthritis
    M. -Strümpell spondylitis
    M. syndrome
    M. -Tooth atrophy ▸ Charcot-
    M. -Tooth disease
    M. -Tooth disease ▸ Charcot-
    M. -Tooth-Hoffman syndrome, Charcot-
marijuana
    m. (Bang/Bhang)
    m. (Bo/Boo)
    m. (Cannabis)
    m. (Charas)
    m. (Colombian)
    m. (Doobie) cigarette
    m. (Ganja)
    m. (Gold)
    m. (Grass)
    m. (Griffa)
    m. (Hashish/Hash)
    m. (Hawaiian)
    m. (Hay)
    m. (Hemp)
    m. (Herb)
    m. (Indian Hay)
    m. (Jamaican)
    m. (J/Jay)
    m. (Locoweed)
    m. (Mary Jane)
    m. (Mexican)
    m. (Mota/Mutah)
    m. (Pot)

marijuana—*continued*
- m. (Ragweed)
- m. (Sativa)
- m. (Sinsemilla)
- m. (Tea)
- m. (Weed)
- m. (Yerba)
- m. cigarette
- m. cigarette (Ace)
- m. cigarette (Joint)
- m. cigarette (Number)
- m. cigarette (Reefer)
- m. cigarette (Roach)
- m. cigarette (Smoke)
- m. cigarette (Stick)
- m. contamination
- m. dependence treatment
- m. economy
- m. (Acapulco Gold), grade of
- m. (Berkeley Boo), grade of
- m. (Panama Red), grade of
- m. -induced affect
- m. ingested
- m., inhalation of
- m. intoxication
- m. mix (Kiff), tobacco and
- m. smoked
- m. use, chronic

marilandica, Spigelia
marina, Spirochaeta
marine
- m. infection
- m. -life sting
- m. organisms

Marinesco
- M. -Radovici, palmomental reflex of
- M. -Radovici reflex
- M. -Sjögren syndrome
- M. succulent hand

marinum, Mycobacterium
Marion-Clatworthy side-to-end vena
 caval shunt
Mariotte's blind spot
Mariotte's spot
marismortui, Chromobacterium
marismortui, Halobacterium
marital
- m. adjustment
- m. communication
- m. conflict
- m. counseling
- m. discord
- m. dynamics
- m. dysfunction
- m. history (MH)

- m. introitus
- m. outlet
- m. problem
- m. reconciliation
- m. separation
- m. status
- m. therapy
- m. violence

maritima, Urginea
mark(s) (Mark)
- m., alignment
- m., beauty
- m., birth
- m. dermatitis, dhobie
- M. IV antireflux procedure, Belsey
- m. from cirrhosis ▸ spider
- m. from defibrillator ▸ paddle
- m. from pregnancy ▸ abdominal
 stretch
- m. from pregnancy ▸ breast stretch
- m. ▸ multiple needle puncture
- m., needle
- m., needle puncture
- m. on arms, needle
- m. on arm ▸ spider
- m., paddle burn
- m., pock◊
- m., Pohl's
- m., port wine
- m., raspberry
- m., scalp electrode
- m., strawberry
- m., stretch
- M. VIII implant, Choyce

marked
- m., abdominal area previously
- m. acute congestion
- m. arms, needle
- m. atrophy of upper extremities
- m., breast area previously
- m. confusion
- m. congestion
- m. degenerative change of hip
- m. density
- m. diffuse congestion
- m. dilation
- m. disorientation
- m. drop in blood pressure (BP)
- m. fatigue
- m. fibrinous pleuritis
- m. giant cell pneumonitis
- m. hyaline deposition
- m. icterus
- m. impulsivity
- m. jaundice

- m. left ventricular hypertrophy
- m. malnutrition
- m. mood shifts
- m. mosaicism
- m. muscular thickening
- m., myelofibrosis
- m. narrowing
- m. observed tremor
- m., operative site previously
- m. plasmocytic infiltrate
- m. reactivity of mood
- m. respiratory stimulation
- m. retardation of mental and
 physical development
- m. skin pallor
- m. squamous metaplasia
- m. veins, previously
- m. weakness

markedly
- m. comminuted
- m. dilated
- m. dilated heart
- m. enlarged
- m. icteric, sclerae
- m. increased energy level
- m. inflamed, trachea
- m. reduced ▸ cardiac output

marker(s)
- m., antibody
- m. catheter
- m. channel
- m., genetic
- m., gold
- m., Gonnin-Amsler
- m. ▸ lead letter
- m., needle
- m., nipple
- m. of disease, serological
- m., sclera
- m., time
- m., tumor
- m. ▸ vein graft ring

Markin position, Feist-
marking(s)
- m. ▸ bilateral patchy alveolar
- m., bronchial
- m., bronchovesicular
- m., convolutional
- m., fibrotic
- m., haustral
- m., interstitial
- m., linear
- m., lung
- m. pencil
- m., peribronchial

m., perihilar
m., prominence of pulmonary
m., pulmonary
m., pulmonary vascular
m., superficial venous
m., template
m., vascular
Marlex
  M. atraumatic tenaculum
  M. graft
  M. mesh
  M. mesh implant
  M. mesh implant material
  M. mesh implant material ▸ Usher's
  M. mesh implant ▸ Usher's
  M. mesh prosthesis ▸ Usher's
  M. suture
Marlow's test
Marmor prosthesis
Marmo's method
Maroteaux-Lamy syndrome
Marquette electrocardiograph (ECG)
Marquez's operation, Gomez-
marriage
  m., abusive
  m. counseling
  m., dysfunctional
marrow
  m. ablation
  m. aplasia, bone
  m. aplasia, fatal bone
  m. aspiration, bone
  m. biopsy, bone
  m., bone
  m., Buffy layer bone
  m., cancerous bone
  m. cavity
  m. cavity, bone
  m. cell
  m. cell, bone
  m. cell ▸ corrected bone
  m. cell ▸ defective bone
  m., dark red bone
  m. depression
  m. depression, bone
  m. depression, late bone
  m. disease, degenerative bone
  m., diseased
  m. donor match, bone
  m. emboli, bone
  m. embolism, bone
  m. engrafting
  m., enriched
  m. examination, bone
  m. failure ▸ bone

m., fat
m. fibrosis
m., gelatinous
m. ▸ genetically matched
m. harvest
m. harvest, bone
m., hypocellular bone
m., incompatible bone
m. infection, bone
m., infuse
m. infusion, bone
m. injections
m. invasion, bone
m. invasion by tumor ▸ bone
m. malfunction ▸ bone
m. malignancy, bone
m. metastases, bone
m. ▸ mildly hyperplastic bone
m., mismatched
m. problem, bone
m. puncture, bone
m., recipient's bone
m., red
m., red bone
m., reinfusing
m. ▸ reinfusion of stored
m. removed and stored, bone
m. scanning, bone
m., sibling
m. smear, bone
m. space
m., spinal
m. stem cells, bone
m. stromal cells
m. suppression, bone
m. tap, bone
m. tissue
m. toxicity, bone
m. transplant
m. transplant, autologous bone
m. transplant, bone
m. transplant rejection, bone
m. transplantation, allogeneic
m. transplantation ▸ blood and
m. transplantation, bone
m., transplanted
m., treated
m., yellow
m., yellow bone
Marshall('s)
  M. fall
  M. fold
  M. ligament
  M. -Marchetti-Krantz operation
  M. -Marchetti operation

M. -Marchetti procedure
M. oblique vein
M. test
M. vein of
marshallii, Alcaligenes
marsupial flap
marsupial notch
marsupialization Bartholin gland cyst
marsupialization of lesion
marsupium, Pterocarpus
martial arts ▸ tai-chi
Martin('s)
  M. operation
  M. pelvimeter
  M. reduction technique
  M. tube
Martius' operation
Mary Jane (marijuana)
Marzinkowsky operation, Filatov-
mas (milliampere second)
masculina, urethra
masculine protest
masculine pubic hair
masculinus, uterus
MASER (microwave amplification by
  stimulated emission of radiation)
MASH (make arthritis stop hurting)
mask(s)
  m., BLB (Boothby, Lovelace,
    Bulbulian)
  m., Curschmann's
  m., death
  m. depression
  m., ecchymotic
  m., face
  m. for electron beam therapy,
    plastic
  m., full-face
  m., Hutchinson's
  m., Kuhn's
  m. -like expression
  m. -like face
  m. -like facial appearance
  m., meter
  m. -mode cardiac imaging
  m. -mode subtraction
  m., nasal
  m., nonrebreathing
  m. of pregnancy
  m., oxygen
  m. pain
  m., Parkinson's
  m. ▸ partial rebreathing
  m., rebreathing
  m. ▸ reservoir face

mask(s)—*continued*
   m., steam-sterilized gowns and
   m., tabetic
   m. ventilation
   m., Wanscher's
masked
   m. depression
   m. face
   m. fat
   m. virus
masker, electronic
masking test
masochism, sexual
Mason (mason) ('s)
   M. dressing, Koch-
   M. incision, Yorke-
   m. lung
   M. vertical banded gastroplasty
mass(es)
   m., abdominal
   m., abnormal
   m., abnormal tissue
   m. absorption coefficient
   m., achromatic
   m., adnexal
   m., appendiceal
   m., appendix
   m., atomic
   m. attenuation coefficient
   m., benign
   m., benign congenital
   m., bisected
   m., black fibrotic
   m., blue
   m., body
   m., body cell
   m., bone
   m., brain
   m., breast
   m., calcified
   m., cancerous
   m., cardiac
   m. causing obstruction ▸ thyroid
   m., cavitary
   m., cell
   m., cellular
   m., central gray
   m., cervical
   m., cicatricial
   m., critical
   m., cystic
   m., cystic ovarian
   m., decreased fat
   m., decreased muscle
   m., definite

m., degenerating fibroid
m. ▸ density and strength bone
m. disaster
m., discernible
m., discrete
m., echodense
m., echogenic
m., electronic
m. ▸ embedded in tumor
m. energy equivalence
m., enlarged
m., erythrocyte
m. ▸ excisional biopsy of tumor
m., extensive bone
m., extrauterine pelvic
m., extrinsic
m., fat-free
m., fecal
m., ferrous carbonate
m., fibrous
m., fibrous cell
m., firm
m., firm cell
m., fluctuant
m., fluid-filled cystic
m. formation, paravertebral
m., friable tumor
m., fungating
m. ▸ hard, indurated colon
m. ▸ high dose radiation to tumor
m., hilar
m. in bone ▸ stimulate formation and increase
m. in chest
m. ▸ increased bone
m. ▸ increased muscle
m. index (BMI), body
m., indurated
m., induration, or tenderness
m. infection
m. ▸ infiltrating irregular tumor
m., inflammatory
m., injection
m., inner cell
m., intermediate
m., intermediate cell
m., intra-abdominal
m., intra-atrial
m., intracardiac
m., intraluminal
m., intravascular
m., intrinsic
m. lab workup ▸ mobile
m., lean body
m. ▸ lean muscle

m. ▸ left ventricular (LV)
m. lesion
m. lesion ▸ intracranial
m., lobulated
m., lobulated tumor
m., localized
m., loss of bone
m. ▸ loss of muscle
m., lymphoid
m., mediastinal
m., mercury
m. miniature radiography
m., movable
m., movable cell
m., muscle
m., myocardial
m., necrotic fungating
m., neoplastic
m. number
m., obstructing
m. of atlas, lateral
m. of blood, localized
m. of ethmoid bone ▸ lateral
m. of Flemming, fibrillar
m. of mucus ▸ oyster
m. of sacrum, lateral
m. of tissue growth, abnormal
m. of vertebrae, lateral
m., or induration ▸ tenderness,
m. or organs, palpable
m., organs or tenderness on palpation
m., ovarian
m., ovarian cell
m., palpable
m., palpable abdominal
m. ▸ palpable extra-uterine
m., palpable organs or
m., parametrial
m., paravertebral
m., peak bone
m., pelvic
m., peripheral
m. peristalsis
m., pill
m., pilular
m., pleural
m., posterior brain
m., posterior mediastinal
m. pressure, extrinsic
m. protoplasm
m. psychogenic illness
m., pulsatile
m., pulsating
m., Priestley's

m., questionable
m., rectal
m., red cell
m. reduction, bone
m. reflex
m. reflex, Riddoch's
m., relativistic
m. ▸ resection of tumor
m., rest
m., retroperitoneal
m. roentgenography
m., ropy
m. sampling
m., Schultze's granular
m. screenings
m., scrotal
m. shadows
m. ▸ small fungating mucosa
m., soft tissue
m., solid appearing
m., solid bone
m., sonolucent
m. spectrometer
m., spherical
m. ▸ spinal bone
m., Stent's
m. stopping power, total
m., strength and balance ▸ muscle
m., strengthening bone
m., subcutaneous
m., subcutaneous perineal
m., subpleural
m. suicide
m., superior perihilar
m., supraclavicular node
m., suprahilar
m., suspicious
m., tender
m., tigroid
m., tissue
m. transfusion, cell
m., transparent jelly-like
m., tubal
m., tumor
m., umbilicated
m., unilateral
m. unit (a.m.u.), atomic
m., Vallet's
m., ventricular muscle
m., ventrolateral
m. x-ray, mobile

massage
m., auditory
m. ▸ basic kneading maneuver during

m., biofeedback and
m., cardiac
m., carotid
m., carotid pulse obtained by
m., carotid sinus
m., cat stroking maneuver during
m., Cederschiold's
m., circular pressure ▸ maneuver during
m., classic
m., closed chest cardiac
m., cranial
m., deep
m. ▸ deep and stretching
m. ▸ deep muscle
m., deep pressure
m., deep tissue
m., diathermy and
m. ▸ direct cardiac
m., douche
m., electrovibratory
m., esthetic
m. ▸ fan stroking maneuver during
m., foot
m. for relaxation
m. ▸ full body
m., heart
m. ▸ holding maneuver during
m., Hubbard tank
m., hydropneumatic
m., ice
m., infant
m., internal cardiac
m. ▸ knuckling maneuver during
m., myofascial
m. ▸ open chest cardiac
m., Oriental
m., periodic
m., relaxing
m., scalp and facial
m., Shiatsu
m. ▸ smooth and repetitive stroke during
m. ▸ soft tissue
m., sports
m., Swedish
m., swelling reduced by
m., therapeutic
m. therapist
m. therapist, deep tissue
m. therapy
m. therapy, deep tissue
m. therapy, heat and
m. ▸ thumb stroking maneuver during

m., tremolo
m. trigger point
m., vapor
m., vibratory
massaged, uterus
massaging gums
massaging motion, circular
massauah, Vibrio
masse, en
Masselon's spectacles
masseter
m. muscle
m. muscle, trismus of
m. muscle, voluntary relaxation of
masseteric
m. area
m. nerve
m. reflex
m. space
m. vein
Massini's maneuver
massive [*passive*]
m. anasarca
m. arousal
m. ascites
m. bleeding
m. brain damage
m. brain tumor
m. cardiac enlargement (CE)
m. centrilobular bile stasis
m. centrilobular necrosis
m. collapse
m. dose technique
m. doses of chemotherapy
m. doses of steroids
m. edema
m. fibrinous pleuritis and emphysema
m. fibrosis, progressive
m. gastrointestinal (GI) hemorrhage
m. hemorrhage
m. hepatic failure
m. hepatic necrosis
m. heart attack
m. herniation
m. infarct of brain stem
m. infarctions
m. infection
m. infiltration
m. intestinal bleeding
m. intra-abdominal bleeding
m. intracerebral bleed
m. intracerebral hemorrhage
m. involvement
m. jerking movements

massive—*continued*
- m. midbrain hemorrhage
- m. multiple trauma
- m. obesity
- m. particle (WIMP) ▸ weakly interacting
- m. pleural effusion
- m. pneumonia
- m. pseudocyst of pancreas
- m. pulmonary embolus
- m. pulmonary thromboemboli
- m. radiation
- m. recent infarction
- m. rectal bleeding
- m. resection
- m. retroperitoneal involvement
- m. scar tissue
- m. sliding graft
- m. spasm
- m. transference shift
- m. transfusion
- m. transfusions
- m. trauma to chest
- m. tumor
- m. upper GI bleed
- m. vitreous retraction
- m. water drinking

massively dilated, abdomen

Masson bodies

mast (MAST)
- M. (medical antishock trousers)
- M. (military antishock trousers)
- M. (military antishock trousers) pants
- M. (military antishock trousers) suit
- m. cell
- m. cell enhancing activity
- m. cell inhibitor
- m. cell leukemia
- m. cells ▸ pulmonary

mastalgia
- m., cyclical
- m., frequent
- m., noncyclical
- m., patient has

mastectomy
- m., bilateral
- m., breast reconstruction after
- m., elective
- m., Halsted radical
- m., keyhole
- m., left radical
- m., modified radical
- m., partial
- m., Patey modified

- m., Patey radical
- m., preventive
- m., primary
- m. products
- m., prophylactic
- m. ▸ prophylactic double
- m., radiation and chemotherapy after
- m., radical
- m. reconstruction
- m., right radical
- m. scar, bilateral
- m. scar, transverse
- m., segmental
- m., simple
- m. ▸ skin sparing
- m., subcutaneous
- m. support
- m., total
- m. ▸ wide excision
- m., Will Meyer Radical

Master('s)
- M. exercise stress test
- M. exercise tolerance test
- M. ▸ SpaceLabs Event
- M. syndrome, Allen
- M. Treatment Plan
- M. "2-step" exercise test

mastery
- m. fantasy ▸ trauma-based
- m. imagery
- m., reparative

mastic test

masticating cycle

masticating surface

masticatory movements

masticatory muscle

mastitis
- m., acute
- m., chronic
- m., chronic cystic
- m., cystic
- m., gargantuan
- m., glandular
- m., interstitial
- m., neonatorum
- m., lactational
- m., parenchymatous
- m., periductal
- m., postpartum
- m., puerperal
- m., phlegmonous
- m., plasma cell
- m., retromammary
- m., stagnation

- m., submammary
- m., suppurative
- m. with breast-feeding

mastitoides, carcinoma

mastocytosis
- m., diffuse cutaneous
- m. syndrome
- m., systemic

mastoid
- m. air cells
- m. angle conchal
- m. antrum
- m. bone
- m. canaliculus
- m. cavity
- m. cavity packed
- m. cells
- m. cortex
- m. dressing
- m. emissary vein
- m. fontanelle
- m. incision ▸ coronary mastoid-to-
- m. notch
- m. osteitis
- m. osteitis, acute
- m. process
- m. process, external
- m. region
- m. searcher
- m. sinus
- m. suture
- m. -to-mastoid incision ▸ coronary
- m. wall

mastoidea, otitis

mastoidectomy
- m. (Type I, II, III) ▸ Bondy
- m., complete simple
- m., modified
- m., radical
- m., simple

mastoideum
- m. antrum
- m. foramen
- m., os

mastoideus, canaliculus

mastoiditis
- m., Bezold's
- m. externa
- m. interna
- m., sclerosing
- m., silent

mastopathia cystica

mastopathy, cystic

mastopexy, Goulain

Masuda-Kitahara disease

MAT (multifocal atrial tachycardia)
mat
    m. activities
    m. activities, bed
    m. mobility, bed
    m., no-skid
Matas(')
    M. aneurysmectomy
    M. operation
    M. test
match
    m., blood and tissue
    m., bone marrow donor
    m., cross-
    m. defect
    m., genetic
    m., organ
    m. organ and recipient
matched
    m. bone marrow donor
    m. control studies
    m. control studies in clinical trials
    m. donor
    m. marrow ▸ genetically
Matchett
    M. -Brown femoral head
        replacement
    M. -Brown prosthesis
    M. prosthesis
matching
    m., afterload
    m., cross
    m. donors
    m. organ transplant recipients
    m. supraclavicular and tangential
        fields
    m. tangential field with internal
        mammary field
matchline fibrosis
mater
    m., arachnoid
    m., dura
    m. encephali, dura
    m. encephali, pia
    m. of brain, dura
    m. of brain, pia
    m. of spinal cord ▸ dura
    m., pia
    m. spinalis, dura
    m. spinalis, pia
material(s)
    m. (heroin)
    m., abnormal sac containing
        semisolid
    m., acrylic ball implant

m., adhesive silicone implant
m. artifact ▸ foreign
m., artifactual
m., artificial joint implant
m., aspirated
m., aspirated foreign
m., aspiration of bloody
m., augmentation with implant
m., autograft
m., base
m., Berens implant
m., blood-tinged mucoid
m., bone implant
m., calcified
m., cellular
m., chromosomal
m., clinical
m., clotted
m., contrast
m., copious mucoid
m., cores of atheromatous
m., cross-reacting
m., dark bloody
m. deposit, foreign
m., diffluent yellow
m., drainage (dr'ge) of purulent
m., dried plant
m., edematous
m. ▸ embolized foreign
m., emesis of fecal
m., equivalent
m., Ethibond synthetic suture
m., Ethiflex synthetic suture
m., excretion of contrast
m. expressed, lens
m., extrachromosomal
m., fatty
m., fecal
m., fibrinohematic
m., fibrinous
m., fibrocartilaginous
m., flame retardant
m., fluorescein
m., gelatinous
m., genetic
m., gold implant
m., gonadotropin-inhibitory
m., granular
m., granular eosinophilic
m. gratification
m., grossly purulent
m., grumous
m., hemorrhagic
m., hemostatic
m., hollow sphere implant

m., homograft implant
m., human genetic
m., impacted fecal
m., impression
m., ingested
m., injection of radiopaque
m., intra-alveolar fibrinous
m., intrathecal contrast
m., intravenous (IV) contrast
m., Ivalon sponge implant
m., lipoid
m., loop of suture
m. ▸ low osmolality contrast
m., Marlex mesh implant
m. ▸ microinjection of genetic
m., mucilaginous
m. ▸ MycroMesh graft
m., necrotic cellular
m., necrotic purulent
m., neurosecretory
m., nonabsorbent
m., non-ionic contrast
m., opaque
m., paraffin implant
m., particulate
m., passing fecal
m., passing flatus
m., PermaMesh
m., plastic implant
m., polyethylene implant
m., polytetrafluoroethylene (PTFE)
    arterial graft
m., poor excretion of contrast
m., Porocaot
m., potentially infectious
m., prompt excretion of contrast
m., proteinaceous
m., Protoplast
m., purulent
m., radioactive
m., reaction to contrast
m., red cells tagged with radioactive
m., Renografin-76 contrast
m., residual contrast
m., retained fecal
m., retention of contrast
m., sanguineous/sanguinous
m., sebaceous
m., sensitized
m., shiny
m., Silastic corneal implant
m., Silastic Cronin implant
m., Silastic implant
m., Silastic subdermal implant
m., silicone implant

material(s)—*continued*
- m., soupy
- m., stained smear of clinical
- m., subdermal implant
- m., subjective
- m., subperiosteal implant
- m., Supramid implant
- m., surrounding graft
- m., suture
- m., synthetic bone
- m., synthetic graft
- m., synthetic suture
- m., tantalum implant
- m., tantalum mesh implant
- m., Teflon
- m., Teflon implant
- m., Teflon mesh implant
- m., Tensilon implant
- m., ▸ thick mucoid
- m., tissue
- m., Tucron suture
- m., ureteral implant
- m., Usher's Marlex mesh implant
- m., vasodepressor
- m., vasoexcitor
- m., vein filled with contrast
- m., verbalizable
- m., Vicryl suture
- m., Vitallium implant
- m., Vivosil implant
- m., Wheeler's implant
- m., wire mesh implant
- m., wound oozing purulent

maternal (Maternal)
- m. age
- m. age ▸ advanced
- m. antibodies
- m. anxiety
- m. behavior, normal active
- m. bleed, fetal
- m. blood typing
- m. brain death
- m. conditions, relevant
- m. death
- m. death after cesarean section
- m. depression
- m. deprivation
- m. dystocia
- m. effect
- m. exercise ▸ vigorous
- m. febrile morbidity
- m. fetal hemorrhage
- m. -fetal medicine
- M. Health Drugs Advisory Committee ▸ Fertility

- m. health risks
- m. hemoglobin, fetal-
- m. immunity
- m. infant
- m. infectious morbidity
- m. left
- m. methadone dosage
- m. morbidity
- m. mortality
- m. mortality and morbidity
- m. mortality, incidence of
- m. mortality rate
- m. -neonatal methadone levels
- m. -neonatal transmission of viral hepatitis
- m. nutrition
- m. placenta
- m. resuscitation
- m. right
- m. smoking during pregnancy
- m. stress
- m. touch, temporary deprivation
- m. treatment
- m. weight gain

maternity leave
mathematical ability, declining
Mathieu's disease
matris, sinus durae
matrix (Matrix)
- m., bony
- m. calculus
- m. carcinoma, hair-
- m. cells
- m., cholesteatoma
- m., extracellular
- m. ▸ extracellular collagen
- m., hair
- m. mode
- m. ▸ myocardial collagen
- m., nail
- m. proteins (NMP) ▸ nuclear
- m., Raven's
- m., research
- m., subependymal glial
- m. technique ▸ wax
- M. Test, Raven's Progressive
- M. (TRAM) ▸ Treatment Rating Assessment
- M. (TRAM) ▸ Treatment Response Assessment
- m. unguis
- m., vacuolization of cerebral

Matsner episiotomy
matte colony

matted with tumor metastases ▸ membranes
matter
- m. echogenicity of periventricular white
- m. embedded ▸ foreign
- m., gray
- m., intrabronchial vegetable
- m. loss due to aging ▸ white
- m. of brain, gray
- m. of spinal cord, gray
- m. of brain, white
- m., particulate
- m., retained particulate
- m., white
- m., withdrawal of purulent

Matthews eave flap, Cronin-
Mattingly disease
mattress
- m., apnea alarm
- m., egg crate
- m., hypothermia
- m., hypothermic
- m., rotating aid
- m. suture
- m. sutures, chromic catgut
- m. sutures, continuous
- m. sutures, double-armed
- m. sutures, everting
- m. sutures, horizontal
- m. sutures, insert
- m. sutures, interrupted
- m. sutures, intradermal
- m. sutures ▸ pledgeted
- m. sutures, right-angle
- m. sutures, silk interrupted
- m. sutures ▸ subannular
- m. sutures ▸ through-the-wall
- m. sutures, vertical
- m., Therm-O-Rite
- m., water

M-A (Miller-Abbott) tube
maturation [*saturation*]
- m., accelerate bone
- m., affinity
- m. arrest
- m., cognitive
- m. division
- m., emotional
- m. ▸ epiphyseal chondroblastic growth and
- m. factor (EMF), erythrocyte
- m., GALT (gut-associated lymphoid tissue)
- m. immunity

m. in humans ▸ sexual
m. index
maturation
m., normal
m., normal bone
m., nuclear and cytoplasmic
m. of breast cells
m. of new skin ▸ growth and
m., psychological
m., skeletal
maturational
m. enuresis
m. normalcy
m. unfolding ▸ normal
m. vicissitudes of superego
mature(s)
m. bone
m. cataract
m. cell
m. cystic teratoma
m. ▸ develops new blood supply and
m. egg
m. granulocytes
m. lymphocytes
m. molecule
m. myelocytes
m. nerve cells
m. neutrophil
m. onset diabetes
m. ovum
m. realism
m. red blood cell ▸ spiculed
m. stump
m. transformation zone
matured skin cells
maturing in donor cell ▸ phage particle
maturity (Maturity)
m., emotional
m., fetal
m., fetal lung
m., filial
m., onset
m., physical
m. ▸ premature fetal
m. ▸ premature sexual
m., pulmonary
m. rating
m. rating, newborn
M. Scale, Columbia Mental
m., secondary to severe
m., sexual
m., skeletal

matutinal
m. and diurnal variation
m. epilepsy
m. variation, diurnal and
Maugeri's syndrome
Mauksch's operation
Mauldsley Medical Questionnaire
Maunoir's hydrocele
Maurer's stippling
Mauriceau('s)
M. maneuver
M. method
M. Smellie maneuver
M. -Smellie-Veit maneuver
Mauthner's test
mauve factor
maw worm
maxi-vessel loops
Maxilith pacemaker, CPI
maxilla [*axilla*]
m., frontal process of
m., alveolar yokes of
m., lacrimal notch of
m., LeFort's fracture of
m., malformed
m., nasal notch of
m., palatine spine of
maxillae, alveoli dentales
maxillae, septa interalveolaria
maxillary
m. alveolectomy
m. alveoloplasty
m. anchorage
m. antrotomy, radical
m. antrum
m. antrum, falx of
m. arch
m. artery
m. bone
m. crest
m. deformities
m. excision
m. fracture, transverse
m. ganglion
m. impression
m. nerve
m. paranasal sinus
m. protraction
m. recontouring alveolectomy
m. ridge
m. sinus
m. sinus cancer
m. sinus roentgenogram
m. teeth
m. torus

m. tuberosity
m. tuberosity deformities
m. tuberosity resectional ostectomies
m. vein
maxillofacial
m. injury
m. prosthesis
m. region
maximal
m. acid output
m. breathing capacity
m. comfort level
m. exercise
m. expiratory flow rate (MEFR)
m. expiratory flow volume (MEFV)
m. fecal excretion
m. forced expiratory flow (MFEF)
m. heart rate
m. in proximity of vertex ▸ amplitude
m. inspiratory flow rate (MIFR)
m. intensity
m. mid-expiratory flow (MMEF)
m. mid-expiratory flow rate (MMEFR)
m. midflow rate (MMFR)
m. potential field
m. sustainable ventilatory capacity (MSVC)
m. tension line
m. therapy
m. tubular excretory capacity
m. velocity
m. ventilation
m. ventilation rate (MVR)
m. vital capacity (MVC)
maximum (Maximum)
m accessibility
m. aerobic capacity
m. allowable concentration
m. amplitude of wave, point of
m. assistance
m. assistance for lower body dressing
m. assistance for upper body dressing
m. assisted transfer
m. breathing capacity
m. breathing capacity ▸ indirect
m. cardiovascular benefit
m. concentration
m. conduction velocity of nerve
m. containment lab
m. dimension

maximum—*continued*
m. dosage
m. expiratory flow rate (MEFR)
m. extension
m. flow rate
m. flow ▸ respirator on
m. (FWHM), full width at half
m. heart rate
m. hospital benefit (MHB)
m. hospital benefit (MHB) ▸ patient reached
m. impulse fifth intercostal space (PMI 5th ICS) ▸ point of
m. impulse (PMI) ▸ point of
m. independence of living
m. inhibiting dilution (MID)
m. inspiratory force
m. inspiratory pressure (MIP)
m. intensity (PMI) ▸ point of
m. isolation
m. level of independence
m. level of independent mobility
m. loudness
m. magnitude of QRS
m. mid-expiratory flow rate (MMEFR)
m. negative potential
m. oxygen (O_2) consumption
m. oxygen (O_2) uptake
m. permissible concentration (MPC)
m. permissible dose (MPD)
m. predicted heart rate (MPHR)
m. pressure
m. QRS vector
m. ratio, scatter
m. ratio, tissue
M. Security Unit (MSU)
m. target absorbed dose
m. terminal flow (MTF)
m. tolerated dose (MTD)
m. total dosage
m. urinary concentration
m. ventricular elastance
m. voluntary ventilation (MVV)
m. walking time
maximus, gluteus
maximus muscle, gluteus
maxi-vessel loops
maxwellian distribution
Maxwell's ring
Maxwell's spot
Maydi's hernia
May-Grunwald-Giemsa stain
May-Hegglin's anomaly

May sign
Mayaro virus
maydis, Ustilago
Mayer('s)
M. position
M. reflex
M. -ray view
Mayfield-Kees headrest
Maylard incision
Mayneord F factor
Mayo
M. -Fueth operation
M. operation
M. sacroiliac belt
M. vaginal hysterectomy, Ward-
M. -Ward vaginal hysterectomy
Mayor's sign
Mayou disease ▸ Batten-
Maxur's operation
Maze
M. procedure
M. procedure, catheter-based
M. procedure ▸ modified left atrial
Mazlin Spring
MB
MB (mesiobuccal)
MB Bands
MB fraction, CK/
MBO (mesiobucco-occlusal)
MBP (mean blood pressure)
MBP (mesiobuccopulpal)
MBTI (Myers-Briggs Type Indicator) test
MC (mc)
Mc (megacurie)
Mc (megacycle)
mc (millicurie)
MCA (middle cerebral artery)
McArdle's disease
McArthur's incision
McArthur's method
MCBR (minimum concentration of bilirubin)
McBride('s)
M. bunionectomy
M. operation
M. tripod pin traction
McBurney('s)
M. incision
M. operation
M. point
M. point ▸ rebound in region of
M. sign
MCC (mutated colorectal cancer)

MCC/MCHC (mean corpuscular hemoglobin concentration)
McCall-Schuman operation
McCall's operation
McCarey-Kaufman (M-K) medium
McCarroll's operation
McCarthy's electrode
McCarthy's reflex
McConckey cocktail
McCormac's reflex
McCune-Albright syndrome
MCD (mean cell diameter)
MCD (mean corpuscular diameter)
McDonald('s)
M. maneuver
M. operation
M. procedure
McDowall reflex
McDowell's operation
MCE (myocardial contrast echocardiography)
McFarland approach, Kocher-
mcg (microgram)
McGavic type operation
McGaw volumetric pump
McGhan intraocular lens (IOL)
McGhan's implant
McGinn-White sign
McGregor's forehead flap
McGregor's line
McGuire's operation
MCH (mean corpuscular hemoglobin concentration)
MCI (mean cardiac index)
mci (millicuries of iodine)
McIndoe operation
McKee-Farrar
M. prosthesis
M. total hip arthroplasty
M. total hip prosthesis
McKeever('s)
M. arthrodesis
M. operation
M. operation ▸ Wilson-
M. patella cap prosthesis
M. patellar prosthesis
M. Vitallium cap prosthesis
McKissock mammoplasty
MCL (midclavicular line)
McLaughlin('s)
M. operation
M. plate
M. plate and screws
M. screw

McLean('s)
- M. manner
- M. suture
- M. tonometer

McMurray
- M. maneuver
- M. sign
- M. test

McNaghten (M'Naghten/ McNaughtren) Rule

McNaught keel

McNeer classification

Mc.p.s. (megacycles per second)

MCR (message competition ratio)

McReynolds operation

McReynolds pterygium transplant

mcs (millicurie seconds) of beta radiation

MCT (mean circulation time)

MCT (mean corpuscular thickness)

MCTD (mixed connective tissue disease)

MCV (mean clinical value)

MCV (mean corpuscular volume)

McVay operation

McVay repair of hernia

MD (muscular dystrophy)

MD (Doctor of Medicine), primary

MDA (mentodextra anterior)

MDD (major depressive disorder)

MDD (mean daily dose)

M-Dip contrast medium, Reno-

M disc

MDP (mentodextra posterior)

MDT (mentodextra transverse)

MDTR (mean diameter–thickness ratio)

MEA (multiple endocrine abnormalities)

MEA (multiple endocrine adenomatosis)

Mead operation ▸ Majorner-

Meadox
- M. graft sizer
- M. Microvet Dacron graft
- M. Teflon felt pledget

meal(s) (Meals)
- m. (pc) ▸ after
- m., after fatty
- m., barium
- m. (ac) ▸ before
- m., Boas test
- m., Boyden's test
- m., Dock's test
- m., dumping of barium

- m., Ehrmann's alcohol test
- m., Ewald's test
- m., fat
- m., fat-free
- m., fatty
- m., Fischer's test
- m., home delivered
- m., Leube's test
- m. lung disease ▸ fish
- m. lung ▸ fish
- m., motor test
- M. on Wheels
- m. (p.p. or postprandial), after
- m. planning
- m. response, fat
- m., Riegel's test
- m., Slazer's test
- m. stimulation test
- m. study barium
- m. worm

mean(s)
- m. aortic pressure (MAP)
- m. arterial blood pressure (MABP)
- m. arterial pressure (MAP)
- m. arterial pressure ▸ systemic
- m., artificial
- m. blood pressure (MBP)
- m. cardiac index (MCI)
- m. capillary pressure
- m. cell diameter (MCD)
- m. circulation time (MCT)
- m. circulatory hematocrit (HCT)
- m. clinical value (MCV)
- m. contrast enhancement
- m. corpuscular diameter (MCD)
- m. corpuscular hemoglobin (MCH)
- m. corpuscular hemoglobin concentration (MCC/MCHC)
- m. corpuscular thickness (MCT)
- m. corpuscular volume (MCV)
- m. daily dose (MDD)
- m. deflection, microvolts
- m. diameter–thickness ratio (MDTR)
- m. diastolic left ventricular pressure
- m. distribution
- m. dominant frequency (MDF)
- m. ejection rate (MER)
- m. electrical axis
- m. forced midexpiratory flow
- m. free path
- m. (GM) ▸ geometric
- m. gradient
- m. hemolytic dose (MHD)
- m. incident energy

- m. incubation period (MIP)
- m., instrumental
- m. left atrial pressure (MLAP)
- m. (LVM) ▸ left ventricular
- m. life span (MLS)
- m. line, arterial
- m. manifest vector
- m., manual
- m. midexpiratory flow rate
- m. normalized systolic ejection rate
- m. of self-destruction
- m. of transmission, efficient
- m., physical
- m. posterior wall velocity, normal
- m. pressure (MP)
- m. pressure (AMP) ▸ average
- m. pressure (PAMP) ▸ pulmonary artery
- m. pressure (PWMP) ▸ pulmonary wedge
- m. pulmonary artery pressure
- m. pulmonary artery wedge pressure
- m. (PWM) ▸ pulmonary wedge
- m. QRS axis
- m. right atrial pressure (MRAP)
- m. (RVM) ▸ right ventricular
- m. right ventricular pressure (MRVP)
- m. square
- m. -square (RMS) ▸ root-
- m. -square voltage ▸ root-
- m. (SDM) ▸ standard deviation of the
- m. (SEM) ▸ standard error of the
- m. survival
- m. survival time
- m. (SM) ▸ systolic
- m. systolic ejection rate (MSER)
- m. systolic left ventricular pressure
- m. temperature
- m. titer (GMT) ▸ geometric
- m. values
- m. velocity
- m. venous pressure (MVP)

meaningful
- m. activity
- m. brain function
- m. relationship

meaningless repetitive motions

Means scratch ▸ Lerman-

measles
- m., atypical
- m., bastard
- m., black

measles—*continued*
- m., confluent
- m., coughing from
- m. encephalitis
- m., German
- m., hemorrhagic
- m. immune globulin
- m. immune globulin (human)
- m. incubation period
- m., mumps, rubella immunization (MMR)
- m. neuroretinitis
- m. pneumonia
- m., pork
- m. virus

measure(s)
- m., adaptive
- m. blood flow
- m. bone density
- m., chemotherapeutic
- m., comfort
- m., conservative
- m., control
- m., curative
- m., emergency
- m., general supportive
- m., heroic
- m. impedance
- m. instituted, emergency
- m., isolation
- m., less restrictive
- m., life-prolonging
- m., life saving
- m. life support
- m., life-sustaining
- m. of arousability
- m. of personality ▸ psychological
- m. of treatment ▸ nonpharmacologic
- m., palliative
- m., personality
- m., precautionary
- m., preventive
- m., prolonged resuscitative
- m., psychotherapeutic
- m. rate of blood flow
- m. resistance
- m., resuscitative
- m., routine preventive
- m. ▸ self-care
- m., self-report
- m. sound
- m., supportive
- m., therapeutic
- m., x-ray immunosuppressive

measured
- m. and recorded ▸ thresholds and sensitiveness
- m. between pairs of electrodes
- m. in microvolts
- m. in picofarads
- m., peripheral vision

measurement(s)
- m., absolute physical
- m., aggregate
- m., anatomical
- m., baseline
- m., bipartial
- m., blood flow
- m., blood gas
- m., blood lactate
- m., blood volume
- m., cardiac output
- m., conjugate
- m., coronary blood flow
- m., crown rump
- m., density
- m., digital pressure
- m., Doppler
- m. for exotropia, Krimsky
- m. ▸ gas clearance
- m., hemodynamic
- m., home blood pressure (BP)
- m. ▸ invasive pressure
- m. of blood pressure ▸ intra-arterial
- m. of electrode resistance
- m. of patient, topography and anatomic
- m. of vital capacity
- m., pain
- m., pelvic
- m., perceptual
- m., physical density
- m., physiologic
- m., plasma testosterone
- m., pressure
- m., pulse wave velocity
- m., quantitative
- m. recorded, pressure
- m. ▸ Reid index
- m., semiquantitative
- m. ▸ shock wave pressure
- m., stereotactic
- m., thermodilution
- m., traditional enzyme
- m. ▸ transstenotic pressure gradient
- m. ▸ venous flow

measuring
- m. blood pressure

- m. device
- m. heart function
- m. stress

meat
- m. exchange
- m. ▸ irradiation of raw
- m. -wrapper's asthma

meatal stenosis
meatal stenosis, urethral
meatoantrotomy, exploratory
meatotomy electrode, ureteral
meatus
- m., acoustic
- m., auditory
- m., external
- m., external acoustic
- m. (EAM) ▸ external auditory
- m., inferior
- m., internal acoustic
- m. (IAM) ▸ internal auditory
- m. media, atrium
- m., middle
- m., nasal
- m., nerve of external acoustic
- m. (EAM) reflex ▸ external auditory
- m., superior
- m., urethral
- m., urinary

mecalil provocation test
mechanic(s)
- m., body
- m., bronchitis
- m., fluid
- m., lung
- m., proper body

mechanica, acne
mechanical
- m. ability
- m. alternation
- m. alternation of heart
- m. assistance ▸ long-term
- m. bowel obstruction
- m. cough
- m. CPR (cardiopulmonary resuscitation)
- m. deflection
- m. devices
- m. diarrhea
- m. diet ▸ soft
- m. dissociation, electrical
- m. dysmenorrhea
- m. emetic
- m. heart
- m. heart pump
- m. heart valve

m. insulin pump
m. kidney, portable
m. knee prosthesis ‣ Walldius Vitallium
m. motion
m. obstruction
m. patterns of speech
m. perforation
m. pleurodesis
m. pump, Jarvik-7
m. relief
m. respirator
m. respirator ‣ breathing supported by
m. soft diet
m. stage
m. sterilization
m. stimulation
m. stimulus
m. strabismus
m. styptic
m. tomograph
m. valve
m. vector
m. ventilation
m. ventilation ‣ long-term
m. ventilator
m. ventilatory assistance ‣ continuous
m. ventricular actuation ‣ direct

mechanism(s)
m., absorptive
m. ‣ activating specific compensatory
m., adaptive
m., balance
m., body defense
m., body temperature
m., calcium homeostatic
m., cognitive
m., compensatory
m., compensatory behavior
m., contractile
m., coping
m., coronary steal
m., countercurrent
m., defense
m., deglutition
m., Douglas'
m., Duncan
m., escape
m. ‣ exposing plaque to cutting
m. for ventilator breathing ‣ sign
m., Frank-Starling
m., gating

m., homeostatic reflex
m. ‣ individual defense
m. ‣ ineffective coping
m., inherent
m., mental
m., metabolic control
m., natural defense
m. ‣ neurogenetic adaptive
m., neutralizing
m., normal response
m., oculogyric
m. of action
m. of denial ‣ defense
m. of hormonal control, feedback
m. of inner ear, balance
m. of labor
m. of taste aversion
m. of testicular injury
m. of tolerance
m., outgoing
m., parenteral
m., pathogenic
m. ‣ peeling back
m., physiologic
m., pinchcock
m., ping-pong
m. ‣ pulmonary sensory
m., quadriceps
m., radiation
m., re-entrant
m., rejection
m., Schultze's
m., sinus
m., somatic
m., splanchnic
m., Starling
m., steal
m., stimulus response
m., stress control
m., swallowing
m., thermoregulatory
m. to brain ‣ balance
m. ‣ utilization and quality review
m. ‣ wave speed

mechanoelectrical feedback
mechlorethamine chemotherapy, topical
Meckel('s)
M. band
M. cavity
M. diverticulectomy
M. diverticulum
M. ganglion
M. ganglionectomy
M., lesser ganglion of

M. rod
meconium
m. aspiration
m. aspiration syndrome
m. discharge
m. fluid
m. ileus
m., late passage of
m. ‣ newborn aspirates
m. peritonitis
m. plug syndrome
m. stained
m. stained amniotic fluid
m. stained fluid
m. staining
m. stool
MED (minimum effective dosage)
Med II, Gamma
Medallion Lens ‣ Worst
media
m., acute otitis
m., acute bacterial otitis
m., acute purulent otitis
m. ‣ acute serous otitis
m., adhesive otitis
m., aerotitis
m., aortic tunica
m., arterial
m., auris
m., barotitis
m., bilateral otitis
m. blitz
m., chronic otitis
m., chronic suppurative otitis
m., contrast
m., culture
m., dioptric
m., fossa cranii
m. fragments
m., gastric pars
m., hydrophilic filter
m., hydrophobic filter
m. influence
m., injection of contrast
m., installation of diagnostic
m. instilled ‣ x-ray contrast
m., iodinated contrast
m., mottling of contrast
m., mucoserous otitis
m. ossea, concha nasalis
m., otitis
m., poor excretion of contrast
m. pressure
m., purulent otitis
m., refracting

media—*continued*
- m., scala
- m., secretory otitis
- m. (SOM) ▸ serous otitis
- m. surrounding brain ▸ alterations of
- m., tunica
- m. violence
- m. with effusion, otitis

medial
- m. anconeus muscle
- m. and lateral tangential breast
- m. angle
- m. ankle sprain
- m. aperture
- m. arch
- m. arteriole of retina
- m. aspect
- m. basal
- m. bundle, longitudinal
- m. calcification of cerebral vessels
- m. capsular reefing
- m. capsule
- m. capsule, reefing of
- m. circumflex femoral veins
- m. collateral ligament
- m. commissure of eyelids
- m. compartment of knee
- m. condyle
- m. cortex
- m. crus
- m. cutaneous nerve
- m. cutaneous nerve of arm
- m. cutaneous nerve of calf
- m. cutaneous nerve of forearm
- m. degeneration ▸ mucoid
- m. deviation
- m. dorsal cutaneous nerve of foot
- m. elbow injury
- m. eminence
- m. epicondyle
- m. femoral condyle
- m. flap
- m. forebrain bundle
- m. gastrocnemius muscle
- m. geniculate body
- m. hypertrophy of pulmonary vessels
- m. incisor
- m. joint level
- m. joint line
- m. lemniscus
- m. malleolus
- m. malleolus of tibia
- m. meniscectomy

- m. meniscus
- m. meniscus, detachment of
- m. meniscus, dislocated
- m. meniscus of knee joint
- m. meniscus, posterior horn of
- m. meniscus, torn
- m. nasi, crus
- m. necrosis, cystic
- m. necrosis of ascending aorta ▸ cystic
- m. neurovascular bundles
- m. oblique axial projection
- m. occipitotemporal gyrus
- m. ossified edge
- m. palatine nerve
- m. palpebral ligament
- m. patellar facet cartilage
- m. pectoral nerve
- m. planter nerve
- m. planter nerve ▸ common planter digital nerves of
- m. planter nerve ▸ proper planter digital nerves of
- m. plateau
- m. popliteal nerve
- m. portion
- m. protrusion
- m. pterygoid muscle
- m. pterygoid nerve
- m. puboprostatic ligament
- m. quadriceps retinaculum
- m. rectus muscle
- m. rectus muscle ▸ advancement of
- m. supraclavicular nerves
- m. surface occipital lobe
- m. surface of cerebral hemisphere
- m. surface of second toe ▸ dorsal digital nerves of
- m. tear
- m. tegmental region
- m. therapy ▸ ischemia-guided
- m. thickness ▸ intimal
- m. tissue ▸ fragments of
- m. umbilical fold
- m. venule of retina
- m. wall
- m. wall of orbit

medialis
- m., gyrus frontalis
- m., gyrus occipitotemporalis
- m., gyrus olfactorius
- m. muscle, rectus
- m. muscle, vastus
- m., musculus rectus
- m. of Retzius ▸ gyrus olfactorius

- m., reefing of vastus
- m. retinae, venula
- m., vastus

medially, reflected

median
- m. antebrachial vein
- m. aspect
- m. bar formation
- m. basilic vein
- m. cephalic vein
- m. cubital vein
- m. curative dose
- m. detection threshold
- m. distribution
- m. effective dose
- m. fatal dose
- m. fissure, anterior
- m. fissure, posterior
- m. harelip
- m. incision
- m. infective dose
- m. lethal dose (MLD or LD$_{50}$)
- m. lethal dose ▸ ratio of
- m. line
- m. lobe decompression
- m. nerve
- m. nerve ▸ common palmar digital nerves of
- m. nerve compression
- m. nerve damage
- m. nerve decompression
- m. nerve distribution
- m. nerve entrapment
- m. nerve hypesthesia
- m. nerve injury
- m. nerve ▸ proper palmar digital nerves of▸
- m. nerve transmits sensation
- m. palatine suture
- m. plane
- m. raphe
- m. recognition threshold
- m. -sagittal plane
- m. sternotomy
- m. sternotomy incision
- m. strumectomy
- m. sulcus
- m. sulcus, posterior
- m. survival time
- m. tissue culture dose
- m. tissue culture infective dose
- m. vein of elbow
- m. vein of forearm
- m. vein of neck

medianus, ramus

mediastinal
- m. abscess
- m. adenoma
- m. adenopathy
- m. adenopathy ▸ tuberculous
- m. air
- m. amyloidosis
- m. amyloidosis ▸ pseudotumoral
- m. bleeding
- m. cavity
- m. crunch
- m. emphysema
- m. fat ▸ indentation for thymus and
- m. fat ▸ thymus and
- m. fatty tissue
- m. fibrosis
- m. flutter
- m. lymph node biopsy
- m. lymph nodes
- m. lymph nodes, anterior
- m. lymph nodes, posterior
- m. mass
- m. mass, posterior
- m. metastases
- m. node
- m. node biopsy
- m. organs
- m. pericarditis
- m. pleura
- m. pleura closed
- m. pleura exposed
- m. pleura incised
- m. pleurisy
- m. plexus
- m. plexus, subpleural
- m. port
- m. seminoma
- m. shadow
- m. shift
- m. shift to the left
- m. shift to the right
- m. space
- m. structures
- m. sump filter
- m. tumor
- m. tumor excision
- m. tumor, malignant
- m. tumor, malignant germ cell
- m. tumor ▸ resection of
- m. tumors, myasthenia gravis and
- m. vein
- m. volume rotation
- m. wedge
- m. widening
- m. widening, decrease in

mediastinale, septum
mediastinitis, descending necrotizing
mediastinitis, fibrous
mediastinum
- m., anterior
- m., bronchogenic cyst of
- m., chest
- m., metastases of
- m., posterior
- m., superior
- m., tomography of upper
- m. volume rotation therapy
- m., widening of
- m., widening of superior

mediate agglutination
mediate auscultation
mediated
- m. antibody, cell-
- m. behavior, automatically
- m. cytotoxicity, cell
- m. cytotoxicity, macrophage-
- m. disease ▸ immune-
- m. endothelial injury ▸ neutrophil-
- m. gene transfer, adenovirus
- m. hypotension (NMH) ▸ neurally
- m. immune reactions, cell
- m. immune response, cellular
- m. immunity, cell
- m. lung injury ▸ neutrophil-
- m. lung injury ▸ oxygen (O₂)-
- m. membranous nephritis ▸
  immune-
- m. relaxation, biofeedback
- m. relaxation ▸ endothelium-
- m. resistance, chromosomal
- m. resistance, plasmin
- m. syncope ▸ mixed neurally
- m. syncope ▸ neurally
- m. tachycardia (PMT), pacemaker

mediation, cognitive
mediation, respiratory
mediator release, allergen-induced
Medicaid
- M. claim
- M. coverage
- M. payment
- M. program

**Medical Literature Analysis and
  Retrieval System (MEDLARS)**
medical (Medical) [*pedicle*]
- m. acupuncture
- m. adhesive silicone implant ▸
  Silastic
- m. admission, elective
- m. advances, significant

- m. advice (AMA) form signed ▸
  against
- m. advice, seek
- m. aid (RMA) ▸ refusal of
- m. alert necklace or bracelet
- m. alert wallet card
- m. anatomy
- m. and diet center
- m. and lateral menisci
- m. and radiation oncology
- m. and surgical, general
- m. antishock pants
- m. antishock suit
- m. antishock trousers (MAST)
- m. aortic valve prosthesis, St. Jude
- m. armamentarium
- m. assessment
- m. assistance, provide
- m. assistant
- M. Association (WMA), World
- m. attention, appropriate
- m. audit
- m. authority
- m. capabilities
- m. care
- m. care, aggressive
- m. care, definitive
- m. care, emergency
- m. care facility ▸ external acute
- m. care ▸ high-quality
- m. care, lack of
- m. care, life-saving
- m. care, patient avoids
- m. care, state-of-the-art
- M. Care Unit (IMCU) ▸ Intermediate
- m. care utilization
- M. Center ▸ Veterans Affair
- m. channels, diversion of drugs
  from licit
- m. chemistry
- m. complications
- m. complications ▸ drug-related
- m. condition
- m. condition, chronic
- m. condition, coexisting
- m. condition, fatal
- m. condition, irreversible
- m. condition, stable
- m. consumers
- m. contraindications
- m. credentials
- m. crisis
- m. criteria
- m. criteria, strict
- m. curettage

medical—*continued*

m. decisions
m. detoxification
m. device ▸ indwelling prosthetic
m. devices
m. diagnosis
m. directives
m. director
m. disciplines
m. disorder
m. education
m. education, continuing
m. emergency
m. emergency, environmental
m. environment
m. epicondylitis
m. equipment
m. equipment or tubing
m. ethics
m. ethics, "outdated"
m. ethics, Western
m. evaluation
m. evaluation ▸ auditory and
m. evaluation, patient admitted for
m. evaluation, urological
m. evidence
m. examination
m. examination, extensive
m. examination ▸ group
m. examiner, chief
m. expertise
m. experts
M. Eye Bank
m. facilities
m. facilities ▸ inpatient non-psychiatric
m. facilities ▸ outpatient non-psychiatric
m. factor
m., general
m. generic screening criteria
m. genes
m. geneticist
m. genetics
m. gloves
m. group, multispecialty
m. health care
m. history (MH)
m. history as screening device for drug abuse
m. history (MH), detailed
m. history (PMH) ▸ past
m. history (MH), patient's
m. illness
m. illness, acute

m. illness, chronic
m. implants
m. indications
m. induction
m. information
m. information identification
m. information system
m. insurance, private
m. intensity
M. Intensive Care Unit (MICU)
m. internal radiation dose
m. intervention
m. jargon
m. knowledge
m. -legal interaction
m. limitations
m. maintenance
m. malpractice
m. maltreatment
m. management
m. management ▸ aggressive
m. management, current
m. management/intervention ▸ acute
m. management of eating disorders
m. management of patient
m. model ▸ middle-class
m. monitoring
m. mortality
m. necessity, determination of
m. needs, prenatal
m. neglect
m. /nursing care ▸ supportive
m. /nursing supervision
m. nutrition therapy
m. observation
m. oncologist
m. oncology
m. ophthalmoscopy
m. options
m. order
m. origin
m. overuse of drugs
m. pain management, advanced
m. paradigm ▸ personalized
m. person
m. personnel
M. Phrase Index (MPI)
m. pion generators
m. practices
m. practice, modern
m. practice, sound
m. problem, chronic
m. problems, coexisting
m. problems in drug abusers

m. problems, related
m. problem ▸ underestimate severity of
m. procedure
m. procedure, invasive
m. process
m. progress
m., psychological, spiritual, physical and nutritional component
M. Questionnaire, Mauldsley
m. reassessment ▸ patient admitted for
m. record
m. record documentation
m. record, electronic
m. regimen
m. remedies
m. research
m. review
m. risk
m. risk factor
m. risk, increased
m. rounds
m. schemes
m. science
m. screening
m. screening, free
m. self-care
m. self-determination
m. self-help
m. service (EMS) ▸ emergency
M. Shock Trauma Acute Resuscitation (MedSTAR)
m. side-effects
m. social services
M. Sonulator
m. stability
m. stabilization
m. staff
m. staff, hospital
m. stressors
m. student's disease
m. study design
m. supplies
m. symptoms
m. syndrome
M. Technician (EMT), Emergency
m. test kits, home
m. therapeutics
m. therapy
m. therapy, adjuvant
m. therapy, aggressive
m. therapy, recommend continued
m. thyroidectomy
m. toxicologist

m. training
m. treatment
m. treatment ▸ accept or reject
m. treatment, aggressive
m. treatment, choice of
m. treatment, court ordered
m. treatment ▸ denial of lifesaving
m. treatment, extended
m. treatment, lifesaving
m. treatment ▸ noncompliance with
m. treatment ▸ right to reject
m. treatment ▸ standard
m. treatment studies
m. unit, acute care
m. unit ▸ self-contained,
   transportable
m. update
m. waste
m. workup, thoracic
m. yoga
medically
m. dependent patients
m. inactive placebos
m. managed intensive addiction
   treatment unit
m., patient managed
m., patient related
m. supervised fasting protocol
m. supervised withdrawal
medicamentosa
m., conjunctivitis
m., dermatitis
m., stomatitis
Medicare
M. assignment
M. benefits
M., certified for
M. claim
M. coverage
M. eligible
M. payment
M. program
M. recipients
medicate patient with azidothymidine
   (AZT)
medicated bath ▸ iodine-
medicated corn pads
medicating ▸ patient self-
medication(s)
m., analgesic
m. ▸ action, dose, route and
   method of administering
m., active
m., acute withdrawal
m., adjunctive

m. adjustment
m., alternative
m., amount of
m. and diet
m. and modification of behavior
   and environment
m. and therapy, pain
m., anti-allergic
m., antianxiety
m. ▸ antianxiety and antidepressant
m., anticholinergic
m., anticoagulant
m., anticonvulsant
m., antidepressant
m., antidiarrheal
m., antiemetic
m., antifungal
m., antiglaucoma
m., antihistamine
m., antihypertensive
m., anti-inflammatory
m., anti-itch
m., antipsychotic
m., antispasmodic
m., antirejection
m., antiseizure
m., antithyroid
m., anti-tissue
m., antiviral
m., approved
m. -assisted detoxification
m., blood pressure (BP)
m., blood-thinning
m., bone preserving
m., brain-shrinking
m., bronchodilator
m., cardiovascular
m. cart
m., cholesterol lowering
m., cocaine blocking
m. compliance, consistent
m., condition induced by
m., continuation of
m., conventional
m., corticosteroid
m., current
m., current pain
m., daily
m., daily schedule of
m. ▸ deteriorating effect on
m. ▸ direct push of
m., discharge
m., discontinuation of
m., dispense
m., dispenser

m. distribution and control
m., diuretic
m. dosage
m., dummy
m. during dialysis
m. ▸ elder misuse of
m. flow sheet
m., frequency of
m., headache
m. ▸ hormone replacement
m., hypnotherapy and
m., immune-suppressive
m., immunosuppressive
m., inactive
m. incompatibilities
m. ▸ increased compliance with
m. -induced stress
m., initiation of
m. injected under conjunctiva
m., inotropic
m., intracardiac
m., intramuscular
m., intratracheal
m., intravenous (IV) administration
   of
m., level of
m., life-long
m. management
m. ▸ migraine prophylactic
m., monitor prescribed
m. ▸ multiple oral
m. ▸ muscle relaxant
m., neuroactive
m., neuroleptic
m., non-narcotic
m., nonprescription
m. ▸ off label use of
m. on discharge
m., oral
m. ▸ oral pain
m., overdose of
m. ▸ over-the-counter (OTC)
m., pain
m., pain control
m. ▸ pain relief
m., parenteral analgesic
m., patient noncompliant with
m., patient pain
m., patient responds to
m., post-menopause
m., preanesthetic
m., preliminary
m., prepackaged
m., prescription
m., preventive pain

medication(s)—*continued*
- m. problems, potential
- m. profile, personalized
- m., prosyncopal
- m., psychiatric
- m., psychoactive
- m., psychotherapeutic
- m., psychotropic
- m. regimen
- m., regular dosage of
- m. release consent
- m. renewal
- m. review
- m., routine
- m. ▸ self administration of
- m., side-effects from
- m., steroid
- m., stimulant
- m., storing
- m., suppressive
- m. ▸ sustained release
- m., symptomatic
- m. ▸ synthetic thyroid
- m. system (PIMS) ▸ programmable implantable
- m., systemic
- m., tapering schedule of
- m. ▸ therapeutic effects of
- m. therapy
- m., thrombolytic
- m. tolerance
- m., topical
- m., topical eye
- m. ▸ topical prescription
- m. ▸ topical skin
- m. treatment
- m. treatment, current
- m. tube ▸ surgically implanted
- m., ulcerogenic
- m., vasodilator
- m. ▸ weight loss
- m. withdrawn

medicinal benefits of garlic
medicinal herbalism
medicinalis, Hirudo
medicine (Medicine)
- m., academic
- m., administrative
- m., advancement of
- m., aerospace
- m., alternative
- M. ▸ American Society of Addiction
- m. and rehabilitation
- M. and Surgery (ASLMS) ▸ American Society of Laser

- m., antibiotic
- m., anticlotting
- m., auricular
- m., aviation
- m., behavioral
- m. cabinet
- m. clinic, emergency
- m. clinic, sports
- m., clinical
- m., comparative
- m., complementary
- m., compound
- m., conventional
- m., cough
- m., critical care
- m., decongestant
- m., domestic
- m., dosimetric
- m., emergency
- m., environmental
- m., experimental
- M., Family
- m., fetal
- m. ▸ finger-stick
- m., folk
- m., forensic
- m., functional
- m., galenic
- m., general
- m., genetic
- m., geriatric
- m., group
- m., herbal
- m., hermetic
- m., holistic
- m., homeopathic
- m., hyperbaric
- m., Indian
- m., industrial
- m., integrated
- m., internal
- m., ionic
- m., laboratory animal
- m., legal
- m., maternal-fetal
- m. ▸ mind-body
- m., molecular
- m., natural
- m., neo-hypocratic
- M., Nuclear
- m., occupational
- m., oral
- m., orthomolecular
- m., over-the-counter
- m., palliative

- m., patent
- m., physical
- m. physician ▸ complementary
- m. physician, emergency
- m., preclinical
- m., prenatal
- m., prescription
- m., preventative
- m., preventive
- M. (MD), primary Doctor of
- m. program, sports
- m., proprietary
- m., psychocutaneous
- m., psychological
- m., psychosomatic
- m., rational
- m., rehabilitation
- m. rehabilitation, physical
- m., response to
- m. scanning, nuclear
- m., scientific
- m. service ▸ hospital's addiction
- m., social
- m., socialized
- m., somatic
- m., space
- m., spagyric
- m. specialist ▸ pediatric emergency
- m. specialist, preventive
- m., sports
- m., state
- m., statis
- m., suggestive
- m., sympathetic
- m., topical
- m., transfusion
- m., transpersonal
- m., trauma
- m., tropical
- m., veterinary

medicolegal emergency
medicolegal interaction
Medicophysics Department
Medigap coverage
Medi-graft vascular prosthesis
medii, atrium meatus
Medi-Kit
Medi-Lifter, portable
Medina worm
medinensis, Dracunculus
mediocanellata, Taenia
mediocollateral ligament of knee ▸ calcification
mediolateral
- m. episiotomy, left

m. episiotomy, right
m. projection
m. view
m. view, supine
medionecrosis of aorta
mediotarsal amputation
Mediport machine
meditating ▸ stretching exercises and
meditation
m. and biofeedback
m., mindfulness
m. ▸ stress reducing
m. (TM) ▸ transcendental
mediterranea, Acetabularia
Mediterranean
M. anemia
M. diet
M. fever
M. kala-azar
MEDI-THERM, Auto-
medium
m., acetrizoate sodium contrast
m., Amipaque contrast
m., Angioconray contrast
m., assay
m., barium sulfate contrast
m., Bilopaque contrast
m., Brun's glucose
m., build-down region of irradiated
m., build-up region of irradiated
m., bunamiodyl contrast
m., Cardiografin contrast
m. chain fatty acid
m. chain triglyceride
m. chain triglyceride diet
m., Cholebrine contrast
m., Cholografin contrast
m., clearing
m., Clysodrast contrast
m., Conray contrast
m., contrast
m., culture
m. culture, charcoal blood
m., Cystografin contrast
m., Cystokon contrast
m. delivery, contrast
m., diatrizoate meglumine contrast
m., diatrizoate sodium contrast
m., Diodrast contrast
m., Dionosil contrast
m., diprotrizoate contrast
m., disperse
m., dispersion
m., dispersive
m. dosage

m., Duografin contrast
m., Ethiodane contrast
m., Ethiodol contrast
m. frequency
m., Gastrografin contrast
m., Hippuran contrast
m., Hypaque contrast
m., Hypaque-Cysto contrast
m., Hypaque M contrast
m., Hypaque Meglumine contrast
m., Hypaque sodium contrast
m., injection of radiopaque contrast
m., intravenous (IV) bolus injection
    of contrast
m., Intropaque contrast
m., iodalphionic acid contrast
m., iodipamide contrast
m., iodomethamate contrast
m., iodophthalein sodium contrast
m., iodopyracet contrast
m., iophdone contrast
m., iophendylate contrast
m., iophenoxic acid contrast
m., iopydol contrast
m., iothalamate contrast
m., ipodate calcium contrast
m., irradiated
m., Isopaque contrast
m., Lipiodol contrast
m., Liquipake contrast
m., Löwenstein's culture
m., meglumine diatrizoate contrast
m., meglumine iodipamide contrast
m., meglumine iothalamate contrast
m., metrizamide contrast
m., metrizoate sodium contrast
m. (MEM) ▸ minimum essential
m., M-K (McCarey-Kaufman)
m., mounting
m., Neo-lopax contrast
m. ▸ non-ionic contrast
m., Novopaque contrast
m., nutrient
m., opanoic acid contrast
m., opaque
m., Orabilex contrast
m., oragrafin calcium contrast
m., oragrafin sodium contrast
m., Pantopaque contrast
m., patient ingested contrast
m., phentetiothalein contrast
m. ▸ polygelin colloid contrast
m., Priodax contrast
m., propyliodone contrast
m., radiopaque contrast

m., Renografin contrast
m., Reno-M-Dip contrast
m., Reno-M-30 contrast
m., Reno-M-60 contrast
m., Renosvist contrast
m., Sabourand's
m., Salpix contrast
m., separating
m., Sinografin contrast
m. size conformer
m., Skiodan Acacia contrast
m., Skiodan contrast
m. smear, Nickerson's
m. smear, Pagano-Levin
m., sodium diatrizoate contrast
m., sodium iodipamide contrast
m., sodium iodohippurate contrast
m., sodium iodomethamate contrast
m., sodium iothalamate contrast
m., sodium ipodate contrast
m., sodium methiodal contrast
m., sodium thorium tartrate contrast
m., sodium tyropanoate contrast
m., Telepaque contrast
m., Thixokon contrast
m., thorium dioxide (TH-0$_2$) contrast
m., tissue culture
m. voltage activity
m. voltage slow wave
m. voltage slowing
m., Wickersheimer's
medius
m., gyrus frontalis
m., gyrus temporalis
m. muscle, gluteus
Medlar bodies
MEDLARS (Medical Literature
    Analysis and Retrieval System)
medronate sodium kit, Tc
    (technetium) 99m
medroxyprogesterone acetate
    (DMPA) ▸ depot-
MedSTAR (Medical Shock Trauma
    Acute Resuscitation)
Medtronic
M. Activitrax rate responsive
    unipolar ventricular pacemaker
M. cardiac cooling jacket
M. defibrillator implant support
    device
M. demand pacemaker
M. Elite DDDR pacemaker
M. Elite II pacemaker
M. external cardioverter defibrillator
M. -Hall device

Medtronic—*continued*

    M. -Hall heart valve prosthesis
    M. -Hall tilting disk valve prosthesis
    M. interventional vascular stent
    M. -Laurens-Alcatel pacemaker
    M. leads
    M. pacemaker, bipolar
    M. pacemaker, SpecTrax
      programmable
    M. Pacette pacemaker
    M. PCD implantable cardioverter
      defibrillator
    M. pulse generator
    M. Pulsor Intrasound pain reliever
    M. radiofrequency receiver
    M. SPO pacemaker
    M. synchroMed pump
    M. temporary pacemaker
    M. transvene endocardial lead
      system

medulla
    m., adrenal
    m. ▸ focally cystic gray
    m., hemorrhage in
    m. ▸ marked congestion of renal
    m. oblongata
    m. of adrenal gland
    m., pons and
    m., pons and cerebellum
    m., renal
    m. spinalis
    m., suprarenal

medullae oblongatae, nucleus
    lateralis

medullaris
    m., conus
    m. nerve, conus
    m. thalami optici, taenia

medullary
    m. adenoma
    m. artery
    m. bone graft
    m. callus
    m. canal
    m. canal, reamer for
    m. cancer
    m. carcinoma
    m. carcinoma of thyroid
    m. cardiorespiratory centers ▸
      paralysis of
    m. cavity
    m. cavity ▸ cancellous bone
      curetted out of
    m. cells
    m. center of cerebellum

    m. chromaffinoma
    m. collecting duct
    m. concentration, minimal
    m. cords
    m. cystic disease
    m. disease
    m. fold
    m. graft
    m. infarct
    m., intra◊
    m. junction, cortical
    m. junction, pontine
    m. nail
    m. nail, Schneider
    m. nailing of tibia
    m. pin, Street-type
    m. paraganglioma
    m. pin, von Saal
    m. ray
    m. respiratory center
    m. segment
    m. sponge kidney
    m. streak
    m. substance
    m. substance of bones
    m. substance of bones, red
    m. substance of kidney
    m. substance of suprarenal gland
    m. tube
    m. tumor
    m. velum
    m. velum, anterior

medullated
    m. fibers and sheaths
    m. nerve fibers
    m. neuroma

medulloblastoma, Cushing's
medusae, caput
Medx camera
Medx scanner
Meese's position
Meesmann's dystrophy
meeting, interdisciplinary team (IDT)
meeting, peer group
MEF (maximal expiratory flow)
MEFR (maximum expiratory flow
    rate)
MEFV (maximal expiratory flow
    volume)
MEG (magnetoencephalography)
    technique
megacolon
    m., acquired
    m., acquired functional
    m., acute

    m., aganglionic
    m., congenital
    m., congenitum
    m., idiopathic
    m., toxic
megacycles per second (Mc. p.s.)
megadose of vitamins
megadose vitamin therapy
megaelectron volt (MeV)
megakaryocytes, atypical appearing
megakaryocytes, circulating
megakaryocytic aplasia ▸ idiopathic
megakaryocytic leukemia
megaloblastic anemia
megaloblastic anemia of pregnancy
megalocephala, Ascaris
megalosplenica, erythrocytosis
megaly, spleno◊
megaly, ventriculo◊
megatherium, Bacillus
megavitamin therapy
megavolt therapy
megista, Trypanosoma
meglumine
    m. contrast medium, diatrizoate
    m. contrast medium, Hypaque
    m. diatrizoate contrast medium
    m. iodipamide contrast medium
    m. iothalamate contrast medium
megohm (M)
megohms, expressed in
meibomian
    m. cyst
    m. foramen
    m. froth
    m. gland
    m. gland carcinoma
    m. glands, dysfunctional
    m. stye
Meier test, Porges-
Meigs'
    M. capillaries
    M. syndrome
    M. test
Meinicke test
Meinicke turbidity reaction
meiosis [*miosis*]
Meissner's
    M. corpuscles
    M. ganglion
    M. plexus
melancholia
    m., acute
    m., affective
    m., agitated

m. attonita
m., flatuous
m. hypochondriaca
m., involutional
m., recurrent
m. religiosa
m., severe
m. simplex
m. stuporous
m. with delirium
melancholic depression
melancholicum, omega
melancholy, feelings of
melancholy, winter
melanin
m. granules
m. pigment
m. -pigmented cells
m. production
m. test
melaninogenicus, Bacteroides
melanocephala, Wyeomyia
melanocyte-stimulating hormone (MSH)
melanocytic nevus
melanocytoma, compound
melanocytoma, dermal
melanoderma, parasitic
melanoderma, senile
melanodes, carcinoma
melanogenus, Acetobacter
Melanolestes picipes
melanoleukoderma colli
melanoma
m., acral lentiginous
m., amelanotic
m. -associated antigens
m., balloon cell
m., benign
m., choroidal
m., Clark's level of malignant
m., cutaneous malignant
m. death
m., disseminated
m., familial
m., juvenile
m., lentigo maligna
m., localized malignant
m., malignant
m., metastatic
m., metastatic malignant
m., mucosal
m., nonlentiginous
m. of extremity, malignant
m. of meninges

m. of skin
m., primary
m., recurrence of
m., skin
m., subungual
m., suburethral
m., terminal-stage
m., unpigmented malignant
m., uveal
m. vaccine
melanophore-stimulating hormone (MSH)
melanosis
m. coli
m. of cornea, diabetic
m. sclerae
melanotic
m. ameloblastoma
m. cancer
m. carcinoma
m. neuroectodermal tumor
m. stool
m. whitlow
melanovogenes, Proteus
melanura, Culiseta
melas, icterus
melasma
m. addisonii
m. gravidarum
m. suprarenale
melatonin
m. level
m. secretion
m. supplement
meleagridis, Amoeba
meleagridis, Histomonas
Meleda disease
melena ▸ hematemesis and/or
melena, hematochezia or hematemesis
melena neonatorum
melenic stools
melioidosis, pulmonary
Melkersson-Rosenthal syndrome
melitensis, Brucella
melitensis, gram-negative Brucella
mellamine, hexamethyl
Meller's operation
mellifcae, Malpighamoeba
mellis, Saccharomyces
mellitus
m. (DM) ▸ adult onset diabetes
m. (DM) ▸ borderline diabetes
m. (DM) controlled ▸ diabetes
m. (DM) ▸ diabetes

m. (GDM) ▸ gestational diabetes
m. (IDDM), insulin dependent diabetes
m. (DM) ▸ juvenile onset diabetes
m. (DM), longstanding ▸ diabetes
m. (NIDDM), noninsulin dependent diabetes
m. (NIDM), noninsulin diabetes
m. ▸ nonketotic diabetes
m. (DM) secondary to endocrine disease, diabetes
m. (DM) secondary to pancreatic disease, diabetes
m. (IDDM), Type I, insulin dependent diabetes
m. (NIDD), Type II, noninsulin dependent diabetes
melting out temperature
melting point
Meltzer sign
MEM (minimum essential medium)
member
m., clinical staff
m., family
m., house staff
m., trauma team
membrana tympani
membranacea, pars
membranacea, placenta
membranaceus bronchi, paries
membranaceus tracheas, paries
membrane(s)
m. abnormalities, mucous
m. abnormality ▸ nuclear
m. activity ▸ cell
m. adjustments ▸ secondary cataract
m., altered oral mucous
m., alveolar capillary
m., alveolocapillary
m., amnion
m., anal mucous
m., anterior mallear fold of tympanic
m., antibasement
m. antibodies ▸ glomerular
m. antibody, antibasement
m. antibody, antiglomerular basement
m. antibody, basement
m. antigen, cell-
m. antigen, cytokeratin
m. antigen, epithelial
m. antigen (PSMA) ▸ prostate specific
m. antigen ▸ surface

membrane(s)—*continued*
m., arachnoid
m., artificial rupture of
m., bacterial cell
m., basement
m., basilar
m., blue mucous
m. -bound antigens
m., Bowman's
m., bronchial mucous
m., Bruch's
m., buccopharyngeal
m. ‣ bulging red tympanic
m. ‣ bulging yellow tympanic
m., capillary basement
m., cell
m., cellular
m. channel
m., choroidal new vessel
m., chorioallantoic
m., chorion
m., conjunctival
m., cricothyroid
m., cuprophane
m. current
m., cystic
m., Debove's
m., Demour's
m., Descemet's
m. disease ‣ extensive hyaline
m. disease (HMD) ‣ hyaline
m. disease ‣ pulmonary hypoplasia
m., drum
m., dryness of mucous
m., dural
m. dysfunction
m., egg's inner
m. electrical potential ‣ cell
m. elution
m., embryonic
m. enucleated, follicular
m., epiretinal
m., false
m., fatty cell
m., fenestrated
m., fetal
m., fetal placental
m., fibrous
m. fluidization
m., follicular
m. function
m., glial
m., glomerular basement
m. graft, mucous
m. gray, tympanic

m. ‣ Henle elastic
m. ‣ Henle fenestrated
m., Henle's
m., hyaline
m., hyaloid
m., hydration of mucous
m., hyoglossal
m., hyothyroid
m., hyperemic
m., hyperplastic
m. in brain, damaged cell
m., inflammation ‣ tympanic
m., infected
m., infected mucous
m., inflammation synovial
m. injected, tympanic
m., inner mucous
m., intermediate
m., internal elastic
m., Jacob's
m., labyrinth
m. lining alveolar spaces ‣ hyaline
m. lining, mucous
m. lining, pleural
m., loose rectal mucous
m. matted with tumor metastases
m., memory cell
m., microvascular
m., microvillus
m., mucous
m. ‣ myocardial basement
m., nasal
m., nasal mucous
m., Nasmyth's
m., nerve cell
m., nuclear
m. of brain, dural
m. of cell
m. of cervix uteri ‣ partial excision mucous
m. of 4th ventricle ‣ glial
m. of joint, synovial
m. of Liliequist
m. of lips ‣ pink mucous
m. of meninges, innermost
m. of nose ‣ inflammation of mucous
m. of tympanum ‣ anterior mallear fold of mucous
m. oxygenation (ECMO) ‣ extracorporeal
m. oxygenator
m. oxygenator ‣ extracorporeal
m. (TM) ‣ perforation of tympanic
m. perforation, tympanic

m., peridental
m., periodontal
m., peritoneal
m. permeability
m., pink mucous
m., placental
m., posterior mallear fold of tympanic
m. potential
m. potential of nerve cell
m. potential ‣ resting
m. (PROM), premature rupture of
m., premature ruptured
m., prolonged rupture of
m., prolonged rupture of fetal
m., pulmonary hyaline
m., pupillary
m., Ranvier's
m., Reissner's
m., retention of
m., Rivinus'
m., rupture of
m., rupture of tympanic
m., ruptured
m. ruptured spontaneously
m., sarcolemmal
m., Scarpa's
m. ‣ schneiderian respiratory
m., secondary tympanic
m., semipermeable
m., serous
m., Shrapnell's
m. ‣ spontaneous rupture of
m., spontaneously ruptured
m. stabilizing activity
m., sterilized
m. ‣ swollen nasal
m., syncytiovascular
m., synovial
m., tectorial
m. temperature ‣ tympanic
m., Tenon's
m., tensor muscle of tympanic
m. ‣ thickened synovial
m. thickening
m., thin plastic
m., thyreohyoid
m. (TM) ‣ tympanic
m., umbo of tympanic
m., venous
m., vitreous
membranoproliferative glomerulonephritis
membranous
m. bronchitis

m. canal
m. cataract
m. conjunctivitis
m. croup
m. cytoplasmic body
m. dysmenorrhea
m. endometritis
m. glomerulonephritis
m. glomerulonephritis, chronic
m. interventricular septum, high
m. labyrinth
m. laryngitis
m. lining, periosteal
m. nephritis ▸ immune-mediated
m. nephropathy
m. pharyngitis
m. pregnancy
m. rhinitis
m. septum
m. stomatitis
m. tissue
m. tube
m. urethra
m. urethra ▸ sphincter muscle of
m. wall
m. wall, lateral
memoriae, lapsus
memory(-ies) (Memory)
m. ability
m., abnormal
m., abstract conceptual
m., abuse
m., affect
m. aids
m., alertness and
m., alterations of
M. and Aging (OPTIMA) ▸ Oxford
    Project to Investigate
m. and attention ▸ verbal
m. and concentration test
m., and distortion ▸ hypnosis,
m., anterograde
m., auditory verbal
m., autobiographical
m. bank in brain
m. capacity
m., cardiac
m. cell membranes
m. cells
m., cellular
m., coast
m. complaint
m., concentration and
m. ▸ confused or faulty

m. ▸ confusion and poor judgment,
    loss of recent
m., conscious
m. consolidation process
m., core
m., corroborated
m., declarative
m. decline
m., decreased
m. defect
m., defective
m. deficit
m. deficit (JMD) ▸ juvenile
m., delayed abstract conceptual
m. disorder
m. disruption ▸ short-term
m. distortion
m. disturbance
m. dulled
m. dysfunction
m. ▸ endless alters, endless
m., episodic
m. exercises
m., false
m. falsification ▸ retroactive
m., faulty
m., feelings and perceptions
m., fleeting
m. flooding, manage
m. for distant events ▸ loss of
m. for past events
m. for recent events
m. for recent events ▸ impaired
m. for recent events ▸ loss of
m. for smell ▸ loss of
m. for trauma
m. for words ▸ loss of
m. ▸ fragmentary sensory
m. function
m. function ▸ long-term
m. function ▸ low
m. function ▸ nondistorting
m., functional
m. gaps
m. gating ▸ in-
m. ▸ hyperarousal and intrusive
m., immediate
m., immediate auditory
m., impaired
m. impaired assisted living
m. ▸ impaired short-term
m. impairment
M. Impairment (AAMI), Age-
    Associated

m. impairment and confabulation ▸
    recent
m., impairment of
m., implanted
m., implicit
m., increased
m., induced
m. ▸ intellectual function or
m., invalidate
m. ▸ involuntary intrusive
m., judge
m., label
m., lack of
m. lapse
m. ▸ lapse in short term
m. (LTM), long-term
m. loop
m. loss
m. loss, age-related
m. loss and confusion
m. loss ▸ dissociative
m. loss from brain
m. loss from depression
m. loss from pernicious anemia
m. loss, gradual
m. loss ▸ partial or complete
m. loss, patient has
m. loss ▸ permanent
m. loss ▸ progressive
m. loss, recent
m. loss ▸ severe
m. loss, short-term
m. loss ▸ slowly progressing
m. loss, temporary
m. loss ▸ total
m. malleability
m., mobility and strength
m. moiety
m., nonverbal
m., normal
m. of abuse, continuous and
    confirmed
m. of child abuse
m. of incest
m. of incest ▸ unverifiable
m. of unknown cause ▸ impaired
m. organization
m. organization, affectomotor
m. organization, competent
    abstract conceptual
m. organization, conceptual
m. organization ▸ verbal conceptual
m., painful
m., pathologic loss of
m. ▸ patient has decreased

memory(-ies)—*continued*
m. ▸ patient has pseudo-
m. ▸ patient has poor
m., patient's short term
m., perception and sensation ▸ intelligence,
m., perceptual
m. persistence
m., persistent
m., photographic
m. ▸ poor attention and
m. problems
m. process
m., progressive loss of
m. quest
m. quotient
m. recall
m. recall, slowed
m., recent
m., recognition
m., reconstruct repressed
m., recovered
m., remote
m. ▸ repetition enhances
m., repressed
m. repression
m. research
m. retention
M. Scale (WMS) ▸ Wechsler
m., screen
m., selective
m., semantic
m. (STM), short term
m. ▸ short-term verbal
m. skills ▸ functional
m., spatial
m. stent ▸ thermal
m. storage
m. storage location
m. ▸ superior rote
m. syndrome, false
m., temporary loss of
m. test
m. test ▸ functional
m. test ▸ nonverbal
m. test ▸ verbal
m. therapist ▸ recovered
m. therapy ▸ recovered
m. trace
m., traumatic
m., true
m., unconscious
m., uncorroborated
m., validate
m., verbal

m., visual
m. ▸ word-list
m., working
men (MEN)
M. (multiple endocrine neoplasia)
m. ▸ alcohol abuse among
m. ▸ estrogen therapy for
m., heterosexual
m., sexually active bisexual
m., sexually active homosexual
m. with alcohol abuse problems
menarche, onset of
menarcheal/menarchial
Mendel('s)
M. -Bekhterev reflex
M. dorsal reflex of foot
M. reflex
M. reflex, Bekhterev-
mendelian
m. characters
m. disease
m. disorder
m. ratio
Mendelson's syndrome
Menetrier's disease
Mengert's index
Menge's operation
Menge's pessary
Mengo encephalomyelitis
Mengo virus
Meniere's disease
Meniere's syndrome
meningeal
m. adhesions
m. anthrax
m. apoplexy
m. artery
m. artery, laceration middle
m. artery, ligation middle
m. carcinomatosis
m. cells
m. fibroblastoma
m. granules
m. hemorrhage
m. hydrops
m. hydrops, hypertensive
m. inflammation
m. irritation
m. leukemia
m. nerve
m. neurosyphilis
m. sarcoma
m. streak
m. vein
m. vein, middle

m. vessel, injury to
m. vessels
m. vessels, hemangioma
m. vessels, hemangiomatosis
m. vessels, ligation of
méningéale, tache
meninges
m., adjacent
m., angioma of
m., bacterial infection of
m., biopsy of
m. ▸ cord and
m., cyst of
m., drainage (dr'ge) of
m., exploration of
m., glistening transparent
m., impedances of
m., inflammation of
m., innermost membrane of
m., melanoma of
m., ossification of
m., suture of
meningioma
m., angioblastic
m., olfactory groove
m., parasagittal
meningitic respiration
meningitic striae
meningitidis, Cryptococcus
meningitidis, Neisseria
meningitis
m., acute
m., acute aseptic
m., acute bacterial
m., adult bacterial
m., African
m., amebic
m., aseptic
m., bacterial
m., basilar
m., benign lymphocytic
m., cerebral
m., cerebrospinal
m., child bacterial
m., chronic serous
m., community-acquired
m., cryptococcal
m., drowsiness from
m., Enteroviral
m., eosinophilic
m., epidemic cerebrospinal
m., external
m., gonococcal
m., gummatous
m., Haemophilus influenzae

m., internal
m., leukemic
m., Listeria monocytogenes
m., lymphocytic
m., meningococcal
m. ▸ meningococcal bacterial
m., meningococcic
m., metastatic
m., metastatic malignant
m., Mollaret's
m., mumps
m. necrotoxica reactiva
m., neonatal
m., neonatal streptococcal
m., nosocomial
m., occlusive
m. ossificans
m., otitic
m., parameningococcus
m., pediatric
m., plague
m., pneumococcal
m., posterior
m., purulent
m., pyogenic
m., Quincke's
m., recurrent
m. sepsis syndrome
m., septicemic
m. serosa
m. serosa circumscripta cystica
m., serous
m., simple
m., spinal
m., staphylococcal
m., sterile
m., streptococcal
m. sympathica
m., syphilitic
m., torula
m., tubercular
m., tuberculous
m., viral

meningocele ▸ repair of spina bifida with

meningococcal
m. bacterial meningitis
m. disease
m. infection
m. meningitis
m. pericarditis
m. vaccine

meningococcemia, acute fulminating
meningococcic meningitis
meningococcus conjunctivitis

meningoencephalitis
m., amebic
m., herpes
m., primary amoebic
m., viral

meningohypophyseal artery
meningomyelocele ▸ repair of spina bifida with
meningosepticum, Flavobacterium
meningovascular
m. neurosis
m. neurosyphilis
m. syphilis

meniscal tear
meniscal test
meniscectomy
m., lateral
m., medial
m., total

menisci ▸ medical and lateral
meniscoid occlusion
menisculocapsular attachment
meniscus
m. articularis
m. bone
m. bone, lateral
m. sign, bronchial
m., bucket-handle tear of
m., detachment of medial
m., dislocated medial
m. fluid
m., lateral
m. lens
m., medial
m. of acromioclavicular (AC) joint
m. of knee, cyst
m. of knee joint ▸ medial
m. of temporomaxillary joint
m., posterior horn of medial
m. sign
m. sign ▸ pleural
m. sign ▸ pulmonary
m., slipped
m., tear of
m., torn lateral
m., torn medial
m. transplant

Mennell's sign
menometrorrhagia, uncontrolled
menopausal
m. depresion
m. distress
m. gonadotropin (HMG), human
m. hot flashes
m. irritants

m. metrorrhagia
m. symptoms
m. symptoms, acute
m. syndrome
m. woman
m. years

menopause
m., artificial
m., atrophic
m., late
m., male
m. medication, post
m., natural
m., physiology of
m., stress
m., surgical
m., symptoms of
m., temporary

menorrhagia [*metrorrhagia*]
menorrhagia, intermittent
menorrhagia, painless
menorrhea
m., oligo◊
m., oligohyper◊
m., oligohypo◊

menses
m., absent
m., anovulatory
m., delayed
m. inducer
m., irregular
m., onset of

menstrual
m. age
m. anxiety
m. bleeding
m. bleeding, excessive
m. blood
m. changes
m. cramps
m. cramps ▸ diarrhea with
m. cycle
m. cycle, cessation of
m. cycles ▸ irregular
m. decidua
m. disorder
m. distress
m. epilepsy
m. extraction
m. flow
m. flow, heavy
m. flow, moderate
m. flow ▸ ovulation and
m. flow, scanty
m. flux

menstrual—*continued*
- m. function
- m. irregularities
- m. leukorrhea
- m. -like bleeding
- m. pain
- m. pain, functional
- m. pain ▸ severe
- m. period (MP)
- m. period ▸ absence of
- m. period from anemia ▸ heavy
- m. period from diabetes ▸ absent
- m. period (LMP) ▸ last
- m. period (LNMP) ▸ last normal
- m. period, late
- m. period, missed
- m. period (NMP) ▸ normal
- m. period (PMP), previous
- m. period with birth control pill
- m. periods ▸ erratic
- m. periods, heavy
- m. periods, irregular
- m. periods ▸ painful
- m. periods, prolonged
- m. periods, regular
- m. periods, scanty
- m. stage
- m. syndrome
- m. toxic shock syndrome (TSS)

menstrualis, decidua
menstrualis, herpes
menstruating, patient
menstruation
- m., anovular
- m., anovulatory
- m., delayed
- m., difficult
- m. disorder
- m., early onset of
- m., excessive
- m., infrequent
- m., irregular
- m., nonovulational
- m., onset of
- m., ovulatory
- m., painful
- m., profuse
- m., regurgitant
- m., retrograde
- m., scanty
- m., supplementary
- m., suppressed
- m., vicarious

mentagrophytes, Trichophyton

mental (Mental) [*dental*]
- m. aberration
- m. abilities and judgment
- m. ability
- m. ability impairment
- m. abnormality
- m. abuse
- m. action, slowness of
- m. activity
- m. activity, concentrated
- m. activity, coordination of
- m. activity, excessive
- m. activity ▸ subject engaged in
- m. acuity
- m. addiction
- m. affliction
- m. age
- m. agility
- m. agraphia
- m. alertness
- m. alterations
- m. and physical abilities
- m. and physical development, marked retardation of
- m. and psychological
- m. anguish
- m. anguish, depression or
- m. anguish, severe
- m. assessments
- m. attitude (PMA), positive
- m. attitudes
- m. bewilderment
- m. block
- m. blocking
- m. burnout
- m. capability
- m. capacity
- m. challenge
- m. characteristics
- m. clarity
- m. clouding
- m. collapse
- m. competence
- m. complex
- m. compulsions
- m. concept
- m. condition
- m. condition ▸ physical and
- m. confusion
- m. control, conscious
- m. decline
- m. defect
- m. defenses
- m. deficiency
- m. deficiency, idiopathic

- m. deficiency ▸ varying
- m. deficit
- m. degeneration
- m. degeneration ▸ progressive
- m. degradation
- m. depression
- m. derangement, temporary
- m. deterioration
- m. deterioration ▸ gradual
- m. deterioration ▸ rapid
- m. deterioration, severe
- m. development
- m. development, arrested
- m. dexterity
- m. disabilities
- m. disabilities, physical or
- m. disease
- m. disease, treatable
- m. disorder
- m. disorder, acute
- m. disorder, drug-induced
- m. disorder, major
- m. disorder ▸ methamphetamine-induced organic
- m. disorder, (nonorganic) ▸ insomnia related to another
- m. disorder, nonpsychotic
- m. disorder, organic
- m. disorder ▸ phencyclidine (PCP) organic
- m. disorder, progressive
- m. disorder ▸ psychoactive substance-induced organic
- m. disorder ▸ psychoactive substance organic
- m. disorder ▸ substance induced organic
- m. disorder ▸ transient organic
- m. disorder, transitory
- m. disorder, unspecified
- m. disorders, comorbidity of
- m. disorientation
- m. distress
- m. disturbance
- m. disturbance, acute
- m. dulling
- m. dullness
- m. dynamism
- m. dysfunction
- m. efficiency
- m. effort
- m. -emotional shift
- m. energy
- m. equilibrium
- m. equilibrium, disturbance of

m. exercise
m. exhaustion
m. faculties
m. faculties ▸ gradual loss of
m. failure
m. fatigue
m. fitness
m. flexibility
m. fluctuation
m. fogginess
m. foramen
m. function
m. function, alteration of
m. function ▸ decline in
m. function, dulling of
m. function ▸ episodic disturbance of
m. functions, higher
m. function, organized
m. function, overall level of
m. function ▸ stimulate
m. functioning
m. functioning, impaired
m. healing
m. health
m. health benefits
m. health care
m. health care ▸ effective
m. health center, community
m. health, comprehensive
m. health coverage ▸ mandated
m. health delivery system
M. Health, Department of
m. health, general
m. health, managed
m. health patients
m. health patients ▸ public
m. health practitioner
m. health problems ▸ nature of
m. health professional
m. health program
m. health provider
m. health service
m. health services ▸ outpatient
m. health status
m. health treatment
m. hygiene
m. illness
m. illness ▸ delusional
m. illness ▸ disabling
m. illness, employee
m. illness, level and degree of
m. illness ▸ major
m. illness, persistent
m. illness ▸ pervasive

m. illness, prevention of
m. illness ▸ previously unrecognized
m. illness ▸ severe
m. illness ▸ severe and persistent
m. illness, treatment of
m. image
m. imagery
m. impairment
m. inactivity
m. laziness
m. life
m. malfunctioning
M. Maturity Scale, Columbia
m. mechanism
m. nerve
m. neuropsychological
m. object
m. obtundity, state of
m. or physical condition ▸ irreversible
m. performance
m. predisposition
m. problems
m. problems ▸ warning signs of
m. process
m. proficiency
m. range
m. region
m. relaxation
m. reorganization
m. retardation
m. retardation, care of child
m. retardation, mild
m. retardation, moderate
m. retardation, profound
m. retardation, severe
m. retardation, undifferentiated
m. retraining
m. ritual
m. ▸ severe retardation,
m. skills, basic
m. skills ▸ progressive loss of
m. sluggishness
m. stability
m. state
m. state, altered
m. status
m. status ▸ alteration in
m. status changes
m. status evaluation
m. status examination
M. Status Examination (BNMSE), Brief Neuropsychological
m. status examination ▸ psychiatric

m. status ▸ fluctuating
m. status ▸ psychiatric
m. status ▸ rapid change in
m. status test
m. status test, mini-
m. status waxed and waned
m. stimulation
m. stress
m. stress, cardiac rehabilitation
m. stress test
m. subnormality
m. subnormality, profound
m. subnormality, severe
m. suffering
m. suggestion
m. symptoms, clearing of
m. syndrome disorder ▸ organic
m. syndrome, organic
m. tension
m. tension, decreased
m. tension, increased
m. therapy
m. toughness
m. word
mentalis muscle
mentalis muscle, ipsilateral
mentality
m., fortress
m. ▸ problem-solving
m. ▸ total blackout
mentally
m. active
m. alert, patient
m. challenged
m. challenged children
m. clear ▸ patient
m. cloudy, patient
m. competent, conscious and
m. confused
m. deranged, patient
m. disordered, patient
m. disordered person
m. disturbed individuals
m. disturbed patient
m. exhausting
m. handicapped
m. handicapped (EMH), educable
m. handicapped (TMH) ▸ trainable
m. ill, patient
m. impaired
m. incapacitated
m. retarded
m. retarded ▸ educable
m. retarded, halfway house for the
m. retarded, patient

mentally—*continued*
- m. retarded patient, trainable
- m. retarded patient, untrainable
- m. retarded ▸ profoundly
- m. retarded range of abilities
- m. stimulating activity
- m. unstimulating occupation

mentation
- m., aberration of
- m., dreaming
- m. or physical status ▸ altered
- m., sleep
- m., slow

Mentha canadensis
mentis, non compos
mentoanterior, left
mentoanterior, right
mentodextra
- m. anterior
- m. posterior
- m. transverse

mentolaeva transverse
mento-occipital diameter
mentoparietal diameter
mentoposterior, left
mentoposterior, right
mentotransverse, left
mentotransverse, right
menu planning, computer assisted
MEP (multimodality evoked potential)
mEq (milliequivalents)
mEq/L (milliequivalents per liter)
MER (mer)
- M. (mean ejection rate)
- M. (methanol extraction residue)
- m., mal de

meralgia paresthetica
mercaptomerin sodium
mercaptopurine (MP)
- m. and prednisone (VAMP) ▸ vincristine, amethopterin, 6-
- m. (POMP) ▸ prednisone, Oncovin, methotrexate, 6-
- m. therapy

Mercedes Benz sign
mercurial stomatitis
mercurialis, cachexia
mercurialis, tremor
mercury
- m. amalgam filling
- m. artifact
- m. lamp, Hildreth
- m. mass
- m. (mmHg) ▸ millimeters of
- m. pressure

- m. vapor lamp
- m. vapor lamp, cold quartz

Mercy Killing
meridian
- m., bladder
- m. degrees
- m. echocardiogram
- m. echocardiography
- m., gallbladder
- m., heart
- m., kidney
- m. ▸ large intestine
- m., liver
- m., lung
- m. of cornea, vertical
- m., pericardium
- m. ▸ small intestine
- m., spleen
- m., stomach
- m. ▸ triple burner
- m., vertical
- m., yang
- m., yin

meridional
- m. aberration
- m. sections
- m. wall stress

Merindino procedure
Mering reflex, von
Merkel's discs
Merkel's muscle
MERRF (myoclonic epilepsy and ragged red fiber) disease
Merritt syndrome, Kasabach
Merseburg triad
Mersilene
- M. graft
- M. sutures
- M. tape

Merculius lacrymans
Merzbacher disease, Pelizaeus
Merzbacher-Pelizaeus disease
mesangial cells
mesangial immune injury
mesaraica, tabes
mesatipellic pelvis
mesaugral proliferation
Mesc (mescaline)
Mescaline (Mescal) (mescaline)
- M. (Big Chief)
- M. (Buttons)
- M. (Cactus)
- M. (Mesc)
- M. (Mescal)
- M. (Nutmeg)

- M. (Peyote)
- M. ingested
- M. inhaled
- M. injected
- M. smoked
- M. sniffed
- M. snorted

mesencephalic
- m. flexure
- m. reticular formation
- m. tractomy

mesencephalon (*same as* meso-cephalon)
mesencephalon, superior portion of
mesenchymal
- m. cell
- m. cell, undifferentiated
- m. chondrosarcoma
- m. -derived tumor
- m. epithelium
- m. form
- m. intimal cell
- m. stem cells
- m. tissue
- m. tumor

mesenteria resection, wide
mesenteric
- m. adenitis
- m. angiogram, inferior
- m. angiogram, superior

m. angiography
- m. arteriography
- m. arterial thrombosis
- m. arteritis
- m. artery
- m. artery bypass ▸ superior
- m. artery (IMA), inferior
- m. artery line
- m. artery occlusion
- m. artery (SMA), superior
- m. artery syndrome ▸ superior
- m. blood vessel
- m. bypass graft
- m. cyst
- m. ganglion, inferior
- m. ganglion, superior
- m. hernia
- m. infarction
- m. ischemia
- m. ischemia ▸ acute
- m. ischemia ▸ chronic
- m. ischemia ▸ recurrent
- m. ischemia ▸ transient
- m. ischemia ▸ nonocclusive
- m. lymph nodes

m. lymph nodes, inferior
m. lymph nodes, superior
m. lymphadenitis
m. lymphadenopathy
m. node
m. node, calcified
m. obstruction
m. pregnancy
m. thrombosis
m. vascular occlusion
m. vascular occlusion ▸ inferior
m. vascular occlusion ▸ recurrent
m. vascular occlusion ▸ superior
m. vascular occlusion ▸ venous
m. vein, inferior
m. vein, superior
m. vein thrombosis
m. venous thrombosis

mesenterica
m., Candida
m., pseudotabes
m., tabes

mesentericus, Saccharomyces
mesentery
m., appendiceal
m. atrophic ▸ omentum and
m., dorsal
m., leaves of
m. of appendix
m. ▸ soft tissue hemorrhage into
m., ventral

mesh
m. gauze, fine
m. graft, tantalum
m. implant, Marlex
m. implant material, Marlex
m. implant material, tantalum
m. implant material, Teflon
m. implant material ▸ Usher's
   Marlex
m. implant material, wire
m. implant, tantalum
m. implant, Teflon
m. implant, Usher's Madex
m. implant, wire
m., Marlex
m. prosthesis, Harrison interlocked
m. prosthesis, House stainless
   steel
m. prosthesis, Teflon
m. prosthesis, Usher's Madex
m. skin
m. stent
m. stent ▸ Schatz-Palmaz tubular
m. stent ▸ stainless steel

m., tantalum
m., Teflon
m., titanium
meshed ball implant
mesher, Tanner
meshwork, trabecular
mesial [*medial*]
m. occlusion
m. surface
m. surface of occipital lobe of brain
m. surface of tooth
mesially ▸ vein ligated and retracted
mesnili, Chilomastix
mesnili, Macrostoma
mesoappendix, isolating
mesoappendix serially clamped, cut
   and ligated
mesoblastic
m. nephroma
m. segment
m. sensibility
mesocardia malposition
mesocaval shunt
mesocaval shunt, Drapanas
mesocephalic hemianesthesia
mesocephalon (*see* mesencephalon)
mesocolic hernia
mesocolic lymph nodes, cecal
mesocolon
m., ascending
m., descending
m., sigmoid
m., transverse
mesocortical pathways
Mesocretus auratus
mesocuneiform bone
mesoderm formation
mesoderm, precardiac
mesodermal
m. sarcoma, mixed
m. segment
m. structures
m. tumor
m. tumor, advanced uterine mixed
mesodermogenic neurosis
mesodermogenic neurosyphilis
mesolateral fold
mesolimbic system
mesonephric adenocarcinoma
mesothelial
m. cells
m. cells, microvilli in
m. hyperplasia
m. surface ▸ fibrinolytic activity of

mesothelioma
m., benign fibrous
m. ▸ benign pleural fibrous
m., malignant
m., malignant fibrous
m. of peritoneum
m. of pleura
m., pericardial
mesothenar muscle
mesouterine fold
message(s)
m., anti-alcohol
m., brain
m. competition ratio (MCR)
m., genetic
m., pain
m. to brain ▸ transmitting
   electrochemical
m. ▸ transmission of electric signals
   or
messenger
m. cells, chemical
m. hormones
m., chemical
m. ribonucleic acid (mRNA)
m., second
MET (minimal exposure transfusion)
MET (motivational enhancement
   therapy)
Meta rate responsive pacemaker
metabolic
m. abnormalities
m. abnormality ▸ genetic
m. acidosis
m. acidosis and coma, severe
m. acidosis, anion gap
m. acidosis, cannulation-induced
m. action
m. activation
m. activity, abnormal
m. activity, brains'
m. activity, normal
m. alkalosis
m. anomaly
m. antagonism
m. antagonist
m. aspect of alcoholism
m. balance
m. balance of heart
m. bone disease
m. cart
m. changes
m. chemistry
m. cirrhosis
m. clearance rate

metabolic—*continued*
- m. coma
- m. complication
- m. control
- m. control mechanisms
- m. defects
- m. demands
- m. detoxification
- m. disease
- m. disorder
- m. disorder ‣ asymptomatic
- m. disorder, chronic
- m. disorder ‣ inherited
- m. disturbance
- m. effect
- m. efficiency, enhanced
- m. emergency
- m. encephalopathy
- m. encephalopathy, toxic
- m. equivalents of task
- m. etiology, toxic
- m. function
- m. function, cerebral
- m. function ‣ regenerative
- m. heat production
- m. heat production ‣ increase
- m. hypoglycemia
- m. imbalance
- m. neuropathy
- m. or electrode disturbance
- m. parameter determination
- m. product
- m. rate
- m. rate (BMR) ‣ basal
- m. rate, cerebral
- m. rate meter
- m. rate, myocardial
- m. rate of glucose ‣ cerebral
- m. rate of oxygen ‣ cerebral
- m. rate (RMR) ‣ resting
- m. rate, somnolent
- m. rate, work
- m. renal syndrome
- m. screening ‣ mandated
- m. stone
- m. syndrome
- m. syndrome ‣ myonephropathic
- m. syndrome ‣ myonephrotic
- m. temperature graph, basal
- m. therapy
- m. transformation
- m. vasodilatory capacity
- m. waste ‣ diffusion of
- m. waste product lactic acid

metabolically active tissue

metabolism
- m., abnormal
- m., aerobic
- m., alcohol
- m., amino acid
- m., anaerobic
- m., arachidonate
- m., assess cardiac
- m., basal
- m., body
- m., bone
- m., brain
- m., calcium
- m., carbohydrate
- m., catecholamine
- m., cell
- m., cellular
- m., cocaine
- m., copper
- m. ‣ decrease in mitochondrial
- m., decreased
- m. disease ‣ iron
- m., disorders of amino acid
- m., fetal
- m., glucose
- m., hepatic
- m. ‣ hepatic drug
- m. in brain, glucose
- m., inborn error of
- m., increased
- m., independent
- m. index (CMI) ‣ carbohydrate
- m., lipid
- m., myocardial
- m., neuronal
- m., neurotransmitter
- m. of fat
- m., polyamine
- m., porphyrin
- m., protein
- m., rapid
- m. ‣ rapid bone
- m., slow
- m. /stress perfusion protocol ‣ rest
- m. syndrome ‣ myonephropathic

metabolite(s)
- m., arachidonic acid
- m., cocaine
- m., prostacyclin

metabolize certain drugs ‣ slowly
metabolize phenylalanine
metabolizing enzymes ‣ microsomal drug
metabolizer, rapid
metabolizer, slow

metabolizing enzyme, altered
metacarpal [*metatarsal*]
- m. bones
- m. epiphyseal centers
- m. fracture
- m. head
- m., neck of
- m. of wrist, first
- m. splint, Lytie's
- m. vein, dorsal
- m. vein, dorsal interosseous
- m. vein, palmar

metacarpophalangeal (MP)
- m. articulations
- m. joint (MPJ)
- m. joint (MPJ), silastic

metachromatic
- m. granules
- m. leukodystrophy (MLD)
- m. stain
- m. substance

metachronal rhythm
metachronous lung cancer
Metagonimus
- M. ovatus
- M., trematoda
- M. yokogawai

metaherpetic keratitis
metal
- m. braces, traditional
- m. disease ‣ hard
- m. electrode
- m. heart valve
- m. implant, polyethylene
- m. insert teeth
- m. -on-metal hip replacement
- m. -on-plastic hip replacement
- m. partial dentures, cast
- m. plate
- m. poisoning, heavy
- m. prosthesis
- m. resonance, bell-
- m. sewing ring
- m. sieve implanted surgically
- m. stain, heavy
- m. stent
- m., trace

Metalase copper vapor laser
metalcaligenes, Alcaligenes
metallic
- m. artifact
- m. breath sounds
- m. clicks
- m. density
- m. echo

m. fixation device
m. foreign body (MFB)
m. fragments
m. implant
m. plate and screws
m. rales
m. sound
m. taste
m. tinkle
m. tremor
metallicum, Simulium
metameric syndrome
metamorphosing respiration, Seitz's
metamorphosis
  m., fatty
  m., mild fatty
  m. of liver ▸ fatty
metanephric caps
metanephrogenic tissue
metaphyseal
  m. bands
  m. bands, dense
  m. dysplasia
metaphysis, distal radial
metaphysis of femur, proximal
metaplasia
  m., agnogenic myeloid
  m., apocrine
  m. ▸ focal areas of squamous
  m. ▸ goblet cell
  m., intestinal
  m., marked squamous
  m., myeloid
  m. of mucosa ▸ squamous
  m. of pulp
  m., osseous
  m., patchy
  m., squamous
  m. with myelofibrosis, myeloid
metaplastic mucus-secreting cell
metapneumonic empyema
metapneumonic pleurisy
metastable state
metastasectomy, pulmonary
metastasis(-es) (mets)
  m., adnexal
  m., adrenal
  m., advanced
  m., axillary
  m., axillary lymph node
  m., biochemical
  m., blastic
  m., blood-borne
  m., bone
  m., bone marrow

m., brain
m., calcareous
m., cannonball
m., cardiac
m., cerebral
m., cervical lymphatic
m., chest wall
m., choriocarcinoma lung with brain
m., choroidal
m. (TNM) classification ▸ tumor/nodes
m., contact
m., contralateral axillary
m., crossed
m., direct
m., distant
m., extensive intra-abdominal
m. ▸ focal infiltrating tumor
m., generalized
m., hematogenous
m. hemorrhagic
m., hemorrhagic tumor
m., hepatic
m. ▸ hepatosplenomegaly with liver
m., hilar node
m., implantation
m. in breast carcinoma, axillary nodal
m. in lung carcinoma, supraclavicular node
m. in ribs ▸ osteoblastic
m., intra-abdominal
m., intracranial
m., intraocular
m., intrapulmonary
m., intrapulmonary nodular
m., iris
m. left adrenal gland ▸ focal
m., liver
m., local
m., lung
m., lung and bone
m. ▸ lymph node
m., lymphangitic
m., lymphatic
m., mediastinal
m. ▸ membranes matted with tumor
m., miliary
m., multiple
m., multiple bone
m., multiple brain
m., multiple tumor
m., multiple widespread
m., neck
m., necrotic

m., necrotic tumor
m., nodular
m., nodular tumor
m., occult
m. of lung
m. ▸ optic disc
m., orbital
m., osseous
m., painful bone
m., painful local and regional
m., palliation in brain
m., paradoxical
m., (mets), patient has brain
m., pelvic
m., periaortic lymph node
m., pleural
m. ▸ primary ovarian carcinoma with
m., pulmonary
m., questionable
m., regional
m., retinal
m., retrograde
m., retroperitoneal liver and lung
m., scapular
m., skeletal
m., skin
m., soft tissue
m., solitary pulmonary
m., spinal epidural
m. (TNM) staging system ▸ tumor, nodes,
m., subcutaneous
m. syndrome, occipital condyle
m. syndrome, orbital
m. syndrome ▸ parasellar and middle fossa
m. system, remote
m. throughout serosa ▸ tumor
m. to bone
m. to chest wall
m. to diaphragm
m. to liver
m. to lung
m. to lung ▸ cannonball
m. to mediastinum
m. to pericardium
m. to pleurae
m. to spleen ▸ focal
m. to thyroid
m., transplantation
m., tumor
m. (TNM) ▸ tumor, nodes,
m., vaginal
m., vertebral

metastasis(-es)—*continued*
  m., widespread
  m., widespread bony
  m., widespread osseous
metastasizing tumor
metastatic
  m. adenocarcinoma
  m. adenocarcinoma pancreas
  m. adenopathy
  m. bladder carcinoma
  m. bone lesion
  m. brain disease
  m. brain tumor
  m. breast cancer
  m. cancer
  m. carcinoid, syndrome
  m. carcinoma
  m. carcinoma, advanced
  m. carcinoma liver
  m. cardiac tumors
  m. cholangiocarcinoma
  m. colon cancer
  m. colorectal cancer
  m. deposits
  m. disease
  m. disease, advanced
  m. disease, clinical evidence of
  m. disease, distant
  m. disease, extensive
  m. disease, extradural
  m. disease, general
  m. disease, occult
  m. disease of liver
  m. disease of lung
  m. disease, osseous
  m. disease, palliation in advanced
  m. disease, palliation in early
  m. disease, presumptive
  m. disease, surgical management
    of
  m. edema
  m. endometrial carcinoma
  m. endometrial stromal sarcoma
  m. factor, anti-
  m. focus, known
  m. implants
  m. involvement
  m. involvement, extensive
  m. large cells undifferentiated
    carcinoma
  m. lesion
  m. liver nodule
  m. lung cancer ▸ inoperable
  m. lung carcinoma
  m. lung disease

  m. malignancy of liver ▸ carcinoid
  m. malignant melanoma
  m. malignant meningitis
  m. mammary cancer
  m. melanoma
  m. meningitis
  m. neoplasia
  m. nodes
  m. nodules
  m. nodules, multiple
  m. ophthalmia
  m. or benign lesion ▸ malignant,
  m. orbital tumor
  m. orchitis
  m. papillary adenocarcinoma
  m. pericardial tumor
  m. phenotype
  m. pneumonia
  m. pulmonary carcinoma
  m. pulmonary lesions, early
  m. recurrence
  m. retinitis
  m. sarcoma
  m. site
  m. spinal cord tumor
  m. spread
  m. testicular cancer
  m. tumor
metatarsal [*metacarpal***]**
  m. arch
  m. area ▸ relieve pressure on
  m. bones
  m. cuneiform joint
  m. fracture
  m. head
  m. osteotomy
  m. pad
  m. splint, Baylor
  m. vein, dorsal
  m. vein, plantar
metatarsalgia, pain of
metatarsophalangeal
  m. articulations
  m. joint (MPJ)
  m. joint arthritis
  m. joint disorder
metatarsus
  m. adductocavus
  m. adductovarus
  m. adductus
  m. adductus, bilateral
  m. atavicus
  m. latus
  m. primus varus deformity
  m. varus

metazoal myocarditis
metchnikovii, Vibrio
meter(s)
  m., analog rate
  m. -angle (ma)
  m., counting rate
  m., decibel
  m. (FM) ▸ Doppler flow◊
  m. (fcm) ▸ foot-candle
  m. (gm-m) ▸ gram-
  m. ▸ home blood glucose
  m., impedance
  m. lens
  m. mask
  m. ▸ metabolic rate
  m. (OSM) ▸ oxygen saturation
  m. per second (m/sec) squared
  m., pulse
  m., rate
  m. (rhm) ▸ roentgens per hour at
    one
  m. run
  m., sanguino◊
  m. spirometer, Venturi's
  m. squared (kg/m^2) ▸ kilogram per
  m. squared ▸ liters per minute per
  m. squared, milligrams per
  m., Statham electromagnetic flow
metered-dose inhaler (MDI)
metered-dose spray
Meth (amphetamines)
Meth (crystal methamphetamine)
methacholine bronchoprovocation
  challenge
methacrylate
  m. cement, methyl
  m. glue, methyl
  m., glycerol
  m., glycol
  m., methyl
methadone
  m. abstinence
  m. detoxification clinic
  m. dosage ▸ maternal
  m. levels ▸ maternal neonatal
  m. maintenance
  m. maintenance treatment program
  m. program
  m. program, outpatient
  m. treatment
  m. treatment units
  m. use in detoxification
methamphetamine
  m. (Speed) (Crank)
  m. abuser

m. addiction
m. (Crank) addiction
m. ▸ cardiovascular effects of
m., crystal
m. (Crank), crystal
m. (Crystal), crystal
m. (Glass), crystal
m. (Ice), crystal
m. (Meth), crystal
m. (Speed), crystal
m. dependents
m. -induced disorder
m. -induced organic mental
    disorder
m. intoxication, chronic
m., neurotoxicity of
m. psychosis
m., pure
m. -related deaths
m., smokable
m. ▸ smokable form of
m. ▸ smoking of crystal
methanol extraction residue (MER)
methaqualone (Quads)
methedrine intoxication, chronic
methemoglobinemic cyanosis ▸
    hereditary
methicillin-resistant Staphylococcus
    aureus (MR-SA)
methicillin sodium
methiodal contrast medium, sodium
methiodal, sodium
methionine diet ▸ low
methionine malabsorption syndrome
method(s) (Method)
m., access
m., Addis
m. anterior shoulder repair, Mosley
m., area length
m., atrial extrastimulus
m., Ball's
m., barrier
m., Bence-Jones protein
m., bench
m., Beuttner's
m. bleeding time, Ivy's
m., bone healing
m., Bonnaire's
m., Borges
m., Bradley
m. bronchography, Cope-
m., Byrd-Dew
m., Caldwell-Moloy
m., Camp-Gianturco
m., cancer detection

m., case
m., Chaput's
m., chromogenic
m., Cobb's
m., Colcher-Sussman
m., conventional
m., Crede's
m., Danforth's
m., Delore's
m., diagnostic
m., disc diffusion
m., Douglas'
m., Dubois'
m ▸ edge detection
m., electromagnetic field
m., Essex-Lopresti
m. ▸ evaluation of behavioral
m., Ferguson's
m. for air gap correction, isodose
    shift
m., Forlanini's
m., Freiburg
m., Freud's cathartic
m., Gabastou's hydraulic
m., Gartner
m ▸ gas clearance
m., Girout's
m., goal attainment
m., gram stain
m., group
m. ▸ half-time
m., Hamilton's
m., Harris' staining
m., Harrison's
m., Harter's
m. ▸ head tilt
m., Heublein's
m., Hirschberg's
m., Hunt's
m., Hyland's
m. ▸ indocyanine green
m., invasive
m., Ionescu
m., iron hematoxylin
m., Isaac's differential distortion
    divergent
m., isodose shift
m., Jung's
m., Kluge's
m., Kristeller's
m., LaLeche
m., Lee-White
m., Lee-White clotting time
m., LeMesuriers
m., Lerous

m., Marmo's
m., Mauriceau
m., McArthur's
m., micro-Kjeldahl
m. ▸ moderation-oriented treatment
m., Monte Carlo
m., Morison's
m., natural healing
m., noninvasive
m. of administering medication ▸
    action, dose, route and
m. of artificial respiration ▸ Schafer
m. of childbirth, Lamaze
m. of delivery, Leboyer
m. of Kaperansky
m. of skin closure
m. of treatment
m. of treatment, alternative
m. of treatment, multidisciplinary
m., Ottonello's
m., Pajot's
m., parallax
m., Parama's
m., Pavlov's
m., peek-and-see
m., Permutit
m., Pfeiffer-Comberg
m., phacoemulsification
m., point-dose prescription
m. ▸ prick test
m., prism
m., Puzo's
m., pyramid
m. ▸ Raff Glantz derivative
m., rhythm
m., routine
m., Scarpa
m., Schiller
m., Schüller
m., Schultze's
m., Schuman's
m., screening
m., selecting treatment
m., self-rescue
m., Sigma
m. ▸ sliding scale
m., Smellie
m., Smellie-Veit
m., Sommer-Foegella
m., Somogyi
m. ▸ Stanford biopsy
m. ▸ stimulus control
m. ▸ stress relief
m., suction
m., Sweet's

method(s)—*continued*
- m., thermodilution
- m., Thoms'
- m., treatment
- M. (TRAM) ▸ Treatment Response Assessment
- m. ▸ visualization and relaxation
- m., Watson's
- m., weight loss
- m., Westergren
- m., Wolf's
- m., wrinkle
- m., Ziehl-Neelsen
- m., Zieve's
- m., Zimmer's

methodic chorea
methodological requirements
methodology
- m., assay
- m., biofeedback
- m., hemapheresis
- m. of clinical trials
- m., research
- m., scientific

methotrexate (MTX)
- m. and cistoplatin, high dose
- m. and 5-fluorouracil ▸ high dose
- m., 5-fluorouracil (CMF) ▸ Cytoxan,
- m. intrathecally
- m., 6-mercaptopurine, and prednisone (VAMP) therapy ▸ vincristine,
- m., 6-mercaptopurine (POMP) ▸ prednisone, Oncovin

methyl
- m. alcohol poisoning
- m. benzoate
- m. ether, ethinylestradiol
- m. group
- m. methacrylate
- m. methacrylate cement
- m. methacrylate glue
- m. red
- m. test-butyl ether (MTBE)

methylcrotonylglycinuria, beta-
methyldopa, alpha
methylene blue
- m.b. active substance
- m.b. agar, eosin
- m.b., carbolic
- m.b. dye test
- m.b., eosin
- m.b. insufflation

methylglucamine, Cholografin
methylmalonic academia

methylmalonic acidosis
methylmercaptopurine riboside
methylprednisolone sodium succinate
methyltyrosine, alpha-
metopic suture
Metopirone test
Metrazol shock therapy
metric ophthalmoscopy
metric system
metritis
- m. dissecans
- m., dissecting
- m., puerperal

metrizamide cisternography
metrizamide contrast medium
metrizoate sodium contrast medium
metrogram, electro◊
metrorrhagia [*menorrhagia*]
metrorrhagia, menopausal
metrorrhagia myopathica
mets (*same as* metastases)
mets (metastases), patient has brain
Meulengracht's diet
MeV (megaelectron volt)
Mev. (million electron volts)
Mexican
- "M. hat" erythrocyte
- M. (marijuana)
- M. Mud (heroin)
- M. patient
- M. Reds (barbiturates)

mexicana, Psilocybe
mexicana, Trypanosoma
mexicanum, Ambystoma
Meyer('s)
- M. hockey stick incision
- M. loop
- M. radical mastectomy, Willy
- M. sinus
- M. theory

Meynert('s)
- M. bundle
- M. commissure
- M. decussation
- M., fountain decussation of
- M., nucleus basalis of
- M. tract

Meynet's nodes
Mezei granules
MF (medium frequency)
MF (microflocculation)
M/F (male-female) ratio
MFB (metallic foreign body)

MFEF (maximal forced expiratory flow)
MFR (mucous flow rate)
MG (mesiogingival)
MG (myasthenia gravis) ▸ muscle-weakening
Mgb assay ▸ serum
mg/mgm (milligram)
mgh (milligram-hour)
M globulin (IgM) deficiency, gamma
mg% (milligrams per 100 milliliters)
MG, streptococcus
MGR (modified gain ratio)
MH (marital history)
MH (medical history)
MHB (maximum hospital benefit)
MHB (maximum hospital benefit) ▸ patient reached
MHD (mean hemolytic dose)
MHD (minimum hemolytic dose)
mHg (millimeters of mercury)
MI (mitral incompetence)
MI (mitral insufficiency)
MI (myocardial infarction)
- MI. ▸ acute
- MI., anterior
- MI., atrial
- MI., inferior
- MI., old
- MI., old inferior wall

MIBG scintigraphy ▸ iodine 131
MIBI imaging ▸ technetium-99m
MIC (minimum inhibitory concentration)
mica pneumoconiosis
micdadei, Legionella
micdadei, Tatlockia
mice, joint
micellar concentration, critical
micelles in vitreous
Michaelis' rhomboid
Michel deformity
Michel technique
Micheli syndrome, Marchiafavas-
micro [*macro*]
microabscesses, multiple
microadenoma, pituitary
microaerophilic cocci
microaerophilic organism
microaneurysm ▸ funduscopic examination revealed
microangiopathic hemolytic anemia
microangiopathy
- m., diabetic
- m. (IRMA), intraretinal

m., thrombotic
microangioplasty, coronary
microbe(s)
m., air
m. genes
m., pneumonia
m. to host ▸ transmission of
microbial
m. action
m. cells
m. contaminants
m. contamination
m. contamination ▸ life-threatening
m. infections, cancer-linked
m. mutants
m. resistance
microbicidal spectrum
microbiologic assessment
microbiologic sampling
microbiological assay
microbiological cure
microbiology, molecular
microcalcifications, breast
microcalcifications, subtle
microcautery unit
microcellular organisms
microcephalic idiocy
microchemical environment
microchip technology
microcirculation
m., coronary
m., normal tissue
m., pulmonary
m., tumor
Micrococcus (micrococcus)
M. lysodeikticus
m. organism
M. pyogenes variety aureus
microcrimped prosthesis
microcystic adenoma
**microcystic pilocytic cerebellar
astrocytoma**
microcytic anemia
microcytic, hyperchromic
microcytotoxicity assay
**microdensitophotometric
quantification**
microdentium, Treponema
microdermabrasion treatment
microdetector, ceramic
microdialysis study ▸ in vivo
microdiscectomy, arthroscopic laser
Microdots (LSD)
microelectrode technique
microembolic disease of lung

microencapsulation assay
microfiche records
microfilament structures
microfilaria
m. bancrofti
m. diurna
m. streptocerca
microflocculation, cardiolipin
microfold cell
microfollicular adenoma
microfolliculoid carcinoma
microglandular adenosis
microglial cell
micrognathia-glossoptosis syndrome
micrografting hair
micrograph, electron
micrographic surgery ▸ Mohs
microhair transplant
**microhemagglutination Treponema
pallidum**
microinjection of genetic material
microinjection therapy
microinvasion, tumor with
microinvasive carcinoma
microinvasive cervical cancer
micro-Kjeldahl method
Microknit patch graft
microlipo injection
Microlith pacemaker pulse generator
microlithiasis, pulmonary alveolar
micromaniacal delirium
micromelic dwarf
micrometer disc
micromillimeter (mm)
Micromonospora purpurea
micromyeloblastic leukemia
microneurosurgical procedure
micronodular cirrhosis
micronodular cirrhosis, severe
microorganism(s)
m., active
m. contamination
m., enterococcus
m., exogenous group of
m., gonococcus
m., mixture of
m., pathogenic
m., pneumococcus
m., Siderobacter
m., susceptible
microphages, fat-laden
microphone, cardiac catheter
microphonic, cochlear
micropigmentation, dermal
micropins, Pischel's

Micropore Tape
microptic delirium
microscope (Microscope)
m., acoustic
m., atomic force
m., beta ray
m., binocular
m., capillary
m., centrifuge
m., comparison
m., compound
m., corneal
m., darkfield
m., electron
m., epic
m., fluorescence
m., Greenough
m., hypodermic
m., infrared
m., integrating
m., interference
m., ion
m., laser
m., Leitz
m., light
m., Omni operating
m., opaque
M., Oto-
m., phase
m., phase-contrast
m., polarizing
m., projection x-ray
m., rectified polarizing
m., reflecting
m., Rheinberg
m. ▸ scanning electron
m., scanning probe
m. (STM) ▸ scanning tunneling
m., schlieren
m., Shambaugh-Derlocki operating
m., simple
m., slit-lamp
m., split lamp
m., stereoscopic
m., stroboscopic
m., trinocular
m., ultrasonic
m., ultraviolet
m., ultraviolet color-translating
television
m., x-ray
m., Zeiss operating
microscopic/macroscopic
m. agglutination
m. air sacs ▸ vital

microscopic—*continued*
- m. analysis
- m. analysis of secretion
- m. anatomy
- m. blood vessels
- m. cancer cells
- m. central nervous system (CNS) lesion
- m. cervical involvement
- m. changes
- m. channels
- m. diagnosis
- m. discectomy
- m. disease ▸ undetected
- m., electron-
- m. evaluation
- m. examination
- m. examination, autopsy
- m. examination, electron
- m. examination of cells
- m. fibroadenoma
- m. findings
- m. findings, negative
- m. findings, positive
- m. focus
- m. focus of cells
- m. glasses
- m. granular cell tumor
- m. hematuria
- m. intestinal parasites
- m. invasion of duodenal wall
- m. level
- m. nerves
- m. plaques
- m. polyangiitis
- m. polymers
- m. section
- m. sensors
- m. slide
- m. slide, concave
- m. strep bacteria
- m. stricture
- m. study
- m. test, filter paper
- m. tumor cells
- m. tumors

microscopically
- m. congested
- m. congested, spleen
- m. immature
- m. immature brain

microscopy
- m., clinical
- m., darkfield

- m. (EM) ▸ definitive diagnosis by electron
- m., electron
- m., fluorescence
- m., fundus
- m., immune electron
- m., immunoelectron
- m., immunofluorescent
- m., light
- m. (RIM) ▸ reflection interference
- m., scanning electron
- m., specular
- m., television
- m., transmission electron

microsection
- m. examination
- m., specimen submitted for
- m., tissue prepared for

microsomal drug-metabolizing enzymes
microsomal TRC (tanned red cells) antibody titer
microsphere(s)
- m. kit, Tc (technetium) -99m albumin
- m. perfusion scintigraphy
- m. ▸ polystyrene latex
- m., radiolabeled
- m. technique

Microsporum
- M. audouini
- M. canis
- M. felineum
- M. fulvum
- M. furfur
- M. gypseum
- M. lanosum

microsurgery
- m., computer assisted stereotactic laser
- m. of ear
- m., reconstructive
- m. technique

microsurgical
- m. conization
- m. instrument
- m. technique

microsurgically implanted graft
microti, Mycobacterium
microtome
- m., freezing
- m., rocking
- m., rotary
- m., sliding

Microtrombidium akamushi

Microtus montebelli
microvascular
- m. abnormalities (IRMA), intraretinal
- m. angina
- m. bone grafting
- m. complication
- m. decompression surgery
- m. disease
- m. disease, coronary
- m. disease ▸ diabetic
- m. free flap
- m. injury
- m. membrane
- m. neurosurgery
- m. permeability ▸ pulmonary
- m. pressure, pulmonary
- m. surgery

Microvel Dacron graft, Meadox
Microvel double velour graft
microvilli in mesothelial cells
microvillus membrane
microvolt(s) (mv/μV)
- m. mean deflection
- m., measured in
- m. per millimeter

microwave(s)
- m. ablation system
- m. (mw) amplification
- m. amplification by stimulated emission of radiation (MASER)
- m., beaming of
- m. dysfunction
- m. hyperthermia
- m. radiation
- m. radiation, hazard of
- m. ▸ shrink prostate with
- m., superficially applied
- m. technology ▸ Adaptive Phased Array
- m. therapy
- m. thermotherapy (TUMT) ▸ transurethral

microwaveable heat packs
micturition
- m. center
- m., control of
- m. cystourethrogram
- m. reflex center in brain
- m. reflex center ▸ spinal
- m. syncope

MICU (Medical Intensive Care Unit)
mid
- m. -cycle phase
- m. -depth ▸ dose calculated as

m. -diastolic heart murmur ▸ apical
m. -diastolic murmur
m. -diastolic rumble
m. -expiratory flow ▸ forced
m. -expiratory flow (MMEF) ▸ maximal
m. -expiratory flow (MMEF) ▸ maximum
m. -expiratory flow rate (MMEFR) ▸ maximal
m. -expiratory flow ▸ mean forced
m. -expiratory flow rate ▸ mean
m. -infrared pulsed laser
m. -parental height
MID (maximum inhibiting dilution)
MID (mesioincisodistal)
MID (minimum infective dose)
midaxillary line (MAL)
midbrain
m. and pons, diminished attenuation
m., aqueduct of
m. deafness
m. ▸ dissection hemorrhage of
m. hemorrhage, massive
m. resistance
MIDCAB (minimally invasive direct coronary artery bypass)
midcarpal joint
midcervical apophyseal joint
midclavicular line (MCL)
midcostal line
midday sleepiness
Middeldorpf's triangle
middle
m. -age spread
m. back ▸ pain in
m. cardiac nerve
m. cardiac vein
m. cerebellar peduncle
m. cerebral artery, accessory
m. cerebral artery (MCA)
m. cerebral artery, clipping
m. cerebral artery thrombosis ▸ acute
m. cerebral peduncle
m. cerebral vein, deep
m. cerebral vein, superficial
m. cervical cardiac nerve
m. cervical ganglion
m. -class medical model
m. clunial nerves
m. colic lymph nodes
m. colic vein
m. commissure of cerebrum

m. cranial fossa
m. ear
m. ear, acute
m. ear bone
m. ear cavity
m. ear cleft
m. ear deafness
m. ear disease
m. ear effusion
m. ear effusion and drainage
m. ear effusion ▸ persistent
m. ear infection
m. ear infection, chronic
m. ear, inflammation of
m. ear, malformed
m. ear ▸ ventilate
m. finger
m. fossa
m. fossa metastasis syndrome ▸ parasellar and
m. frontal gyrus
m. gluteal nerve
m. hemiblock ▸ left
m. hemorrhoidal vein
m. lobe
m. lobe (RML) bronchial orifice ▸ right
m. lobe bronchus
m. lobe collapse
m. lobe (RML) of lung ▸ right
m. lobe of right lung
m. lobe orifice
m. lobe (RML) ▸ right
m. lobe syndrome
m. lobe (RML) syndrome ▸ right
m. meatus
m. meningeal artery, laceration
m. meningeal artery, ligation
m. meningeal vein
m. pain
m. palatine nerve
m. palatine suture
m. petrosal nerve, superficial
m. phalanx
m. portion of stroma
m. rectal vein
m. sacral vein
m. scalene muscle
m. supraclavicular nerves
m. temporal gyrus
m. temporal vein
m. third
m. third, junction of
m. thyroid vein
m. turbinate

m. umbilical fold
m. umbilical ligament
midepigastric pain, severe
midepigastric tenderness
midepigastrium to pubis, scar from
midesophageal diverticulum
midflow rate (MMFR) ▸ maximal
midforceps operative delivery
midgut ischemia
midlife
m. brain degeneration
m. depression
m. sexuality
m. transition
midline
m. episiotomy
m. granuloma
m. incision
m. malignant polymorphic reticulosis
m., movable in
m. scar
m., septum in
m. sharp and mobile ▸ carina
m. shift
m. skin incision
m. structures
m. structures, shift of
m., tongue protrudes in
m., trachea
m. tumor, deep
midlung field
midnodal extrasystole
midnodal rhythm
midoccipital electrode, low
midplane doses, identical
midsacral region
midsagittal plane
midsagittal plane dose of rads in fractions
midshaft of bone
midsternal incision
midsternal line
midstream culture, urine
midsystolic
m. buckling
m. click syndrome
m. clicks
m. dip
m. murmur
m. notching
midtemporal
m. area
m. focus
m. focus of slow activity

midtemporal—*continued*
  m. slow wave focus
  m. spike focus
  m. spiking
midthoracic esophagus
midtibial perforator
midtrimester bleeding
Miege's syndrome
Miescher('s)
  M. corpuscles
  M. elastoma
  M. tubes
  M. tubules
MIF (migration inhibition factor)
MIFR (maximal inspiratory flow rate)
mignon lamp
Mignon's eosinophilic granuloma
migraine
  m., abdominal
  m. aborting drug
  m. -associated vertigo
  m. attack
  m., atypical
  m. aura
  m., basilar
  m., basilar hemiplegic
  m., biofeedback therapy of
  m., classic
  m., common
  m. equivalent
  m., fulgurating
  m. headache
  m. headache, autogenic training for
  m. headache, childhood
  m. headache ▸ confusion from
  m. headache from birth control pill
  m. headache ▸ syncopal
  m. headache ▸ weather-related
  m. headaches, chronic
  m., hormone
  m. (ECM) lesion ▸ erythema chronicum
  m., ophthalmic
  m., ophthalmoplegic
  m., oro-cheiro
  m. pain control
  m. ▸ painful and disabling
  m. personality
  m. ▸ postdrome of
  m. ▸ prodrome of
  m. prophylactic medication
  m., recurrence of
  m. syncope
  m. therapy, acute
  m. ▸ trigger factors for

  m., variants of
  m., vertebrobasilar
  m., vestibular
migrainous neuralgia
migrainous neuralgia, Harris,
migrans
  m., Agamonematodum
  m., erythema
  m., erythema chronicum
  m. ▸ ocular larva
  m., thrombophlebitis
  m. visceral larva
migrate [*ligate, plicate*]
migrated tumor
migrating
  m. cheilitis
  m. pacemaker
  m. phlebitis
migration
  m. inhibition factor (MIF)
  m., larval
  m. ▸ neural crest
  m., pigmentary
migratory
  m. cells
  m. deep vein thrombophlebitis
  m. ophthalmia
  m. pain
  m. pneumonia
  m. polyarthritis
  m. pulmonary infiltrate
  m. thrombus
Migula's classification
mika operation
Mikity syndrome, Wilson-
Mikity-Wilson syndrome
Mikulicz('s)
  M. amputation, Wladimiroff-
  M. cells
  M. disease
  M. operation
  M. pyloroplasty, Heineke-
  M. syndrome
  M. variance
milammeter (*see* milliammeter)
Milch's operation
mild
  m. abnormality
  m. analgesic
  m. arterial and arteriolonephrosclerosis
  m. arteriosclerosis with arteriolonephrosclerosis
  m. atherosclerosis
  m. atherosclerotic vascular disease

  m. bibasilar atelectasis
  m. ▸ bipolar disorder, depressed,
  m. ▸ bipolar disorder, manic,
  m. ▸ bipolar disorder, mixed,
  m. biventricular dilatation and hypertrophy
  m. centri-acinar emphysema
  m. chronic pancreatic exocrine insufficiency
  m. cognitive impairment
  m. colloid depletion
  m. concussion
  m. cortical damage
  m. dependent lividity
  m. depression
  m. depressive reaction
  m. dilatation, diffuse
  m. dysplasia, cells indicative of
  m. edema upper and lower extremities
  m. euphoria ▸ temporary
  m. eye correction
  m. fatty metamorphosis
  m. focal chronic inflammatory infiltrate
  m. focal cortical nodular hyperplasia
  m. focal interstitial scarring
  m. hemophilia
  m. hypertension
  m. hypoxic neuronal changes
  m. illness
  m. increase in motor activity
  m. leaking of aortic valve
  m. loss of appetite
  m. ▸ major depression,
  m. ▸ major depression, recurrent
  m. ▸ major depression, single episode
  m. mental retardation
  m. myopia
  m. observed tremor
  m. pain, patient in
  m. pancreatitis
  m. pulmonary edema
  m. pulmonary valve disorder
  m. residual defect
  m. skin irritation
  m. sodium restricted diet
  m. steatorrhea
  m. subcostal retractions
  m. symptoms of dementia
  m. systemic atherosclerosis
  m. thyroid failure
  m. tinnitus

m. -to-moderate levels of depression
m. -to-moderate pain
m. -to-moderately impaired
m. trabeculation
m. tremor
m. vertigo
m. weakness

mildly
m. dilated ▸ renal pelves
m. hyperplastic bone marrow
m. icteric, infant
m. inflamed ▸ eye
m. inflamed, pleura

Miles' abdominoperineal resection
Miles' operation
Milian's syndrome
miliaria rubra
miliaris disseminata ▸ tuberculosis
miliaris, lupus
miliary
m. aneurysm
m. embolism
m. gumma
m. metastases
m. plaques, Redlich-Fisher
m. punctation
m. sclerosis
m. tuberculosis
m. tuberculosis, acute

milieu
m., cognitive
m. management
m. management interventions
m. management protocol
m. management strategy ▸ therapeutic
m. programming
m., therapeutic
m. therapy
m., ward

military
m. anti-shock pants
m. anti-shock suit
m. anti-shock trousers (MAST)
m. attitude
m. press
m. tuberculosis

milk
m., acidophilus
m. ▸ alcohol in breast
m. -alkali syndrome
m. based tube feeding
m., breast
m., certified

m., condensed
m. consumption, limit
m., corn-soy
m., cow's
m. ducts
m. ducts ▸ flush
m. ducts, infection in
m. exchange
m. fat
m. fever
m. -free bland diet
m. glands
m. globule
m., homogenized
m. intolerance
m., lactase-treated
m. lactose allergy
m. leg
m. letdown
m. letdown reflex
m., litmus
m. ▸ low fat
m. lysozyme, human
m., modified
m., mother's
m., nonfat
m. of bismuth
m. of magnesia
m. of sulfur
m. -producing cells
m. production, abnormal
m. production, suppression of
m. ring test
m. scan
m. -secreting alveoli, clusters of
m. -secreting glands
m. sensitivity
m. sickness
m., skim
m. spots
m. spots ▸ ventricular
m., soy
m. sugar
m. syndrome, inspissated
m. teeth
m., uterine
m., vegetable
m. ▸ vitamin D
m., whole
m., witch's

milked out, lesion
milked superiorly
milker's nodules
Milkman syndrome, Looser-
Milkman's syndrome

milky
m. ascites
m. cataract
m. fluid, turbid
m. urine

mill-wheel murmur
Millard-Gubler syndrome
Millard's island flap
mille-feuilles effect
millefolium, Achillea
Millen technique
Millerian capsule
Miller's (millers')
M. -Abbott tube
m. asthma
M. operation
M. position
M. syndrome
M. tube, Abbott

milleri, Streptococcus
mill-house murmur
milliammeter (*same as* milammeter)
milliampere (ma)
m. hour (mah)
m. minute (mam)
m. second (mas)

millicurie(s)
m. hour (mch)
m. seconds (mcs) of beta radiation
m. of iodine (mcl)

milliequivalents (Meq)
milliequivalents per liter (Meq/L)
milligram(s) (mg/mgm)
m. -hour (mgh)
m. per meter squared
m. per 100 milliliters (mg%)

Millikan rays
Milliknit
M. graft
M. vascular graft
M. vascular graft prosthesis

milliliter(s) (ml)
m. (colonies/mi) ▸ colonies per
m. (mg%) ▸ milligrams per 100
m. of nutrient broth

millimeter(s) (mm)
m. (mm)
m. (cmm/cu mm) ▸ cubic
m., microvolts per
m. of mercury (mHg)
m. partial pressure (mmpp)
m. (r/mm) ▸ roentgens per

millimole (Mm)
millimoles per liter (Mm/L)
Millin-Read operation

millinormal (mN)
million electron volts
million international units (MIU)
millisecond (msec)
millisecond (msec) slow wave
millivolt (MV)
millivoltage (mv) slow wave
Milroy's disease
Mils' cautery
Miltner rotary bone rasp
Milton's edema
Milwaukee brace
Milwaukee shoulder syndrome
mimetic
    m. chorea
    m. convulsion
    m. labor
mimic convulsion
mimic tic
mimica, asemia
M immunoglobulin
    M. (IgM) deficiency, gamma
    M. (IgM) determination ▸ gamma
    M., gamma
mind('s)
    m. activity
    m. -altering drugs
    m. -altering effects
    m. blind
    m. -body interaction
    m. –body medicine
    m. -body phenomenon
    m. -body therapy
    m. -brain function
    m. clarity
    m. -clearing repetitious activity
    m. control
    m. control, delusions of
    m. eye orientation
    m. function, disordered
    m. pain
    m., preconscious
    m., unsoundness of
minded, broad-
minded ▸ patient tough-
mindfulness, core
mindfulness meditation
mine amputees ▸ land
mineral(s)
    m. balance
    m. chemistry
    m. composition, bone
    m. density (BMD), bone
    m. density, decreased bone
    m. density scan, bone-

    m. depletion
    m. deposits
    m. imbalance
    m. loss, bone-
    m. ▸ malabsorption of vitamins and
    m. oil aspiration
    m. oil emulsion
    m. replacement therapy
    m. supplement
    m. test, bone
    m. therapy
mineralocorticoid hormone
miner's(s')
    m. anemia
    m. asthma
    m. elbow
    m. headache
    m. lung, coal
    m. nystagmus
    m. phthisis
Minerva jacket
Minerva jacket case
mini-
    m- dose herapin
    m- mental status test
    m- nursing services
    m- peel, patient had
    m- stroke ▸ patient had
    m- thoracotomy ▸ patient had
miniature
    m. end-plate potential
    m. petit mal discharges
    m. radiography, mass
    m. roentgenography
    m. stomach
Minibennies (amphetamines)
mini-invasive vascular study
Minilith pacemaker, CPI
Minilith pacemaker pulse generator
minimal [*liminal*]
    m. arterionephrosclerosis
    m. assist, ambulates with
    m. assistance
    m. assistance for lower body
        dressing
    m. assistance for transfers
    m. assistance for upper body
        dressing
    m. assistance in lower body
        dressing
    m. assistance in upper body
        dressing
    m. assisted transfer
    m. bactericidal concentration
    m. bactericidal level

    m. bleeding
    m. blood loss
    m. brain dysfunction (MBD)
    m. calcific changes
    m. caliectasis
    m. cardiomegaly
    m. degenerative changes
    m. dust exposure
    m. effective dose
    m. erythema dose
    m. exercise
    m. exertion
    m. exposure transfusion (MET)
    m. fatal dose
    m. fibrosis ▸ focal areas of
    m. focus
    m. inhibitory concentration (MIC)
    m. leak technique
    m. level, bone pain at
    m. luminal diameter
    m. medullary concentration
    m. mitral regurgitation
    m. potential field
    m. residual disease
    m. spontaneous breathing
    m. stringy density
    m. supportive therapy
    m. tension line
    m. tolerance dose
minimally
    m. active, infant
    m. invasive biopsy technique
    m. invasive brain surgery
    m. invasive breast biopsy
        procedure
    m. invasive direct coronary artery
        bypass (MIDCAB)
    m. invasive laparoscopy surgery
    m. invasive procedure
    m. invasive technique
    m. invasive valve replacement
        surgery
minimi muscle ▸ extensor digiti
minimization of alcohol symptoms
minimize
    m. fluid retention
    m. normal brain dose
    m. or delay urinary incontinence
    m. risk of transfusion-related
        disease
    m. stress and strain
minimizing discomfort of withdrawal
minimum
    m. aerobic activity
    m. alveolar concentration (MAC)

m. concentration of bilirubin (MCBR)
m. deviation
m. effective dosage (MED)
m. essential medium (MEM)
m. extensibility line
m. hemolytic dose (MHD)
m. infective dose (MID)
m. inhibitory concentration (MIC)
m. isolation
m. lethal dose (MLD)
m. morbidostatic dose (MMD)
m. mycoplasmacidal concentration
m. reacting dose (MRD)
m. stage
m. target absorbed dose
m. time interval (MTI)
m. wavelength
minimus
   m., digitus
   m. muscle, gluteus
   m., Scopulariopsis
minin rays
minister, bereavement
ministry, pastoral
mink encephalopathy
Minkowski-Chauffard syndrome
Minnesota
   M. code
   M. Multiphasic Personality Inventory (MMPI)
   M. Multiphasic Personality Inventory (MMPI) test
minor(s) (Minor's)
   m. alpha asymmetry
   m. amputation
   m., anulus iridis
   m., authorization for treatment of a
   m. burns
   m. calyces
   m., chorea
   m. delusions
   m. discomfort
   m. epididymidis, globus
   m. epilepsy
   m. fissure
   m. fissure, bulging of
   m. focal epilepsy
   m. hallucinations
   m. hearing loss
   m. hemopericardium
   m. hysteria
   m. impairment
   m. infection, chronic
   m. injury

m., intoxicated
m. laceration
m., Lagochilascaris
m. light sensitivity
m. muscle, pectoralis
m., musculus helicis
m., musculus pectoralis
m., musculus teres
m., Naumanniella
m. painful discomfort
m., pectoralis
m., pelvis aequabiliter justo
m. procedure
m. shoe adaption
m. side effects
M. sign
m. skin wound
m. stroke
m., thalassemia
m. tranquilizers
m. vessel
m. wound
minora, labia
minores, calyces renals
Minotaur's labyrinth
minoxidil and hair loss
minoxidil-based Rogaine
Minsky's operation
mint, mountain
mint, wild
Mintweed (phencyclidine)
minuscule blood vessels
minuscule clumps of tumor cells
minuta, Plasmodium vivax
minute
   m., alveolar ventilation per
   m. anatomy
   m., beats per
   m. (cpm) ▸ counts per
   m. (c/min) ▸ cycles per
   m. (dpm) ▸ disintegrations per
   m. embryonic structures
   m. gun cough
   m. interval, 30-
   m. (lpm) ▸ liters per
   m., lymphatic nodules
   m. (mam) ▸ milliampere
   m. output
   m. output (CMO) ▸ cardiac
   m., oxygen (O_2) consumption per
   m. per meter squared ▸ liters per
   m. (RRpm) ▸ respiratory rate per
   m. (rpm) ▸ revolutions per
   m. studies
   m. ventilation

m. ventilation, alveolar
m. volume (MV)
m. volume, mandatory
m. volume (RMV) ▸ respiratory
minutissima, Nocardia
minutissimum, Corynebacterium
miosis [*meiosis*]
   m., irritative
   m., paralytic
   m., spastic
MIP (maximum inspiratory pressure)
MIP (mean incubation period)
Mira cautery
mirabilis, Proteus
miracle cure
miracle match
mires, images of
mirror
   m. focus
   m. hands
   m. image dextrocardia
   m. image laryngoscopy
   m. images, Purkinje-Sanson
   m., laryngeal
   m. image lung syndrome
   m. reflection
   m. speech
   m. twins
   m. writing
mirroring of extremities
misaligned
   m. eyes
   m. jaw
   m. tooth
   m. vertebrae
misalignment
   m. of eyes
   m. of knees
   m., spinal
   m., spine
   m. of bone
   m. of rotator cuff
   m. of teeth
miscarriage(s)
   m., incomplete
   m., increased risk of
   m., inevitable
   m., missed
   m., multiple
   m., patient admitted with
   m., recurrent
   m., repeated
   m., spontaneous
   m. support group
   m., threatened

miscarried, patient
misery and unhappiness disorder
misfiring ▸ brain cells
misfortune to others, anticipation of
misfortune to self, anticipation of
misidentification, delusional
mismanagement, pain
mismatch
    m., neurosensory
    m. pattern ▸ uptake
    m. ▸ ventilation/perfusion
mismatched marrow
mismatching, afterload
misplacing things ▸ patient
misregistration artifact
missed beat
missed miscarriage
misshapen, brittle toenails
missing
    m. chromosome
    m. digits
    m. enzyme
mist humidifier, cold
mist vaporizer, cool
mistreatment, past
mistreats others ▸ patient
mistrust ▸ feeling of
misunderstood ▸ feeling of isolation
    and being
misuse
    m., alcohol
    m. of medication ▸ elder
    m. of nonprescription drugs
    m. of prescription drugs
    m. ▸ psychotherapeutic drug
    m., substance
misusers of drugs
Mitchell's disease, Weir
mite(s)
    m. dermatitis, cat
    m., dust
    m., harvest
    m., itch
mitochondria ▸ abnormalities
    structure and function of
mitochondria, skeletal muscle
mitochondrial
    m. antibody
    m. calcium deposition
    m. cardiomyopathy
    m. damage
    m. diseases
    m. enlargement
    m. enzymes
    m. function

m. gene
m. gene, mutant
m. genetics
m. genome
m. metabolism ▸ decrease in
m. mutations
m. myopathies
m. myopathy ▸ dysautonomic
m. proteins
mitral
m. annular calcification
m. arcade, anomalous
m. atresia
m. balloon commissurotomy
m. balloon commissurotomy ▸
    percutaneous
m. balloon valve
m. balloon valvotomy ▸
    percutaneous
m. balloon valvuloplasty (PMB) ▸
    percutaneous
m. buttonhole
m. click
m. combined disease murmur,
    aortic-
m. commissurotomy, balloon
m. commissurotomy, closed
    transventricular
m. commissurotomy ▸
    percutaneous
m. commissurotomy ▸
    percutaneous transatrial
m. commissurotomy ▸
    percutaneous transvenous
m. cusp syndrome, ballooning
m. E to F slope
m. facies
m. first sound (M_1)
m. funnel
m. inflow ▸ turbulent diastolic
m. insufficiency ▸ rheumatic
m. leaflet, calcified
m. leaflet ▸ hammocking of
    posterior
m. leaflet ▸ posterior
m. opening snap (MOS)
m. prolapse
m. prolapse murmur
m. prolapse, pan
m. prolapse, systolic
m. prosthesis
m. prosthesis ▸ Starr-Edwards
m. regurgitant jet
m. regurgitation
m. regurgitation artifact

m. regurgitation ▸ ischemic
m. regurgitation, minimal
m. regurgitation murmur
m. restenosis
m. rim
m. ring prosthesis, Carpentier
    Rhone Poulenc
m. second sound (M2)
m. -septal apposition
m. stenosis
m. stenosis, buttonhole
m. stenosis, calcific
m. stenosis, congenital
m. stenosis ▸ fish-mouth
m. stenosis murmur
m. stenosis ▸ silent
m. stenosis ▸ subvalvular
m. tap
m. tricuspid
m. valve (MV)
m. valve aneurysm
m. valve area (MVA)
m. valve, cleft
m. valve, closed
m. valve closure index
m. valve commissurotomy
m. valve commissurotomy ▸
    transventricular
m. valve, congenital anomaly of
m. valve disease ▸ severe
m. valve ▸ diseased
m. valve disorder
m. valve dysautonomia
m. valve echocardiography
m. valve endocarditis
m. valve ▸ fibrous thickening
m. valve, flail
m. valve, floppy
m. valve hypoplasia
m. valve insufficiency
m. valve leaflet
m. valve leaflet, bowing of
m. valve ▸ leaky
m. valve ▸ moderate leaking of
m. valve ▸ myxomatous
    degeneration of
m. valve ▸ parachute
m. valve prolapse
m. valve prolapse syndrome
m. valve prosthesis, Barnard
m. valve prosthesis, Beall
m. valve prosthesis, Cooley-
    Bloodwell
m. valve prosthesis ▸ Hancock

m. valve prosthesis ▸ Lillehei-Kaster
m. valve prosthesis ▸ Sorin
m. valve regurgitation
m. valve repair
m. valve replacement
m. valve replacement, Cosgrove
m. valve ▸ replacement of
m. valve replacement ▸ supra-annular
m. valve ring
m. valve ▸ Starr-Edwards
m. valve stenosis
m. valve stenosis ▸ rheumatic
m. valve syndrome, billowing
m. valve syndrome ▸ prolapsed
m. valvotomy, balloon
m. valvotomy ▸ repeat balloon
m. valvulitis
m. valvuloplasty
m. valvuloplasty, balloon
m. valvuloplasty ▸ percutaneous
m. valvuloplasty ▸ percutaneous balloon

mitrale, P
mittelschmerz, symptoms of
mitten

m. discharge
m. hand
m. pattern
m. pattern, fast
m. pattern, slow

Mittendorf's dot
MIU (million international units)
mix, oncology
mix (Kiff), tobacco and marijuana
mixed

m. abscess
m. aerobic-anaerobic infections
m. amputation
m. aneurysm
m. angina
m. aphasia
m. apnea
m. asthma
m. astigmatism
m. bacterial flora
m. bacterial infection
m. bacterial infiltrate
m. beat
m. ▸ bipolar affective disorder,
m. ▸ bipolar disorder,
m. capillary cavernous hemangioma
m. cataract

m. cell agglutination reaction
m. comedo
m. common flora
m. connective tissue disease (MCTD)
m. cryoglobulin (EMC) ▸ essential
m. culture
m. deafness
m. development disorder
m. disorders as reaction to stress
m. disturbance of conduct and emotions
m. disturbance of emotions and conduct
m. disturbance of emotions and conduct ▸ adjustment disorder with
m. emotional disturbances of adolescence
m. emotional disturbances of childhood
m. emotional features
m. emotional features ▸ adjustment disorder with
m. emotional features ▸ adjustment reaction with
m. feelings
m. flora, sputum showed
m. fungal infection
m. glioma
m. hemadsorption
m. hemorrhoids
m. immunity
m. immunofluorescence
m., in full remission ▸ bipolar disorder,
m., in partial remission ▸ bipolar disorder,
m. infection
m. joint
m. lesion
m. leukocyte culture (MLC)
m. leukocyte reaction
m. levocardia
m. lymphocyte culture
m. mammary tumor
m. mesodermal sarcoma
m. mesodermal tumor, advanced uterine
m., mild ▸ bipolar disorder,
m., moderate ▸ bipolar disorder,
m. nerve
m. neurally mediated syncope
m. nodular tumor
m. nystagmus

m. odontoma
m. origin ▸ organic, emotional or
m. rheumatoid and degenerative arthritis
m. rhythm
m., severe, without psychotic features ▸ bipolar disorder,
m. sleep apnea
m. spasm
m. stones
m. terminal tumor
m. thrombus
m. tissue transplant
m. tissue tumors
m. tumor
m. tumor of lacrimal gland
m. type epilepsy
m. type nodules
m., unspecified ▸ bipolar disorder,
m. vaginitis
m. venous
m. venous blood
m. venous oxygen (O_2)
m. venous oxygen (O_2) saturation
m. with plasma, red cells
m., with psychotic features ▸ bipolar disorder,

MixEvac machine
mixture

m., anaerobic gas
m., barium
m., Brompton
m., dextrose solution
m. of microorganisms

Miyagawanella

M. bovis
M. bronchopneumoniae
M. felis
M. illinii
M. louisianae
M. lymphogranulomatosis
M. opossumi
M. ovis
M. pecoris
M. pneumoniae
M. psittaci

M-K (McCarey-Kaufman) medium
MKS (meter-kilogram-second)
MK 3 Holter scanner, CardioData
ML (mesiolingual)
ml (milliliter)
ml (colonies per milliliter) ▸ colonies/
M:L (monocyte-lymphocyte ratio)
Mla (mesiolabial)
Mladick ear reconstruction

MLal (mesiolabioincisal)
MLAP (mean left atrial pressure)
MLC (mixed leukocyte culture)
MLC (multileaf collimator)
MLD (minimum lethal dose)
MLD or LD$_{50}$ (median lethal dose)
MLI (mesiolinguoincisal)
M lignocaine
M-line protein
M-lines
MLNS (mucocutaneous lymph node syndrome)
MLO (mesiolinguo-occlusal)
MLP (mentolaeva posterior)
MLP (mesiolinguopulpal)
MLS (mean lifespan)
MM bands
MM virus
Mm (millimole)
mm (millimeter)
MMD (minimum morbidostatic dose)
MMEF (maximum mid-expiratory flow)
MMEFR (maximal mid-expiratory flow rate)
MMEFR (maximum mid-expiratory flow rate)
MMFR (maximal midflow rate)
Mm/L (millimoles per liter)
mmm (micromillimeter)
mmm (millimicron)
M-mode
  M.m. (motion mode)
  M.m. echocardiogram
  M.m. recording
  M.m. (motion modulation) scanning
MMPI (Minnesota Multiphasic Personality Inventory) test
mmpp (millimeters partial pressure)
MMR (measles, mumps, rubella immunization)
Mn (millinormal)
MN (motor neuron)
  MN. (motor neuron), degeneration of
  MN. (motor neuron) disease ▸ inherited
  MN. (motor neuron) dysfunction ▸ lower
MNCV (motor nerve conduction velocity)
mnemonic
  m. children
  m. dementia
  m. device

m. instructions
m., loci
m. programming
M 90%, hypaque-
MO (mesio-occlusal)
moan test
mobile (Mobile)
  m. arm support
  m. ▸ carina midline sharp and
  m. cecum
  m. chart carrier
  m., cor
  m., cords
  M. Coronary Care Unit (MCCU)
  m. hospital
  M. Intensive Care Unit (MICU)
  m. kidney
  m. mammography unit
  m. mass lab workup
  m. mass x-ray
  m. meals
  m. nasal, septum
  m. portion of tongue
  M. -Standing Frame
  m. testicle
  m. testing unit
  m. tissues
  m., uterus freely
  m. x-ray unit ▸ AMX 110
mobilis, Macromonas
mobility [*motility*]
  m. aids
  m. and cognition
  m. and reduce pain ▸ restore
  m. and strength ▸ memory,
  m., assistance and
  m., bed
  m., bed/mat
  m., electrophoretic
  m., impaired
  m., impaired physical
  m., joint
  m. ▸ knee joint
  m. ▸ level of
  m. ▸ maximum level of independent
  m., muscle strength and walking
  m. of ossicular chain
  m. of patient, maintain
  m., pain and limited
  m., patient needs minimal assistance for wheelchair
  m., postsurgical
  m. problems
  m. reduced
  m. ▸ relieve pain and restore

m., restore finger
m., restored
m. shift assay
m. skills
m. spine
m. ▸ stiffness, pain and lack of
m., strength and
m., subject
m., thumb
m., wheelchair
mobilization
  m., cervical
  m., gentle active
  m., localized leukocyte
  m., stapes
mobilize knee
mobilized, cecum
mobilized, uterus
mobilizing substance, fat
Mobitz
  M. heart block
  M. I
  M. II
Möbius(')
  M. disease
  M. sign
  M. syndrome
MOD (mesio-occlusodistal)
modal
  m. effects, cross-
  m. target absorbed dose
  m. test, cross-
modality(ies)
  m. and duration
  m., chemotherapeutic
  m., combined drug and radiation
  m., group
  m., individual sensory
  m., major treatment
  m., nonverbal
  m. of sensation
  m. of treatment
  m., pacing
  m. ▸ psychiatric treatment
  m., sensory
  m., specific
  m., therapeutic
  m. therapy, combination
  m. therapy, combined
  m. therapy, independent toxicity in combined
  m. therapy, protocol design in combined
  m. therapy, research design in combined

m. therapy, response and combined
m. therapy, spatial cooperation in combined
m. therapy, survival rates with combined
m. therapy, temporal consolidation in combined
m. treatment

mode
m. Acquisition and Targeting (BAT) ▸ B-
m. alternative atrial pacing
m. amplification, common
m., atrial pacing
m. (brightness modulation), B
m. cardiac imaging ▸ mask-
m., decay
m., dual pacing, dual sensing (DDD) ▸ dual
m. echocardiogram, M-
m. echo-tracking device, A-
m. echocardiography, A-
m. ergometer ▸ pedal
m., evocative
m., expressive
m. ▸ fight or flight
m. ▸ fixed rate
m., flow
m. ▸ gated list
m., histogram
m., list
m., magnet
m., matrix
m. (M mode) ▸ motion
m., multiplanar
m. of action
m. of administration with cannabinoids
m. of administration with depressants
m. of administration with hallucinogens
m. of administration with inhalants
m. of administration with opioids
m. of administration with phencyclidines
m. of administration with stimulants
m. of behavior
m. of behavior ▸ present
m. of communication
m. of function
m. of ineffective functioning
m. of spread of infection
m. of transmission

m. pacemaker, committed
m., pacing
m., passive
m. (RPM), rapid processing
m., receptive
m. recording ▸ M-
m. rejection, common
m. rejection ratio, common
m. (amplitude modulation) scanning, A-
m. (brightness modulation) scanning, B-
m. (motion modulation) scanning, M-
m. signal, common
m. subtraction ▸ mask-
m. switching
m. switching (AMS), automatic
m. (amplitude modulation) ultrasonography, A-
m. ultrasonography, B-
m. ultrasonography ▸ high resolution B-
m. ultrasound, B-
m. ventilation, control

model(s)
m. behavior
m., developmental
m. GTF-A gastrocamera ▸ Olympus
m. ▸ middle-class medical
m. of atomic structure, Bohr
m. of motivation
m. of reentry ▸ Schmitt-Erlanger
m., program
m., receptor binding
m., role

modeling, positive
moderate
m. aerobic activity
m. amounts of alcohol
m. arthritic condition
m. assistance
m. atherosclerosis
m. atherosclerosis with calcification
m. ▸ bipolar disorder, depressed,
m. ▸ bipolar disorder, manic,
m. ▸ bipolar disorder, mixed,
m. calcified atheroma
m. cardiomegaly
m. chronic depression
m. chronic pancreatic exocrine insufficiency
m. contraction
m. decrease in voltage ▸ localized

m. degree of involution
m. depression
m. drinkers
m. dysplasia, cells indicative of
m. exercise
m. exercise, daily
m. exercise program
m. infiltrate
m. intensity exercise
m. leaking of aortic valve
m. leaking of mitral valve
m. levels of depression ▸ mild-to-
m. ▸ major depression
m. ▸ major depression, recurrent
m. ▸ major depression, single episode
m. menstrual flow
m. mental retardation
m. myopia
m. narrowing
m. nystagmus on gaze to right
m. pain
m. pain, mild to
m. physical activity
m. post-surgical pain
m. respiratory disease
m. salt reduction
m. recent activity
m. shift to left
m. shift to right
m. sodium restricted diet
m. steatorrhea
m. voltage
m. walking

moderately
m., drink
m., drinking
m. impaired ▸ mild-to-
m. prominent generalized atrophy
m. slow activity, focal

moderating alcohol consumption
moderating factors ▸ stress
moderation of drug use, abstention versus
moderation-oriented treatment methods
modern medical practice
modifiable risk factors
modification
m., activity
m., Astler-Coller
m., AV node
m., behavior
m., behavioral
m., cardiac risk factor

modification—*continued*
- m., cognitive
- m., dialect
- m., dietary
- m., environmental
- m. factor, dose
- m. ▸ gradual lifestyle
- m., home
- m. hypothesis
- m., lifestyle
- m. of behavior and environment, medication and
- m. of electroencephalogram (EEG)
- m. of Nissen fundoplication ▸ Rossetti
- m. of radiation beam
- m. of target enzyme
- m. of Waterson anastomosis, Cooley
- m., pain
- m. patterns of dose fractionation
- m., physiological
- m., possible receptor
- m. program, behavioral
- m., radiation field
- m. ▸ risk factor
- m. technique, behavior
- m. therapy, behavior

modified
- m. activity
- m. anesthesia
- m. arthroplasty, Magnuson
- m. behavior
- m. blue loop intraocular lens (IOL), Sinskey/Sinskey
- m. brachial technique
- m. Bruce protocol
- m. diet
- m. Ellestad protocol
- m. gain, ratio
- m. Hibbs' technique
- m. incus
- m. job
- m. left atrial Maze procedure
- m. mantled rads
- m. mastectomy, Patey
- m. mastoidectomy
- m. milk
- m. Moore hip locking prosthesis
- m. multifactorial index of cardiac risk
- m. myectomy
- m., procedure
- m. push-ups

- m. radiation
- m. radical hysterectomy
- m. radical mastectomy
- m. Richardson technique
- m. surgical procedure
- m. Thal fundoplasty
- m. tone decay test
- m. upper mantle radiation treatment
- m. viruses

modifiers, biological response
modifiers, chemical
modify
- m. body's response to pain
- m. hearing patterns
- m. pain
- m. protocol
- m. stress
- m. stressful living habits
- m. therapy

modifying
- m. antirheumatic drug (DMARD) ▸ disease
- m. drug, mood-
- m. drugs ▸ suppressive or disease
- m. substance ▸ mood-
- m. the incus

modiolus, spiral vein of
modular tube, glow
modulate emotional reactions
modulated pacemaker ▸ rate
Modulated Radiation Therapy (IMRT) ▸ Intensity
modulation
- m. (A-mode), amplitude
- m., autonomic
- m. (B-mode), brightness
- m., frequency
- m., image
- m., object
- m. procedure, immune
- m. (A-mode) scanning, amplitude
- m. (B-mode) scanning, brightness
- m. (M-mode) scanning, motion
- m. transfer function (MTF)
- m. (A-mode) ultrasonography, amplitude

modulator, immune
modulators (SERM) ▸ selective estrogen receptor
module(s)
- m., lighting
- m., recovery
- m., skill
Moe plate

Moe procedure
Moebius syndrome
Mohs'
- M. chemosurgery
- M. correct
- M. micrographic surgery
- M. procedure
- M. surgery
- M. technique

moiety
- m., carbohydrate
- m., corrin
- m., memory

moist
- m. compress
- m. compresses, hot
- m. cotton
- m. dressing
- m. gangrene
- m. heat
- m. heat pad
- m. heat treatment
- m. heat, warm
- m. lap packs
- m., mouth pink and
- m., mucosa pink and
- m. packs, hot
- m. poultice, hot
- m. rales
- m. rales, fine
- m., skin
- m. skin, cold

moistened cornea
moisture
- m. content
- m. evaporation
- m. exchanger ▸ heat/

moisturizing lotion
Mol wt (molecular weight)
molal solution
molar(s)
- m., impacted
- m., Moon's
- m., mulberry
- m., permanent
- m. pregnancy
- m., sixth-year
- m. socket
- m. teeth
- m. teeth, impacted
- m., third
- m. tooth
- m., twelfth-year
- m. volume

mold(s)
- m. and bacteria ▸ airborne
- m., cesium
- m., endolaryngeal brachytherapy
- m. fungus
- m., heat
- m., intraoral dental
- m. spores
- m., toxic

molded plastic splint
molded Teflon
molding, knotted
molding of head
mole
- m., breast cancer
- m., Breu's
- m. hair
- m., hydatidiform
- m., pigmented
- m., suspicious

molecular
- m. analysis
- m. approach
- m. biology
- m. breast cancer therapy
- m. change
- m. code
- m. death
- m. fat
- m. genetic analysis
- m. genetics
- m. genetics ▸ human
- m. heat
- m. layer
- m. lesion
- m. level
- m. medicine
- m. microbiology
- m. neuroscience
- m. pharmacology
- m. science
- m. sequence
- m. structure
- m. substance
- m. synthesis
- m. vibrations
- m. weight
- m. weight dextran, low
- m. weight (GMW) ▸ gram-
- m. weight, high
- m. weight, low

molecule(s)
- m., alcohol
- m., aminoglycoside
- m., antibody

- m., calcium
- m., dopamine
- m., DNA (deoxyribonucleic acid)
- m., disease fighting
- m., effector
- m. (ELAM) ▸ endothelial leukocyte adhesion
- m., enhancer
- m. ▸ family of organic
- m. ▸ filamentous actin and myosis
- m. ▸ free radical
- m., HCG
- m., icon
- m., inactivate the
- m., insulin
- m., mature
- m. of synthetic DNA
- m. ▸ oxidized fatty
- m. ▸ oxygen (O_2)
- m., phosphate
- m., postsynaptic
- m., protein
- m., reactive
- m., receptor
- m., repressant
- m., repressor
- m., serotonin
- m., sugar
- m., tau
- m., toxic
- m. ▸ unstable oxygen (O_2)

moles on skin ▸ multiple
molestus, Culex
Moll, gland of
Mollaret's meningitis
molle, carcinoma
Mollies (amphetamines), Black
mollis, chorea
molluscum conjunctivitis
molluscum contagiosum
Maloney leukemogenic virus
Maloney sarcoma virus
Moloy classification, Caldwell-
Moloy method, Caldwell-
molybdenum radiation therapy
moment, magnetic
momentary
- m. awakening
- m. falling asleep
- m. lapse in normal breathing
- m. lapse of awareness
- m. loss

- m. loss of skeletal muscular tone
- m. loss of strength
- m. paralysis ▸ cyclic,
- m. passion
- m. recognition
- m. vertigo

Monaghan respirator
Monakow's bundle, von
Monakow's fibers, von
Monaldi's drainage (dr'ge) system
Monaldi's operation
monamine oxidase
monarthritis caused by tuberculosis ▸ knee
monaural
- m. bifrequency loudness balance
- m. hearing
- m. hearing loss

Mönckeberg's
- M. arrhythmia
- M. arteriosclerosis
- M. deformity
- M. degeneration
- M. sclerosis

Moncrieff's operation
Mondonesi's reflex
M₁ (mitral first sound)
Monday
- M. disease
- M. dyspnea
- M. fever
- M. morning headache
- M. morning heart attack

Mondini malformation
Mondini pulmonary arteriovenous malformation
Mondor's disease
money ▸ repeated squandering of
Monge's disease
mongol opacification
mongolian idiocy
mongolian idiot
mongolism, double-trisomy
mongolism, translocation
mongoloid features
mongoloid, patient
Monilia albicans
Monilia vaginitis
monilial
- m. esophagitis
- m. granuloma
- m. infection
- m. vaginitis
- m. vulvitis

moniliform hair
moniliformis, Streptobacillus
monitor (Monitor)
  m., air
  m. (ABPM), ambulatory blood
    pressure
  m., ambulatory Holter
  m., apnea
  m., automated
  m., beam
  m., blood glucose
  m., blood perfusion
  m., blood pressure (BP)
  m. cancer
  m., cardiac
  m. catheter placement, arterial
    line
  m. (CFM), cerebral function
  m. changes
  m. changes in pressure
  M. (CFM) ▸ Corometrics Fetal
  m., deceleration of
  m. educational needs
  m. ▸ electrocardiographic (ECG)
    transtelephonic
  m., electronic fetal
  m., electronic glucose
  m. evaluation, Holter
  m., event
  m. ▸ event activated
  m., fetal
  m., fetal heart
  m. fluid intake and output
  m. function
  m., glucose
  m., heart
  m., heart rate
  m., Holter
  M., Huntleigh Domiciliary Fetal
  m. in skull, intracranial pressure
  m., intracranial
  M. ▸ King of Hearts
  m., labor
  m. leads
  m. liver function
  m. ▸ noninvasive glucose
  m. ▸ oxygen (O₂)
  m. patient care activities
  m., perinatal
  m. prescribed medication
  m. progression of disorder
  m. pulmonary capillary wedge
    pressure
  m., radiation
  m. recalibrated regularly

  m. ▸ SpaceLabs Holter
  m. stone disintegration
  m. technician
  m. telemetry
  m. television
  m. therapy
  m., 3 channel Holter
  m. tracing
  m. tracing, fetal heart
  m., transcutaneous oxygen (O₂)
  m. ▸ transtelephonic ECG
    (electrocardiograph)
  m. ▸ transtelephonic exercise
  m., video
  m. vital functions
monitored
  m. baby, apnea
  m., fetus continuously
  m. for contamination, nebulizer
  m., heart rate
  m. in office ▸ blood counts
  m. program, well-
  m., routinely
  m. with electrocardiogram
    (ECG/EKG)
monitoring
  m., advanced fetal
  m. (AEM), ambulatory electro-
    cardiographic
  m., ambulatory electrocardiography
    (AECG)
  m. (AHM), ambulatory Holter
  m., ambulatory ischemia
  m., anesthesia feedback
  m., arterial
  m. arterial blood pressure
  m., automatic blood pressure
    (BP)
  m., biochemical
  m., blood-
  m., blood coagulation
  m., blood pressure (BP)
  m. blood pressure ▸ self-
  m. breathing patterns
  m., cardiac
  m., cardiac hemodynamic
  m. cart
  m., central venous pressure
  m., constant
  m., continuous
  m., continuous invasive
  m. device
  m. device, electronic
  m. device, pressure
  m. ▸ electrocardiographic (ECG)

  m. ▸ electrophysiologic vs electro-
    cardiographic
  m., environmental
  m., feedback
  m., fetal
  m. ▸ fetal heart
  m., frequent
  m., full
  m., glucose
  m., glucose self-
  m. heartbeat
  m., hemodynamic
  m., home
  m., home blood sugar
  m., home glucose
  m. in hyperthermia, thermometer
  m., industrial
  m., internal fetal heart rate
  m., intracranial pressure
  m., intraocular pressure
  m., laboratory
  m. lines inserted and positioned
  m., medical
  m., multiple-bed
  m., observation and
  m. of blood pressure (BP)
  m. of deep tendon reflexes (DTR)
  m. of eighth nerve function
  m. of fetal heart tones (FHT),
    Doptone
  m. of fetus, Doppler
  m. of patient ▸ formal
  m. of renal function
  m. of signals
  m. of sterilizers
  m. of sterilizers, biological
  m., ongoing
  m., ophthalmologic
  m., pacemaker
  m., performance
  m., periodic
  m., physiological
  m., plasma
  m. practices
  m. process, random
  m. ▸ pulse oximetry
  m., radiation
  m., rejection
  m. respiratory equipment
  m., simultaneous
  m. situation
  m. skills ▸ self-
  m. sleep patterns
  m. sucking pattern
  m. system

m. system, fetal
m. system, pediatric
m. system ▸ quality information
m. system ▸ transtelephonic ambulatory
m., systematic
m., systems in drug abuse
m. techniques
m., telemetric
m. ▸ transtelephonic arrhythmia
m. ▸ transtelephonic pacemaker
m., 24 hour
m. venous blood pressure
m. ▸ weight/electrolyte
Moniz carotid siphon
monkey (Monkey)
M. Dust (phencyclidine)
m. hand
m. orphan (ECMO) virus ▸ enteric cytopathic
m. paw
m., Rhesus
m. virus
Monks-Esser island flap
Monneret's pulse
monoamine (Monoamine)
m. oxidase
m. oxidase activity ▸ platelet
m. oxidase inhibitor (MAOI)
M. Oxidase (MAO) inhibitor diet ▸ restricted tyramine and
monoblastic leukemia (AMOL), acute
monochromatic
m. eye
m. radiation
m. rays
monoclonal
m. antibodies
m. antibodies, anti-anesthetic
m. antibody ▸ humanized
m. antibody therapy
m. band
m. gammopathy, IgA
m. hypothesis
m. theory of atherogenesis
monocrotic pulse
monocular
m. diplopia
m. eye dressing
m. rotations
m. strabismus
m. vision
monocyte(s)
m. cells

m. lineage antigen
m. ▸ embryonic cardiac
monocytic
m. angina
m. ehrlichiosis (HME) ▸ human
m. leukemia
m. leukemia (AML), acute
m. leukemia ▸ Schilling-type
monocytogenes
m., Listeria
m. meningitis, Listeria
m. strain ▸ Listeria
monocytoid reticuloendothelial cell
monocytolysis of heart
monocytosis inducing factor
monoeca, Siderocapsa
monofilament(s)
m. absorbable suture
m. polypropylene suture
m. stainless steel wire
m. suture
monofocal lenses
monoform tachycardia
monogamous relationship
monogamous sexual relationship
monogenic disorder
Monokow, fasciculus abberans of
monolateral strabismus
monomorphic
m. adenoma
m. ventricular tachycardia
m. ventricular tachycardia ▸ repetitive
m. ventricular tachycardia ▸ sustained
mononeuritis multiplex
mononeuritis, viral
mononuclear
m. cell
m. cells, atypical
m. phagocyte system
mononucleosis
m. ▸ acute infectious
m., chronic
m. ▸ heterophile negative
m., infectious
m. -like illness
m., post-transfusion
m. syndrome, acute
m. virus
mononucleotide, flavin
monophasic
m. action potential
m. action potential duration

m. complex
m. wave
monophonic wheeze
monophosphate
m., adenosine
m. (CAMP), cyclic adenosine
m., cytidine
m. shunt, hexose
m., thymidine
m., uridine
monophthalmica, polyopia/ polyopsia
monoplace chamber
monoplane ultrasound scanner ▸ Biosound wide-angle
monopolar
m. montage
m. needle electrode
m. temporary electrode
monoproliferative disorders
monorhythmic sinusoidal delta activity
monosodium glutamate
monosodium urate
monosomy 7 syndrome
Monosporium apiospermum
Monospot Slide Test
monosymptomatic hysteria
monosynaptic reflex
monotherapy ▸ oral
monotherapy treatment
monotypic lesion
monounsaturated fats
monotone, speak in rapid
monotonous stimulation
monotonous voice pitch
monovalent influenza vaccine
monovalent oral poliovirus vaccine
monoxide
m., carbon
m., dinitrogen
m., nitrogen
m. (CO) poisoning, carbon
monoxime, diacetyl
monozygotic twins
Monro, foramen of
Monro's abscess
mons
m. pubis
m. uteris
m. veneris
montage(s) (Montage)
m., bipolar
m., circumferential bipolar

montage(s)—*continued*
  m., common reference
  m., coronal bipolar
  M., International
  m., monopolar
  m., posterior scalp to scalp
  m., referential
  m., transverse bipolar
  m., triangular bipolar
  m., unipolar
montanus, Ceratophyllus
montanus, Diamanus
montebelli, Microtus
Monte Carlo method
Monteggia's dislocation
Monteggia's fracture
montevideo, Salmonella
Montevideo unit
Montezuma's revenge
Montgomery strap
monthly
  m. /bimonthly contraceptive
    injections
  m. breast self-exams
  m. intervals
  m. period
  m. self-examination
months, gestational
monticulus cerebelli
montoyai, Penicillium
mood(s) (Mood)
  m. adjustment ▸ disorder with
    anxious
  m. adjustment ▸ disorder with
    depressed
  m. alteration
  m. altering capacity
  m. altering chemical transmitters
  m. altering chemicals
  m. altering drug
  m. altering substances
  m. and energy swings
  m. and perceptions, altered
  m., anxious
  m., basic dysphoric
  m., blue
  m. change
  m. change, abrupt
  m. change ▸ rapid
  m. changes apathy, loss of
    energy
  m. changes ▸ frequent
  m. cycles
  m., depressed
  m. ▸ depressed or irritable

m. disorder
m. disorder, co-occurring
m. disorder, delusional
m. disorder, hallucinogen
m. disorder ▸ long-term
m. disorder ▸ major
m., disorder of
m. disorder, organic
m. disorder ▸ phencyclidine
  (PCP)
m. disorder ▸ psychoactive
  substance
m. disorder ▸ seasonal
m. disturbance
m. disturbance, persistent
m., elevated
m. elevating drug
m. elevating effect
m. elevator
m. enhancing drug
m. enhancing effect
m., erratic
m., euphoric
m. fluctuations
m., hypomanic
m. instability
m., irritable
m., labile
m. lability
m. ▸ marked reactivity of
m. -modifying drug
m. -modifying substance
m. or behavior, changes in
m. ▸ persistent elevation of
m., positive
m., pure
m. regulator
M. Scale, Clyde
m. ▸ severe premenstrual changes
  in
m. shifts, marked
m., stabilization of
m. stabilizer
m. -stabilizing drugs
m. swings
m. swings and depression
m. swings, disruptive
m. swings, dizzying
m. swings, extreme
m. swings ▸ frequent
m. swings ▸ irritability and
m. swings ▸ rapid
m. swings ▸ seasonal
m. swings ▸ sudden
m. swing ▸ volatile

m. swings, wide-ranging
m., temporary alterations in
m. unpredictable
m., unstable
moodiness ▸ intense, short-term
moody
  m., irritable and aggressive
  m., patient
  m. ▸ patient glum and
moon (Moon)('s)
  m. (hallucinogen)
  M. -Biedl syndrome ▸ Laurence-
  m. face
  M. molars
  m. -shaped face
  m. -shaped facies
  M. teeth
Moore('s)
  M. and Chong sandwich flap
  M. electrode, Neil-
  M. endoprosthetic arthroplasty ▸
    Austin-
  M. fracture
  M. hip locking prosthesis ▸
    modified
  M. hip prosthesis
  M. hip prosthesis, Austin-
  M. operation
  M. pin
  M. pin, Austin-
  M. plate
  M. prosthesis
  M. reamer
  M. reamer, Austin-
  M. self-locking prosthesis ▸
    Vitallium
  M. template
  M. tracheostomy buttons
Mooren's ulcer
mooseri, Rickettsia
MOPP (nitrogen mustard, Oncovin,
  prednisone, procarbazine)
moral
  m. behavior
  m. code
  m. consideration
  m. imbecile
  m. imbecility
  m. implications
  m. insanity
  m. judgment
  m. language
  m. obligation
  m. oligophrenia
  m. persuasion

m. philosophy
m. reasoning
m. treatment
moralism, symbolic
morally acceptable
morally rigid
Moran procedure, Ruiz-
Morax('s)
  M. -Axenfeld bacillus
  M. -Axenfeld conjunctivitis
  M. -Axenfeld diplococcus
  M. -Axenfeld haemophilus
  M. diplobacillus
  M. operation
Moraxella
  M. catarrhalis
  M. lacunata
  M. liquefaciens
morbi, genius
morbid
  m. dread of night
  m. excrescence
  m. obesity
morbidity (Morbidity)
  m. and mortality
  m. and mortality ▸ cardiovascular
  m. and mortality, fetal
  m. and mortality, infant
  m. and mortality ▸ long-term
  m. and mortality ▸ operative
  m. and mortality ▸ perioperative
  m. and mortality rate
  m., baseline
  m., febrile
  m., infectious
  m., infective
  m. ▸ long-term psychological
  m., maternal
  m. ▸ maternal febrile
  m., maternal infectious
  m. ▸ maternal mortality and
  m., mortality and
  M. -Mortality Rate
  m., neonatal
  m., postoperative
  m. ▸ puerperal febrile
  m. rate
  m. ratio, proportionate
  m., septic
  m., tuberculosis
morbidly obese
morbidostatic dose (MMD) ▸
  minimum
morbilliform rash
morbillorum, Diplococcus

morbus, cholera
morcellement operation
Mörch('s)
  M. respirator
  M. respirator, Mueller-
  M. tracheostomy tube
mordens, Physaloptera
Morel-Kraepelin disease
Morel's ear
Morestin's operation
Morf (Percodan)
Morfina (Percodan)
Morgagni('s)
  M. -Adams-Stokes syndrome
  M. appendix
  M. caruncle
  M. column
  M. crypt
  M., cyst of
  M., disease of
  M. foramen
  M., fossa of
  M. globule
  M. hernia
  M. hernia, foramen of
  M., hydatid of
  M., hyperostosis of
  M., lacunae of
  M., liquor of
  M. nodules
  M., prolapse of
  M., sinus of
  M. ventricle
morgagnian cataract
morgagnian cyst
Morganelli morganii
morgani, Proteus
Morganii, Morganelli
Morgan's bacillus
morgue, body transferred to
Morison('s)
  M. incision
  M. method
  M. pouch
Morley's peritoneocutaneous
  reflex
morning (Morning)
  m. arousal, early
  m. awakening, early
  m. awakening, premature
  m. diarrhea
  m. drowsiness, drug-induced
  m. eye pain
  m. glory seeds (flying saucers)
  M. glory seeds (hallucinogen)

m. glory seeds (heavenly blue)
m. glory seeds (licorice drops)
m. glory seeds (pearly gates)
m. glory seeds injected
m. headache
m. headache, Monday
m. heart attack ▸ Monday
m. lark riser
m. sickness
m. sputum, early
m. stiffness
Moro('s)
  M. embrace reflex
  M. grasp
  M. -Heisler diet
  M. reaction
  M. reflex
  M. reflex, incomplete
  M. reflex, negative
  M. test
Morphine (morphine)
  M. (Cube)
  M. (First Line)
  m. (hocus)
  m. abstinence
  m. addiction
  m. cocktail
  m., lethal overdose of
  m. sulfate
  m. tolerance and dependence
Morpho (Percodan)
morphogenesis of heart ▸ secondary
morphogenetic activity, bone
morphologic feature
morphologic synthesis
morphological aspect
morphology
  m., bacterial
  m., blood
  m., cellular
  m., ductal
  m., gross
  m. of individual organisms
  m., QRS
  m., splenic
  m., tumor
morphonuclear, poly◊
Morphy (Percodan)
Morquio's
  M. disease
  M. sign
  M. syndrome
  M. Ullrich syndrome
morrhuate, sodium
morsal teeth

Morsier-Gauthier syndrome, de
mortality (Mortality)
- m. and body fat
- m. and chemotherapy
- m. and morbidity
- m. and morbidity ▸ maternal
- m., cardiac
- m., cardiovascular
- m. ▸ cardiovascular morbidity and
- m. ▸ coronary artery disease
- m., fetal morbidity and
- m., flu
- m., incidence of maternal
- m., infant
- m., infant morbidity and
- m. ▸ long-term morbidity and
- m., maternal
- m., medical
- m. ▸ morbidity and
- m. ▸ operative morbidity and
- m., opioid
- m., perinatal
- m. ▸ perioperative morbidity and
- m., postcoronary
- m. rate
- m. rate, infant
- m. rate ▸ maternal
- M. Rate, Morbidity-
- m. rate, perinatal
- m. rate, predicted
- m. rates, short-term
- m. ratio
- m. ratio, crude
- m. ratio, standard
- m., reproductive
- m. risk
- m. ▸ ruptured aneurysm
- m. statistics ▸ alcohol-related
- m. study
- m., surgical

mortar kidney
mortem decomposition, post-
mortice [*mortise*]
mortice, ankle
mortis
- m., articulo
- m., livor
- m. ▸ myocardial rigor
- m., rigor

mortise [*mortice*]
- m., ankle
- m. of joint
- m., tibiofibular

Morton('s)
- M. cough
- M. fluid
- M. neuralgia
- M. neuroma
- M. neuroma ▸ excision
- M. operation, Taussig-
- M. toe

mortuary gown, disposable
morular cell
moruloid fat
Morvan's chorea
mOs (milliosmole)
MOS (mitral opening snap)
mosaic (Mosaic)
- M. cardiac bioprosthesis
- m. development
- m. fungus
- m. jet
- m. jet signals
- m. perfusion
- m. trisomy C
- m. virus, tobacco

mosaicism
- m., marked
- m., Turner's
- m. ▸ white epithelium, punctuation, and

moschata, nux
Moschcowitz's operation
Mosher('s)
- M. esophagoscope tube
- M. operation, Toti-
- M. -Toti operation

Moskowitz procedure
Mosley method anterior shoulder repair
mOsm (milliosmole)
mosquito-borne hemorrhagic fever ▸ Southeast Asian
moss-agate sputum
Moss' classification
Mosso's ergograph
Mossuril virus
mossy cell
Mota (marijuana) (*same as* Muta)
Mota (hashish), Goma de
mother(s) ('s) (Mothers)
- m., addicted
- M. Against Drunk Driving (MADD)
- m. breast milk
- m. cell
- m., Colle's
- m., diabetic
- m., drug abusing

- m. figure
- m., high risk
- m. ▸ identified high-risk
- m. -infant bonding
- m. -infant interaction
- m. (IDM), infant of diabetic
- m., infant of high risk
- m., infant of infected
- m. infected with AIDS (acquired immune deficiency syndrome) virus
- m. instinct
- m. milk
- m. ▸ narcotic-addicted
- m., short-term separation from
- m., substance abusing
- m., surrogate
- m. thumb-printed in delivery room
- m. to infant, transmission from infected
- m. touch
- m. womb, penetrated

motile
- m. organism
- m. protozoa
- m. sperm, healthy

motility [*mobility*]
- m., abnormal
- m., body
- m., degree of
- m. disorder
- m. disorder, esophageal
- m. dysfunction ▸ esophageal
- m., esophageal
- m. esophagoscopy
- m. factor (AMF), autocrine
- m. ▸ irregular esophageal
- m., normal
- m. ▸ postoperative gastrointestinal (GI)
- m. ▸ size, shape and
- m., sperm
- m. studies
- m. study, esophageal
- m. test, esophageal
- m., visual

motion(s) Motion
- m. abnormality ▸ left ventricular (LV)
- m. abnormality ▸ regional wall
- m. abnormality, wall
- m. ▸ absence of
- m., active
- m., active head
- m. (ROM), active range of

m. analysis ▸ wall
m. and suppleness ▸ adequate range of
m., arm
m. artifact
m. artifact, aortic
m., asynchrony of
m. at fracture site
m., atrioventricular (AV) junction
m., body
m. clinic, balance
m., circular
m., circular massaging
m., cogwheel
m., continuous
m. -controlling nerve cells
m., cusp
m., decrease spinal
m. ▸ detection of
m., diastolic
m. display echo
m. disorder, repetitive
m. disorders
m. distress
m., exaggerated
m. exercise
m. exercise ▸ gentle range-of-
m. exercise ▸ range-of-
m., extremes of
m., fetal
m., finger
m. (ROM) ▸ full range of
m. (ROM) ▸ functional range of
m., gentle rocking
m., gliding
m., head
m., heel-toe
m., hip
m. in the joint ▸ repetitive
m. in spine ▸ restricted excess
m. injury, repetitive
m. ▸ interventricular septal
m., jarring
m., joint
m. ▸ joint range of
m. (ROM) ▸ left ankle full range of
m. (ROM) ▸ left elbow full range of
m. (ROM) ▸ left femur full range of
m. (ROM) ▸ left knee full range of
m. (ROM) ▸ left lower extremity full range of
m. (ROM) ▸ left shoulder full range of
m. (ROM) ▸ left upper extremity full range of

m., left ventricular wall
m. (ROM) ▸ left wrist full range of
m., leg
m. (LOM) ▸ limitation of
m., limited joint
m. (ROM) ▸ limited range of
m., loss of
m., lumbar spine
m., macular
m. ▸ maintaining joint range of
m. ▸ meaningless repetitive
m., mechanical
m. -mode (M mode)
m. modulation (M-mode) scanning
m., muscle
m., neck
m. (ROM) ▸ neck full range of
m. ▸ normal range of (ROM)
m. of extremity, limited
m. of spine
m. of wrist joint ▸ repetitive
m. on muscles ▸ excessive repetitive
m., pain aggravated by
m., pain-free
m. ▸ paradoxic wall
m., passive
m. (ROM), passive range of
m., pedaling
m., peristaltic
m. pictures of operation ▸ authorization form for taking of
m. pictures of operation ▸ consent form for taking of
m., pill rolling
m., posterior leaflet
m., precordial
m. (ROM) ▸ range of
m., range of knee
m., rapid repetitive
m. ▸ regional wall
m., repetitive
m. ▸ repetitive hand
m. ▸ repetitive wrist
m. (ROM) ▸ restricted range of
m., restriction of
m. (ROM) ▸ right ankle full range of
m. (ROM) ▸ right elbow full range of
m. (ROM) ▸ right femur full range of
m. (ROM) ▸ right knee full range of
m. (ROM) ▸ right lower extremity full range of
m. (ROM) ▸ right shoulder full range of

m. (ROM) ▸ right upper extremity full range of
m., right ventricular wall
m. (ROM) ▸ right wrist full range of
m., rotatory
m., rowing
m. scaling
m., scapulothoracic
m. score index ▸ wall
m. ▸ segmental wall
m. ▸ septal wall
m. severely restricted
m., shoulder
m. sickness
m. sickness skin patch
m. sickness syndrome
m. study ▸ floating wall
M. Study Laboratory
m. study ▸ wall
m., subtalar
m., systolic
m. (SAM) ▸ systolic anterior
m., task related
m. (TM), time
m., uterus tender to
m. ▸ ventricular wall
m. ▸ violent and irregular jerking
m., wall
m., whorl
motional averaging
motivated
m. behavior
m. for treatment
m., highly
m. individual
m. patient
m., patient self-
motivating factor
motivation
m., altruistic
m., burst of
m. for change
m., lack of
m., lack of drive or
m. ▸ lack of pleasure or
m. ▸ learning and
m., loss of
m. ▸ loss of ambition and
m., low
m., model of
m. ▸ patient renews
m., personal
m., poor

motivation—*continued*
- m. programs
- m., stress and
- m., suicide
- m., visualization and concentration

motivational
- m. counseling
- m. development
- m. enhancement therapy (MET)
- m. impairment
- m. interviewing
- m. problem, patient is
- m. process
- m. specialist
- m. syndrome
- m. technique

motivator, major

motives, concealed

motofacient tremor

motoneuron(s) (*same as* motor neuron)
- m., alpha
- m., gamma
- m., heteronymous
- m., homonymous
- m., lower
- m., peripheral
- m., upper

motor
- m. abilities
- m. abreaction
- m. activation
- m. activities, patient perseverates in
- m. activity
- m. activity, dysjunctive
- m. activity ▸ mild increase in
- m. activity ▸ potentiation of
- m. activity, undesired
- m. agitation, intense
- m. agraphia
- m. amusia
- m. and sensory changes
- m. and sensory deficits
- m. and sensory function
- m. and sensory nerve conduction study
- m. aphasia
- m. apraxia
- m. area
- m. area, supplementary
- m. -assisted device
- m. ataxia
- m. behavior
- m. behavior, fine

- m. cell
- m. center
- m. control center of brain
- m. changes, cognitive and
- m. cognitive disorder ▸ human immunodeficiency virus (HIV) associated
- m. component, somatic
- m. component, splanchnic
- m. control
- m. control ▸ lack of
- m. control ▸ loss of consciousness and
- m. control system, brain's
- m. coordination
- m. coordination, fine
- m. coordination ▸ gross and fine
- m. coordination ▸ impaired
- m. coordination ▸ lack of
- m. coordination ▸ loss of
- m. coordination, visual-
- m. cortex
- m. defect
- m. deficit
- m. deficit ▸ visual-
- m. deterioration, irreversible
- m. development
- m. discriminative acuity
- m. disease ▸ sensory
- m. disorder
- m. disturbance
- m. dysfunction
- m. endings
- m. examination ▸ oral
- m. expressive aphasia
- m. fibers
- m. function
- m. function, diminished
- m. function disorder
- m. function, impaired
- m. function ▸ loss of
- m. function ▸ partial loss of
- m. function ▸ sensation and
- m. function ▸ total loss of
- m. function, unimpaired
- m. function, visual-
- m. function waxed and waned ▸ left
- m. function waxed and waned ▸ right
- m. group, major
- m. impulses
- m. incoordination
- m. inhibition, psycho-
- m. innervation of bladder ▸ normal

- m. involvement
- m. movement, involuntary
- m. movements, abnormal
- m. movements, bilateral fine
- m. nerve
- m. nerve action potential
- m. nerve conduction velocity (MNCV)
- m. nerve fibers
- m. nerve of tongue
- m. nerve, peripheral
- m. nerve root
- m. neuron (MN) (*see* motoneuron)
- m. neuron (MN), degeneration of
- m. neuron (MN) disease
- m. neuron (MN) disease, infantile
- m. neuron (MN) disease ▸ inherited
- m. neuron (MN) disease, juvenile hereditary
- m. neuron (MN) dysfunction ▸ lower
- m. neuron (MN) dysfunction ▸ superimposed upper
- m. neuron (MN), lower
- m. neuron (MN) paralysis
- m. neuron (MN), upper
- m. neuropathy
- m. nuclei
- m. oculi
- m. or vocal tic disorder ▸ chronic
- m. organization and analysis, perceptual-
- m. organization, complex
- m. paralysis
- m. paralysis, complete
- m. paralytic bladder
- m. parasomnias
- m. pathway
- m., pen
- m. performance
- m. planning
- m. planning deficit
- m., plastic
- m. power
- m. power and coordination
- m. power, defective
- m. power, disorder of
- m. power, episodic loss of
- m. premonitory symptoms
- m. program, central
- m. recognition, visual
- m. reflexes
- m. region
- m. response
- m. response, clonic
- m. response, slowing of

m. response, tetanic
m. restlessness
m. retardation
m. saw ▸ fragments pared with
m. seizure
m. signs, focal
m. skills
m. skills ▸ awkward
m. skills, cognitive perceptual
m. skills, control
m. skills ▸ intact
m. skills ▸ intellectual and
m. skills ▸ loss of
m. skills, oral
m. skills, perceptual and
m. skills ▸ slow
m. skills ▸ slowing down of
m. speech
m. speech center
m. speed test
m. strip
m. stroke
m. syndrome ▸ sensory
m. system
m. task, visual-
m. test meal
m. tic
m. tic disorder, chronic
m. tics ▸ involuntary
m. tics ▸ simple
m. tics ▸ transient
m. tract, descending
m. tract intact
m. unit action potential
m. unit action potentials, individual
m. unit potentials
m. unit, single
m. units ▸ conscious control of
m. vehicle crash ▸ injurious
m. vehicle injury
m. weakness

motorized wheelchair
Mott cell
mottled
m. appearance
m. appearance ▸ spleen had
m. area
m. calcification
m. density
m. enamel
m. hemorrhagic appearance
m. hemorrhagic area
m. in appearance
m. infiltration
m., myocardium extensively

m. shadows
m. skin
m. skin, dry
m. teeth

mottling
m., areas of
m. of contrast media
m. of extremities
m. of retina, nonspecific

moulin, bruit de
moulin, bruit de la roue de
mountain (Mountain)
m. anemia
m. fever, American
m. mint
m. sickness
m. sickness, acute
m. sickness, chronic
M. spotted fever, Rocky

mounted allograft valve ▸ stent-
mounted heterograft valve ▸ stent-
mounting medium
mourning
m. ▸ children's grief and
m., grief and
m., period of

mouse
m. cell
m. encephalomyelitis
m. encephalomyelitis, Theiler's
m. interferon
m., joint
m., patient is house
m., peritoneal
m., pleural
m. retrovirus
m. tail pulse
m. unit (MU)
m. uterine units (MUU)

mouth
m., acid taste in
m. anaerobes
m. -and-hand synkinesis
m. and throat ▸ infection of
m. at bedtime (npo/h.s.) ▸ nothing by
m., bad taste in
m., bitter sour taste in
m., bitter taste in
m. breather
m. breathing
m. breathing, mouth-to-
m. (PO or per os), by
m. cancer
m., carcinoma of floor of

m. care
m. care before and after chemotherapy ▸ lip and
m. cells
m., Ceylon sore
m., commissure of lips of
m. corners ▸ down-turned
m. corners from sagging cheek ▸ cracked
m. cusp ▸ fish
m. dentures, full
m., depressor muscle of angle of
m., diaphragm of
m. discomfort
m. disease, foot-in-
m. disease ▸ hand, foot and
m. disorder
m., drooling from
m., drooping of
m., dry
m., dryness of
m. ▸ dryness of eyes and
m. dryness ▸ severe
m. extraction, full
m. ▸ extreme dryness of
m., floor of
m. from antihistamine ▸ dry
m. from anxiety ▸ trench
m. from aspirin ▸ burning
m. from cold sore ▸ burning
m. from coughing ▸ blue
m. from dentures ▸ burning
m. from depression ▸ burning
m. from diabetes ▸ burning
m., frothing at
m., fungal infection in
m. incision ▸ fish
m. infection
m., levator muscle of angle of
m. mitral stenosis ▸ fish-
m. movement, hand-to-
m. ▸ mucous lining of
m. (npo) ▸ nothing by
m. ▸ numbness and tingling around
m., orbicular muscle of
m., patient has dry
m. ▸ permanent drooping
m. ▸ permanent dry
m. pink and moist
m. position, closed
m. position, open
m. prop

mouth—*continued*

m. resuscitation, emergency mouth-to-
m. resuscitation, mouth-to-
m. rinse
m., roof of
m. ▸ saliva bubbling from
m. series, full
m. sores
m. sores ▸ recurring
m. syndrome, burning
m., tight seal over victim's
m. ▸ tingling sensation in
m. -to-mouth breathing
m. -to-mouth respiration
m. -to-mouth resuscitation
m. -to-mouth resuscitation, emergency
m. -to-mouth ventilation
m. -to-nose resuscitation
m., trench
m., ulceration of
m. ulcers
m. ulcers, develop
m., ulcers in
m. ventilation ▸ mouth-to-
m., vestibule of
m. x-rays, full

mouthed cervix, fish-
mouthpiece, breathes with
mouthpiece ▸ sip-and-puff
mouthwash, saline
movable

m., carina freely
m. cell mass
m., freely
m. heart
m. in midline
m. joint, freely
m. mass
m. pulse
m. subcutaneous nodule
m., uterus freely

move normally, cords
move tongue ▸ inability to
moved and positioned, patient
movement(s)

m., abnormal
m., abnormal body
m., abnormal eye
m., abnormal motor
m., abnormal muscle
m. ▸ abnormal rhythmic eye
m. abnormality ▸ severe
m., abrupt

m., absence of
m., absence of voluntary muscle
m., active
m., active muscle
m., ameboid
m., agitated
m., air
m. ▸ altered bowel
m. arousal
m. artifact
m. artifact, eye
m. artifact potential ▸ asymmetric eyeball
m., associated
m., asymmetric
m., athetoid
m., automatic
m., automatic repetitive
m., backward
m., bilateral face
m., bilateral fine motor
m., bilateral limb
m., binocular voluntary
m., bodily
m., body
m., border
m., bowel
m., characteristic
m., choreic athetoid
m., choreiform
m., ciliary
m. ▸ colloid osmotic pressure
m., comfortable bowel
m., complex rotational
m., conjugate
m., conjugate eye
m., contralateral
m., contralateral associated
m. control
m. ▸ control head
m., convulsive
m., coordinate muscle
m., coordination of
m. (NREM) cycle, nonrapid eye
m. (NREM-REM) cycle, nonrapid eye movement-rapid eye
m., decomposition of
m. (REM) density, rapid eye
m. desensitization and reprocessing (EMDR) ▸ eye
m. desensitization ▸ eye
m., diminished bowel
m. ▸ diminished intensity of
m., directional
m. disabilities

m., disjointed
m. ▸ disjointed, agitated
m. disorder
m. disorder, body
m. disorder, involuntary
m. disorder, progressive
m., disorganized muscular
m. disorder (PLMD) ▸ periodic limb
m. disorder ▸ rhythmic
m. ▸ disordered muscular
m., downward
m. ▸ drug-related involuntary
m., dystonic
m., excessive
m. exercises ▸ desensitizing
m. ▸ exhibits constant
m. (EOM) ▸ extraocular
m., eye
m., eyeball
m., fetal
m. ▸ fiber and bowel
m., fine hair
m., fluid
m., forced
m., forward
m. ▸ frequent bowel
m. ▸ general slowing of
m., gravitational
m., hand
m., hand-to-mouth
m., harmonious
m., head
m., hypoactive
m., hypokinetic
m., impaired
m. ▸ impairment of power of
m., imprecise eye
m. in sleep (PLMS) ▸ periodic limb
m., inability to perform purposeful
m., incessant
m. ▸ incoordination of all voluntary
m., infant tracks
m. injury
m. intact (EOMI), extraocular
m., interference
m., intestinal
m. (NREM) intrusion, nonrapid eye
m., involuntary
m. ▸ involuntary body
m. ▸ involuntary eye
m., involuntary motor
m., involuntary muscular

m., involuntary rapid
m., involuntary repetitive
m., inward
m. ▸ irregular bowel
m., irregular involuntary
m., irregular jerky
m. ▸ irregular, spasmodic, involuntary
m., jaw
m., jerking
m., jerking eye
m., jerky
m. ▸ jerky step-wise
m. ▸ labile muscle
m. (REM) latency, rapid eye
m., lateral
m., lateral eye
m., limb
m., limitation of
m., limited
m., limited joint
m., lip
m., loose bowel
m., loss of
m., loss of associated
m., loss of automatic
m., loss of joint
m., loss of power of voluntary
m., low impact
m. ▸ major body
m., mandibular
m., maniacal
m., manual
m. ▸ massive jerking
m., masticatory
m., muscle
m., muscular
m., myoclonic
m., natural purposeful
m. (NREM) ▸ nonrapid eye
m., normal bone
m. of arm ▸ repetitive overhead
m. of bradykinesia ▸ slow diminished
m. of chorea, involuntary
m. of cupula ▸ gravity-dependent
m. of electroencephalogram (EEG) paper ▸ velocity of
m. of extremity ▸ limited
m. of eyeball ▸ involuntary
m. of eyes and eyelids, sluggish
m. of heart
m. of legs ▸ involuntary jerking
m. of limbs and face ▸ uncontrolled
m. of limbs ▸ no spontaneous

m. of others ▸ imitating
m. of thumb ▸ control
m. of tongue and lips ▸ smacking
m. (REM) onset, rapid eye
m., opening
m., organized
m. ▸ outstretched arm
m., outward
m. ▸ overhead arm
m., pain aggravated by
m. ▸ painful and restricted
m., passive
m., passive limb
m., patient has no purposeful
m., pattern
m., pendular
m. (NREM) period, nonrapid eye
m. (REM) period, rapid eye
m. (REM) period, sleep onset rapid eye
m., periodic leg
m. ▸ periodic limb
m., periodic spasmodic athetoid
m., peristaltic
m. ▸ persistent dyskinetic
m. (NREM) physiology, nonrapid eye
m., precordial
m., purposeful
m. ▸ purposeless, uncontrolled sinuous
m., random
m. (RAM), rapid alternating
m. (REM), rapid eye
m. -rapid eye movement (NREM-REM) cycle, nonrapid eye
m. ▸ rapid head
m. (REM) rebound, rapid eye
m., reflex
m., repetitious automatic
m., repetitive
m. ▸ repetitive body
m. ▸ repetitive twisting
m. (RM), respiratory
m., restless
m., restricted
m. ▸ restricted eye
m. ▸ reversible oppositional
m., rhythmic jerking
m., right-to-die
m., rolling
m., saccadic eye
m., scissors
m., segmentation
m. ▸ sequential oppositional

m., skilled
m. sleep (NREMS), nonrapid eye
m. (REM) sleep anxiety dreams ▸ rapid eye
m. (REM) sleep ▸ increased rapid eye
m. (REM) sleep interruption insomnia ▸ rapid eye
m. (REM) sleep ▸ rapid eye
m. (REM) sleep-related hypoxemia ▸ rapid eye
m., slow
m. ▸ slow, controlled
m., slowed
m. ▸ slowness of
m. (SPEM) ▸ smooth pursuit eye
m., spasmodic
m., spasticity with shoulder
m. (REM), spindle rapid eye
m., spontaneous
m., stereotyped repetitive
m. ▸ stiffness and restriction of
m. ▸ straining on bowel
m. ▸ sucking or chewing
m., sudden
m., synkinetic
m. tachycardia ▸ antidromic circus
m. tachycardia, circus
m. ▸ tarry black bowel
m. ▸ therapeutic eye
m. ▸ therapeutic humor
m. therapy ▸ constraint-induced
m. therapy ▸ eye
m., thoracic respiratory
m. time
m., tonic-clonic
m. ▸ tremors and jerky
m., trunk
m. ▸ twitches and involuntary
m. ▸ uncontrollable body
m., uncontrolled
m., uncontrolled rhythmic limb
m., uncoordinated
m. ▸ uncoordinated arm
m. ▸ uncoordinated leg
m., unintentional
m., upward
m. ▸ urgent bowel
m., ventilatory
m., vermicular
m., vertical eye
m., vigorous
m. ▸ violent repetitive

movement(s)—*continued*
- m., volitional
- m., voluntary
- m., voluntary muscular
- m., watery bowel
- m. ▸ weak arm
- m. within functional limits

moving
- m. boundary electrophoresis
- m. grid
- m. spots before eyes

moyamoya disease
Moynihan respirator
Moynihan's test
Mozart ear
MP
- MP (mean pressure)
- MP (menstrual period)
- MP (mercaptopurine)
- MP (mesiopulpal)
- MP (metacarpophalangeal)

MPAP (mean pulmonary arterial pressure)
MPC (maximum permissible concentration)
MPD (maximum permissible dose)
MPD (multiple personality disorder)
MPD (myofascial pain dysfunction) syndrome
M period
M-protein serotype
M syndrome ▸ X-linked immunoglobulin
MPHR (maximum predicted heart rate)
MPI (Medical Phrase Index)
MPI (metacarpophalangeal joint), silastic
MPJ (metacarpophalangeal joint)
MPL (mesiopulpolingual)
MPLa (mesiopulpolabial)
MR (mr) (Mr.)
- mr (milliroentgen)
- MR (mitral reflux)
- MR (mitral regurgitation)
- MR (magnetic resonance) brain scan
- Mr. Natural (LSD)

MRA (magnetic resonance angiography)
- MRA ▸ intracranial
- MRA ▸ selective arterial
- MRA ▸ selective venous

MRAP (mean right atrial pressure)
MRD (minimum reacting dose)

MRF (magnetic resonance flow-metry)
MRF (mitral regurgitant flow)
MRFIT (Multiple Risk Factor Intervention Trial)
MRI (magnetic resonance imaging)
- MRI (magnetic resonance imaging) ▸ conventional
- MRI (magnetic resonance imaging) ▸ diffusion weighted
- MRI (magnetic resonance imaging) ▸ enhancement of
- MRI (magnetic resonance imaging) ▸ functional
- MRI (magnetic resonance imaging) scan, enhanced
- MRI (magnetic resonance imaging) scan, side-view
- MRI (magnetic resonance imaging) scanner
- MRI (magnetic resonance imaging) spectrometer
- MRI (magnetic resonance imaging) ▸ spin-echo

mRNA (messenger ribonucleic acid)
MR-SA (methicillin-resistant Staphylococcus aureus)
MRSI (magnetic resonance spectroscopy imaging)
MRVP (mean right ventricular pressure)
MS (mitral stenosis)
MS (morphine sulfate)
MS (multiple sclerosis)
- MS (multiple sclerosis), chronic progressive
- MS (multiple sclerosis) ▸ nerve degeneration in
- MS (multiple sclerosis) ▸ primary progressive
- MS (multiple sclerosis) ▸ progressive relapsing
- MS (multiple sclerosis) ▸ relapsing, remitting
- MS (multiple sclerosis) ▸ worsening, relapsing-remitting

MSAS (Mandel Social Adjustment Scale)
msec (millisecond)
msec (millisecond) slow wave
m/sec (meters per second)
MSER (mean systolic ejection rate)
M 75%, hypaque-
MSH (melanocyte-stimulating hormone)

MSH (melanophore-stimulating hormone)
MSHIF (melanocyte-stimulating hormone inhibiting factor)
MSI (magnetic source imaging)
M-60 contrast medium, Reno-
MSL (midsternal line)
MSU (Maximum Security Unit)
MSUD (maple syrup urine disease)
MSVC (maximal sustainable ventilatory capacity)
MTBE (methyl test-butyl ether)
MTD (maximum tolerated dose)
MTF (maximum terminal flow)
MTF (modulation transfer function)
M-30 contrast medium, Reno-
MTI (minimum time interval)
M-25 virus
M2 (mitral second sound)
M₂ (second mitral sound) M_2 (second mitral sound)
MTX (methotrexate)
MU (mouse unit)
Mu (milliunit)
mu (machine units)
mu/μ (micron)
mu/μ rhythm
mu/μ rhythm, reactivity of
MUC (maximum urinary concentration)
mucedo, Mucor
Much granules, Schrön-
Much's granules
mucicarmine stain
mucilaginous material
mucin
- m., focal
- m., intracytoplasmic
- m. negative
- m. -producing adenocarcinoma

mucinosa, alopecia
mucinous
- m. adenocarcinoma
- m. carcinoma
- m. cyst ▸ fluid
- m. cystadenoma
- m. layer of valve
- m. neoplasm (IPMN) ▸ intraductal papillary
- m. tumor

muciparum, carcinoma
mucobuccal fold
mucocellulare, carcinoma
mucociliary clearance
mucocutaneous
- m. candidiasis, chronic

m. hemorrhoid
m. junction
m. leishmaniasis
m. lymph node syndrome (MLNS)
m. pigmentation
m. wart

mucoepidermoid carcinoma
mucogenicum, Mycobacterium
mucoid
m. adenocarcinoma
m. bile
m. colony
m. discharge
m. exopolysaccharide
m. expectoration
m. impaction
m. material, blood tinged
m. material, copious
m. material ▸ thick
m. medial degeneration
m. plexus
m. secretion
m. secretion, tenacious
m. softening
m., urine

mucolabial fold
mucoperiosteal
m. fibromatosis
m. flap
m. flap trimming
m. flap ▸ von Langenbeck's bipedicle
m. implant placement

mucopolysaccharide, acid
mucoprotein test
mucopurulent
m. discharge
m. exudate
m. sputum
m. vaginal discharge

Mucor
M. corymbifer
M. mucedo
M. pusillus
M. racemosus
M. ramosus
M. rhizopodiformis

mucoretention cyst
mucormycosis, pulmonary
mucoroides, Aspergillus
mucosa
m. and submucosa, carcinoma invading
m., antral

m. appeared inflamed
m., arytenoid
m. at cardioesophageal junction, tear in
m., bladder
m., bowel
m., bronchial
m., buccal
m., Cellfalcicula
m. closure, mucosa-to-
m., colonic
m., columnar
m., congested
m., congestion of
m. ▸ congestion of bladder
m. ▸ denudation of normal
m., denuded bladder
m., duodenal
m., edema of bronchial
m., effacement of
m., endocervical
m., endocervical columnar
m., eroded
m., erythmatous
m., esophageal
m. ▸ extensive hemorrhage bronchial
m. (GM), gastric
m., gastroduodenal
m., gastrosuccorrhea
m., hemorrhagic
m., hyperemic laryngeal
m. ▸ hyperemic nasal
m. ▸ inflammation of oral
m., intestinal
m., jejunal
m., laryngeal
m., lower lip
m. masses ▸ small fungating
m. muscularis
m., nasal
m., necrosis of
m. necrotic
m., necrotic bladder
m. of bowel
m. of stomach ▸ congestion of
m. of stomach ▸ small, flat, white patches on
m. of trachea
m. of urinary bladder
m., oral
m., parietal
m., pharyngeal
m. pigmentation ▸ gingival and oral
m. pink and moist

m., retromolar
m., retrotuberous
m. slightly nodular
m., small bowel
m., squamous cell carcinoma buccal
m. ▸ squamous metaplasia of
m., swelling nasal
m., throat
m. -to-mucosa closure
m., tracheal
m., ulcerated buccal
m., ulceration of
m., upper lip
m., uterine
m., vaginal
m., vesical

mucosal
m. abnormalities
m. atrophy, gastric
m. autolysis, diffuse
m. autolysis, focal
m. barrier
m. coarsening
m. cuff
m. defect
m. edema
m. erosions, gastric
m. erythema
m. exposure ▸ eye
m. exudate
m. fold pattern
m. fold pattern, coarsened
m. glands, autolysis of
m. graft
m. hemorrhage
m. hemorrhage, bladder
m. hemorrhage, gastric
m. hernia
m. hyperkeratosis
m. inflammation, colonic
m. inflammatory hyperplasia
m. irregularity
m. irritant
m. layer
m. lesion
m. lesions ▸ multiple punctate
m. lining
m. melanoma
m. muscle
m. necrosis
m. pattern
m. pattern, hyperemic
m. pattern, spastic
m. reddening

mucosal—*continued*
- m. reflection
- m. relief roentgenography
- m. secretions
- m. stump
- m. surface
- m. surface, atrophic
- m. surfaces of duodenum
- m. surfaces of esophagus
- m. surfaces of large intestine
- m. surfaces of small intestine
- m. surfaces of stomach
- m. thickening
- m. tumor
- m. ulceration
- m. ulceration, focal
- m. ulceration ▸ foci of
- m. walls

mucoserous cells
mucoserous otitis media
mucosis (*same as* mucosus)
mucosis otitis
mucositis necroticans agranulocytica
mucositis, oral
mucosum, carcinoma
mucosum, Treponema
mucosus
- m., Diplococcus
- m. otitis
- m., Streptococcus

mucous (mucus)
- m. blanket, bronchial
- m., blood stained
- m., bloody
- m. build-up
- m. carcinoma
- m. cells
- m., cervical
- m. colic
- m. colitis
- m. cyst
- m. dessication
- m. diarrhea
- m. discharge
- m. drainage
- m., esophageal
- m., excessive
- m. fistula
- m. flow rate (MFR)
- m. fluid
- m. fluid streaked with blood
- m. glands
- m. hypersecretion
- m. in lungs
- m. in stools
- m. in throat
- m. inhibitor
- m. inhibitor, bronchial
- m. lining of mouth
- m. membrane
- m. membrane abnormalities
- m. membrane, altered oral
- m. membrane, anal
- m. membranes, blue
- m. membrane, bronchial
- m. membrane, dryness of
- m. membrane exposure
- m. membrane graft
- m. membrane, hydration of
- m. membrane, infected
- m. membrane, inner
- m. membrane lining
- m. membrane, loose rectal
- m. membrane, nasal
- m. membrane of cervix uteri ▸ partial excision
- m. membrane of lips ▸ pink
- m. membrane of nose ▸ inflammation of
- m. membrane, pink
- m., nasal
- m. ophthalmia
- m. ▸ oyster mass of
- m. particles
- m. ▸ passage of
- m. plaque
- m. plug
- m. plugging
- m. plugging of bronchial tree
- m. -producing cough ▸ chronic
- m. rales
- m. -secreting cell ▸ metaplastic
- m. secretion
- m. secretions
- m. secretions ▸ excess
- m. sheets
- m., shreds of
- m. ▸ stomach's protective lining of
- m. stool
- m. test, cervical
- m. ▸ thick, sticky
- m. threads
- m. tissue
- m. traps
- m., uterine
- m. velocity ▸ tracheal
- m., viscid

Mud
- M. (heroin)
- M. (Percodan)
- M. (heroin), Mexican

muddled thinking
Mueller('s)
- M. arthroplasty, Charnley-
- M. cautery
- M. Duo-Lock hip prosthesis
- M. maneuver

muenchen, Salmonella
muffled heart sounds
MUGA (multiple-gated acquisition)
- MUGA angiography scan
- MUGA blood pool radionuclide scan
- MUGA electrocardiogram (ECG) ▸ stress

Muir valve ▸ Passy-
Mujer (cocaine)
mulatta, Macaca
mulberry
- m. calculus
- m. cell
- m. fat
- m. molar
- m. tooth
- m. type papilloma

Mules(') (mule)
- M. implant
- M. operation
- m. -spinner's cancer

muliebre, pudendum
muliebris
- m., corpus spongiosum urethrae
- m., crista urethralis
- m., hydrocele
- m., urethra

Müller('s)
- M. counter, Geiger-
- M. fibers
- M. fluid
- M. fluid, formol-
- M. -Hillis maneuver
- M. horopter, Vieth-
- M. muscle
- M. operation
- M. test
- M. trigone

müllerian
- m. adenosarcoma
- m. duct
- m. duct anomaly

Mulligan Silastic prosthesis
multangular
- m. bone
- m. bone, greater

m. bone, lesser
m. torsion
multi-access catheter
multiaxial joint
multiaxial system
multicellular organism
multicellular tissues
Multicenter (multicenter)(s)
m. clinical trial
M., Digital Vascular Imager (DVI)
m. trial
Multiceps
multichannel analyzers
multichannel implant
multicolor data analysis
multicolored spots
multicomponent analysis
multicomponent protocol
multicrystal gamma camera
multicultural assessment
multicuspid teeth
multidisciplinary
m. activities, daily
m. approach
m. approach to pain management
m. assessment
m. care
m. evaluation
m. group
m. method of treatment
m. pain clinics
m. palliative care
m. plan
m. response
m. team
m. treatment
m. treatment planning
m. treatment team
m. treatment team approach
multidrug
m. abuse
m. abusers, assessing needs of
m. resistant
m. -resistant TB (tuberculosis)
multi-electrode lead
multifaceted personality disorder
multifaceted syndrome
**multifactorial index of cardiac risk ▸
modified**
**multifactorially inherited
predisposition**
multifamily group counseling
multifernentans, Clostridium
multifidus muscle
multifilament wire

multifocal
m. anaplastic astrocytoma
m. atrial tachycardia (MAT)
m. contractions
m. ectopic beats
m. fibrosis
m. heartbeats
m. infiltrated duct cell carcinoma
m. lens implants
m. leukoencephalopathy,
progressive
m. PVCs (premature ventricular
contractions)
**multiform premature ventricular
complex**
multiform tachycardia
multiforme
m., erythema
m., glioblastoma
m., granuloma
m., spongioblastoma
multiformis endemica, urticaria
multiformis, Haverhillia
multifraction survival curves
multifractionated radiation
multifunctional defibrillator
multigated angiography
**multigated radionuclide
ventriculography ▸ equilibrium**
multigenerational drug use
multigenerational studies
multihandicapped support
multihit injury
multihole collimator
multihospital systems
multi-infarct
m. dementia
m. dementia, uncomplicated
m. dementia, with delirium
m. dementia, with delusions
m. dementia, with depression
m. disease
multi-institutional clinical trials
multilamellar body
multilamellar cytosome
multilead electrode
multileaf collimator (MLC)
multilevel spinal fusion
multilinear regression analysis
multilobe infiltrate
multilobate placenta
multilobed placenta
multilobular cirrhosis
multilobular cyst
multilocular cyst

multilocularis, Echinococcus
multilumen catheter
multimodal
m. therapies
m. therapy
m. treatment protocol
multimodality
m. approach
m. evoked potential (MEP)
m. therapy
multinodular
m. goiter
m. goiter, benign
m. liver
m. thyroid
m. thyroid gland
multinucleated
m. cells
m. giant cells
m. plasma cells
multiparity, grand
multiparous [*nulliparous*]
multiparous female
multiparous, patient
multipartita, placenta
multiphasic (Multiphasic)
M. Personality Inventory (MMPI) ▸
Minnesota
M. Personality Inventory (MMPI)
test ▸ Minnesota
m. pill
m. screening
m. screening, automated
multiphilia, Stentotrophomonas
multiplanar mode
multiplanar technique
multiplane scanner, tomographic
multiple (Multiple)
m. abdominal scars
m. abrasions
m. abscesses
m. adenomatous polyps
m. admissions
m. air fluid levels
m. amputation
M. Analyzer Computer (SMAC) ▸
Sequential
m. analyzer (SMA-6) test,
sequential
m. analyzer (SMA-1 2) test,
sequential
m. apertures
m. apical fibrous adhesions
m. arrhythmia
m. balloon valvuloplasty

multiple—*continued*

m. -bed monitoring
m. benign cystic epithelioma
m. biopsies taken
m. bipolar derivations
m. births
m. births, abortions, live births (GPMAL) ▸ Gravida, para,
m. body sites
m. bone metastases
m. brain metastases
m. branching
m. calcifications
m. cancers
m. cardiac risk factors
m. caries, foul sputum ▸ malnourished
m. cartilaginous exostosis
m. channel implants
m. cholesterol emboli
m. clicks
m. clinical syndrome
m. complaints
m. complaints, patient admitted with
m. congenital anomalies
m. congenital defects
m. coronal sections
m. cultures
m. disabilities, severe
m. disorders
m. drug chemotherapy
m. drug dependent
m. drug program
m. drug program, patient on
m. drug protocol
m. drug therapies
m. drugs
m. drugs, abuse potential of
m. drugs, acute intoxication with
m. drugs, detoxification from
m. drugs, flashback reactions with
m. drugs, organic brain syndrome with
m. drugs, panic reactions with
m. drugs, patient OD (overdosed) with
m. drugs, psychotic reactions with
m. drugs, toxicity of
m. drugs, treatment of acute drug reactions to
m. drugs, withdrawal from
m. ecchymoses
m. ecchymoses on skin
m. embolisms

m. endocrine abnormalities (MEA)
m. endocrine adenomatosis
m. endocrine adenopathies (MEA)
m. endocrine neoplasia (MEN)
m. endocrine neoplasia syndromes
m. epiphyseal dysplasia
m. exostosis
m. exostosis, hereditary
m. facetted stones
m. family therapy
m. fibrinous adhesions
m. focal calcified granulomata
m. foci
m. fractures
m. fragment wounds
m. fragmentations
m. gallstones
m. -gated acquisition (MUGA)
m. -gated acquisition (MUGA) blood pool radionuclide scan
m. -gated acquisition (MUGA) electrocardiogram (ECG) ▸ stress
m. -gated angiography (MUGA) scan
m. genes
m. handicapped (P/MH), physically/
m. handicaps
m. hemorrhage, traumatic
m. hospitalizations
m. hyaloserositis ▸ progressive
m. infarcts
m. interstitial pulmonary hemorrhages
m. intrauterine pregnancy
m. keratoses
m. leiomyomata
m. lentigines syndrome
m. lesions
m. loops of small bowel
m. metastases
m. metastatic nodules
m. microabscesses
m. miscarriages
m. moles on skin
m. myeloma
m. myeloma with leukemic transformation
m. needle puncture marks
m. needle puncture wounds
m. needle punctures
m. neuropathy
m. nuclide
m. offenses
m. old nasal fractures

m. oral medications
m. organ damage
m. organ donor
m. organ transplants
m. parameter technique
m. pathologic fractures
m. pelvic adhesions
m. pericardial adhesions
m. perpetrators
m. personality
m. personality disorder (MPD)
m. personality, dissociative disorders
m. petechiae
m. plasmacytomas of bone
m. point electrode
m. pregnancies
m. prescriptions
m. pressure transducer system
m. previous infarctions
m. problem behaviors
m. pulmonary abscesses
m. pulmonary emboli
m. pulmonary infarcts
m. punctate hemorrhages
m. punctate mucosal lesions
m. puncture wounds
m. regression
m. relapses
m. rheumatic symptoms
m. rib fractures
m. risk factors
M. Risk Factor Intervention Trial (MRFIT)
m. sclerosis (MS)
m. sclerosis (MS), acute
m. sclerosis (MS), benign
m. sclerosis (MS) ▸ chronic progressive
m. sclerosis (MS) ▸ nerve degeneration in
m. sclerosis (MS) ▸ plaques of
m. sclerosis (MS) ▸ primary progressive
m. sclerosis (MS) ▸ progressive
m. sclerosis (MS) ▸ progressive relapsing
m. sclerosis ▸ relapsing-remitting
m. sclerosis (MS) virus
m. sclerosis (MS) ▸ worsening, relapsing-remitting
m. screening
m. seborrheic keratoses
m. sections of aorta
m. sex partners

m. sexual partners
m. sheets of skin
m. shunt levels
m. sites
m. sites ▸ bleeding from
m. skills group
M. Sleep Latency Test
m. slits in cornea
m. small calcified leiomyomas
m. spike-and-slow wave complex
m. spike complex
m. spike foci
m. spike waves
m. staining
m. stripping
m. subpial transection
m. surgical excisions
m. symptom clusters
m. symptoms
m. system atrophy
m. tendons
m. thoracenteses
m. thrombi in vessels of heart
m. trauma
m. trauma, massive
m. trauma, patient has
m. tumor metastases
m. ulcerations
m. ulcers of esophagus
m. ulcers of stomach
m. uninflammed diverticula
m. vague symptoms
m. victim situation
m. washings taken for examination
m. widespread metastases

multiplex
m., dysostosis
m., mononeuritis
m., paramyoclonus
m. personality disorder
m., trichoepithelioma papillosum
m., xanthoma
m., xanthoma tuberosum

multiplication, viral
multiplier
m. effect
m. phototube
m. tube, electron

Multipoise headrest
multipolar
m. catheter
m. catheter electrode
m. coagulation

multipotential cells

multipurpose catheter, angulated
multireactive patients
multirisk programs
multirooted tooth
multisensor catheter
multisensory perceptions
multisided Z-plasty closure
multislice imaging
multispecialty medical group
multisystem
m. disease
m. disorder
m. occlusive disease
m. organ failure
m. trauma

multivalve insufficiency
multivalvular disease
multivalvular disease murmur
multivariant analysis
multivariant regressional analysis
multivariate analysis of variance
multivessel disease
multivitamin supplements
multiware proportional chamber
multocida, Pasteurella
Mummery's pink tooth
mummified fetus
mummified pulp
mumps
m. incubation period
m. meningitis
m., orchitis due to
m., postsurgical
m. skin test antigen
m. virus

Munchausen's syndrome
Munnell's operation
Munro-Kerr maneuver
muqueux, rale
mural
m. aneurysm
m. atheroma
m. atherosclerosis, calcific
m. endocarditis
m. endocardium
m. endocardium, overlying
m. endocardium, smooth
m. fibrosing alveolitis
m. kidney
m. leaflet
m. pregnancy
m. salpingitis
m. thrombi
m. thrombi, antemortem
m. thrombosis

m. thrombus
Murdoch wrist sign ▸ **Walker-Muret sign, Quénu-**
Murgo pressure contours
muricola, Rickettsia
murina, Hymenolepis
murine
m. encephalomyelitis
m. encephalomyelitis virus
m. interferon
m. leukemia virus
m. sarcoma virus

muris
m., Actinomyces
m., Haemobartonella
m. -ratti, Actinomyces
m., Trichomonas

muriseptica ▸ **gram-positive Erysipelothrix**
murisepticum, Corynebacterium
murium, Mycobacterium leprae
murmur(s)
m., abnormal
m., accidental
m., amphoric
m., anemic
m., aneurysmal
m., aortic
m., aortic incompetent
m., aortic left ventricular (LV) tunnel
m., aortic-mitral combined disease
m., aortic regurgitation
m., aortic stenosis
m., apex
m., apical
m., apical diastolic
m. ▸ apical mid-diastolic heart
m., apical systolic heart
m., arterial
m., atrioventricular (AV) flow rumbling
m., attrition
m., Austin Flint
m., basal diastolic
m., bellows
m., benign
m. ▸ benign heart
m., blood
m., blowing
m., blowing ejection systolic
m., blowing systolic
m., blubbery diastolic
m., brain
m., Bright's

murmur(s)—*continued*
- m., bronchial
- m., bronchial collateral artery
- m., carcinoid
- m., cardiac
- m., cardiopulmonary
- m., cardiorespiratory
- m., Carey-Coombs
- m., carotid artery
- m., click
- m., coarse
- m., congenital
- m., continuous
- m., continuous heart
- m., cooing
- m., crescendo
- m., crescendo-decrescendo
- m., Cruveilhier-Baumgarten
- m., decrescendo early systolic
- m., deglutition
- m. ▸ diamond ejection
- m., diamond-shaped
- m. (DM), diastolic
- m., diastolic decrescendo
- m., direct
- m., Docke's
- m., Duroziez's
- m., dynamic
- m., early diastolic
- m. ▸ early peaking systolic
- m. (EM), ejection
- m. (ESM), ejection systolic
- m., end-diastolic
- m., end-systolic
- m., endocardial
- m. ▸ enlargement, thrill or
- m., Eustace Smith's
- m. ▸ exit block
- m., exocardial
- m., expiratory
- m., extracardiac
- m., faint diastolic
- m., Fisher's
- m., Flint's
- m., flow
- m., Fraentzel's
- m., friction
- m., functional
- m., functional heart
- m., Gibson
- m. ▸ goose honk
- m., Grade 1 through 6
- m., Graham Steell
- m., groaning
- m., Hamman's

- m., harsh systolic
- m., heart
- m., hemic
- m. ▸ high frequency
- m. ▸ high-pitched
- m., holodiastolic
- m., holosystolic
- m., honking
- m., hour-glass
- m., humming
- m., humming-top
- m., incidental
- m., indirect
- m., innocent
- m. ▸ innocent heart
- m., inorganic
- m., inspiratory
- m., lapping
- m. ▸ late apical systolic
- m. ▸ late peaking systolic
- m. (LSM), late systolic
- m. ▸ left ventricular-right atrial communication
- m., loud systolic
- m. ▸ low frequency
- m. ▸ low pitched
- m., machinery
- m., Makin's
- m., mammary souffle
- m. ▸ mid-diastolic
- m., midsystolic
- m., mill-house
- m. ▸ mill wheel
- m., mitral
- m., mitral prolapse
- m. ▸ mitral regurgitation
- m. ▸ mitral stenosis
- m. ▸ multivalvular disease
- m., muscle
- m., muscular
- m., musical
- m., noninvasive
- m., nun's
- m., obstructive
- m. of elderly ▸ innocent
- m. of heart, Graham-Steell
- m. or rubs
- m., organic
- m., outflow
- m., pansystolic
- m., Parrot's
- m., pathologic
- m. ▸ patent ductus arteriosus
- m., pericardial
- m., physiologic

- m., pleuropericardial
- m., prediastolic
- m., presystolic
- m. ▸ primary pulmonary hypertension
- m., prominent
- m., protodiastolic
- m., pulmonary
- m., pulmonic
- m., rasping
- m., reduplication
- m., regurgitant
- m., respiratory
- m., Roger's
- m., rubs or
- m. ▸ rumbling diastolic
- m., scratchy
- m., seagull
- m., seesaw
- m., soft blowing diastolic
- m., Steell's
- m., stenosal
- m., Still's
- m., subclavian
- m., subclavicular
- m. syndrome, click-
- m. syndrome ▸ systolic click
- m., systolic
- m., systolic apical
- m., systolic ejection
- m. (SEM) ▸ systolic ejection
- m. ▸ systolic regurgitant
- m., to-and-fro
- m., transmission of
- m., transmitted
- m., Traube's
- m., tricuspid
- m., vascular
- m., venous
- m., vesicular
- m., water-wheel
- m., whooshing

Murphy('s)
- M. -Pattee test
- M. percussion
- M. sign

Murray Valley encephalitis virus

Mus
- M. alexandrinus
- M. decumanus
- M. musculus
- M. norvegicus
- M. rattus

Musca
- M. autumnalis

M. domestica
M. domestica nebulo
M. domestica vicina
M. luteola
M. sorbens
M. vomitoria
muscae, Entomophthora
muscaria, Amanita
muscarinic agonist
muscarinic receptor
muscarius, Agaricus
muscle(s) (*see also* musculus)
m. ability
m., abductor digiti quinti
m., abductor pollicis brevis
m., abductor pollicis longus
m. abnormality, heart
m. abscess ▸ papillary
m., accessory
m., accessory flexor
m. ache ▸ generalized
m. ache, joint and
m. aches
m. aches and pains ▸ fatigue,
m. aching and stiffness ▸
    widespread
m. action potential
m. activity
m. activity and awareness
m. activity ▸ chaotic heart
m. activity ▸ energy for
m. activity, feedback of speech
m. activity, jaw
m., activity of voluntary
m. activity, resting
m. activity, scalp
m. activity, skeletal
m. activity, spastic
m., adductor hallucis
m., adductor longus
m., adductor magnus
m., adductor pollicis
m., advancement external rectus
m., advancement inferior oblique
m., advancement inferior rectus
m., advancement internal rectus
m., advancement lateral rectus
m., advancement medial rectus
m., advancement ocular
m., advancement of eye
m., advancement superior oblique
m., advancement superior rectus
m., Aeby's
m., affected facial
m. ▸ age-related loss of

m., agonistic
m., Albinus'
m. ▸ alternating contracting and
    relaxing of
m. ▸ anal sphincter
m., anconeus
m. and joints ▸ pain in
m. and tendons ▸ fatigue,
m., anesthesia of leg
m., antagonistic
m., anterior auricular
m., anterior intertransverse
m., anterior papillary
m., anterior sacrococcygeal
m., anterior scalene
m., anterior serratus
m., anterior sheath of rectus
m., anterior tibial
m., antigravity
m., appendicular
m., arrectores pilorum
m., articular
m. artifact
m. artifact, eye
m., aryepiglottic
m., atrophic
m., atrophied abdominal
m. atrophy
m. atrophy, denervated
m., atrophy of abdominal
m., atrophy of leg
m., atrophy of skeletal
m., atrophy of thenar
m., avoid overuse of
m. avulsion ▸ peroneus longus
m., back
m. balance check
m. balance, normal
m., beating heart
m. behavior
m. behavior and emotions
m., Bell's
m., biceps brachii
m., biceps femoris
m. biopsy
m., bipennate
m., bladder
m., bladder control
m. bleeding points
m. bleeding points individually
    clamped and coagulated
m. ▸ block in normal
    communication between nerves
    and
m., blood diffuses into heart

m., body
m., Bowman's
m., brachial
m., brachioradial
m. breakdown
m. breathing
m. bridging
m., bronchoesophageal
m., Brücke's
m., bruised
m., buccinator
m., buccopharyngeal
m., build
m. building
m. -building drug
m., bulbocavernous
m. bulk
m. bundle
m., calf
m., canine
m., capillary
m., cardiac
m., casserian
m., Casser's
m. cell
m. cell contraction
m. cell ▸ degeneration of
m. cell, heart
m. cell necrosis
m. cell nuclei
m. cell ▸ patch quilt degeneration
    of
m. cell, smooth
m. cell ▸ transferring immature
m. cells, autorhythmic heart
m. cells ▸ vascular smooth
m., ceratocricoid
m., ceratopharyngeal
m., Chassaignac's axillary
m., chondroglossus
m., chondropharyngeal
m., chronic pain in
m., ciliaris
m., ciliary
m., circular
m., circular Santorini's
m., clonic spasm of voluntary
m., coccygeal
m. ▸ compensatory hypertrophy of
    heart
m. compliance ▸ left ventricular
m., congenerous
m. constrict urethra
m. contract
m. contract, bladder

muscle(s)—*continued*

m. contracted
m. contractility of heart
m. contracting
m. contraction
m. contraction, force of
m. contraction headaches
m. contraction, improve
m. contraction, involuntary
m. contraction of bowel
m., contraction of calf
m., contraction of heart
m., contraction of uterine
m. contraction, painful
m. contraction ▸ stimulation of
m. contraction, thenar
m. contraction ▸ vascular smooth
m. contractions, bursts of uncontrolled
m. contractions of esophagus
m. contractions ▸ repeated
m. contracture ▸ ischemic
m. control
m. control, cognition and
m. control ▸ loss of
m., cool working
m. coordination
m. coordination ▸ small
m., coracobrachial
m. cramp
m. cramping
m. cramps and spasms
m. cramps ▸ heart
m., Crampton's
m., cremasteric
m., cricoarytenoid
m., cricopharyngeal
m., cricopharyngeus
m., cricothyroid
m., crushed
m., cuff
m., cutaneous
m. damage, heart
m., dead area of heart
m. death, heart
m. degeneration ▸ acute heart
m. degeneration ▸ skeletal
m., deltoid
m., depressor septi nasi
m. deteriorate, heart
m., deterioration of heart
m., detrusor urinae
m., diaphragmatic
m., diastasis of
m., digastric

m. discomfort
m. disease ▸ alcoholic heart
m. disease, cardiac
m. disease ▸ chronic alcoholic heart
m. disease, heart
m. disease ▸ left ventricular
m. disease ▸ preclinical heart
m. disease ▸ respiratory
m. disease ▸ symptomatic alcohol heart
m. ▸ diseased heart
m. ▸ disintegration of
m. disorder
m. disorder ▸ anxiety-related
m. disorder, degenerative
m. disorder ▸ skeletal
m. dissected free, inferior rectus
m. distress, silent heart
m. disuse atrophy
m., dorsal sacrococcygeal
m. dysfunction
m. dysfunction ▸ enhanced
m. dysfunction, papillary
m. dysfunction ▸ respiratory
m. dystrophy, ocular
m. effort
m. ▸ electrical activity in nerve and
m. electrical interference ▸ extraneous scalp
m. ▸ elongated papillary
m. ▸ embryonic cardiac
m., emergency
m. endurance
m., enlarged heart
m., epicranial
m., epimeric
m., epitrochleoanconeus
m. erotism
m., eustachian
m. ▸ excess skin and
m. ▸ excessive repetitive motion on
m. ▸ excessive stretching of ventricular
m. ▸ excessive use of involved
m. exercise, pelvic
m. exercise ▸ pelvic floor
m. exertion
m. extensor carpi radialis brevis
m. extensor carpi radialis longus
m., extensor carpi ulnaris
m., extensor digiti minimi
m., extensor digiti quinti proprius
m., extensor digitorum brevis

m., extensor digitorum communis
m., extensor digitorum longus
m., extensor hallucis brevis
m., extensor hallucis longus
m., extensor indicis
m., extensor pollicis brevis
m., extensor pollicis longus
m., external intercostal
m., external oblique
m., external obturator
m., external pterygoid
m. ▸ external sphincter
m., extracostal
m., extraocular
m. ▸ extraocular eye
m., extrinsic
m. fascia
m. fasciculation
m. fatigue
m., feedback training of parts of buccinator
m., femoral
m. fiber
m. fiber, atrial
m. fiber, cardiac
m. fiber, heart
m. fiber ▸ loss of
m. fibers
m. fibers, atrophic
m. fibers ▸ disorganized
m. fibers, heart
m. fibers, hyperplastic
m. fibers ▸ inflamed
m. fibers ▸ ischemic
m. fibers, skeletal
m. fibers, striated
m. fibrosis, papillary
m., finger
m., fixation
m., fixator
m., flap
m., flexed
m. flexibility
m. flexibility, maintain
m., flexor carpi radialis
m., flexor carpi ulnaris
m., flexor digitorum brevis
m., flexor digitorum longus
m., flexor digitorum profundus
m., flexor digitorum sublimis
m., flexor digitorum superficialis
m., flexor hallucis brevis
m., flexor hallucis longus
m., flexor pollicis brevis
m., flexor pollicis longus

m., Folius'
m., frontalis
m., full voluntary contraction of
m. function
m., fusiform
m., gastrocnemius
m., Gavard's
m., gemellus
m., genioglossus
m., geniohyoideus
m., glossopalatine
m., glossopharyngeal
m., gluteal
m., gluteus maximus
m., gluteus medius
m., gluteus minimus
m., gracilis
m. graft
m., great adductor
m., greater pectoral
m., greater psoas
m., greater rhomboid
m., greater trochanter
m., greater zygomatic
m. group
m. groups ▸ strengthen and tone
m. growth, rapid
m. guarding
m. guarding, abdominal
m., Guthrie's
m., hamstring
m., heart
m., helicis
m. hemoglobin
m., herniation of
m., Hilton's
m., Homer's
m., Houston's
m., hyoglossal
m., hyoglossus
m., hypaxial
m. hypertrophy
m., hypomeric
m., hypotonia of
m., iliac
m. iliacus
m., iliococcygeal
m., iliocostal
m., iliocostalis cervicis
m., iliocostalis lumborum
m., iliocostalis thoracis
m., iliopsoas
m. imbalance
m. imbalance ▸ eye
m. immunocytochemical study

m. ▸ impaired contactibility of
    hypertrophied
m. in head and neck, clenched
m., inactive
m. in neck ▸ weak
m. incoordination
m., increased blood flow to heart
m., inferior constrictor
m., inferior gemellus
m., inferior oblique
m., inferior posterior serratus
m., inferior rectus
m., inferior tarsal
m., inflammation of
m. ▸ inflammation of heart
m., infrahyoid
m., infraspinous
m. ▸ injured heart
m. injuries
m. injury, abdominal
m., innermost intercostal
m. innervated
m. irritation
m., inspiratory
m., intact chest
m., interarytenoid
m., intercostal
m., interfoveolar
m., internal intercostal
m., internal oblique
m., internal obturator
m., internal pterygoid
m. ▸ internal sphincter
m., internal thyroarytenoid
m., interosseous
m., interspinal
m., intertransverse
m., intra-auricular
m., intraocular
m., intrinsic
m., involuntary
m., ipsilateral mentalis
m., iridic
m. ischemia ▸ skeletal
m., ischemic
m. ▸ ischemic heart
m. ▸ ischemic skeletal
m., ischiocavernous
m. isolated and tagged
m., Jarjavay's
m. joint evaluation, computerized
m. junctions, nerve-
m., Jung's
m., Koyter's
m., lack of oxygen (O₂) to cardiac

m., Landström's
m., Langer's
m., lateral anconeus
m., lateral cricoarytenoid
m., lateral gastrocnemius
m., lateral malleolus
m., lateral pterygoid
m., lateral rectus
m., latissimus dorsi
m., lax facial
m. layer ▸ hypertrophic smooth
m. layers
m., layers of
m., least gluteal
m., lesser rhomboid
m., lesser zygomatic
m., levator
m., levator ani
m., levator palpebrae superior
m., levator veli palatine
m. level
m., long adductor
m., long fibular
m., long palmar
m., long peroneal
m., long rotator
m., longissimus
m., longitudinal
m., Luschka's
m. malfunction ▸ age-related
m. mass
m. mass ▸ decreased
m. mass ▸ increased
m. mass ▸ lean
m. mass ▸ loss of
m. mass, strength and balance
m. mass, ventricular
m. massage ▸ deep
m., masseter
m., masticatory
m., medial anconeus
m., medial gastrocnemius
m., medial pterygoid
m., medial rectus
m., mentalis
m., Merkel's
m., mesothenar
m., middle scalene
m. mitochondria, skeletal
m. motion
m. movement
m. movement, abnormal
m. movement, absence of
    voluntary

muscle(s)—*continued*

m. movement, active
m. movement, coordinate
m. movements ▸ labile
m., mucosal
m., Müller's
m., multifidus
m. murmur
m., myectomy of ocular
m., mylohyoid
m., mylopharyngeal
m., myotomy of ocular
m., nasal
m., neck
m. necrosis
m. necrosis, cardiac
m. necrosis ▸ ischemic
m., necrotic
m. ▸ nerve deprived
m., nonspastic
m., nonstriated
m., oblique
m., oblique arytenoid
m., obliquus inferior
m., obliquus superior
m., occipital
m., occipitofrontal
m., Ochsner's
m., ocular
m. of abdomen, external oblique
m. of abdomen, internal oblique
m. of abdomen, transverse
m. of affected side
m. of angle of mouth ▸ depressor
m. of angle of mouth ▸ levator
m. of antitragus
m. of anus, external sphincter
m. of anus, internal sphincter
m. of arm, biceps
m. of arm, triceps
m. of auditory ossicles
m. of auricle, oblique
m. of auricle, pyramidal
m. of auricle, transverse
m. of back, longissimus
m. of base of stapes ▸ fixator
m. of bile duct, sphincter
m. of calf, triceps
m. of chin, transverse
m. of digits, common extensor
m. of duodenum, suspensory
m. of elbow, articular
m. of evacuation ▸ strengthen
m. of eye
m. of eye, orbicular

m. of eyeball, inferior oblique
m. of eyeball, superior oblique
m. of fascia lata, tensor
m. of fauces
m. of fifth digit ▸ proper extensor
m. of fingers, deep flexor
m. of fingers, extensor
m. of fingers, superficial flexor
m. of foot, dorsal interosseous
m. of foot, lumbrical
m. of great toe, abductor
m. of great toe, adductor
m. of great toe, long extensor
m. of great toe, long flexor
m. of great toe, short extensor
m. of great toe, short flexor
m. of hair, arrector
m. of hand, dorsal interosseous
m. of hand, lumbrical
m. of head, longissimus
m. of head, semispinal
m. of head, splenius
m. of hepatopancreatic ampulla ▸
    sphincter
m. of hyoid bone
m. of index finger, extensor
m. of inferior lip, incisive
m. of knee, articular
m. of left ventricle ▸ anterior
    papillary
m. of left ventricle ▸ posterior
    papillary
m. of little finger, abductor
m. of little finger, extensor
m. of little finger, opposing
m. of little finger, short flexor
m. of little toe, abductor
m. of little toe, short flexor
m. of lower lip, depressor
m. of lower lip, incisive
m. of lower lip, quadrate
m. of membranous urethra,
    sphincter
m. of mouth, orbicular
m. of nape, transverse
m. of naris, compressor
m. of neck
m. of neck, anterior intertransverse
m. of neck, longissimus
m. of neck, posterior
    intertransverse
m. of neck, rotator
m. of neck, semispinal
m. of neck, splenius
m. of nose, dilator

m. of palate and fauces
m. of palatine velum ▸ levator
m. of penis, erector
m. of perineum
m. of perineum, deep transverse
m. of perineum, superficial
    transverse
m. of pharynx, constrictor
m. of pharynx, superior constrictor
m. of prostate, levator
m. of pupil, dilator
m. of pupil, sphincter
m. of pylorus, sphincter
m. of respiration
m. of respiration, accessory
m. of ribs, levator
m. of ribs, long levator
m. of ribs, short levator
m. of right ventricle ▸ septal
    papillary
m. of scapula, levator
m. of scrotum, dartos
m. of septum of nose ▸ depressor
m. of sole, quadrate
m. of spine, erector
m. of superior lip ▸ incisive
m. of the left ventricle ▸ papillary
m. of thigh, biceps
m. of thigh, quadriceps
m. of thorax, interspinal
m. of thorax, intertransverse
m. of thorax, longissimus
m. of thorax, rotator
m. of thorax, semispinal
m. of thorax, transverse
m. of thumb, adductor
m. of thumb, long abductor
m. of thumb, long extensor
m. of thumb, long flexor
m. of thumb, opposing
m. of thumb, short abductor
m. of thumb, short extensor
m. of thumb, short flexor
m. of thyroid glando-levator
m. of toes, long extensor
m. of toes, long flexor
m. of toes, short extensor
m. of toes, short flexor
m. of tongue, inferior longitudinal
m. of tongue, superior longitudinal
m. of tongue, transverse
m. of tongue, vertical
m. of tragus
m. of Treitz
m. of tympanic membrane ▸ tensor

m. of tympanum, tensor
m. of upper extremities atrophic
m. of upper eyelid, levator
m. of upper lip and ala of nose ▸ levator
m. of upper lip, incisive
m. of upper lip, levator
m. of upper lip, quadrate
m. of urethra, sphincter
m. of urinary bladder ▸ sphincter
m. of uvula
m. of velum palatine, levator
m. of velum palatine, tensor
m., omohyoid
m., opened, chest
m., opponens pollicis
m., orbicular
m., orbital
m., organic
m. ▸ overcontraction of
m., overgrown
m. ▸ oxygen (O_2) -deprived leg
m. ▸ oxygen (O_2) -starved heart
m. pain
m. pain and chills
m., pain and spasm of
m. pain, chronic
m. pain, general
m. ▸ pain in calf
m. pain ▸ soft tissue
m. pain syndrome ▸ chronic
m. pain, tenderness or weakness
m., palatoglossus
m., palatopharyngeal
m., palmar interosseous
m., palmaris brevis
m., palmaris longus
m., papillary
m. paralysis
m. paralysis, chronic
m., paralysis of eye
m., paralysis of eyelid
m., paralysis of facial
m., paralyzed
m. paralyzing disease
m. paraspinal
m. paresis
m. pattern
m. pectinate
m., pectineal
m., pectineus
m., pectoral
m., pectoralis major
m., pectoralis minor
m., pelvic

m. ▸ pelvic floor
m., penniform
m., peroneus brevis
m., peroneus longus
m., peroneus tertius
m., pharyngeal constrictor
m., pharyngopalatine
m., Phillips'
m. ▸ physical elasticity of
m. ▸ physiologic elasticity of
m., piriform
m., planter
m., planter interosseous
m. plasticity ▸ skeletal
m., platysma
m., pleuroesophageal
m., popliteal
m., postaxial
m., posterior auricular
m., posterior cricoarytenoid
m., posterior papillary
m., posterior sacrococcygeal
m., posterior scalene
m., posterior sheath of rectus
m., posterior tibial
m. potential, resting
m., preaxial
m., procerus
m., pronator quadratus
m., pronator teres
m. protein
m., psoas
m., pterygoid
m., pterygopharyngeal
m., pubicoperitoneal
m., pubococcygeal
m., pubococcygeus
m., puboprostatic
m., puborectal
m., pubovaginal
m., pubovesical
m., pulled
m., pyramidal
m., quadrate pronator
m., quadriceps
m., recession of ocular
m. reconditioners
m. ▸ reconstruct heart
m., rectococcygeus
m., rectourethral
m., rectouterine
m., rectovesical
m., rectus
m. ▸ rectus abdominis
m., rectus inferior

m., rectus lateralis
m., rectus medialis
m., rectus superior
m., red
m. reflected from insertion
m. reflexes
m., Reisseisen's
m. related pain
m. relax periodically
m., relax prostate
m. relaxant
m. relaxant effect, residual
m. relaxant medication
m. relaxant ▸ nondepolarizing
m. relaxant, skeletal
m. relaxation
m. relaxation, deep
m. relaxation exercise
m. relaxation, feedback-induced
m. relaxation in normal persons
m. relaxation in patients with neck injuries
m. relaxation, induced
m., relaxation of
m., relaxation of heart
m. ▸ relaxation of pelvic
m. relaxation, progressive
m. relaxation ▸ smooth
m. -relaxation splints
m. relaxing drug
m. removed ▸ slice of heart
m. repaired
m. reperfusion injury ▸ postischemia skeletal
m., resection levator
m., respiratory
m. response
m. rest ▸ respiratory
m. retracted, chest
m., retraction of rectus
m., retraining
m. ▸ revascularize heart
m., ribbon
m., rider's
m., rigid
m. rigidity
m. rigidity and tremor
m., Riolan's
m., risorius
m. rod
m., rotator
m. ▸ rotator cuff
m., Rouget's
m., round pronator
m., rupture of

muscle(s)—*continued*

m. rupture ▸ papillary
m., Ruysch's
m., sacrospinal
m., salpingopharyngeal
m., Santorini's
m., scalene
m., scalenus
m., scarring of heart
m. seated cold
m., semimembranous
m., semispinal
m., semitendinous
m. sense
m. ▸ sense of fatigue in leg
m., serratus
m. -setting exercise
m., short adductor
m., short anconeus
m., short fibular
m., short palmar
m., short peroneal
m., short rotator
m. sites ▸ tender
m. size, increase in
m., skeletal
m., smaller pectoral
m., smaller psoas
m., smallest adductor
m., smallest scalene
m., smooth
m., soleus
m., somatic
m. soreness, delayed onset
m. sound
m., sore calf
m. soreness
m. soreness, delayed
m. spasm
m. spasm, cervical
m. spasm ▸ involuntary
m. spasm, painful
m. spasm, paraspinal
m. spasm, rectal sphincter
m. spasm, relieve
m. spasm, severe
m. spasm ▸ severe back
m. spasm ▸ uncontrollable
m. spasms and cramps
m. spasms and twitches
m. spasms, occupational
m. spasms of eyes
m. spastic
m. spasticity
m., sphincter

m., sphincter ani
m., spinal
m., splenius
m. split longitudinally
m. split, rectus
m. splitting incision
m. splitting incision, rectus
m. splitting technique
m. ▸ spontaneous spasm of airway
m. stamp
m., stapedius
m. status
m., sternal
m., sternocleidomastoid (SCM)
m., sternohyoid
m., sternomastoid
m., sternothyroid
m. stiffness
m. ▸ stiffness and discomfort in
m. stiffness and soreness
m., stimulate heart
m. stimulation
m. stimulation (EMS) ▸ electrical
m. stimulator
m. strain
m. strain ▸ reduce stress and
m. strain ▸ acute
m. strain, relieve
m., strained
m. strand
m., strap
m. strength
m. strength, abdominal
m. strength and endurance
m. strength and flexibility
m. strength and flexibility ▸ regain
m. strength and walking ▸ mobility,
m. strength, bolster
m. strength, decreased
m. strength ▸ increased
m. strength ▸ long-term restoration of
m. strength, loss of
m. strength, maintain
m. strength ▸ shoulder
m. strength test
m., strengthen back
m. strengthening
m. strengthening exercise
m., stretch
m. stretch reflexes
m., stretched
m. stretches, calf
m., stretching key

m., stretching of
m., striated
m., striped
m. structure
m., styloglossus
m., stylohyoid
m., stylopharyngeus
m., subclavius
m., subcostal
m., subscapular
m., subvertebral
m. ▸ sudden, involuntary contraction of
m. sugar
m., superciliary depressor
m., superior auricular
m., superior gemellus
m., superior oblique
m., superior posterior serratus
m., superior rectus
m., supinator
m., suprahyoid
m., supraspinous
m. sympathetic nerve activity
m. syndrome ▸ papillary
m. syndrome ▸ single papillary
m., synergic
m., synergistic
m. ▸ taut bands of
m., tear of
m., temporal
m., temporoparietal
m. ▸ tender joint and
m. tenderness, calf
m. ▸ tenderness of jaw
m. tendons
m. tension
m. tension, aching, pain and stiffness
m. tension and anxiety
m. tension artifact
m. tension, chronic
m. tension, frontalis
m. tension headache
m. tension overload
m. tension variability
m., tensor fasciae latae
m., tensor veli palatini
m., teres
m. test, manual
m. testing for strength
m. testing, manual
m., thenar
m. thermodynamics
m. therapy ▸ deep

m., thickened heart
m., thickening of colon
m., third fibular
m., third peroneal
m., thyroarytenoid
m., thyroepiglottic
m., thyrohyoid
m., thyropharyngeal
m., tibial
m., tibialis
m., tight
m. ▸ tight calf
m. ▸ tight, knotted
m. tightness
m. tip ▸ papillary
m. tissue
m. tissue, blood-starved heart
m. tissue, death of heart muscle
m. tissue ▸ heart
m. tissue, lost
m. tissue viability
m. to digitalis toxicity ▸ sensitize heart
m. tone
m. tone, abdominal
m. tone, alteration of
m. tone and collapse ▸ loss of
m. tone ▸ disordered
m. tone, enhance
m. tone, improved
m. tone ▸ increased
m. tone ▸ lack of
m. tone, loss of
m. tone of uterus
m. tone ▸ persistent abnormal
m. tone ▸ poor
m. tone, smooth bronchial
m., tonic spasm of voluntary
m. tonicity
m., toning
m. tonus
m., tonus of extrinsic laryngeal
m., torn
m. ▸ total elasticity of
m., tracheal
m., trachelomastoid
m. training ▸ respiratory
m., transplantation of ocular
m. ▸ transplanted skeletal
m., transversalis
m., transverse
m., transverse arytenoid
m., transversus perinei
m., transversospinal
m., trapezius

m., Treitz's
m. tremors
m., triangular
m., triceps brachii
m., triceps surae
m., trismus of masseter
m., trunk
m. tumor
m. twitches
m. twitching
m., underlying
m., underlying chest
m. ▸ undue retraction of
m., unipennate
m., unstriated
m., vaginal
m., vastus intermedius
m., vastus lateralis
m., vastus medialis
m. ▸ venous smooth
m., ventral sacrococcygeal
m., ventricular papillary
m., vestigial
m., visceral
m., vocal
m., volar interosseous
m., voluntary
m., voluntary pelvic
m., voluntary relaxation of masseter
m. wall
m. wall defect
m. wall, thickening of
m., wasted
m. wasting
m. wasting and fasciculations
m. wasting disease
m. wasting disease, childhood
m., wasting of skeletal
m., weakened
m. ▸ weakened heart
m. ▸ weakened pelvic
m., weakening calf
m. -weakening myasthenia gravis (MG)
m. ▸ weakening of pelvic
m. weakness
m. ▸ weakness and wasting of
m. weakness cataplexy
m. weakness, focal
m. weakness ▸ general
m. weakness, generalized
m. weakness ▸ heart
m. weakness in leg
m. ▸ weakness of facial
m. ▸ weakness of foot

m. weakness ▸ residual
m. weakness, serious
m., white
m., Wilson's
m. with aerobic exercise ▸ condition
m. wrap, cardiac
m., yoked
m., zygomatic
musculaire, folie
muscular
m. aches
m. action
m. action ▸ voluntary
m. activity ▸ impaired
m. artifact
m. asthenopia
m. atrophy
m. atrophy and cyanosis
m. atrophy, Aran-Duchenne
m. atrophy, Duchenne
m. atrophy, long lasting
m. atrophy, myelopathic
m. atrophy, neurogenic
m. atrophy ▸ peroneal
m. atrophy, progressive
m. atrophy, progressive neuropathic
m. atrophy, progressive spinal
m. atrophy, pseudohypertrophic
m. atrophy, spinal
m. atrophy ▸ Type I spinal
m. attachment
m. canal
m. contraction
m. contraction, respiratory
m. contraction, involuntary
m. contraction ▸ spasmodic
m. contractions, intermittent tonic
m. contractions of bowel ▸ cyclic
m. contractions ▸ rhythmic
m. control
m. control exercises
m. control, poor
m. coordination
m. coordination, disorder of
m. coordination, failure of
m. defect, skeletal
m. defense
m. development
m. disability
m. disease
m. disease, Aran-Duchenne
m. disorder
m. dystrophy (MD)

muscular—*continued*
- m. dystrophy ▸ Becker-type tardive
- m. dystrophy (MD) ▸ Duchenne's
- m. dystrophy ▸ limb-girdle
- m. dystrophy ▸ myotonic
- m. dystrophy (MD) ▸ progressive
- m. dystrophy (MD) ▸ pseudohypertrophic
- m. dystrophy ▸ pseudohypertrophic infantile
- m. exercise
- m. endurance
- m. endurance exercises
- m. fitness
- m. hypertrophy
- m. imbalance
- m. incompetence
- m. incoordination
- m. jerks
- m. layer
- m. movements
- m. movements ▸ disordered
- m. movements, disorganized
- m. movements, involuntary
- m. movements, voluntary
- m. murmur
- m. necrosis
- m. pain and fatigue
- m. pain and tension
- m. pain, chronic
- m. pains
- m. paralysis
- m. pouch
- m. receptors
- m. reflex
- m. relaxation
- m. relaxation training ▸ biofeedback-assisted
- m. resistance, severe
- m. rheumatism
- m. rigidity
- m. rigidity, abdominal
- m. rigidity, diffuse
- m. ring
- m. senses
- m. spasm
- m. spasm, chronic
- m. strabismus
- m. strain
- m. strength
- m. structure
- m. subaortic stenosis, hypertrophic
- m. substance of prostate
- m. system

- m. tension
- m. thickening, marked
- m. tightness
- m. tissue of myocardium ▸ striated
- m. tissues
- m. tone
- m. tone, momentary loss of skeletal
- m. tone, skeletal
- m. trabeculation
- m. tremors
- m. twitching
- m. twitchings, continuous
- m. veins
- m. venous pump
- m. wall
- m. wall of bladder
- m. wall of stomach
- m. wastage, severe
- m. weakness
- m. weakness and stupor
- m. weakness of bladder
- m. weakness, one side of body
- m. weakness, severe

muscularis, carcinoma invading
muscularis, mucosa
musculature
- m., abdominal wall
- m., cervical
- m., conus
- m., facial
- m., hip
- m., homogeneous
- m., lumbar
- m. of face, discrete jerking
- m., paravertebral
- m., pelvic
- m., pharyngeal
- m., rigidity, abdominal
- m., spastic
- m., suprahyoid
- m., thickened
- m., uterine
- m., ventricular

musculi, Leptopsylla
musculo-aponeurotic system (SMAS), superficial
musculocartilaginous structure
musculocutaneous
- m. amputation
- m. flap
- m. nerve
- m. nerve of foot
- m. nerve of leg

musculofascially, incision closed
musculophrenic veins

musculoskeletal
- m. cancer
- m. department
- m. disorder
- m. evaluation
- m. function
- m. in origin
- m. infection
- m. limitations
- m. pain
- m. pain ▸ debilitating
- m. problems
- m. reaction
- m. reaction ▸ physiological
- m. soft tissue aging
- m. stress and strain
- m. tissue
- m. tumor

musculospiral nerve
musculotendinous cuff
musculus (*see also* muscle)
- m. abductor pollicis longus
- m. adductor pollicis
- m. extensor pollicis brevis
- m. extensor pollicis longus
- m. flexor digitorum sublimis, tendinous chiasm of
- m. flexor pollicis brevis
- m. flexor pollicis longus
- m. helicis major
- m. helicis minor
- m. levator palpebrae superioris
- m., Mus
- m. obliquus inferior
- m. obliquus superior
- m. orbicularis oculi
- m. pectineus
- m. pectoralis major
- m. pectoralis minor
- m. rectus inferior
- m. rectus lateralis
- m. rectus medialis
- m. scalenus posterior
- m. temporalis
- m. tensor tympani
- m. teres major
- m. teres minor
- m. transversalis
- m. vastus lateralis

mush heart
Mushroom (mushroom)
- m. (psilocybin)
- M. (Psilocyn)
- m. catheter
- m. catheter, Silastic

m. dust
M. (hallucinogen), Magic
M. (psilocybin) ▸ magic
m. poisoning
m. (hallucinogen), sacred
m. (psilocybin) ▸ sacred
m. -shaped polyp
m. worker's lung
music therapy
Musical (musical)
m. bruit
M. Industries (EMI) brain scanner, Electric and
m. rales
musician's cramp
musicogenic epilepsy
Musset's sign, de
mussitans, delirium
MUST (medical unit, self-contained, transportable)
mustache dressing
mustard (Mustard's)
M. atrial baffle
m., nitrogen
m., Oncovin, prednisone, procarbazine (MOPP) ▸ nitrogen
M. operation
m., phenylalanine
m. poultice
M. procedure
m. therapy, nitrogen
m., uracil
Mustarde procedure
Mutah (marijuana), Mota/
mutans, streptococcus
mutant
m. adenovirus
m. allele
m. chromosomal genes
m. cold virus
m. mitochondrial gene
mutation(s)
m. assay ▸ lymphoblast
m., cell
m., chromosomal gene
m., collagen
m., familial
m., gene
m., genetic
m., germline
m., inherited
m., mitochondrial
m., new
m., somatic

m. to drug resistance
mute
m., deaf-
m., patient
m. ▸ patient rigid, nonresponsive and
m. reflexes
m. ▸ rigid, nonresponsive and
m. toe signs
mutilans, arthritis
mutilates self ▸ patient
mutilating behavior, self-
mutilation, act of self-
mutilation ▸ thoughts of self-
mutilative acts ▸ self-
mutilative behavior, self-
mutism
m., akinetic
m., elective
m., hysterical
muttering delirium
mutton fat KPs (keratic precipitates)
mutual
m. aid group
m. self-help course
m. trust
muzzled sperm
MV (minute volume)
mv/μV (microvolt)
mv (millivolt)
MV (mitral valve)
mv (millivoltage) slow wave
MVA (mitral valve area)
MVC (maximal vital capacity)
MVP (mean venous pressure)
MVP (mitral valve prolapse)
MVR (maximal ventilation rate)
MVV (maximum voluntary ventilation)
MVV (maximum voluntary ventilation) ▸ estimated
mw (microwave)
mw (microwave) amplification
MW (molecular weight)
M wave
My (myopia)
myalgia
m., eosinophilic
m., epidemic
m. gravis
m., intercostal
m. syndrome (EMS), ▸ eosinophilia
m., systemic
m., tension
myalgic encephalomyelitis, benign
Myà's disease

myasthenia
m. cordis
m. gastrica
m. gravis
m. gravis and mediastinal tumors
m. gravis ▸ double vision from
m. gravis (MG) ▸ muscle-weakening
m. gravis, Tensilon test for
m. laryngis
myasthenic crisis
mycelial fungus
mycetogenetica, stomatitis
mycetoides, Corynebacterium
mycetomi, Madurella
mycobacteria infection, atypical
mycobacterial
m. colonization, atypical
m. disease ▸ nontuberculous
m. obstruction, atypical
Mycobacterium
M. abscessus
M. avium
M. avium complex (MAC)
M. avium complex (MAC) infection
M. avium intracellular (MAI)
M. avium intracellulare (MAI) complex
M. avium intracellulare (MAI) infection
M. berolinenis
M. bovis
M. butyricum
M. chelonae
M. fortuitum
M. gordonae
M. intracellularis
M. kansasii
M. leprae
M. leprae murium
M. luciflavum
M. lymphadenitis
M. marinum
M. microti
M. mucogenicum
M. organism
M. paratuberculosis
M. peregrinum
M. phlei
M. pneumonia infection
M. scrofulaceum
M. smegmatis
M. species
M. thermoresistable

Mycobacterium—*continued*
   M. tuberculosis
   M. tuberculosis, gram-positive
   M. ulcerans
   M. vaccae
Mycoderma (mycoderma)
   M. aceti
   M. dermatitidis
   M. immite
   m., Saccharomyces
mycoides, Asterococcus
mycoides, Mycoplasma
mycology data, clinical
Myconostoc gregarium
Mycoplana bullata
Mycoplana dimorpha
Mycoplasma
   M. faucium
   M. hominis
   M. incognitus
   M. infection
   M. mycoides
   M. pharyngis
   M. pneumoniae
   M. xenopi
mycoplasms, genital
mycoplasmacidal concentration,
   minimum
mycoplasmal pneumonia
mycosis
   m., candida
   m. fungoides
   m. fungoides dermatitis
   m., Gilchrist's
   m., intestinalis
   m., Posada
   m., pulmonary
   m., splenic
   m., systemic
   m., toxigenic
mycotic
   m. aneurysm
   m. aortic aneurysm
   m. aortography
   m. endocarditis
   m. infection
   m. infection, systemic
   m. nail, debridement
mycotic tonsillitis
mycotica, colpitis
MycroMesh graft material
mydriasis, spinal
mydriatic eye drops
mydriatic rigidity

myectomy
   m., modified
   m. of ocular muscle
   m., partial
   m., septal
   m. -septal resection ▸ myotomy-
myelin
   m. debris
   m. globules
   m. kidney
   m. sheath
myelinated nerve fibers
myelinic neuroma
myelinoclasis
   m., acute perivascular
   m., central pontine
   m., postinfection perivenous
myelitis
   m., acute ascending
   m., acute transverse
   m., chronic
   m., disseminated
   m. of cord
   m., transverse
myeloblastic
   m. leukemia
   m. leukemia (AML), acute
   m. leukosis
myeloblastoma (*same as*
   myoblastoma)
myelocytes
   m., basophilic
   m., eosinophilic
   m., mature
   m., neutrophilic
myelocytic
   m. anemia, chronic
   m. erythrocytic ratio
   m. erythrocytic ration ▸ normal
   m. leukemia
   m. leukemia (AML), acute
   m. leukemia (CML), chronic
   m. leukosis
myelocytoma, cutaneous
myelodysplasia ▸ spina bifida with
myelodysplastic syndrome
myelofibrosis
   m. and myelosclerosis ▸ severe
   m., marked
   m., myeloid metaplasia with
myelogenous
   m. disease, chronic
   m. leukemia (CML), chronic
   m. pseudoleukemia
myelogram [*pyelogram*]

myelogram, lumbar
myelography, opaque
myeloid
   m. -associated antigen
   m. cell
   m. -erythroid ratio
   m. leukemia
   m. leukemia, chronic
   m. lineage antigen
   m. metaplasia
   m. metaplasia, agnogenic
   m. metaplasia, myelosclerosis with
   m. metaplasia with myelofibrosis
   m. precursors
   m. tissue
myeloma
   m. cell
   m. -cell protein
   m. cells, destroying
   m., giant cell
   m., malignant
   m., multiple
   m., smoldering
   m. with leukemic transformation ▸
      multiple
myelomonoblastic leukemia
   (AMMOL), acute
myelomonocytic
   m. antigen
   m. leukemia (AMML), acute
   m. leukemia, chronic
   m. leukemia, subacute
myelon, ventricle of
myelo-opticoneuropathy, subacute
myelopathic
   m. anemia
   m. muscular atrophy
   m. polycythemia
myelopathy, radiation
myelophthisic anemia
myelophthisic splenomegaly
myeloproliferative
   m. disease
   m. disorder
   m. syndrome
myeloradicular dysplasia/
   myeloradiculodysplasia
myelosclerosis ▸ severe
   myelofibrosis and
myelosclerosis with myeloid
   metaplasia
myelosis
   m., aleukemic
   m., chronic nonleukemic
   m., erythremic

m., nonleukemic
myelosuppressed patient
myelotomy, commissural
Myers-Briggs Type Indicator (MBTI) test
Myerson's sign
MyG (myasthenia gravis)
myiasis, cutaneous
myiasis, dermal
mylohyoid
   m. line
   m. muscle
   m. nerve
   m. region
mylopharyngeal muscle
myoblast transfer therapy
myoblasts, skeletal
myoblastoma (*same as* myeloblastoma)
myocardial
   m. abscess
   m. anoxia
   m. band
   m. basement membrane
   m. bed
   m. biopsy
   m. blood flow
   m. blood flow ▸ abnormal
   m. blood flow ▸ regional
   m. blush
   m. bridge
   m. bridging
   m. cell
   m. cell, chicken wire
   m. cell ▸ foamy
   m. cell remnants
   m. cells ▸ death of
   m. circulation
   m. cold spot perfusion scintigraphy
   m. collagen matrix
   m. concussion
   m. conduction defect
   m. contractility
   m. contraction ▸ inherent strength of
   m. contrast echocardiography (MCE)
   m. contusion
   m. cytoskeleton
   m. damage
   m. depolarization
   m. depressant factor
   m. depressant ▸ substance
   m. depression
   m. disease

m. disease ▸ ischemic
m. disease, primary
m. disease, progression of
m. disease, unknown origin
m. dysfunction
m. dysfunction, reversible
m. edema
m. electrode, bipolar
m. failure
m. fiber bundles
m. fiber shortening
m. fibers
m. fibers ▸ striations of
m. fibers, surrounding
m. fibrosis
m. fibrosis, Davies
m. fibrosis, focal
m. fibrosis ▸ interstitial left ventricular
m. fibrosis, patchy
m. function
m. function assessment
m. hamartoma
m. hibernation
m. hypertrophy
m. hypertrophy (IMH), idiopathic
m. imaging
m. imaging ▸ planar
m. infarct (MI)
m. infarct (MI) ▸ acute subendocardial
m. infarct (MI) ▸ anterior lateral
m. infarct (ASMI), anteroseptal
m. infarct (MI), healed
m. infarct (MI), recent
m. infarction (MI)
m. infarction (MI) ▸ acute
m. infarction (MI) ▸ acute anterolateral
m. infarction (MI) ▸ acute anteroseptal
m. infarction (MI), age-undetermined
m. infarction (MI) ▸ anterior
m. infarction (AWMI) ▸ anterior wall
m. infarction (MI), anteroinferior
m. infarction (MI), anterolateral
m. infarction (MI), atrial
m. infarction (MI) ▸ chills from
m. infarction (MI), complete
m. infarction (MI), complicated
m. infarction (MI), conduction defects in acute
m. infarction (MI), diaphragmatic

m. infarction (MI), evolving
m. infarction (MI), extension of
m. infarction (MI), healed
m. infarction (MI) ▸ impending
m. infarction (MI) in dumbbell form
m. infarction (MI) in H-form
m. infarction (MI), inferior
m. infarction (IWMI) ▸ inferior wall
m. infarction (MI) ▸ inferolateral,
m. infarction (MI) ▸ lateral
m. infarction (MI) ▸ nontransmural
m. infarction (MI) ▸ old
m. infarction (MI) ▸ old healed
m. infarction (MI) ▸ old inferior wall
m. infarction (MI), pathogenesis of acute
m. infarction (MI) ▸ patient candidate for
m. infarction (MI) ▸ posterior
m. infarction (MI) ▸ previous posterior
m. infarction (MI) ▸ primary angioplasty in
m. infarction (MI) ▸ Q-wave
m. infarction (MI), recurrent
m. infarction (MI) research unit
m. infarction (MI) ▸ rule out
m. infarction (MI) ▸ silent
m. infarction (MI) ▸ stuttering
m. infarction (MI) ▸ subacute
m. infarction (MI) ▸ subendocardial
m. infarction (MI) therapy
m. infarction (MI) ▸ through-and-through
m. infarction (MI) ▸ transmural
m. infarction (MI) ▸ non-Q-wave
m. infundibular stenosis
m. injury
m. injury strain
m. insufficiency
m. insufficiency ▸ Sternberg
m. ischemia
m. ischemia, acute
m. ischemia, clandestine
m. ischemia ▸ exercise-induced silent
m. ischemia ▸ silent
m. ischemic disease
m. ischemic syndrome
m. jeopardy index
m. layer ▸ superficial
m. lead
m. lesions

myocardial—*continued*
- m. malnutrition
- m. mass
- m. metabolic rate
- m. metabolism
- m. necrosis
- m. oxygen (O_2) consumption
- m. oxygen (O_2) demand
- m. oxygen (O_2) supply
- m. oxygen (O_2) unit
- m. oxygen (O_2) uptake
- m. perforation
- m. perfusion image ▸ stress washout
- m. perfusion imaging
- m. perfusion imaging ▸ stress thallium-201
- m. perfusion scintigraphy
- m. perfusion scintigraphy ▸ thallium-201
- m. perfusion
- m. perfusion study
- m. protection
- m. protection pouch, Cardio-Cool
- m. reperfusion injury
- m. reserve
- m. revascularization
- m. revascularization, direct
- m. revascularization, elective
- m. revascularization (PMR) ▸ percutaneous
- m. rigor
- m. rigor mortis
- m. rupture
- m. salvage
- m. scan
- m. scintigraphy ▸ infarct avid
- m. segment, dyssynergic
- m. shortening ▸ fractional
- m. sinusoids
- m. sparing
- m. stiffness
- m. stimulation in pacing
- m. stunning
- m. subendocardial infarct
- m. tension
- m. tissue
- m. transit time
- m. tumors
- m. tumors, benign
- m. viability
- m. viability scintigraphy
- m. wall tension
- m. wall thickness

myocardiopathy
- m., alcoholic
- m., chagasic
- m., idiopathic

myocarditis
- m., acute
- m., acute bacterial
- m., acute isolated
- m., bacterial
- m., cardiac sarcoidosis
- m., chronic
- m., clostridial
- m., coxsackievirus
- m., cryptococcal
- m., diphtheritic
- m., echovirus
- m., fibrous
- m., Fiedler's
- m., fragmentation
- m., giant cell
- m., Histoplasma
- m., hypersensitivity
- m., idiopathic
- m., indurative
- m., interstitial
- m., metazoal
- m., parenchymatous
- m., peripartum
- m., protozoal
- m. ▸ Ratliff criteria for
- m., rheumatic
- m., rickettsial
- m. scarlatinosa
- m., spirochetal
- m. syndrome ▸ pericarditis-
- m., syphilitic
- m., toxic
- m., tuberculoid
- m., tuberculous
- m., viral

myocardium
- m., consistency of
- m. ▸ contractile function in cells of
- m., contraction of
- m. contracture
- m., degeneration of
- m., dysfunctional
- m. electrical system
- m., embryonic
- m. extensively mottled
- m. following infarction ▸ rupture of
- m., fragmentation of
- m., hibernating
- m. ▸ infarct of

- m. ▸ ischemia of
- m., ischemic
- m., jeopardized
- m. ▸ left ventricular (LV)
- m. ▸ patchy fibrosis of ventricular
- m., postischemic
- m., rupture of
- m., senescent
- m. ▸ striated muscular tissue of
- m., stunned
- m., underperfused
- m., ventricular
- m., viable

myocardosis, Riesman's
myocervical collar
myoclonal antibodies
myoclonal jerks
myoclonic
- m. encephalopathy of childhood
- m. epilepsy
- m. epilepsy and ragged red fiber (MERRF) disease
- m. epilepsy, progressive familial
- m. jerk
- m. movements
- m. petit mal epilepsy
- m. seizure

myoclonus
- m., benign neonatal
- m. encephalopathy, infantile
- m. epilepsy
- m., facial
- m., nocturnal
- m., ocular
- m., palatal
- m., pharyngeal
- m., spinal

myo-control signals
myocytes(s)
- m., cardiac
- m., heart
- m. hypertrophy

myocytolysis, coagulative
myocytolysis of heart
myoelectric
- m. arm
- m. hand
- m. output ▸ visual feedback of

myoepithelial cells
myofascial
- m. massage
- m. pain
- m. pain and dysfunction
- m. pain dysfunction (MPD) syndrome

m. pain syndrome
m. release
m. syndrome
myofiber necrosis
myofibril breakdown
myofibril necrosis
myofibrosis cordis
myofilament contractive activation
myogenic theory
myoglobin
  m. assay
  m., serum
  m., urine
myoglobinuria
  m., acute
  m., fatal
  m., nontraumatic
  m. ▸ paroxysmal paralytic
  m., radioimmunodiffusion
  m. ▸ rhabdomyolysis with
  m., rhabdomyolytic
myoglobinuric nephrosis
myoglobinuric renal failure
myoglobulin ▸ radioimmunoassay human
myography, electro◊
myoid cells
myoides, platysma
myointimal plaque
myolysis cardiotoxica
myoma
  m., atrial
  m., rhabdo◊
  m., uterine
myomalacia cordia
myomata
  m., submucous
  m. uteri
  m., uterine
myomectomy
  m., laparoscopic
  m., uterine
  m., vaginal
myometrial
  m. cycle
  m. invasion
  m. invasion, adenocarcinoma with
  m. invasion in endometrial carcinoma
  m. surface
  m. wall
myonecrosis, severe
myonephropathic metabolic syndrome

myonephropathic metabolism syndrome
myonephrotic metabolic syndrome
myoneural junction
myoneuronal function
myoneurosis, colic
myoneurosis, intestinal
myopathia cordis
myopathic disorder
myopathica, metrorrhagia
myopathy(-ies)
  m., alcoholic
  m., centronuclear
  m., chronic fibrosing
  m. ▸ dysautonomic mitochondrial
  m., hypertrophic
  m., inflammatory
  m., ischemic
  m., mitochondrial
  m., myotonic
  m., myotubular
  m., steroid
myopia
  m., axial
  m. corrective surgery
  m., index
  m., mild
  m., moderate
  m. night
  m., pernicious
  m., prodromal
  m., reduce
myopic
  m. astigmatism (As.M.)
  m. astigmatism, compound
  m. crescent
  m. eye
  m. keratomileusis
  m., patient
  m. reflex
myosin
  m., cardiac
  m. complex and relaxation of cell ▸ actin-
  m. heavy chain
  m. heavy chain gene, beta
  m. light chain
myosis molecule ▸ filamentous actin and
myositis
  m., acute progressive
  m., epidemic
  m. fibrosa
  m., lumbar

m. ossificans
m., progressive ossifying
m., rheumatoid
m. serosa
m., suppurative
m. syndrome
myotatic contraction
myotatic reflex
myotomy
  m., Heller's
  m. -myectomy-septal resection
  m. of ocular muscle
  m., septal
myotonia
  m. acquisita
  m. atrophica
  m., chondrodystrophic
  m. congenita
  m. dystrophica
  m. neonatorum
  m., weakness and
myotonic
  m. dystrophy
  m. muscular dystrophy
  m. myopathy
  m. reflexes
  m. response
myotubular myopathy
myringis, arcus lipoides
myringis bullosa
myringoplasty (VGM) ▸ vein graft
myringotomy tubes
myringotomy ▸ tympanocentesis and
Myrtophyllum hepatis
mystax, Ascaris
myxedema
  m. coma
  m., pretibial
myxedematosus, lichen
myxoid cystoma
  m. heart
  m., infantile
  m., primary
myxoid cyst
myxoid stroma ▸ valvular
myxoma
  m., atrial
  m., cardiac
  m., infected
  m. ▸ left atrial
  m. ▸ left ventricular (LV)
  m. ▸ right atrial
  m. ▸ right ventricular (RV)
  m. tumor

myxoma—*continued*
- m., ventricular
- m. virus, rabbit

myxomatodes, carcinoma

myxomatosis, infectious

myxomatous
- m. change
- m. degeneration
- m. degeneration of heart valve
- m. degeneration of mitral valve
- m. degenerative change
- m. proliferation
- m. pulmonary embolism
- m. soft connective tissue
- m. tissue

myxomembranous colitis

myxoneurosis, intestinal

N

N and V (nausea and vomiting)
n rays
NA (Na)
    NA (Narcotics Anonymous)
    Na (sodium)
    Na (sodium) atom
nabothian
    n. cyst
    n. follicle
    n. gland
    n. ovules
Naboth's
    N. cysts
    N. follicles
    N. glands
    N. ovules
    N. vesicles
NaCl (sodium chloride)
Nadbath akinesia
Naden-Rieth femoral prosthetic head
nafcillin sodium
Naffziger('s)
    N. operation
    N. sign
    N. syndrome
    N. test
Nagamatsu incision
Nägele's
    N. obliquity
    N. pelvis
    N. rule
Nägele's maneuver
nagging
    n. cough
    n. cough or hoarseness
    n., fleeting pain
nail(s)
    n., Augustine's
    n. bed
    n. bed angle ▸ nail-to-
    n. bed infection
    n. bed lesions
    n. bed ▸ nail plate of
    n. beds, blue
    n. beds, bluish tinge to lips and
    n. beds, cyanosis of
    n. beds, cyanotic

n. beds, pale
n. -biter, patient
n. -biting
n. -biting habit ▸ severe
n., bowing of
n. breaking from athlete's foot
n. breaking from circulatory
    problem
n., brittle
n., brittle grooved
n., cannulated
n., cyanosis of finger◊
n., debridement mycotic
n. ▸ dermatophyte infections of
n. disease ▸ fungal
n. dystrophy
n. extension
n., finger◊
n. fold, proximal
n. fracture
n., fragility of
n. from anemia ▸ white or pale
n. from chemical ▸ spooned
n. from cirrhosis ▸ white or pale
n. fungus
n. ▸ fungus infected
n., hang◊
n., Hansen-Street intramedullary
n., Harrington's
n. ▸ horizontal ridging of
n., I-beam
n. infection and care
n. infection ▸ fungal
n., ingrown
n. injury
n. inserted into neck and head of
    femur
n., intramedullary
n., Jewett
n., K
n., Ken
n., Küntscher's
n., Lottes'
n. lunula
n., malformed
n., Massie's
n., matrix

n., medullary
n., Neufeld
n., perionyx on newborn
n. plate
n. plate of nail bed
n., psoriatic
n., Pugh's
n. pulse
n., retropulsion of
n., Rush intramedullary
n., Schneider intramedullary
n., Schneider medullary
n., Smillie
n., Smith-Petersen
n. syndrome ▸ yellow
n., Thornton's
n., threaded portion of
n. -to-nail bed angle
n., toe◊
n. trimming, improper
n. unit ▸ fungal infection of
n., Venable-Stuck
n. ▸ vertical ridging of
n., Vesely-Street
n. wedge section
nailing
    n., hip
    n., intramedullary
    n. of tibia, medullary
Nairobi eye
naive optimism
Najjar syndrome, Crigler-
Nakayama anastomosis
naked vision (NV)
Naloxone test
name drug, brand
name, generic
names for drugs, street
naming, confrontation
nana
    n., Endolimax
    n., Entamoeba
    n., Hymenolepis
    n., Taenia
nanism, Paltauf's
nanocephalic dwarf
nanocurie (nc. or nCi)

nanograms per cubic centimeter (ng/cc)
nanoliter (nl)
nanometer (nm)
Nanta disease, Gandy-
nap
n. behavior
n., pressure
n., recreational
NAPARE (National Association for Perinatal Addiction Research Education)
nape, region of
nape, transverse muscle of
naphthalinic cataract
napkin
n. erythema
n. -ring calcification
n. -ring defect
n. -ring stenosis
nappiformis, placenta
narcissism, primary
narcissistic
n. disturbance
n. exhibitionism
n. personality
n. personality disorder
n. rage
n. sensitivity and vulnerability ▸ extreme
n. trait
narcolepsy syndrome
narcoleptic sleep
narcoleptic tetrad
narcosis, nitrogen
narcotic(s) (Narcotics)
n. (Miss Emma)
n. abuse
n. -addicted mother
n. addicts
n. agents, oral
n. analgesics
N. Anonymous (NA)
n. dependent
n. drug
n. effect
n. -induced respiratory depression
n. lollipop
n. medication, non-
n. overdose
n. prescription
n. ▸ preset amount of
n. requirement reduced
n. reversal
n., sedative

n. treatment facilities
n. withdrawal
n. withdrawal scale
naris(-es)
n., anterior
n., blood in
n., compressor muscle of
n., external
n., internal
n. not obstructed
n. obstructed
n. packed
n., posterior
narium, choana
narrow
n. -angle glaucoma
n. -angle glaucoma ▸ chronic
n. band frequency analysis
n. beam half-thickness
n. complex tachycardia
n. cone
n. duodenal opening
n. frequency band
n. rim of cytoplasm
n. spinal channel
narrowed
n. arteries
n. artery
n. atrial ventricle valve
n. blood vessels
n. coronary artery
n. disc space
n. duct, dilate
n. field of vision
n. heart valve
n. portion
n. pulmonary valve
n. pulse
n. renal artery
n. urethra
n. valve
n. valve, expand
narrowing
n., airway
n. and lipping
n., arteriosclerotic
n., artery
n. at lumbosacral level
n., atherosclerotic
n., carotid artery
n., eccentric
n., esophageal
n., fusiform
n., luminal
n., marked

n., moderate
n. of aorta
n. of aortic valve
n. of arteries
n. of artery ▸ severe
n. of blood vessels
n. of carotid arteries
n. of common duct
n. of coronary arteries
n. of coronary arteries ▸ repeated
n. of disc space
n. of esophagus ▸ scarring and
n. of gastric outlet
n. of heart valve
n. of interspace
n. of intervertebral disc space
n. of joint space
n. of lumen
n. of ostia of coronary arteries ▸ severe
n. of outlet
n. of perceptions
n. of spinal canal
n. of visual field
n., outlet
n., severe heart valve
n., tubular
n., vaginal
NAS (no added salt) diet
nasal
n. airway
n. airway obstruction
n. airways clear
n. airways obstructed
n. airways unobstructed
n. allergy
n. aperture
n. application, intra◊
n. arch
n. arteriole of retina
n. asthma
n. blockage
n. blood, shrink
n. bone
n. bone, contour of
n. bone, depression of
n. bone fragments
n. border of optic disc
n. breathing
n. breathing ▸ difficulty in
n. bridge
n. bridge, broad
n. burning
n. canal
n. cannula

n. cannula ▸ oxygen (O_2) by
n. canthus
n. capsule
n. cartilage
n. catarrh
n. cavity
n. cavity cancer
n. cell
n. chamber
n. conchae
n. congestion
n. congestion ▸ rebound
n. continuous positive airway pressure (NCPAP)
n. contour
n. crest
n. culture
n. decongestant
n. discharge
n. discharge, bloody
n. douche
n. drainage
n. drainage (PND) ▸ purulent
n. drip pad
n. duct
n. elevator
n. eminence
n. endoscopy
n. feeding
n. field
n. field of vision
n. flaring
n. fossa
n. fracture
n. fracture, old
n. fracture reduced
n. fractures, multiple old
n. gavage
n. glioma
n. hairs
n. hemianopia
n. hemorrhage
n. hydrorrhea
n. infection
n. injection
n. insulin
n. intubation
n. irritation
n. laceration
n. lead
n. mask
n. meatus
n. membranes
n. membranes ▸ swollen
n. mucosa

n. mucosa ▸ hyperemic
n. mucosa, swelling of
n. mucosa, swollen
n. mucous membrane
n. mucus
n. muscle
n. nicotine spray
n. notch of maxilla
n. obstruction
n. obstruction, unilateral
n. pack, MacKenty
n. packing
n. pancreatogram
n. passage, blocked
n. passage inflammation
n. passage ▸ obstructed
n. passages
n. passages, irritate
n. passages ▸ lining of
n. passageway
n. polyp
n. polypectomy
n. polyposis
n. problem from aspirin
n. pyramid
n. pyramid compressed
n. pyramid realigned
n. reconstruction, Taglicozzi's
n. refinement
n. reflex
n. region
n. retina
n. ridge
n. secretion
n. secretions ▸ virus contaminated
n. septum
n. septum, deflection of
n. septum, deviated
n. septum subluxation
n. septum ulceration
n. sinus
n. sinus disease
n. smear
n. speech
n. spine
n. spray
n. spray flu vaccine
n. spray, insulin
n. spray ▸ nicotine
n. spray ▸ steroid
n. spur
n. step, Rönne's
n. stuffiness
n. surgery, cosmetic
n. suture

n. swelling
n. tampon
n. tip cautery
n. tissues
n. tissues, destroyed
n. turbinate
n. turbinates, conchae
n. veins, external
n. venule of retina ▸ inferior
n. venule of retina ▸ superior
n. vestibule
n. vestibule cancer
n. washings
n. washings, culture of

nasale, os
nasalis
n. inferior ossea, concha
n. media ossea, concha
n. retinae inferior, venula
n. retinae superior, venula
n. superior ossea, concha
n. suprema ossea, concha

nascentium, trismus
NASH (nonalcoholic steatohepatitis)
nasi
n., agar
n., ala
n., apex
n., cancrum
n., cavum
n., columella
n., crus mediale
n., dorsum
n., limen
n. muscle, depressor septi
n., plica
n., septum mobile
n., vestibulum

Nasmyth's membrane
nasoantral window
nasobiliary catheter cholangiogram
nasobiliary pigtail catheter placement
nasociliary nerve
nasoendotracheal anesthesia
nasoendotracheal intubation
nasoesophageal feeding tube
nasofrontal suture
nasofrontal vein
nasogastric (NG)
n. (NG) aspirate
n. feeding tube
n. intubation
n. suction
n. tube

nasogastric—*continued*
- n. tube in stomach
- n. tube suctioning

nasojejunal (NJ) feeding

nasolabial
- n. crease
- n. droop
- n. fold
- n. junction
- n. reflex

nasolabialis, sulcus

nasolacrimal duct

nasolacrimal system

nasomaxillary fracture

nasomaxillary suture

nasomental reflex

naso-oral leishmaniasis

nasopalatine
- n. injection
- n. nerve
- n. recess

nasopharyngeal (NP)
- n. airway
- n. angiofibroma
- n. applicator
- n. bursa
- n. cancer
- n. carcinoma (NPC)
- n. carcinoma, lymph node involvement in
- n. carcinoma, lymphatic spread of
- n. culture
- n. electrode
- n. electrode recording
- n. fold
- n. leishmaniasis
- n. lymphoepithelioma
- n. smear
- n. specimen
- n. swab
- n. tissue
- n. wall
- n. washings

nasopharynx
- n. (NP), carcinoma of
- n. (NP), lymphoepithelioma of
- n. (NP), palpitation of
- n. (NP), posterior

nasoseptal deviation

nasoseptal reconstruction

nasotracheal (NT)
- n. catheter
- n. intubation
- n. intubation anesthesia
- n. suction

- n. suctioning
- n. tube

nasoturbinal concha

natal class, pre-

natal life, ante◊

Nathan pacemaker

Nathan's test

nation's blood supply

National (national)
- N. Association for Perinatal Addiction Research and Education (NAPARE)
- N. Association for Private Psychiatric Hospitals
- N. Cancer Institute (NCI)
- N. Cholesterol Education Program (NCEP)
- n. clinical trials
- N. Health Discharge Survey (NHDS)
- n. health insurance
- N. Hospice Organization (NHO)
- N. Institute on Drug Abuse (NIDA)
- N. Nosocomial Infection Study (NNIS)
- N. Poison Control Network
- n. practice patterns

native
- n. aorta
- n. coarctation
- n. coronary anatomy
- n. immunity
- n. valve
- n. vessel

natriuresis curve ▸ pressure

natriuretic
- n. factor (ANF) ▸ atrial
- n. factor ▸ proatrial
- n. hormone
- n. peptide
- n. peptide, brain
- n. peptide ▸ human atrial
- n. polypeptide, atrial

natural (Natural)
- n. aging process
- n. air exchange
- n. amputation
- n. antibody
- n. anticancer agent
- n. background radiation
- n. bacterial flora
- n. balance of bacteria, body's
- n. barrier
- n. bypass

- n. causes, patient expired due to
- n. chemicals, brain's
- n. childbirth
- n. coping mechanism
- n. course, disease to pursue
- n. crown
- n. death
- n. death, patient died
- n. defense against infection
- n. defense mechanism
- n. defenses, body's
- n. delivery
- n. digestive enzymes
- n. disaster
- n. Dopamine production, brain's
- n. environments
- n. family planning
- n. food fiber
- n. frequency
- n. growth hormone
- n. healing ability ▸ body's
- n. healing method
- n. healing power, body's
- n. hemostatic processes
- n. history
- n. history of congestive heart failure (CHF)
- n. holistic technique
- n. immunity
- n. immunity to hepatitis B virus, patient has
- n. joint
- n. killer (NK) cell
- n. killer (NK) cell antigen
- n. lecithin, cardiolipin
- n. line
- n. medicine
- n. menopause
- N. (LSD), Mr.
- n. nap
- n. or synthetic hormones
- n. pacemaker
- n. process of bereavement
- n. purposeful movements
- n. sleep
- n. sodium content
- n. stress level
- n. stress reducer
- n. teeth
- n. trance capacity
- n. vegetable laxative

naturalistic evaluation studies

nature
- n., beneficial therapeutic
- n., chest pain exertional in

n., degenerative
n., homogeneous
n. of mental health problems
n. of pain
n. unknown, exact
n. -versus-nurture controversy
naturopathic manipulative therapy
naturopathic physician
Naughton treadmill protocol
Naumanniella
N. catenata
N. elliptica
N. minor
N. neustonica
N. pygmaea
nausea
n., abdominal cramping
n. and anxiety
n. and diarrhea, frequent
n. and emesis ‣ anorexia, pain,
n. and emesis ‣ dysphagia,
n. and emesis postprandially
n. and vomiting (N and V)
n. and vomiting (N and V) after presedation
n. and vomiting ‣ chills,
n., chemotherapy-induced
n., chest discomfort with
n., constant
n., cyclical
n. ‣ diarrhea, weakness and
n. ‣ dizziness and
n. ‣ dizziness, weakness and
n. -emesis reaction to chemotherapy
n. ‣ fatigue and
n. ‣ fever and
n. from appendicitis
n. from cirrhosis
n. ‣ hair loss and
n., heartburn and
n. in pregnancy
n., induce
n., onset of
n., pain and
n. ‣ pain in abdomen with
n., persistent
n., postoperative
n. producing drugs
n. ‣ severe postchemotherapy
n., vomiting and abdominal pain
n., vomiting and diarrhea
n., vomiting and lethargy
n., vomiting and nystagmus
n., vomiting and visual disturbance

n., vomiting with
n., vomiting without
nauseated
n. and dizzy
n., patient
n. ‣ patient weak and
navel piercing
navicular
n. arthritis
n. bone
n. cell
n. fossa
n. fossa of male urethra
n. fracture
n. projection
navicularis, fossa
navicularis urethrae, fossa
navigation (ISN) ‣ interactive surgical
NB (newborn)
nc. (nanocurie)
nc. or nCi (nanocurie)
NCEP (National Cholesterol Education Program)
NCI (National Cancer Institute)
nCi (nanocurie), nc. or
NCP (NeuroCybernetic Prosthesis) generator
NCPB (neurolytic celiac plexus block)
NDE (near death experience)
NDV (Newcastle disease virus)
Nd:YAG laser (neodymium:yttrium-aluminum-garnet)
NE (Nurse Epidemiologist)
near
n. death experience (NDE)
n. delusions
n. -drowning victim, patient
n. edge of incision ‣ brought out
n. -fainting spell
n. field
n. -gain
n. -infrared spectroscopy
n. -normal quality of life
n. object, viewing a
n. point of convergence (NPC)
n. point reaction
n. sight
n. -syncope
n. -term gestation
n. -vegetative state
n. vision
n. vision test
n. visual acuity (NVA)
nearsighted eye

nearsighted, patient
nearsightedness corrective surgery
nearsightedness, extreme
NEAT (nonexercise activity thermo-genesis)
Nebbies (barbiturates)
Nebraska Test, Luria-
nebulized solution
nebulizer
n., air powered
n., Albuterol
n., contaminated reservoir
n., home
n. monitored for contamination
n., reservoir
n., ultrasonic
nebulo, Musca domestica
nebulous urine
Necator americanus
necessary, no treatment
necessary (prn) ‣ whenever
necessitatis, empyema
necessity, determination of medical
neck
n. ache
n. adenoma, bladder
n. and head of femur ‣ nail inserted into
n. and shoulder pain from disc
n. and shoulders ‣ tension in
n., anterior
n., anterior intertransverse muscles of
n., anterior region of
n. artery, clogged
n., auscultation of
n., base of
n., bladder
n., broken
n., bruit in base of
n. cancer
n. cane, swan-
n., clenched muscles in head and
n. compression ‣ asphyxia by
n. contracture, bladder
n. contracture, vesical
n., cord around infant's
n. deformity, swan-
n. dissection, Bocca
n. dissection, radical
n. dissection, standard radical
n. dissection, supraomohyoid
n. droop
n., extension of
n., femoral

neck—*continued*

n. flap, MacFee
n. flap, Wookey's
n. flexion
n. flexors
n. fracture, basal
n. fracture, displaced femoral
n. fracture site, femoral
n. full range of motion (ROM)
n. in extended position ▸ head and
n. injuries ▸ muscle relaxation in patients with
n. injury
n. injury ▸ immobilization of
n. irradiation, elective
n. isometrics
n. isometrics ▸ stretching and
n. lesion
n. -lift
n. lift ▸ face and
n. lift, head tilt with
n. lift surgery
n., longissimus muscle of
n. lymph nodes
n. lymphadenopathy
n., median vein of
n. metastasis
n. motion
n. muscles
n. normal, head and
n. obstruction, bladder
n. of bladder
n. of cervix
n. of femur
n. of femur, anteversion
n. of humerus, anatomical
n. of humerus, surgical
n. of infant, cord about
n. of metacarpal
n. of radius, fracture
n. of scapula
n. of tooth
n. of tooth, surgical
n. operation, radical
n. pain
n. ▸ pain in upper back and in
n. pain, persistent
n. ▸ pain spreading to
n. pain ▸ throbbing
n. palpable
n. passively flexed
n. ▸ posterior intertransverse muscles of
n., posterior region of
n. push up

n., radial
n. reflex ▸ Magnus and de Kleijn
n. reflex, tonic
n., rhabdomyosarcoma of head and
n., rotator muscles of
n., semispinal muscle of
n. sign
n. soft
n. ▸ spasm one side of
n., splenius muscle of
n. stenosis, bottle
n., stiff
n. -strengthening exercise
n. stretching exercise
n. supple
n., surgical
n. swelling ▸ breathing with
n. tension
n., tight bladder
n., transverse nerve of
n., transverse veins of
n. twist of
n. vein distended
n. vein distention
n. vein engorged
n. vein engorgement
n. vein not distended
n. vein not pulsating
n. vein, turgescence of
n., vesical
n. ▸ weak muscles in
n., webbing of
n., whiplash injury to
n. without palpable lesion
n. wound, penetrating
n., wry
necklace, lifeline
necklace or bracelet ▸ medical alert
necrobiosis lipoidica
necrobiosis lipoidica diabeticorum
necrobiotic nodules
necrobiotic rays
necrogenic wart
necrolysis, toxic epidermal
necrophorus, Actinomyces
necrophorus, Fusiformis
necrosing arteritis
necrosis
n., active
n., acute hepatocellular
n., acute retinal
n. (ATN), acute tubular
n. and ulceration
n. ▸ areas of hemorrhage and
n., aseptic

n., avascular
n., Balser's fatty
n., bone
n., bone aseptic
n., calcification
n., cardiac muscle
n., caseous
n., central
n., centrilobular
n., cheesy
n., coagulative
n., contraction band
n., cortical
n., cystic medial
n., decubital
n., digital
n., dirty
n., extensive acute
n. factor
n. factor (TNF) ▸ tumor
n., fat
n., fibrinoid
n., hepatic
n., icteric
n. in astrocytoma
n. in skin cancer therapy, radiation
n., ischemic
n. ▸ ischemic muscle
n. ▸ ischemic pressure
n. ▸ liver congested with central
n., massive centrilobular
n., massive hepatic
n., mucosal
n., muscle
n. ▸ muscle cell
n., muscular
n., myocardial
n., myofiber
n. of ascending aorta ▸ cystic medial
n. of brain
n. of brain ▸ cortical
n. of brain tissue
n. of bowel
n. of liver ▸ centrilobular
n. of liver, submassive
n. of mucosa
n. of pancreatic tissue
n. of tumor
n., Paget's quiet
n. ▸ postinjectional fat
n., premortem tubular
n., pseudolaminar
n., pulmonary
n., pulmonary hemorrhagic

n., radiation
n., renal cortical
n., renal papillary
n. ▸ renal tubular
n., skin
n. ▸ small focus of hepatic
n., spinal cord
n., subendocardial
n., tissue
n., traumatogenic pulpal
n., tubular
n., vascular
n., vessel
n., Zenker's

necrotic [*neurotic*]
n. arachnidism
n. areas
n. bladder mucosa
n. cellular material
n. centers
n. cyst
n. debris
n. fungating masses
n. gangrenous tissue
n. infarction, large
n. inflammatory cells
n. kidney tissue
n. lesion
n. lung tissue
n. metastases
n. mucosa
n. muscle
n. pancreatic tissue
n. placental tissue
n. pulp
n. purulent material
n. ▸ tail of pancreas
n. tissue
n. tissue, debridement of
n. tissue, friable
n. tissue, postirradiation
n. tissue, residual
n. toes
n. tumor
n. tumor metastases
n. ulcers

necroticans
n. agranulocytica, mucositis
n., enteritis
n. infectiosus, conjunctivitis

necrotized chilblain
necrotizing
n. angiitis
n. arteriolitis

n. arteritis
n. bronchopneumonia
n. bronchopneumonia ▸ bilateral
diffuse
n. colitis
n. cystitis ▸ focal hemorrhagic
n. encephalitis, acute
n. encephalomyelopathy, infant
n. enterocolitis
n. fasciitis
n. mediastinitis, descending
n. nephrosis
n. panangiitis, diffuse
n. pancreatitis
n. pancreatitis, acute
n. pneumonia
n. pseudomembranous colitis
n. respiratory granulomatosis
n. scleritis
n. ulcerative gingivitis
n. ulcerative gingivostomatitis
n. ulcerative stomatitis
n. vasculitis
n. vasculitis ▸ systemic

necrotoxica reactive, meningitis
NED (no evidence of disease)
need(s)
n., assessing pastoral
n., assessing patient
n. assistance, patient
n., clinical
n., create physical
n., dependency
n., emotional
n. for sleep ▸ decreased
n. for touch
n., homebound
n., human
n. ▸ independent living
n. minimal assistance for
wheelchair mobility, patient
n., monitor educational
n., nutritional
n. of cannabinoid abusers,
assessing
n. of hallucinogen abusers,
assessing
n. of inhalant abusers, assessing
n. of multi-drug abusers, assessing
n. of opioid abusers, assessing
n. of phencyclidine abusers,
assessing
n. of stimulant abusers, assessing
n., palliative
n., patient's identified

n., physical
n., physiological
n., prenatal medical
n., special
n., spiritual
n. to be with people ▸ patient's
n. to void ▸ immediate, intense
n., unique recovery
n., vital

needle(s)
n. ablation (TUNA) ▸ transurethral
n. -and-pins sensation
n. and syringe exchange
n. and syringes, contaminated
n. aspirate
n. aspiration
n. aspiration biopsy ▸ fine
n. aspiration biopsy, thoracic fine
n. aspiration biopsy ▸ transthoracic
n. aspiration (FNA), fine
n. aspiration of lung
n. aspiration of pancreatic
pseudocyst
n. aspiration, percutaneous
n. aspiration, skinny
n. biopsy
n. biopsy, bronchoscopic
n. biopsy, closed
n. biopsy, core
n. biopsy, fine
n. biopsy investigation, fine
n. biopsy of liver
n. biopsy of prostate
n. biopsy ▸ percutaneous
n. biopsy ▸ stereotactic
n. biopsy, transrectal
n. brachytherapy, radium
n. cholangiogram, percutaneous
n. contact
n., contaminated drug
n. ▸ contamination from unsterile
n. count correct ▸ sponge and
n. cricothyroid puncture
n. electrode
n. electrode, bipolar
n. electrode, concentric
n. electrode, monopolar
n. exchanges
n. ▸ feeling of pins and
n., hypodermic
n. implant, two plane
n., inadequately sterilized
n., infected IV (intravenous) drug
n. -like probe

needle(s)—*continued*
- n. localization
- n. marked arms
- n. markers
- n. marks
- n. marks on arm
- n. precaution
- n. puncture marks
- n. puncture marks ▸ multiple
- n. puncture wounds
- n. puncture wounds ▸ multiple
- n. punctures, multiple
- n. punctures, therapeutic
- n., puncturing of skin by contaminated
- n., radium
- n., recapping used
- n. scarred arm
- n. scope
- n. sensation ▸ pins-and-
- n., shared
- n. sharing
- n. sharing behaviors ▸ universality of
- n., sharing drug
- n. sharing, history of
- n. ▸ sharing infected intravenous drug
- n. sharing, intravenous (IV)
- n. site
- n. site care, intravenous (IV)
- n. stick
- n. stick ▸ accidental
- n. stick, contaminated
- n. stick exposure
- n. stick injury
- n. stick ▸ intravenous
- n. stick transmission
- n. stick, user
- n., stress on
- n. tracks, patient has
- n. transhepatic cholangiography (FNTC) ▸ fine
- n., ultrasonic
- n., unsterilized
- n., venous

needlepoint electrocautery
needling of cataract
needling of lens
Neelsen method, Ziehl-
Neelsen stain, Ziehl-
neencephalon (*same as*** neoencephalon)**
Neer prosthesis
Neer shoulder prosthesis

NEFA scintigraphy
negation, delusion of
negation emission
negative(s)
- n. accommodation
- n., adnexa
- n. Aerobacter aerogenes ▸ gram-
- n. aerobes ▸ gram-
- n. aerobic bacilli ▸ gram-
- n. afterimage
- n. airflow system
- n. association
- n. bacilli ▸ enteric gram-
- n. bacilli, gram-
- n. bacilli infection ▸ gram-
- n. bacteria, gram-
- n. bacteremias ▸ gram's stain
- n. bean-shaped diplococci ▸ gram-
- n. behaviors
- n. biopsy
- n. blood, antigen
- n. (Rh-) blood ▸ Rh
- n. bone scan
- n. brain scan
- n. Brucella abortus ▸ gram-
- n. Brucella melitensis ▸ gram-
- n. Brucella suis ▸ gram-
- n. calorie food group
- n. cardiogram
- n. charge
- n. chemotaxis
- n. chronotropism
- n. cigar-shaped rods ▸ gram-
- n., coagulase
- n. cocci, gram-
- n. coccobacilli Acinetobacter ▸ gram-
- n. coccobacilli ▸ lightly staining gram-
- n. coccobacilli ▸ pleomorphic gram-
- n. coccobacilli, small gram-
- n. contrast
- n. culture
- n. cytology
- n. deflection
- n. discharge
- n. ▸ dye-injected
- n. Eberthella typhi ▸ gram-
- n. effect
- n. emotional context
- n. emotions
- n. end-expiratory pressure
- n. endocarditis, culture
- n. enteric bacilli ▸ gram-
- n. enteric bacilli ▸ gram's stain

- n. Escherichia (E.) coli ▸ gram-
- n. Escherichia communior ▸ gram-
- n., essentially
- n. ▸ estrogen receptor
- n. eugenics
- n. examination, essentially
- n. exercise test
- n. extracellular bean-shaped diplococci ▸ gram-
- n. extracellular kidney-shaped diplococci ▸ gram-
- n. evaluation
- n. (Rh-) factor ▸ Rh
- n., false-
- n. feedback
- n. feelings
- n. filling defects in bladder
- n. findings
- n., findings essentially
- n. flu diagnoses ▸ false-
- n. for cancer ▸ node
- n. for growth, culture
- n. for malignancy, tissue
- n. for pathogens, culture
- n. for pathogens, stool culture
- n. for pathology
- n., fundi
- n. (GN) ▸ gram-
- n. Haemophilus influenzae ▸ gram-
- n. Haemophilus pertussis ▸ gram-
- n., hemoculture
- n. image
- n. imagery
- n., indole-
- n. inotrope
- n. inotropy
- n. inspiratory force (NIF)
- n. intracellular bean-shaped diplococci ▸ gram-
- n. intracellular diplococci ▸ gram-
- n. intracellular kidney-shaped diplococci ▸ gram-
- n. ion therapy
- n. kidney-shaped diplococci ▸ gram-
- n. Klebsiella ozogenes ▸ gram-
- n. Klebsiella pneumoniae ▸ gram-
- n. laparotomy
- n. Malleomyces mallei ▸ gram-
- n. microscopic findings
- n. mononucleosis ▸ heterophile
- n. Moro reflex
- n., mucin
- n. Neisseria gonorrhoeae ▸ gram-
- n. Neisseria intracellularis ▸ gram-

n. node
n. organism, gram-
n. organism, nosocomial gram-
n. organism, proteolytic gram-
n. output terminal
n., Pap (Papanicolaou) smear
n. Pasteurella lepiseptica ▸ gram-
n. Pasteurella pestis ▸ gram-
n. Pasteurella tularensis ▸ gram-
n. patient outcome
n., patient response is
n. (Rh-), patient Rh
n. pelvic
n. pericarditis ▸ gram-
n. pneumonia, gram-
n. pole
n. politzerization
n. potential ▸ maximum
n. predictive value
n. pressure
n. -pressure assisted ventilation (INPAV) ▸ intermittent
n. pressure (LBNP) ▸ lower-body
n. pressure respirator
n. Proteus vulgaris ▸ gram-
n. Pseudomonas aeuruginosa ▸ gram-
n. P wave
n. reaction
n. reinforcement
n. results
n. results, false-
n. results in clinical trials, false-
n. (Rh-) ▸ Rh
n., Rhesus factor
n. rod, aerobic gram-
n. rods and cocci ▸ gram-
n. rods, anaerobic gram-
n. rods, cluster of short gram-
n. rods, encapsulated gram-
n. rods, gram-
n. rods, pleomorphic gram-
n. Salmonella aertrycke ▸ gram-
n. Salmonella enteritidis ▸ gram-
n. Salmonella schottmülleri ▸ gram-
n. Salmonella suipestifer ▸ gram-
n. scotoma
n., scout
n. self-image
n. self-perceptions
n. sensation
n. sepsis, gram-
n. septicemia, gram-
n. Shigella paradysenteriae ▸ gram-
n. species, gram-

n. spherical aberration
n. spiking
n. spiking dysrhythmia
n. spiking, sporadic
n. spirilla, gram-
n. staining
n. Staphylococci, coagulase
n. stool, guaiac
n. straight leg raising (SLR)
n. stress
n. stressor
n. style of behaving
n. style of thinking
n. surgical pathogens, gram-
n. test, false
n. test result ▸ true
n. therapeutic reaction
n. thinking
n. thinking, distorted
n. thinking process
n. thoughts
n. torsion
n. (TN) ▸ total
n. treppe
n., true
n. tumor ▸ hormone receptor
n. undetected disease ▸ true-
n. variation
n. variation, conative
n. variation (CNV), contingent
n. Vibrio comma ▸ gram-
n. wave
n. x-ray findings
negativism ▸ exhibits irritable
negativistic, patient
negativistic personality disorder
neglect (Neglect)
  n., apathy and disorientation ▸ self-
  n., child
  n., child abuse or
  n., emotional
  n. of personal appearance
  n., functional
  n., mistreatment and
  N. (SCAN), Stop Child Abuse and
  n., unilateral
neglectful, caregiver
negligent conduct
negligible blood loss
negotiate therapeutic impasses
Negri bodies
neighboring tissue
Neil-Moore electrode
Neisser, diplococcus of

Neisseria
  N. catarrhalis
  N. flava
  N. gonorrhea
  N. gonorrhoeae
  N. gonorrhoeae, gram-negative
  N. intracellularis
  N. intracellularis, gram-negative
  N. meningitidis
  N. pharyngis
  N. sicca
  N. species
Neisserian culture
Neisserian species
Nélaton's
  N. dislocation
  N. fold
  N. line
  N. operation
  N. sphincter
nemaline myopathy
nematode
  n. infection
  n. infestation
  n. larvae
neoadjuvant chemotherapy
neocortex, atrophy of
neocortex ▸ severe atrophy of
neodymium:yttrium-aluminum-garnet (Nd:YAG) laser
neoencephalon (*see* **neencephalon**)
neoendothrix, Trichophyton
neoformans, Cryptococcus
neoformans, Saccharomyces
neo-hippocratic medicine
neointimal
  n. hyperplastic response
  n. proliferation
  n. tear
Neo-iopax contrast medium
neon ion therapy
neon laser, helium
neonatal (Neonatal)
  n. ascites
  n. asphyxia
  n. center
  n. complications of drug abuse
  n. conjunctivitis
  n. course
  n. death
  n. death, early
  n. death ▸ premature birth,
  n. death ▸ term delivery,
  n. diarrhea
  n. distress

neonatal—continued
- n. gastrointestinal hemorrhage
- n. giant cell hepatitis
- n. hemochromotosis
- n. hepatitis
- N. ICU (Intensive Care Unit)
- n. infection control
- N. Intensive Care (NIC)
- N. Intensive Care Unit (NICU)
- n. jaundice
- n. lung edema
- n. lung ▸ fluid balance in
- n. meningitis
- n. methadone levels ▸ maternal
- n. morbidity
- n. myoclonus, benign
- n. oxygen (O₂) exposure
- n. phototherapy
- n. resuscitation
- n. seizures
- n. sepsis
- n. septicemia
- n. sleep pattern
- n. stabilization
- n. streptococcal meningitis
- n. syphilis
- n. teeth
- n. thermoregulation
- n. toxoplasmosis
- n. transfusion
- n. transmission of viral hepatitis ▸ maternal-
- n. withdrawal syndrome

neonate
- n. ▸ large for gestational age
- n. respiratory failure
- n. ▸ small for gestational age
- n., term AGA (appropriate for gestational age) female
- n., term AGA (appropriate for gestational age) male

neonatorum
- n., acne
- n., anemia
- n., anoxia
- n., apnea
- n., asphyxia
- n., blennorrhea
- n., eczema
- n., edema
- n., encephalitis
- n., erythema
- n., erythema toxicum
- n., erythroblastosis
- n., icterus gravis

- n., impetigo
- n., mastitis
- n., melena
- n., myotonia
- n., ophthalmia
- n., pemphigus
- n., scleredema
- n., sclerema
- n. toxicum, erythema
- n., trismus
- n., volvulus

neoplasia
- n., cerebral
- n., cervical
- n. (CIN), cervical intraepithelial
- n., estrogen dependent
- n., intraepidermal
- n., laser destruction of intraepithelial
- n., laser treatment of cervical
- n., laser treatment of vaginal
- n., lobular
- n., metastatic
- n. (MEN), multiple endocrine
- n. syndromes, multiple endocrine
- n., vaginal intraepithelial
- n., vulvar
- n., vulvar intraepithelial

neoplasm
- n., advanced
- n., bronchogenic
- n., extrathoracic
- n. headache, intracranial
- n., hemianopsia in intracranial
- n., intracranial
- n. (IPMN) ▸ intraductal papillary mucinous
- n., local
- n., malignant
- n. ▸ nervous system
- n., pancreatic
- n., papillary
- n. ▸ primary cerebral
- n., primary intracranial
- n., rapidly growing
- n., sebaceous gland
- n., seizures in intracranial
- n., slow growing cortical
- n., undifferentiated
- n., vascular
- n., vulvar intraepithelial

neoplastic
- n. arachnoiditis
- n. cells
- n. change
- n. destruction of rib

- n. disease
- n. disorder
- n. erosion
- n. fracture
- n. growth
- n. hyperplasia
- n. lesion
- n. lymphocytes
- n. mass
- n. proliferating angioendothelio-matosis

neoplasticum, Gongylonema
neoprecipitin test
neopterin, serum
neosalpingostomy, cuff
Neosporin powder (Pwd)
neovascular glaucoma
nephralgia, idiopathic
nephrectomy
- n., abdominal
- n., adjunctive
- n., anterior
- n., bilateral
- n., lumbar
- n., paraperitoneal
- n., posterior
- n., pretransplant bilateral
- n., radical

nephritic calculus
nephritica, retinitis
nephritis
- n., albuminous
- n., allergic tubulointerstitial
- n., arteriosclerotic
- n., azotemic
- n., bacterial
- n., capsular
- n. caseosa
- n., catarrhal
- n., cheesy
- n., chloroazotemic
- n., chronic
- n., clostridial
- n., congenital
- n., croupous
- n., degenerative
- n., desquamative
- n., diffuse
- n., diffuse bacterial
- n., dolorosa
- n., dropsical
- n., exudative
- n., familia juvenile
- n., familial
- n., fibrolipomatous

n., fibrous
n., focal
n., glomerular
n., glomerulocapsular
n. gravidarum
n., hemorrhagic
n., hereditary
n., hydremic
n., hydropigenous
n., hypogenetic
n., idiopathic
n. ▸ immune-mediated membranous
n., indurative
n., interstitial
n., Lancereaux's
n., lipomatous
n., Löhlein's
n., lupus
n. mitis
n., nephrotoxic
n. of pregnancy
n., parenchymatous
n., phenacetin
n., pneumococcus
n., potassium-losing
n., productive
n., radiation
n. repens
n., salt-losing
n., saturnine
n., scarlatinal
n., subacute
n., suppurative
n., syphilitic
n., tartrate
n., transfusion
n., trench
n., tubal
n., tuberculous
n., vascular
n., Volhard's
n., war
nephrogenic
n. adenoma
n. diabetes insipidus
n. tissue
n. zone ▸ active cortical
nephrogenous albuminuria
nephrogenous proteinuria
nephrolithotomy, percutaneous
nephrolumbar ganglion
nephroma
n., embryonal
n., hyper◊

n., mesoblastic
nephron nephrosis, lower
nephropathic cardiomyopathy
nephropathic cardiopathy
nephropathy
n., analgesic
n., Balkan
n., diabetic
n., dropsical
n., gouty
n., hypazoturic
n., hypercalcemic
n., hypertensive
n., hyperuricemic
n., hypochloruric
n., membranous
n., obstructive
n., reflux
n., toxic
nephrophthisis (FJN), familial juvenile
Nephros bioartificial kidney
nephrosclerosis
n., anteriolar
n., arterial
n., benign
n., hyaline arteriolar
n., hyperplastic arteriolar
n., intercapillary
n., malignant
n., senile
n. with azotemia
nephrosis
n., amyloid
n., cholemic
n., Epstein's
n., glycogen
n., hydropic
n., hydroureteral
n., hypokalemic
n., larval
n., lipid
n., lipoid
n., lower nephron
n., myoglobinuric
n., necrotizing
n., osmotic
n., toxic
n., vacuolar
nephrosonephritis, hemorrhagic
nephrosonephritis, Korean hemorrhagic
nephrostomy drain, pigtail
nephrostomy, percutaneous
nephrotic syndrome

nephrotic syndrome, idiopathic
nephrotomography, infusion
nephrotomy, lumbar
nephrotomy, radial
nephrotoxic
n. agent
n. antibody
n. drug
n. nephritis
nephrotoxicity, potential
NER (no evidence of recurrence)
NERD (no evidence of recurrent disease)
nerve(s)
n., abducens
n., abducent
n., accelerator
n., accessory
n., accessory deep peroneal
n., accessory phrenic
n., accessory spinal
n. accommodation
n., accompanying vein of hypoglossal
n., acoustic
n. action potential
n. action potential, motor
n. action potential (SNAP), sensory
n. activity, eighth
n. activity ▸ muscle sympathetic
n. activity ▸ sympathetic
n., afferent
n., affliction
n., alveolar
n., anabolic
n. and muscle ▸ electrical activity in
n. and muscles ▸ block-in normal communication between
n. and muscle study
n., Andersch's
n., anococcygeal
n., anterior ampullar
n., anterior auricular
n., anterior ethmoidal
n., anterior labial
n., anterior palatine
n., anterior scrotal
n., anterior supraclavicular
n., Arnold's
n., articular
n., association
n. atrophy, optical
n. atrophy of optic
n. atrophy ▸ toxic optic
n. attachment, optic

nerve(s)—*continued*

n., auditory
n., auricular branch of vagus
n., auricular nerve of vagus
n., auriculotemporal
n., autonomic
n., avulsion of optic
n., axillary
n., Bell's
n., biopsy of
n. block
n. block, axillary
n. block, cervical
n. block, cervical plexus
n. block ▸ continuous
n. block, cranial
n. block, digital
n. block, facial
n. block ▸ femoral
n. block, intercostal
n. block ▸ interscalene
n. block, neurosurgical
n. block, peripheral
n. block ▸ sciatic
n. block ▸ stellate
n. block, stellate ganglion
n. block ▸ supraclavicular
n. block, sympathetic
n. block technique
n. blocking anesthesia
n., blunting of
n., Bock's
n., buccal
n., buccinator
n. bundle
n. canal
n., cardiac sensory
n., cardioaccelerator
n., caroticotympanic
n., carotid sinus
n., celiac
n. cell
n. cell body
n. cell degeneration
n. cell disorder
n. cell fibers, twisted
n. cell function
n. cell growth ▸ inhibit
n. cell loss
n. cell membrane
n. cell, membrane potential of
n. cell ▸ normal
n. cell transplant
n. cell transplant ▸ fetal
n. cells, age-related loss of

n. cells, behavior of
n. cells, degeneration of
n. cells, degeneration of dopamine-producing
n. cells, destruction of
n. cells ▸ healthy
n. cells, mature
n. cells ▸ motion-controlling
n. cells of cerebral cortex
n. cells ▸ regrow damaged
n. cells, regrowth of
n. cells ▸ selective degeneration of
n. cells, sensory
n. cells ▸ structure of
n. cells with brain
n. center
n. center, respiratory
n., centrifugal
n., centripetal
n., cerebral
n., cervical
n., cervical sympathetic
n., chorda tympani
n., circulation to optic
n., circumflex
n., coccygeal
n., cochlear
n., colloid deposits in optic
n., coloboma of optic
n., common fibular
n., common palmar digital
n., common palmar digital nerves of median
n., common palmar digital nerves of ulnar
n., common peroneal
n., common plantar digital nerves of lateral plantar
n., common plantar digital nerves of medial plantar
n. compression
n. compression, median
n. ▸ compression of spinal
n. compression, ulnar
n. conduction
n. conduction deafness
n. conduction, sensory
n. conduction studies
n. conduction study ▸ motor and sensory
n. conduction velocity (MNCV) ▸ motor
n. conduction velocity study
n. conduction velocity tests
n., conus medullaris

n. cord ▸ spinal
n., cranial
n. (first through twelfth) ▸ cranial
n., crotaphitic
n. crush, obturator
n. crushed, phrenic
n., crushing of
n., crushing of optic
n., cubital
n., cupping of disc or
n., cut, intercostal
n., cutaneous
n., Cyon's
n. damage
n. damage, eighth
n. damage, incapacitating
n. damage, median
n. damage, peripheral
n. damage, phrenic
n. damage ▸ postfundoplication vagal
n. damage ▸ vagal
n. damaging disease
n. deafness
n. deafness, total
n. death in stroke victim
n. decompression
n. decompression, median
n., deep fibular
n., deep petrosal
n., deep radial
n., deep temporal
n., deep vidian
n. deficit
n. deficit ▸ cranial
n. deficit, facial
n. deficit, functional tendon
n. deflection, sensory
n. degeneration
n. degeneration, eighth
n. degeneration in multiple sclerosis (MS)
n. ▸ degeneration of optic
n., depressor
n. deprived muscles
n., derangement of vasomotor
n., descending cervical
n. deterioration
n., diaphragmatic
n., digastric
n., digital
n. disease
n. disease, diabetic
n. disorder
n. disorder ▸ extrapyramidal

n. disorder ▸ inherited
n. ▸ disorder of facial
n. disorder, optic
n. disorder, painful
n. disorder, peripheral
n. dissection, facial
n. distribution
n. distribution, median
n. distribution, sciatic
n. distribution, ulnar
n., dorsal branch of ulnar
n., dorsal digital nerves of radial
n., dorsal digital nerves of ulnar
n. ▸ dysfunction of peripheral
n., efferent
n., eighth
n., eighth cranial
n. ▸ electrical stimulation of
    auditory
n., electrical stimulation to
n., eleventh
n., eleventh cranial
n. ending
n. ending, peripheral
n. ending, skin
n. endings, sensory
n. endings, severed
n. endings ▸ stimulation of
n. endings ▸ truncated
n. ends, severed
n. entrapment
n. entrapment, median
n. entrapment, ulnar
n., entrapped
n., esodic
n., ethmoidal
n., exciter
n., excitoreflex
n., exodic
n., exploration of
n., external
n., external carotid
n., external popliteal
n., external pterygoid
n., external spermatic
n., facial
n., FB (foreign body) in optic
n., femoral
n. fiber
n. fiber bundles
n. fiber, motor
n. fiber, peripheral
n. fibers, afferent spinal
n. fibers, brain
n. fibers, bundle of

n. fibers, bundles of nonmyelinated
n. fibers, damage to
n. fibers, demyelinated
n. fibers, deterioration of
n. fibers, large
n. fibers, medullated
n. fibers, motor
n. fibers, myelinated
n. fibers, pain bearing
n. fibers ▸ parasympathetic
n. fibers, regeneration after
    damage to
n. fibers, sensory
n. fibers, small
n. fibers, sympathetic
n. fibers, unmyelinated
n., fifth
n., fifth cranial
n., fifth trigeminal
n., filaments
n., filaments of spinal
n., first
n., first cranial
n., foreign body (FB) in optic
n., fourth
n., fourth cranial
n., frontal
n. function, facial
n. function, impair
n. function, monitoring of eighth
n. function, radial
n. function, recurrent laryngeal
n., furcal
n., gangliated
n. ganglionectomy, cerebral
n. gas
n. gas poisoning
n., gastric
n., genitofemoral
n., gland of trigeminal
n. glioma, optic
n., glossopharyngeal
n. graft
n. graft ▸ peripheral
n. graft, Seddon's
n., great auricular
n., greater occipital
n., greater palatine
n., greater petrosal
n., greater splanchnic
n., greater superficial
n. grossly intact, cranial
n. growth factors (NGF)
n. growth inhibitor
n. head analysis ▸ optic

n. head, choking of optic
n. head, optic
n., hearing
n., hereditary atrophy optic
n., Hering's
n. hyperactivity ▸ peripheral
n. hypesthesia, median
n., hypogastric
n., hypoglossal
n., Hyrtl's
n., iliohypogastric
n., ilioinguinal
n. impairment, cranial
n. impingement
n. ▸ impingement on spinal
n. implant
n. implantation
n. impulse
n. impulse, loss of
n. impulse, stimulate
n. impulses, conduction of
n. impulses ▸ interrupting conduc-
    tion of
n. impulses, transmission of
n. in foot, sensory
n. in spinal cord ▸ regenerating
n. in tooth, dead
n. ▸ increased pressure on
n., inferior alveolar
n., inferior ampullar
n., inferior cardiac
n., inferior cervical cardiac
n., inferior clunial
n., inferior dental
n., inferior ganglion of
    glossopharyngeal
n., inferior gluteal
n., inferior hemorrhoidal
n., inferior laryngeal
n., inferior rectal
n., inferior splanchnic
n., inflamed
n., inflamed spinal
n., inflammation of
n., inflammation of optic
n., infraoccipital
n., infraorbital
n., infratrochlear
n., inhibitory
n. injections
n. injury
n. injury ▸ median
n. injury, peripheral
n. injury, radial
n. ▸ intact auditory

nerve(s)—*continued*

n. intact, cranial
n. intact, radial
n., intercostal
n., intercostobrachial
n., intermediary
n., intermediate
n., intermediate dorsal cutaneous
n., intermediate supraclavicular
n., intermedius
n., internal auricular
n., internal carotid
n., internal occipital
n., internal popliteal
n., internal pterygoid
n. involvement
n. involvement, cranial
n. irritation
n. ▸ irritation of sciatic
n. irritation, trigeminal
n., ischiadic
n., Jacobson's
n., jangled
n., jugular ganglion of glosso-pharyngeal
n., jugular ganglion of vagus
n. junction
n., junction of optic
n., labioglossopharyngeal
n., lacrimal
n., Langley's
n., laryngeal
n., lateral ampullar
n., lateral femoral cutaneous
n., lateral pectoral
n., lateral plantar
n., lateral popliteal
n., lateral pterygoid
n., lateral supraclavicular
n., least occipital
n. lesions, peripheral
n., lesser occipital
n., lesser palatine
n., lesser petrosal
n., levator
n., lingual
n., long ciliary
n., long thoracic
n., loop of hypoglossal
n., loops of spinal
n., lower ganglion of glossopharyn-geal
n., lower ganglion of vagus
n., lowest splanchnic
n., lumbar

n., lumbar splanchnic
n., lumboinguinal
n., major spinal
n. malfunction
n. malfunction, peripheral
n., mandibular
n., masseteric
n., maxillary
n., maximum conduction velocity of
n., medial cutaneous
n., medial palatine
n., medial pectoral
n., medial plantar
n., medial popliteal
n., medial pterygoid
n., medial supraclavicular
n., median
n., meningeal
n., mental
n., microscopic
n., middle cardiac
n., middle cervical cardiac
n., middle clunial
n., middle gluteal
n., middle palatine
n., middle supraclavicular
n., mixed
n., motor
n. -muscle junctions
n., musculocutaneous
n., musculospiral
n., mylohyoid
n., nasociliary
n., nasopalatine
n. neuritis, optic
n. neurotomy, cranial
n. neurotomy, spinal
n., ninth
n., ninth cranial
n., nonfunctioning
n., nuclei, cranial
n. -numbing drug
n., obturator
n., oculomotor
n. of abdomen ▸ anterior cutaneous
n. of arm ▸ inferior lateral cutaneous
n. of arm ▸ medial cutaneous
n. of arm ▸ posterior cutaneous
n. of arm ▸ superior lateral cutaneous
n. of calf ▸ lateral cutaneous
n. of calf ▸ medial cutaneous
n. of clitoris ▸ cavernous
n. of clitoris ▸ dorsal

n. of Cotunnius
n. of external acoustic meatus
n. of foot ▸ dorsal digital
n. of foot ▸ intermediate dorsal cutaneous
n. of foot ▸ lateral dorsal cutaneous
n. of foot ▸ medial dorsal cutaneous
n. of foot ▸ musculocutaneous
n. of forearm ▸ anterior interos-seous
n. of forearm ▸ dorsal cutaneous
n. of forearm ▸ lateral cutaneous
n. of forearm ▸ medial cutaneous
n. of forearm ▸ posterior cutaneous
n. of forearm ▸ posterior interosseous
n. of hearing, sensory
n. of Hering
n. of Kuntz
n. of Lancisi
n. of Lancisi ▸ longitudinal
n. of lateral plantar nerve ▸ common plantar digital
n. of lateral plantar nerve ▸ proper plantar digital
n. of lateral surface of great toe ▸ dorsal digital
n. of leg ▸ interosseous
n. of leg ▸ musculocutaneous
n. of lung
n. of lung ▸ sensory
n. of Luschka
n. of medial plantar nerve ▸ common plantar digital
n. of medial plantar nerve ▸ proper plantar digital
n. of medial surface of second toe ▸ dorsal digital
n. of median nerve ▸ common palmar digital
n. of median nerve ▸ proper palmar digital
n. of neck ▸ transverse
n. of penis ▸ cavernous
n. of penis ▸ dorsal
n. of pterygoid canal
n. of radial nerve ▸ dorsal digital
n. of scapula ▸ dorsal
n. of tensor tympani
n. of tensor veli palatini
n. of thigh ▸ lateral cutaneous
n. of thigh ▸ posterior cutaneous
n. of tongue ▸ motor

n. of ulnar nerve ▸ common palmar digital
n. of ulnar nerve ▸ dorsal digital
n. of ulnar nerve ▸ proper digital
n. of vagus nerve ▸ auricular
n. of Willis
n. of Wrisberg
n., olfactory
n., ophthalmic
n., ophthalmic recurrent
n., optic
n. pain
n. pain, chronic
n. pain, diabetic
n. pain ▸ facial
n., palatine
n. palsy, cranial
n. palsy ▸ facial
n. palsy, peroneal
n. palsy, sixth
n. palsy, ulnar
n., papilla of optic
n. paralysis
n. paralysis, laryngeal
n. paralysis, phrenic
n., parasympathetic
n., parotid
n. path, afferent
n. pathway
n. pathways ▸ infection of
n., pelvic splanchnic
n., perineal
n., peripheral
n., peripheral motor
n., peripheral sensory
n., peroneal
n., petrosal
n., phrenic
n., phrenicoabdominal
n., pilomotor
n., pinched
n., pinched sciatic
n., pneumogastric
n., posterior ampullar
n., posterior auricular
n., posterior ethmoidal
n., posterior labial
n., posterior palatine
n., posterior scrotal
n., posterior supraclavicular
n., pressor
n. pressure on optic
n. pressure, relieve
n. problem ▸ taste abnormalities from cranial

n. procedure ▸ peripheral
n., proper
n., proper digital nerves of ulnar
n., proper palmar digital
n., proper palmar digital nerves of median
n., proper plantar digital nerves of lateral plantar
n., proper plantar digital nerves of medial plantar
n., pterygopalatine
n., pudendal
n., radial
n. radiation, sciatic
n. receptors
n. receptors ▸ serotonin
n., recurrent
n., recurrent laryngeal
n. reflex
n. reflex, auriculocervical
n. ▸ regenerate damaged
n. regeneration
n. regeneration ▸ spinal
n. repair
n. resected, intercostals
n. responsiveness
n., retinal
n. root
n. root anomaly, conjoined
n. root, anterior
n. root ▸ compressed
n. root compression
n. root, demyelinated
n. root ▸ demyelinization of
n. root, dorsal
n. root elevator ▸ Campbell's
n. root irritation
n. root, motor
n. root, posterior
n. root retractor ▸ Campbell's
n. root retractor ▸ Love
n. root rhizotomy ▸ dorsal
n. root rhizotomy ▸ ventral
n. root, sacral
n. root, sensory
n. root, spinal
n. root, ventral
n. rootlet
n., saccular
n., sacral
n., sacral splanchnic
n., saphenous
n., Scarpa's
n., sciatic
n., second

n., second cranial
n., secretory
n. section, recurrent
n. section ▸ translabyrinthine vestibular
n., sedative
n. sensation
n., sensory
n., sensory receptor or
n., seventh
n., seventh cranial
n., sheaths of optic
n., short ciliary
n. signals
n. signals, defective
n. signs, abducens
n. signs, accessory
n. signs, acoustic
n. signs, cranial
n. signs, facial
n. signs, glossopharyngeal
n. signs, hypoglossal
n. signs, oculomotor
n. signs, olfactory
n. signs, trigeminal
n. signs, trochlear
n. signs, vagus
n., sinu-vertebral
n., sinus
n., sixth
n., sixth cranial
n., small sciatic
n., somatic
n. -sparing radical retropubic prostatectomy
n. -sparing surgery
n., spinal
n., spiral ganglion of cochlear
n., splanchnic
n., stapedial
n., stapedius
n. stimulant
n. stimulation
n. stimulation, electrical
n., stimulation of peripheral
n. stimulation (TENS), transcutaneous electrical
n. stimulation, transcutaneous
n. stimulation ▸ vagus
n. stimulator, Hilger facial
n. stimulator (TENS), transcutaneous electronic
n. stimulator (VNS) ▸ vagus
n., stomach
n., stretching of

nerve(s)—*continued*

n., stretching of supratrochlear
n. structures
n., stylohyoid
n., stylopharyngeal
n., subclavian
n., subcostal
n., subcutaneous temporal
n., sublingual
n., submaxillary
n., suboccipital
n., subscapular
n., sudomotor
n., superficial branch of radial
n., superficial branch of ulnar
n., superficial fibular
n., superficial middle petrosal
n., superficial peroneal
n., superficial radial
n., superior alveolar
n., superior cardiac
n., superior cervical cardiac
n., superior clunial
n., superior ganglion of glossopharyngeal
n., superior ganglion of vagus
n., superior gluteal
n., superior internal laryngeal
n., superior laryngeal
n. supply, unimpaired
n., supraclavicular
n., supraorbital
n., suprascapular
n., supratrochlear
n., supreme cardiac
n., sural
n. ▸ surgical treatment for severed
n. suture
n., swollen
n., sympathetic
n. tabes
n., temporal facial
n., tenth
n., tenth cranial
n., tentorial
n., terminal
n. terminal ▸ central dopaminergic
  serotinergic
n., third
n., third cranial
n., third occipital
n., thoracic
n., thoracic cardiac
n., thoracodorsal
n., tibial

n., Tiedemann's
n. tissue
n. tissue regrowth
n., tonsillar
n. toxicity, eighth
n., transection cranial
n. transmission
n. transmits sensation ▸ median
n. transplant
n., transplanted
n., transverse cervical
n., trigeminal
n., trochlear
n., trophic
n. trunks, sympathetic
n. tumor, peripheral
n., twelfth
n., twelfth cranial
n., tympanic
n. -type deafness
n., ulnar
n., uterine
n., utricular
n., utriculoampullar
n., vagal
n., vagal accessory
n., vaginal
n., vagus
n., vascular
n., vasoconstrictor
n., vasodilator
n., vasomotor
n., vasosensory
n., vertebral
n., vestibular
n., vestibulocochlear
n., vidian
n. ▸ viral destruction of
n., viral inflammation of
n., Wrisberg's
n., zygomatic
n., zygomaticofacial
n., zygomaticotemporal
nervea of Brücke, tunica
nervi facialis, genu
nervi laryngei, plica
nervorum, rigor
nervorum, vasa
nervosa
n., angina
n., anorexia
n., bulimia
n., dysphagia
n., lues
nervosus, singultus gastricus

nervous

n. and apprehensive
n. asthenopia
n. asthma
n. bladder
n. breakdown
n. chill
n. degenerative disease, chronic
n. depression
n. discharge
n. disorder
n. disorder treatment
n. disturbance
n. dyspepsia
n. energy
n. eructation
n. exhaustion
n. exhaustion, chronic
n. impulses
n. indigestion
n. instability
n. pathways, sympathetic
n., patient
n. personality
n. respiration
n. responses
n. stimulant
n. supportive tissue ▸ overgrowth of
  non-
n. symptoms, varied
n. system
n. system (CNS) activity ▸ central
n. system, adrenergic
n. system and anxiety ▸ autonomic
n. system, autonomic
n. system ▸ breathing difficulty with
  problem from central
n. system cancer
n. system (CNS) ▸ central
n. system ▸ constipation with
  problem of central
n. system, damage to central
n. system (CNS) defect, central
n. system, degenerative disorder of
n. system (CNS) depressant ▸
  central
n. system (CNS) depression ▸
  central
n. system (CNS) deterioration,
  organic central
n. system (CNS) disease ▸ central
n. system disease ▸ peripheral
n. system (CNS) disorder ▸ central
n. system, disorders of brain and
n. system dysfunction, autonomic

n. system (CNS) dysfunction ▸ central

n. system, dysplasia of

n. system effect ▸ peripheral autonomic

n. system, enteric

n. system flatworm

n. system from AIDS ▸ problems with central

n. system from alcoholism ▸ problem with central

n. system from diet pill ▸ problem with central

n. system from sleep apnea ▸ problem with central

n. system from vomiting ▸ problem with central

n. system function ▸ perturbed autonomic

n. system ▸ fungal infection of

n. system, hereditary disease of

n. system (CNS) hypersomnolence ▸ idiopathic central

n. system ▸ incomplete development of autonomic

n. system (CNS) infarction ▸ central

n. system (CNS) infection ▸ nosocomial central

n. system (CNS), infratentorial parts of central

n. system, intracranial

n. system (CNS), intracranial part of central

n. system, involuntary

n. system (CNS) lesion ▸ macroscopic central

n. system (CNS) lesion ▸ microscopic central

n. system (CNS) lymphoma, primary central

n. system ▸ maintenance of

n. system, maldeveloped

n. system neoplasm

n. system, parasympathetic

n. system, peripheral

n. system, poisoning of

n. system relaxation techniques ▸ autonomic

n. system, sensory

n. system (CNS) sequelae, central

n. system (CNS) shunt ▸ central

n. system side-effects

n. system, somatic

n. system (CNS) stimulant, central

n. system stimulation, block

n. system ▸ strep throat and problem with central

n. system, supratentorial parts of central

n. system, sympathetic

n. system (CNS) therapy, central

n. system tolerance to radiation therapy, central

n. system (CNS) trauma, central

n. system, trypanosomiasis of

n. system, vegetative

n. system, visceral

n. tachypnea

n. tension

n. tension headache

n. tics

n. tissues

n. tunic

n. urine

n. vomiting

nervousness

n. and anxiety

n. and irritability

n., confusion and suspicion

n., dizziness with

n. from caffeine

n. from depression

n. from pain in back

nest(s)

n. in bladder carcinoma ▸ von Brunn's

n. lesions, birds'

n. of veins

n. syndrome, empty

nesting on plates ▸ wet

net

n. ▸ geodesic sensor

n. gradient of fluid outflow

n. protein utilization

nettle rash

Nettleship's syndrome

network (Network)

n., care

n., Chiari

n., community

N. (DAWN), Drug Abuse Warning

n. ▸ fibrillary collagen

N. for Organ Sharing, United

n. ▸ interstitial and perivascular collagen

n. ▸ local area

N., National Poison Control

n. of support

N. ▸ Organ Procurement and Transplantation

N., Organ Sharing

n., Purkinje's

n., referral

n. structure ▸ social support

n. therapy

neuf, bruit de cuir

Neufeld nail

Neufeld plate and screws

Neumann's cells

neural

n. activity

n. arch

n. arch defect

n. atrophy

n. block

n. canal

n. canal, cervical

n. claudication

n. crest, cardiac

n. crest malformation

n. crest migration

n. crest tumor

n. crest ▸ vagal

n. deafness

n. discharge

n. ectoderm

n. efficiency

n. fold

n. foramen

n. foramina

n. hearing loss ▸ sensory

n. impulse

n. parenchyma

n. pathway

n. reflexes

n. stalk

n. stimuli

n. structures

n. therapy

n. thread protein (NTP)

n. thread protein level

n. tissue

n. transmission

n. transmitter

n. transplantation

n. tube

n. tube defects (NTD)

n. tube disorder

n. tube, embryonic

neuralgia

n., brachial

n., cervicobrachial

n., cranial

n., facial

n., Fothergill's

neuralgia—*continued*
- n., geniculate
- n., glossopharyngeal
- n., hallucinatory
- n., Harris' migrainous
- n., Hunt's
- n., migrainous
- n., Morton's
- n. of bladder
- n. (PHN) ▸ post-herpetic
- n., postshingles
- n., retrobulbar
- n., sphenopalatine
- n., trigeminal
- n., vidian

neuralgic amyotrophia
neuralgic amyotrophy
neurally
- n. mediated hypotension (NMH)
- n. mediated syncope
- n. mediated syncope ▸ mixed

neuraminidase spike
neurasthenic vertigo
neurasthenica intermittens ▸ dysbasia
neuraxis irradiation
neuraxis irradiation in radiation therapy
neurectomy
- n., gastric
- n., obturator
- n., opticociliary
- n., presacral

neurenteric cyst
neurilemma/neurolemma
neurilemmal cell nucleus
neurilemmal cytoplasm
neurilemmoma/neurilemoma/ neurolemmoma
neurinoma, acoustic
neuritic
- n. muscular atrophy
- n. plaques
- n. senile plaques

neuritis
- n., acoustic
- n., brachial
- n., diabetes
- n., diabetic
- n., optic
- n., optic nerve
- n. ▸ optic or retrobulbar
- n., paralytic brachial
- n., peripheral
- n. plaque

- n., retrobulbar
- n., sciatic

neuroactive medication
neuroanastomosis
- n., hypoglossal-facial
- n., spinal accessory-facial
- n., spinal accessory-hypoglossal

neuroanatomy, chemical
neuroanatomy, sensory
neurobehavioral
- n. approach
- n. approach ▸ integrative
- n. assessment
- n. impairment
- n. sexual differentiation ▸ process of
- n. therapy

neurobiological level
neuroblastoma, adult
neuroblastoma sympathicum
neurocardiogenic syncope
neurochemical(s)
- n. imbalance
- n. impulse
- n. perspective
- n. sensitization

neurocirculatory asthenia
neurocutaneous syndrome
NeuroCybernetic Prosthesis (NCP) generator
neurodegenerative diseases
neurodegenerative disorder
neurodermatitis circumscripta
neurodermatitis disseminata
neurodevelopmental dysfunction disorder, childhood
neurodiagnostic procedure
neurodiagnostic scanner
neuroectodermal
- n. origin
- n. tumor, melanotic
- n. tumor (PNET) ▸ peripheral primitive

neuroemergency, pediatric
neuroencephalomyelopathy, optic
neuroendocrine theory
neuroendocrine tumor
neuroendocrinological disease
neuroepithelial
- n. bodies in lung
- n. cells
- n. elements of the retina

neurofibrillary tangles (NFT)
neurofibroma of pleura
neurofibroma, ulcerated

neurofibromatosis (NF) patient
neurofilament(s)
- n., function of
- n. kinase
- n. subunits
- n. subunits ▸ structure of

neuroforamina, patent
neurogenetic adaptive mechanism
neurogenic
- n. abnormalities
- n. atrophy
- n. bladder
- n. bladder, atonic
- n. bladder disorder
- n. bladder, uninhibited
- n. breathing pattern ▸ central
- n. component
- n. fracture
- n. hypertension
- n. muscular atrophy
- n. pulmonary edema
- n. shock
- n. theory
- n. tonus
- n. tumor

neurogenous tumor
neuroglia, fascicular
neuroglia, peripheral
neuroglial cells
neurohearing loss ▸ sensory
neurohormonal function
neurohormonal stimulation
neurohormones, activating
neurohumoral
- n. control of pulmonary vessels
- n. factors
- n. stimulus

neuroimaging study
neuroimaging technique
neurolabyrinthitis, viral
neurolemma/neurilemma
neurolemmoma/neurilemmoma/ neurilemoma
neuroleptic
- n. agent
- n. drug
- n. medication
- n. syndrome, malignant
- n. therapy

neurolinguistic programming
neurologic
- n. complications
- n. complications of systemic cancer
- n. defect ▸ reversible ischemic

n. deficit
n. deficit, acute
n. deficit, focal
n. deterioration
n. disease
n. disease, degenerative
n. disease ▸ long-term
n. disorder, active
n. disorder, chronic
n. disturbance, transient
n. dysfunction
n. dysfunction ▸ generalized
n. evaluation
n. examination
n. function
n. function ▸ sensory
n. function ▸ sensory aspect of
n. handicap
n. instability
n. rehabilitation
n. signs ▸ focal
n. signs, focal and lateralizing
n. signs ▸ objective
n. status
n. survey
n. symptomatology
n. symptoms
n. syndrome
n. voice disorder

neurological
n. activity
n. apnea
n. assessment
n. basis
n. complication
n. damage
n. damage, debilitating
n. damage ▸ irreversible
n. defect
n. deficit
n. deficit, focal
n. deficits, severe
n. disability
n. disease
n. disease, diffuse
n. disease ▸ genetic
n. disorder
n. disorder, deteriorating
n. disorder ▸ progressive
n. disorder, symptoms of
n. disturbance, diffuse
n. effects
n. emergency
n. evaluation
n. evoked responses

n. examination
n. examination of extremities
n. footdrop
n. function
n. function, impaired
n. impairment
n. impairment, severe
n. instrument, Yasargil
n. irregularity
n. lesion ▸ evolving
n. nursing care
n. parameters, gross
n. rehabilitation
n. seizure ▸ postoperative
n. signs
n. signs, localized
n. signs, localizing
n. symptoms
n. syndrome
n. testing
n. trauma, acute

neurologically
n. evoked responses
n. impaired
n. intact
n. over-responsive to stimulation

Neurology ▸ American Academy of neurology and biochemistry
Neurolon suture
neurolytic celiac plexus block (NCPB)
neuroma
n., acoustic
n. ▸ excision of Morton's
n., excision of
n., foot
n., interdigital
n., medullated
n., Morton's
n., myelinic
n., painful
n., peripheral
n., plantar
n., plexiform
n. ▸ slow-growing acoustic
n. tumor
n., Verneuil's

neuromediated syncope
neuromuscular
n. atrophy
n. atrophy, progressive
n. blocking agents
n. cell
n. complications of drug abuse
n. contractility

n. control
n. control exercises
n. deficit
n. development of speech
n. disease
n. disease ▸ degenerative
n. disease, fatal
n. disease ▸ inherited
n. disease ▸ lethal
n. disease ▸ numeroperoneal
n. disease, progressive
n. disease ▸ progressive idiopathic
n. disorder
n. electrical stimulation
n. facilitation (PNF) ▸ proprioceptive
n. feedback training
n. firing
n. firing in normal subjects
n. firing in spastic subjects
n. hypertension
n. integration
n. junction
n. maturity
n. physical characteristics
n. problems related to drug abuse
n. re-education of the hemiplegic
n. therapy
n. thermography

neuromuscularly handicapped
neuromyasthenia, epidemic
neuromyelitis optica
neuromyography, electro◊
neuromyopathic disease
neuromyopathic disorder
neuron(s)
n., affected
n., afferent
n. bodies
n., central
n., cerebral
n., connecting
n., correlation
n., degeneration of hippocampal
n. (MN), degeneration of motor
n. destroying plaques in brain
n. disease, infantile motor
n. (MN) disease ▸ inherited motor
n. disease, juvenile hereditary motor
n. disease, motor
n., dopaminergic
n. (MN) dysfunction ▸ lower motor
n. (MN) dysfunction ▸ superimposed upper motor

neuron(s)—*continued*
n., efferent
n. in spinal cord
n., inside
n., intact
n. (MN), lower motor
n. (MN), motor
n., multiform
n., normal
n. of brain
n., outside
n. paralysis, lower motor
n. paralysis, motor
n., peripheral
n., peripheral sensory
n., polymorphic
n., postganglionic
n., premotor
n., presynaptic
n. ▸ primary afferent
n., projection
n., pyramidal
n., receptive
n., receptor
n., sensory
n., short
n. ▸ shrunken atrophied
n. ▸ synaptic branching of
n., upper motor
n. with eosinophilic cytoplasm
neuronal
n. activity
n. changes ▸ mild hypoxic
n. connections, abnormal growth of
n. discharge, excessive
n. discharge, recurring excessive
n. function, disorganization of
n. hyperexcitability
n. impulses
n. interconnection
n. metabolism
n. signaling
n. tangles
neuronitis ▸ acute vestibular
neuro-oncologist, pediatric
neuro-ophthalmic examination
neuroparalytic
n. congestion
n. keratitis
n. ophthalmia
neuropathic
n. arthropathy
n. atrophy
n. central pain
n. diathesis

n. disorder
n. edema
n. eschar
n. muscular atrophy, progressive
n. pain
n. pain, chronic diabetic
neuropathy(-ies)
n., anterior ischemic optic
n., autonomic
n., compressive
n., cranial
n., diabetic
n., diabetic peripheral
n. ▸ drug-induced
n., familial
n. ▸ hypertensive optic
n. improvement, diabetic
n., intestinal
n., ischemic
n. ▸ ischemic optic
n., Leber's
n. ▸ Leber's hereditary optic
n., metabolic
n., motor
n., multiple
n., obstructive
n. of chemotherapy
n. of feet
n. pain
n., painful
n. ▸ painful diabetic
n., peripheral
n., postherpetic
n., progressive hypertrophic interstitial
n. ▸ radiation optic
n., subacute myelo-optico◊
n., toxic
n. ▸ ulnar compression
neuroperfusion pump
neurophysiologic factor
neurophysiology of enlightenment
neuroprotective agent
neuroprotective therapy
neuropsychiatric disorder
neuropsychological (Neuropsychological)
n. assessment
n. defect
n. deficiencies
n. deficits
n. evaluation
n. function
n. impairment

N. Mental Status Examination (BNMSE), Brief
n. research
N. Test Battery for Adults or Children ▸ Halstead
n. testing
neuropsychologist, clinical
neuropsychology
n., clinical
n., forensic
n. therapist
neurorehabilitation facility
neuroretinitis, measles
neuroretinopathy, acute macular
neuroretinopathy, hypertensive
neuroscience
n., cellular
n., cognitive
n., molecular
neurosecretory material
neurosecretory substance
neurosensory
n. cell
n. film
n. mismatch
neurosis(-es)
n., accident
n., acute anxiety
n., anxiety
n., association
n., biofeedback
n., biofeedback in
n., cardiac
n., character
n., combat
n., compensation
n., compulsion
n., conversion
n., craft
n., depersonalization
n., depressive
n., deprivation
n., existential
n., expectation
n., experimental
n., fatigue
n., fixation
n., gastric
n., homosexual
n., hypochondriacal
n., hysterical
n., intestinal
n., meningovascular
n., mesodermogenic
n., obsessional

n., obsessive-compulsive
n., occupation
n., paretic
n., pension
n., phobic
n., professional
n., rectal
n., regression
n., sexual
n., tabetic
n., torsion
n., transference
n., traumatic
n., true
n., vegetative
n., war
neurostimulator, surgically implanted
neurosurgery, microvascular
neurosurgery, stereotaxic
neurosurgical
  n. approach
  n. evaluation
  n. gamma knife
  n. headrest
  n. intervention
  n. nerve block
neurosyphilis
  n., ectodermogenic
  n., meningeal
  n., meningovascular
  n., mesodermogenic
  n., paretic
  n., tabetic
neurotic [*necrotic*]
  n. atrophy
  n. denial
  n. depression
  n. disorder
  n. excoriation
  n. fatigue
  n. illness
  n., obsessive
  n. overlay
  n., patient
  n. syndrome, severe
neurotica, alopecia
neuroticum, papilloma
neurotomy
  n., acoustic
  n., cranial nerve
  n., glossopharyngeal
  n., opticociliary
  n., retrogasserian
  n., spinal nerve
neurotonic reaction

neurotoxic drug
neurotoxic effect
neurotoxicity of chemotherapy
neurotoxicity of methamphetamine
neurotransmitter
  n. action, inhibitory
  n. activity
  n., brain's system of
  n., chemical
  n. depletion
  n. glutamate
  n. level ▸ imbalance in
  n. metabolism
  n. substance
neurotrauma services
neurotropic (neurotrophic)
  n. angina
  n. atrophy
  n. factor
  n. keratitis
  n. variant
  n. virus
neurovascular
  n. bundle
  n. bundles, medial
  n. compression
  n. compromise
  n. structure
neurovital signs
neuroxonal dystrophy, infantile
neustonica, Naumanniella
Neusser's granules
neutral
  n. AP (anteroposterior)
  n. dyes
  n. electrode
  n. fat
  n. occlusion
  n. or gray area
  n. or stretched position
  n. pelvis position
  n. position
  n. reaction
  n. red
  n. stain
neutralization
  n., acid
  n., enzyme
  n. equivalent
  n. test
  n., toxin
  n., viral
  n., virus
neutralize free radicals
neutralize stomach acidity

neutralizing
  n. acid in stomach
  n. antibody
  n. capacity, virus
  n. mechanism
  n., virus
neutron(s)
  n. absorption process
  n. activation analysis
  n. beam therapy, fast
  n., epithermal
  n., fast
  n., intermediate
  n. number
  n. radiation
  n. radiography
  n., thermal
  n., unit for fast
neutropenia, febrile
neutropenia, severe
neutropenic
  n. angina
  n. patient
  n. patient ▸ febrile
neutrophic cyctoplasmic
  autoantibody ▸ anti-
neutrophil/neutrophile(s)
  n. activity
  n., band
  n., decrease in
  n. defects
  n. elastase
  n. granules
  n., intra-alveolar
  n., juvenile
  n., mature
  n. -mediated endothelial injury
  n. -mediated lung injury
  n., polymorphonuclear
  n. recruitment ▸ host generated
  n., segmented
  n., stab
  n. steroid, stabnuclear
neutrophilic
  n. cell
  n. leukemia, chronic
  n. leukocytes
  n. myelocytes
  n. polymorphonuclear leukocyte
never starting food and fluid ▸
  stopping or
Neviaser's operation
Nevin syndrome, Kiloh-
nevoblasts, embryonal

nevoid
- n. amentia
- n. basalioma syndrome
- n. lesion

nevus (nevi)
- n., amelanotic
- n. araneus
- n., blue
- n. cell
- n., cellular blue
- n., compound
- n., dysplastic
- n. flammeus
- n., hairy
- n., halo
- n., intradermal
- n., junctional
- n., melanocytic
- n. ▸ nonfamilial dysplastic
- n., pigmented
- n. pilosus
- n., spider
- n. spilus
- n., spindle cell
- n., Spitz
- n. syndrome, basal cell
- n. syndrome, dysplastic
- n., verrucous

Neville tracheal prosthesis

new (New)('s)
- n. blood supply and matures ▸ develops
- n. bone formation
- n. bone formation ▸ extensive
- n. bone ▸ replaced with
- n. brain
- n. column of bone
- n. drug therapy
- n. growth, circumscribed
- n. host cell
- n. host cell ▸ phage particle infects
- n. identity ▸ assumption of a
- n. information, retaining
- n. lesion formation
- n. mutation
- n. needle
- n. sensation
- n. sickle flap
- n. skin ▸ growth and maturation of
- n. tube
- n. vessel growth, stimulate
- n. vessel membranes, choroidal
- N. York Heart Association (NYHA) classification

newborn (Newborn)
- n. appearance
- n. aspirates meconium
- n., aspiration of
- n. care
- n. circumcision
- n., congenital anemia of
- n., cytomegalic inclusion disease (CMID) of
- n. drug toxicity
- n., epidemic diarrhea of
- n. footprinted in delivery room
- n. for galactosemia ▸ testing of
- n. (HDN), hemolytic disease of the
- n., hemorrhagic disease of
- n., idiopathic respiratory distress of
- n. in delivery room ▸ footprint taken of
- n. infant
- n. infant care
- n., lamellar exfoliation of
- n. maturity rating
- n. nails, perionyx on
- N. Nursery
- n., Parrot's artery of the
- n., Parrot's atrophy of the
- n. ▸ persistent pulmonary hypertension of
- n., physical assessment of
- n., premature
- n., resuscitation of depressed
- n. screening program
- n. syndrome, drowned
- n. ▸ transient tachypnea of

Newcastle (newcastle)
- N. disease
- N. disease virus (NDV)
- N. -Manchester bacillus
- n., Shigella

newly
- n. acquired disease
- n. diagnosed diabetes
- n. recovering alcoholic

newtonian aberration

Newton's disc

next
- n. -of-kin
- n. -of-kin authorization form to use eyes
- n. -of-kin, permission of

Nezelof's syndrome

NF (neurofibromatosis) patient

NFT (neurofibrillary tangles)

NG (nasogastric)

NG (nasogastric) aspirate

NG (nasogastric) tube

ng (nanogram)

N$_{gas}$ (cavity-gas calibration factor)

ng/cc (nanograms per cubic centimeter)

NH region

NHDS (National Health Discharge Survey)

NHO (National Hospice Organization)

NI NR (no-infection no-rejection)

niacin therapy

nibbled colony

NIC (Neonatal Intensive Care)

niche
- n. cell
- n., oval window
- n., round window
- n., ulcer

Nichol's procedure

nickel dermatitis

Nickerson's medium smear

nicking, arteriovenous (AV)

nicking of retinal vein

Nicol prism

Nicoladoni-Branham sign

Nicolas-Favre disease

Nicolas-Favre disease ▸ Durand-

Nicola's operation

nicotina, stomatitis

nicotine
- n., absorption of
- n. acid
- n. addict
- n. addiction
- n., addiction liability of
- n. (T/N) cigarette, low tar/
- n. consumption ▸ caffeine or
- n. dependence
- n. fit
- n. gum
- n. gum ▸ physical dependence on
- n. inhaler
- n. level
- n. nasal spray
- n. patch
- n. patch ▸ stick-on
- n. patch, transdermal
- n. patch treatment
- n. receptors
- n. replacement therapy
- n. skin patch
- n. spray ▸ nasal
- n. therapy ▸ non-
- n. threshold
- n. transdermal patches

n. transdermal system
n. withdrawal
n. withdrawal ▸ alleviate symptoms of
n. withdrawal syndrome
nicotinic receptor blockade therapy
NICU (Neonatal Intensive Care Unit)
Nida's operation
NIDDM (noninsulin dependent diabetes mellitus)
NIDM (noninsulin diabetes mellitus)
nidulans, Aspergillus
Niebauer prosthesis
Nielsen syndrome ▸ Jervell and Lange-
Niewenglowski's rays
NIF (negative inspiratory force)
nifedipine enzyme immunoassay
nificornis, Sarcophaga
niger
n., Aspergillus
n., Rhizopus
n., Vibrio
night (Night)
n. blindness
n. cramps
n. cycle, day-
n. electroencephalogram (EEG) recording ▸ all-
n. ▸ excessive urination at
n. grinding of teeth
n. hospital
N. Hospital Program
n. ▸ morbid dread of
n. myopia
n. sight
n. sleep recording, all
n. sweats
n. sweats ▸ chills, fever and
n. sweats, cough, foul sputum ▸ fever,
n. sweats, drenching
n. sweats ▸ shaking chills and
n. terrors
n. terrors, somnambulism or
n. vision
n. vision, decreased
n. vision, poor
n. voiding
n. wandering
nightguard, plastic
nightmare(s)
n., adult

n. and flashbacks
n. disorder
n. disorder (dream anxiety disorder)
n. ▸ insomnia and
n. ▸ patient has
n., rescripting
nightstick fracture
nighttime
n. calf cramps
n. heartburn
n. leg cramps
n. sleep
n. urination ▸ frequent
n. voiding
nightwalker, patient
nigra
n., cardiopathia
n. cells, loss of substantia
n., dermatosis papulosa
n., lingua
n., lingua villosa
n., substantia
nigral degeneration, striatal
nigricans
n., acanthosis
n., pseudoacanthosis
n., Rhizopus
nigrovarius, Trypanosoma
nigrum, carcinoma
nigrum, tapetum
nihilistic delusion
Nikolsky's sign
Nile
N. encephalitis, West
N. fever, West
N. -like fever ▸ West
N. -like viral encephalitis ▸ West
N. -like virus ▸ West
N. virus, West
Nimbles (barbiturates)
IX antigen, factor
99m
99m aggregated albumin kit, Tc (technetium)
99m albumin microspheres kit, Tc (technetium)
99m etidronate sodium kit, Tc (technetium)
99m generator, Tc (technetium)
99m hexamibi ▸ Tc (technetium)
99m imaging ▸ Tc (technetium)
99m medronate sodium kit, Tc (technetium)

99m MIBI imaging ▸ Tc (technetium)
99m pentetate sodium kit, Tc (technetium)
99m pyrophosphate ▸ Tc (technetium)
99m scan, Tc (technetium)
99m serum albumin kit, Tc (technetium)
99m sestamibi scintigraphy ▸ Tc (technetium)
99m stannous pyrophosphate/ polyphosphate, Tc (technetium)
99m sulfur colloid, Tc (technetium)
90%, hypaque-M
ninth cranial nerve
ninth nerve
nipple(s)
n. abnormalities
n., adenoma of
n., aortic
n., areola of
n., dark skin surrounding
n., darkening of
n. discharge
n. discharge from antidepressant
n. discharge from birth control pill
n. discharge from breast injury
n. ▸ distortion or retraction of
n. ducts
n. everted
n. feeding
n., flattened
n. fluid
n. from breast ▸ retracted
n., inflamed
n., invaginated
n., inverted
n., jogger's
n. marker
n., numb
n., oversensitive
n. problem from breastfeeding
n. reconstruction
n. retraction
n., retraction of breast
n. ▸ retraction of the
n., scaliness of
n. shadow
n. site
n. transplants
n., undersensitive
nipponica, Rickettsia
Nissen fundoplication

Nissen fundoplication
- ▸ **Rossetti modification of**

Nissl('s)
- N. bodies
- N. granules
- N., substance of

niter paper

nitidus, lichen

nitrate
- n., amyl
- n., peroxyacetyl
- n. (AgNO₃) ▸ silver
- n. (Sr 85), strontium

nitrazine test

nitric oxide hemoglobin

nitrite, sodium

Nitro 5, Transderm-

nitrogen
- n., alkali-soluble
- n., alpha amino
- n. (BUN) ▸ blood urea
- n. curve ▸ single breath
- n. (BUN) ▸ elevated blood urea
- n. excretion
- n. (BUN) fluctuation ▸ blood urea
- n. ▸ freezing with liquid
- n. lag
- n., liquid
- n. monoxide
- n. mustard
- n. mustard, Oncovin, prednisone, procarbazine (MOPP)
- n. mustard therapy
- n. narcosis
- n., nonprotein
- n. (D-N) ratio ▸ dextrose-
- n. (G-N) ratio ▸ glucose-
- n. retention test
- n. (SUN) ▸ serum urea
- n. test, alpha amino
- n. (BUN) test ▸ blood urea
- n. test, nonprotein
- n. test, urea
- n. unit (PNU) ▸ protein
- n., urea
- n. (UUN) ▸ urine urea
- n. washout test ▸ single breath

nitroglycerin
- n. patch
- n. (NTG) patch ▸ transdermal
- n. sublingual
- n. therapy

nitrol ointment

nitrol paste

nitroprusside
- n. infusion
- n. poisoning
- n., sodium

nitrous
- n. oxide (N₂O)
- n. oxide (N₂O) barbiturate
- n. oxide (N₂O) tank

nits, and pubic lice ▸ eggs,

nivialis, ophthalmia

Nizetic's operation

NJ (nasojejunal) feeding

NK (natural killer) cells

nl (nanoliter)

NLP (no light perception)

nm (nanometer)

NMH (neurally mediated hypotension)

NMP (normal menstrual period)

NMP (nuclear matrix proteins)

NMR (nuclear magnetic resonance)

NMR (nuclear magnetic resonance) imaging

NMR (nuclear magnetic resonance) spectroscopy

NMRS (Nuclear Magnetic Resonance Scanner)

NNIS (National Nosocomial Infection Study)

no
- n. abnormality of fetus
- n. added salt (NAS) diet
- n. appreciable change
- n. appreciable disease
- n. evidence of active disease
- n. evidence of disease (NED)
- n. evidence of pathology
- n. evidence of recurrence (NER)
- n. evidence of recurrent disease (NERD)
- n. -infection no-rejection (NI NR)
- n. interest in surroundings, patient has
- n. known cure
- n. -leak technique
- n. light perception (NLP)
- n. line of demarcation
- n. palpable thrill
- n. -patch cataract removal, no-stitch and
- n. -phase wrap
- n. reflow phenomenon
- n. -rejection (NI NR) ▸ no-infection
- n. significant abnormality
- n. significant change

- n. significant disease
- n. skid mat
- n. smoking clinic
- n. spontaneous movement of limbs
- n. -stitch and no-patch cataract removal
- n. -stitch cataract surgery
- n. -stitch, no-patch cataract surgery
- n. -threshold substances
- n. touch technique
- n. touch technique ▸ en bloc
- n. treatment necessary
- n. voluntary activity
- n. weight bearing

No. 1 ▸ Stahl's ear,

No. 2 ▸ Stahl's ear,

Nobelpharma Implant System

noble cells

Nocard bacillus, Preisz-

Nocardia
- N. asteroides
- N. brasiliensis
- N. caviae
- N. farcinica
- N. israelii
- N. lurida
- N. madurae
- N. minutissima
- N. pulmonalis
- N. transvalensis

nocardiosis/nocardiasis

nocardiosis, pulmonary

Nocard's bacillus

nociceptive
- n. pathway
- n. reflexes
- n. stimuli
- n. threshold

noctuae, Haemoproteus

nocturia, patient has

nocturna, chorea

nocturnal
- n. amaurosis
- n. angina
- n. asthma
- n. awakening
- n. confusion
- n. dyspnea
- n. dyspnea (PND) ▸ paroxysmal
- n. emission
- n. enuresis
- n. enuresis, primary
- n. epilepsy
- n. heartburn

n. hemoglobinuria (PNH) ▸ paroxysmal
n. leg cramps
n. myoclonus
n. regurgitation
n. seizure
n. sleep
n. teeth grinding

nocturnus, pavor

nodal

n. arrhythmia
n. artery
n. automaticity
n. automaticity ▸ sinus
n. beat
n. bigeminy
n. bradycardia
n. cell
n. conduction AV (atrioventricular)
n. drainage
n. dysfunction ▸ sinus
n. escape
n. escape rhythm
n. extrasystole
n. extrasystole ▸ lower
n. extrasystole ▸ upper
n. involvement
n. involvement in breast carcinoma, survival relative to
n. irradiation (TNI) ▸ total
n. metastasis in breast carcinoma, axillary
n. metastasis, intrapulmonary
n. paroxysmal tachycardia
n. pathways, atrioventricular (AV)
n. pathways ▸ dual atrioventricular
n. point
n. premature beat (NPB)
n. premature contraction
n. reentrant paroxysmal tachycardia ▸ atrioventricular (AV)
n. reentrant tachycardia
n. reentrant tachycardia ▸ atrioventricular (AV)
n. reentrant tachycardia ▸ S-A
n. reentrant tachycardia ▸ sinus
n. reentry, atrioventricular (AV)
n. reentry ▸ sinus
n. rhythm
n. rhythm, atrioventricular (AV)
n. rhythm, coronary
n. rhythm ▸ lower
n. rhythm, nonparoxysmal
n. rhythm, paroxysmal

n. stage radiograph ▸ 24-hour delayed lymph
n. systole, atrioventricular (AV)
n. tachycardia
n. tachycardia, atrioventricular (AV)
n. tachycardia, nonparoxysmal
n. tissue

nodding of head

nodding spasm

node(s)

n., abdominal lymph
n. ablation, AV
n., anterior lymph
n., anterior mediastinal lymph
n., anterior tibial lymph
n., anthracotic hilar
n., anthracotic lymph
n., aplastic lymph
n. area, popliteal
n. artery ▸ sinoatrial (S-A)
n. artery ▸ sinus
n., Aschoff-Tawara
n., Aschoff's
n. aspiration, retromandibular
n., AV
n. (AVN) ▸ atrioventricular
n., axillary
n., axillary lymph
n., azygos
n. bearing area of lymph nodes, regional
n. biopsies, selected retroperitoneal lymph
n. biopsy, abdominal lymph
n. biopsy, lymph
n. biopsy, mediastinal
n. biopsy ▸ mediastinal lymph
n. biopsy, scalene
n. biopsy, scalene lymph
n. biopsy ▸ sentinel
n. biopsy, supraclavicular
n. biopsy ▸ supraclavicular lymph
n., Bouchard's
n., bronchial lymph
n., bronchopulmonary lymph
n., buccal lymph
n., calcified
n., calcified hilar
n., calcified lymph
n., calcified mesenteric
n. cancer of lymph
n., cancer-positive
n., cecal mesocolic lymph
n., celiac
n., celiac lymph

n., cervical
n., cervical lymph
n. classification in squamous cell carcinoma, cervical lymph
n., clinical status of
n., Cloquet's
n., common iliac lymph
n. ▸ cortical substance of lymph
n., cubital lymph
n., deep cervical lymph
n., deep inguinal lymph
n., Delphian lymph
n. disease, lymph
n. disease ▸ sinus
n. dissection
n. dissection, axillary lymph
n. dissection ▸ lymph
n. dissection, radical inguinal
n. dissection, radical retroperitoneal
n. drainage (dr'ge) ▸ pelvic lymph
n., Dürck's
n. dysfunction, sinus
n., enlarged lymph
n., enlarged periaortic
n., enlarged retromandibular
n. enlargement, lymph
n. enlargement, periaortic lymph
n. enlargement ▸ residual axillary lymph
n., epigastric lymph
n., Ewald's
n., external iliac lymph
n., femoral
n., Féréol's
n. ▸ first or second echelon lymph
n. ▸ first or second station lymph
n., Flack's
n. function ▸ sinus
n., gastroepiploic lymph
n., gouty
n., Haygarth's
n., Heberden's
n., hemal
n., hemolymph
n. ▸ hemorrhagic omental lymph
n., Hensen's
n., hepatic lymph
n., hilar
n., hilar lymph
n., His-Tawara
n., histiocytic hyperplasia of lymph
n. hyperplasia ▸ lymph
n., ileocolic lymph
n., iliac lymph
n. impulse, sinus

node(s)—*continued*

n., inferior mesenteric lymph
n., inferior tracheobronchial lymph
n., inguinal
n., inguinal lymph
n., intercostal lymph
n., internal iliac lymph
n., internal jugular lymph
n., internal mammary lymph
n. involvement
n. involvement, axillary lymph
n. involvement in nasopharyngeal carcinoma, lymph
n. involvement, internal
n. involvement, primary
n. involvement, regional
n. involvement, regional lymph
n. involvement, serial lymph
n. irradiation, axillary lymph
n. irradiation ▸ total axial
n., jugular lymph
n., jugulodigastric
n., junctional lymph
n., juxta-articular
n., Keith-Flack
n., Keith's
n., Koch's
n., left colic lymph
n., left gastric lymph
n., left hilar lymph
n., Legendré's
n., lumbar lymph
n., lymph
n., lymph paratracheal
n. ▸ lymphoid depletion of lymph
n., mandibular lymph
n. masses, supraclavicular
n., mediastinal
n., mediastinal lymph
n., mesenteric
n., mesenteric lymph
n. metastases, axillary lymph
n., metastases (TNM) classification ▸ tumor,
n. metastases, hilar
n. metastases in lung carcinoma, supraclavicular
n., metastases, periaortic lymph
n., metastases (TNM) staging system ▸ tumor,
n., metastases (TNM) ▸ tumor,
n. metastasis ▸ lymph
n., metastatic
n., Meynet's
n., middle colic lymph

n. modification, AV
n., neck lymph
n., negative
n. negative for cancer
n., nonmovable
n., occipital lymph
n. of Ranvier
n. of Tawara
n., Osler's
n. ▸ pacemaking sinus
n. ▸ painless lymph
n., palpable
n., pancreaticosplenic lymph
n., pancreatoduodenal lymph
n., parapharyngeal lymph
n., paraportal lymph
n., parasternal lymph
n., paratracheal
n., paratracheal lymph
n., Parrot's
n. pathway ▸ slow AV
n. (AVN) pathways, atrioventricular
n., pelvic lymph
n., periaortic infrarenal
n., periaortic lymph
n., perigastric lymph
n. ▸ perihilar lymph
n., peripancreatic
n., peripancreatic lymph
n. permeability factor, lymph
n., pharyngeal lymph
n., phrenic lymph
n., pleural lymph
n., popliteal lymph
n., positive
n. ▸ positive lymph
n., positive pelvic
n., positive periaortic
n., posterior mediastinal lymph
n., prelaryngeal
n., pretracheal
n. ▸ pretracheal lymph
n., primitive
n., pulmonary lymph
n., pyloric lymph
n., questionable
n. recovery time, corrected sinus
n. recovery time, sinus
n. reentrant, AV
n. reentry ▸ sinus
n. reentry tachycardia ▸ atrial ventricular (AV)
n., regional
n., regional lymph

n., regional node bearing area of lymph
n. resection
n., retroperitoneal
n., retroperitoneal lymph
n. ▸ retropharyngeal lymph
n. ▸ rhythmic pattern sinoatrial (S-A)
n., right colic lymph
n., right gastric lymph
n., right hilar lymph
n., S-A (sinoatrial)
n. sampling, pelvic
n. sampling, periaortic
n., scalene
n., scalene lymph
n., Schmorl's
n. scintigraphy ▸ thyroidal lymph
n. ▸ second atrioventricular
n., sentinel
n., shotty lymph
n., shotty residual
n., shotty residual lymph
n., signal
n., singer's
n., sinoatrial (S-A)
n., sinoauricular
n. (SN) ▸ sinus
n. ▸ small, tender lymph
n., spinal accessory chain lymph
n., spindle-shaped
n., subcutaneous intraocular
n., subdigastric lymph
n., submandibular lymph
n., submental lymph
n., superficial and deep parotid lymph
n., superficial cervical lymph
n., superficial inguinal lymph
n., superior mesenteric lymph
n., superior tracheobronchial lymph
n., supraclavicular
n., supraclavicular lymph
n. swelling ▸ generalized lymph
n., swollen lymph
n. syndrome (MLNS), mucocutaneous lymph
n., syphilitic
n. system, lymph
n., teacher's
n. ▸ tender, soft, nonmovable
n. tenderness, lymph
n., tracheal lymph
n., tracheobronchial lymph
n., triticeous

n., Troisier's
n. ▸ underarm lymph
n., Virchow's
n., vital

nodi
n. lymphatici, hilus
n. lymphatici ▸ vasa afferentia
n. lymphatici ▸ vasa efferentia

nodo-Hisian bypass tract

nodosa
n., arteritis
n., arthritis
n., chorditis
n., isthmica
n., ophthalmia
n., periarteritis
n. phthisis
n., polyarteritis
n., salpingitis isthmica
n., trichomycosis
n., trichorrhexis
n., trichosporosis

nodose arteriosclerosis
nodosum
n., erythema
n., ganglion
n., infantile periarteritis
n. leproticum, erythema
n. syphiliticum, erythema

nodosus, Streptomyces
nodoventricular
n. fiber
n. fibers, accessory
n. tract

nodular
n. aortic stenosis, calcific
n. arteriosclerosis
n. consistency
n. corneal dystrophy, Salzmann's
n. cortical adrenal hyperplasia
n. density
n. density ▸ benign appearing
n. fasciitis
n. ▸ fluid-filled
n. gliosis, hypertrophic
n. goiter
n. growth of tissue
n. hyperplasia
n. hyperplasia, focal
n. hyperplasia ▸ mild focal cortical
n. hyperplasia of prostate gland
n. lesion
n. lesions ▸ soft fluctuant
n., liver
n. liver ▸ firm, irregular,

n., lung
n. lymphoma
n. metastases
n. metastasis, intrapulmonary
n., mucosa slightly
n. non-Hodgkin's lymphoma
n. or flat growth ▸ firm, red
n. pattern ▸ diffuse reticular
n., poorly differentiated lymphocytes (NPDL)
n. prostatic hypertrophy
n. pulmonary amyloidosis
n. salpingitis
n. scarring
n. sclerosis
n. silicosis
n. stromal hyperplasia of ovary
n. thyroid, residual
n. tumor metastasis
n. tumor, mixed
n. type Hodgkin's disease ▸ mixed
n. vasculitis

nodularis, enteritis
nodularity, focal
nodularity, underlying
nodulation
n., discrete
n., irregular with
n. of lung, discrete

nodule(s) [*globule, lobule*]
n. ablation ▸ thyroid
n., accessory thymic
n., acinar
n., aggregate
n., Albini's
n., antihelix elastic
n., apple jelly
n., Aschoff's
n., benign
n., Bianchi's
n., Bohn's
n., Bouchard's
n., breast
n., Busacca
n., calcareous
n., calcified
n., cancerous thyroid
n., chest
n., cold
n., colloid
n., confluence of
n., Cruveilhier's
n., Dalen-Fuchs
n., discrete
n., encapsulated

n., erythematous
n., fibrocystic
n., fibrous
n., focal colloid
n. formation
n., Fraenkel's
n., Gamna
n., Gandy-Gamna
n., granular inflammatory
n., Guatamahri's
n., hard subcutaneous
n., Hoboken's
n., hyperplastic
n., hyperplastic cortical
n., Jeanselme's
n., juxta-articular
n., Koeppe
n., Koester's
n., Leishman's
n., lentiform
n. ▸ liver studies with
n., Lutz-Jeanselme
n., lymph
n., lymphatic
n., lymphosarcomatous
n., malignant thyroid
n., metastatic
n., metastatic liver
n., milker's
n. ▸ minute, lymphatic
n., mixed type
n., Morgagni's
n., movable subcutaneous
n., multiple metastatic
n., necrobiotic
n. of aortic valve
n. of Arantius
n. of Kerckring
n. of large intestine ▸ solitary lymphatic
n. of pulmonary trunk valves
n. of residual tumor ▸ focal
n. of small intestine ▸ solitary lymphatic
n. of stomach, lymphatic
n. of thyroid ▸ colloid
n. of vermis
n. on liver ▸ tumor
n., palpable
n., Paterson's
n., pearly
n., pedunculated
n., peritoneal tumor
n. ▸ peritoneum studded with tumor
n., pigmented

nodule(s)—*continued*
- n., primary
- n., pulmonary
- n., pulp
- n., regenerated
- n., retrosternal
- n., rheumatic
- n., satellite
- n., satellite tumor
- n., scattered lymphocytic
- n., Schmorl's
- n., secondary
- n., shiny
- n., siderotic
- n., singers'
- n. ‣ small firm circumscribed
- n., solitary
- n., solitary pulmonary
- n. ‣ studded with numerous tumor
- n., subcutaneous
- n., surfers'
- n. tabac
- n., teachers'
- n., tendon
- n., thyroid
- n., triticeous
- n., tumor
- n., typhoid
- n., typhus
- n., ulcerated
- n., vestigial
- n., violaceous
- n., vocal cord
- n., warm

nodus sinuatrialis echo

noise(s)
- n., average peak
- n., clicking
- n., environmental
- n., heterogeneous
- n. in ear
- n. -induced deafness
- n. -induced hearing loss
- n. ‣ irreversible ear damage from
- n. level
- n. level, low
- n. level ‣ noxious
- n. ‣ loud, high-pitched
- n. (S/N) ratio, signal-to-
- n. reduction
- n., ringing
- n. ‣ sensitivity to light and
- n. signal
- n., sonorous
- n. spike artifact

- n., ultrasensitive to
- n., whooshing

noisy chest
Nölke's position
noma vulvae
nominal
- n. aphasia
- n. single dose
- n. standard dose (NSD)

nomotopic stimulus
non ‣ conditio sine qua
non-A, non-B hepatitis
nonablative laser
nonablative laser technique
nonabsorbable surgical suture
nonabsorbent material
nonacidic diet ‣ low fat,
nonacute total occlusion
nonaddictive painkillers
nonaddictive way
nonaffective psychotic disorder
nonagglutinating vibrios
nonalcoholic
- n. fatty liver
- n. psychiatric outpatient
- n. steatohepatitis (NASH)

non-Alzheimer's disease-related pattern
nonarticular arthritis
nonassertive, patient
non-B hepatitis
non-B hepatitis ‣ non-A,
nonbacterial
- n. cystitis
- n. thrombotic endocardial lesion
- n. thrombotic endocarditis
- n. verrucous endocarditis

nonbarbiturate therapy
nonbiological signal
nonbizarre delusions
noncalcified valve
noncancerous
- n. enlargement of prostate gland
- n. polyp
- n. skin growth
- n. sun-induced keratosis
- n. tumor

noncardiac
- n. angiography
- n. chest pain
- n. pulmonary edema
- n. surgery
- n. syncope

noncardiogenic origin
noncardiogenic pulmonary edema

noncaseating granuloma
noncausal association
noncephalic lead
nonchew diet, bland
nonchromaffin paraganglioma
noncleaved cell lymphoma
nonclinical services
noncollagenous pneumoconiosis
noncomitant squint
noncomitant strabismus
noncommittal, patient
noncommunicating hydrocele
noncommunicating hydrocephalus
noncompensatory pause
noncompliance with medical treatment
noncompliant, patient
noncompliant with medication, patient
nonconducted premature atrial contraction
nonconfrontational cognitive restructuring
noncongestive glaucoma
noncontributory
- n., family history (FH)
- n., past history (PH)
- n. to present illness (PI)

nonconversive, patient
noncoronary cusp
noncoronary sinus
noncovered benefits
noncurarized state
noncyclical breast pain
noncyclical mastalgia
noncystic acne
nondeciduous placenta
nondependent abuse of drugs
nondepolarizing muscle relaxant
nondiabetic personality
nondialysis time
nondirective psychotherapy
nondirective therapy
nondisabled peer
nondisabling stroke
nondisplaced
- n. crack fracture
- n. fracture
- n. zygmatic arch fracture

nondistorting memory
nondistorting memory function
nondouloureux, tic
nondrinker, patient
nondrinking behaviors
none law, all or

nonejection systolic click
nonemergency transportation
   services
nonenhancing lesion
nonepithelial tumor
nonexercise activity thermogenesis
   (NEAT)
nonexertional angina
nonexpansional dyspnea
nonfade scope
nonfamilial dysplastic nevi
nonfat milk
nonfatal
   n. attempt at suicide
   n. heart attack
   n. injury
   n. stroke
nonfever-related seizure
nonfiberoptic bronchoscopy
nonfilament polymorphonuclear
nonfilamented form
nonflotation catheter
nonfluent aphasia
nonfunctional
   n. return
   n. tooth
   n., totally
   n., written language
nonfunctioning
   n. catheter
   n. cerebral cortex
   n. gallbladder
   n. kidney
   n. lung ▸ unilateral
   n. nerves
   n. retina
nonglycoside inotropic agent
nongonococcal cervicitis
nongonococcal urethritis
nongranulomatous ileojejunitis
nonhealing
   n. open sore, persistent
   n. ulceration
   n. ulceration, superficial
nonhemodynamic effect
nonhemolytic jaundice, chronic
   familial
nonhemolytic streptococcus
nonhereditary breast cancer
nonhereditary chorea, chronic
   progressive
nonhistiocytic type lymphoma
non-Hodgkin's lymphoma
   n.-H. lymphoma, diffuse
   n.-H. lymphoma, nodular

   n.-H. lymphoma, null-type
   n.-H. lymphoma of stomach
nonhostile confrontation ▸ realistic
nonictal psychiatric disorder
nonicteric hepatitis
nonicteric, sclerae
nonidentical twin transplants
nonidentical twins
nonidentity, reaction of
nonimmunocompromised host
nonimpact aerobic activities
noninfectious
   n. cause
   n. disease
   n. disorder
   n. entities
   n. ulcer
noninfective state
noninfiltrating cancer
noninfiltrating intraductal carcinoma
noninflamed diverticula
noninflammatory disease ▸ primary
noninsulin
   n. dependent diabetes mellitus
      (NIDDM)
   n. dependent diabetes mellitus
      (NIDDM), Type II-
   n. diabetes mellitus (NIDM)
nonintegrated transvenous
   defibrillation lead
nonintegrated tripolar lead
noninterferon immunomodulators
nonintervention ▸ point of
nonintrusive procedure
nonintrusive test
noninvasive
   n. aspergillosis
   n. assessment
   n. brain test
   n. cancer
   n. cardiac assessment
   n. cardiac evaluation
   n. cervical cancer
   n. coronary angiography
   n. diagnostic procedure
   n. diagnostic test
   n. evaluation
   n. examination
   n. glucose monitor
   n. lesion
   n. lithotripsy
   n. method
   n. murmur
   n. pain management
   n. procedure

   n. programmed stimulation
   n. screening
   n. surgery
   n. technique
   n. temporary pacemaker
   n. temporary pacing
   n. test
   n. testing
   n. therapy
   n. thymoma
   n. treatment
   n. vascular laboratory assessment
nonionic contrast material
nonionic contrast medium
nonionizing radiation
nonirritating diet
nonischemic dilated cardiomyopathy
nonjudgmental attitude ▸ calm,
   assured,
nonkeratinizing stratified squamous
   epithelium
nonketotic
   n. coma, hyperglycemic
   n. coma, hyperosmolar
   n. diabetes mellitus
   n. hyperosmotic
nonlentiginous melanoma
nonlethal underlying disease
nonleukemic myelosis
nonleukemic myelosis, chronic
nonlife-threatening disorder
nonliquefaciens, Pseudomonas
nonlocalized inflammation
nonlymphocytic leukemia (ANLL),
   acute
nonlymphoid leukemia (ANLL),
   acute
nonmalignant
   n. chest disease
   n. chest lesions
   n. disorder
   n. lesion of uterus
   n. tissue
nonmannite fermenting
nonmarital introitus
nonmatching donor relative
nonmedical approach
nonmedical support
nonmedicine placebo
nonmelanoma skin cancer
nonmeningeal cryptococcal disease
nonmetastatic carcinoma, advanced
nonmovable node
nonmovable node ▸ tender, soft,
nonmutated gene

nonmyelinated nerve fibers
▸ bundles of
nonnarcotic analgesic
nonnecrotizing angiitis
nonnervous supportive tissue ▸
overgrowth of
Nonne's syndrome
nonnicotine therapy
nonoat cell carcinoma
nonobese diabetic
nonocclusive arterial
rhabdomyolysis
nonocclusive mesenteric ischemia
nononcogenic polyomavirus
nononcogenic virus
nonopaque calculi
nonoperable cancer
nonoperable tumor
nonoperative closure
nonopioid analgesic
nonorganic
n. failure to thrive
n. ▸ hypersomnia related to mental
disorder
n. ▸ insomnia related to mental
disorder
n. psychosis
n. sleep disorder
nonosteogenic fibromata
nonovulational menstruation
nonpalpable abnormality
nonpalpable thyroid
nonpancreatic etiology
nonpapillary hyperplasia
nonparalytic strabismus
nonparoxysmal
n. atrioventricular (AV) junctional
tachycardia
n. junctional tachycardia
n. nodal rhythm
n. nodal tachycardia
nonpathogenic fungi
nonpathogenic saprophyte
nonpenetrating rupture
nonpenetrating wound
nonpenicillinase producing staph
nonperforated ulcer
nonperforated ulcers, acute
nonphagocytic squamous cells
nonpharmacologic
n. intervention
n. measure of treatment
n. therapy ▸ conservative
nonphasic sinus arrhythmia
nonpitting edema

nonpolio enterovirus
nonpolyposis colon cancer (HNPCC)
▸ hereditary
nonpolyposis colorectal cancer ▸
hereditary
nonprescription
n. drugs, misuse of
n. medication
n. pain reliever
nonpressor doses
nonproductive cough
nonprogressive disturbance, chronic
nonproliferative diabetic retinopathy
(NPDR)
nonproliferative retinopathy
nonprotein nitrogen
nonprotein nitrogen test
nonpsychiatric medical facilities ▸
inpatient
nonpsychiatric medical facilities ▸
outpatient
nonpsychotic
n. distorted thinking
n. mental disorders
n. psychiatric disorder
n. ▸ unspecified mental disorder
nonpumping scar tissue
non-Q-wave myocardial infarction
nonradiating pain
nonradioactive hydrogen isotopes
nonrandomized clinical trials
nonrandomized clinical trials,
randomized vs
nonrapid eye movement (NREM)
n. eye movement (NREM) cycle
n. eye movement (NREM) intrusion
n. eye movement (NREM) period
n. eye movement (NREM)
physiology
n. eye movement–rapid eye
movement (NREM–REM) cycle
n. eye movement sleep (NREMS)
nonreactive
n., pupils
n., serology
n. VDRL (Venereal Disease
Research Laboratories)
nonrebreathing mask
nonreflective glass screen
nonreflex bladder
nonrefractory patient
nonrenal death
nonrenewal cellular systems
nonrenewal systems of cells, slow
renewal and

nonresidue liquid diet
nonrespiratory acidosis
nonresponsive
n. and mute ▸ patient rigid,
n. patient
n. to oral penicillin
n. tumor
nonresponsiveness, profound
nonreversible virus
nonrhythmic electroencephalogram
(EEG) activity
nonroughage diet
nonseasonal allergic rhinitis
nonseasonal hay fever
nonsecretory phase
nonsedating relief
nonselective coronary angiography
nonsensical speech ▸ exhibit
nonsensing, atrial
nonserous leptomeningitis
nonsex chromosomes
nonsimultaneous occurrence of
electroencephalogram (EEG)
activities
nonsmall
n. cell carcinoma
n. cell lung cancer
n. lung cancer
nonsmoker, patient
nonsmoking section
nonspastic muscles
nonspecific
n. chronic lymphocytic thyroiditis
n. complaints
n. depressant effect ▸ EEG
(electroencephalogram)
n. depressive reaction
n. diffuse spike discharges
n. etiology
n. hepatocellular abnormality
n. histologic pattern
n. immunity
n. intraventricular conduction defect
n. irritant in airway
n. mottling of retina
n. peripheral activity
n. pneumonitis
n. repolarization changes
n. sialadenitis, chronic
n. stimulation
n. stomatitis
n. ST-T wave changes
n. symptoms ▸ subtle and
n. ulcers
n. urethritis (NSU)

nonspherocytic hemolytic anemia, congenital
nonspherocytic, hereditary
nonsterile
- n. catheterization techniques
- n. environmental surface
- n. irrigation techniques
- n. surface

nonsteroidal
- n. anti-inflammatory
- n. anti-inflammatory agent
- n. anti-inflammatory drug (NSAID)

nonstrenuous activity
nonstrenuous contact sports
nonstreptococcal pharyngitis
nonstress test
nonstress testing, perinatal
nonstriated muscle
nonsubstance induced disorder
nonsurgical
- n. alternative
- n. angioplasty
- n. biliary drainage
- n. cardiology procedure
- n. electroencephalogram (EEG)
- n. face lift
- n. personnel
- n. procedure
- n. therapy
- n. treatment

nonsustained ventricular tachycardia
nonsustained ventricular tachycardia ▸ rapid
nonsymptomatic hemorrhoids
nonsyphilitic pneumopathy ▸ seropositive
nontarget ratio, target-to-
nonterminal situation
nontherapeutic drugs
nonthermal laser
nonthoracotomy
- n. defibrillation lead syndrome
- n. implantable cardioverter-defibrillator
- n. implantable cardioverter-defibrillator ▸ Transvene
- n. lead implantable cardioverter defibrillator
- n. lead placement

nonthreatening
- n. activities, resume
- n. atmosphere
- n. environment

nontoxic goiter
nontoxic treatment

nontraditional treatment
nontransmural myocardial infarction
nontranssexual type of adolescence
nontranssexual type of adulthood
nontraumatic
- n. arterial rhabdomyolysis
- n. cardiac arrest
- n. cardiac tamponade
- n. coma
- n. myoglobinuria
- n. rhabdomyolysis
- n. tap

nontraumatizing catheter
nontropical sprue
nontuberculous mycobacterial disease
nontuberculous species
nonulcer dyspepsia
nonuniform rotational defect
nonuniformity factor
nonunion of fracture
nonverbal
- n. behavior
- n. communication
- n. language of body posture
- n. learning
- n. memory
- n. memory test
- n. modalities
- n. social comprehension
- n. social cues
- n. support, provide appropriate

nonvertebral osteoporotic fracture
nonviable fetus
nonviable tissue
nonvigorous activity
nonviolent depression
nonviral hepatitis
nonvirus infected cells
nonvisualization of gallbladder
nonvisualized kidney
nonvital tooth
nonvoluntary active euthanasia
nonweight
- n. bearing
- n. bearing brace
- n. bearing ▸ patient ambulating with walker

Noonan's syndrome
noothymopsychic ataxia
nootropic effect
norepinephrine and dopamine
norethindrone test
norethynodrel test

Norland-Cameron photon densitometry
normal
- n. abdomen
- n. ability level ▸ difficulty functioning at
- n. acceptable behavior
- n. activities, impaired
- n. activity
- n. adult respiration
- n. affect
- n. aging
- n. aging process
- n. alpha rhythm
- n. anatomic alignment ▸ restoration of
- n. anatomic position
- n. anatomic situation
- n., anatomically
- n. AP (anteroposterior) view
- n. appearing stomach
- n. architecture ▸ loss of
- n. artery
- n. assay volume
- n. atrial rhythm
- n. atrioventricular (AV) septation
- n. atrioventricular (AV) synchrony
- n. atrophy of old age
- n. axis deviation
- n. bacterial flora
- n., balanced alignment
- n. behavior
- n. behavior and attitude
- n. birth weight
- n. blood circulation
- n. blood flow
- n. blood indices
- n. blood pressure (BP)
- n. body or facial contours
- n. body weight
- n. bone chemistry
- n. bone maturation
- n. bone movement
- n. bone scan
- n. bowel action
- n. bowel control
- n. bowel function
- n. brain dose, minimize
- n. brain tissue
- n. breast structures
- n. breast tissue cells
- n., breasts and axillary contents
- n. breathing, enhancing
- n. breathing ▸ momentary lapse in
- n. bronchial pattern

normal—*continued*

n. capacity
n. capacity ▸ patient functioning at ___%
n., cardiac sounds
n. cardiomegaly
n. cell
n. cell function
n. cervical curvature
n. chemical reactions in body
n. chest
n. child development
n. childhood fantasy
n. color and texture
n. color vision
n. communication between nerves and muscles ▸ block in
n. comprehension of spoken language
n. consent requirement
n. contour of heart
n. control subjects
n. curve of development
n. delivery
n. delivery (FTND), full term
n. delivery, term
n., deviation from
n. dialysis solution
n. differential
n. distribution of hair
n. dwarf
n. ejection fraction
n. electrical axis
n. electroencephalogram (EEG) activity
n. electrolytes
n. emotional behavior
n. emptying
n. epithelial tissue ▸ functioning of
n. evacuation
n. evacuation of barium
n. exercise study
n. feces
n. female adult genitalia
n. female genitalia
n. fetal growth
n. fetal lobulations
n. fetal tolerance
n. flexibility
n. flexion of great toe
n. flora
n. flora, stools showed
n. flow
n. full term delivery
n. function

n. functioning ileal transverse colostomy
n. functioning of GI tract
n. gene
n. general cognitive impairment
n. geometry
n. gigantism
n. grief
n. grieving process
n. gross appearance
n., grossly
n. growth and development
n., head and neck
n. hearing
n. heart activity
n. heart function
n. heart rhythm
n. heart size
n. heartbeat
n. histologic pattern
n. histology
n. hormonal balance
n. hospital air
n. host
n. human development
n. human serum
n. human serum albumin
n. hydration
n. hypertrophic changes
n. immature brain tissue
n. immune system function
n. in anteroposterior (AP) diameter ▸ uterus
n. in appearance
n. in length, uterus
n. in size
n. in size and shape ▸ uterus
n. in size, heart
n. in size, uterus
n. infant, patient delivered
n. innervation, disruption of
n. intraocular tension
n. intravascular pressure
n. jaw function
n., kidneys anatomically
n. lifestyle
n. lifestyle, resume
n. limits (WNL) ▸ hematology within
n. limits, speech and language within
n. limits (WNL) ▸ within
n. lumbar curvature ▸ flattening of
n. lymphocyte transfer test
n. male adult genitalia
n. male genitalia

n. maturation
n. maturational unfolding
n. mean posterior wall velocity
n. memory
n. menstrual period (NMP)
n. menstrual period (LNMP) ▸ last
n. metabolic activity
n. mobility and function
n. motility
n. motor innervation of bladder
n. mucosa ▸ denudation of
n. muscle balance
n. myelocytic-erythrocytic ratio
n. nerve cell
n. neurons
n. occlusion
n. opacification
n. organ function
n. oropharyngeal flora
n. P wave
n., palate and pharynx
n. pattern
n. pattern ▸ electrocardiogram (ECG/EKG) showed
n. pelvis
n., percentage of
n. perfusion
n. personality
n. persons ▸ muscle relaxation in
n. physical function
n. physiologic function
n. plantar response
n. plasma
n. position ▸ scope reverted to
n. position ▸ uterus shifts to
n. postoperative course
n. pregnancy
n. pregnancy and delivery ▸ product of
n. pressure hydrocephalus (NPH)
n. process of digestion
n. proprioception
n. psychomotor functioning ▸ retardation in
n. pulmonary function
n. pulmonary function screen
n. pulse rate
n. quality of life ▸ near-
n. range
n. range of abilities, bright/
n. range of motion (ROM)
n. reaction
n. reactivity
n. record, borderline
n. recovery

n. reference serum
n. reflex
n., reflux into terminal ileum
n. renal function
n. respiration
n. response, lack of
n. response mechanism
n. resting electroencephalogram (EEG) pattern development
n. resting pulse rate
n. retinal correspondence
n. rhythm of heart
n. rhythm ▸ patient shocked back into
n. rhythm ▸ reboot faulty heart's
n. rhythm, shock heart into
n. risk
n. ROM (range of motion)
n. saline (N/S)
n. saline (N/S) enema
n. saline (N/S) solution
n. saline (N/S) ▸ wound irrigated with
n., sella turcica
n. sexual development
n. sinus heart rhythm
n. sinus rhythm (NSR)
n. sinus rhythm (NSR) ▸ resumption of
n. size
n. size and condition
n. size and configuration
n. size and shape
n. size heart
n. size ▸ heart reduced to
n. sleep, drifts into
n. sleeping pattern
n. solution, hundredth-
n. spectrum
n. sperm production
n. spinal fluid
n. spindles of sleep
n. spontaneous delivery (NSD)
n. spontaneous vaginal delivery (NSVD)
n. sputum
n. stance
n. stimulus environment
n. stomach and bowel functions
n. structural relationship
n. subject, patient
n. subjects ▸ neuromuscular firing in
n. substrate of enzyme
n. tachycardia

n. temperature
n. temperature and pressure (NTP)
n. tension glaucoma
n. texture, hair
n. tissue
n. tissue considerations in radiation therapy
n. tissue effects of dose fractionation
n. tissue microcirculation
n. to palpation
n. tremor
n. triglyceride levels
n., upper limits of
n. urinary function
n. urination ▸ disruption in
n. urine flow
n. urine output
n. uterine endometrium
n. vaginal birth
n. vaginal flora
n. value
n. variability
n. variability, range of
n. variant
n. ventricular contraction
n. vital capacity
n., vital signs
n. waking activity
n. waking electroencephalogram (EEG)
n. waking electroencephalogram (EEG) pattern
n. walk, alteration in
normalcy, maturational
normalcy ▸ socially defined behavioral
normality ▸ traditional standard of
normalize thyroxin level
normalized
n., hearing
n. ratio (INR) ▸ international
n. systolic ejection rate ▸ mean
normally
n., bladder empties
n., cords move
n. functioning kidney
n. outlined
n. potent
normative
n. base rates ▸ establishing
n. study
n. symptoms
normoactive
n. bowel sounds

n. bowel tones
n., reflexes
normoblast
n., acidophilic
n., basophilic
n., early
n., eosinophilic
n., intermediate
n., orthochromatic
n., oxyphilic
n., polychromatic
normocephalic, head
normochromic anemia
normochromic erythrocyte
normocytic anemia
normophysiological reflexes
normopressure hydrocephalus
normotensive hydrocephalus
normothermic cardioplegia
norms
n., conforms to social
n., social
n., textbook
Norrie's disease
North American blastomycosis
norvegicus, Mus
norvegicus, Rattus
Norwalk viruses
Norwegian scabies
Norwood univentricular heart probe
nose (Nose)
n. (cocaine)
n. and eyes ▸ itchy, runny
n. and throat (ENT) ▸ ears,
n. and throat (ENT) emergency ▸ ear,
n. and throat (HEENT) ▸ head, eyes, ears,
n. and throat (HEENT) not remarkable ▸ head, eyes, ears,
n. and throat (ENT) trauma ▸ ear,
n., arch of
n., basal cell carcinoma of ear and
n., beaked
n., beak-like protrusion of
n., bleeding from
n. ▸ body pain with runny
n., brandy
n., bridge of
n. bridge prosthesis ▸ Rosi L-type
N. Candy (cocaine)
n. carcinoma
n. ▸ chronic stuffy
n., cleft
n., constantly running

nose—*continued*
n. deformity ▸ external
n. deformity, saddle
n., depressor muscle of septum of
n., dilator muscle of
n., drippy
n. drops
n., external
n., FB (foreign body) in
n., finger-to-
n., flattened
n., frostbite of
n., hairs of
n., hammer
n. ▸ inflammation of mucous membrane of
n., irrigation of
n., levator muscle of upper lip and ala of
n. packed
n. piercing
n., potato
n. problem from cold
n. reshaping
n. resuscitation ▸ mouth-to-
n., runny
n. ▸ runny, itchy
n., saddle
n., saddle-back
n., saddle deformity of
n. shut, pinch
n., squamous cell carcinoma ear and
n. strategy ▸ hard-
n. stuffiness from Actifed
n. stuffiness from birth control pill
n., stuffy
n., summit of
n., swayback
n. ▸ swollen, bulbous
n. (F-N) test ▸ finger-to-
n., underside of
n., vestibule of
n. while breathing ▸ whistling in
nosebleed(s)
n., anterior
n., chronic
n., uncontrollable
nosecone spasm
nosocomial (Nosocomial)
n. anemia
n. bacteremia
n. bacterial infection ▸ control of
n. bacterial infection ▸ prevention of
n. Candidemia

n. central nervous system (CNS) infection
n. cutaneous infection
n. diarrhea
n. endocarditis
n. fungal infection
n. gastrointestinal (GI) infection
n. gram-positive organism
n. gynecological (GYN) infection
n. infection
n. infection control program
N. Infection Control (SENIC) ▸ Study on the Efficacy of
n. infection, fatal
n. infection, gram-positive
n. infection outbreak
n. infection, preventable
n. infection, site of
N. Infection Study (NNIS) ▸ National
n. infections, gastrointestinal (GI)
n. meningitis
n. organisms
n. pathogen
n. pneumonia
n. postpartum endometritis
n. respiratory tract infection
n. scabies
n. transmission of organism
n. vascular infection
n. wound infection
nosocomii, angina
Nosopsyllus fasciatus
nostalgia paresthetica
nostras, cholera
nostras, influenza
nostril(s)
n., blood in
n., flaring of
n. obstructed by foreign body (FB)
n. oozing blood
n. packed
n. reflex
n., stuffed
n. ▸ stuffed or runny
not
n. appear enlarged ▸ adenoids do
n. appear enlarged ▸ heart does
n. appear enlarged ▸ liver does
n. appear enlarged ▸ lump in left breast does
n. appear enlarged ▸ lump in right breast does
n. appear enlarged ▸ spleen does
n. appear enlarged ▸ tonsils do

n. dilated ▸ ureters patent and
n. isolated
n. obstructed, nares
n. palpable ▸ liver, spleen, kidneys (LSK)
n. remarkable ▸ family history (FH)
n. remarkable ▸ head, eyes, ears, nose and throat (HEENT)
n. remarkable ▸ past history (PH)
n. resuscitate (DNR) patient ▸ do
n. yet diagnosed (NYD)
notation, summary
notatum, Penicillium
notch(es)
n., acetabular
n., anacrotic
n., antegonial
n., anterior cerebellar
n., aortic
n., arterial
n., atrial
n., auricular
n., cardiac
n., cerebellar
n., clavicular
n., coracoid
n., cotyloid
n. deformity
n., dicrotic
n., early asterixis
n., fibular
n., filter
n., frontal
n., gastric
n., greater ischiatic
n., greater sacrosciatic
n., greater sciatic
n., inferior thyroid
n., inferior vertebral
n., interarytenoid
n., interclavicular
n., intercondylar
n., interlobar
n., intertragic
n., intervertebral
n., Kemohan's
n. lesser ischiatic
n., lesser sacrosciatic
n., lesser sciatic
n., mandibular
n., marsupial
n., mastoid
n. of femur, intercondylar
n. of frontal bone ▸ ethmoidal
n. of gallbladder

n. of left lung ▸ cardiac
n. of ligamentum teres
n. of mandible, semilunar
n. of maxilla, lacrimal
n. of maxilla, nasal
n. of occipital bone ▸ interclavicular
n. of occipital bone ▸ jugular
n. of palatine bone ▸ palatine
n. of palatine bone ▸ sphenopalatine
n. of radius, ulnar
n. of Rivinus
n. of scapula, semilunar
n. of sternum, clavicular
n. of sternum, costal
n. of sternum, jugular
n. of stomach, cardiac
n. of temporal bone ▸ interclavicular
n. of temporal bone ▸ jugular
n. of temporal bone ▸ parietal
n. of ulna, radial
n. of ulna, trochlear
n., palatine
n., pancreatic
n., parotid
n., posterior cerebellar
n., preoccipital
n., presternal
n., pterygoid
n., radial
n., radical
n., rib
n., rivinian
n., sacroiliac
n., scapular
n., sciatic
n., semilunar
n., Sibson's
n., sigmoid
n. sign ▸ pulmonary
n., sternal
n., superior thyroid
n., superior vertebral
n., supraorbital
n., suprascapular
n., suprasternal
n., tentorial
n., thyroid
n., trigeminal
n., trochlear
n., tympanic
n., ulnar
n., umbilical
n., vertebral
n. views

notched wave
notching, midsystolic
notching, rib
note(s)
    n., clinical
    n., percussion
    n., tympanic percussion
notha, angina
notha, peripneumonia
nothing by mouth (npo)
nothing by mouth at bedtime (npo/h.s.)
Nothnagel's sign
Nothnagel's syndrome
notice, death
notification
    n., advance
    n., funeral home
    n. of death
notions, grandiose
notochord, vestigial
nourished (W/N) ▸ patient well-
nourishing oral supplement
novemcincta, Dasypus
noverca, Amphimerus
novo lesion, de
Novopaque contrast medium
novyi, Clostridium
noxious
    n. bacilli
    n. noise level
    n. process
    n. stimulus
    n. stimulus, perception of
    n. substance
NP (nasopharyngeal)
NP (nasopharynx)
NPB (nodal premature beat)
NPC (nasopharyngeal carcinoma)
NPC (near point of convergence)
NPDL (nodular, poorly differentiated lymphocytes)
NPDR (nonproliferative diabetic retinopathy)
NPH (normal pressure hydro-cephalus)
NPI (nucleoplasmic index)
NPN (nonprotein nitrogen)
npo (nothing by mouth)
npo/h.s. (nothing by mouth at bedtime)
NREM (non rapid eye movement)
    N. cycle
    N. intrusion
    N. period

N. physiology
N/S (normal saline)
    N/S enema
    N/S solution
NSAID (nonsteroidal anti-inflammatory drug)
NSD (normal spontaneous delivery)
NSQ (not sufficient quantity)
NSR (normal sinus rhythm)
NSR (normal sinus rhythm) ▸ resumption of
NSU (nonspecific urethritis)
NT (nasotracheal)
NTD (neural tube defects)
NTG (nitroglycerin) Patch ▸ Transdermal
NTP (neural thread protein)
NTP (normal temperature and pressure)
N₂O (nitrous oxide)
Nu Gauze packing material
Nu Gauze dressing
nuchal
    n. cord
    n. flexure
    n. fluid, fetal
    n. line
    n. region
    n. rigidity
nuchofrontal projection
Nuck, canal of
Nuck's hydrocele
nuclear (Nuclear)
    n. abnormality
    n. accelerator
    n. accident
    n. agenesis
    n. and cytoplasmic maturation
    n. angiogram ▸ gated
    n. angiography
    n. angiography ▸ rest and exercise-gated
    n. anomaly, Pelger-Huet
    n. antibodies (ENA), extractable
    n. antigen
    n. antigen, extractable
    n. antigen ▸ proliferating cell
    n. aplasia
    n. bronzing
    n. cardiac scanning
    n. cardiology equipment
    n. cataract
    n. cataract, embryonal
    n. changes
    n. chromatin

nuclear—*continued*
- n. community
- n. detection, ambulatory
- n. detector, ambulatory
- n. differentiation
- n. dust, background
- n. element
- n. emulsion
- n. energy
- n. envelope
- n. facial palsy
- n. family
- n. fusion
- n. heart scan
- n. imaging
- n. lymphoscintigraphy
- n. magnetic resonance (NMR)
- N. Magnetic Resonance (NMR) Imaging
- N. Magnetic Resonance Scanner (NMRS)
- N. Magnetic Resonance (NMR) Spectroscopy
- n. matrix proteins (NMP)
- N. Medicine
- n. medicine physician
- n. medicine scanning
- n. medicine technology
- n. membrane
- n. membrane abnormality
- n. ophthalmoplegia
- n. pacemaker
- n. particles
- n. pleomorphism
- n. probe
- n. proliferation antigen
- n. pulse amplifier
- n. reaction
- n. reactor
- n. scan
- n. scanner
- n. scanning techniques
- n. sclerosis
- n. stain
- n. stress test
- n. structure, atomic and
- n. tau
- n. tracer
- n. variability
- n. ventricular function study
- n. waste

nucleated [*enucleated*]
- n. cells
- n. contractile fiber cell
- n. epithelial cells
- n. erythrocytes
- n. fusiform cells
- n. red blood cell
- n. red cells

nuclei
- n., anterior thalamic
- n. ▸ basophilic pleomorphic irregularly shaped
- n., bland
- n., brain stem
- n., cell
- n., cranial nerve
- n., dark-staining
- n. dentati, hilus
- n., droplet
- n., flattened
- n., free
- n., hyperchromatic
- n., hyperchromatic ovoid
- n., hyperobulated
- n., interstitial
- n., large irregular
- n., liver cell
- n., motor
- n., muscle cell
- n., oculomotor
- n. of anterior hypothalamus (INAH), interstitial
- n. of dividing cells
- n. olivaris, hilus
- n. ▸ paired vestibular
- n., pale-staining
- n., pleomorphic
- n., pleomorphic hyperchromatic
- n., pyknotic
- n., raphe
- n., subcortical
- n., subthalamic
- n., tritium
- n., vesicular
- n., vestibular

nucleic
- n. acid
- n. acid core
- n. acid technology

nucleocytoplasmic ratio

nucleolar satellite

nucleolus(-i)
- n. ▸ chromatin clumps and
- n. ▸ coarse chromatin clumps and
- n. organizer
- n., prominent
- n., small prominent

nucleoplasmic (NP) index

nucleoplasmic (NP) ratio

nucleoplasty procedure

nucleoprotein, viral

nucleoside reverse transcriptase inhibitors

nucleotide
- n., diphosphopyridine
- n. polymorphisms (SNPs) ▸ single
- n. sequence of gene
- n., triphosphopyridine

nucleotidyltransferase activity

nucleotidyltransferase, aminoglycoside

nucleus
- n., abducens
- n., accessory cuneate
- n. ambiguus
- n. arcuatus
- n. basalis of Meynert
- n., Bechterew's
- n., caudate
- n., cell
- n., cochlear
- n., cuneate
- n. cuneatus
- n., Darkshevich's
- n., deeply staining
- n., Deiters'
- n., dentate
- n., Edinger-Westphal
- n. gracilis
- n. ▸ head of caudate
- n., hilus of olivary
- n., human cell
- n. implant ▸ subthalamic
- n. lacrimalis
- n., large oval
- n. lateralis medullae oblongatae
- n. lateralis of Le Gros Clark
- n., lenticular
- n., neurilemmal cell
- n. of cell
- n. of Darkshevich
- n. of Gudden
- n. of Luys
- n. of Perlia
- n. of personality ▸ heredocongenital
- n. of Rose, lateral mammillary
- n. of thalamus, ventroposterolateral
- n., olivary
- n., oval
- n., parafascicular (PF)
- n., parasympathetic
- n., Perlia's
- n., primary
- n. pulposus

n. pulposus, extrusion of
n. pulposus (HNP) ▸ herniated
n. pulposus (HNP) ▸ herniation of
n., round
n. salivatorius
n., Schwalbe's
n., Stilling's
n., subthalamic
n. -to-cytoplasm ratio

nuclide(s)
n., daughter
n., multiple
n., radioactive

NUG (necrotizing ulcerative gingivitis)

null
n. cell adenoma
n. cell lymphoblastic leukemia
n. cells
n. hypothesis
n. point
n. type non-Hodgkins lymphoma
n., vision

nulligravida, patient
nulliparous introitus
nulliparous, patient
numb
n., feeling
n. fingers
n. hands
n. nipple
n. parts, anesthetics

Number (number)
N. (marijuana cigarette)
n., atomic
n., Avogadro's
n., Euler's
n., laboratory ID
n., mass
n., neutron
n., slow
n., thermal

numbing
n. and amnesia ▸ emotional
n., emotional

numbness
n., aching and
n. and disbelief ▸ shock
n. and hypesthesia
n. and tingling
n. and tingling around mouth
n. and tingling in fingers
n. and weakness ▸ tingling,
n., arm
n. ▸ cold, burning, pain and

n., emotional
n., episode of
n., hypesthesia and
n. in arm
n. in extremities ▸ tingling or
n. in feet
n. in feet ▸ tingling and
n. in fingers and/or toes
n. in lower back
n. in lower leg
n., localized
n. ▸ localized tingling or
n. of arm ▸ sudden
n. of arm ▸ sudden weakness or
n. of arm ▸ weakness or
n. of extremities
n. of extremity ▸ sudden weakness or
n. of face ▸ sudden weakness or
n. of face ▸ weakness or
n. of feet
n. of fingers
n. of leg ▸ sudden
n. of leg ▸ weakness or
n. of lips
n. of lower leg
n. of tongue
n. one side of body
n. one side of body ▸ sudden weakness or
n. one side of face ▸ sudden
n. or paralysis ▸ sudden weakness,
n. or tingling
n. or weakness, temporary
n., penile
n., prolonged
n. ▸ sense of disbelief, shock,
n., skin
n., sudden
n. tingling and burning
n. tingling and pain
n., tingling or weakness
n. ▸ tingling, prickling, or
n., weakness and paralysis of arm
n., weakness and paralysis of face
n., weakness and paralysis of leg

numerary renal anomaly
numeric
n. abilities
n. atrophy
n. hypertrophy

numerical scale, Borg
numerous
n. adhesions
n. compression fractures

n. physicians ▸ patient sees
n. to count (TNTC) ▸ too
n. tumor nodules ▸ studded with

nummular
n. aortitis
n. eczema
n. eczematous dermatitis
n. sputum

nummularis, keratitis
Numorphan (Goma)
nun's murmur
nurse (Nurse)('s)
n. aide
N. Association (VNA) ▸ Visiting
n. cells
n., charge
n., circulating
n., clinical
n. clinician, psychiatric
n. consultant
n., critical care
N. (ESN) ▸ Environmental Surveillance
N. Epidemiologist (NE)
N., Head
N., Health
n., hospice
N. (ICN) ▸ Infection Control
N. (LPN) ▸ Licensed Practical
n. manager
n. manager, clinical
n. -on-call ▸ surgical
n. practitioner
n., primary
N. (PHN) ▸ Public Health
N. (QCN) ▸ Quality Control
n. ▸ radiation therapy
n. screening criteria
n., scrub
n. service, visiting
n. specialist
n. specialist, clinical
n., specialty care
n., staff
n., surgical
n. therapist, rehabilitation
N. (TPN) ▸ Trained Practical
N. (VN) ▸ Visiting
N. (VRN), Visiting Registered

nursemaids' elbow
nursery (Nursery)
n. exposure
n., hand-washing in
N. (ICN) ▸ Intermediate Care
N., Newborn

nursery—*continued*
   N., Observation
   N. (SCN), Special Care
nursing (Nursing)
   n. assessment and diagnosis
   n. assessment and intervention ▸
     psychiatric
   n. assistance (GNA) ▸ general
   n. assistant
   n., behavioral science
   n. bottle syndrome
   n. bottle tooth decay
   n., cardiovascular
   n. care (GNC) ▸ general
   n. care, home
   n. care, intensive
   n. care, intermediate
   n. care ▸ intermittent skilled
   n. care ▸ long-term skilled
   n. care, neurological
   n. care, orthopedic
   n. care plan
   n. care, psychiatric
   n. care, respiratory
   n. care ▸ short-term
   n. care, skilled
   n. care ▸ specialized
   n. care, supportive
   n. care ▸ supportive medical/
   n. cells
   n., coronary care
   n. diagnosis
   N., Director of
   n. equipment
   n. facility
   n. facility, alternate care
   n. facility, certified skilled
   n. facility, skilled
   n., functional
   n. goals
   n., holistic
   n. home
   n. home assessment
   n. home bacteriuria
   n. home ▸ patient discharged to
   n. home ▸ patient transferred to
   n. home placement
   n. home, transfer to
   n. intervention strategies ▸
     innovative psychiatric
   n. interventions
   n. management
   n. observations
   n., primary
   n. procedure

   n. protocol
   n. service
   n. services, mini-
   n. services, psychiatric
   n. staff
   n. students, instructing
   n. supervision, general
   n. supervision, medical/
   N. Supervisor
   n. treatment
   N. Triage
nurturance
   n. and tenderness ▸ restoring
   n., eliciting
   n. ▸ manipulates to gain
nurture controversy ▸ nature-versus-nurtures patient, caregiver
nurturing
   n. activities ▸ self-
   n. ▸ lack of
   n. qualities
   n. qualities idealized
nutans, chorea
nutcracker esophagus
nutmeg
   n. (mescaline)
   n. (trimethoxy amphetamine)
   n. architecture
   n. (trimethoxy amphetamine)
     ingested
   n. (trimethoxy amphetamine)
     sniffed
nutrient(s)
   n. absorption
   n. analysis
   n., antioxidant
   n. artery
   n., brain
   n. broth
   n. broth, milliliter of
   n. cardioplegia
   n. cells
   n., conversion into
   n. deficiency
   n. deficits
   n. density
   n. ▸ diffusion of oxygen and
   n. enema
   n. intakes
   n. malabsorption
   n. medium
   n. ▸ oral chelating
   n. poisoning
   n. transfer
   n., transfer to blood

   n. vessels
nutritia, vasa
nutrition
   n., adequate
   n., altered
   n. analysis
   n. and exercise ▸ proper
   n. and weight control
   n., artificial
   n., cachexia and
   n. (TPN) catheter, total parenteral
   n. counselor
   n., elemental diet in
   n., enteral
   n., human
   n. (TPN) hyperalimentation ▸ total
     parenteral
   n., infant
   n. intake, alteration in
   n. (TPN) line, total parenteral
   n., maternal
   n. of lungs
   n., parenteral
   n. plan
   n., poor
   n., postnatal
   n., postoperative
   n., prenatal
   n., proper
   n. quackery
   n. repletion
   n. screening initiative
   n., sensible
   n., supplemental
   n. therapy
   n. therapy ▸ medical
   n. (TPN) therapy, total parenteral
   n. to recovery
   n. (TPN) ▸ total parenteral
   n. (TPPN), total peripheral
     parenteral
nutritional
   n. abnormality
   n. assessment
   n. behavior
   n. biochemistry
   n. biotherapy
   n. blindness
   n. care
   n. component ▸ medical, psycho-
     logical, spiritual, physical and
   n. consultation
   n. counseling
   n. data
   n. deficiency

n. deficit
n. deficit, potential
n. disorders
n. disturbance
n. factor
n. imbalance
n. immunity
n. intake, therapeutic
n. needs
n. planning, balanced
n. services
n. siderosis
n. status
n. supplementation
n. supplements
n. support
n. sweetener
n. therapy
n. therapy, intravenous (IV)
nutritionally balanced diet
nutritive
n. enema
n. ratio
n. yolk
Nuttallia equi
Nuttallia gibsoni
nux moschata
nux vomica
NV (naked vision)
NVA (near visual acuity)
NVD (nausea, vomiting and diarrhea)
nycthemeral rhythm
NYD (not yet diagnosed)
NYHA (New York Heart Association)
   classification
Nyhan syndrome ▸ Lesch-
Nylen-Barany maneuver
Nylmerate douche solution
nylon
n. retention suture
n., skin closed with running
   subcuticular suture of
n. suture
n. suture, intracuticular
nyong virus, O'nyong-
nystagmograph, electro◊
nystagmus
n., aural
n., associated
n., Baer's
n., Bekhterev
n., caloric
n., central
n., Cheyne
n., disjunctive

n., end-position
n., fine type
n., halting
n., horizontal
n. ▸ inner ear
n., labyrinthine
n., lateral
n., miner's
n., mixed
n. -myoclonus
n. ▸ nausea, vomiting and
n. on gaze to right ▸ moderate
n. on upward gaze ▸ slight
n. (OKN), optokinetic
n., oscillating
n., paretic
n., pendular
n. (PAN), periodic alternating
n., peripheral
n., positional
n., ptosis and/or
n., retraction
n., rotary
n., spontaneous
n., sustained horizontal
n. ▸ thermally induced
n. ▸ torsional, upbeat
n., undulatory
n., vertical
n., vestibular
n., vibratory

O

O (occipital)
O (oral)
O agglutination
O agglutinin
O. (ohne Hauch) colony
O point of cardiac apex pulse
O, streptolysin
O (ASO) titer, antistreptolysin
O, toluidine blue
OA
    OA (occipital artery)
    OA (occipitoanterior)
    OA (osteoarthritis)
    OA (Overeaters Anonymous)
oak, poison
oakridgensis, Legionella
oat
    o. cell
    o. cell carcinoma
    o. cell carcinoma, bronchogenic
    o. cell pathology
    o. cell tumor
    o. cell variety
    o. seed cell
    o. seed cell carcinoma
    o. -shaped cells
Oath, Hippocratic
OAV (oculoauriculovertebral
    dysplasia)
OB (obstetrics)
OB and GYN (obstetrics and
    gynecology)
OBE (out-of-body experience)
Obermeyer's test
Ober's
    O. operation
    O. sign
    O. test
Obersteiner-Redlich area
obese
    o. abdomen
    o., morbidly
    o. patient
obesity
    o., abdominal
    o., alimentary
    o. and inactivity
    o., central

o., chronic
o., constitutional
o. drug, anti-
o., endogenous
o., exogenous
o. gene
o., hyperinsulinar
o., hyperinterrenal
o., hyperplasmic
o., hypogonad
o., hypoplasmic
o., hypothyroid
o. hypoventilation syndrome
o. ▸ male pattern
o., massive
o., morbid
o. -related causes
o. -related disease
o., severe
o., simple
o., striae from
o. surgery
o., truncal
obeys commands, patient
OBG (obstetrics and gynecology)
object(s)
    o. amalgam, emotional-
    o. blurry, distant
    o., distant
    o. embedded
    o. /face recognition
    o. ▸ fixation on a single
    o., foreign
    o. fuzzy, distant
    o. in wound ▸ foreign
    o., inability to recognize
    o. ▸ inappropriate attachment to
    o., lightweight
    o. lodged in ear
    o., mental
    o. modulation
    o., ocular pursuit of
    o., patient ▸ swallowed foreign
    o., potentially dangerous
    o. relations psychotherapy
    o. relations theory
    o. relationship

o. sorting test
o., transitional
o., viewing a near
o. vision system
objection, conscientious
objective
    o., achromatic
    o., apochromatic
    o. assessment
    o. baseline data
    o. basis
    o. change
    o. decision
    o., dry
    o., establish treatment
    o. evidence
    o., fluorite
    o., immersion
    o. improvement
    o., interpersonally
    o. neurologic signs
    o. personality testing
    o. response
    o., semiapochromatic
    o. sensation
    o. sign
    o. symptoms
    o. tinnitus
oblation (*same as* ablation)
obligate
    o. aerobes
    o. anaerobes
    o. carrier
    o. intercellular organisms
obligation(s)
    o. ▸ honor financial
    o., moral
    o., primary
obligatory alkalinization
obligatory parasite
obliqua pelvis, diameter
oblique
    o. amputation
    o. (RAO) angulation ▸ right
        anterior
    o., anterior
    o. approach ▸ supine

oblique—*continued*
- o. approximated, internal
- o. arytenoid muscle
- o. astigmatism
- o. axial projection, lateral
- o. axial projection, medial
- o. conus
- o. diameter of pelvis
- o., external
- o. fascia, external
- o. film
- o. fissure
- o. fracture
- o. hernia
- o. illumination
- o. incision
- o., internal
- o., isocentric
- o. jaw roentgenogram, lateral
- o. lateral projection
- o. (LAO), left anterior
- o. (LPO), left posterior
- o. muscle
- o. muscle ▸ advancement of inferior
- o. muscle ▸ advancement of superior
- o. muscle, external
- o. muscle, inferior
- o. muscle, internal
- o. muscle of abdomen ▸ external
- o. muscle of abdomen ▸ internal
- o. muscle of auricle
- o. muscle of eyeball ▸ inferior
- o. muscle of eyeball ▸ superior
- o. muscle, superior
- o. position
- o. (RAO) position ▸ right anterior
- o. presentation
- o. projection, anterior
- o. projection, lateromedial
- o. projection, left anterior
- o. ridge
- o., right anterior
- o. (RAO) ▸ right anterior
- o. (RPO), right posterior
- o. sinus
- o. spot view
- o. study
- o. tendon, superior
- o. vein, Marshall's
- o. vein of left atrium
- o. view
- o. view ▸ long axial

obliquity
- o. inferior muscle

- o. inferior, musculus
- o., Litzmann's
- o., Nagele's
- o. reflex
- o., Roederer's obliquus
- o. superior muscle
- o. superior, musculus

obliterans
- o. (ASO), arteriosclerosis
- o., arteriosclerotic
- o., arteritis
- o., balanitis xerotica
- o., bronchiolitis
- o., bronchiolitis fibrosa
- o., bronchitis
- o., cerebrospinal thromboangiitis
- o., endarteritis
- o. organizing pneumonia, bronchiolitis
- o., pericarditis
- o., thromboangiitis
- o., thromboarteriosclerosis
- o., xerotica

obliterated, costophrenic angle
obliterating
- o. bronchiolitis, acute
- o. pericarditis
- o. phlebitis

obliteration
- o., cortical
- o. of cavity
- o. of cul-de-sac
- o. of vein
- o., temporary

obliterative
- o. bronchiolitis
- o. cardiomyopathy
- o. pleuritis
- o. vascular disease

oblongata, medulla
oblongata, pons
oblongatae, nucleus lateralis medullae
O'Brien('s)
- O. akinesia
- O. block
- O. cataract

OBS (organic brain syndrome)
obscene
- o. gestures ▸ makes
- o. gestures ▸ patient displays
- o. statements ▸ makes

obscenities, spewing
obscure
- o. detail

- o. etiology, fever of
- o. vision

obscured, details
observation(s) (Observation)
- o. and examination
- o. and hydration ▸ 24 hour period of
- o. and monitoring
- o. and treatment
- o. and treatment ▸ patient admitted for
- o., conservative
- o., constant
- o., continuous
- o. for rejection, daily
- o. form ▸ seclusion/restraint
- o., medical
- O. Nursery
- o., nursing
- o., patient admitted for
- o., patient discharged after brief
- o., patient discharged after period of
- o., period of
- o., preliminary
- O. Radio (COR) ▸ Coronary
- o., skilled
- o., treatment and
- O. Unit (ITOU) ▸ Intensive Therapy

observational learning
observational study
observed
- o. heart
- o. therapy, directly
- o. tremor, marked
- o. tremor, mild
- o. value

observers ▸ authorization form to admit
obsessed culture ▸ success-
obsession(s)
- o. and rituals ▸ idiosyncratic
- o., bizarre
- o. focus
- o., germ
- o., jealousy and control
- o. with imagined ugliness ▸ irrational

obsessional
- o. and compulsive symptoms
- o. constitution ▸ ideo-
- o. ideas ▸ overvalued
- o. neurosis
- o. slowness ▸ primary
- o. speech
- o. symptoms
- o. thoughts

o. thoughts ▸ vague
o. urges ▸ violent

obsessive
o. behavior
o. -compulsive
o. -compulsive behavior (OCB)
o. -compulsive conduct disorder
o. -compulsive disorder (OCD)
o. -compulsive disorder ▸ treatment-resistant
o. -compulsive neurosis
o. -compulsive overeating
o. -compulsive personality
o. -compulsive personality disorder
o. -compulsive reaction
o. -compulsive spectrum disorder
o. dieting
o. exercise
o. neurotic
o., patient
o. personality
o. rumination
o. symptoms
o. -type personality

obsoleta, placenta
obstacle course, wheelchair
obstetric (OB)
o. analgesia
o. anesthesia
o. auscultation
o. complications of drug abuse
o. conjugate diameter
o. disorder
o. disorder, cocaine-related
o. stethoscope ▸ DeLee-Hillis

obstetrical (Obstetrical)
o. binder
o. history
o. infection
o. injury
o. management of drug abuser
o. position
O. Service
o. stethoscope
O. Unit

obstetrician's hand
obstetrics and gynecology (OB and GYN/OBG)
obstetrics, psychoprophylaxis in
obstipated, patient
obstipation [*constipation*]
obstruct flow of air
obstructed
o., airway
o. airway skills

o. arteries
o. bile duct
o. blood flow
o. by foreign body (FB) ▸ nostril
o. common duct
o. labor
o., nares
o., nares not
o. nasal airways
o. nasal passage
o. pulmonary artery
o., shunt
o., testis
o. throat
o., tube
o. upper airway
o., urethra completely

obstructing
o. adhesions, bowel
o. airway ▸ FB (foreign body)
o. airway, food
o. airway, tongue
o. artery ▸ fracture plaque
o. bolus of food
o. lesion
o. mass

obstruction
o., abdominal
o., airway
o., aortic valve
o., arterial
o., bile duct
o., biliary
o., biliary tract
o., bladder
o., bladder neck
o. ▸ bladder outlet
o., bowel
o., bronchial
o., cardiac
o. carotid vessels, major
o., central retinal vein
o., chronic airway
o., chronic bile
o., chronic outlet
o., complete
o., complete bowel
o. ▸ congenital lacrimal
o. ▸ constipation from intestinal
o. ▸ diarrhea from intestinal
o. disease, airway
o., eustachian tube
o., extrahepatic
o., extrahepatic venous
o., extrinsic

o., false colonic
o., fecalith
o. ▸ fixed airflow
o., forearm
o., foreign body
o. ▸ foreign body airway
o., gastric outlet
o., hepatic
o. in syncope, cardiac
o., inferior vena caval (IVC)
o., infundibular
o. ▸ intermittent small bowel
o., internal
o., intestinal
o., intestinal pseudo-
o., intrahepatic
o., intrinsic
o., kidney
o., large bowel
o. ▸ left ventricular (LV) low outflow tract
o. ▸ left ventricular (LV) low tract
o., lower airway
o., lymphatic
o., mechanical
o., mechanical bowel
o., mesenteric
o., mitral
o., nasal
o., nasal airway
o. of air passages
o. of airflow
o. of airway
o. of airway, complete
o. of bladder ▸ partial
o. of ear
o. of esophagus ▸ major
o. of esophagus ▸ slight
o. of fallopian tube
o. of flow
o. of major organs
o. of pancreatic duct
o. of renal artery ▸ progressive
o. of ureter
o. of urethra
o., outflow
o. ▸ outflow tract
o., outlet
o., pain and
o., partial
o., partial intestinal
o., plaque
o., proximal
o. ▸ pulmonary vascular
o., pyloric

obstruction—*continued*
- o., reduced outflow
- o., renal
- o., respiratory
- o. ▸ right ventricular (RV) inflow
- o. ▸ right ventricular (RV) outflow
- o. ▸ saphenous vein
- o. secondary to carcinoma ▸ extrahepatic binary
- o. ▸ shock due to
- o., small bowel
- o. ▸ stop-valve airway
- o., subpulmonary
- o., subvalvular
- o., suprahepatic venous
- o. syndrome ▸ distal intestinal
- o., temporary
- o. ▸ thyroid mass causing
- o., total
- o., tracheal
- o., transverse colon
- o., tubal
- o., tube free of
- o. ▸ unconscious airway
- o., unilateral nasal
- o. ▸ unilateral ureteral
- o., upper airway
- o., ureteral
- o., ureteropelvic
- o., ureteropelvic junction
- o., urinary
- o., vascular
- o., vena caval
- o., venous
- o. with ascites ▸ small bowel

obstructive
- o. airway defect
- o. airway disease
- o. airway disease, chronic
- o. airway disease, lower
- o. airway disease ▸ reversible
- o. anuria
- o. apnea
- o. atelectasis
- o. bronchitis, chronic
- o. cardiomyopathy, familial hypertrophic
- o. cardiomyopathy, hypertrophic
- o. coronary disease ▸ underlying
- o. defect
- o. defect, chronic
- o. disease
- o. disease (AIOD), aortoiliac
- o. disease, carotid
- o. disease (CVOD) ▸ cerebrovascular

- o. disease ▸ pulmonary vascular
- o. dysmenorrhea
- o. emphysema
- o. emphysema ▸ localized
- o. glaucoma
- o. hydrocephalus
- o. jaundice
- o. lesion
- o. lung disease
- o. lung disease, chronic
- o. lung disease ▸ cigarette-induced
- o. lung disease, lower
- o. murmur
- o. neuropathy
- o. phenomenon
- o. phlebitis
- o. physiology
- o. pneumonia
- o. problems, vocal
- o. prostatism
- o. pulmonary disease
- o. pulmonary disease (COPD), chronic
- o. pulmonary emphysema
- o. pulmonary emphysema (COPE), chronic
- o. respiratory disease, chronic
- o. rushes
- o. shock
- o. site
- o. sleep apnea
- o. symptoms
- o. thrombus
- o. uropathy
- o. ventilatory defect

obtain [*attain*]
obtain physician order
obtained
- o. by massage ▸ carotid pulse
- o., good exposure
- o., hemostasis
- o., limited exposure
- o. with Doptone, FHT (fetal heart tones)

obtundation, increased
obtunded, patient
obtundity, state of mental
obturating embolus
obturator
- o. airway ▸ esophageal
- o. artery
- o. crest
- o. foramen
- o. fossa
- o. hernia

- o. muscle, external
- o. muscle, internal
- o. nerve
- o. nerve crush
- o. neurectomy
- o. sign
- o., Timberlake
- o. veins

obtuse
- o. marginal (OM)
- o. marginal artery
- o. marginal artery ▸ first
- o. marginal artery ▸ second
- o. marginal branch
- o. marginal, first
- o. marginal lymphatic
- o. marginal, second
- o., patient

obvelata, Syphacia
OC (occlusocervical)
occasional
- o. anxiety
- o. assistance, patient requires
- o. auditory hallucinations
- o. confusion
- o. drink
- o. drug use
- o. drug user, patient
- o. late filling wave
- o. palpitations, patient has
- o. parasite
- o. premature beat
- o. seizure activity
- o. synesthesia
- o. tactile hallucinations

occidentalis, Dermacentor
occidentalis, Prunus
occipital
- o. aphasia, parieto-
- o. area
- o. artery (OA)
- o. artery ▸ parieto-
- o. bone
- o. bone ▸ interclavicular notch of
- o. bone ▸ jugular notch of
- o. condyle metastasis syndrome
- o. cortex
- o. diameter, fronto-
- o. diameter, mento-
- o. diploic vein
- o. dysfunction ▸ localized
- o. emissary vein
- o. fontanelle
- o. foramen
- o. fracture

o., fronto-
o. gyri, lateral
o. gyrus, inferior
o. gyrus, superior
o. headache
o. intermittent rhythmical delta activity (OIRDA)
o. lobe
o. lobe infarcts, bilateral
o. lobe, medial surface
o. lobe of brain
o. lobe of brain ▸ excision
o. lobe of brain, mesial surface of
o. lobes ▸ sulci of
o. lymph nodes
o. muscle
o. nerve, greater
o. nerve, internal
o. nerve, least
o. nerve, lesser
o. nerve, third
o., parieto-
o. placement, parieto-
o., postero-
o. protuberance
o. protuberance, external
o. protuberance, transverse
o. region
o. region, parieto-
o. regions of head
o. rhythm, basic
o. segment
o. sharp transient, positive
o. sharp transients of sleep ▸ positive
o. sinus
o. slow wave foci
o. slow wave focus
o. spike focus
o. spur
o. suture
o. vein

occipitale magnum, foramen
occipitale, os
occipitalis, arcus parieto-
occipitoanterior (OA)
o. (LOA) ▸ left
o. position
o., right
occipitoatlantoaxial anomaly
occipitodextra (OD)
o. anterior (ODA)
o. posterior (ODP)
o. transverse (ODT)

occipitofrontal
o. circumference (OFC)
o. diameter
o. muscle
occipitolaeva anterior (OLA)
occipitolaeva posterior (OLP)
occipitomastoid suture
occipitomastoid suture lines
occipitomental diameter
occipitoparietal suture
occipitoposterior
o., left
o. position
o., right
occipitosacral position
occipitosphenoidal suture
occipitotemporal
o. convolution
o. gyrus, lateral
o. gyrus, medial
occipitotemporalis lateralis, gyrus
occipitotemporalis medians, gyrus
occipitotransverse
o., left
o. position
o., right
occiput posterior, persistent
occlude blood vessel in vital organs
occluded
o. artery
o., blood vessel
o., bronchi
o. carotid vessels
o. common bile duct stent
o. coronary vessels
o., fistula site
o., renal artery
o. segments, bypass
occludens, zonula
occluder prosthesis ▸ Rashkind double-disk
occluding
o. agent ▸ fluid vascular
o. frame
o. ligature
o. thrombus
occlusal
o., axio-
o., axiomesio-
o. balance
o., bucco-
o. contact
o., disto-
o., distobucco-
o., distolinguo-

o. embrasure
o. equilibration
o. glide
o. harmony
o. harmony, functional
o. level
o., linguo-
o., mesio-
o., mesiobucco-
o., mesiolinguo-
o. pattern
o. position
o. pressure
o. relationship
o. surface
o. surface of tooth
occlusion (Occlusion)
o., abnormal
o., acentric
o., acute
o., acute abdominal aortic
o., acute aortic
o., acute arterial
o., afunctional
o., anatomic
o., angioplasty-related vessel
o., anterior
o., aortic
o., aortic bifurcation
o., arterial
o., arteriosclerotic
o., balanced
o. basilar artery ▸ total
o., branch retinal vein
o., branch vessel
o., buccal
o., capsular
o., central
o. ▸ central retinal artery
o., centric
o., cerebrovascular
o., chronic
o., complete
o., components of
o., coronary
o., coronary artery
O. Device ▸ Prima Total
o., distal
o., disto-
o., eccentric
o., edge-to-edge
o., embolic
o., end-to-end
o., enteromesenteric
o. ▸ femoral artery

occlusion—*continued*
- o. ▸ femoral vein
- o. ▸ femoropopliteal artery
- o., functional
- o., graft
- o., habitual
- o., high
- o., hyperfunctional
- o., hypogastric
- o., ideal
- o. ▸ iliac artery
- o. ▸ inferior mesenteric vascular
- o. ▸ inferior vena cava
- o. ▸ intermittent coronary sinus
- o. (ICAO), internal carotid artery
- o., lateral
- o. left bronchus
- o., liminal
- o., line of
- o., lingual
- o. main bronchus, partial
- o., meniscoid
- o. ▸ mesenteric artery
- o. ▸ mesenteric vascular
- o., mesial
- o., neutral
- o. ▸ nonacute total
- o., normal
- o. of arterial supply
- o. of arteries
- o. of bronchus
- o. of internal carotid arteries
- o. of intramuscular arteries
- o. of left bronchus
- o. of left carotid artery
- o. of mainstem bronchus
- o. of pupil
- o. of retinal arterioles
- o. of right carotid artery
- o. of right coronary trunk ▸ complete
- o., partial
- o., pathogenic
- o., physiologic
- o. plethysmography ▸ venous
- o., posterior
- o., postnormal
- o., prenormal
- o. pressure ▸ pulmonary artery
- o., protrusive
- o. pulmonary angiography, balloon
- o., punctal
- o. ▸ recurrent mesenteric vascular
- o. ▸ retinal artery
- o. ▸ retinal vein
- o. ▸ retinal vessel
- o., retrusive
- o., severe cerebrovascular
- o. ▸ side branch
- o., spherical form of
- o. ▸ straight protrusive
- o. ▸ superior mesenteric vascular
- o. system ▸ vessel
- o. technique, airway
- o. ▸ temporary unilateral pulmonary artery
- o., terminal
- o. test, ear
- o., thrombotic
- o. time
- o., total outlet
- o., traumatic
- o., traumatogenic
- o. ▸ treatable vascular
- o., tubal
- o., vascular
- o. ▸ venous mesenteric vascular
- o., working

occlusive
- o. arteriopathies
- o. atherosclerosis
- o. disease
- o. disease, aortoiliac
- o. disease, arterial
- o. disease, arteriosclerotic
- o. disease, carotid
- o. disease, carotid vaso-
- o. disease, chronic
- o. disease, coronary
- o. disease, coronary artery
- o. disease, femoral popliteal
- o. disease ▸ multisystem
- o. disease of liver ▸ veno-
- o. disease, peripheral arterial
- o. disease, peripheral arteriosclerotic
- o. disease ▸ pulmonary veno-
- o. disease, severe
- o. disease ▸ vertebrobasilar
- o. dressing
- o., dressing dry and
- o. emboli, aortic
- o. lesion
- o. meningitis
- o. thromboaortopathy
- o. thrombus
- o. vascular disease
- o. wedge pressure ▸ pulmonary artery

occlusodistal, mesio-

occult
- o. abscess
- o. aortic stenosis
- o. bleeding
- o. blood
- o. blood in stool
- o. blood, positive
- o. blood, stool positive for
- o. blood test
- o. blood test (FOBT) ▸ fecal
- o. blood test ▸ focal
- o. blood testing ▸ fecal
- o. cancer
- o. fracture
- o. immunization
- o. infection
- o. lesions
- o. lung cancer
- o. metastasis
- o. metastatic disease
- o. pericardial constriction
- o. pericarditis
- o. pulmonary emboli

occulta, amentia
occulta, spina bifida
occupancy rate
occupation
- o. functioning ▸ impairment in
- o. ▸ mentally unstimulating
- o. neurosis
- o. tic

occupational (Occupational)
- o. activity
- o. activity ▸ increase in
- o. and social impairment
- o. asthma
- o. compensation
- o. disorder
- o. dyskinesia
- o. exposure
- o. exposure to chemicals
- o. hazards
- o. health
- o. health risk
- o. history
- o. jet lag
- o. limitation
- o. lung disease
- o. lung disorder
- o. medicine
- o. muscle spasms
- o. problem
- o. psychiatry
- o. rehabilitation

o., sexual activity ▸ increase in social,
o. stressors
O. Therapist (OT)
O. Therapy (OT)
o. therapy evaluation
o. therapy, psychosocial
o. therapy ▸ rehabilitation
occupied ▸ patient self-
occupying change, space
occupying lesion, space
occur bilaterally synchronously
occurrence(s)
o., fictitious
o., local
o. of electroencephalogram (EEG) activity ▸ non-simultaneous
o. ▸ transient spontaneous
occurring sporadically
OCD (obsessive compulsive disorder)
ocellata, Trichobilharzia
OCG (oral cholecystogram)
ochracea, Leptothrix
ochraceum, Trichophyton
ochraceus, Aspergillus
ochraceus, Cellvibrio
Ochrobium tectum
Ochromyia anthropophaga
ochronosis, exogenous
ochronosis, ocular
Ochsenbein's gingivectomy
Ochsner('s)
O. -Mahorner echocardiogram
O. muscle
O. treatment
Ocimum basilicum
o'clock position ▸ 1 (2, 3, etc.)
o'clock ▸ tear at 1 (2, 3, etc.)
O'Connor('s) operation
O'Connor('s)-Peter operation
Octomitus hominis
Octomyces etiennei
octopus test
ocular
o. abnormality
o. adnexa
o. adnexa ▸ lymphoma of
o. adnexal malignancy
o. albinism
o. and cerebellar dysfunction
o. anesthesia
o. ataxia
o. ballottement
o., cerebro-

o. chart (AOC) ▸ abridged
o. complications
o. cup
o. cytopathology
o. density (OD) values
o. disease
o. disease, herpetic
o. disease, hypertensive
o. disorder
o. effects, toxic
o. emergency
o. etiology of headache
o. fluid pressure
o. fundi
o. fundus
o. globe
o. herpes infection
o. histoplasmosis syndrome
o. humor
o. hypertelorism
o. hypertension
o. implant, BioMatrix
o. infection
o. inflammation ▸ ischemic
o. ischemic syndrome
o. larva migrans
o. lesion ▸ pathogenesis of
o. metastasis, intra-
o. muscle
o. muscle, advancement of
o. muscle dystrophy
o. muscle, myectomy of
o. muscle, myotomy of
o. muscle, recession of
o. muscle, transplantation of
o. myoclonus
o. ochronosis
o. pain
o. palsy
o. phthisis
o. pressure
o. proptosis
o. prosthesis
o. pursuit of objects
o. reflex, vestibular
o. refraction
o. region
o., retro-
o. rosacea
o. scoliosis
o. tendon, tenotomy of
o. tension
o. tissue
o. tremor
o. tremor artifact

o. vesicle
oculi
o., adnexa
o., albuginea
o., bulbus
o., fundus
o., hypertonia
o., hypotonia
o., motor
o., musculus orbicularis
o., orbicularis
o., sphincter
o., tapetum
o., tunica adnata
o., tunica vasculosa
oculoauriculovertebral (OAV) dysplasia
oculocardiac reflex
oculocephalic reflex
oculocephalic reflex, absent
oculocephalogyric reflex
oculocutaneous telangiectasia
oculodentodigital (ODD) dysplasia
oculogenitalis, Chlamydia
oculogram (EOG), electro-
oculogyric
o. crisis
o. mechanism
o. reflex, audito-
oculomotor
o. deficit
o. hemiplegia, alternating
o. nerve
o. nerve signs
o. nuclei
o. sulcus
oculomucocutaneous syndrome
oculopathy, pituitarigenic
oculopharyngeal reflex
oculoplastic reconstruction
oculoplastic surgery
oculopupillary reflex
oculosensory cell reflex
oculovagal reflex
OD
OD (occipitodextra)
OD (ocular density)
OD (overdosed)
OD (overdosed) ▸ patient
OD (overdosed) with cannabinoids, patient
OD (overdosed) with depressants, patient
OD (overdosed) with hallucinogens, patient

OD—*continued*
OD (overdosed) with inhalants, patient
OD (overdosed) with multiple drugs, patient
OD (overdosed) with opioids, patient
OD (overdosed) with phencyclidines, patient
OD (overdosed) with stimulants, patient
OD (right eye)
ODA (occipitodextra anterior)
ODD (oculodentodigital) dysplasia
ODD (oppositional defiant disorder)
odd play ▸ sustained
odd repetitive behavior
Oddi('s)
O. dysmotility disorder ▸ sphincter of
O. manometry, sphincter of
O. muscle
O. spasm, sphincter of
O., sphincter of
OD$_{450}$ delta
odontalgia, phantom
odontectomies, mandibular dentitional
odontogenic fibrosarcoma
odontogenic infection
odontoid process
odontoid, syndesmo-
odontoma
o. adamantinum
o., ameloblastic
o., complex composite
o., composite
o., compound composite
o., coronary
o., dilated
o., embryoplastic
o., fibrous
o., mixed
o., radicular
odontotomy, prophylactic
odor(s)
o., anodal closing
o., body
o., breath
o. -causing bacteria
o. -causing plaque
o., fetid
o., foot
o., hallucinatory
o., heightened sensitivity to

o. of body, locker room
o., pelvic
o., recurrent pungent
odorata, Cananga
odorous amniotic fluid
ODP (occipitodextra posterior)
ODT (occipitodextra transversa)
Oeciacus hirudinis
Oeciacus vicarius
oedematiens, Bacillus
oedematiens, Clostridium
oedematis maligni No. II ▸ Bacillus
oedematosa, coryza
Oedipal conflict
Oedipal feelings
Oedipus complex
Oehler's symptom
Oertel's treatment
oesophageal veins
Oestrus hominis
Oestrus ovis
OFC (occipitofrontal circumference)
off (Off)
o. -axis factors
o. -balance ▸ feeling
o., blood vessel sealed
o. calories, burn
o. -center ratios
o., emotional stand-
o., frozen skin sloughs
o. label use of drugs
o. label use of medication
o., peeled
o. pump coronary artery bypass (OPCAB)
O. Pounds Sensibly (TOPS) diet ▸ Take
o., sharp dose fall-
o. skin ▸ sloughed-
o. -the-job accidents
o. tissue, burn
o. -trial treatment
o. ▸ ventilator pop-
o. violence, hands-
offender(s)
o., delinquent status
o., repeat drug
o., sex
offending artery
offending organism
offense(s)
o., alcohol-related
o., drug-related
o., multiple
o., sexual

Office (office)
O., admission orders sent to Admitting
O., Admissions
O., Admitting
o. angina
o., blood counts monitored in
o. follow-up
o. follow-up ▸ patient discharged to
o. follow-up visit
o. hypertension
o., patient followed in
o. visit, postnatal
o. visit, postoperative
o. visit, postsurgical
o. visit, prenatal
Officer
O. (EO) ▸ Environmental
O. (ECO) ▸ Environmental Control
O. (ESO) ▸ Environmental Surveillance
O. (ICO) ▸ Infection Control
O. (SO) ▸ Surveillance
officinalis
o., Althaea
o., Cochlearia
o., Haementeria
officinarum, Saccharum
Offner electroencephalogram (EEG) machine
offset, E-zero
offspring
o., drug-exposed
o., unborn
o., viable
Ogston's line
Ogston's operation
ohm(s) (Ohm's)
o., expressed in
O. law
o. resistance
ohmic heating
ohmmeter, volt
ohne Hauch (O.) colony
Öhnell, X wave of
Ohnishi disease ▸ Takayasu-
OI (opportunistic infection)
oil (Oil)
o. aspiration ▸ mineral
o. breakfast
o. embolism
o. emersion field
o. emulsion, mineral
O. (hashish oil), Hash
o. (Hash Oil), hashish

o. (hashish) ▸ Honey
o. immersion
o., polyunsaturated vegetable
o., residual iodized
o., scalp
o. study, iodized
o. sugar
o. supplements, fish
o. (hashish) ▸ Weed

oily skin
oily stools
ointment
o., antibiotic
o., enzyme
o., nitrol
o., ophthalmic
o., steroid
o., topical

OIRDA (occipital intermittent rhythmical delta activity)
Okamura-Brockhurst technique, Schepens-
OKN (optokinetic nystagmus)
OKT₃ drug
OLA (occipitolaeva anterior)
old
o. age
o. age ▸ benign forgetfulness of
o. age, debilitating effects of
o. age ▸ normal atrophy of
o. age, phenomena of
o. age, premature
o. age, problems of
o. balloon angioplasty (POBA) ▸ plain
o. brain
o. burn scars
o. cystic infarct
o. dislocation
o. fibrous adhesions
o. fracture
o. healed fracture
o. healed myocardial infarction
o. incision excised
o. infarct
o. inferior wall myocardial infarction (MI)
o. myocardial infarction (MI)
o. nasal fracture
o. nasal fractures, multiple
o. pocket ▸ electrode reimplanted in
o. pseudocyst ▸ outpouching of
o. scarring
o. sight
o. subcortical infarction

o. triggers
oleate, ethanolamine
olecranal region
olecranon
o. bursa
o. fossa
o. ligament
o. process
o. spur

Oleson technique, Ritter-
olfactoria, crus
olfactorius
o. lateralis of Retzius ▸ gyrus
o. medialis, gyrus
o. medialis of Retzius ▸ gyrus

olfactory
o. amnesia
o. aura
o. brain
o. bulb
o. cells
o. esthesioneurocytoma
o. esthesioneuroepithelioma
o. ganglion
o. groove meningioma
o. hallucinations
o. hallucinations ▸ vivid visual, auditory and
o. lobe of brain
o. nerve
o. nerve signs
o. peduncle
o. perceptual changes
o. receptor cells
o. region
o. stria

oligemic shock
oligoclonal bands
oligodendroglial cell
oligo-ovulation
oligophrenia
o., moral
o., phenylpyruvic
o. phenylpyruvica
o., polydystrophic

oliva cerebellaris
olivaris, hilus nuclei
olivary
o. body
o. nucleus
o. nucleus, hilus of
o. peduncle of Schwalbe

olive tip catheter
Oliver's sign
olivocerebellar tract

olivocochlear bundle of Rasmussen
olivopontocerebellar atrophy
Ollendorff syndrome, Buschke-
Ollier('s)
O. disease
O. dyschondroplasia
O. law
O. layer
O. operation
O. syndrome
O. -Thiersch graft
O. -Thiersch operation

OLP (occipitolaeva posterior)
Olsen syndrome, Alström-
Olshausen's operation
Olshausen's sign
OM (obtuse marginal)
Omaya reservoir
omega melancholicum
omental
o. adhesions
o. adhesive band
o. apron
o. cyst
o. fat
o. grafts
o. hernia
o. lymph nodes ▸ hemorrhagic

omentectomy, total
omentum
o. and mesentery atrophic
o., colic
o., gastrocolic
o., gastrohepatic
o., gastrosplenic
o., greater
o., lesser
o. majus
o. minus
o., pancreaticosplenic
o., splenogastric
o., varicosity of

omissions, acts of
Omni
O. -Atricor pacemaker
O. -cor pacemaker
O. -Ectocor pacemaker
O. operating microscope
O. -Stanicor pacemaker

omnifocal lens
omnipotence of thought
Omniscience single leaflet cardiac valve prosthesis
Omniscience tilting disk valve prosthesis

omohyoid muscle
omphalitis, infant
omphalomesenteric duct
omphalomesenteric veins
Omsk hemorrhagic fever
Onchocerca
    O. caecutiens
    O. cervicalis
    O. gibsoni
    O. volvulus
oncofetal antigen
oncofetal antigen ▸ pancreatic
oncogene activation
oncogene expression, blocking
oncogenesis and teratogenesis
oncogenesis theory, viral
oncogenic
    o. agent
    o. effect ▸ proto-
    o. factor, anti-
oncologic anatomy
oncologic therapy protocols,
    complex
oncological radiation
oncologist
    o., clinical
    o., gynecological
    o., medical
    o., pediatric neuro-
    o., surgical
    o., urologic
Oncology (oncology)
    O. Clinic
    o., clinical
    o., gynecologic
    o., human
    o., medical
    o., mix
    o., pediatric
    o. physicist, radiation
    o., radiation
    o. rehabilitation
    O. Service
oncotic
    o. fluid
    o. pressure
    o. pressure, colloid
    o. pressure, increasing
    o. pressure (POP) ▸ plasma
    o. therapy
Oncovin
    O., methotrexate, 6-mercaptopurine
        (POMP) ▸ prednisone
    O., prednisone (COP) ▸ Cytoxan,

    O., prednisone, procarbazine
        (MOPP) ▸ nitrogen mustard,
Ondine curse breathing
Ondine's curse
I(1)
    I alcoholic, Type
    1 -antitrypsin deficiency, alpha-
    1 -antitrypsin serum ▸ alpha-
    I apertognathia repair, LeFort
    1 beta ▸ interleukin
    I gastrostomy, Billroth
    1 gene ▸ human preproendothelin-
    1 hypertension ▸ Stage
    1, grid
    1 hemadsorption virus (HA1) ▸ type
    1, input terminal
    1 (2, 3, etc.) o'clock position
    1 (2, 3, etc.) o'clock ▸ tear at
    1, parainfluenza virus
    1 ▸ Stahl ear, No.
    1, 3-glucosidase deficiency ▸ a-
    1 through 6 murmur ▸ Grade
    1 through 6 ▸ V leads
100 milliliters (mg%) ▸ milligrams per
110 mobile x-ray unit ▸ AMX
111 scintigraphy ▸ indium
^{113m}In-transferrin
125 serum albumin, iodinated I
131 MIBG scintigraphy ▸ iodine
132, tantalum-
137 bougie tube brachytherapy,
    cesium
137, cesium
137 teletherapy machine, cesium
195m radionuclide ▸ gold
197, chlormerodrin Hg
one (One)
    o. and two rescuer CPR
        (cardiopulmonary resuscitation)
    o. block claudication
    o. -celled organisms
    o. -child sterility
    o. counseling ▸ one-to-
    O. Diet ▸ Step-
    o. eye, blurred vision in
    o. eye ▸ dimmed vision in
    o. eye ▸ double vision in
    o. -flight exertional dyspnea
    o. hole angiographic catheter
    o. meter (rhm) ▸ roentgens per
        hour at
    o. -on-one patient care
    o. -on-one personal care
    o. -on-one therapy

    o. person CPR (cardiopulmonary
        resuscitation)
    o. personal care, one-on-
    o. -rescuer CPR (cardiopulmonary
        resuscitation)
    o. second ▸ forced expiratory
        volume in
    o. side of body ▸ muscular
        weakness
    o. side of body ▸ numbness
    o. side of body ▸ progressive
        weakness
    o. side of body ▸ sudden weakness
    o. side of body ▸ sudden weakness
        or numbness
    o. side of body ▸ temporary
        weakness
    o. side of face ▸ sudden numbness
    o. side of face ▸ sudden paralysis
    o. side of face ▸ sudden weakness
    o. side of neck ▸ spasm
    o. -sided chorea
    o. -sided headaches
    o. spinal muscular atrophy ▸ Type
    o. -stage esophagectomy in benign
        disease
    o. -stage retrosternal bypass
        coloplasty
    o. -stitch cataract procedure
    o. -stitch technique
    o. -to-one counseling
    o. ventricle heart
    o. -year survival rate
ongoing
    o. assessment ▸ complete and
    o. clinical trials
    o. monitoring
    o. pastoral care
    o. relationship
    o. stress
    o. surveillance
    o. treatment of patient
onion scale lesion
onionskin lesion
onlay
    o. bone graft
    o. cortical graft, single
    o. graft
    o. graft, dual
online stress test
only (LPO) ▸ light perception
only ▸ patient treated for comfort
onset
    o., abrupt
    o., acute

o., adult
o. adult diabetes, acute
o. Alzheimer's disease ▸ early
o. asthma ▸ late
o. crack dependence ▸ late-
o., crisis
o. diabetes, adult
o. diabetes, juvenile-
o. diabetes ▸ mature
o. diabetes mellitus (DM) ▸ adult
o. diabetes mellitus (DM) ▸ juvenile
o. familial Alzheimer's disease ▸ early
o., focal
o., gradual
o. insomnia, sleep
o., juvenile
o., maturity
o. muscle soreness, delayed
o. of atrial fibrillation ▸ acute
o. of chills and fever
o. of cycle
o. of dyspnea ▸ insidious
o. of facial weakness
o. of fever, sudden
o. of flashes and floaters ▸ recent
o. of jaundice, rapid
o. of labor
o. of labor, spontaneous
o. of menarche
o. of menses
o. of menstruation
o. of menstruation, early
o. of nausea
o. of overt heart failure
o. of pain ▸ spontaneous
o. of paralysis
o. of senility ▸ early
o. of stimulus
o. of symptoms
o. of unconsciousness, sudden
o. of weakness ▸ progressive
o. (PO), period of
o., rapid eye movements (REM)
o. REM (rapid eye movements) period, sleep
o., severe
o., sleep
o., sudden
o. ▸ symptoms of stroke
o., uncomplicated ▸ primary degenerative dementia of Alzheimer type, presenile

o., uncomplicated ▸ primary degenerative dementia of Alzheimer type, senile
o. (WASO), wake after sleep
o., with delirium ▸ primary degenerative dementia of Alzheimer type, senile
o., with delusions ▸ primary degenerative dementia of Alzheimer type, senile
o., with depression ▸ primary degenerative dementia of Alzheimer type, presenile
o., with depression ▸ primary degenerative dementia of Alzheimer type, senile
onychogenic substance
onychomycosis ▸ distal subungual
onychomycosis, fingernail
O'nyong-nyong virus
oogenetic cycle
oophorectomy
o., bilateral prophylactic
o. (s-o) ▸ bilateral salpingo-
o. ▸ laparoscopic salpingo-
o., prophylactic
o. (s-o) ▸ salpingo-
o. (s-o) ▸ unilateral salpingo-
oophoretic cyst
oophoritis, fetal
oophoritis parotidea
oophorus, cumulus
Oort, bundle of
ooze, capillary points of
ooze, graft
oozed blood, shunt
oozing
o. about shunt site
o., bleeding and
o. blood, nostril
o. fistula
o. fluid
o. from dermatitis
o. from eczema
o. from os, blood
o. from site, active
o. from wound
o. from wound, active
o. of blood
o. purulent material, wound
OP (Op)
OP (opening pressure)
OP (opium)
OP (osmotic pressure)
opaca, cornea

opacification
o., alveolar
o., amorphous parenchymal
o., apical
o., coronary
o., cortical
o., faint
o. ▸ ground-glass
o., lens
o., mongol
o., normal
o., opaque linear
o., stringy
o. study
opacity(-ies)
o., capsular
o., Caspar's ring
o., corneal
o., early lens
o., left chest
o., linear
o., stromal
o., subcapsular
o., vitreous
opaline plaque
opaque
o. arthrography
o. calculi
o. contact lens
o. enema
o. foreign body (FB)
o. free bodies
o. linear opacification
o. material
o. medium
o. microscope
o. myelography
o. shadows
OPCAB (off pump coronary artery bypass)
OPD (Outpatient Department)
open
o. -air drying
o. airway
o. amputation
o. angle glaucoma
o. angle glaucoma, chronic
o. angle glaucoma ▸ primary
o. biopsy
o. biopsy ▸ imaging-guided
o. biopsy of lung and pleura
o. bite
o. -bite malocclusion
o. bladder brachytherapy implant
o. blocked fallopian tubes

open—*continued*
- o., bracing vessel walls
- o. bronchus sign
- o. -chain chain
- o. chest cardiac massage
- o. chest cardiac resuscitation
- o. crib
- o. dislocation
- o. drainage (dr'ge)
- o. drainage (dr'ge) ▸ thoracotomy with
- o. drop anesthesia
- o. -ended support group
- o. ends of stomach and duodenum ▸ closure
- o. eye procedure
- o. -face crown
- o. fistula
- o., fontanelle
- o. fracture
- o. fresh traumatic wounds
- o. genital sores
- o. glottis
- o. heart surgery
- o. heart table ▸ Siemens
- o. hospital
- o. injury
- o. label study
- o. lung biopsy
- o. mouth position
- o. pneumothorax
- o. practice of euthanasia
- o. prostatectomy
- o. pubic arch
- o. reduction
- o. reduction and internal fixation (ORIF)
- o. reduction of fracture
- o. reduction of humerus
- o. reduction of skull fracture
- o. rib cage ▸ splaying
- o. sore, persistent nonhealing
- o. sores
- o. spine
- o. spontaneously, eyes
- o. surgical biopsy
- o., teased
- o. technique
- o. to pain, eyes
- o. to speech, eyes
- o. tuberculosis
- o. womb operation
- o. womb surgery
- o. wound
- o. wound of skin

opened
- o., capsule
- o., chest
- o., chest cavity
- o., chest muscles
- o., pericardium
- o., pleura
- o. posteriorly, lumbodorsal fascia
- o. transversely, skin

opening
- o., abdominal
- o. airway
- o., anal
- o. (AO), anodal
- o. (AO), aortic
- o., aortic valve
- o., artificial
- o., bile duct
- o., bite
- o. clonus, cathodal
- o. contraction
- o. contraction (AOC), anodal
- o. contraction, cathodal
- o., duodenal
- o. for bile drainage, patent
- o. in joint, temporary
- o., incomplete
- o. movement
- o. narrow, duodenal
- o. of atrioventricular valves
- o., oval-shaped
- o., patent
- o., peritoneal
- o., permanent urinary
- o., pilosebaceous
- o., piriform
- o. pressure (OP)
- o., sheath
- o., sinus
- o. snap
- o. snap (MOS) ▸ mitral
- o. snap ▸ tricuspid
- o., surgically created
- o., temporary
- o., temporary urinary
- o. tetanus (AOT), anodal
- o. through lens
- o., urethral
- o., vertical
- o. wedge-type osteotomy

opera-glass hand
operable
- o. breast cancer
- o. cancer
- o. case

operant
- o. acceleration of heart rate
- o. cardiac conditioning
- o. conditioning
- o. deceleration of heart rate
- o. heart rate conditioning ▸ human

operated
- o. calcium channel ▸ receptor
- o. on, patient
- o. penile implant, pump-

operating (Operating)
- o. microscope
- o. microscope, Omni
- o. microscope, Shambaugh-Derlacki
- o. microscope, Zeiss
- O. Room
- O. Room, Director of
- o. scope
- o. voltage

operation
- o., Abbe's
- o., Abbott
- o., Abbott-Lucas
- o., Abell's
- o., Abernethy's
- o., Aburel's
- o., Adams'
- o., Adelmann's
- o., Agnew's
- o., Albee-Delbet
- o., Albee's
- o., Albert's
- o., Aldrich's
- o., Alexander-Adams
- o., Alexander's
- o., Ammon's
- o., Anagnostakis'
- o. and grafting of tissue ▸ authorization form for
- o. and grafting of tissue ▸ consent form for
- o., Anderson's
- o., Andrews
- o., Anel's
- o., Annandale's
- o., Argyll Robertson
- o., Arlt-Jaesche
- o., Arlt's
- o., Arruga's
- o., arterial switch
- o., atrial baffle
- o., authorization form for
- o., authorization form for taking of motion pictures of

o., authorization form for televising of
o., Avila's
o., Axer's
o., Badal's
o., Badgley's
o., Baldwin's
o., Baldy-Webster
o., Baldy's
o., Ball's
o., Bancroft-Plenk
o., Bankart's
o., Bardelli's
o., Barkan's
o., Barker's
o., Barraquer's
o., Barrio's
o., Barton's
o., Barwell's
o., basiotripsy
o., Basset's
o., Bassini's
o., Basterra's
o., Bateman's
o., Baudelocque's
o., Beatson's
o., Beck-Jianu
o., Beer's
o., Bent's
o., Berens'
o., Berke
o., Bielschowsky's
o., Bigelow's
o., Billroth I
o., Billroth II
o., Bischoff's
o., Bissell's
o., Blair's
o., Blalock-Hanlon
o., Blalock-Taussig
o., Blasius'
o., Blaskovics'
o., Blatt's
o., Blount's
o., Blundell-Jones
o., Bobroff's
o., Bodinger's
o., Böhm's
o., Bonnet
o., Bonaccolto-Flieringa
o., Bonzel's
o., Borthen
o., Bossalino's
o., Bosworth's
o., Bouilly's

o., Bowman's
o., Boyd's
o., Bozeman's
o., Brailey
o., Brauer
o., Brenner's
o., Brett's
o., Bricker's
o., Briggs'
o., Bristow's
o., Brittain's
o., Brockman's
o., Brock's
o., Brophy's
o., Brunschwig's
o., Buck's
o., Bunnell's
o., Burch's
o., Burow's
o., Buzzi's
o., Cairns'
o., Caldwell-Luc
o., Callahan's
o., Campbell's
o., cardiopulmonary bypass
o., Carrell's
o., Carter's
o., Casanellas'
o., Castroviejo's
o., cataract flap
o., Cave
o., Cave-Rowe
o., Celsus'
o., Chiene's
o., Cloward's
o., Codivilla's
o., Coffey's
o., Cole's
o., Collin-Beard
o., Colonna's
o., Commando's
o., Compere's
o., computer-assisted
o., Conn's
o. consent form
o., consent form for
o., consent form for taking of motion pictures of
o., consent form for televising of
o., Cotte's
o., Crafoord's
o., Credo's
o., Critchett's
o., Crutchfield
o., Csapody's

o., Cubbins
o., Custodis'
o., Cutler-Beard
o., Czermak's
o., Dana's
o., Daniel's
o., Darrach's
o., Davier's
o., Davies-Colley
o., Davis'
o., de Grandmont's
o., Decker's
o., Del Toro's
o., Delorme's
o., Denuse's
o. DeWecker
o., Dickson-Diveley
o., Dickson's
o., Dieffenbach's
o., Doderlein's
o., Doléris'
o., Donald-Fothergill
o., Donald's
o., Doyen's
o., Dudley's
o., Dührssen's
o., Dunn-Brittain
o., Dupuy-Dutemps
o., Durman's
o., Durr's
o., Duverger and Velter's
o., Eden-Hybbinette
o., Eggers'
o., Elliot's
o., Ellis-Jones
o., Elmslie-Cholmeley
o., Eloesser's
o., Elschnig's
o., Ely's
o., Emmet's
o., equilibrating
o., Estes'
o., Estlander's
o., Evans'
o., Eversbusch's
o., eyelid ptosis
o., Eyler's
o., Fahey's
o., Falk-Shukuds
o., Falk's
o., Fasanella
o., Fasanella-Servat
o., fenestration
o., Filatov-Marzinkowsky
o., Filatov's

operation—*continued*

o., Flajani's
o., Fleming's
o., foraminotomy
o., Förster-Penfield
o., Förster's
o., Fothergill's
o., Fowler's
o., Fox's
o., Franceshetti's
o. ▸ Frangenheim-Goebell-Stoeckel
o., Frazier-Spiller
o., Freund's
o., Fricke's
o., Friedenwald's
o., Friede's
o., Friedrich's
o., Fritsch's
o., Fritz-Lange
o., Frommel's
o., Frost-Lang
o., Fuchs'
o., Fukala's
o., Gant's
o., Gardner's
o. ▸ gastric band
o., gastric bypass
o., Gatellier's
o., Gayet's
o., Georgariou's
o., Ghormley's
o., Gibson's
o., Gifford's
o., Gigli's
o., Gillespie's
o., Gilliam-Doléris
o., Gilliam's
o., Gillies'
o., Gill's
o., Giordano's
o., Girard's
o., Girdlestone
o., Glenn
o., Goebell-Stoeckel
o., Goffe's
o., Goldthwait's
o., Gomez-Marquez
o., Gonin's
o., goniopuncture
o., Goodall-Power
o., Gottschalk's
o., Graber-Duvernay
o., Gradle's
o., Graefe's
o., Grant-Ward

o., Grice-Green
o., Guleke-Stookey
o., Gutzeit's
o., Haas'
o., Halpin's
o., Halsted's
o., Hammond's
o., Hark's
o., Harmon's
o., Harrington's
o., Harris-Beath
o., Hasner's
o., Haultaim's
o., Hauser's
o., Haynes'
o., Hegar's
o., Heifitz's
o., Heine's
o., Henderson's
o., Hendry's
o., Henry-Geist
o., Herbert's
o., Hess
o., Heuter's
o., Heyman
o., Hibbs'
o., Hippel's
o., Hirst's
o., Hoffa-Lorenz
o., Hoffa's
o., Hogan's
o., Hohmann's
o., Holme's
o., Holth's
o., Horay's
o., Horsley's
o., Horvath's
o., Horwitz-Adams
o., hospital
o., Hotz's
o., Houston's
o., Howorth
o., Hufnagel's
o., Hughes'
o., Huntington's
o., Hyam's
o., Imre
o., intermediate
o., interposition
o., iris stretching
o., Irving's
o., Jaboulay's
o., Jacobaeus
o., Jaesche-Arlt
o., Jameson's

o., Jones'
o., Joplin's
o., Kapel's
o., Kellogg-Speed
o., Kelly's
o., Kennedy's
o., Kessler's
o., Key's
o., Kidner's
o., Killian's
o., King-Richards
o., Kirby's
o., Kirkaldy-Willis
o., Kirmisson's
o., Knapp-Imre
o., Knapp's
o., Kocher's
o., Kocks'
o., Koenig-Wittek
o., Kofler's
o., Kolomnin's
o., König's
o., Köstner's
o., Kraupa's
o., Krause's
o., Kreibig's
o., Kreiker's
o., Kreuscher's
o., Kroener's
o., Krönlein-Berke
o., Krönlein's
o., Krukenberg's
o., Kuhnt
o., Kuhnt-Szymanowski
o., Lacarrere's
o., Lagleyze's
o., Lagrange's
o., Lambrinudi's
o., Landolt's
o., Langenbeck's
o., Lange's
o., Lash's
o., Latzko's
o., Le Fort's
o., Lefiche's
o., Leopold's
o., L'Episcopo's
o., Levine's
o. ▸ limb lengthening
o., Lincoff's
o., Lindner's
o., Littler's
o., Littlewood's
o., Lohlein's
o., Londermann's

o., Lopez-Enriquez
o., Lorenz's
o., Lottes'
o., Lowenstein's
o., Lucas-Cottrell
o., Luck's
o., Ludloff's
o., Lund's
o., Lyon-Horgan
o., MacAusland's
o., Macewen's
o., Machek-Blaskovics
o., Machek-Gifford
o., Machek's
o., Mackenrodt's
o., Madlener
o., Magitot's
o., magnet
o., Magnuson
o., Magnuson-Stack
o., Majewsky's
o., Majorner-Mead
o., Manchester
o., Marckwald's
o., Marshall-Marchetti
o., Marshall-Marchetti-Krantz
o., Martin's
o., Martius'
o., Matas'
o., Mauksch's
o., Mayo-Fueth
o., Mayo's
o., Mazur's
o., McBride's
o., McBurney's
o., McCall-Schuman
o., McCall's
o., McCarroll's
o., McDonald's
o., McDowell's
o., McGavic type
o., McGuire's
o., McIndoe
o., McKeever's
o., McLaughlin's
o., McReynold's
o., McVay's
o., Meller's
o., Menge's
o., mika
o., Mikulicz's
o., Milch's
o., Mile's
o., Millers
o., Millin-Read

o., Minsky's
o., Mitchell's
o., Monaldi's
o., Moncrieff's
o., Moore's
o., Morax's
o., morcellement
o., Morestin's
o., Moschcowitz's
o., Mosher-Toti
o., Mules'
o., Müllers
o., Mumford-Gurd
o., Munnell's
o., Mustard
o., Naffziger's
o., Nélaton's
o., Neviaser's
o., Nicola's
o., Nida's
o., Nizetic's
o., Ober's
o., O'Connor
o., O'Connor-Peter
o. of filter controls
o. of sensitivity controls
o., Ogston's
o., Ollier
o., Ollier-Thiersch
o., Olshausen's
o. on canaliculi, plastic
o. on cataract, double needle
o. on eyeball, plastic
o., open-womb
o., Osborne's
o., Osgood's
o., O'Sullivan's
o., Overholt's
o., Oxford's
o., Pact's
o., palliative
o., Palmer-Widen
o., Panas'
o., Pancoast's
o., Paufique's
o., Pauwel
o., Péan's
o., Peter's
o., Peterson's
o., Pheasant's
o., Phelps'
o., Phemister
o., Physick's
o., plastic
o., Pollock's

o., Polya's
o., Pomeroy's
o., Poncet's
o., Porro-Veit
o., Porro's
o., Potts
o., Potts-Smith-Gibson
o., Poulard's
o., Power's
o., Pozzi's
o., Putti-Platt
o., Puusepp's
o., Quaglino's
o., radical
o., radical antrum
o., radical neck
o., Ransohoff's
o., Rastelli's
o., Raverdino's
o., Récamier's
o., reconstruction
o., reconstructive
o., Reichenheim-King
o., Reis-Wertheim
o., Reverdin's
o., Richet's
o., Ridlon's
o., Rizzoli's
o., Routier's
o., Roux-Goldthwait
o., Rovsing's
o., Rowinski's
o., Rubbrecht's
o., Rubin's
o., Saemisch's
o., Saenger's
o., Salter's
o., Sayre's
o., Scanzoni's
o., Scarpa's
o., Schanz's
o., Schauffler's
o., Schauta-Wertheim
o., Schauta's
o., Schede's
o., Scheie's
o., Schmalz's
o., Schröder's
o., Schuchardt's
o., scleral fistula
o. ▸ second look
o., Semb's
o., Senning
o., shelf
o., shelving

operation—*continued*
- o., Shirodkar
- o., shunt
- o., Silva-Costa
- o., Simon's
- o., simple
- o., sling
- o., Slocum's
- o., Smith-Kuhnt-Szymanowski
- o., Smith-Petersen
- o., Smith's
- o., Smithwick's
- o., Snelien's
- o., Sofia's
- o., Sofield's
- o., Sonneberg's
- o., Sordille's
- o., Spaeth's
- o., Spalding-Richardson
- o., Speas'
- o., Speed-Boyd
- o., Spencer-Watson
- o., Spinelli's
- o., Stallard's
- o., Stamm's
- o., Steindler's
- o., Stock's
- o., Strap
- o., Strassman-Jones
- o., Sturmdorf's
- o., Suarez-Villafranca
- o., Sugiura
- o., Swanson's
- o., switch
- o., Szymanowski-Kuhnt
- o., Szymanowski's
- o., tagliacotian
- o., talc
- o., Tanner's
- o., Tansley's
- o., Taussig's
- o., Te Linde
- o., Terson's
- o., Thomas'
- o., Thomson's
- o., Torkildsen's
- o., Torpin's
- o., ► total hip replacement
- o., Toti-Mosher
- o., Toti's
- o., Trantas'
- o., Trendelenburg's
- o., Troutman's
- o., Turko's
- o., Twombly-Ulfelder

- o., Twombly's
- o., uneventful
- o., Van Gorder's
- o., Vernoeff's
- o., Vernon-David
- o., Verwey's
- o., Vineberg's
- o., von Graefe's
- o., Wagner's
- o., Waldhauer's
- o., Warren's
- o., Water's
- o., Watkins'
- o., Watkins-Wertheim
- o., Watson-Jones
- o., Webster's
- o., Weeker's
- o., Wees'
- o., Weiner's
- o., Wertheim-Schauta
- o., Wertheim's
- o., West's
- o., Weve's
- o., Wharton's
- o., Wheeler's
- o., Whitacre's
- o., Whitman's
- o., Wicherkiewicz'
- o., William's
- o., Williams-Richardson
- o., Wilmer's
- o., Wilms'
- o., Wilson
- o., Wilson-McKeever
- o., window
- o., Wladimiroff's
- o., Wolfe's
- o., Worth's
- o., Wyeth's
- o., Wylie's
- o., Young's
- o., Yount's
- o., Zahradnicek's
- o., Zancolli's
- o., Ziegler's

operational
- o. error
- o. technique
- o. thinking, abstract

operative
- o. ablation
- o. amputation
- o. area irrigated with saline
- o. bronchoscopy
- o. bronchoscopy and dilatation

- o. cholangiogram
- o. cholangiography
- o. cholangiography, delayed
- o. consent
- o. damage
- o. delivery, midforceps
- o. delivery, rotation
- o. delivery, vacuum extraction
- o. field
- o. field anesthetized
- o. field prepared and draped
- o. field, sterile
- o. findings
- o. incision
- o. management
- o. morbidity and mortality
- o. pancreatography
- o. permit signed
- o. procedure
- o. repair
- o. risk
- o. scar
- o. site
- o. site infection
- o. site irrigated
- o. suite
- o. therapy
- o. wound
- o. wound clean and healed
- o. wound, delayed closure of
- o. wound, disruption of
- o. wound, resuture disrupted

opercular fold
operculofrontal artery
operculum, dental
operculum, orbital
operti, gyri
Ophthaine anesthesia
ophthalmia
- o., actinic ray
- o., catarrhal
- o., caterpillar
- o. eczematosa
- o., Egyptian
- o., electric
- o., flash
- o., gonococcal
- o., gonorrheal
- o., granular
- o., jequirity
- o., metastatic
- o., migratory
- o., mucous
- o. neonatorum
- o., neuroparalytic

o. nivialis
o. nodosa
o., phlyctenular
o., purulent
o., scrofulous
o., strumous
o., sympathetic
o., transferred
o., ultraviolet ray
o., varicose

ophthalmic
o. aneurysm, carotid
o. artery
o. artery thrombosis
o. brachytherapy
o. cautery, Scheie's
o. cholinergic
o. cup
o. examination ▸ neuro-
o. ganglion
o. laser
o. lens, Volk conoid
o. migraine
o. nerve
o. ointment
o. plexus
o. reaction
o. recurrent nerve
o. scoliosis
o. solution, sterile
o. tumors
o. ultrasound
o. vein, inferior
o. vein, superior
o. vesicle

ophthalmica, vesicula
ophthalmicus
o., caliculus
o., herpes
o., plexus

ophthalmobium, Agamodistomum
ophthalmodynamometry test
ophthalmography, echo-
ophthalmologic function
ophthalmologic monitoring
Ophthalmologist, Pediatric
ophthalmologist's laser
ophthalmomandibulomelic dysplasia
ophthalmomeningeal vein
ophthalmometer, Javal's
ophthalmopathy, Graves'
ophthalmoplegia
o., chronic external
o., exophthalmic
o. externa

o., fascicular
o., interna
o. (INO), intranuclear
o., nuclear
o., Parinaud's
o. partialis
o. progressive
o. progressive external
o., Sauvineau's
o. totalis

ophthalmoplegic migraine
ophthalmoscope, scanning
ophthalmoscope (SLO) ▸ scanning laser
ophthalmoscopic examination
ophthalmoscopy
o., binocular indirect
o., direct
o., indirect
o., medical
o., metric
o. test

ophthalmovascular choke
opiate
o. abuse, chronic
o. addict
o. addict, detoxified
o. addict ▸ treatment of
o. binding site
o. -dependent patient ▸ pregnant
o. detoxification, ambulatory
o. drugs
o. intoxication
o. receptors
o., synthetic
o. use
o. withdrawal
o. withdrawal symptomatology
o. withdrawal symptoms
o. withdrawal syndrome

Opie paradox
opinion, second
opinionated, excessively
opioid(s)
o. (China White)
o. abuse
o. abuse, comorbid
o. abuse, pattern of
o. abuse, physical effects of
o., abuse potential of
o. abuse, prevalence of
o. abusers, assessing needs of
o. -abusing women
o., acute intoxication with
o. addiction, history of

o. analgesic
o. antagonist
o., blood level of
o., dependence on
o. -dependent cocaine user
o. -dependent patient
o., detoxification from
o. ▸ duration of effects of
o., effects of
o., flashback reactions with
o. intoxification
o., kappa
o. ▸ long-term self-administration of
o. maintenance
o., mode of administration with
o. mortality
o., organic brain syndrome with
o. overdose
o., panic reactions with
o., patient OD (overdosed) with
o., potential tolerance to
o., psychoactive doses of
o., psychoactive properties of
o., psychological effects of
o., psychotic reactions with
o., receptor sites for
o., tolerance to
o., toxicity of
o., treatment of acute drug reactions to
o. -type dependence
o., urine level of
o., withdrawal from

opiophagorum, tremor
Opisthorchis
O. felineus
O. noverca
O., Trematoda
O. viverrini

opisthotonos/opisthotonus
opisthotonos fetalis
opisthotonos position
Opitz syndrome ▸ Smith-Lemli-
opium
o. (OP)
o. (Poppy)
o. addiction
o. habit
o. smoking
o., tincture of

opossumi, Miyagawanella
Oppenheim('s)
O. brace
O. disease
O. disease, Ziehen-

Oppenheim('s)—*continued*
- O. gait
- O. reflex
- O. sign

Oppler bacillus, Boas-
Oppler ▸ lactobacillus of Boas-
opponens pollicis, muscle
opportunistic
- o. diseases
- o. infection (OI)
- o. infection prevention
- o. pathogen
- o. pneumonia

opposed parallel beam
opposing
- o. lateral fields
- o. margins
- o. muscle of little finger
- o. muscle of thumb
- o. parallel portals
- o. portals, anterior and posterior
- o. skull portals
- o. tangential fields, parallel
- o. vocal cord

opposite
- o. phases, waves of
- o. sex, decline in interest of
- o. sides of head
- o., warm to the same (COWS) ▸ cold to the

opposition [*apposition*]
- o. exercises, finger
- o. of flow of alternating current (AC)
- o. of flow of direct current (DC)
- o., rhythmic

oppositional
- o. behavior
- o. defiant disorder (ODD)
- o. disorder
- o. movements ▸ reversible
- o. movements ▸ sequential

oppression, fat
oppressive pain
opsonic immunity
opsonin, serum
opsonizing antibody
OPTACON (OPtical TActile CONverter)
optic
- o. agraphia
- o. aphasia
- o. ataxia
- o. atrophy
- o. atrophy, hereditary
- o. atrophy, Leber's

- o. atrophy ▸ permanent
- o. atrophy, primary
- o. atrophy, secondary
- o. axis
- o. center
- o. chiasm
- o. chiasm, sulcus for
- o. commissure
- o. cup
- o. cupping
- o. diaphragm
- o. disc/disk
- o. disc, edema of
- o. disc metastasis
- o. disc, nasal border of
- o. foramen of sclera
- o. fundi
- o. ganglion
- o. glioma
- o. iridectomy
- o. keratoplasty
- o. nerve
- o. nerve, atrophy of
- o. nerve atrophy ▸ toxic
- o. nerve attachment
- o. nerve, avulsion of
- o. nerve, circulation to
- o. nerve, colloid deposits in
- o. nerve, coloboma of
- o. nerve, crushing of
- o. nerve damage
- o. nerve ▸ degeneration of
- o. nerve disorder
- o. nerve ▸ foreign body (FB) in
- o. nerve glioma
- o. nerve head
- o. nerve head analysis
- o. nerve head, choking of
- o. nerve, hereditary atrophy of
- o. nerve, inflammation of
- o. nerve, junction of
- o. nerve neuritis
- o. nerve, papilla of
- o. nerve, pressure on
- o. nerve, sheaths of
- o. neuritis
- o. neuroencephalomyelopathy
- o. neuropathy, anterior ischemic
- o. neuropathy ▸ hypertensive
- o. neuropathy ▸ ischemic
- o. neuropathy ▸ Leber's hereditary
- o. neuropathy ▸ radiation
- o., or retrobulbar neuritis
- o. papilla
- o. papilla, cavity of

- o. papilla, cysticercosis of
- o. pathway
- o. radiation
- o. reflex
- o. stalk
- o. stroke
- o. thalamus
- o. tract
- o. vesicle

optica, neuromyelitis
optical (Optical)
- o. activity
- o. alexia
- o. axis ▸ rotation of eye around
- o. coherence tomography
- o. colonoscopy
- o. density
- o. density (OD) values
- o. disk stamper
- o. error, correct
- o. fiber
- o. fiber catheter
- o. illusion
- o. immunoassay
- o. nerve atrophy
- o. scanner
- o. sensor
- O. TActile CONverter (OPTACON)
- O. Tracking System (OTS)

optically inactive
optici, taenia medullaris thalami
opticociliary
- o. neurectomy
- o. neurotomy
- o. vessels, anomaly

opticofacial winking reflex
opticomalacia, Kreibig's
opticoneuropathy, subacute myelo-
opticostriate region
opticum, chiasma
Optiflex intraocular lenses (IOL)
OPTIMA (Oxford Project to Investi-gate Memory and Aging)
optimal (Optimal)
- o. bone production
- o. care
- o. control system
- o. diastolic pressure
- o. dose of chemotherapy
- o. dose selection
- o. intensity
- o. level
- o. level of independence
- o. levels of functioning
- o. management

o. physiological functioning
o. stimulation sites
O. Treatment (HOT), Hypertension
o. treatment study ▸ hypertension
o. weight
optimally, shunt functioning
optimism, extreme
optimism, naive
optimum calorie intake
optimum care of patient
option(s)
    o., contraceptive
    o., curative
    o., medical
    o. of consent
    o., surgical
    o., therapeutic
    o., treatment
optional exchange
optional rhythm, basic
Optiray contrast
optochiasmatic arachnoiditis
optokinetic nystagmus (OKN)
OPV (oral polio vaccine)
OR
    OR (operating room)
    OR (orienting reflex)
    OR (Operating Room) Director
ora
    o., scope passed per
    o. serrata
    o. serrata retinae
Orabilex contrast medium
Oragrafin
    O. calcium
    O. calcium contrast medium
    O. sodium
    O. sodium contrast medium
oral [*aural*]
    o. aerobics
    o. agent
    o. airway
    o. allergy syndrome
    o. analgesic
    o. anesthesia
    o. antiarrhythmic therapy
    o. antibiotic
    o. anticoagulant therapy
    o. antifungal
    o. antifungal agent
    o. antihistamine
    o. appliance, extra
    o. arch
    o. bacteria
    o. biology specialist

o. cancer
o. cancer screening
o. cancer ▸ warning signs of
o. candidiasis
o. carcinoma
o. cavity
o. cavity cancer
o. chelating nutrients
o. chelation therapy
o. chemotherapy
o. cholecystogram (OCG)
o. cholecystography
o. communication
o. contents
o. contraceptive
o. contraceptive-induced hypertension
o. contraceptive, sequential type
o. decongestant
o. diabetes drugs
o. diaphragm
o. digitalization
o. dissolution therapy
o. disulfiram treatment
o. dosage
o. dose
o. drug therapy
o. enzyme
o. eroticism
o. estrogen therapy
o. facial infections
o. feedings
o. flora
o. function, restoration of
o. glucose tolerance test
o. habit
o. hairy leukoplakia
o. hematinic
o. herpes, dermal or
o. hormone tablets
o. hydration
o. hygiene
o. hygiene, daily
o. implantology
o. infection
o. ingestion
o. insulin
o. intake
o. intake, poor
o. intubation
o. language skill
o. leishmaniasis, naso-
o. lesions
o. leukoplakia
o. medication

o. medications ▸ multiple
o. medicine
o. monotherapy
o. motor examination
o. motor skills
o. mucosa
o. mucosa ▸ inflammation of
o. mucosa pigmentation ▸ gingival and
o. mucositis
o. mucous membrane
o. narcotic agents
o. -oral transmission by saliva
o. pain medication
o. passages
o. pathology
o. pemphigus
o. penicillin ▸ nonresponsive to
o. polio immunization
o. polio vaccine (OPV)
o. poliovirus vaccine
o. poliovirus vaccine ▸ monovalent
o. poliovirus vaccine ▸ trivalent
o. radiation
o. radiography, pan-
o. region
o. rehabilitation
o. route
o. route, fecal-
o. route of infection ▸ fecal-
o. secretions
o. secretions, direct contact with contaminated
o. sedative
o. stage
o. steroid
o. steroid drug
o. stomatitis
o. supplement, nourishing
o. surgeon
o. surgery
o. temperature
o., tetravalent rotavirus vaccine
o. therapy
o. thermometer
o. thrush
o. tissues
o. tissues, soft
o. transmission by saliva ▸ oral-
o. transmission of viral hepatitis
o. treatment
o. tuberculosis
o. ulcer
o. urography
o. vasodilator

oral—*continued*
- o. virus
- o. yeast infection

oralis, Bacteroides
oralis, Prevotella
orally ingested
orally ▸ peyote ingested
Oram syndrome, Holt-
Orange
- O. (amphetamines)
- O., Agent
- O. Sunshine (LSD)
- O. syndrome, Agent

orbicular
- o. alignment
- o. muscle
- o. muscle of eye
- o. muscle of mouth
- o. reflex, cochleo-
- o. ring
- o. zone of hip

orbiculare, os
orbiculare, Pityrosporon
orbicularis
- o., alopecia
- o. atrophy
- o. ciliaris
- o. oculi
- o. oculi, musculus
- o. oris
- o. reaction
- o. reflex

orbiculus ciliaris
orbiculus, Veillonella
orbit
- o., abscess of
- o., aneurysm in
- o., biopsy of
- o., decompression of
- o., emphysema of
- o., facial
- o., fibroma of
- o., fibrosarcoma of
- o., filariasis of
- o., fistula of
- o., floor of
- o., granuloma of
- o., hemangioma of
- o., hematoma of
- o., hemorrhage in
- o., leiomyoma of
- o., lymphoma of
- o., medial wall of
- o., plastic repair of
- o., recession of eyeball into

- o., rhabdomyosarcoma of

orbitae, aditus
orbitae, corpus adiposum
orbital
- o. abscess
- o. aneurysm
- o. bone
- o. cavity
- o. cellulitis
- o. contents, exenteration of
- o. decompression
- o. fat ▸ excessive
- o. floor
- o. floor prosthesis
- o. fracture
- o. ganglion
- o. gyri
- o. hypertelorism
- o. hypotelorism
- o. implant
- o., infra◊
- o. injury
- o. lamina
- o. margin
- o. metastasis
- o. metastasis syndrome
- o. muscle
- o. myositis
- o. operculum
- o. plate
- o. projections, parieto-
- o. prosthesis, solid silicone
- o. pseudolymphoma
- o. pseudotumor
- o. region
- o. ridge
- o. rim
- o. rim, lateral
- o. rim, periosteum of
- o. septum
- o. septum, tarsus
- o. structures
- o., supra◊
- o. surgery
- o. tumor
- o. tumor, metastatic
- o. tumor, rhabdomyosarcoma

orbitales, gyri
orbitofrontal cortex
orbitosphenoidal bone
orchalis, adiposis
orchidorrhaphy/orchiorrhaphy
orchidotomy/orchiotomy
orchiectomy, bilateral
orchiectomy, inguinal

orchiopexy/orchidopexy
orchioplasty/orchidoplasty
orchitis
- o., acute
- o. due to mumps
- o., metastatic
- o. parotidea
- o., spermatogenic granulomatous
- o., traumatic
- o. variolosa

order(s)
- o. accompanying patient on admission
- o., birth
- o. (KVO) ▸ constant verbal
- o. kinetics, first
- o. kinetics ▸ zero-
- o. mailed in prior to admission
- o., medical
- o., obtain physician
- o. on admission postal
- o. on admission ▸ standing
- o. on chart
- o. on routine admission, standing
- o. (PO) ▸ phone
- o., physician
- o., postdischarge
- o., postoperative
- o., preoperative
- o. ▸ putting affairs in
- o., restraining
- o. sent to Admitting Office ▸ admission
- o., standard
- o., standing
- o., stat
- o., telephone
- o. (VO), verbal
- o., written

ordered
- o. assessment, court
- o. medical treatment, court
- o. phase encoding ▸ respiratory

orderly-on-call
ore, fetor ex
organ(s) (Organ)
- o., abdominal
- o. ablation
- o. activity
- o. and recipient ▸ match
- o. and tissue recovery
- o. and tissues, distribution of donor
- o. and tissues, preservation of donor

o. and tissues, procurement of donor
o. and tissues, surgical recovery of donated
o., atrophy of endocrine
o. availability
o. ▸ block rejection of transplanted
o. blood flow to transplanted
o., bodily rejection of
o., cadaver
o., cadaveric
o., colorectal
o. ▸ combat rejection of transplanted
o., congenital eversion of
o., cornea and tissue
o. damage, end-
o. damage, enzymatic
o. damage ▸ multiple
o. disease, end stage
o. disease, target
o., diseased
o. distribution
o., donated
o., donated human
o. donation
o. donation, cadaver
o. donation, consent for
o. donation, criteria for
o. donation, directed
o. donation, solid
o. donation, vital
o., donor
O. Donor Awareness Program
o. donor candidate, vital
o. donor card
o. donor, deceased
o. donor ▸ identify potential
o. donor, infected
o. donor, living related
o. donor, multiple
o. donor, potential
o. donor, vital
o., end-
o., endocrine
o. exenteration, pelvic
o. failure
o. failure ▸ major
o. failure ▸ multisystem
o. for transplant ▸ authorization form for removal of
o. for transplant ▸ consent form for removal of
o. for transplantation ▸ procurement of cadaver

o., foreign
o. -forming substances
o. function
o. function, normal
o. graft ▸ solid
o. grafts
o., harvest
o. harvesting
o., healthy appearing
o., hollow
o., hollow viscus
o., human
o., images of body
o., inferior
o. ▸ inflammation of lining of
o. ischemic time ▸ donor
o. isolated
o., life-saving
o. malformation
o. malfunction
o. match
o., mediastinal
o., obstruction of major
o. ▸ occlude blood vessel in vital
o. of Corti
o. of Giraldés
o. of hearing
o. of hearing, receptor
o. of special sense
o. or masses, palpable
o. ▸ oxygen deprivation in critical
o., oxygenation of
o., palpable
o., pelvic
o. perfusion, artificial
o., peripheral sense
o., pillar of Corti's
o. preservation
o. preservation fluid
o. ▸ procure and allocate donated
o. procurement
O. Procurement and Transplantation Network
o. readily available ▸ donor
o. recipient
o. recipient candidate
o. recipient, potential
o. recovery
o. recovery coordinator
o. recovery team
o. rejection
o., rejection of transplantation
o., removal of rejected
o. replacement ▸ major
o., reproductive

o. retrieval
o. retrieval and preservation
o. sharing
O. Sharing Network
O. Sharing, United Network for
o. shielding blocks
o. shielding blocks, critical
o., shielding of
o. ▸ shortage of donor
o., sold
o. source
o. specific antigen
o. support
o., surgical excision of
o., surgical removal of
o., surgical removal of donated
o. system
o. system malfunctions ▸ major
o., T categories in hollow
o. -tissue procurement
o. -tissue recovery
o. tolerance dose (OTD)
o., total system failure of vital
o. transplant
o. transplant ▸ authorization form for recipient of
o. transplant center
o. transplant ▸ consent form for recipient of
o. transplant recipient
o. transplant recipients ▸ matching
o. transplant ▸ solid
o. transplant, whole
o. ▸ transplantable cadaver
o. transplantation
o. transplantation, human
o. transplantation surgery
o. transplantation, total lymphoid irradiation in
o., transplanted
o. transplants, multiple
o. transplants, vascular
o., vascular
o. viability
o., viable
o., visceral
o., vital
o., wall of
o. with defective development
organic
o. affective syndrome
o. affective syndrome ▸ drug-induced
o. amnesia
o. anxiety disorder

organic—*continued*
- o. brain changes
- o. brain disease
- o. brain disease, progressive
- o. brain disorder
- o. brain syndrome
- o. brain syndrome, acute
- o. brain syndrome, acute treatment for
- o. brain syndrome, chronic
- o. brain syndrome, clinical manifestations of
- o. brain syndrome, differential diagnosis in
- o. brain syndrome, drug reactions in
- o. brain syndrome, subacute treatment
- o. brain syndrome, treatment of
- o. brain syndrome with cannabinoids
- o. brain syndrome with depressants
- o. brain syndrome with hallucinogens
- o. brain syndrome with inhalants
- o. brain syndrome with multiple drugs
- o. brain syndrome with opioids
- o. brain syndrome with phencyclidines
- o. brain syndrome with stimulants
- o. cardiac lesion
- o. cause
- o. chemistry
- o. CNS (central nervous system) deterioration
- o. colon pathology
- o. contracture
- o. damage to brain
- o. deafness
- o. defects
- o. delusional disorder
- o. delusional syndrome
- o. delusional syndrome ▸ drug-induced
- o. dementia
- o. deterioration
- o. disease
- o. disorder
- o. dust exposure
- o. dust pneumoconiosis
- o. dust pneumonoconiosis
- o. dysfunction
- o. emotional lability
- o., emotional or mixed origin

- o., epilepsy
- o. factor ▸ hypersomnia related to a known
- o. factor ▸ insomnia related to a known
- o. hallucinosis
- o. hallucinosis syndrome
- o., headache
- o. heart disease
- o. lesion
- o. mental disorder
- o. mental disorder ▸ methamphetamine-induced
- o. mental disorder ▸ phencyclidine (PCP)
- o. mental disorder ▸ psychoactive substance
- o. mental disorder ▸ psychoactive substance-induced
- o. mental disorder ▸ substance-induced
- o. mental disorder ▸ transient
- o. mental syndrome
- o. mental syndrome disorder
- o. molecules
- o. mood disorder
- o. murmur
- o. muscle
- o. origin
- o. pain
- o. personality disorder
- o. personality syndrome
- o. psychosis
- o. psychotic condition
- o. psychotic condition ▸ presenile
- o. psychotic condition ▸ senile
- o. psychotic condition ▸ transient
- o. radical
- o. reaction type
- o. stricture

organically impaired brain function
organism(s)
- o., acid-fast
- o., aerobic
- o., amoeba
- o., anaerobic
- o., anaerobic bacillus
- o., antibiotic-resistant
- o., Arizona
- o. aspirated into lungs ▸ drug-resistant
- o. ▸ aspiration of gastrointestinal
- o., bacterial
- o., benign
- o., Borrelia

- o., Campylobacter
- o., causative
- o., cell wall of
- o., coliform
- o., colonies of
- o., cryptosporidiosis
- o., culturable
- o., culture
- o., culture grew
- o., disease-causing
- o., dormant
- o., drug-resistant
- o. dwarfs
- o., E. (Escherichia) coli
- o., encapsulated
- o., endemic hospital
- o., etiologic
- o., extracellular
- o., fungal
- o. ▸ fungi and protozoal
- o., gram-negative
- o., gram-positive
- o., gutless
- o., hospital-acquired
- o. /hpf (per high power field)
- o. identification
- o. identified, causative
- o. in sputum ▸ rod shaped
- o., infecting
- o., infectious
- o., intracellular
- o. isolated after 72 hours
- o., lethal
- o., living
- o., marine
- o., microaerophilic
- o., microcellular
- o., micrococcus
- o., morphology of individual
- o., motile
- o., multicellular
- o., mycobacterium
- o., nosocomial
- o., nosocomial gram-negative
- o., nosocomial gram-positive
- o., nosocomial transmission of
- o., obligate intercellular
- o., offending
- o., one-celled
- o., parasitic
- o., pathogenic
- o., pathological
- o. per high power field (organisms/hpf)
- o., phage typing of

o. (PPLO), pleuropneumonia-like
o., pneumonia-causing
o., predominant
o., predominating
o., proteolytic gram-negative
o., pus-producing
o., resistant
o., Rickett's
o., salmonella
o., Shigella
o., single celled
o., skin test for fungus
o., staphylococcus
o., streptothrix
o., taenia/tenia
o., tatlock
o., toxin producing common
o., unicellular
o., vibrio
o., Vincent's
o., viral producing common
o., virulent
o., yeast

organization(s) (Organization)
o., affectomotor memory
o. and analysis, perceptual-motor
o., competent abstract conceptual
   memory
o., conceptual memory
o. (HMO), health maintenance
o., memory
O. (NHO), National Hospice
o. (PPO), preferred provider
o. ▸ verbal conceptual memory
O. (WHO), World Health

organizational structure
organized
o. mental functions
o. movement
o. thrombus
o. transport protocol

organizer
o., nucleolar
o., nucleolus
o., primary
o., secondary
o., tertiary

organizing
o. aspiration pneumonia
o. hemorrhagic cyst
o. interstitial pneumonia oxygen
   (O_2) therapy
o. pneumonia, bronchiolitis
   obliterans
o. pneumonia, interstitial

o. pneumonitis, chronic
o. thrombus
o. thrombus of basilar artery

organogenesis, abnormal cardiac
organogenesis, cardiac
organoids, cytoplasmic
organotropic drugs
orgasm, inhibited female
orgasm, inhibited male
oriental (Oriental)
o. diet
O. female, patient
o. hemoptysis
O. male, patient
O. massage

orientalis
o., Phlebotomus
o., Rickettsia
o., Trichostrongylus

orientation (Orientation)
o., admission
O. and Amnesia Test (GOAT) ▸
   Galveston
o., attention and recent recall ▸
   evaluate
o., conflict ▸ sexual
o., disturbance of
o., false spatial
o. in space ▸ sensation of
o., language skills and perception ▸
   attention,
o., level of
o. ▸ mind's eye
o. or perception ▸ spatial
o., patient
o., poor
o. program
o., psychological
o., reality
o. reflex audiometry ▸ conditioned
o., sexual
o., spatial
o., spiritual
o., staff
o. to hospital

oriented
o. activities, family
o. activity ▸ prolonged task-
o., alert and
o. as to person, place and time ▸
   patient
o. behavior ▸ goal-
o. behavior, spatially
o. group ▸ interactive process-
o., image-

o. in all spheres
o. issues, family
o., patient
o., patient alert and
o. process group ▸ topic-
o. psychotherapy ▸ goal-
o. psychotherapy, intensive insight
o. psychotherapy, reality
o., speech
o. tasks ▸ goal-
o. therapy ▸ insight-
o. therapy ▸ psychodynamically
o. to time, place, and person
o. treatment, abstinence
o. treatment methods ▸
   moderation-

orienting reflex (OR)
**ORIF (open reduction and internal
   fixation)**
orifice(s)
o., abdominal
o., adequately visualized
o., anal
o., anorectal
o., aortic
o., atrioventricular (AV)
o., bronchial
o., cardiac
o. ▸ effective regurgitant
o. electrogram, coronary sinus
o., external
o., external urethral
o., floor of
o. ▸ flow across
o., hymenal
o., internal
o., internal urethral
o., LLL (left lower lobe) bronchial
o., LUL (left upper lobe) bronchial
o., middle lobe
o., mitral
o. of male urethra
o. of ureter
o. of uterine tube, abdominal
o., patent
o., pharyngeal
o., pulmonary
o., RLL (right lower lobe) bronchial
o., RML (right middle lobe)
   bronchial
o., RUL (right upper lobe) bronchial
o., segmental
o., tricuspid
o., tympanic
o., ureteral

orifice(s)—*continued*
   o., urethral
   o., uterine
   o., vaginal
   o., valve
   o., valvular
   o., vesicourethral
   o. widely patent
orificial stenosis
orificial tuberculosis
orificii externi, urethritis
origin
   o., adenocarcinoma pancreatic
   o. and distribution, anatomic
   o. ▸ anemia of undetermined
   o., anomalous
   o., bacterial
   o., biological
   o., cardiac
   o., cerebral
   o., chemical
   o., common psychobiological
   o., emotional
   o. empowerment sessions ▸ family-
   o. (FUO) ▸ fever of undetermined
   o. (FUO) ▸ fever of unknown
   o., genetic
   o., hospital
   o., illness of emotional
   o., lumbar spinal root
   o., medical
   o., musculoskeletal
   o. ▸ myocardial disease, unknown
   o., noncardiogenic
   o. of the renal artery
   o. of virus
   o., organic
   o. ▸ organic, emotional or mixed
   o., pain of central
   o., physical
   o., psychiatric
   o., psychogenic
   o., psychological
   o., pyrexia of unknown
   o., site of
   o. specific to childhood ▸
      psychoses with
   o. ▸ tissue of prostatic
   o., traumatic
   o., undetermined
   o., unknown
   o., vascular in
original
   o. dosage
   o. host cell

   o. incision
   o. injection site
   o. rectal lesion
   o. signal
   o. site, cancer localized in
   o. tuberculin
   o. tumor site
originaria, paranoia
originating extrapyramidal system
   (COEPS) ▸ cortically
originating infection
oris
   o., cancrum
   o., fetor
   o., Filaria hominis
   o., orbicularis
   o., sphincter
   o., vestibulum
ornithosis virus
oroantral fistula
oro-cheiro migraine
orodigitofacial dysostosis
oroendotracheal tube
orofacial dyskinesia
oromandibular dystonia ▸ blepharo-
   spasm and
oronasal fistula
oropharyngeal
   o. airway
   o. Candidiasis
   o. carcinoma
   o. disease, suppurative
   o. dysphagia
   o. flora, normal
   o. pack
   o. tularemia
Oropouche virus
Oropsylla idahoensis
Oropsylla silantiewi
orotic aciduria
orotracheal
   o. intubation
   o. intubation ▸ rapid sequence,
      induction (RSI)
   o. tube
Oroya fever
orphan (Orphan)
   o. (CELO) ▸ chicken-embryo-lethal
   o. drugs
   O. Drugs Program
   o. (ECHO) ▸ enterocytopathogenic
      human
   o. (ECHO) virus ▸ enteric
      cytopathic human
   o. virus

   o. virus, enteric
   o. (ECBO) virus ▸ enteric cyto-
      pathic bovine
   o. (ECHO) virus ▸ enteric cyto-
      pathic human
   o. (ECMO) virus ▸ enteric cyto-
      pathic monkey
   o. (ECSO) virus ▸ enteric cyto-
      pathic swine
Orr technique
Orr treatment
orthocardiac reflex
orthochromatic
   o. erythroblast
   o. erythrocyte
   o. normoblast
orthodontic
   o. appliance
   o. correction
   o. treatment
orthodox sleep
orthodromic
   o. AV reentrant tachycardia
   o. reciprocating tachycardia
   o. tachycardia
   o. tachycardia ▸ reciprocating
      macroreentry
orthogonal
   o. angiography, biplane
   o. delivery
   o. electrocardiogram (ECG)
   o. fields, beam overlap in
   o. lead system
   o. plane
   o. radiography
   o. thesis
   o. view
orthograde conduction
orthomolecular medicine
orthomolecular psychiatry
Orthomyxoviridae virus
orthopedic (Orthopedic)
   o. emergency
   o. emergency, pediatric
   o. grafting
   o. impairment, chronic
   o. implant infection
   o. limitations
   o. nursing care
   o. problems
   o. rehabilitation
   O. Shoes, Child Life
   o. surgeon
   o. surgery
orthophoria, asthenic

orthophosphate, calcium
orthoplastic rhinoplasty
orthopnea
- o. ▸ breathlessness, insomnia and
- o. position
- o., three-pillow
- o., two- or three-pillow
- o., two-pillow

orthoptic hepatic transplant
orthoptic training
orthorexia nervosa
orthoscopic lens
Orthosis, Servo-Driven
orthostatic
- o. blood pressure (BP)
- o. drainage (dr'ge)
- o. dyspnea
- o. hypertension
- o. hypopiesis
- o. hypotension
- o. hypotension, chronic
- o. hypotension, chronic idiopathic
- o. hypotension ▸ idiopathic
- o. lightheadedness
- o. line
- o. proteinuria
- o. purpura
- o. syncope
- o. tachycardia
- o. tachycardia syndrome (POTS) ▸ postular
- o. vital signs

orthotic(s)
- o., custom
- o. ▸ custom designed foot
- o. device
- o., foot
- o. ▸ foot control corrective
- o. shoes
- o. system

orthotonos position
orthotopic
- o. biventricular artificial heart
- o. cardiac transplant
- o. hepatic transplant
- o. transplantation
- o. univentricular artificial heart

orthovoltage units
Ortolani's
- O. click
- O. sign
- O. test

oryzae, Rhizopus
os
- o. (left eye)

o. acetabuli
o., blood exuding from external
o., blood oozing from
o. calcis
o., cervical
o. cuboideum
o. epitympanicum
o. ethmoidale
o., external
o. frontale
o. hyoideum
o., incompetent cervical
o., internal
o., internal cervical
o. interparietale
o. lacrimale
o. lunatum
o. magnum
o. mastoideum
o. nasale
o. occipitale
o. orbiculare
o. palatinum
o. parietale
o. penis
o., per
o., pinpoint
o. (by mouth), PO or per
o. pubis
o. sphenoidale
o. temporale
o., tissue extruding at cervical
o., tissue in
o. trigonum tarsi
o. triquetrum
o. unguis
o. uteri
o. uteri ▸ dilation of
o. zygomaticum

OSA (obstructive sleep apnea)
osazone test
Osborne's operation
oscillating
- o. grid
- o. nystagmus
- o. vision

oscillation
- o., double
- o. ▸ high frequency
- o., involuntary rhythmic
- o. of baseline
- o. of eyeballs, rhythmic horizontal
- o. of eyeballs, rhythmic vertical
- o., periodic
- o. technique ▸ forced

o. ventilator ▸ high frequency
o. wave

oscillatory afterpotential
oscillatory electricity
oscillometric blood pressure (BP) monitor ▸ automatic
oscillopsia ▸ gait, balance and
Osgood('s)
- O. operation
- O. -Schlatter disease
- O. -Schlatter syndrome

osial lesion
Osiander's sign
Osler('s)
- O. disease
- O. disease, Vaquez-
- O. nodes
- O. phenomenon
- O. sign
- O. syndrome
- O. triad
- O. -Vaquez disease
- O. -Weber disease ▸ Rendu-
- O. -Weber syndrome ▸ Sutton-Rendu-

OSM (oxygen saturation meter)
osmolality
- o. contrast material ▸ low
- o., decreased serum
- o., increased urine
- o., plasma
- o., serum
- o., urine

osmolar dehydration
osmolarity
- o. of blood
- o. of blood and urine ▸ hypo-
- o., serum

Osmolite feedings
osmophore group
osmophoresis, immunoelectro-
osmoregulatory center
osmosis, electro-
osmosis (RO) ▸ reverse
osmotic
- o. diarrhea
- o. diuresis
- o. diuretic
- o. fragility
- o. laxative
- o. nephrosis
- o. pressure (OP)
- o. pressure (COP) ▸ colloid
- o. pressure (COP) measurement ▸ colloid

osmotic—*continued*
- o. pressure (OP) movement ▸ colloid
- o. pressure (COP) of plasma ▸ colloid
- o. shock

ossea
- o., concha nasalis inferior
- o., concha nasalis media
- o., concha nasalis superior
- o., concha nasalis suprema
- o. dentis, substantia
- o., lymphadenia

ossei, vertex cranii
osseocartilaginous arch
osseointegrated implant
osseointegration procedure
osseointegration process
osseoligamentous arch
osseous
- o. abnormality
- o. cell
- o. fragments, irregular
- o. graft
- o. labyrinth
- o. metaplasia
- o. metastases, widespread
- o. metastasis
- o. metastatic disease
- o. portion
- o. structures
- o. tissue

ossicles
- o., articulations of auditory
- o., auditory
- o., muscles of auditory

ossicular
- o. chain
- o. chain, mobility of
- o. chain, palpation of
- o. chain, superior
- o. replacement prosthesis (PORP), partial
- o. replacement prosthesis (TORP), Plastiport total
- o. replacement prosthesis (TORP), total

ossificans
- o., carcinoma
- o., meningitis
- o., myositis
- o., osteitis
- o., pelvospondylitis
- o. traumatics, tendinitis

ossification
- o. centers
- o. of meninges
- o., pulmonary

ossified edge, medial
ossified papillary thyroid carcinoma
ossifying
- o. diathesis
- o. myositis, progressive
- o. pneumonitis

ossis sphenoidalis, forament ovale
ossium, fragilitas
ossium, xanthomatosis generalisata
ostearthrotomy/osteo-arthrotomy
ostectomies ▸ maxillary tuberosity resectional
ostectomy/osteectomy/osteo-ectomy
osteitis
- o., acute mastoid
- o., alveolar
- o. condensans generalisata
- o. condensans ilii
- o. deformans
- o. fibrosa cystica
- o., localized alveolar
- o., mastoid
- o. ossificans
- o., periapical rarefied

osteoarthritic
- o. changes
- o. hypertrophic spur formation
- o. lipping

osteoarthritis (OA)
- o., cervical
- o., debilitating
- o. gait
- o., generalized
- o. knee pain
- o. of hip
- o. of knee ▸ painful
- o. of spine
- o. temporomandibular joints

osteoarthropathy
- o., hypertrophic pulmonary
- o., idiopathic hypertrophic
- o., pulmonary
- o. ▸ pulmonary hypertrophic

osteoblastic
- o. activity
- o. lesions
- o. metastases in ribs

osteocapsular arthroplasty
osteocartilaginous body
osteocartilaginous growths
osteochondral exostosis

osteochondral junction
osteochondritis
- o. deformans
- o. deformans juvenilis
- o. dissecans
- o. ischiopubica

osteochondrodystrophy, familial
osteochondromatosis, synovial
osteoclast
- o., Collins
- o., Phelps-Gocht
- o., Rizzoli's

osteodysplastica, geroderma
osteodystrophy, azotemic
osteodystrophy, renal
osteogenesis
- o., fixation with
- o. imperfecta
- o. imperfecta cystica

osteogenic
- o. imperfecta
- o. sarcoma
- o. tissue

osteoid
- o. carcinoma
- o. osteoma
- o. tissue

osteolytic
- o. calvarial lesion
- o. lesion
- o. lesions ▸ widespread bony

osteoma
- o., cavalryman's
- o., choroidal
- o. dentale
- o., osteoid
- o. sarcomatosum
- o. spongiosum

osteomalacia, juvenile
osteomyelitis
- o., acute hematogenous
- o., chronic
- o., chronic petrous
- o., chronic refractory
- o., Garré's
- o. of skull, post-traumatic
- o., staphylococcal
- o., vertebral

osteonecrosis
- o., knee
- o. of femur
- o. of joint
- o. of knee
- o., radiation

osteo-onychodysplasia, hereditary

osteopathic manipulation
osteopathic scoliosis
osteopenia of disuse
osteoperiosteal
- o. bone graft
- o. graft
- o. iliac bone graft

osteoperiostitis, alveolodental
osteophyte
- o. formation
- o. formation, dorsal
- o. production

osteophytosis, intra-articular
osteoplastic
- o. amputation
- o. craniotomy
- o. flap
- o. rhinoplasty

osteoplasty, hetero-
osteoporosis
- o., at risk for
- o., bone weakening
- o., clinical
- o., debilitating
- o., disuse
- o. ▸ estrogen replacement for
- o., generalized
- o., idiopathic
- o. management
- o., postmenopausal
- o., post-traumatic
- o. prevention
- o. -related spine fractures
- o. screening
- o., spinal
- o. ▸ steroid-induced
- o. therapy

osteoporotic
- o. bone
- o. compression fractures
- o. fracture
- o. fracture ▸ nonvertebral
- o. thinning of vertebral column

Osteo-Stim apparatus
osteotomized, femur
osteotomy
- o., block
- o., Coventry's
- o., cuneiform
- o., cup-and-ball
- o., derotation
- o., femoral shortening
- o., innominate
- o., Keller bunion
- o., linear

- o., Lorenz's
- o., Macewen's
- o., metatarsal
- o., opening wedge-type
- o., plane, wire
- o., Salter
- o. site
- o., Smith-Petersen
- o., Southwick
- o., subtrochanteric
- o., transtrochanteric
- o., truncated
- o., Z-cut

osteotopic pain
osteotympanic conduction
Ostertag, Streptococcus of
ostial dimple, coronary
ostial lesion, aorto-
ostium(-a)
- o. abdominale tubae uterinae
- o., coronary
- o. of coronary artery ▸ severe narrowing
- o. primum
- o. primum defect
- o. primum defect, atrial
- o. primum ▸ persistent
- o. secundum
- o. secundum defect
- o. ▸ solitary coronary
- o. uteri
- o. uterinum tubae uterinae
- o. vaginae

ostomy (Ostomy)
- o. care
- O. Club
- o., continence (WOC) nurse ▸ wound,
- o. procedure
- o. products
- o. rehabilitation
- O. Rehabilitation Program
- o., temporary

ostosclerosis
- o., clinical
- o., early
- o. of ear

ostosclerotic fixation
ostoscopic examination
ostracea, parakeratosis
Ostwald viscosimeter
O'Sullivan's operation
Osypka rotational angioplasty
OT (Occupational Therapist)
OT (Occupational Therapy)

otalgia
- o. dentalis
- o. intermittens
- o., reflex

OTC (over-the-counter) drugs
OTC (over-the-counter) medication
OTD (organ tolerance dose)
other(s)
- o., alienation of
- o., anticipation of misfortune to
- o. characteristic symptoms
- o., conning
- o., conscious exploitation of
- o. ▸ disregard rights of
- o. ▸ echoing words of
- o., exploits
- o. ▸ imitating movements of
- o. ▸ indifferent to feelings of
- o. ▸ insensitive to
- o., interact with
- o. interpersonal problem
- o. ▸ lack of interest in
- o. or unspecified psychoactive substance delusional disorder
- o. or unspecified psychoactive substance intoxication
- o., patient has good rapport with
- o. ▸ patient mistreats
- o. ▸ pervasive pattern of disregard for
- o. ▸ potential for violence to
- o. ▸ reckless disregard for safety of
- o. ▸ relative disregard for sensitivity of
- o. sensitivities ▸ disdain for
- o., significant
- o. specified family circumstances
- o. ▸ suspicious of
- o., threat to self or
- o. ▸ unreasonable expectations of
- o. ▸ unwitting exploitation of
- o. ▸ violates rights of

otic
- o. capsule
- o. depression
- o. ganglion

oticus, herpes zoster
otitic
- o. barotrauma
- o. hydrocephalus
- o. meningitis

otitis
- o., acute
- o. desquamativa
- o. externa

otitis—*continued*
- o., furuncular
- o. haemorrhagica
- o. ▸ invasive external
- o. ▸ malignant external
- o. mastoidea
- o. media
- o. media, acute
- o. media, acute bacterial
- o. media ▸ acute purulent
- o. media ▸ acute serous
- o. media, adhesive
- o. media, bilateral
- o. media, chronic
- o. media, chronic suppurative
- o. media, mucoserous
- o. media, purulent
- o. media, secretory
- o. media (SOM) ▸ serous
- o. media with effusion
- o., mucosis
- O., mucosus
- o., serous

otoacoustic emissions
otoconia, dislocated
otoconia ▸ free-floating
otoconial debris
otogenous/otogenic
otogenous pyemia
otologic surgery
otomicroscope
Otomyces hageni
Otomyces purpureus
otomycosis aspergillina
otopharyngeal tube
otoplasty, Crikelair
otoplasty, flap
otorhinolaryngological evaluation
otorrhea
- o., cerebrospinal
- o., chronic
- o., intermittent

otoscopic ear canal inspection ▸
video
otoscopy, pneumatic
ototoxic agent
OTS (Optical Tracking System)
Otto pelvis
Ottonello's method
Otto's disease
O₂ (oxygen)
- O₂ (oxygen) catheter, intratracheal
- O₂ (oxygen) cisternography
- O₂ (oxygen) consumption, systemic
- O₂ (oxygen) deficiency, severe

O₂ (oxygen) dependent, patient
O₂ (oxygen) difference, arterio-
  venous
O₂ (oxygen) effect
O₂ (oxygen) enhancement ratio
O₂ (oxygen), home
O₂ (oxygen), hyperbaric
O₂ (oxygen), infant with
O₂ (oxygen) monitor, transcuta-
  neous
O₂ (oxygen) saturation
O₂ (oxygen) saturation testing
O₂ (oxygen), supplemental inspired
O₂ (oxygen) tank, portable
O₂ (oxygen) therapy, hyperbaric
O₂ (oxygen), transcutaneous
O₂ (oxygen), transtracheal
O₂ (oxygen) uptake, maximum

OU (both eyes/each eye)
ou de rape, bruit de scie
Ouchterlony technique
ounce (fl oz) ▸ fluid
out
- o., acting in and acting
- o. (r/o) appendicitis ▸ rule
- o. area ▸ punched-
- o. ▸ arterial wall balloons
- o. behaviors, acting
- o., blacking
- o., bottomed
- o., burn-
- o. (r/o CA) ▸ carcinoma to be ruled
- o. cheek flap, over-and-
- o., client drop-
- o., criminal acting
- o., crying
- o., echo drop-
- o. exercises ▸ push-
- o., extremity vessels washed
- o. eyelid, turned
- o. fantasies, act
- o. ▸ feeling spaced
- o. ▸ feeling washed
- o. -flare shoes
- o. fracture
- o. fracture, blow-
- o. germinal centers ▸ hyalinized
  burned
- o., in and
- o., job burn
- o. kidneys, flush
- o. knee
- o., lesion milked
- o. myocardial infarction ▸ rule
- o. near edge of incision ▸ brought

o. of artery wall, ballooning-
o. of blood vessel, ballooning-
o. -of-body experiences (OBE)
o. -of-control ▸ feeling
o. -of-control ▸ patient
o. of medullary cavity ▸ cancellous
  bone curetted
o. -of-phase
o. -of-phase signals
o. of sync ▸ patient
o., patient acting
o., patient pulled catheter
o., patient spaced
o., patient stressed
o., pelvic clean-
o. plaque ▸ flush
o., remnants of lens washed
o. (r/o) ▸ rule
o., sexual acting
o., shallow breathing with forced
  blowing
o. shoe, swing-
o., suturing cyst inside
o. technique ▸ time-
o. temperature, melting
o. tendencies ▸ rebellious,
  aggressive acting
o. through stab wound ▸ drain
  brought
o. through wound ▸ tissue brought
o. -toeing
o. -toeing, infant has
o., white
o. wire, Bunnell pull-

outbreak(s)
- o., disease
- o., dysentery
- o. ▸ Ebola virus
- o., food-borne
- o., food-borne illness
- o., Hantavirus
- o. investigation
- o., nosocomial infection
- o., potential
- o., prevent further
- o., staphylococcal
- o., waterborne illness

outburst(s)
- o., angry
- o. ▸ displays verbal
- o., emotional
- o. of aggression or rage
- o., patient experiences emotional
- o., sudden
- o., violent

outcome(s) (Outcome)
- o., adverse fetal
- o., diagnosis and therapeutic
- o. ▸ negative patient
- o. of resuscitation
- O. Prospective Study (TOPS) ▸ Treatment
- o., psychological
- o. rate, average
- o. research
- o. research, patient-
- o. research, treatment
- o. study, controlled
- o. ▸ substance abuse treatment
- o., successful treatment

outcropping of lesions
outdated medical ethics
outdated prescription
outer
- o. aspect
- o. border
- o. canthus
- o. canthus, left
- o. canthus of eye
- o. canthus, right
- o. cell wall
- o. convexity
- o. dimension
- o. ear
- o. ear infection
- o. ear, malformed
- o. hair cell
- o. hamstring
- o. interrupted silk sutures
- o. layer of alveolar wall
- o. layer of eyeball
- o. layer of skin
- o. malleolus
- o. phalangeal cells
- o. pillar
- o. pillar cells
- o. quadrant, lower
- o. quadrant, upper
- o. rim, intact
- o. rods
- o. surface of eye
- o. surface of eye, protective
- o. table bones of skull
- o. table frontal bone
- o. table graft
- o. tables of skull

Outerbridge scale
Outerbridge's ridge
outermost
- o. covering of brain

- o. covering of spinal cord
- o. layer of skin

outflow
- o. conduit
- o., decreased penile
- o. murmur
- o. ▸ net gradient of fluid
- o. obstruction
- o. obstruction, reduced
- o. obstruction ▸ right ventricular (RV)
- o. of bile
- o. resistance
- o., revision of
- o. tract
- o. tract, biliary
- o. tract ▸ left ventricular
- o. tract obstruction
- o. tract obstruction ▸ left ventricular (LV)
- o. tract, pulmonary
- o. tract ▸ right ventricular (RV)
- o. tract tachycardia ▸ right ventricular (RV)
- o. tract velocity ▸ left ventricular (LV)
- o. tract, ventricular

outgoing mechanism
outgoing, patient is
outgrowth, bony
outlet
- o., bladder
- o. decompression, thoracic
- o., deformity of gastric
- o. forceps delivery
- o., gastric
- o. irritability, gastric
- o. left ventricle (LV), double
- o. left ventricle (LV) malposition ▸ double
- o., marital
- o., narrowing of
- o., narrowing of gastric
- o. obstruction
- o. obstruction ▸ bladder
- o. obstruction, chronic
- o. obstruction, gastric
- o. occlusion, total
- o., pelvic
- o., relaxed vaginal
- o. right ventricle, double-
- o. right ventricle (RV) malposition ▸ double
- o. strut fracture
- o. syndrome ▸ recurrent thoracic

- o. syndrome, thoracic
- o., transverse diameter of pelvic
- o., vaginal

outline
- o., heart size and
- o. of discs
- o., ovoid

outlined
- o., cytoplasmic borders well
- o., discs well
- o., normally
- o. with brilliant green

outlining amniotic cavity
outpatient (Outpatient)
- o. admission, potential
- o. basis
- o. basis, chemotherapy continued on
- o. basis, patient followed on
- o. basis, treated on an
- o. basis, weekly
- o. care
- O. Chemical Dependency Clinic
- O. Clinic
- O. Community Clinic
- o. counselor
- O. Department (OPD)
- o. detoxification
- o. drug-free program
- o. drug-free treatment
- o. drug treatment system
- o. evaluation
- o. facility
- o. follow-up
- o. mental health services
- o. methadone program
- o. ▸ non-alcoholic psychiatric
- o. non-psychiatric medical facilities
- o., patient followed as
- o. phlebectomy
- o. procedure
- O. Program ▸ Day Intensive
- O. Program, Intensive
- o. psychiatric treatment
- o. psychotherapy
- o., return as
- o. satisfaction assessment
- O. Service
- o. sessions
- o. setting
- o. surgery
- o. surgical suite
- o. therapeutic suspension status
- o. therapy
- o. transfer, inpatient to

outpatient—*continued*
- o. treatment
- o. treatment, long-term
- o. treatment program ▸ intense
- o. treatment program ▸ intensive
- o. visits

outplacement counseling

outpocketing, embryonic

outpouching of old pseudocyst

outpouchings, sacular

output
- o., adequate cardiac
- o., alteration in cardiac
- o. and intake
- o., basal acid
- o., bile
- o., bladder
- o., cardiac
- o. (CMO) ▸ cardiac minute
- o. circuit, phototube
- o., current
- o., decreased cardiac
- o. decreased, renal
- o., decreased urinary
- o., decreasing cardiac
- o. device
- o. factor
- o. failure ▸ low
- o., fluid
- o. ▸ fluid intake/
- o. frequency, amplifier
- o. heart failure, high
- o. heart failure ▸ low-
- o. impedance, low
- o., inadequate cardiac
- o., increased urinary
- o. index, cardiac
- o., insensible fluid
- o., intake and
- o. ▸ left ventricular (LV)
- o. ▸ low cardiac
- o., marginal cardiac
- o. markedly reduced ▸ cardiac
- o., maximal acid
- o. measurement, cardiac
- o., minute
- o. ▸ monitor fluid intake and
- o., normal urine
- o. of pituitary gland, hormone
- o., pacemaker
- o. pen deflection
- o. pen deflection ▸ percent reduction of
- o., positive
- o., reduced cardiac

- o., resting cardiac
- o., saliva
- o. signal voltage, ratio of
- o., sperm
- o., stroke
- o., systemic cardiac
- o. terminal, negative
- o. ▸ thermodilution cardiac
- o., urinary
- o. ▸ vasodilators increase cardiac
- o., visual feedback of myoelectric
- o. voltage

outreach program, family

outreach sessions, family

outside
- o. diameter
- o. neurons
- o. of body experience
- o. stimulation

outstretched arm movement

outstretched hand or tongue

outward movement

outward rotation

ova
- o. and parasites
- o. and parasites, stools for
- o., primordial
- o., unfertilized

oval
- o. amputation
- o. cell
- o. center, greater
- o. foramen, closed
- o. lesions with small white centers
- o. nucleus
- o. nucleus, large
- o. -shaped
- o. -shaped opening
- o. window
- o. window defect
- o. window niche
- o. window reflex

ovale
- o., Amblyomma
- o. basis crania, foramen
- o. closed, foramen
- o. cordis, foramen
- o., foramen
- o. ossis sphenoidalis, foramen
- o., patent foramen
- o., Pityrosporon
- o., Plasmodium

ovalis
- o., annulus
- o. cordis, fossa

- o., fenestra
- o., fossa

ovalocytary anemia

ovarian (Ovarian)
- o. ablation
- o. abnormality, congenital
- o. abscess, tubo-
- o. agenesis
- o. amenorrhea
- o. appendage
- o. artery
- o. ascorbic acid depletion
- o. atrophy
- o. calculus
- o. cancer
- o. cancer cells
- o. cancer, inoperable
- o. cancer syndrome ▸ hereditary breast-
- o. carcinoma
- o. carcinoma, primary
- o. carcinoma with ascites
- o. carcinoma with metastases ▸ primary
- o. castration, radiation for
- o. cell mass
- o. cumulus
- o. cycle
- o. cyst
- o. cyst, malignant
- o. cyst torsion
- o. cyst, tubo-
- o. cystectomy
- o. duct
- o. dysfunction
- o. dysgerminoma
- o. dysmenorrhea
- o. dyspepsia
- o. endodermal sinus tumor
- o. endometriosis
- o. epithelial cancer
- o. estrogen
- o. failure
- o. fimbria
- o. follicle
- o. fossa
- o. fragment
- o. function
- o. hernia
- o. inflammatory cysts
- o. ligament
- o. mass
- o. mass, cystic
- o. plexus
- o. pregnancy

o. pregnancy, tubo-
o. pregnancy, utero-
o. remnant
o. salpingolysis, salpingo-
o. seminoma
o. serous cystadenocarcinoma
o. stroma
o. stromal hyperplasia
o. syndrome (PCOS) ▸ polycystic
o. teratoma, immature
o. tissue banking
o. transposition
o. tube
o. tubular adenoma
o. tumor
O. Tumor Registry
o. varicocele
o. varicocele, utero-
o. vein
o. vein, left
o. vein, right
ovarica, fimbria
ovarica, fossa
ovaricus cumulus
ovaricus, plexus
ovarii
o., adenoma endometrioides
o., adenoma tubulare testiculare
o., endometriosis
o., stroma
o. testiculare, adenoma
o., testiculoma
ovarioabdominal pregnancy
ovariopariva, cachexia
ovary(-ies)
o., adenocystic
o., aplasia of
o. atrophic, left
o. atrophic, right
o., carcinoma of
o., cystadenocarcinoma of
o. dermoid cyst of
o. disease ▸ polycystic
o. ▸ enzymatic abnormality of
o., fetal
o., function of
o., hilus of
o., inflamed
o. involutional changes of
o. ▸ nodular hyperplasia of
o., papillary cystadenocarcinoma of
o., papillary serous cystadeno-
    carcinoma
o., polycystic
o. protection in radiation therapy

o., pseudomucinous cystadeno-
    carcinoma
o., release of eggs from
o., right and/or left
o., sclerotic
o., serocystadenoma of
o., streaked
o., stroma of
o. ▸ surgical absence of
o., swelling of
o. syndrome (PCOS) ▸ polycystic
o., wandering
o., white scar of
ovatus, Metagonimus
Ovenstone factor
over
o. alcohol, powerless
o. -and-out cheek flap
o. -and-over suture
o. -attentiveness, parental
o. cerebral cortex ▸ electrodes
    applied
o. cotton, sutures tied down
o., cross-
o., crossing
o. disloyalty ▸ guilt
o. -end running technique ▸ end-
o. -excretion of sodium in urine
o. graft, bolus tie-
o. left lung ▸ dullness
o. perforation, sealed
o. periosteum, sheath reflected
o. posture ▸ stooped
o. -responsive to stimulation,
    neurologically
o. right lung ▸ dullness
o. rubber shoes, sutures tied
o., sealed
o. -stent, tie-
o. -the-counter (OTC) antihist-
    amines
o. -the-counter (OTC) drugs
o. -the-counter (OTC) medication
o. -the-counter (OTC) products
o. victim's mouth, tight seal
o., wound closed
overactive
o. behavior
o. bladder
o. bladder syndrome
o. child
o. glands
o. immune system
o. parathyroid glands
o. thyroid

o. thyroid disorder
o. thyroid gland
overactivity
o., emotional
o., physical
o., psychomotor
overall
o. alignment
o. assessment, rapid
o. body strength
o. fitness
o. functional progress
o. functioning
o. functioning, improved
o. level of mental function
o. seroprevalence rate
o. size
o. therapeutic goals
o. treatment duration, increased
o. treatments
o. weakness
overanxious disorder
overbed table
overbreathing, patient
overburdened heart
overcoming denial
overcontraction of muscles
overcontrolled hostility scale
overconvergence, adult
overdistention of bladder
overdistention, uterine
overdosage
o., acute
o., digitalis
o., drug
overdose (OD)
o., accidental
o., alcohol
o., anticholinergic
o., cocaine
o., drug
o., fatal
o., habituation and
o., intended
o., intentional
o., narcotic
o. of medication
o. of morphine, lethal
o., opioid
o., patient took
o., poisonings and
o. potential
o. state
o., sympathomimetic
o., toxic

overdose—*continued*
- o., treatment of
- o., vitamin
- o. with hallucinogens

overdosed (OD)
- o. ▸ patient
- o. with cannabinoids, patient
- o. with depressants, patient
- o. with hallucinogens, patient
- o. with inhalants, patient
- o. with multiple drugs, patient
- o. with opioids, patient
- o. with phencyclidines, patient
- o. with stimulants, patient

overdosing
- o., acute treatment for
- o., clinical manifestations of
- o., differential diagnosis with
- o., psychological state with
- o., subacute treatment for
- o., symptoms of

overdrive
- o. atrial pacing
- o. pacing
- o. suppression

Overeaters Anonymous (OA)

overeating
- o., compulsive
- o. disorder
- o. ▸ obsessive, compulsive
- o., repetitive

overestimates abilities

overexcited, easily

overexposed to sun

overexposure to heat

overexposure to sunlight

overflex knee

overflow
- o. incontinence
- o. of tears
- o. wave

overgrown muscle

overgrowth
- o., arthritic
- o., bacterial
- o., bony
- o. of non-nervous supportive tissue
- o. of uterine lining ▸ precancerous

overhang, bony

overhead arm movement

overhead movement of arm ▸ repetitive

overheated, smear

Overholt's operation

overhydrated, patient

overinflation, congenital lobar

overinflation of lungs

overinvolvement, emotional

overjet, excess

overkill phenomenon

overlap
- o., horizontal
- o. in orthogonal fields, beam
- o. shadow
- o., vertical

overlapping suture

overlapping visits ▸ stress of

overlay
- o. and depression, psychological
- o., anxiety
- o., emotional
- o., functional
- o., neurotic
- o., psychogenic
- o., psychological
- o. sign ▸ hilum
- o., significant functional

overload
- o., activity
- o., circulatory
- o., diastolic
- o. disease, iron
- o., fluid
- o., fluid volume
- o., major
- o., muscle tension
- o., pressure
- o., stress
- o., volume

overloading, cardiac

overly impressionistic speech

overlying
- o. gas shadows
- o. intestinal gas
- o. mural endocardium
- o. pneumonitis
- o. skin

overmedicated, patient

overnight pass, patient released on

overnight sleep evaluation

overproduction of mucus

overproduction of saliva

overreactive airway disease

overreactive patient

overreactivity, physiological

override, aortic

overriding aorta

overripe cataract

oversedated, patient

oversensing, afterpotential

oversensing pacemaker

oversensitive nipple

oversensitivity to pain

overstimulated ▸ patient

overstimulation
- o. and resulting confusion
- o. of breasts
- o. of salivary glands

Overstreet syndrome, Gordan-

overstressed body

overt
- o. anger ▸ inappropriate
- o. behavior
- o. competition
- o. congestive failure
- o. diabetes
- o. heart failure
- o. heart failure ▸ onset of
- o. homosexuality
- o. hostility, patient exhibits
- o. left ventricular dysfunction
- o. responses
- o. symptom of heart disease

overtly symptomatic

overtone, psychic

overtone, psychological

overtures, suicidal

overuse
- o. injury
- o. of drugs
- o. of drugs, medical
- o. of joint
- o. of muscles, avoid
- o. strain injury
- o. syndrome
- o. tendinitis

overutilization, bed

overvalued
- o. false idea
- o. ideas
- o. obsessional ideas

overwhelmed, feeling

overwhelming
- o. episode of terror
- o. exhaustion
- o. fatigue
- o. feelings of sadness and grief
- o. infection
- o. sense of panic

oviduct, fimbriated end of

oviduct, pavilion of the

oviductal pregnancy

ovigerous cords

ovine lactogenic hormone

ovis
- o., Anaplasma
- o., Ascaris
- o., Corynebacterium
- o., Cysticercus
- o., Miyagawanella
- o., Oestrus
- o., Psoroptes
- o., Taenia

ovitoxicus, Clostridium
ovo vegetarian diet ▸ lacto-
ovoid [*avoid*]
- o. cells, elongated
- o., Manchester
- o. nuclei, hyperchromatic
- o. outline

ovulating, patient
ovulation
- o., abnormal
- o. and menstrual flow
- o. and spermatogenesis
- o., cessation of
- o. cycle
- o. disorder
- o., escape
- o. failure of
- o., irregular
- o., oligo-
- o. ▸ pituitary hormone trigger
- o. problem
- o. test

ovulatory
- o. agent
- o. failure
- o. menstruation

ovule(s)
- o., graafian
- o., nabothian
- o., Naboth's
- o., primitive
- o., primordial

ovum (Ovum)
- o., blighted
- o., fertilize
- o. ▸ implantation of fertilized
- o., mature
- o., release of
- o., ripe
- O. Transfer (TOT), Tubal

OVWI (Operating Vehicle While Intoxicated)
OVWI (Operating Vehicle While Intoxicated) Program
Owen's view
own defense mechanism, body's

owned clinics ▸ physician-
ox cell hemolysis test
ox heart
oxacillin sodium
oxalate
- o., calcium
- o. calculus
- o. calculus, calcium
- o. crystals, calcium
- o. diet
- o., sodium
- o. stone, calcium

oxalic
- o. acid
- o. diathesis
- o. gout
- o. transaminase (SGOT), serum glutamic-

oxaloacetic
- o. transaminase (EGOT) ▸ erythrocyte glutamic-
- o. transaminase (GOT) ▸ glutamic-
- o. transaminase (SGOT) ▸ serum glutamic-

Oxford Project to Investigate Memory and Aging (OPTIMA)
Oxford's operation
oxidant-induced lung injury
oxidants (FRO) ▸ free radical
oxidase (Oxidase)
- o. activity ▸ platelet monoamine
- o., diamine
- O. (MAO) inhibitor diet ▸ restricted tyramine and monoamine
- o. inhibitor (MAOI) ▸ monoamine
- o., monoamine
- o. reaction ▸ xanthine

oxidate respiration
oxidating stress
oxidation of cholesterol
oxidative
- o. damage
- o. process in tissues
- o. reaction
- o. reaction ▸ adverse
- o. reaction ▸ photo-

oxide
- o. barbiturate, nitrous
- o., ethylene
- o. hemoglobin, nitric
- o., magnesium
- o. (N₂O), nitrous
- o. tank, nitrous

oxidized
- o. cellulose

- o. fat ▸ rancid
- o. fatty molecules
- o. glutathione

oximeter, pulse
oximeter ▸ SpaceLabs pulse
oximetric catheter
oximetry
- o. device ▸ pulse
- o., finger
- o. monitoring ▸ pulse
- o., pulse
- o., reflectance
- o., transcutaneous

oxogenic steroid
oxybutyric acids (BOBA), beta-
Oxycel pack
oxydans, Acetobacter
oxygen (O₂)
- o. administered
- o. and carbon dioxide (CO₂) levels
- o. and ether gas
- o. and humidity
- o. and nutrients ▸ diffusion of
- o. -binding capacity
- o., blood
- o. by nasal cannula
- o., capacity
- o., carbon dioxide with
- o. -carrying capacity
- o. -carrying red cells
- o. catheter, intratracheal
- o., cerebral metabolic rate of
- o. (HBO) chamber, hyperbaric
- o. cisternography
- o., compressed
- o. concentration
- o. concentration, high
- o. concentrator
- o. conditions, low
- o. consumption
- o. consumption computer
- o. consumption index
- o. consumption ▸ maximum
- o. consumption ▸ myocardial
- o. consumption ▸ peak exercise
- o. consumption per minute
- o. consumption, systemic
- o. consumption ▸ volume
- o. content
- o. content determination
- o. content of blood decreases
- o., continuous
- o. deficiency
- o. deficiency, severe
- o. deficit

oxygen—*continued*
- o. delivery
- o. demand ▸ myocardial
- o. -dependent, patient
- o. -depleted blood
- o. deprivation
- o. deprivation ▸ control of heart rate during
- o. deprivation in critical organs
- o. -deprived leg muscles
- o. -derived free radicals
- o. difference (AV DO$_2$), arterio-venous
- o. -diffusing capacity
- o. dissociation curve
- o. dissociation curve ▸ hemoglobin
- o. effect
- o. enhancement ratio
- o. exchange in lung
- o. filter
- o. flow to tumor
- o. (FIO$_2$) ▸ fraction of inspired
- o. -free radicals
- o., high
- o., high pressure
- o., home
- o. ▸ humidifier and
- o., humidity and
- o., hyperbaric
- o., imbalance of
- o., infant with
- o. inhalation
- o. insufficiency
- o. (IPPO), intermittent positive pressure inflation with
- o., lack of
- o. level
- o. level, blood
- o., liquid
- o., liters of
- o. mask
- o. -mediated lung injury
- o., mixed venous
- o. molecules
- o. molecules ▸ unstable
- o. monitor
- o. monitor, transcutaneous
- o. paradox
- o. partial pressure, alveolar
- o. (PO$_2$) ▸ partial pressure of
- o., portable supplemental
- o. pressure (PO$_2$)
- o. pressure (HOP) ▸ high
- o. quotient
- o. quotient, cerebral glucose
- o. radical
- o. -rich blood
- o. -rich blood ▸ starved for
- o. saturation
- o. saturation (SaO$_2$), arterial
- o. saturation (SaO$_2$), blood arterial
- o. saturation level
- o. saturation meter (SM)
- o. saturation ▸ mixed venous
- o. saturation ▸ step-up in
- o. saturation testing
- o. -starved brain
- o. -starved heart muscle
- o. -starved tissue
- o., supplemental
- o., supplemental inspired
- o. supply
- o. supply critical
- o. supply ▸ myocardial
- o. tank, portable
- o. tension
- o. tension, alveolar
- o. tension/concentration
- o. tension gradient, alveoloarterial
- o. tension, reduced
- o. tent
- o. therapy
- o. therapy, home
- o. therapy, hyperbaric
- o. therapy ▸ long-term
- o. therapy ▸ organizing interstitial pneumonia
- o. therapy ▸ supplemental
- o., tissue
- o. to brain ▸ lack of
- o. (O$_2$) to cardiac muscle ▸ lack of
- o. to heart ▸ flow of blood and
- o. toxicity
- o. toxicity in immature lung
- o., transcutaneous
- o. transport
- o. transport ▸ deficit in
- o. transtracheal
- o. treatment ▸ hyperbaric
- o. under high pressure
- o. unit
- o. unit ▸ myocardial
- o. uptake, maximum
- o. uptake ▸ myocardial
- o. vapor

oxygenated
- o. blood
- o. blood supply
- o. hemoglobin

oxygenation
- o. before recirculation
- o. blood
- o., bubble
- o., disc
- o., disk
- o., efficiency of
- o. (ECMO) ▸ extracorporeal membrane
- o., film
- o., hyperbaric
- o. of blood
- o. of blood, deficient
- o. of organs
- o., proper
- o., pump
- o. ▸ rotating disk
- o., screen
- o., tissue

oxygenator
- o., bubble
- o., disc
- o. ▸ extracorporeal membrane
- o., intravascular
- o., membrane
- o. pump

oxyhemoglobin dissociation curve

OXY-Hood

oxyphil
- o., amphophilic-
- o. cells
- o. granules

oxyphilic
- o. adenoma
- o. cells
- o. erythroblast
- o. normoblast

oxytoca, Klebsiella

oxytocic rupture

oxytocin augmentation

Oxyuris incognita

Oxyuris vermicularis

oyster mass of mucus

oyster shuckers' keratitis

ozaenae, Klebsiella

ozogenes, gram-negative Klebsiella

Ozone (ozone)
- O. (phencyclidine)
- o. layer damage
- o. ▸ lung injury from

ozzardi, Mansonella

Ozzard's filariasis

P

p (P)
   p. (after)
   p. (parietal)
   P., substance
p. ae. (in equal parts)
P and A (percussion and auscultation)
P and A (percussion and auscultation) ▸ chest clear to
P and A (percussion and auscultation) ▸ lungs clear to
P congenitale
P loop
P mitrale
P terminal force
P 32, chromic phosphate
P 32, sodium phosphate
P vector
P wave
   Pw. axis
   Pw., bifid
   Pw., diphasic
   Pw. ▸ peaked
   Pw. ▸ retrograde
   Pw. triggered ventricular pacemaker
PA (physician's assistant)
PA (posteroanterior)
   PA and lateral projections
   PA film
   PA lordotic projection
   PA position
   PA projection
   PA projection, transtabular AP/
   PA study
   PA view
PA (pulpoaxial)
P-A interval
Pabry's disease
PAC (papular acrodermatitis of childhood)
PAC (premature atrial/auricular contraction)
PACAB (port-access coronary artery bypass)
pacchionian
   p. bodies

p. depressions
p. foramen
p. glands
p. granulations
pace
   p. mapping
   p. therapy, ablative
   p. ▸ ventricular lead
paced
   p. breathing
   p. cycle length
   p. cycle length, atrial-
   p. rhythm
   p. rhythm ▸ ventricular
   p. ventricular evoked response
pacemaker
   p., activity sensing
   p. adaptive rate
   p. afterpotential
   p., alternating atrial
   p. amplifier refractory period
   p., Amtech-Killeen
   p., antitachycardia
   p., Arco
   p., Arco lithium
   p. artifact
   p., artificial
   p., artificial cardiac
   p., asynchronous
   p., asynchronous atrial
   p., atrial asynchronous
   p., atrial demand inhibited
   p., atrial demand triggered
   p., atrial tracking
   p. ▸ atrial triggered ventricular inhibited
   p., atrial VOO
   p., Atricor Cordis
   p., atrioventricular (AV) junctional
   p., atrioventricular (AV) sequential
   p., Aurora dual chamber
   p., Autima II dual chamber
   p., automatic
   p. automaticity
   p., AV sequential
   p., AV synchronous
   p., Avius sequential

p. battery change, cardiac
p., bifocal demand
p., Biotronik
p., bipolar
p., bipolar Medtronic
p., biventricular
p., body's circadian
p., brain
p. breathing
p. burst pacing
p. capture
p., cardiac
p. catheter
p. cell electrophysiology
p. cells
p., Chardack-Greatbatch
p., cilium
p. code
p. code system
p. committed mode
p. complex sinoatrial (SA)
p., Coratomic
p., Cordis
p., Cordis Atricor
p., Cordis-Ectocor
p., Cordis fixed rate
p., Cordis Ventricor
p., CPI Maxilith
p., CPI Minilith
p., cross-talk
p. damage
p., Dash single-chamber rate adaptic
p., decremental atrial
p., demand
p. ▸ dual chamber AV (atrioventricular)
p. ▸ dual chamber cardiac
p., dual demand
p., dual pass
p., Durapulse
p., Ectocor
p., ectopic
p., Elecath
p., electric cardiac
p. electrode
p., Electrodyne

pacemaker—*continued*

p., electronic
p., endocardial bipolar
p. ▸ end-of-life
p., epicardial
p., escape
p. escape interval
p., external
p., external asynchronous
p., external demand
p., external-internal
p. failure
p., fixed rate
p. for brain ▸ permanent
p., fully automatic
p. function
p., gastric
p., GE (General Electric)
p., General Electric (GE)
p. generator, unipolar
p., heart
p., hysteresis
p. impedance
p. implant
p. implant temporary
p., implantable
p. implantation ▸ dual chamber
p. implantation of
p. implantation permanent
p., implanted
p. implanted under skin
p. infection
p. insertion
p. insertion, permanent
p., Intermedics
p., Intermedics Thinlith II
p., internal
p., junctional
p. lag time
p., Lambda
p., latent
p. lead
p. lead finned
p. lead fracture
p. lead steroid eluting
p. line, transvenous
p., lithium
p. load electronic
p. ▸ Maestro implantable cardiac
p. malfunction
p., Mallory
p. management, permanent
p. management, temporary
p., Maxilith
p. mediated tachycardia (PMT)

p. ▸ Medtronic Activitrax rate responsive unipolar ventricular
p., Medtronic demand
p., Medtronic Elite DDDR
p. ▸ Medtronic Elite II
p., Medtronic-Laurens-Alcatel
p., Medtronic Pacette
p. ▸ Medtronic SPO
p. ▸ Medtronic temporary
p. ▸ Meta rate responsive
p., migrating
p., Minilith
p. monitoring
p. monitoring transtelephonic
p., Nathan
p., natural
p. ▸ noninvasive temporary
p., nuclear
p. of heart
p., Omni-Atricor
p., Omni-cor
p., Omni-Ectocor
p., Omni-Stanicor
p. output
p., oversensing
p. ▸ P wave triggered ventricular
p., Pacesetter
p. ▸ Paragon II
p., Pasar tachycardia reversion
p. patient testing system complete
p., permanent
p. ▸ permanent cardiac
p., permanent myocardial
p., permanent transvenous
p., pervenous
p., phantom
p. placement permanent
p. placement, temporary transvenous
p. pocket
p. potential
p., Prima
p., programmable
p., programming
p. pulse generator ▸ Microlith
p. pulse generator ▸ Minilith
p. ▸ Q-T interval sensing
p., Quantum
p., radio-frequency
p., rate-adaptive
p. ▸ rate-modulated
p. ▸ rate-responsive
p. reedswitch
p. ▸ refractory period of electronic
p. ▸ Relay cardiac

p. replacement
p. ▸ reprogram dual
p. ▸ reprogram single
p., respiratory
p., runaway
p., Schuletz
p., secondary
p., Seecor
p. sensitivity
p. ▸ sensor-driven
p., Shaldach
p., shifting
p. ▸ single chamber
p., single-pass
p., sinus
p. sound
p. spike
p., Stanicor
p., Starr-Edwards
p. stimulus
p. strategy
p. ▸ Stride cardiac
p. study (VPS) ▸ vasovagal
p. ▸ subsidiary atrial
p. support group
p., synchronous
p. syndrome
p., Tachylog
p., Telectronic
p. ▸ temperature-sensing
p., temporary
p., temporary cardiac
p., temporary transvenous
p. therapy
p., Thermos
p. threshold
p., transthoracic
p., transvenous
p., transvenous catheter
p. twiddler's syndrome
p. undersensing
p., unipolar
p. unit, Cordis
p., universal
p., Ventricor
p. ▸ ventricular asynchronous
p. ▸ ventricular demand inhibited
p. ▸ ventricular demand triggered
p., ventricular suppressed
p., ventricular-triggered
p., Versatex cardiac
p., Vitatron
p., Vivalith-10
p., wandering
p., Xoll

p., Xytron
p., Zyrel's
p., Zytron
pacemaking cells
pacemaking sinus node
pacer
    p. cardioverter defibrillator
    p. cardioverter ▸ Jewell
    p. ▸ Intertach II
    p. spike, double counting of
    p. spikes
Pacesetter pacemaker
Pacette pacemaker, Medtronic
pachometer instrument
pachydermic cachexia
pacificus, Ixodes
pacing
    p., access atrial
    p. and sensing thresholds
    p., antitachycardia
    p., asynchronous
    p., atrial
    p., atrial overdrive
    p., atrial synchronous
    p., atrioventricular sequential
    p., autodecremental
    p., bipolar
    p., biventricular
    p. box ▸ digital constant current
    p., bradyarrhythmia
    p., burst
    p., burst atrial
    p. cable
    p., cardiac
    p. catheter
    p. catheter, bipolar
    p. code
    p. cycle length
    p., decremental atrial
    p. device ▸ implantable
    p., diaphragmatic
    p. digital ventriculography
    p., dual chamber
    p., dual sensing (DDD) ▸ dual
      mode, dual
    p., dual-site atrial
    p. electrode ▸ Stockert cardiac
    p. electrode, temporary atrial
    p. electrode, temporary epicardial
    p. electrode wire
    p. function
    p. hysteresis
    p. impulse
    p. ▸ incremental atrial
    p. ▸ incremental ventricular

p. -induced angina
p., inhibited
p. interval ▸ magnet
p., intracardiac
p. lead barbed epicardial
p. lead ▸ permanent cardiac
p. modalities
p. mode
p. mode alternative atrial
p. mode atrial
p. ▸ myocardial stimulation in
p. ▸ noninvasive temporary
p., overdrive
p., overdrive atrial
p. ▸ pacemaker burst
p., patient
p., permanent
p., physiologic
p. protocol ▸ SCAN antitachycardia
p., ramp
p. ▸ rapid atrial
p. ▸ rapid burst
p. ▸ rate responsive
p., restless
p. stimulus
p. stress test atrial
p. system analyzer
p. system, malfunction of
  permanent demand ventricular
p. systems, permanent cardiac
p. systems, permanent demand
  ventricular
p., tachyarrhythmia
p. techniques
p., temporary
p. threshold
p. ▸ trains of ventricular
p., transatrial
p. ▸ transesophageal atrial
p. ▸ transesophageal echocardiography with
p., triggered
p. underdrive
p. unipolar
p. ventricular
p. wire, atrial
p. withdrawal
Pacini's corpuscles
Paci's operation
pack(s)
    p. and bed rest, hot
    p., antral
    p., battery
    p., Bellow's

p., chemical snap
p., cold
p., drains or
p., film
p., gas
p., Gelfoam
p. ▸ hot, moist
p., hydrocollator
p., ice
p., lap
p., MacKenty nasal
p. ▸ microwaveable heat
p., moist lap
p. or drains
p., oropharyngeal
p., Oxycel
p., pharyngeal
p., platelet
p., vaginal
packaged irrigating solution ▸
    pre◊
packed
    p. beads
    p. cell volume
    p. cells, unit of
    p. erythrocytes
    p. human blood cells
    p., inferiorly, viscera
    p., mastoid cavity
    p., nares
    p., nose
    p., nostril
    p. red blood cell transfusions
    p. red blood cells
    p. red cells, volume of
    p., uterus
    p., vagina
    p. with gauze, uterus
    p., wound
packing
    p. fraction
    p., Gelfoam
    p., iodoform gauze
    p., nasal
    p. of paracolic gutters
    p., surgical
    p., vaginal
pact, suicide
PAD (peripheral arterial disease)
pad(s)
    p., alcohol
    p. and shield applied, eye
    p., Aqua-K
    p. biopsy, scalene fat
    p., breast sensor

pad(s)—*continued*
- p., cotton gauze
- p., electrode
- p. enlargement ▸ dorsocervical fat
- p., eye
- p., fat
- p., felt gauze
- p., geriatric chair
- p., heel
- p., hydrocollator
- p., Kotex
- p. ▸ Littman defibrillation
- p., medicated corn
- p., metatarsal
- p., nasal drip
- p. of pleura, fat
- p., peri (perineal)
- p., periarterial
- p., pericardial fat
- p., prep
- p., protective eye
- p., retropatellar fat
- p. sign
- p. sign, fat
- p., thumb
- p., vag (vaginal)
- p., viable tissue
- p., volar
- p., wheelchair

padding ▸ displacement of cartilage

paddle(s)
- p., anteroposterior
- p. burn marks
- p. burns present
- p., cardioversion
- p., compression
- p., defibrillation
- p., defibrillator
- p., electrode
- p. marks from defibrillation

Padgett's graft

Paecilomyces variotii

Paessler syndrome, Romberg-

Pagano-Levin medium smear

Paget's
- P. abscess
- P. cell
- P. disease
- P. disease, extramammary
- P. disease of bone
- P. disease of breast
- P. quiet necrosis

paging beeper, pocket

paging receiver, pocket

PAH (pulmonary artery hypertension)

pain (Pain) [*gain, stain*]
- p., abdominal
- p., abdominal cramping
- p., abdominal swelling and
- p., absence of sensibility to
- p., aching
- p., acute
- p., acute back
- p., acute flank
- p., acute intrascrotal
- p., acute stabbing
- p. after childbirth ▸ back
- p. after childbirth ▸ breast
- p., afterbirth
- p. aggravated by motion
- p. aggravated by movement
- p. alleviated
- p., ameliorate
- p., anal
- p. and anxiety
- p. and chills ▸ muscle
- p. and debility, severe
- p. and discomfort
- p. and discomfort ▸ joint
- p. and dysfunction ▸ myofascial
- p. and exertion
- p. and fatigue ▸ muscular
- p. and fatigue ▸ severe joint
- p. and fever ▸ diarrhea, abdominal
- p. and inactivity ▸ cycle of
- p. and lack of mobility ▸ stiffness,
- p. and limited mobility
- p. and nausea
- p. and numbness ▸ cold, burning,
- p. and obstruction
- p. and restore mobility ▸ relieve
- p. and soreness ▸ rectal
- p. and spasm of muscles
- p. and stiffness
- p. and stiffness ▸ aches,
- p. and stiffness ▸ joint
- p. and stiffness ▸ muscle tension, aching,
- p. and swelling
- p. and swelling ▸ diarrhea with abdominal
- p. and swelling, joint
- p. and swelling of leg
- p. and symptom management
- p. and temperature ▸ diminished perception of
- p. and tenderness
- p. and tension ▸ muscular
- p. and tightness, chest
- p. and trauma

- p. and twitching ▸ facial
- p. and vomiting ▸ stomach
- p. and weakness, back
- p., angina chest
- p., ankle
- p., anxiety induced
- p., arm
- p., arthritic
- p., assessment of
- p. associated with blood loss ▸ abdominal
- p. at incision site
- p. at minimal level, bone
- p., atypical chest
- p., back
- p., beefing-down
- p. beefing nerve fibers
- p. behavior
- p. behavior decondition
- p. between shoulders
- p. ▸ bilateral pleuritic chest
- p., biofeedback and
- p., bladder
- p., blinding
- p., blinding head
- p. blocking illusion
- p., bodily
- p., body's response to
- p., bone
- p., boring
- p., breakthrough
- p., breast
- p. ▸ breathing with back, chest or abdomen
- p., Broudie's
- p., burning
- p., burning abdominal
- p., burning knife-like
- p., burning or freezing
- p. causation and management
- p., central
- p., cessation of
- p., Charcot's
- p., chest
- p., chest wall
- p., childbirth without (CWP)
- p. ▸ chill with back
- p. ▸ chills with swollen scrotum and
- p., chronic
- p., chronic aches and
- p., chronic and widespread
- p., chronic back
- p., chronic bone
- p., chronic chest

p., chronic debilitating knee
p., chronic diabetic neuropathic
p., chronic headache
p., chronic intermittent low back
p., chronic joint
p., chronic leg
p., chronic muscle
p., chronic muscular
p., chronic nerve
p., chronic pelvic
p., chronic vulvar
p., circular interaction between anxiety and
p., claudication limb
p. clinic program
p. clinics, multidisciplinary
p., colicky
p., colicky abdominal
p., constant
p., constant abdominal
p. ‣ constant buttock
p. ‣ constant, harsh
p. control
p. control, brain-based
p. control, chronic
p. control clinic
p. control, effective
p. control medication
p. control ‣ migraine
p. control system ‣ SKY epidural
p., coping with
p., costochondritis
p. ‣ coughing up blood with chest
p., cramp-like pelvic
p., cramping
p., cramping abdominal
p. cramps ‣ cyclic abdominal
p., crampy abdominal
p. cripple
p. crisis
p., crushing chest
p. cycle
p. cycle ‣ fear-tension-
p. ‣ cyclic back
p., cyclical
p., cyclical breast
p., debilitating
p., debilitating back
p. ‣ debilitating musculoskeletal
p., decrease
p., deep aching
p., deep-seated
p., desultory
p. determined by expectation
p. determined by level of anxiety

p. determined by suggestion
p., diabetic nerve
p., dilating
p. ‣ diminished responsiveness to
p., diminution in chest
p., diminution of
p., disabling
p. ‣ disease-induced
p. disorder
p. disorder, somatoform
p. down legs
p., dream
p., dull
p., dull abdominal
p., dull aching
p. ‣ dull chest
p., dull epigastric
p. dulled, sense of
p. during urination
p. dysfunction
p. dysfunction syndrome (MPD) ‣ myofacial
p., ear
p. ‣ edema, stiffness and
p., electric-like
p., emotional
p. ‣ emotional and psychological aspect of
p. ‣ emotional effects of
p., epigastric
p., episodic
p., evaluation of
p., exacerbate the
p., exacerbated by coughing
p., exacerbation of
p., excruciating
p., exertional chest
p. exertional in nature ‣ chest
p., expulsive
p., exquisite
p. extends down legs ‣ back
p., extreme
p., eye
p., eyes open
p., facial
p. ‣ facial nerve
p. factor
p., false
p., false labor
p., fatigue, and insomnia
p. ‣ fatigue, muscle aches and
p. fibers
p., flank
p., fleeting
p., fleeting chest

p., foot
p. -free
p. -free motion
p. -free, patient
p. -free period
p. -free state
p. -free surgery
p. -free walking time
p. -free zone
p. from arteriosclerosis ‣ calf
p. from arthritis
p. from arthritis ‣ facial
p. from breastfeeding ‣ breast
p. from caffeine ‣ breast
p. from cancer
p. from cold ‣ eye
p. from conjunctivitis
p. from cyst ‣ pilonidal, tailbone
p. from dentures ‣ tongue
p. from disc ‣ back
p. from disc ‣ neck and shoulder
p. from heart problem ‣ chest
p. from pneumonia ‣ chest
p. from shingles
p. from TMJ (temporomandibular joint) disorder ‣ chest
p., fulgurant
p., functional
p., functional menstrual
p. ‣ gastroesophageal-related chest
p., general aches and
p., general body
p., general joint
p., general muscle
p., generalized
p., generalized abdominal
p., girdle
p., gnawing
p., grating
p., grimacing in
p., grinding
p., growing
p. ‣ hammering head
p., head
p., headaches
p. ‣ heel stick
p., hemorrhoid
p., herpes
p., heterotopic
p., hip
p., homotopic
p., hunger
p., idiogenous
p., imperative

pain—*continued*
- p. impulse
- p. impulses, block
- p. impulses transmitted
- p. in abdomen ▸ appetite loss from
- p. in abdomen from Addison's disease
- p. in abdomen from appendicitis
- p. in abdomen from colic
- p. in abdomen from Crohn's disease
- p. in abdomen from diverticulitis
- p. in abdomen from diverticulosis
- p. in abdomen from food poisoning
- p. in abdomen from gallstones
- p. in abdomen from gastritis
- p. in abdomen from hepatitis
- p. in abdomen from hernia
- p. in abdomen from indigestion
- p. in abdomen from insect sting
- p. in abdomen from irritable bowel syndrome
- p. in abdomen from lactose intolerance
- p. in abdomen from pancreatitis
- p. in abdomen from peritonitis
- p. in abdomen from proctitis
- p. in abdomen from ulcers
- p. in abdomen with back pain
- p. in abdomen with constipation
- p. in abdomen with diarrhea
- p. in abdomen with fever
- p. in abdomen with nausea
- p. in abdomen with vaginal discharge
- p. in abdomen with vomiting
- p. in anus
- p. in back
- p. in back and abdomen
- p. in back from cancer
- p. in back from pyelonephritis
- p. in back from slipped or ruptured disc
- p. in back from TMJ (temporomandibular joint) disorder
- p. in back from whiplash injury
- p. in back ▸ nervousness from
- p. in back with inability to straighten
- p. in ball of foot
- p. in bone
- p. in breast
- p. in breast ▸ localized
- p. in calf muscles
- p. in chest, jaw or extremities
- p. in chest ▸ squeezing

- p. in ear from sore throat
- p. in ear from TMJ (temporomandibular joint) disorder
- p. in ear from tongue problem
- p. in ear from tonsil problem
- p. in ear from tooth decay
- p. in head ▸ throbbing
- p. in joints
- p. in ligaments, chronic
- p. in lower back
- p. in lower back ▸ persistent
- p. in males ▸ chills with genital
- p. in middle back
- p. in muscles and joints
- p. in muscles, chronic
- p. in pancreas
- p. in runner, knee
- p. in upper back and in neck
- p. incapability, foot
- p., incapacitating
- p. ▸ incapacitating chest
- p., incisional
- p., incompletely treated
- p., increased tolerance of
- p. increasing in severity
- p. ▸ indifference to
- p., insensitivity to
- p., insufferable
- p., intense
- p. ▸ intense back
- p., intense burning
- p., intense headache
- p. ▸ intense, prolonged chest
- p. ▸ intense stabbing
- p. ▸ intense throbbing
- p., intensity of
- p., interacting determinants of
- p., intermenstrual
- p., intermittent
- p., intermittent episodes of
- p., intermittent episodes of acute abdominal
- p., intermittent heart
- p., intolerable
- p., intra-abdominal
- p., intractable
- p., intractable bone
- p. ▸ intractable facial
- p. ▸ intractable head
- p., intractable pelvic
- p., involuntary facial
- p., irreversible
- p., jaw
- p., joint
- p., jumping

- p. killer
- p., labor
- p., lancinating
- p., leg
- p., lessening of
- p., level of
- p., lightening
- p., localized
- p., localized aching
- p. ▸ long-term
- p. ▸ long-term chronic
- p. ▸ loss of sensation of
- p., low back
- p., lower abdominal
- p., lumbar
- p. management
- p. management, advanced medical
- p. management, cancer
- p. management control (PMC)
- p. management, multidisciplinary approach to
- p. management ▸ noninvasive
- p., management of chronic
- p. management, postoperative
- p. management program
- p. management specialist
- p. management strategy
- p., managing
- p., mask
- p. measurements
- p. medication
- p. medication and therapy
- p. medication, current
- p. medication ▸ oral
- p. medication, patient
- p. medication, preventive
- p., menstrual
- p. message
- p., middle
- p., migratory
- p., mild to moderate
- p., mind
- p. mismanagement
- p., moderate
- p. ▸ moderate, post-surgical
- p. modification
- p., modify
- p. ▸ modify body's response to
- p. ▸ morning eye
- p., muscle
- p. ▸ muscle-related
- p., muscular
- p., musculoskeletal
- p., myofascial
- p. ▸ nagging, fleeting

p., nature of
p., nausea and emesis ▸ anorexia,
p. ▸ nausea, vomiting and
   abdominal
p., neck
p. nerve
p., neuropathic
p. ▸ neuropathic central
p., neuropathy
p. ▸ noncardiac chest
p., noncyclical breast
p., nonradiating
p., numbing
p. ▸ numbness, tingling and
p., ocular
p. of central origin
p. of fibromyalgia
p. of generalized distribution
p. of heart attack
p. of localized distribution
p. of metatarsalgia
p. of tendons, chronic
p. on affected side of face
p. on chewing
p. on deep breathing ▸ chest
p. on defecation
p. on exertion, chest
p. on palpation
p. on speaking
p. on swallowing
p. on the whole person, effects of
p. on urination
p. on walking
p., oppressive
p., organic
p. ▸ osteoarthritis knee
p., osteotopic
p., oversensitivity to
p. ▸ pain in abdomen with back
p., palliation in pelvic
p., paraplegic
p. ▸ paroxysm of
p., paroxysmal
p. pathways
p., patient experiences remissions
   and exacerbations of
p. ▸ patient has persistent
p., patient in chronic
p., patient's perception of
p. pattern, radicular
p., pelvic
p. perception
p. perception ▸ reduced
p. ▸ periodic abdominal
p., peripatellar

p., peripheral
p. ▸ peripheral joint
p., persistent
p., persistent aching
p., persistent chest
p., persistent epigastric
p., persistent neck
p. ▸ persistent shingles
p., phantom
p., phantom limb
p., pinching
p., pleuritic
p., pleuritic chest
p. point
p. postcesarean (PPC) section
p., postherpetic
p., postlaminectomy
p., postoperative
p., postorbital
p., postpartum low back
p., postprandial
p., postshingles
p., postsurgical
p., potential
p., precordial chest
p., predominant
p., pre-heart attack
p., premonitory
p., preventing
p. prevention
p. primarily localized
p. profile
p., prolonged
p. ▸ prolonged episodes of chest
p., psychogenic
p. ▸ psychogenic aversion to labor
p., psychological
p. ▸ psychological management of
   chronic
p., psychosomatic
p. ▸ psychosomatic aches and
p., pulmonary
p., pulsatile
p., pulsating
p. radiates
p., radiating
p. radiating down leg
p. radiating into back
p. radiating to jaw and shoulder ▸
   chest
p. radiation
p. radiation, chest
p. radiation therapy for bone
p., radicular
p., rasping

p. reaction
p. receptor
p., recurrent
p., recurrent abdominal
p., recurrent chest
p., reduce
p., referred
p. reflex
p. rehabilitation
p. related to exertion
p. relief
p. relief, arthritis
p. relief ▸ electrical stimulator for
p., relief from
p. relief medication
p. relief ▸ symptomatic
p., reliever
p. reliever ▸ Medtronic Pulsor
   Intrasound
p. reliever ▸ nonprescription
p. reliever ▸ topical
p. relieving effects
p. relieving injection
p. relieving potential
p. relieving remedy
p. relieving ▸ sleep-enhancing and
p. ▸ repeated paroxysms of
p. research, cancer
p., residual
p. ▸ residual facial
p. response
p. response, chronic
p., rest
p. ▸ restore mobility and reduce
p., retrosternal
p., retrosternal chest
p., rheumatoid
p. ▸ right pleuritis chest
p., root
p., sacroiliac joint
p., sciatic
p., searing
p., self-limiting
p. sensation
p. sensation, diminution of
p. sensation, reduction in
p. sense
p. sense of touch and
p., sensitive to
p. sensory pathways ▸ referred
p., severe
p. severe back
p., severe chest
p., severe constricting
p., severe cramping

pain—*continued*
p. ▸ severe, jabbing facial
p., severe joint
p. ▸ severe menstrual
p., severe midepigastric
p. ▸ severe, searing facial
p. ▸ severe, stabbing
p. ▸ severe throbbing
p., sharp
p. ▸ sharp cutting
p. ▸ sharp, jabbing
p. ▸ sharp, jabbing or electric
p. ▸ sharp, localized
p., sharp retrosternal
p. ▸ sharp, stabbing
p. ▸ sharp substernal
p., shift of
p., shooting
p., short-lived
p., short-term
p., shoulder
p. signals
p. signals, incoming
p., significant level of perceived
p., sinus
p. site
p., site unspecified ▸ psychogenic
p., skeletal
p., slipped disc
p. ▸ soft tissue muscle
p., somatoform
p., soul
p. specialists
p., spiritual
p. ▸ spontaneous onset of
p., spot
p. spreading to arms
p. spreading to neck
p. spreading to shoulder
p. ▸ spurious labor
p., stabbing
p., stabbing chest
p. ▸ stabbing joint
p., staccato
p., starting
p. state, acute
p. ▸ stiffness, aching and burning
p. stimuli
p., stimulus-induced
p., stomach
p., stress action
p. ▸ stress-induced chest
p. study
p. study, biofeedback
p., subjective

p., substernal pressing
p., subxiphoid
p., sudden
p. sufferers
p. support group
p. suppressing drug
p. swelling and
p. symptoms ▸ persistent chest
p. syndrome
p. syndrome, chronic
p. syndrome ▸ chronic muscle
p. syndrome ▸ chronic reflex
p. syndrome ▸ complex regional
p. syndrome ▸ myofascial
p. syndrome ▸ post-thalamic stroke
p. syndrome ▸ thalamic
p., tailbone
p., tearing
p. ▸ temporary relief of headache
p., tenderness and
p., tenderness or weakness ▸ muscle
p., terebrant
p., terminal cancer
p., thalamic
p. threshold
p. threshold ▸ increased
p. threshold ▸ low
p., throbbing
p. ▸ throbbing neck
p. ▸ throbbing, pulsating
p., tingling
p. tolerance
p. tolerance ▸ increased
p. ▸ tolerance level for
p., total relief of
p., transient
p., transient joint
p., traumatic
p. treatment
P. Treatment Center
p. treatment ▸ emergency
p. treatment ▸ intractable
p., treatment of chronic
p. treatment program
p., trigger
p., twinge of
p., ulcer
p., uncontrollable
p., undermedication for
p. ▸ undersensitivity to
p., undertreatment of
p., unexplained
p., unilateral
p., unilateral head

P. Unit, Chest
p., unmanageable
p., unrelieved
p., vague abdominal
p. ▸ vague aches and
p., vascular
p., violent
p., visceral
p., viscerosomatic
p., vise-like
p., voluntary control of
p., wandering
p., waves of
p., waxing and waning chest
p. ▸ weakness, dizziness and joint
p. well controlled
p., whiplash
p., widespread
p. with breathing difficulty ▸ chest
p. with colitis ▸ recurrent abdominal
p. with Crohn's disease ▸ abdominal
p. with hoarseness ▸ chest
p. with palpitation ▸ chest
p. with runny nose ▸ body
p. with sweating ▸ chest
p., wrenching
painful
p. and debilitating
p. and disabling migraines
p. and restricted movement
p. area
p. arthritis ▸ chronic
p. blister
p., blister-type lesion
p. blistering rash
p. bone metastases
p. bruises
p. burning of feet
p., burning sensation in chest
p. callus
p. claudication of legs
p. condition ▸ chronic
p. contraceptive spasms
p. corn
p. diabetic neuropathy
p. discomfort, minor
p. dislocation
p., extremely
p. heel
p. heel spur
p. heel syndrome
p. hemorrhagic glaucoma
p., inflamed area
p. inflammation

p. inflammation of joints
p. intercourse
p. intestinal contraction
p. joints
p. joints, swollen and
p. knee, chronically
p. leg cramps
p. lesion
p. local and regional metastases
p. memory
p. menstrual periods
p. menstruation
p. muscle contraction
p. muscle spasm
p. nerve disorder
p. nerve spasms
p. neuroma
p. neuropathy
p. osteoarthritis of knee
p. sensations
p. sexual intercourse
p. skin rash ▸ severe,
p. spasm
p. stimuli
p. stimuli ▸ excessive sensitivity to
p. swallowing
p. swelling of breast
p. swollen gland
p. swollen joints
p. symptoms
p. syndrome
p., tingling sensation
p. ulcer
p. urination
p. vision
p. withdrawal reaction
painfully slow death
painfully swollen glands
painkiller, effective
painkillers, nonaddictive
painkilling drug
painkilling ingredients, active
painless
p. bleeding
p. hematuria
p. increased pressure inside the eye
p. intermittent hematuria
p. intestinal bleeding
p. jaundice
p. labor, accelerated
p. lymph node
p. menorrhagia
p. sclerotherapy
p., small, intact blister

p. spasm
p. steatorrhea
p. swelling
p. ulcer
painted with gentian violet ▸ area
painting base of tumor
pair(s) (PAIRS)
p. and chains ▸ gram-positive cocci in
p., base
p., electrode
p. of electrodes ▸ measured between
p. of electrodes ▸ spacing between
p. of electroencephalogram (EEG) electrodes
p. production
P. (Psychiatric Alcohol Inpatient Review System) program
p., stimulating electrode
paired
p. beats
p. cocci
p. donor exchange
p. electrical stimulation
p. response
p. vertebral arches
p. vestibular nuclei
Pajao Rojo (barbiturates)
Pajot's
P. law
P. maneuver
P. method
PAL (posterior axillary line)
palatal
p. arch
p. linguoplate
p. myoclonus
p. reflex
p. seal, posterior
palate(s)
p. and fauces ▸ muscles of
p. and pharynx normal
p., arch of
p., artificial
p., bony
p., bony hard
p., brachygnathia and cleft
p., carcinoma of hard
p., cleft
p. ▸ cleft lip and
p., congenital cleft
p., cutaneous suture of
p., falling
p., hard

p. ▸ hard and soft
p., high arched
p. impression, cleft
p., longitudinal suture of
p., pendulous
p., pillars of soft
p., posterior cleft
p., primary
p. prosthesis, cleft
p., secondary
p., smoker's
p., soft
p., vault of
palatine
p. arch
p. bone
p. bone ▸ palatine notch of
p. bone ▸ sphenopalatine notch of
p. canals
p. cells
p. folds
p. folds, transverse
p. nerve
p. nerve, anterior
p. nerve, greater
p. nerve, medial
p. nerve, middle
p. nerve, posterior
p. nerve, lesser
p. notch
p. notch of palatine bone
p. process
p. protuberance
p. raphe
p. reflex
p. spine of maxilla
p. suture, anterior
p. suture, median
p. suture, middle
p. suture, posterior
p. suture, transverse
p. tonsil
p. tonsil calculus
p. tonsil, crypts of
p. uvula
p. vein, external
p. velum ▸ levator muscle of
palatini
p., arcus
p., levator muscle of velum
p. muscle, levator veli
p. muscle, tensor veli
p. nerve of tensor veli
palatinum, os
palatinum, velum

palatinus, torsus
palatoethmoidal suture
palatoglossal arch
palatoglossus, arcus
palatoglossus muscle
palatomaxillary arch
palatomaxillary suture
palatopharyngeal arch
palatopharyngeal muscle
palatopharyngeus, arcus
palatoplasty
    p. (LAUP), laser-assisted uvula
    p., Veau-Wardill
    p., Wardill
palatum, globus
pale
    p. and clammy skin
    p. and diaphoretic, skin
    p. and malodorous stools
    p. and swollen ▸ kidneys
    p. cytoplasm, scanty
    p. facial appearance
    p. hypertension
    p. nail beds
    p. nails from anemia ▸ white or
    p. nails from cirrhosis ▸ white or
    p., patient
    p. shrunken torso
    p., skin
    p. -staining nuclei
    p. -staining polyhedral cells
    p. stool with Crohn's disease
    p. thrombus
    p. transparent granules
    p. unstained ring
    p. white, brain
paleencephalon/paleoencephal
paleocerebellar dysfunction
paleopneumoniae, Diplococcus
paleopneumoniae, Peptostrepto-
    coccus
palestinensis, Acanthamoeba
Pali determinations
Pali panel
palialic speech
palidromic rheumatism
palisade worm
palisading, peripheral
pallesthetic sensibility
palliation
    p. ▸ emotional considerations in
    p., endoscopic
    p. in advanced metastatic disease
    p. in brain metastasis
    p. in early metastatic disease

    p. in pelvic pain
    p., intraluminal
    p. of malignant esophageal
      stenosis
    p., physical considerations in
    p. purposes
palliative
    p. capabilities
    p. care
    p. care ▸ advance
    p. care, elected
    p. care, multidisciplinary
    p. drugs
    p. effects
    p. gastrojejunostomy
    p. home care
    p. management
    p. measures
    p. medicine
    p. needs
    p. operation
    p. procedure
    p. program
    p. radiation therapy
    p. radiotherapy
    p. resection
    p. service
    p. surgery
    p. therapy
    p. treatment
pallid and shocky
pallid skin
pallida, asphyxia
pallida, Spirochaeta
pallidotomy procedure
pallidotomy, stereotactic
pallidum
    p. immobilization (TPI), Treponema
    p. ▸ microhemagglutination
      Treponema
    p., Treponema
pallidus, globus
pallisading histiocytes
pallor
    p. and cyanosis
    p., fatigue and
    p. from anemia
    p., marked skin
    p. of disc
    p. of skin
    p., perinuclear
palm(s)
    p. and soles, erythematous
      macules of
    p. -chin reflex

    p. -heel strike
    p., liver
    p. of hand
    p., simian crease of
    p. sugar
    p. ▸ sweating forehead, armpits
      and
    p., sweaty
palmar
    p. angulation
    p. aponeurosis, transverse bundles
      of
    p. arch
    p. arch flow
    p. contraction
    p. crease
    p. crease, abnormal
    p. desquamation
    p. digital nerve, common
    p. digital nerve, proper
    p. digital nerves of median nerve ▸
      common
    p. digital nerves of median nerve ▸
      proper
    p. digital nerves of ulnar nerve ▸
      common
    p. digital vein
    p. erythema
    p. fascia
    p. fasciitis
    p. flexion
    p. grasp reflex
    p. interosseous muscle
    p. metacarpal vein
    p. muscle, long
    p. muscle, short
    p. space
    p. surface
    p. xanthoma
palmare, xanthoma striatum
palmaris
    p. brevis muscle
    p., keratosis
    p. longus muscle
    p. longus tendon
palmatae, plicae
palmate folds
Palmaz
    P. intravascular stent ▸ Schatz-
    P. -Schatz stent
    P. tubular mesh stent ▸ Schatz-
palmellina, trichomycosis
Palmer-Widen operation
palmesthetic sensation
palmesthetic sensibility

palmomental reflex
palmomental reflex of Marinesco-
   Radovici
palpable
   p. abdominal mass
   p. abnormality
   p. aorta
   p. breast pump
   p. calyx
   p. carotid pulse
   p. extra-uterine mass
   p. femoral lymphadenopathy
   p. femoral pulse
   p. fibroid
   p. inguinal lymphadenopathy
   p. lesion
   p. lesion ► calvarium without
   p. lesion ► scalp without
   p. lesion, without
   p., liver edge
   p. ► liver, spleen, kidneys (LSK)
      not
   p. lymphadenopathy
   p. mass
   p. masses
   p., neck
   p. nodes
   p. nodule
   p. organs
   p. organs or masses
   p., pedal pulses
   p., pulses
   p. radial pulse
   p., spleen not
   p. stone
   p. stones in gallbladder
   p. thrill
   p. thrill, no
   p. thyomegaly
   p., thyroid
   p. venous cord
palpably enlarged, liver not
palpably enlarged, spleen not
palpated
   p. regularly, prostate
   p., spleen
   p., tibial crest
palpating finger
palpation(s) [*palpitation*]
   p. ► abdomen tender to
   p., bimanual precordial
   p., breathing with
   p. ► chest pain with
   p., deep
   p., dyspnea and fatigue

   p. from alcohol
   p. from anxiety
   p. from caffeine
   p., heart
   p., kidney
   p., manual
   p. ► masses, organs or tenderness
      on
   p. of nasopharynx
   p. of ossicular chain
   p. or percussion ► tenderness to
   p., pain on
   p., patient has occasional
   p., rectal
   p. ► weakness, sweating and
palpatory percussion
palpatory proteinuria
palpebra tertius
palpebrae
   p. superior muscle, levator
   p. superiors, musculus levator
   p., tarsus inferior
   p., tarsus superior
palpebral
   p. aperture
   p. commissure
   p. conjunctive
   p. fissure
   p. fold
   p. furrow
   p. ligament, medial
   p. raphe
   p. region, inferior
   p. region, superior
   p. vein
   p. vein, inferior
   p. vein, superior
palpebrale, coloboma
palpebralis
   p., Filaria
   p. inferior, arcus
   p. superior, arcus
palpebrarum
   p., pediculosis
   p., xanthelasma
   p., xanthoma
palpebronasal fold
palpebronasalis, plica
palpitation(s)
   p. and shortness of breath
      (SOB)
   p. cordis
   p., heart
   p., paroxysmal
   p. ► patient has occasional

   p., premonitory
   p., recurring
palsied child, deaf cerebral
palsy
   p., Bell's
   p., brachial
   p., brachial plexus
   p., bulbar
   p. (CP), cerebral
   p., cranial nerve
   p., deltoid
   p., Erb's
   p., facial
   p. ► facial nerve
   p., gaze
   p., hemiplegic form of cerebral
   p., nuclear facial
   p., ocular
   p., paraplegic form of cerebral
   p. ► permanent Bell's
   p., peroneal nerve
   p., progressive supranuclear
   p., radial
   p., shaking
   p., sixth nerve
   p. ► temporary Bell's
   p., Todd's
   p., ulnar nerve
   p. ► vertical gaze
Paltauf's dwarf
Paltauf's nanism
paludis, Clostridium
paludum, Haemopis
PAMP (pulmonary artery mean
   pressure)
pampiniform plexus
pampiniformis, plexus
PAN (pan)
   P. (periodic alternating nystagmus)
   p., bed◊
   p. mitral prolapse
   p. -oral radiography
   p. -sensitive
   p. T cell antigen
panacinar emphysema
Panama
   P. fever
   P. larvicide
   P. Red (grade of marijuana)
panangiitis, diffuse necrotizing
Panas' operation
panchamber enlargement
Pancoast('s)
   P. operation
   P. suture

Pancoast('s)—*continued*
- P. syndrome
- P. tumor
- P. -type tumor ▸ bronchogenic

panconduction defect

pancreas
- p., aberrant
- p. accessorium
- p., accessory
- p., activity of
- p. ▸ adenocarcinoma in head of
- p. and duodenum
- p., annular
- p., artificial
- p., Aselli's
- p. atrophic
- p. autolytic
- p., bionic
- p. cancer
- p., carcinoma head of
- p., carcinoma of
- p. cells
- p., chronic inflammation of
- p. ▸ chronic inflammatory disease of
- p., cystic fibrosis of
- p. divisum
- p., donated
- p., dorsal
- p. enzyme
- p., excision head of
- p., external secretion of
- p., external secretory activity of
- p., fibrosis of
- p. fibrotic
- p., head of
- p. ▸ histologic sections of
- p., incision of
- p., inflammation of
- p., lesser
- p. lobulated
- p., metastatic adenocarcinoma
- p. necrotic ▸ tail of
- p., pain in
- p., parenchyma of
- p., perfusion in tail of
- p., pseudocyst of
- p., purulent inflammation of
- p., resection head of
- p., rudiments of
- p. secretes insulin
- p. soft ▸ tail of
- p., swelling of
- p. syndrome, ulcerogenic tumor of

- p., tail of
- p., thromboembolism in
- p., transected
- p. transplant
- p. transplant ▸ human fetal
- p. transplant, partial
- p. transplantation
- p. transplants, kidney-
- p., traumatic transection of
- p., tumor of
- p., ulceration of
- p., ventral
- p., Willis'
- p., Winslow's

pancreatic
- p. abscess
- p. abscess formation
- p. adenocarcinoma
- p. allograft
- p. amylase
- p. ascites
- p. ascites, pseudocyst
- p. atrophy
- p. beta cells
- p. biopsy
- p. calcification
- p. calculus
- p. cancer
- p. cancer, human
- p. cancer ▸ inoperable
- p. carcinoma
- p. cell transplant technique
- p. colic
- p. cyst
- p. cystitis
- p. cytology
- p. density ▸ diffuse increase in
- p. diabetes
- p. diastase
- p. digestive juices ▸ elimination of
- p. disease
- p. disease, diabetes mellitus (DM) secondary to
- p. disorder
- p. duct
- p. duct ▸ disruption of
- p. duct hyperplasia
- p. duct ▸ obstruction of
- p. duct patent
- p. duct ▸ stones present in
- p. duct, surgical anastomosis of
- p. edema
- p. enema
- p. enzymes
- p. etiology

- p. exocrine function
- p. exocrine function test
- p. exocrine insufficiency
- p. exocrine insufficiency ▸ mild chronic
- p. exocrine insufficiency ▸ moderate chronic
- p. exocrine secretion
- p. exocrine secretion tests
- p. extract
- p. fibrosis
- p. fistula
- p. function test
- p. inflammation
- p. insufficiency
- p. insufficiency, exocrine
- p. insufficiency, severe
- p. insufficiency syndrome
- p. insufficiency with malabsorption
- p. islet cell
- p. isomylase levels
- p. juice
- p. lesion
- p. lipase
- p. liver scan
- p. neoplasm
- p. notch
- p. oncofetal antigen
- p. origin, adenocarcinoma
- p., patent
- p. polypeptide
- p. procedure
- p. pseudocyst
- p. ranula
- p. reaction
- p. replacement therapy
- p. scan
- p. secretions
- p. secretory function test
- p. tissue
- p. tissue, autodigestion of
- p. tissue, autolysis of
- p. tissue ▸ necrosis of
- p. tissue, necrotic
- p. tumor
- p. tumor syndrome
- p. veins

pancreatica
- p., achylia
- p., diarrhea
- p., sialorrhea

pancreaticobiliary ductography, peroral retrograde
pancreaticobiliary tract
pancreaticoduodenal artery

pancreaticoduodenal veins
pancreaticoduodenectomy proce-
    dure
pancreaticoduodenography,
    retrograde
pancreaticogastric folds
pancreaticohepatic syndrome
pancreaticojejunostomy
    p., caudal
    p., distal
    p., longitudinal
    p. with roux-en-y
pancreaticosplenic lymph nodes
pancreaticosplenic omentum
pancreatitis
    p., acute
    p., acute hemorrhagic
    p., acute necrotizing
    p., alcohol-induced
    p., alcoholic
    p., biliary
    p., calcareous
    p., calcific
    p., centrilobar
    p., chronic
    p., chronic calcific
    p., chronic relapsing
    p., colonic
    p. ▸ drug-associated primary
        acute
    p., estrogen-induced
    p. ▸ etiology of chronic
    p. ▸ fatal hemorrhagic
    p., focal
    p. from alcohol
    p., gallstone
    p., hemorrhagic
    p., hereditary
    p., interstitial
    p., isolated
    p., localized
    p. ▸ management of acute
    p. ▸ management of chronic
    p., mild
    p., necrotizing
    p. ▸ pain in abdomen from
    p., perilobar
    p., post-traumatic
    p., purulent
    p., redevelopment of
    p., relapsing
    p. secondary to gallstones
    p., severe hemorrhagic
    p., steroid
    p. ▸ tenderness in abdomen from

p., traumatic
pancreatoduodenal lymph nodes
pancreatogenous fatty diarrhea
pancreatogram, nasal
pancreatography, endoscopic
    retrograde
pancreatography, operative
pancytopenia
    p., congenital
    p., Fanconi's
    p., secondary
pancytopenic and septic ▸ patient
pandemic disease
pandemic influenza
panduriform placenta
panduriformis, placenta
Pandy's reaction
Pandy's test
panel [*channel*]
    p., chemistry
    p., consensus
    p., drug screening
    p., lipid
    p., Pali
    p., personality
    p., thyroid
    p., toxin
    p,. viral hepatitis
panencephalitis, Pette-Doring
panencephalitis (SSPE) ▸ subacute
    sclerosing
panendoscopic examination
Paneth's cells
pang(s)
    p., breast
    p., brow
    p., hunger
panhematopenia, primary splenic
panhematopoietic cell antigen
panhypopituitarism, prepubertal
panic [*manic*]
    p., acute homosexual
    p. anxiety disorder
    p. attack
    p. attack, active
    p. attack ▸ agoraphobia with
    p. attack ▸ agoraphobia without
    p. attack, alleviate
    p. attack, cannabis-induced
    p. attack ▸ fear of
    p. attack, repeated
    p. attacks ▸ spontaneous
    p. ▸ depression, anxiety and
    p. disorder
    p. disorder ▸ full-blown

p. disorder patient
p. disorder with agoraphobia
p. disorder without agoraphobia
p. episode
p., homosexual
p. -like symptoms
p. or despair ▸ periods of anger,
p. or fury
p. ▸ overwhelming sense of
p., pot
p. reaction
p. reaction, acute
p. reactions, acute treatment for
p. reactions, clinical manifestations
    of
p. reactions, differential diagnosis
    in
p. reactions, psychological state in
p. reactions, subacute treatment of
p. reactions, symptoms of
p. reactions, treatment of
p. reactions with cannabinoids
p. reactions with depressants
p. reactions with hallucinogens
p. reactions with inhalants
p. reactions with multiple drugs
p. reactions with opioids
p. reactions with phencyclidines
p. reactions with stimulants
p. ▸ sense of
Panje voice button
panleukopenia virus
panlobular emphysema
panmyelopathy, constitutional
    infantile
panneuritis epidemica
panniculus
    p., abdominal
    p. adiposus
    p. carnosus
    p., fatty
    p., thin
pannus, allergic
pannus, eczematous
panophthalmitis/panophthalmia
panoramic
    p. radiograph
    p. tomography
    p. view
panphobia/pantophobia
panretinal photocoagulation
Pansch's fissure
Panstrongylus geniculatus
pansystolic flow
pansystolic murmur

pant(s)
  p. ▸ medical antishock
  p. ▸ military antishock
pantaloon
  p. embolism
  p. hernia
  p. inguinal hernia
  p. patch
pantherina, Amanita
panting center
pantomographic view
pantomography, concentric
pantomography, eccentric
Pantopaque
  P. column
  P. column, cervical
  P. column, lumbar
  P. contrast medium
pantothenate synthetase
pantothenic acid
PAP
  PAP (positive airway pressure)
  PAP (primary atypical pneumonia)
  PAP (pulmonary artery pressure)
Pap (Papanicolaou)
  P. screenings
  P. smear
  P. smear, abnormal
  P. smear, atypical
  P. smear, cervical
  P. smear, lung
  P. smear negative
  P. smear, Richart
  P. smear ▸ vaginal cuff
  P. smears ▸ Richart and VCE
    (vaginal, cervical, endocervical)
  P. smears ▸ vaginal, cervical,
    endocervical (VCE)
  P. stain
  P. study of cells
  P. test
papatasii, Phlebotomus
Paper(s) (paper)
  P. Acid (LSD)
  p., asthma
  p. chromatography
  p. chromatography, filter
  p. -doll fetus
  p. electrophoresis
  p. microscopic test, filter
  p., niter
  p. patch, cigarette
  p., rolling
  p. speed
  p. syndrome, carbonless

  p., velocity of movement of EEG
    (electroencephalogram)
  p. work, admission
papilla
  p., acoustic
  p., anomalous vessels of
  p., Bergmeister's
  p., capillary loop in dermal
  p., capillary loop in hair
  p., cavity of optic
  p., cysticercosis of optic
  p. diameter
  p., duodenal
  p., hair
  p., hypertrophied
  p., lacrimal
  p. lacrimalis
  p. of optic nerve
  p. of Vater
  p., optic
  p. parotidea
  p., splitting of lacrimal
papillae
  p. blunted
  p., circumvallate
  p., filiform
  p., foliate
  p. fungiform
  p., fusiform
  p., lingual
  p., renal
papillaris, areola
papillary [*capillary*]
  p. adenocarcinoma
  p. adenocarcinoma, metastatic
  p. adenocystoma lymphomatosum
  p. adenoma
  p. area
  p. carcinoma
  p. conjunctivitis (GPC) ▸ giant
  p. cystadenocarcinoma
  p. cystadenocarcinoma of ovary
  p. cystic adenoma
  p. dermis
  p. duct
  p. ectasia
  p. fibroelastoma
  p. hemangioma
  p. hypertrophy
  p. mucinous neoplasm (IPMN) ▸
    intraductal
  p. muscle
  p. muscle abscess
  p. muscle, anterior
  p. muscle dysfunction

  p. muscle, elongated
  p. muscle fibrosis
  p. muscle of left ventricle ▸ anterior
  p. muscle of left ventricle ▸
    posterior
  p. muscle of left ventricle ▸ septal
  p. muscle, posterior
  p. muscle rupture
  p. muscle syndrome
  p. muscle syndrome ▸ single
  p. muscle tip
  p. muscle, ventricular
  p. necrosis, renal
  p. neoplasms
  p. serous cystadenocarcinoma
  p. serous cystadenocarcinoma
    ovary
  p. stasis
  p. stenosis
  p. thyroid carcinoma
  p. thyroid carcinoma ▸ ossified
  p. tumor
  p. wave
papilledema, diopters of
papilliform rash
papilloma
  p. acuminatum
  p., benign
  p., benign intraductal
  p., conjunctival
  p., ductal
  p., mulberry type
  p. neuroticum
  p. of breast ▸ intraductal
  p., squamous cell
  p., trachea
  p., transitional cell
  p. virus
  p. virus (HPV), human
papillomatosis
  p., intraductal
  p., laryngeal
  p. ▸ recurrent respiratory
  p. ▸ subareolar duct
papillomatous goiter
papillomavirus infection ▸ genital
papillomavirus (HPV) infection ▸
  human
papillosum multiplex,
  trichoepithelioma
papillotomy
  p. diet
  p., endoscopic
  p. patient, test diet for
pappataci fever virus

pappataci viruses
Pappenheim's stain
papular acrodermatitis, infantile
papular acrodermatitis of childhood (PAC)
papule, fibrous
papule, foreign body (FB)
papulonecrotic tuberculosis
papulosa
    p., acne
    p., endometritis tuberosa
    p. infantum, acrodermatitis
    p., iritis
    p. nigra, dermatosis
    p., urticaria
papulosis, atrophic
papulosis, bowenoid
papulous vaginitis
PAPVR (partial anomalous pulmonary venous return)
papyraceous/papyraceus
papyraceous fetus
papyraceous layer
papyraceus, fetus
PAQ (Personal Attributes Questionnaire)
Paquelin's cautery
par glissement, hernia
para
    p. -aminohippurate clearance
    p. -aortic bodies
    p. -aortic lymphatic channels
    p., multiple births, abortions, live births (GPMAL) ▸ Gravida,
    p. I (II, III, etc.)
parabasal cell
parabasals, WBC
parabotulinum, Clostridium
parabotulinum equi, Clostridium
paracathodic rays
paracentesis
    p., abdominal
    p. cordis
    p., diagnostic
    p., electro◊
    p. pulmonis
    p., therapeutic
    p. thoracis
paracentral
    p. gyrus
    p. lobule
    p. scotoma
paracentralis, gyrus
paracervical anesthetic
paracervical block

paracholera vibrios
parachute deformity
parachute mitral valve
paracicatricial emphysema
paracoccidioidal granuloma
Paracoccidioides brasiliensis
paracolic gutter
paracolic gutters ▸ packing of
Paracolobactrum
    P. aerogenoides
    P. arizonae
    P. coliforme
    P. intermedium
paracolon
    p. aerogenes
    p. bacilli
    p. bacillus
    p. coliform
    p. intermedium
paracorporeal heart
paracostal incision
paradental pyorrhea
paradigm(s)
    p. ▸ personalized medical
    p. shift
    p., unrecognized transference
Paradise (cocaine)
paradox
    p., calcium
    p., French
    p. image
    p. of Kretz
    p., Opie
    p., oxygen (O_2)
    p., thoracoabdominal
    p., Weber's
paradoxic
    p. condition
    p. deafness
    p. pupillary reflex
    p. wall motion
paradoxical
    p. aberrancy
    p. cerebral embolism
    p. contraction
    p. diarrhea
    p. diplopia
    p. drug effect
    p. embolism
    p. embolization
    p. flexor reflex
    p. incontinence
    p. lateralization
    p. metastasis
    p. phenomenon, Hunt's

    p. pulse
    p. pulse ▸ Kussmaul
    p. pulse ▸ reversed
    p. reflex
    p. respiration
    p. response
    p. rocking impulse
    p. sleep
    p. stimulation
paradoxically split S2 sound
paraduodenal fold
paraduodenal hernia
paradysenteriae, gram-negative Shigella
paradysenteriae, Shigella
paraesophageal hernia
parafascicular (PF) nucleus
parafascicular thalamotomy (PFT)
paraffin
    p. bath
    p. block, embedded tissue in
    p. cancer
    p. implant
    p. implant material
    p. section
    p. therapy
Parafossarulus manchouricus
paraganglioma
    p., jugulotympanic
    p., medullary
    p., nonchromaffin
    p. tumor
Paragon II pacemaker
Paragonimus
    P. africanus
    P. heterotrema
    P. kellicotti
    P. ringeri
    P., Trematoda
    P. westermani
Paragordius
    P. cintus
    P. tricuspidatus
    P. varius
parahemolyticus, Haemophilus
parahemolyticus, Vibrio
parahippocampal cortex
parahippocampal gyrus
parahippocampalis, gyrus
parahormone level
parainfluenza
    p. virus
    p. virus 1
    p. virus 2
parainfluenzae, Haemophilus

parakeratosis
p. ostracea
p., patches of
p. psoriasiformis
p. scutularis
p. variegata
parakrusei, Candida
parallax
p., binocular
p., crossed
p., direct
p., heteronymous
p., homonymous
p. method
p., vertical
parallel
p. bars, patient ambulates on
p. beam, opposed
p., electrodes connected in
p. grid
p. -hole collimator
p. incision
p. opposing tangential fields
p. plate dialyzer
p. portals, opposing
p. rays
p. reaction
p. shunt
p. striae, Retzius'
p. to the spine
p. transcription
p. with edges of wound ▸ sutured
paralogia, thematic
paralogism, thematic
paralunate dislocation
paralysis
p., abducens
p., acute facial
p. (AFP), acute flaccid
p. agitans
p. and coma, sudden
p., ascending
p. attacks, sleep
p., bulbar
p., chronic muscle
p., complete
p., complete motor
p., congenital abducens-facial
p., conjugate
p., cortical
p. ▸ cyclic, momentary
p., diphtheritic
p., Duchenne-Erb
p., Duchenne's
p., emotional

p., Erb's
p., eye muscle
p., facial
p., flaccid
p., general
p., hypesthesia and
p., hysterical
p. ▸ idiopathic facial
p., incomplete
p., infantile
p., infectious bulbar
p., initial
p., ischemic
p., Klumpke's
p., Landry's
p., laryngeal nerve
p., Lissauer's
p., long-term
p., lower motor neuron
p., motor
p., motor neuron
p., muscle
p., muscular
p., nerve
p. of accommodation of eye
p. of arm
p. of arm ▸ numbness, weakness and
p. of arm ▸ sudden
p. of eyelid muscles
p. of face
p. of face ▸ numbness, weakness and
p. of facial muscles
p. of leg
p. of leg ▸ numbness, weakness and
p. of leg ▸ sudden
p. of medullary cardiorespiratory centers
p. of upward gaze
p. of vocal cord
p. one side of body
p. one side of face ▸ sudden
p. ▸ onset of
p., partial
p. ▸ partial facial
p., partial or complete
p., periodic
p., permanent
p., phrenic nerve
p., post-injury
p., Potts
p., progressive

p., progressive labioglosso-pharyngeal
p., pseudobulbar
p., quickening
p., residual
p., residual peripheral
p., respiratory
p., rigid
p., secondary partial
p. ▸ selective blindness and
p., sensory
p., sleep
p., spastic
p., spinal
p. ▸ spinal cord injury
p., sudden
p. ▸ sudden weakness, numbness or
p., temporary
p., tick
p., Todd's
p., total
p., transient
p. ▸ trauma-induced hysterical
p. ▸ uncontrollable seizures and
p. ▸ varying degrees of
p., vasomotor
p., vocal
p. ▸ Volkmann ischemic
p., weakness and
paralytic
p. abasia
p. bladder
p. bladder, motor
p. bladder, sensory
p. brachial neuritis
p. chest
p. chorea
p. dementia
p. disease
p. drugs
p. idiocy
p. ileus
p. illness ▸ severe
p. incontinence
p. miosis
p. myoglobinuria ▸ paroxysmal
p. polio
p. polio (VAPP) ▸ vaccine-associated
p. poliomyelitis, spinal
p. scoliosis
p. shock
p. strabismus
p. strabismus, acute

p. stroke
paralytica
    p., aphonia
    p., dementia
    p., dysphagia
paralyticum, ectropion
paralyticus
    p., ictus
    p., laryngismus
    p., thorax
paralyzed
    p. limb, rigidity of
    p. muscles
    p., patient
    p. vocal cord
paralyzing
    p. disease ▸ muscle
    p. injury
    p. phobia
    p. vertigo
Parama's method
paramagnetic
    p. artifact
    p. resonance spectroscopy ▸ electron
    p. substance
paramecia compound
paramedial sulcus
paramedian incision
paramediastinal shadow
Paramedic(s) (paramedic)
    P. Rescue Team
    P. Team
    p. training
    P. Unit
parameningeal rhabdomyosarcoma
parameningococcus meningitis
paramesonephric duct
parameter(s) [*perimeter*]
    p., actual behavioral
    p., clinical
    p. determination ▸ metabolic
    p., gross neurological
    p., hemodynamic
    p., hemologic
    p. initialization
    p., serologic
    p. status, system
    p. ▸ systemic hemodynamic
    p. technique ▸ multiple
parametrial
    p. invasion
    p. mass
    p. thickening

parametric
    p. hematocele
    p. image
    p. imaging
paramnesia, reduplicative
Paramphistomum cervi
paramuscular incision
paramyoclonus multiplex
Paramyxoviridae virus
paranasal erythema
paranasal sinus
    p.s. cancer
    p.s., ethmoidal
    p.s., frontal
    p.s., maxillary
    p.s., sphenoidal
paranemic coil
paraneoplastic
    p. anemia
    p. anorexia
    p. syndrome
paranephritis, lipomatous
paraneural block
paranoia
    p., acute hallucinatory
    p., alcoholic
    p. ▸ hallucinations, delusions and
    p., hallucinatory
    p., heboid
    p. ▸ insomnia and
    p., litigious
    p. originaria
    p., querulous
    p. simplex
    p. ▸ suspicion and
paranoic in thinking, patient
paranoic psychosis
paranoica, aphonia
paranoid
    p. delusions
    p. depressive attitudes
    p. disorder
    p. disorder, shared
    p. group, heboid-
    p. ideation
    p. individual
    p. insomniac
    p., patient
    p. personality
    p. personality disorder
    p. psychoneurosis
    p. psychosis
    p. psychosis, psychogenic
    p. psychotic state ▸ amphetamine-induced

    p. psychotic state ▸ relapse of
    p. reaction, acute
    p. schizophrenia
    p. schizophrenia ▸ chronic
    p. state
    p. state induced by drugs
    p. state, simple
    p. thinking
    p. trend
    p. type
    p. type, chronic ▸ schizophrenia
    p. type, chronic with acute exacerbation ▸ schizophrenia
    p. type, subchronic ▸ schizophrenia
    p. type, subchronic with acute exacerbation ▸ schizophrenia
    p. type, unspecified ▸ schizophrenia
paranoides, amentia
paranoides, dementia
paranormal claims
paranosic gain
Paranthenus apicalis
paranuclear body
paraparesis (TSP) ▸ tropical spastic
paraperitoneal hernia
paraperitoneal nephrectomy
parapertussis
    p., Acinetobacter
    p., Bordetella
    p., Haemophilus
parapharyngeal abscess
parapharyngeal lymph nodes
paraphasia
    p., central
    p., literal
    p., verbal
paraphrenia
    p. confabulans
    p. expansiva
    p., late
    p. phantastica
    p. systematica
paraphyseal arch
paraplane echocardiography
paraplegia
    p., ataxic
    p., cerebral
    p., flaccid
    p. in spinal cord tumor
    p., senile
    p., spastic
paraplegic(s)
    p. form of cerebral palsy
    p. idiocy

paraplegic(s)—*continued*
p. pain
p., patient
p. rehabilitation
p. ▸ support groups for
parapneumonic effusion
paraportal lymph nodes
paraprofessional health workers
parapsilosis, Candida
parapsychological techniques
pararectus incision
Parasaccharomyces ashfordi
parasaccular hernia
parasacral block
parasagittal
p. lesion
p. meningioma
p. plane
p. zones
**parasellar and middle fossa
metastasis syndrome**
paraseptal emphysema
paraserum reflex
parashigae, Shigella
parasite(s)
p., accidental
p., allantoic
p., animal
p., blood-borne
p., celled
p., celozoic
p., cytozoic
p. diarrhea, Giardia
p., ectozoic
p., endophytic
p., entozoic
p., eurytrophic
p., facultative
p., hematozoic
p., incidental
p., intercellular
p., intermittent
p., intestinal
p., karyozoic
p., malarial
p. ▸ microscopic intestinal
p., obligatory
p., occasional
p., ova and
p., periodic
p., permanent
p., plant
p., protozoan
p., skin
p., specific

p., sporozoan
p., spurious
p., stenotrophic
p., stools for ova and
p., temporary
p., teratoid
p., trematode
p., vegetable
parasitic
p. cardiomyopathy
p. disease
p. fetus
p. fungi
p. hemoptysis
p. infection
p. infection in pregnancy
p. infestation
p. melanoderma
p. organism
p. worm
parasitica, dermatorrhagia
parasiticus, Aspergillus
parasiticus, craniphagus
parasitovorax, Cheyletiella
parasomnias, autonomic
parasomnias, motor
paraspecific stimulation
paraspinal
p. abscess
p. muscle
p. muscle spasm
paraspinous fascia
Paraspirillum vejdovskii
parasternal
p. examination
p. heave
p. impulses, left
p. impulses, right
p. intercostal tenderness
p. long-axis view
p. long-axis view echocardiogram
p. lymph nodes
p. short-axis view
p. short-axis view echocardiogram
p. systolic lift
p. systolic thrill
p. tissue
p. view
p. view echocardiogram ▸ long-axis
p. view ▸ short-axis
parasympathetic
p. fiber
p. function
p. innervation of lung
p. nerve

p. nerve fibers
p. nervous system
p. nucleus
p. stimulation
p. system
parasystole
p., atrial
p., pure
p., ventricular
parasystolic ventricular tachycardia
parataxic/paratactic
parataxic distortion
paratenon [*peritenon*]
paraterminal gyrus
paraterminalis, gyrus
paratesticular rhabdomyosarcoma
parathormone (PTH)
parathyreoprivus, status
parathyroid
p. adenoma
p. adenoma, ectopic
p. aplasia, thymic-
p. disease
p. dysfunction
p. extract
p. gland
p. gland function
p. glands ▸ overactive
p. hormone (PTH)
p. hormone deficiency
p. hormone (IPTH),
immunoreactive
p. hormone secretion rate
p. ▸ increased secretion of
p. insufficiency
p. tetany
p. tissue
p. tumor ablation
parathyroprival tetany
paratracheal
p. adenopathy
p. chain
p. region
paratrigeminal syndrome
paratrooper fracture
paratuberculosis, Mycobacterium
paratuberculous lymphadenitis
paratubular adhesions
paratyphi
p. A, Salmonella
p. B, Salmonella
p. C, Salmonella
paratyphoid
p. A
p. B

p. -enteritidis group
p. fever
p. infection
p. vaccine, typhoid-
paratyphosa B ▸ gastroenteritis
paraumbilical (*same as* **parumbilical**)
paraurethral duct
paraurethral gland
paravaginal hysterectomy
paravaginal incision
paraventricular veins
paravertebral
p. block
p. mass
p. mass formation
p. musculature
paravertex waves
paravesical extraperitoneal cesarean section
paravesical fossa
parchemin, bruit de
parchment heart
parchment induration
pared with motor saw ▸ fragments
parenchyma
p., beefy red
p., brain
p. congested
p. congested, liver
p. ▸ cut section of liver
p., defective renal
p. edematous
p. extremely congested
p., hepatic
p., incised renal
p. infiltration
p., kidney
p., liver
p. ▸ lobulated, firm, tan
p., lung
p., neural
p. of lens
p. of pancreas
p. pattern
p., pulmonary
p., renal
p., surrounding lung
p., testicular
p. testis
parenchymal [*parenteral*]
p. amyloidosis
p. atrophy
p. change, active
p. density
p. disease, active

p. disease ▸ primary pulmonary
p. disease, renal
p. fibrosis
p. hemorrhage
p. infiltrate
p. lung disease
p. opacification, amorphous
p. restriction ▸ progressive
p. scarring
p. softening, diffuse
p. window ▸ pulmonary
parenchymatosus, xerosis
parenchymatous
p., carcinoma
p. center
p. change
p. goiter
p. hemorrhage
p. keratitis
p. mastitis
p. myocarditis
p. nephritis
p. pneumonia
p. salpingitis
p. tissue
p. tonsillitis, acute
parent(s) (Parent)
p. abuse
p., abused
p. -adolescent communication
p., adoptive
p. artery
p. authority figure
p., bereaved
p., biological
p. cell
p. -child interaction
p. -child interaction evaluation
p. ▸ child of alcoholic
p. -child problem
p., children of incarcerated
p., chronic disability in
p. class, expectant
p., clinging to
p., controlling
p. counseling, single
p. ▸ daughter of alcoholic
p. effectiveness training
p. element
p., expectant
p. fixation
p., foster
p., impaired
p. -infant bonding
p. of short stature

p., protector/provider for
p. relationships, child-
p. ▸ son of alcoholic
p. status, single-
P. Support Group ▸ Tough Love
p. support group ▸ youth/
p. syndrome, battered
parentage of chromosomes
parental
p. alcoholism
p. alienation
p. antisocial behavior
p. authorization
p. bereavement
p. consent
p. discipline ▸ inconsistent
p. donor
p. empowerment
p. figure
p. flexibility
p. habits of blame
p. habits of praise
p. height, mid-
p. influence
p. kidney
p. loss, early
p. over-attentiveness
p. psychopathology
p. Rh (Rhesus) incompatibility
p. role conflict
p. role, quasi-
p. separation, early
p. stress
p. transplants
parenteral [*parenchymal*]
p. administration
p. alimentation
p. analgesic medication
p. antimicrobial agent
p. diarrhea
p. diuretics
p. feedings
p. fluids
p. hyperalimentation
p. injection
p. inoculation
p. mechanism
p. nutrition
p. nutrition (TPN) catheter, total
p. nutrition (TPN) hyperalimentation ▸ total
p. nutrition (TPN) line, total
p. nutrition (TPN) therapy, total
p. nutrition, total
p. nutrition (TPPN), total peripheral

parenteral—*continued*
    p. prophylactic therapy
    p. therapy
    p. transmission
    p. treatment
Parenthood, Planned
parenting
    p., altered
    p. behavior
    p. classes
    p. education
    p. issues
    p. skills, effective
    p. style, dysfunctional
    p., surrogate
    p. ▸ unstable or erratic
paresis
    p., cerebral
    p., facial
    p., galloping
    p., general
    p., muscle
    p., residual
    p., stationary
paresthesia(s)
    p., Berger's
    p., Bernhardt's
    p. of extremity
    p. of feet
    p. of limbs
    p., paroxysmal
    p., visceral
paresthetic feeling
paresthetica
    p., cheiralgia
    p., macromelia
    p., meralgia
    p., nostalgia
    p., pseudomelia
paretic
    p. dementia
    p. impotence
    p. neurosis
    p. neurosyphilis
    p. nystagmus
Parham band
paries
    p. anterior vaginae
    p. jugularis
    p. membranaceus bronchi
    p. membranaceus tracheas
    p. tegmentalis
    p. tracheae
parietal
    p. area

p. area left wave-spike
p. area right wave-spike
p. area sharp wave-spike
p. bone flap
p. boss
p. cells
p. damage ▸ right hemispheric
p. decidua
p. diameter
p. dysfunction
p. dysfunction ▸ right
p. electrode
p. emissary vein
p. endocarditis
p. endocarditis ▸ isolated
p. eye
p. fibroplastic endocarditis,
    Löffler's
p. gyrus
p. headache
p. hernia
p. hump
p. lead
p. lobe
p. lobe of brain
p. lobe of brain ▸ excision
p. lobule, inferior
p. lobule, superior
p. mucosa
p. notch of temporal bone
p. -occipital placement
p. pericardiectomy
p. pericardium
p. peritoneum
p. pleura
p. pleura, resection of
p. pregnancy
p. presentation
p. region
p. segment
p. shunt
p. slow wave focus
p. spike
p. spike focus
p. stroke, evolving right
p. suture
p. thrombus
p. vein of Santorini
parietale, os
parietalis, decidua
parietalis fibroplastica, endocarditis
parietocolic fold
parietography, gastric
parietomastoid suture
parietomastoid suture lines

parieto-occipital
    p. aphasia
    p. area
    p. artery
    p. placement
    p. region
    p. suture
parieto-occipitalis, arcus
parieto-orbital projection
parietoperitoneal adhesions
parietoperitoneal fold
parietotemporal region
Parinaud's
    P. conjunctivitis
    P. ophthalmoplegia
    P. syndrome
paring of lesion
paring of wart
Paris
    P. cast, plaster of
    P. dose distribution system
    P. jacket, plaster of
**Parker dose distribution ▸ Paterson
and**
parkeri, Borrelia
Parker's fluid
parking for handicapped
Parkinson('s)
    P. dementia complex
    P. disease
    P. disease ▸ surgical treatment for
    P. facies
    P. -like tremor
    P. mask
    P. syndrome
    P. syndrome, drug-induced
    P. tremor disorder
    P. -White bypass tract ▸ Wolff-
    P. -White reentrant tachycardia ▸
        Wolff-
    P. -White (WPW) syndrome, Wolff-
parkinsonian syndrome
parkinsonian-like disturbances
parkinsonism, drug-induced
parkinsonism, postencephalitic
Park's aneurysm
Parlett serologic test ▸ Youman-
parlor syncope ▸ beauty
Parona's space
paronychia tendinosa
paroophoritic cyst
parotid [*carotid*]
    p. abscess
    p. adenocarcinoma
    p. duct

p. enlargement
p. function
p. gland
p. lymph nodes ▸ superficial and deep
p. nerves
p. notch
p. saliva
p. tumor
p. tumor, malignant
p. vein
p. vein, anterior
p. vein, posterior

parotidea
  p., oophoritis
  p., orchitis
  p., papilla
parotideomasseteric region
parotitis [*parotiditis*] phlegmonosa
parotitis [*parotiditis*], radiation for
parous cervix
parous introitus
parovarian cyst
paroxysm(s)
  p., febrile
  p., involuntary general
  p. of artery
  p. of cough
  p. of pain
  p. of pain ▸ repeated
paroxysmal
  p. activity
  p. activity, cerebral
  p. activity, interictal
  p. activity, latent
  p. aggressive behavior ▸ positive
  p. atrial fibrillation
  p. atrial tachycardia (PAT)
  p. atrial tachycardia (PAT) aborted
  p. atrial tachycardia (PAT) with aberrancy
  p. burst
  p. cerebral dysrhythmia (PCD)
  p. cerebral phenomena
  p. cold hemoglobinuria
  p. contraction
  p. cortical activity
  p. cough
  p. coughing spasm
  p. discharge
  p. disease
  p. dyspnea
  p. high voltage discharge
  p. high voltage slow waves
  p. hypertension

p. junctional tachycardia
p. nocturnal dyspnea (PND)
p. nocturnal hemoglobinuria (PNH)
p. nodal rhythm
p. nodal tachycardia
p. pain
p. palpitation
p. paralytic myoglobinuria
p. paresthesias
p. patterns
p. positional vertigo
p. positional vertigo (BPPV) ▸ benign
p. positional vertigo ▸ recalcitrant benign
p. pulmonary edema
p. reentrant supraventricular tachycardia
p. response, photo◊
p. sinus tachycardia
p. sleep
p. slow activity
p. slow waves
p. slowing
p. slowing, diffuse
p. supraventricular arrhythmia
p. supraventricular tachycardia (PSVT)
p. tachycardia
p. tachycardia, atrial
p. tachycardia ▸ atrioventricular (AV) nodal reentrant
p. tachycardia ▸ nodal
p. tachycardia ▸ recurrent
p. trepidant abasia
p. ventricular tachycardia (PVT)
p. ventricular tachycardia ▸ repetitive
p. vertigo

Parrot's (parrot)
  P. artery of the newborn
  P. atrophy of the newborn
  P. disease
  p. fever
  P. murmur
  P. node
  P. pseudoparalysis
  P. sign
  P. tongue
  P. ulcer
  p. virus
parry fracture
Parry's disease
pars
  p. articularis

p. centralis
p. fetalis placentae
p. flaccida
p. frontalis
p. inarticularis
p. intermedia
p. marginalis
p. media, gastric
p. membranacea
p. sulci cinguli
p. tensa
p. uterina placentae
p. uterine tubae uterinae

parse information
Parsonnet pulse generator pouch
Parsons' disease
part(s)
  p. A benefits
  p. B benefits
  p. breath, three-
  p. ▸ liposuction of body
  p. of body ▸ rhythmic shaking of
  p. of bone, spongy
  p. of central nervous system (CNS), intracranial
  p. of central nervous system, supratentorial
  p.. of CNS (central nervous system), infratentorial
  p. of pons, tegmental
  p. ▸ protrusion of fetal
  p. sarcoma, alveolar soft
  p. ▸ wear resistant artificial joint
partial (Partial)
  p. agglutinin
  p. amputation
  p. anesthesia
  p. ankylosis
  p. anomalous pulmonary venous connection
  p. anomalous pulmonary venous drainage
  p. anomalous pulmonary venous return (PAPVR)
  p. artificial airway
  p. asphyxia ▸ repeated
  p. atrioventricular (AV) canal
  p. autolysis
  p. avulsion
  p. awakening
  p. baldness
  p. birth abortion
  p. blindness
  p. blockage in artery
  p. bowel blockage

partial—*continued*
- p. breast amputation
- p. breech delivery
- p. breech extraction
- p. bypass
- p. bypass procedure ▸ robotic
- p. cardiopulmonary bypass
- p. cataract
- p. clearing
- p. colectomy
- p. collapse ▸ right lower lobe (RLL)
- p. denture
- p. denture impression
- p. dentures, acrylic
- p. dentures, cast metal
- p. disability
- p. dislocation
- p. emission
- p. emptying of stomach
- p. encircling endocardial ventriculotomy
- p. epileptic seizure
- p. excision
- p. excision mucous membrane of cervix uteri
- p. facial paralysis
- p. food irradiation
- p. function
- p. gastrectomy
- p. hearing loss
- p. heart block
- p. hospital treatment program
- P. Hospitalization ▸ American Association for
- p. hospitalization programs
- p. hysterectomy
- p. ileal bypass
- p. impairment of conduction
- p. inability to urinate
- p. intermixed fibrosis
- p. intestinal obstruction
- p. isolation
- p. keratectomy
- p. knee placement
- p. laryngectomy
- p. left ventriculectomy
- p. lesion
- p. ligament tear
- p. liquid ventilation (PLV)
- p. lobectomy
- p. loss of motor function
- p. loss of vision
- p. lower denture
- p. mastectomy

- p. myectomy
- p. obstruction
- p. obstruction of bladder
- p. occlusion
- p. occlusion inferior vena cava clip
- p. occlusion main bronchus
- p. omentectomy
- p. or complete memory loss
- p. or complete paralysis
- p. ossicular replacement prosthesis (PORP)
- p. pancreas transplant
- p. paralysis
- p. paralysis, secondary
- p. penetrating keratoplasty
- p., permanent
- p. phalangectomy
- p. placenta previa
- p. plate
- p. pneumonectomy
- p. pressure (PP)
- p. pressure, arterial
- p. pressure gradient, alveolo-capillary
- p. pressure (mmpp) ▸ millimeters
- p. pressure of carbon dioxide (PCO_2)
- p. pressure of inhalational anesthetic, alveolar
- p. pressure of oxygen (PO_2)
- p. pressure ▸ postanesthetic arterial
- p. push-up
- p. quadriplegia
- p. reaction of degeneration
- p. rebreathing anesthesia
- p. rebreathing mask
- p. remission
- p. remission ▸ bipolar disorder, depressed, in
- p. remission ▸ bipolar disorder, manic, in
- p. remission ▸ bipolar disorder, mixed, in
- p. remission ▸ major depression, in
- p. remission ▸ major depression, single episode, in
- p. removal
- p. resection of stomach
- p. residual
- p. restraints
- p. restraints, patient in
- p. salpingectomy, bilateral
- p. seizure
- p. seizure, complex

- p. seizure, simple
- p. severance
- p. skinning vulvovaginectomy
- p. tearing of ligament
- p. thickness skin graft
- p. thickness transplant
- p. thoracoplasty
- p. thromboplastin time
- p. thromboplastin time (APTT), activated
- p. thromboplastin time ▸ kaolin
- p. thromboplastin time test
- p. thyroidectomy
- p. ulnar deviation
- p. union of fracture
- p. upper denture
- p. veneered crown
- p. vision
- p. weight bearing
- p. zona drilling (PZD)

partialis
- p. continua, epilepsia
- p. fugax, amaurosis
- p., ophthalmoplegia
- p., placenta previa

partially
- p. amputated, toe
- p. clogged artery
- p. dilated, cervix
- p. disabled, patient
- p. improved, patient
- p. suspended, bodily functions

participation, condition of
particle(s)
- p., alpha
- p., aspiration of food
- p., atherogenic
- p., bacteriophagic
- p. beams, physical effects of
- p. bean therapy, heavy charged
- p., benign calcium
- p., beta
- p., charged
- p., clot
- p., electronic
- p., elementary
- p., food
- p., foreign
- p. ▸ human intracisternal A type retroviral
- p. infects new host cell ▸ phage
- p., ingested food
- p. ▸ loose cartilage
- p. maturing in donor cell ▸ phage
- p., mucus

p., nuclear
p., patient vomited undigested food
p., phage
p., radioactive
p., regurgitated food
p., retained fecal
p., subatomic
p. therapy
p. therapy, heavy
p. therapy in eye tumors, heavy charged
p. transport time
p., undigested food
p., viral
p., virus
p. (WIMP) ‣ weakly interacting massive

particulate(s)
p. air, high efficiency
p. contaminants
p., entrained air and
p. material
p. matter
p. matter, retained
p. radiation

partita, patella
partition
p. chromatography
p. coefficient
p. coefficient, blood gas
p. coefficient, brain-blood

partitioning ‣ left atrial
partner(s)
p. abuse
p., multiple sexual
p., phobic
p., sexual

parts
p., affected
p., component
p., divide in equal
p. (p. ae.) ‣ in equal
p. of buccinator muscle ‣ feedback training of

parturient women ‣ infected
party payor, third
parumbilical (*same as* **paraumbilical**)
p. cutaneous circulation
p. hernia
p. vein

parvicollis, uterus
parvovirus infection
parvula, Veillonella
parvum
p., Corynebacterium

p., Cryptosporidium
p., Diphyllobothrium
parvus alternans
parvus et tardus pulse
PAS (Physicians Activities Study)
PAS (Professional Activities Study)
Pasar tachycardia reversion pacemaker
Pascheff's conjunctivitis
Paschen's granules
pass
p. filter, high
p. filter, low
p. lead ‣ single
p. pacemaker, dual
p. pacemaker, single-
p., patient released on overnight
p. radionuclide angiocardiography ‣ first-
p. technique ‣ first-
p. ‣ therapeutic home
p. urine ‣ inability to

passage(s)
p., air
p., atresia of lacrimal
p. become inflamed, air
p., blocked breathing
p., blocked nasal
p., bronchial
p. ‣ constriction of breathing
p., foreign body (FB) in air
p. ‣ hard stool
p. inflammation ‣ nasal
p., irritate nasal
p. ‣ lining of nasal
p., nasal
p. ‣ obstructed nasal
p., obstruction of air
p. of bile ‣ block
p. of blood
p. of catheter
p. of cerebrospinal fluid (CSF) ‣ blocking of
p. of clots
p. of dark brown urine
p. of flatus
p. of instrument, attempted
p. of instrument, successful
p. of meconium
p. of meconium, late
p. of mucus
p. of sound
p. of stone
p. of tissue
p. of tissue, spontaneous

p. of urine ‣ free
p., oral
p., respiratory
p., sinus
p., stenosis of lacrimal
passageway, air
passageway, nasal
Passavant's bar
passed
p., bronchoscope
p., foreign body (FB)
p., guide wire
p. per ora, scope
p., scope
p., speculum
p. through esophagus into stomach ‣ barium
p. up through incision ‣ forceps
p. with ease, catheter
p. with ease, instrument
p. without difficulty ‣ instrument

passeris, Haemoproteus
passing
p. faradic current into larynx
p. fecal material
p. flatus material
p. flatus, patient
p. gas
p. of kidney stone

passion, momentary
passive [*massive*]
p. activities
p. -aggressive
p. -aggressive personality
p. -aggressive personality disorder
p. alignment
p. atelectasis
p. clot
p. collusion
p. congestion
p. congestion, acute
p. congestion, chronic
p. congestion of liver ‣ acute
p. congestion of liver ‣ chronic
p. congestion of lung
p. congestion of lungs ‣ chronic
p. congestion ‣ severe acute
p. congestive changes
p. contraction
p. cutaneous anaphylaxis
p. -dependent
p. -dependent personality
p. edema
p. euthanasia
p. exercise

passive—*continued*
- p. flexion
- p. flexion of leg
- p. hyperemia
- p. hyperemia of retina
- p. illusion
- p. immunity
- p. immunization
- p. incontinence
- p. interval
- p. limb movements
- p. lingual arch
- p. loneliness ▸ displays
- p. mode
- p. motion
- p. movement
- p., patient
- p. placement
- p. range of motion (ROM)
- p. relaxation
- p. smoke
- p. smoke exposure
- p. smoking
- p. stretching
- p. stretching ▸ resistance to
- p. therapy
- p. tobacco smoke
- p. treatments
- p. tremor
- p. vaccine
- p. venous congestion
- p. volition versus consciousness

passively flexed, neck
passivity and inaction
passover humidifier
passularum, Carpoglyphus
Passy-Muir valve
past
- p. activity ▸ vigorous
- p. conditioning
- p. events, memory for
- p. events, recalling
- p. experience, unrecognized
- p. history (PH)
- p. history (PH) noncontributory
- p. history (PH) not remarkable
- p. medical history (PMH)
- p. mistreatment
- p. pathway ▸ selective
- p. -pointing
- p. -pointing test
- p. psychiatric disorder
- p., relinquishing the
- p. surgical history (PSH)

paste
- p. boot ▸ Unna's
- p., cocaine
- p., electrode
- p., Lassar's
- p., Lassar's betanaphthol
- p., Lassar's plain zinc
- p., nitrol
- p., smoking cocaine
- p., Unna's

Pasteurella
- P. aerogenes
- P. lepiseptica, gram-negative
- P. multocida
- P. pestis
- P. pestis, gram-negative
- P. pseudotuberculosis
- P. tularensis
- P. tularensis, gram-negative

pasteurianum, Clostridium
pasteurianus, Acetobacter
pasteurization, wet
Pasteur's fluid
Pastia's sign
pastille radiometer
pastoral
- p. care
- p. care, ongoing
- p. counseling
- p. follow-up
- p. ministry
- p. need, assessing
- p. visitation

pastorianum, Clostridium
pastorianus, Saccharomyces
pasty looking, patient
PAT (paroxysmal atrial tachycardia)
Patau's syndrome
patch(es) (Patch)
- p. ▸ abdominal testosterone
- p., alcohol
- p. aneurysm ▸ ventricular
- p. angioplasty
- p., autologous pericardial
- p., cardiac
- p., Carrel
- p. cataract removal, no stitch and no
- p. cataract surgery ▸ no-stitch, no-
- p., cigarette paper
- p. closure of defect
- p. compression dressing, eye
- p., Dacron
- p., Dacron intracardiac
- p., defibrillation

- p. dressing
- p., Edwards'
- p., electrical lead
- p., electrode
- p. electrode, cutaneous thoracic
- p. enlargement of ascending aorta
- p. ▸ epicardial defibrillator
- p., estrogen
- p., eye
- p., felt
- p. from anemia ▸ white
- p. from diabetes ▸ white
- p., gel
- p. ▸ Gore-Tex cardiovascular
- p. ▸ Gore-Tex surgical
- p. graft
- p. graft angioplasty
- p. graft, compressed Ivalon
- p. graft ▸ Microknit
- p. graft, Weavenit
- p., gray
- p., herald
- p. implant ▸ Edwards Teflon intracardiac
- p. injection, blood
- p., intracardiac
- p. ▸ Ionescu-Shiley pericardial
- p., Ivalon
- p. ▸ motion sickness skin
- p., nicotine
- p. ▸ nicotine skin
- p., nicotine transdermal
- p., nitroglycerin
- p. of atelectasis ▸ lobular
- p. of parakeratosis
- p. of pigmentation ▸ symmetrical
- p. of skin ▸ thick, red, itchy
- p. on mucosa of stomach ▸ small, flat, white
- p. or blister on arm ▸ red
- p., pantaloon
- p., pericardial
- p., persistent reddish
- p., Peyer's
- p. plasty ▸ endoventricular circular
- p. ▸ polypropylene intracardiac
- p. prosthesis ▸ Edwards Teflon intracardiac
- p., psoriatic
- p. quilt degeneration of muscle cells
- p., red scaly
- p., sandwich
- p., sclerotic
- p., Silastic

p., skin
p. skin test
p. ▸ small adhesive skin
p., smoker's
p., soldiers'
p. ▸ stick-on nicotine
p. technique
p. technique, anterior sandwich
p. technique ▸ two-
p., Teflon
p. ▸ Teflon intracardiac
p. test
p. test for allergy
p. test for tuberculosis (TB)
p. testing
p. therapy
p., transdermal nicotine
P. ▸ Transdermal NTG (nitroglycerin)
p. treatment ▸ nicotine

patchy
p. alveolar making ▸ bilateral
p. amnesia
p. area
p. area of bronchopneumonia
p. area of consolidation
p. area of old fibrosis
p. area of pneumonic consolidation
p. atelectasis
p. baldness
p. chronic inflammatory infiltrate
p. demineralization
p. depigmentation of skin
p. early bilateral
   bronchopneumonia
p. fibrosis
p. fibrosis, diffuse
p. fibrosis of ventricular
   myocardium
p. friability
p. infiltrate
p. infiltration
p. infiltrative process
p. interstitial fibrosis
p. metaplasia
p. myocardial fibrosis
p. perisplenitis
p. pneumonia
p. pneumonic infiltrate
p. purpuric hemorrhage
p. rash

Patein's albumin

patella
p. alta
p., ballotable

p. bipartita
p. bone
p. cap prosthesis ▸ McKeever
p., chondromalacia of
p. cubiti
p. disease
p., dislocated
p., dislocation of
p., floating
p., fracture of
p. partita
p., retinacular release of
p., slipping
p., tripartite fracture of

patellae, chondromalacia

patellar
p. chondromalacia
p. dome
p. facet cartilage, medial
p. femoral arthritis
p. ligament
p. prosthesis
p. prosthesis, McKeever
p. reflex
p. release
p. retinaculum
p. subluxation ▸ chronic
p. synovial fold
p. tendon
p. tendon advancement
p. tendon bearing
p. tendon insertion
p. tendon insertion, medial
   transplantation of
p. tendon reflex
p. tendon transfer
p. tendon transplant
p. tendon transposition

patello-adductor reflex

patellofemoral
p. arthritis
p. articulation
p. degenerative arthritis

patency [*latency*]
p. and spill
p., catheter
p., epicardial vessel
p. of veins
p., postoperative tubal
p., probe

patent [*latent*]
p. airway
p. and not dilated ▸ ureters
p. anus
p., arteries

p., biliary system
p. branches
p. bronchus sign
p., coronary arteries
p. ▸ coronary arteries widely
p. duct
p. ductus
p. ductus arteriosus (PDA)
p. ductus arteriosus murmur
p. ductus arteriosus umbrella
p. ductus renal agenesis with
   associated stigmata
p. fallopian tubes
p. foramen ovale
p. gastrojejunostomy
p. glottis
p. lumen
p. medicine
p. neuroforamina
p., normally
p. opening
p. opening for bile drainage
p. orifice
p., orifices widely
p. os
p. pancreatic
p., pancreatic duct
p., tube
p. urachus
p., ureters
p. vessels
p. vitelline duct

paternal deprivation
paternity studies
paternity testing
Paterson('s)
P. and Parker dose distribution
P. –Brown-Kelly syndrome
P. nodules
Patey modified mastectomy
Patey radical mastectomy
path, afferent nerve
path, mean free
pathematic aphasia
pathogen(s)
p., acquired immune deficiency
   syndrome (AIDS) primary
p., activation of endogenous
p., airborne
p., animal
p., bacterial
p., blood-borne
p. carrier, asymptomatic
p., culture negative for
p., enteric

pathogen(s)—_continued_
p. free (SPF) ▸ specific
p., fungal intracellular
p., gram-negative surgical
p., gram-positive surgical
p., nosocomial
p., opportunistic
p., stool culture negative for
pathogenesis
p. of acute myocardial infarction
p. of infection, bacterial
p. of ocular lesion
p. of pulmonary artery stenosis
p. of the disease
pathogenic
p. agent
p. bacteria
p. fungi
p. mechanism
p. micro-organisms
p. occlusion
p. organism
p. species
p. vibrios
pathogenesis of infection
pathogens, resistant
pathologic
p. abnormality
p. alcohol use ▸ pattern
p. anatomy
p. atrophy
p. cell
p. classification
p. compression fracture
p. diagnosis
p. diagnosis, final
p. dislocation
p. drug intoxication
p. examination
p. fracture
p. fractures, multiple
p. gambling
p. histology
p. insult
p. loss of memory
p. murmur
p. perforation
p. prognostic factors
p. reflex
p. rigidity
p. stress
pathological
p. alterations
p. amputation
p. anatomy

p. change
p. conditions
p. delusion
p. depression
p. diagnosis
p. diagnosis, final
p. doubts
p. examination, tissue removed for
p. fracture
p. gambling
p. hair pulling
p. left-handedness
p. liar
p. organism
p. process
p. process, gross
p. report
p. scars
p. specimen
p. stool
p. temper
p. test
p. tissue examination
p. use
p. use, history of
pathologist
p. -on-call
p., speech
p., speech and language
p., tissue submitted to
pathology (Pathology)
p., active pulmonary
p. and staging
P. (AFIP) ▸ Armed Forces Institute of
p., benign
p., bone
p., bone or joint
p., brain
p., coexistent
P. Department
p., electro◊
p., evidence of
p., joint
p., negative for
p., no evidence of
p., oat cell
p., oral
p., organic colon
p., psychoanalytic
p., rotator cuff
p. service, language
p. service, speech
p., significant
p., speech

p., structural
pathophysiologic correlates
pathway(s)
p. ablation ▸ slow
p., accelerated
p., accessory
p., accessory atrioventricular
p., afferent
p., air
p., antegrade internodal
p., anterior internodal
p., ascending
p., atrial preferential
p., atrio-His
p., atrioventricular (AV) nodal
p., atrioventricular node (AVN)
p., auditory
p., biochemical
p., cerebellar
p., conduction
p., descending
p. ▸ dual atrioventricular (AV) nodal
p. effective refractory period (APERP), accessory
p., energy
p., fascicular ventricular
p., fast
p. ▸ final common
p. ▸ ground-glass
p., hourglass
p. ▸ infection of nerve
p., internodal
p., main sensory
p. mapping ▸ tachycardia
p., mesocortical
p., motor
p., nerve
p., neural
p., nociceptive
p., optic
p., pain
p. potential ▸ purative slow
p. radiofrequency ablation ▸ fast
p., reentrant
p. ▸ referred pain sensory
p. ▸ retrograde fast
p. ▸ scavenger cell
p. ▸ selective past
p., sensory
p., septal
p., shunt
p. ▸ slow AV node
p., spinal
p., subarachnoid
p., sympathetic nervous

p., Thorel
p., visual
patient(s) ('s) (Patient)
p. abdomen distended
p. ability to perform
p. absentminded
p. abusive and hostile
p. accident prone
p. achieve independence ▸ help
p., acquired immune deficiency
  syndrome (AIDS)
p. acting inappropriately
p. acting out
p. active carrier
p. actively hallucinating
p. actively terminated
p. acts before thinking
p., acute alcoholic
p. acutely ill
p., addicted
p. admitted
p. admitted and transfused with
  fresh frozen plasma
p. admitted and transfused with
  whole blood
p. admitted crowning
p. admitted for complete checkup
p. admitted for evaluation and
  workup
p. admitted for medical evaluation
p. admitted for medical reassessment
p. admitted for observation
p. admitted for observation and
  treatment
p. admitted for terminal care
p. admitted in dazed condition
p. admitted with active infection
p. admitted with disguised infection
p. admitted with miscarriage
p. admitted with multiple complaints
p. afebrile
p. affect dull
p. affirmation
p., aggressive
p., agitated
p. agitated and confused
p. AIDS (acquired immune
  deficiency syndrome) carrier
p. aimlessly agitated
p., air evacuation of trauma
p., air transport of
p. alcohol dependent
p., alcoholic

p., alert
p. alert and cooperative
p. alert and oriented
p. alert to space, time and persons
p. allergic to _____
p., Alzheimer's
p., ambivalent
p. ambulated
p. ambulates on parallel bars
p. ambulates with assistance
p. ambulates with walker
p. ambulating with walker
p. ambulating with walker nonweight bearing
p., ambulatory
p., ambulatory peritoneal dialysis
p. Ambulift
p. amnesic
p. analyzed
p. anemic
p. anephric
p. anergic
p. anesthetized
p. angry
p. angry at God
p. anorectic
p. anorexic
p., antihypertensive coronary
p. anuretic
p. anxiety
p., anxious
p. apathetic
p. apneic
p. appetite good
p. appetite poor
p. apprehensive
p. arousable
p. ▸ artery-clogging plaque in
  atherosclerosis
p. arthritic
p. articulate
p. ▸ aspirin-sensitive
p., asplenic
p. assault on staff
p. assaultive
p., assess the
p. ▸ assessing and referring
p. assessment
p. asthmatic
p., asymptomatic
p. at complete bed rest
p. at high risk of exposure
p. at risk
p. at risk for AIDS (acquired
  immune deficiency syndrome)

p. at risk ▸ identify
p. at risk ▸ intervene with
p. at risk ▸ manage
p. at strict bed rest
p., autistic
p. avoids medical care
p. awake, alert and cooperative
p. awakes fatigued
p. aware of surroundings
p. awareness
p., basilar artery
p. basis ▸ treated on out◊
p., bedfast
p. bedridden
p. bedwetter
p. behavior
p. behavior as a screening device
p. behavior as a screening device
  for drug abuse
p. behavior problem
p., belligerent
p. bilateral lower limb amputee
p. bilateral upper limb amputee
p. black female (b/fe)
p. black male (b/m)
p. blames self
p. bloated
p. blood circulated to machine for
  cleansing
p. blushing
p. body donated to _____
p. body habitus
p. body temperature cooled
p. borderline
p., brain damaged
p. brain dead
p., breast cancer
p. breast-feeding
p. breathing circuit
p. breathless
p. brittle diabetic
p. burned beyond recognition
p. cachectic
p. calm and relaxed
p. calmed down
p. candidate for coronary attack
p. candidate for myocardial
  infarction (MI)
p. candidate for surgery
p. cannot be roused
p. cardiac cripple
p. cardioverted
p. care
p. care activities, monitor
p. care, adequate

patient(s)—*continued*

p. care, clinical
p. care ▸ collaborative
p. care conference
p. care coordinator
p. care, direct
p. care equipment
p. care experience
p. care, immediate
p. care, one-on-one
p. care practices
p. care procedures
p. care, progressive
p. care record
p. care techniques
p. care, total
p., caregiver abandoning
p., caregiver nurtures
p. catatonic
p. catheterized
p. Caucasian female
p. Caucasian male
p. -centered care
p. chart
p. chemical history
p., chemical restraint of
p., chemotherapy
p. choked to death
p. chronic carrier
p., chronic pain
p., chronic relapsing schizophrenic
p. chronically ill
p. circumcised
p. clinical condition
p. clinically stable
p. clumsy
p., cocaine dependent
p. cocky
p., codependent
p. cognitive abilities
p. coherent
p. cold and clammy
p. collapsed
p., comatose
p., combative
p. combative and agitated
p. combative to stimuli
p. committed
p. communicating
p. communicative
p., competent
p., complainant
p. completely disabled
p. completes basic transfer
p. completes independent transfer

p. completes toilet transfer
p. compliance with drug regimens
p. compliant
p., compulsive
p. concealed illness
p. condition, assessment of
p. condition deteriorated
p. condition precipitated by external factors
p. condition stabilized
p. condition stable
p. conditioned
p. confined to bed
p. confused
p. confused and dyspneic
p. conscious
p., conservative management of
p. constipated
p. contact, direct
p. contemplated suicide
p. continent
p. control of symptomatology
p. -controlled analgesia
p. convalescing
p. conversant
p. convulsing
p. cooperative
p., crack addicted
p. craving drugs
p. cries easily
p. crippled with arthritis
p. critical
p. crowning
p. crying
p. currently infectious
p. cyanotic
p., dangerous
p., dark-skinned
p. daydreams
p. dazed
p. dead on arrival (DOA)
p. death
p. debilitated
p. deceitful
p. deceptive
p. deeply anesthetized
p. deeply comatose
p. defervesced
p., defiant
p. defibrillating
p. dehydrated
p. dehydrated and debilitated
p. dejected
p. delirious

p. delivered by cesarean section (C-section)
p. delivered congenitally deformed infant
p. delivered macerated fetus
p. delivered normal infant
p. delivered prematurely
p. delivered stillborn
p. delivered triplets
p. delivered twins
p. delusional
p., demented
p., demise of
p. demoralized
p. dentulous
p. dependent
p. depressed
p., depressed cancer
p., depressed heart attack
p. deranged
p. desperate
p. despondent
p. deteriorating
p. diabetic
p. diagnosed and treated
p., dialysis
p. dialyzed
p. diaphoretic
p. died accidental death
p. died in sleep
p. died natural death
p. died suddenly
p. died unexpectedly
p. died unnatural death
p. dieting
p. dieting with exercise
p. difficult to arouse
p. digitalized
p. ▸ direct contact with
p., directly kill
p. disabled
p. discharge
p. discharged
p. discharged after period of observation
p. discharged ambulatory
p. discharged from hospital
p. discharged improved
p. discharged in good condition
p. discharged to care of relatives
p. discharged to convalescent treatment center
p. discharged to Coordinated Home Care Program
p. discharged to follow-up

p. discharged to home
p. discharged to home care
p. discharged to nursing home
p. discharged to office follow-up
p. discharged to treatment
p. discomfort
p. disillusioned
p. disoriented
p. disoriented and dysfunctional
p. displays obscene gestures
p. disrupting ward
p., disruptive
p., dissociative
p. distraught
p. distressed
p. disturbed
p. diuresed
p. dizzy
p. DNR (do not resuscitate)
p. DOA (dead on arrival)
p. does ADL (activities of daily living) with supervision
p. donor, autologous
p. ▸ dose distribution and heterogeneity of
p. drags left/right lower extremity
p. drooling
p. drowsy
p., drug controlling
p. drug dependent
p. drug-free treatment ▸ out-
p. drug history
p. "drying out"
p., dual diagnosis
p. dull and lethargic
p. dumping
p., duodenal ulcer
p. dysarthric
p. dysphagic
p. dysphoric
p. dyspneic
p., eating disorders
p. edentulous
p. education
p. education coordinator
p. education instruction sheet
p. education on drug abuse
p. egocentric
p. elbow, Heelbo used on
p. emaciated
p., emergency care of
p. emotional status
p., emotional support to
p. emotionally ill
p. emotionally stable

p. emotionally unstable
p. empirically treated
p. endurance deteriorated
p., enraged
p. enuretic
p. epileptic
p., escort
p., essential hypertensive
p. euphoric
p. evaluated
p., evaluation of
p. evasive
p. examined
p. excessively thirsty
p. excited
p., exercises for heart
p. exercising
p. exhausted
p. exhibited muscle guarding
p. exhibitionist
p. exhibits overt hostility
p. exhibits spasticity
p. expelled flatus
p. experiences emotional outbursts
p. experiences flashbacks
p. experiences remissions and exacerbations of pain
p. experiences weakness
p. experiencing withdrawal symptoms
p. expired
p. expired due to natural causes
p. expired in sleep
p. expired quietly
p. expired suddenly
p. expired, time
p. expired unexpectedly
p. exploding
p. exploitative
p. exposed to asbestos
p. exposed to tuberculosis
p. expressed guilt feelings
p. extroverted
p. extubated
p. failed to respond
p. fair-skinned
p. faking illness
p. -family advocate
p. farsighted
p. fearful
p. febrile
p. ▸ febrile neutropenic
p. feebleminded
p. feeling hostile
p. feeling stressed

p. feels abandoned
p. feels blue
p. feels damaged
p. feels demoralized
p. feels down
p. feels empty
p. feels estranged
p. feels giddy
p. feels guilty
p. feels isolated
p. feels rejected or ridiculed
p. fertile
p. feverish
p. fidgets
p. filled with self-pity
p. financial services (PFS)
p. flaccid
p. flaked out
p. flamboyant
p. flexed lower back
p. flexed upper back
p. ▸ fluid repletion of shock
p. -focused care
p. followed as outpatient
p. followed in office
p. followed on outpatient basis
p. forgetful
p. forgetful and confused
p. ▸ formal monitoring of
p. ▸ frail elderly
p. friendly
p. frustrated
p. fully roused
p. functional ability
p. functionally blind
p. functionally illiterate
p. functioning alcoholic
p. functioning at _____% normal capacity
p. fussy about details
p. gags reflexively
p. gainfully employed
p. gasping and cyanotic
p., geriatric
p. given enema
p. given enema prior to delivery
p. given enema prior to examination
p. given enema prior to surgery
p. given enema prior to x-ray
p. given placebo
p. glib
p. glum and moody
p. goals
p. gravida I (II, III, etc.)

patient(s)—*continued*

p. grimacing
p. grinds teeth
p. grunts and squeals
p. had elevated temperature
p. had evidence of show
p. had face lift
p. had fit
p. had flare-up of _____
p. had flashback reactions from drug abuse
p. had gastrocystostomy
p. had mini-peel
p. had mini-stroke
p. had mini-thoracotomy
p. had previous workup
p. had quadrantectomy
p. had relapse of disease
p. had respiratory arrest
p. had sclerotherapy
p. had seizure
p. had steady downhill course
p. had stillbirth
p. had stormy course
p. had uneventful postoperative course
p. hallucinating
p. handicapped
p. has adrenoleukodystrophy
p. has agoraphobia
p. has brain mets (metastases)
p. has bulimia
p. has character problems
p. has chills
p. has colostomy
p. has croup
p. has decreased memory
p. has diarrhea
p. has difficulty swallowing
p. has disorientation and hallucinations
p. has dry mouth
p. has disequilibrium
p. has dysuria
p. has endotracheal tube in place
p. has eyestrain
p. has fear of doctors
p. has fear of hospitals
p. has fibromyalgia
p. has flashbacks
p. has flat affect
p. has floating feeling
p. has forgetfulness, irritability and confusion
p. has frequency of urination

p. has generalized weakness
p. has good rapport with others
p. has headache
p. has heartburn
p. has hyperhidrosis
p. has indigestion
p. has insomnia
p. has interest in surroundings
p. has labored breathing
p. has lack of concentration
p. has leathery skin
p. has lipedema
p. has lockjaw
p. has low energy
p. has lump in throat
p. has lymphedema
p. has mastalgia
p. has memory loss
p. has multiple trauma
p. has natural immunity to hepatitis B virus
p. has needle tracks
p. has neuropathy
p. has nightmares
p. has no interest in surroundings
p. has no purposeful movement
p. has nocturia
p. has occasional palpitations
p. has persistent pain
p. has phlebothrombosis
p. has phobias
p. has polydipsia
p. has polyuria
p. has poor concentration
p. has poor insight
p. has poor memory
p. has potential for violence
p. has progeria
p. has pseudo-memory
p. has quinsy
p. has rash
p. has religious values
p. has scanning speech
p. has sense of doom
p. has stretchmarks
p. has suicidal tendencies
p. has swelling of upper arm
p. has tachycardia
p. has tantrums
p. has the shakes
p. has toothache
p. has tremors
p. has urinary retention
p. has urostomy
p. has vertigo

p. has vertigo and unsteadiness
p. has whiplash injury
p. hears voices
p., heart
p. ▸ heart attack
p., heart transplant
p. heavy drinker
p. heavy smoker
p. heel, Heelbo used on
p. hemiplegic
p. hemorrhaging
p. heparinized
p. heterogeneities
p. hiccoughing
p., high-risk
p. high-strung
p. highly compulsive
p. home environment
p., homebound
p., homosexual
p. hospital course turbulent
p. hospitalized
p. hospitalized for workup
p. hostile
p. housebound
p. humiliated
p. hustlers
p. hyperactive
p. hyperglycemic
p. hyperopic
p. hypersalivating
p. hypersensitive
p. hypersensitive to aspirin
p., hypertensive
p., hyperventilating
p. hypnotized
p. hypochondriacal
p. hypoglycemic
p. hyponatremic
p. hypotensive
p., hypoventilating
p. hysterical
p. ID (identification) bracelet
p. identified needs
p., identifying drug-abusing
p. imbibes
p. immature
p. immobile
p. immobilized
p., immune-depressed
p. immune response
p. ▸ immune system of cancer
p. immune to hepatitis B infection
p. immunocompetent
p., immunocompromised

p., immunocompromised cancer
p., immunodepressed
p., immunosuppressed
p. impacted
p. impatient
p., implant
p. impotent
p. improved
p. impulsive
p. in cardiac arrest
p. in cardiogenic shock
p. in catatonic state
p. in chronic pain
p. in coma
p. in complete relapse
p. in complete remission
p. in complete restraints
p. in continuous remission
p. in control
p. in crisis
p. in critical condition
p. in dazed state
p. in deep sleep
p. in delirium
p. in extreme distress
p. in extremis
p. in fetal position
p. in full leathers
p. in great distress
p. in home ▸ exercises for
p. in insulin shock
p. in isolation
p. in labor
p. in mild pain
p. in partial restraints
p. in postnatal depression
p. in psychoeducation
p. in psychotherapy
p. in rage
p. in remission
p. in respiratory distress
p. in restraints
p. in shock
p. in stable condition
p. in state of physical decay
p. in stupor
p. in vegetative state
p. inappropriate
p. inarticulate
p. incapable of caring for self
p. incapacitated
p. inclusion criteria
p. incoherent
p. incompetent
p. incontinent of feces

p. incontinent of stool
p. incontinent of urine
p., increase active extension in stroke
p. incurably ill
p. indecisive
p. independent in ambulation
p. independent in bathing with cueing
p. independent in bedmatic activities
p. independent in boosting and rolling
p. independent in feeding
p. independent in lower body dressing
p. independent in transfers
p. independent in upper body dressing
p. independent with small-based quad cane
p. Indian female
p. Indian male
p. indifferent
p., indigent
p., infectious
p. ingested contrast medium
p. injected with lethal substance
p. injected with liposomes
p. insecure
p. insomniac
p., institutionalized adult
p. intense
p. interaction ▸ staff-
p. interview as a screening device
p. interview as a screening device for drug abuse
p. intimidated
p. intolerant to aspirin therapy
p. intoxicated
p. introverted
p., intubate
p. intubated
p. intubated with bronchoscope
p., involuntary
p. irrational
p. irritable
p. irritable and jumpy
p. irritable and tense
p. irritable ▸ clinical pharmacology
p. is bow-legged
p. isolated
p. jogs
p. juvenile diabetic
p. Kardex card

p. kept comfortable
p. keyed up
p., kidney transplant
p. known asthmatic
p. lactating
p., lanthanic
p. lapsed into coma
p. latent diabetic
p. laughs inappropriately
p. left-handed
p. legal guardian
p., legally competent
p., legally incompetent
p. lethargic
p. level of anxiety
p. level of consciousness
p. level of disability
p. lifestyle
p. lift chair
p. lift, electric
p., liver transplant
p. load, average daily
p. lower extremity strength
p. lucid
p., maintain mobility of
p. makes deliberate actions
p. makes full fist
p. malingering
p. malnourished
p. managed medically
p. management, combination therapy in
p. management, decision trees in
p. management issues
p. manic-depressive
p. manifests suicidal tendencies
p. manipulative
p. medical history
p., medical management of
p., medically dependent
p. menopausal
p. menstruating
p., mental health
p. mentally alert
p. mentally clear
p. mentally cloudy
p. mentally deranged
p. mentally disordered
p. mentally disturbed
p. mentally ill
p. mentally retarded
p., Mexican
p. miscarried
p. misplacing things
p. mistreats others

patient(s)—*continued*

p. mongoloid
p. moody
p., motivated
p. moved and positioned
p. multiparous
p., multireactive
p. mute
p. mutilates self
p., myelosuppressed
p. myopic
p. nail-biter
p. nauseated
p. near-drowning victim
p. nearsighted
p. need to be with people
p. needs, assessing
p. needs assistance
p. needs minimal assistance for wheelchair mobility
p. negativistic
p. nervous
p. neurotic
p. neutropenic
p., NF (neurofibromatosis)
p. nightwalker
p. nonassertive
p. noncommittal
p. noncompliant
p. noncompliant with medication
p. nonconversive
p. nondrinker
p., nonrefractory
p. nonresponsive
p. nonsmoker
p. normal subject
p. not circumcised
p. nulligravida
p. nulliparous
p. nursing
p. obese
p. obeys commands
p. obsessive
p. obstipated
p. obstreperous
p. obtunded
p. obtuse
p. OD'd (overdosed)
p. on a high
p. on admission, orders accompanying
p. on back, reposition
p. on bail ▸ hospitalized
p. on continuing chemotherapy
p. on critical list

p. on edge
p. on fluid restriction
p. on multiple drug program
p. on respirator
p. on side, reposition
p. on ventilator
p. on waiting list
p., ongoing treatment of
p. operated on
p. ▸ opioid-dependent
p., optimum care of
p. Oriental female
p. Oriental male
p. orientation
p. oriented
p. oriented as to person, place and time
p. out of control
p. out of sync
p. outcome ▸ negative
p. outcome research
p. overbreathing
p. overdosed (OD'd)
p. overdosed (OD) with cannabinoids
p. overdosed (OD) with depressants
p. overdosed (OD) with hallucinogens
p. overdosed (OD) with inhalants
p. overdosed (OD) with multiple drugs
p. overdosed (OD) with opioids
p. overdosed (OD) with phencyclidines
p. overdosed (OD) with stimulants
p. overhydrated
p. overmedicated
p., overreactive
p. oversedated
p. overstimulated
p. ovulating
p. oxygen (O₂) dependent
p. pacing
p. pain-free
p. pain medication
p. pale
p. pancytopenic and septic
p. ▸ panic disorder
p. paralyzed
p. paranoic in thinking
p. paranoid
p. paraplegic
p. partially disabled
p. partially improved

p. passing flatus
p. passive
p. pasty looking
p. perceived suffering
p. perception of pain
p. perception of problem areas
p. perfectionist
p. perfectionist in self-defeating way
p. performance status
p. perplexed
p. perseverates in motor activities
p. perseverates in speech
p. perseverating ▸ schizophrenic
p. ▸ personality of
p. pessimistic
p. physically active
p. physically impaired
p. physically weak
p. physiologically unstable
p. picks at skin
p. placed at bed rest
p. placed in Croupette
p. placed in isolation
p. placed in traction
p. placement
p. placement program
p. placement program for adolescents
p. placement program for adults
p., polycystic
p. poor risk
p. poor surgical risk
p. population
p. population ▸ prevalence of drug abuse in general
p. positioning
p., postcystoscopy
p., postinfarct
p., postlaryngectomy
p., postmenopausal
p., postnatal
p., postoperative
p., postpartum
p. ▸ post-transplant
p. potentially infectious
p., pregnant
p. ▸ pregnant opiate-dependent
p. premedicated
p. premenarche
p., premenopausal
p. premenstrual
p., premorbid personality traits of
p., prenatal
p. preoccupied

p., preoperative
p. prepared and draped
p. prepped and draped in routine manner
p. prepped for surgery
p. presenile
p. previously hospitalized
p. primiparous
p. privacy
p. private pay
p. privilege, psychologist-
p. productive
p. progress
p. progress record
p. progressing satisfactorily
p. pronounced dead
p. propels wheelchair
p. ▸ prospective transplant
p. provides excuses
p. ▸ psychoactive substance-dependent
p. psychologic index
p., psychosomatic
p., psychotic
p. ▸ public mental health
p. pulled catheter out
p. pulls hair
p. pulseless and breathless
p. pursued rapid downhill course
p. quadriplegic
p. quality assurance
p. quarantined
p. questionnaire as a screening device
p. questionnaire as a screening device for drug abuse
p. quitting cold turkey
p. randomized
p. rapidly dehydrated
p. rapidly deteriorated
p. rapidly intubated
p. rationalizes
p. reached maximum hospital benefit (MHB)
p. reacting
p. reacts with disdain
p. reacts with rage
p. readmitted
p. receiving respiratory assistance
p. reckless
p. record
p. recovered
p. ▸ recovering stroke
p., recycle
p. re-evaluated

p. referred to follow-up
p., refractory
p. regained active status
p. regained consciousness
P. Registration
p. regresses emotionally
p. regurgitated
p. rehabilitation
p. rehospitalized
p. rehydrated
p. rejected
p. relationship, doctor-
p. relationship, physician-
p. relatively asymptomatic
p. release
p. release form
p. released
p. released against medical advice (AMA)
p. released in care of relatives
p. released on overnight pass
p. remained in asystole
p. remorseful
p. ▸ renal impaired
p. renews motivation
p. repeats ritualistic acts
p. repositioned
p. requesting admission
p. requires occasional assistance
p., residential
p. resigned
p. responded to care
p. responded to treatment
p. responded verbally
p. responds to medication
p. response is negative
p. responsive
p. rest, disrupt
p. restless
p. restrained with vest
p., restrictive cardiomyopathy
p. resuscitated
p. retarded
p. retching and vomiting
p. returned to room
p. Rh− (negative)
p. Rh+ (positive)
p. rheumatoid arthritic
p. right-handed
p. rights
p. rigid, nonresponsive and mute
p. ritualistic
p. rolls independently
p. rooming-in
p. routinely fatigued

p. safety
p. safety awareness
p. sarcastic
p. satisfaction
p. satisfaction assessment
p., satisfactory positioning of
p. schedule
p., schizophrenic
p. ▸ secretion spills from hepatitis
p. sedated
p., sedentary
p. seductive
p. seen in consultation
p. sees numerous physicians
p. sees visions
p., seizure disorder
p., selected population of
p. selection
p. self-absorbed
p. self-assertive
p. self-assured
p. self-conscious
p. self-deprecating
P. Self-Determination Act (PSDA)
p. self-disciplined
p. self-dramatizes
p. self-esteem is fragile
p. ▸ self-esteem of
p. self-image
p. self-medicating
p. self-motivated
p. self-occupied
p. self-preoccupied
p. self-regulates
p. self-righteous
p. self-sufficient
p., semiambulatory
p. semicomatose
p. semistuporous
p. senile
p. sensitive to _____
p. sent to Recovery Room
p. seriously ill
p. seriously retarded
p. serum magnesium
p., severely affected
p. severely cachectic
p., severely debilitated
p. severely dehydrated
p. ▸ severely self abusive
p. shock count ▸ total
p. shocked back into normal rhythm
p. shocky
p. short in stature

patient(s)—*continued*

p. short of breath
p. short term memory
p. short-winded
p. shouts
p. showed subjective improvement
p. ▸ sleep deprived
p. sleeptalking
p. sleepwalker
p. smokes
p. sober
p. social environment
p. socially withdrawn
p. spaced out
p., Spanish
p. spiked fever
p. spiked temperature
p. spilled protein
p. spilled sugar
p., split-brain
p. spread, patient-to-
p. stabilized
p. -staff relationship
p. staggers
p. stares
p. status
p. steadily deteriorated
p. sterile
p. ▸ stress disorder
p., stress in hypertensive
p., stress reactions in dental
p. stressed out
p. strung-out
p. stubborn
p. stuporous
p. subgroups
p., substance abusing
p. successfully resuscitated
p. succumbed
p. suctioned
p. suffered respiratory arrest
p. suffering from malnutrition
p., suicidal
p. ▸ suicide-prone
p. suicides
p. sundowning
p. superficial
p., supportive care of
p. survival rate
p. susceptibility
p. suspicious
p. sustained first degree burns
p. sustained second degree burns
p. sustained third degree burns
p. swallowed foreign object

p. sweating and disoriented
p. symptomatic
p. symptomatically improved
p. symptom-free
p. tachypneic
p. talkative
p. taught deep breathing
p. taught leg exercises
p. tearful
p. teenager
p. tends to self-diagnose
p. tense
p. tensed up
p. tentatively scheduled
p. terminal
p. terminally ill
p., test diet for papillotomy
p. tested cognitively
p. testing system, complete pacemaker
p. theatrical
p. -therapist confidentiality
p. thinks about ending life
p. thirsty and tired
p. threatening
p. threw an embolus
p. to push fluids
p. to receive weekly injections
p. to resume previous diet
p. -to-patient spread
p. -to-patient transmission
p. -to-staff transmission
p., toe tag on
p. tolerance and endurance
p. tolerated diagnostic procedures well
p. tolerated full course of radiation
p. tolerated procedure well
p. tolerated therapy
p. took overdose
p., topography and anatomic measurements of
p. totally dependent
p. totally disabled
p. totally inoperable
p. tough-minded
p. toxic
p. tranquilized
p. transferred
p. transferred to custodial care
p. transferred to nursing home
p. transfers with walker
p. transfused
p. transfused and treated with supportive care

p. transmission ▸ patient-to-
p. transmission ▸ staff-to-
p., transplant
p. transport
p. transported on gurney
p., trauma
p. treated conservatively
p. treated for comfort only
p. treated for smoke inhalation
p. treated in hospital
p. treated initially
p. treated initially with intravenous (IV) fluids
p. treated medically
p. treated with placebo
p. treated with radiation and chemotherapy
p. treated with radiation therapy
p. treated with supportive care
p. treated with tamoxifen
p. treated with thermotherapy
p., treatment of acute drug reactions in violent
p., treatment of suicidal
p. trembling
p. tremulous
p., triage
p. turned from side to side
p. turned on side
p., ultra low risk category
p. unable to cope
p. unable to perform basic activity
p. unable to relax
p., unable to resuscitate
p. unable to sit still
p. unable to void
p. unable to walk
p. unconscious
p. uncontrollable
p. under constant stress
p. under psychiatric care
p. under sedation
p. under self-hypnosis
p. undergoing personality change
p. underlying disease
p. unempathetic
p. unimproved
p. unknown AIDS (acquired immune deficiency syndrome) carrier
p. unresponsive
p. unstable
p. unsteady in gait
p. up ad lib
p. up in chair

p. upper extremity strength
p. uptight
p. uses cane
p. uses cocaine (Ice)
p. uses inappropriate words
p. uses quad cane with verbal cueing
p. uses walker
p. utilization
p. ventricular response
p. verbalizes slowly
p. verbalizing
p., vertiginous
p. very vocal
p. victim of drowning
p., viruses isolated from
p. vomited large quantities of blood
p. vomited undigested food particles
p. vomiting
p. vomiting blood
p. walks alone
p. walks straight line
p. warrior white cells, cancer
p. weak
p. weak and nauseated
p. weak, hypotensive and unresponsive
p. weaned from respirator
p. wears dentures
p. well being
p. well-developed
p. well-hydrated
p. well-nourished (W/N)
p. went full term
p. wheezing
p. wh/fe (white female)
p. wh/m (white male)
p. with azidothymidine (AZT) ▸ medicate
p. with chronic disease ▸ malnourished
p. with neck injuries ▸ muscle relaxation in
p. withdrawn
p. withdrawn, depressed and apathetic
p. withdrawn from life
p. W/N (well-nourished)
p. work perfunctory
p. worked up
p., writhing
p. zombie-like
Patrick's
  P. maneuver

P. sign
P. test
patronizing attitude
Pattee test, Murphy-
pattern(s)
  p., abnormal
  p., abnormal excitation
  p., abnormal heat
  p., abnormal sleep
  p., abusive
  p., action
  p., activity
  p. after surgical resection, failure
  p., alpha
  p., alteration in rest
  p., alteration in sleep
  p., altered sexuality
  p., alveolar filling
  p., antibiotic sensitivity
  p., antibiotic susceptibility
  p., antimicrobial sensitivity
  p., associative thought
  p., atheromatous
  p., autogenic training and EEG (electroencephalogram)
  p. ▸ autosomal dominant
  p., background
  p., baldness, female
  p., baldness, male
  p., behavior
  p., behavioral family
  p., beta
  p., biphasic
  p., bizarre eating
  p., bizarre gait
  p., bowel
  p., bowel gas
  p., brain wave
  p., breathing
  p., burst-suppression
  p., calyceal
  p., cell
  p., cellular
  p. ▸ central neurogenic breathing
  p. ▸ change in bladder
  p., change in bleeding
  p. ▸ change in bowel
  p., change in sleeping
  p. change, sleep/wake
  p., chemical usage
  p., circadian
  p., clinical
  p., coarsened mucosal fold
  p., compulsive work
  p., contraction

  p., coping
  p., crista
  p., cystometric
  p., defensive
  p., destructive
  p., destructive thought
  p., detrusor
  p., develop behavioral
  p. development ▸ normal resting EEG (electroencephalogram)
  p., dietary
  p., diffuse
  p. ▸ diffuse reticular nodular
  p., disordered sleep
  p. ▸ disruptive sleep
  p. ▸ disturbance in sleep
  p. ▸ disturbed sleep
  p., dominant
  p., ductal
  p., ECG/EKG (electrocardiogram) showed normal
  p., echo
  p., EEG (electroencephalogram)
  p., EEG (electroencephalogram) seizure
  p., EEG (electroencephalogram) sleep
  p., eggshell
  p., electrocardiogram (ECG/EKG) showed normal
  p., electrophoretic
  p., embolic
  p., epileptic
  p., epileptiform
  p. ▸ erratic sleep-wake
  p. evoked potentials
  p., fast mitten
  p., fishnet
  p., fixed action
  p., follicular
  p., gait
  p., gas
  p., genetic
  p., growth
  p., habitual
  p. hair loss ▸ female-
  p., haustral
  p., headache
  p., heat
  p., high voltage
  p., honeycomb
  p., hyperemic mucosal
  p., hypsarrhythmia
  p., identical
  p., inconclusive

pattern(s)—*continued*

p. ‣ ineffective breathing
p., interference
p., interstitial
p., intestinal gas
p. ‣ intraventricular conduction
p., irregular breathing
p., ischemic
p., juvenile
p., lifestyle
p., lobular
p., maladaptive
p., mitten
p., modify hearing
p., monitoring breathing
p., monitoring sleep
p., monitoring sucking
p. movement
p., mucosal
p., mucosal fold
p., muscle
p., national practice
p., neonatal sleep
p. ‣ non-Alzheimer's disease-related
p., nonspecific histologic
p., normal
p., normal bronchial
p., normal histologic
p., normal sleeping
p., normal waking electroencephalogram (EEG)
p. obesity ‣ male
p., occlusal
p. of addiction, family
p. of anxiety, image
p. of behavior ‣ repetitive and persistent
p. of binge eating ‣ episodic
p. of brain electrical activity ‣ shift in direction and
p. of cancer spread, lymphangitic
p. of cannabinoid abuse
p. of depressant abuse
p. of disregard for others ‣ pervasive
p. of dose fractionation, modification
p. of drinking
p. of drug use
p. of electrical activity, recruitment
p. of excretion ‣ significant variation in
p. of hallucinogen abuse
p. of impulsivity

p. of inhalant abuse
p. of insomniacs, sleep
p. of instability ‣ pervasive
p. of light ‣ irregular, flashing
p. of lung carcinoma, extrathoracic spread
p. of lung carcinoma, local spread
p. of lung carcinoma, lymphatic spread
p. of opioid abuse
p. of pathologic alcohol use
p. of phencyclidine abuse
p. of speech ‣ mechanical
p. of speech ‣ robotic
p. of stimulant abuse
p. of stomach, rugal
p. of stress physiology
p. of urinary elimination
p. of urinary elimination, alteration in
p. of use
p. of waves, total
p. on breast self-exam, concentric circle
p. on breast self-exam ‣ vertical
p. on breast self-exam ‣ wedge section
p., parenchymal
p., paroxysmal
p., perception of form and
p., personality
p., pervasive
p., phage
p., positive spike
p., preseizure
p., projected
p., psychomotor variant
p., pulmonary fibrotic
p., QR
p., QS
p., radicular pain
p. ‣ recessive inheritance
p., recorded brain wave
p., recruitment
p., reduced interference
p., regression
p. release ‣ physiologic
p. resemblance ‣ biofeedback EMG (electromyogram)
p., respiratory
p., reticular
p. reversal stimulation
p., sawtooth
p. ‣ scintillating speckle
p., seizure

p. ‣ self-defeating behavior
p., shift of total
p., sigma
p. ‣ sine-wave
p. sinoatrial (SA) node ‣ rhythmic
p., sleep
p., sleep-wake
p., slow mitten
p., slow wave
p., social
p., spastic mucosal
p., speckled
p., speech
p., spike
p., spike-and-wave
p., spindling
p., startle
p., stimulus
p., storiform
p. strabismus, A-
p., strain
p., submucosal vascular
p., symmetrical sleep
p., tangential speech
p. test, dot
p., therapeutic sleep
p. therapy
p. thermography, heat
p., theta
p., thought
p. ‣ torpedo-shaped
p., trabecular
p., trait
p., treatment failure
p., unhealthy eating
p. ‣ uptake mismatch
p., variations of
p., variety of abuse
p., vascular
p., ventricular strain
p., walking
p., wave-like
p., wax
p., weight
p., whorled
patterned alopecia
patterned visual stimulation
patulous introitus
patulous urethral wall
patulum, Penicillium
paucity of findings
Paufique's operation
Paufique's trephine
Paul('s)
    P. -Bunnell-Barrett test

P. -Bunnell test
P. pulsator, Bragg-
P. treatment
Pauli's exclusion principle
pause [*gauze*]
p., compensatory
p. -dependent arrhythmia
p., end-expiratory
p., noncompensatory
p., postextrasystolic
p., sinus
p. ▸ sinus exit
Pautrier's abscess
Pauwel fracture
Pauwel operation
Pauzat's disease
pavement cells
pavilion of the oviduct
paving stent ▸ polymeric endo-
luminal
paving stone degeneration
Pavlik harness
Pavlov('s)
P. dog
P. method
P. reflex
P. stomach
pavor diurnus
pavor nocturnus
Pavy's disease
paw, monkey
paw-like hand
Pawlik's fold
Pawlik's triangle
Pawlow's position
pay, patient private
Paykel scale
payment(s)
p., diagnostic-related groups
(DRG)
p., Medicaid
p., Medicare
p. system, prospective
payor, third party
Payr's disease
PB (pubococcygeal) muscle
P.B. test, Harvard
PBA (pulpobuccoaxial)
PBC (primary biliary cirrhosis)
PBF (pulmonary blood flow)
PBI (protein-bound iodine)
PB% (phonetic balanced percent)
PBT (protein-bound thyroxide)
PBV (pulmonary blood volume)

pc (PC)
pc (after meals)
PC (pentose cycle)
pc (picocurie)
pc./pCi (picocurie)
PCA (patient-controlled analgesic)
PCD (paroxysmal cerebral
dysrhythmia)
PCD (programmable cardioverter
defibrillator)
PCD ▸ Medtronic implantable
PCOS (polycystic ovarian syndrome)
pCO₂ (carbon dioxide partial
pressure)
PCP (phencyclidine)
PCP (hallucinogen)
PCP (phencyclidine)
PCP (phencyclidine) abuse
PCP (phencyclidine) delirium
PCP (phencyclidine) delusional
disorder
PCP (phencyclidine) dependence
PCP (phencyclidine) ingested
PCP (phencyclidine) injected
PCP (phencyclidine) intoxication
PCP (phencyclidine) mood disorder
PCP (phencyclidine) organic
mental disorder
PCP (phencyclidine) smoked
PCP (phencyclidine) snorted
PCP /PeaCe Pill (hallucinogen)
PCP /PeaCe Pill (phencyclidine)
PCP (primary care physician)
PCPB (percutaneous cardiopul-
monary bypass)
PCPy/PHP (phencyclidine analog)
PCR (polymerase chain reaction)
machine
PCR (polymerase chain reaction)
technique
PCRA (percutaneous coronary
rotational angioplasty)
PCT (porphyria cutanea tarda)
PCT (progesterone challenge test)
PCV (packed cell volume)
PCW (pulmonary capillary wedge)
PD
PD (interpupillary distance)
PD (prism diopter)
PD (pulpodistal)
PDA (patent ductus arteriosus)
PDGF (platelet derived growth factor)
PDT (photodynamic therapy)
PDT (photodynamic therapy)
treatment for cancer

PE
PE (pharyngoesophageal)
PE (physical examination)
PE (pleural effusion)
PE (pressure equalizing) tube
PE (pulmonary edema)
PE (pulmonary embolism)
pea soup stool
Peace pill LSD (lysergic acid
diethylamide)
PeaCe Pill/PCP (hallucinogen)
PeaCe Pill/PCP (phencyclidine)
Peace (STP) pill ▸ Serenity-
Tranquility-
Peaches (amphetamines)
peak(s)
p. A velocity
p., adaptive
p. amplitude period
p. and trough levels
p. area
p., backscatter
p. bone mass
p., Bragg
p., coincidence sum
p. deflection ▸ peak-to-
p. diastolic filling rate
p. E velocity
p. emptying rate
p. exercise
p. exercise oxygen (O₂)
consumption
p. exertion level
p. expiratory flow (PEF)
p. expiratory flow rate (PEFR)
p. filling rate (PFR)
p. flow of urinary bladder
p. flow rate (PFR)
p. flowmeter
p. gradient ▸ aortic valve
p. heart rate
p. heart rate ▸ expected
p. incidence
p. inspiratory flow (PIF)
p. inspiratory flow rate (PIFR)
p. instantaneous gradient
p. jet flow rate
p. (KVP) ▸ kilovolt
p. levels ▸ trough and
p. magnitude
p. noise, average
p. of component waves, sharp
p. powered, high
p. scatter factor
p. serum concentration

peak(s)—*continued*
- p. serum level
- p., sharp Bragg
- p., spread Bragg
- p. systolic aortic pressure (PSAP)
- p. systolic gradient (PSG)
- p. systolic gradient, peak-to-
- p. systolic velocity
- p. temperature
- p. therapy, psychedelic-
- p. tidal inspiratory flow
- p. -to-peak deflection
- p. -to-peak systolic gradient
- p. transaortic valve gradient
- p. twitch force
- p. velocity ▸ instantaneous spectral
- p. velocity ▸ time-averaged
- p. weight
- p. withdrawal
- p. work load
- p., work-tolerance

peaked P wave
peaked pulses
peaking systolic murmur ▸ early
peaking systolic murmur ▸ late
Pean's operation
PEAP (positive end-airway pressure)
pear-shaped body
pear-shaped heart
Pearce Tripod implant cataract lens
pearl(s)
- p., Elschnig's
- p., Epstein's
- p. fashion ▸ string of
- p. formation
- p., Laennec's

pearly
- p. gates (morning glory seeds)
- p. lesion
- p. nodule

Pearson('s)
- P. attachment to splint
- P. correlation coefficient
- P. position

peau
- p. de chagrin
- p. d'orange
- p. d'orange appearance
- p. d'orange in breast carcinoma

pecoris, Miyagawanella
Pecquet's cistern
pectate line
pectinate
- p. ligament
- p. line

- p. muscle

pectineal
- p. crural hernia
- p. hernia
- p. line
- p. muscle

pectineus muscle
pectineus, musculus
pectiniforme, septum
pectoral
- p. fascia
- p. girdle
- p. groove
- p. heart
- p. muscle, greater
- p. muscle, smaller
- p. nerve, lateral
- p. nerve, medial
- p. reflex
- p. regions
- p. tea

pectoralis
- p. major muscle
- p. major, musculus
- p. minor
- p. minor muscle
- p. minor, musculus

pectoriloquous bronchophony
pectoriloquy, aphonic
pectoriloquy, whispering
pectoris
- p. (AP), angina
- p. decubitus, angina
- p., disabling angina
- p., variant angina
- p. vasomotoria, angina

pectus
- p. carinatum
- p. deformity
- p. excavatum
- p. excavatum of anterior chest
- p. excavatum repair ▸ pericardioplasty in
- p. gallinatum
- p. recurvatum

pecuarium, Simulium
peculiar
- p. behavior
- p. taste, aura of
- p. unblinking stare

pedal
- p. edema
- p. mode ergometer
- p. pulse
- p. pulses palpable

- p. pulses strong
- p. pulses weak

pedaling motion
pediatric (Pediatric)
- p. allergy
- p. arrhythmias
- p. cardiology
- p. cardiomyopathy
- p. dentistry
- p. digital angiography
- p. disease
- p. eczema
- p. emergency medicine specialist
- p. endocrinologist
- p. eye care
- p. heart syndrome
- p. hypertension
- p. meningitis
- p. monitoring system
- p. neuroemergency
- p. oncology
- P. Ophthalmologist
- p. orthopedic emergency
- p. psychopharmacology, clinical
- p. resuscitation
- p. rheumatology
- p. trauma
- p. trauma center
- p. trauma units
- p. venous return anomaly

pediatrician, developmental
Pedic Cushions, Pedifix's
pedicle [*medical*]
- p., absence of
- p., dermal
- p. flap
- p. flap, double
- p. flap, tubed
- p. graft
- p., inferior
- p. intact
- p., inverted Y and spleen
- p. of vertebral arch
- p., pulmonary
- p., renal
- p., stump of
- p., superior
- p., tissue
- p., vascular

pedicled cyst
pediculated cells
pediculi, Rickettsia
Pediculoides ventricosus
pediculosis
- p. capillitii

p. capitis
p. corporis
p. inguinalis
p. palpebrarum
p. pubis
p. vestimenti
p. vestimentorum
pediculus (Pediculus)
    p. arcus vertebrae
    P. capitis
    P. corporis
    P. humanus
    P. humanus var. capitis
    P. humanus var. corporis
    P. humanus var. vestimentorum
    P. inguinalis
    P. pubis
Pedifix's Pedic Cushions
Pediococcus acidilactici
Pediococcus cerevisiae
pedis
    p. arteries, dorsalis
    p., calcar
    p. (DP) pulsation ‣ dorsalis
    p. (DP) pulse ‣ dorsalis
    p., tinea
pedrosianum, Trichosporon
pedrosoi
    p., Acrotheca
    p., Fonsecaea
    p., Hormodendrum
peduncle
    p., cerebral
    p., inferior cerebellar
    p., middle cerebellar
    p., middle cerebral
    p. of flocculus
    p. of hypophysis
    p. of pineal body
    p. of Schwalbe, olivary
    p. of thalamus, inferior
    p., olfactory
    p., pineal
    p., superior cerebellar
peduncular loop
pedunculated
    p. adenoma
    p. adenomatous polyp
    p. adenomatous polyps ‣ small
    p. fibroid
    p. growth
    p. juvenile polyp
    p. lesion
    p. nodules
pedunculated thrombus

peek-and-see method
peel
    p., chemical
    p., cortical
    p., freshening
    p., laser
    p. ‣ patient had mini-
    p., pericardial
    p., pleural
    p., thick visceral
    p., visceral
peeled off
peeling
    p. -back mechanism
    p. from athlete's foot ‣ skin
    p. of hands and feet
    p. of skin
    p. or blistering of skin ‣ cracking,
    p. skin from dermatitis
    p. skin from eczema
PEEP (positive and expiratory
    pressure)
peer(s)
    p. counseling
    p., difficulty with
    p. -driven intervention
    p. environment
    p. group
    p. group meeting
    p. groups, drug-using
    p. influence
    p., interaction with
    p., nondisabled
    p. pressure
    p., recovering
    p. relations
    p. review
    p. review program
    p. social activities ‣ loss of interest
      in
    p. stressors
    p. support
PEF (peak expiratory flow)
PEFR (peak expiratory flow rate)
PEG (percutaneous endoscopic
    gastrostomy)
PEG (pneumoencephalogram)
peg (Peg)(s)
    p. bone graft
    p. cells
    p. graft
    p., rete
    p. teeth
    P. Test
PEI (phosphate excretion index)

PEI (physical efficiency index)
pejorative attitude
Pel-Ebstein pyrexia
PELCA (percutaneous excimer laser
    coronary angioplasty)
Pelger-Huet
    P. anomaly
    P. cells
    P. nuclear anomaly
Pelizaeus-Merzbacher disease
Pell sectioning technique, Gregory
pellagra-preventing (P-P) substance
pellagra preventive
Pellegrini-Stieda calcification
Pellegrini-Stieda disease
pellet(s)
    p. artifact
    p. ‣ implanted radioactive
    p., radioactive
pelletieri, Streptomyces
pelletierii, Actinomadura
pellicular enteritis
pellio, Leptodera
pellio, Rhabditis
Pellizzi's syndrome
pellucida, zona
pellucidi, cavum septi
pellucidum, vein of septum
Pelomyxa carolinesis
Pel's crises
pelves
    p. and/or calyces
    p., calyces and ureters
    p. mildly dilated ‣ renal
    p., renal
pelvic
    p. abscess
    p. abscess, gram stain of
    p. adhesions, lysis
    p. adhesions, multiple
    p. adnexa
    p. aneurysm
    p. arteriogram
    p. artery
    p. basin
    p. blood clots
    p. bone
    p. brim
    p. canal
    p. carcinoma
    p. cavity
    p. cellulitis
    p. clean-out
    p. colon
    p. device, exterior

pelvic—*continued*
- p. diameter
- p. diaphragm
- p. diathermy
- p. disease (IPD) ▸ inflammatory
- p. drainage
- p. endometriosis
- p. endoscopy
- p. exam inconclusive
- p. examination
- p. examination, bimanual
- p. examination, routine
- p. examination, sterile
- p. examination under anesthesia
- p. exenteration
- p. exenteration, anterior
- p. exenteration, posterior
- p. exenteration, total
- p. findings
- p. floor
- p. floor electromyography
- p. floor, female
- p. floor, laceration of
- p. floor muscle exercise
- p. floor muscles
- p. floor pressure
- p. floor, relaxed
- p. floor weakness
- p. fossa
- p. fracture
- p. ganglia
- p. girdle
- p. gutter
- p. hematoma
- p. infections
- p. inflammatory disease (PID)
- p. inflammatory disease (PID) ▸ chronic
- p. inflammatory disease (PID) from chlamydia
- p. inflammatory disease (PID) residues
- p. inflammatory disease (PID) ▸ sexually transmitted
- p. inlet
- p. inlet, conjugate diameter of
- p. irradiation
- p. irradiation, preoperative
- p. laparoscopy
- p. laparotomy
- p. lymph nodes
- p. lymph nodes ▸ drainage (d'rge) of
- p. malignancy
- p. ▸ manual examination of

- p. mass
- p. mass, extrauterine
- p. measurements
- p. metastases
- p. muscle exercises
- p. muscle ▸ relaxation of
- p. muscle, voluntary
- p. muscle ▸ weakening of
- p. muscles
- p. musculature
- p., negative
- p. node sampling
- p. nodes, positive
- p. odor
- p. organ exenteration
- p. organs
- p. outlet
- p. outlet, transverse diameter of
- p. pain
- p. pain, chronic
- p. pain, cramp-like
- p. pain, intractable
- p. pain, palliation in
- p. peritoneal cavity
- p. peritonitis
- p. -phalangeal dystrophy ▸ thoracic-
- p. presentation
- p. pressure
- p. protrusion of acetabulum
- p. radiation imaging studies
- p. radiation treatments
- p. relaxation
- p. rock
- p. scanography
- p. splanchnic nerves
- p. strait
- p. strait ▸ entrance of fetal head into superior
- p. stress fracture
- p. support
- p. support defect
- p. support, good
- p. support problem
- p. thrombophlebitis, septic
- p. tilt exercise
- p. tone-up
- p. traction
- p. traction, halo-
- p. tumor
- p. ultrasound
- p. ultrasound sonarography
- p. version
- p. viscera

- p. viscera surrounded by hematoma
- p. wall
- p. washings, postoperative

pelvimeter
- p., Breisky's
- p., Collin's
- p., Collyer's
- p., DeLee's
- p., Martin's
- p., Thoms'
- p., William's

pelvimetry study
pelvimetry, x-ray
pelviolithotomy/pelvilithotomy
pelvioprostatic capsule
pelviradiography study
pelvirectal achalasia
pelvis
- p., acetabulum of
- p., adequate gynecoid
- p. aequabiliter justo major
- p. aequabiliter justo minor
- p. and hips
- p., android
- p. angusta
- p., anthropoid
- p., beaked
- p., bifid
- p., bony
- p., borderline
- p., brachypellic
- p., brim of
- p. cancer, renal
- p., contracted
- p., Deventer's
- p., diameter oblique
- p., diameter transverse
- p., diaphragm of
- p., dolichopellic
- p., false
- p., flat
- p., frozen
- p., funnel-shaped
- p., greater
- p., gynecoid
- p., hips and
- p., hyperthermia in
- p., inadequate
- p., infantile
- p. inspected
- p., intrapelvic kidney
- p., irrigated
- p., large
- p., left renal

p., lesser
p., linea terminalis
p., mesatipellic
p., Nagele's
p., normal
p., oblique diameter of
p. of kidney
p. of ureter
p., Otto
p., pithecoid
p. plana
p., platypellic
p., platypelloid
p. position ▸ neutral
p., pubic segment of
p. radiation, whole
p., redundant
p., renal
p., reperitonealize the
p., rhabdomyosarcoma of
p., right renal
p., Robert's
p., rostrate
p., rotation of
p., small
p. ▸ transitional cell carcinoma of renal
p., transverse diameter of
p., true
pelvospondylitis ossificans
Pemco valve prosthesis
PEMF (pulsing electromagnetic fields)
pemphigoid, bullous
pemphigus
p. acutus
p. disseminatus
p. erythematosus
p. foliaceus
p. malignus
p. neonatorum
p., oral
p. syphiliticus
p. vegetans
p. vulgaris
pen (Pen)
p. deflection
p. deflection, downward
p. deflection ▸ percent reduction of output
p. deflection, upward
p. deflections, simultaneous
p. galvanometer
p. injector ▸ insulin
p., light

p. motor
P. Pump Infuser
p. pump, insulin
p., Skin Skribe
p. writer
penal rehabilitation ▸ halfway house for
pencil
p., Blaisdell skin
p. dosimeter
p., electrosurgery
p., flexible
p., Handtrol electrosurgical
p., marking
p. percussion
p. -shaped stools
p., skin
p. -thin stools
pendelluft syndrome
pen-determined ejection fraction ▸ light
pending, results still
Pendred's syndrome
pendular movement
pendular nystagmus
pendulous
p. abdomen
p. and atrophic, breast
p., breasts
p. heart
p. palate
p. urethra
pendulum
p., cor
p. exercise
p. rhythm
penetate sodium, Yb (ytterbium)
penetrability, source
penetrans
p., Dermatophilus
p., Sarcopsylla
p., Tunga
penetrated bone ▸ infection
penetrated mother's womb
penetrating
p. abdominal wound
p. arterial lesions
p. bundle
p. cardiac wound
p. graft
p. injury
p. injury of major airway
p. keratoplasty, partial
p. neck wound
p. renal injury

p. rupture
p. trauma
p. ulcer
p. wound
p. wound, deep-
p. wound of abdomen
p. wound of heart
p. wounds of great vessels
penetration
p., extensive
p. fraction
p., vitreous
Penfield operation, Förster-
penicillic acid
penicillin(s)
p., acid- and penicillinase-resistant
p., acid-resistant
p., aqueous
p. binding protein
p. derivatives
p., dimethoxyphenyl
p., extended-spectrum
p. ▸ fatal allergic reaction to
p. G benzathine
p. G potassium
p. G procaine
p. G sodium
p., isoxazolyl
p. ▸ nonresponsive to oral
p., penicillinase-resistant
p., (Pen-Vee K) ▸ potassium phenoxymethyl
p., prophylactic
p., repository form of
p. -resistant pneumococci
p., semisynthetic
p. sensitive coccus, gram-positive
penicillinase
p., extracellular
p. -resistant penicillins
p. -resistant penicillins ▸ acid-and
p., Staph aureus
Penicillium
P. barbae
P. bouffardi
P. charlesii
P. crustaceum
P. glaucum
P. minimum
P. montoyai
P. notatum
P. patulum
P. spinulosum

penile
- p. artery
- p. -brachial pressure index
- p. cancer
- p. discharge
- p. discharge from chlamydia
- p. edema
- p. episadias
- p. herpes
- p. injury
- p. implant
- p. implant ▸ pump-operated
- p. induration
- p. inflow, increased
- p. lesion
- p. numbness
- p. outflow, decreased
- p. problems from diabetes
- p. prosthesis, Silastic
- p. prosthesis, Small-Cardon
- p. prosthesis, Surgitek
- p. reflex
- p. shaft
- p. shaft, verrucous
- p. skin

penis
- p., bulbus
- p. carcinoma
- p., cavernous nerve of
- p., cavernous vein of
- p., clubbed
- p., crus
- p., deep dorsal vein of
- p., dorsal nerve of
- p., erector muscle of
- p., frenulum of prepuce of
- p., glans
- p., kraurosis
- p., leukoplakia
- p., ligamentum fundiforme
- p., os
- p. plastica
- p., prepuce of
- p., raphe
- p., reflex
- p., septum
- p., septum glandis
- p., septum of glans
- p., superficial dorsal veins of
- p., vein of bulb of

Penn State total artificial heart
penniform muscle
pennsylvanica, Epicauta
pennsylvanicum, Xanthium
penopubic epispadias

penoscrotal fistulas
pen-r cells
Penrose drain
pens cells
pensé, déjà
pensée, tic de
pension, disability
pension neurosis
pentagastric stimulation test
pentagastrin stimulated analysis
pentalogy of Fallot
pentandra, Ceiba
pentane test, breath
Pentastoma
- P. constrictum
- P. denticulatum
- P. taenioides

Pentatrichomonas ardin delteili
Pentatrichomonas hominis
penta-X chromosomal aberration
pentazocine, detoxification from
pentetate sodium kit, Tc (technetium) 99m
pentose
- p. cycle (PC)
- p., Krebs
- p. shunt

Pentothal
- P. and Anectine
- P. anesthesia
- P. anesthesia, sodium
- P., sodium

pent-up
- p. feelings
- p. frustration
- p. hostility
- p. tension, release

Pen-Vee K (potassium phenoxy-methyl penicillin)
people
- p., inability to relate to
- p. ▸ patient's need to be with
- p., street

Pep Pills (amphetamines)
PEPI (postmenopausal estrogen/progestin interventions)
pepo, Cucurbita
PEPP (positive expiratory pressure plateau)
pepper grains, cayenne
pepper, spicy (CAPS) foods-free diet ▸ caffeine, alcohol,
peppermint test
peptic
- p. aspiration pneumonia

- p. aspiration pneumonitis
- p. cells
- p. esophagitis
- p. inflammatory disease
- p. stricture
- p. ulcer (PU)
- p. ulcer disease (PUD)
- p. ulcer, low incidence of
- p. ulcer, perforated
- p. ulceration

peptidase (GGP) ▸ gamma glutamine
peptidases, intestinal
peptide(s)
- p., brain gut
- p., brain natriuretic
- p. group
- p. hormone
- p. ▸ human atrial natriuretic
- p., natriuretic
- p., neuro◇
- p. T
- p. (VIP) ▸ vasoactive intestinal
- p., vasoconstrictor

Peptococcus constellatus
peptone
- p. infusion, duodenal
- p. infusion, intraduodenal
- p. shock

Peptostreptococcus
- P. anaerobius
- P. asaccharolyticus
- P. evolutus
- P. paleopneumoniae
- P. prevotii
- P. productus
- P. saccharolyticus

PER (protein efficiency ratio)
percavus, talipes
perceived (Perceived)
- p. exertion
- p. exertion (RPE) ▸ ratings of
- P. Exertion Scale (PES)
- P. Exertion Scale (BPES), Borg
- p. loss, actual or
- p. pain ▸ significant level of
- p. worthlessness ▸ self-

percent
- p. (PB%) ▸ phonetic balanced
- p. reduction of output pen deflection
- p. time
- p., volume

percentage depth dose
percentage of normal

perception(s)
p., alteration in time
p., alteration of
p., altered
p. ▸ altered mood and
p., altered time
p. and association
p. and tonus
p. ▸ attention, orientation skills and
p., bizarre
p., blurred sensory
p., change in
p. check, depth
p., cognitive
p., color
p., confused
p. deficiency, color
p. deficiency ▸ red-green color
p., depth
p. disorder ▸ hallucinogen persisting
p. disorder, posthallucinogen
p., distorted depth
p. ▸ distorted sense of time and
p. distorted ▸ time-
p. ▸ distorted visual
p. ▸ distortion of
p. ▸ distortion of sensory
p., disturbance of
p., emotional
p., enhanced somatosensory
p. (ESP) ▸ extrasensory
p., false
p., false sensory
p., health
p., heart rate
p., hypnagogic
p. illusion
p. impaired
p. (LP) ▸ light
p., light and color
p., load
p. ▸ memories, feelings and
p., multisensory
p. ▸ narrowing of
p., negative self-
p. (NLP), no light
p. of colors ▸ heightened
p. of environment
p. of feeling
p. of form and pattern
p. of impending separation
p. of noxious stimulus
p. of pain and temperature ▸ diminished

p. of pain, patient's
p. of physical sensations
p. of problem areas, patient's
p. of rejection
p. of self
p. of situation
p. of speech
p. of speech sounds, auditory
p. of symptoms
p. of temperature
p. of time and distance, poor
p. of touch
p. only (LPO) ▸ light
p., pain
p. ▸ permanent absence of depth
p., poor
p. ▸ reduced pain
p. reflex
p. ▸ restriction of
p., sense
p., spatial
p. ▸ special orientation or
p., tension
p., thought and recognition of information
p. unimpaired
p., visual
perceptional insanity
perceptive
p. deafness
p. disorders
p. loss
perceptual
p. alterations ▸ sensory
p. and motor skills
p. aspect
p. changes
p. changes, olfactory
p. cut
p. data, spatial-
p. deficit
p. deficit ▸ visual
p. disorder
p. distortion
p. distortions ▸ illusions or
p. disturbance ▸ persisting
p. disturbances, color and space
p. functioning
p. functions
p. losses ▸ visual and
p. measurement
p. memory
p. motor organization and analysis
p. motor skills, cognitive
p. status

p. threshold, anginal
percha, gutta-
perchlorate, potassium
Percodan
P. (Morf)
P. (Morfina)
P. (Morpho)
P. (Morphy)
P. (Mud)
percreta, placenta
percussed, liver
percussion
p. abdomen
p. and auscultation (P and A)
p. and auscultation (P and A) ▸ chest clear to
p. and auscultation (P and A) ▸ lungs clear to
p. and postural drainage
p. and vibration, chest
p. (A and P) ▸ auscultation and
p., auscultatory
p., bimanual
p., chest
p., clear to
p., coin
p., compression and
p., deep
p., digital
p., direct
p. (DTP) ▸ distal tingling on
p., dullness to
p., finger
p., fist
p., instrumental
p., Krönig's
p., lungs revealed to hyper-resonance to
p., Murphy
p. note
p. note, tympanic
p. of bone
p. of suprapubic area ▸ manual
p. of tendon
p. of the abdomen
p., palpatory
p., pencil
p., piano
p. ▸ postural drainage and
p., resonant to
p., respiratory
p., right apex clear to
p., shifting on
p., slapping
p. sound

percussion—*continued*
- p., strip
- p., tangential
- p., tenderness to
- p., tenderness to palpation or
- p. tenderness, vertebral
- p., thorax resonant on
- p., threshold
- p. wave

percutaneous
- p. absorption
- p. antegrade biliary drainage
- p. antegrade pyelography
- p. antegrade urography
- p. approach
- p. arteriogram
- p. arteriography
- p. aspiration
- p. atherectomy
- p. automated diskectomy
- p. balloon angioplasty
- p. balloon aortic valvuloplasty
- p. balloon mitral valvuloplasty
- p. balloon pulmonic valvuloplasty
- p. balloon valvuloplasty
- p. biopsy
- p., bronchography
- p. cardiopulmonary bypass (PCPB)
- p. cardiopulmonary bypass support
- p. cardiopulmonary support
- p. catheter ‣ straight flush
- p. cholangiography
- p. cholecystolithotomy
- p. cholecystostomy
- p. coronary rotational angioplasty (PCRA)
- p. coronary rotational atherectomy
- p. dilational tracheostomy
- p. diskectomy
- p. dissolution therapy
- p. endoscopic gastrostomy (PEG)
- p. enterostomy
- p. ethanol ablation
- p. excimer laser coronary angioplasty (PELCA)
- p. exposure
- p. hepatobiliary cholangiography
- p. intervention
- p. laser disk decompression
- p. left heart bypass
- p. liver biopsy
- p. low stress angioplasty
- p. lumbar diskectomy, automated
- p. mitral balloon commissurotomy
- p. mitral balloon valvotomy

- p. mitral balloon (PMB) valvuloplasty
- p. mitral commissurotomy
- p. mitral valvuloplasty
- p. myocardial revascularization (PMR)
- p. needle aspiration
- p. needle biopsy
- p. needle cholangiogram
- p. nephrolithotomy
- p. nephrostomy
- p. peritoneal biopsy
- p. portocaval anastomosis
- p. reaction
- p. revascularization
- p. rhizotomy
- p. rotational thrombectomy
- p. route
- p. stent
- p. stone manipulation
- p. technique
- p. transatrial mitral commissurotomy
- p. transhepatic catheterization
- p. transhepatic cholangiogram (PTC)
- p. transhepatic cholangiography (PTC)
- p. transhepatic cholangiography, direct
- p. transhepatic drainage
- p. transhepatic portography
- p. transluminal angioplasty (PTA)
- p. transluminal angioscopy
- p. transluminal balloon valvuloplasty
- p. transluminal coronary angiography (PTCA)
- p. transluminal coronary angioplasty (PTCA)
- p. transluminal coronary revascularization (PTCR)
- p. transmyocardial revascularization
- p. transtracheal bronchography
- p. transvenous mitral commissurotomy
- p. tumor ablation
- p. tunnel
- p. umbilical blood sampling (PUBS)
- p. vertebroplasty

percutaneously, cannulated
Percy's cautery
peregrinum, Mycobacterium

perennial
- p. allergic conjunctivitis
- p. allergic rhinitis
- p. asthma
- p. hay fever
- p. rhinitis

Pereyra procedure
Perez cassette, Sanchez-
Perez's sign
perfect fungus
perfecta, osteogenic
perfection of surgical skills
perfectionist in self-defeating way ‣ patient
perfectionist, patient
perfluorochemical emulsion ‣ intravascular
perfoliatum, Echinostoma
perfoliatus, Echinochasmus
perforated
- p. appendicitis
- p. appendix
- p. corneal ulcers
- p. eardrum
- p. eye shield
- p. gallbladder
- p. peptic ulcer
- p. septum
- p., shot-
- p. substance, anterior
- p. substance, posterior
- p. ulcer
- p. uterus
- p. viscus

perforating
- p. acute ulceration
- p. arteries
- p. arteries ‣ septal
- p. corneal wound
- p. fracture
- p. hyperplasia of pulp, chronic
- p. ulcer
- p. vein, Boyd
- p. vein, incompetent
- p. veins
- p. wound

perforation
- p. and bleeding
- p., anterior
- p., attic
- p., Bezold's
- p., bowel
- p., cardiac
- p., colonic
- p., drum

p., ear drum
p., esophageal
p., gastrointestinal (GI)
p. ▸ gross bleeding or
p., guidewire
p., healed
p. in colonoscopic polypectomy
p. in endarterectomy
p., intestinal
p. ▸ intestinal wall
p., mechanical
p., myocardial
p. of bowel
p. of colon
p. of esophagus, traumatic
p. of tympanic membrane (TM)
p., pathologic
p. pocket, attic
p., pyloroduodenal
p. ▸ reconstruction of esophageal
p., root
p., sealed over
p., septal
p., tympanic membrane
p., ventricular
p., wall
perforative peritonitis
perforator(s)
p. and tributaries
p., midtibial
p., septal
p. tied
perform
p. basic activity ▸ patient unable to
p. first aid
p., patient ability to
p. purposeful movements ▸ inability to
p. routine tasks, decline in ability to
performance
p., altered
p., altered role
p., altered school
p. and tolerance ▸ improved
p. anxiety
p., athletic
p., automaticity of
p., baseline
p., cardiac
p., cognitive
p., declining job
p., diminished job
p. ▸ drop in academic
p. enhancement
p., impaired cognitive

p. ▸ impairing exercise
p. ▸ impairment of systolic and diastolic
p. index
p., instrument
p. intensity
p. IQ (intelligence quotient)
p., job
p. ▸ left ventricular (LV) systolic
p., mental
p. monitoring
p., motor
p. of tasks, efficient
p., poor
p. potential
p. problem, sexual
p. ▸ rationalizing poor
p., role
p. scale
p. score, clinical
p. status of patients
p., ventricular
performed, copious lavage
performed in routine fashion ▸ appendectomy
performing familiar tasks ▸ difficulty
performing scale
perfringens, Clostridium
perfunctory
p. and cooled, kidneys
p., kidneys
p., patient is
p. with fresh blood, extremity vessels
perfusion [*profusion*]
p., alteration of tissue
p., altered cerebral tissue
p., altered renal tissue
p., arterial
p., artificial organ
p. assessment
p. balloon angioplasty (TPBA) ▸ thermal/
p. bed
p., blood
p. cannula ▸ femoral
p., cardiac
p. catheter, coronary
p., cerebral
p. defect
p. defect ▸ fixed
p. defect ▸ scintigraphic
p. defect, ventilation
p. defection ▸ scintigraphic
p. deficit

p. deficit, protracted
p., extracorporeal
p. image ▸ stress washout myocardial
p. imaging, adenosine radionuclide
p. imaging ▸ myocardial
p. imaging ▸ pharmacologic stress
p. imaging ▸ stress thallium-201 myocardial
p. imaging ▸ thallium
p. imaging ▸ ventilation/
p. in tail of pancreas
p., isolated
p. ▸ isolated heat
p. ▸ isolated hyperthermic limb
p., lung
p. lung scan, ventilation-
p. mismatch ▸ ventilation/
p. monitor, blood
p., mosaic
p., myocardial
p., normal
p. of an extremity, isolated heat
p. of heart
p. of tissues
p. pressure
p. pressure, cerebral
p. pressure, coronary
p. pressure ▸ transmyocardial
p. protocol ▸ rest metabolism/stress
p. rate
p. rate, cerebral cortex
p. ratio ▸ ventilation/
p., regional
p. relation ▸ ventilation/
p., root
p. scan
p. scan ▸ ventilation/
p. scanning ▸ exercise
p. scanning, pulmonary
p. scintigraphy
p. scintigraphy ▸ microsphere
p. scintigraphy ▸ myocardial
p. scintigraphy ▸ myocardial cold spot
p. scintigraphy ▸ thallium-201
p. scintigraphy ▸ thallium-201 myocardial
p. ▸ splanchnic bed
p. study
p. study ▸ myocardial
p. ▸ stuttering of
p. system ▸ regulated
p. /ventilation
peri (perineal) pad

periaccretio pericardii
peri-adrenal hemorrhage
perianal
- p. abscess
- p. adenoma
- p. area
- p. condyloma acuminatum
- p. discomfort
- p. erythema
- p. hematoma
- p. irritation
- p. itching
- p. maceration
- p. reflex
- p. skin
- p. squamous cell carcinoma
- p. wart ▸ excisional biopsy

periaortic
- p. atelectasis
- p. chain
- p. infrarenal node
- p. irradiation
- p. lymph involvement
- p. lymph node metastases
- p. lymph nodes
- p. lymph nodes, enlargement of
- p. lymphadenopathy
- p. nodes, enlarged
- p. nodes, positive
- p. node sampling

periapical
- p. abscess
- p. bone structure
- p. curettage
- p. lesion
- p. rarefied osteitis

periaqueductal gray electrode
periarterial pad
periarterial sympathectomy
periarteritis
- p. gummosa
- p. nodosa
- p. nodusa, infantile

periarticular
- p. calcification
- p. fracture
- p. soft tissues

peribronchial
- p. chronic inflammatory infiltrates
- p. cuffing
- p. desquamation
- p. fibrosis
- p. infiltrate, lymphocytic
- p. markings
- p. pneumonia

peribronchiolar connective tissue
pericallosal artery
pericallosal artery and veins
pericapillary cells
pericapillary encephalorrhagia
pericardectomy (*see* pericardi-ectomy)
pericardiac
- p. tamponade
- p. tumor
- p. veins

pericardiacophrenic veins
pericardial
- p. adhesions, multiple
- p. baffle
- p. biopsy
- p. calcification
- p. cavity
- p. constriction
- p. constriction ▸ occult
- p. cyst
- p. disease
- p. diverticula
- p. echo
- p. effusion
- p. effusion and tamponade
- p. effusion, chylous
- p. effusion ▸ silent
- p. fat pads
- p. fibrinous adhesions
- p. flap
- p. fluid
- p. fluid ▸ straw-colored
- p. fremitus
- p. friction rub
- p. friction rub ▸ systolic
- p. friction sound
- p. fusion
- p. hemangioma
- p. knock
- p. lavage
- p. lavage, continuous
- p. leiomyoma
- p. mesothelioma
- p. murmur
- p. patch
- p. patch, autologous
- p. patch ▸ Ionescu-Shiley
- p. peel
- p. pleura
- p. poudrage
- p. pressure
- p. puncture
- p. reflex
- p. rub

- p. rupture
- p. sac
- p. sac discolored
- p. sac distended
- p. sling
- p. space
- p. splenosis
- p. surfaces, friction of
- p. tamponade
- p. tap
- p. teratoma
- p. thickening
- p. tissue ▸ porcine
- p. tumor
- p. tumor, metastatic
- p. valve, bovine
- p. valve graft ▸ Hancock
- p. well
- p. window
- p. xenograft, Ionescu-Shiley

pericardicentesis/pericardiocentesis
pericardiectomy (*same as* pericardectomy)
pericardiectomy, visceral
pericardii
- p., accretio
- p., concretio
- p., hydrops
- p., periaccretio
- p. ▸ sinus transversus
- p., synechia

pericardiocentesis ▸ echo-guided
pericardiocentesis procedure
pericardiophrenic artery
pericardioplasty in pectus excavatum repair
pericardiosternal ligament
pericardiotomy (*same as* pericardotomy)
pericardiotomy ▸ subxiphoid limited
pericarditis
- p., acute fibrinous
- p., adhesive
- p., amebic
- p., bacterial
- p., calcific
- p. calculosa
- p. callosa
- p., carcinomatous
- p., cholesterol
- p., chronic constrictive
- p., constrictive
- p., drug-associated
- p., drug-induced
- p., dry

p. effusion, chronic
p. ▸ effusive constrictive
p. epistenocardiaca
p. externa et interna
p., fibrinous
p., fibrous
p., focal acute
p. ▸ gram-negative
p., hemorrhagic
p., histoplasmic
p., idiopathic
p., infective
p., inflammatory
p. ▸ internal adhesive
p., ischemic
p., localized
p., mediastinal
p., meningococcal
p. -myocarditis syndrome
p., neoplastic
p., obliterans
p., obliterating
p., occult
p., pleural
p., postinfarction
p., postoperative
p., purulent
p. ▸ radiation-induced
p., rheumatic
p., serofibrinous
p., serous
p. sicca
p., Sternberg
p., subacute
p., suppurative
p., transient
p., traumatic
p., tuberculous
p., uremic
p. villosa
p., viral
p. with effusion
pericardium
p., absent
p., adherent
p. around heart, adhesions of
p., bleeding into
p., bread-and-butter
p., calcified
p., congenitally absent
p., decompression of
p., diaphragmatic
p., dropsy of
p., empyema of
p. externum

p. fibrosum
p., fibrous
p., heart with
p. ▸ inflammation of
p. internum
p. meridian
p. ▸ metastases to the
p. opened
p., parietal
p., petechial hemorrhages of
p. serosum
p., serous
p., shaggy
p. strips, bovine
p., thickened
p., visceral
pericardotomy (*see* pericardiotomy)
pericellular cells
pericellular edema
pericementitis, apical
pericementitis, chronic suppurative
pericholecystic abscess
pericholecystitis, gaseous
perichondrial elevator
perichondrial graft
perichondrium, tragal
Perico (cocaine)
pericolonic
p. fat
p. lymph nodes
p. penetration
pericoronal flap
pericranii, sinus
pericular infection ▸ treatment of
peridental/peridontal (*see* periodontal)
peridental membrane
peridicrotic wave
periductal mastitis
peridural anesthesia
perielectrode fibrosis
peri-esophageal hemorrhage
perifollicular elastolysis
perigastric lymph nodes
perihepatic abscess
perihilar
p. area
p. lymph nodes
p. markings
p. mass, superior
p. scarring
peri-infarct zone, ischemia in
peri-infarction block
peri-infarctional disturbance

peri-infarctional ventricular arrhythmias
perilimbal incision
perilobar pancreatitis
perilunate dislocation
perilunate fracture
periluteal phase dysphoric disorder
perilymph fistula
perilymph fluid
perilymphatic
p. fistula (PLF)
p. fistulization
p. infiltration
perilymphatici, ductus
perimembranous ventricular septal defect
perimenopausal
p. period
p. phase
p. symptoms
perimeter [*parameter*]
perimeter, Ferree-Rand
perimeter, Schweigger's
perimuscular plexus
perimysial plexus
Perinatal (perinatal)
P. Addiction Research and Education (NAPARE) ▸ National Association for
p. anoxia
p. asphyxia
p. condition
p. death
p. distress
p. grief
p. injury
p. loss
p. monitor
p. mortality
p. mortality rate
p. non-stress testing
p. stress testing
p. substance abuse
p. transmission
perinatally infected
perineal [*perioneal, peroneal*]
p. area
p. area, radiation therapy
p. artery
p. body, relaxed
p. care
p. contamination
p. exercises
p. flexure of rectum
p. mass, subcutaneous

perineal—*continued*
- p. nerves
- p. (peri) pad
- p. prep and drape
- p. prostatectomy
- p. prostatosemino-vesiculectomy
- p. region
- p. skin tags
- p. support
- p. support stitches
- p. support sutures
- p. tear
- p. tissue

perinei muscle, transverse
perineoplastic syndromes
perineorrhaphy ▸ Emmet-Studdiford
perinephric
- p. abscess
- p. air injection
- p. capsule
- p. fascia
- p. fat

perinephritic fat
perineum
- p., deep transverse muscle of
- p., lacerated
- p., muscles of
- p., raphe of
- p., superficial transverse muscle of

perineural
- p. anesthesia
- p. block
- p. infiltration

perinodal tissue
perinuclear
- p. cataract
- p. cataract, lamellar zonular
- p. pallor

period(s)
- p. ▸ absence of menstrual
- p. (ARP), absolute refractory
- p. (APERP), accessory pathway effective refractory
- p., active
- p., active treatment
- p. analysis
- p., antegrade refractory
- p., apneic
- p., association
- p. ▸ at-home recovery
- p., atrial effective refractory
- p. (AVRP), atrioventricular refractory
- p., cardiac refractory
- p., child-bearing

- p., cool-down
- p., developmental
- p., dialysis
- p., diastolic filling
- p., disease-free
- p. ▸ effective refractory
- p., ejection
- p., embryonic
- p. ▸ erratic menstrual
- p., fertile
- p., follow-up
- p. from anemia ▸ heavy menstrual
- p. from diabetes ▸ absent menstrual
- p., functional refractory
- p., gestational
- p., guarded postoperative
- p., heavy
- p., heavy menstrual
- p., hypotensive
- p., inconstant
- p., incubation
- p., infantile
- p., initial dose
- p., interim
- p., interseizure
- p., intersystolic
- p., intervening
- p., intrapartum
- p. ▸ intrinsic refractory
- p., irregular
- p., irregular menstrual
- p., isoelectric
- p. ▸ isometric contraction
- p. ▸ isometric relaxation
- p. ▸ isovolumetric relaxation
- p. ▸ isovolumic relaxation
- p. (LMP) ▸ last menstrual
- p. (LNMP) ▸ last normal menstrual
- p., late
- p., late menstrual
- p., latency
- p. ▸ latency age
- p., latent
- p. length
- p., long-term survival
- p., M
- p., manic
- p. (MIP) ▸ mean incubation
- p. (MP) ▸ menstrual
- p., missed menstrual
- p., monthly
- p., nonrapid eye movement (NREM)
- p. (NMP) ▸ normal menstrual
- p. of absent breathing

- p. of abstinence
- p. of alertness and lucidity
- p. of anger, panic or despair
- p. of anoxia, prolonged
- p. of bereavement
- p. of cardiac cycle ▸ isometric
- p. of confinement
- p. of depression, intermittent
- p. of dysfluency
- p. of electronic pacemaker ▸ refractory
- p. of enforced inactivity
- p. of extreme stress
- p. of fluency
- p. of grandiosity ▸ sustained
- p. of lucidity
- p. of mourning
- p. of observation
- p. of observation and hydration, 24-hour
- p. of observation ▸ patient discharged after
- p. of onset (PO)
- p. of pyrexia
- p. of quarantine
- p. of relative quiescence
- p. of remission
- p. of remission and relapse
- p. of remission and relapse ▸ fluctuating
- p. of reorientation
- p. of rest
- p. of satisfaction
- p. of sleep, longer
- p. of sobriety and sanity
- p. of suppuration
- p. of the complex
- p. of the wave
- p. of unconsciousness
- p. of well-being
- p. ▸ pacemaker amplifier refractory
- p., pain-free
- p. ▸ painful menstrual
- p., peak amplitude
- p., perimenopausal
- p., postembryonic
- p., postinfarction
- p., postpartum
- p., postsphygmic
- p., practice
- p., preejection
- p., presphygmic
- p. (PMP), previous menstrual
- p., prolonged menstrual
- p., pulse

p., quiescent
p., reaction
p., recovery
p., recuperative
p., refractory
p., regular, menstrual
p., relative refractory
p., REMS (rapid eye movements)
p. (REMP), roentgen-equivalent-man
p., safe
p., scanty menstrual
p., sequence of waves of inconstant
p., sleep onset rapid eye movement (REM)
p., sleep stage
p., systolic ejection
p., total infusion
p., trial
p. ▸ ventricular effective refractory
p., vulnerable
p., warm-up
p., washout
p., Wenckebach's
p. with birth control pill ▸ menstrual

periodic
p. abdominal pain
p. abstinence from chemicals
p. alternating nystagmus (PAN)
p. blood transfusions
p. bloodletting
p. breathing
p. bursts of high voltage
p. cessation of breathing
p. confusion
p. dilatation
p. dropped beat
p. edema
p. electrical stimulation to brain
p. exam
p. examination
p. exotropia
p. fever
p. health examination
p. heterotropia
p. inoculations
p. insanity
p. lateral epileptiform discharges
p. lateralized epileptiform discharges (PLED)
p. leg movements
p. leukorrhea
p. limb movement
p. limb movement disorder (PLMD)

p. limb movements in sleep (PLMS)
p. loss of consciousness
p. mammography screening
p. massages
p. monitoring
p. muscle twitching of face
p. oscillation
p. paralysis
p. parasite
p. positional vertigo
p. proctosigmoidoscopy
p., pseudo◊
p., psychosis
p., quasi◊
p. respiration
p. reversal
p. review
p. short pulse
p. slow bursts
p. slowing
p. spasmodic athetoid movements
p. strabismus
p. swelling
p. syndrome
p. table
p. vomiting
p. x-rays
p. yeast infection

periodical mania
periodically, muscles relax
periodicity block ▸ Wenckebach
periodontal (*same as* **peridental, peridontal**)
p. abscess
p. anesthesia
p. disease
p. grafting
p. gum care
p. infection ▸ chronic
p. membrane
p. tissue

periodontitis, compound
periodontitis, development of
periodontosis, terminal
perionyx on newborn nails
perioperative
p. antimicrobial prophylaxis
p. antimicrobial therapy
p. arrhythmias
p. diagnosis
p. management
p. morbidity and mortality
p. problem
p. red cell transfusion

perioral dermatitis
perioral tremor
periorbital
p. cellulitis
p. ecchymosis
p. edema
p. hematoma
p. soft tissue
p. swelling

periosteal
p. artery
p. bone
p. bone collar
p. cyst
p. elevator
p. flaps raised
p. ganglion
p. graft
p. implantation
p. irregularity
p. level
p. membranous lining
p. procedure
p. reflexes
p. sarcoma
p. thickening
p. transplantation

periosteitis (*see* **periostitis**)
periosteoplastic amputation
periosteotome, Alexander-Farabeuf
periosteotome, Alexander's
periosteotomy/periostotomy
periosteum
p. alveolare
p. closed with plain catgut
p. incised
p. incised and retracted
p. of orbital rim
p. reflected, flap of
p. sheath reflected over
p. stripped away
p., thickening of

periostitis (*same as* **periosteitis**)
peripancreatic lymph nodes
peripancreatic nodes
peripapillary retinal edema
peripapillary scotoma
peripartum cardiomyopathy
peripartum myocarditis
peripatellar incision
peripatellar pain
peripelvic cyst
peripheral
p. access system
p. activity, nonspecific

peripheral—*continued*
p. air leak
p. airspaces
p. angiography
p. angioplasty
p. apnea
p. arterial disease
p. arterial disease screening
p. arterial occlusive disease
p. arteriography
p. arteriosclerosis
p. arteriosclerotic occlusive disease
p. artery disease
p. aspect
p. atherectomy system
p. atherosclerotic disease
p. autonomic nervous system effect
p. autonomic toxicity
p. blood
p. blood cell count
p. blood eosinophilia
p. blood smear
p. blood studies
p. callus
p. cataract
p. chemoreceptors
p. circulation
p. circulation, good
p. circulation, poor
p. circulatory system
p. circulatory values
p. culture
p. cyanosis
p. cyanosis of all extremities
p. deficiency
p. dilation of bronchi
p. disease
p. edema
p. edema, dependent
p. embolic phenomena
p. eosinophilia
p. fields
p. fremitus
p. giant cell reparative granuloma
p. glioma
p. infusion
p. innervation, aberrant
p. intravenous (IV) administration
p. iridectomy
p. IV (intravenous)
p. joint pain
p. laser angioplasty (PLA)
p. lesion
p. limbs
p. lines

p. lung fields
p. lung problem
p. lymphocyte count
p. lymphocyte count, decreased
p. margin
p. mass
p. motoneurons
p. motor nerves
p. nerve
p. nerve block
p. nerve damage
p. nerve disorder
p. nerve ending
p. nerve fiber
p. nerve graft
p. nerve hyperactivity
p. nerve injury
p. nerve lesions
p. nerve malfunction
p. nerve procedure
p. nerve tumor
p. nerves
p. nerves ▸ dysfunction of
p. nerves, stimulation of
p. nervous system
p. nervous system disease
p. neuritis
p. neuroglia
p. neuroma
p. neurons
p. neuropathy
p. neuropathy, diabetic
p. nystagmus
p. pain
p. palisading
p. paralysis, residual
p. parenteral nutrition (TPPN), total
p. plasmacytoma
p. primitive neuroectodermal tumor
p. pulmonary emboli
p. pulmonic stenosis
p. pulsations, arterial
p. pulses
p. pulses, diminution of
p. pulses full and equal bilaterally
p. pulses intact
p. reflex
p. resistance
p. resistance index ▸ total
p. resistance (TPR), total
p. resistance unit (PRU)
p. resistance ▸ vascular
p. retina
p. ring of hemoglobin
p. saturation

p. sense organs
p. sensory nerves
p. sensory neuron
p. somatic effect
p. stem cells
p. stigmata
p. sympathetic system
p. system
p. thrombosis
p. total resistance (PTR)
p. type
p. vascular collapse
p. vascular disease
p. vascular disease, arteriosclerotic
p. vascular implications
p. vascular laboratory
p. vascular resistance
p. vascular resistance, decreasing
p. vascularity
p. vasodilation and hypotension ▸ increased
p. vasodilator
p. vein
p. vein plasma
p. venography
p. vessel
p. vessel spasm, catheter-related
p. vessels ▸ endarterectomy in
p. vestibulopathy
p. vision
p. vision check
p. vision ▸ loss of
p. vision measured
peripherica, pseudotabes
periphery
p. cell
p. of cornea
p. of eye
p. of retina
peripneumonia notha
periportal
p. carcinoma
p. cirrhosis
p. fibrosis
periprocedural evidence
perirectal abscess
perirenal
p. air study
p. fascia
p. fasciitis
p. fat
p. insufflation
p. space
p. tissues
periscapular incision

periscapular incision, curved
periscleral space
periscopic
- p. concave
- p. convex
- p. lens

perispinal area
peri-splenitis, patchy
perispondylitis, Gibney's
peristalsis
- p., accelerated
- p., active
- p., bowel
- p., esophageal
- p., intestinal
- p., mass
- p. of abdomen
- p., primary
- p., retrograde
- p., reversed
- p. ▸ uncoordinated esophageal

peristaltic
- p. actions of colon ▸ abnormal
- p. activity
- p. activity, tertiary
- p. anastomosis
- p. hyperemia
- p. motion
- p. movements
- p. rushes
- p. sounds
- p. unrest
- p. waves

peritendinitis
- p., adhesive
- p. calcarea
- p. crepitans

peritenon [*peratenon*]
perithelial cell
perithelium
peritomy, total
peritoneal [*perineal, peroneal*]
- p. abscess
- p. adhesion
- p. ari, free
- p. biopsy
- p. biopsy ▸ percutaneous
- p. carcinoma ▸ primary
- p. carcinomatosis
- p. catheter
- p. cavity
- p. cavity ▸ blood fluid in
- p. cavity, general
- p. cavity insufflated
- p. cavity, lesser

- p. cavity, pelvic
- p. closure
- p. closure accomplished
- p. contents
- p. cyst
- p. cytology
- p. cytology, positive
- p. dialysis
- p. dialysis, ambulatory
- p. dialysis (CAPD), continuous ambulatory
- p. dialysis (CCPD), continuous cyclical
- p. dialysis patient, ambulatory
- p. dialysis solution
- p. drainage (dr'ge)
- p. dropsy
- p. edge
- p. edge ▸ lower
- p. edge ▸ upper
- p. effusion
- p. fibrinolytic activity
- p. flap ▸ lower
- p. flap ▸ upper
- p. floor
- p. fluid
- p. fluid, bloody
- p. fluid ▸ gram stain of
- p. incision
- p. inflammatory reaction
- p. injury and repair
- p. insert of shunt
- p. irritation
- p. lavage
- p. membranes
- p. mouse
- p. opening
- p. reflection
- p., retro◇
- p. seeding in endometrial carcinoma
- p. shunt
- p. shunt, LeVeen
- p. shunt, Silastic ventriculo-
- p. space
- p. stitching
- p. stripping
- p. surface
- p. surface ▸ remesothelialization of
- p. surfaces ▸ dry serosal
- p. surfaces smooth and glistening
- p. tap
- p. transudate
- p. trauma
- p. tumor nodules

- p. venous shunt
- p. venous shunt, Denver

peritonei, carcinomatosis
peritonei, pseudomyxoma
peritoneocutaneous reflex, Morley's
peritoneointestinal reflex
peritoneopericardial hernia
peritoneoscopy examination
peritoneovenous shunt
peritoneovenous shunt, LeVeen
peritoneum
- p., abdominal
- p., bladder
- p., caudal
- p. closed
- p., closure of
- p. entered
- p., exposing
- p., fold of
- p., incise
- p. incised
- p., intestinal
- p., loose
- p., mesothelioma of
- p., parietal
- p., pelvic
- p. ▸ petechial hemorrhages of
- p. reflected ▸ vesicouterine
- p. smooth and glistening
- p. studded with tumor nodules
- p., tumor seeded
- p., vesicouterine
- p., visceral

peritonitis
- p., acute
- p., asymptomatic
- p., bacterial
- p., chronic
- p., chylous
- p., diffuse
- p. due to enterococci
- p. ▸ E. (Escherichia) coli sepsis
- p., fibrinopurulent
- p., focal fibrinous
- p. from appendix ▸ ruptured
- p. from cirrhosis
- p., generalized
- p., hemorrhagic
- p., localized
- p., meconium
- p. ▸ pain in abdomen from
- p., pelvic
- p., perforative
- p., septic
- p., serous

peritonitis—*continued*
- p., silent
- p. (SBP), spontaneous bacterial
- p. ▸ tenderness in abdomen from
- p., terminal
- p., tuberculous

peritonsillar
- p. abscess
- p. abscess, ruptured
- p. cellulitis
- p. tags

periungual desquamation
periungual wart
periurethral duct carcinoma
perivaginal fascia
perivalvular leak
perivascular
- p. canal
- p. cells
- p. collagen network ▸ interstitial and
- p. edema
- p. eosinophilic infiltrates
- p. fibrosis
- p. gliosis
- p. infiltrate of lymphocytes
- p. infiltration
- p. lymph spaces
- p. myelinoclasis, acute
- p. space ▸ His
- p. spaces

perivenous myelinoclasis, post-infection
periventricular
- p. gray substance
- p. hemorrhage
- p. white matter ▸ echogenicity of

perivesical abscess
perivesical fascia
periwinkle alkaloid
PERK (prospective evaluation of radial keratotomy) protocol
Perkins Brailler
PERL (pupils equal, react to light)
PERLA (pupils equal, react to light and accommodation)
Perlia's nucleus
Perma-Flow coronary graft
Perma-Hand suture
PermaMesh material
permanent
- p. absence of depth perception
- p. addiction
- p. adrenocortical insufficiency
- p. behavioral changes

- p. Bell's palsy
- p. biopsy
- p. blindness
- p. brain damage
- p. bridge
- p. callus
- p. cardiac pacemaker
- p. cardiac pacing lead
- p. cardiac pacing systems
- p. colostomy
- p. damage
- p. decline in intellectual function
- p. deformation, residual
- p. demand ventricular pacing system, malfunction of
- p. demand ventricular pacing systems
- p. disability
- p. disfigurement
- p. drooping mouth
- p. dry mouth
- p. functional losses
- p. hardness
- p. hearing loss
- p. ileostomy
- p. impairment
- p. implant therapy
- p. implants
- p. incisor
- p. joint damage
- p. junctional reciprocating tachycardia (PJRT)
- p. kidney damage
- p. lip enhancement
- p. loss of vision
- p. memory loss
- p. molars
- p. myocardial pacemaker
- p. optic atrophy
- p. pacemaker
- p. pacemaker for brain
- p. pacemaker implantation
- p. pacemaker insertion
- p. pacemaker management
- p. pacemaker placement
- p. pacing
- p. paralysis
- p. parasite
- p. partial
- p., pervasive effects
- p. prosthetic teeth
- p. regression
- p. remission
- p. section
- p. seed technique

- p. sterility
- p. stricture
- p. teeth
- p. teeth replacement
- p. tracheotomy
- p. transvenous pacemaker
- p. urinary opening
- p. vegetative state
- p. vision loss
- p. visual impairment
- p. weight control

permanently
- p., arms contracted
- p. implanted ventricular assist device (VAD)
- p. unconscoius

permanganate, potassium
permeability
- p., artery wall
- p. constant
- p. factor, lymph node
- p., increased lung
- p., increasing capillary
- p., membrane
- p. pulmonary edema
- p. ▸ pulmonary microvascular
- p. ▸ pulmonary vascular
- p. quotient
- p., vascular

permeable (RGP) contact lenses ▸ rigid gas
permissible concentration (MPC) ▸ maximum
permissible dose (MPD) ▸ maximum
permission
- p. for autopsy denied
- p. for autopsy granted
- p. for blood transfusion ▸ form refusing
- p. of next-of-kin

permissive hypercapnia
permit
- p. signed, autopsy
- p. signed, operative
- p. signed, surgical

permitting safe expression of anger
permutit method
pernicious
- p. anemia
- p. anemia ▸ appetite loss from
- p. anemia ▸ dementia from
- p. anemia, juvenile
- p. anemia ▸ memory loss from
- p. anemia ▸ tongue inflammation from

p. anemia ▸ weight loss from
p. maculation
p. myopia
p. vomiting
pernio, erythema
pernio, lupus
peromysci, Grahamella
peroneal [*perineal, peritoneal*]
p. artery
p. atrophy
p. bypass ▸ femoral-tibial-
p. groove
p. muscle, long
p. muscle, short
p. muscle, third
p. muscular atrophy
p. nerve
p. nerve, accessory deep
p. nerve, common
p. nerve, deep
p. nerve palsy
p. nerve, superficial
p. sheath
p. sign
p. tendon
p. tendonitis
p. vein
peroneus
p. brevis muscle
p. brevis transplant
p. longus muscle
p. longus muscle avulsion
p. tertius muscle
peroral endoscopy
peroral retrograde pancreaticobiliary ductography
peroxidase/peroxydase
p. activity ▸ endogenous
p. deficiency ▸ erythrocyte glutathione
peroxidation product ▸ lipid
peroxide, hydrogen
peroxyacetyl nitrate
perpendicular, incised
perpendicular plate of ethmoid
perpetrator, acquaintance rape
perpetrators, multiple
perpetual arrhythmia
perplexed, patient
perplexing, clinical nightmare
Perrin-Ferraton disease
PERRLA (pupils equal, round, react to light and accommodation)
PERS (personal emergency response system)

Persea americana
Persea gratissima
persecution
p. complex
p., delusions of
p. ▸ delusions of jealousy and
persecutory
p. delusional disorder
p. delusions
p. delusions, conspiratorial
perseverated letters and punctuation
perseverates in motor activities, patient
perseverates in speech, patient
perseverating ▸ schizophrenic patient
perseveration
p., clonic
p. of strategies
p., speech
p., tonic
Persian (Iranian heroin)
Persian Brown (Iranian heroin)
persica, Borrelia
persistence, memory
persistence scope
persistent
p. abnormal muscle tone
p. aching pain
p. aching sensation
p. alpha activity
p. anger
p. antisocial personality traits
p. asthma
p. back pain
p. backache
p. chest pain
p. chest pain symptoms
p. cilioretinal vein
p. common atrioventricular (AV) canal
p. cough
p. cough with hemoptysis
p. diarrhea
p. disorder initiating sleep
p. disorder of initiating wakefulness
p. disorder of maintaining sleep
p. disorder of maintaining wakefulness
p. ductus arteriosus
p. dyskinetic movements
p. elevation of blood pressure (BP)
p. elevation of mood
p. enuresis
p. epigastric pain

p. fatigue
p. feelings
p. feelings of anxiety
p. feelings of guilt
p. feelings of hopelessness
p. feelings of sadness
p. fetal circulation
p. fever
p. foot ulcer
p. hacking cough
p. headache
p. headache, vomiting or confusion
p. heartburn
p. hoarseness
p. hyperplastic primary vitreous (PHPV)
p. hyperplastic vitreous, primary
p. identity disturbance
p. illness
p. incontinence
p. indigestion
p. inflammation
p. inflammation of stomach
p. inflammatory stimulation
p. injury by chronic alcoholism
p., intrusive thoughts and compulsions
p. irritability
p. irritated area
p. ischemia
p. macular edema
p. memories
p. mental illness
p. mental illness ▸ severe and
p. middle ear effusion
p. mood disturbance
p. nausea
p. neck pain
p. nonhealing open sore
p. ostium primum
p. pain
p. pain in lower back
p. pain ▸ patient has
p. pattern of behavior ▸ repetitive
p. primitive trigeminal artery
p. psychosis, acute or
p. pulmonary hypertension of newborn
p. occiput posterior
p. reddish patch
p. remorse
p. shingles pain
p. snoring
p. S-T segment elevation
p. swelling of feet

persistent—*continued*
- p. symptoms
- p. thoughts
- p. tinnitus
- p. tissue inflammation
- p. tolerant infection
- p. tremor
- p. truncus arteriosus
- p. vegetative state
- p. vertigo
- p. viremia
- p. vomiting
- p. vomiting, severe or
- p. wave

persistently sad

persistently unstable self-image

persisting
- p. hepatitis, chronic
- p. perception disorder ▸ hallucinogen
- p. perceptual disturbances

person(s) (Person)(s)
- p., abnormally undersized
- p., abusive invasive
- p., addicted
- p., alcoholic drug dependent
- P. (AARP), American Association of Retired
- p., bereaved
- p., chemically dependent
- p., clergy
- p. CPR (cardiopulmonary resuscitation), one
- p., dependent
- p., disabled
- p., effects of pain on the whole
- p., homebound
- p. (HTP) ▸ house-tree-
- p., human concerns
- p., immunocompromised
- p., immunosuppressed
- p., medical
- p., mentally disordered
- p., muscle relaxation in normal
- p. ▸ oriented to time, place and
- p. ▸ patient alert to space, time and
- p., place and time ▸ patient oriented as to
- p., primary care
- p., sexually active
- p. susceptibility to cancer
- P. Test, Color-a-
- P. Test, Draw-a-
- P., Tree, House Test ▸ Draw
- p., unconscious

personal (Personal)
- p. abandonment
- p. affirmation
- p. agenda
- p. appearance, disinterest in
- p. appearance ▸ neglect of
- p. assistive listening device (ALD)
- p. asthma triggers
- P. Attributes Questionnaire (PAQ)
- p. behavior
- p. behavior, altered
- p. belief, false
- p. care
- p. care, one-on-one
- p. cleanliness
- p. contact, direct
- p. contact, indirect
- p. creativity
- p. decision-making
- p. emergency response system (PERS)
- p. fulfillment
- p. gain, desire for
- p. goals
- p. goals ▸ apathy and lack of interest in
- p. grooming ▸ loss of interest in
- p. growth
- p. harm ▸ fear of
- p. hearing loss profile
- p. hygiene
- p. identity disturbance
- p. indifference
- p. injury
- p. lifestyle change
- p. motivation
- p. perspective
- p. physician
- p. pleasure
- p. presence
- p. profit
- p. reaction
- p. recovery program
- p. relationship
- p. relationship, disturbed
- p. relationship ▸ tumultuous
- p. risk factor
- p. stability
- p. stress management
- p. therapy
- p. triggers

personality(-ies) (Personality)
- p., abnormal
- p., addictive
- p., affective

- p., alcoholic
- p., alternating
- p., amoral
- p., anancastic
- p. and depression, borderline
- p. and drug abuse, antisocial
- p., antisocial
- p. assessment
- p. assessment findings
- p., asthenic
- p., authoritarian
- p., avoidant
- p., borderline
- p., cancer
- p. change
- p. change, disorientation and
- p. changes ▸ irritability, depression and
- p. changes ▸ psychotic
- p. changes ▸ subtle
- p. changes ▸ unexplained
- p. characteristics
- p., codependent
- p., cognitive therapy of
- p., compulsive
- p., control-dominated
- p., core
- p., cycloid
- p., cyclothymic
- p., dependent
- p., derangement of
- p. deterioration
- p. deterioration, generalized
- p. development, level of
- p. differences, inborn
- p., disease-prone
- p. disintegration ▸ increased
- p. ▸ disintegration of
- p. disorder
- p. disorder, affective
- p. disorder, anancastic
- p. disorder, antisocial
- p. disorder, avoidant
- p. disorder (BPD), borderline
- p. disorder ▸ chronic depressive
- p. disorder ▸ chronic hypomanic
- p. disorder, compulsive
- p. disorder, dependent
- p. disorder, epileptoid
- p. disorder, explosive
- p. disorder, histrionic
- p. disorder ▸ intermittent explosive
- p. disorder, multifaceted
- p. disorder, multiple
- p. disorder ▸ multiplex

p. disorder, narcissistic
p. disorder ▸ negativistic
p. disorder ▸ obsessive compulsive
p. disorder, organic
p. disorder, paranoid
p. disorder ▸ passive aggressive
p. disorder ▸ psychoactive
    substance
p. disorder, schizoid
p. disorder, schizotypal
p. disorder ▸ self-defeating
p. disorder ▸ severe
p., dissociative disorders ▸
    multiple
p. disturbance
p., double
p., dual
p. dysfunction and stress
p., dyssocial
p. evaluation
p., explosive
p. factor
p. features
p. function
p. ▸ fusing of
p. ▸ heredocongenital nucleus of
p., histrionic
p., hostile
p., hypertensive
p., hypochondriacal
p., hypomanic
p., hysterical
p. ▸ impulse dominated
p., inadequate
p., introverted
P. Inventory (MMPI), Minnesota
    Multiphasic
P. Inventory (MMPI) Test,
    Minnesota Multiphasic
p., labile
p., manic-depressive
p., manipulative
p. measures
p., migraine
p., multiple
p., narcissistic
p., nervous
p., nondiabetic
p., normal
p., obsessive
p., obsessive-compulsive
p., obsessive-type
p. of patient
p. panel
p., paranoid

p., passive-aggressive
p., passive-dependent
p. pattern
p., premorbid
p. problems, biofeedback and
p. profile
p. ▸ psychological measures of
p., psychology of
p., psychopathic
p., sadistic
p., schizoid
p., schizotypal
p., seclusive
p. ▸ self-defeating
p. ▸ self-healing
p., shut-in
p., sociopathic
p., split
p., subdued
p. syndrome, organic
p. test
p. test, Guilford-Zimmerman
p. testing, objective
p. traits
p. traits, antisocial
p. traits ▸ histrionic
p. traits in alcoholics
p. traits ▸ inflexible antisocial
p. traits ▸ maladaptive antisocial
p. traits of patient, premorbid
p. traits ▸ persistent antisocial
p., Type A
p., Type B
p., violent alter
p., workaholic
personalized medical paradigm
personalized medication profile
personnel
p., emergency
p. health care
p. health program
p., infected
p., medical
p., nonsurgical
perspective
p., behavioral
p., biopsychological
p., clinical
p., cultural
p., ecological
p., gain
p., holistic
p., in-depth
p., neurochemical
p., personal

p., professional
p., psychodynamic
p., psychosocial
p., realistic
perspiration
p., excessive
p., excessive foot
p., profuse
perstans
p., Acanthocheilonema
p., acrodermatitis
p., Dipetalonema
p., xanthoerythrodermia
persuasion, moral
persulcatus, Ixodes
pertechnetate Tc 99m, sodium
pertenue, Treponema
Perthes(')
P. disease
P. disease ▸ Calvé-
P. incision
P. syndrome ▸ Calvé-Legg-
pertinent laboratory findings
pertinent physical findings
pertrochanteric fracture
**perturbation in cardiovascular
    system**
**perturbed autonomic nervous system
    function**
pertussis
p., Bacillus
p., Bordetella
p., gram-negative Haemophilus
p., Haemophilus
p., Hemophilus
p. immune globulin
p. immune globulin (human)
p., tetanus ▸ (DPT) diphtheria,
p. toxin
p. vaccine
p. vaccine ▸ diphtheria, tetanus
    toxoids and acellular
p. vaccine ▸ diphtheria, tetanus
    toxoids and whole cell
p. vaccine, Haemophilus
peruana, verruga
Peruvian Flake (cocaine)
**PERV (porcine endogenous
    retrovirus)**
pervasive
p. anxiety
p. developmental disorder
p. effects ▸ permanent,
p. mental illness
p. pattern

pervasive—*continued*
- p. pattern of disregard for others
- p. pattern of instability

pervenous pacemaker
perversion, sexual
PES (Perceived Exertion Scale)
pes
- p. abductus
- p. adductus
- p. anserine transfer
- p. anserinus
- p. arcuatus
- p. calcaneus
- p. cavus
- p. equinovarus
- p. excavatum
- p. planus
- p. pronatus
- p. supinatus
- p. tendonitis
- p. valgus
- p. varus

pesco-vegetarian diet
pessary
- p. cell
- p., cup
- p., diaphragm
- p. donut, vaginal
- p., doughnut
- p., Emmert-Gellhorn
- p., Gariel's
- p., Gehrung
- p., Gellhorn's
- p., gynefold
- p., Hodge's
- p., lever
- p., Menge's
- p., ring
- p., Smith-Hodge
- p., Smith's
- p., stem
- p., Thomas'
- p., Wylie's
- p., Zwanck's

pessimistic, patient
pessimistic ruminations
pesticide poisoning
pestis
- p. ambulans
- p., Bacillus
- p. bubonica
- p. bubonicae, Bacterium
- p., gram-negative Pasteurella
- p., Pasteurella

- p. siderans
- p., Yersinia

PET (positron emission tomography)
petal-fugal flow
pet-borne illness
petechiae
- p., focal
- p., hemorrhagic
- p. in conjunctive
- p., multiple
- p. of tongue
- p., serosal

petechial
- p. capillary cordeolum
- p. fever
- p. hemorrhage
- p. hemorrhages, diffuse
- p. hemorrhages, focal
- p. hemorrhages of bowel
- p. hemorrhages of epicardium
- p. hemorrhages of kidneys
- p. hemorrhages of pericardium
- p. hemorrhages of peritoneum
- p. hemorrhages of skin
- p. hemorrhages, subendocardial
- p. lesions

Peter operation, O'Connor-
Peter's anomaly
Petersen
- P. approach, Smith-
- P. hip cup prosthesis ▸ Smith-
- P. nail, Smith-
- P. operation, Smith-
- P. osteotome ▸ Carroll-Smith-
- P. osteotomy, Smith-
- P. prosthesis, Smith-

Peterson's operation
Pethadol (Cube), Demerol/
petit mal
- p.m., compatible with
- p.m. convulsion
- p.m. discharge
- p.m. discharge, pseudo
- p.m. discharges, miniature
- p.m. epilepsy
- p.m. epilepsy, myoclonic
- p.m., pseudo
- p.m. status
- p.m. substances, anti◇
- p.m., true
- p.m. variant
- p.m. variant ▸ compatible with
- p.m. variant discharge

Petit's
- P. canal

- P. hernia
- P. sinus

Petrassi syndrome, Fanconi-
Petri dish
Petri test
petrificans
- p., conjunctivitis
- p., keratitis
- p., urethritis

petrobasilar suture
petrolatum emulsion, liquid
petroleum distillate poisoning
petroleum ether
petrosa, crusta
petrosa dentis, crusta
petrosal
- p. cells, deep
- p. ganglion
- p. ganglion, inferior
- p. nerve
- p. nerve, deep
- p. nerve, greater
- p. nerve, lesser
- p. nerve, superficial middle

petrosphenobasilar suture
petrosphenoidal syndrome
petrosphenooccipital suture of Gruber
petrosquamosal/petrosquamou
petrosquamous suture
petrotympanic fissure
petrous
- p. apex
- p. apices
- p. bone
- p. bone, caries of
- p. osteomyelitis, chronic
- p. pyramid
- p. ridge
- p. tips

PETT (positron emission transaxial tomography)
PETT (positron emission transverse tomography)
Pette-Döring panencephalitis
Petzetaki-Takos syndrome
Peutz-Jeghers syndrome
Peyers' patches
Peyers' plaques
Peyote (peyote)
- P. (Mescaline)
- p. chewed and swallowed
- p. ingested orally
- p. intoxication
- p. smoked

Peyronie's disease
Peyrot's thorax
pf (picofarad)
PF (parafascicular) nucleus
Pfannenstiel's incision
Pfeiffer('s)
    P. bacillus
    P. -Comberg method
    P. procedure
PFG (pressure flow gradient)
PFR (peak filling rate)
PFR (peak flow rate)
PFS (patient financial services)
PFT (parafascicular thalamotomy)
PFT (pulmonary function test)
PFU (plaque-forming units)
Pfuhl-Jaffe sign
Pfuhl's sign
PG (pneumogram)
PGR (psychogalvanic reflex)
PH (past history)
PH (past history) noncontributory
PH (past history) not remarkable
pH
    pH (hydrogen ion concentration)
    pH determination
    pH, scalp
    pH test
P-H interval
phacoemulsification
    p., Kelman
    p. method
    p. procedure
    p. surgery
Phaenicia sericata
phage(s) [*stage*]
    p., defective
    p., immature
    p. particle
    p. particle infects new host cell
    p. particle maturing in donor cell
    p. pattern
    p. type
    p. -typing
    p. typing of organisms
phagedenic
    p. chancroid
    p. gingivitis
    p. ulcer
    p. ulcer, tropical
phagocyte, alveolar
phagocyte system, mononuclear
phagocytic
    p. cells
    p. dysfunction

    p. function
    p. immunity
    p. index
    p. receptor
phagocytosis ▸ impaired Kupffer's
    cell
phagocytosis, splenic
phakogenic glaucoma
phakolytic glaucoma
phalange [*flange*]
phalangeal
    p. articulations
    p. bones
    p. cells
    p. cells, inner
    p. cells, outer
    p. dystrophy ▸ thoracic-pelvic-
    p. epiphyseal centers
    p. fracture
    p. joints, metatarsal-
    p. tuft
    p. wall cancer
phalangectomy, partial
phalanges, clubbing of distal
phalangophalangeal amputation
phalanx
    p., distal
    p., middle
    p., proximal
    p., shaft of proximal
    p., terminal
Phalen('s)
    P. maneuver
    P. sign
    P. sign test
    P. test
phallic stage
phallic symbol
phalloides, Amanita
Phaneuf's maneuver
phantastica, paraphrenia
phantom
    p. aneurysm
    p. hand
    p. illness
    p. limb
    p. limb pain
    p. odontalgia
    p. pacemaker
    p. pain
    p. pregnancy
    p. ratio, tissue
    p. spike-and-waves
    p. sponge
    p. tumor

pharmaceutical (Pharmaceutical)
    p. chemistry
    p. management
    P. Powder (cocaine)
    p. rounds
pharmacist-on-call
pharmacokinetic factor
pharmacologic
    p. addiction
    p. agents
    p. aspect
    p. interventions
    p. management
    p. relief
    p. stress
    p. stress echocardiography
    p. stress perfusion imaging
    p. syndromes, toxicologic-
    p. therapy
pharmacological
    p. actions
    p. cardioversion
    p. data
    p. interactions, clinical and
    p. intervention
    p. strategy
    p. therapy
    p. therapy of arrhythmias
    p. treatment
pharmacology
    p., experimental
    p., human
    p. in trauma
    p., molecular
    p. patient irritable, clinical
pharmacotherapy
    p. for alcoholism
    p. for hyperactivity
    p. of substance abuse
pharmacy, hospital
pharyngea, keratosis
pharyngeal [*laryngeal*]
    p. abscess
    p. adenoids
    p. airway, binasal
    p. arch
    p. artery
    p. artery, ascending
    p. bursa
    p. candidiasis
    p. clefts
    p. constrictor muscle
    p. crisis
    p. diverticulum

pharyngeal—*continued*
- p. diverticulum ▸ small saccular posterior
- p. dysphagia
- p. flap repair
- p. hemisphincter
- p. injection
- p. lead
- p. lymph nodes
- p. mucosa
- p. musculature
- p. myoclonus
- p. orifice
- p. pack
- p. plexus
- p. pouch syndrome
- p. pouches
- p. reflex
- p. reflexes, protective
- p. tonsil
- p. tonsil, crypts of
- p. veins
- p. wall ▸ posterior

pharyngectomy [*laryngectomy*]

pharyngis
- p., globus
- p., Mycoplasma
- p., Neisseria

pharyngitis
- p., acute
- p., acute catarrhal
- p., arcanobacterial
- p., atrophic
- p., bacterial
- p., catarrhal
- p., chronic
- p., croupous
- p., diphtheric
- p., follicular
- p., gangrenous
- p., glandular
- p., granular
- p. ▸ Group A beta streptococcal
- p., herpangina
- p. herpetica
- p., hypertrophic
- p. keratosa
- p., lymphonodular
- p., membranous
- p., nonstreptococcal
- p., phlegmonous
- p., plaque
- p., purulent
- p., pustular
- p. sicca
- p., streptococcal
- p. syndrome, acute
- p. tonsillitis
- p. ulcerosa
- p., viral

pharyngoconjunctival fever
pharyngoconjunctival fever virus
pharyngoepiglottic arch
pharyngoepiglottic fold
pharyngoesophageal (PE) diverticulum
pharyngoesophageal (PE) reconstruction, Wookey's
pharyngopalatine arch
pharyngopalatine muscle
pharyngopalatinus, arcus
pharyngotympanic cephalalgia
pharyngotympanic tube

pharynx [*larynx*]
- p., cancer of
- p., constrictor muscle of
- p., inflamed
- p. injected
- p., junction of
- p., larynx and trachea anesthetized
- p. level
- p. normal, palate and
- p. not injected
- p. not injected, posterior
- p., oral
- p. ▸ raphe of
- p., regurgitated food in
- p., superior constrictor muscle of

phase(s) [*gaze*]
- p., acute
- p. advance
- p. advance syndrome
- p. angle
- p. angle of displacement
- p., chronic
- p., clonic
- p. contrast angiography
- p. -contrast microscope
- p., crucial
- p. current, single-
- p. current, three-
- p. delay
- p. delay syndrome
- p., delayed sleep
- p., depressive
- p. detoxification
- p. discrimination, in-
- p. dysphoric disorder ▸ late luteal
- p. dysphoric disorder, periluteal
- p., ejection
- p. encoded velocity image
- p. encoding ▸ respiratory ordered
- p. endometrium, proliferative
- p. endometrium, secretory
- p., follicular
- p. generator, three-
- p., heart's relaxed
- p., hyperacute
- p. image
- p. image analysis
- p. imaging
- p. index, ejection
- p. index ▸ isovolumetric
- p. index ▸ left ventricular (LV) diastolic
- p., initial assessment
- p., latent
- p., luteal
- p., manic
- p. mapping, digital
- p. microscope
- p., mid-cycle
- p., nonsecretory
- p. of bipolar disorder ▸ manic
- p. of cardiac cycle (cc) ▸ resting
- p. of facial hair ▸ growth
- p. of facial hair ▸ resting
- p. of life problem
- p. of sleep, early
- p. of treatment
- p. of treatment ▸ acute
- p. of treatment ▸ initial stabilization
- p., out of
- p., perimenopausal
- p., plateau
- p., postacute
- p., premenstrual
- p., prodromal
- p. reaction, late
- p., relaxation
- p. reversal
- p. reversal, instrumental
- p. reversal, true
- p., shedding
- p. shift artifact
- p. -shift disruption of 24-hour sleep-wake cycle
- p. signal, in-
- p. signal, out-of-
- p. ▸ supernormal recovery
- p. syndrome (DSPS) ▸ delayed sleep
- p. syndrome (FASPS) ▸ familial advanced sleep
- p. system, three-

p., tonic
p., transition
p., venous
p., vulnerable
p., washout
p., waves of opposite
p. wrap ▸ no-
phased
p. array
p. array microwave technology ▸ adaptive
p. array sector scanner
p. array study
p. array ▸ symmetrical
p. array system
p. array system, annular
p. array technology
Phaseolus limensis
phasic
p. activity
p. arrhythmia
p. event
p. reflex
p. sinus arrhythmia
Pheasant's operation
Phelps' operation
Phelps-Gocht osteoclast
Phemister graft
Phemister operation
phenacetin nephritis
phencyclidine(s)
p. (Angel Dust)
p. (animal tranquilizer)
p. (CJ)
p. (Coon)
p. (Crystal)
p. (Cyclone)
p. (Dummy Dust)
p. (Dust of Angels)
p. (elephant tranquilizer)
p. (Embalming Fluid)
p. (Hog)
p. (horse tranquilizer)
p. (Killer Weed)
p. (Krystal)
p. (Mintweed)
p. (Monkey Dust)
p. (Ozone)
p. (PCP)
p. (PCP/PeaCe Pill)
p. (Scuffle)
p. (Sherman)
p. (Supergrass)
p. abuse
p. abuse, pattern of

p. abuse, physical effects of
p., abuse potential of
p. abuse, prevalence of
p., abusers, assessing needs of
p., acute intoxication with
p. analog (PCPy/PHP)
p. analog (Rocket Fuel)
p. analog (TCP/TPCP)
p., blood level of
p. delirium
p. dependence
p., dependence on
p., effects of
p., flashback reactions with
p. (PCP) ingested
p. (PCP) injected
p. intoxication
p., mode of administration with
p. mood disorder
p., organic brain syndrome with
p., panic reactions with
p., patient OD (overdosed) with
p., potential tolerance to
p., psychoactive doses of
p., psychoactive properties of
p., psychological effects of
p., psychotic reactions with
p. smoked
p. (PCP) snorted
p., tolerance to
p., toxicity of
p., treatment of acute drug reactions to
p., withdrawal from
phenol
p. liquefactum
p. red
p. salicylate
phenolics, quats and
phenolized and inverted, stump
phenolized, stump
phenolphthalein test
phenolsulfonphthalein test
phenomenology, psychotic
phenomenon(-a)
p. ▸ age-related
p., Arias-Stella
p., Ashman
p., autoimmune
p., Bell's
p., blush
p., booster
p., cascade
p., cerebral
p., coagulation

p., coronary steal
p., Cushing's
p., déjà vu
p., diaphragm
p., diaphragmatic
p., dip
p., EEG (electroencephalogram)
p., embolic
p., emotional
p., fern
p., flicker
p. ▸ gap conduction
p. ▸ Gartner's vein
p., Hering's
p., Hoffmann's
p., Hunt's
p., Hunt's paradoxical
p., hypnagogic
p., immature
p., interference
p. (ISP) ▸ interesting sociological
p., Jacoud's
p., Katz-Wachtel
p., Kindling
p., Koebner
p., lateral constriction
p., Magendie's
p., Marcus Gunn
p. ▸ mind-body
p. ▸ no reflow
p., obstructive
p. of old age
p., Osler's
p., overkill
p., paroxysmal cerebral
p., peripheral embolic
p., psychological
p., Raynaud's
p., reentry
p., regeneration
p., relatively primitive
p. ▸ R-on-T
p., Rumpel-Leede
p., scleroderma, telangiectasia (CRST) syndrome ▸ calcification, Raynaud's
p., sensory
p., spike
p., spike-and-slow wave
p., spiking
p., staircase
p., steal
p., Strassmann's
p., treppe
p., Trousseau's

phenomenon(-a)—*continued*
   p., Twort-d'Herelle
   p., vacuum
   p., vascular
   p. ▸ warm-up
   p., washout
   p., Wenckeback
   p. ▸ white coat
phenothiazine poisoning
phenotype, metastatic
phentetiothalein contrast medium
phenylalanine, metabolize
phenylalanine mustard
phenylisopropylamine (Love Pill)
phenylketonuria test
phenylpyruvic
   p. acid (PPA)
   p. amentia
   p. oligophrenia
phenylpyruvica, oligophrenia
pheochrome bodies
pheochrome cells
Phialophora verrucosa
Philadelphia
   P. chromosome
   P. cocktail
   P. collar
philippina, Taenia
philippinensis, Filaria
philippinensis, Mallotus
Philippson's reflex
Philip's glands
Phillips' muscle
Phillips' screw
philosophical intellectualization
philosophy
   p., hospice
   p., moral
   p., therapeutic
   p., treatment
philtrum, long
phimosis vaginalis
pHisoHex scrub
phlebectasia laryngis
phlebectomy, ambulatory
phlebectomy, outpatient
phlebitic induration
phlebitis
   p., adhesive
   p., anemic
   p., bacterial
   p. ▸ blood clot in
   p., blue
   p., chlorotic
   p. from birth control pill

   p. from cancer
   p., gouty
   p., infusion
   p., IV (intravenous) infusion
   p., migrating
   p., obliterating
   p., obstructive
   p. of cavernous sinus
   p. of cranial sinus
   p. of cranial sinus, septic
   p. of lateral sinus
   p., plastic
   p., productive
   p., proliferative
   p., puerperal
   p., recurrent
   p., sclerosing
   p., septic
   p., sinus
   p., superficial
   p., suppurative
phlebogram examination
phlebothrombosis ▸ patient has
Phlebotomus (phlebotomus)
   P. argentipes
   P. chinensis
   p. fever
   P. intermedius
   P. macedonicum
   P. noguchi
   P. orientalis
   P. papatasii
   P. sergenti
   P. verrucarum
   P. vexator
phlebotomy
   p., bloodless
   p., layer
   p., therapeutic
phlegm
   p., blood specked
   p. ▸ foul-smelling
   p., increased
   p., yellowish
phlegmasia
   p. alba dolens
   p. alba dolens puerperarum
   p., cellulitic
   p. cerulea dolens
phlegmonosa, angina
phlegmonosa, parotitis
phlegmonous
   p. adenitis
   p. dacryocystitis
   p. enteritis

   p. gastritis
   p. laryngitis
   p. mastitis
   p. pharyngitis
   p. vulvitis
phlei, Mycobacterium
phlyctenular
   p. conjunctivitis
   p. keratitis
   p. ophthalmia
PHN (post-herpetic neuralgia)
PHN (Public Health Nurse)
phobia(s)
   p., and anxieties ▸ fears,
   p., cancer◇
   p., cancers◇
   p., carcino◇
   p., childhood
   p., dental
   p., flight
   p. in children ▸ school
   p., irrational
   p., isolated
   p., paralyzing
   p. ▸ patient has
   p., school
   p., simple
   p., social
   p., waking
   p., water
   p. ▸ white coat
phobic
   p. anxiety
   p. anxiety and desensitization
   p. disorder
   p. neurosis
   p. partner
   p. reaction
   p. reactions ▸ systematic
     desensitization of
   p. response
   p. stimuli
phocomelic dwarf
Phoenix total artificial heart
Phonate speaking valve ▸ Shiley
phonating edge
phonating structure
phonation [*pronation*]
phonation, approximate on
phonation study
phone order (PO)
phone radiation ▸ cell
phonemic awareness
phonetic [*phrenetic, frenetic*]
phonetic analysis, acoustic and

phonetic balanced percent (PB%)
phonetically balanced
phonocardiogram study
phonocardiograph
   p., linear
   p., logarithmic
   p., spectral
   p., stethoscopic
phonocardiographic study
phonocardiographic transducer
phonocardiography
   p., intracardiac
   p., linear
   p., spectral
   p. study
phonocatheterization, intracardiac
phoretogram, electro◊
Phormia regina
phosphatase
   p., acid
   p. (ALP), alkaline
   p., heat stable alkaline
   p., leukocyte alkaline
   p., prostatic acid
   p., serum
   p., serum alkaline
   p. test
   p. test, acid
   p. test, alkaline
   p. (LAP) test, leukocyte alkaline
   p. (TSPAP) ▸ total serum prostatic
     acid
phosphate
   p. acid, histamine
   p. -buffered saline
   p., calcium
   p. crystals, amorphous
   p. crystals, triple
   p. cycle
   p. dehydrogenase
   p. dehydrogenase deficiency
     anemia ▸ glucose-6-
   p. dehydrogenase deficiency,
     glucose-6-
   p. dehydrogenase, glucose
   p. dehydrogenase, glyceraldehyde
   p., dihydroxyacetone
   p., diisopropyl
   p. excretion index (PEI)
   p., histamine
   p. isomerase, glucose
   p. isomerase, triose
   p., Krebs-Ringer
   p. laser ▸ potassium titanyl
   p. molecule

p. P 32, chromic
p. P 32, sodium
p. scan
p., triorthocresyl
p., tubular reabsorption of
p. uridyl transferase, galactose
phosphogluconate dehydrogenase
phosphoglyceraldehyde dehydrogenase
phosphoglycerate kinase
phosphohexokinase, platelet
phosphokinase, creatine
phosphokinase, serum creatine
phospholipid ratio, cholesterol-
phospholipid test
phosphorescens, Vibrio
phosphorescent sweat
phosphoribose isomerase
phosphoribosyl transferase,
   hypoxanthine guanine
phosphoric acid test
phosphorus
   p., calcium and
   p. level, blood
   p. (p^{32}) ▸ radioactive
   p., serum
   p. test, serum
   p. 32 (p^{32})
   p. threshold, theoretical renal
phosphorylated, proteins abnormally
phosphorylating enzyme
phosphorylation of proteins
phosphotransferase activity
photic
   p., driving
   p. epilepsy
   p. sneeze reflex
   p. stimulation
   p. stimulation, intermittent
   p. stimulation procedure
   p. stimulation, repetitive
   p. stimulator
photo
   p. acoustic shock wave
   p. image
   p. -oxidative reaction
photoaging, roughness of
photochemical transformation
photocoagulation
   p., ialo
   p., infrared
   p., panretinal
   p. procedure
   p. (PRP), proliferative retinopathy
   p. repair of detached retina

p. scatter
photocoagulator
   p., laser
   p., xenon (Xe) arch
   p., Zeiss
photoconvulsive activity
photoconvulsive response
photodisplay unit
photodisruptive laser
photodynamic
   p. therapy (PDT)
   p. therapy (PDT) treatment for
     cancer
   p. therapy ▸ tumor
   p. tumor therapy
photoelectric
   p. absorption
   p. effect
   p. emission
   p. interaction
   p. sensor
photofluorographic examination
photofluorographic study
photogenic epilepsy
photogenic seizure
photographic
   p. emulsion
   p. memory
   p. plate
   p. radiometer
photographs ▸ authorization form for
   taking and publication of
photographs ▸ consent form for
   taking and publication of
photography, retinal fundus
photometer, electro◊
photomultiplier tube
photomyoclonic activity
photomyoclonic response
photomyogenic activity
photomyogenic response
photon
   p., Compton
   p., degraded
   p. densitometry, Norland-Cameron
   p. detection ▸ single
   p. emission computed tomography
     (SPECT) scan ▸ single
   p. emission computed tomography
     (SPECT), single
   p. emission ▸ single
   p. emission tomography (SPET)
     imaging ▸ single
   p. energy
   p. energy accelerators ▸ dual

photon—*continued*
- p. gamma scintigraphy ▸ single
- p. irradiation technique in radiation therapy
- p. linear accelerator ▸ dual-
- p. therapy
- p. therapy, combination electron and

photonuclear effect
photonuclear reaction
photo-ophthalmia/photophthalmia
photoparoxysmal response
photopenic area
photopic vision
photoplethysmography, digital
photoreactive agent
photorefractive keratectomy (PRK)
photorejuvenation procedure
photoselective vaporization of prostate (PVP)
photosensitive epilepsy
photosensitivity ▸ extreme skin
photosensitivity reaction
photosensitization technique
phototherapy, neonatal
photothermolysis, selective
phototube, multiplier
phototube output circuit
PHPD (post-hallucinogenic perceptual disorder)
PHPV (persistent hyperplastic primary vitreous)
phrase(s) (Phrase)
- p., autosuggestion
- *P. Index* (MPI), *Medical*
- p. length speech
- p. length utterance

phrenetic [*phonetic, frenetic*]
phrenic [*splenic*]
- p. ampulla
- p. artery
- p. center
- p. ganglion
- p. lymph nodes
- p. nerve
- p. nerve crushed
- p. nerve damage
- p. nerve paralysis
- p. nerves, accessory
- p. veins, inferior
- p. veins, superior
- p. wave

phrenicoabdominal nerves
PHRT (procarbazine hydroxyurea radiotherapy)

phrygian [*pterygium*]
phrygian cap
phthinoid
- p. bronchitis
- p. chest
- p. type

phthiriasis inguinalis
phthiriasis, pubic
Phthirus pubis
phthisic type
phthisica, spes
phthisis
- p., aneurysmal
- p., bacillary
- p., black
- p. bulbi
- p., colliers'
- p. corneas
- p., diabetic
- p., fibroid
- p., flax dressers'
- p., grinders'
- p., miner's
- p., nodosa
- p., ocular
- p., potters'
- p., pulmonary
- p., stone cutters'

phycomycetous fungi
phycomycosis entomophthorae
phylloides, cystosarcoma
Phymatosorus scolopendrium
Physaloptera
- P. caucasica
- P. mordens
- P. rara
- P. truncata

physeal bar
Physeter catodon
physical (Physical)
- p. abilities ▸ mental and
- p. ability
- p. ability to react, brain's
- p. abnormalities
- p. abnormalities in drug abusers
- p. abuse
- p. activity
- p. activity, aerobic
- p. activity, daily
- p. activity ▸ excessive
- p. activity, increased
- p. activity, limitations of
- p. activity, limited
- p. activity ▸ moderate
- p. activity program

- p. activity ▸ reduced tolerance for
- p. activity ▸ regular
- p. activity, restricted
- p. activity ▸ strenuous
- p. activity ▸ vigorous
- p. addiction
- p. adjustment
- p. affliction
- p. agent
- p. agents and techniques
- p. ailment
- p. and biochemical effects
- p. and emotional aspects of cancer
- p. and emotional changes
- p. and emotional support
- p. and mental condition
- p. and nutritional component ▸ medical, psychological, spiritual,
- p. and psychological dependence
- p. aspect
- p. aspects of cancer
- p. aspects of heart
- p. assault
- p. assaults ▸ repeated
- p. assessment
- p. assessment of newborn
- p. barrier
- p. brain damage
- p. burnout
- p. capabilities ▸ alteration in
- p. capability
- p. challenge
- p. change in brain
- p. characteristics
- p. characteristics, neuromuscular
- p. chemistry
- p. comforting
- p. complaints
- p. complaints ▸ adjustment disorder with
- p. complications of problem feet
- p. compulsion
- p. condition
- p. condition ▸ irreversible mental or
- p. condition ▸ psychological factors affecting
- p. conditioning
- p. considerations in palliation
- p. coordination
- p. cravings
- p. cues of stress
- p. cycle
- p. decay
- p. decay, patient in state of
- p. deficits

p. deformity
p. degradation
p. density measurement
p. dependence on drugs
p. dependence on nicotine gum
p. dependency
p. deterioration
p. deterioration ▸ prevention of
p. development, marked retardation
   of mental and
p. diagnosis
p. disabilities
p. disability evaluation
p. discomfort
p. discomfort, undue
p. disease ▸ psychological
   manifestations of
p. disorder
p. disorder of brain
p. disruption of cell
p. drive
p. drug dependence
p. effects
p. effects of AIDS (acquired
   immune deficiency syndrome)
p. effects of cannabinoid abuse
p. effects of depressant abuse
p. effects of drug abuse
p. effects of hallucinogen abuse
p. effects of heavy ions
p. effects of inhalant abuse
p. effects of opioid abuse
p. effects of particle beams
p. effects of phencyclidine abuse
p. effects of stimulant abuse
p. efficiency index (PEI)
p. elasticity of muscle
p. /emotional care
p. energy
p. evaluation
p. evaluation, complete
p. evaluation, executive
p. evidence of trauma
p. examination (PE)
p. examination, admission
p. examination, annual
p. examination as a screening
   device for drug abuse
p. examination, complete
p. examination, entrance
p. examination, executive
p. examination (HPE), history and
p. examination, initial
p. examination, preoperative
   screening

p. examination, routine
p. examination, screening
p. exercise
p. exercise, lack of
p. exercise ▸ regular
p. exertion
p. exhaustion
p. fights ▸ repeated
p. findings, pertinent
p. findings, radiographic
p. fitness
p. fitness ▸ lack of
p. fitness program
p. forces
p. function, normal
p. functioning
p. functioning, degree of
p. growth
p. half-life
p. handicap
p. harm or violence
p. harm ▸ threats of
p. health
p. (H and P) ▸ history and
p. hyperactivity
p. illness, depression triggered by
p. illness ▸ underlying
p. immaturity
p. inactivity
p. incapacity
p. injury
p. inoculation
p. intervention
p. limitations
p. malady
p. maneuver
p. manifestation of disease
p. manipulation
p. maturity
p. means
p. measurement, absolute
p. medicine
p. medicine and rehabilitation
   (PMR)
p. mobility, impaired
p. need, create
p. needs
p. or emotional factors
p. or mental disabilities
p. origin
p. overactivity
p. power ▸ feeling of intellectual
   and
p. predisposition
p., preemployment

p. pressure
p. profile, balanced
p. reaction
p. reaction ▸ severe
p. reactions ▸ slowing of
p. rehabilitation
p. relaxation
p. repercussions
p. restlessness
p. restoration
p. restraint
p. restrictions
p. retardation
p. risk
p. (REP) ▸ roentgen equivalent
p. self-endangerment
p. sensation
p. sensations ▸ perception of
p. sign
p. skills, basic
p. standpoint
p. status
p. status ▸ altered mentation of
p. stimulation
p. stimuli
p. stimulus
p. strain
p. strain ▸ stress and
p. strength and endurance
p. stress
p. stress disorders
p. stress, work-related
p. suffering
p. support
p. symptom control
p. symptom relief
p. symptoms
p. symptoms ▸ adjustment react
   with
p. symptoms ▸ chronic factitious
   illness with
p. symptoms ▸ factitious disorder
   with
p. symptoms in grief
p. symptoms, uncontrolled
p. tension
p. therapist
p. therapy
P. Therapy (PT)
p. therapy ▸ conventional
P. Therapy (PT) Department
p. therapy ▸ rehabilitative
p. therapy services
p., thorough
p. threatening and aggression

physical—*continued*
p. tiredness
p. touch stretch
p. training
p. trait
p. trauma
p. trauma, major
p. triggers
p. unattractiveness, delusions of
p. violence ▸ threats of
p. weakness
p. well being
p. withdrawal symptoms
p. work activity
p. work capacity
P. Work Capacity exercise stress test
p. work environment

physically
p. active ▸ patient
p. addictive
p. aggressive
p. and emotionally stressful
p., brain changes
p. challenged
p. coated stents
p. debilitated
p. declining
p. devastating
p. disabled
p. disabled, rehabilitation center for
p. drained
p. exhausted
p. handicapped
p. handicapped, halfway house for
p. handicapped, rehabilitation center for
p. impaired
p. impaired, patient
p. inactive
p. inactive lifestyle
p. stressful
p. /multiple handicapped (P/MH)
p. weak, patient

physician('s)
p., admitting
p. advisor
p. assessment
p. assistant (PA)
p. assisted suicide
p., attending
p. authority
p., authorization for delivery by alternate
p. -based intervention

p. care
p., clinical
p. ▸ complementary medicine
p., consent form to delivery by alternate
p., contact
p. directed interdisciplinary care
p. drug abuse
p. drug abusers, attitudes of
p., emergency medicine
p., family
p. ▸ frequent visits to
p. ▸ hospital-based
p., house
p., naturopathic
p. -on-call
p. order
p. order, obtain
p. owned clinics
p., patient discharged to care of family
p. -patient relationship
p. ▸ patient sees numerous
p., personal
p. population, prevalence of drug abuse in
p., primary
p. (PCP) ▸ primary care
p., private
p., procurement
p., radiation oncology
p. referral service
p., referring
p., rehabilitation
p., reviewing
p. services
p. ▸ site-based
p., transplant
P. ▸ Urgent Care
p. who abuse drugs, treatment of

Physicians Activities Study (PAS)
physicist, radiation
Physick's operation
physics, solid state
physics, source
physiognomonic anatomy
physiologic
p. action
p. activity
p. activity, selected
p. alterations in body
p. amenorrhea
p. anemia
p. atrophy
p. basis

p. congestion
p. cup
p. cup, large
p. disorder
p. dwarf
p. effect
p. elasticity of muscle
p. electroencephalogram (EEG) rhythms
p. epilepsy
p. function
p. function, normal
p. habit
p. hypogammaglobulinemia
p. incompatibility
p. jaundice
p. limits, within
p. low stress angioplasty (PLSA)
p. measurement
p. mechanism
p. murmur
p. occlusion
p. pacing
p. pattern release
p. psychology
p. reflexes
p. response
p. rest position
p. scotoma
p. third heart sound
p. tremor
p. zero

physiological
p. addiction
p. age
p. anatomy
p. arousal
p. arousal, reducing
p. awakening
p. change
p. chemistry
p. cravings
p. crown
p. dead space
p. dependence
p. disturbance
p. factor
p. factors ▸ genetic and
p. factors in drug abuse
p. faint
p. function
p. function of cell
p. functioning
p. functioning, optimal
p. malfunction

p. modification
p. monitoring
p. musculoskeletal reaction
p. needs
p. overreactivity
p. problems ▸ underlying
p. process
p. psychology
p. ramifications
p. response
p. response to relaxation training
p. retina
p. saline
p. saline solution
p. saline, sterile
p. sounds
p. state, voluntary control of
p. stimuli
p. stress
p. third heart sound
p. variables
p. variant
p. withdrawal
physiologically unstable ▸ patient
physiologist, exercise
physiology
p. acid base
p., body
p., cardiovascular
p., cellular
p., disease and treatment
p., electro◇
p., exercise
p., NREM (nonrapid eye movement)
p., obstructive
p. of heart contraction
p. of menopause
p. of sleep
p., pattern of stress
p., pulmonary
p., respiratory
p., restrictive
p., sensory
physiopathology of fatigue
physiotherapy (PT)
physiotherapy, chest
physiotherapy, gentle
physique anxiety
Physocephalus sexalatus
Physotigma venenosum
phytohemagglutinin, lymphocyte
   irradiation and
PI (pulmonary incompetence)
PI (pulmonary infarction)
pi cell

pia
p. arachnoid
p. intima
p. mater encephali
p. mater of brain
p. mater spinalis
pian bois
piano percussion
piaulement, bruit de
Piazza's fluid
Piazza's test
Pic syndrome ▸ Bard-
PICA (pica)
P. (posterior inferior cerebellar
   artery)
P. (posterior inferior communicating
   artery)
P. (posterior inferior cerebellar
   artery) aneurysm
p. artifact
picipes, Melanolestes
pick(s) (Pick)
p. at skin
p. at skin ▸ patient
P. body
p., Burch's
P. cells
P. cells, Niemann-
P. convolutional artery
P. convolutional atrophy
P. disease
P. disease, Niemann-
P. retinitis
P., Rhein's
P. syndrome
p. view ▸ ice-
P. vision
Picker Vanguard deep therapy unit
picker's disease, apple
picking and excoriating of skin
picking, skin
pickup toe exercise ▸ marble
pickwickian syndrome
picocurie (pCi/pc)
picofarad (pf)
picofarads, measured in
Picornaviridae virus
picornavirus
pictor, Aspergillus
pictorial aphasia
picture(s) (Picture)
p., anodal closing
p., clinical
p., digital recorded
p. element (pixel)

p. of operation ▸ authorization form
   for taking of motion
p. of operation ▸ consent form for
   taking of motion
P. -Story Test ▸ Make-A-
p. test, Blacky
PICU (Prenatal Intensive Care Unit)
**PICU (Pulmonary Intensive Care
Unit)**
Pic-Ups, Surgical Lint
PID (pelvic inflammatory disease)
PID (pelvic inflammatory disease) ▸
   chronic
PID (pelvic inflammatory disease)
   residues ▸ chronic
PID (pelvic inflammatory disease) ▸
   sexually transmitted
**PIE (pulmonary infiltration and
eosinophilia)**
**PIE (pulmonary interstitial
emphysema)**
piece of tissue, wedge-shaped
piecemeal, lesion resected
piecemeal removal of kidney
pieces, fragments splintered to
piechaudii, Alcaligenes
Piedmont fracture
Piedraia hortae
pierced ear
piercing
p., body
p., cheek
p., ear
p., eyebrow
p., navel
p., nose
p., tongue
Pierquin position, Laquerriere-
Pierre Robin syndrome
Pierson attachment
Pietrie's cast
PIF (peak inspiratory flow)
PIFR (peak inspiratory flow rate)
Pig (pig)
P. ABS, Guinea
p. bronchus
p. cell implant
p. cell transplant ▸ fetal
p. inoculation, guinea
p. insulin
pigeon
p. breast
p. breast deformity
p. breeder's disease
p. breeder's lung

pigeon—*continued*
p. chest
p. toe
piggyback lens
piggy-backing IV (intravenous) fluids
pigment(s)
p., accumulation of bile
p., bile
p., blood
p., carbon
p. cell
p. cell ▸ retinal
p., cirrhosis
p., color
p., composition
p., deposit of
p., derangement
p., disruption
p., epithelium
p., epithelium, dysfunctional
p., epithelium, retinal
p., gallstones ▸ prone to developing
p., granules
p., hemofuscin
p., implantation
p., laded macrophages, brown
p., Lake's
p., lipochrome
p., lipofuscin
p., melanin
p. ▸ produce excess bile
p. -producing cells
p. -producing rays
p., regenerate hair
p., rejection
p., seam
p., skin
p., stones
p. test, bile
pigmentary
p. atrophy
p. changes
p. cirrhosis
p. deposits on lens
p. glaucoma
p. migration
p. retinopathy
pigmentation(s)
p., area of increased
p. ▸ blemishes, eruptions or
p. changes
p. changes, radiation
p., dark
p., foreign
p. ▸ gingival and oral mucosa

p., hematogenous
p., liver
p., mucocutaneous
p. of fundus
p. ▸ scattered fibrosis without
p., scleral
p., skin
p., stasis
p. ▸ symmetrical patches of
p., tourniquet
pigmented
p. ameloblastoma
p. basal cell carcinoma
p. cells, melanin-
p. epithelium, senile atrophy of
p. growth
p. lesion
p. lesion of skin
p. mole
p. nevus
p. nodule
p. tunic, vascular
pigmentosa
p., pseudoretinitis
p., psilosis
p., retinitis
p. syndrome ▸ retinitis
p., urticaria
pigmentosum, xeroderma
Pignet's standard
pigskin, split thickness graft of
pigtail
p. catheter
p. catheter placement, nasobiliary
p. curl, stent tube with
p. nephrostomy drain
Pila conica
pilaris, keratosis
pilaris, pityriasis rubra
pile, sentinel
pill(s) (Pill)
p. amenorrhea, post-
p. and capsules
p., birth control
p., calcium
p. ▸ chlamydia from birth control
p., contraceptive
p. ▸ fatigue from birth control
p. ▸ hair loss from birth control
p. ▸ hepatitis from birth control
p. ▸ high blood pressure (BP) from birth control
P. (phenylisopropylamine), Love
P., LSD (lysergic acid diethylamide) Peace

p. mass
p. ▸ menstrual period with birth control
p. ▸ migraine headache from birth control
p., multiphasic
p. ▸ nipple discharge from birth control
p. ▸ nose stuffiness from birth control
P. (amphetamines), Pep
p. ▸ phlebitis from birth control
p. ▸ problem with central nervous system from diet
p., radio
p. rolling motion
p. ▸ skin disorder from birth control
P. (barbiturates), Sleeping
p. ▸ slow-dissolving fluoride
P., STP (Serenity-Tranquility-Peace)
p. ▸ swelling from birth control
p., tanning
p. ▸ wireless video
pillar(s)
p., anterior
p., anterior faucial
p. cells
p. cells, inner
p. cells, outer
p., inner
p., iris
p. of Corti's organ
p. of diaphragm
p. of fauces
p. of fauces, anterior
p. of fauces, posterior
p. of fornix, anterior
p. of fornix, posterior
p. of iris replaced with spatula
p. of soft palate
p., outer
p. projection
p. replaced, iris
p., tonsillar
p., Uskow's
Pillat's dystrophy
Pilling's tube
pillion fracture
pillow
p. inserted under shoulder
p. orthopnea, three-
p. orthopnea, two-
pilocarpine iontophoresis sweat test ▸ quantitative

pilocystic astrocytoma
pilocystic astrocytoma ▸ juvenile
pilocytic cerebellar astrocytoma ▸
    macrocystic
pilocytic cerebellar astrocytoma ▸
    microcystic
piloid astrocytoma
pilomotor
    p. disturbance
    p. erection
    p. nerves
    p. reflex
pilonidal
    p. area
    p. cyst
    p. cyst, infected
    p. cystectomy
    p. infection
    p. sinus
    p., tailbone pain from cyst
pilorum muscles, arrectores
pilosebaceous opening
pilosebaceous unit
pilosellus, Cimex
pilosus
    p., Damalinia
    p., Ixodes
    p., nevus
    p., Trichodectes
pilot study
pilot study in clinical trials
Piltz reflex, Westphal-
Piltz's reflex
pilular mass
pilus, sex
pilus tortus
pimprina, Streptomyces
PIMS (programmable implantable
    medication system)
pin(s)
    p. and needles ▸ feeling of
    p. -and-needles sensation
    p., Austin-Moore
    p., Bohlman
    p., Compete's
    p. -cushion distortion
    p., Deyerle
    p., guide
    p., Hagie hip
    p., Hansen-Street
    p., Hatcher's
    p. hole collimator
    p. implant
    p., Knowles'
    p., Lottes'

p., Moore
p., Pischel's
p., Pischel's micro◇
p., Rush intramedullary
p. sensation, needles-and-
p. sensation, touch-and-
p., Steinmann's
p., Street-type medullary
p. teeth, cross-
p. teeth, straight-
p. tract
p. tract infection
p. traction, McBride tripod
p., Turner's
p., von Saal medullary
p., Walker's
p., Zimmer
Pinard's maneuver
Pinard's sign
pince, main en
pinch
    p. bruises, devil's
    p. graft
    p. graft technique, Braun
    p. nose shut
pinchcock mechanism
pinched nerve
pinched sciatic nerve
pinching pain
pine resin colophony
pineal
    p. body
    p. body, peduncle of
    p. eye
    p. gland
    p. gland calcification
    p. gland calcified
    p. peduncle
    p. tumor
pineale, corpus
Pinel's system
ping-pong fracture
ping-pong mechanism
pinheaded sperm
pinhole
    p. goggles
    p. pupil
    p. tomography ▸ seven
pining, yearning and sadness
pink(s) (Pink)
    p. and moist, mouth
    p. and moist, mucosa
    p. and warm, skin tone
    p. disease
    P. Ladies (barbiturates)

p. mucous membranes
p. mucous membranes of lips
p. puffers (PP)
P., Reds and Blues (barbiturates)
p. sputum
p. tetralogy of Fallot
p. tooth, Mummery's
p. white, lungs
pinked up
pinkish
    p., blood-tinged sputum
    p. lesion
    p. vaginal discharge
pinna
    p., bifid
    p., malformation of
    p., pointed
    p. prosthesis, ear
pinned, femur
pinning, hip
pinning, root canal silver
Pinoyella simii
pinpoint
    p. os
    p. pupils
    p. subpleural blebs
pinprick analgesia
pinprick, diminished sensation to
pintae, Treponema
pinworm infection
pion
    p. beam
    p. dosimetry
    p. generator, medical
Piotrowski's sign
PIP (proximal interphalangeal)
pipe
    p. ▸ artificial tear
    p. colon, lead
    p., glass
    p. rigidity, lead
    p. stem cirrhosis
    p. -stem stool
    p., tear
PIPIDA Scan
pipiens, Culex
piping rales, loud
pipistrella, Cimex
PIPJ (proximal interphalangeal joint)
Pirenella conica
PIRI (postischemic reperfusion
    injury)
Pirie transoral projection
Pirie's bone

piriform (*same as* **pyriform**)
- p. aperture
- p. crest
- p. fossa
- p. muscle
- p. opening
- p. process
- p. sinus
- p. thorax

piriformis syndrome
Pirogoff's amputation
Pirogoff's edema
Pirquet reaction ▸ quanti-
piscatorum, Serratia
Pisces Sigma ▸ unipolar
Pischel's
- P. electrode
- P. micropins
- P. pin

pisiform bone
pisiformis, Taenia
Piskacek's sign
pisohamate ligament
pisometacarpal ligament
pistol-shot femoral sound
pistol-shot pulse
piston
- p. prosthesis, ear
- p. prosthesis ▸ Schuknecht Teflon wire
- p. pulse
- p. strut
- p. -type prosthesis

PIT (plasma iron turnover)
Pitanguy mammaplasty, Aries-
Pitanguy mammary ptosis procedure, Aries-
pitch
- p., absolute
- p., monotonous voice
- p. warts
- p. -workers' cancer

pitched
- p. murmur ▸ high-
- p. murmur ▸ low-
- p. noises ▸ loud, high-
- p. ringing in ear ▸ low
- p. sounds ▸ high

pitchers' elbow, baseball
Pitcher's hemostatic bag
pithecoid idiot
pithecoid pelvis
Pithomyces chartarum
Pitney thromboplastin generation test ▸ Hicks-

Pitocin
- P. augmentation of labor
- P. (DIVP) ▸ dilute intravenous
- P. drip
- P. drip ▸ intravenous (IV)

pitressin spray, lysine
pits, gastric
Pitt talking tracheostomy tube
pitting
- p., acne
- p. edema
- p. edema all extremities ▸ severe
- p. edema lower extremities
- p. edema of ankles
- p. edema, severe
- p. of the skin

Pittsburgh pneumonia
pituitarigenic oculopathy
pituitary
- p. acromicria
- p. adamantinoma
- p. adenoma
- p. adenoma, cystic
- p. adrenal axis ▸ hypophyseal
- p. -adrenal (HPA) axis ▸ hypothalamic-
- p. adrenocortical axis (HPAA) ▸ hypothalamic
- p. ameloblastoma
- p. amenorrhea
- p., anterior
- p. apoplexy
- p. cachexia
- p. cells ▸ entrapped anterior
- p. Cushing's disease
- p. disorder
- p. dwarf
- p. dwarfism
- p. eunuchism
- p. extract
- p. extract, anterior
- p. folds
- p. fossa
- p. gigantism
- p. gland
- p. gland, anterior
- p. gland, anterior lobe of
- p. gland, anterior lobule of
- p. gland, hormone output of
- p. gland, intermediate lobe of
- p. gland, posterior lobe of
- p. gland, stimulate
- p. gonadotropin, human
- p. growth hormone
- p. hormone

- p. hormone, posterior
- p. hormone trigger ovulation
- p. hormones, circulating
- p., human
- p. hyperfunction
- p. lesion
- p. microadenoma
- p. reproductive hormones
- p. secretion
- p. stalk
- p. stimulation
- p. synergist
- p. tumor
- p. tumor ▸ endocrine inactive
- p. tumor, hyperfunctional
- p. tumor, prolactin secreting

Pituitrin injected into uterus
pity ▸ full of self-
pity ▸ patient filled with self-
pityriasis [*psoriasis*]
- p. rosea
- p. rubra pilaris
- p. simplex
- p. versicolor

Pityrosporon orbiculare
Pityrosporon ovale
pivot
- p. joint
- p. shift test
- p. shift test in lateral position
- p. shift test of MacIntosh
- p. transfer
- p. transfer of wheelchair

pixel (picture element)
P-J interval
PJRT (permanent junctional reciprocating tachycardia)
PKD (polycystic kidney disease)
PKD (polycystic kidney disease), autosomal dominant
PKU (phenylketonuria)
PL (pulpolingual)
PLA (peripiheral laser angioplasty)
PLa (pulpolabial)
PLA (pulpolinguoaxial)
place
- p. and person ▸ oriented to time,
- p. and time, disorientation in
- p. and time ▸ patient oriented as to person,
- p., catheter in
- p., confusion about time and
- p., drainage (dr'ge) tube in
- p. ▸ endotracheal tubes in
- p., graft sutured in

p. ▸ patient has endotracheal tube in
p., screw plate in
p. ▸ subclavian line in
p., thoracotomy tube in
p., tracheostomy tube in

placebo
p., alternating
p. control group
p. control prophylactic study ▸ double-blind
p. control study ▸ double-blind
p. controlled clinical trial
p. controlled experiment
p. controlled study
p. controlled study, crossover
p. controlled trial
p. controlled trial ▸ randomized,
p. controlled trial ▸ randomized double-blinded
p. controls
p. effect
p., inactive
p. injection
p., medically inactive
p., nonmedicine
p., patient given
p., patient treated with
p., pure lactose
p. regimen
p. relief
p. therapy
p. trial, double-blind

placed
p. at bed rest, patient
p. for support, sandbag
p. graft ▸ catheter
p. graft ▸ surgically
p. in Croupette, patient
p. in incubator, infant
p. in isolation, patient
p. in isolette, infant
p. in position, electrodes
p. in traction, patient
p. in warmer, infant
p. into wound, drain
p. on scalp, electrodes
p. on surface of head, electrodes
p., tracheostomy tube
p. under Bili-Lites ▸ infant

placei, Haemonchus
placement
p., adoption
p. and prognosis
p., arterial line

p., arterial line monitor catheter
p., biofeedback electrode
p., catheter
p., chest tube
p., clinical
p. consideration
p. ▸ coronary stent
p. decisions, treatment
p., demographic
p., discharge
p., EEG (electroencephalogram) electrode
p., effects of
p., electrode
p., esophageal prosthesis
p., foster
p., foster home
p., halfway house
p., implant
p. in radiation therapy, block
p., intracavitary container
p., lead
p., mucoperiosteal implant
p., nasobiliary pigtail catheter
p., nonthoracotomy lead
p., nursing home
p. of electrodes, bipolar
p. of stent
p. on forehead, electrode
p., parietal-occipital (parietooccipital)
p., passive
p., patient
p., permanent pacemaker
p. program
p. program for adolescents ▸ patient
p. program for adults ▸ patient
p. program, patient
p., protective
p. ▸ rational/empirical clinical
p., residential
p., retropubic
p., site of electrode
p., standard electrode
p., status postfistula
p., stent
p., Surgicel gauze implant
p., Surgicel implant
p., temporary transvenous pacemaker
p., tube
p., vertex
p., walker

placenta
p., accessory
p. accreta
p., adherent
p., annular
p., battledore
p., bidiscoidal
p., bilobate
p., bilobed
p., biopsy of
p. bipartita
p., bipartite
p., chorioallantoic
p., choriovitelline
p. circumvallata
p., circumvallate
p., cirsoid
p. cirsoides
p., cyst of
p., deciduous
p. delivered
p. delivered intact
p. delivered manually
p. diffusa
p. dimidiata
p., discoid
p. discoidea
p., duplex
p., endotheliochorial
p., epitheliochorial
p. expelled
p. extracted
p. febrilis
p. fenestrata
p., fetal
p., fibrosis of
p. foetalis
p., fundal
p., furcate
p., hematoma of
p., hemochorial
p., hemoendothelial
p., horseshoe
p., incarcerated
p. increta
p., infarction of
p. inflamed
p. intact
p., labyrinthine
p., lobed
p., low insertion of
p., low lying
p., manual delivery of
p., manual removal of
p. marginalis

placenta—*continued*
- p. marginata
- p., maternal
- p. membranacea
- p., multilobate
- p., multilobed
- p. multipartita
- p. nappiformis
- p., nondeciduous
- p. obsoleta
- p., panduriform
- p., panduriformis
- p. percreta
- p. praevia
- p. praevia, marginal
- p., premature separation of
- p. previa
- p. previa centralis
- p. previa marginalis
- p. previa partialis
- p. previa, total
- p. reflexa
- p. removed manually
- p. reniformis
- p., retained
- p., retention of
- p. scan
- p., Schultze's
- p. spuria
- p., stone
- p. succenturiata
- p., succenturiate
- p., syndesmochorial
- p. triloba
- p., trilobate
- p. tripartita
- p., tripartite
- p. triplex
- p. truffée
- p. uterina
- p., uterine
- p., velamentous
- p., villous
- p., yolk sac
- p., zonary
- p., zonular

placentae
- p., ablatio
- p., abruptio
- p., marginal abruptio
- p. marginalis, abruptio
- p., pars fetalis
- p., pars uterina

placentaire, bruit

placental
- p. abruption
- p. barrier
- p. bleeding
- p. bruit
- p. circulation
- p. cotyledon
- p. dysfunction
- p. dysfunction syndrome
- p. dystocia
- p. epithelium
- p. forceps
- p. fragment
- p. fragments, retention of
- p. growth hormone
- p. immunity
- p. insufficiency
- p. lactogen
- p. lactogen (HPL) and plasma, human
- p. lactogen, human
- p. membrane, fetal
- p. membranes
- p. presentation
- p. residual blood volume
- p. respiration
- p. septum
- p. site
- p. souffle
- p. stage
- p. thrombosis
- p. tissue
- p. tissue, necrotic
- p. tissue, retained
- p. tissue tumor
- p. transfusion
- p. transport
- p. villi

placentogram, displacement
Placido's disc
placing of clamps
placoides, Leptotrichia
plagarumbelli, Diplococcus
plagiocephalic idiocy
plague
- p., bubonic
- p. conjunctivitis, squirrel
- p., heroin
- p., human
- p., meningitis
- p. pharyngitis
- p. pneumonia
- p., pneumonic

plain [*plane*]
- p. catgut

- p. catgut, fine
- p. catgut, interrupted
- p. catgut, periosteum closed with
- p. catgut sutures
- p. film
- p. gut
- p. gut suture
- p. old balloon angioplasty (POBA)
- p. view
- p. x-ray
- p. zinc paste, Lassar's

plan(s) (Plan)
- p., aftercare
- p. ahead, failure to
- p. ahead ▸ impulsivity to
- p., comprehensive health
- p., developing treatment
- p., development of discharge
- p. ▸ health care rationing
- p., individual treatment
- p., individualized treatment
- p., initial psychiatric treatment
- p., low fat eating
- p. ▸ managed behavioral health
- P., Master Treatment
- p., multidisciplinary
- p., nursing care
- p., nutrition
- p., process of treatment
- p., relapse prevention
- p. review, treatment
- p., suicidal
- p., suicide
- p. ▸ unavoidable changes in

plana
- p., cornea
- p., coxa
- p. juvenilis, verruca
- p., pelvis
- p., verruca
- p., vertebra

planar
- p. imaging ▸ echo
- p. myocardial imaging
- p. scintigraphy ▸ thallium-201
- p. thallium scintigraphy
- p. thallium test

Planck's constant
Planck's quantum theory
plane(s) [*plain*]
- p., Addison's
- p., Aeby's
- p. aortography ▸ single
- p., axial
- p., coronal

p., cove
p., cross-sectional
p., dose calculated in a tangential
p. dose of rads in fractions, mid-
   sagittal
p., fascial
p., fracture bilaterally in a horizontal
p., frontal
p., horizontal
p., intra-aural
p. joint
p. lens, iris
p., longitudinal
p., median
p., median-sagittal
p., midsagittal
p. needle, implant, two
p. of body
p. of contact lens
p. of iris
p., orthogonal
p., parasagittal
p. radium implant, two
p., sagittal
p. sensitivity
p., short-axis
p., sternal
p., sternoxiphoid
p., subcutaneous
p. tomography, focal
p., transaxial
p., transverse
p., vertical
p. wart
p., wire osteotomy
p. xanthoma
p. xanthoma, generalized
planing, root
planned dose of rads
Planned Parenthood
planning
p., aftercare
p. and simulation, treatment
p., anticipatory
p., balanced nutritional
p., complete aftercare
p., computer assisted menu
p. deficit, motor
p., discharge
p., family
p. format, treatment
p. ▸ joint treatment
p., meal
p., motor
p., multidisciplinary treatment

p., natural family
p. process, discharge
p., quality assurance in treatment
p., treatment
plano lens, Coquille
planoconcave lens
planoconvex lens
planographic examination
planovalgus feet
planovalgus, taipes
plant(s)
p. alkaloid
p., allergy to
p. genome
p., Indian hemp
p. material, dried
p. parasite
p. poisoning
p. protease test
p. toxicity
p. viruses
plantanoides, Acer
plantar
p. arch
p. aspect
p. aspect of foot
p. calcaneal spur
p. compartmental anatomy
p. desquamation
p. digital nerves of lateral plantar
   nerve ▸ common
p. digital nerves of lateral plantar
   nerve ▸ proper
p. digital nerves of medial plantar
   nerve ▸ common
p. digital nerves of medial plantar
   nerve ▸ proper
p. digital veins
p. erythema
p. extensor responses
p. fascia
p. fascia ▸ irritated
p. fascia, release of
p. fasciitis
p. fibroma
p. flexion
p. flexors
p. flexors, weakness of
p. interosseous muscles
p. ischemia
p. ischemia test
p. ligament
p. metatarsal vein
p. nerve ▸ common plantar digital
   nerves of lateral

p. nerve ▸ common plantar digital
   nerves of medial
p. nerve, lateral
p. nerve, medial
p. nerve ▸ proper plantar digital
   nerves of lateral
p. nerve ▸ proper plantar digital
   nerves of medial
p. neuroma
p. puncture wound
p. reflex
p. reflexes flexor
p. regions of toes
p. response
p. response, extensor
p. response, flexor
p. response, normal
p. surface
p. thallium scintigraphy
p. verrucae
p. view
p. wart
plantaris, keratosis
plantaris, verruca
plantarum, Lactobacillus
plantodorsal projection
planum temporalis
planum, xanthoma
planus
p. from dentures ▸ lichen
p., lichen
p., pes
plaque(s)
p. accumulation
p., amyloid
p. and tangles
p. and tangles of Alzheimer's
   disease, brain
p., argyrophile
p., arterial
p., arteriosclerotic
p. assay ▸ hemolytic
p., atheromatous
p., atherosclerotic
p. bacteria
p., bacterial
p., bacteriophage
p., blockage of
p. blockage, vaporize
p., brain
p. buildup
p. buildup ▸ fatty
p. buildup, reversing
p., calcified
p., calcium

plaque(s)—*continued*

p., carcinoid
p., carotid
p., cholesterol
p. ▸ cholesterol-filled
p., cholesterol-laden
p., chorionic
p. -cleaning agent
p., cobalt-60 eye
p., coronary
p. cracker ▸ Leveen
p., dental
p. deposit
p. deposits, abnormal
p., diaphragmatic
p., disease
p. disruption
p., echolucent
p., endocardial
p., fat-laden
p., fatty
p., fatty thickened
p., fibrofatty
p., fibromyelinic
p., fibrous
p. fissuring
p. ▸ flush out
p., foamy interstitial
p. formation
p. formation, localized
p. -forming cell
p. forming units (PFU)
p. fracture
p., fragmented
p., Hollenhorst
p. in arteries, fatty
p. in atherosclerosis patient ▸
   artery-clogging
p. in blood vessels, fatty
p. in brain ▸ neuron destroying
p. in the brain
p. in vessel walls ▸ fatty
p. inhibitor
p., intimal foamy
p., intraluminal
p., laser vaporized
p., Lichtheim's
p. -like lesion
p. ▸ lipid-filled atherosclerotic
p. ▸ lipid-rich
p., microscopic
p., mucous
p., myointimal
p., neuritic
p. ▸ neuritic senile

p., neuritis
p. obstructing artery ▸ fracture
p. obstruction
p. ▸ odor-causing
p. of Alzheimer's disease
p. of multiple sclerosis
p., opaline
p., Peyer's
p., pleural
p., Randall's
p., Redlich-Fisher miliary
p. regression
p. removal devices
p. rupture
p. rupture, atherosclerotic
p., residual
p., senile
p., septicemic
p., shaved
p. ▸ shelf of
p., stable
p., sticky
p. strutting
p., subintimal
p., submucosal
p., talc
p. therapy ▸ arterial
p., thickened whitish
p. to cutting mechanism ▸ exposing
p., ulcerated
p., ulcerating
p., unstable
p., vaporized
p. victims
p. ▸ wheals and
p., white
p., whitish

plaquing, candida
plaquing, pleural
plasm, germ
plasma

p., acetone
p. aldosterone, urine and
p., antilymphocyte
p., antipseudomonas human
p., blood
p. catecholamines
p. cell antigen
p. cell ▸ bizarre giant
p. cell count
p. cell granuloma
p. cell hepatitis
p. cell infiltrate
p. cell leukemia
p. cell mastitis

p. cell pneumonia
p. cell pneumonia, interstitial
p. cell tumors
p. cell vulvitis
p. cells
p. cells, multinucleated
p. cells, proliferating
p. cells, vacuolated
p. cholesterol, fasting
p. coagulation system
p. ▸ colloid osmotic pressure of
p. component therapy
p. concentration
p. defect
p. depletion
p., deuterium
p. ▸ donated human
p., donor
p. endothelin concentration
p. erythropoietin
p. exchange
p. exchange column
p. exchange therapy
p. expander
p. expander ▸ hetastarch
p. flow (ERPF) ▸ effective renal
p. flow (RPF) ▸ renal
p. fraction
p., fresh frozen
p., frozen
p. glucose disappearance rate
p. glucose, fasting
p. glucose ▸ postprandial
p. glucose tolerance test
p. hemorrhage
p., honey colored
p., human placental lactogen (HPL)
   and
p., infectious blood
p. infusion
p. infusion ▸ fresh frozen
p. inorganic iodine
p. insulin activity
p. iron disappearance
p. iron disappearance time
p. iron turnover (PIT)
p. iron turnover rate
p. level ▸ human
p. levels
p., lymphoid
p., magnetically confined
p. monitoring
p., normal
p. oncotic pressure (POP)
p. osmolality

p. ▸ patient admitted and transfused with fresh frozen
p., peripheral vein
p. ▸ platelet-poor
p., platelet-rich
p. (U/P) ratio ▸ urine
p. reagin (RPR) ▸ rapid
p. reagin (RPR) test, rapid
p., red cells mixed with
p. renin
p. renin activity
p. renin assay
p. renin levels
p. skimming
p. sodium concentration
p. testosterone measurement
p. thromboplastin antecedent (PTA)
p. thromboplastin component (PTC)
p. transfusion
p., transfusion of fresh frozen
p. triglyceride
p. triglyceride, fasting
p. viscosity
p. volume
p. volume expander
p. volume expander ▸ Hespan
p. volume ▸ reduction in
p. water

plasmacytic leukemia
plasmacytoid lymphocyte
plasmacytoid reticulum cells
plasmacytoma(s)
p., extramedullary
p. of bone, multiple
p., peripheral
plasmapheresis
p. center
p. research
p. treatment
plasmatic stain
plasmatic vascular destruction
plasmic stain
plasmid(s)
p., autonomous
p. -carrying cell
p., episomes and
plasmin mediated resistance
plasminogen
p. activation (TPA) ▸ tissue
p. activator (TPA) infusion ▸ tissue
p. activator inhibitor
p. activator (TPA) ▸ tissue
p. activator ▸ urokinase-type

p. complex ▸ streptokinase
p. -streptokinase complex
plasmocrine vacuole
plasmodium (Plasmodium)
p. embolism
p., exoerythrocytic
p. falciparum
p. malariae
p. ovale
p. pleurodyniae
P. species
p. vivax
p. vivax minuta
Plasmolyte solution
plasmycytic infiltrate, marked
plaster
p. bandage
p. boot
p. cast
p. cast, application of
p. cast, immobilized in
p. dressing
p., encased in
p. of Paris cast
p. of Paris jacket
plastic
p. achillotenotomy
p. anatomy
p. and reconstructive surgery
p. ball, insertion
p. bonding compound
p. braces ▸ ceramic or
p. bronchitis
p. closure
p. endocarditis
p. gel, flexible
p. heart valve
p. hip replacement ▸ metal-on-
p. implant
p. implant material
p. induration
p. iritis
p. lens
p. lens, Thorpe
p. mask for electron beam therapy
p. membrane, thin
p. motor
p. nightguard
p. operation
p. operation on canaliculi
p. operation on eyeball
p. phlebitis
p. pleurisy
p. polymer
p. procedure, reconstructive

p. reconstruction
p. reconstruction of bronchus
p. reconstructive surgeon
p. reconstructive surgery
p. repair
p. repair of anus
p. repair of bronchus
p. repair of defects
p. repair of eyelid
p. repair of orbit
p. revision
p. sewing ring
p. sphere implant
p. splint, molded
p. state
p. surgery
p. surgery, aesthetic
p. surgery, endoscopic
p. surgery ▸ facial
p. surgery ▸ injectable fillers in
p. suture
p. tent isolator
p. tone
plastica, linitis
plastica, penis
plasticity ▸ skeletal muscle
Plasticor torque-type prosthesis
Plastiport TORP (total ossicular replacement prosthesis)
Plastizote collar
plasty
p. closure, multi-sided Z-
p. ▸ endoventricular circular patch
p., eyelid
p. incision, Z-
p. repair, L-
p. revision, W-
p. revision, Z-
p. scar, Z-
p., sliding
p., W-
plate(s) [*state*]
p., affix
p. affixed
p. and screws, bone
p. and screws, Eggers'
p. and screws, McLaughlin
p. and screws, metallic
p. and screws, Neufeld
p. and screws, Sherman
p., Badgley's
p., blade
p., blood agar
p., Blount's
p., blue portion of foot-

plate(s)—*continued*
p., bone
p. ▸ bone growth
p., Brophy's
p., cell
p., cloverleaf
p., complete
p., cribriform
p. culture
p., dental
p., Deyerle
p. dialyzer, parallel
p., dural
p., Eggers'
p., Elliott
p., end
p., epiphyseal
p., epiphyseal growth
p., fracture
p. fracture ▸ volar
p., Fresnel zone
p. hemorrhages ▸ subependymal germinal
p., Hoen's skull
p. in place, screw
p., injury, volar
p., intertrochanteric
p., lower
p., Ishihara's
p., Jaeger's lid
p., Jewett
p., Kessel's
p., Laing's
p., Lane
p., Lawson-Thornton
p. -like atelectasis
p., Massie's
p., McLaughlin
p., metal
p., Moe
p., Moore
p., nail
p. of abdomen, flat
p. of ethmoid, cribriform
p. of ethmoid, perpendicular
p. of nail bed ▸ nail
p., orbital
p., partial
p., photographic
p. potential ▸ miniature end-
p., serpentine
p., Sherman
p., slotted
p., tarsal
p., Thornton

p. thrombosis
p. thrombus
p. thrombus, blood
p., upper
p., vulcanite dental
p. ▸ wet nesting on
p., Wilson's
p., Wright's
p., Zueler hook

plateau
p. fracture, tibial
p., h
p. joint surface, lateral
p., lateral tibial
p., medial
p. phase
p. (PEPP) ▸ positive expiratory pressure
p. prosthesis, Macintosh tibial
p. pulse
p. response
p. speech
p., tibial
p., ventricular

platelet(s)
p. activating factor
p. activity
p. adhesiveness
p. agglutination
p. agglutinin
p. -aggregating factor
p. aggregation
p. aggregation alteration
p., blood
p., circulating
p. clumping in blood
p., clumping of
p. concentrate
p. count
p. count, direct
p. count, indirect
p. count, interval
p. count, low
p. count, reduction of
p., decreased
p. defect
p. derived growth factor (PDGF)
p. destruction
p. disorder
p. disorder, blood
p. dysfunction
p. dysfunction syndrome
p. estimates
p. factor
p. factor 4

p. function
p. imaging
p., in vivo adhesive
p., increased
p. inhibitors
p. level
p. monoamine oxidase activity
p. packs
p. phosphohexokinase
p. plug formation
p. -poor blood
p. -poor plasma
p. ▸ produce blood cells and
p. receptor glycoprotein
p. -rich plasma
p. skimming
p. ▸ stickiness of
p. thrombi
p. thrombosis
p. thrombus
p. thrombus, blood
p. transfusion
p., units of
p. (ZIP) ▸ zoster immune

platform
p. lift
p., posturography
p. walker

Platina Clip implant cataract lens
platinum
p. filter
p. iridium capsule
p. loop

Platt operation, Putti-
platypellic pelvis
platypelloid pelvis
platysma
p. incised
p. muscle
p. myoides

platysmal reflex
plautivincenti, Fusobacterium
Plaut's angina
Plaut-Vincent's angina
play
p., abnormal social
p. ▸ absent or abnormal social
p., absent social
p., evocative
p., fantasy
p. in groups ▸ inability to
p. preference
p. ▸ pretend/imaginative
p. re-enactment
p. ▸ sustained odd

p. therapy
p. therapy ▸ directive group
p. therapy ▸ psychodynamic
playing and response ▸ role-playing, systematic role-
pleasure
p. centers in brain
p. centers of brain, activate
p., end-
p. ▸ inability to feel
p., libidinous
p. or motivation ▸ lack of
p., personal
p., principle
p., sensual
plectonemic coil
PLED (periodic lateralized epileptiform discharges)
pledge card, donor
pledget(s)
p., Dacron
p. ▸ Meadox Teflon felt
p., polypropylene
p. suture buttress ▸ Teflon
p., Teflon
pledgeted mattress suture
PLEDS (periodic lateral epileptiform discharges)
Plenk operation, Bancroft-
pleomorphic
p. adenocarcinoma
p. adenoma
p. adenoma, carcinoma ex
p. cells
p. gram-negative coccobacilli
p. gram-negative rod
p. hyperchromatic nuclei
p. irregularly shaped nuclei ▸ basophilic
p. nuclei
p. premature ventricular complex
p. rod-shaped cells
p. tachycardia
pleomorphism, nuclear
plesiosectional tomography
plethoric dysmenorrhea
plethysmograph
p., body
p., digital
p., finger
p., jerkin
plethysmography
p., air cuff
p., body
p., cuff

p., dynamic venous
p. (IPG), impedance
p., strain gauge
p., thermistor
p., venous
p. ▸ venous occlusion
pleura(-ae)
p., black
p., cervical
p. closed, mediastinal
p., costal
p., costodiaphragmatic recess of
p., costomediastinal recess of
p., cupula of
p., diaphragmatic
p., discission of
p. exposed, mediastinal
p., fat pads of
p. ▸ fibrin bodies of
p., hydrops of
p. incised, mediastinal
p. incised, visceral
p. ▸ inflammation of
p., laceration of
p. ▸ malignant disease of
p., mediastinal
p., mesothelioma of
p., metastases to the
p. mildly inflamed
p., neurofibroma of
p. opened
p., parietal
p., pericardial
p., pulmonary
p., resection of parietal
p. sign, black
p., thickened
p., thickening of
p., visceral
pleural [*plural*]
p. abrasion
p. adhesions
p. adhesions ▸ bilateral apical fibrous
p. adhesions, fibrinous
p. adhesions ▸ fibrinous intraseptal
p. amyloidosis
p. aspergillosis
p. -based tumor
p. biopsy
p. biopsy, closed
p. biopsy punch, Abrams'
p. blebs
p. cap
p. cavity

p. cavity, air in
p. cavity, aspiration
p. cavity, block in
p. cavity entered
p. cavity, fluid in
p. cavity ▸ watery fluid in
p. crackles
p. diaphragmatic adhesions
p. disease
p. drainage (dr'ge) ▸ closed
p. edges approximated
p. effusion (PE)
p. effusion, bilateral
p. effusion ▸ bilateral and right serosanguinous
p. effusion, chyliform
p. effusion ▸ cultures of
p. effusion ▸ exudative
p. effusion, loculated
p. effusion ▸ malignant
p. effusion, massive
p. effusion, recurrent
p. effusion, serosanguinous
p. effusion, serous
p. effusion ▸ transudative
p. empyema
p. exudate
p. fibrin balls
p. fibrosis
p. fibrosis, apical
p. fibrosis, focal
p. fibrous mesothelioma ▸ benign
p. fluid
p. fluid aspiration
p. fluid changes
p. fluid, encapsulated
p. fremitus
p. friction rub
p. inflammatory change
p. involvement, extensive
p. lavage
p. layer, visceral
p. lymph nodes
p. lymphatics
p. mass
p. membrane lining
p. meniscus sign
p. metastases
p. mouse
p., parietal
p. peel
p. pericarditis
p. plaquing
p. poudrage
p. pressure gradients ▸ vertical

pleural—*continued*
- p. pressure ▸ juxtacardiac
- p. rale
- p. reaction
- p. reflection
- p. rings
- p. rub
- p. rub, right
- p. rubs, bilateral
- p. sac
- p. sac free of fluid
- p. sac, left
- p. sac, right
- p. scarring
- p. shock
- p. space
- p. surfaces
- p. symphysis
- p. tag
- p. tap
- p. tear
- p. tents
- p. thickening
- p. thickening, apical
- p. thickening, focal
- p. tube
- p. tube, angled
- p. villi

pleurectomy ▸ thorascopic apical
pleuripotential cells
pleuripotential stem cell
pleurisy
- p., acute
- p., adhesive
- p., blocked
- p., cholesterol
- p., chronic
- p., chyliform
- p., chylous
- p., circumscribed
- p., costal
- p., diaphragmatic
- p., diffuse
- p., double
- p., dry
- p., encysted
- p., exudative
- p., fibrinous
- p., hemorrhagic
- p., ichorous
- p., indurative
- p., interlobar
- p., interlobular
- p., latent
- p., mediastinal

- p., metapneumonic
- p., plastic
- p., primary
- p., proliferating
- p., pulmonary
- p., pulsating
- p., purulent
- p., sacculated
- p., secondary
- p., serofibrinous
- p., serous
- p., single
- p., suppurative
- p., tuberculous
- p., typhoid
- p., visceral
- p., wet
- p. with effusion

pleuritic [*pruritic*]
- p. chest pain
- p. chest pain ▸ bilateral
- p. chest pain ▸ right
- p. effusion
- p. pain
- p. pneumonia
- p. respiration
- p. rub

pleuritis
- p. and emphysema ▸ massive fibrinous
- p., chronic
- p. ▸ fibrinous acute
- p., fibrous
- p. ▸ fibrous and fibrinous
- p., lupus
- p., marked fibrinous
- p., obliterative
- p., severe fibrinous

pleurodesis
- p., mechanical
- p., talc
- p. ▸ thorascopic talc

pleurodynia, epidemic
pleurodyniae, Plasmodium
pleuroesophageal fistula
pleuroesophageal muscle
pleurogenic pneumonia
pleuropericardial
- p. adhesion
- p. rub
- p. window

pleuroperitoneal hernia
pleuroperitoneal shunt, Denver
pleuropneumonia-like organism (PPLO)

pleuropulmonary congestion
plexiform lesion
plexiform neuroma
Plexiglas implant
plexogenic pulmonary arteriopathy
plexopathy, brachial
plexus(es)
- p. activity, brachial
- p., annular
- p., Auerbach's
- p. block, celiac
- p. block (NCPB) ▸ neurolytic celiac
- p., brachial
- p., calcification of choroid
- p., carcinoma of choroid
- p., cardiac
- p., carotid
- p. cavernosus clitoridis
- p., cervical
- p., cholesteatoma of choroid
- p., choroid
- p., enteric
- p., esophageal
- p., excision of choroid
- p., ganglia of sympathetic
- p., hypogastric
- p., intraepithelial
- p. involvement, brachial
- p., Kiesselbach's
- p., laryngeal
- p., lumbar
- p., mediastinal
- p., Meissner's
- p., mucoid
- p., myenteric
- p. nerve block, cervical
- p. of clitoris, cavernosus
- p. of Santorini
- p. of ventricles, choroid
- p., ophthalmic
- p., ophthalmicus
- p., ovarian
- p. ovaricus
- p. palsy, brachial
- p., pampiniform
- p. pampiniformis
- p., perimuscular
- p., perimysial
- p., pharyngeal
- p., prostatic
- p., prostaticovesical
- p., pulmonary
- p., renal
- p., sacral

p., Santorini's
p., solar
p., spermatic
p., subepithelial
p., subpleural mediastinal
p., suprarenal
p., testicular
p., tympanic
p., ureteric
p., uterine
p., uterovaginal
p. uterovaginalis
p., vaginal
p., vascular
p. venosus vaginalis
p., venous
p., vertebral
p., vesical
p., vesicoprostatic
PLF (perilymphatic fistula)
pliable, skin
pliable, vagina soft and
plica
p. isthmicae tubae uterinae
p. nasi
p. nervi laryngei
p. palpebronasalis
p. pubovesicalis
p. rectouterina
p. salpingopharyngea
p. stapedis
p. supratonsillaris
p., synovial
p. triangularis
p. vesicalis transversa
p. vocalis
plicae
p. ampullares tubae uterinae
p. ciliares
p. iridis
p. palmatae
p. tubariae tubae uterinae
p. vaginae
plicata, lingua
plicate [*ligate*]
plicated tongue
plicatilis, Spirochaeta
plication [*ligation*]
plication, fundal
plication sutures
pliers, Allen's root
pliers, crown-crimping
PLMD (periodic limb movement disorder)

PLMS (periodic limb movements in sleep)
plombage/plumbage
plombage, extraperiosteal
plop sound ▸ tumor
PLSA (physiologic low stress angioplasty)
plug(s)
p., bile
p., bone
p., cotton
p., Dittrich's
p. formation, platelet
p., Imlach's fat
p., Mackenty's choanal
p., mucous
p., mucus
p. of tumor
p., punctal
p. syndrome, meconium
p. tear ducts
plugged
p. artery
p. ear
p., endoprosthesis
p. tube
plugging
p., mucus
p. of bronchial tree ▸ mucus
p., stent
plumb line sign
Plummer('s)
P. disease
P. -Vinson applicator
P. -Vinson radium applicator
P. -Vinson syndrome
plunger CPR (cardiopulmonary resuscitation) ▸ toilet
plunging goiter
plural [*pleural*]
plural pregnancy
pluripotent state
PLV (partial liquid ventilation)
plymuthica, Serratia
PMB (percutaneous mitral balloon) valvuloplasty
PMC (pain management control)
PMH (past medical history)
P/MH (physically/multiple handicapped)
PMI
PMI (point of maximum impulse)
PMI (point of maximum intensity)
PMI 5th ICS (point of maximum impulse fifth intercostal space)

PMN/LPF (polymorphonuclears per low powered field)
PMP (previous menstrual period)
PMR (percutaneous myocardial revascularization)
PMR (polymyalgia rheumatica)
PMS (premenstrual syndrome)
PMT (pacemaker-mediated tachycardia)
PMT (premenstrual tension)
PMZ (postmenopausal zest)
PND
PND (paroxysmal nocturnal dyspnea)
PND (postnasal discharge)
PND (postnasal drainage)
PND (postnasal drip)
PND (purulent nasal drainage)
pneocardiac reflex
pneumatic
p. antishock garment
p. antishock trousers
p. cells
p. compression boots ▸ intermittent
p. compression ▸ intermittent
p. compression stockings
p. conveying system
p. cuff
p. dilatation of esophagus
p. dilation
p. dilation and cardiomyotomy
p. larynx
p. lesion
p. otoscopy
p. retinopexy
p. space
p. tourniquet
p. tourniquet control
p. tourniquet controlled bleeding
p. tube conveyor
pneumatotherapy, electro◊
pneumobacillus, Friedländer's
pneumococcal
p. bacteria
p. bloodstream infection
p. conjugate vaccine
p. disease
p. disease ▸ invasive
p. empyema
p. infection
p. meningitis
p. pneumonia
p., polyvalent

pneumococcal—*continued*
  p. vaccination
  p. vaccine
pneumococci
  ‣ penicillin-resistant
pneumococcus
  p. bacteria
  p. in vitro fetal anomalies
  p. microorganism
  p. nephritis
  p., resistant
  p. ‣ resistant strains of
pneumoconiosis
  p., asbestos
  p., coal workers'
  p., collagenous
  p., fibrogenic
  p., mica
  p., noncollagenous
  p. ‣ organic dust
  p., rheumatoid
  p. siderotica
  p., silicotic
  p., talc
  p. type disease
Pneumocystis
  P. carinii
  P. carinii pneumonia (PCP)
  P. carinii pneumonitis
  P. choroiditis
  P. pneumonitis
pneumoencephalogram (PEG)
pneumoencephalomyelogram study
pneumogastric nerve
pneumogram (PG)
pneumography, cerebral
pneumography, retroperitoneal
pneumonectomy
  p., complete
  p., left radical
  p., partial
  p., radical
  p., right radical
  p., total
pneumonia
  p., abortive
  p. ‣ acquired immune deficiency
    syndrome (AIDS) related
  p., acute
  p. ‣ acute bronchial
  p., acute interstitial
  p., adenoviral
  p. alba
  p., alcohol
  p., alcoholic

p., amebic
p., anthrax
p., apex
p., apical
p. apostematosa
p., aspiration
p., atypical
p., bacterial
p., bilious
p., bronchial
p., bronchiolitis obliterans
  organizing
p., Buhl's desquamative
p., Candida
p., Carrington
p., caseous
p., catarrhal
p. -causing bacterium
p. -causing organism
p., central
p., cerebral
p., cheesy
p. ‣ chest pain from
p., chills with
p., Chlamydia
p., chronic
p., chronic eosinophilic
p., chronic fibrous
p., cold agglutinin
p. community-acquired
p. ‣ community-acquired lobar
p., confluent
p., congenital aspiration
p., core
p., Corrigan's
p., coughing from
p., croupous
p., deglutition
p., Desnos'
p., desquamative
p., desquamative interstitial
p. dissecans
p., double
p., Eaton agent
p., embolic
p., eosinophilic
p., ephemeral
p., ether
p., extensive aspiration
p., fibrinous
p. ‣ fibrinous acute lobar
p., fibrous
p., focal acute
p., Friedländer's
p., Friedländer's bacillus

p., gangrenous
p. ‣ gelatinous acute
p., giant cell
p., gram-negative
p., Haemophilus influenzae
p., Hecht's
p., herpes
p., hospital-acquired
p., hypersensitivity
p., hypostatic
p. ‣ idiopathic acute eosinophilic
p. ‣ idiopathic interstitial
p., indurative
p. infection ‣ Mycobacterium
p. ‣ influenza virus
p., influenzal
p., inhalation
p. inoculation
p., interlobularis purulenta
p., interstitial
p., interstitial organizing
p., interstitial plasma cell
p., intrauterine
p., Kaufman's
p., Klebsiella
p., left upper lobe (LUL)
p., Legionella
p., Legionnaire's
p., lingular
p., lipoid
p., lobar
p., lobular
p., Löffler's
p., Louisiana
p. ‣ lymphoid interstitial
p., massive
p., measles
p., metastatic
p. microbes
p., migratory
p., mycoplasmal
p., necrotizing
p., nosocomial
p., obstructive
p. ‣ oil aspiration
p., opportunistic
p., organizing aspiration
p. oxygen (O₂) therapy ‣ organizing
  interstitial
p., parenchymatous
p., patchy
p. ‣ peptic aspiration
p., peribronchial
p., Pittsburgh
p. ‣ plasma cell

p., pleuritic
p., pleurogenic
p., pneumococcal
p., Pneumocystis carinii
p., polymicrobial
p. (PAP), primary atypical
p. ▸ primary eosinophilic
p., progressive
p., Proteus
p. protocol ▸ community-acquired
p., purulent
p., radiation
p., rheumatic
p., rickettsial
p., Riesman's
p., right upper lobe (RUL)
p., running
p., secondary
p., septic
p., Serratia
p., smoldering
p., staphylococcal
p., Stoll's
p., streptococcal
p., superficial
p., suppurative
p., susceptibility to
p. syndrome, atypical
p., terminal
p., Torulopsis glabrata
p., toxemic
p., transplant
p., transplantation
p., traumatic
p., tuberculous
p., tularemic
p., typhoid
p., unresolved
p., uremic
p. vaccination
p. vaccination booster
p., vagus
p., varicella
p. ▸ ventilator-associated
p., viral
p., walking
p., wandering
p., white
p., woolsorter's
pneumoniae
p., Bacillus
p., Chlamydia
p., Diplococcus
p. ▸ drug-resistant Streptococcus
p., gram-negative Klebsiella

p., gram-positive Diplococcus
p. infection, Chlamydia
p., Klebsiella
p., Miyagawanella
p., Mycoplasma
p., Streptococcus
pneumonic
p. consolidation
p. consolidation ▸ patchy areas of
p. fever
p. infiltrate
p. infiltrate, patchy
p. infiltration
p. involvement
p. plague
p. process
pneumonitis
p., acute interstitial
p., acute radiation
p., anaerobic
p., aspiration
p., atelectatic
p., chemical
p., cholesterol
p., chronic organizing
p., cytomegalovirus
p. (DIP) ▸ desquamative interstitial
p., diffuse
p., eosinophilic
p., granulomatous
p. ▸ herpes simplex
p., hypersensitivity
p., interstitial
p., interstitial hypersensitivity
p. ▸ lymphocytic interstitial
p., malarial
p. ▸ marked giant cell
p., nonspecific
p., ossifying
p., overlying
p. ▸ peptic aspiration
p., Pneumocystis
p., Pneumocystis carinii
p., postobstructive
p., radiation
p., radiation therapy
p., recurrent
p. virus
pneumonoconiosis, bauxite
pneumonoconiosis, rheumatoid
pneumonocyte, granular
pneumonopathy, eosinophilic
pneumopathy ▸ seropositive nonsyphilitic
pneumopericardium, tension

pneumopericardium ▸ ventilator-induced
pneumophila, Legionella
pneumoradiography, retroperitoneal
pneumosintes, Bacteroides
pneumosintes, Dialister
pneumotaxic center
pneumothoraces, bilateral
pneumothorax (PX)
p., artificial
p., clicking
p., closed
p., closed chest
p., diagnostic
p., extrapleural
p. formation
p., iatrogenic
p., induced
p., left
p., open
p., pressure
p., right
p., spontaneous
p., tension
p., therapeutic
p., traumatic
p., valvular
p. ▸ ventilator-induced
PNF (proprioceptive neuromuscular facilitation)
PNH (paroxysmal nocturnal hemoglobinuria)
PNU (protein nitrogen unit)
PO
PO (by mouth/per os)
PO (period of onset)
PO (phone order)
PO (postoperative)
pO$_2$ (partial pressure of oxygen)
POBA (plain old balloon angioplasty)
POC (products of conception)
pocket(s)
p., abdominal
p., air
p., attic perforation
p., attic retraction
p., breast
p. chamber
p., conjunctival
p. dosimeter
p., electrode reimplanted in old
p. erosion ▸ pulse generator
p., gingival
p. infection ▸ pulse generator
p. of pus, separate

pocket(s)—*continued*
  p. of Zahn
  p., pacemaker
  p. paging beeper
  p. paging receiver
  p., pus
  p., Rathke's
  p., regurgitant
  p., retropectoral
  p., subpleural air
  p., tooth
pocketing of barium
podalic version
Poehl's test, von
Pohl's mark
point(s) [*joint*]
  p., acupressure
  p. assay ▸ four
  p. average, grade
  p., axial
  p. ▸ beam intersection
  p., bifurcation
  p. biopsy, four-
  p., bleeding
  p., boiling
  p., Boyd
  p. coagulated, bleeding
  p. controlled, bleeding
  p. cut
  p., diathermy
  p. -dose prescription methods
  p. electrical axis ▸ joule
  p. electrocoagulated, bleeding
  p. electrode
  p. electrode, multiple
  p., end-
  p., Erb's
  p. exercise ▸ toe
  p., exit
  p. ▸ facial artery pressure
  p. ▸ femoral artery pressure
  p. fixation
  p., focal
  p., freezing
  p. gait, four-
  p. gait, three-
  p. gait, two-
  p. hair, exclamation
  p., Hartmann's
  p. individually clamped and
    coagulated ▸ muscle bleeding
  p. injection ▸ trigger
  p., isoelectric
  p., joule
  p. leather restraints, four-

  p. ▸ massage trigger
  p., McBurney's
  p., melting
  p., muscle bleeding
  p., nodal
  p., null
  p. of application
  p. of cardiac apex pulse ▸ F
  p. of cardiac apex pulse ▸ O
  p. of convergence (NPC) ▸ near
  p. of critical stenosis
  p. of incidence
  p. of intervention
  p. of intoxification
  p. of maximum amplitude of wave
  p. of maximum impulse (PMI)
  p. of maximum impulse fifth
    intercostal space (PMI 5th ICS)
  p. of maximum intensity (PMI)
  p. of nonintervention
  p. of ooze, capillary
  p. of radiation beam exit
  p. of stimulation
  p. of tenderness
  p. on artery ▸ pressure
  p. os, pin◊
  p., pain
  p., pin◊
  p. ▸ popliteal artery pressure
  p., pressure
  p. pressure ▸ z
  p. ▸ radial artery pressure
  p. reaction, near-
  p., rebound in region of McBurney's
  p. score, tender
  p. secured, bleeding
  p. sensitivity
  p. specific areas of body ▸ tender
  p., stand◊
  p. ▸ stimulation of pressure
  p. subpleural blebs ▸ pin-
  p., Sudeck's
  p. ▸ superficial temporal artery
    pressure
  p., sylvian
  p. tenderness
  p. therapy ▸ trigger
  p., tissue saturation
  p. to septal separation, E
  p. treadmill test ▸ J
  p., trigger
pointed pinna
pointer, hip
Pointes
  P., source of acquired Torsades de

  P., Torsades de
  P., ventricular tachycardia with
    Torsades de
pointing
  p. board, alphabet
  p., past-
  p. test, Barony's
  p. test, past-
pointless side-to-side swinging of
  head
poison (Poison)
  p., absorbed
  p., cell
  p. control
  P. Control Network, National
  p., corrosive
  p., ingested
  p., inhalable
  p., inhaled
  p. ivy
  p. ivy blisters
  p. oak
  p., systemic
  p., toxic
poisoned wound
poisoning(s)
  p., accidental
  p. and overdose
  p., arsenic
  p., aspirin
  p., Bacillus cereus food
  p., barbiturate
  p., beryllium
  p., blood
  p., caffeine
  p., carbon monoxide (CO)
  p., ciguatera
  p., clostridial food
  p., death by
  p. ▸ diarrhea from food
  p. ▸ drug-related fatal
  p., enterococcal food
  p., fluorocarbon
  p., food
  p. ▸ free radical
  p., heavy metal
  p., insecticide
  p., lead
  p., lithium
  p., magnesium
  p., methyl alcohol
  p., mushroom
  p. ▸ nerve gas
  p., nitroprusside
  p., nutrient

p. of adolescent, treatment of
p. of children, treatment of
p. of nervous system
p. ▸ pain in abdomen from food
p., pesticide
p., petroleum distillate
p., phenothiazine
p., plant
p., radium
p., salicylate
p., salmonella
p., scombroid
p., scopolamine
p., seafood
p., selenium
p., strychnine
p., succinylcholine
p., thallium
p., therapeutic
p., toluene
p., toxic
p., uremic

poisonous
p. gas
p. substance
p. substance, ingestion of
p. substance, ingestion of
potentially

Poisson
P. distribution
P. -Pearson formula
P. statistical formula

poker back
poker spine
pokewheat mitogens
polar
p. anemia
p. bodies
p. cataract
p. cataract, anterior
p. cataract, diabetic
p. cataract, posterior
p. cells
p. coordinate map
p. coordinate mapping, bull's eye
p. globule
p. granules
p. hyperplasia
p. presentation
p. ray
p. staining

polarity
p. and hyperchromatism ▸ loss of
p. convention
p., dynamic

p. EEG (electroencephalogram)
wave
polarization
p., electrochemical
p., electrode
p., varying degrees of electrode
polarized glasses
polarizing
p. microscope
p. microscope, rectified
p. therapy
pole(s)
p., apical
p. calyx, lower
p., caudal
p. left kidney, scar lower
p., negative
p. of calyces, superior
p. of incision, lower
p. of uterine incision, upper
p., positive
p. right kidney, scar lower
p. striding ▸ fitness
p. walking ▸ fitness
Polgár syndrome, Bársony-
police interview
police-assisted suicide
policeman's heel
polichinelle ▸ voix de
policy
p., hospital
p., infection control
p., insurance
p., isolation
p., program
p., required request
p., smoking
polio
p. immunization, oral
p., paralytic
p. vaccine
p. vaccine (IPV) ▸ inactivated
p. vaccine (OPV), oral
p. (VAPP) ▸ vaccine-associated
paralytic
p. virus
polioencephalitis
p., acute bulbar
p., bulbar
p., inferior
p., superior hemorrhagic
poliomyelitis
p., abortive
p., acute bulbospinal
p., anterior

p., bulbar
p., cerebral
p. immunization
p., posterior
p., spinal
p., spinal paralytic
p. vaccine, killed
p. vaccine, live
p. virus
poliovaccine, inactivated
poliovaccine, oral
poliovirus
p. vaccine ▸ inactivated
p. vaccine, monovalent oral
p. vaccine, oral
p. vaccine, trivalent oral
polisher, posterior capsule
polishing disc
political fanatic
Politzer('s)
P. air bag
P. test
P. treatment
politzerization, negative
pollen
p. antigen
p. asthma
p. induced allergies
pollicis
p. artery, princeps
p. brevis muscle, abductor
p. brevis muscle, extensor
p. brevis muscle, flexor
p. brevis, musculus extensor
p. brevis, musculus flexor
p. brevis tendon, extensor
p. longus muscle, abductor
p. longus muscle, extensor
p. longus muscle, flexor
p. longus, musculus abductor
p. longus, musculus extensor
p. longus, musculus flexor
p. muscle, adductor
p., muscle opponens
p., musculus adductor
pollinotic rhinitis
Pollock's operation
pollo-vegetarian diet
pollutants, toxic air
pollution
p., air
p., environmental
p. risk, lead
Polvo (heroin)
Polvo Blanco (cocaine)

Poly (polymorphonuclear leukocyte)
polyamine metabolism
polyangiitis, essential
polyangiitis, microscopic
poly-antiviral treatment
polyarcuate diaphragm
polyarteritis, disseminated
polyarteritis nodosa
polyarthritis, juvenile chronic
polyarthritis, migratory
polyarticular gout
Polya's operation
polyaxial joint
polychondritis, relapsing
polychromatic
    p. cells
    p. erythroblast
    p. erythrocyte
    p. normoblast
polychromatophil cells
polyclonal
    p. antibody
    p. gammopathy
    p. hypergammaglobulinemia
polycoria spuria
polycoria vera
polycrotic pulse
polycyclic aromatic hydrocarbon
polycycloidal tomography
polycystic
    p. cyst
    p. disease
    p. disease ▸ infantile
    p. kidney
    p. kidney disease (PKD)
    p. kidney disease (PKD), adult
    p. kidney disease (PKD) ▸
      autosomal dominant
    p. lung
    p. ovarian syndrome (PCOS)
    p. ovary
    p. ovary disease
    p. ovary syndrome (PCOS)
    p. patient
    p. renal disease
    p. tumor
polycysticum, adamantinoma
polycythaemica, polyemia
polycythemia
    p., absolute
    p., appropriate
    p., benign
    p., compensatory
    p. hypertonica
    p., inappropriate

    p., myelopathic
    p., primary
    p., relative
    p. rubra
    p. rubra vera
    p., secondary
    p., splenomegalic
    p., spurious
    p., stress
    p. vera
Polydek suture
polydipsia ▸ patient has
polydipsia, psychogenic
polydrug
    p. dependency
    p. use
    p. use, adolescent
polydysplasia, hereditary ectodermal
polydystrophic oligophrenia
polydystrophy, pseudo-Hurler
polyemia
    p. aquosa
    p. hyperalbuminosa
    p. polycythaemica
    p. serosa
polyester
    p. fiber suture
    p. suture, coated
    p. suture, Ethibond
polyethylene
    p. ball
    p. collar button
    p. drainage (dr'ge) tube ▸ Shea
    p. (HDPE) ▸ high density
    p. implant
    p. implant, insertion
    p. implant material
    p. metal implant
    p. snare
    p. stent
    p. strut
    p. suture
    p. tube
polyfunctional alkylating agent
polygelin colloid contrast medium
polygenic
    p. disease
    p. disorder
    p. hypercholesterolemia
polyglandular syndrome
polygonal cell
polygonal cells ▸ squamous-like
polygraph
    p. machine
    p. test

    p. tracings
polygraphic recording
polyhedral
    p. cells
    p. cells, pale-staining
    p. epithelial cells
    p. -shaped forms
    p. surface reconstruction
polymavirus/polyoma virus
polymer, plastic
polymerase
    p. activity ▸ deoxyribonucleic acid
      (DNA)
    p. chain reaction (PCR)
    p. chain reaction assay
    p. chain reaction (PCR) machine
    p. chain reaction (PCR) technique
    p. chain reaction test ▸ reverse
      transcriptase
    p. ▸ RNA (ribonucleic acid)
      dependent DNA
      (deoxyribonucleic acid)
polymeric endoluminal paving stent
polymerizing tissue adhesive
polymers, microscopic
polymicrobial
    p. bacteriuria
    p. infection
    p. pneumonia
polymorphic
    p. activity
    p. layer
    p. neuron
    p. premature ventricular complex
    p. reticulosis, midline malignant
    p. slow wave
    p. ventricular tachycardia
    p. ventricular tachycardia ▸
      inducible
polymorphism(s)
    p. (RFLPs) ▸ restriction fragment
      length
    p. (SNPs) ▸ single nucleotide
    p. (SSCP) ▸ single strand
      conformational
polymorphonuclear
    p. basophil
    p. cell
    p. cell response
    p. eosinophil
    p., filament
    p. infiltration
    p. leukocyte
    p. leukocyte count
    p. leukocyte infiltrate ▸ interstitial

p. leukocyte infiltration
p. leukocyte, neutrophilic
p. leukocyte response
p. leukocytes
p. leukocytes ▸ increase in
p. leukocytes, interstitial
p. leukocytes ▸ sequestration of
p. neutrophil
p., nonfilament
p. per low-powered field
    (PMN/LPF)
polymorphous
p. dystrophy, Schlichting posterior
p. macular rash
p. ventricular tachycardia
p. wave formation
polymyalgia rheumatica syndrome
polymyxa, Bacillus
polynesiensis, Aedes
polyneuritic insanity
polyneuritic psychosis
polyneuritica, psychosis
polyneuritis
p., acute febrile
p., acute idiopathic
p., acute infective
p., acute postinfectious
p., anemic
p., Guillain-Barré
p., infectious
p., postinfectious
polyneuropathy
p., ascending
p., erythredema
p. ▸ Roussy-Lëvy
p., sensorimotor
polyomavirus, nononcogenic
polyophia monophthalmica
polyopia/polyopsia
polyopia, binocular
polyostotic fibrous dysplasia
polyp(s)
p., adenomatous
p., benign adenomatous
p., benign rectal
p., bladder
p., cardiac
p., cervical
p., choanal
p., colon
p., colonic
p., colorectal
p. detection
p., endocervical
p., endometrial

p., fibrinous
p., fibroepithelial
p., flat
p., Hopmann's
p. hyperplastic rectal
p. in canaliculus
p. in lacrimal sac
p., inflammatory
p., intestinal
p., intrauterine
p., juvenile
p., large
p., lymphoid
p., malignant
p., multiple adenomatous
p., mushroom-shaped
p., nasal
p., noncancerous
p. of cervix
p. of large intestine, benign
p. of larynx
p. or tumors ▸ ulcers,
p., pedunculated
p., pedunculated adenomatous
p., precancerous
p. ▸ pre-malignant
p., rectal
p., retention
p., sentinel
p., sessile
p., sinus
p. ▸ small pedunculated
    adenomatous
p., stomach
p., unilateral
p., uterine
p. ▸ vocal cord
polypectomy
p., colonscopic
p., endocervical
p., nasal
p. ▸ perforation in colonoscopic
p. procedure
polypeptide
p., adrenocorticotropic
p., atrial natriuretic
p. chain
p., pancreatic
polyphaga, Acanthamoeba
polyphase generator
polyphasic
p. action potential
p. activity
p. wave

**polyphosphate, Tc (technetium) 99m
    stannous pyrophosphate**
polypi, endometrial
polyplastic cell
polypneic center
polypoid
p. adenocarcinoma of colon
p. adenoma
p. adenoma, benign
p. anorectal lesion, fibroepithelial
p. bronchitis
p. cystic structure
p. hyperplasia
p. lesion
p. lesion, rectosigmoid
p. tissue
p. urethritis
polypoidal lesion
polyposa, colitis
polyposa, enteritis
polyposis
p. and cancer ▸ familial
p., cervical
p. coli syndrome
p., colonic
p., familial
p. (FAP) ▸ familial adenomatous
p., familial gastrointestinal
p., nasal
polypous endocarditis
polypous gastritis
polypropylene
p. intracardiac patch
p. pledget
p. suture ▸ monofilament
polyradicular joint disease
**polyradiculoneuropathy, acute
    inflammatory**
polyreactive antibody
polysaccharide
p. iron complex
p. storage disease
p. substance
p. substance tumor
polyserositis, idiopathic
polysomnographic diagnosis
polysomnographic study
polyspike and slow wave complex
polyspike complex
polysplenia syndrome
Polystan cardiotomy reservoir
Polystan shunt
polystyrene latex microspheres
polysubstance
p. abuse

polysubstance—*continued*
   p. abuse in pregnancy
   p. abuse vulnerability
   p. dependence
   p. use and abuse
polysurgical addiction
polytetrafluoroethylene (PTFE)
   p. arterial graft material
   p. Gore-Tex graft
   p. Impra graft
polytropous enteronitis
polyunsaturated
   p. fat
   p. fatty acids
   p. vegetable oils
polyurethane
   p. foam
   p. foam embolus
   p. implant
   p. sheath
polyuria ▸ patient has
polyuria syndrome ▸ tachycardia-
polyvalent pneumococcal
polyvinyl
   p. alcohol
   p. chloride
   p. drain
   p. prosthesis
   p. sponge implant
polyvinylpyrrolidone (PVP), iodine
Pomeroy('s)
   P. manner
   P. operation
   P. tuboligation
pomona, Leptospira
POMP (prednisone, Oncovin,
   methotrexate, 6-mercaptopurine)
Pompe's disease
Poncet's operation
Poncet's rheumatism
pond fracture
ponderal index
ponderance, ventricular
pong fracture, ping-
pong mechanism, ping-
pons
   p. and cerebellum ▸ medulla,
   p. and medulla
   p. cerebelli
   p., cerebellum and
   p., diminished attenuation midbrain
     and
   p., dissolution of
   p. oblongata
   p. hepatis

   p. ▸ histologic sections of
   p. oblongata
   p. tarini
   p., tegmental part of
   p. varolii
   p., ventral portion of
pontile apoplexy
pontile hemianesthesia
pontine
   p. angle, cerebellar
   p. flexure
   p. junction
   p. lesions
   p. medullary junction
   p. myelinoclasis, central
   p. tumor
pontis, basis
pontis, taenia
pool(s)
   p. activity, blood
   p. angiography ▸ gated blood
   p., blood
   p., circulating granulocyte
   p. granuloma, swimming
   p. imaging, blood
   p. imaging, cardiac blood
   p. imaging ▸ gated blood
   p. in legs, blood
   p., marginal granulocyte
   p. radionuclide scan ▸ multiple
     gated acquisition (MUGA) blood
   p. scan, blood
   p. scanning ▸ gated blood
   p. scintigraphy ▸ gated blood
   p. study ▸ equilibrium-gated blood
   p. study ▸ gated blood
   p., therapeutic
   p., total blood granulocyte
pooled rat feces
poor
   p. academic achievement
   p. air exchange
   p. appetite
   p. arterial circulation
   p. articulation
   p. attention and memory
   p. attention span
   p. balance
   p. balance, tremor, weakness and
     rigidity
   p. bite
   p. bladder control
   p. blood circulation
   p. blood, iron-
   p. blood, platelet-

   p. body image
   p. circulation
   p. circulation in hands
   p. circulation in toes
   p. circulation to the feet
   p. color vision
   p. concentration
   p. concentration/forgetfulness
   p. concentration, patient has
   p. contact with skin
   p. coordination
   p. dental hygiene
   p. dental repair, teeth in
   p. dietary habits
   p. dietary intake
   p. distal runoff
   p. excretion of contrast material
   p. excretion of contrast media
   p. functional status
   p. habituation
   p. impulse control
   p., infant suck is
   p. insight, patient has
   p. intellectual focus
   p. judgment
   p. judgment ▸ loss of recent
     memory, confusion and
   p. liver function
   p. management skills
   p. memory, patient has
   p. motivation
   p. muscle tone
   p. muscular control
   p. nutrition
   p. oral intake
   p. orientation
   p., patient's appetite
   p. perception
   p. perception of time and distance
   p. performance
   p. performance ▸ rationalizing
   p. -plasma ▸ platelet
   p. posture
   p. pulmonary air exchange
   p. R wave progression
   p. repair, dentition in
   p. respiratory effort
   p. response
   p. risk, patient
   p. school adjustment
   p. self-esteem
   p. self-image
   p. surgical risk, patient
   p. tissue ▸ vascular
   p. venous circulation

p. vision, enhancing
p. visualization
p. wound healing

poorly
p. defined
p. defined borders
p. developed spike
p. differentiated
p. differentiated adenocarcinoma
p. differentiated anaplastic
carcinoma
p. differentiated carcinoma
p. differentiated ductal carcinoma
p. differentiated large-cell
carcinoma
p. differentiated lymphocytes
(NPDL), nodular
p. differentiated lymphocytic
lymphoma
p. differentiated squamous cell
carcinoma
p. differentiated squamous cell
carcinoma ▸ bronchogenic
p. expanded, lungs
p. fitting dentures
p. reversible asthma
p. visualizing gallbladder

POP (plasma oncotic pressure)
pop scars
popliteal
p. aneurysm
p. arch
p. artery
p. artery aneurysm
p. artery pressure point
p. bypass, femoral
p. bypass surgery, femoral
p. cyst
p. fossa
p. fossa tumor
p. joint
p. ligament
p. lymph nodes
p. muscle
p. nerve, external
p. nerve, internal
p. nerve, lateral
p. nerve, medial
p. node area
p. notch
p. occlusive disease, femoral
p. pulse
p. space
p. tibial bypass vein graft
p. vein

popliteus tendon
pop-off ▸ ventilator
popping sensation
Poppy (opium)
population
p., alcoholic
p., cellular
p., clinical
p., control
p., general
p., heroin-using
p., high-risk
p., high-risk adolescent
p., homeless
p., indigent
p. of patients, selected
p., patient
p., prevalence of drug abuse in
general patient
p., prevalence of drug abuse in
physician

porcelain
p. aorta
p. dentures
p. gallbladder
p. inlay
p. laminate
p. veneer
p. veneers, etched

porch lifts
porcine
p. aortic valve prosthesis ▸
stentless
p. bioprosthesis
p. encephalomyelitis, infectious
p. endogenous retrovirus (PERV)
p. graft
p. heart valve
p. heterograft
p. pericardial tissue
p. prosthesis
p. prosthetic valve
p. small intestinal submucosa
p. valve
p. valve bioprostheses
p. xenograft
p. xenograft ▸ stentless

pore(s)
p., acne-prone
p., prominent
p., sieve-like
p. size
p., sweat

porencephalic cyst
Porges-Meier test

Porges-Salomon test
pork
p. insulin
p. insulin ▸ regular purified
p. measles
p. tapeworm
p. worm

Porocephalus
P. armillatus
P. clavatus
P. constrictus
P. denticulatus

Porocoat material
porosity, bone
porous
p. and spongy, bone
p. bones
p. implant

**PORP (partial ossicular replacement
prosthesis)**
porphobilinogen test
porphyria
p., acute
p. (CEP), congenital erythropoietic
p. cutanea tarda (PCT)
p. (HEP) ▸ hepatoerythropoietic
p., variegata

porphyrin
p. biosynthesis
p. in urine
p. metabolism
p. screening
p. test

Porphyromonas asaccharolytica
Porphyromonas gingivalis
Porro('s)
P. cesarean (C-) section
P. hysterectomy
P. operation
P. -Veit operation

port
p., abdominal
p. -access bypass procedure
p. -access coronary artery bypass
(PACAB)
p. -access coronary artery bypass
grafting
p., chemotherapy
p., chest
p., infuse-a-
p., injection
p., mandibular
p., mediastinal
p. of entry
p. pump, angle

port—*continued*
- p., Q
- p., side
- p., supraclavicular
- p. surgery ▸ heart
- p. wine hemangioma
- p. wine mark
- p. wine stain

porta
- p. hepatis
- p. lienis
- p. pulmonaris

portable
- p. analyzing machine
- p. aspirator
- p. biofeedback unit
- p. blood drainage
- p. defibrillator
- p. defibrillator unit
- p. dialysis unit
- p. electrocardiogram (ECG/EKG) machine
- p. film
- p. film of abdomen
- p. insulin infusion system
- p. mechanical kidney
- p. Medi-Lifter
- p. oxygen (O₂) tank
- p. recumbent AP (anteroposterior) and lateral films
- p. recumbent film
- p. respirator
- p. scooter
- p. semi-upright film of chest
- p. supplemental oxygen
- p. x-ray machine

portacaval
- p. anastomosis
- p. H graft
- p. shunt
- p. transposition

Portagen diet

portal(s)
- p., anterior and posterior opposing
- p., anteromediastinal
- p. area
- p. block
- p. circulation
- p. cirrhosis
- p. connective tissue
- p., direct
- p. fibrosis of liver
- p., hepatic
- p. hypertension
- p. hypertension, intrahepatic

- p. hypertension of the liver
- p. hypertension with ascites
- p. inflammation
- p. localization
- p., opposing parallel
- p., opposing skull
- p. portography
- p. pyemia
- p. shunt
- p., single direct
- p. sinus
- p. system
- p. -systemic encephalopathy
- p. systemic shunt
- p. technique, four
- p. to systemic venous shunt
- p. tracts
- p. tracts ▸ extensive fibrosis of
- p. tracts of liver
- p., treatment
- p. triad
- p. vein (PV)
- p. vein aneurysm
- p. vein (HPV) ▸ hepatic
- p. vein thrombosis (PVT)
- p., velopharyngeal
- p. venography
- p. venous access
- p. venous flow (PVF)
- p. venous gas (HPVG) ▸ hepatic
- p. venous pressure (PVP)

portarenal shunt
portasystemic encephalopathy
Portex tracheostomy tube
portio and stroma
portio, vaginal
portion [*torsion*]
- p., cartilaginous
- p., conchal
- p., dependent
- p., diseased
- p., distal
- p., infradiaphragmatic
- p. main circumflex, distal
- p., marginal
- p., medial
- p., mid◇
- p., narrowed
- p. of blood vessel, excision of
- p. of cerebrum, posterior
- p. of chest wall, excision of
- p. of colon ▸ dysfunctional
- p. of duodenum, second
- p. of foot-plate, blue
- p. of incision, lateral

- p. of ligament, shelving
- p. of lung, artificial collapse of upper
- p. of lung, basilar
- p. of mesencephalon, superior
- p. of nail, threaded
- p. of pons, ventral
- p. of root, apical
- p. of small intestine, distal
- p. of stroma, middle
- p. of tongue, mobile
- p. of uterus, cornual
- p. of uterus, fundal
- p. of ventricle, excision ischemic
- p., osseous
- p., tumorous

portional, posterior direct
portocaval anastomosis ▸ percutaneous
portogram, splenic
portography
- p., computed tomography angiographic
- p., percutaneous transhepatic
- p., portal
- p., splenic

portoportal anastomosis
portopulmonary shunt
portopulmonary venous anastomosis
portosystemic anastomosis
portosystemic shunt ▸ transjugular intrahepatic
portoumbilical circulation
portrait dentures
portwine stain
Posada mycosis
Posada-Wernicke disease
Posey restraints
position
- p., abduction
- p., adduction
- p., Albers-Schönberg
- p. ametropia
- p., anatomical
- p. and alignment
- p. and alignment, anatomical
- p. and alignment of fracture
- p., anteverted
- p., AP (anteroposterior)
- p., atypical
- p., Bécléres
- p., Benassi's
- p., Blackett-Healy
- p., body
- p., Bonner's

p., Brickner
p., Broden's
p., brow-down
p., brow-up
p., Buie
p., Caldwell's
p., calibrate
p., Camp-Coventry
p., change of
p., claw toe
p., Cleaves'
p., closed mouth
p., complete breech
p., conversion of
p., cross-table lateral
p., decubitus
p., dorsal
p., dorsal decubitus
p., dorsal elevated
p., dorsal lithotomy
p., dorsal recumbent
p., dorsal rigid
p., dorsolithotomy
p., dorsorecumbent
p., dorsosacral
p., dorsosupine
p. ▸ electrical heart
p., electrodes placed in
p., energy of
p., erect
p., eversion
p., extension
p., face-down
p., Feist-Markin
p., fetal
p., Fick's
p., Fleischner's
p., flexion
p., Fowler's
p., frequent changes in body
p., Friedman's
p., frog-legged
p., frontoanterior
p., frontoposterior
p., frontotransverse
p., functional
p., Gaynor-Hart
p., Grashey's
p., gravity free
p., Haas
p., head
p., head and neck in extended
p., head dependent
p. ▸ head down
p., heart

p., Hickey's
p., high
p., horizontal
p., incomplete breech
p., inlet
p., inversion
p., Isherwood's
p., jackknife
p., Johnson's
p., Jones
p., juxta◊
p., knee-chest
p., knee-elbow
p., Kurzbauer's
p., Lange's
p., Laquerrière-Pierquin
p., Larkin's
p., lateral decubitus
p., lateral recumbent
p., Lawrence's
p., Law's
p. ▸ left anterior oblique (LAO)
p., left decubitus
p., left lateral
p., Leonard-George
p., levotransposed
p., Lewis'
p., Lilienfeld's
p., Lindblom's
p., lithotomy
p., Lorenz'
p., Mayer's
p., Meese's
p., Miller's
p., neutral
p. ▸ neutral or stretched
p. ▸ neutral pelvis
p., Nölke's
p., normal anatomic
p. nystagmus, end-
p., oblique
p., obstetrical
p., occipitoanterior
p., occipitoposterior
p., occipitosacral
p., occipitotransverse
p., occlusal
p. of extension, hand held in
p. of eyeball, shift in
p. of fetus
p. of infant, abnormal
p., 1 (2, 3, etc.) o'clock
p., open mouth
p., opisthotonos
p., orthopnea

p., orthotonos
p., PA (posteroanterior)
p. ▸ patient in fetal
p., Pawlow's
p., Pearson's
p., physiologic rest
p., pivot shift test in lateral
p., Proetz's
p., prone
p., pulmonary wedge
p., recumbent
p., rescuer's
p., rest
p. ▸ right anterior oblique (RAO)
p., right decubitus
p., right lateral
p., Rose's
p., sacroanterior
p., sacroposterior
p., sacrotransverse
p. satisfactory, postreduction
p., scapuloanterior
p., scapuloposterior
p., Schüller's
p., scope reverted to normal
p., scorbutic
p., Scultetus'
p., semierect
p., semiprone
p., semireclining
p., semirecumbent
p. sensation ▸ impaired
  discriminatory, vibratory
p. sensation, joint
p. sense
p. sense, decreased
p. sense (JPS), joint
p., Settegast's
p., shift in
p., shock
p., Sims'
p., sitting
p. ▸ size, shape and
p., sleep cycle
p. ▸ spine in flexed
p., Staunig's
p., Stecher's
p., Stenver's
p., supine
p., Tarrant's
p., Taylor's
p., Titterington's
p., Towne's
p., Trendelenburg
p., tricuspid

position—*continued*
- p., 12 o'clock
- p., Twining
- p., upright
- p., usual anatomic
- p. ▸ uterus shifts from normal
- p., Waters'
- p., Wigby-Taylor
- p., Williams'
- p., Zanelli's

positional
- p. asophyxia ▸ accidental
- p. dyspnea
- p. lightheadedness
- p. nystagmus
- p. return
- p. vertigo (BPV), benign
- p. vertigo ▸ paroxysmal
- p. vertigo ▸ periodic
- p. vertigo ▸ recalcitrant benign paroxysmal

positioned
- p. and bonded ▸ reimplanted,
- p. and draped ▸ prepped,
- p., catheter
- p. in stirrups, legs
- p., monitoring lines inserted and
- p., patient moved and

positioner ▸ starfish heart

positioning
- p. controls, tube
- p. of patient, satisfactory
- p., patient
- p., quick lateral
- p., rapid manual
- p. vertigo
- p. vertigo, disabling
- p. vertigo, episodic

positive
- p. accommodation
- p. Actinomyces bovis ▸ gram-
- p. activities
- p. afterimage
- p. afterpotential
- p. airway pressure (PAP)
- p. airway pressure, bi-level
- p. airway pressure (CPAP) ▸ continuous
- p. airway pressure ▸ expiratory
- p. airway pressure ▸ inspiratory
- p. airway pressure (NCPAP) ▸ nasal continuous
- p. airway pressure ▸ variable
- p. alternatives
- p. attitude

- p. Bacillus anthracis ▸ gram-
- p. bacteria, gram-
- p. behavior change
- p., biologic false-
- p. biopsy
- p. blood, antigen
- p. blood culture
- p. (Rh+) blood ▸ Rh
- p. body language
- p. bone scan
- p. bowel sounds
- p. brain scan
- p. bursts ▸ 14 and six hertz (Hz)
- p. charge
- p. chemotaxis
- p., chronic false-
- p. chronotropism
- p. Clostridium butyricum ▸ gram-
- p. Clostridium septicum ▸ gram-
- p. Clostridium sordellii ▸ gram-
- p. Clostridium tetani ▸ gram-
- p. Clostridium welchii ▸ gram-
- p., coagulase
- p. cocci ▸ aerobic gram-
- p. cocci ▸ clusters of gram-
- p. cocci, gram-
- p. cocci in clusters ▸ gram-
- p. cocci in pairs and chains ▸ gram-
- p. cocci ▸ short-chain gram-
- p. component, late
- p. Corynebacterium diphtheriae ▸ gram-
- p. culture
- p. cytology
- p. deflection
- p. diagnosis
- p. diplococci ▸ helmet-shaped gram-
- p. diplococci ▸ lancet-shaped gram-
- p. Diplococcus pneumoniae ▸ gram-
- p. discharge
- p. E. (Escherichia) coli infection ▸ gram-
- p. effect
- p. emotional expression
- p. end airway pressure (PEAP)
- p. end expiratory pressure (PEEP)
- p. endometrial biopsy
- p. Erysipelothrix muriseptica ▸ gram-
- p. eugenics
- p. expiratory pressure
- p. expiratory pressure plateau (PEPP)

- p. (Rh+) factor ▸ Rh
- p. factor ▸ Rh (Rhesus)
- p., false-
- p. family history
- p. feedback
- p. feeling
- p. fetal blood cells, Rh
- p. findings
- p. findings, reporting
- p. for drugs ▸ testing
- p. for tuberculosis, patch test
- p., gram-
- p., HIV
- p., indole-
- p. inspiratory pressure
- p. lymph node
- p. maneuver
- p. mental attitude (PMA)
- p. microscopic findings
- p. modeling
- p. mood
- p. Mycobacterium tuberculosis ▸ gram-
- p. node
- p. nodes, cancer-
- p. nosocomial infection ▸ gram-
- p. occipital sharp transient
- p. occipital sharp transients of sleep
- p. occult blood
- p. organism, gram-
- p. organism ▸ nosocomial gram-
- p. output
- p. paroxysmal aggressive behavior
- p. (Rh+) ▸ patient Rh
- p., patient Rh (Rhesus)
- p. pelvic nodes
- p. penicillin-sensitive coccus ▸ gram-
- p. periaortic nodes
- p. peritoneal cytology
- p. pole
- p. pressure
- p. pressure airway, continuous
- p. pressure breathing (PPB)
- p. pressure breathing (CPPB) ▸ continuous
- p. pressure breathing (IPPB) ▸ intermittent
- p. pressure, continuous
- p. pressure inflation with oxygen (IPPO), intermittent
- p. pressure infusion device
- p. pressure (IPP) ▸ intermittent

p. pressure respiration (IPPR) ▸ intermittent
p. pressure ventilation (PPV)
p. pressure ventilation ▸ high-frequency
p. pressure ventilation (IPPV) ▸ intermittent
p. pulmonary infiltrate ▸ Wasserman-
p. rays
p. reaction
p. reaction, false-
p. reactor, biologic false-
p., reappraisal
p. reinforcement
p. relationships
p. relationships, building
p. results, false-
p. results in clinical trials, false-
p. (Rh+) ▸ Rh
p., Rh (Rhesus)
p., Rhesus factor
p. rods and cocci ▸ gram-
p. rods, gram-
p. rods ▸ large, darkly staining gram-
p., scout
p. screening test ▸ false-
p. self-image
p. self-introspection
p. serology, false-
p. sharp wave
p. species, gram-
p. spherical aberration
p. spike pattern
p. spikes ▸ 14 and six hertz (Hz)
p. spikes ▸ 14 and six per second
p. spikes, six and 14
p. spiking, sporadic
p., Staph aureus coagulase
p. Staphylococcus aureus ▸ gram-
p. stools, guaiac
p. stools, hemocult
p. strains, ingrown
p. Streptococcus faecalis ▸ gram-
p. Streptococcus hemolyticus ▸ gram-
p. Streptococcus lactis ▸ gram-
p. Streptococcus salivarius ▸ gram-
p. Streptococcus viridans ▸ gram-
p. stressor
p. support systems
p. surgical pathogens, gram-
p. syphilis serology, false-
p. test ▸ false-

p. test result ▸ true-
p. therapeutic effect
p. torsion
p. treppe
p., true
p. tumor ▸ hormone receptor
p. urine drug screen
p. values of sobriety
p. VDRL (Venereal Disease Research Laboratories)
p. washout test
p. wave
p. wave, exaggerated
p. (W+) ▸ weakly
p. x-ray findings

positron(s)
p. coincidence
p. computed tomography
p. decay
p. emission tomographic scanning ▸ fluorodopamine
p. emission tomography (PET)
p. emission transaxial tomography (PETT)
p. emission transverse tomography (PETT)
p. scanning technique
p. scintillation camera
p., x-rays or

Posner-Schlossman syndrome
possession, inanimate
possible
p. diagnosis
p. hallucinations
p. psychological addiction
p. receptor modification
p. source of bleeding

post
p. balloon angioplasty restenosis
p. cesarean hemorrhage
p. coitum
p. C-section
p. divorce family
p. heart attack apoptosis
p. hoc analysis
p. injury paralysis
p. ischemia skeletal muscle reperfusion injury
p. pericardotomy syndrome
p. -term birth
p. -term infant
p. -thalamic stroke pain syndrome
p. -therapy evaluation
p. -thoracentesis chest film
p. -thoracotomy changes

p. -thromboaneurysmectomy
p. -tonsillectomy hemorrhage
p. -trail feedback, discrete
p. -training testing
p. -transfusion hepatitis
p. -transfusion mononucleosis
p. -transfusion purpura
p. -transfusion syndrome
p. -transplant astigmatism
p. -transplant isolation
p. -transplant patient
p. -transplantation
p. -trauma response
p. -trauma response syndrome
p. -traumatic acute renal failure (PTARF)
p. -traumatic amnesia
p. -traumatic arthritis
p. -traumatic atrophy of bone
p. -traumatic epilepsy
p. -traumatic flashbacks
p. -traumatic headache
p. -traumatic osteomyelitis of skull
p. -traumatic osteoporosis
p. -traumatic pancreatitis
p. -traumatic seizures
p. -traumatic stress disorder (PTSD)
p. -traumatic stress disorder ▸ prolonged
p. -traumatic stress disorder ▸ psychotherapy of
p. -traumatic symptoms
p. -traumatic syndrome
p. -traumatic vertigo
p. -traumatic vertigo, chronic
p. -treatment abstinence
p. -treatment alcohol use
p. -treatment bleeding
p. -treatment drug use
p. -treatment environment
p. -tussive suction
p. -tussive vomiting
p. -Vietnam syndrome
postabortal infection
postabortion
p. healing
p. syndrome
p. trauma
postabsorptive state
postactivation depression
postactivation facilitation
postacute phase
postanal gut

postanesthesia
  p. hemodynamics
  p. pulmonary edema
  p. recovery area
  p. room
postanesthetic
  p. apnea
  p. arterial partial pressure
  p. depression, drug-induced
  p. respiratory depression ▸ drug-induced
postapical segment
postaural arch
postauricular
  p. area
  p. graft, full-thickness
  p. incision
  p. sulcus
postaxial muscle
postballoon angioplasty restenosis
postbrain stem stroke syndrome
postbulbar diverticula
postbulbar ulcer
postcannulation findings and diagnosis
postcardinal veins
postcardiopulmonary bypass
postcardiotomy syndrome
postcardioversion pulmonary edema
postcaval shunt
postcaval ureter
postcentral area
postcentral vein, Kuhnt's
postcentralis, gyrus
postcerebrovascular accident chorea
postcesarean
  p. hemorrhage
  p. section
  p. section, abscess formation
  p. section, pain
  p. sepsis
postchemotherapy nausea ▸ severe
postchemotherapy vomiting ▸ severe
postcholecystogastrostomy, status
postcoital
  p. birth control
  p. bleeding
  p. distress
  p. headache
  p. spotting
  p. test
postcommissurotomy syndrome
postconcussion syndrome
postconcussive headache
postconvulsive stupor

postcoronary mortality
postcorrosive stricture ▸ pharyngoesophageal (PE)
postcostal anastomosis
postcricoid cancer
postcricoid region
postcystoscopy patient
postdelivery headache
postdiphtheritic stenosis
postdischarge instructions
postdischarge orders
postdivorce family
postdormital depression
postdrive depression
postdrome of migraine
postembryonic period
postencephalitic behavior disorder
postencephalitis parkinsonism
poster cervical brace ▸ four-
posterior
  p. ampullar nerve
  p. angle of wound
  p. antebrachial region
  p. (A and P) ▸ anterior and
  p. approach
  p. arch
  p. aspect
  p. asynclitism
  p. auricular muscle
  p. auricular nerve
  p. auricular vein
  p. axial embryonal cataract
  p. axillary line
  p. basal
  p. bending
  p. boundary
  p. brain mass
  p. canal
  p. capsule
  p. capsule polisher
  p. cavity
  p. central gyrus
  p. centriole
  p. cerebellar notch
  p. cerebral artery
  p. cerebral artery, choroidal branches of
  p. cerebral artery ▸ left
  p. cerebral artery ▸ right
  p. chamber of eye
  p. ciliary artery, long
  p. ciliary artery, short
  p. ciliary axis, long
  p. ciliary axis, short
  p. circumflex artery

  p. cistern
  p. cleft palate
  p. colporrhaphy
  p. colpotomy
  p. commissure
  p. commissure, chiasmatic
  p. commissure of labia
  p. communicating artery
  p. communicating artery aneurysm
  p. conjunctival artery
  p. conjunctival vein
  p. corneal deposits
  p. cranial fossa
  p. crest of ilium
  p. cricoarytenoid muscle
  p. cruciate ligament
  p. crural region
  p. crus of stapes
  p. cubital region
  p. cul-de-sac of vagina
  p. cutaneous nerve of arm
  p. cutaneous nerve of forearm
  p. cutaneous nerve of thigh
  p. descending artery
  p. direct portional
  p. discission
  p. displacement
  p. drawer test
  p. ethmoidal nerve
  p. facial height
  p. facial vein
  p. fontanelle
  p. fornix
  p. fossa
  p. fossa ▸ chondrosarcoma of
  p., fossa cranii
  p. fossa tumor
  p. fovea
  p., frontodextra
  p., frontolaeva
  p. gastrojejunostomy
  p. gray column
  p. gray commissure
  p., gyrus centralis
  p. hemiblock ▸ left
  p. horn of medial meniscus
  p. impaction
  p. incision, Boyd's
  p. infarction
  p. inferior cerebellar artery (PICA)
  p. inferior cerebellar artery (PICA) aneurysm
  p. inferior communicating artery (PICA)
  p. inferior defect

p. intercostal vein (IV-XI)
p. interosseous nerve of forearm
p. intertransverse muscles of neck
p. intervertebral ganglion of head
p. labial hernia
p. labial nerves
p. labial veins
p. leaflet
p. leaflet, mitral valve
p. leaflet motion
p. ligament
p. ligament of incus
p. lipping
p. lobe of pituitary gland
p. longitudinal bundle
p. longitudinal ligaments ▸ rupture of anterior and
p. mallear fold of tympanic membrane
p. median fissure
p. median sulcus
p. mediastinal lymph nodes
p. mediastinal mass
p. mediastinotomy
p. mediastinum
p. meningitis
p., mentodextra
p., mentolaeva
p. mitral leaflet
p. mitral leaflet ▸ hammocking
p., musculus scalenus
p. myocardial infarction (MI)
p. myocardial infarction (MI) ▸ previous
p. nares
p. nasopharynx
p. nephrectomy
p. nerve roots
p. oblique (LPO), left
p. oblique (RPO), right
p., occipitodextra
p., occipitolaeva
p. occlusion
p. opposing portals, anterior and
p. palatal seal
p. palatine nerve
p. palatine suture
p. papillary muscle
p. papillary muscle of left ventricle
p. parotid veins
p. pelvic exenteration
p. ▸ perforated substance,
p., persistent occiput
p. pharyngeal diverticulum ▸ small saccular

p. pharyngeal wall
p. pharynx not injected
p. pillar of fauces
p. pillar of fornix
p. pituitary hormone
p. polar cataract
p. poliomyelitis
p. polymorphous dystrophy, Schlichting
p. portion of cerebrum
p. presentation
p. region of head
p. region of neck
p. (A and P) repair ▸ anterior and
p. sacrococcygeal muscle
p., sacrodextra
p., sacrolaeva
p. scalene muscle
p. scalp to scalp montage
p., scapulodextra
p., scapulolaeva
p. sclerosis
p. scrotal nerves
p. scrotal veins
p. segment of lung
p. septum apex
p. serratus muscle, inferior
p. serratus muscle, superior
p. sheath of rectus muscle
p. ▸ spina bifida
p. splint
p. staphyloma
p. subcapsular cataract (PSC)
p. sulcus
p. superior annulus
p. supraclavicular nerves
p. surface
p. surfaces, concave
p. symblepharon
p. teeth
p. temporal slow activity
p. thalamus
p. tibial artery
p. tibial dysfunction
p. tibial muscle
p. tibial pulses
p. tibial tendon
p. tibial vein
p. urethrovesical angle
p. vaginal hernia
p. vaginal wall lesion
p. vein of left ventricle
p. ventricle septal wall
p. view
p. vitreous detachment (PVD)

p. wall
p. wall excursion
p. wall excursion, left ventricular
p. wall infarct
p. wall infarction
p. wall thickness, left ventricular
p. wall thickness—diastole
p. wall thickness—systole
p. wall velocity
p. wall velocity, normal mean
posteriorly, antero◊
posteriorly, lumbodorsal fascia opened
posterius stapedis, crus
posteroanterior (PA)
  p. film
  p. lordotic projection
  p. position
  p. study
  p. view
posteroinferior
  p. aspect
  p. division of left branch ▸ block in
  p. dyskinesis
posterointermediate sulcus
posterolateral
  p. aspect
  p. flap
  p. fontanelle
  p. infarction
  p. sclerosis
  p. sulcus
posteromedial aspect
posteromedian lobule
posterotemporal
  p. region
  p. slow activity
  p. slow waves
posterotransverse diameter
posteroseptal wall
postevacuation film
postexchange bilirubin
postexercise flexibility stretches
postexercise hypotension
postexposure management
postexposure prophylaxis
postextraction bleeding
postextrasystolic
  p. aberrancy
  p. beat
  p. pause
  p. potentiation
  p. T wave
postfistula placement, status

postfundoplication vagal nerve damage
postgamma proteinuria
postganglionic neurons
postgastrectomy dumping syndrome
postglomerular arteriole
posthallucinogen perception disorder
posthallucinogenic perceptual disorder (PHPD)
postheart attack shock
posthemiplegic chorea
postheparin lipolytic activity
posthepatic cirrhosis
postherpetic
    p. neuralgia (PHN)
    p. neuropathy
    p. pain
posthospital care
posthyperventilation reactivity
posthypnotic amnesia
posthypnotic suggestion
postictal
    p. activity
    p. confusion
    p. depression
    p. EEG (electroencephalogram)
    p. slowing
    p. state
    p. stupor
posticum, staphyloma
postinfarct edema
postinfarct patient
postinfarction
    p. angina
    p. pericarditis
    p. period
    p. syndrome
postinfection
    p. encephalitis
    p. encephalomyelopathy
    p. perivenous myelinoclasis
postinfectious
    p. bradycardia
    p. encephalomyelitis
    p. polyneuritis, acute
postinfective bradycardia
postinflammatory adenopathy
postinflammatory renal atrophy
postinjection reaction
postinjectional fat necrosis
postirradiation
    p. necrotic tissue
    p. residual tumor
    p. tanning

postischemia skeletal muscle reperfusion injury
postischemic
    p. biochemical changes
    p. changes
    p. heart
    p. myocardium
    p. reperfusion injury (PIRI)
    p. revascularization
postlaminectomy pain
postlaryngectomy patient
postlaryngectomy speech
postlaser
    p. conization
    p. edema
    p. treatment
postlumbar puncture headache
postmantle radiation therapy
postmarital amaurosis
postmastectomy reconstructive surgery
postmature infant
postmeal blood sugar surge
postmenopausal
    p. atrophy
    p. bleeding
    p. breast architecture
    p. breast cancer
    p. depression
    p. estrogen
    p. estrogen/progestin interventions (PEPI)
    p. estrogen replacement
    p. estrogen therapy
    p. heart disease
    p. hormonal status
    p. hormone therapy
    p. hormones
    p. hyperplasia
    p. levels
    p. osteoporosis
    p. patient
    p. women
    p. zest (PMZ)
postmenopause medicine
postmenopause weight gain
postmicturition syncope
postmicturitional adrenergic attack
postmortem
    p. autolysis
    p. blood clot
    p. blood cultures
    p. cardiac blood culture
    p. clot
    p. cultures

    p. decomposition
    p. diagnosis
    p. examination
    p. findings
    p. fingerprints
    p. fractures
    p. induced fractures
    p. intussusception
    p. lividity
    p. putrefaction
    p. rigidity
    p. rigidity, severe
    p. studies
    p. thrombus
    p. tissue
postmyocardial infarction
postmyocardial infarction syndrome
postnasal [*postnatal*]
    p. bleeding
    p. catarrh
    p. discharge (PND)
    p. drainage (PND)
    p. dressing
    p. drip (PND)
    p. drip, chronic
    p. intervention, intensive
    p. tube
postnatal [*postnasal*]
    p. care
    p. checks
    p. classes
    p. condition
    p. course
    p. depression, patient has
    p. development
    p. follow-up
    p. growth deficiency
    p. nutrition
    p. office visits
    p. patient
postnecrotic cirrhosis
postnecrotic tissue
postneonatal problem
postnormal occlusion
postnuclear cap
postobstructive
    p. atelectasis
    p. pneumonitis
    p. renal atrophy
postoncolytic immunity
postoperative (post-op)
    p. abdominal distention
    p. analgesia
    p. arrhythmia
    p. atelectasis

p. atrial fibrillation
p. bladder dysfunction
p. bleeding
p. bowel resection
p. care
p. changes
p. cholangiography
p. coloboma left iris
p. coloboma right iris
p. complication
p. convalescence
p. convalescence, uneventful
p. coronary revascularization
p. course
p. course complicated
p. course normal
p. course, patient had uneventful
p. day
p. discomfort
p. fever
p. follow-up
p. gastrointestinal motility
p. ileus
p. incontinence
p. infection
p. inflammation
p. irradiation
p. irrigation
p. lung complication
p. morbidity
p. nausea
p. neurological seizure
p. nutrition
p. office visit
p. orders
p. pain
p. pain management
p. patient
p. pelvic washings
p. pericarditis
p. period, guarded
p. progress
p. pulmonary function
p. pulmonary problems
p. radiation
p. radiation therapy
p. radiotherapy
p. reaction
p. recovery
p. recovery and rehabilitation
p. reduction
p. relief
p. retching
p. rise in temperature
p. scan

p. shock
p. skin closure
p. status
p. tubal patency
p. vomiting
p. withdrawal
p. wound infection
postoperatively, stormy course
postorbital pain
postovulation hormone changes
postpartum
p. alopecia
p. bleeding
p. blues
p. cardiomyopathy
p. care
p. classes
p. course
p. depression
p. endometritis
p. endometritis, nosocomial
p. examination
p. follow-up
p. hemorrhage
p. hemorrhage ▸ intractable
p. hypertension
p. infection
p. low back pain
p. mastitis
p. patient
p. period
p. psychosis
p. reaction
p. shock
p. state
p. voiding dysfunction
p. women
postperfusion
p. lung
p. psychosis
p. syndrome
postpericardiotomy syndrome
postpharyngeal abscess
postphlebitis syndrome
postpill amenorrhea
postplaced sutures
postpneumonectomy tuberculous empyema
postpolio syndrome
postpoliomyelitic contracture
postponed labor
postprandial (p.p. or after meals)
p. angina
p. blood sugar
p. discomfort

p. glucose
p. hypotension
p. levels
p. lipemia
p. pain
p. plasma glucose
p., two hours
postprandially ▸ nausea and emesis
postprimary tuberculosis
postprocedural management
postprostatectomy incontinence
postpump syndrome
postradiation
p. dysplasia
p. endometritis
p. flexible sigmoidoscopy
p. follow-up
p. therapy
postreduction
p. films
p. position satisfactory
p. status
postrenal
p. albuminuria
p. anuria
p. azotemia
p. proteinuria
postseizure stupor
postseizure stupor, localized
postshingles neuralgia
postshingles pain
postsphygmic interval
postsphygmic period
postspinal headache
poststatus augmentation mammoplasty
poststenotic dilatation
poststenotic dilation
poststimulation respiratory depression
poststreptococcal glomerulonephritis
poststroke depression
poststyloid space
postsurgery exercises
postsurgical
p. aphakia
p. aphakia left eye
p. aphakia right eye
p. bowel requirements
p. colon
p. course
p. discomfort
p. follow-up
p. healing

postsurgical—*continued*
- p. infection
- p. mobility
- p. mumps
- p. office visits
- p. pain
- p. pain ▸ moderate
- p. radiation therapy
- p. state
- p. treatment
- p. use ▸ short-term

postsynaptic
- p. molecules
- p. potential (EPSP), excitatory
- p. potential (IPSP), inhibitory
- p. receptor sensitivity
- p. site
- p. terminal

posttransfusion syndrome
posttraumatic symptoms
posttreatment symptoms
posttussive emesis
posttussive syncope
postural
- p. abnormalities
- p. adjustments
- p. back problem
- p. blood pressure
- p. changes
- p. contraction
- p. deformity, breech
- p. drainage (dr'ge)
- p. drainage ▸ percussion and
- p. drainage system
- p. epilepsy, tonic
- p. hypertension
- p. hypotension
- p. instability
- p. kyphosis
- p. low blood pressure
- p. orthostatic tachycardia syndrome (POTS)
- p. proteinuria
- p. reflex
- p. reflux symptoms
- p. righting reflexes
- p. sensation, loss of
- p. sensation ▸ vibratory, discriminatory and
- p. stability
- p. syncope
- p. tone
- p. tone, loss of
- p. vertigo

posture(s)
- p. and balance ▸ impaired
- p. and maneuvers ▸ hyperextension
- p., change in gait and
- p. continuously
- p., coordination and
- p. defect
- p., developmental sequence
- p., forward flexed
- p. ▸ nonverbal language of body
- p., poor
- p., relaxed body
- p., rigid
- p. screening, free
- p. sense
- p., sitting
- p., sleeping
- p., stooped
- p. ▸ stooped over
- p., upright

posturing, decerebrate
posturing, decorticate
posturography platform
postvaccinal
- p. encephalitis
- p. encephalomyelitis
- p. encephalomyelopathy

postvaccination encephalitis
postvention of suicide
postviral asthenia
postviral syndrome
postvital staining
postvoiding
- p. cystogram (PVC)
- p. film
- p. residual (PVR)
- p. residual volume

Pot (pot)
- P. (marijuana)
- p. belly
- p. felé, bruit de
- p. panic
- p. resonance, cracked-
- p. smoke
- p., smoking
- p. sound, cracked-

potassium
- p. and magnesium ▸ depletion of
- p. arsenite
- p. cardioplegia, cold
- p. cardioplegia, crystalloid
- p. chloride
- p. deficiency
- p. depletion

- p. diet ▸ low sodium, high
- p. exchange ▸ sodium
- p. gluconate
- p. ▸ glucose, insulin and
- p. inhibition
- p. intake
- p. iodide (SSKI), saturated solution of
- p. ion
- p. leg cramps
- p. level
- p. level, abnormal
- p. level ▸ low blood
- p. -losing nephritis
- p. penicillin C
- p. perchlorate
- p. permanganate
- p. restriction
- p., serum
- p. -sparing diuretic
- p. supplement
- p. test
- p. titanyl phosphate laser
- p., total body
- p. wasting
- p. -wasting diuretic

potato, couch
potato nose
potatorum, tremor
potency
- p., biologic
- p., estrogen
- p., immunologic
- p., progestational
- p., prospective
- p., reactive
- p., sexual
- p., social
- p., steroidgenic
- p. test, tubal
- p. vitamin, high

potent
- p. drugs
- p. hormone angiotensin II
- p. inhalant
- p. synthetic form of limonene

potential(s)
- p. ability
- p., abuse
- p., action
- p., addiction
- p., addictive
- p. alcoholic
- p., asymmetric eyeball movement artifact

p., auditory evoked
p., average
p. (AEP), average evoked
p. benefits of supportive care
p., bioelectric
p., biphasic action
p., bizarre high frequency
p. blood donor
p. blood recipient
p. brain resuscitation
p. (BAEP), brain stem auditory evoked
p. breast cancer link
p., cardiac action
p. caregivers ▸ idealize
p., cautery
p. ▸ cell membrane electrical
p. cell replication
p. change, biological
p. change, sequence of
p. change, source of
p., children with regressive
p. clinical virological efficacy
p., cochlear
p. complications
p. difference, electrical
p. differences
p. donor
p. donors, testing
p. drug interaction
p., drug's addictive
p. duration, action
p. duration ▸ monophasic action
p., electric
p., electrical
p. electrode, average
p. ▸ electrodispersive skin
p. energy
p., event-related
p. ▸ event-related brain
p. (EP), evoked
p., evoked action
p. (EPSP), excitatory postsynaptic
p., extracerebral
p., extraneous electrode
p., fasciculation
p. fetal hypertensive crisis
p. (FAP), fibrillating action
p. field
p. field, maximal
p. field, minimal
p. ▸ fire-setting
p. for human betterment
p. for infection
p. for self-harm

p. for surgery
p. for tolerance
p. for violence, patient has
p. for violence ▸ self-directed
p. for violence to others
p. gradient
p., hypertensive crisis
p., immune
p., individual motor unit action
p. (IPSP), inhibitory postsynaptic
p. injury
p. inpatient admission
p., intellectual
p. intrapersonal determinants of relapse
p. isolation
p., Kent
p. latex sensitivity
p. level, skin
p. ▸ maximum negative
p. medication problems
p., membrane
p., miniature end-plate
p., monophasic action
p., motor nerve action
p., motor unit action
p. (MEP), multimodality evoked
p., muscle action
p. nephrotoxicity
p., nerve action
p. nutritional deficit
p. of cannabinoids, abuse
p. of cannabinoids, therapeutic
p. of delayed recall ▸ therapeutic
p. of depressants, abuse
p. of hallucinogens, abuse
p. of inhalants, abuse
p. of multiple drugs, abuse
p. of nerve cell, membrane
p. of opioids, abuse
p. of phencyclidines, abuse
p. of stimulants, abuse
p. organ donor
p. organ donor ▸ identify
p. organ recipient
p. outbreak
p. outpatient admission
p., overdose
p., pacemaker
p. pain
p., pain-relieving
p., pattern evoked
p., performance
p., polyphasic action
p. prevention of jet lag

p. ▸ purative slow pathway
p. recipient
p. reference, average
p. reference electrode, zero
p., rehabilitation
p., repetitive fibrillation
p. response, skin
p., resting
p. ▸ resting membrane
p., resting muscle
p., risk
p. risks and benefits
p., sensory evoked
p. (SNAP), sensory nerve action
p. side-effect
p. signal averaging (EPSA), evoked
p. site of blockage
p., skin
p. (SEP or SSEP), somatosensory evoked
p. source of infection
p., steady
p. stroke victim
p., summating
p., teratogenic
p., tetraphasic action
p., therapeutic
p. therapy
p. tissue damage
p. tolerance to cannabinoids
p. tolerance to depressants
p. tolerance to hallucinogens
p. tolerance to inhalants
p. tolerance to opioids
p. tolerance to phencyclidines
p. tolerance to stimulants
p. toxic effects
p. toxicity
p., transient evoked
p., transmembrane
p. triggers
p., triphasic action
p. victims, high-risk
p. virus carrier
p. (VEP), visual evoked
p., vocational

potentially
p. dangerous
p. dangerous objects
p. fatal condition
p. fatal disease
p. harmful stimulation
p. hazardous substance
p. infectious
p. infectious blood specimen

potentially—*continued*
p. infectious material
p. infectious patient
p. infective
p. infective bodily fluids
p. irreversible psychosis
p. life-threatening illness
p. poisonous substance ▸ ingestion of
p. serious psychological disorder
p. sight-threatening problems
p. suitable donor
p. terminal disease
potentiation of motor activity
potentiation, postextrasystolic
POTS (postular orthostatic tachycardia syndrome)
Pottenger's sign
potter(s) (Potter)('s)
p. asthma
P. -Bucky diaphragm
P. -Bucky grid
P. diaphragm, Bucky-
p. phthisis
P. syndrome
P. version
Potts (Pott's)
P. anastomosis
P. aneurysm
P. disease
P. fracture
P. gangrene
P. operation
P. paralysis
P. procedure
P. puffy tumor
P. shunt
P. -Smith anastomosis
P. -Smith-Gibson operation
pouch(es)
p., Broca's
p., Cardio-Cool myocardial protection
p., colostomy
p., Douglas'
p., Hartmann's
p., ileoanal
p., ileostomy
p., intestinal
p., J
p., laryngeal
p., Morrison's
p., muscular
p. ▸ Parsonnet pulse generator
p., pharyngeal

p., Prussak's
p., Rathke's
p., rectal
p., renal
p., suprapatellar
p. syndrome ▸ pharyngeal
p., vaginal
p., vallecular
p., vesicouterine
poudrage
p., Beck epicardial
p., pericardial
p., pleural
p., talc
Poulard's operation
Poulencmitral ring prosthesis, Carpentier-Rhone-
Poulet's disease
poultice, hot moist
poultice, mustard
pounding heart
pounding heartbeat ▸ rapid
pounds (Pounds)
p. of traction ▸ _____
p. per square inch (psi)
P. Sensibly (TOPS) diet ▸ Take Off
Poupart's ligament [*Cooper's ligament*]
pourquoi, folie du
poverty guidelines, income
poverty of ideas
povidone-iodine solution
Powassan virus
powder (Powder) (pwd)
p. and liquid ▸ hypaque sodium
p., Domeboro
p., Gelfoam
p., licorice
p., Neosporin
p., Pan Alba
P. (cocaine), Pharmaceutical
p., snorting
p. test, Seiditz
p., white crystalline
powdered
p. digitalis
p. stomach
p. tantalum
power(s) (Power)('s)
p. and coordination, motor
p. and endurance exercises
p. angiography, color
p., body's recuperative
p. bounds
p., brain

p., carbon dioxide (CO_2) combining
p., cognitive
p., combining
p., defective motor
p. deposition
p., disorder of motor
p. distance ▸ half-
p. Doppler ultrasound
p., episodic loss of motor
p. factor, intellectual
p. ▸ feeling of intellectual and physical
p. field (hpf) ▸ high-
p. field (lpf) ▸ low-
p. field (organisms/hpf) ▸ organisms per high-
p. field (wbc/hpf) ▸ white blood cells per high-
p. injector
p. ▸ left ventricular (LV)
p. ▸ manipulates to gain
p., motor
P. of Attorney (POA)
p. of attorney decision ▸ durable
P. of Attorney (POA) health care document
p. of reason
p. of suggestion
p. of voluntary movement ▸ impairment
p. of voluntary movement ▸ loss of
p. of warm baths ▸ healing
P. operation
P. operation, Goodall-
p., resolving
p. source, primary
p., spectral
p. to visualize
p., total mass stopping
p., ventricular
p., visual
powered
p. field (PMN/LPF), polymorphonuclears per low-
p., high peak
p. magnification ▸ high-
p. nebulizer, air-
p. treadmill ▸ self-
powerless over alcohol
powerless over chemicals
poxvirus/pox virus
PP
PP (partial pressure)
PP (pink puffers)
PP (postpartum)

PP (postprandial or p.p., after meals)
PP (pulse pressure)
P-P interval
P-P (pellagra-preventing) substance
PPA (phenylpyruvic acid)
PPB (positive pressure breathing)
PPC (pain post-Cesarean) section
PPD (Purified Protein Derivative)
PPD (Purified Protein Derivative) intermediate
PPD (Purified Protein Derivative) skin testing
ppg (picopicogram)
PPLO (pleuropneumonia-like organism)
PPO (preferred provider organization)
P-pulmonale
P-pulmonale ▸ pseudo
PPV (positive pressure ventilation)
PQ (permeability quotient)
P-Q interval
P-Q segment depression
P-R interval
P-R interval, fixed
P-R interval, short
P-R segment
Practical (practical)
    P. Nurse (LPN) ▸ Licensed
    P. Nurse (TPN) ▸ Trained
    p. psychology
practice(s)
    p., admission
    p., aseptic
    p., clinical
    p., cultural beliefs and
    p., current standards of
    p., deceptive cult
    p., discharge
    p., effective surveillance
    p., family
    p., general
    p., hospital-wide
    p., independent
    p. issues, clinical
    p., medical
    p., modern medical
    p., monitoring
    p. of euthanasia, open
    p., patient care
    p. patterns, national
    p. period
    p., psychotherapy
    p. ▸ risk-related

    p. session
    p., sexual
    p., sound medical
    p., spiritual
    p., standard hygienic
    p., standards of clinical
    p., treatment
practicing professional
practitioner (Practitioner)
    p. ▸ advanced level
    p. care ▸ routine general
    p., family
    p., general
    P. (ICP) ▸ Infection Control
    p., mental health
    p., nurse
    p., unethical
praecox
    p., ascites
    p., climacterium
    p., dementia
    p., icterus
    p., lymphedema
praeputialis, herpes
praesens, status
praevia (*see* **previa)**
    p., marginal placenta
    p., placenta
    p., vasa
Prague maneuver
prairie conjunctivitis
praise or admiration ▸ constantly seeking
praise ▸ parental habits of
prandial rhinorrhea
pravastatin sodium
preacher's hand
preadmission information
preadmission screening summary
preadolescent children ▸ depression in
preadolescents, behavioral problems of
preagonal ascites
preagonal staining
preanesthetic medication
preantibiotic era
prearteriolar vessel ▸ intramyocardial
preauricular radiation therapy
preaxial muscle
pre-beta lipoprotein
precancerous
    p. abnormality
    p. actinic keratosis
    p. cells

    p. cervical growth
    p. condition
    p. dermatosis
    p. growth
    p. keratoses
    p. lesion
    p. overgrowth of uterine lining
    p. polyps
    p. skin spots
    p. spots
precannulation antibiotic
precapillary
    p. anastomosis
    p. arterioles
    p. sphincter
precardiac mesoderm
precardinal veins
precatheterization laboratory studies
precatorius, Arbrus
precaution(s)
    p., barrier
    p., body fluid
    p., dressing
    p., enteric
    p., enteric infectious
    p., excreta
    p., isolation
    p., needle
    p., proper
    p., safety
    p., specific isolation
    p., stringent technical
    p., suicide
precautionary measures
preceded by aura, classic headache
precentral artery
precentral gyrus
precentralis, gyrus
precerebral arteries
precertification review
precession angle
precession angle ▸ magnetization
precipitable fraction, heparin
precipitable iodine, serum
precipitant urination
precipitate(s)
    p., granular
    p. (KP) ▸ keratic
    p. labor
    p. (KP), mutton fat keratic
    p. urgency
precipitated
    p. by exertion

precipitated—*continued*
- p. by external factors ▸ patient's condition
- p. psychosis ▸ drug-

precipitating
- p. cause
- p. factor
- p. stress

precipitation
- p., immune complex
- p. reaction, Price
- p., tuberculin

precipitin test
precipitin tube
precipitous labor
precipitous thrombocytopenia
precise match
precision high dose
preclinical
- p., acute and chronic ▸ alcoholic cardiomyopathy:
- p. heart muscle disease
- p. medicine
- p. studies

preclotted, graft
precocious dentition
precocious puberty
preconception counseling
preconceptional care
preconscious mind
precontractile heart
precordial
- p. A wave
- p. bulge
- p. cardiogram
- p. catch
- p. catch syndrome
- p. chest pain
- p. depression
- p. distress
- p. electrocardiography
- p. heart rate
- p. heave
- p. honk
- p. lead
- p. lead ▸ unipolar
- p. motion
- p. movement
- p. pain
- p. palpation, bimanual
- p. pulse
- p. region
- p. thrill
- p. thump

precordium, quiet

precornified cell
precornified superficial cells
precostal anastomosis
pre-crisis behavior
precursor(s)
- p., erythroid
- p., myeloid
- p. protein, amyloid
- p. protein ▸ thrombus
- p. ▸ red and white cell
- p., red cell

precystic stage
predeposit donation, autologous
predetermined biological factors
predetermined intervals of time
prediastolic murmur
predicrotic wave
predicted
- p. blood volume
- p. heart rate (MPHR), maximum
- p. mortality rate

predicting response, indices
predictive
- p. relapse
- p. value
- p. value ▸ negative

predisposed, genetically
predisposing
- p. cause
- p. factor
- p. gene

predisposition
- p., biological
- p., congenital
- p., familial
- p., genetic
- p., hereditary
- p., mental
- p. ▸ multifactorially inherited
- p., physical
- p. testing ▸ genetic
- p. thesis, characterological
- p. to alcohol, genetic
- p. to disease
- p. to psychiatric illness ▸ genetic
- p. toward illness

prednisone (Prednisone)
- p., and chlorambucil (APC) chemotherapy ▸ AMSA,
- P. (COP) ▸ Cytoxan, Oncovin,
- p. (CVP) ▸ Cytoxan, vincristine,
- p., Oncovin, methotrexate, 6-mercaptopurine (POMP)
- p., procarbazine (MOPP) ▸ nitrogen mustard, Oncovin,

- p. (VAMP) therapy ▸ vincristine, methotrexate, 6-mercaptopurine, and
- p. (VAMP) ▸ vincristine, amethopterin, 6-mercaptopurine, and
- p. ▸ vincristine, daunorubicin,

predominance of major affective disorder
predominant
- p. disturbance of conduct
- p. disturbance of consciousness
- p. disturbance of emotions
- p. emphysema
- p. figure
- p. manifestation
- p. organism
- p. pain
- p. psychomotor disturbance
- p. resistant bacteria
- p. strain

predominating cells
predominating organism
predonation of blood
predorsal bundle
predose level
preeclampsia of pregnancy
preeclamptic toxemia
pre-ejection period
pre-ejection time
pre-embryotic genetic testing
pre-employment
- p. evaluation
- p. examination
- p. physical

preemptive immunity
pre-epidemic stage
pre-eruptive cough
pre-evacuation film
pre-excitation
- p., combined forms of
- p. syndrome
- p., ventricular
- p. wave

pre-exercise ultrasound
pre-existing
- p. bipolar disorder
- p. breast tumor
- p. condition
- p. coronary disease
- p. disorder, exacerbation of
- p. hepatic disease
- p. illness
- p. psychiatric illness ▸ exacerbation of

p. renal damage
p. temporal bone fracture
preference
p., food
p., idiosyncratic food
p., individual
p., play
p., story
preferential
p. anosmia
p. pathways, atrial
p. rape
preferred
p. language
p. provider organization (PPO)
p. therapy
p. treatment
p. treatment in cancer
prefollicle cells
prefrontal
p. area
p. artery
p. cortex
p. cortex, dorsolateral
p. cortex ▸ left
p. cortex ▸ right
p. leukotomy
p. lobotomy
p. region
preganglionic cells
preganglionic neurons
preglomerular arteriole
preglottic tonsillitis
pregnancy
p., abdominal
p., abdominal stretch marks from
p., abdominal striae of
p., afetal
p. and abortion ▸ ectopic
p. and childbirth diet
p. and delivery, product of normal
p. at term
p. at term, intrauterine
p., bigeminal
p., bleeding during
p. blood (Biocept-G), radio-receptor assay
p., breast stretch marks from
p., care and treatment during
p. cell
p., cervical
p., cocaine-related complications in
p., combined
p., complication of
p., cornual

p., crisis
p. cycle
p., delayed
p., delayed first
p., diabetic
p. disorder
p. ▸ drinking alcohol during
p., drinking during
p., early
p., ectopic
p., exochorial
p., extrauterine
p., fallopian
p., false
p., first
p., first trimester of
p., full-term
p., gemellary
p., heterotopic
p., high risk
p., human
p., hydatid
p., hypertension in
p., hysteric
p., incomplete
p. -induced hypertension
p., interstitial
p., intraligamentous
p., intramural
p., intraperitoneal
p. (IUP), intrauterine
p., labor and delivery
p., mask of
p. ▸ maternal smoking during
p., megaloblastic anemia of
p., membranous
p., mesenteric
p., molar
p., multiple
p., multiple intrauterine
p., mural
p., nausea in
p., nephritis of
p., normal
p., ovarian
p., ovarioabdominal
p., oviductal
p. ▸ parasitic infection in
p., parietal
p., phantom
p., plural
p. ▸ polysubstance abuse in
p., preeclampsia of
p., prevent
p., prolonged

p. rate
p. -related anemia
p. ▸ ruptured tubal ectopic
p., sacrofetal
p., sacrohysteric
p., second trimester of
p., single intrauterine
p., spurious
p., striae of
p., stump
p. ▸ substance abuse during
p., teenage
p., term
p. terminated
p. test
p. test, direct agglutination
p., third trimester of
p. ▸ thromboembolism in
p., toxemia of
p. (tubopregnancy) ▸ tubal
p., tuboabdominal
p., tuboligamentary
p., tubo-ovarian
p., tubouterine
p., twin
p., twin intrauterine
p., unintended
p., unruptured ectopic
p., unwanted
p., uremia of
p. urine (PU)
p. ▸ uterine bleeding during
p., uteroabdominal
p., utero-ovarian
p., uterotubal
p. ▸ vaginal bleeding in
p., vomiting of
p. weight, pre-
pregnanediol level
pregnant
p. abdomen
p. addict
p. asthmatic
p. opiate-dependent patient
p. patient
p. uterus, abdominal removal of
p. women ▸ drug-abusing
p. women, healthy
pre-heart attack pain
prehemiplegic chorea
prehepatic coma
prehepatic edema
prehospital
p. emergency care
p. evaluation

prehospital—*continued*
- p. management
- p. trauma care
- p. triage

preinfarction angina
preinfarction syndrome
preinsular gyri
pre-intake interview
preinvasive carcinoma
preinvasive lesions
Preiser's disease
Preisz-Nocard bacillus
prejudice and discrimination
prelaryngeal node
prelatency behavior
preliminary
- p. diagnosis
- p. film
- p. film of abdomen
- p. findings
- p. impression
- p. iridectomy
- p. match
- p. medication
- p. observations
- p. simulation
- p. studies

prelipid substance
preload
- p. reduction
- p. reserve
- p., ventricular

premalignant
- p. disorder
- p. lesion
- p. polyp
- p. tissue changes

premammillary artery
premarital counseling
premarital screening
premasseteric space abscess
premature
- p. aging
- p. arteriosclerosis
- p. arthritis
- p. atherosclerosis
- p. atrial beat
- p. atrial complex
- p. atrial contraction, nonconducted
- p. atrial contractions (PAC)
- p. atrioventricular (AV) junctional complex
- p. auricular beats
- p. auricular contraction
- p. beat

- p. beat (APB), atrial
- p. beat, auricular
- p. beat (NPB), nodal
- p. beat, occasional
- p. beat (VPB), ventricular
- p. beats, isolated
- p. beats, sinus
- p. birth
- p. birth, living child
- p. birth, neonatal death
- p. calcification of costal cartilages
- p. cardiovascular disease
- p. complex ▸ ventricular
- p. complexes, atrial
- p. contraction
- p. contraction (APC), atrial
- p. contraction, nodal
- p. contraction, supraventricular
- p. coronary disease
- p. death
- p. delivery
- p. delivery, threatened
- p. depolarization contractions (APDC) ▸ atrial
- p. depolarization contractions (VPDC) ▸ ventricular
- p. disability
- p. discharge
- p. disease
- p. ejaculation
- p. excitation
- p. extrastimulation ▸ single
- p. farsightedness
- p. fetal maturity
- p. heart disease
- p. infant
- p. junctional beats
- p. junctional systoles
- p. labor
- p. labor, spontaneous
- p. male genitalia
- p. morning awakening
- p. newborn
- p. old age
- p. reproductive failure
- p. rupture of membranes (PROM)
- p. ruptured membranes
- p. separation of placenta
- p. sexual maturity
- p. skin wrinkles
- p. systole
- p. vascular disease
- p. ventricular beat
- p. ventricular complex
- p. ventricular complex ▸ multiform

- p. ventricular complex ▸ pleomorphic
- p. ventricular complex ▸ polymorphic
- p. ventricular complex ▸ R-on-T
- p. ventricular complex trigger hypothesis
- p. ventricular contractions (PVC)
- p. ventricular contractions (PVC) with coupling
- p. ventricular systole

prematurely aging skin
prematurely, patient delivered
prematurity
- p., chronic pulmonary insufficiency of
- p., complications of
- p., retinopathy of

premaxillary suture
premedicated, patient
premeditated death ▸ calculated,
premenarche, patient
premenopausal
- p. amenorrhea
- p. calcium intake
- p. diabetic women
- p. patient

premenstrual
- p. breast tenderness
- p. changes in mood ▸ severe
- p. dysphoric disorder
- p. patient
- p. phase
- p. symptoms
- p. syndrome (PMS)
- p. syndrome ▸ bloating from
- p. syndrome ▸ depression from
- p. tension (PMT)

premixed insulin
premolar teeth
premonitory
- p. contractions
- p. pain
- p. palpitation
- p. subjective sensation
- p. symptoms ▸ absence of
- p. symptoms, motor
- p. syndrome

premorbid
- p. personality
- p. personality traits
- p. psychopathology

premortem
- p. bronchial biopsy
- p. cultures

p. sputum cultures
p. tubular necrosis
premotor area
premotor neuron
prenatal (Prenatal)
p. abuse of illicit drug
p. abuse of licit drugs
p. alcohol exposure
p. care
p. care, good
p. care, increased
p. care, intensive
p. care, routine
p. checks
p. classes
p. cocaine exposure
p. condition
p. counseling session
p. course
p. course, uneventful
p. development
p. diagnosis
p. diagnosis of birth defects
p. diagnosis of esophageal atresia
p. diagnostic technology
p. diagnostic tests
p. drug
p. effects, cocaine
p. effects of alcohol
p. effects of cocaine
p. effects of smoking
p. exercises
p. influence
p. injury
P. Intensive Care Unit (PICU)
p. medical needs
p. medicine
p. nutrition
p. office visits
p. patient
p. screening
p. screening test
p. support
p. testing
p. transplants
p. ultrasonography
prenatally, diagnose disease
prenormal occlusion
preoccipital notch
preoccupation
p., sexual
p. with crisis
p. with death
p. with fantasies
p. with fantasies of grandeur

p. with food
p. with incident
p. with self
preoccupied
p. ▸ patient self-
p. with details
p. with fantasies
preoedipal fantasies
preoperative (preop)
p. anesthesia
p. antibiotics
p. assessment
p. care
p. chemotherapy
p. contraindications to surgery
p. cystoscopy
p. diagnosis
p. enema
p. evaluation
p. examination
p. gastric aspiration
p. irradiation
p. irrigation
p. laboratory workup
p. orders
p. patient
p. pelvic irradiation
p. radiation therapy
p. screening physical examination
p. screening ▸ routine
p. sedation
p. skin preparation
p. staging
p. status
p. therapy
p. visit
preoral gut
preorbital cellulitis
prep
p. and drape, perineal
p., Betadine
p., bowel
p. for delivery
p., iodo
p. pad
p., surgical
prepackaged irrigating solution
prepackaged medication
prepaid health care
preparation
p. and draping
p. and draping of field, sterile
p., anticancer
p. classes, childbirth
p., commercial

p., food
p., insulin
p. ▸ Langendorff heart
p. ▸ liquid bowel
p. of body
p. of drugs
p., preoperative skin
p., red cell
p., skin
p., Tzenck
p., vitamin
preparative immunofiltration
preparatory iridectomy
prepare body for viewing
prepare family to view body
prepared
p. and draped in routine manner, patient
p. and draped, operative field
p. and draped, patient
p. digitalis
p. for microsection, tissue
p. sterilely, area
p. with Septisol, area
prepatellar bursitis
preperitoneal bleeders
preperitoneal space
preplaced suture
preponderance, directional
preponderance, ventricular
prepotential reflexes
prepped
p. and draped, abdomen
p. and draped ▸ abdomen scrubbed,
p. and draped, area
p. and draped in routine manner ▸ area
p. and draped in routine manner ▸ patient
p. and draped, skin
p. and draped, sterilely
p. and infiltrated ▸ washed,
p. for surgery, patient
p. in routine fashion
p., positioned and draped
p., skin
p., vagina
pre-pregnancy weight
preproendothelin-1 gene ▸ human
preprogrammed insulin delivery system
prepsychotic level of development
prepubertal children
prepubertal panhypopituitarism

prepubescent
  p. female
  p. male
  p. schizophrenia
prepuce
  p. of clitoris
  p. of penis
  p. of penis, frenulum of
  p., redundant
prepulmonary screen
preputial gland
prepyloric
  p. ulcer
  p. ulcer, chronic
  p. vein
prereduction film
prerenal
  p. anuria
  p. azotemia
  p. uremia
presacral
  p. anomaly
  p. block
  p. edema
  p. insufflation
  p. neurectomy
presbyopia check
preschool sexual abuse
preschool vision screening
prescribe and administer
prescribed
  p. dose
  p. drugs
  p. drugs, abuse of
  p. exercise
  p. medication, monitor
  p. regimen
prescription(s)
  p. bottle
  p., dose
  p. drug
  p. drug abuse
  p. drug therapy
  p. drugs ▸ misuse of
  p., exercise
  p. eyeglasses
  p., faulty
  p. gum
  p., illegible
  p. ▸ improper use of
  p. medication
  p. medication ▸ topical
  p. medicine
  p. methods, point-dose
  p., multiple

  p., narcotic
  p., outdated
presection suture
preseizure pattern
presence
  p. of distinctive symptoms
  p. of edema
  p. of infection
  p. of xanthochromia
  p., personal
presenile
  p. arteriosclerosis
  p. dementia
  p. onset, with delirium ▸ primary
    degenerative dementia of
    Alzheimer type,
  p. onset, with delusions ▸ primary
    degenerative dementia of
    Alzheimer type,
  p. onset, with depression ▸ primary
    degenerative dementia of
    Alzheimer type,
  p. organic psychotic condition
  p., patient
  p. sclerosis
presenilis, anxietas
present
  p. at birth ▸ respiratory distress
  p. at time of death, family
  p. at time of demise, family
  p., clots
  p. effects of weight ▸ ever-
  p. functioning ▸ level of
  p. illness (PI)
  p. illness (HPI) ▸ history of
  p. illness (PI) ▸ noncontributory to
  p. in abdomen ▸ chest tubes
  p. in pancreatic duct ▸ stones
  p. mode of behavior
  p., paddle burns
presentation
  p., breech
  p., brow
  p., case
  p., cephalic
  p., clinical
  p., complete breech
  p., compound
  p., face
  p., footling
  p., footling breech
  p., frank breech
  p., full breech
  p., funis
  p., head down

  p., knee breech
  p., longitudinal
  p., oblique
  p., parietal
  p., pelvic
  p., placental
  p., polar
  p., posterior
  p., roentgenographic
  p., shoulder
  p., torso
  p., transverse
  p., trunk
  p., vertex
presenting
  p. diagnosis
  p. psychiatric diagnosis ▸
    primary
  p. symptoms
preservation
  p. fluid, organ
  p. of donor organs and tissues
  p. of health
  p. of quality of life
  p., organ
  p. ▸ organ retrieval and
  p., self-
  p., tissue
preservative, cold
preserved
  p. ▸ amniotic fluid drained and
  p. cornea
  p. for anatomical study, cadaver
  p. ▸ generic skin growth and
  p., grossly
  p., landmarks
  p. sclera
  p. vitreous fluid
preserving
  p. alternatives, breast
  p. functions, basic life-
  p. medication, bone
preset amount of narcotic
presomite embryo
presphygmic interval
presphygmic period
press
  p., bench
  p. exercise, chest
  p. exercise, leg
  p. exercise, shoulder
  p. exercises, bench
  p., military
pressing, breast lump
pressing pain, substernal

pressor
- p. dose
- p. drug
- p. effect, synergistic
- p. nerve
- p. reflex
- p. substance
- p. substance, renal
- p. test, cold
- p. testing maneuver, cold

pressoreceptor reflex
pressosensitivity, reflexogenic
pressure(s)
- p., abdominal
- p., abnormal intraluminal
- p., actual
- p. airway, continuous positive
- p. ▸ alveolar carbon dioxide (CO_2)
- p., ambient
- p. (ATP) ▸ ambient temperature and
- p. amplitude
- p. amplitude, acoustic
- p. and volume ▸ presystolic
- p. anesthesia
- p., ankle brachial blood
- p., aortic blood
- p., aortic pullback
- p. applied
- p. (ASP) ▸ area systolic
- p. (AP) ▸ arterial
- p. (ABP) ▸ arterial blood
- p., arterial partial
- p. artifact ▸ end-
- p., ascending aortic
- p. assisted ventilation (INPAV) ▸ intermittent negative-
- p., atmospheres of
- p., atrial
- p., atrial filling
- p. atrophy
- p. atrophy deformity
- p., aural
- p. (AIP) ▸ average intravascular
- p. (AMP) ▸ average mean
- p., back
- p. bandage
- p. bandage applied, gentle
- p., barometric
- p. (BP), basic blood
- p., bi-level positive airway
- p., biting
- p., bladder
- p. bleed, low
- p. (BP) ▸ blood

- p. (BP) ▸ borderline high blood
- p. breathing (CPPB) ▸ continuous positive
- p. breathing (IPPB) ▸ intermittent positive
- p. breathing (PPB) ▸ positive
- p., capillary
- p., capillary hydrostatic
- p., capillary wedge
- p., carbon dioxide
- p., cardiovascular
- p. (ICP) catheter, intracranial
- p. catheter, intrauterine
- p. (CVP) ▸ central venous
- p., cerebral perfusion
- p. (CSP) ▸ cerebrospinal
- p. (CSFP) ▸ cerebrospinal fluid
- p. chamber, high
- p. chamber, walk-in high
- p. changes
- p. (BP) check ▸ blood
- p., chemical
- p., chest
- p. (BP) ▸ chronic high blood
- p. circulatory assist (EPCA) ▸ external
- p. (BP) clinic ▸ blood
- p. (CP) ▸ closing
- p., coaxial
- p., colloid oncotic
- p. (COP) ▸ colloid osmotic
- p., continuous positive
- p. (CPAP) ▸ continuous positive airway
- p. contours ▸ Murgo
- p. (BP) control, blood
- p., controlled high blood
- p. controlled inverse ratio ventilation
- p., controlling eye
- p. conversion
- p., coronary perfusion
- p., coronary venous
- p. ▸ crushing chest
- p., cuff-
- p. cuff, automated blood
- p. cuff, blood
- p. cuff deflated ▸ blood
- p. curve ▸ intracardiac
- p. cycled ventilator
- p., damp
- p. decay
- p. (BP), decreased blood
- p. (SBP) ▸ decreased systolic blood

- p., depressed diastolic
- p., depressed systolic
- p. (DP) ▸ diastolic
- p. (DBP) ▸ diastolic blood
- p., diastolic filling
- p. differential
- p., differential blood
- p., directional
- p. discomfort ▸ diffuse, dull aching
- p. ▸ disorder from blood
- p. ▸ dizziness from blood
- p., downstream venous
- p. dressing
- p. dressing applied
- p. (BP) dropped ▸ blood
- p., dynamic
- p., ear
- p., effective
- p. electrogram dissociation ▸ intracavitary
- p. (BP) ▸ elevated blood
- p. ▸ elevated eye
- p. ▸ elevated pulmonary artery
- p. ▸ elevated venous blood
- p. (BP) elevation, blood
- p. elevator
- p., emotional
- p. (EDP) ▸ end-diastolic
- p. ▸ end-diastolic left ventricular (LV)
- p., endocardial
- p., endolymphatic
- p., equalize
- p., equalize air
- p. equalizing (PE) tube
- p., esophageal
- p. eustachian tube
- p., exophthalmos due to
- p. ▸ expiratory positive airway
- p., extrinsic
- p., extrinsic mass
- p., eye
- p., feeling
- p. (BP) fell ▸ blood
- p. (FBP) ▸ femoral blood
- p. flow gradient (PFG)
- p. flow relationship
- p. (BP) fluctuated ▸ blood
- p. fluctuating, blood
- p. (BP) fluctuations, blood
- p., fluid
- p. fracture
- p. from birth control pill ▸ high blood
- p. garment ▸ Jobst
- p., gastric

pressure(s)—*continued*

p. gauge
p. gradient
p. gradient, alveolocapillary partial
p. gradient, aortic
p. gradient ▸ colloid hydrostatic
p. gradient, Doppler
p. gradient ▸ intracavitary
p. gradient measurement ▸ transstenotic
p. gradient support stockings ▸ venous
p. gradients ▸ vertical pleural
p. gun injury
p. half-time
p. half-time technique
p. (BP) ▸ high blood
p., high intracranial
p. (HOP) ▸ high oxygen
p. ▸ high risk systolic
p., higher air
p. hydrocephalus (NPH), normal
p., hydrostatic
p., hyperbaric
p., hypogastric
p. in abdomen
p. in blood vessel of lung
p. in ear
p. in eye ▸ fluid
p. in eyeball, elevated
p. in rectum
p. in the eye
p. (BP) ▸ inability to control blood
p., increased
p., increased blood
p. ▸ increased central venous
p. ▸ increased fluid
p., increased intracranial
p., increased intraocular
p. ▸ increased pulmonary artery
p. ▸ increased venous
p., increasing oncotic
p. index ▸ penile-brachial
p. index ▸ segmental
p. (IVCP) ▸ inferior vena cava
p. inflation with oxygen (IPPO), intermittent positive
p. infusion device
p. infusion device, positive
p. ▸ inner eye
p. inside the eye, painless increased
p. ▸ inspiratory positive airway
p. (IP) ▸ instantaneous

p. (DBP) ▸ instrumental conditioning of diastolic blood
p., interabdominal
p. (BP) ▸ intermittent elevation of blood
p. (IPP) ▸ intermittent positive
p. ▸ internal eye
p. (IJP) ▸ internal jugular
p., intra-abdominal
p. ▸ intra-arterial measurement of blood
p., intracardiac
p., intracranial
p. (BP) ▸ intracranial blood
p., intraluminal
p. (IOP) ▸ intraocular
p., intrapleural
p., intrathoracic
p., intrauterine
p. ▸ intravascular hydrostatic
p., intraventricular
p., intrinsic
p., isometric
p. ▸ jugular venous
p. ▸ juxtacardiac pleural
p. kept at _____ torr, dropped to _____ torr
p. (BP) ▸ labile blood
p., lateral
p. (LAP) ▸ left atrial
p. (LVP) ▸ left ventricular
p. (LVDP) ▸ left ventricular diastolic
p. (LVEDP) ▸ left ventricular end-diastolic
p. ▸ left ventricular (LV) filling
p. (LVSP) ▸ left ventricular systolic
p. level (SPL) ▸ sound
p. ▸ light tactile
p. (AP) line ▸ insertion of arterial
p. (LBP) ▸ low blood
p., lower air
p., lower esophageal sphincter
p. (LBNP) ▸ lower-body negative
p. lowered in Addison's disease ▸ blood
p. lowering drug, blood
p., lowering eye
p., lung
p., maintain systolic
p. maintained
p. management, expiratory
p. maneuver during massage, circular
p., manometric
p. (BP) ▸ marked drop in blood

p. massage, deep
p., maximum
p. (MIP) ▸ maximum inspiratory
p. (MP) ▸ mean
p. (MAP) ▸ mean aortic
p. (MAP) ▸ mean arterial
p. (MABP) ▸ mean arterial blood
p. (MBP) ▸ mean blood
p., mean capillary
p. ▸ mean diastolic left ventricular (LV)
p. (MLAP) ▸ mean left atrial
p. (MPAP) ▸ mean pulmonary artery
p. ▸ mean pulmonary artery wedge
p. (MRAP) ▸ mean right atrial
p. (MRVP) ▸ mean right ventricular
p. ▸ mean systolic left ventricular
p. (MVP) ▸ mean venous
p. measurement
p. (COP) measurement ▸ colloid osmotic
p. measurement, digital
p. (BP) measurement ▸ home blood
p. measurement ▸ invasive
p. measurement ▸ shock wave
p. measurements recorded
p., measuring blood
p., media
p. (BP) medication, blood
p., mercury
p. (mmpp) ▸ millimeters partial
p. monitor (ABPM), ambulatory blood
p. (BP) monitor ▸ automatic oscillometric blood
p. (BP), monitor blood
p., monitor changes in
p. (BP) monitor ▸ electronic finger blood
p., monitor pulmonary capillary wedge
p. (ABP) ▸ monitoring arterial blood
p. (BP) monitoring, automatic blood
p. (BP) monitoring, blood
p. monitoring, central venous
p. monitoring device
p. (BP) monitoring ▸ home blood
p. monitoring, intracranial
p. monitoring, intraocular
p. (BP) ▸ monitoring of blood
p., monitoring venous blood
p. movement ▸ colloid osmotic
p. nap

p. (NCPAP) ‣ nasal continuous positive airway
p., natriuresis curve
p. necrosis ‣ ischemic
p., negative
p. ‣ negative end-expiratory
p. (BP) ‣ normal blood
p. ‣ normal intravascular
p. (NTP), normal temperature and
p., occlusal
p., ocular
p., ocular fluid
p. of blood ‣ increased
p. of carbon dioxide (PCO$_2$) ‣ partial
p. of inhalational anesthetic, alveolar partial
p. of oxygen (PO$_2$) ‣ partial
p. (COP) of plasma ‣ colloid osmotic
p. of urethra ‣ relieve
p. on discs
p. on metatarsal area ‣ relieve
p. on nerves ‣ increased
p. on optic nerve
p. on primary suture line ‣ relieve
p. on spinal cord
p. on the brain
p. on toe joint
p. on urethra
p., oncotic
p. (OP) ‣ opening
p., optimal diastolic
p. (BP) ‣ orthostatic blood
p. (OP) ‣ osmotic
p. overload
p. (PO$_2$), oxygen
p. (PP) ‣ partial
p. (PSAP) ‣ peak systolic aortic
p. ‣ peak systolic gradient
p., peer
p., pelvic
p., pelvic floor
p., perfusion
p., pericardial
p. (BP) ‣ persistent elevation of blood
p., physical
p. (POP) ‣ plasma oncotic
p. plateau (PEPP) ‣ positive expiratory
p. pneumothorax
p. point
p. point ‣ facial artery
p. point ‣ femoral artery

p. point on artery
p. point ‣ popliteal artery
p. point ‣ radial artery
p. point ‣ stimulation of
p. point ‣ superficial temporal artery
p. (PVP) ‣ portal venous
p., positive
p. (PAP), positive airway
p. (PEAP), positive end-airway
p. (PEEP), positive end-expiratory
p. ‣ positive expiratory
p. ‣ positive inspiratory
p. ‣ postanesthetic arterial partial
p. ‣ postural blood
p. ‣ postural low blood
p. (BP) ‣ primary high blood
p. product ‣ rate
p., pullback
p., pulmonary
p., pulmonary arterial
p. (PAP) ‣ pulmonary artery
p. (PAMP) ‣ pulmonary artery mean
p. ‣ pulmonary artery occlusion
p. ‣ pulmonary artery occlusive wedge
p. ‣ pulmonary artery wedge
p., pulmonary capillary
p. ‣ pulmonary capillary wedge
p. ‣ pulmonary hypertension
p., pulmonary microvascular
p. ‣ pulmonary vascular
p. (PWP) ‣ pulmonary wedge
p. (PWMP) ‣ pulmonary wedge mean
p. (PP) ‣ pulse
p. pulse ‣ triple-humped
p. pump
p. ‣ rapid buildup of
p. ratio ‣ ankle brachial blood
p. (BP) reaction ‣ blood
p. (BP) reading ‣ blood
p. recovery
p., rectal
p., reduced air
p. reducer, Honan
p. (BP) reduction ‣ blood
p. (BP) reduction ‣ correlates of blood
p., regulate
p. -regulated volume control ventilation

p. release ventilation (APRV) ‣ airway
p., relief of intracranial
p., relieve nerve
p. respiration (IPPR) ‣ intermittent positive
p. respirator, negative
p. response, Cushing
p. (RP) ‣ resting
p., rhythmic
p. (RAP) ‣ right atrial
p. ‣ right ventricular (RV) diastolic
p. (RVEDP) ‣ right ventricular end-diastolic
p. ‣ right ventricular (RV) systolic
p., right-sided filling
p. (BP) ‣ rise in blood
p., screen filtration
p. (BP) screening, blood
p. (BP) screening, free blood
p. (BP) ‣ secondary high blood
p. (BP) ‣ self-monitoring blood
p. sensation
p. sensation in chest
p. sense
p. sensitive cells
p. sensor
p. sensor, telemetric
p. ‣ sitting blood
p. sling
p., social
p. sore
p., sphincter
p. (SFP) ‣ spinal fluid
p. spot films
p. (BP) stabilized ‣ blood
p. (STP) ‣ standard temperature and
p. stasis
p. study, esophageal
p., stump
p. support ventilation
p. support ‣ volume-assured
p., suprapubic
p., systemic
p. (SAP) ‣ systemic arterial
p. (SBP) ‣ systemic blood
p. ‣ systemic mean arterial
p. (SP), systolic
p. (SBP) ‣ systolic blood
p. ‣ systolic left ventricular (LV)
p. tamponade ‣ low
p., tenderness on
p. (BP) test ‣ blood
p. (BP) therapy, blood

pressure(s)—*continued*
p. (TDP) ▸ thoracic duct
p. time index, diastolic
p. time index ▸ systolic
p., tissue water
p. to control bleeding
p., torr
p. tracing
p. (BP) track ▸ blood
p. transducer
p. transducer, Statham
p. transducer system, multiple
p. transducer system, single
p. (TMP), transmembrane
p., transmural
p. ▸ transmyocardial perfusion
p., transpulmonary
p. treatment, high
p. ulcer
p., uncontrolled high blood
p. (BP), unstable blood
p., ureteral
p., urethral profile
p. urgency
p. urticaria
p., vaginal
p. ▸ variable positive airway
p. variations, intrathoracic
p., venous
p. ventilation ▸ high frequency
     positive
p. ventilation (IPPV) ▸ intermittent
     positive
p. ventilation (PPV) ▸ positive
p. ventilator
p. ▸ ventricular diastolic
p., ventricular filling
p. (VFP) ▸ ventricular fluid
p. (VP) ▸ volume
p. volume analysis
p. volume curve
p. volume curve ▸ left ventricular
     (LV)
p. volume diagram
p. volume loop ▸ ventricular
p. volume relation
p. volume relation ▸ diastolic
p. volume relation ▸ end-systolic
p. volume relation ▸ ventricular
     end-systolic
p. wave
p. wave form
p. wave form, pulmonary
p. (WP) ▸ wedge
p. ▸ z point

p. ▸ zero-end expiratory
p. ▸ zero-end inspiratory
pressured speech
pressurized air
presternal notch
prestige ▸ loss of
prestyloid space
presumed consent
presumptive
p. carcinoma
p. cause
p. diagnosis
p. diagnosis of etiologic agent
p. disability
p. etiologic diagnosis
p. metastatic disease
p. region
presurgical laboratory workup
presurgical testing
presynaptic
p. neuron
p. site
p. terminals
presyncopal episode
presyncopal spell
presystolic
p. gallop
p. murmur
p. pressure and volume
p. rumble
p. thrill
preteens and adolescents
pretend/imaginative play
pretentious, boastful and
preterm
p. birth
p. birth, reduced risks of
p. contractions
p. infant
p. labor
prethreaded Teflon pledgets
pretibial
p. edema
p. fever
p. myxedema
pretracheal
p. fascia
p. lymph nodes
p. node
pretransfusion testing
pretransplant
p. bilateral nephrectomy
p. pulmonary function tests
p. surgery

pretreatment
p., antioxidant vitamin
p. assessment
p. evaluation
p. level
p., Mannitol
p. therapeutic instructions
prevalence
p. of cannabinoid abuse
p. of depressant abuse
p. of drug abuse
p. of drug abuse in alcoholics
p. of drug abuse in general patient
     population
p. of drug abuse in physician
     population
p. of hallucinogen abuse
p. of inhalant abuse
p. of opioid abuse
p. of phencyclidine abuse
p. of prostate cancer
p. of stimulant abuse
p. rate, amebic
p. rounds
p. survey
prevalent illnesses
prevent
p. baldness
p. exercise-induced asthma
p. further outbreak
p. heart disease
p. pregnancy
p. reinjury
p. rejection
p. spread of infection
p., stop or reverse complication of
     diabetes
p. transmission of disease
p. withdrawal symptoms
preventable
p. birth defect ▸ folate
p. death
p. disease
p. disease, vaccine
p. nosocomial infection
preventing
p. adequate flow of blood
p. disease
p. frostbite
p. pain
p. reinjury
p. (P-P) substance ▸ pellagra-
prevention
p., accident

p. ▸ acquired immune deficiency syndrome (AIDS)
p., alcohol
p. and control ▸ cause,
p. and control ▸ HIV
p. and control ▸ infection
p. and control of disease
p. and control of infection
p. and early detection, cancer
p. and early intervention
p. and screening ▸ cancer detection,
p. and treatment ▸ cancer detection,
p. and treatment ▸ diagnosis
p., anger management relapse
p., breast cancer
p., cancer
p., cardiovascular disease
p., clot
p., colon-cancer
p., crisis
p., diagnosis and implementation
p., disease
p., drug abuse
p. /education programs
p. (ERP) ▸ exposure and response
p., failures in
p. in crush injury ▸ infection
p., infection
p. of anginal attacks, relief and
p. of arrest
p. of child abuse
p. of hospital infections
p. of infection
p. of mental illness
p. of nosocomial bacterial infection
p. of physical deterioration
p. of re-bleeding
p. of reinfection
p. of stroke ▸ surgical
p. ▸ opportunistic infection
p., osteoporosis
p., pain
p. plan, relapse
p., pro-active relapse
p. program ▸ drug education and
p. program ▸ treatment and
p., relapse
p., response
p., secondary
p., selective
p. services
p. services, better
p. skills ▸ relapse

p. strategy, alcohol
p., stroke
p., suicide
p., surgical infection
p. ▸ treatment, recovery, and relapse

preventive
p. antibiotic(s)
p. aspirin therapy
p. assessment
p. behavior
p. breast removal
p. care
p. dental care
p. knee brace
p. lifestyles, disease
p. maintenance
p. mastectomy
p. measure
p. measures, routine
p. medication
p. medicine
p. medicine specialist
p. pain medication
p., pellagra
p. substance
p. therapy
p. therapy, daily
p. treatment
preventricular artery
preventricular stenosis
prevertebral
p. fascia level
p. ganglia
p. space
prevesical prostatectomy, retropubic
prevesical space
previa (*same as* **praevia**)
p. centralis, placenta
p. marginalis, placenta
p. partialis, placenta
p., placenta
p., total placenta
previllous embryo
previous
p. admission, refer to
p. behavior ▸ disruptions in
p. excisional scars, well healed
p. infarctions, multiple
p. menstrual period (PMP)
p. posterior myocardial infarction
p. records, refer to
p. seizure disorder
p. studies
p. studies, compared with

p. therapy
p. tracings
p. treatment experience
p. treatment experience criteria
p. workup, patient had
previously
p. demonstrated
p. hospitalized, patient
p. marked, breast area
p. marked veins
p. split lid
p. unrecognized mental illness
Prevotella
P. buccae
P. intermedius
P. melinogenica
P. oralis
prevotii, Peptostreptococcus
Preyer's reflex
PRICE (protection, rest, ice compression and elevation)
Price precipitation reaction
prick
p. skin test
p. test, finger
p. test method
prickle
p. cell
p. cell cancer
p. cell carcinoma
prickling, or numbness ▸ tingling,
prickling sensation ▸ tingling or
prickly
p. feeling, burning, tingling
p. heat
p. heat rash
p. sensation ▸ sharp,
Priessnitz bandage
Priessnitz compress
Priestley's mass
prima (Prima)
p., fissura
P. pacemaker
P. Total Occlusion Device
primal scene
primam
p., foramen
p. healing, per
p., incision healed per
p. intentionem, per
p., per
p., wound healed per
primarily localized, pain
primary
p. -acquired immunodeficiency

primary—*continued*

p. acute care
p. acute pancreatitis ▸ drug-associated
p. addiction
p. adenocarcinoma of gallbladder
p. adrenocortical insufficiency
p. afferent neurons
p. aldosteronism
p. amenorrhea
p. amine
p. amoebic meningoencephalitis
p. amputation
p. amyloidosis
p. anastomosis
p. anemia
p. angioplasty in myocardial infarction
p. aplastic anemia
p. approach
p. aspergillosis
p. atelectasis
p. atrial arrhythmia
p. atypical pneumonia (PAP)
p. auditory cortex
p. bacteremia
p. biliary cirrhosis (PBC)
p. bone cancer
p. bone sarcoma
p. brain tumor
p. bronchus, right
p. bundles of tendons
p. cancer (CA)
p. carcinoma unknown
p. cardiomyopathy
p. care
p. care giver
p. care intervention
p. care person
p. care physician (PCP)
p. care provider
p. care setting
p. carina
p. carrier
p. cataract
p. cause
p. cell
p. cerebral neoplasm
p. cesarean (C-) section
p. chemical of abuse
p. chemoprophylaxis
p. choana
p. closure
p. closure, delayed

p. CNS (central nervous system) lymphoma
p. coccidioidomycosis
p. complex
p. constriction
p. cytomegalovirus infection
p. defect
p. degenerative dementia of Alzheimer type, presenile onset, with delirium
p. degenerative dementia of Alzheimer type, presenile onset, with delusions
p. degenerative dementia of Alzheimer type, presenile onset, with depression
p. degenerative dementia of Alzheimer type, senile onset, uncomplicated
p. degenerative dementia of Alzheimer type, senile onset, with delirium
p. degenerative dementia of Alzheimer type, senile onset, with delusions
p. degenerative dementia of Alzheimer type, senile onset, with depression
p. dementia
p. deviation
p. diagnosis
p. disease
p. disorder
p. dysfunctional labor
p. dysmenorrhea
p. eosinophilic pneumonia
p. extrapulmonary coccidioidomycosis
p. eye care
p. eye disorder
p. failure rate
p. familial xanthomatosis
p. fissure
p. focus
p. follicle
p. function, abnormal
p. gain
p. ganglion
p. generalized seizure disorder
p. glaucoma
p. glioma
p. goal
p. growth
p. head veins
p. headache

p. headache disorder
p. healing
p. hemorrhage
p. hepatic disease
p. high blood pressure (BP)
p. hip replacement surgery
p. hydrocephalus
p. hypernephroma
p. hyperoxaluria
p. hyperparathyroidism
p. hypersomnia
p. hypertension
p. implant
p. impression
p. infection
p. infection, site of
p. infertility
p. insanity
p. insomnia
p. integration
p. interpretation
p. intracranial neoplasm
p. lateral sclerosis
p. lesion
p. lesion, Ghon's
p. liver cancer
p. lobule of lung
p. lung disease
p. malignant cardiac tumor
p. mastectomy
p. M.D. (Doctor of Medicine)
p. melanoma
p. myocardial disease
p. myxedema
p. narcissism
p. nocturnal enuresis
p. node involvement
p. nodule
p. noninflammatory disease
p. nucleus
p. nurse
p. nursing
p. obligation
p. obsessional slowness
p. open angle glaucoma
p. optic atrophy
p. organizer
p. ovarian carcinoma
p. ovarian carcinoma with metastases
p. palate
p. pathogen ▸ acquired immune deficiency syndrome (AIDS)
p. peristalsis
p. peritoneal carcinoma

p. persistent hyperplastic vitreous
p. physician
p. pleurisy
p. polycythemia
p. power source
p. presenting psychiatric diagnosis
p. process
p. progressive multiple sclerosis (MS)
p. pulmonary fibrosis
p. pulmonary histiocytosis X
p. pulmonary hypertension
p. pulmonary hypertension murmur
p. pulmonary hypertension risk factor
p. pulmonary parenchymal disease
p. puncture wounds
p. radiation therapy
p. ray
p. reconstruction
p. referral
p. regimen
p. renal disease
p. respiratory alkalosis
p. respiratory lobule
p. retinal detachment
p. risk factor
p. sclerosing cholangitis
p. sensation
p. sensory area
p. sex characteristics
p. signal
p. site
p. site ▸ residual tumor at
p. Sjogren's syndrome
p. source
p. source unknown
p. splenic panhematopenia
p. sterility
p. stimuli
p. suture
p. suture line
p. suture line, relieve pressure on
p. syndrome
p. systemic amyloidosis
p. teeth
p. tenorrhaphy
p. therapeutic theories
p. therapy
p. thrombus
p. thyroid disease
p. transformer coil
p. treatment
p. tuberculosis
p. tumor

p. tumor site
p. tumor site unknown
p. tumor, unknown
p. vector
p. ventricular fibrillation
p. ventricular tachycardia
p. vitreous
p. vitreous (PHPV), persistent hyperplastic

prime

p. coil, blood used to
p. complexes, R-
p. interval, R-R
p., R-R
p., RSR
p. site

primed lymphocyte test
primed, pump
priming

p. dose
p. effect
p. of artificial kidney
p. of infusing solutions
p. solution

primiparous, patient
primitive

p. acoustic artery
p. aorta
p. cells
p. circulation
p. disc, Bardeen's
p. dislocation
p. drives
p. ectoderm
p. entoderm
p. erythroblasts
p. fold
p. gut
p. hypoglossal artery
p. neuroectodermal tumor, peripheral
p. node
p. ovule
p. phenomena, relatively
p. pulp tissue
p. segment
p. streak
p. trigeminal artery ▸ persistent
p. tumor cells
p. wandering cell

primordial

p. cells
p. dwarf
p. germ cells
p. kidney

p. ova
p. ovule

primum

p. atrial septal defect
p., ostium
p. ▸ persistent ostium
p., septum

primus varus deformity, metatarsus
princeps pollicis artery
principal cells
principalis dexter, bronchus
principalis sinister, bronchus
principle(s)

p., behavioral
p., Fick's
p. ▸ Frank-Straub-Wiggers-Starling
p., hemodynamic
p. of donor maintenance
p., Pauli's exclusion
p., pleasure
p., psychological
p., reality-
p., Talion law or
p., uncertainty

print disability
print, finger◇
Prinzmetal('s)

P. angina
P. effect
P. variant angina

Priodax contrast medium
prior

p. detoxification
p. suicidal behavior
p. to admission
p. to admission, orders mailed in
p. to arrival
p. to birth
p. to delivery
p. to delivery, patient given enema
p. to discharge
p. to discharge, home evaluation
p. to examination, patient given enema
p. to surgery, patient given enema
p. to treatment
p. to x-ray, patient given enema

prism

p. balloon
p. degree
p. diopter (PD)
p. diopter (PD) distance
p. eyeglass lenses
p. glasses
p., Goldmann's contact lens

prism—*continued*
- p., Maddox
- p. method
- p., Nicol
- p., Risley's rotary
- p., Ziegler's

prison psychosis
Pritikin Longevity Center
privacy, patient's
private (Private)
- p. antigen
- p. duty care
- p. hospital
- p. medical insurance
- p. pay, patient
- p. physician
- p. psychiatric facility ▸ free-standing
- p. psychiatric hospitals
- P. Psychiatric Hospitals ▸ American Association of
- p. ritual, bizarre
- p. -sector addiction program
- p. -sector program
- p. toilet facilities

privet cough
privilege(s)
- p., admitting
- p. (BRP) ▸ bathroom
- p., psychologist-patient
- p., visitation

prizefighter ear
PRL (prolactin)
PRLA (pupils react to light and accommodation)
prn (whenever necessary)
Pro time (prothrombin time)
proacrosomal granule
proactive relapse prevention
proarrhythmic effect
proarrhythmic effect ▸ late
proatrial natriuretic factor
probability
- p. analysis
- p. curves, complication
- p. density function
- p. of recovery, low
- p. of survival, high
- p., survival
- p., tumor control

probe
- p., blood flow
- p., cardiac
- p. cauterization, heater
- p., coronary artery

p., Doppler velocity
p., esophageal temperature
p. ▸ hot tip laser
p. ▸ Jatene arterial switch
p. localization ▸ intraoperative gamma
p. microscopes, scanning
p., needle-like
p. ▸ Norwood univentricular heart
p., nuclear
p., patency
p., scintillation
p. shield
p., transcranial Doppler
p., transesophageal
p. ▸ transesophageal echo
p., transrectal

probed, depths of wound
probing
- p. finger
- p. of lacrimonasal duct
- p. of tendon sheath
- p. of wound

problem(s)
- p., academic
- p., activity-related heart
- p., adolescent behavior
- p. ▸ age-related weight
- p., alcohol
- p., alcohol-related
- p. ▸ allergic asthma airway
- p., anesthesia-related
- p., ankle
- p. areas, patient's perception of
- p., associated
- p., autogenic training and stress-related
- p., behavior
- p. behaviors, multiple
- p., biobehavioral
- p., biofeedback and behavior
- p., biofeedback and personality
- p., blood-circulation
- p., blood vessel
- p., bone marrow
- p., cervical disc
- p. ▸ chest pain from heart
- p., child behavior
- p., child has sleep
- p., childhood behavior
- p. children
- p. ▸ children with alcohol abuse
- p., chronic breathing
- p., chronic health
- p., chronic medical

p., chronic respiratory
p., circulatory
p. ▸ clamminess from circulatory
p., clinical
p., cocaine
p., coexisting medical
p., complex
p., coping with
p., cornea
p., cross-generational
p., crush injury renal
p., defective gene
p. derived from entitlement
p., dietary
p., disciplinary
p., diverse psychosomatic
p. drinker
p. drinker ▸ early-stage
p., drinking
p. -drinking client
p., drug
p., emotional
p., exhibit emotional
p., experiencing
p., extremity-threatening
p. ▸ eyelid-related
p. feet ▸ physical complications of
p., feigned psychological
p., fertility
p., financial
p. ▸ foot problem from circulatory
p. from aging ▸ gum
p. from anemia ▸ tongue
p. from arthritis ▸ foot
p. from arthritis ▸ joint
p. from aspirin ▸ nasal
p. from atherosclerosis
p. from breastfeeding ▸ nipple
p. from central nervous system ▸ breathing difficulty with
p. from circulatory problem ▸ foot
p. from cold ▸ ear
p. from cold ▸ nose
p. from constipation ▸ anorectal
p. from Crohn's disease ▸ anorectal
p. from diabetes ▸ circulatory
p. from diabetes ▸ foot
p. from diabetes ▸ penile
p. from diarrhea ▸ anorectal
p., general health
p., hearing
p., heart
p. ▸ heart rhythm
p., identity
p. ▸ immune dysfunction

p. in drug abusers, medical
p. in Raynaud's disease ▸ blood vessel
p. ▸ intermittent functional bowel
p., interpersonal
p., intestinal
p. ▸ language-based learning
p. ▸ learning and behavior
p., life circumstance
p., life-threatening
p., limb-threatening
p., male infertility
p., marital
p. ▸ men with alcohol abuse
p., mental
p., mobility
p., musculoskeletal
p. ▸ nails breaking from circulatory
p. ▸ nature of mental health
p., occupational
p. of adolescents, behavioral
p. of aging
p. of central nervous system ▸ constipation with
p. of drug abusers, psychological
p. of old age
p. of pre-adolescents ▸ behavioral
p., orthopedic
p., other interpersonal
p., ovulation
p. ▸ pain in ear from tongue
p. ▸ pain in ear from tonsil
p., parent-child
p., patient behavior
p., patient has character
p., patient has motivational
p., pelvic support
p., perioperative
p., peripheral lung
p. ▸ phase of life
p., postneonatal
p., postoperative pulmonary
p., postural back
p., potential medication
p. ▸ potentially sight-threatening
p., psychological
p., psychosocial
p., public health
p., recognize
p. ▸ reduce risk of back
p., reframing
p., related medical
p. related to drug abuse, cardiovascular

p. related to drug abuse, endocrinologic
p. related to drug abuse, genitourinary (GU)
p. related to drug abuse, GI (gastrointestinal)
p. related to drug abuse, hematopoietic
p. related to drug abuse, hepatic
p. related to drug abuse, neuromuscular
p. related to drug abuse, psychological
p. related to drug abuse, renal
p. related to drug abuse, septic
p., relationship
p., respiratory
p., rethinking the
p., retrieval
p., school behavioral
p., self-created
p. ▸ sensory integrative
p., severe respiratory
p., sexual performance
p., sleep
p., social
p. -solving
p. -solving ability
p. -solving capacity
p. -solving, critical
p. -solving, daily
p. -solving devices
p. -solving mentality
p. -solving skills
p. -solving skills training
p. -solving therapy
p., sperm allergy
p. ▸ stress caused health
p., stress-related
p. ▸ stroke produces speech
p., studies to serve as baselines for future
p. ▸ sudden vision
p. ▸ taste abnormalities from cranial nerve
p. ▸ tear-related
p., treatment
p. ▸ underestimate severity of medical
p. ▸ underlying physiological
p., urinary
p., vision
p., vocal obstructive
p. ▸ warning signs of mental

p. ▸ warning signs of smoking-related
p., weight
p. ▸ weight-related health
p. with central nervous system from AIDS
p. with central nervous system from alcoholism
p. with central nervous system from diet pill
p. with central nervous system from sleep apnea
p. with central nervous system from vomiting
p. with central nervous system ▸ strep throat and
p. with cold sensitivity ▸ circulatory
p. ▸ women with alcohol abuse
problematic behavior
problematic life-threatening behavior
probolurus, Trichostrongylus
procaine penicillin G
procaine toxicity
procarbazine hydroxyurea radiotherapy (PHRT)
procarbazine (MOPP) ▸ nitrogen mustard, Oncovin, prednisone,
procedure(s)
p., abdominoplasty
p., activation
p., adjunctive
p., adrenalectomy
p., alternative
p. and apparatus
p. and treatment, diagnostic
p., angiogenesis
p., angioplasty
p., aortography
p., apicolysis
p., Aries-Pitanguy mammary ptosis
p., arterial switch
p., arteriectomy
p., arthrectomy
p., arthrocentesis
p., arthroscopy
p., aspiration
p., atherectomy
p., Bankart
p., baseline
p., Battista
p., Belfield
p., Belsey Mark IV antireflux
p., Bergenhem
p., bilateral augmentation
p., biliary

procedure(s)—*continued*
- p. biobypass
- p., Blalock-Hanlen
- p., Blalock-Taussig
- p., blepharoplasty
- p., Blount's staple
- p., Bouilly
- p., brachytherapy
- p., Brailey
- p., Bricker
- p., Brock
- p., browlift
- p., Caldwell-Luc
- p., calibration
- p., capsulotomy
- p. (CIP), cardiac invasive
- p., cardiac revascularization
- p., cardiocentesis
- p., cardiodiagnostic
- p., cardiomyoplasty
- p., catheter-based maze
- p., cerclage
- p., cingulotomy
- p., clinical
- p., closed eye
- p., closed womb
- p., Cloward
- p., Collin-Beard
- p., colonoscopy
- p., colostomy
- p., compartment
- p., controlled
- p., coordination of surveillance
- p., coronary bypass
- p., corrective
- p., corridor
- p., cosmetic
- p., Cotton
- p., cryodestruction
- p., cryothalamotomy
- p., culdocentesis
- p., Damian graft
- p., Darrach's
- p., de-airing
- p., debubbling
- p., debulking
- p., defibrillation
- p., denervation
- p., dental
- p., departmental
- p., dermabrasion
- p., desensitization
- p., destructive
- p., DeVries
- p., diagnostic
- p., diagnostic tests and
- p., dialysis
- p., diaphanography
- p., diaphanoscopy
- p., domino
- p., double-blind
- p., drop-foot
- p., ductogram
- p., Duhamel
- p., DuVal
- p., egg retrieval
- p., Eggers'
- p., elective
- p., electrical counterconditional
- p., electroencephalogram (EEG) biofeedback
- p., electroparacentesis
- p., emergency
- p., endoscopic
- p., endosurgery
- p., escharotomy
- p., esophageal sling
- p. evaluated, sterilization
- p., experimental
- p., Faden
- p., flap advancement
- p., Fontan
- p. for shoulder dislocation, Bankart
- p. for subarachnoid hemorrhage ▸ surgical
- p., foraminotomy
- p., four-flap
- p., frenoplasty
- p., fundoplication
- p., fusion
- p. ▸ gamma knife
- p., Garden
- p. ▸ gastric band
- p. ▸ gastric bypass
- p., gastric stapling
- p., gene therapy
- p., Girdlestone-Taylor
- p. ▸ gluteal-free flap
- p., goniopuncture
- p., gram stain
- p., grievance
- p., Hauser
- p. ▸ heart trimming
- p. ▸ hemi-arthroplasty
- p., hemispherectomy
- p., high-risk
- p., hyperventilation
- p., hypnotic-alpha
- p., hypothermic
- p., ileostomy
- p. ▸ image-guided
- p., imaging
- p., immune modulation
- p. ▸ immunohematologic diagnostic
- p. in cardiac arrest, field
- p., infection control
- p., Inge
- p., intra-abdominal
- p., intra-abdominal laser
- p., invasive
- p., invasive diagnostic
- p., invasive medical
- p., iontophoresis
- p., iridencleisis
- p. ▸ islet cell transplant
- p., Jones
- p., Kasai
- p., Keller
- p., Kestenbach-Anderson
- p., Kono
- p., Kraske
- p., Kuhnt-Szymanowsky
- p., kyphoplasty
- p., Lam
- p., laminotomy
- p., LASEK (laser-assisted subepithelial keratectomy)
- p. ▸ latissimus dorsi
- p. ▸ Lawman's single
- p. ▸ left atrial isolation
- p., Lempert's
- p., lens delivered by tumbling
- p., lesionectomy
- p., life-sustaining
- p., liposuction
- p., lithotripsy
- p. ▸ loop electrosurgical excision
- p., lower GI (gastrointestinal)
- p., Lowman's sling
- p., lumpectomy
- p. ▸ lung reduction
- p. ▸ lung redux
- p., mammotome
- p., mammotomography
- p., Marshall-Marchetti
- p., maze
- p., McDonald
- p., medical
- p., Merindino
- p., microneurosurgical
- p. ▸ minimally invasive
- p. ▸ minimally invasive breast biopsy
- p., minor
- p., modified

p. ▸ modified left atrial maze
p., modified surgical
p., Moe
p., Mohs'
p., Moskowitz
p., Mustard
p., Mustarde
p., neurodiagnostic
p., Nichol's
p., nonintrusive
p., noninvasive
p. ▸ noninvasive diagnostic
p., nonsurgical
p. ▸ nonsurgical cardiology
p., nucleoplasty
p., nursing
p. of rigorous analysis ▸ standard
p. ▸ one-stitch cataract
p. ▸ open eye
p., operative
p., osseointegration
p., ostomy
p., outpatient
p., palliative
p., pallidotomy
p., pancreatic
p., pancreaticoduodenectomy
p., patient care
p., Pereyra
p., pericardiocentesis
p., periosteal
p. ▸ peripheral nerve
p., Pfeiffer's
p., phacoemulsification
p., photic stimulation
p., photocoagulation
p., photorejuvenation
p., polypectomy
p. ▸ port-access bypass
p., Potts
p., proper sterilization
p. ▸ prostate cancer screening
p., provocation
p., Puestow
p., push-back
p., quarantine
p., radical
p., radical surgical
p., radical Wertheim
p., radiological
p., Rashkind
p., Rastelli
p., reconstruction
p., reconstructive
p., reconstructive plastic

p., reconstructive surgical
p., referral
p., reimbursement
p., restenosis
p., restorative
p., retrosternal
p., revascularization
p., rhinoseptoplasty
p., rhytidectomy
p. ▸ robotic partial bypass
p., rotoblator
p., Ruiz-Moran
p., Schonander
p., scleral buckling
p., sclerotherapy
p., Senning
p. ▸ Senning transposition
p., septation
p., shelf
p., Shirodkar
p., shunt
p., simple
p. site
p., Skoog
p. skull of fetus, crushing
p., Soave abdominal pull-through
p., Sondergaard
p., standard
p., stent
p., sterile
p., sterilization
p., sternal spitting
p., strap
p., strategy
p., Strayer
p., surgical
p. ▸ surgical and dental
p. ▸ surgical revascularization
p., surveillance
p., Swenson pull-through
p., switch
p., systematic desensitization
p. ▸ systematic follow-up
p., teletherapy
p., Temple
p., termination of
p., thalamotomy
p., therapeutic
p., therapeutic endoscopic
p. ▸ Therma Choice
p., thoracotomy
p., Torkildsen's shunt
p. ▸ total hip replacement
p., transfusion
p., transillumination

p., transplantation
p., tumbling
p., urostomy
p., uvulopalatopharyngoplasty
p., vaginal suspension
p., Valsalva's
p., valvuloplasty
p., ventrosuspension
p., vertebroplasty
p., Vineberg
p., vitrectomy
p., Weiss
p. well, patient tolerated
p. well, patient tolerated diagnostic
p., Whipple
p., withdraw life-sustaining
p., withhold life-sustaining
p., xenotransplantation
p., Young's
procerus muscle
process(es) [*progress*]
p., abnormal growth
p., absorption
p., accessory
p., acromion
p., active disease
p., active infiltrative
p. ▸ active invasive infectious
p., acute
p., acute infectious
p., admission
p., aging
p., alteration in thought
p., altered family
p., altered thought
p. and imaging, staging
p., angiogenesis
p., anterior
p., appropriate educational
p., articular
p., atrophic
p., attenuation
p., atypical reactive
p., awareness
p., axis cylinder
p., balding
p., benign
p., biological
p., birth
p., blocking of thought
p., blood-purifying
p., body's vital
p., bonding
p., bone
p. bone, cribriform

process(es)—*continued*

p., bony destructive
p., bremsstrahlung
p., capitular
p., chronic
p., chronic inflammatory granulomatous
p., chronic pulmonic
p., ciliary
p., clinoid
p., cochleariform
p., complex psychophysiological
p., condyloid
p., conoid
p., consolidative
p., contraction
p., control disease
p., coping
p., coracoid
p., coronoid
p., decision-making
p., defense
p., degenerative
p. ► derangement in thought
p., destructive
p., discharge
p., discharge planning
p., disease
p. ► disoriented or slow thought
p. drilled, tip of coracoid
p., dying
p., dysfunctional
p., ego
p., emotional
p., endocrine
p., endothelial transformation
p., exfoliation
p., external mastoid
p. ► family services intake
p., fibrous
p., focal cortical
p., fragmentation
p., frontonasal
p., genetic
p., glenoid
p., grieving
p., gross pathological
p. group ► thematic
p. group ► topic-oriented
p., hamular
p., healing
p., hemolytic
p., highly active epileptic
p., immune destructive
p., improved thought

p. in tissues ► oxidative
p., infectious
p., infiltrative
p., inflammatory
p. ► inflammatory disease
p., intercondylar
p., internal learning
p., irradiation
p. ► islet isolation
p., learning
p. ► life-threatening disease
p., malignant
p., mastoid
p., medical
p., memory
p. ► memory consolidation
p., mental
p., motivational
p., natural aging
p., natural hemostatic
p. ► negative thinking
p., neutron absorption
p., normal aging
p. ► normal grieving
p., noxious
p., odontoid
p. of bereavement, natural
p. of bone, thinning
p. of digestion
p. of digestion, normal
p. of incus, lenticular
p. of incus, long
p. of malleus, lateral
p. of maxilla, frontal
p. of neurobehavioral sexual differentiation
p. of radius, styloid
p. of ramus, coronoid
p. of recovery
p. of scapula, coracoid
p. of treatment plan
p. of ulna, styloid
p., olecranon
p. or metabolize drugs
p. -oriented group ► interactive
p., osseointegration
p., palatine
p., patchy infiltrative
p., pathological
p., physiological
p., piriform
p., pneumonic
p., primary
p., progressive degenerative disease

p., prolong dying
p., protoplasmic
p., psychiatric
p., psychophysiological growth
p., pyriform
p., random monitoring
p., randomization
p., recombination
p., regression of disease
p., relapse
p., research
p., respiratory
p., retrieval
p., rhabdomyolytic
p., scanning
p. schizophrenia
p., seclusion
p., secondary
p., self-actuated learning
p., septal
p., septic
p., sphenoidal
p., spinous
p. ► stall the healing
p., stenotic
p., styloid
p., superior articulating
p., therapeutic
p., therapeutic grieving
p., thought
p., Todd's
p., transverse
p., treatment
p., uncinate
p. ► underlying disease
p., ungual
p., vegetative
p., vocal
p., xiphisternal
p., xiphoid/xyphoid
p., zygomatic
processing
p. (ADP), automatic data
p., cross-temporal
p. deficits, auditory
p. film, rapid
p. information
p. mode (RPM), rapid
p. of words, brain
p., signal
p. unit (CPU), central
p., word
processor, image
processor, speech
processus vaginalis

procidentia of uterus
procoagulant deficiency ▸ inherited
procrastination, repeated
procrastination skills
procreative years
proctalgia fugax
proctitis
    p., chronic
    p., diagnosis of
    p., epidemic gangrenous
    p. ▸ pain in abdomen from
    p., radiation
    p., symptoms of
    p., ulcerative
proctoscopic air
proctoscopic examination
proctoscopy, flexible
proctosigmoidoscopic evaluation
proctosigmoidoscopic examination
proctosigmoidoscopy, periodic
procure and allocate donated organ
Procurement (procurement)
    P. and Transplantation Network,
      Organ
    p. coordinator
    p., donor
    p. of cadaver organs for
      transplantation
    p. of donor organs and tissues
    p., organ
    p., organ-tissue
    p. physician
    p., tissue
procursive chorea
procursive epilepsy
procyonis, Baylisascaris
prodromal
    p. labor
    p. myopia
    p. phase
    p. stage
    p. stages, early
    p. symptom
prodrome of migraine
produce(s)
    p. blood cells and platelets
    p. cancer
    p. excess bile pigment
    p. speech problem ▸ stroke
produced by computerized
    tomography (CT) ▸ images
producing
    p. adenocarcinoma ▸ mucin-
    p. adenoma, aldosterone-
    p. areas of brain ▸ seizure-

p. bacteria, disease-
p. beta cells, insulin-
p. cancer cells, antigen-
p. cells, insulin-
p. cells, milk-
p. cells ▸ pigment
p. common organisms, toxin
p. common organisms, viral
p. corpus luteum cells ▸
    progesterone-
p. cough ▸ chronic mucus-
p. cough, sputum-
p. drug ▸ addictive disease-
p. drugs, nausea-
p. factor, exophthalmos
p. factor ▸ stress
p. gland ▸ atrophy of tear
p. nerve cells, degeneration of
    dopamine-
p. organisms, pus-
p. rays, erytherma-
p. rays, pigment-
p. region, hair
p. situations, anxiety-
p. staph, nonpenicillinase-
p. substance, exophthalmos-
p. substances, dependence-
Product(s) (product)
    P. (heroin)
    p. ▸ allergy to dairy
    p., aspirin
    p., blood
    p., calcium
    p. contaminated by AIDS (acquired
      immune deficiency syndrome)
      virus ▸ blood
    p., decay
    p., diabetic
    p., diagnostic
    p. ▸ digestion of dairy
    p., double
    p., drug
    p., end
    p. evaluation
    p. excretes waste
    p., fibrin degradation
    p., fibrinogen breakdown
    p. ▸ fibrinogen fibrin degradation
    p., fibrinogen-split
    p., fibrinsplint
    p. ▸ flatulence from dairy
    p., health care
    p., incontinence
    p., lactic acid ▸ metabolic waste
    p. ▸ lipid peroxidation

p., mastectomy
p., metabolic
p. of conception (POC)
p. of fibrin, split
p. of normal pregnancy and
    delivery
p., ostomy
p., over-the-counter
p. ▸ rate pressure
p. /solution ▸ quaternary-amine
    type
p., special rehabilitation
p., therapeutic
p. transfusion, blood
p., waste
production
    p., abnormal milk
    p., acid
    p., alpha
    p., beta amyloid
    p., bile
    p., brain's natural dopamine
    p., carbon dioxide (CO_2)
    p., Cerenkov radiation
    p., control of alpha
    p. ▸ decreasing tear
    p. ▸ depress cellular energy
    p., ectopic hormone
    p., energy
    p., enhance sperm
    p., excessive heat
    p., excessive sputum
    p. ▸ expanded cell
    p. ▸ fetal lung liquid
    p., fluid
    p., free fatty acid
    p., hemoglobin
    p., histidine
    p., hormone
    p. in brain, stimulate dopamine
    p., increase heart
    p. ▸ increase metabolic heat
    p., insulin
    p., liver cholesterol
    p., male hormone
    p., melanin
    p., normal sperm
    p. of adrenalin ▸ excess
    p. of angiotensin ▸ decrease
    p. of female sex estrogen hormone
      ▸ stimulate
    p. of progesterone ▸ stimulate
    p. of protein in brain, diminished
    p. of red blood cells (RBC)
    p. of sex hormones

production—*continued*
- p. of various brain wave components
- p., optimal bone
- p., osteophyte
- p., pair
- p. rate
- p. rate, cortisol
- p. rate, estradiol
- p. rate, testosterone
- p., saliva
- p., sputum
- p., stimulate prolactin
- p., suppression of milk
- p., sweat
- p. ▸ thyroid hormone
- p., trigger testosterone
- p., urea
- p., voltage

productive
- p. bronchitis
- p. cough
- p. coughing and expectoration
- p. nephritis
- p. of bloody sputum ▸ cough
- p. of sputum, cough
- p., patient
- p. phlebitis
- p. sputum
- p. tuberculosis

productus, Peptostreptococcus
Proetz's position
Proetz's treatment
Professional (professional)(s)
- P. Activities Study (PAS)
- p. ▸ alcohol and substance abuse treatment
- p., allied health
- p. and public tolerance
- p. ataxia
- p. caregiver
- p., chemical dependency
- p. facials
- p., health care
- p. help
- p., mental health
- p. neurosis
- p. perspective
- p., practicing
- p. staff
- p., treatment

Profeta's immunity
proficiency, mental
profile (Profile)
- p., aortic valve velocity

- p., automated chemistry
- p., balanced physical
- p., behavioral
- p., blood fat
- p., bony
- p., cardiac
- p., cell volume
- p., chemical
- p., chemical enzyme
- p., chemistry
- p., cholesterol
- p., clinical
- p., deflated
- p., detoxification
- p., dose
- p., drug
- p., drug safety
- p., electrolyte
- p., electrophoretic
- p., emotional
- p., fat
- p., gene
- p., genetic
- p., heart valve prosthesis ▸ Hufnagel low
- p., hepatitis
- p., Hood chemistry
- P., Hypnotic Induction
- p., lipid
- p., liver
- p., pain
- p. ▸ personal hearing loss
- p., personality
- p., personalized medication
- p. pressure, urethral
- p., prognathic
- p. prosthesis, Gott low
- p., psychosocial
- P., Psychotic Reaction
- p., Renin
- p. research, high-
- p., retrognathic
- p. ▸ serum lipid
- p. ▸ side-effect
- p. test, SMA-12
- p., thyroid
- p. ▸ thyroid function
- p., total lipid
- p. ▸ ultra-low

profit ▸ manipulates to gain
profit, personal
profluens, salpingitis
profound
- p. change in affect
- p. change in behavior

- p. change in cognition
- p. change in self-image
- p. depression
- p. hearing loss
- p. idiocy
- p. idiot
- p. mental retardation
- p. mental subnormality
- p. nonresponsiveness
- p. weakness

profoundly mentally retarded
profunda
- p. brachii artery
- p., colitis cystica
- p. femoris artery
- p. femoris vein
- p., keratitis
- p., keratitis pustuliformis

profundi cerebri, gyri
profundum ▸ vas lymphaticum
profundus
- p., flexor digitorum
- p. function
- p. muscle, flexor digitorum
- p. tendon, flexor digitorum

profuse
- p. bleeding
- p. diarrhea ▸ watery,
- p. hemorrhage
- p. menstruation
- p. perspiration
- p. sweating

profusely, sweating
profusion [*perfusion*]
profusion ▸ Laser Doppler blood
progenitalis, herpes
progenitor cell antigen
progeria, patient has
progestational
- p. agent
- p. hormones
- p. potency
- p. stage
- p. steroids

progesterone
- p. challenge test (PCT)
- p. -producing corpus luteum cells
- p. ▸ stimulate production of
- p. withdrawal test

progestin interventions (PEPI) ▸ postmenopausal estrogen/
progestin, synthetic estrogen and
prognathic
- p. dilatation
- p. mandible

p. profile

prognosis

p., case

p., diagnosis-

p. for carcinoma

p., functional

p., genetic

p., grave

p. guarded

p. ▸ incidence, risk, and

p., limited

p. ▸ long-term

p., management and

p., placement and

prognostic

p. analysis

p. evaluation

p. factor, cytolysis

p. factors

p. factors, pathologic

p. index (CPI) ▸ coronary

p. indicators, diagnostic and

p. scale

p. score ▸ Duke treadmill

p. score ▸ initial

p. score ▸ VAMC

program(s) (Program)

p., active management of labor

p., aftercare

p. ▸ aggressive rehabilitative

p., alcohol dependency

p., alcoholism/chemical dependency

p., Antabuse

p., aquacise

p., aspects of

p., assembly

p., awareness

p., background

p., balanced exercise

p., behavioral

p., behavioral modification

p. ▸ bowel management

p., bowel training

P., Breast Cancer Detection Awareness

P., Breast Screening

p., cardiac rehabilitation

p., central motor

p., chemical dependency

p., clinical drug evaluation

p., clinical research

p., community bereavement

p., computer therapy

p., conditioning

p., continuing education

P., Coordinated Home Care

p. ▸ coronary gene therapy

p., day care

P. ▸ Day Intensive Outpatient

p., detoxification

p. development, clinical

p., diagnostic

p. ▸ diet-and-exercise

p., drug abuse

p., drug education

p. ▸ drug education and prevention

p., drug interdiction

p., drug intervention

p., drug screening

p., drug treatment

p., drug-free treatment

p., early detection

p., egg donor

p. ▸ electrophysiology diagnostic

P. (EAP), Employee Assistance

p., employee health

P., ESRD (End Stage Renal Disease)

p., exercise

p., experimental treatment

p., extensive treatment

p., family

p. ▸ family day educational

p., family intervention

p., family outreach

p., federal immunization

p. for adolescents ▸ patient placement

p. for adults ▸ patient placement

p. for caregivers

p., foreground

P. ▸ Forensic Urine Drug Testing

p. ▸ gender-specific treatment

p. ▸ heart rehabilitation

P., Home Care

p., home exercise

p., hospice

p., hospice home care

p., hospital inservice

p., hospital residency

p., hypertension screening

p., infant stimulation

p., in-house

p., Inservice Education

p., intense outpatient

p., intensive

P., Intensive Cocaine

P., Intensive Outpatient

p. ▸ intensive outpatient treatment

p., intensive supportive

P. (IDP), Intoxicated Driver

p., liquid diet

p., maintenance

p., mall walking

p., management

p. ▸ mandatory vaccination

p., Medicaid

p., Medicare

p., mental health

p., methadone

p. ▸ methadone maintenance treatment

p., models

p., moderate exercise

p., motivation

p., multiple drug

p., multi-risk

P. (NCEP) ▸ National Cholesterol Education

p., newborn screening

P., Night Hospital

p., nosocomial infection control

P. ▸ Organ Donor Awareness

p., orientation

P., Orphan Drugs

p. ▸ outpatient drug-free

p., outpatient methadone

P., OVWI (Operating Vehicle While Intoxicated)

p., pain clinic

p., pain management

p. ▸ pain treatment

p., palliative

p. ▸ partial hospital treatment

p., partial hospitalization

P., patient discharged to Coordinated Home Care

p., patient on multiple drug

p., patient placement

p., peer review

p., personal recovery

p., personnel health

p., physical activity

p., physical fitness

p., placement

p. policies

p., private sector

p. ▸ private sector addiction

p. ▸ psychiatric case management

p., public health

p. ▸ public health education

p. ▸ publicly assisted drug abuse treatment

p. ▸ pulmonary rehabilitation

p., quality of

program(s)—*continued*
p., rehabilitation
p., remediation
p., residential
p. ▸ residential drug-free
p., respite care
p., rigid treatment
p., screening
p., self-help
p., self-improvement
p., smoke-free
p., smoking cessation
p. ▸ specialized AIDS home care
p., specialized exercise
p., sports medicine
p., state-funded
p. stimulation
p., strength-training
p., stress management
p., stress reduction
p. ▸ supervised exercise
P., Surveillance
p., terminal care
p., tetanus and rabies control
p., total fitness
p., traditional
p., traditional drug
p., treatment
p. ▸ treatment and prevention
p. ▸ 12-step
p., ulcer
p., utilization review
p. ▸ vestibular rehabilitation
p. ▸ vigorous exercise
p. ▸ vigorous inflight exercise
p., voluntary testing
p., walking
P., Weekend Family
p., weight control
p., weight loss
p., weight reduction
p., well-monitored
p., wellness
p., work hardening
p., written home exercise
Programalith III pulse generator
programmable
p. analog hearing aid
p. cardioverter-defibrillator (PCD)
p. device
p. pacemaker
programmatic changes
programmed
p. behavior therapy techniques
p. cell death

p. electrical stimulation
p. electrical stimulation ▸ slaved
p. stimulation, noninvasive
p. stimulation ▸ ventricular
p. yeast, genetically
programmer
p., application
p., system
p., utility
programming
p., Antabuse
p., appropriateness for
p., binary
p., milieu
p., mnemonic
p., neurolinguistic
p. pacemaker
progress [*process*]
p., academic
p., failure to
p. film
p., medical
p., overall functional
p., patient
p., postoperative
p. record, patient
p. studies
p., therapy
progressed, labor
progressed slowly, disease
progressing
p. bilateral hearing loss ▸ rapidly
p. memory loss ▸ slowly
p. satisfactorily, patient
progression
p., delay disease
p., gradual exercise
p. of activity
p. of addiction
p. of atherosclerosis
p. of disease
p. of disease, biological
p. of disease, rate of
p. of disease ▸ symptomatic
p. of disorder ▸ monitor
p. of myocardial disease
p. of symptoms
p. ▸ poor R wave
p. ▸ R wave
p., rapid
p., slow
p., tumor
progressiva
p., amyotrophia spinalis
p. ▸ dysbasia lordotica

p., ophthalmoplegia
progressive (Progressive)
p. ambulation
p. amnesia
p. and incurable condition
p. anorexia
p. arthritis
p. ataxia, hereditary
p. atrophy
p. azotemia
p. blindness
p. brain deterioration
p. brain disease
p. brain disorder
p. cataract
p. chorea, chronic
p. choreic tic
p. choroidal atrophy
p. clinical deterioration
p. clouding of the lens
p. cognitive deterioration
p. condition
p. course ▸ acute, rapidly
p. course, chronic
p. course ▸ relapsing-
p. crippling
p. crushing of vertebral bones
p. curvature of radius
p., debilitating, incurable brain
   disease
p. decline in function
p. decline in intellectual function
p. deep relaxation
p. degenerative disease
p. degenerative disease process
p. dementia
p. deterioration
p. deterioration of retina
p. dialysis encephalopathy
p. difficulty in walking
p. disease
p. disease ▸ incurable,
p. disorder
p. downhill course
p. dysfunction
p. edema
p. encephalitis
p. enlargement
p. exercise
p. external ophthalmoplegia
p. familial myoclonic epilepsy
p. fatigue
p. fatigue and weakness
p. gait imbalance
p. glomerulonephritis, rapidly

p. growth of cells
p. growth of tissues
p. headache, chronic
p. hearing loss
p. hearing loss, bilateral
p. hereditary chorea, chronic
p. hereditary disorder ▸ slowly
p. hoarseness
p. hypertrophic interstitial neuropathy
p. idiopathic neuromuscular disease
p. illness, chronic and
p. impairment of vision
p. improvement
p. inability to walk
p. increase in voltage
p. inflammation
p. intellectual deterioration
p. interstitial pulmonary fibrosis
p. irreversible disorder
p. jaundice
p. kidney damage
p. kidney failure
p. labioglossopharyngeal paralysis
p. laryngitis
p. lenticular degeneration
p. lingual hemiatrophy
p. liver disease
p. loss of cerebral function
p. loss of memory
p. loss of mental skills
p. lung disease ▸ chronic
p. malignancy
p. massive fibrosis
P. Matrix Test, Raven's
p. memory loss
p. mental degeneration
p. mental disorder
p. movement disorder
p. multifocal leukoencephalopathy
p. multiple hyaloserositis
p. multiple sclerosis (MS)
p. multiple sclerosis (MS) ▸ chronic
p. multiple sclerosis (MS) ▸ primary
p. multiple sclerosis (MS) ▸ secondary
p. muscle relaxation
p. muscular atrophy
p. muscular dystrophy
p. myositis, acute
p. neurological disease
p. neurological disorder
p. neuromuscular atrophy
p. neuromuscular disease

p. neuropathic muscular atrophy
p. nonhereditary chorea, chronic
p. obstruction of renal artery
p. onset of weakness
p. organic brain disease
p. ossifying myositis
p. paralysis
p. parenchymal restriction
p. patient care
p. pneumonia
p. pulmonary disease, rapidly
p. relapsing multiple sclerosis (MS)
p. relaxation
p. relaxation, brief
p. relaxation for insomnia
p. relaxation training
p. relaxation under hyperactivity
p. resistant quadriceps exercises
p. respiratory failure
p. retardation
p. retinal degeneration
p. rheumatic diseases
p. rigidity
p. scanning
p. sclerosis ▸ systemic
p. shortness of breath (SOB)
p. spinal muscular atrophy
p. stiffness
p. subcortical encephalopathy
p. supranuclear palsy
p. symptoms
p. systemic sclerosis (PSS)
p. thrombus
p. torsion spasm
p. tumor
p. unilateral facial atrophy
p. unilateral hearing loss
p. vision loss
p. weakness
p. weakness of extremity
p. weakness one side of body
p. weakness ▸ slowly
progressively downhill course
progressively shaky, handwriting
prohealthy functioning change
proinflammatory substance
project, coronary drug
Project to Investigate Memory and Aging (OPTIMA) ▸ Oxford
projected patterns
projectile vomiting
projectile vomitus
projecting staphyloma
projection(s)
   p., anterior oblique

p., anteroposterior lordotic
p., AP (anteroposterior)
p., apical lordotic
p., axial
p., axillary
p., ball-catcher's
p., basilar
p., basovertical
p., biplane
p., blowout
p., bony
p., Chassard-Lapine
p., cone
p., coned AP (anteroposterior)
p., cone-down
p., craniocaudad
p., cross-sectional transverse
p., dorsoplantar
p., erect fluoro spot
p., flexion-extension
p., frog-leg
p., frontal
p., half-axial
p., inferior-superior
p., inferior-superior tangential
p., inferosuperior axial
p., intraoral
p., lateral
p., lateral oblique axial
p., lateral transcranial
p., lateral transfascial
p., lateromedial oblique
p., Lauenstein and Hickey
p., left anterior oblique
p. ▸ left lateral
p., L5 S1
p., Low-Beer
p., lumbosacral
p., medial oblique axial
p., mediolateral
p., navicular
p., neuron
p., nuchofrontal
p., oblique lateral
p., PA (posteroanterior)
p., PA (posteroanterior) and lateral
p., PA (posteroanterior) lordotic
p., parieto-orbital
p., pillar
p., Pirie transoral
p., plantodorsal
p., recumbent lateral
p., right anterior oblique
p. roentgenogram, Towne
p., Ruström

projection(s)—*continued*
- p., scaphoid
- p., semiaxial
- p., semiaxial anteroposterior (AP)
- p., semiaxial transcranial
- p., skyline
- p., spider
- p., spiny
- p., stereo left lateral
- p., stereo right lateral
- p., submentovertical axial
- p., sunrise
- p., superoinferior
- p., tangential
- p., Templeton and Zim carpal tunnel
- p., transtabular AP/PA
- p., transthoracic
- p., tunnel
- p., verticosubmental
- p., Water's
- p. x-ray microscope

projective (Projective)
- p. assessment
- P. Human Figure Drawing Test
- p. tests

prolactin
- p. (PRL)
- p. cells, adenomatous
- p. inhibiting factor
- p. level
- p. production, stimulate
- p., secrete
- p. secreting pituitary tumor

prolapse
- p., anal
- p., aortic valve leaflet
- p., bladder
- p., cord
- p. ▸ coronary spasm and
- p., first-degree uterine
- p., frank
- p. into vagina ▸ rectum
- p., iris
- p., mitral
- p. (MVP), mitral valve
- p. murmur, mitral
- p. of cord
- p. of iris
- p. of iris, late
- p. of Morgagni
- p. of urethra and bladder
- p. of uterus
- p., pan mitral
- p., rectal
- p. repair, LeFort uterine

- p., second-degree uterine
- p. syndrome ▸ mitral valve
- p., systolic mitral
- p., third-degree uterine
- p. ▸ tricuspid valve
- p., uterine
- p., vaginal
- p., valvular

prolapsed
- p. bladder
- p., cord
- p. disc
- p. fibroid
- p. fitness
- p. hemorrhoid
- p. mitral valve
- p. mitral valve syndrome
- p. rectum, redundant
- p. vaginal wall
- p. valve

prolapsing hemorrhoids
Prolene suture
proliferans
- p., angiocholitis
- p., cholecystitis glandularis
- p., endarteritis
- p., retinitis

proliferating
- p. angioendotheliomatosis ▸ neoplastic
- p. angioendotheliomatosis ▸ reactive
- p., bony
- p., cellular
- p. of bone
- p. of glia
- p. plasma cells
- p. pleurisy
- p. tumor, rapidly

proliferation
- p. ▸ actual cell
- p. antigen
- p. antigen ▸ nuclear
- p. area
- p. assay ▸ lymphocyte
- p. -associated antigen
- p., bile duct
- p., cell
- p., fibroglandular
- p., fibrous tumor
- p., mesaugral
- p., myxomatous
- p. of atypical alveolar cells
- p. of cuboidal cells
- p. of cuboidal cells, abnormal

- p. of esophageal cancer
- p. of fibroblasts
- p. of syncytial cells, abnormal
- p., vascular

proliferative
- p., acute
- p. diabetic retinopathy
- p. diabetic retinopathy, advanced
- p. endometrium
- p. endophlebitis
- p. fasciitis
- p. hyperplasia
- p. phase endometrium
- p. phlebitis
- p. retinitis
- p. retinopathy
- p. retinopathy photocoagulation (PRP)
- p. skin lesion
- p. stage

proligerous disc
prolong
- p. dying process
- p. life
- p. pregnancy

prolongation
- p. of air flow
- p. of air flow during expiration
- p. of expiration
- p. of life, artificial

prolonged
- p. abuse
- p. activity
- p. and deep ▸ breathing
- p. anesthetic effect
- p. antibiotic therapy
- p. anxiety
- p. bedrest
- p. cerebral apnea
- p. chest pain ▸ intense,
- p. contact
- p. deep inspiration
- p. depressive reaction
- p. disability
- p. drug therapy
- p. ear drainage
- p. eating disorder
- p. emotional stress
- p. episodes of chest pain
- p. expiration
- p. exposure, extreme
- p. generalized fatigue
- p. grief
- p. heavy drinking
- p. hiccups

p. hospital care
p. hospitalization
p. hypotension
p. illness
p. inactivity
p. indigestion
p. indwelling catheter
p. intensive hyperventilation
p. irreversible coma
p. labor
p. lassitude
p., life
p. menstrual periods
p. numbness
p. or repeated exposure
p. pain
p. period of anoxia
p. post-traumatic stress disorder
p. pregnancy
p. psychotic reactions
p. psychotic symptoms
p. Q-T interval
p. Q-T interval syndrome
p. Q-T syndrome
p. remission
p. resuscitative measures
p. rupture of fetal membranes
p. rupture of membranes
p. sleep
p. standing
p. steroid therapy
p. stress
p. symptomatic illness
p. task-oriented activity
p. therapy
p. thumbsucking
p. time to sustained respiration
p. tissue concentration
p. unconsciousness
p. unexplained hyperbilirubinemia
p. uterine bleeding
p. uveitis
p. vasospastic reaction
p. vertigo
p. vigorous exercise
prolonging
p. death
p. life
p. machine, life-
p. measures, life-
p. treatment, life-
prolotherapy technique
PROM (premature rupture of membranes)

prominence
p., anterior
p., bony
p., central vascular
p., chamber
p., facial canal
p., gastric rugal
p., hilar
p., laryngeal
p. of bone
p. of canal
p. of facial canal
p. of forehead
p. of left hilum
p. of pulmonary markings
p. of pulmonary vasculature
p. of pulmonary vessels
p. of right hilum
p., pulmonary
p., sacral
p., ventricular
p., vertebral
prominens ductus cochlearis ▸ vas
prominens reflex, vertebra
prominent
p. acryocyanosis
p. anthelix
p. bruit
p. delusions ▸ schizophrenia with
p. elevation
p. eyes
p. findings
p. forehead
p. generalized atrophy ▸ moderately
p. hallucinations
p. heel
p. murmur
p. nucleoli
p. nucleolus, small
p. pore
p. scoliosis
p. shoulder blades
p. thrill
promiscuity, sexual
promiscuous behavior
promiscuous behavior in child
promontory of tympanum
promoting factor ▸ leukocytosis-
prompt
p. appearance of dye
p. emptying
p. excretion of contrast material
p. excretion of dye
p. spill into duodenum

p. surgical closure
promptly, dye appears
promptly, stomach empties
promyelocytic leukemia
promyelocytic leukemia (APL), acute
pronated arches
pronated, hand
pronation [*phonation*]
p., abnormal
p. and supination
p., excessive
p. exercise, elbow
p. sign
pronator
p. drift
p. muscle, quadrate
p. muscle, round
p. quadratus muscle
p. teres muscle
pronatus, pes
prone
p., accident-
p. addicts, relapse-
p., behavioral
p., cancer-
p. families, cancer-
p. feet, blister-
p. film
p., patient accident-
p. patient ▸ suicide-
p. personality, disease-
p. pores, acne-
p. position
p., seizure-
p. to developing pigment gallstones
p. to diabetes ▸ genetically
p. to fantasy ▸ highly
p. virus, error-
proneness and absorption, fantasy
prong, hemilaminectomy
prong stem finger prosthesis ▸ two-
pronged cane, four-
pronounced dead, patient
pronouncement of brain death
pronouncement of death
proof
p. of concept
p. suction unit, explosion-
p. tank, sound-
prop
p. cells
p. graft
p., mouth
propagated thrombus
propagating thrombosis

propagation, impulse
propagation of R wave
propels wheelchair, patient
proper
    p. alignment and apposition of
       fracture
    p. alignment of temporomandibular
       joint (TMJ)
    p. balancing of ligaments
    p. balancing of tendons
    p. body mechanisms
    p. digital nerves of ulnar nerve
    p. exercise walking technique
    p. extensor muscle of fifth digit
    p. flow of blood ▸ ensure
    p. fungus
    p. nerve
    p. nutrition
    p. nutrition and exercise
    p. oxygenation
    p. palmar digital nerve
    p. palmar digital nerves of median
       nerve
    p. plantar digital nerves of lateral
       plantar nerve
    p. plantar digital nerves of medial
       plantar nerve
    p. precautions
    p. realignment of teeth
    p. rest
    p. station
    p. sterilization procedure
    p. substance of cornea
    p. substance of sclera
    p. substance of tooth
properitoneal hernia
properties
    p., direct anticancer
    p., dopamine receptor agonist
    p. of abused drugs, psychoactive
    p. of cannabinoids, psychoactive
    p. of depressants, psychoactive
    p. of hallucinogens, psychoactive
    p. of inhalants, psychoactive
    p. of lipophilicity
    p. of opioids, psychoactive
    p. of phencyclidines, psychoactive
    p. of stimulants, psychoactive
prophage, site of
prophesies, self-fulfilling
prophetic dimension of grief
prophylactic
    p. agent
    p. antibiotic(s)
    p. antibody

    p. antimicrobial drugs
    p. basis
    p. basis ▸ radiation therapy on
    p. braces
    p. bracing
    p. breast surgery
    p. course
    p. cranial irradiation
    p. cranial radiation
    p. destruction of transformation
       zone
    p. dose
    p. double mastectomy
    p. drip, Lidocaine
    p. gamma globulin
    p. hysterectomy
    p. knee brace
    p. mastectomy
    p. medication ▸ migraine
    p. odototomy
    p. oophorectomy
    p. oophorectomy, bilateral
    p. penicillin
    p. radiation
    p. study ▸ double-blind placebo
       control
    p. therapy
    p. therapy, parenteral
    p. urethritis
prophylaxis
    p., antibiotic
    p., antimicrobial
    p., calcium removal
    p., chemotherapy
    p., Crede's
    p., endocarditis
    p., local
    p., malaria
    p. ▸ perioperative antimicrobial
    p., postexposure
    p., primary
    p., routine
    p., stroke
    p. ▸ subacute bacterial endocarditis
       (SBE)
    p., surgical
propiolactone, beta
Propionibacterium acnes
proportion to age, in
proportional
    p. assist ventilation
    p. chamber, multiwire
    p. counter
    p. sensitivity
proportionate morbidity ratio

proposed treatment
propoxyphene, detoxification from
propria
    p. ▸ chronic inflammation of
    p. corneas, substantia
    p., lamina
    p. of Jungbluth, vasa
    p., tunica
proprietary medicine
proprioception
    p., decreased
    p. in control of behavior ▸ role of
    p., loss of
    p., normal
proprioceptive
    p. discrimination
    p. influence
    p. neuromuscular facilitation (PNF)
    p. reflex
    p. sense
    p. sensibility
    p. stimuli
Proprioni bacterium
proprius
    p., extensor indicis
    p. muscle, extensor digiti quinti
    p., sacculus
proptosis, ocular
propulsion, wheelchair
propylhexedrine abuse
propyliodone contrast medium
prospective (Prospective)
    p. evaluation of radial keratotomy
       (PERK) protocol
    p. payment system
    p. potency
    p. randomized study
    p. recipient
    p. study
    P. Study (TOPS) ▸ Treatment
       Outcome
    p. surveillance
    p. survey
    p. transplant patient
    p. transplant recipient
prostacyclin metabolite
prostaglandin synthesis
prostaglandins, synthetic
prostate [*prostrate*]
    p., adenocarcinoma
    p., apex
    p., benign hypertrophy of
    p. cancer, advanced
    p. cancer cells
    p. cancer detection

p. cancer ▸ early-stage
p. cancer ▸ hereditary
p. cancer ▸ localized
p., cancer of
p. cancer ▸ prevalence of
p. cancer screening
p. cancer screening procedure
p. cancer treatment
p. carcinoma
p. cell growth
p., digital examination of
p. disease
p., enlarged
p. enlargement
p. enlargement, relax
p. gland
p. gland, cancer of
p. gland, chronic infection in
p. gland ▸ enlarged, inflamed
p. gland, fibroadenomatous
   hyperplasia of
p. gland ▸ nodular hyperplasia of
p. gland ▸ noncancerous
   enlargement of
p. gland ▸ shrink enlarged
p., histologic sections of
p. hormone therapy
p. hyperplasia
p., immature
p. ▸ inflammation of
p., levator muscle of
p., lobe of
p. muscles, relax
p. ▸ muscular substance of
p. needle biopsy
p. palpated regularly
p. (PVP) ▸ photoselective
   vaporization of
p. ▸ radioactive seeding of
p. radiotherapy
p., rhabdomyosarcoma of
p. screening
p. size, reduce
p. specific antigen (PSA)
p. specific membrane antigen
   (PSMA)
p. ▸ stimulate growth of
p. surgery ▸ radical
p. tissue
p. tissue ▸ excess
p. tissue ▸ transurethral
   vaporization of
p. (TUIP) ▸ transurethral incision of
p. (TURP), transurethral resection
   of

p. treatment drug
p. tumor
p., ultrasound of
p. volume
p. with microwave ▸ shrink
prostatectomy
p. ▸ laparoscopic radical
p., nerve-sparing radical retropubic
p., open
p., perineal
p., radical
p., retropubic
p., retropubic prevesical
p., suprapubic
p., suprapubic transvesical
p., transurethral
p. (TULIP) ▸ transurethral
   ultrasound-guided laser-induced
prostatic
p. abscess
p. acid phosphatase
p. acid phosphatase (TSPAP) ▸
   total serum
p. adenocarcinoma ▸ lymphangitic
   spread of
p. adenoma
p. balloon dilation
p. biopsy
p. calculi
p. calculus
p. cancer
p. carcinoma
p. diverticulum
p. duct
p. enlargement
p. fossa
p. fraction
p. ganglion
p. hyperplasia
p. hyperplasia, benign
p. hypertrophy
p. hypertrophy (BPH) ▸ benign
p. hypertrophy, nodular
p. infection
p. lobe
p. origin ▸ tissue of
p. plexus
p. sinus
p. specific antigen (PSA)
p. tissue
p. tissue, intravesical
p. urethra
p. utricle
p. varices
p. vesicle

prostaticovesical plexus
prostaticus, liquor
prostaticus, sinus
prostatism, obstructive
prostatism, vesical
prostatitis
p., acute
p., acute bacterial
p., bacterial
p., chronic
p., chronic bacterial
p., granulomatous
p., tuberculous
prostatoseminovesiculectomy,
   perineal
prostatron thermotherapy
prosthesis (Prosthesis)
p., Alvarez valve
p., Angelchik anti-reflux
p., antireflux
p., aortic
p., aortic valve
p., Ashley's breast
p., Aufranc-Turner
p., Austin-Moore hip
p. ▸ ball and socket
p., ball valve
p., Barnard mitral valve
p., Bateman universal proximal
   femur (UPF)
p., Bateman's
p., Beall disk valve
p., Beall mitral valve
p., Bechtal
p., Bentall cardiovascular
p., bifurcated seamless
p., biliary duct
p., Bjork-Shiley aortic valve
p., Bjork-Shiley mitral valve
p., bone ingrowth
p., Braunwald's
p., breast
p., Buckholz
p., caged-ball
p., Cape Town aortic valve
p., cardiac valve
p., Carpentier annuloplasty ring
p., Carpentier-Edwards aortic valve
p., Carpentier-Rhone-Poulencmitral
   ring
p., Cartwright heart
p., Cartwright valve
p., cleft palate
p., collagen tape
p., collar

prosthesis—*continued*

p., computerized assisted design (CAD)
p., Cooley-Bloodwell mitral valve
p., crimped Dacron
p., Cross-Jones valve
p., Cutter SCDK
p. ▸ Cutter-Smeloff cardiac valve
p., Dacron
p., Dacron arterial
p., Dacron bifurcation
p., Dacron valve
p., Dacron vessel
p., DeBakey
p., DeBakey ball valve
p., DeBakey valve
p., DeBakey Vasculour II vascular
p., dental
p., DePalma hip
p., DePuy's
p., disc valve
p., discoid aortic
p., duckbill voice
p., ear pinna
p., ear piston
p., Edwards
p., Edwards seamless
p., Edwards Teflon intracardiac patch
p., Eicher hip
p., endoluminal
p., esophageal
p., fascia lata
p., femur repaired with
p. fitting, breast
p., 4-A Magovern valve
P. (NCP) generator ▸ NeuroCybernetic
p., geometric knee
p., Gott and Daggett valve
p., Gott low profile
p., Gott's
p., Guepar hinge knee
p., Hall-Kaster mitral valve
p. ▸ Hancock mitral valve
p., Harkins valve
p., Harris HD hip
p., Harrison interlocked mesh
p., HD II total hip
p., heart
p. ▸ heart valve
p., Helanca seamless tube
p., hollow sphere
p., House stainless steel mesh
p., Howmedica

p., Hufnagel low-profile heart valve
p., Hufnagel valve
p., insertion of
p., insertion of vascular
p., Ionescu-Shiley aortic valve
p., Joplin toe
p., Judet's
p., Kastec mitral valve
p., Kay-Shiley valve
p., Kay-Suzuki disc valve
p., Kinematic rotating hinge knee
p. ▸ knitted vascular
p., laryngeal
p., left hip
p., Leinbach's
p. ▸ Lillehei-Cruz-Kaster
p. ▸ Lillehei-Kaster
p. ▸ Lillehei-Kaster cardiac valve
p. ▸ Lillehei-Kaster mitral valve
p., Lippman hip
p., Lorenzo SMO
p., MacIntosh tibial plateau
p., Mackler intraluminal tube
p., Magovern-Cromie valve
p., mammary
p., Marmor
p., Matchett
p., Matchett-Brown
p., maxillofacial
p., McKee-Farrar
p., McKeever patella cap
p., McKeever Vitallium cap
p., Medi-graft vascular
p. ▸ Medtronic-Hall heart valve
p. ▸ Medtronic-Hall tilting disk valve
p., metal
p., microcrimped
p. ▸ Milliknit vascular graft
p., mitral
p., modified Moore hip locking
p., Moore hip
p., Mueller Duo-Lock hip
p., Mulligan Silastic
p., Neer
p., Neer shoulder
p. ▸ Neville tracheal
p., Niebauer
p., ocular
p. ▸ Omniscience single-leaflet cardiac valve
p. ▸ Omniscience tilting disk valve
p., orbital floor
p. (PORP), partial ossicular replacement
p., patellar

p., Pemco valve
p., piston-type
p. placement, esophageal
p., Plasticor torque-type
p. (TORP), Plastiport total ossicular replacement
p., polyvinyl
p., porcine
p. ▸ Rashkind double-disk occluder
p., re-anchor
p. retention, debridement and
p., right hip
p., Rosi L-type nose bridge
p., Sauerbruch's
p. ▸ Sauvage filamentous
p., SCDT heart valve
p., Schuknecht Teflon wire piston
p. ▸ sea leg
p., Sheehy-House incus replacement
p., Shier's total knee
p., Silastic
p., Silastic penile
p., Silastic testicular
p., silicone
p., Small-Carrion penile
p., Smeloff-Cutter valve
p., Smith-Petersen hip cup
p., solid silicone orbital
p. ▸ Sorin mitral valve
p., Speed radius cap
p. ▸ St. Jude heart valve
p., St. Jude Medical aortic valve
p., stabilizing
p., Starr-Edwards aortic valve
p. ▸ Starr-Edwards ball valve
p. ▸ Starr-Edwards cardiac valve
p. ▸ Starr-Edwards disk valve
p. ▸ Starr-Edwards heart valve
p. ▸ Starr-Edwards mitral
p. ▸ stentless porcine aortic valve
p., Stenzel rod
p. ▸ supra-annular
p., Surgitek penile
p., Teflon
p., Teflon mesh
p., Teflon sheeting
p., Teflon tri-leaflet
p., Thompson's
p., tibial
p. ▸ tilting disk aortic valve
p. (TORP), total ossicular replacement
p., Townley
p., tri-leaflet aortic

p., two-prong stem finger
p. ▸ Ultra-Low resistance voice
p. ▸ unicompartmental knee
p., Usher's Marlex mesh
p., Vanghetti's
p., vascular
p. ▸ vascular graft
p., Vitallium hip
p., Vitallium Moore self-locking
p., Wada hingeless heart valve
p., Walldius Vitallium mechanical
   knee
p., Weavenit
p., Wesolowski Weavenit vascular
p. ▸ woven Teflon
p., Xenophor femoral
p., Zimaloy femoral head
prosthetic
p. aortic valve
p. appliance
p. ball valve
p. ball valve ▸ Starr-Edwards
p. cardiac valve
p. device
p. device infection
p. device, manipulation of
p. failure
p. glenohumeral joint
p. group
p. head, Eicher femoral
p. head ▸ Judet-type femoral
p. head ▸ Naden-Rieth femoral
p. heart valve
p. heart valve surgery
p. joint
p. joint ▸ indwelling
p. joint infection
p. joint infection ▸ staph aureus
p. lens
p. limb
p. medical device ▸ indwelling
p. ring annuloplasty
p. system
p. teeth, permanent
p. training
p. valve, caged ball
p. valve endocarditis
p. valve ▸ porcine
p. valve sewing ring
p. valve ▸ Starr-Edwards
p. valve thrombosis
p. valve ▸ tilting disk
p. valve vegetation
p. vegetation
prostration and diaphoresis

prostration, heat
prosyncopal medication
protamine insulin
protean [*protein*]
protease
p. -antiprotease imbalance
p. inhibitor
p. inhibitor therapy
protect and stabilize injured knees
protection
p. activity, radiation
p., birth control
p. capacity, radiation
p. factor (SPF), sun
p. factor (SPF) ▸ sunscreen
p. in radiation therapy, ovary
p., lack ultraviolet
p., myocardial
p. pouch, Cardio-Cool myocardial
p. ▸ radiation-leukemia-
p., rest, ice compression and
   elevation (PRICE)
p., sun
p., sunscreen
p., white cell
protective (Protective)
p. agent
p. antibody
p. bandage
p. block
p. brace
p. chemical
p. custody
p. dressing
p. eye pad
p. eye shield
p. eye wear
p. gloves
p. inoculation
P. Isolation
p. laryngeal reflexes
p. layer of brain
p. layer of spinal cord
p. lining of mucous ▸ stomach's
p. outer surface of eye
p. pharyngeal reflexes
p. placement
p. spasm
p. survival strategy
p. therapy, cerebral
p. zone
protector
p., Arruga's
p., disposable elbow
p., disposable heel

p., elbow
p., heel
p. /provider for parent
proteidin, pyocyanase
protein(s) (Protein) [*protean*]
p., abnormal filament
p. abnormally phosphorylated
p. activity index (SPAI) ▸ steroid
p., acyl-carrier
p. allergy ▸ latex
p., amyloid
p., amyloid precursor
p., anticancer
p. antigens
p., anti-inflammatory
p., bacterial
p., beta amyloid
p. -binding
p. binding abnormality
p., blood-clotting
p. -bound iodine (PBI)
p. -bound iodine (SPBI) ▸ serum
p. -bound thyroxine (PBT)
p. -calorie deficiency
p. calorie malnutrition
p., cardiac gap junction
p., coagulation
p., coat
p., common core
p. complement fixation test ▸ Reiter
p., complex
p., contractile
p. (CRP), C-reactive
p., cytosolic
p. decomposition
p. deficiency
p., dephosphorylation of
P. Derivative (PPD) intermediate ▸
   Purified
P. Derivative (PPD) ▸ Purified
P. Derivative (PPD) skin testing ▸
   Purified
p. diet
p. diet, high
p. diet, low
p. digestion absorption
p. efficiency ratio (PER)
p. electrolyte
p. electrophoresis
p., electrophoretic
p., eosinophil cationic
p., extracellular
p. filaments
p. ▸ genetically engineered
p. granules

protein(s)—*continued*
- p., heat shock
- p., high
- p. (hs-CRP) ▸ high-sensitivity C-reactive
- p. immunoelectrophoresis
- p. in brain, diminished production of
- p., increased excretion of
- p., inflammatory
- p. intake
- p. interactions ▸ protein-
- p. kinase
- p. level, neural thread
- p. levels, serum
- p. levels test
- p. -losing enteropathy
- p. loss in hepatic disease
- p. loss test, gastrointestinal (GI)
- p., low
- p., M line
- p. metabolism
- p. method, Bence-Jones
- p., mitochondrial
- p., mitotic control
- p. molecule
- p., muscle
- p., myeloma-cell
- p. (NTP) ▸ neural thread
- p. nitrogen unit (PNU)
- p. (NMP) ▸ nuclear matrix
- p., patient spilled
- p., penicillin-binding
- p., phosphorylation of
- p. -protein interactions
- p. ▸ rat urine
- p., reactive
- p., recognition
- p. renin, high levels of kidney
- p. restricted diet
- p. restriction
- p. (RNP), ribonuclear
- p. S
- p. S deficiency
- p. ▸ secretory leukoprotease inhibitor
- p. serotype ▸ M-
- p., serum
- p. shell
- p. shock
- p. sickness
- p., single-celled
- p., sticky
- p. stimulate growth
- p. syndrome ▸ M-
- p. synthesis
- p. synthesis, decreased
- p. synthesis, impair
- p. synthesis inhibition
- p., synthetic
- p. test
- p. test, alpha fetal
- p. test, Bence-Jones
- p. test, C-reactive
- p. ▸ thrombus precursor
- p., thyroxine-binding
- p. (TP) ▸ total
- p. (TSP) ▸ total serum
- p., total urine
- p., transmembrane
- p. utilization, net

proteinaceous
- p. debris
- p. fluid
- p. material

proteinosis, pulmonary alveolar
proteinuria
- p., adventitious
- p., Bence Jones
- p., cardiac
- p., colliquative
- p., cyclic
- p., decreased
- p., emulsion
- p., enterogenic
- p., febrile
- p., globular
- p., gouty
- p., hematogenous
- p., intrinsic
- p., nephrogenous
- p., orthostatic
- p., palpatory
- p., postgamma
- p., postrenal
- p., postural
- p., residual
- p. test

proteoglycan binding
proteolytic
- p. digestion
- p. enzymes
- p. gram-negative organism

protest, masculine
proteus (Proteus)
- p., Amoeba
- p., Bacillus
- p. group
- P. hydrophilus
- P. inconstans
- P. melanovogenes
- P. mirabilis
- P. morgani
- P. pneumonia
- P. rettgeri
- P. species
- p., Vibrio
- P. vulgaris
- P. vulgaris, gram-negative

prothrombin (Pro)
- p. activity
- p. consumption time
- p. conversion accelerator (SPCA) ▸ serum
- p. test
- p. time
- p. time ▸ quick

prothrombinase complex
protocol(s)
- p., advanced cardiac life support (ACLS)
- p., antirejection
- p., Bruce
- p., Bruce treadmill
- p., chemotherapeutic
- p., chemotherapy
- p., clinical
- p. ▸ community-acquired pneumonia
- p., complex oncologic therapy
- p., continuous ramp
- p., Cornell exercise
- p., Dartmouth
- p. design in combined modality therapy
- p., discharge
- p. dose, recommended
- p., Ellestad
- p., evaluate
- p. exercise test, Bruce
- p. exercise test, Davidson
- p., experimental drug
- p., exsanguination
- p., field
- p. for clinical trials
- p., formal
- p., hospital
- p., inpatient treatment
- p., management
- p., medically supervised fasting
- p. ▸ milieu management
- p. ▸ modified Bruce
- p. ▸ modified Ellestad
- p., modify
- p., multicomponent
- p. ▸ multimodal treatment

p. ▸ Naughton treadmill
p., nursing
p., organized transport
p. ▸ Reeves treadmill
p., reinjection
p., research
p. ▸ rest metabolism/stress
　　perfusion
p. ▸ SCAN antitachycardia pacing
p. ▸ Sheffield treadmill
p. ▸ standard Bruce
p., standardized treatment
p., three-drug
p., transfusion
p. ▸ Westminster drug-free
p., written treatment
protodiastolic
p. gallop
p. murmur
p. rumble
proton (Proton)
p. beam therapy
p. beams
p. density
P. pump blockers
p. pump inhibitor
p. spectroscopy
proto-oncogenic effect
protopathic sensibility
protoplasm
p., degenerated
p., functional
p., granular
p., mass of
p. of a cell
p., superior
p., totipotential
p., undifferentiated
protoplasmic
p. astrocyte
p. astrocytoma
p. process
p. stain
Protoplast material
protoporphyria, erythrohepatic
protoporphyrin, erythrocyte
protoporphyrin, free erythrocyte
Protostrongylus rufescens
prototype strain
protovertebral segment
protozoa, intestinal
protozoa, motile
protozoal
p. dysentery
p. infections

p. myocarditis
p. organisms ▸ fungi and
protozoan
p. enteritis
p. parasite
p., trypanosome
protracta, Trypanosoma
protracted
p. descent
p. labor
p. perfusion deficit
p. treatment, tumor regeneration
　　and
p. withdrawal syndrome
protraction, mandibular
protraction, maxillary
protruded eyeball
protrudes down, hernia
protrudes in midline, tongue
protruding
p. cystocele
p. ears
p. growth
p. lumbosacral disc
p. mandible
p. spine
p. tongue
protrusio shill
protrusion
p., abnormal
p., bimaxillary
p., bimaxillary dentoalveolar
p., bone
p., bony
p., disc
p., eyeball
p., hernial
p., interior epidural
p., intervertebral disc
p., intrapelvic
p., lumbosacral disc
p., medial
p. of acetabulum, pelvic
p. of center of cornea, conical
p. of disc
p. of eyeball, abnormal
p. of eyes
p. of fetal part
p. of iris
p. of nose, beak-like
p., sac-like
p., tongue
p., unexplained
protrusive
p. excursion

p. excursion ▸ lateral
p. occlusion
p. occlusion ▸ straight
protuberance
p., external occipital
p., laryngeal
p., occipital
p. of chin
p., palatine
p., transverse occipital
p., tubal
protuberans, dermatofibrosarcoma
protuberant, abdomen
proven safe and effective
Proverbs Test
provide(s)
p. appropriate nonverbal support
p. excuses ▸ patient
p. gentle resistance ▸ water
p. medical assistance
p. reality base
Providencia rettgeri
provider
p. for parent, protector/
p., health care
p., mental health
p. organization (PPO), preferred
p., primary care
provirus, visna
provisional
p. callus
p. diagnosis
p. ligature
**provocation angina ▸ ergonovine
　　maleate**
provocation, bronchial
provocative
p. behavior
p. behavior ▸ inappropriate sexually
p. factor
provoked response, electronically
provoked seizure
provoking choice, anxiety-
provoking situation, anxiety-
Provox speaking valve
Prowazek-Greeff bodies
Prowazek-Halberstaedter bodies
prowazekii, Rickettsia
**Prower factor deficiency disease ▸
　　Stuart-**
Prower factor ▸ Stuart-
proximal
p. antrum
p. cervical spinal cord
p. colon

proximal—*continued*
- p. convoluted tubule
- p. coronary sinus
- p. duodenum
- p. duodenum ▸ traumatic transection of
- p. electrode
- p. ends of tendon identified
- p. esophagus
- p. femora
- p. femur (UPF) prosthesis, Bateman universal
- p. focal femoral deficiency
- p. humeri
- p. interphalangeal (PIP)
- p. interphalangeal joint (PIPJ)
- p. isovelocity surface area
- p. ligation
- p. ligatures
- p. loop of roux-en-y
- p. metaphysis of femur
- p. nail fold
- p. obstruction
- p. phalanx
- p. phalanx, shaft of
- p. revision
- p. shaft
- p. small bowel
- p. space
- p. stump doubly ligated
- p. third
- p. tibia
- p. to shunt
- p. tubular adenoma
- p. tubular degeneration
- p. ureter
- p. ureterolithiasis
- p. ureterolithotomy

proximally retracted
proximate cause
proximity of vertex ▸ amplitude maximal in
PRP (proliferative retinopathy photocoagulation)
PRP (Psychotic Reaction Profile)
PRR (pupils round and regular)
PRU (peripheral resistance unit)
prudent diet
prudent heart living
Pruitt-Inahara carotid shunt
Pruitt vascular shunt
prune juice sputum
prune-belly syndrome
pruned
- p. hilum

- p. -tree appearance
- p. -tree arteriogram

pruning, branch vessel
Prunus occidentalis
pruritic [*pleuritic*]
pruritic keratoses
pruritic rash
pruritus
- p. ani
- p., anogenital
- p., generalized
- p., jaundice
- p. vulvae

Prussak's
- P. fibers
- P. pouch
- P. space

Prussian helmet sign
ps (per second)
PSA (prostate specific antigen)
psammoma bodies
PSAP (peak systolic aortic pressure)
PSC (posterior subcapsular cataract)
PSDA (Patient Self-Determination Act)
pseudacacia, Robinia
Pseudallescheria
- P. boydii
- P. maltophilia
- P. stutzeri

pseudarthrosis of leg, congenital
pseudo petit mal
pseudo petit mal discharge
pseudo P-pulmonale
pseudoacanthosis nigricans
pseudoalternating current
Pseudoamphistomum truncatum
pseudoanemia angiospastica
pseudoaortic insufficiency
pseudobulbar paralysis
pseudocele/pseudocoele
pseudocholinesterase level
pseudochylous ascites
pseudocoarctation of aorta
pseudocylindrical bronchiectasis
pseudocyst
- p. abscessed
- p. formation
- p. gastrocystostomy
- p., infected
- p., leaking
- p. of pancreas
- p. ▸ outpouching of old
- p., pancreatic
- p. pancreatic ascites

pseudodiphtheriticum, Bacillus
pseudodiphtheriticum, Corynebacterium
pseudodisappearance criterion
pseudoendometrium, decidual
pseudoepileptic convulsions
pseudoepitheliomatous hyperplasia
pseudoexfoliation syndrome
pseudofelineus, Amphimerus
pseudofollicular salpingitis
pseudofracture artifact
pseudofusion beat
pseudogout crystals
pseudogout in knees
pseudohemophilia hepatica
pseudo-Hurler polydystrophy
pseudohypertrophic
- p. infantile muscular dystrophy
- p. muscular atrophy
- p. muscular dystrophy

pseudohypoparathyroidism
pseudohypoparathyroidism, pseudo-
pseudoicterogenes, Spirochaeta
pseudojoint formation
pseudo-Kaposi sarcoma
pseudolaminar necrosis
pseudoleukemia
- p. cutis
- p. gastrointestinalis
- p., infantile
- p. lymphatica
- p., myelogenous

pseudoleukemica infantum, anemia
pseudoleukoplakic vulvitis
pseudologia fantastica
pseudolymphocytic choriomeningitis
pseudolymphoma, orbital
Pseudolynchia canariensis
Pseudolynchia maurah
pseudomallei
- p., Actinobacillus
- p., Bacillus
- p. group
- p., Mallemyces
- p., Pseudomonas

pseudomedical therapy
pseudomelia paraesthetica
pseudomembranous
- p. angina
- p. bronchitis
- p. colic
- p. colitis
- p. colitis ▸ necrotizing,
- p. conjunctivitis
- p. croup

p. enteritis
p. enterocolitis
p. gastritis
p. rhinitis
pseudomemory ▸ patient has
Pseudomonas (pseudomonas)
P. aeruginosa
P. aeruginosa ▸ gram-negative
P. aeruginosa infections
p. aeruginosa, sepsis
P. bacteremia
p. bacteria
P. cepacia
P. eisenbergii
P. elastase
P. exotoxin
P. fluorescens
p. folliculitis
P. fragi
P. infection
P. mallei
P. maltophilia
P. nonliquefaciens
P. pseudomallei
P. pyocyanea
P. reptilivora
P. septica
P. stutzeri
P. syncyanea
P. viscosa
pseudomotor cerebri
pseudomucinous
p. cystadenocarcinoma
p. cystadenocarcinoma ovary
p. cystadenoma
pseudomuscular hypertrophy
pseudomyxoma peritonei
pseudoneurotic-type schizophrenia
pseudonormalization of T wave
pseudo-obstruction, intestinal
pseudoparalysis
p. agitans
p., arthritic general
p., congenital atonic
p., Parrot's
p., syphilitic
pseudoparalytica, myasthenia gravis
pseudophakia adiposa
pseudophakia fibrosa
pseudopolypoid changes
pseudo-pseudohypoparathyroidism
pseudoretinitis pigmentosa
pseudosacralization, lumbar
pseudosarcomatous fasciitis
pseudoscopic vision

pseudoscutellaris, Aedes
pseudoscutellaris, Aedes scutellaris
pseudotabes
p. mesenterica
p. peripherica
p., pupillotonic
pseudotriculare biatriatum, cor
pseudotropicalis, Candida
pseudotruncus arteriosus
pseudotuberculosis
p., Corynebacterium
p. hominis streptothrica
p., Pasteurella
p., Yersinia
pseudotumor
p. cerebri
p. effect
p., orgital
pseudotumoral mediastinal
amyloidosis
pseudovacuolata, Leptothrix
pseudoxanthoma elasticum
syndrome
PSG (peak systolic gradient)
PSH (past surgical history)
psi (pounds per square inch)
Psidium guajava
psilocybin
p. (magic mushrooms)
p. (mushroom)
p. (sacred mushrooms)
p. (shroom)
p. eaten raw
p. ingested
p. injected
Psilocyn (Mushroom)
psilosis stomatitis intertropica
psittaci, Chlamydia
psittaci, Miyagawanella
psittacosis
p., cocci triad ▸ Q fever,
p. infection ▸ lympho-granuloma
venereum
p. virus
PSMA (prostate specific membrane
antigen)
psoas
p. abscess
p. margin
p. muscle
p. muscle, greater
p. muscle, smaller
p. shadow
Psoralea corylifolia

psoralens
p. plus ultraviolet light (PUVA)
regimen
p. plus ultraviolet light (PUVA)
treatment
p., repigmentation with
psoriasiformis, parakeratosis
psoriasis [*pityriasis*]
p. buccalis
p., facial
p. from anxiety
p. linguae
p., pustular
p., scalp
p. treatment
psoriatic
p. arthritis
p. nails
p. patches
Psorophora ferox
Psorophora lutzii
Psoroptes
P. bovis
P. cuniculi
P. equi
P. ovis
psoroptic mange
PSP (phenolsulfonphthalein)
PSS (progressive systemic sclerosis)
PSVT (paroxysmal supraventricular
tachycardia)
psychedelic
p. drug
p. drug ingestion
p. experience
p. experience ▸ distressing
psychiatric (Psychiatric)
p. admission, emergent
P. and Alcohol Inpatient Review
System (PAIRS) Program
p. and substance abuse services
p. assessment
P. Association (APA) ▸ American
p. care
p. care, inpatient
p. care, patient under
p. case management program
p. comorbidity
p. complications of drug abuse
p. condition
p. condition, stabilized
p. conditions, various
p. consultation, inpatient
p. criteria
p. diagnosis

psychiatric—*continued*
- p. diagnosis ▸ primary presenting
- p. diagnostic interview
- p. disease
- p. disorder
- p. disorder, acute
- p. disorder, adolescent
- p. disorder, childhood
- p. disorder, distinct
- p. disorder ▸ heterogeneity of
- p. disorder, nonictal
- p. disorder ▸ past
- p. disorder, treatable
- p. disorder ▸ underlying
- p. disorders in drug abusers
- p. disorders, nonpsychotic
- p. dysfunction, acute
- p. effects ▸ drug-induced
- p. emergency
- p. emergency service
- p. evaluation
- p. evaluation, standardized
- p. facilities ▸ free-standing private
- p. facility ▸ free-standing
- p. hospital
- p. hospital, accredited
- p. hospitalization
- P. Hospitals ▸ American Association of Private
- p. hospitals, private
- p. illness
- p. illness ▸ exacerbation of pre-existing
- p. illness ▸ genetic predisposition to
- p. instability
- p. intervention
- p. manifestations
- p. medical facilities ▸ inpatient non-
- p. medication
- p. mental status
- p. mental status examination
- p. nurse clinician
- p. nursing assessment and intervention
- p. nursing care
- p. nursing intervention strategies ▸ innovative
- p. nursing services
- p. origin
- p. outpatient ▸ non-alcoholic
- p. process
- P. Rating Scale Test, Wittenborn
- P. Rating Scale (WPRS) ▸ Wittenborn
- p. reaction

- p. reaction, adverse
- p. residents
- p. services
- p. services ▸ management of
- p. social worker
- p. symptoms
- p. symptoms, alleviating
- p. symptoms ▸ severe
- p. syndrome
- p. syndrome ▸ identifiable
- p. therapy
- p. treatment, childhood
- p. treatment, inpatient
- p. treatment modalities
- p. treatment of delusions
- p. treatment, outpatient
- p. treatment plan, initial
- p. treatment, supportive

psychiatrically impaired

psychiatrist
- p., adolescent
- p., criminal
- p., independent
- p., supervising

psychiatry (Psychiatry)
- p., adult
- P. ▸ American Academy of Child and Adolescent
- p., biological
- p., child
- p., clinical
- p., community
- p., consultation-liaison
- p., descriptive
- p., dynamic
- p., existential
- p., forensic
- p., geriatric
- p., industrial
- p. ▸ managed care-based
- p., occupational
- p., orthomolecular
- p. residency
- p., social
- p., transcultural

psychic
- p. ability
- p. blindness
- p. blindness, cortical
- p. cells
- p. censor
- p. conflict, extra◇
- p. conflict, intra◇
- p. dependence
- p. determinism

- p. dysfunction
- p. dysuria
- p. effect
- p. energizer
- p. energy level
- p. epilepsy
- p. equivalent
- p. factors
- p. impotence
- p. influence
- p. insomnia
- p. level
- p. life
- p. overtone
- p. reflex
- p. retardation
- p. seizure
- p. shock
- p. stigma
- p. syndrome
- p. trauma

psychoactive
- p. doses of depressants
- p. doses of hallucinogens
- p. doses of inhalants
- p. doses of opioids
- p. doses of phencyclidines
- p. doses of stimulants
- p. drug
- p. drug effect ▸ intense
- p. effect
- p. medications
- p. properties of abused drugs
- p. properties of cannabinoids
- p. properties of depressants
- p. properties of hallucinogens
- p. properties of inhalants
- p. properties of opioids
- p. properties of phencyclidines
- p. properties of stimulants
- p. substance
- p. substance abuse
- p. substance abuse disorder
- p. substance amnestic disorder
- p. substance anxiety disorder
- p. substance delirium
- p. substance delusional disorder ▸ other or unspecified
- p. substance dependence
- p. substance intoxication ▸ other or unspecified
- p. substance mood disorder
- p. substance organic mental disorder
- p. substance personality disorder

p. substance use
p. substance use disorders
p. substance withdrawal
p. substance-dependent patient
p. substance-induced organic
  mental disorder
psychoanalysis, clinical
psychoanalysis therapy
psychoanalytic
p. concept of repression
p. evaluation
p. insight
p. pathology
psychobiological origin, common
psychocardiac reflex
psychocutaneous medicine
psychodynamic
p. concepts
p. evaluation
p. explanation
p. factor
p. perspective
p. play therapy
p. psychotherapy
p. psychotherapy ▸ individual
p. reductionism
p. theory
p. therapy
p. therapy ▸ short-term
p. treatment
psychodynamically oriented therapy
psychoeducation ▸ patient in
psychoeducational group therapy
psychogalvanic reaction
psychogalvanic reflex
psychogenic
p. amnesia
p. aversion to labor pains
p. basis
p. coma
p. disorder
p. dysmenorrhea
p. dyspnea
p. dysuria
p. factors
p. fugue
p. gastrointestinal (GI) reaction
p. genitourinary malfunction
p. illness, mass
p. impotence
p. origin
p. overlay
p. pain
p. pain, site unspecified
p. paranoid psychosis

p. polydipsia
p. reaction, gastrointestinal (GI)
p. rheumatism
p. rumination
p. skin reaction
p. stress
p. vaginismus
p. vomiting
psycholeptic episode
psychologic
p. adjustment
p. distress
p., emotional, somatic support
p. factor
p. impact
p. index, patient
p. relief
psychological
p. abnormality
p. abuse
p. addiction
p. addiction ▸ possible
p. adjustment
p. adjustment, improved
p. allergic reaction
p. and emotional effects
p. approach
p. approach, self
p. aspect
p. aspect of pain ▸ emotional and
p. assessment
p. autopsy
p. barrier
p. battering
p. battery ▸ emotional and
p. calm
p. changes
p. complications
p. component
p. conflict ▸ internal
p. cost of euthanasia
p. counseling
p. craving
p. defense
p. dependence
p. dependence, physical and
p. dependency
p. discomfort
p. disorder
p. disorder ▸ potentially serious
p. dissociation
p. disturbance
p. drug dependence
p. dysfunction
p., educational and social therapy

p. effects
p. effects, adverse
p. effects of cannabinoid abuse
p. effects of depressants
p. effects of drug abuse
p. effects of hallucinogens
p. effects of hypnotic suggestion
p. effects of inhalants
p. effects of opioids
p. effects of phencyclidines
p. effects of relaxation training
p. effects of stimulants
p. emergency, behavioral
p. evaluation
p. evaluation, compulsory
p. factor
p. factors affecting physical
  condition
p. factors in drug abuse
p. factors of longevity
p. functioning
p. gender
p. growth
p. health
p. history as a screening device
p. history as a screening device for
  drug abuse
p. illness
p. impact
p. impotence
p. inaccessibility
p. make-up
p. maladjustment
p. management of chronic pain
p. manifestations
p. manifestations of acute drug
  reactions
p. manifestations of physical
  disease
p. maturation
p. measures of personality
p. medicine
p., mental and
p. morbidity ▸ long-term
p. orientation
p. origin
p. outcome
p. overlay
p. overlay and depression
p. overtones
p. pain
p. phenomenon
p. principle
p. problems
p. problems, feigned

psychological—*continued*
p. problems of drug abusers
p. problems related to drug abuse
p. reaction
p. reaction, acute adverse
p. reactions ▸ slowing of
p. recovery
p. reports
p. resources
p. risk
p. scars
p. screening
p. self-exploration
p. services
p. skills
p. sophistication
p., spiritual, physical and nutritional component ▸ medical,
p. stability
p. state during withdrawal
p. state in acute drug intoxication
p. state in flashback reactions
p. state in panic reactions
p. state, voluntary control of
p. state with overdosing
p. status
p. stimuli
p. strain
p. stress
p. stress of hospitalization
p. stress ▸ sudden
p. studies
p. study, clinical
p. suffering
p. support
p. support, augmented
p. symptoms ▸ factitious disorder with
p. symptoms ▸ factitious illness with
p. technique
p. technique, behavioral
p. terror
p. testing
p. tests, standard
p. therapy
p. traits
p. trauma
p. treatment
p. treatment, supportive
p. turmoil
p. variables
psychologically
p. abusive
p. addicting

p. disabled
p. impaired
p. stable
psychologist
p., clinical
p., licensed consulting
p. -patient privilege
p., rehabilitation
p., trained adolescent
psychology
p., abnormal
p., analytic
p., applied
p., behavioristic
p., child
p., clinical
p., cognitive
p., comparative
p., constitutional
p., correctional
p., counseling
p., criminal
p., depth
p., developmental
p., disaster
p., dreaming self-
p., dynamic
p., educational
p., ego
p. ▸ ego deficit
p., evolutionary
p., experimental
p., experimental social
p., forensic
p., genetic
p., gestalt
p., holistic
p., humanistic
p., individual
p., industrial
p. of addictive behavior
p. of dreaming, self-
p. of personality
p., physiologic
p., physiological
p., practical
p., reverse
p., self-
p., social
p., theoretical
psychometric
p. evaluation
p. examination
p. testing
psychomimetic agent

psychomotor
p. activity
p. activity ▸ increased
p. agitation
p. coordination
p. disturbance, predominant
p. epilepsy
p. excitement
p. functioning ▸ retardation of normal
p. impairment
p. inhibition
p. overactivity
p. retardation
p. retardation, functional
p. seizure
p. skills
p. skills ▸ evaluation of
p. variant
p. variant ▸ compatible with
p. variant discharge
p. variant pattern
psychoneurosis, paranoid
psychoneurotic disorders
psychoneurotic reaction
psychopath, dull
psychopath, serial sexual
psychopathic
p. constitution
p. diathesis
p. inferiority ▸ constitutional
p. personality
p. state, constitutional
psychopathological reaction to stress
psychopathology
p., child
p., childhood
p., deep-seated
p. ▸ human
p. of holocaust survivors
p., premorbid
psychopharmacological treatment
psychopharmacology, clinical
psychopharmacology, clinical pediatric
psychophysical technique
psychophysics, respiratory
psychophysics, sensory
psychophysiologic disorder
psychophysiological
p. background
p. effects of relaxation
p. gastrointestinal (GI) reaction
p. growth process

p. insomnia
p. malfunction
p. process, complex
psychoprophylaxis in obstetrics
psychosensory aphasia
psychosensory disturbance
psychoses, hereditary
psychosexual
    p. development
    p. development ▸ regression and
    p. disorder
    p. dysfunction
    p. dysfunction ▸ inhibited sexual
       desire
    p., hereditary
    p. identity ▸ disorders of
    p. sphere
    p. stage
psychosis(-es)
    p., acute or persistent
    p., affective
    p., alcoholic
    p., amphetamine
    p., battle
    p., biofeedback in
    p., bipolar
    p., brief reactive
    p., Cheyne-Stokes
    p., circular
    p., debilitating
    p., depressive
    p., depressive type
    p., disintegrative
    p., drug
    p., drug-induced
    p., drug-precipitated
    p., early childhood
    p., epileptic
    p., excitative type
    p., exhaustion
    p., existing
    p., famine
    p., febrile
    p. ▸ full-blown
    p., functional
    p., gestational
    p., idiophrenic
    p., impending
    p. in the elderly
    p. induced by cocaine
    p., infantile
    p., infection exhaustion
    p., involutional
    p., Korsakoff's
    p. -like state

p. ▸ lysergic acid diethylamide
    (LSD) -induced
p., manic
p., manic-depressive
p., methamphetamine
p., nonorganic
p., organic
p., paranoiac
p., paranoid
p., periodic
p., polyneuritic
p., polyneuritica
p., postpartum
p., postperfusion
p. ▸ potentially irreversible
p., prison
p., psychogenic paranoid
p., puerperal
p., purpose
p., reactive
p., schizoaffective
p. ▸ schizophrenia-like
p., senile
p., severe
p., situational
p., symbiotic
p., syphilitic
p., toxic
p., unipolar
p., unipolar depression with
p., Wernicke's
p. with origin specific to childhood
p., zoophil
psychosocial (Psychosocial)
    p. adjustment
    P. Adjustment to Illness Scale
    p. aspect
    p. development
    p. dysfunction
    p. evaluation
    p. factor
    p. functioning
    p. history, complete
    p. influences
    p. intervention
    p. occupational therapy
    p. perspective
    p. problem
    p. profile
    p. risk assessment
    p. stigma
    p. strategy
    p. stress
    p. stressors
    p. technique

p. therapy
p. treatment
p. variables
psychosomatic
    p. aches and pains
    p. complaint
    p. disease
    p. disorder
    p. hysteria
    p. illness
    p. medicine
    p. pain
    p. patient
    p. problems, diverse
    p. symptoms
psychospiritual disorder
psychostimulant dependence
psychostimulant dysfunction
psychotherapeutic
    p. and educational activities
    p. drug misuse
    p. intervention
    p. measures
    p. medications
    p. strategy
    p. treatment
psychotherapist, infant
psychotherapy
    p., adolescent
    p. by somatic alteration
    p., child
    p., dynamic
    p., eclectic
    p., emotional release
    p., focused
    p. for anxiety, analytical
    p. for depression, analytical
    p. ▸ goal-oriented
    p., group
    p. group ▸ structured adolescent
    p. ▸ harm reduction
    p., individual
    p. ▸ individual psychodynamic
    p., insight
    p., integrated
    p., intensive insight-oriented
    p., interpersonal
    p., long-term
    p., nondirective
    p. ▸ object relations
    p. of post-traumatic stress disorder
    p., outpatient
    p. ▸ patient in
    p. practice
    p., psychodynamic

psychotherapy—*continued*
  p., rational
  p., reality-oriented
  p., short-term
  p., split
  p., supportive
  p., systemic
  p., traditional
  p. ‣ trauma-focused approach to
psychotic (Psychotic)
  p. attack
  p. behavior
  p. condition, organic
  p. condition ‣ presenile organic
  p. condition ‣ senile organic
  p. condition ‣ transient organic
  p. delusions
  p. depression
  p. depressive reaction
  p. depth ‣ severe disorder of
  p. disorder
  p. disorder, induced
  p. disorder ‣ nonaffective
  p. disorder ‣ shared
  p. epileptic
  p. episode
  p. features ‣ bipolar disorder, depressed, severe, without
  p. features ‣ bipolar disorder, depressed, with
  p. features ‣ bipolar disorder, manic, severe, without
  p. features ‣ bipolar disorder, manic, with
  p. features ‣ bipolar disorder, mixed,
  p. features ‣ bipolar disorder, mixed, severe, without
  p. features ‣ bipolar disorder, mixed, with
  p. features ‣ major depression, recurrent, severe, without
  p. features ‣ major depression, recurrent, with
  p. features ‣ major depression, severe, without
  p. features ‣ major depression, single-episode severe
  p. features ‣ major depression, single-episode, with
  p. features ‣ major depression, with
  p. illness
  p. individual
  p. -like symptoms
  p. patient

  p. personality changes
  p. phenomenology
  p. reaction
  p. reaction, acute
  P. Reaction Profile
  p. reaction ‣ prolonged
  p. reactions, acute treatment for
  p. reactions, clinical manifestations of
  p. reactions, differential diagnosis of
  p. reactions, subacute treatment of
  p. reactions, symptoms of
  p. reactions, treatment of
  p. reactions with cannabinoids
  p. reactions with depressants
  p. reactions with hallucinogens
  p. reactions with inhalants
  p. reactions with multiple drugs
  p. reactions with opioids
  p. reactions with phencyclidines
  p. reactions with stimulants
  p. shock
  p. state
  p. state, acute
  p. state ‣ amphetamine-induced paranoid
  p. state ‣ relapse of paranoid
  p. state ‣ schizophrenic-like
  p. symptoms
  p. symptoms ‣ prolonged
  p. symptoms ‣ recurrent
  p. syndrome
  p. theory
  p. thought disorder
  p. thought disorder ‣ acute
psychotoxic effect
psychotoxic manifestation
psychotropic
  p. agents
  p. drug
  p. medication
psyllium-based laxative
PT (physical therapy/physiotherapy)
PT (Physical Therapy) Department
PTA (percutaneous transluminal angioplasty)
PTA (plasma thromboplastin antecedent)
PTARF (post-traumatic acute renal failure)
PTC (percutaneous transhepatic cholangiogram)
PTC (plasma thromboplastin component)

PTCA (percutaneous transluminal coronary angiography)
PTCA (percutaneous transluminal coronary angioplasty)
PTCR (percutaneous transluminal coronary revascularization)
pteriotic center
Pterocarpus marsupium
pteroylglutamic acid
pterygium [*phrygian*]
  p. buried
  p. colli
  p., congenital
  p., encroachment of
  p., head of
  p. transplant
  p. transplant ‣ McReynolds'
  p. undermined
  p. unguis
pterygoid
  p. artery
  p. canal, nerve of
  p. canal, vein of
  p. depression
  p. muscle
  p. muscle, external
  p. muscle, internal
  p. muscle, lateral
  p. nerve, external
  p. nerve, internal
  p. nerve, lateral
  p. nerve, medial
  p. notch
pterygomandibular raphe
pterygomaxillary region
pterygopalatine ganglion
pterygopalatine nerves
PTFE
  PTFE (polytetrafluoroethylene) arterial graft material
  PTFE (polytetrafluoroethylene) Gore-Tex graft
  PTFE (polytetrafluoroethylene) Impra graft
PTH (parathormone)
PTH (parathyroid hormone)
p^{32} (phosphorus 32/radioactive phosphorus)
ptosis
  p., acquired
  p. adiposa
  p. and/or nystagmus
  p., breast
  p., brow
  p., congenital

p., Horner's
p., hypomastia with
p., lid
p. lipomatosis
p. of eyelid
p. of eyelid, unilateral
p. of kidney
p. operation, eyelid
p. procedure, Aries-Pitanguy
  mammary
p., renal
p. repair ▸ brow
p. sling, Supramid
p. sympathica
p. ▸ upper eyelid
ptotic kidney
PTR (peripheral total resistance)
**PTSD (post-traumatic stress
  disorder)**
PTT (partial thromboplastin time)
P₂ (pulmonic second sound)
P₂ (pulmonic second sound) split
PU (peptic ulcer)
PU (pregnancy urine)
pubarche and thelarche
pubcoccygeus muscle
puberty ▸ idiopathic isosexual
puberty, precocious
pubes [*tubes*]
pubescent uterus
pubic
p. arch
p. arch ▸ open
p. area
p. bone
p. hair
p. hair, absence of facial and
p. hair, masculine
p. lice
p. lice ▸ eggs, nits, and
p. louse
p. phthiriasis
p. ramus, left
p. ramus, right
p. region
p. region of abdomen
p. ridge
p. segment of pelvis
p. symphysis
p. tubercle
pubica, symphysis
pubicoperitoneal muscle
pubis
p., hairs of
p., mons

p., Os
p., pediculosis
p., Pediculus
p., Phthirus
p. ▸ scar from midepigastrium to
p., symphysis
p., xiphoid to
public (Public)
p. antigen
p. health
p. health education programs
p. health hazard
P. Health Nurse (PHN)
p. health program
P. Health Service (PHS)
p. mental health patients
p. relations
p. tolerance, professional and
**publication of photographs ▸
  authorization form for taking and**
**publication of photographs ▸ consent
  form for taking and**
**publicly assisted drug abuse
  treatment program**
pubocapsular ligament
pubocervical fascia
pubococcygeal line
pubococcygeal muscle
pubofemoral ligament
puboprostatic
p. ligament, lateral
p. ligament, medial
p. muscle
puborectal muscle
pubosacral diameter
pubotuberous diameter
pubovaginal muscle
pubovesical ligament
pubovesicalis, plica
pubovesicocervical fascia
**PUBS (percutaneous umbilical blood
  sampling)**
puckering of skin
PUD (peptic ulcer disease)
puddler's cataract
**pudenda ▸ ulcerating granuloma of
  the**
pudendal
p. artery
p. block
p. block anesthesia
p. hematocele
p. hernia
p. nerve
p. vein, external

p. vein, internal
pudendi, frenulum labiorum
pudendi, granuloma
pudendum femininum
pudendum muliebre
pudente tropicum, granuloma
Pudenz's
P. reservoir
P. shunt
P. tube
P. valve
P. valve, Sheldon-
P. ventriculoatrial shunt
puerile respiration
puerperal
p. convulsion
p. eclampsia
p. endometritis
p. febrile morbidity
p. fever
p. hemiplegia
p. insanity
p. mania
p. mastitis
p. metritis
p. phlebitis
p. psychosis
p. pyelonephritis
p. sepsis
p. thrombophlebitis
p. thrombosis
p. uremia
puerperarum, colostrum
**puerperarum, phlegmasia alba
  dolens**
Puestow procedure
puff
p. mouthpiece ▸ sip-and-
p. of smoke
p. tonometer ▸ air-
p., veiled
puffers (PP), pink
puffiness
p. of abdomen
p. of face
p. of feet
p. of hands
puffing sound
puffy
p. ankles
p. face, bruised and
p. gums, red and
p., swollen eyelids
p. tumor, Potts
Pugh's nail

pugilistica, dementia
Puig-Massana-Shiley annuloplasty
   ring
pulchrum, Gongylonema
Pulex cheopis
Pulex irritans
pull(s)
   p. down exercise
   p. exercise ▸ toe
   p. hair ▸ patient
   p. -out wire, Bunnell
   p. -out wire sutures
   p. -through procedure, Soave
     abdominal
   p. -through procedure, Swenson
   p. -ups
pullback
   p., aortic
   p. pressure
   p. pressure, aortic
pulled
   p. catheter out, patient
   p. elbow
   p. muscle
   p. taut, strand
pulley tendon
pulling
   p. and separation ▸ vitreous
   p., compulsive hair
   p. or itching feeling ▸ fidgeting,
     aching,
   p. ▸ pathological hair
   p. skills, pushing and
pullorum, Aegyptianella
pullorum, Salmonella
pullulans, Aureobasidium
Pullularia pullulans
pulmoaortic canal
pulmonale
   p., atrium
   p., cor
   p., Distoma
   p., P-
   p. ▸ pseudo P-
pulmonalis
   p., lunulae valvularum semilunarium
     arteriae
   p., lunulae valvularum semilunarium
     trunci
   p., Norcardia
   p., Trichomonas
pulmonaris, porta
pulmonary (Pulmonary)
   p. abnormality
   p. abscess

p. abscesses, multiple
p. acid aspiration syndrome
p. actinomycosis
p. adenomatosis
p. adenopathy
p. agenesis
p. agenesis ▸ unilateral
p. air exchange ▸ poor
p. airways, clearing of
p. alterations
p. alveolar hemorrhage
p. alveolar hemorrhage ▸ diffuse
p. alveolar microlithiasis
p. alveolar proteinosis
p. alveoli
p. amebiasis
p. amyloidosis
p. amyloidosis ▸ nodular
p. aneurysm ▸ arteriovenous (AV)
p. angiitis
p. angio-aortic arch study ▸
  cardiac-
p. angiogram
p. angiography
p. angiography, balloon occlusion
p. angiography ▸ wedge
p. angioma
p. anthrax
p. apex, left
p. aplasia
p. arches
p. arterial pressure
p. arterial vasculature
p. arterial web
p. arteries, coarctation of
p. arteriography
p. arteriolar resistance
p. arteriole
p. arteriopathy ▸ plexogenic
p. arteriovenous aneurysm
p. arteriovenous (AV) fistula
p. arteriovenous fistula ▸ solitary
p. arteriovenous malformation
p. arteriovenous malformation ▸
  Mondini
p. artery
p. artery anastomosis ▸ systemic to
p. artery aneurysm
p. artery band
p. artery banding
p. artery branches
p. artery catheter ▸ flow-directed
p. artery catheterization
p. artery, congenital absence of
p. artery, congenital aneurysm of

p. artery, dilated
p. artery hypertension (PAH)
p. artery ▸ invisible main
p. artery, left
p. artery, main
p. artery mean pressure (PAMP)
p. artery ▸ obstructed
p. artery occlusion pressure
p. artery occlusion ▸ temporary
  unilateral
p. artery occlusive wedge pressure
p. artery pressure (PAP)
p. artery pressure ▸ increased
p. artery, right
p. artery, right main
p. artery shunt ▸ ascending aorta-
  to-
p. artery sling
p. artery steal
p. artery stenosis
p. artery stenosis, branch
p. artery stenosis ▸ pathogenesis of
p. artery syndrome ▸ epibronchial
  right
p. artery tumor
p. artery wedge
p. artery wedge pressure
p. artery wedge pressure ▸ mean
p. asbestosis
p. aspects in esophageal atresia
p. aspergillosis
p. aspergillosis ▸ invasive
p. atelectasis
p. atelectasis, basal
p. atelectasis, bilateral
p. atresia
p. atrium
p. barotrauma
p. bed
p. blastoma
p. bleeding
p. blood clots
p. blood flow (PBF)
p. blood flow study
p. blood flow (TPBF) ▸ total
p. blood volume (PBV)
p. botryomycosis
p. branch stenosis
p. bypass
p. candidiasis
p. capillaries
p. capillaries, leaking
p. capillary pressure
p. capillary wedge (PCW)

p. capillary wedge pressure, monitor
p. carcinoma ▸ metastatic
p. cavitation
p. circulation
p. cirrhosis
p. coccidioidomycosis
p. collapse
p. commissurotomy
p. compliance
p. complications
p. complications of drug abuse
p. concussion
p. congestion
p. congestion, bilateral
p. contusion
p. conus
p. cyanosis
p. cystic lymphangiectasis, chronic
p. diffusion capacity
p. diffusion study
p. disease
p. disease, active
p. disease, advanced
p. disease anemia syndrome
p. disease (COPD), chronic obstructive
p. disease, congestive
p. disease, diffuse
p. disease, obstructive
p. disease, rapidly progressive
p. disorder
p. disorder ▸ chronic
p. disorder ▸ chronic cyclic
p. drainage (dr'ge)
p. dysmaturity syndrome
p. edema (PE)
p. edema, acute
p. edema (ACPE), acute cardiogenic
p. edema, asbestosis
p. edema, cardiogenic
p. edema, chronic
p. edema ▸ fatal acute
p. edema ▸ flash
p. edema ▸ florid
p. edema, focal
p. edema, fulminant
p. edema (HAPE) ▸ high-altitude
p. edema, interstitial
p. edema, mild
p. edema ▸ neurogenic
p. edema, noncardiac
p. edema, noncardiogenic
p. edema ▸ paroxysmal

p. edema, permeability
p. edema ▸ postanesthesia
p. edema ▸ postcardioversion
p. edema, resolving
p. edema, uremic
p. effusion
p. embolectomy
p. emboli
p. emboli, multiple
p. emboli ▸ occult
p. emboli, peripheral
p. emboli, recurrent
p. emboli with small infarct
p. embolism (PE)
p. embolism, acute
p. embolism, air
p. embolism ▸ myxomatous
p. embolism ▸ submassive
p. embolization
p. embolus
p. embolus, massive
p. emphysema
p. emphysema, chronic
p. emphysema (COPE), chronic obstructive
p. emphysema, obstructive
p. endocrine cells
p. endothelium
p. eosinophilia ▸ tropical
p. epithelial cells
p. evaluation
p. excretions
p. exercises
p. failure
p. fever
p. fibrosis
p. fibrosis, chronic interstitial
p. fibrosis, diffuse interstitial
p. fibrosis, familial
p. fibrosis (IPF) ▸ idiopathic
p. fibrosis, interstitial
p. fibrosis ▸ primary
p. fibrosis ▸ progressive interstitial
p. fibrosis ▸ rejection-associated
p. fibrotic pattern
p. fibrotic scarring
p. fields
p. fields, clear
p. flow
p. form
p. function
p. function, abnormal
p. function laboratory
p. function, normal
p. function ▸ postoperative

p. function screen ▸ normal
p. function screening
p. function studies
p. function test (PFT)
p. function testing
p. function tests ▸ pretransplant
p. function ventilation studies
p. gas exchange
p. granulomatosis
p. hamartoma
p. heart
p. heart valve disorder
p. hemorrhage
p. hemorrhage, acute
p. hemorrhage, fatal
p. hemorrhages ▸ multiple interstitial
p. hemorrhagic necrosis
p. hemosiderosis
p. hemosiderosis ▸ essential
p. hemosiderosis, idiopathic
p. hemosiderosis, secondary
p. hilus
p. histiocytosis X ▸ primary
p. histoplasmosis
p. hyaline membrane
p. hypertension
p. hypertension ▸ chronic thromboembolic
p. hypertension, hypercorbia
p. hypertension ▸ hypoxic
p. hypertension murmur ▸ primary
p. hypertension of newborn ▸ persistent
p. hypertension pressure
p. hypertension, primary
p. hypertension risk factor ▸ primary
p. hypertension, secondary
p. hypertrophic osteoarthropathy
p. hypoplasia
p. hypoplasia membrane disease
p. hypoplasia, secondary
p. hypothalamic stimulation
p. immaturity and atelectasis
p. incompetence (PI)
p. infarct
p. infarct, diaphragmatic
p. infarction (PI)
p. infarction syndrome
p. infarcts, multiple
p. infection
p. infection, benign
p. infection, chronic
p. infiltrate fever

pulmonary—*continued*

p. infiltrate ‣ migratory
p. infiltrate ‣ Wasserman-positive
p. infiltrates
p. infiltrates, bibasilar
p. infiltrates ‣ bilateral alveolar
p. infiltration
p. infiltration and eosinophilia (PIE)
p. insufficiency
p. insufficiency revascularization syndrome
P. Intensive Care Unit (PICU)
p. interstitial disorder
p. interstitial edema
p. interstitial emphysema (PIE)
p. interstitial fibrosis
p. interstitial fibrosis ‣ chronic
p. irradiation, adjuvant
p. lesion
p. lesions, early metastatic
p. ligament
p. lobules
p. lymph nodes
p. lymphangiectasis, congenital
p. lymphoma
p. markings
p. markings, prominence of
p. mast cells
p. maturity
p. melioidosis
p. meniscus sign
p. metastasectomy
p. metastases
p. microcirculation
p. microvascular permeability
p. microvascular pressure
p. mucormycosis
p. murmur
p. mycosis
p. necrosis
p. nocardiosis
p. nodule, solitary
p. nodules
p. notch sign
p. orifice
p. ossification
p. osteoarthropathy
p. osteoarthropathy, hypertrophic
p. outflow tract
p. pain
p. parenchyma
p. parenchymal disease ‣ primary
p. parenchymal window
p. pathology, active
p. pedicle

p. perfusion scanning
p. phthisis
p. physiology
p. pleura
p. pleurisy
p. plexus
p. pressure
p. pressure wave form
p. problems, postoperative
p. prominence
p. pulse
p. rales
p. rales ‣ bilateral diffuse
p. regurgitation
p. rehabilitation
p. rehabilitation program
p. resection, segmental
p. resistance
p. resistance (TPR) ‣ total
p. sarcoidosis
p. schistosomiasis
p. scintigraphy
p. scleroderma
p. screen, pre◇
p. secretions
p. segment
p. sensory mechanism
p. sequestration
p. services
p. shunt, cardiac
p. shunt ‣ systemic to
p. siderosis
p. sling syndrome
p. stenosis
p. surface tensions ‣ altered
p. surfactant
p. syndrome, eosinophilic
p. syndrome ‣ Hantavirus
p. systemic blood flow ratio
p. target sign
p. technology
p. test
p. thromboemboli
p. thromboemboli, massive
p. thromboembolic disease
p. thromboembolism
p. thromboembolism, acute
p. thromboembolus
p. thromboendarterectomy
p. thrombosis
p. tissue ‣ compression of
p. toilet
p. toilet, vigorous
p. trunk
p. trunk ‣ base of

p. trunk, bifurcation of
p. trunk valves ‣ lunulae of
p. trunk valves ‣ nodules of
p. tuberculosis (TB)
p. tuberculosis (TB), active
p. valve
p. valve anomaly
p. valve area
p. valve ‣ carcinoid involving
p. valve disease
p. valve disorder
p. valve disorder, asymptomatic
p. valve disorder ‣ mild
p. valve echocardiography
p. valve gradient
p. valve ‣ narrowed
p. valve restenosis
p. valve stenosis
p. valve ‣ stenosis in
p. valve vegetation
p. valvotomy
p. valvotomy, balloon
p. valvular regurgitation
p. valvuloplasty
p. valvuloplasty, balloon
p. valvulotomy
p. vascular disease
p. vascular disease, hypertensive
p. vascular disorder
p. vascular hyperplasia
p. vascular markings
p. vascular obstruction
p. vascular obstructive disease
p. vascular permeability
p. vascular pressure
p. vascular pulsations
p. vascular reactivity
p. vascular redistribution
p. vascular resistance
p. vascular resistance index
p. vascular resistance (TPVR) ‣ total
p. vascularity
p. vasculature
p. vasculature free of emboli
p. vasculature, prominence of
p. vasculatures, central
p. vasculitis
p. vasoconstriction
p. vasoconstriction, hypoxic
p. vein
p. vein, anomalous
p. vein isolated, superior
p. vein, left
p. vein, left inferior

p. vein, left superior
p. vein, right
p. vein, right inferior
p. vein, right superior
p. vein transplant, right
p. veno-occlusive disease
p. venous congestion
p. venous connection
p. venous connection anomaly
p. venous connection ▸ partial anomalous
p. venous connection ▸ total anomalous
p. venous drainage (dr'ge)
p. venous drainage ▸ partial anomalous
p. venous drainage (dr'ge) ▸ total anomalous
p. venous return
p. venous return, anomalous
p. venous return anomaly
p. venous return (PAPVR) ▸ partial anomalous
p. venous return ▸ total anomalous
p. ventilation
p. ventilation, cessation of
p. ventilation impairment
p. ventilation, initiate
p. venule
p. vesicles
p. vessels ▸ engorgement of
p. vessels ▸ medial hypertrophy of
p. vessels ▸ neurohumoral control of
p. vessels ▸ prominence of
p. wedge
p. wedge angiography
p. wedge mean (PWM)
p. wedge mean pressure (PWMP)
p. wedge position
p. wedge pressure (PWP)
p. Wegener's granulomatosis

pulmonic
p. area
p. closure
p. closure sound
p. endocarditis
p. incompetence
p. insufficiency
p. murmur
p. process, chronic
p. regurgitation
p. scarring
p. second sound (P_2)
p. second sound (P_2) split

p. sound
p. stenosis
p. stenosis ▸ peripheral
p. stenosis ▸ severe
p. stenosis, valvular
p. valve
p. valve closure sound
p. valve gradient (PVG)
p. valve ▸ quadricuspid
p. valvular stenosis
p. valvuloplasty ▸ percutaneous balloon

pulmonis
p., alveoli
p., basis
p., paracentesis

pulmonocoronary reflex
pulmonum, aluminosis
pulp
p. atrophy
p. canal
p. capping
p. cavity
p. chamber
p., chronic perforating hyperplasis of
p., coronal
p., dental
p. disease
p., hernia of
p. horns
p. hyperemia
p., metaplasia of
p., mummified
p., necrotic
p. nodule
p., radicular
p., rudimentary white
p., splenic red
p. stage, transitional
p. stone
p. tissue, primitive
p. vein
p. worker's lung ▸ wood

pulpa dentis
pulpa lienis
pulpal
p. devitalization
p. excavations
p. necrosis, traumatogenic
p. wall

pulpar cells
pulpless tooth
pulposus
p., extrusion of nucleus

p. (HNP) ▸ herniated nucleus
p. (HNP) ▸ herniation of nucleus
p., nucleus

pulpy testis
pulsatile
p. assist-device
p. flow
p. pain
p. tinnitus

pulsating
p. aneurysm
p. aorta
p. bulge in abdomen
p. current
p. empyema
p. mass
p., neck veins not
p. pain
p. pain ▸ throbbing,
p. pleurisy
p. sensation

pulsation(s)
p., arterial peripheral
p., carotid
p., dorsalis pedis (DP)
p., expansile
p. in esophagus
p., low-frequency
p., pulmonary vascular
p. rate
p. ▸ spontaneous retinal arterial
p., suprasternal
p. ▸ transmitted carotid

pulsator, Bragg-Paul
pulse(s) (Pulse)
p., abdominal
p., abrupt
p. absent
p., allorhythmic
p., alternating
p. amplifier
p. amplifier, nuclear
p. amplitude
p. amplitude, atrial
p. amplitude ▸ ventricular
p., anacrotic
p., anadicrotic
p., anatricrotic
p. and respiration
p. and respiration (TPR) ▸ temperature,
p., ankle
p., apical
p., arachnoid
p., arterial

pulse(s)—*continued*

p., arteriovenous (AV)
p., atrial liver
p., atrial venous
p., atriovenous
p., auriculovenous
p., Bamberger's bulbar
p., biferious
p., bifid
p., bigeminal
p., bigeminal bisferious
p., bisferious
p., bounding
p., brachial
p., bronchial
p., bulbar
p., cannonball
p., capillary
p., carotid
p., catacrotic
p., catadicrotic
p., catatricrotic
p., centripetal venous
p., collapsing
p., cordy
p., Corrigans'
p., coupled
p. curve
p., CV wave of jugular venous
p., decreased
p., decurtate
p. deficit
p., dicrotic
p., digitalate
p., diminution of peripheral
p., dorsalis pedis (DP)
p., dropped beat
p. duration
p. duration ▸ half amplitude
p., ear
pulse, effective carotid
p., elastic
p., electric
p., entoptic
p., epigastric
p., equal
p., equal, carotid
p. ▸ F point of cardiac apex
p. ▸ f wave of jugular venous
p., febrile
p., feeble
p., femoral
p., filiform
p., flickering
p. flip angle

p., fluttering
p., formicant
p., frequent
p., full
p. full and equal bilaterally ▸
  peripheral
p. ▸ full, strong
p., funic
p., gaseous
p. generator
p. generator, asynchronous
p. generator, atrial synchronous
p. generator, atrial triggered
p. generator, Aurora
P. Generator, Chardack-Greatbatch
  Implantable Cardiac
p. generator, demand
p. generator ▸ elective replacement
p. generator ▸ fixed rate
p. generator ▸ Medtronic
p. generator ▸ Microlith pacemaker
p. generator ▸ Minilith pacemaker
p. generator pocket erosion
p. generator pocket infection
p. generator pouch ▸ Parsonnet
p. generator ▸ Programalith III
p. generator ▸ standby
p. generator ▸ ventricular inhibited
p. generator ▸ ventricular
  synchronous
p., guttural
p., hard
p. height analyzer
p. height spectrometry
p. -height spectrum
p., hepatic
p., high-tension
p., hyperdicrotic
p., hyperkinetic
p., hypokinetic
p., iliac
p. imperceptible
p., incisura
p., increased
p. indicator, xylol
p., infrequent
p. intact, peripheral
p., intermittent
p., irregular
p., irregularity of
p. ▸ irregularly irregular
p., jerky
p., jugular
p. (JVP) ▸ jugular venous
p. ▸ Kussmaul paradoxical

p., Kussmaul's paradoxical
p., labile
p., long
p., low-tension
p. magnitude, average
p. meter
p., Monneret's
p., monocrotic
p., mouse tail
p., movable
p., nail
p., narrowed
p. ▸ O point of cardiac apex
p. obtained by massage ▸ carotid
p. oximeter
p. oximeter ▸ SpaceLabs
p. oximetry
p. oximetry device
p. oximetry monitoring
p. palpable
p., palpable carotid
p., palpable femoral
p., palpable, pedal
p., palpable, radial
p., paradoxical
p. ▸ parvus et tardus
p., peaked
p., pedal
p. period
p., periodic short
p., peripheral
p., pistol-shot
p., piston
p., plateau
p., polycrotic
p., popliteal
p., posterior tibial
p., precordial
p. pressure (PP)
p., pulmonary
p., quadrigeminal
p., quick
p., Quincke's capillary
p., racing
p., radial
p. ▸ radial artery
p., rapid
p., rapidly rising
p. rate
p. rate control
p. rate, effective
p. rate, increased
p. rate, normal
p. rate, normal resting
p. rate, rapid

p. regular
p. repetition
p. repetition frequency
p., respirations and
p., respiratory
p., resting
p., retrosternal
p. ▸ reversed paradoxical
p., Riegel's
p., runaway
p., running
p., saphenous
p. ▸ SF wave of cardiac apex
p., sharp
p., short
p., slow
p., slowed
p., slowing of
p., soft
p. ▸ spike-and-dome
p. ▸ square wave
p. stabilized
p., stimulus
p., strong
p. strong and regular
p. strong, pedal
p. system, cine
p., tense
p., thready
p., tibial
p. ▸ tidal wave
p. tracing
p. tracing, carotid
p. tracing ▸ jugular venous
p. tracing, venous
p., trembling
p., tremulous
p., tricrotic
p., trigeminal
p., trip-hammer
p. ▸ triple-humped pressure
p. trisection
p., ulnar
p., undulating
p., unequal
p., vagus
p., venous
p., ventricular venous
p., vermicular
p., vibrating
p. volume recorder
p. volume recording
p., water-hammer
p. wave
p. wave velocity measurement

p., weak
p., weak and rapid
p., weak and thready
p., weak pedal
p. width
p. width, atrial
p. width ▸ ventricular
p., wiry
p. ▸ y depression of jugular venous
p. ▸ y descent of jugular venous

pulsed
p. ablation
p. Doppler echocardiography
p. Doppler flowmetry
p. Doppler ultrasonography ▸
  duplex
p. dye laser
p. dye laser, coumarin
p. -field gel electrophoresis
p. idioventricular rhythm
p. laser ablation
p. laser ▸ infrared
p. laser ▸ mid-infrared
p. laser, short
p. light therapy
p. ruby laser ▸ high-energy
p. wave Doppler echocardiography
p. wave Doppler mapping

pulseless
p. and breathless ▸ patient
p. bradycardia
p. disease
p. electrical activity
p. idioventricular rhythm
p. nonbreather

pulsing electrical activity ▸ rapidly
**pulsing electromagnetic fields
  (PEMF)**
pulsion hernia
**Pulsor Intrasound pain reliever ▸
  Medtronic**
pulsus
p. cordis
p. duplex
p. heterochronicus
p. respiratione intermittens
p. vacuus
p. venosus
pultaceous carcinoma
pultaceous debris
pulverize stone
pumilus, Bacillus
pump(s) (Pump)
p., Abbott infusion
p., abdominothoracic

p., acupressure infusion
p., air
p. ▸ angle port
p., aortic balloon
p., artificial heart left
p., Autosyringe insulin
p., balloon
p., Barron
p. blockers, Proton
p. blood
p. bump
p. ▸ cardiopulmonary bypass
p., closed-loop insulin
p. coronary artery bypass
  (OPCAB), off
p. current
p. /drive unit
p., external insulin
p., extracorporeal
p. failure
p., Felig insulin
p. function
p., fuser
p., Graseby
p., Hakim-Cordis
p., Harvard infusion
p., heart
p., implantable
p., implantable drug infusion
p. ▸ implantable insulin infusion
p. inefficiency, chronic
P. Infuser, Pen
p. inhibitor ▸ proton
p., insulin pen
p., interaortic balloon
p., internal insulin
p., intra-aortic balloon
p., intrathecal
p., intravenous
p., ion
p., IVAC volumetric infusion
p., Jarvik-7 mechanical
p. ▸ Jobst extremity
p., kidney perfusion
p. ▸ left ventricular bypass
P., Life Care
p. lung
p., McGaw volumetric
p., mechanical heart
p., mechanical insulin
p. ▸ Medtronic synchroMed
p. ▸ muscular venous
p., neuroperfusion
p. -operated penile implant
p. oxygenation

pump(s)—*continued*
  p. oxygenator
  p., pressure
  p. primed
  p., pulmonary
  p., respiratory
  p., roller
  p., strap-on
  p., surgically implanted
  p., syringe
  p., venous
pumping
  p. ability ▸ impaired
  p. ability of failing heart
  p. ability of weakened heart
  p. action, heart's
  p. capacity ▸ weakened
  p. chamber
  p. chamber, heart's
  p. chamber to lungs
  p. function of heart
  p., heart
  p. heart ▸ weakly
  p. (IABP) ▸ intra-aortic balloon
  p. of blood ▸ inefficient
  p. stomach
pumpkin seeding
pumpkin vessel
punch(-es)
  p., Abrams' pleural biopsy
  p. biopsy
  p. biopsy, colposcopic directed
  p. biopsy, directed cervical
  p. biopsy, Kevorkian
  p., kidney
  p., straight front
  p. tenderness
punched-out area
puncta calcific stones
punctal occlusion
punctal plug
punctata
  p., Aeromonas
  p. albescens, retinitis
  p., chondrodysplasia
  p. ▸ dysplasia epiphysealis
  p., Haemaphysalis
  p., hyalitis
  p., keratitis
  p., keratosis
  p. subepithelialis, keratitis
punctate
  p. basophilia
  p. cataract
  p. hemorrhage

  p. keratitis
  p. mucosal lesions ▸ multiple
  p. retinitis
  p. wound
punctation
  p., and mosaicism ▸ white
    epithelium,
  p., coalescing
  p., miliary
punctiform lesion
punctor, Aedes
punctual stimulation
punctuate hemorrhages, multiple
punctuation, perseverated letters and
punctum
  p. caecum
  p., dilation of
  p., eversion of
  p., lacrimal
  p., senile eversion of
puncture
  p., acu◇
  p. ▸ apical left ventricular (LV)
  p., aqua◇
  p., arterial
  p., bone marrow
  p., cardiac
  p., cisternal
  p., Corning
  p., cranial
  p., diathermy
  p., direct cardiac
  p., epigastric
  p., exploratory
  p. fracture
  p. headache
  p. headache, lumbar
  p. headache, postlumbar
  p. laceration
  p. laparoscopy, double
  p. ▸ left ventricular (LV)
  p. (LP), lumbar
  p., lung
  p. marks ▸ multiple needle
  p. marks, needle
  p., multiple needle
  p., needle cricothyroid
  p. of brain
  p. of subarachnoid space
  p. of ventricles
  p., pericardial
  p. reaction
  p. -resistant container
  p. -resistant container, rigid
  p., retinal cautery

  p., secondary
  p. site
  p., skin
  p., spinal
  p., splenic
  p., sternal
  p., subdural
  p., thecal
  p., therapeutic needle
  p., tonsil
  p., tracheoesophageal
  p., transseptal
  p., vena
  p., venous
  p., ventricular
  p. wound
  p. wound, deep
  p. wound, plantar
  p. wounds endocervical canal,
    secondary
  p. wounds, multiple
  p. wounds ▸ multiple needle
  p. wounds, needle
  p. wounds, primary
punctured lung
puncturing
  p., blister
  p. of skin by contaminated
    instruments
  p. of skin by contaminated needle
pungent odor, recurrent
punicifolia, Malpighia
punishing behavior of anorexic
punishing behavior of bulimic
punjabensis, Ceratophyllus
punktal lens
PUO (pyrexia of unknown origin)
pup cell
pupil(s)
  p., Adie's
  p. and hypothermia ▸ dilated
  p., Argyll Robertson
  p., attention reflex of
  p., Behr's
  p., bounding
  p., brisk reactive
  p., Bumke's
  p., cat's eye
  p. constricted
  p., constriction of
  p. contracted
  p., contraction of
  p., cornpicker's
  p., diameter of
  p., dilatation of

p., dilated
p., dilation of
p., dilator muscle of
p. equal
p. equal, react to light (PERL)
p. equal, react to light and
  accommodation (PERLA)
p. equal, round, react to light and
  accommodation (PERRLA)
p., fixed
p. fixed and dilated
p., Horner's
p., Hutchinson's
p., keyhole
p., lower border of
p. nonreactive
p., occlusion of
p., pinhole
p., pinpoint
p. react
p. react sluggishly
p. react to light and
  accommodation (PRLA)
p. reaction
p. reaction and size
p. reflex
p. reflex check
p. round and regular (PRR)
p. size
p. size or shape ▸ unequal
p., skew
p. sluggish to light
p., sphincter muscle of
p., stiff
p., sudden dilation of
p., tonic
p. unequal
p. unreactive
p., updrawn
p., upper border of
pupillae
p., caligo
p. congenita, ectopia
p., sphincter
p., synizesis
pupillary
p. aperture
p. area
p. border
p. changes
p. constriction
p. dilatation
p. dilation
p. distance
p. fatigue

p. membrane
p. reaction, hemiopic
p. reaction, vestibular
p. reaction, Wernicke's
p. reflex
p. reflex, cutaneous
p. reflex, paradoxic
p. reflex, retrobulbar
p. reflex, skin
p. reflex, Westphal's
p. size
pupillotonic pseudotabes
puppet syndrome, happy
purative slow pathway potential
pure
p., chemically
p. cocaine rock
p. culture
p. dwarf
p. flutter
p. lactose placebo
p. methamphetamine
p. mood
p. parasystole
p. red cell agenesis
p. red cell aplasia
p. tone audiometric findings
p. tone test
p. water
pureed diet
purge syndrome, binge and
purging
p. behavior
p. behavior of anorexic
p. behavior of bulimic
p., bingeing and
p. disorder
p., eating and
p., self-induced
p. (bulimarexia), starvation and
purification system, ultraviolet
purification system, water-
purified (Purified)
p. fetal cells
p. pork insulin ▸ regular
P. Protein Derivative (PPD)
P. Protein Derivative (PPD)
  intermediate
P. Protein Derivative (PPD) skin
  testing
purify blood-clotting factors
purifying process, blood-
purine
p. base
p. bodies test

p. diet, low
p. -free diet
Purinethol (6 MP/6 mercaptopurine)
purity, radiochemical
purity, radionuclide
Purkinje('s)
P. cells
P. cells, degeneration of
P. conduction, His-
P. corpuscles
P. fiber
P. fibers ▸ His-
P. fibers ▸ terminal
P. image
P. network
P. -Sanson mirror images
P. system
P. system ▸ His-
P. tissue ▸ His-
P. tumor
puromycin aminonucleoside
Purple (purple)
P. Haze (LSD)
P. Hearts (barbiturates)
p., visual
purplish hemorrhagic spots on skin
purpose(s)
p., cosmetic
p. ▸ cosmetic and functional
p., diagnostic
p. lens, general
p. lens, special
p., palliation
p. psychosis
purposeful
p. movements
p. movements ▸ inability to perform
p. movements, natural
p. movements, patient has no
p. response
purposefully, withdraws
purposeless, uncontrolled sinuous
  movements
purpura
p. abdominalis
p., allergic
p., anaphylactoid
p. angioneurotica
p. annularis telangiectodes
p. (AIP) ▸ autoimmune
  thrombocytopenic
p. bullosa
p. cachectica
p. fulminans
p., gin and tonic

purpura—*continued*
- p., hemorrhagic
- p. hemorrhagica
- p., Henoch's
- p. hyperglobulinemica
- p., idiopathic
- p., idiopathic thrombocytopenic
- p., Landouzy's
- p. maculosa
- p., orthostatic
- p. ▸ post-transfusion
- p. rheumatica
- p., Schönlein-Henoch
- p., senile
- p. simplex
- p., symptomatic
- p. (TTP), thrombic thrombocytopenic
- p., thrombocytopenic
- p. (TP), thrombotic
- p., toxic
- p. urticans
- p. variolosa

purpurea
- p., Claviceps
- p., Digitalis
- p., Micromonospora

purpureus, Otomyces
purpuric hemorrhage, patchy
purpuric lesion
purring thrill
purring tremor
pursed-lip style of breathing
pursestring of black silk
pursestring suture
pursing, lip
pursue natural course ▸ disease to
pursued rapid downhill course ▸ patient
pursuit(s)
- p. eye movement (SPEM) ▸ smooth-
- p., goal
- p., social

Purtscher's angiopathic retinopathy
Purtscher's disease
purulent
- p. and foul smelling ▸ sputum
- p. ascites
- p. conjunctivitis
- p. cyclitis
- p. discharge
- p. discharge, gram stain of
- p. drainage (dr'ge)
- p. encephalitis
- p. exudate
- p. fluid
- p. gastritis
- p. inflammation of pancreas
- p. iritis
- p. labyrinthitis
- p. labyrinthitis, acute
- p. malodorous discharge
- p. material
- p. material ▸ drainage (dr'ge) of
- p. material, grossly
- p. material, necrotic
- p. material, wound oozing
- p. matter, withdrawal of
- p. meningitis
- p. nasal drainage (dr'ge)
- p. ophthalmia
- p. otitis media
- p. otitis media ▸ acute
- p. pancreatitis
- p. pharyngitis
- p. pleurisy
- p. pneumonia
- p. rhinitis
- p. salpingitis
- p. sputum
- p., sputum grossly
- p. wound

purulenta
- p., lochia
- p., pneumonia interlobularis
- p., thromboarteritis

pus
- p. accumulation
- p. at incision site
- p. cells
- p. cells, absence of
- p. coating stool
- p., drainage of
- p. -filled blisters
- p. from conjunctivitis
- p. from the ear ▸ discharge of
- p. in ear
- p. in urine
- p. -like blisters
- p. pocket
- p. -producing organisms
- p., release of
- p., separate pockets of
- p. tube

Pusey's emulsion
push
- p. -back procedure
- p. fluids
- p. fluids, patient to
- p. of medication ▸ direct
- p. -out exercises
- p., syringe
- p. therapy, total
- p. -up, classic
- p. -up exercise ▸ wall
- p. -up ▸ modified
- p. -up ▸ neck

pushdowns, tricep
pushing and pulling skills
pusillus, Mucor
pustular
- p. ecthyma
- p. lesion
- p. pharyngitis
- p. psoriasis
- p. tonsillitis
- p. varicella

pustules, rash
pustuliformis profunda, keratitis
pustulosa
- p., acne
- p., trichomycosis
- p., varicella

pustulous endocarditis
putrefaction, bacterial
putrefaction, postmortem
putrefactive diarrhea
putrid bronchitis
putrid empyema
Putti
- P. bone rasp
- P. frame
- P. -Platt operation

putting affairs in order
putty kidney
Putty (hallucinogen), Silly
Puusepp's operation
Puusepp's reflex
PUVA (psora-lens plus ultraviolet light) regimen
PUVA (psora-lens plus ultraviolet light) treatment
Puzo's method
puzzle, body image
PV (portal vein)
PVC
- PVC (postvoiding cystogram)
- PVC (premature ventricular contractions) ▸ multifocal
- PVC (premature ventricular contractions) ▸ unifocal
- PVC with coupling ▸ premature ventricular contractions

PVD (peripheral vascular disease)

PVD (posterior vitreous detachment)
PVF (portal venous flow)
PVG (pulmonic valve gradient)
PVP (photoselective vaporization of prostate)
PVP (portal venous pressure)
PVP (polyvinylpyrrolidone), iodine
PVR (postvoiding residual)
PVS (persistent vegetative state)
PVS (premature ventricular systole)
PVT (paroxysmal ventricular tachycardia)
PVT (portal vein thrombosis)
PW contact lens, Sauflon
Pwd (powder)
PWM (pulmonary wedge mean)
PWMP (pulmonary wedge mean pressure)
PWP (pulmonary wedge pressure)
PX (pneumothorax)
pyaemia (*see* pyemia)
pycnic (*same as* pyknic)
pycnic habit
pyelitic [*pyretic*]
pyelitis
    p., calculous
    p. cystica
    p., defloration
    p., encrusted
    p. glandularis
    p. granulosa
    p. gravidarum
    p., hematogenous
    p., hemorrhagic
    p., suppurative
    p., urethritis and cystitis cystica
    p., urogenous
pyelocaliectasis, ureteral
pyelocalyceal system
pyelogram [*myelogram*]
    p., dragon
    p., excretory
    p., hydrated
    p., infusion
    p. (IVP) ‣ intravenous
    p., rapid sequence
    p. (IVP) ‣ rapid sequence intravenous
    p. (RP), retrograde
pyelographic
    p. roentgen studies
    p. study, infusion
    p. study, retrograde
pyelography
    p., air

p., ascending
p., drip infusion
p., excretion
p., infusion
p. (IVP), intravenous
p., percutaneous antegrade
p., respiration
p., retrograde ureteral
p., washout
pyeloileocutaneous anastomosis
pyelolithotomy, coagulum
pyelolymphatic backflow
pyelomorphic cells, atypical
pyelonephritis
    p., acute
    p., bilateral chronic
    p., chronic
    p., localized
    p., pain in back from
    p., puerperal
    p., xanthogranulomatous
pyelorenal backflow
pyelotomy incision
pyelotomy wound
pyelotubular backflow
pyeloureteritis cystica
pyelovenous backflow
pyemia (*same as* pyaemia)
    p., arterial
    p., cryptogenic
    p., otogenous
    p., portal
pyemic embolism
Pyemotes ventricosus
pygmaea, Naumanniella
pyknic (*see* pycnic)
pyknic type
pyknoepilepsy/pyknolepsy
pyknotic index
pyknotic nuclei
Pyle, bone age according to Greulich and
Pyle, Greulich and
pylori
    p. bacterium, Helicobacter
    p., Campylobacter
    p., H. (Helicobacter)
    p. infection ‣ Helicobacter
pyloric
    p. antrum
    p. atresia
    p. cap
    p. channel ulcer
    p. incompetence
    p. lymph nodes

p. obstruction
p. region
p. sphincter
p. stenosis
p. stenosis, congenital
p. stenosis, hypertrophic
p. vein
pyloroduodenal perforation
pyloromyotomy, Ramstedt
pyloroplasty
    p. and vagotomy
    p., Finney's
    p., Heineke-Mikulicz
    p., Jaboulay's
    p., Judd's
    p., vagotomy and
pylorus
    p., gastric
    p. of stomach
    p., resection of
    p., sphincter muscle of
pyocyanase proteidin
pyocyanea, Pseudomonas
pyocyaneus, Bacillus
pyoderma gangrenosum
pyoderma, infant
pyogenes
    p., Corynebacterium
    p. infection, Streptococcus
    p., Staphylococcus
    p., Streptococcus
    p. var. aureus, Micrococcus
pyogenic [*pyrogenic*]
    p. abscess
    p. albumosuria
    p. arthritis
    p. bacteria
    p. encephalitis
    p. granuloma
    p. infection
    p. meningitis
pyorrhea
    p. alveolaris
    p. around lower teeth
    p. around upper teeth
    p., paradental
    p., Schmutz
PYP scan
pyramid
    p., bony
    p., cartilaginous
    p. compressed, nasal
    p. method
    p., nasal
    p. of kidney

pyramid—*continued*
- p., petrous
- p. realigned, nasal
- p., renal

pyramidal
- p., anterior
- p. cataract
- p. cell
- p. cells, solitary
- p. decussation
- p. eminence
- p. eye implant
- p. fracture
- p. functions
- p. implant, Berens
- p. muscle
- p. muscle of auricle
- p. neuron
- p. sign, Barre's
- p. tract
- p. tube

pyretic [*pyelitic*]
pyretogenic stage
pyrexia
- p. of unknown etiology
- p. of unknown origin
- p., Pel-Ebstein
- p., period of

pyrexial headache
pyridoxilated stroma-free hemoglobin
pyridoxine-deficient diet
pyridoxine-responsive anemia
pyriform (*see* piriform)
pyriform thorax
pyrimidine antagonist
pyrimidine base
pyrogenes, Leptospira
pyrogenes, Toxoplasma
pyrogenetic stage
pyrogenic [*pyogenic*]
pyrogenic reaction
pyrolytic chemistry
pyroninophilic granulations
pyrophosphate
- p. imaging
- p., lipothiamide
- p. /polyphosphate, Tc (technetium) 99m stannous
- p. scintigram
- p. scintigraphy
- p. ▸ technetium-99m
- p., tetraethyl
- p., thiamine

pyruvate dehydrogenase

pyruvic
- p. acid
- p. transaminase (GPT) ▸ glutamic-
- p. transaminase (SGPT) ▸ serum glutamic-

pyuria
- p. and hematuria
- p., asymptomatic
- p., gross

Q-R

q (every)

Q
- Q disc
- Q (query) fever
- Q fever, Australian
- Q fever, psittacosis, cocci triad
- Q treatment, compound-

Q port

Q wave
- Qw. myocardial infarction
- Qw. myocardial infarction ▸ non-
- Qw. regression

QCA (quantitative coronary angiography)

QCN (Quality Control Nurse)

QCT (Quantitative Computed Tomography)

q.d. (every day)

q.h. (every hour)

Q-H interval

q.i.d. (four times a day)

Q-M interval

q.o.d. (every other day)

qO₂ (oxygen quotient)

q.q.h. (every four hours)

Q-R interval

QR pattern

Q-RB interval

QRS
- QRS alternans
- QRS angle
- QRS axis
- QRS axis ▸ mean
- QRS axis ▸ superior
- QRS changes
- QRS complex
- QRS complex, aberrant
- QRS complex, short
- QRS complex, widening of
- QRS configuration
- QRS duration
- QRS interval
- QRS loop
- QRS maximum, magnitude of
- QRS morphology
- QRS ▸ slurring of
- QRS -ST junction

- QRS synchronous atrial defibrillation shocks
- QRS tachycardia ▸ regular, wide
- QRS tachycardia ▸ wide
- QRS vector
- QRS vector, maximum
- QRS voltage
- QRS wave

QRS-T
- QRS-T angle
- QRS-T complex
- QRS-T interval
- QRS-T value

q.s. (sufficient quantity)

QS
- QS complex
- QS pattern
- QS wave

Q-Stress

Q-Stress treadmill

Q-S2

Q-S2 interval

QT (Q-T)
- QT corrected for heart rate
- QT dispersion
- Q-T interval
- Q-T interval, prolonged
- Q-T interval sensing pacemaker
- Q-T interval syndrome ▸ idiopathic long
- QT /QTc dispersion
- QT syndrome ▸ congenital long
- Q-T syndrome ▸ long
- QT syndrome, prolonged

Q-T_c interval

Q-TU interval syndrome

Q-TU syndrome ▸ long

QU interval

qua non, conditio sine

quack drugs

quack theories

quackery
- q., arthritis
- q., cancer
- q., nutrition

quad
- q. atrophy

- q. cane
- q. cane, large base
- q. cane, patient independent with small based
- q. cane with verbal cueing, patient uses
- q. cough
- q. coughing
- q. exercises
- q. screen format
- q. strengthening exercises
- q. strengthening exercises, active
- q. strengthening exercises, isometric

quadrangular lobule of cerebellum

quadrant
- q. anopsia
- q. biopsy, four
- q. field
- q. hemianopia
- q. (LLQ) ▸ left lower
- q. (LLQ) ▸ left upper
- q., lower inner
- q., lower outer
- q. (LLQ) of abdomen ▸ left lower
- q. (LUQ) of abdomen ▸ left upper
- q. (RLQ) of abdomen ▸ right lower
- q. (RUQ) of abdomen ▸ right upper
- q. of breast
- q. (RLQ) ▸ right lower
- q. (RUQ) ▸ right upper
- q. section
- q. (RUQ) tenderness ▸ right upper
- q., upper inner
- q. (ULQ) ▸ upper left
- q., upper outer
- q. (URQ) ▸ upper right

quadrantal cephalalgia

quadrantectomy-axillary dissection-radiotherapy (QUART)

quadrantectomy ▸ patient had

quadrantic hemianopia

quadrate
- q. gyrus
- q. muscle of lower lip
- q. muscle of sole
- q. muscle of thigh**

quadrate—*continued*
  q. muscle of upper lip
  q. pronator muscle
quadratic formula for dose survival, linear
quadratic survival relationship, linear
quadratus muscle, pronator
quadriceps
  q. atrophy
  q. exercise
  q. exercises, progressive resistant
  q. extension exercise
  q. jerk
  q. mechanism
  q. muscle
  q. muscle of thigh
  q. reflex
  q. stretch exercise
  q. tendon
quadricuspid pulmonic valve
quadrigeminal pulse
quadrigeminal rhythm
quadrilateral cartilage
quadrilateral septum
quadriplegia
  q., partial
  q., total
  q., ventilator dependent
quadriplegic
  q., cervical vent-dependent
  q., patient
  q., rehabilitation
  q., spastic
  q. standing frame
  q. ▸ support groups for
  q. ▸ vent dependent
quadripod cane (*see* quadruped cane)
quadrivation test
quadruped cane
quadruple amputation
quadruple rhythm
Quads (barbiturates)
Quads (methaqualone)
Quaglino's operation
Quain's degeneration
Quain's fatty heart
qualifications, training
qualified clinical
qualitative
  q. albumin
  q. fat
  q. sugar
quality(-ies) (Quality)
  q. and effective treatment ▸ high-

q. and quantity
q. assessment
q. assurance
q. assurance for patient
q. assurance in dosimetry
q. assurance in radiation safety
q. assurance in simulators
q. assurance in treatment machines
q. assurance in treatment planning
q., bone
q. care, high-
q. control
Q. Control Nurse (QCN)
q. control standards
q. health care
q. idealized ▸ nurturing
q. image, dissection
q. information monitoring system
q. medical care ▸ high
q., nursing
q. of daily life
q. of ice ▸ therapeutic
q. of life
q. of life, enhance
q. of life ▸ improve
q. of life issues
q. of life, low
q. of life ▸ near-normal
q. of life, preservation of
q. of program
q. of service
q. of treatment
Q. of Well Being Index
q. of work ▸ deteriorating
q. relaxation
q. review mechanisms ▸ utilization and
q. staining
q., subjective sleep
q. treatment, cost-effective
q., ultraviolet absorbing
q. versus quantity of life
q. vision, adult
quantification
  q., acoustic
  q., microdensitophotometric
  q., shunt
quanti-Pirquet reaction
quantitative (Quantitative)
  q. albumin
  q. analysis
  q. arteriography
  Q. beta sub unit
  Q. Computed Tomography (QCT)

q. coronary angiographic
q. coronary angiographic analysis
q. coronary angiography (QCA)
q. coronary arteriography
q. Doppler
q. evaluation ▸ sequential
q. hyperplasia
q. inhalation challenge apparatus
q. left ventriculography
q. measurements
q. pilocarpine iontophoresis sweat test
q. regional lung function study
q. risk assessment
q. study
q. sugar
q. two-dimensional echocardiography
quantity(-ies)
  q. of blood ▸ patient vomited large
  q. of life ▸ quality versus
  q. ▸ quality and
  q. (q.s.) ▸ sufficient
quantum (Quantum)
  q. energy, high
  q. interference devise (SQUID) ▸ superconducting
  Q. pacemaker
  q. theory
  q. theory, Planck's
quarantine period
quarantine procedure
quarantined, patient
QUART (quadrantectomy/axillary dissection/radiotherapy)
quartan ague
quartan fever
quarter [*border*]
quarter run
quartile range
quartz
  q. lamp
  q. mercury vapor lamp, cold
  q. transducer
Quas (barbiturates)
quasi-parental role
quasi-sinusoidal biphasic wave form
quaternary germicides
quaternary-amine type product/solution
quats and phenolics
queasiness, intestinal
Quebec beer drinker's cardiomyopathy
Queckenstedt's
  Q. maneuver

Q. sign
Q. test
Queensland tick typhus
quellung reaction
Quénu-Muret sign
querulous paranoia
Quervain's disease, de
Quervain's fracture
query (Q) fever
quest, memory
questionable
q. Babinski sign
q. diverticulum
q. epilepsy
q. etiology ▸ anemia of
q. lesion
q. mass
q. metastases
q. nodes
q. retinopathy
q. seizure activity
q. significance
questioning, dull on
questionnaire (Questionnaire)
q. as a screening device for drug abuse, patient
q. as a screening device, patient
q., bladder
q., Coping Strategies
q., health care
q., Kellner
Q., Mauldsley Medical
Q. (PAQ), Personal Attributes
q. ▸ Seattle angina
questions ▸ delay in responding to
Questran Light
Queyrat's erythroplasia
quick (Quick)
q. breaths, four
q. fix
q. lateral positioning
q. prothrombin time
q. pulse
Q. test
q. to anger, child
q. upward thrust
quickening, fetal
quickening paralysis
Quicker-Dryden probe
quiescence, period of relative
quiescent period
quiet
q. -alert state
q. breath sounds
q. chest

q. heart sounds
q. necrosis, Paget's
q. precordium
q. sleep
quietly, patient expired
quilt degeneration of muscle cells ▸
patch
quilt suture
Quimby dose distribution system
Quincke's
Q. capillary pulse
Q. disease
Q. edema
Q. sign
quinidine effect
quinidine gluconate
quinine amaurosis
quinine fever
quinquefasciatus, Culex
quinquestriata, Hirudo
quinsy
q., lingual
q., patient has
q. throat
quintan ague
Quintana
Q. bacteremia, Bartonella
Q. fever
Q., Rickettsia
quinti muscle, abductor digiti
quinti proprius muscle, extensor
digiti
Quinton suction biopsy instrument
Quinton-Scribner shunt
Quintuple bypass surgery
quit "cold turkey"
quit smoking clinic
quivering spells, brief
quotidian ague
quotidian fever
quotient (Quotient)
q., achievement
q., cerebral glucose oxygen
q., circadian
q., developmental
q. (IQ) ▸ intelligence
q., memory
q., oxygen
q., permeability
q., respiratory
Q. (IQ) Test, full-scale Intelligence
q. (TLQ) ▸ total living
q. (IQ), verbal intelligence
q., V/Q
****

R (r) (R.)
R (rectally)
R (roentgen)
R analysis, Spenco
R (rough) cells
r cells, pen-
R. (rough) colony
R and E (rest and exercise)
R and R (rest and recuperation)
R interval ▸ flutter
R unit
R wave
Rw. amplitude
Rw. gating
Rw. progression
Rw. progression ▸ poor
Rw. ▸ propagating of
Rw. ▸ propagation of
RA
RA (rheumatoid arthritis)
RA (right atrial)
RA (right atrium)
RA cell
RA (rheumatoid factor) cell
rabbit
r. -ear sign
r. fever
r. fibroma virus
r. myxoma virus
r. syndrome
rabiei, Encephalitozoon
rabies
r. control programs, tetanus and
r. immune globulin, human
r. virus
raccoon eyes
race effect ▸ horse
race walking
racemic epinephrine
racemosa, Cimicifuga
racemosa, livedo
racemose aneurysm
racemosum
r., angioma arteriale
r., angioma venosum
r., staphyloma corneae
racemosus, Mucor
racetrack microton
rachitic dwarf
rachitic scoliosis
racial fanatic
racial unconscious
racing
r. atria
r., carotid

racing—*continued*
  r. heart
  r. heart rhythm
  r. heartbeat
  r. pulse
  r. thoughts
  r. thoughts ▸ disconnected and
racket [*raquet*]
racket amputation
raconté déjà
racquet incision
rad(s) (RAD)
  r. (radiation absorbed dose)
  R. (reactive attention disorder)
  R. (right axis deviation)
  r. ▸ daily fractionation rate of
  r. equivalent therapy (RET)
  r. in fractions, mid-sagittal plane
    dose of
  r. in fractions, total dose of
  r. modified mantled
radial
  r. and astigmatic keratotomy
  r. antebrachial region
  r. aplasia
  r. artery
  r. artery bypass surgery
  r. artery pressure point
  r. artery pulse
  r. aspect
  r. bone
  r. depression
  r. deviation
  r. epiphysis, distal
  r. fossa
  r. fracture site
  r. head
  r. head epiphysis
  r. head implant, Swanson
  r. head subluxation
  r. immunity
  r. incision
  r. keratotomy (RK)
  r. keratotomy (PERK) protocol,
    prospective evaluation of
  r. keratotomy (RK) technique
  r. malleolus
  r. metaphysis, distal
  r. neck
  r. nerve
  r. nerve, deep
  r. nerve ▸ dorsal digital nerves of
  r. nerve function
  r. nerve injury
  r. nerve splint

  r. nerve, superficial
  r. nerve, superficial branch of
  r. notch
  r. notch of ulna
  r. palsy
  r. pulse, palpable
  r. pulses
  r. reflex
  r. reflex, inverted
  r. shaft
  r. shortening
  r. steal syndrome
  r. subtraction imaging system
  r. sutures, direct
  r. symmetry
  r. traction
  r. tuberosity
radialis
  r. brevis muscle, extensor carpi
  r., flexor carpi
  r. indicis artery
  r. longus muscle, extensor carpi
  r. muscle, flexor carpi
  r. sign
  r. tendon, flexor carpi
radians, Trichophyton
radiant
  r. energy
  r. heat
  r. heat device
  r. stones
radiated by breast, heat
radiates, pain
radiatic doses
radiatic doses, computation of
radiating
  r. chest pain
  r. down leg, pain
  r. heat
  r. into back, pain
  r. pain
  r. to jaw and shoulder ▸ chest pain
radiation (Radiation)
  r., abdominal
  r., abdominal wall
  r. absorbed dose (rad)
  r., accumulative
  r., acoustic
  r., adaptive
  r., airline flight
  r. alopecia
  r., alpha
  r. and chemotherapy
  r. and chemotherapy after
    mastectomy

  r. and chemotherapy ▸ patient
    treated with
  r. and 5-fluorouracil, combined
  r., annihilation
  r. arc, simulated
  r., artery
  r. assaults on tumors
  r., atomic
  r. attack on tumor
  r., auditory
  r., background
  r. beam
  r. beam, collimation of
  r. beam, direction of
  r. beam, exit point of
  r. beam, lead beads for
  r. (laser) beam ▸ light amplification
    by stimulated emission of
  r. beam, modification of
  r. beam, secondary shaping blocks for
  r., beamlet of
  r., benefits
  r., beta
  r., betatron
  r. biologist
  r., boost
  r. (bremsstrahlung), braking
  r. burn
  r., burst of
  r., cell
  r., cell destruction by
  r. ▸ cell phone
  r., Cerenkov
  r., cesium
  r., cesium tube
  r. change
  r., chest pain
  r. chimera
  r., cobalt
  r. colitis
  r., concentrate
  r., contralateral
  r. counter
  r., cranial
  r. damage
  r. damage ▸ susceptible to
  r., debilitating
  r. dosage
  r. dose
  r. dose, medical internal
  r. dosimetry ▸ external
  r. dosimetry ▸ internal
  r. effect (CRE), cumulative
  r. (EDR), effective direct
  r., effectiveness of

r. effects
r., electromagnetic
r. emission
r., emitted
r. enterocolitis
r. equivalent in man (REM)
r. exposure
r. exposure, excessive
r., external
r., external beam
r. fibrosis
r. field
r. field, limited
r. field modification
r., field of
r. fields ▸ virtual
r. fluence
r. for ovarian castration
r. for parotitis
r. ▸ full body
r., full brain
r., full course of
r., gamma
r. gastritis
r., generalized body
r. hazard
r., heat
r. ▸ heat loss by
r., high dose
r., high energy
r., high linear energy transfer
r. imaging studies ▸ pelvic
r., immunology
r. implant
r. -induced cancer
r. -induced carcinogenesis
r. -induced disease
r. -induced heart changes
r. -induced immunoenhancement
r. -induced malignancy
r. -induced pericarditis
r., infrared
r., injected
r. injury of target cells
r. injury of vascular system
r., internal
r., interstitial
r. intoxication
r., intracavitary
r., ionizing
r., irritative
r., laser
r., lead shielding in
r., left sciatic
r. -leukemia-protection

r. level
r. (laser) ▸ light amplification by stimulated emission of
r. linked antibodies
r. linked disease
r. ▸ loss of fertility from
r., low
r., low dose
r., low level
r. ▸ lumpectomy and
r. lung disease
r., mammography
r. mantle technique
r., massive
r., mcs (millicurie seconds) of beta
r. mechanism
r., microwave
r. (MASER) ▸ microwave amplification by stimulated emission of
r., millicurie seconds (mcs) of beta
r. modality, combined drug and
r., modified
r. monitor
r. monitoring
r., monochromatic
r., multifractionated
r. myelopathy
r., natural background
r. necrosis
r. necrosis in skin cancer therapy
r. nephritis
r., neutron
r., nonionizing
r. of pain
r., oncological
r. oncology
r. oncology, medical and
r. oncology physicist
r., optic
r. optic neuropathy
r., oral
r. osteonecrosis
r., pain
r., particulate
r., patient tolerated full course of
r. physicist
r. pigment changes
r. pigmentation changes
r. pleuritis and pericarditis
r. pneumonia
r. pneumonitis
r., pneumonitis, acute
r., postoperative
r. proctitis

r. production, Cerenkov
r. prophylactic
r. protection activity
r. protection capacity
r. rash
r. related
r. response
r. restenosis
r. retinopathy
r., right sciatic
r. safety
r. safety, quality assurance in
r. scattered
r., sciatic nerve
r., secondary
r. sickness
r., small boost dose of
r., solar
r. source
r. source, artificial
r., sources, intracavitary
r., spectral distribution curve for
r. ▸ spinal deterioration due to
r., spot
r., stimulated emission of
r., sun's ultraviolet
r. surgery, intraoperative
r., targeted
r. technologist
r., thalamic
r. ▸ therapeutic ionizing
r. therapy
r. therapy, acute reaction to
r. therapy, anatomical considerations in
r. therapy, biologic basis of
r. therapy, block placement in
r. therapy, cancer
r. therapy, central nervous system tolerance to
r. therapy, chemotherapy and
r. therapy, clinical
r. therapy, combined chemotherapy/
r. therapy, complications of
r. therapy ▸ conformal
r. therapy, delayed reaction to
r. therapy, dosimetry in
r. therapy, emergency
r. therapy, endocavitary
r. therapy ▸ endoluminal
r. therapy, external
r. therapy, eyebrow and eyelash loss in
r. therapy, focal
r. therapy, follow-up

radiation—*continued*
r. therapy for bone pain
r. therapy for carcinoma
r. therapy for intact breast
r. therapy, full brain
r. therapy, full course
r. therapy, hemibody
r. therapy, high dose
r. therapy ▸ high dose fractionation
r. therapy, humeral block in
r. therapy in acromegaly, conventional
R. Therapy (IMRT) ▸ Intensity Modulated
r. therapy, intermittent
r. therapy, internal
r. therapy ▸ intracavitary
r. therapy, intraluminal
r. therapy, intraoperative
r. therapy, laryngeal block in
r. therapy, late reactions to
r. therapy, limitations of
r. therapy, local
r. therapy, local recurrence after
r. therapy, lumbosacral fields for
r. therapy, lung
r. therapy, mantle field in
r. therapy, mantle technique in
r. therapy, molybdenum
r. therapy, neuraxis irradiation in
r. therapy, normal tissue considerations in
r. therapy nurse
r. therapy of tumor
r. therapy on prophylactic basis
r. therapy, ovary protection in
r. therapy, palliative
r. therapy, patient treated with
r. therapy perineal area
r. therapy, photon irradiation technique in
r. therapy pneumonitis
r. therapy, postmantle
r. therapy, postoperative
r. therapy ▸ postsurgical
r. therapy, preauricular
r. therapy, preoperative
r. therapy, primary
r. therapy, radical
r. therapy resumed in full course
r. therapy ▸ secondary to
r. therapy, sequelae of
r. therapy, spinal cord block in
r. therapy, spinal cord tolerance in
r. therapy, staging systems in

r. therapy, steroid therapy in
r. therapy, subdiaphragmatic
r. therapy, subdiaphragmatic fields in
r. therapy, supramediastinal mantle in
r. therapy, systemic
r. therapy technique
r. therapy, therapeutic ratio in
r. therapy, therapy complications in
r. therapy, thin liver block in
r. therapy, thin lung blocks in
r. therapy ▸ three-dimensional
r. therapy ▸ three-dimensional conformal
r. therapy, thymic
r. therapy, total body
r. therapy treatment
r. therapy, treatment volume in
r. therapy, whole abdomen
r. therapy, whole abdominal treatment in
r. therapy, whole brain
r. therapy, whole brain vs local brain
r., tissue absorption by
r. to tumor mass ▸ high dose
r., total body
r., toxic
r. treatment
r. treatment ▸ combined hyperthermia and
r. treatment ▸ conformed
r. treatment ▸ conventional
r. treatment for bursitis
r. treatment, modified upper mantle
r. treatment of glandular tissue
r. treatment of tendinitis
r. treatment, standard
r. treatments ▸ pelvic
r., upper abdominal
r., upper mantle
r., UV (ultraviolet)
r., whole brain
r., whole pelvis
r. within body ▸ scattered
radiational effect
radiative interactions
radical(s) [*radicle*]
r. abdominal hysterectomy
r. antrum operation
r. axillary dissection
r. behavior change
r. brain surgery
r. cancer surgery
r. change in lifestyle
r. damage, free-
r. enucleation

r. excision
r. excision of tumor
r. fossa
r., free
r. frontal antrotomy
r., hepatic
r., hydroxyl
r. hysterectomy
r. hysterectomy, Latzko's
r. hysterectomy, modified
r. hysterectomy, Wertheim's
r. inguinal node dissection
r. lobotomy
r. mastectomy
r. mastectomy, Halsted
r. mastectomy, left
r. mastectomy, modified
r. mastectomy, Patey
r. mastectomy, right
r. mastectomy, Willy Meyer
r. mastoidectomy
r. mastoidectomy ▸ modified
r. maxillary antrotomy
r. molecules ▸ free
r. neck dissection
r. neck dissection, standard
r. neck operation
r. nephrectomy
r. notch
r. operation
r., organic
r. oxidants (FRO) ▸ free
r. ▸ oxygen (O₂)
r. ▸ oxygen (O₂) derived free
r. ▸ oxygen (O₂) -free
r. pneumonectomy, left
r. pneumonectomy, right
r. poisoning ▸ free
r. procedure
r. prostate surgery
r. prostatectomy
r. prostatectomy ▸ laparoscopic
r. radiation therapy
r. retroperitoneal node dissection
r. retropubic prostatectomy, nerve sparing
r. surgery
r. surgical procedure
r. theory, free
r. toenail excision
r. treatment
r. vaginal hysterectomy, Schauta's
r. vulvectomy
r. Wertheim procedure
radicle (*same as* radical)

radicular
  r. artery
  r. artery, great anterior
  r. cyst
  r. odontoma
  r. pain
  r. pain pattern
  r. pulp
radiculitis, cervical
radiculopathy
  r., cervical
  r., lumbar
  r., lumbosacral
radii (TAR) ▸ thrombocytopenia with absent
Radio (radio)
  R. (COR) ▸ Coronary Observation
  r. pill
  r. waves
radioactive
  r. antibodies
  r. applicator
  r. beads
  r. brain scan
  r. colloids
  r. compound
  r. decay
  r. elements
  r. equilibrium
  r. fallout
  r. fibrinogen uptake test
  r. gallium (Ga)
  r. glucose
  r. gold
  r. gold grains
  r. Hippuran (RAH) test
  r. hydrogen isotope
  r. implant
  r. implant, insert
  r. injection
  r. iodinated human serum albumin
  r. iodinated serum albumin (RISA) study
  r. iodine (I^{131})
  r. iodine treatment
  r. iodine (RAI) uptake
  r. iodine (RAI) uptake test
  r. iron
  r. isotope
  r. isotopes ▸ injected
  r. isotopes, interstitial implantation of
  r. labeled isotopes
  r. material
  r. material, red cells tagged with
  r. nuclides

  r. particles
  r. pellets
  r. pellets ▸ implanted
  r. phosphorus (P^{32})
  r. poisoning
  r. rays
  r. rods
  r. scans
  r. seed implant
  r. seeding of prostate
  r. seeds
  r. series
  r. sources, implanting
  r. stents
  r. substance
  r. tag
  r. technetium (Tc^{99})
  r. thallium exercise test
  r. toxins
  r. tracer
  r. tracer, low level
  r. treadmill test
  r. waste
  r. water
radioactivity administration ▸ intralymphatic
radioactivity, unit of
radioallergoabsorbent test (RAST)
radiobiologic concepts
radiobiology (Radiobiology)
  r. and tumor response in antibodies
  R. Research Lab
  r., tissue
radiocarpal
  r. angle
  r. articulations
  r. implant, Swanson
  r. ligament
radiochemical purity
radiocontrast dye
radiocurable tumor
radiodensity area
radiodensity data
radiodermatitis, chronic
radioencephalogram study
radiofrequency (RF)
  r. ablater
  r. ablation (RFA)
  r. ablation ▸ catheter
  r. ablation ▸ fast pathway
  r. absorption
  r., capacitive
  r. catheter ablation
  r. current
  r. delivery

  r. denervation
  r. electric field, conductive
  r. electric field, dielectric
  r. electric field hyperthermia
  r. electric field, inductive
  r. electric field, interstitial
  r. electric field, resistive
  r. electrophrenic respiration
  r. energy
  r. hot balloon
  r., inductive
  r. interference (RFI)
  r., interstitial
  r. lesioning, stereotactic
  r. pacemaker
  r. receiver ▸ Medtronic
  r. thalamotomy
  r. waves
radiograph
  r., Brasfield chest
  r., cephalometric
  r., panoramic
  r. ▸ 24-hour delayed lymph nodal stage
radiographic
  r. anatomy
  r. assessment
  r. density
  r. effect
  r. evidence
  r. healing
  r. lesion
  r. physical findings
  r. stability of lesion
  r. studies
  r. technique
  r. tests
radiographically not determined, etiology
radiography
  r., biomedical
  r., body section
  r. ▸ comparative dental
  r., diagnostic
  r. invasion depth
  r., mass miniature
  r., neutron
  r., orthogonal
  r., pan-oral
  r., spot film
  r., stereoscopic
  r., urine
radiohumeral bursitis
radioimmunoassay
  r., Coat-a-Count

radioimmunoassay—*continued*
  r. human myoglobulin
  r., Mallinckrodt
  r. of hair (RIAH)
radioimmunodiffusion myoglobinuria
radioimmunometric technique
radioimmunoglobulin research
radioimmunoglobulin therapy
radioimmunoprecipitation test
radioiodide, sodium
radioiodinated
  r. fatty acid
  r. serum
  r. serum albumin
radioiodine test
**radioiodinized serum albumin (RISA)
  scan**
radioisotope(s)
  r., activity of
  r. angiogram
  r. applicator
  r. bone scan
  r. calibrator
  r. camera
  r., carrier-free
  r., cobalt 60 (Co^{60})
  r., gold 198 (Au^{198})
  r. imaging
  r. implants
  r., iodine 131 (I^{131})
  r., iodine 131 with triiodothyronine
    (I^{131} T$_3$)
  r., iridium 192 (Ir^{192})
  r., phosphorus 32 (P^{32})
  r., radium 226 (Ra^{226})
  r., radon 222 (Rn^{222})
  r. renogram test
  r. scanner
  r. scanning
  r. scanning studies
  r., tantalum 182 (Ta^{182})
  r., technetium (Tc^{99})
  r., unsealed
  r. uptake studies
radioisotopic study
radiolabeled
  r. antigen
  r. fibrinogen
  r. iodine
  r. microsphere
radioligand assay
radiologic
  r. assessment
  r. examination
  r. magnification study

  r. procedure
  r. scimitar syndrome
  r. studies
  r. technique ▸ interventional
radiological
  r. anatomy
  r. diagnosis
  r. evaluation
  r. procedure
  r. studies
  r. technologist
radiology
  r., diagnostic
  r., interventional
  r., therapeutic
  r., ultrasound
radiolucent
  r. bed
  r. calculus
  r. defect
  r. density
  r. line
  r. stone
radiometer, pastille
radiometer, photographic
radiometric analysis
radiononopaque stone
radionuclear bone scan
radionuclear dynamics
radionuclide
  r. angiocardiography
  r. angiocardiography ▸ exercise
  r. angiocardiography (ACG) ▸ first-
    pass
  r. angiocardiography ▸ gated
  r. angiogram
  r. angiography
  r. angiography (ERNA) ▸
    equilibrium
  r. angiography ▸ gated
  r. angiography ▸ rest
  r. cineangiocardiography
  r. cisternography
  r. cystography
  r. emission computerized
    tomographic (ECT) system
  r. esophageal transit study
  r. ▸ gold 195m
  r. imaging
  r. kinetics
  r. perfusion imaging, adenosine
  r. purity
  r. scan ▸ multigated acquisition
    (MUGA) blood pool

  r. scan, multiple gated acquisition
    blood (MUGA) pool
  r. scanning
  r. study
  r. technique
  r. thyroid imaging
  r. transit
  r. ventriculogram (RNV)
  r. ventriculography
  r. ventriculography ▸ equilibrium
    multigated
  r. ventriculography ▸ rest exercise
    equilibrium
  r. ventriculography ▸ tomographic
  r. voiding cystourethrography
radiopaque
  r. bone cement, Surgical Simplex P
  r. catheter
  r. contrast medium
  r. contrast medium, injection of
  r. density
  r. dye
  r. lesion
  r. material, injection of
  r. medium
  r. substance
  r. substance, injection of
  r. tantalum stent
  r. tantalum stent, Cordis
radiopharmaceutical, high energy
radiopharmaceutical, standard
radioprotective drugs
**radioreceptor assay pregnancy blood
  (Biocept-G)**
radioresistant tumor
radiosensitivity
  r. and cell cycle redistribution
  r., relative
  r. test
radiosensitizing drugs
**radiosurgery ▸ gamma knife
  stereotactic**
radiosurgery, stereotactic
radiotherapy (Radiotherapy)
  r., chemotherapy combined with
  r. consultation
  r., extensive
  r., 5-fluorouracil combined with
  r., fractionated
  r., implant
  r., interstitial
  r., intracavitary
  r., intraoperative
  r., localized
  r., palliative

r., postoperative
r. (PHRT), procarbazine hydroxyurea
r., prostate
r. (QUART) ▸ quadrantectomy-
    axillary dissection-
R. Service
r. treatment
radioulnar synostosis, congenital
radium
r. applicator, Ernst
r. applicator, Plummer-Vinson
r. bomb
r. capsule
r. capsule, Ernst
r., cervical insertion of
r. emanation
r., exposure to
r. implant
r. implant, two plane
r. implantation
r. insertion
r. needle
r. needle brachytherapy
r. poisoning
r. seeds
r. tandem, Ernst
r. therapy
r. 226 (Ra^{226})
radius
r. at wrist, fracture of
r., Bohr
r. cap prosthesis, Speed
r., curvature of
r., dislocation head of
r., distal
r., fracture neck of
r., Galeazzi's fracture of
r., head of
r., progressive curvature of
r., resection head of
r., styloid process of
r. syndrome ▸ thrombocytopenia-
    absent
r., ulnar notch of
radix
r. arcus vertebrae
r. dentis
r. two algorithm
radon
r. concentration
r. contamination
r. level
r. risk
r. seed implantation
r. 222 (Rn^{222})

Radovici, palmomental reflex of
    Marinesco-
RADS (reactive airways disease
    syndrome)
RAE (right atrial enlargement)
RAEB (refractory anemia with excess
    blasts) ▸ syndrome of
Raeder's syndrome
Raff-Glantz derivative method
rage
r., aggression or
r. and fear
r. and resistance ▸ anger,
r. attacks ▸ unprovoked
r., consumed by
r. disorder
r. disorder ▸ road
r., excessive
r. ▸ exhibits road
r., frustration and belligerency
r., harboring deep
r., impotent
r., lucid
r., narcissistic
r. ▸ outbursts of aggression or
r. ▸ patient in
r. ▸ patient reacts with
r. reduction technique
r. reduction therapy
r., senseless
r. ▸ senseless laughter, weeping or
r., sports
r., violent
ragged red fiber (MERRF) disease ▸
    myoclonic epilepsy and
Raggedy Ann (LSD)
ragpicker's disease
ragsorter's disease
Ragweed (marijuana)
RAH (right atrial hypertrophy)
RAH (radioactive Hippuran) test
Rahe Scale ▸ Holmes-
RAI (radioactive iodine)
RAI (radioactive iodine) uptake
RAI (radioactive iodine) uptake test
raid, drug
Raillietina demarariensis
Raillietina madagascariensis
railroad
r. sickness
r. track appearance
r. track ductus arteriosus
r. track sign
Raimondi ventricular catheter
rain of collaterals

Rainbows (rainbow)
R. (barbiturates)
r., regular insulin
r. vision
Rainey's tubes
Rainier, hemoglobin
Rainville test
raise
r. exercise ▸ arm
r. exercise ▸ side leg
r. exercise ▸ toe
r. exercise ▸ toe-heel
raised
r. edges
r. lesions
r., periosteal flaps
r., skin flaps
raises, calf
raising
r. appliance, bite-
r., bite-
r. denture, bite-
r., leg
r. (SLR) ▸ negative straight leg
r. (SLR) ▸ straight leg
r. tenderness (SLRT), straight leg
r. test (SLRT), straight leg
raisonnante, folie
rake teeth
rale(s)
r., amphoric
r. and rhonchi
r., atelectatic
r., audible
r. audible at bases
r., basilar
r., bibasilar
r., bilateral
r. ▸ bilateral diffuse pulmonary
r., border
r., bronchial
r., bronchiectatic
r., bubbling
r., cavernous
r., cellophane
r., clicking
r., coarse
r., collapse
r., consonating
r., crackling
r., crepitant
r. de retour
r., dry
r., extrathoracic
r., fine

rale(s)—*continued*
  r., fine crepitant
  r. ▸ fine, moist
  r., frank
  r., gurgling
  r., guttural
  r., Hirtz's
  r. in chest
  r. indux
  r., inspiratory
  r., laryngeal
  r., localized
  r., loud piping
  r., marginal
  r., metallic
  r., moist
  r., mucous
  r., muqueux
  r., musical
  r. or wheezes
  r., pleural
  r., pulmonary
  r. redux
  r., respiratory
  r., rhonchi and
  r., scattered
  r., sibilant
  r., Skoda's
  r., snoring
  r., sonorous
  r., subcrepitant
  r., tracheal
  r., transitory
  r., Velcro
  r., vesicular
  r., wet
  r., whistling
RAM (rapid alternating movements)
Raman spectography
Raman spectroscopy
rami, suprapubic
ramificata superficialis, keratitis
ramifications, bronchial
ramifications, physiological
Ramirez shunt
ramollitio retinae
Ramon flocculation
Ramond's sign
ramosa, Absidia
ramosus, Bacteroides
ramosus, Mucor
ramp
  r. pacing
  r. protocol, continuous
  r., wheelchair

rampant dental caries
Ramsay Hunt syndrome
Ramses' diaphragm
Ramstedt pyloromyotomy
ramus (rami)
  r., ascending
  r. bone
  r., coronoid process of
  r., descending
  r., inferior
  r. intermedius artery
  r., ischial
  r., ischiopubic
  r., left pubic
  r. medianus
  r., right pubic
  r. roentgenogram, lateral
  r., superior
ranarum, Lankesterella
rancens, Acetobacter
rancid oxidized fat
Rand perimeter, Ferree-
Randall('s)
  R. plaques
  R. repair, Tennison-
  R. sign
random
  r. access
  r. basis
  r. control clinical trial
  r. drug testing
  r. homologous donation
  r. monitoring process
  r. movement
  r. specimen
  r. surveillance
  r. uncontrollable behavior
  r. variation
  r. waves
randomization process
randomized
  r., blinded, controlled study
  r. clinical trial
  r. controlled assessment
  r. controlled clinical trial
  r. controlled trials
  r. double-blind comparison
  r. double-blinded placebo controlled
    trial
  r., patients
  r., placebo-controlled trial
  r. prospective trials
  r. study
  r. study, prospective
  r. treatment trial

  r. trial
  r. vs nonrandomized clinical trials
Range (range)
  R. Achievement Test, Wide
  r., alpha-theta electroencephalo-
    gram (EEG) frequency
  r. -alternating current
  r., brain wave frequency
  r., dosage
  r., dynamic
  r., electroencephalogram (EEG)
    frequency
  r., frequency
  r., interquartile
  r., inversion
  r., limited activity
  r. ▸ logarithmic dynamic
  r., mental
  r., normal
  r. of abilities, bright/normal
  r. of abilities ▸ low average
  r. of abilities ▸ mentally retarded
  r. of accommodation
  r. of disorders
  r. of effects, broad
  r. of flexion and extension ▸ full
  r. of frequency
  r. of knee motion
  r. of normal variability
  r. of symptoms, full
  r., quartile
  r., speech
range of motion (ROM)
  ROM, active
  ROM and suppleness ▸ adequate
  ROM exercises
  ROM exercises ▸ gentle
  ROM, full
  ROM, functional
  ROM ▸ joint
  ROM, left ankle full
  ROM, left elbow full
  ROM, left femur full
  ROM, left knee full
  ROM, left lower extremity full
  ROM, left shoulder full
  ROM, left upper extremity full
  ROM, left wrist full
  ROM, limited
  ROM ▸ maintaining joint
  ROM, neck full
  ROM, normal
  ROM, passive
  ROM, restricted
  ROM, right ankle full

ROM, right elbow full
ROM, right femur full
ROM, right knee full
ROM, right lower extremity full
ROM, right shoulder full
ROM, right upper extremity full
ROM, right wrist full
ranging mood swings, wide
rank test ▸ log
Ranke complex
Ranke's stage
Rankine scale
Ransohoff's operation
ranula, pancreatic
Ranvier('s)
  R. crosses
  R. membrane
  R., nodes of
  R. segments
  R. tactile discs
RAO (right anterior oblique)
  RAO (right anterior oblique) angulation
  RAO (right anterior oblique) equivalent
  RAO (right anterior oblique) position
  RAO (right anterior oblique) view
RAP (right atrial pressure)
rap session
rape
  r., acquaintance
  r., allegation of
  r., alleged
  r., bruit de
  r., bruit de scie ou de
  r. intervention
  r. perpetrator, acquaintance
  r., preferential
  r., reality of
  r. trauma
  r. trauma syndrome
  r. trauma syndrome, compound reaction
  r. trauma syndrome, silent reaction
  r. victim
  r. victim, acquaintance
raphe (*same as* **rhaphe**)
  r. cells
  r., linear
  r., median
  r. nuclei
  r. of perineum
  r. of pharynx
  r. of scrotum

r., palatine
r., palpebral
r. penis
r., pterygomandibular
r. scroti
r., septal
rapid
  r. acquisition computed axial tomography
  r. aging
  r. alternating movements (RAM)
  r. and chaotic thinking and speech
  r. and deep breathing ▸ dizziness from
  r. atrial pacing
  r. beating of heart
  r. bone loss
  r. bone metabolism
  r. breathing
  r. breathing and limpness
  r. breathing ▸ shallow,
  r. build up of pressure
  r. burst pacing
  r. change in mental status
  r. contractions
  r. deep relaxation
  r. depolarization
  r. deterioration
  r. detox (detoxification)
  r. dissemination of disease
  r. downhill course
  r. downhill course, patient pursued
  r. dyssynchronous depolarization
  r. ejection
  r. exercise
  r. extinction
  r. eye movement (REM)
  r. eye movement (NREM-REM) cycle, nonrapid eye movement-
  r. eye movement (REM) density
  r. eye movement (REM) latency
  r. eye movement (REM) period, sleep onset
  r. eye movement (REM) rebound
  r. eye movement (REM) sleep anxiety dreams
  r. eye movement (REM) sleep ▸ increased
  r. eye movement (REM) sleep interruption insomnia
  r. eye movement (REM) sleep-related hypoxemia
  r. eye movements (REMS) onset
  r. eye movements (REMS) period
  r. eye movements (REM) sleep

r. eye movements (REMS), spindle
r. filling wave
r. flow brain scan
r. freeze, slow thaw treatment
r. head movement
r. heart action
r., heart rate
r. heart rate, abnormally
r. heart rate ▸ excessively
r. heart rhythms
r. heartbeat
r. high
r. ingestion
r. ingestion of large amounts of food
r. manual positioning
r. mental deterioration
r. metabolism
r. metabolizer
r. monotone, speak in
r. mood change
r. mood swings
r. movement, involuntary
r. muscle growth
r. nonsustained ventricular tachycardia
r. onset of jaundice
r. overall assessment
r. plasma reagin (RPR)
r. plasma reagin (RPR) test
r. pounding heartbeat
r. processing film
r. processing mode (RPM)
r. progression
r. pulse
r. pulse rate
r. pulse, weak and
r. recovery
r. remission
r. renewal cell system
r. repetitive motion
r. repolarization ▸ early
r. repolarization ▸ final
r. respiration
r. rhythms
r. sequence excretory urography
r. sequence filming
r. sequence induction (RSI)
r. sequence induction (RSI) orotracheal intubation
r. sequence intravenous pyelogram (IVP)
r. sequence pyelogram
r. sequential CT (computerized tomography) scanning
r. shallow breathing

rapid—*continued*
   r., shallow respirations
   r. speech
   r. standing
   r. talking
   r. transit
   r. ventricular filling
   r. ventricular response
   r. weight gain
   r. weight loss
rapidly
   r. accumulating ascites
   r. advancing disease
   r. dehydrated, patient
   r. descent
   r. deteriorating, patient
   r. disseminating disease
   r. growing brain tumor
   r. growing lesion
   r. growing tumor
   r. intubated, patient
   r. progressing bilateral hearing loss
   r. progressive course ▸ acute
   r. progressive glomerulonephritis
   r. progressive pulmonary disease
   r. proliferating tumor
   r. pulsing electrical activity
   r. rising pulse
   r. shifting emotions
rapist, serial
rappel, bruit de
rapport with others, patient has good
raptoria, Scaptocosa
rara, Physaloptera
rare
   r. cancers
   r. contractions
   r. disease
   r. lentivirus
   r. skin disorder
rarefaction click
rarefied area
rarefied osteitis, periapical
Rasch's sign
rash(es)
   r. and blisters
   r., chills with
   r., confluent
   r., contact skin
   r., diaper
   r. discoid
   r. ▸ erythematous, maculopapular
   r., facial
   r. from diuretics
   r., heat

r., intractable skin
r., itching
r., itchy skin
r. ▸ lacy red
r., macular
r., maculopapular
r., morbilliform
r., nettle
r. on abdomen
r. on chest
r. on face, red butterfly-shaped
r. ▸ painful blistering
r., papilliform
r., patchy
r. ▸ patient has
r., polymorphous macular
r., prickly heat
r., pruritic
r. pustules
r., radiation
r., recurring skin
r. ▸ red, ring-shaped
r. ▸ relapsing skin
r. ▸ scaly, disc-shaped
r. ▸ severe, painful skin
r., skin
r., urticarial
r., warm weather
Rashkind
   R. balloon catheter
   R. balloon technique
   R. cardiac device
   R. double-disk occluder prosthesis
   R. double umbrella
   R. procedure
Rasmussen's
   R. aneurysm
   R. encephalitis
   R. ▸ olivocochlear bundle of
   R. syndrome
Rasmuten's encephalitis
rasp [*grasp, clasp*]
   r., bone
   r., frontal sinus
   r., Lundsgaard's
   r., Miltner rotary bone
   r., nasal
   r., Putti bone
   r., sinus
   r., Wiener-Pierce
raspatory, Kirmission's
raspberry mark
raspberry tongue
rasping murmur
rasping pain

RAST (radioallergoabsorbent test)
Rastelli('s)
   R. conduit
   R. operation
   R. procedure
rasus, Ixodes
rat
   r. -bite fever
   r. brain
   r. brain, female
   r. brain, male
   r. feces, pooled
   r. -tailed larva
   r. unit (RU)
   r. urine protein
rate(s) (Rate)
   r., abnormality in heart
   r., abnormally rapid heart
   r., accelerating heart
   r. adaptic pacemaker ▸ Dash single-chamber
   r. adaptive device
   r. -adaptive pacemaker
   r., aldosterone excretion
   r., aldosterone secretion
   r., amebic prevalence
   r. and clinical trials, exclusion
   r. and force of contraction
   r. and rhythm regular (RRR)
   r., apical
   r., apneic infant with decreased heart
   r., arousal heart
   r., arterial blood flow
   r., attack
   r., average outcome
   r. (BMR) ▸ basal metabolic
   r., baseline variability of fetal heart
   r. (BFR) ▸ blood flow
   r., blood sedimentation
   r., bone formation
   r., breast cancer
   r., breast cancer fatality
   r., caloric burn
   r., cancer fatality
   r., cardiac
   r., cerebral cortex perfusion
   r., cerebral metabolic
   r., change in heart
   r. changes ▸ large magnitude voluntary heart
   r., clearance
   r., coil flow
   r., complication
   r. conditionability, heart

r. conditioning ▸ human operant heart
r. constant, air kerma
r., constant dose
r. constant, exposure
r. constant, filtered exposure
r. control, heart
r. control learning and awareness ▸ heart
r. control, pulse
r. control, voluntary heart
r. (SR) ▸ corrected sedimentation
r., cortisol production
r., cortisol secretion
r., count
r., critical
r., cure
r., death
r., decreased heart
r. -dependent angina
r. dependent conduction delay
r., diadochokinesia
r. ▸ differentials in abstinence
r., disease-free survival
r., disintegration
r. disorder, heart
r., dose
r. during oxygen deprivation ▸ control of heart
r., effective pulse
r., ejection
r. ▸ elevated heart
r. elevated ▸ sed (sedimentation)
r. eradication
r., error
r. (ESR) ▸ erythrocyte sedimentation
r. ▸ establishing normative base
r., estradiol production
r. ▸ excessively rapid heart
r., exercise heart
r. ▸ expected peak heart
r. ▸ expiratory flow
r., failure
r., fast growth
r. ▸ fast heart
r., fatality
r. feedback, anticipatory bogus heart
r. feedback, heart
r., fetal heart
r., five year survival
r., flow
r., fractionated high dose
r., fracture
r. (GFR), glomerular filtration

r., growth
r., heart
r., high
r., high cure
r., high death
r., high dose
r., hourly dose
r. hysteresis
r. immunonephelometry
r. in coil, flow
r., increased flow
r., increased heart
r. ▸ increased heart and breathing
r., increased pulse
r., increased respiratory
r., increasing heart
r., infant mortality
r., infection
r., infectivity
r., infusion
r. (IFR) ▸ inspiratory flow
r., intrinsic heart
r. irradiation, low dose
r., irregular
r., leukemia relapse
r. ▸ long-term survival
r., low
r., low birth
r., low cure
r. ▸ low flow
r., magnet
r. ▸ maternal mortality
r., maximal heart
r. (MIFR) ▸ maximal inspiratory flow
r. (MMEFR) ▸ maximal midexpiratory flow
r. (MMFR) ▸ maximal midflow
r. (MVR) ▸ maximal ventilation
r. (MEFR) ▸ maximum expiratory flow
r. ▸ maximum flow
r., maximum heart
r. (MIFR) ▸ maximum inspiratory flow
r. (MMEFR) ▸ maximum midexpiratory flow
r. (MPHR), maximum predicted heart
r. (MER) ▸ mean ejection
r. ▸ mean midexpiratory flow
r. ▸ mean normalized systolic ejection
r. (MSER) ▸ mean systolic ejection
r., metabolic
r., metabolic clearance

r. meter
r. meter, analog
r. meter, counting
r. meter ▸ metabolic
r. mode ▸ fixed
r. -modulated pacemaker
r. monitor, heart
r. monitored, heart
r. monitoring, internal fetal heart
r., morbidity
R., Morbidity-Mortality
r., mortality
r. (MFR) ▸ mucus flow
r., myocardial metabolic
r., normal resting pulse
r., occupancy
r. of accuracy
r. of blood flow ▸ measure
r. of blood ▸ shear
r. of change ▸ variation in
r. of glucose, cerebral metabolic
r. of growth
r. of healing
r. of incidence of infection
r. of infection
r. of infusion, drip
r. of learning
r. of oxygen, cerebral metabolic
r. of progression of disease
r. of rads ▸ daily fractionation
r. of recidivism
r. of red blood cells (RBC) ▸ sedimentation
r. of respiration
r. ▸ one-year survival
r., operant acceleration of heart
r., operant deceleration of heart
r., overall seroprevalence
r. ▸ pacemaker adaptive
r. pacemaker, Cordis' fixed
r. pacemaker, fixed
r., parathyroid hormone secretion
r., patient survival
r. ▸ peak diastolic filling
r. ▸ peak emptying
r. (PEFR) ▸ peak expiratory flow
r. (PFR) ▸ peak filling
r. (PFR) ▸ peak flow
r. ▸ peak heart
r. (PIFR) ▸ peak inspiratory flow
r. ▸ peak jet flow
r. per minute (RRpm) ▸ respiratory
r. perception, heart
r., perfusion
r., perinatal mortality

rate(s)—*continued*

r., plasma glucose disappearance
r., plasma iron turnover
r., precordial heart
r., predicted mortality
r., pregnancy
r. pressure product
r., primary failure
r., production
r., pulsating
r., pulse
r. pulse generator ▸ fixed
r. ▸ QT corrected for heart
r. rapid, heart
r., rapid pulse
r. reading, fetal heart
r., recovery
r. recovery ▸ heart
r., recurrence
r., reduced heart
r., regular, heart
r., reinfection
r., rejection
r., relapse
r., remission
r., renin-release
r., repetition
r. reserve ▸ heart
r., respiratory
r., response
r. responses, heart
r. responses, instrumental heart
r. responsive ▸ dual chamber
r. responsive pacemaker
r. responsive pacemaker ▸ Meta
r. responsive pacing
r. responsive ▸ single chamber
r. responsive unipolar ventricular
    pacemaker ▸ Medtronic
    Activitrax
r. ▸ resting heart
r. (RMR) ▸ resting metabolic
r. ▸ rising heart
r. (SR) ▸ Rourke-Ernstein
    sedimentation
r. sampling
r., secretion
r. (SR) ▸ sedimentation
r., self-control of heart
r., short-term mortality
r., sleep respiratory
r., slew
r., slow growth
r., slow heart
r., somnolent metabolic

r. ▸ standing heart
r. ▸ stroke ejection
r., success
r., success and failure
r., suicide
r., survival
r. ▸ sustained response
r. (SER) ▸ systolic ejection
r., tachycardia detection
r., target heart
r. test, erythrocyte sedimentation
r., testosterone production
r. ▸ training heart
r. variability, heart
r., variable
r., varying flow
r., ventricular
r., ventricular conductive
r. (SR) ▸ Westergren's sedimentation
r. (SR) ▸ Wintrobe's sedimentation
r. with combined modality therapy,
    survival
r., work metabolic
r. zone (THRZ) ▸ target heart

Rathke's

R. folds
R. pocket
R. pouch
R. tumor

rathouisi, Fasciolopsis

rating (Rating)(s)

r., Apgar
R. Assessment Matrix (TRAM) ▸
    Treatment
r. (20/20, 20/50, etc.) ▸ eye
r., maturity
r., newborn maturity
r. of perceived exertion (RPE)
R. Scale, Hamilton
R. Scale, Himmelsbach
R. Scale, Karnofsky
R. Scale Test, Wittenborn
    Psychiatric
R. Scale (VDRS) ▸ Verdun
    Depression
R. Scale (VTSRS) ▸ Verdun Target
    Symptom
R. Scale (WPRS) ▸ Wittenborn
    Psychiatric
r., strength
r., vision

ratio

r., acid-base
r., albumin/globulin (A/G)
r., aortic root

r., arm
r. (AVR) ▸ arteriovenous
r., birth-death
r. ▸ body hematocrit/venous
    hematocrit
r., body-weight
r., bone age
r., bound-free
r., branching
r. (CTR), cardiothoracic
r., cell color
r., cholesterol-phospholipid
r., common mode rejection
r., concentration
r., conduction
r., contrast
r., crude mortality
r., CT (cardiothoracic)
r., cytoplasmic
r., dextrose-nitrogen (D-N)
r., discrimination
r. ▸ E:A wave
r. ▸ E:I
r., estimated thyroid (ETR)
r., expiration-inspiration
r., expiratory exchange
r., flow
r. ▸ forced vital capacity
r., glucose-nitrogen (G-N)
r., granulocyte-erythroid
r., grid
r., hand
r., holdaway
r., I:E
r. in radiation therapy, therapeutic
r., inspiratory-expiratory (I/E)
r. (INR) ▸ international normalized
r., karyoplasmic
r., ketogenic-antiketogenic
r., La:A
r., lactate-pyruvate
r., lecithin sphingomyelin (LS)
r., light-dark
r., L/S
r. (MDTR) ▸ mean diameter
    thickness
r., mendelian
r. (MCR) ▸ message competition
r., modified gain
r., monocyte-lymphocyte
r., mortality
r., myeloid-erythroid
r., nucleocytoplasmic
r., nucleoplasmic
r., nucleus-to-cytoplasm

r., nutritive
r. of amplifications
r. of input signal voltage
r. of median lethal dose
r. of output signal voltage
r., off-center
r., oxygen (O_2) enhancement
r., proportionate morbidity
r. (PER) ▸ protein efficiency
r. ▸ pulmonary systemic blood flow
r. ▸ renal vein renin
r., resin-uptake
r., resistance
r., respiratory control
r., respiratory exchange
r., shunt
r., risk
r., risk-benefit
r., R/S
r., scatter air
r., scatter maximum
r., sensitizer enhancement
r., sex
r., S/N (signal-to-noise)
r., standard mortality
r. ▸ systolic velocity
r., target-to-nontarget
r. test ▸ albumin/globulin (A/G)
r., therapeutic
r., thyroid to serum
r., tissue air
r., tissue maximum
r., tissue phantom
r., transformer
r. ▸ transmitral Doppler E:A
r. ▸ transmitral E:A
r., U/P (urine plasma)
r., urea excretion
r., urine plasma (U/P)
r. (VR) ▸ ventilation
r., ventilation ▸ inverse
r., ventilation ▸ pressure controlled inverse
r. ▸ ventilation/perfusion
r. (WHR) ▸ waist-hip

ration
r., myelocytic erythrocytic
r., normal myelocytic erythrocytic
r., V/C

rational
r. control
r. /empirical clinical placement
r. hypertensive therapy
r. medicine
r. psychotherapy

r. thinking
r. thinking skills
rationality, irrational
rationalization ▸ level of
rationalization, superficial
rationalizes, patient
rationalizing poor performance
rationing plan ▸ health care
Ratliff criteria for myocarditis
ratti ▸ Actinomyces muris-
rattle of return
rattling sound in lungs
rattus (Rattus)
r. alexandrinus, Rattus
r., Mus
R. norvegicus
Rauchfuss' sling
Rauchfuss triangle
raucous murmur
Rauwolfia
R. alkaloid
R. extract
R. serpentina
RAV (Rous-associated virus)
ravaged body, cancer
rave, fracture en
Raven's matrix
Raven's Progressive Matrix Test
Raverdino's operation
raw
r. area
r. meat ▸ irradiation of
r. ▸ psilocybin eaten
ray(s) (Ray)('s)
r., actinic
r., alpha
r., anode
r., antirachitic
r., astral
r., bactericidal
r. beam filtration ▸ x-
r., Becquerel
r., beta
r., Blondlot
r., border
r., borderline
r., Bucky
r., caloric
r., canal
r., capture gamma
r. cataract, heat-
r., cathode
r., central
r., characteristic
r., chemical

r., constant, specific gamma
r., convergent
r., corresponding
r., cosmic
r., delta
r., detection of gamma
r. diffraction analysis ▸ x-
r., digital
r., direct
r., direction
r., divergent
r., Dorno's
r. dosage ▸ unit of roentgen
r., dynamic
r., electromagnetic
r., erythema-producing
r. exposure, x-
r., Finsen
r., fluorescent
r. fungus
r., gamma
r. generator ▸ x-
r., glass
r., Goldstein's
R. Greenfield filter, Kim-
r., grenz
r., H
r., hard
r., heat
r., hertzian
r., incident
r., indirect
r., infrared
r., infra-roentgen
r. ▸ intensity of roentgen
r., intermediate
r., laser light
r., Lenard
r. -like fashion
r., luminous
r., Lyman
r. magnification ▸ x-
R. mania
r., medullary
r. microscope, beta
r., Millikan
r., minin
r., monochromatic
r., n
r., necrobiotic
r., Niewenglowski's
r. ophthalmia, actinic
r. ophthalmia, ultraviolet
r., paracathodic
r., parallel

ray(s)—*continued*
r., pigment-producing
r., polar
r., positive
r., primary
r., radioactive
r., refracted
r., roentgen
r., s
r., Sagnac
r., scattered
r., Schumann
r., secondary
r., soft
r. spectra, gamma-
r. spectrometer, beta-
r. spectrometer, gamma-
r. sum
r., supersonic
r. surgery, gamma
r. therapy, deep roentgen
r. therapy, gamma
r., titanium
r., transition
r. treatment, grenz
r. tube (CRT), cathode
r., ultraviolet
r., vertical
r., vital
r., W
r., x-
Rayleigh scattering law
Raymond's apoplexy
Raynaud's
R. disease
R. disease ▸ blood vessel problem in
R. disease ▸ idiopathic
R. gangrene
R. phenomenon
R. phenomenon, scleroderma, telangiectasia (CRST) syndrome ▸ calcification,
R. sign
R. symptoms
R. syndrome
Rayner-Choyce implant
rayon gauze
rayon strip
RayTec sponge
RBBB (right bundle branch block)
RBC
RBC (red blood cell count)
RBC (red blood cells)
RBC (red blood cells), transfusion of

RBC/hpf (red blood cells per high power field)
RBF (renal blood flow)
RC (root canal)
R-C (resistance-capacitance)
R-C (resistance-capacitance) coupled amplifier
RCA
RCA (right circumflex coronary artery)
RCA (right coronary angiogram)
RCA (right coronary artery)
RCD (relative cardiac dullness)
RCM (right costal margin)
RCU (Respiratory Care Unit)
rd (rutherford)
RDA
RDA (recommended daily allowances)
RDA (recommended dietary allowances)
RDA (right dorsoanterior)
RDP (right dorsoposterior)
RDS (respiratory distress syndrome)
RE (relationship enhancement) family therapy
RE (relationship enhancement) therapy
reabsorbable suture
reabsorbed, volume
reabsorption
r., altered tubular
r. of amylase ▸ decreased tubular
r. of blood
r. of glucose, tubular
r. of phosphate, tubular
r., subchondral bony
reaccumulation, fluid
reach (Reach)
r. and sway ▸ sweep and glide,
r. test ▸ stretch-and-
R. to Recovery
R. to Recovery Program
reached maximum hospital benefit (MHB) ▸ patient
reaching behavior
react(s)
r., brain's physical ability to
r., pupils
r. sluggishly, pupils
r. to light and accommodation (PRLA) ▸ pupils
r. to light and accommodation (PERLA) ▸ pupils equal,
r. to light and accommodation (PERRLA) ▸ pupils equal, round,

r. to light (PERL) ▸ pupils equal,
r. with defiant counterattack
r. with disdain ▸ patient
r. with physical symptoms ▸ adjustment
r. with rage ▸ patient
reacting
r. dose (MRD) ▸ minimum
r. material, cross-
r., patient
r. substance of anaphylaxis ▸ slow-
r. substance, slow
reaction(s) (Reaction)
r., accelerated
r., acetic acid
r., acid
r., acute adverse psychological
r., acute anxiety
r., acute drug
r., acute dystonic
r., acute febrile
r., acute panic
r., acute paranoid
r., acute psychotic
r., acute situational
r., acute situational or stress
r., acute stress
r., acute treatment for flashback
r., acute treatment for panic
r., acute treatment for psychotic
r., adjustment
r., adult situational stress
r., adult traumatic
r., adverse
r., adverse drug
r. ▸ adverse oxidative
r., adverse psychiatric
r., adverse therapy
r. after chemotherapy, adverse
r., agglutinoid
r., alarm
r., alkaline
r., allergic
r., allergic cosmetic
r., allergic skin
r., allergic-type
r., allograft
r., anamnestic
r., anaphylactic
r., anaphylactic transfusion
r., anaphylactoid
r., anaphylaxis allergic
r., anatoxin
r. and size, pupil
r., angiophylactic

r., anosmic conversion
r., antiemetic drug
r., antigen-antibody
r., antigen-antiglobulin
r., antiglobulin
r., antitryptic
r., anxiety
r., anxiety depression
r. assay ▸ polymerase chain
r., associated
r., associative
r., autoimmune
r., axonal
r., bacteriolytic
r., behavioral
r., biomolecular
r., biphasic
r., biuret
r., blanching
r., blood pressure (BP)
r., brief depressive
r., cachexia
r., cadaveric
r., Calmette
r., cancer
r., Casoni's
r., catastrophic
r., cell mediated immune
r., cellular
r. center
r., chain
r., characteristic inflammatory
r., chemical
r., chemotherapy nausea-emesis
r., cholera vaccine
r., clinical manifestations of drug
r., clinical manifestations of
    flashback
r., clinical manifestations of panic
r., clinical manifestations of
    psychotic
r., coagulation
r., common
r., complement fixation
r., conglobation
r., conglutination
r., conjunctival
r., consensual
r., consensual light
r., conversion
r., coping
r., countertransference
r., coupled
r., cross
r., Cushing's

r., cutaneous
r., cytotoxic
r., dark
r., defense
r., delayed
r., delayed asthmatic
r., delayed hemolytic
r., delayed-blanch
r., delayed-type hypersensitivity
r., depot
r., depressive
r., desmoid
r., desmoplastic
r., diagnosis of acute drug
r., dietary thermogenesis
r., differential diagnosis in panic
r., differential diagnosis of psychotic
r., displacement
r., dissociative
r., dual
r., dysergastic
r. ▸ dyskinetic and dystonic
r., dystonic
r. ▸ egg yellow
r., Ehrlich
r., Eisenmenger
r., emotional
r., endoergic
r., enzymatic
r., enzyme
r., erysipeloid
r., erythematous-edematous
r. (ESR) ▸ erythrocyte
    sedimentation
r., exoergic
r., false-positive
r. ▸ fatal allergic
r. ▸ fatal hypersensitivity
r., fatal transfusion
r., fatigue
r. ▸ febrile transfusion
r., Felix-Weil
r., fibrinolytic
r. ▸ fight-or-flight
r., flocculation
r., flushing
r., focal
r., foreign body
r., foreign body granulomatous
r. formation
r., fright
r. from drug abuse, patient had
    flashback
r., gastrointestinal (GI) psychogenic
r., generalized Shwartzman's

r., giant cell
r. (GVHR) ▸ graft-versus-host
r., gram
r., grief
r., gross stress
r., group
r., Gruber-Widal
r., guilt
r., healthy
r. ▸ heightened startle
r., hemagglutination-inhibition
r., hemiopic pupillary
r., hemoclastic
r., Henle's
r., Herxheimer's
r., heterophil antibody
r., hexokinase
r., homograft
r., hormonal
r., hunting
r., Hunt's
r., hypersensitivity
r., hysterical
r., id
r., idiosyncratic
r., immediate
r., immediate transfusion
r., immune
r., immune complex
r., immunity
r., immunologic hypersensitivity
r. in body ▸ normal chemical
r. in dental patient, stress
r. in organic brain syndrome, drug
r. in violent patients, treatment of
    acute drug
r. ▸ incapacitating insulin
r., inflammatory
r., initial
r. ▸ injection site
r., insulin
r., intracutaneous
r., intradermal
r., irritant cosmetic
r., irritative
r., Jolly's
r., Kveim
r., late phase
r., lengthening
r., leukemic
r., leukoagglutinin
r., life-threatening
r. ▸ life-threatening allergic
r., local
r. ▸ local adverse

reaction(s)—*continued*

r., localized depressive
r., localized immune
r., localized irritative
r., long-term
r. machine (PCR) ▸ polymerase chain
r., Meinicke turbidity
r., mild depressive
r., mixed cell agglutination
r., mixed leukocyte
r. ▸ modulate emotional
r., Moro's
r., myasthenic
r., myotonic
r., near-point
r., negative
r., negative therapeutic
r., neurotonic
r., neutral
r., nonspecific depressive
r., normal
r., nuclear
r., obsessive-compulsive
r. of childhood ▸ hyperkinetic
r. of degeneration ▸
r. of degeneration, partial
r. of exhaustion
r. of identity
r. of nonidentity
r., ophthalmic
r., orbicularis
r., oxidative
r., pain
r., painful withdrawal
r., pancreatic
r., Pandy's
r., panic
r., parallel
r., percutaneous
r. period
r., peritoneal inflammatory
r., personal
r., phobic
r., photonuclear
r. ▸ photo-oxidative
r., photosensitivity
r., physical
r. ▸ physiological musculoskeletal
r., pleural
r. (PCR) ▸ polymerase chain
r., positive
r., postoperative
r., postpartum
r., Price precipitation

R. Profile, Psychotic
r., prolonged depressive
r. ▸ prolonged psychotic
r. ▸ prolonged vasospastic
r., psychiatric
r., psychogalvanic
r., psychogenic gastrointestinal (GI)
r., psychogenic skin
r., psychological
r. ▸ psychological allergic
r., psychological manifestations of acute drug
r., psychological state in flashback
r., psychological state in panic
r., psychoneurotic
r., psychotic
r., psychotic depressive
r., puncture
r., pupil
r., pyrogenic
r. ▸ quanti-Pirquet
r., quellung
r. ▸ rape trauma syndrome, compound
r. ▸ rape trauma syndrome, silent
r., recurrence of dystonic
r., reflex-like
r., reversible
r., schizophrenic
r., sedimentation
r., seizure
r., Selivanoff's
r., Seliwanow's
r., sensitivity
r., seroenzyme
r., seropositive
r., severe
r. ▸ severe allergic
r., severe depressive
r. ▸ severe physical
r., severe systemic
r., severe withdrawal
r., Sgambati's
r., sharpened
r., shock
r., shortening
r., sigma
r., skin
r. ▸ slowing of physical
r. ▸ slowing of psychological
r., sluggish
r. ▸ smallpox vaccine
r., somatic
r., somatization
r., staining

r., startled
r., stress
r., stress-induced
r., stress-type leukemoid
r., subacute treatment of flashback
r., subacute treatment of panic
r., subacute treatment of psychotic
r. ▸ suppress immune
r., suspected transfusion
r., sympathetic
r., symptoms of acute drug
r., symptoms of panic
r., symptoms of psychotic
r., systematic desensitization of phobic
r., systemic allergic
r. (PCR) technique ▸ polymerase chain
r., tendon
r. test, interpersonal
r. test ▸ reverse transcriptase polymerase chain
r., thermonuclear
r., thyroid function
r., tibial stress
r. time
r. times, slowed
r. to adulthood, adjustment
r. to aversive stimulation
r. to cannabinoids, treatment of acute drug
r. to contrast material
r. to crisis, emotional
r. to depressants, treatment of acute drug
r. to drug
r. to drug ▸ idiosyncratic
r. to dye, allergic
r. to electron beam therapy, skin
r. to hallucinogens, treatment of acute drug
r. to illness, family
r. to inhalants, treatment of acute drug
r. to local anesthesia ▸ toxic
r. to multiple drugs, treatment of acute drug
r. to opioids, treatment of acute drug
r. to penicillin ▸ fatal allergic
r. to phencyclidines, treatment of acute drug
r. to radiation therapy, acute
r. to radiation therapy, delayed
r. to radiation therapy, late

r. to stimulants, treatment of acute drug
r. to stings ▸ allergic
r. to stress ▸ acute
r. to stress ▸ mixed disorders as
r. to stress, psychopathological
r. to therapy, adverse
r. to transfusion, delayed
r. to transfusion, untoward
r., toxic
r., toxin-antitoxin
r., transfusion
r., treatment of acute drug
r., treatment of flashback
r., treatment of panic
r., treatment of psychotic
r., trigger
r., tuberculin
r. type, organic
r., uniphasic
r., untoward
r., urine
r., urticarial
r., vaccination
r., vagal
r., vasovagal
r., vestibular
r., violent
r., Wassermann
r., Weil-Felix
r., Wernicke's pupillary
r., wheal-flare
r., white-graft
r., Widal's
r. ▸ widespread allergic skin
r. with cannabinoids, flashback
r. with cannabinoids, panic
r. with cannabinoids, psychotic
r. with depressants, flashback
r. with depressants, panic
r. with depressants, psychotic
r. with depression, grief
r. with hallucinogens, flashback
r. with hallucinogens, panic
r. with hallucinogens, psychotic
r. with inhalants, flashback
r. with inhalants, panic
r. with inhalants, psychotic
r. with mixed emotional features ▸ adjustment
r. with multiple drugs, flashback
r. with multiple drugs, panic
r. with multiple drugs, psychotic
r. with opioids, flashback
r. with opioids, panic

r. with opioids, psychotic
r. with phencyclidines, flashback
r. with phencyclidines, panic
r. with phencyclidines, psychotic
r. with stimulants, flashback
r. with stimulants, panic
r. with stimulants, psychotic
r. with withdrawal ▸ adjustment
r., withdrawal
r. withdrawal, treatment of acute drug
r. ▸ xanthine oxidase
reactiva, meningitis necrotoxica
reactivated TB (tuberculosis)
reactivation, cross-
reactivation tuberculosis
reactive
r. airway disease
r. airway disease ▸ over-
r. airways disease syndrome (RADS)
r. arthritis
r. attachment disorder
r. attachment disorder of early childhood
r. attachment disorder of infancy
r. attachment disorder of infancy or early childhood
r. attention disorder (RAD)
r. behavior, abuse
r. cells
r. change
r. confusion
r. depression
r. dilation
r. disorder
r. hyperemia
r. hyperemia blood flow
r. hyperplasia
r. hypoglycemia
r. molecules
r. potency
r. process, atypical
r. proliferating angioendotheliomatosis
r. protein
r. protein (CRP) C-
r. protein (hs-CRP) ▸ high sensitivity C-
r. protein test ▸ C-
r. psychosis
r. psychosis, brief
r. pupils, brisk
r. schizophrenia
r. sera
r. substance, slow-
r. type of depression

r. VDRL (Venereal Disease Research Laboratories)
r., weakly
reactivity
r., cellular immunologic
r., emotional
r. ▸ hepatitis B surface antigen (HBsAG)
r., humoral immunologic
r. index (ARI) ▸ airway
r., normal
r. of brain, electrical
r. of mood ▸ marked
r. of mu/F rhythm
r., posthyperventilation
r. ▸ pulmonary vascular
r. to interpersonal stresses ▸ extreme
r. to tendon reflexes ▸ excessive
r., topography and/or
reactor
r., anniversary
r., biologic false-positive
r., breeder
r., nuclear
r. syndrome ▸ hot
Read operation, Millin-
read time
readable image
readily available ▸ donor organs
reading
r. ability
r., blood pressure (BP)
r. chart
r. comprehension
r., diastolic
r. difficulty
r. disability
r. disorder
r. disorder, developmental
r., fetal heart rate
r., lip
r. of x-rays ▸ wet
r. skills
r., speech
r., systolic
r. unit, Aloe
readmitted, patient
readout, accurate digital
readout, digital
reagent, Watson
reagin
r., atopic
r. (RPR) ▸ rapid plasma
r. (RPR) test, rapid plasma

real
   r. abandonment
   r. thirst
   r. -time three-dimensional
      echocardiography
   r. -time ultrasonography
   r. -time ultrasound
realigned, nasal pyramid
realignment
   r., bit
   r. of fracture fragments
   r. of teeth ▸ proper
realism, depressed
realism, mature
realistic
   r. commitment
   r. goals
   r. nonhostile confrontation
   r. perspective
   r. self-concept
   r. self-talk
   r. support and reassurance
   r. time-limited separation
reality
   r., awareness of
   r. base
   r. base, provide
   r. contact, break in
   r., contact with
   r., distortion of
   r., escape
   r. ▸ fantasy and
   r. ▸ feeling removed from
   r. focus ▸ strengthen
   r. ▸ hallucinations and loss of
   r. ▸ imagination and
   r. ▸ interpretation of
   r., loss of contact with
   r. of death
   r. of injury
   r. of loss
   r. of rape
   r. orientation
   r. oriented psychotherapy
   r. -principle
   r., relation to
   r. ▸ severe impairment in
      interpretation of
   r. testing
   r. testing ▸ impaired
   r. therapy
reanastomosis, limb
re-anchor prosthesis
reaper's keratitis
reapplication, cast

reappraisal, positive
reapproximate skin edges
reapproximated, subcutaneous
   tissues
rearing difficulties, child-
reason ▸ power of
reason, referral
reasoning
   r. ability
   r. ability adequate
   r., abstract
   r., arithmetical
   r., deductive
   r., inductive
   r., logical
   r., moral
   r., verbal
reassessment of cardiac rhythm
reassessment ▸ patient admitted for
   medical
reassurance, verbal
reassuring and calm
reattached
   r., extremity
   r. severed digit
   r. surgically, severed digit
   r. surgically, severed extremity
   r. surgically, severed limb
reattaching severed limb
reattachment
   r. of choroid
   r. of retina
   r. of tendon
   r., retinal
Réaumur scale
rebellion in home
rebellious, aggressive acting-out
   tendencies
rebellious behavior ▸ aggressive
rebels against authority
rebleeding, prevention of
rebleeding risk, decreased
re-blockage, aortic
reboot faulty heart's normal rhythm
rebound
   r., analgesic
   r. angina
   r. congestion
   r., guarding and/or
   r., guarding or rigidity
   r. headaches
   r. in region of McBurney's point
   r. in region of umbilicus
   r. nasal congestion
   r., rapid eye movement (REM)

   r. rhinitis
   r. tenderness
   r., tenderness without
   r., viral
rebreathing
   r. anesthesia, partial
   r. mask
   r. mask ▸ partial
Rebuck skin window technique
recalcitrant benign paroxysmal
   positional vertigo
recalcitrant hypertension
recalibrated regularly, monitor
recall
   r. ability
   r. and listening skills
   r., auditory
   r., autobiographical
   r., delayed
   r., dream
   r., enhanced
   r. ▸ evaluate orientation, attention
      and recent
   r. events, inability to
   r., failure of immediate
   r., immediate
   r. ▸ immediate and delayed
   r., immediate auditory
   r., immediate sensory trace
   r., inability to
   r., intentional
   r., memory
   r. of lung ▸ elastic
   r. of traumatic experiences
   r., recognition
   r., selective
   r., short-term
   r., slowed memory
   r., spontaneous
   r. test ▸ delayed word
   r. ▸ therapeutic limitations of delayed
   r. ▸ therapeutic potential of delayed
recalling past events
recalling recent events
Récamier's operation
recanalization ▸ excimer laser
recanalization, intraoperative
recanalizing thrombosis
recantation and self-blame ▸
   symptoms of
recapping used needles
receded gums
receding hairline
receding lower jaw
receive weekly injections ▸ patient to

receiver
- r. bandwidth
- r., implanted
- r. ▸ Medtronic radiofrequency
- r., pocket paging
- r. -stimulator
- r. /stimulator ▸ 22 channel
- r., transmitter-

recent
- r. activity ▸ moderate
- r. acute infection
- r. alcohol or drug use
- r. bereavement
- r. bleeding in retina
- r. contusion
- r. dislocation
- r. events ▸ impaired memory for
- r. events ▸ loss of memory for
- r. events, memory for
- r. events, recalling
- r. exposure
- r. fracture
- r. hemorrhage ▸ area of
- r. infarct
- r. infarction, massive
- r. memory
- r. memory ▸ confusion and poor judgment, loss of
- r. memory impairment and confabulation
- r. memory loss
- r. myocardial infarct
- r. onset of flashes and floaters
- r. recall ▸ evaluate orientation, attention and
- r. soft tissue hemorrhage
- r. surgery
- r. thromboembolization
- r. trauma

reception
- r., auditory
- r., expression and
- r., speech
- r. test, speech
- r. threshold (SRT) ▸ speech

receptive
- r. aphasia
- r. aphasia, expressive-
- r. cell
- r. disorder
- r. language disorder ▸ developmental
- r. language function
- r. mode
- r. neuron
- r. substance

receptivity to suggestion and direction
receptor(s)
- r., acetyl choline
- r., adrenergic
- r. agonist properties, dopamine
- r., alpha
- r., alpha 2
- r. antagonist ▸ thromboxane
- r., anti-estrogen
- r. assay, estrogen
- r. (ER) assay test, estrogen
- r., beta
- r., beta adrenergic
- r. binding model
- r. binding sites
- r. blockade therapy ▸ nicotinic
- r. blocker, angiotensin
- r., brain
- r., catecholamine
- r., cell
- r. cells ▸ malfunctioning insulin-
- r. cells of hearing
- r. cells, olfactory
- r., cholinergic
- r., chylomicron remnant
- r. ▸ damaged hair cell
- r. destroying enzymes
- r., dopamine
- r. dysfunction ▸ glutamate
- r. (ER), estrogen
- r. function, impair
- r. gene, estrogen
- r. glycoprotein ▸ platelet
- r., hormonal
- r., hormone
- r. in cancer cells ▸ suppress estrogen
- r. in heart ▸ stimulate calcium
- r., insulin
- r., irritant
- r., juxtacapillary
- r. kinase activity
- r. modification, possible
- r. modulators (SERM) ▸ selective estrogen
- r. molecules
- r., muscarinic
- r., muscular
- r. negative ▸ estrogen
- r. negative tumor ▸ hormone
- r., nerve
- r., neurons
- r., nicotine
- r. of ear ▸ sensory

- r. operated calcium channel
- r., opiate
- r. or nerve, sensory
- r. organ of hearing
- r., pain
- r., phagocytic
- r. positive tumor ▸ hormone
- r., ryanodine
- r. sensitivity ▸ postsynaptic
- r., sensory
- r. ▸ serotonin nerve
- r. site
- r. sites for opioids
- r. sites lose function
- r., skin
- r., somatosensory
- r., sound
- r. stimulated by injury
- r. ▸ stimulation of
- r., stimulation of beta
- r., stretch
- r. study, estrogen
- r., temperature-sensitive
- r. test ▸ hormone
- r., testosterone
- r. tumor estradiol
- r., uncoupling of
- r. ▸ upper airway
- r., vestibular

receptoric atrophy
recess
- r., epitympanic
- r., nasopalatine
- r. of pleura, costodiaphragmatic
- r. of pleura, costomediastinal
- r., sphenoethmoidal

recession [*resection*]
- r. glaucoma, angle-
- r., gum
- r. of eye muscle
- r. of eyeball
- r. of eyeball into orbit
- r. of ocular muscles

recessive
- r. chamber
- r. character
- r. characteristics
- r. gene, defective
- r. genes
- r. inheritance
- r. inheritance pattern

rechannelization of coronary artery
recharging of ventricles
rechecked, approximation
recidivism, rate of

recipient(s) ('s)
r. aorta
r., artificial heart
r., blood
r., blood transfusion
r. body
r. bone marrow
r. candidate, organ
r. cardiac transplant
r. cell
r., corneal transplant
r., donor's chromosome transferred to
r. eye
r. facility
r., heart
r., heart transplant
r. hospital
r. institution
r., kidney
r., liver
r. lymphocytes, donor and
r. ▸ matching organ transplant
r., medicare
r. of organ transplant ▸ authorization form for
r. of organ transplant ▸ consent form for
r., organ
r., organ transplant
r., potential
r., potential blood
r., potential organ
r., prospective
r. ▸ prospective transplant
r. selection
r., seropositive
r. site
r., transient contact between donor and
r., transplant
r., waiting
reciprocal
r. altruism
r. beat
r. bigeminy
r. innervation
r. interest ▸ lack of
r. rhythm
r. rhythm ▸ reversed
r. ST depression
r. transfusion
reciprocating
r. macroreentry orthodromic tachycardia
r. rhythm

r. tachycardia
r. tachycardia ▸ antidromic atrioventricular (AV)
r. tachycardia (AVRT), atrioventricular
r. tachycardia, atrioventricular (AV) junctional
r. tachycardia ▸ junctional
r. tachycardia ▸ junctioning
r. tachycardia ▸ orthodromic
r. tachycardia ▸ orthodromic atrioventricular (AV)
r. tachycardia (PJRT) ▸ permanent junctional
reciprocity, law of
reciprocity theorem, dose
recirculation, oxygenation before
reckless
r. activities ▸ involvement in
r. activity
r. and impulsive activity
r. behavior
r. disregard for safety of others
r. disregard for safety of self
r., patient
recklessness, adolescent
Recklinghausen's disease, von
reclamped, aorta
reclogged, artery
reclogged blood vessel
recoarctation of aorta
Recognition (recognition)
R. and Treatment (D/ART) ▸ Depression/Awareness
r., color
r., face
r., failure of
r. ▸ immediate and delayed
r., lucid
r. memory
r., momentary
r. ▸ object/face
r. of information ▸ perception, thought and
r., patient burned beyond
r. protein
r. recall
r. threshold, median
r., visual motor
r., word
recognize
r. authority
r. objects, inability to
r. problem

recoil
r., elastic
r., increased
r. of arterial wall ▸ elastic
r. tendency, elastic
r. wave
recollection
r., conscious
r. of incident ▸ distressing
r., temporary
recombinant
r. deoxyribonucleic acid (DNA)
r. DNA technology
r. interferon
r. interferon alpha
r., intertypic
r. technology
recombination frequency
recombination process
recombined set
recommend continued medical therapy
recommendations, treatment team
recommended
r. daily allowance
r. daily dietary allowance
r. dietary allowances (RDA)
r. dosage
r. protocol dose
recompression chamber
reconciliation, marital
reconditioned heart
reconditioners, muscle
reconditum, Dipetalonema
reconnected, tissue
reconstitution, homocollateral
reconstruct
r. heart muscle
r. knee
r. repressed memory
reconstructed breast
reconstructed limb
reconstruction
r. accomplished
r. after mastectomy, breast
r., arterial
r. ▸ bifurcated vein graft for vascular
r., breast
r., Brent's eyebrow
r., Cabral coronary
r., cosmetic
r., esophageal
r., facial
r., in vitro

r., Landolt's eyelid
r., laryngeal
r., mastectomy
r., Mladick ear
r., nasoseptal
r., nipple
r., oculoplastic
r. of artery
r. of blood vessel
r. of breast, tissue
r. of bronchus, plastic
r. of esophageal perforation
r. of eyelid
r. of joint
r. of wound
r. operation
r., plastic
r. ▸ polyhedral surface
r., primary
r. procedure
r. ▸ Sheen airway
r., shoulder
r., Steffanoff's ear
r. surgery, breast
r., Tanzer's auricle
r. technique, algebraic
r. ▸ total joint
r., tubal
r., vascular
r., Wookey's pharyno-esophageal

reconstructive
r. arthroplasty
r. breast surgery
r. cosmetic surgery
r. dentistry
r. eyelid surgery
r. hip surgery
r. microsurgery
r. operation
r. plastic procedure
r. procedure
r. surgeon, plastic
r. surgery
r. surgery ▸ general
r. surgery, plastic and
r. surgery, postmastectomy
r. surgical procedures
r. technique

recontouring
r. alveolectomy, mandibular
r. alveolectomy, maxillary
r., body

record(s)
r. analyst, health
r., biotelemetric

r., borderline normal
r., clinical
r., confidentiality of
r. documentation, medical
r., electronic medical
r., low voltage
r., medical
r. of electrocerebral inactivity
r. of electrocerebral silence
r., patient
r., patient care
r., patient progress
r., refer to previous
r., resting
r., treatment
r., wake

recorded
r. activity, diminution of
r. brain wave pattern
r. electrical brain activity
r. picture, digital
r., pressure measurements
r., thresholds and sensitivities
    measured and

recorder
r., circadian event
r., event
r. ▸ external loop recorder
r. ▸ implantable loop
r., loop
r., pulse volume
r., videotape

recording
r., all night sleep
r., all-night electroencephalogram
    (EEG)
r., awake
r., bipolar esophageal
r., cine loop
r., Doppler
r., ECS (electrocerebral silence)
r., EEG (electroencephalogram)
r. electrode
r. electrodes, scalp
r., electronystagmographic (ENG)
r. from cortex, direct
r., graphic
r., high frequencies of
r. ▸ His bundle
r. instrument ▸ electroencephalo-
    gram (EEG)
r. ▸ M-mode
r., nasopharyngeal electrode
r. of electrical activity
r., polygraphic

r. ▸ pulse wave
r., referential
r. site
r., sleep
r., technique of

recovered
r. memory
r. memory therapist
r. memory therapy

recovering
r. addicts
r. alcoholic
r. alcoholic ▸ newly
r. community
r. from surgery
r. peer
r. stroke patient

recovery (Recovery)
r., adolescents in family
r. and confirmation
r. and rehabilitation ▸ postoperative
r., and relapse prevention ▸
    treatment,
r. area, postanesthesia
r., barrier to
r. complicated
r. coordinator, organ
r. ▸ diagnosis, treatment and
r. function, auditory
r., functional
r., grief
r. group, bereavement
r. groups
r. ▸ heart rate
r. heat
r. incision
r. ▸ long-term
r., low probability of
r. module
r. needs, unique
r., normal
r., nutrition to
r. of alcohol or drug use
r. of donated organs and tissues,
    surgical
r., organ-tissue
r. period
r. period ▸ at-home
r. phase ▸ supernormal
r., postoperative
r., pressure
r. process
r. program, personal
r., psychological
r., rapid

recovery—*continued*
- r. rate
- R., Reach to
- R. Room
- R. Room, patient sent to
- r., satisfactory
- r., stages of
- r. status
- r. stroke
- r. ▸ support long-term
- r., supportive therapeutic
- r., sustained
- r. team ▸ organ
- r. technique
- r. time
- r. time, corrected sinus node
- r. time ▸ sinoatrial (SA)
- r. time, sinus node
- r., trauma
- r., visual
- r., vital organ

recreating heart tissue
recreation, structured
recreation therapy
recreational
- r. activities
- r. drug abuse
- r. drugs
- r. injury
- r. nap
- r. therapy
- r. use
- r. use, social/

recriminatory, self-
recruitable collateral vessel
recruitment
- r. ▸ host-generated neutrophils
- r. pattern
- r. pattern of electrical activity
- r. studies
- r., Tschiassny

recrystallized form
recta, vasa
rectal
- r. abscess
- r. abscess drained
- r. ampulla
- r. anesthesia
- r. arteries, bulging
- r. bleeding
- r. bleeding, massive
- r. bleeding secondary to hemorrhoids
- r. branch, superior
- r. burning
- r. burning from bisacodyl

- r. canal
- r. cancer
- r. carcinoma
- r. enema
- r. deferred
- r. discharge
- r. evacuant
- r. examination
- r. examination, digital
- r. fistula
- r. fistula drained
- r. folds
- r. hemorrhage, acute
- r. hemorrhoids
- r. hernia
- r. incontinence
- r. irritation
- r. itching
- r. lesion
- r. lesion, original
- r. manometry
- r. margins
- r. mass
- r. mucous membrane, loose
- r. nerves, inferior
- r. neurosis
- r. pain and soreness
- r. palpation
- r. polyp
- r. polyp, benign
- r. polyp, hyperplastic
- r. pouch
- r. pressure
- r. prolapse
- r. reflex
- r. shelf
- r. site
- r. skin tags
- r. sphincter
- r. sphincter muscle spasm
- r. sphincter tone
- r. sphincterotomy
- r. suppository
- r. swab
- r. tags
- r. tear
- r. temperature
- r. tenesmus
- r. test, digital
- r. thermometer
- r. tumor
- r. tumor ▸ local resection of
- r. vein, superior
- r. veins, inferior
- r. veins, middle

- r. verge
- r. warts

rectally (Rectally)
rectangular
- r. amputation
- r. flap, long
- r. flap, short
- r. wave form

rectangulare, Ferribacterium
recti
- r. abdomis, diastasis
- r., Alcaligenes
- r., diastasis

rectification
- r., anomalous
- r. ▸ inward-going
- r., synchronous

rectified polarizing microscope
rectilinear scanner
recto, hernia in
rectocardiac reflex
rectococcygeus muscle
rectocutaneous fistula
rectolabial fistula
rectosigmoid
- r. carcinoma
- r. junction
- r. polypoid lesion

rectourethral muscle
rectouterina, plica
rectouterine
- r. fold
- r. ligament
- r. muscle

rectovaginal
- r. dose
- r. examination
- r. fascia
- r. fistula
- r. fold
- r. septum
- r. septum tumors

rectovesical
- r. center
- r. fascia
- r. fold
- r. muscle
- r. septum

rectovesicale, septum
rectum
- r., adenocarcinoma of
- r., bleeding from
- r. cancer
- r., carcinoma of
- r., decompression of

r. defecation
r. development
r., displacement of
r., horizontal folds of
r., implantation of ureter into
r. ▸ internal hemorrhoids of
r., mucous folds of
r., per
r., perineal flexure of
r. ▸ pressure in
r., redundant prolapsed
r., sacral flexure of
r., stool in
r., transverse folds of

rectus
r. abdominis
r. abdominis muscle
r. bridle suture, superior
r. fascia
r. femoris
r. femoris tendon
r., gyrus
r. incision, lateral
r. inferior muscle
r. inferior, musculus
r. lateralis muscle
r. lateralis, musculus
r. medialis muscle
r. medialis, musculus
r. muscle, advancement of external
r. muscle, advancement of inferior
r. muscle, advancement of internal
r. muscle, advancement of lateral
r. muscle, advancement of medial
r. muscle, advancement of superior
r. muscle, anterior sheath of
r. muscle dissected free, inferior
r. muscle, inferior
r. muscle, lateral
r. muscle, medial
r. muscle, posterior sheath of
r. muscle, retraction of
r. muscle split
r. muscle splitting incision
r. muscle, superior
r. sheath
r. superior muscle
r. traction suture, superior

recumbency cramps
recumbent
r. AP (anteroposterior) and lateral
    films, portable
r. film, portable
r. lateral projection
r., left arm

r. position
r. position, dorsal
r. position, lateral
r., right arm

recumbivax injections
recuperation
r., lengthy
r. (R and R) ▸ rest and
r. time

recuperative period
recuperative power, body's
recurrence
r., abrupt
r. after radiation therapy, local
r., cancer
r., central
r., fulminant
r. ▸ ipsilateral breast tumor
r., local
r., metastatic
r. (NER), no evidence of
r. of cancer
r. of carcinoma, local
r. of disease
r. of dystonic reactions
r. of melanoma
r. of migraines
r. of pain
r. of tumor ▸ local
r. of tumor ▸ regional
r. rate
r., regional
r. risk

recurrens, herpes
recurrent
r. abdominal pain
r. abdominal pain with colitis
r. adenocarcinoma
r. angina
r. apneic attack
r. aspiration
r. atrial flutter
r. bleed
r. bleeding
r. brain tumor
r. breast cancer
r. breast carcinoma
r. bronchogenic carcinoma
r. bronchospasm
r. cancer
r. carcinoma
r. chest pain
r. congestive heart failure (CHF)
r. depression
r. disease

r. disease ▸ intrastent
r. disease (NERD), no evidence of
r. dislocation
r. embolism
r. episode
r. episode ▸ major depressive
    disorder,
r. excruciating headache
r. eye twitch
r. fever
r. fibrosarcoma
r. fibrosarcoma of uterus
r. genital herpes
r. heart attack
r. hemorrhage from aneurysm
r. hernia
r. Hodgkin's disease
r. illness
r., in full remission ▸ major
    depression
r. infections
r. insanity
r. kidney infections
r. laryngeal nerve
r. laryngeal nerve function
r. lesion
r. lung destruction
r. ▸ major depression
r. malignant ventricular tachycardia
r. melancholia
r. meningitis
r. mesenteric ischemia
r. mesenteric vascular occlusion
r., mild ▸ major depression,
r. miscarriages
r., moderate ▸ major depression,
r. myocardial infarction
r. nerve
r. nerve, ophthalmic
r. nerve section
r. pain
r. paroxysmal tachycardia
r. phlebitis
r. pleural effusion
r. pneumonitis
r. psychotic symptoms
r. pulmonary emboli
r. pungent odor
r. respiratory papillomatosis
r. salpingitis
r. seizures ▸ brief
r. sensibility
r., severe, without psychotic
    features ▸ major depression
r. shortness of breath

recurrent—*continued*
- r. sinusitis
- r. skin tumors
- r. sneezing
- r. stricture
- r. stroke
- r. stroke, risk of
- r. suicidal behavior
- r. symptoms
- r. thoracic outlet syndrome
- r. thoughts of death
- r. thoughts of suicide
- r. thromboemboli
- r. tumor
- r. ulcerative blepharitis
- r., unspecified ▸ major depression,
- r. upper respiratory tract infection
- r. urinary tract infection
- r. vaginal bleeding
- r. vaginal yeast infection
- r. variceal hemorrhage
- r. ventricular ectopy
- r. vertigo
- r. vestibulopathy
- r. vomiting
- r., with psychotic features ▸ major depression

recurrentis, Borrelia

recurring
- r. blackouts
- r. bladder infections
- r. colon cancer
- r. depression, chronic
- r. excessive neuronal discharge
- r. hallucinations
- r. headaches
- r. hemorrhage
- r. infections
- r. mouth sores
- r. palpitations
- r. pneumonia
- r. sense of loss
- r. skin rashes
- r. thoughts of death or suicide
- r. venereal warts
- r. ventricular tachycardia
- r. yeast vaginitis

recurva, Trypanosoma

recurvatum
- r. deformity
- r., genu
- r., pectus

recycle patient

recycled human blood substitute

Red(s) (red)
- R. (barbiturates)
- R. and Blues (barbiturates) ▸ Pinks,
- r. and puffy gums
- r. and swollen eyelids
- r. and swollen ▸ irritated,
- r. and swollen ▸ itchy,
- r. and warm breast
- r. and white cell precursors
- r. atrophy
- r. blood, bright
- r. blood cell antigen
- r. blood cell aplasia ▸ pure
- r. blood ▸ copious bright
- r. blood corpuscle
- r. bone marrow
- r. bone marrow, dark
- r. butterfly-shaped rash on face
- r. cell antigen
- r. cell therapy
- r. cell transfusion ▸ perioperative
- R. Code
- r. corpuscle
- r., cracked and itchy hands ▸ dry,
- R. Devils (barbiturates)
- r. discharge, brownish-
- R. Dragon (LSD)
- r. ears from dermatitis
- r. ears from eczema
- r. eyes
- r. fiber (MERRF) disease ▸ myoclonic epilepsy and ragged
- r. glass test
- r. -green color perception deficiency
- r. -green test for diplopia ▸ Lancaster's
- r. gums from dentures
- r. hemorrhagic fluid
- r. herring
- r. hypertension
- r. induration
- r. infarct
- r. infection
- r., itchy patches of skin ▸ thick,
- r. kidney, large
- r. laser illumination
- r. light therapy
- r. line up arm
- r. marrow
- r. ▸ medullary substances of bones
- r., methyl
- R. (barbiturates), Mexican
- r. muscle
- r., neutral

- r., nodular or flat growth ▸ firm,
- R. (grade of marijuana), Panama
- r., parenchyma beefy
- r. patch or blister on arm
- r., phenol
- r. pulp, splenic
- r. rash ▸ lacy
- r. reflex
- r., ring-shaped rash
- r., scaly and itchy ▸ blister
- r., scaly patch
- r. skin
- r. softening
- r. spider veins
- r. spot, cherry
- r. spot on breast
- r. stain, Congo
- r. "strawberry" tongue
- r. substance of spleen
- r. swollen joint
- r., swollen, tender gums
- r. test, Congo
- r. thrombus
- r. tympanic membrane ▸ bulging
- r. venous blood
- r. vermilion lip line

red blood cell(s) (RBC)
- RBC ▸ abnormal
- RBC ▸ accelerated destruction of
- RBC count
- RBC deficiency
- RBC ▸ destruction of
- RBC loss
- RBC mass
- RBC, nucleated
- RBC, packed
- RBC per high power field (RBC/hpf)
- RBC ▸ production of
- RBC returned to donor
- RBC ▸ sedimentation rate of
- RBC, spiculed mature
- RBC survival
- RBC, transfusion of
- RBC transfusions ▸ packed
- RBC volume

red cell(s)
- r.c. agenesis, pure
- r.c. (TRC) antibody titer, microsomal tanned
- r.c. casts
- r.c. count
- r.c. drained
- r.c. folate
- r.c. fragility
- r.c., frozen

r.c. gravitate to bottom of container
r.c. indices
r.c. mass
r.c. mixed with plasma
r.c., nucleated
r.c. ▸ O₂ (oxygen) carrying
r.c., packed
r.c. precursors
r.c. preparations
r.c., sedimented
r.c. tagged with radioactive material
r.c. (TRC), tanned
r.c. transfused back into donor
r.c. transfusion
r.c. volume
r.c., volume of packed
r.c., washed

Redbirds (barbiturates)
reddened
r. areas of skin
r., dry, fissured lips
r., flushed skin
reddening, mucosal
reddish macules
reddish patch, persistent
redefining family's values
redevelopment of pancreatitis
rediscovering a sense of self-worth
redistribution
r. and dose fractionation, cell cycle
r. and dose hyperfractionation, cell cycle
r., cell cycle
r. imaging
r. ▸ pulmonary vascular
r., radiosensitivity and cell cycle
r., smoking
r. thallium 201 imaging ▸ rest
r., transcellular
r., vascular
Redlich-Fisher miliary plaques
redness
r. along incision site
r. and flakiness from athlete's foot
r. and inflammation
r. and warmth in joint
r. at incision site
r. ▸ double vision with eye
r., dryness and itching
r. ▸ light feathering or
r. of skin
r. of skin ▸ burning, itching and
r., warmth and
redraped skin

redressed, wound
redressing, sterile
reduce
r. alertness and coordination
r. astigmatism
r. blinking
r. blood clotting
r. blood flow
r. blood pressure (BP)
r. circulating volume
r. fever
r. fluid formation
r. intake
r. myopia
r. pain
r. pain ▸ restore mobility and
r. prostate size
r. risk of back problems
r. risk of hospital-associated infections
r. salt intake
r. size of tumor
r. sodium intake
r. stress and muscle strain
r. swelling in brain
r. swelling in legs
r. tension
r. tension and distress
r. tension headache frequency
r. tissue swelling
reduced (Reduced)
r. activity
r. activity therapy
r. activity to emotional situations
r. air pressure
r. alcohol consumption
r. amplification
r. appetite
r. awareness
r. bladder capacity
r. blood flow
r. blood flow to brain
r. blood supply to heart
r. blood temperature
r. body temperature
r. by massage, swelling
r. cardiac output
r. ▸ cardiac output markedly
r. cerebral blood flow
r. circulation
r. cognitive function
r. concentration
r. cranial capacity
r. diet, lactose
r. distance vision

r. effectiveness of mammograms
r. ejection
r. elasticity, blood vessels with
R. Environmental Stimulation Therapy (REST)
r. eyesight
r. fat diet
r. flow of saliva
r., fracture
r. glutathione
r. hearing at high frequency
r. heart rate
r. hemoglobin
r. inhibitions
r. interference pattern
r. kidney function
r. libido
r. lung capacity
r., mobility
r., narcotic requirement
r., nasal fracture
r. outflow obstruction
r. oxygen tension
r. pain perception
r. renal function
r. risks to pre-term birth
r. spasticity
r. spontaneity, curiosity, and initiative
r. stimulation
r. to normal size ▸ heart
r. tolerance for physical activity
r. urinary flow
r. ventricular filling
r. vision
r. voltage, generalized
r. voltage, symmetrically
r. weight bearing
r. white blood count (WBC)
reducer(s)
r., afterload
r., Honan pressure
r., natural stress
reducible hernia
reducing
r. alcohol consumption
r. clot formation
r. drugs, fever-
r. effects, stress-
r. frequency of seizures
r. meditation ▸ stress
r. physiological arousal
r. saturated fats
r. sugar
r. techniques, stress

reducing—*continued*
- r. tumor
- r. unit (TRU) ▸ turbidity

reductase, glutathione

reduction
- r. abnormality ▸ limb
- r., acid
- r., afterload
- r. and internal fixation (ORIF), open
- r. anomaly ▸ limb
- r., blood pressure (BP)
- r., bone mass
- r., breast
- r., cardiac risk
- r., cholesterol
- r., closed
- r., coronary risk
- r., correlates of blood pressure (BP)
- r. diet
- r. diet, weight
- r. division
- r. ▸ exercise and weight
- r. facial fracture
- r. factor, dose
- r. ▸ female breast
- r. films, post◊
- r., gradient
- r., harm
- r., headache
- r. ▸ health care cost
- r. in amplitude
- r. in amplitude ▸ extreme lateralized
- r. in cost
- r. in pain sensation
- r. in plasma volume
- r. in seizure
- r. in voltage, bilateral
- r. in volume of air
- r. inhibition, tetrazolium-
- r. ▸ left ventricular
- r. ▸ male breast
- r. mammoplasty
- r., manual
- r., moderate salt
- r., noise
- r. of anxiety
- r. of blood fats
- r. of examination anxiety
- r. of fracture
- r. of fracture, closed
- r. of fracture, open
- r. of fracture ▸ rotation and
- r. of humerus, open
- r. of output pen deflection ▸ percent
- r. of platelet count

- r. of salt intake
- r. of sensitivity of an electroencephalogram (EEC) channel
- r. of sensitivity, relative
- r. of skull fracture ▸ open
- r. of tumor size
- r. of voltage, lateralized
- r. of voltage, localized
- r., open
- r. position satisfactory, post◊
- r., post◊
- r., postoperative
- r., preload
- r. procedure ▸ lung
- r. program, stress
- r. program, weight
- r. psychotherapy ▸ harm
- r. ▸ relaxation and stress
- r. rhinoplasty, standard
- r., risk
- r. ▸ risk factor
- r., smoking
- r. ▸ stapled lung
- r. status, post◊
- r., stress
- r. surgery, breast
- r. surgery, double lung
- r. surgery ▸ heart
- r. surgery ▸ left ventricular (LV)
- r. surgery ▸ lung
- r. surgery ▸ lung volume
- r. surgery ▸ single lung
- r. surgery ▸ unilateral lung
- r. surgery ▸ weight
- r., symptom
- r. technique, Crutchfield
- r. technique, Essex-Lopresti
- r. technique, Lottes'
- r. technique, Magnuson
- r. technique, Martin
- r. technique ▸ rage
- r. technique ▸ Speed and Boyd
- r. technique, stress
- r. technique, Thomson
- r. technique, Wagner
- r., tetrazolium
- r. therapy ▸ rage
- r. ▸ trauma incident
- r., tremor
- r. verified by x-ray
- r., weight

reductionism, biological
reductionism, psychodynamic
redundancy, aneurysm
redundancy of colon

redundant
- r. cusp syndrome
- r. foreskin
- r. pelvis
- r. prepuce
- r. prolapsed rectum
- r. skin
- r. tissue

reduplication cataract
reduplication murmur
reduplicative paramnesia
redux
- r. procedure ▸ lung
- r., rale
- r., testis

reed electrometer, vibrating
Reed-Sternberg cells
reedswitch, pacemaker
**re-education of the hemiplegic ▸
  neuromuscular**
reefed, vaginal cuff
Reefer (marijuana cigarette)
reefing
- r., medial capsular
- r. of medial capsule
- r. of vastus medialis

reeling, staggering gait
reemergent symptoms
reemerging infection
reenactment(s)
- r. /flashbacks
- r., play
- r., traumatic

**reentrance supraventricular
  tachycardia**
reentrant
- r. arrhythmia
- r. atrial tachycardia
- r., AV node
- r. circuit
- r. loop
- r. mechanism
- r. paroxysmal tachycardia,
  atrioventricular (AV)
- r. pathway
- r. rhythm
- r. ▸ supraventricular tachycardia
- r. supraventricular tachycardia ▸
  paroxysmal
- r. sustained ventricular tachycardia
  ▸ spontaneous
- r. tachycardia
- r. tachycardia ▸ atrial
  atrioventricular nodal

r. tachycardia, atrioventricular (AV) nodal
r. tachycardia, bundle branch
r. tachycardia ▸ intra-atrial
r. tachycardia ▸ nodal
r. tachycardia ▸ orthodromi A-V
r. tachycardia ▸ S-A nodal
r. tachycardia ▸ sinus
r. tachycardia ▸ sinus nodal
r. tachycardia ▸ Wolff-Parkinson-White

reentry
r., atrioventricular (AV) nodal
r., atrioventricular node (AVN)
r., AV nodal
r., bundle branch
r. phenomenon
r. ▸ Schmitt-Erlanger model of
r. ▸ sinus nodal
r. ▸ sinus node
r. tachycardia, atrial
r. tachycardia ▸ atrial ventricular nodal
r. theory
r., ventricular

Rees and Ecker diluting fluid
Reese('s)
R. Ellsworth classification
R. stimulator
R. syndrome
re-evaluate patient
re-evaluation of existing drug therapy
Reeves treadmill protocol
re-excision surgery
re-excision, tumor
re-expansion of lung
refer to previous admission
refer to previous records
reference
r., average
r., average potential
r., delusion of
r. ▸ delusion or idea of
r. electrode
r. electrode, common
r. electrode, common average
r. electrode, single
r. electrode, sternospinal
r. electrode, zero potential
r. electrodes
r., idea of
r. montage, common
r. serum, normal
r. system ▸ hexaxial
r. system ▸ triaxial

r. ▸ transient ideas of
r. value
referential
r. derivations
r. montage
r. recording
r. thinking
referral
r., cultural
r. for incest, court
r., language
r. network
r., primary
r. procedure
r. reason
r. resource service
r., selective
r., self-
r. service, physician
r. services
r. source
r. to community agencies
r. to support group
r. transplant center
referred
r. pain
r. pain sensory pathways
r. sensation
r. to follow-up ▸ patient
referring
r. doctor
r. patients ▸ assessing and
r. physician
refill, capillary
refill, transcapillary
refine bone storage technique
refined wool fat
refinement, facial
refinement, nasal
reflect [*respect*]
reflectance oximetry
reflected [*rejected*]
r., flap of periosteum
r. from insertion, muscle
r. laterally
r. medially
r. over periosteum, sheath
r., scalp
r., skin flaps
r. upward
r., vesicouterine peritoneum
reflecting level
reflecting microscope
reflection [*resection*]
r., bladder

r. interference microscopy (RIM)
r., mirror
r., mucosal
r. of scalp
r. of sound waves
r. of sternum
r., peritoneal
r., pleural
r. rheography (LRR), light
r., serosal
r. ▸ shock wave
r., uterine
reflective reverie
reflective self-awareness
reflector, dental
reflex(es) [*reflux*]
r., abdominal
r., abdominocardiac
r., Abrams'
r., Abrams' heart
r. absent
r., absent corneal
r., absent oculocephalic
r., accommodation
r., Achilles tendon
r., acquired
r. action
r. activity
r. activity, depressed
r., adductor
r., afferent
r., allied
r., anal
r. angina
r., ankle
r., antagonistic
r., anticus
r., aortic
r. arc, simple
r., arteriolar light
r., Aschner's
r. asthma
r. asymmetry
r., atriopressor
r., attitudinal
r. audiometry, conditioned orientation
r., audito-oculogyric
r., auditory
r., aural
r., auricle
r., auricular
r., auriculocervical nerve
r., auriculopalpebral
r., auriculopressor

reflex(es)—*continued*

r., autonomic
r., axon
r., Babinski
r., Bainbridge
r., Barkman's
r., baroreceptor
r. barrier ▸ gastric component
r., basal joint
r., Bechterew-Mendel
r., Bechterew's
r., behavior
r., Bekhterev-Mendel
r., Bekhterev's
r., Bezold-type
r., biceps
r. bilaterally equal
r., black
r., bladder
r. bladder, automatic
r., bladder control
r., blink
r., bradycardia and absent corneal
r., (Russell) Brain
r., brain stem
r., bregmocardiac
r., Breuer-Hering inflation
r., brisk
r., Brissaud
r., Brudzinski's
r., bulbocavernous
r., bulbomimic
r., cardiac
r., cardiac depressor
r., carotid sinus
r., cat's eye
r. center
r. center in brain ▸ micturition
r. center ▸ spinal micturition
r., cerebral cortex
r., Chaddock's
r., chain
r. changes
r. check, pupil
r., chemoreceptor
r., chin
r., chocked
r., ciliary
r., ciliospinal
r., clasp-knife
r., cochleo-orbicular
r., cochleopalpebral
r., cochleopupillary
r., cochleostapedial
r., concealed

r., conditional
r., conditioned
r., conjunctival
r., consensual
r., consensual light
r. contractions, suppress
r. control
r., convergency
r., convulsive
r., coordinated
r., corneal
r., corneal blink
r., corneomandibular
r., corneomental
r., corneopterygoid
r., coronary
r. cough
r., cranial
r., craniocardiac
r., cremasteric
r., crossed
r., cuboidodigital
r., Cushing
r., cutaneous pupillary
r., dartos
r., Davidson's
r., dazzle
r. decidua
r., decreased
r., deep
r., deep abdominal
r. (DTR) ▸ deep tendon
r., defecation
r., defense
r., delayed
r., depressed
r., depressor
r., digital
r., diminished
r., direct
r., direct light
r. disease (GERD) ▸
    gastroesophageal
r., diving
r., doll's eye
r., domino
r., dorsal
r., dorsocuboidal
r., duodenocolic
r. dyspepsia
r. dystrophy
r., elbow
r., embrace
r., emergency light
r., enterogastric

r., epigastric
r. epilepsy
r. equal
r. equal and active bilaterally
r. (DTR) equal and active bilaterally
    ▸ deep tendon
r. equal and brisk
r. equal bilaterally
r., Erben's
r., erector spinae
r., Escherich's
r., esophagosalivary
r., ether
r. evaluation
r., exaggerated
r., exaggerated blink
r., excessive reactivity to tendon
r., eyeball compression
r., eyeball-heart
r., eyelid closure
r., facial
r., fainting
r., faucial
r., femoral
r., finger flexion
r., finger-thumb
r. flexor, plantar
r., fontanel
r., foveolar
r., front-tap
r., fusion
r., gag
r., galvanic skin
r., gasp
r., gastrocnemius
r., gastrocolic
r., gastroileal
r., gastropancreatic
r., Gault's cochleopalpebral
r., Geigel's
r., genital
r., Gifford-Galassi
r., Gifford's
r., gluteal
r., Gordon's
r., grasp
r., grasping
r., Grünfelder's
r., gustolacrimal
r., H-
r., Haab's
r., hair-trigger gag
r. hallucination
r. headache
r., heart

r., heel-tap
r., hepatojugular
r., Hering-Breuer
r., Hirschberg's
r., Hoffmann's
r., Hughes'
r., hyperactive
r., hyperactive carotid sinus
r., hypoactive
r. (DTR) ▸ hypoactive deep tendon
r., hypochondrial
r., ileogastric
r. ileus
r., inborn
r., incomplete Moro
r. incontinence
r., increased
r. ▸ increased action of
r. (DTR) ▸ increased deep tendon
r., indirect
r., inflation
r., infraspinatus
r., inguinal
r., interscapular
r., intestinointestinal
r., inverted
r., inverted radial
r., iris contraction
r. irritability
r., ischemic
r., jaw
r., jaw jerk
r., Joffroy's
r., Juster
r., juvenile
r., Kehrer's
r., Kisch's
r., knee
r., knee jerk
r., Kocher's
r., lacrimal
r., Landau
r., laryngeal
r., laryngopharyngeal
r., lash
r., laughter
r., letdown
r., lid
r., Liddel and Sherrington
r., light
r. -like reaction
r., lip
r., Livierato's
r., local spinal
r., Lovén

r., lumbar
r., Lust's
r., Magnus and de Kleijn neck
r., mandibular
r., Marinesco-Radovici
r., mass
r., masseteric
r., Mayer's
r., McCarthy's
r., McCormac's
r., McDowall
r. mechanism, hemostatic
r., Mendel-Bekhterev
r., Mendel's
r., milk letdown
r., Mondonesi's
r. (DTR) ▸ monitoring of deep
  tendon
r., Morley's peritoneocutaneous
r., Moro embrace
r., Moro's
r., motor
r. movement
r., muscle
r., muscle stretch
r., muscular
r., mute
r., myenteric
r., myopic
r., myotatic
r., myotonic
r., nasal
r., nasolabial
r., nasomental
r., negative Moro
r., nerve
r., neural
r., nociceptive
r., normal
r. normoactive
r., normophysiological
r., nostril
r., obliquus
r., oculocardiac
r., oculocephalic
r., oculocephalogyric
r., oculopharyngeal
r., oculopupillary
r., oculosensory cell
r., oculovagal
r. of foot, adductor
r. of foot, Mendel's dorsal
r. of leg, flexion
r. of Marinesco-Radovici,
  palmomental

r. of pupil, attention
r., Oppenheim's
r., optic
r., opticofacial winking
r., orbicularis
r. (OR) ▸ orienting
r., orthocardiac
r. otalgia
r., oval window
r., pain
r. pain syndrome ▸ chronic
r., palatal
r., palatine
r., palmar grasp
r., palm-chin
r., palmomental
r., paradoxic pupillary
r., paradoxical
r., paradoxical flexor
r., paraserum
r., patellar
r., patellar tendon
r., patelloadductor
r., pathologic
r., Pavlov
r., pectoral
r., penile
r., penis
r., perception
r., perianal
r., pericardial
r., periosteal
r., peripheral
r., peritoneointestinal
r., pharyngeal
r., phasic
r., Philippson's
r. ▸ photic sneeze
r., physiologic
r., pilomotor
r., Piltz's
r., plantar
r., platysmal
r., pneocardiac
r., postural
r. ▸ postural righting
r., prepotential
r., pressor
r., pressoreceptor
r., Preyer's
r., proprioceptive
r., protective laryngeal
r., protective pharyngeal
r., psychic
r., psychocardiac

reflex(es)—*continued*
r., psychogalvanic
r., pulmonocoronary
r., pupillary
r., Puusepp's
r., quadriceps
r., quadrupedal extensor
r., radial
r., rectal
r., rectocardiac
r., red
r., regional
r., Remak's
r., renointestinal
r., renorenal
r., respiratory
r. response
r., retrobulbar pupillary
r., retrocardiac
r., Riddoch's mass
r., righting
r., Roger's
r., Romberg
r., rooting
r., Rossolimo's
r., round window
r., Ruggeri's
r., Russell Brain
r., sacral
r., Saenger's
r., scapular
r., scapulohumeral
r., Schäffer's
r., scratch
r., scrotal
r., segmental
r., senile
r. sensation
r., sexual
r., shot-silk
r., simple
r., sinus
r. skills, conditioned
r., skin
r., skin pupillary
r., slowed
r., sneeze
r., Snellen's
r., sole
r., Somagyi's
r., somatointestinal
r., spinal
r., startle
r., static
r., statotomic

r., stepping
r. stimulation
r., Stookey
r., stretch
r. strong and equal bilaterally
r., Strümpell's
r., suck
r., sucking
r., superficial
r., superficial abdominal
r., supinator longus
r., supraorbital
r., suprapatellar
r., suprapubic
r., supraumbilical
r., swallowing
r. (DTR) symmetrical ▸ deep tendon
r. sympathetic dystrophy (RSD)
r. sympathetic dystrophy (RSD)
    syndrome
r. sympathoexcitation
r. tachycardia
r., tapetal light
r., tarsophalangeal
r. tearing
r., tendon
r. testing, acoustic
r. testing ▸ strength, sensation and
r. (CR) therapy, conditioned
r., threat
r., Throckmorton's
r., tibioadductor
r., timed Achilles tendon
r., toe
r., tonic
r., tonic neck
r., tracheal
r., trained
r., transient loss of respiratory
r., triceps
r., triceps surae
r., trigeminus
r. -type ileus
r., ulnar
r. (UCR) ▸ unconditioned
r., urinary
r., vaccinoid
r., vagal
r., vagus
r., vascular
r. vasculospastic activity
r. vasodilation
r., vasopressor
r., vasovagal
r., venorespiratory

r., vertebra prominens
r., vesical
r., vesicointestinal
r., vestibular ocular
r., virile
r., visceral
r., viscerocardiac
r., visceromotor
r., viscerosensory
r., viscerotrophic
r. voiding, induced
r., vomiting
r., von Mering
r., water-silk
r., Weiss'
r., Westphal-Piltz
r., Westphal's pupillary
r., wrist clonus
r., zygomatic
reflexa, decidua
reflexa, placenta
reflexive
r. activities
r. ileus
r. response
reflexively, patient gags
reflexogenic pressosensitivity
reflexology, art of
reflexology treatment
reflow phenomenon ▸ no
reflux [*reflex*]
r., abdominojugular
r., acid
r., blood
r., cardioesophageal
r. disease, acid
r. disease (GERD),
    gastroesophageal
r. dissecting abdominal aortic
    aneurysm
r. drug, anti◇
r., erosive
r. esophageal
r. esophagitis
r. esophagitis ▸ chronic
r. esophagitis ▸ erosive
r. filling
r., free esophageal
r. from stomach
r., gastroesophageal
r., hepatojugular
r. -induced esophageal stricture
r., intermittent
r. into terminal ileum normal
r. (MR), mitral

r. nephropathy
r. of barium
r. of bile
r. of gastric contents
r. of urine, ureteral
r. prosthesis, Angelchik anti-
r. sympathetic dystrophy (RSD)
r. symptoms, postural
r. test ▸ hepatojugular
r., urethrovesiculo-differential
r., urinary
r., vesicoureteral
refluxing veins, eradicate
refocus your attention
reform
r. eye implant, conventional
r. eye, Snellen's
r. implant, Snellen conventional
reformation of chamber, delayed
refractability, cell
refracted ray
refracting media
refraction [*retraction*]
r., double
r., dynamic
r., fogging system of
r., homatropine
r., index of
r., light
r., manifest
r., ocular
r. of eye
r. of lens, asymmetric
r., relative index of
r., static
r. test
refractive
r. ametropia
r. care
r. disease
r. error
r. examination
r. eye surgery
r. index (RI)
r. keratectomy, photo-
r. surgery
r. surgery ▸ laser
r. to treatment
refractory
r. anemia
r. anemia, chronic
r. anemia with excess blasts
   (RAEB) ▸ syndrome of
r. angina ▸ severe,
r. depression

r. edema
r. ergonovine-induced vasospasm
r. heart failure
r. osteomyelitis, chronic
r. patient
r. period
r. period (ARP), absolute
r. period (APERP), accessory
   pathway effective
r. period, antegrade
r. period, atrial effective
r. period (AVRP), atrioventricular
r. period, effective
r. period, functional
r. period ▸ intrinsic
r. period of electronic pacemaker
r. period ▸ pacemaker amplifier
r. period, relative
r. period ▸ ventricular effective
r. periods, cardiac
r. state
r. supraventricular arrhythmias
r. tachycardia
r. tachycardia, drug-
r. to treatment
r. ulcer
refractured, bone
reframing problems
refrigerant diuretic
refringens, Borrelia
refringens, Treponema
Refsum's disease
Refsum's syndrome
refusal
r. form, blood transfusion
r. intervention ▸ right to
r. of medical aid (RMA)
r. to do chores
r. to speak
r. to submit to treatment, form for
refused admission
**refusing permission for blood
   transfusion ▸ form**
regain muscle strength and flexibility
regained active status, patient
regained consciousness, patient
regenerate
r. blood cells
r. cartilage
r. damaged nerves
r. spinal cord
regenerated
r., axon
r., nodules
r. rib

regenerating nerves in spinal cord
regeneration
r., accelerated tissue
r. after damage to nerve fibers
r. and apoptosis ▸ cellular
r. and protracted treatment, tumor
r., bone
r., cartilage
r., cell
r., cellular
r., linear
r., nerve
r. of cervical epithelium
r. phenomena
r. ▸ renal tubular epithelial
r. research
r. ▸ spinal nerve
r., spiritual
r., tissue
r., tumor
regenerative
r. activity
r. cells, atypical
r. heart therapy
r. metabolic function
r. therapy
Regen's flexion exercises
regime
r., chemotherapy
r., exercise
r., Smith and Smith
r., ulcer
regimen(s)
r., antibacterial
r., antihypertensive
r., antiretroviral
r., chemoprophylactic
r., chemotherapeutic
r., detoxification
r., dosage
r., drug
r., medical
r., medication
r. of chemotherapy, Einhorn
r., patient compliance with drug
r., placebo
r., prescribed
r., primary
r., psoralens plus ultraviolet light
   (PUVA)
r., regular exercise
r., split course
r. ▸ stepped care antihypertensive
r., therapeutic
r., treatment

region(s) [*lesion*]
r., abdominal
r., adnexal
r., anal
r., anterior antebrachial
r., anterior crural
r., anterior cubital
r., anterolateral
r., auricular
r., axillary
r., brachial
r., Broca's
r., buccal
r., build-down
r., build-up
r., calcaneal
r., cancerous
r., central
r., cervical
r., ciliary
r., clavicular
r., cortical
r., deltoid
r., dorsal lip
r., encephalic
r., epigastric
r., external abdominal
r., extrapolar
r., facial
r., falcine
r. fracture ▸ intertrochanteric
r., frontal
r., frontocentral
r., genitourinary (GU)
r., gluteal
r., hair producing
r., hilar
r., homologous
r., hyoid
r., hypochondriac
r., hypogastric
r., ileocecal
r., iliac
r., inferior labial
r., inferior palpebral
r., infraclavicular
r., inframammary
r., infraorbital
r., infrascapular
r., infratemporal
r., inguinal
r., interscapular
r., intertrochanteric
r., laryngeal
r., lateral abdominal

r., left acetabular
r., limbic
r., lower cervical
r., lumbar
r., mammary
r., mastoid
r., maxillofacial
r., medial tegmental
r., mental
r., mid-sacral
r., motor
r., mylohyoid
r., nasal
r., nuchal
r., occipital
r., ocular
r. of abdomen, epigastric
r. of abdomen, hypogastric
r. of abdomen, left hypochondriac
r. of abdomen, left iliac
r. of abdomen, left inguinal
r. of abdomen, left lateral
r. of abdomen, left lumbar
r. of abdomen, pubic
r. of abdomen, right hypochondriac
r. of abdomen, right iliac
r. of abdomen, right inguinal
r. of abdomen, right lateral
r. of abdomen, right lumbar
r. of abdomen, umbilical
r. of accommodation
r. of fingers, dorsal
r. of fingers, volar
r. of hand, volar
r. of head, occipital
r. of head, posterior
r. of irradiated medium, build-down
r. of irradiated medium, build-up
r. of McBurney's point, rebound in
r. of nape
r. of neck, anterior
r. of neck, posterior
r. of scalp, centroparietal
r. of spinal cord, lateral
r. of toes, dorsal
r. of toes, plantar
r. of umbilicus, rebound in
r., olecranal
r., olfactory
r., opticostriate
r., oral
r., orbital
r., paratracheal
r., parietal
r., parieto-occipital

r., parietotemporal
r., parotideomasseteric
r., pectoral
r., perineal
r., postcricoid
r., posterior antebrachial
r., posterior crural
r., posterior cubital
r., posterotemporal
r., precordial
r., prefrontal
r., presumptive
r., pterygomaxillary
r., pubic
r., pyloric
r., radial antebrachial
r., respiratory
r., retrocardiac
r., right acetabular
r., rolandic
r., sacral
r., scapular
r., self-transmissibility
r., sensory
r., sharp blow to
r., sternocleidomastoid
r., subareolar
r., subauricular
r., subendocardial
r., subhyoid
r., submaxillary
r., submental
r., superior labial
r., superior palpebral
r., supraclavicular
r., supraorbital
r., suprapubic
r., suprasternal
r., target
r., temporal
r., tenderness of umbilical
r., tentorial
r., thoracic
r., thyroid
r., trabecular
r., ulnar antebrachial
r., umbilical
r., upper cervical
r., urogenital
r., vertebral
r., vestibular
r., volar antebrachial
r., watershed
r., zygomatic

regional
   r. adenopathy
   r. analgesia
   r. anatomy
   r. anesthesia
   r. anesthetic
   r. block
   r. block anesthesia
   r. burn center
   r. cancer
   r. carcinoma, advanced
   r. cerebral blood volume
   r. colitis
   r. control
   r. deep heating
   r. differentiation
   r. enteritis
   r. enterocolitis
   r. epidemic
   r. examination
   r. excision
   r. ileitis
   r. involvement
   r. lung function study, quantitative
   r. lymph involvement
   r. lymph nodes
   r. metastases
   r. metastases, painful local and
   r. myocardial blood flow
   r. node
   r. node bearing area of lymph nodes
   r. node involvement
   r. pain syndrome ▸ complex
   r. perfusion
   r. recurrence
   r. recurrence of tumor
   r. reflex
   r. spread
   r. spread ▸ loco-
   r. sympathectomy
   r. sympathetic blockage
   r. trauma center
   r. wall motion
   r. wall motional abnormality
Registered Nurse (RN)
Registered Nurse (VRN), Visiting
registration, maxillomandibular
Registration, Patient
registry (Registry)
   r. and tissue bank
   R., Cancer
   R., Ovarian Tumor
regitine test
regitine test for hypertension
regloving and regowning carried out

regressed clinically
regresses emotionally ▸ patient
regression
   r. analysis
   r. analysis ▸ multilinear
   r. and psychosexual development
   r., arteriographic
   r., atavistic
   r. coefficient
   r. equation
   r. ▸ least squares
   r., linear
   r., multiple
   r. neurosis
   r. of disease
   r. of disease process
   r. of symptoms
   r. pattern
   r., permanent
   r., plaque
   r. ▸ Q wave
   r., spontaneous
   r., tumor
regressional analysis ▸ multivariant
regressive
   r. behavior
   r. deterioration
   r. potentials, children with
regret factor
regrow damaged nerve cells
regrow hair
regrowth
   r., cataract
   r. ▸ excess tissue
   r., nerve tissue
   r. of nerve cells
   r., tumor
   r., vulvar
regular
   r. aerobic exercise
   r. and equal (RRE) ▸ round,
   r. contractions
   r. diet
   r. discharges ▸ long
   r. dosage of medication
   r. drug use
   r. exercise
   r. exercise regimen
   r. foot hygiene
   r., heart
   r. heart rhythm
   r., heart tones
   r. insulin infusion
   r. insulin rainbow
   r. jogging

   r. mammograms
   r., menstrual periods
   r. physical activity
   r. physical exercise
   r., pulse
   r., pulse strong and
   r. (PRR) ▸ pupils round and
   r. purified pork insulin
   r. (RRR) ▸ rate and rhythm
   r., react to light and accommodation
      (PERRRLA) ▸ pupils equal, round,
   r. respiration, deep and
   r. rhythm
   r. self-inspections
   r. sinus rhythm (RSR)
   r. weight bearing exercise
   r., wide QRS tachycardia
regularity of signal
regularly
   r., exercise
   r. irregular rhythm
   r., monitor recalibrated
   r., prostate palpated
   r. repeated EEG (electroencephalo-
      gram) complexes
   r. repeated EEG (electroencephalo-
      gram) waves
regulate(s)
   r. body temperature
   r. medical wastes
   r., patient self-
   r. pressure
regulated perfusion system
regulated volume control ventilation
   ▸ pressure-
regulating
   r. center, heat-
   r. suggestion, self-
regulation(s)
   r., cardiac self-
   r., confidentiality
   r., drug
   r., emotion
   r. ▸ heart rhythm
   r., insulin
   r. of body temperature
   r. of cardiovascular development ▸
      gene
   r., temperature
   r., volume
regulative development
regulator
   r., cystic fibrosis
   r., electric infusion
   r., mood

regulatory agency
regulatory center, brain's
regurgitant
r. esophagitis
r. flow (MRF), mitral
r. fraction
r. jet area
r. jet ▸ mitral
r. menstruation
r. murmur
r. murmur ▸ systolic
r. orifice ▸ effective
r. pockets
r. wave
regurgitated
r. food
r. food in pharynx
r. food particles
regurgitation
r. (AR), aortic
r., aortic valve
r. artifact ▸ mitral
r., bloating and
r., combined mitral stenosis and
r., esophageal
r. in mitral valve
r. ▸ ischemic mitral
r., minimal mitral
r. (MR), mitral
r. ▸ mitral valve
r. murmur, aortic
r. murmur ▸ mitral
r., nocturnal
r. of bile
r. of food
r., pulmonary
r. ▸ pulmonary valvular
r., pulmonic
r. ▸ semilunar valve
r., tricuspid
r., valvular
rehabilitate injured area ▸ exercise to
rehabilitation (Rehabilitation)
r., adult
r. after stroke
r. and balance ▸ dysmobility,
r., aural
r., cardiac
R. Center, Drug
r. center for alcoholics
r. center for drug addicts
r. center for physically disabled
r. center for physically handicapped
r. clinic
r., cognitive

r. counseling
r. counselor, vocational
r. ▸ elevation bracing and
r. environment
r. exercise ▸ rest and
r. facilities, cardiac
r. ▸ habituation and balance
r., halfway house for penal
r., heart attack
r. hospital
r., impatient
r. ▸ low vision
r. medicine
r. mental stress, cardiac
r., neurologic
r., neurological
r. nurse therapist
r., occupational
r. occupational therapy
r. of disabilities as result of stroke
r. of heart disease
r., oncology
r., oral
r., orthopedic
r., ostomy
r., pain
r., paraplegic
r., patient
r., physical
r. (PMR) ▸ physical medicine and
r. physician
r. ▸ postoperative recovery and
r. potential
r. products, special
r. program
r. program ▸ aggressive
r. program, cardiac
r. program ▸ exercise-based
r. program ▸ heart
r. program ▸ pulmonary
r. program ▸ vestibular
r. psychologist
r., pulmonary
r., quadriplegic
r. service
r., speech
r., substance abuse
r. team
r. team, cardiac
r. team goals
r. technique, standard
r. therapy
r. therapy ▸ vestibular and balance
r., vision
r., vocational

r., work
rehabilitative
r. exercise
r. physical therapy
r. therapy
r. treatment
rehearsal, behavioral
rehospitalized, patient
rehydrate after exercise
rehydrated [*dehydrated*]
rehydrated, patient
rehydration and detoxification
rehydration solutions
Reichel's chondromatosis
Reichel's cloacal duct
Reichenheim-King operation
Reichert's scar
Reichert's substance
Reichmann's disease
Reichmann's rod
Reich-Nechtow curette
Reichstein's substance Fa
Reichstein's substance M.
Reid('s)
R. baseline
R. index
R. index measurement
Reider cell leukemia
Reifenstein's syndrome
Reil, island of
Reil, taeniola corporis callosi of
Reilly granulations
reimbursement procedure
reimplant avulsed teeth
reimplant ureters
reimplantation arthroplasty
reimplantation fingertip ▸ injury and
reimplanted
r. extremity
r. in old pocket ▸ electrode
r. in socket ▸ tooth
r., positioned and bonded
r. tooth
reinfarction, risk for
reinfection
r., prevention of
r. rate
r. tuberculosis
reinflated, lung
reinforce weakened area
reinforcement
r., intermittent
r., negative
r., positive
r., trap

reinforcing stimulus
reinforcing suture
reinfuse blood
reinfusing marrow
reinfusion of stored marrow
Reinhard unit ▸ **Shinowara-Jones-**
reinjection protocol
reinjury, preventing
reintegration, community
reinvigorate brain cells
Reisberg's scale
Reis-Bückler disease
Reisseisen's muscles
Reissner's canal
Reissner's membrane
Reitan test, Halstead-
Reitan-Indiana aphasic screening test
Reiter('s)
   R. disease
   R. protein complement fixation
   R. syndrome
Reitland-Franklin unit (RFU)
reject
   r. control
   r. medical treatment ▸ accept or
   r. medical treatment ▸ right to
rejected [*reflected*]
   r., cell
   r., feeling
   r., heart
   r. or ridiculed ▸ patient feels
   r. organ, removal of
   r., patient
   r. (TGAR) ▸ total graft area
rejection
   r., acute
   r., acute allograft
   r., acute lung
   r. and abandonment
   r. -associated pulmonary fibrosis
   r., bone marrow transplant
   r., bouts of
   r. cardiomyopathy
   r. cardiomyopathy transplant
   r., chronic
   r., classical signs of
   r., common mode
   r., daily observation for
   r. drugs, anti-
   r., early sign of
   r. episode
   r. factors
   r. ▸ fear and
   r. fraction ▸ global left ventricular (LV)

r., graft
r., grafted kidney
r., homograft
r. ▸ hyperacute xenograft
r., immediate graft
r., immune to
r., kidney transplant
r., late graft
r., left ventricular
r. mechanism
r. monitoring
r. (NI NR) ▸ no infection no
r. of grafted kidney
r. of organ, bodily
r. of transplant
r. of transplant, threatened
r. of transplanted heart, immune
r. of transplanted organ
r. of transplanted organ ▸ block
r. of transplanted organ ▸ combat
r. of transplanted tissue
r., organ
r. ▸ perception of
r., pigment
r., prevent
r. rate
r. ratio, common mode
r. responses
r. ▸ signs of
r., tissue
r., transplant
rejuvenate damaged heart
rejuvenation
   r. cosmetic surgery ▸ facial
   r., facial
   r. ▸ laser facial
   r. ▸ laser skin
   r., skin
Rekoss disk
relapse(s)
   r. and life expectancy ▸ remissions,
   r. circumstances
   r., determinants of
   r., early signs of
   r. ▸ fluctuating periods of remission and
   r. hazards
   r., Hodgkin's disease in
   r. in depression
   r. in schizophrenia
   r. -inducing adverse influences
   r., lithium
   r., multiple
   r. of disease ▸ patient had
   r. of paranoid psychotic state

r., patient in complete
r. ▸ periods of remission and
r. ▸ potential intrapersonal determinants of
r., predictive
r. prevention
r. prevention, anger management
r. prevention plan
r. prevention, pro-active
r. prevention skills
r. prevention ▸ treatment, recovery, and
r. process
r. -prone addicts
r. rate
r. rate, leukemia
r. specific strategies
r. testing
r. triggering situations
relapsed, abstinent or
relapsed group
relapsing
   r. disease
   r. disease ▸ life-long,
   r. disorder, chronic
   r. fever
   r. multiple sclerosis (MS) ▸ progressive
   r. pancreatitis
   r. pancreatitis, chronic
   r. polychondritis
   r. -progressive course
   r. -remitting course
   r. -remitting multiple sclerosis
   r. -remitting multiple sclerosis (MS) ▸ worsening,
   r. schizophrenic patient, chronic
   r. skin rash
   r. vestibulopathy
relate to people, inability to
related (Related)
   r. accident, alcohol-
   r. accident, farm-
   r. activities ▸ abnormal dread of school-
   r. activities, home-
   r. activities, job-
   r. activity, child-
   r. affliction, age-
   r. aging of brain ▸ stress-
   r. aggressivity, drinking-
   r. ailment, age-
   r. ailments, job
   r. anemia, pregnancy-
   r. antigen ▸ factor VIII-

related—*continued*

r. arrhythmia ▸ stress-
r. bacteremia ▸ catheter-
r. bacteremia ▸ venous access device-
r. behavior, alcohol-
r. birth defects ▸ alcohol-
r. blood clot ▸ travel
r. brain potential ▸ event-
r. bronchitis ▸ allergy-
r. cancer ▸ tobacco-
r. cataracts, age-
r. causes ▸ obesity-
r. cerebral disorder, alcohol-
r. checkup, cancer-
r. chest pain ▸ gastroesophageal-
r. cognitive decline (ARCD), age-
r. complex, acquired immune deficiency syndrome (AIDS)
r. complex (ARC), acquired immune deficiency syndrome (AIDS)
r. complication ▸ diabetes-
r. complications, anesthetic-
r. complications in pregnancy, cocaine-
r. crisis, drug-
r. crisis, infection-
r. death, alcohol-
r. death, cocaine-
r. death ▸ diabetes-
r. death, disease-
r. death, drug-
r. death, farm-
r. death, lightning-
r. death, methamphetamine
r. defects, alcohol-
r. degeneration of valve, age-
r. dementia, age-
r. dementia, alcohol-
r. depression, abuse-
r. dermatitis ▸ work-
r. diagnostic services ▸ cancer-
r. diarrhea, antibiotic-
r. disability, job-
r. disability ▸ service-
r. disease, age-
r. disease, alcohol-
r. disease, asbestos-
r. disease, bowel-
r. disease, diabetic-
r. disease, fat-
r. disease ▸ minimize risk of transfusion-
r. disease ▸ obesity

r. disease, smoking-
r. disease, stress-
r. disease, transfusion-
r. diseases, blood-
r. disorder
r. disorder, cocaine-
r. disorder ▸ joint-
r. disorder ▸ sleep-
r. disorder ▸ stroke-
r. disorder ▸ substance-
r. disorders, heat-
r. disorders, high altitude-
r. disorders, smoking-
r. disorders, stress-
r. donor, emotionally
r., dose
r. emergency, altitude-
r. emergency room episodes ▸ heroin-
r. emotional stress, work-
r. eye disease ▸ age-
r. factor, stress-
r. fatal poisoning ▸ drug-
r. fatalities, alcohol-
r. fear, age-
r. feelings, crisis-
r. forms, accident
r. gene ▸ abnormal cholesterol
R. Groups (DRG) ▸ Diagnosis
r. groups (DRG) ▸ diagnostic-
r. groups (DRG) payments ▸ diagnostic-
r. headache, alcohol-
r. headache, cold food-
r. headache, stress-
r. health hazards ▸ alcohol-
r. health problems ▸ weight-
r. hearing loss ▸ age-
r. heart attack victim, cocaine-
r. heart condition ▸ stress-
r. heart disorders, alcohol-
r. heart problem, activity-
r. hepatitis, alcohol-
r. homicide, drug-
r. hormones, stress
r. hypertension ▸ stress-
r. hypoxemia ▸ rapid eye movement (REM) sleep-
r. illness, alcohol
r. illness, asbestos-
r. illness ▸ heat-
r. illness ▸ influenza-
r. illness ▸ swimming-
r. illnesses, high altitude
r. immune deficiency (GRID) ▸ gay-

r. impairment, drug-
r. infection, catheter-
r. infection ▸ device-
r. infection, drug-
r. infection ▸ hospital-
r. infection, transfusion
r. injury, alcohol-
r. injury, fire-
r. injury ▸ heat-
r. injury, job-
r. injury, sports-
r. injury, work-
r. involuntary movement ▸ drug-
r. itching ▸ emotion-
r. legislation, health-
r. living donor
r. loss of muscle ▸ age-
r. loss of nerve cells, age-
r. macular degeneration (ARMD) ▸ advanced age-
r. macular degeneration (ARMD), age-
r. macular degeneration (ARMD) ▸ dry, age-
r. macular degeneration (ARMD) ▸ intermediate age-
r. macular degeneration (ARMD) ▸ wet age-
r. medical complications ▸ drug-
r. medical problems
r. memory loss, age-
r. migraine headache ▸ weather-
r. mortality statistics ▸ alcohol
r. motion, task
r. muscle disorder ▸ anxiety-
r. muscle malfunction ▸ age-
r. obstetric disorder, cocaine-
r. offenses, alcohol-
r. offenses, drug-
r. organ donor, living
r. pain ▸ muscle-
r. pattern ▸ non-Alzheimer's disease-
r. peripheral vessel spasm, catheter-
r. phenomenon ▸ age-
r. physical stress, work-
r. pneumonia, acquired immune deficiency syndrome (AIDS)
r. potentials, event-
r. practice ▸ risk-
r. problem, anesthesia-
r. problem ▸ eyelid-
r. problem ▸ tear-
r. problems, alcohol-

r. problems ▸ autogenic training
  and stress-
r. problems, stress-
r. problems ▸ warning signs of
  smoking-
r., radiation
r. seizure
r. seizure ▸ nonfever-
r. sensations, anxiety-
r., shunt
r. site
r. skin disorder, alcohol-
r. sleeplessness ▸ stress-
r. spine fractures, osteoporosis-
r. stress, job-
r. studies
r. symptoms ▸ stress-
r. tension, stress-
r. tissue shrinkage ▸ age-
r. to a known organic factor ▸
  hypersomnia
r. to a known organic factor ▸
  insomnia
r. to another mental disorder
  (nonorganic) ▸ hypersomnia
r. to cancer, dermatomyositis-
r. to chemotherapy, anemia
r. to drug abuse, cardiovascular
  problems
r. to drug abuse, endocrinologic
  problems
r. to drug abuse, genitourinary (GU)
  problems
r. to drug abuse, GI
  (gastrointestinal) problems
r. to drug abuse, hematopoietic
  problems
r. to drug abuse, hepatic problems
r. to drug abuse, neuromuscular
  problems
r. to drug abuse, psychological
  problems
r. to drug abuse, renal problems
r. to drug abuse, septic problems
r. to exertion, pain
r. to mental disorder (nonorganic) ▸
  hypersomnia
r. to mental disorder (nonorganic) ▸
  insomnia
r. to stress, condition
r. tremulousness ▸ stress-
r. urinary tract infection ▸ catheter-
r. vascular headache ▸ cocaine-
r. vertebrate blood systems ▸
  cardiac-

r. vessel, angioplasty-
r. vessel ▸ infarct-
r. vessel occlusion, angioplasty-
r. violence, alcohol-
r. violence, cocaine-
r. violence, drug-
r. visual impairment, age-
r. vitamin deficiency, alcohol-
r. weight problems ▸ age-

relation(s)
r., age
r., causal
r., centric
r., concentration effect-
r. ▸ diastolic pressure volume
r. ▸ end-systolic pressure volume
r. ▸ end-systolic stress dimension
r. ▸ force frequency
r. ▸ force length
r. ▸ force velocity length
r. ▸ force velocity volume
r., human
r. ▸ impaired interpersonal
r. ▸ interval strength
r. ▸ length resting tension
r. ▸ length tension
r., peer
r. ▸ pressure volume
r. psychotherapy ▸ object
r., public
r. ▸ resting length tension
r., spatial
r. technique
r. ▸ tension-length
r. theory ▸ object
r. to reality
r. ▸ ventilation/perfusion
r. ▸ ventricular end-systolic
  pressure volume

relational coil
relational disorder
relationship(s)
r., abusive
r., building a positive
r., causal
r., cause-and-effect
r., child-parent
r., clinical
r., conscious-subconscious
r., constricted
r., decline in social
r. dependence
r. ▸ disturbed personal
r. dynamics
r., dysfunctional

r., economic
r. enhancement (RE) family therapy
r. enhancement (RE) therapy
r. established, satisfying
r., family
r., genetic
r., hostile
r., intense
r. ▸ intense interpersonal
r., interpersonal
r., linear quadratic survival
r. ▸ meaningful
r., monogamous
r., normal structural
r., object
r., occlusal
r. of film, density-exposure
r., ongoing
r., patient-staff
r., personal
r., physician-patient
r., positive
r. ▸ pressure flow
r. problems
r., sexual
r., short-term working
r., social
r., spatial
r. ▸ stress shortening
r. syndrome, addictive
r., therapeutic
r. to deceased
r., trusting
r. ▸ tumultuous personal
r. ▸ unstable and intense
r. ▸ unstable interpersonal
r., violent
r. ▸ withdrawn from
r., working

relative(s)
r. accommodation
r. amenorrhea
r. biological effectiveness
r. blood
r. bradycardia
r. cardiac dullness (RCD)
r. cardiac volume
r. centrifugal force
r. dehydration
r. disregard for sensitivity of others
r. fluorescence
r. hemianopia
r. hepatic dullness
r. humidity
r. incompetence

relative(s)—*continued*
- r. index of refraction
- r. ▸ nonmatching donor
- r., patient discharged to care of
- r., patient released in care of
- r. polycythemia
- r. quiescence, period of
- r. radiosensitivity
- r. reduction of sensitivity
- r. refractory period
- r. risk
- r. scotoma
- r. specific activity
- r. specificities
- r. sterility
- r. strabismus
- r. to nodal involvement in breast carcinoma, survival
- r. value index (RVI)
- r. vertebral density
- r. wall thickness

relatively asymptomatic, patient
relatively primitive phenomena
relativistic mass
relax(es)
- r. heart
- r. ▸ inability to
- r., patient unable to
- r. periodically, muscles
- r. prostate enlargement
- r. prostate muscles
- r. reflex
- r. spasticity

relaxant
- r., colon
- r. effect, residual muscle
- r. medication ▸ muscle
- r., muscle
- r. ▸ nondepolarizing muscle
- r., skeletal muscle

relaxation
- r., active
- r. and biofeedback
- r. and drowsiness
- r. and meditation techniques
- r. and stress reduction
- r., applied
- r. atelectasis
- r., atrial
- r., autogenic
- r., awareness
- r., biofeedback-assisted cue-controlled
- r., biofeedback-mediated
- r., brief progressive

- r., complete
- r., conditioned
- r., controlled
- r. cycle, contraction-
- r., dazed
- r., deep muscle
- r., diastolic
- r. distraction and imagery
- r., drug-induced
- r. during childbirth ▸ biofeedback techniques of
- r., dynamic
- r. ▸ endothelium-mediated
- r. exercise, cool down
- r. exercise ▸ muscle
- r. exercises
- r. exercises, autogenic training
- r. exercises ▸ breathing and
- r. exercises, daily
- r., feedback technique for deep
- r., feedback-induced muscle
- r., focused
- r. for insomnia, hypnotic
- r. for insomnia, progressive
- r., gradual
- r., group desensitization and
- r., guided
- r., hypnotically suggested
- r. in asthma ▸ EMG (electromyogram) biofeedback
- r. in labor, deep
- r. in normal persons, muscle
- r. in systematic desensitization
- r., induced muscle
- r., induced state of
- r. internal sphincter
- r., isometric
- r., isovolumetric
- r., isovolumic
- r., learned
- r. ▸ left ventricular diastolic
- r., ligamentous
- r. loading
- r., massage for
- r., mental
- r. methods ▸ visualization and
- r., muscle
- r., muscular
- r. of cell
- r. of heart ▸ contraction and
- r. of heart muscle
- r. of joint
- r. of masseter muscle, voluntary
- r. of muscle
- r. of pelvic muscle

- r., passive
- r., pelvic
- r. period ▸ isometric
- r. period ▸ isovolumetric
- r. period ▸ isovolumic
- r. phase
- r., physical
- r., progressive
- r. ▸ progressive deep
- r., psychophysiological effects of
- r., quality
- r. ▸ rapid, deep
- r. response
- r. response in headache therapy
- r., rest and
- r., rhythmic
- r. skills
- r. ▸ smooth muscle
- r. splints, muscle-
- r., stress
- r. suture
- r. tapes
- r. technique
- r. technique, alternative
- r. technique, autonomic nervous system
- r. technique, breathing and
- r. technique, electromyographic feedback as
- r. techniques ▸ biofeedback, imagery and
- r., tension and
- r. therapy
- r. therapy, biofeedback
- r. therapy exercise
- r. therapy for hyperactivity
- r. therapy, long-term biofeedback
- r. therapy ▸ response to
- r. time
- r. time index
- r. time ▸ isovolumic
- r. time ▸ magnetic
- r. time ▸ T2
- r. training
- r. training, biofeedback-assisted muscular
- r. training, physiological response to
- r. training, progressive
- r. training, psychological effects of
- r. training sessions
- r. training ▸ stress management
- r. training technique, general
- r. under hyperactivity, progressive
- r., upward

r., ventricular
r., verbal
relaxed
r. and daydreaming
r. anterior wall
r. attitude
r. body posture
r. breathing
r. inhibitions
r. introitus
r. lower esophageal sphincter
r., muscles
r., patient calm and
r. pelvic floor
r. perineal body
r. phase, heart's
r. skin tension lines (RSTL)
r., support
r. vaginal outlet
r. wakefulness
relaxing
r. drug ▸ muscle
r. factor ▸ endothelium-derived
r. massage
Relay cardiac pacemaker
relearn skills of daily living
release
r., adductor tendon
r., allergen-induced mediator
r. and repair ▸ surgical
r., carpal tunnel
r. consent, medication
r., emotional
r. form for ritual circumcision
r. form, patient
r. forms
r. medication ▸ sustained
r., myofascial
r. of biological fluid
r. of egg ▸ irregular
r. of eggs from ovary
r. of energy
r. of hormones
r. of hormones ▸ formation and
r. of hormones ▸ slow
r. of information
r. of ovum
r. of patella, retinacular
r. of plantar fascia
r. of pus
r. of scar tissue ▸ arthroscopic
r., patellar
r., patient's
r. pent-up tension
r. ▸ physiologic pattern

r. psychotherapy, emotional
r. rate, renin-
r., renin
r., sense of
r. slip signed
r. ▸ stimulating insulin
r., sustained
r., syndactylism
r. systems, controlled
r., temporary stress
r. tension
r. ▸ trigger thumb
r. ventilation (APRV) ▸ airway
pressure
released
r. against medical advice (AMA) ▸
patient
r. from anterior chamber ▸ fluid
r. hormones, stress-
r. in care of relatives ▸ patient
r. on overnight pass ▸ patient
r., patient
r., tendon
r., time-
r., tourniquet
releasing
r. agent, gonadotropin
r. drugs, dopamine-
r. exercises ▸ stretching and
r. factor
r. factor, corticotropin
r. factor, growth hormone
r. factor, histamine
r. factor, luteinizing hormone
r. factor, somatotropin
r. factor (TRF) ▸ thyrotropin
r. hormone (CRH), corticotropin-
r. hormone (Gn-RH), gonadotropin-
r. hormone response ▸ thyrotropin-
r. hormone, thyrotropin
relentless
r. child abuse ▸ severe and
r. downhill course
r. fatigue
relevant maternal conditions
reliability ▸ test-retest
reliance, maximum self-
reliant, self-
relief
r. and prevention of anginal attacks
r., arthritis pain
r., electrical stimulator for pain
r. from symptoms
r. ▸ improved symptom
r. incision

r., long-term
r. ▸ long-term pain
r., mechanical
r. medication ▸ pain
r. methods ▸ stress
r., nonsedating
r. of headache pain ▸ temporary
r. of intracranial pressure
r. of pain
r. of pain, total
r. of symptoms, dramatic
r. of symptoms, total
r., pharmacologic
r. physical symptom
r., placebo
r., postoperative
r., psychologic
r. roentgenography, mucosal
r., short-term
r., subjective
r., symptomatic
r. ▸ symptomatic pain
r., temporary
relieve
r. choking
r. fibromyalgia symptoms
r. inhibitions
r. muscle spasms
r. muscle strain
r. nerve pressure
r. pain
r. pain and restore mobility
r. pressure on metatarsal area
r. pressure on primary suture line
r. pressure on urethra
r. stress
r. swelling
r. symptoms, temporarily
r. tension
reliever
r. ▸ Medtronic Pulsor Intrasound pain
r. ▸ nonprescription pain
r., pain
r., stress
r. ▸ topical pain
relieving
r. effects, pain-
r. exercise ▸ tension
r. formula ▸ tension
r. injection ▸ pain-
r. pain or discomfort
r. potential, pain-
r. remedy, pain
r. ▸ sleep enhancing and pain
religiosa, melancholia

religiosity, intrinsic
religious
    r. beliefs
    r. cult involvement
    r. fanatic
    r. hallucinations
    r. mania
    r. services ▸ loss of desire to attend
    r. support
    r. values, patient has
relining of denture
relinquishing the past
reliving ▸ uncontrolled intrusive
reluctance, extreme
REM (radiation equivalent in man)
REM (rem) (roentgen-equivalent-man)
REM(S) (rapid eye movement)(s)
    REM density
    REM latency
    REM onset
    REM period
    REM period, sleep onset
    REM rebound
    REM sleep
    REM sleep anxiety dreams
    REM sleep ▸ increased
    REM sleep interruption insomnia
    REM sleep-related hypoxemia
    REM spindle
remained in asystole, patient
remaining lifetime, average
Remak('s)
    R., fiber of
    R. ganglion
    R. reflex
remarkable
    r., family history (FH) not
    r. ▸ head, eyes, ears, nose and
        throat (HEENT) not
    r., past history (PH) not
remediation program
remedy
    r., herbal
    r., homeopathic
    r., medical
    r., pain-relieving
remember spoken words ▸ inability to
remesothelialization of peritoneal
    surface
Remine speculum, Auvard-
reminiscence ▸ therapeutic exercise
    for
remission(s)
    r., acute exacerbations and
    r. and exacerbation

r. and exacerbations of pain ▸
    patient experiences
r. and relapse ▸ fluctuating periods of
r. and relapse ▸ periods of
r. ▸ bipolar disorder, depressed, in
    full
r. ▸ bipolar disorder, depressed, in
    partial
r. ▸ bipolar disorder, manic, in full
r. ▸ bipolar disorder, manic, in partial
r. ▸ bipolar disorder, mixed, in full
r. ▸ bipolar disorder, mixed, in
    partial
r., cancer in
r., clinical
r., complete
r., complete clinical
r., disease in complete
r., exacerbation and
r., Legroux's
r. ▸ long-term
r. ▸ major depression, in full
r. ▸ major depression, in partial
r. ▸ major depression, recurrent, in
    full
r. ▸ major depression, single
    episode, in full
r. ▸ major depression, single
    episode, in partial
r. of depression
r. of disease
r. of symptoms
r., partial
r., patient in
r., patient in complete
r., period of
r., permanent
r., prolonged
r., rapid
r. rate
r., relapses and life expectancy
r., spontaneous
r., symptom
r., total
remittent disease
remittent fever
remitting
    r. course ▸ relapsing-
    r. multiple sclerosis (MS) ▸ relapsing-
    r. multiple sclerosis (MS) ▸
        worsening, relapsing-
remnant(s)
    r., chylomicron
    r., myocardial cell
    r. of lens washed out

r., ovarian
r. receptor, ▸ chylomicron
remodeling
    r., arterial
    r., bone
    r., concentric
    r., heart
    r., ventricular
remorse ▸ lack of
remorse, persistent
remorseful, patient
remote
    r. cause
    r. clinic
    r. external stimulus
    r. hospital
    r. memory
    r. metastases system
remotivation ▸ therapeutic exercise
    for
remottling fracture site
removable
    r. appliance
    r. bridge
    r. bridgework
    r. dentures
    r. devices, plaque
    r. implants
removal
    r., calculi
    r., cast
    r., cataract
    r. FB (foreign body)
    r. FB (foreign body) from cornea
    r. FB (foreign body) ▸ sclerotomy
        with
    r., first transplant
    r. foreign body (FB) ▸ electromagnetic
    r. foreign body (FB) from cornea
    r. foreign body (FB) ▸ sclerotomy
        with
    r., foreign material
    r., gallstone
    r., hair
    r. ▸ laser face wrinkle
    r. ▸ laser hair
    r., magnetic
    r., no stitch and no patch cataract
    r. of astragalus
    r. of benign thyroid tumor
    r. of blood components
    r. of chest tubes
    r. of dental alveolus
    r. of donated organs, surgical
    r. of foreign body (FB)

r. of foreskin
r. of kidney, piecemeal
r. of life supports
r. of organ for transplant ▸
  authorization form for
r. of organ for transplant ▸ consent
  form for
r. of organ, surgical
r. of placenta, manual
r. of pregnant uterus, abdominal
r. of rejected organ
r. of sample of tissue
r. of stool, digital
r. of thymus gland
r. of tissue for grafting ▸
  authorization form for
r. of tissue for grafting ▸ consent
  form for
r. of tumor, subtotal
r. of tumor, surgical
r. of vermiform appendix
r. ▸ preventive breast
r. prophylaxis, calcium
r., return for suture
r., scar
r., second transplant
r., surgical
r., tattoo
r., tracheoscopy with
r. treatment ▸ hair
r. treatment ▸ laser hair
r. ▸ ureteroscopic stone
r., wart
r., wrinkle

removed
r. and stored, bone marrow
r., calculus
r., cervical stump
r., FB (foreign body)
r. for pathological examination ▸
  tissue
r., foreign body (FB)
r. from reality ▸ feeling
r. in part
r. in toto
r. manually, placenta
r. ▸ slice of heart muscle
r., sutures
r., tourniquet

**REMP (roentgen-equivalent-man
  period)**

renal (Renal)
r. abscess
r. acidosis, hyperchloremic
r. adenocarcinoma

r. agenesis
r. agenesis with associated
  stigmata ▸ patent ductus
r. albuminuria
r. allograft
r. amyloidosis
r. aneurysm
r. aneurysm, congenital
r. angiogram
r. angiography
r. angioplasty
r. anomaly ▸ numerary
r. anuria
r. arteriography
r. arteriography ▸ selective
r. arteriolar sclerosis
r. arteriole
r. artery
r. artery aneurysm
r. artery, blockage of
r. artery ▸ blocked
r. artery bypass graft
r. artery disease
r. artery ▸ narrowed
r. artery occluded
r. artery ▸ origin of the
r. artery ▸ progressive obstruction of
r. artery reverse saphenous vein
  bypass
r. artery stenosis
r. atrophy
r. atrophy ▸ postinflammatory
r. atrophy ▸ postobstructive
r. autoregulation
r. axis
r. azotemia
r. ballottement
r. biopsy
r. blood flow (RBF)
r. blood flow (ERBF) ▸ effective
r. blood flow (TRBF) ▸ total
r. blood vessel
r. bruits
r. calculi
r. calculus
r. cancer
r. capsule
r. capsules adherent
r. capsules stripped easily
r. carcinoma, undifferentiated
r. cell adenocarcinoma
r. cell cancer
r. cell carcinoma
r. cell carcinoma of kidney
r. circulation

r. clearance
r. colic
r. colic, feigned
r. collecting system
r. complications of drug abuse
r. cortex
r. cortical adenoma
r. cortical necrosis
r. cyst
r. cyst ablation
r. cyst ▸ isolated
r. cyst ▸ simple
r. cystic disease
r. damage
r. damage, pre-existing
r. decortication
r. dialysis
R. Dialysis Unit
r. diet
r. disease
r. disease, cardiovascular
r. disease, chronic
r. disease (ESRD), end stage
r. disease, polycystic
r. disease, primary
R. Disease (ESRD) Program, End
  Stage
r. disorder
r. dwarf
r. dysfunction
r. dyspnea
r. ectopia
r. effects
r. epistaxis, Gull's
r. epithelial cells, desquamated
r. erythropoietic factor
r. evaluation
r. excretion
r. failure
r. failure (ARF), acute
r. failure, chronic
r. failure ▸ myoglobinuric
r. failure (PTARF) ▸ post-traumatic
  acute
r. fascia
r. fistula
r. fossa
r. fossa ▸ kidney replaced in
r. function
r. function, bilateral
r. function, compromised
r. function, decreased
r. function ▸ deterioration in
r. function, Hipputope
r. function, impaired

renal—*continued*
- r. function, monitoring of
- r. function, normal
- r. function, reduced
- r. function study
- r. function study, split
- r. fungus ball
- r. ganglia
- r. glycosuria
- r. hamartoma, fetal-
- r. hematuria
- r. hemorrhage
- r. homotransplantation
- r. hyperplasia
- r. hypertension
- r. impaired patient
- r. infarct
- r. infarction
- r. injury, blunt
- r. injury, penetrating
- r. insufficiency
- r. lithiasis
- r. malignancy
- r. medulla
- r. medulla ▸ marked congestion of
- r. obstruction
- r. osteodystrophy
- r. output decreased
- r. papillae
- r. papillary necrosis
- r. parenchyma
- r. parenchyma, defective
- r. parenchyma, incised
- r. parenchymal disease
- r. pedicle
- r. pelves
- r. pelves mildly dilated
- r. pelvis
- r. pelvis cancer
- r. pelvis, left
- r. pelvis, right
- r. pelvis ▸ transitional cell carcinoma of
- r. phosphorus threshold, theoretical
- r. plasma flow (RPF)
- r. plasma flow (ERPF) ▸ effective
- r. plexus
- r. pouch
- r. pressor substance
- r. problem, crush injury
- r. problems related to drug abuse
- r. ptosis
- r. pyramids
- r. retention
- r. retinitis

- r. rhabdosarcoma
- r. rickets
- r. scan
- r. scanning
- r. scarring
- r. sclerosis, vascular
- r. segments
- r. shadow
- r. shutdown
- r. sinus
- r. splanchnic steal
- r. stone fragmentation
- r. surgery ▸ extracorporeal
- r. syndrome ▸ hemorrhagic fever with
- r. syndrome ▸ metabolic
- r. thrombosis
- r. tissue
- r. tissue perfusion, altered
- r. toxicity
- r. transplant
- r. transplant ▸ first, second or third
- r. transplantation
- r. tuberculosis
- r. tubular absorption
- r. tubular acidosis
- r. tubular defect
- r. tubular dysfunction
- r. tubular epithelial regeneration
- r. tubular necrosis
- r. tubule
- r. tubule hypokalemia
- r. tuft
- r. tumor
- r. tumor, malignant
- r. ultrasonogram
- r. ultrasound
- r. vascular disease ▸ severe
- r. vascular hypertension
- r. vascular lesion
- r. vascular resistance
- r. vascular supply
- r. vasculature
- r. vein
- r. vein, main
- r. vein renin
- r. vein renin activity
- r. vein renin concentration
- r. vein renin ratio
- r. vein thrombosis
- r. vein tributaries
- r. venogram
- r. venography
- r. venous renin assay

renale, Corynebacterium
renales minores, calyces

renalis, hilus
renalis, sinus
Rendu('s)
- R. -Osler-Weber disease
- R. -Osler-Weber syndrome ▸ Sutton-
- R. tremor

renewal
- r. and nonrenewal systems of cells, slow
- r. cell system, rapid
- r., medication

renewed tumor activity
renews motivation ▸ patient
reniformis, placenta
reniformis, Veillonella
renin (*same as* rennin)
- r. activity
- r. activity, plasma
- r. activity, renal vein
- r. angiotensin
- r. angiotensin aldosterone cascade
- r. angiotensin aldosterone system
- r. angiotensin blocker
- r. -angiotensin system (RAS)
- r. -angiotensin system (RAS) activity
- r. -angiotensin system (RAS) ▸ tissue
- r. assay, plasma
- r. assay, renal venous
- r. concentration
- r. concentration, renal vein
- r. essential hypertension (HTN) ▸ low
- r., high levels of kidney protein
- r. inhibitor
- r. level ▸ serum
- r. levels, plasma
- r., plasma
- r. profile
- r. ratio ▸ renal vein
- r. release
- r. -release rate
- r., renal vein
- r. substrate
- r. vein assay

renis
- r., capsula adiposa
- r., capsula fibrosa
- r., septum

Renografin-76 contrast material
renogram
- r., isotope
- r. study
- r. test, radioisotope

renointestinal reflex

Reno-M
R. -Dip contrast medium
R. -60 contrast medium
R. -30 contrast medium
renomedullary lipid
Rénon-Delille syndrome
renopelvic hemorrhages
renoprival hypertension
renorenal reflex
renovascular
r. angiography
r. disease
r. hypertension
Renovist contrast medium
rent in uterus
rent of intestine
rental equipment
reopened, temporary closure
reorganization, mental
reorientation, period of
reoxygenated blood
reoxygenation
r. and brachytherapy
r. and dose fractionation
r. and dose hyperfractionation
REP (roentgen equivalent physical)
repair
r., Allison hiatal hernia
r. ▸ anal surgical
r., aneurysm
r., anterior and posterior (A and P)
r., anteroposterior (AP) vaginal vault
r., aortic aneurysm
r., arterial
r., arterioplasty
r., Bassini inguinal hernia
r., Bassini's
r., Bassini-type hernia
r., Belsey's
r., bladder
r., Boerema hernia
r., Brom
r., bronchoplasty
r., bronchorrhaphy
r. ▸ brow ptosis
r., cartilage
r., cheiloplasty
r., congenital deformity
r., customized joint
r., DeBakey-Creech aneurysm
r., dentition in poor
r., DuVries hammer toe
r. ▸ Effler hiatal hernia
r., elective
r., endovascular

r. ▸ femoral artery
r., Fontan
r. for vesicovaginal fistula, Latzko
r. ▸ gastrointestinal (GI) tract tissue
r., hernia
r. ▸ inadequate tissue
r., Jones' toe
r. ▸ knee ligament
r. ▸ laparoscopic hernia
r., LeFort uterine prolapse
r., L-plasty
r. ▸ mitral valve
r., Mosley method anterior shoulder
r., nerve
r. of anus, plastic
r. of artery
r. of blood vessel
r. of bronchus
r. of bronchus, plastic
r. of defect
r. of defects, plastic
r. of detached retina, photocoagulation
r. of eyelid, plastic
r. of hernia
r. of hernia, McVay
r. of joint
r. of lip ▸ Abbe flap
r. of orbit, plastic
r. of shoulder, Sever-L'Episcopo
r. of spina bifida
r. of spina bifida with meningocele
r. of spina bifida with meningomyelocele
r., operative
r. or replace damaged valve
r. ▸ pericardioplasty in pectus excavatum
r. ▸ peritoneal injury and
r., pharyngeal flap
r., plastic
r., retinal
r., retinal detachment
r., Rose-Thompson
r. ▸ rotator cuff
r., secondary
r., sublethal damage
r., surgical
r. ▸ surgical release and
r., teeth in good dental
r., teeth in poor dental
r., Tennison-Randall
r., tissue
r., vaginal
r., valve

r., vlistow
repaired muscles
repaired with prosthesis, femur
reparative
r. cardiac surgery
r. closure, alveoloplasty
r. granuloma ▸ central giant cell
r. granuloma, giant cell
r. granuloma ▸ peripheral giant cell
r. mastery
r. surgery
repeat(s)
r. angioplasty
r. balloon mitral valvotomy
r. cesarean section (CS)
r. chest x-ray
r. drug offenders
r. examination
r. films
r. heart attack
r. hip replacement surgery
r. revascularization
r. ritualistic acts ▸ patient
r. smear
r. study
r. venous hematocrit (Hct)
r. water study
r. words, ability to
repeated
r. ear infections
r. electrical stimulation
r. electroencephalogram (EEG) complexes ▸ regularly
r. electroencephalogram (EEG) waves ▸ regularly
r. exposure, prolonged or
r. failure
r. fainting spells
r., involuntary sinuous movements ▸ slow,
r. lying
r. miscarriages
r. muscle contractions
r. narrowing of coronary arteries
r. panic attacks
r. paroxysms of pain
r. partial asphyxia
r. physical assaults
r. physical fights
r. procrastination
r. skin grafting
r. spontaneous abortions
r. squandering of money
r. stress on tendon
r. stress to tissue lining

repeated—*continued*
- r. strokes
- r. treatment

repens
- r., Aspergillus
- r., Dirofilaria
- r., Eurotium
- r., nephritis

repercussions, physical

reperitonealize the pelvis

reperfusion
- r. arrhythmia
- r. catheter
- r., coronary artery
- r., emergency
- r. -induced hemorrhage
- r. injury
- r. injury ‣ ischemic
- r. injury ‣ myocardial
- r. injury ‣ postischemia skeletal muscle
- r. injury (PIRI) ‣ postischemic
- r. ‣ ischemic tissue
- r., late
- r. syndrome
- r. transition ‣ forced ischemia
- r., vascular

repertoire ‣ identical genetic

repetition
- r. compulsion
- r., compulsive
- r. enhances memory
- r. frequency ‣ pulse
- r. of words
- r., pulse
- r. rate
- r. time (RT)

repetitious
- r. activity ‣ mind clearing
- r. automatic movements
- r. behavior
- r. behavior and tantrums

repetitive
- r. action
- r. activities
- r. acts
- r. and persistent pattern of behavior
- r. behavior
- r. behavior ‣ odd
- r. body movements
- r. carotid damage
- r. complexes
- r. compulsions
- r. EEG (electroencephalogram) discharges

- r. electrical stimulation
- r. exercises
- r. fibrillation potentials
- r. force
- r. hand motion
- r. intrusions of sleep
- r. monomorphic ventricular tachycardia
- r. motion
- r. motion disorder
- r. motion in the joint
- r. motion injury
- r. motion of wrist joint
- r. motion on muscles ‣ excessive
- r. motion, rapid
- r. motions ‣ meaningless
- r. movement
- r. movement, automatic
- r. movement, involuntary
- r. movement, stereotyped
- r. movement ‣ violent
- r. overeating
- r. overhead movement of arm
- r. paroxysmal ventricular tachycardia
- r. photic stimulation
- r. ritualized behavior
- r. rituals
- r. sharp-and-slow waves
- r. skills, structured
- r. sound stimulation
- r. speech
- r. spike-and-slow waves ‣ atypical
- r. stereotyped behavior
- r. stimulus
- r. strain injury (RSI)
- r. stress
- r. stress disorder
- r. stress injury (RSI)
- r. stress syndrome
- r. stroke during massage ‣ smooth and
- r. tasks
- r. twisting movement
- r. waves
- r., weight-bearing, strenuous activity
- r. words and actions
- r. wrist motion

repigmentation with psoralens

replaced
- r. damaged valve ‣ repair or
- r. fluid losses
- r. in cast, window
- r. in renal fossa ‣ kidney
- r., iris pillars

- r. with new bone
- r. with spatula ‣ pillars of iris

replacement (Replacement)
- r., adequate fluid
- r., ankle
- r. ‣ aortic graft
- r. (AVR), aortic valve
- R. Arthroplasty (TARA), Total Articular
- r. atrophy, fat
- r., blood
- r. bone
- r. donation
- r. ‣ dual lock total hip
- r., elbow
- r., elbow joint
- r., elective
- r., endoprosthetic femoral head
- r., enzyme
- r., esophagus
- r., estrogen
- r., fibrous
- r., finger
- r., fluid
- r., fluid and electrolyte
- r. for osteoporosis ‣ estrogen
- r. graft
- r., hair
- r. ‣ heart valve
- r., hip
- r., hormone
- r. indicators ‣ elective
- r., knee joint
- r. ‣ major organ
- r., Matchett-Brown femoral head
- r. medication ‣ hormone
- r. ‣ metal-on-metal hip
- r. ‣ metal-on-plastic
- r., mitral valve
- r. of cerebrospinal fluid (CSF)
- r. of damaged joint
- r. of diseased joint
- r. of generators
- r. of heart valve
- r. of joint
- r. of lung tissue
- r. of mitral valve
- r. operation ‣ total hip
- r., pacemaker
- r. ‣ partial knee
- r. ‣ permanent teeth
- r. ‣ postmenopausal estrogen
- r. procedure ‣ total hip
- r. prosthesis (PORP), partial ossicular

r. prosthesis (TORP), Plastiport total ossicular
r. prosthesis ▸ Sheehy-House incus
r. prosthesis (TORP), total ossicular
r. pulse generator ▸ elective
r., self-articulating femoral hip
r., shoulder
r., skin
r. solution, colloid
r. ▸ stem cell
r. ▸ supra-annular mitral valve
r. surgery ▸ hair
r. surgery ▸ hip
r. surgery, joint
r. surgery ▸ knee
r. surgery ▸ minimally invasive valve
r. surgery ▸ primary hip
r. surgery ▸ repeat hip
r. surgery ▸ revision hip
r. surgery, valve
r. teeth ▸ artificial
r. therapy
r. therapy, blood component
r. therapy (ERT) ▸ estrogen
r. therapy, fluid
r. therapy (HRT) ▸ hormone
r. therapy ▸ mineral
r. therapy, nicotine
r. therapy, pancreatic
r. therapy ▸ testosterone
r. (THR) ▸ thyroid hormone
r. tissue
r., total hip
r., total joint
r., total knee
r. ▸ trach (tracheostomy) tube
r. transfusion
r., valve
r. valve leakage
r. with colon in children ▸ esophagus
r., wrist
replacer, Green's
replant, limb
replantation, intentional
replantation, surgical
repletion
r., fluid
r., nutrition
r. of shock patients ▸ fluid
r., volume
replica of donor tissue
replicated set
replication
r. ability

r. and transfer
r., genetic
r. life ▸ cell
r. potential, cell
r., self-
r. ▸ stimulate viral
r., viral
repolarization
r., benign early
r. changes, nonspecific
r. ▸ early rapid
r. effect
r. ▸ final rapid
r. wave, atrial
report [*record*]
r., autopsy
r., case
r. cause of death (COD) ▸ autopsy
r., daily status
r. measures, self-
r., pathological
r., psychological
reportable diseases
reported history, self-
reporting positive findings
reposited, iris
reposition
r. patient on back
r. patient on side
r. tissue
repositioned, patient
repositioning
r., canalith
r. of eyelid
r. of incus
Repository (CDR), Clinical Data
repository form of penicillin
representation
r., character
r., distorted
r., schematic
repressant molecules
repressed
r. desires
r. emotions
r. memories
r. memory, reconstruct
repression
r. ▸ dissociation and
r., memory
r. of emotions
r. ▸ psychoanalytic concept of
r., secondary
repressor molecules
repressor site

reprocessing (EMDR) ▸ eye movement desensitization
reproducible skill building resources
reproduction, cell
reproductive
r. ability
r. behavior
r. cancers
r. capacity
r. complications of drug abuse
r. cycle
r. endocrinologist
r. endocrinology
r. failure ▸ premature
r. function
r. genes
r. genetics
r. hormones
r. hormones ▸ pituitary
r. immunology
r. mortality
r. organs
r. system
r. system ▸ cancer of
r. system impairment ▸ sexual/
r. systems, malformed
r. techniques, assisted
r. technology
r. toxicity study
r. tract
r. tract, cancer of male
r. tract, female
r. tract infection
reprogram dual pacemaker
reprogram single pacemaker
reptilivora, Pseudomonas
request (Request)
r., consultation
r. form
R. Law, Required
r. policy, required
r., required
requested, autopsy
requesting admission, patient
required (Required)
r. consent
r. request
R. Request Law
r. request policy
requirement(s)
r., analgesic
r., fiber dietary
r., legal
r., methodological
r., normal consent

requirement(s)—*continued*
 r., postsurgical bowel
 r. reduced, narcotic
requires occasional assistance, patient
reroute blood
reroute digestive system
rerouting of blood flow
rescreening, annual
rescripting nightmares
rescue (Rescue)
 r., air
 r. angioplasty
 r. breathing
 r. chemotherapy, citrovorum
 r., citrovorum
 r. coronary bypass surgery
 r. factor
 r. factor, citrovorum
 r., leucovorin
 r. method, self-
 R. Team, Paramedic
rescuer('s)
 r. CPR (cardiopulmonary resuscitation), one-
 r. CPR (cardiopulmonary resuscitation), two-
 r. position
research (Research)
 r., addiction
 r., alcohol
 r., alpha-epilepsy
 R., Alzheimer's Disease
 r., anatomical
 r., antioxidant
 r. associate
 r., authorization for body to be donated for scientific
 r., basic
 r., behavioral
 r., biological
 r., biomedical
 r., brain tumor
 r., breast cancer
 r., cancer
 r., cancer pain
 r. center, genetic
 r. cholesterol embolization
 r., clinical
 r., clinical cancer
 r., consent form for body to be donated for scientific
 r., contraceptive
 r. design for immunology

 r. design in combined modality therapy
 r., drug
 r. ethics
 r., ethnographic
 r. ▸ gene therapy
 r., genetic
 r., genomics
 r., history of
 R. Lab, Radiobiology
 R. Laboratories (VDRL) Test, Venereal Disease
 R. Laboratories (VDRL) ▸ Venereal Disease
 r. logic linear array
 r. matrix
 r., medical
 r., memory
 r. methodology
 r., neuropsychological
 r., oncologist
 r., outcome
 r., patient-outcome
 r., plasmapheresis
 r. process
 r. program, clinical
 r. protocols
 r., radioimmunoglobulin
 r., regeneration
 r. results
 r., sleep
 r. study
 r. study, collaborative
 r. subject
 r. subject, clinical
 r., systems
 r., tissue
 r., treatment outcome
 r. trial, clinical
 r. unit, clinical
 r. unit, myocardial
researcher, trauma
resectable lesion
resectable, tumor
resected
 r. aneurysm
 r. end-to-end ileal colostomy
 r., estimated tissue
 r., intercostal nerve
 r. piecemeal, lesion
 r. rib subperiosteally
 r. tonsil
resecting fracture
resection [*recession, reflection*]
 r., abdominoperineal

 r., activation map-guided surgical
 r. and rhinoplasty (SMRR), submucous
 r., anterior
 r., antral
 r., arthroscopic
 r., Balfour gastric
 r., block
 r., bronchial sleeve
 r., colon
 r., curative
 r., Darrach's
 r., electro◇
 r., en bloc
 r., endocardial
 r., extensive
 r., failure patterns after surgical
 r., gastric
 r., Girdlestone joint
 r. head of pancreas
 r. head of radius
 r. in acromegaly, transsphenoidal
 r. ▸ infundibular wedge
 r., lesser
 r. levator muscle
 r., liver
 r., low anterior
 r., lung
 r., massive
 r., Miles' abdominoperineal
 r. ▸ myotomy-myectomy-septal
 r., node
 r. (TUR) of bladder ▸ transurethral
 r. of eyelid
 r. of intestines
 r. of lung
 r. of mediastinal tumor
 r. of parietal pleura
 r. of prostate (TURP), transurethral
 r. of pylorus
 r. of rectal tumor ▸ local
 r. of stomach, partial
 r. of thoracic esophagus ▸ Torek
 r. of tumor mass
 r., palliative
 r. ▸ postoperative bowel
 r., rib
 r., scleral
 r., segmental
 r., segmental colon
 r. ▸ segmental lung
 r., segmental pulmonary
 r., septal
 r., small bowel
 r. (SMR), submucous

r., surgical
r. (TUR) ▸ transurethral
r., wedge
r., wedge colon
r., wide
r., wide mesenteric

resectional ostectomies ▸ maxillary tuberosity

resemblance ▸ biofeedback EMG (electromyogram) pattern

resentment
r., anger and
r. ▸ feeling of
r. of criticism

reserve(s)
r. air
r., breathing
r. capacity, functional
r. capacity ▸ inspiratory
r., cardiac
r., cardiopulmonary
r. cell carcinoma
r. cells
r., cochlear
r., cognitive
r., coronary arterial
r., coronary flow
r., coronary vascular
r., coronary vasodilator
r. days, lifetime
r., diastolic
r., exocrine functional
r., extraction
r. ▸ Frank Starling
r. ▸ heart rate
r. ▸ impaired coronary vascular
r., myocardial
r., preload
r., respiratory
r., systolic
r. technique, coronary flow
r., vasodilator
r. volume (ERV) ▸ expiratory
r. volume (IRV) ▸ inspiratory

reservoir
r., Cardiometrics cardiotomy
r., cardiotomy
r. chest drainage, cardiotomy
r., Cobe cardiotomy
r., double-bubble flushing
r. face mask
r., fluid
r. ▸ Jostra cardiotomy
r., Koch's
r. nebulizer

r. nebulizer, contaminated
r., Omaya
r. ▸ Polystan cardiotomy
r., Pudenz's
r. ▸ Shiley cardiotomy

resets rhythm, brain

reshaping
r., body
r., heart
r., nose
r., tooth

residence, assisted living

residency program, hospital

residency, psychiatry

resident
r., house
r. -on-call
r. psychiatrist
r., surgical

residential (Residential)
r. care facility
r. care, juvenile
r. cell
r. drug-free program
R. Facility (CBRF), Community Based
r. patient
r. placement
r. program
r. setting
r. treatment
r. treatment facility
r. treatment facility ▸ acquired immune deficiency syndrome (AIDS)
r. treatment for alcohol
r. treatment for drug abuser

residual [*decidual*]
r. acini
r. affinity
r. air
r. albuminuria
r. appendix
r. arch
r. axillary lymph node enlargement
r. barium
r. blood volume, placental
r. capacity, functional
r. Conray
r. contrast material
r. damage
r. defect, mild
r. deformity
r. dental arch
r. disability ▸ schizophrenic behavior with

r. disease
r. disease ▸ minimal
r. drug traces
r. dye
r. enlargement
r. esophagitis
r. facial pain
r. functional vision
r. gradient
r. handicap
r. hematoma
r. immunity
r. infiltrate
r. iodized oil
r. jet
r. lung capacity (RLC)
r. lung disease
r. lymph nodes, shotty
r. lymphoid tissue
r. muscle relaxant effect
r. muscle weakness
r. necrotic tissue
r. neurological impairment
r. nodes, shotty
r. nodular thyroid
r. pain
r. pancreatic tissue
r. paralysis
r. paresis
r., partial
r. peripheral paralysis
r. permanent deformation
r. plaque
r. (PVR), postvoiding
r. proteinuria
r. root
r. scarring
r. scarring of eardrum
r. schizophrenia
r. stenosis
r. stomatitis
r. stool
r. tissue
r. tumor
r. tumor at primary site
r. tumor, extensive
r. tumor ▸ focal nodules of
r. tumor, postirradiation
r. tumor site
r. type, chronic ▸ schizophrenia,
r. type, chronic with acute exacerbation ▸ schizophrenia,
r. type ▸ schizophrenia,
r. type, subchronic ▸ schizophrenia,

residual—*continued*
- r. type, subchronic with acute exacerbation ▸ schizophrenia,
- r. type, unspecified ▸ schizophrenia,
- r. urine
- r. urine volume ▸ low
- r. volume
- r. volume, postvoiding
- r. volume to total lung capacity (RV/TLC) ratio
- r. weakness

residue
- r. diet, low
- r., fecal
- r. (MER), methanol extraction
- r., pelvic inflammatory disease (PID)
- r., tumor

resigned, patient

resilience, experiential

resin
- r., anion exchange
- r. -based composite
- r., bile acid binding
- r., cholestyramine
- r. colophony ▸ pine
- r., IRA-400
- r. teeth, acrylic
- r. test, triiodothyronine
- r., thermosetting
- r. uptake
- r. -uptake ratio

resistance (Resistance)
- r., acid alcohol
- r., afterload
- r., airway
- r., alternating current (AC)
- r. ▸ anger, rage and
- r., antibiotic
- r., aortic valve
- r., arteriolar
- r., bacterial
- r., basal skin
- r. -capacitance (R-C) coupled amplifier
- r., cell
- r., cerebrovascular
- r., chromosomal mediated
- r., coronary vascular
- r., decreasing peripheral vascular
- r., defensive
- r. determinant
- r. determinants, antibiotic
- r., direct current (DC)
- r., drug

R. Education (DARE) Program ▸ Drug Awareness
- r., elastic
- r., electrical
- r., electrode
- r. encountered
- r., essential
- r. exercise
- r., external
- r., external urethral
- r., extraordinary
- r., galvanic skin
- r., genetics of drug
- r., hemolytic
- r., host
- r., increasing airway
- r. index ▸ pulmonary vascular
- r. index ▸ systemic vascular
- r. index ▸ total peripheral
- r. index ▸ vascular
- r., inductive
- r., input
- r., insulin
- r., internal
- r., measure
- r., measurement of electrode
- r., microbial
- r., midbrain
- r., ohm
- r., outflow
- r., peripheral
- r. (PTR) ▸ peripheral total
- r., peripheral vascular
- r., plasmin mediated
- r., protease
- r., pulmonary
- r., pulmonary arteriolar
- r., pulmonary vascular
- r. ratio
- r., renal vascular
- r. response, skin
- r. ▸ severe insulin
- r., severe muscular
- r., skin
- r. strains
- r. syndrome ▸ insulin
- r., systemic
- r., systemic arteriolar
- r., systemic vascular
- r. testing (GART) ▸ genotypic antiretroviral
- r., therapeutic
- r., thyroid hormone
- r. to antibiotic, acquired
- r. to antibiotic, intrinsic

- r. to antibody
- r. to disease
- r. to infection
- r. to infection ▸ lowered
- r. to passive stretching
- r. to venous return
- r. (TR) ▸ total
- r. (TPR) ▸ total peripheral
- r. (TPR) ▸ total pulmonary
- r. (TPVR) ▸ total pulmonary vascular
- r. training
- r. training, gentle
- R. Transfer Factor (RTF)
- r., trichomonas
- r. unit
- r. unit (PRU) ▸ peripheral
- r., vascular
- r. ▸ vascular peripheral
- r. vessel
- r. vessel, coronary
- r., vital
- r. voice prosthesis ▸ Ultra-Low
- r. ▸ water provides gentle

resistant (Resistant)
- r. alcoholism, treatment
- r. antibiotics, aminoglycoside
- r. artificial joint parts ▸ wear-
- r., aspirin
- r. bacteria, antibiotic
- r. bacteria ▸ drug-
- r. bacteria ▸ harmful antibiotic-
- r. bacteria, predominant
- r. container, puncture
- r. container, rigid puncture
- r. depression ▸ treatment-
- r. diabetes ▸ insulin
- r. disease, drug-
- r., drug-
- R. Education (DARE) ▸ Drug Abuse
- r. genes, drug-
- r. hypertension
- r. individual
- r. infection, drug-
- r., isoxazolyl group
- r., multi-drug
- r. obsessive-compulsive disorder ▸ treatment-
- r. organism
- r. organism, antibiotic-
- r. organisms aspirated into lungs ▸ drug-
- r. organisms, drug-
- r. pathogens
- r. penicillins, acid-

r. penicillins ▸ acid- and penicillinase-
r. penicillins, penicillinase-
r. pneumococci ▸ penicillin-
r. pneumococcus
r. quadriceps exercises, progressive
r. rickets ▸ vitamin D
r., salt
r. schizophrenia, drug-
r. Staphylococcus aureus (MR-SA) ▸ methicillin-
r. strain
r. strains, drug-
r. strains of bacteria
r. strains of pneumococcus
r. Streptococcus pneumoniae ▸ drug-
r. sunscreen, water-
r. tachyarrhythmia
r. TB (tuberculosis) ▸ multi-drug
r. to change
r. to drugs, bacteria
r. to stimuli
r. virus ▸ drug-

resistive
r. exercise
r. exercises, active
r. heating
r. radiofrequency electric field

resolution
r. B mode ultrasonography ▸ high
r., complete
r. computed tomography (HRCT) scan ▸ high
r., contrast
r., energy
r. of grief
r., slow
r., spatial
r., temporal

resolving
r. power
r. pulmonary edema
r. time

resonance
r. angiography (carotid MRA) ▸ contrast enhanced carotid magnetic
r. (MR) angiography ▸ intracranial magnetic
r. angiography (MRA) ▸ magnetic
r. (MR) angiography ▸ selective arterial magnetic
r. (MR) angiography ▸ selective venous magnetic
r., bandbox

r., bell-metal
r. (MR) brain scan, magnetic
r. capture
r., cough
r., cracked-pot
r., electron paramagnetic
r. flowmetry (MRF) ▸ magnetic
r. generator
r. image, magnetic
r. imaging (fMRI) brain scan ▸ functional magnetic
r. imaging (EEMRI) coil ▸ endoesophageal magnetic
r. imaging (MRI), conventional magnetic
r. imaging (MRI) ▸ diffusion-weighted magnetic
r. imaging (MRI) ▸ enhancement of magnetic
r. imaging (fMRI/MRI) ▸ functional magnetic
r. imaging ▸ gated sweep magnetic
r. imaging (MRI) machine, magnetic
r. imaging (MRI), magnetic
r. imaging (NMRI) ▸ nuclear magnetic
r. imaging (MRI) scan, magnetic
r. imaging (MRI) scan, sideview magnetic
r. imaging (MRI) scanner, magnetic
r. imaging (MRI) spectrometer, magnetic
r. imaging (MRI) ▸ spin-echo magnetic
r. imaging ▸ velocity encoded cine-magnetic
r. scanner, magnetic
R. Scanner (NMRS), Nuclear Magnetic
r., shoulder-strap
r. signal ▸ magnetic
r., skodaic
r. spectroscopy ▸ electron paramagnetic
r. spectroscopy imaging (MRSI) ▸ magnetic
r. spectroscopy, magnetic
r. (NMR) spectroscopy, nuclear magnetic
r., vesicular
r., vocal
r., whispering
r., wooden

resonant
r. frequency

r. on percussion, thorax
r. to percussion

resonator imaging (MRI) scan, enhanced magnetic

resorption
r. atelectasis
r., bone
r. ▸ bone formation and
r. ▸ inherit bone

resorptive atelectasis

resource(s)
r., addiction treatment
r. available, treatment
r., community
r., counseling
r., health care
r., identifying
r., interior
r., psychological
r. ▸ reproducible skill building
r. service, referral
r., social

respect [*reflect*]
respect, self-
respective input terminals
respiration(s)
r., abdominal
r., absence of
r., absent
r., absent spontaneous
r., accelerated
r., accessory muscles of
r., aerobic
r., agonal
r., amphoric
r., anaerobic
r. and pulse
r., apneustic
r. (AR), artificial
r., assisted
r., asthmoid
r., Austin Flint
r., Biot's
r., Bouchut's
r., bronchial
r., bronchocavernous
r., bronchovesicular
r., cavernous
r., cellular
r., central
r., cerebral
r., cessation of
r., Cheyne-Stokes
r., cogwheel
r., collateral

respiration(s)—*continued*
r., controlled
r., controlled diaphragmatic
r., Corrigan's
r., costal
r., cyclic
r., decreased
r., deep
r., deep and regular
r., depth of
r., diaphragmatic
r., direct
r., divided
r., electrophrenic
r., embarrassed
r., excessive artificial
r., external
r., fetal
r., forced
r., frequent blowing
r., gasping
r., granular
r., grunting
r., harsh
r., hunger
r., impaired
r., inspiratory
r. (IPPR) ▸ intermittent positive
    pressure
r., internal
r., interrupted
r., intrauterine
r., irregular
r., jerky
r., Kussmaul-Kien
r., Kussmaul's
r., labored
r., meningitic
r., mouth-to-mouth
r., muscles of
r., nervous
r., normal
r., normal adult
r., oxidate
r., paradoxical
r., periodic
r., placental
r., pleuritic
r., prolonged time to sustained
r., puerile
r., pulse and
r. pyelography
r. ▸ radiofrequency electrophrenic
r., rapid
r. ▸ rapid, shallow

r., rate of
r., restoration of
r., rude
r. ▸ Schafer method of artificial
r., Seitz's metamorphosing
r., shallow
r., sighing
r., slow
r. slow and shallow
r., slowed
r., sonorous
r., spontaneous
r., stertorous
r., stimulate
r., stridulous
r., supplementary
r., suppressed
r., sustained
r. (TPR) ▸ temperature, pulse and
r., thoracic
r., tissue
r., transitional
r., tubular
r., vesicular
r., vesiculocavernous
r., vicarious
r., wavy
respiratione intermittens ▸ pulsus
respirator
r., Ambu
r., BABYbird (Bird)
r., Bennett
r., Bird
r. brain
r., breathing supported by mechanical
r., cabinet
r., cuirass
r., Emerson cuirass
r., mechanical
r., Monaghan
r., Mörch
r., Moynihan
r., Mueller-Mörch
r., negative pressure
r. on maximum flow
r., patient on
r. ▸ patient weaned from
r., portable
r., volume cycled
respiratoria, anosmia
**respiratory (Respiratory) [*excretory,
    expiratory*]**
r. acidosis
r. acidosis, increasing
r. acidosis, terminal

r. activity
r. ailment
r. airflow
r. alkalosis
r. alkalosis, primarily
r. allergy
r. arrest
r. arrest ▸ patient had
r. arrest ▸ patient suffered
r. arrhythmia
r. assessment
r. assistance
r. assistance, patient receiving
r. bronchioles
r. burst
r. capacity
r. care
r. care technician on-call
R. Care Unit (RCU)
r. cells
r. center
r. center, medullary
r. chain
r. collapse
r. complications ▸ life-threatening
r. congestion, upper
r. control ▸ abnormalities of
r. control ratio
r. depression
r. depression, central
r. depression, drug-induced
    postanesthetic
r. depression inhalation anesthetic
r. depression, narcotic-induced
r. depression, post-stimulation
r. depth
r. difficulty
r. disease
r. disease (ARD), acute
r. disease, chronic obstructive
r. disease, febrile
r. disease, hereditary
r. disease syndrome
r. disease, upper
r. disorder
r. distress
r. distress, acute
r. distress at birth
r. distress ▸ infant in
r. distress ▸ infant in acute
r. distress, moderate
r. distress of newborn ▸ idiopathic
r. distress ▸ patient in
r. distress present at birth
r. distress ▸ serious

r. distress syndrome (RDS)
r. distress syndrome (ARDS), acute
r. distress syndrome (ARDS), adult
r. distress syndrome ▸ early
r. distress syndrome (IRDS), idiopathic
r. distress syndrome ▸ infant
r. distress, transient
r. distress ▸ ventilatory support in
r. disturbance
r. disturbance index
r. drive
r. drive test
r. dysfunction
r. effort
r. effort, decrease in
r. effort, poor
r. embarrassment
r. emergency
r. epithelium
r. equipment, monitoring
r. evaluation
r. exchange
r. exchange rate
r. exchange ratio
r. excursion
r. failure
r. failure, acute
r. failure, chronic
r. failure, cocaine-induced
r. failure, fatal
r. failure, full
r. failure ▸ impending
r. failure ▸ neonate
r. failure, progressive
r. failure syndrome
r. feedback
r. flora
r. function
r. function, alteration in
r. functions, irreversible cessation of circulatory and
r. granulomatosis, necrotizing
r. illness (RI)
r. impairment
r. infection
r. infection, acute
r. infection, anaerobic
r. infection, incipient
r. infection ▸ lower
r. infection ▸ rhinoviral
r. infection (URI) ▸ upper
r. infection, viral
r. inflammation
r. insufficiency

r. insufficiency, severe
r. irritation
R. Isolation
r. jacket ▸ Willock
r. lag
r. lobule, primary
r. mediation
r. membrane ▸ schneiderian
r. minute volume (RMV)
r. movement (RM)
r. movements, thoracic
r. mucous glands
r. murmur
r. murmur, laryngeal
r. muscle disease
r. muscle dysfunction
r. muscle rest
r. muscle training
r. muscles
r. muscular contraction
r. nerve center
r. nursing care
r. obstruction
r. ordered phase encoding
r. pacemaker
r. papillomatosis ▸ recurrent
r. paralysis
r. passage
r. pattern
r. percussion
r. physiology
r. problem
r. problem, chronic
r. problem, severe
r. process
r. psychophysics
r. pulse
r. pump
r. quotient
r. rales
r. rate
r. rate, increased
r. rate per minute (RRpm)
r. rate, sleep
r. reflex ▸ transient loss of
r. reflexes
r. region
r. reserve
r. secretions
r. sensation
r. shock
r. sound
r. spasm
r. standstill
r. status, declining

r. stimulant
r. stimulation, marked
r. stridor
r. support
r. swing
r. symptoms
r. syncytial virus (RSV)
r. syncytial virus (RSV) conduit
r. syncytial virus (RSV) IV immune globulin
r. syndrome ▸ severe, acute
r. system
r. system shock
r. therapist
r. therapy
R. Therapy Department
r. therapy devices
r. therapy devices ▸ effluent gas from
r. tic
r. toilet
r. tract
r. tract discomfort, upper
r. tract fistula
r. tract fistula ▸ esophageal carcinoma with
r. tract fluid (RTF)
r. tract from gases ▸ burns to
r. tract infection
r. tract infection, acute
r. tract infection, concurrent upper
r. tract infection ▸ hospital-associated
r. tract infection, nosocomial
r. tract infection ▸ recurrent upper
r. tract inflammation
r. tract inflammation ▸ lower
r. tract, lower
r. tract, upper
r. transmission
r. tube
R. Unit
r. viral syndrome ▸ upper
r. virus
r. volume (RV)
r. volume (RV), decreased
r. wave
r. wheezes

respite
r. and in-home care
r. care
r. care program
r. care, short-term institutional
r. service

respond(s)
   r. ▸ failure to identify and
   r., patient failed to
   r. to estrogen, cells
   r. to medication ▸ patient
   r. verbally
responded
   r. to care, patient
   r. to treatment, patient
   r. verbally ▸ patient
respondent conditioning
responding
   r. tissue, acute responding vs late
   r. to questions ▸ delay in
   r. tumor, late
   r. vs late responding tissue, acute
response (Response)
   r., abnormal immunologic
   r., abnormal sexual
   r. ▸ active immune
   r., acute
   r., adaptive
   r., agitated
   r., alpha
   r., amplitude of successive
   r., anamnestic
   r. and combined modality therapy
   r., antibody immune
   r., appropriate emotional
   r., arousal
   R. Assessment Matrix (TRAM) ▸
      Treatment
   R. Assessment Method (TRAM) ▸
      Treatment
   r. audiometer, evoked
   R. Audiometry (ERA), Electric
   r. (ABR), auditory brainstem
   r. (AER), auditory evoked
   r., autoimmune
   r., automatic
   r., autonomic
   r., average evoked
   r., behavioral
   r., body's immune
   r., brain wave
   r. (BAER), brainstem auditory
      evoked
   r. (BSER), brainstem evoked
   r., cardiac
   r., cardiovascular
   r., cellular
   r., cellular immune
   r., cellular mediated immune
   r., cholinergic
   r., chronic pain

   r., chronotropic
   r., clonic motor
   r., cocaine
   r., compulsive
   r., conditioned
   r., conditioned behavior
   r., conditioned fear
   r. (CDR) ▸ control domination
   r., controlled ventricular
   r., cortical
   r., cortical evoked
   r., cry
   r., curve, frequency
   r., Cushing pressure
   r., decrementing
   r., defective immune
   r., delayed
   r., denial
   r., dose
   r. ▸ dynamic frequency
   r., electrodermal
   r., electroencephalic
   r., electronically provoked
   r., emotional
   r., equivocal
   r. (ER), evoked
   r., extensor plantar
   r., eye
   r., faradic
   r., fat meal
   r., fight-or-flight
   r., flexor plantar
   r. fluctuations
   r., frequency
   r., frequency following
   r., galvanic
   r., galvanic skin
   r. ▸ giving up
   r., good
   r., grasp
   r., Hallpike caloric stimulation
   r., heart rate
   r., heighten sexual
   r., high frequency
   r., humoral
   r., humoral antibody
   r. imaging ▸ transient
   r., immediate
   r., immune
   r., immunity
   r., implantation
   r. in antibodies, radiobiology and
      tumor
   r. in headache therapy, relaxation
   r., incrementing

   r. (IR) ▸ index of
   r., indices predicting
   r., inflammatory
   r., inhibiting stress
   r., initial immune
   r., instrumental heart rate
   r. interruption
   r., involuntary
   r., irritative
   r. is negative, patient
   r., lack of normal
   r., latency of
   r., libidinal
   r., low frequency
   R. manual resuscitator ▸ First
   R. manual resuscitator ▸ Safe
   r. mechanism, normal
   r. mechanism, stimulus
   r., modifiers, biological
   r., motor
   r., multidisciplinary
   r., muscle
   r., myotonic
   r., nervous
   r., neurological evoked
   r., normal plantar
   r., objective
   r. of brain to electrical stimulation
   r. of cardiovascular system, stress
   r. of skin ▸ electrical
   r., overt
   r. ▸ paced ventricular evoked
   r., pain
   r., paired
   r., paradoxical
   r., patient's immune
   r., patient's ventricular
   r., phobic
   r., photoconvulsive
   r., photomyoclonic
   r., photomyogenic
   r., photoparoxysmal
   r., physical
   r., physiologic
   r., physiological
   r., plantar
   r., plantar extensor
   r., plateau
   r., polymorphonuclear cell
   r., polymorphonuclear leukocyte
   r., poor
   r. ▸ post-trauma
   r. prevention
   r. prevention (ERP) ▸ exposure and
   r., purposeful

r., radiation
r., rapid ventricular
r. rate
r. rate ▸ sustained
r., reflex
r., reflexive
r., rejection
r., relaxation
r. ▸ role-playing and
r., secondary
r., secondary immune
r., sensitization
r., sexual
r. (SER), short latency somatosensory evoked
r., skin
r., skin conductance
r., skin potential
r., skin resistance
r., sleep
r., slow
r., slow immune
r., slowing of motor
r., slowness of
r. (SER), somatosensory evoked
r. ▸ square wave
r., startle
r., stress
r. study ▸ hypoxic
r., subjective
r., sucking
r. ▸ suppress emotional
r., suppressed immune
r., swallow
r. syndrome ▸ post-trauma
r. syndrome ▸ systemic inflammatory
r. system (PERS) ▸ personal emergency
r. test, evoked
r., tetanic motor
r., therapeutic
r. ▸ thyrotropin-releasing hormone
r. time
r. to anxiety-evoking stimuli ▸ autonomic
r. to electromyogram (EMG) biofeedback ▸ hyperkinesis
r. -to-injury hypothesis
r. -to-injury hypothesis of atherogenesis
r. -to-injury theory
r. to light stimulation
r. to medicine
r. to pain

r. to pain, body's
r. to pain ▸ modify body's
r. to relaxation therapy
r. to relaxation training ▸ physiological
r. to social situations
r. to sound
r. to stress, heart
r. to therapy
r. to treatment
r. (TR) ▸ total
r., tumor
r. unit, audio
r., vagal
r., vascular
r., ventricular
r., verbal
r., vigilance
r., visual evoked
r., wake

responsibility(-ies)
r., encourage sense of
r., ethical
r., health
r., legal
r., structured
r., undemanding

responsible clinician

responsive
r. and attentive
r. anemia, pyridoxine-
r. ▸ dual chamber rate
r. pacemaker ▸ Meta rate
r. pacemaker ▸ rate-
r. pacing ▸ rate
r., patient
r. ▸ single chamber rate
r. to stimulation ▸ neurologically over-
r. to systemic therapy ▸ cancer
r. tumor
r. -unipolar ventricular pacemaker ▸ Medtronic Activitrax rate

responsiveness
r., affective
r., nerve
r. to external stimuli
r. to pain, diminished

Rest (rest) (REST)
R. (Reduced Environmental Stimulation Therapy)
r. and exercise (R and E)
r. and exercise balance
r. and exercise study

r. and exercise-gated nuclear angiography
r. and recuperation (R and R)
r. and rehabilitation exercise
r. and relaxation
r. angina
r. angina ▸ ischemic
r., bed
r., Chan wrist
r., disrupt patient's
r. dyspnea
r. ejection fraction
r. elevated, kidney
r., evaluation of denervated heart at
r. exercise equilibrium radionuclide ventriculography
r. gated equilibrium image ▸ supine
r., hot packs and bed
r. hypoxemia
R., Ice, Compression, Elevation (RICE)
r., ice, compression and elevation (PRICE) ▸ protection,
r., Light-Veley head
r. metabolism/stress perfusion protocol
r., padded foot
r. pain
r., patient at complete bed
r., patient placed at bed
r. pattern, alteration in
r. period
r. position
r. position, physiologic
r., proper
r. radionuclide angiography
r. redistribution thallium 201 imaging
r. ▸ respiratory muscle
r. seat
r., subsiding with
r. syndrome ▸ stop and
r., Veley head

restaurant food, tainted
Restaurant Syndrome (CRS) ▸ Chinese
rested state contraction
restenosis
r., aortic valve
r., graft
r., intrastent
r. lesion
r., mitral
r. ▸ postballoon angioplasty
r. procedure

restenosis—*continued*
  r. ▸ pulmonary valve
  r., radiation
  r., tricuspid
restful awareness
resting
  r. activity, evaluation of
  r. cardiac output
  r. cell
  r. electroencephalogram (EEG)
    pattern development ▸ normal
  r. energy
  r. hair
  r., heart
  r. heart rate
  r. length tension relation
  r. membrane potential
  r. metabolic rate (RMR)
  r. muscle activity
  r. muscle potential
  r. phase of cardiac cycle (cc)
  r. phase of facial hair
  r. potential
  r. pressure (RP)
  r. pulse
  r. pulse rate, normal
  r. record
  r. stage
  r. state
  r. tachycardia
  r. tension relation ▸ length
  r. tremor
  r. value
  r. wandering cell
restless
  r. leg from caffeine
  r. leg syndrome
  r. legs
  r. movements
  r. pacing
  r., patient
  r. ▸ vegetative and
restlessness
  r. and drowsiness
  r. and incoherence
  r. and intense craving ▸ irritability,
  r. and pacing ▸ agitation,
  r., anorexia and irritability
  r., feeling of
  r. ▸ irritability, agitation, and
  r., motor
  r., physical
Reston virus
restoration (Restoration)
  r., crown

r., dental
r., electrolyte balance
R., Eye Bank for Sight
r. ▸ laser facial skin
r. of continuity
r. of muscle strength ▸ long-term
r. of normal anatomic alignment
r. of oral function
r. of respiration
r. of sight
r. of tooth
r. of wakefulness
r., physical
r. surgery ▸ hair
restorative
  r. care
  r. dentistry
  r. drug
  r. procedure
  r. sleep
  r. therapy
restore
  r. blood flow
  r. finger mobility
  r. lost movement and function
  r. lost or thinning hair
  r. mobility and reduce pain
  r. mobility ▸ relieve pain and
  r. tissue to affected area
restored cycle
restored mobility
restoring nurturance and tenderness
restrain hernia ▸ supportive device to
restrained
  r. beam
  r., limbs
  r. with vest, patient
restraining order
restraining tape
restraint(s)
  r., ankle
  r., bedspread
  r., chemical
  r., complete
  r. ▸ four-point leather
  r. ▸ full leather
  r., leather
  r. observation form ▸ seclusion/
  r. of patient, chemical
  r., partial
  r., patient in
  r., patient in complete
  r., patient in partial
  r., physical
  r., Posey

r., seclusion or
r., sheet
r., use of
r., vest
r., wrist
restricted
  r. activity
  r. air flow
  r. calories
  r. chest expansion
  r. diet, fat
  r. diet, gluten
  r. diet, lactose
  r. diet, mild sodium
  r. diet, moderate sodium
  r. diet, protein
  r. diet, sodium
  r. diet, strict sodium
  r. environmental stimulation
  r. environmental technique
  r. excess motion in spine
  r. expansion of chest
  r. expression of emotions
  r. eye movements
  r. ▸ motion severity
  r. movement
  r. movement ▸ painful and
  r. physical activity
  r. range of motion (ROM)
  r. sense
  r. transduction
  r. tyramine and MAO (monoamine
    oxidase) inhibitor diet
restricting food intake
restriction(s)
  r., activity
  r., bronchial
  r., caloric
  r., calorie
  r. diet, calorie
  r. diet, salt
  r., dietary
  r. endonuclease
  r. enzyme
  r., fluid
  r. fragment length polymorphisms
    (RFLPs)
  r. in activity
  r. in drug abuse, legal
  r. of lung volume
  r. of motion
  r. of movement ▸ stiffness and
  r. of perceptions
  r. ▸ patient on fluid
  r., physical

r., potassium
r. ▸ progressive parenchymal
r., protein
r., salt
r., sensory
r., smoking
r., sodium
r. therapy ▸ sleep
r., treatment

restrictive
r. abnormality
r. airway defect
r. airway disease
r. cardiomyopathy ▸ idiopathic
r. cardiomyopathy patient
r. diet, less-
r. dieting
r. disease
r. environment
r. functional impairment
r. heart disease (HD)
r. long-term ward
r. lung disease
r. lung disease ▸ interstitial
r. measures, less
r. physiology
r. ventilatory defect

restructuring
r., cognitive
r., confrontational cognitive
r. ▸ nonconfrontational cognitive

result(s)
r., breathalizer
r., curative
r., false-negative
r., false-positive
r., good cosmetic
r. in clinical trials, false-negative
r. in clinical trials, false-positive
r., inconclusive
r., laboratory
r., negative
r. of stroke, rehabilitation of
  disabilities as
r. of testing
r., positive
r., research
r. still pending
r., therapeutic
r., therapy
r., trial
r. ▸ true-negative test
r. ▸ true-positive test

resultant hemopericardium

**resulting confusion ▸ overstimulation
  and**
resume(s)
r. active lifestyle
r. drinking
r. drug use
r. non-strenuous activities
r. normal lifestyle
r. previous diet, patient to
**resumed in full course, radiation
  therapy**
**resumption of normal sinus rhythm
  (NSR)**
resurface skin
resurfacing
r., carbon dioxide (CO$_2$) laser skin
r. ▸ face laser skin
r. for facial wrinkles ▸ laser
r., laser
r. ▸ laser facial
r., skin
resuscitate
r. (DNR) decision, do not
r. (DNR), do not
r. (DNR) patient, do not
r. patient, unable to
resuscitated
r., heart
r., patient
r., patient successfully
resuscitation (Resuscitation)
r. attempt
r. attempt ▸ baby expired following
r., attempted cardiopulmonary
r. attempts unsuccessful
r. bag
r., cardiac
r. (CPR), cardiopulmonary
r. cart
r., emergency
r., emergency mouth-to-mouth
r., fluid
r. ▸ heart-lung
r., initial
r. (CPR) ▸ initiate cardiopulmonary
r., legal aspects of
r., maternal
r. (CPR), mechanical
  cardiopulmonary
R. (MedSTAR), Medical Shock
  Trauma Acute
r., mouth-to-mouth
r. ▸ mouth-to-nose
r., neonatal
r. of depressed newborn

r. (CPR), one and two rescuer
  cardiopulmonary
r. (CPR), one person
  cardiopulmonary
r. (CPR), one rescuer
  cardiopulmonary
r., open chest cardiac
r., outcome of
r., pediatric
r. potential, brain
r. (CPR) techniques ▸
  cardiopulmonary
r. (CPR) ▸ toilet plunger
  cardiopulmonary
r. (CPR), two-rescuer
  cardiopulmonary
resuscitative
r. attempts
r. device (CARD), cardiac
  automatic
r. efforts
r. measures, prolonged
resuscitator
r. ▸ BagEasy disposable manual
r. ▸ First Response manual
r. ▸ infant Ambu
r. ▸ Safe Response manual
resuture disrupted operative wound
resynchronization therapy ▸ cardiac
resynchronizer, cardiac
RET (rad equivalent therapy)
retail therapy
retained
r. alpha activity
r., barium
r. blood
r. FB (foreign body)
r. fecal material
r. fecal particle
r. feces
r. foreign body (FB)
r. gastric antrum
r. lung fluid
r. particulate matter
r. placenta
r. placental tissue
r. root
r. root tip
r. secretions
r. secretions in stomach
r. secundines
r. stool
r. sutures
r. testis
r. urine

retainer arch bar
retaining
   r. catheter, self-
   r. laxative, water-
   r. new information
   r. retractor, self-
retard
   r. bone activity
   r., expiratory
   r. fetal growth
retardant
   r. gowns, flame
   r. linens, flame
   r. material, flame
   r., tumor
retardation
   r., care of child with mental
   r., fetal alcohol
   r., functional psychomotor
   r., growth
   r. in children ▸ growth
   r. (IUGR), intrauterine growth
   r., mental
   r., mild mental
   r., moderate mental
   r., motor
   r. of mental and physical
     development, marked
   r. of normal psychomotor
     functioning
   r., physical
   r., profound mental
   r., progressive
   r., psychic
   r., psychomotor
   r., severe mental
   r. syndrome ▸ alpha thalassemia X-
     linked
   r., undifferentiated mental
retarded
   r. dentition
   r. depression
   r. ▸ educable mentally
   r. growth
   r., halfway house for the mentally
   r., mentally
   r., patient
   r., patient mentally
   r. ▸ patient seriously
   r. patient ▸ trainable mentally
   r. patient ▸ untrainable, mentally
   r. ▸ profoundly mentally
   r. range of abilities ▸ mentally
   r., severely
retch [*wretch*]

retching
   r. and vomiting, patient
   r., postoperative
   r., vomiting and
rete
   r., malpighian
   r. pegs
   r. ridges
retention (Retention)
   r., acute urinary
   r. and swelling ▸ fluid
   r. catheter
   r. cyst
   r. cyst lacrimal gland
   r. cyst of kidney
   r. cyst, urinary
   r., debridement and prosthesis
   r. defect
   r., defective
   r., excess fluid
   r. film
   r., fluid
   r., memory
   r., minimize fluid
   r. of cocaine abusers
   r. of consciousness
   r. of contrast material
   r. of decidual fragment
   r. of membranes
   r. of placenta
   r. of placental fragments
   r. of urine
   r., patient has urinary
   r. polyps
   r., renal
   r., salt
   r. ▸ salt and water
   r., sodium
   r. suture
   r. suture, heavy
   r. suture, nylon
   r., sweat
   R. Test, Benton Visual
   r. test, nitrogen
   r. toxicity
   r. uremia
   r., urinary
   r., water
retentive stabilization
retentive triangles
retest consistency, test-
retest reliability ▸ test-
rethinking the problem
**reticence in social situations ▸
   extreme**

reticular
   r. activating system
   r. cells
   r. dermis
   r. fibers of connective tissue
   r. formation, mesencephalic
   r. formation of brain stem
   r. keratitis
   r. lymphocyte
   r. nodular pattern ▸ diffuse
   r. pattern
   r. substance
reticularis, livedo
**reticulated carbon deposition ▸
   subpleural**
reticulated tissue
reticulocyte count
reticuloendothelial
   r. cell
   r. cell leukemia
   r. cell, monocytoid
   r. malignancy
   r. system
   r. system ▸ impaired
reticuloendotheliosis, leukemic
reticulohistiocytic granuloma
reticuloid dermatitis, actinic
reticulopathy, malignant
**reticulosis, midline malignant
   polymorphic**
reticulum
   r. cell
   r. cell sarcoma
   r. cell sarcoma, lymphosarcoma
   r. cell sarcoma of brain
   r. cells, plasmacytoid
   r., endoplasmic
   r., rough endoplasmic
   r., sarcoplasmic
   r., smooth endoplasmic
   r., striated
retina
   r., active hyperemia of
   r., angiomatosis of
   r., angiopathy of
   r., atrophy of
   r., blood vessels of
   r., central
   r., central vision of
   r., cholesterol in
   r., coarctate
   r., coloboma of
   r., cyanosis of
   r., cyst of
   r., detached

r., electrical activity of
r. examination
r. fatigue
r., hemangioma of
r., hemangiomatosis of
r., hemorrhage in
r., hole in
r., hyperemia of
r., infarction of
r., inferior nasal venule of
r., inferior temporal venule of
r. ▸ inflammation of
r., ischemia of
r., leopard
r., lower
r., macular deterioration of
r., malignant lymphoma of
r., medial arteriole of
r., medial venule of
r., nasal
r., nasal arteriole of
r., neuroepithelial elements of
r., nonfunctioning
r., nonspecific mottling of
r., passive hyperemia of
r., peripheral
r., periphery of
r., photocoagulation repair of
  detached
r., physiological
r. ▸ progressive deterioration of
r., reattachment of
r. ▸ recent bleeding in
r., shot-silk
r. ▸ specialized cells of
r., superior nasal venule of
r., superior temporal venule of
r., temporal
r., temporal arteriole of
r., tigroid
r., torn
r., upper
r. vascular lesion disease
r., watered-silk
r., yellow spot (YS) of

retinacular release of patella
retinae
r., ablatio
r., albedo
r., amotio
r., coloboma
r., commotio
r., cyanosis
r., dialysis
r., fovea centralis

r., ganglion
r., glioma
r., inferior, venula nasalis
r., inferior, venula temporalis
r., ischemia
r., limbus luteus
r., macula
r., macula lutea
r., ora serrata
r., ramollitio
r., rubeosis
r., sublatio
r. superior, venula nasalis
r. superior, venula temporalis
r., torpor
r., vasa sanguinea
r., vena centralis
r., venula medialis

retinal (Retinal)
r. abiotrophy
r. adaptation
r. and choroidal vessels ▸
  anastomosis of
r. aplasia
r. arterial pulsations ▸ spontaneous
r. arteries ▸ silver wiring of
r. arterioles, occlusion of
r. artery
r. artery central
r. artery, embolism of
r. artery occlusion
r. artery occlusion ▸ central
r. asthenopia
r. barrier, blood
r. bleeding
r. blood vessels
r. cautery puncture
r. cells
r. cells, bipolar
r. changes
r. commotio
r. concussion
r. cones
r. correspondence
r. correspondence (ARC) ▸
  anomalous
r. correspondence, harmonious
r. correspondence, normal
r. degeneration
r. degeneration, progressive
r. detachment
r. detachment ▸ floaters, flashes
  and
r. detachment ▸ focal
r. detachment ▸ impending

r. detachment, primary
r. detachment repair
r. detachment, rhegmatogenous
r. detachment ▸ traction
r. disease
r. disease, diabetic
r. disorder
r. disorder ▸ congenital
r. edema, Iwanoff's
r. edema, peripapillary
r. emboli
r. embolism
r. exudative changes
r. fundus photography
r., half-
r. hemorrhage
r. hemorrhages ▸ shaped
r. hole
r. infarction
r. injury
r. lesion
r. metastasis
r. necrosis, acute
r. nerves
r. pigment cell
r. pigment epithelium
r. reattachment
r. repair
r. rods
r. scarring
r. staphyloma
r. tear
r. thinning
r. tissue
R. Vascular Center
r. vascular changes
r. vasculature
r. vasculitis
r. vessel
r. vessel occlusion
r. vessels ▸ leaking

retinal vein(s)
r.v., central
r.v. distended
r.v., endophlebitis of
r.v. engorgement
r.v., nicking of
r.v. obstruction, central
r.v. occlusion
r.v. occlusion, branch

retinalis, lipemia
retinitis
r., actinic
r.,.apoplectic
r., central angiospastic

retinitis—*continued*
- r., central serous
- r., circinate
- r., Coats'
- r., cytomegalovirus
- r., diabetic
- r. disciformans
- r., exudative
- r. gravidarum
- r., gravidic
- r. haemorrhagica
- r., herpes
- r., hypertensive
- r., Jacobson's
- r., Jensen's
- r., leukemic
- r., metastatic
- r. nephritica
- r., Pick's
- r. pigmentosa syndrome
- r. proliferans
- r., proliferative
- r. punctata albescens
- r., punctate
- r., renal
- r., serous
- r., solar
- r., splenic
- r. stellate
- r., striate
- r., suppurative
- r., syphilitica
- r., uremic
- r., Wagener's

retinocerebellar angiomatosis
retinochoroiditis juxtapapillaris
retinochoroiditis, toxoplasmi
retinogram (ERG) ▸ electro◊
retinoids, synthetic
retinopathy
- r., advanced
- r., advanced proliferative diabetic
- r., arteriosclerotic
- r., background
- r., central disk-shaped
- r., central serous
- r., chloroquine
- r., circinate
- r., diabetic
- r., early diabetic
- r., exudative
- r., flecked
- r. (FFDR) ▸ full florid diabetic
- r., hypertensive
- r., hyperviscosity

- r., laser therapy of diabetic
- r., leukemic
- r., nonproliferative
- r. (NPR) ▸ nonproliferative diabetic
- r. of prematurity
- r. photocoagulation (PRP), proliferative
- r., pigmentary
- r., proliferative
- r. ▸ proliferative diabetic
- r., Purtscher's angiopathic
- r., questionable
- r., radiation
- r., talc
- r. ▸ venous stasis

retinopexy, pneumatic
Retired Persons (AARP), American Association of
Retirement Communities (CCRCs), Continuing Care
retour, rale de
retract proximally
retract true accusations
retractable fiberoptic tube
retracted
- r. anteriorly
- r., cartilage
- r., chest muscles
- r., cricoid cartilage
- r. mesially, vein ligated and
- r. nipple from breast
- r., periosteum incised and
- r., wound edges

retracting and grunting
retracting and grunting ▸ infant
retraction(s) [*refraction*]
- r., breast nipple
- r., clot
- r., eardrum
- r., eyelid
- r., grunting or
- r., infrasternal
- r., intercostal
- r., massive vitreous
- r., mild subcostal
- r., nipple
- r. nystagmus
- r. of muscles ▸ undue
- r. of nipple ▸ distortion or
- r. of vena cava
- r. or grunting
- r. pocket, attic
- r., rectus muscle
- r., regular
- r., scar

- r., sternal intercostal
- r., subcostal
- r., suprasternal
- r. syndrome
- r. syndrome, Duane
- r. test, clot
- r. time, clot
- r., vacuum

retractor ▸ Love nerve root
retraining
- r., behavioral
- r., bladder
- r. brain
- r., cognitive
- r., computerized diaphragmatic breathing
- r., mental
- r. muscles
- r. visual capacity

retreat ▸ symptoms of hesitation and
retrieval (Retrieval)
- r. and preservation ▸ organ
- r. ▸ intravascular foreign body
- r., organ
- r. problem
- r. procedure, egg
- r. process
- R. System (MEDLARS) ▸ Medical Literature Analysis and
- r., word

retrieved, donor heart
retroactive amnesia
retroactive memory falsification
retroauricular sulcus
retrobulbar
- r. block
- r. bursitis
- r. neuralgia
- r. neuritis
- r. neuritis ▸ optic or
- r. pupillary reflex

retrocardiac
- r. abnormality
- r. area
- r. reflex
- r. region
- r. space
- r. temperature

retrocaval ureter
retrocecal appendix
retrocecal hernia
retrocedent gout
retrocentral sulcus
retrocession [*retroflexion*]
retrocession of uterus

retrococcygeal air study
retrocochlear hearing loss
retroesophageal
   r. aorta
   r. arch
   r. arch, circumflex
retroflexed uterus
retroflexion [*retrocession*]
retrogasserian neurotomy
retrognathic profile
retrograde
   r. activation mapping
   r. amnesia
   r. amnesia ▸ fractional
   r. aortogram
   r. aortography
   r. arteriogram
   r. atrial activation
   r. atrial activation mapping
   r. beat
   r. block
   r. cancer
   r. cardioangiography
   r. cardioplegia, antegrade-
   r. catheterization
   r. cholangiogram
   r. cholangiogram, endoscopic
   r. cholangiopancreatography
     (ERCP), endoscopic
   r. cystogram
   r. cystourethrogram
   r. cystourethrography
   r. degeneration, transsynaptic
   r. ejaculation
   r. embolism
   r. endoscopic approach
   r. extrasystole
   r. fast pathway
   r. femoral approach
   r. filling
   r. flow of barium
   r. hernia
   r. infection
   r. menstruation
   r. metastasis
   r. P wave
   r. pancreaticobiliary ductography,
     peroral
   r. pancreaticoduodenography
   r. pancreatography, endoscopic
   r. peristalsis
   r. pyelogram (RP)
   r. pyelographic studies
   r. pyelography
   r. ureteral pyelography

   r. urethrogram (RUG)
   r. urogram
   r. urogram study
   r. urography
   r. ventriculoatrial conduction
retroiliac ureter
retrolental fibroplasia (RLF)
retrolental space
retromammary mastitis
retromandibular
   r. node aspiration
   r. node, enlarged
   r. vein
retromolar
   r. mucosa
   r. triangle
   r. trigone
retroparotid space syndrome
retropatellar fat pad
retropectoral pocket
retroperfusion, coronary sinus
retroperitoneal
   r. adenopathy
   r. adhesions
   r. air study
   r. fibrosis
   r. gas insufflation
   r. hemorrhage
   r. hernia
   r. involvement, massive
   r. liver and lung metastasis
   r. lymph node biopsies, selected
   r. lymph nodes
   r. mass
   r. metastasis
   r. node
   r. node dissection, radical
   r. pneumography
   r. pneumoradiography
   r. rhabdomyosarcoma
   r. seminoma
   r. space
   r. space entered
   r. subphrenic metastasis
   r. tumor
retroperitoneum closed
retroperitoneum irrigated
retropharyngeal
   r. abscess
   r. lymph node
   r. space
retropubic
   r. placement
   r. prevesical prostatectomy
   r. prostatectomy

   r. prostatectomy, nerve sparing
     radical
   r. surgery
retropulsion of nail
retroscopic lens
retrospect, historical
retrospective
   r. analysis
   r. diagnosis
   r. falsification
   r. study
   r. surveillance
   r. survey
retrosternal
   r. abnormality
   r. burning sensation
   r. bypass coloplasty ▸ one-stage
   r. chest pain
   r. free space
   r. hematoma
   r. hernia
   r. nodule
   r. pain
   r. pain, sharp
   r. procedure
   r. thyroid
retrotarsal fold
retrotracheal adenoma
retrotracheal space
retrotuberous mucosa
retrourethral catheterization
retrouterine hematocele
retrouterine hematoma
retrovaginal hernia
retrovaginal septum
retroverted uterus
retroviral
   r. infection
   r. particle, human intracisternal A
     type
   r. syndrome, acute
   r. treatment
   r. vaccine
retrovirus
   r., benign
   r., human
   r., mouse
   r. (PERV) ▸ porcine endogenous
retrusive excursion
retrusive occlusion
Rett syndrome
rettgeri, Proteus
rettgeri, Providencia
return
   r., anomalous pulmonary venous

return—*continued*

r. anomaly ▸ pediatric venous
r. anomaly ▸ pulmonary venous
r. as outpatient
r. curve ▸ venous
r. extrasystole
r. flow
r. flow hemostatic catheter
r. for suture removal
r., nonfunctional
r. of appetite
r. of function
r. of sensation and function
r. (PAPVR), partial anomalous pulmonary venous
r., positional
r. ▸ pulmonary venous
r. ▸ rattle of
r. red blood cells to donor
r., resistance to venous
r. ▸ systemic venous
r. to heart, decreased venous
r. to heart ▸ venous
r. ▸ total anomalous pulmonary venous
r., venous

returned

r. to abdomen, cecum
r. to donor ▸ red blood cells
r. to extremity, function
r. to room, patient

returning cycle
retusis, Trichodectes
Retzius(')

R. abscess ▸ space of
R., gyrus olfactorius lateralis of
R., gyrus olfactorius medialis of
R. parallel striae
R., space of
R. veins

Reusner's sign
Reuss's color charts
Reuss's tables
Reuter button
revascularization

r. assessment
r., coronary
r., direct
r., direct myocardial
r., elective myocardial
r., genetic
r. ▸ heart laser
r., laser
r., myocardial
r. of blood vessels of heart

r., percutaneous
r. (PMR) ▸ percutaneous myocardial
r. (PTCR) ▸ percutaneous transluminal coronary
r. ▸ percutaneous transmyocardial
r., postischemic
r., postoperative coronary
r. procedure
r. procedure, cardiac
r. procedure ▸ surgical
r., repeat
r. syndrome ▸ pulmonary insufficiency
r. (TMR) ▸ transmyocardial

revascularize heart muscle
revealed

r. decreased expansion ▸ lungs
r. diminished breath sounds ▸ lungs
r. hyperresonance to percussion ▸ lungs
r. microaneurysms, funduscopic examination

reveals increased activity ▸ bone scan
reveil, cataplexies du
revenge, desires
revenge, Montezuma's
reverberation artifact
reverberation, echo
Reverdin graft
Reverdin's operation
reverie imagery
reverie, reflective
reversal(s)

r., habit
r., instrumental phase
r., lead
r., narcotic
r. of cervical curve
r. of lumbar curve
r., periodic
r., phase
r. stimulation, pattern
r., sudden role
r., temperature
r. time
r., true phase
r., tubal

reverse

r. augmentation
r. complication of diabetes ▸ prevent, stop or
r. coronary disease
r. exercise-induced asthma

r. flow
r. heart disease
r. heart failure
r. isolation
r. osmosis (RO)
r. psychology
r. saphenous vein
r. saphenous vein bypass ▸ renal artery
r. -shape implant
r. tolerance
r. transcriptase
r. transcriptase inhibitors ▸ nucleoside
r. transcriptase polymerase chain reaction test
r. transcriptase ▸ ribonucleic acid (RNA)

reversed

r. arm leads
r. bypass
r. coarctation
r. ductus arteriosus
r. emotions
r. paradoxical pulse
r. peristalsis
r. reciprocal rhythm
r. rhythm
r. saphenous vein graft
r. shunt

reversible

r. aggregation of cells
r. anemia
r. asthma ▸ poorly
r. brain syndrome
r. bronchospasm
r. condition
r. ischemia
r. ischemic neurologic defect
r. myocardial dysfunction
r. obstructive airway disease
r. oppositional movements
r. reaction
r. symptoms

reversing plaque buildup
reversion pacemaker, Pasar tachycardia
reversionary atrophy
reverted to normal position ▸ scope
reverting scope
review (Review)

r., antibiotic utilization
r., arrhythmic
R. Board (IRB), Institutional
r., critical incident

r., episodic
r. mechanisms ▸ utilization and quality
r., medical
r., medication
r., peer
r., periodic
r., precertification
r. program, peer
r. program, utilization
r., system
R. System (PAIRS) program ▸ Psychiatric Alcohol Inpatient
r., treatment plan
r., utilization
reviewing physician
revised, wound margins
revision
r. and debridement
r. (FSR), fusiform skin
r. hip replacement surgery
r. of amputation stump
r. of in-flow
r. of out-flow
r., plastic
r., proximal
r., scar
r., scar tissue
r., surgical
r., W-plasty
r., Z-plasty
revitalization, skin
revitalize hair growth
revival techniques
revolutions per minute (rpm)
revolutum, Echinostoma
Rey Auditory Verbal Learning Test
Reya lamp, Finsen-
Reye's syndrome
Reye's syndrome from aspirin
RF (rheumatic fever)
RF wave
RFA (radiofrequency ablation)
RFA (right frontoanterior)
RFI (radiofrequency interference)
RFLP (restriction fragment length polymorphisms)
RFP (right frontoposterior)
RFT (right frontotransverse)
RFU (Reitland-Franklin unit)
RGP (rigid gas permeable) contact lenses
Rh (Rhesus)
Rh agglutinin
Rh agglutinin, anti-

Rh antibody titer
Rh blood factor
Rh blood group
Rh factor
Rh factor antigen
Rh factor negative
Rh factor positive
Rh immune globulin
Rh immunization
Rh incompatibility ▸ parental
Rh isoimmunization
Rh isosensitization
Rh negative (Rh-)
Rh negative (Rh-) blood
Rh negative (Rh-) factor
Rh negative (Rh-) ▸ patient
Rh positive (Rh+)
Rh positive (Rh+) blood
Rh positive (Rh+) factor
Rh positive fetal blood
Rh positive fetal blood cells
Rh positive (Rh+) ▸ patient
Rh sensitization
Rh$_0$ (D antigen) immune globulin
Rhabditis pellio
rhabdoid
r. suture
r. /teratoid tumor, atypical
r. tumor, atypical
rhabdomyolysis
r., arterial
r., exertional
r., hypokalemic
r. ▸ nonocclusive arterial
r., nontraumatic
r. ▸ nontraumatic arterial
r., traumatic
r. with myoglobinuria
rhabdomyolytic
r. myoglobinuria
r. process
r. syndrome
rhabdomyoma of tongue
rhabdomyosarcoma
r., alveolar
r., embryonal
r. of extremities
r. of head and neck
r. of orbit
r. of pelvis
r. of prostate
r. of soft tissue
r. of urinary bladder
r. of vagina
r. orbital tumor

r., parameningeal
r., paratesticular
r., retroperitoneal
rhabdosarcoma, renal
rhagiocrine vacuole
rhaphe (*see* raphe)
RHD (rheumatic heart disease)
rhegmatogenous detachment
rhegmatogenous retinal detachment
Rheinberg microscope
Rhein's picks
rheography (LRR), light reflection
rheologic
r. change
r. study
r. therapy
Rhesus (*see also* Rh)
R. (Rh) factor antigen
R. (Rh) immunization
R. (Rh) incompatibility ▸ parental
R. monkey
rheumatic
r. aortitis
r. arteritis
r. arthritis, acute
r. atrophy
r. carditis
r. chorea
r. contraction
r. diet
r. disease
r. diseases ▸ progressive
r. endocarditis
r. fever
r. fever, acute
r. fever, treatment of
r. gout
r. granulomas
r. heart disease (RHD)
r. mitral insufficiency
r. mitral valve stenosis
r. myocarditis
r. nodules
r. pericarditis
r. pneumonia
r. scoliosis
r. symptoms ▸ multiple
r. tetany
r. valvular disease
r. valvulitis
r. valvulitis, healed
rheumatica
r., angina
r. (PMR) ▸ polymyalgia
r., purpura

rheumatism
r., Besnier's
r., desert
r., Heberden's
r., MacLeod's capsular
r., muscular
r. of heart
r., palindromic
r., Poncet's
r., psychogenic
r., soft tissue
rheumatoid
r. and degenerative arthritis ▸ mixed
r. arteritis
r. arthritic, patient
r. arthritis (RA)
r. arthritis (RA) cell
r. arthritis (RA), debilitating
r. arthritis (RA) factor
r. arthritis (RA) ▸ inflammatory
r. arthritis (RA), joint
r. arthritis (JRA) ▸ juvenile
r. arthritis (RA) latex fixation test
r. arthritis ▸ total lymphoid irradiation in
r. factor
r. factor, latex
r. factor test
r. lung
r. lung disease
r. myositis
r. pains
r. pneumoconiosis
r. spondylitis
r. synovitis
rheumatology, adolescent
rheumatology, pediatric
rhexis, hemorrhage per
rhinaria, Linguatula
rhinitis
r., allergic
r., anaphylactic
r., atrophic
r. caseosa
r., catarrhal
r., chronic
r., congestive seasonal allergic
r., croupous
r., dyscrinic
r., fibrinous
r., gangrenous
r., hypertrophic
r., membranous
r. ▸ nonseasonal allergic

r., perennial allergic
r., pollinotic
r., pseudomembranous
r., purulent
r., rebound
r., scrofulous
r., seasonal allergic
r. sicca
r., syphilitic
r., tuberculous
r., vasomotor
rhinocerebral infection
Rhinocladium fungi
rhinogenous headache
rhinolalia aperta
rhinolalia, clausa
rhinoplasty
r., Carpue's
r., dactylocostal
r., English
r., Indian
r., Italian
r., orthoplastic
r., osteoplastic
r., standard reduction
r. (SMRR), submucous resection and
r., tagliacotian
rhinorrhea
r., cerebrospinal
r., ipsilateral
r., prandial
r., spinal fluid
rhinoscleroma bacillus
rhinoscleroma lacrimal sac
rhinoscleromatis, Klebsiella
rhinoseptoplasty procedure
rhinosinusitis, acute
Rhinosporidium seeberi
rhinoviral colds
rhinoviral respiratory infection
rhinovirus inhibitor
rhizomelic spondylosis
rhizopodiformis, Mucor
Rhizopus
R. equinus
R. niger
R. nigricans
R. oryzae
rhizotomy
r., anterior
r., dorsal nerve root
r., percutaneous
r., trigeminal
r., ventral nerve root

RHL (rump heel length)
rhm (roentgens per hour at one meter)
rhodesiense, Trypanosoma
Rhodotorula glutinis
Rhodotorula rubra
RhoGAM
R. antepartum
R. cross-match
R. injection
R. test
R. vaccine
rhomboid
r. ligament
r., Michaelis'
r. muscle, greater
r. muscle, lesser
rhonchorous cough
rhonchus(-i)
r. and rales
r., audible
r., bilateral
r., coarse
r., diffuse
r., expiratory
r., inspiratory
r., rales and
r., scattered
r., scattered coarse
r., sibilant
r., sonorous
Rhone-Poulencmitral ring prosthesis ▸ Carpentier-
Rhus
R. diversiloba
R. toxicodendron
R. venenata
rhusiopathiae, Actinomyces
rhusiopathiae, Erysipelothrix
rhythm(s)
r., abnormal cardiac
r., abnormal heart
r., abnormality
r., abnormality, heart
r. abnormality ▸ life-threatening heart
r., abnormally slow
r., accelerated atrioventricular (AV) junctional
r., accelerated idionodal
r., accelerated idioventricular
r., accelerated intraventricular
r., accelerated junctional
r., accelerated ventricular
r. after cardiac surgery ▸ junctional

r., agonal
r., alpha
r., alphoid
r., alternate with alpha
r., analogous
r. and tone
r., arceau
r. ▸ (AV) arteriovenous junctional
r., atrial
r., atrioventricular (AV)
r., atrioventricular (AV) junctional
r., atrioventricular (AV) junctional escape
r., atrioventricular (AV) nodal
r., auriculoventricular
r., AV (atrioventricular) nodal
r., baseline
r., basic occipital
r., basic optional
r., Berger
r., beta
r., bigeminal
r., bio◇
r., biological
r., blocking of electroencephalo-gram (EEG)
r., body
r., brain resets
r., cantering
r., cardiac
r., change in heart
r. change ▸ sudden
r., chaotic
r. ▸ chaotic heart
r. ▸ chaotic useless
r., characteristic
r., circadian
r., circadian biological
r., circus
r., comb
r., concealed
r., converted
r., coordinated
r., coronary nodal
r., coronary sinus
r., coupled
r., decelerate breathing
r., delta
r. disorder ▸ benign
r. disorder, life-threatening
r. ▸ disorder of heartbeat
r. disorder, severe
r., disrupted
r., disturbance
r. disturbance ▸ controlled heart

r. disturbance ▸ fatal heart
r. disturbance, heart
r., disturbance in cardiac
r., disturbance, increased
r., disturbance, life-threatening
r. disturbance syndrome circadian
r., diurnal
r. drug ▸ heart
r., ectopic
r., electroencephalogram (EEG)
r., embryocardia
r. en arceau
r., erratic heart
r., escape
r., fast alpha variant
r., fatal heart
r. ▸ faulty heart
r., fetal
r., fibrillation
r. (F and R), force and
r., frequency of
r., frontocentral beta
r., gallop
r., gamma
r., heart
r., heart's electrical
r., idiojunctional
r., idionodal
r., idioventricular
r., infradian
r., intermixed with alpha
r., irregular
r., irregular heart
r. ▸ irregular heartbeat
r. ▸ irregularly irregular
r., isochronal
r., junctional
r. ▸ junctional escape
r., kappa
r. ▸ lethal heart
r. ▸ life-threatening heart
r. ▸ lower nodal
r. method
r., metachronal
r., midnodal
r., mixed
r., mu/μ
r., nodal
r. ▸ nodal escape
r., nonparoxysmal nodal
r., normal alpha
r., normal atrial
r. ▸ normal heart
r. (NSR) ▸ normal sinus
r. ▸ normal sinus heart

r., nycthemeral
r. of alpha frequency
r. of heart ▸ normal
r., paced
r., paroxysmal nodal
r. ▸ patient shocked back into normal
r., pendulum
r., physiologic electroencephalogram (EEG)
r. problems ▸ heart
r. ▸ pulsed idioventricular
r. ▸ pulseless idioventricular
r., quadrigeminal
r., quadruple
r., racing heart
r., rapid
r. ▸ rapid heart
r., reactivity of mu/μ
r., reassessment of cardiac
r. ▸ reboot faulty heart's normal
r., reciprocal
r., reciprocating
r., reentrant
r., regular
r. regular, heart
r. regular (RRR) ▸ rate and
r. (RSR), regular sinus
r. ▸ regularly irregular
r. regulation ▸ heart
r., resumption of normal sinus
r., reversed
r. ▸ reversed reciprocal
r. (SMR) ▸ sensorimotor
r., shock heart into normal
r., sigma/σ
r., sinoatrial
r., sinoventricular
r., sinus
r., sinus cardiac
r., six and 14 spike
r. sleep disorder ▸ circadian
r. ▸ slow escape
r. ▸ slow heart
r. ▸ slow, steady
r. ▸ speaks in staccato
r., spike-and-slow wave
r., steady alpha
r. strip
r., supraventricular
r., systolic gallop
r., theta
r. ▸ tic-tac
r., trainwheel
r., trigeminal

rhythm(s)—*continued*
- r., triple
- r., ultradian
- r., variable frontocentral beta
- r., ventricular
- r., ventricular paced
- r., vital
- r., waking by
- r., wicket
- r. ▸ wide complex

rhythmic
- r. activity
- r. activity, burst of
- r. activity, wave lengths of
- r. beta
- r. chorea
- r. compression
- r. compression of chest
- r. contractions
- r. cramping
- r. delta activity, frontal intermittent
- r. delta activity, frontal irregular
- r. delta activity, occipital intermittent
- r. electroencephalogram (EEG) activity
- r. exercise
- r. eye movement ▸ abnormal
- r. frequency, basic
- r. horizontal oscillation of eyeballs
- r. instability of head and trunk
- r. irregularities ▸ lethal
- r. jerking movements
- r. limb movements, uncontrolled
- r. movement disorder
- r. muscular contractions
- r. opposition
- r. oscillation, involuntary
- r. pattern sinoatrial (SA) node
- r. pressure
- r. relaxation
- r. shaking of part of body
- r. stimuli
- r. temporal theta burst of drowsiness
- r. trembling
- r. tremor
- r. vertical oscillation of eyeballs
- r. wave frequencies
- r. waves
- r. waxing and waning

rhythmical
- r. breathing
- r. delta activity (OIRDA), occipital intermittent

- r. tremor

rhytidectomy, facial
rhytidectomy procedure
RI (refractive index)
RI (respiratory illness)
RIA (radioimmunoassay)
RIAH (radioimmunoassay of hair)
rib(s)
- r., abdominal
- r. apart, spread
- r., arch of
- r., asternal
- r., bicipital
- r. bones
- r., broken
- r. cage
- r. cage ▸ inflammation of cartilage of
- r. cage intact
- r. cage ▸ splaying open
- r., cervical
- r., component
- r., contiguous
- r. destruction
- r. detail
- r., false
- r. field treatment
- r., first
- r., floating
- r. formation, cervical
- r., fractured
- r. fractures, multiple
- r., gummas of
- r. ▸ hairline fracture of
- r. incision ▸ smaller
- r., inflammation of breastbone and
- r., inner surface of
- r. involvement
- r. lesion
- r., levator muscles of
- r., long levator muscles of
- r. margin
- r., neoplastic destruction of
- r. notches
- r. notching
- r. ▸ osteoblastic metastases in
- r., regenerated
- r. resection
- r. retractor
- r. separations
- r. shears
- r., short levator muscles of
- r., slipping
- r. spreader
- r. spreader inserted

- r. spreaders enlarged wound
- r., sternal
- r. subperiosteally resected
- r., supernumerary
- r., supernumerary cervical
- r. syndrome, cervical
- r. syndrome, costoclavicular
- r. syndrome, slipping
- r. taken, bites of
- r. tenderness
- r. therapy, slipping
- r. thoracic syndrome, anomalous first
- r., true
- r., upper edge of
- r., vertebral
- r., vertebrocostal
- r., vertebrosternal
- r., Zahn's

ribbon
- r. arch
- r. gut
- r. -like keratitis
- r. -like stools ▸ soft and
- r. muscles
- r., safety
- r. shaped stools
- r. worm

Ribes' bag, Champetier de
Ribes' ganglion
riboflavin deficiency
ribonuclear protein (RNP)
ribonucleic
- r. acid (RNA)
- r. acid (DNA) ▸ deoxy◇
- r. acid (RNA) dependent DNA (deoxyribonucleic acid) polymerase
- r. acid (mRNA), messenger
- r. acid (RNA) reverse transcriptase
- r. acid (RNA) ▸ soluble
- r. acid (RNA) virus

riboside (FUR) ▸ fluorouracil
riboside, methylmercaptopurine
ribosomal subunits
ribosome, bacterial
Ricard's amputation
RICE (Rest, Ice, Compression, Elevation)
rice
- r. bodies
- r. diet
- r. water stool

rich (Rich)
- r. blood, oxygen-

r. blood ▸ starved for oxygen-
r. plaque ▸ lipid-
r. plasma, platelet-
R. syndrome, Hamman-
r. tissue ▸ vascular
Richards operation, King-
Richardson
R. hysterectomy, Spaulding-
R. operation, Spalding-
R. operation, Williams-
R. technique
R. technique, modified
Richart and VCE (vaginal, cervical,
endocervical) Pap (Papanicolaou)
smears
Richart Pap (Papanicolaou) smear
Richet's aneurysm
Richet's operation
Richter hernia, Littre-
richteri, Solenopsis saevissima
Richter's hernia
Ricinus communis
ricinus, Ixodes
rickets, renal
rickets ▸ vitamin D resistant
Rickett's organism
Rickettsia
R. akamushi
R. akari
R. australis
R. conorii
R. diaporica
R. mooseri
R. muricola
R. nipponica
R. orientalis
R. pediculi
R. prowazekii
R. quintana
R. rickettsii
R. tsutsugamushi
R. typhi
R. wolhynica
Rickettsial (rickettsial)
R. disorder
R. infection
r. myocarditis
r. pneumonia
rickettsii, Rickettsia
ridden, patient bed◊
Riddoch's mass reflex
Riddoch's syndrome
rider's
r. bone
r. muscles

r. sprain
r. tendon
ridge(s) [*bridge*]
r., alveolar
r., basal
r. -count (TRC) ▸ total
r. extension
r., facial
r., interureteric
r., mandibular
r., marginal
r., maxillary
r., nasal
r., oblique
r., orbital
r., Outerbridge's
r., petrous
r., pubic
r., rete
r. sign ▸ trapezius
r., sphenoid
r., tranverse
r., triangular
r., ureteral
r., ureteric
r., vomerine
ridged, fingernails horizontally
ridged, fingernails vertically
ridging
r., arthritic
r. of nails ▸ horizontal
r. of nails ▸ vertical
ridiculed ▸ patient feels rejected or
riding breech deformity
riding embolus
Ridley implant cataract lens
Ridley's sinus
Ridlon's operation
Riedel('s)
R. disease
R. lobe
R. needle
R. struma
R. thyroiditis
Rieder cell leukemia
Rieder's cell
Riegel's pulse
Riegel's test meal
Rieger's syndrome
Riesman's myocardosis
Riesman's pneumonia
Ries-Wertheim hysterectomy
Ries-Wertheim operation
Rieux's hernia
RIF (right iliac fossa)

Rifkind's sign
Rift Valley fever virus
right(s)
r. acetabular region
r. activists, disability
r. advocated, disability
r. and left heart syndrome ▸
hypoblastic
r. angle chest tube
r. angle clip, Braun-Yasargil
r. -angle lens
r. -angle mattress suture
r. -angle telescope
r. ankle full range of motion (ROM)
r. antecubital fossa
r. anterior aortic cusp
r. anterior chest wall
r. anterior oblique (RAO)
r. anterior oblique (RAO) angulation
r. anterior oblique (RAO) equivalent
r. anterior oblique (RAO) position
r. anterior oblique (RAO) projection
r. anterior oblique (RAO) view
r. aortic arch
r. apex clear to percussion
r. arm
r. arm electrode
r. arm ▸ hemiparesis
r. arm recumbent
r. ascending colon ▸ Dukes C
classification of
r. atrial (RA)
r. atrial (RA) abnormality
r. atrial (RA) appendage
r. atrial (RA) appendage
electrogram
r. atrial (RA) communication
murmur ▸ left ventricular (LV)-
r. atrial (RA) dimension
r. atrial (RA) electrogram ▸ low
septal
r. atrial enlargement (RAE)
r. atrial hypertrophy (RAH)
r. atrial (RA) myxoma
r. atrial pressure (RAP)
r. atrial pressure (MRAP) ▸ mean
r. atrial (RA) thrombus
r. atrium (RA)
r. atrium ▸ catheter stimulation of
r. atrium, contraction of
r. atrium, emptying of
r. atrium, filling of
r. atrium (RA) ▸ high
r. atrium of heart
r. axillary area

right(s)—*continued*

r. axis deviation
r. axis deviation (ARAD), abnormal
r. base, effusion
r. base, fluid
r. base, fluid density in
r. brachiocephalic vein
r. breast does appear enlarged ▸ lump in
r. breast does not appear enlarged ▸ lump in
r. bronchial tree
r. bronchus
r. bundle branch
r. bundle branch block (RBBB)
r. bundle branch block (RBBB) ▸ complete
r. bundle branch block (RBBB) ▸ incomplete
r. buttock ▸ incision and drainage (I and D) of
r. cardiac catheterization
r. carotid aortic dissection
r. carotid artery ▸ occlusion of
r. carotid endarterectomy
r. cataract surgery
r. central cortical area
r. cerebral hemisphere
r. chest opacity
r. circumflex coronary artery (RCA)
r. colic lymph nodes
r. colic vein
r. collecting system, duplication of
r. common carotid artery
r. coronary angiogram (RCA)
r. coronary artery
r. coronary artery angiography
r. coronary artery ▸ severe stenosis
r. coronary cineangiography
r. coronary trunk ▸ complete occlusion of
r. costal margin
r. decubitus position
r. deltoid
r., deviation to the
r. diaphragm
r. discrimination, impaired
r. dorsoanterior
r. dorsoposterior
r. ear (AD)
r. elbow full range of motion (ROM)
r. endobronchial tree
r. esotropia
r. exotropia
r. external canthus, left-

r. eye, deorsumduction of
r. eye, dextroduction of
r. eye, evisceration
r. eye ▸ flapping of conjunctiva,
r. eye ▸ herpes virus of
r. eye, levoduction of
r. eye, postsurgical aphakia
r. eye, sursumduction of
r. eye (TOD) ▸ tension of
r. eye (VOD) ▸ vision,
r. eye, visual acuity
r. facial weakness
r. femoral artery
r. femur
r. flexure of colon
r. flow tract
r. frontal dysfunction
r. frontal hematoma
r. frontal slowing spikes
r. frontoanterior
r. frontoposterior
r. frontotransverse
r. gastric lymph nodes
r. gastric vein
r. gastroepiploic vein
r. gluteal
r. -handed
r. -handed individual
r. -handed, patient
r. handedness
r. heart
r. heart bypass
r. heart catheterization
r. heart failure
r. heart strain
r. hemicolectomy
r. hemiparesis and aphasia
r. hemisphere
r. hemisphere deficit
r. hemisphere of brain
r. hemisphere of brain ▸ dysplastic
r. hemispheric parietal damage
r. hemothorax
r. hemothorax, spontaneous
r. hepatic lobe
r. heterotropia
r. hilar lymph node
r. hilum
r. hilum prominence of
r. hip prosthesis
r. hippocampal
r. hydronephrosis
r. hyperphoria
r. hypertrophia

r. hypochondriac region of abdomen
r. iliac fossa (RIF)
r. iliac region of abdomen
r. inferior pulmonary vein
r. inguinal region of abdomen
r. inner canthus
r. innominate artery
r. internal jugular vein
r. internal mammary artery
r. iris, postoperative coloboma
r. kidney
r. kidney, duplication of
r. kidney, scar lower pole
r. knee full range of motion (ROM)
r. lateral
r. lateral bending
r. lateral position
r. lateral projection, stereo
r. lateral region of abdomen
r. lateral thorax
r. leg
r. leg electrode
r. leg, hypesthesia of
r. lower extremity (RLE)
r. lower extremity (RLE) amputated
r. lower extremity (RLE) flexed
r. lower extremity full range of motion (ROM)
r. lower extremity, patient drags
r. lower lobe (RLL)
r. lower lobe (RLL) bronchial orifice
r. lower lobe (RLL) infiltrate
r. lower lobe (RLL) lesion
r. lower lobe (RLL) of lung
r. lower lobe (RLL) partial collapse
r. lower quadrant (RLQ)
r. lower quadrant (RLQ) of abdomen
r. lumbar region of abdomen
r. lung (RL)
r. lung, adenocarcinoma
r. lung ▸ apex of
r. lung base
r. lung base, atelectasis
r. lung ▸ diaphragmatic surface of
r. lung ▸ dullness over
r. lung ▸ inferior margin of
r. lung infiltrate
r. lung ▸ lower lobe of the
r. lung ▸ middle lobe of
r. lung ▸ sternal margin of
r. lung ▸ upper lobe of
r. main coronary artery
r. main pulmonary artery

r. main stem bronchus
r. major hand
r. mastectomy, radical
r., maternal
r., mediastinal shift to the
r. mediolateral episiotomy
r. mentoanterior
r. mentoposterior
r. mentotransverse
r. middle lobe (RML)
r. middle lobe (RML) bronchial orifice
r. middle lobe (RML) of lung
r. middle lobe (RM) syndrome
r. ▸ moderate nystagmus on gaze to
r., moderate shift to the
r. motor function waxed and waned
r. occipitoanterior
r. occipitoposterior
r. occipitotransverse
r. of others ▸ disregard
r. of others ▸ violates
r. outer canthus
r. ovarian vein
r. ovary atrophic
r. parasternal impulses
r. parietal dysfunction
r. parietal stroke, evolving
r., patient
r. pleural rub
r. pleural sac
r. pleuritic chest pain
r. pneumothorax
r. posterior cerebral artery
r. posterior oblique (RPO)
r. prefrontal cortex
r. primary bronchus
r. pubic ramus
r. pulmonary artery
r. pulmonary artery syndrome, epibronchial
r. pulmonary vein transplant
r. pulmonary veins
r. radical pneumonectomy
r. renal pelvis
r., rotated to
r. sacroanterior
r. sacroposterior
r. sacrotransverse
r. scapuloanterior
r. scapuloposterior
r. sciatic radiation
r., scoliosis with convexity to

r. serosanguinous pleural effusion ▸ bilateral and
r., shift to
r. shoulder full range of motion (ROM)
r. shunt ▸ left-to-
r. side
r. side of body
r. side of brain
r. side of head
r. -sided
r. -sided endocarditis
r. -sided facial droop
r. -sided filling pressures
r. -sided heart failure
r. -sided subclavian catheter
r. -sided weakness
r. stem bonchus
r. sternal border (RSB)
r. subclavian artery
r. subclavian artery, aberrant
r. subclavian vein (RSV)
r. subclavian vein dialysis catheter
r. subcostal area
r. submaxillary salivary gland
r. superior intercostal vein
r. superior pulmonary vein
r. suprarenal vein
r. temporal lobe focus
r. testicular vein
r. thalamus
r. thigh
r. thoracostomy
r. thoracotomy
r. to be assisted to die
r. to die
r. to refuse intervention
r. to reject medical treatment
r. -to-die movement
r. -to-left shunt
r., trachea shifted to
r. upper extremity (RUE)
r. upper extremity (RUE) amputated
r. upper extremity (RUE) flexed
r. upper extremity full range of motion (ROM)
r. upper lobe (RUL)
r. upper lobe (RUL) bronchial orifice
r. upper lobe (RUL) lesion
r. upper lobe (RUL) of lung
r. upper lobe (RUL) pneumonia
r. upper quadrant (RUQ)
r. upper quadrant (RUQ) of abdomen

r. upper quadrant (RUQ) tenderness
r. ureter
r. ureteral calculus
r. ventricle (RV)
r. ventricle (RV), contraction
r. ventricle (RV), double-outlet
r. ventricle (RV) ▸ hypoplasia of
r. ventricle (RV) malposition ▸ double outlet
r. ventricle (RV) of heart
r. ventricle (RV) ▸ septal papillary muscle of
r. ventricular (RV) apex
r. ventricular (RV) apex electrogram
r. ventricular (RV) assist-device
r. ventricular (RV) cardiomyopathy
r. ventricular (RV) conduction defect
r. ventricular (RV) contraction
r. ventricular (RV) decompensation
r. ventricular (RV) diastolic collapse
r. ventricular (RV) diastolic pressure
r. ventricular (RV) dimension
r. ventricular (RV) disease
r. ventricular (RV) dysplasia
r. ventricular (RV) dysplasia ▸ arrhythmogenic
r. ventricular (RV) ejection fraction
r. ventricular ejection time (RVET)
r. ventricular end-diastolic pressure (RVEDP)
r. ventricular end-diastolic volume (RVEDV)
r. ventricular enlargement (RVE)
r. ventricular (RV) failure
r. ventricular (RV) fistula, coronary artery
r. ventricular (RV) fullness ▸ borderline
r. ventricular (RV) function
r. ventricular (RV) heart failure ▸ acute
r. ventricular (RV) heave
r. ventricular hypertrophy (RVH)
r. ventricular (RV) hypoplasia
r. ventricular (RV) infarction
r. ventricular (RV) inflow obstruction
r. ventricular (RV) injection
r. ventricular mean (RVM)
r. ventricular (RV) myxoma

right(s)—*continued*
r. ventricular (RV) outflow
  obstruction
r. ventricular (RV) outflow tract
r. ventricular (RV) outflow tract
  tachycardia
r. ventricular pressure (MRVP) ▸
  mean
r. ventricular (RV) study
r. ventricular (RV) systolic pressure
r. ventricular (RV) systolic time
  interval
r. ventricular (RV) wall
r. ventricular (RV) wall motion
r. wave-spike ▸ parietal area
r. wrist full range of motion (ROM)
righteous avenger
righteous ▸ patient self-
righting reflex
righting reflexes ▸ postural
rightward axis
rigid
r., abdomen
r. and stooped
r., back
r. bronchoscopy
r. chest
r. gas permeable (RGP) contact
  lenses
r. hymen
r. in thinking
r. limb
r., morally
r. muscles
r., nonresponsive and mute ▸
  patient
r. paralysis
r. position, dorsal
r. posture
r. puncture resistant container
r. sigmoidoscopy
r. treatment program
rigidity
r., abdominal
r., abdominal musculature
r., anatomical
r. and tremor ▸ muscle
r. and/or guarding
r., board-like
r., cadaveric
r., cerebellar
r., cervix uteri
r., clasp-knife
r., cogwheel
r., decerebrate

r., diffuse muscular
r., diminish tremor and
r., disabling
r., effect of emotional stress on
r., emotional
r., guarding and/or
r., hemiplegic
r., increased
r., lead pipe
r., muscle
r., muscular
r., mydriatic
r., nuchal
r. of abdomen ▸ board-like
r. of paralyzed limb
r. or rebound ▸ guarding,
r., pathologic
r. ▸ poor balance, tremor,
  weakness and
r., postmortem
r., progressive
r. ▸ rebound, guarding or
r., severe postmortem
r., spasm or tenderness
r., spasmodic
r., spastic
r., tenderness and
r. ▸ tremor, bradykinesia and
r., wax-like
rigidly extended, legs
rigidus, hallux
rigor(s)
r., calcium
r. ▸ dyspnea, cough and
r. mortis
r. mortis ▸ myocardial
r. nervorum
r. tremens
rigorous analysis ▸ standard
  procedure of
rigorous conditioning
Riley-Day syndrome
Riley-Shwachman syndrome
RIM (rim)
R. (reflection interference
  microscopy)
r., atrioventricular (AV)
r., helical
r., intact outer
r., intercartilaginous
r., lateral orbital
r., mitral
r. of cytoplasm, narrow
r., orbital
r., periosteum of orbital

r., scleral
r. sign
Rindfleisch's cell
Rindfleisch's folds
ring(s)
r. abscess
r. and leaflets ▸ valve
r. annuloplasty ▸ prosthetic
r., aortic
r. apophysis
r., atrial
r., atrioventricular (AV)
r., beta lactam
r. bodies, Cabot's
r., Bonaccolto's scleral
r. calcification ▸ napkin
r., Cannon's
r., Carpentier
r., cartilage
r. cataract, Soemmering's
r. cell carcinoma, signet-
r. cells, signet
r., Coats'
r., common tendinous
r. complex ▸ sling
r., corneal
r., coronary
r. defect, napkin-
r. division ▸ vascular
r. ▸ drowsiness from insect
r. ▸ Duran annuloplasty
r. dysphagia, contractile
r. electrode
r. ▸ esophageal A-
r. ▸ esophageal B-
r., esophageal contraction
r., external inguinal
r., Falope
r. finger
r., first cartilaginous
r., Fleischer
r., Flieringa scleral
r. forceps ▸ bleeding controlled with
r. fracture
r. graft
r., hymenal
r. in eyes ▸ implantable
r. incised, cartilaginous
r., inflatable comfort
r., inguinal
r., internal inguinal
r., Kayser-Fleischer
r. ▸ knitted sewing
r., Landolt's broken
r. loop ▸ sewing

r., Löwe's
r. marker ▸ vein graft
r., Maxwell's
r. ▸ metal sewing
r., mitral valve
r., muscular
r., Ochsner's
r. of bone
r. of bone concept
r. of hemoglobin, peripheral
r. opacity, Caspar's
r., orbicular
r., pale unstained
r. pessary
r. ▸ plastic sewing
r., pleural
r. prosthesis, Carpentier
  annuloplasty
r. prosthesis, Carpentier-Rhone-
  Poulencmitral
r. ▸ prosthetic valve sewing
r., rust
r., Schatzki's esophageal
r. scotoma
r., second cartilaginous
r., semicircular
r., sewing
r. shadow
r. -shaped rash ▸ red,
r. sign
r., Soemmering's
r. ▸ St. Jude annuloplasty
r. stage
r. stenosis ▸ napkin
r. stratification
r., tantalum
r. test, milk
r., thiazole
r., third cartilaginous
r., tracheal
r. tripolar lead ▸ segmented
r., tubal
r., vaginal
r., valve
r., vascular
r., Vossius' lenticular
r., Waldeyer's
r. -wall lesion
r., Yoon

Ringer('s)
R. lactate solution
R. lactate stain
R. phosphate, Krebs-
R. solution, lactated
ringeri, Distoma

ringeri, Paragonimus
ringing
r. in affected ear
r. in ear ▸ low pitched
r. in ears
r. noise
r. sound
r. sound in ears
ringworm, blister from
Rinman's sign
Rinne's sign
Rinne's test
rinse, mouth
Riolan('s)
R., anastomosis of
R. arch
R. artery
R. muscle
ripe
r. cataract
r. cervix
r. ovum
ripeness of cataract
ripple effect of alcoholism
ripple voltage
RISA
R. (radioiodinized serum albumin)
R. (radioiodinized serum albumin)
  scan
R. (radioactive iodinated serum
  albumin) study
Risdon approach
Risdon's wire
rise
r., enzyme
r. in blood pressure (BP)
r. in temperature, postoperative
r. time
riser ▸ morning lark
rising
r. health care costs
r. heart rate
r. pulse, rapidly
risk(s) (Risk)
r. adolescent population, high
r. analysis
r. and benefits of treatment
r. and benefits, potential
r., and prognosis ▸ incidence
r. angioplasty ▸ high-
r., antibiotic toxicity
r. appraisal, health
r., assess
r. assessment
r. assessment, computerized

r. assessment, heart
r. assessment interview
r. assessment, psychosocial
r. assessment ▸ quantitative
r. baby, high
r. behavior, high
r. -benefit analysis
r. -benefit estimate
r. -benefit ratio
r. -benefit threshold
r., bladder cancer
r., breast cancer
r., cancer
r. candidate, high
r., cardiovascular
r. category, high-
r. category patient, ultra low
r., coronary
r., death
r., decreased rebleeding
r., disability
r., disease
r., donor infection
r., element of
r., environmental
r., exercise
r. exercise, low
r. factor
r. factor, cardiovascular
r. factor, controlling
r. factor ▸ coronary
r. factor counseling
r. factor, genetic
r. factor ▸ health
r. factor ▸ heart attack
r. factor ▸ heart disease
r. factor ▸ hypermobility as
r. factor ▸ inherited
R. Factor Intervention Trial (MRFIT)
  ▸ Multiple
r. factor, known
r. factor ▸ major
r. factor ▸ medical
r. factor ▸ personal
r. factor ▸ primary
r. factor ▸ primary pulmonary
  hypertension
r. factor modification
r. factor modification, cardiac
r. factor reduction
r. factor, unknown
r. factors for drug abusers
r. factors, genetic transmission of
r. factors ▸ modifiable
r. factors, multiple

risk(s)—*continued*

r. factors ▸ multiple cardiac
r., family at
r. follow-up, high-
r. for addiction, at
r. for AIDS (acquired immune deficiency syndrome), patient at
r. for breast cancer ▸ high
r. for disease ▸ highest
r. for illness ▸ increased
r. for osteoporosis ▸ at
r. for reinfarction
r. ▸ free of significant
r. -free surgery
r., genetic
r., genetically at
r. group, high-
r. groups for infections
r., health
r., heart
r., heart attack
r., high-
r. ▸ high clotting
r., high degree of
r., high genetic
r., homicidal
r. ▸ identified at-
r. ▸ identify patient-at-
r., increased medical
r. index
r. index, cardiac
r. index score ▸ Goldman cardiac
r. infant, high
r., infection
r., inherent
r. ▸ intervene with patient-at-
r. ▸ ischemic stroke
r., known cardiac
r., lead pollution
r., lifestyle, high-
r., lifetime
r., low
r., magnitude of
r. ▸ manage patient-at-
r. management
r., maternal health
r., medical
r. ▸ modified multifactorial index of cardiac
r., mortality
r. mother, high
r. mother ▸ identified high-
r. mother, infant of high-
r., normal
r., occupational health

r. of back problems ▸ reduce
r. of breast cancer ▸ increased
r. of cancer
r. of cardiac death
r. of cardiac rupture
r. of clot formation ▸ increased
r. of colon cancer death
r. of developing alcoholism
r. of developing cervical cancer ▸ high
r. of dying ▸ lower
r. of exposure
r. of exposure, patient at high
r. of falling
r. of first heart attack
r. of heart disease
r. of heart disease ▸ decreased
r. of heart disease ▸ lower
r. of HIV (human immunodeficiency virus) infection ▸ high
r. of hospital-associated infections ▸ reduced
r. of infection
r. of infectious disease
r. of kidney disease
r. of major surgery
r. of miscarriage, increased
r. of pre-term birth, reduced
r. of recurrent stroke
r. of stroke
r. of stroke ▸ increased
r. of sudden death
r. of suicide, high
r. of transfusion-related disease ▸ minimize
r. of transmission
r. of ventricular fibrillation
r., operative
r., patient at
r., patient ▸ high-
r., patient poor
r., patient poor surgical
r., physical
r. population ▸ high-
r., potential
r. potential victims ▸ high-
r. pregnancy, high
r. procedure, high
r. programs, multi-
r., psychological
r., radon
r. ratio
r., recurrence
r. reduction
r. reduction, cardiac

r. reduction, coronary
r. -related practice
r., relative
r., serious health
r. sexual activity ▸ high-
r. sexual behavior ▸ high-
r. situation, high
r. stratification
r., stroke
r., suicide
r., surgical
r. systolic pressure ▸ high
r. -taking behavior
r. ▸ unwillingness to take
r., uterine cancer
risky behavior
risky behavior ▸ unusual
Risley's prism
Risley's rotary prism
risorius muscle
Risser localizer cast
risus caninus
risus sardonicus
Ritgen maneuver
ritodrine hydrochloride
Ritter-Oleson technique
ritual(s) (Ritual)
r. abuse
R. Abuse (SRA), Sadistic
r., action
r. and routines, detailed
r. behavior
r., bizarre private
r. circumcision ▸ release form for
r., cognitive
r., compulsive
r. /cult abuse
r. hazing
r. ▸ idiosyncratic obsessions and
r., mental
r., repetitive
ritualistic
r. acts
r. acts ▸ patient repeats
r. acts ▸ senseless,
r. behavior
r., patient
ritualized behavior ▸ repetitive
rivalry, sibling
river blindness
Rivers' cocktail
Riviere's sign
Rivini, incisura
rivinian
r. foremen

r. notch
r. segment
Rivinus(')
R., duct of
R. gland
R. membrane
R., notch of
R. segment
R., segment of
rivus lacrimalis
Rizzoli's operation
RK (radial keratotomy)
RKY (roentgen kymography)
RL (right lung)
R-L (right to left)
RLC (residual lung capacity)
RLE (right lower extremity)
RLE (right lower extremity) flexed
RLF (retrolental fibroplasia)
RLL
RLL (right lower lobe)
RLL (right lower lobe) bronchial
orifice
RLL (right lower lobe) infiltrate
RLL (right lower lobe) lesion
RLL (right lower lobe) of lung
RLL (right lower lobe) partial
collapse
RLP (radiation-leukemia-protection)
RLQ (right lower quadrant)
RLQ (right lower quadrant) of
abdomen
RM (respiratory movement)
RMA (refusal of medical aid)
RMA (right mentoanterior)
RML
RML (right middle lobe)
RML (right middle lobe) bronchial
orifice
RML (right middle lobe) of lung
RML (right middle lobe) syndrome
r/mm (roentgens per millimeter)
RMP (right mentoposterior)
RMR (resting metabolic rate)
RMS (root-mean-square)
RMT (right mentotransverse)
RMV (respiratory minute volume)
RN (Registered Nurse)
RNA
RNA (ribonucleic acid)
RNA (ribonucleic acid) dependent
DNA (deoxyribonucleic acid)
polymerase
RNA (ribonucleic acid) reverse
transcriptase

RNA (ribonucleic acid) ▸ soluble
RNA (ribonucleic acid) virus
RNP (ribonuclear protein)
Rn²²² (radon 222)
RNV (radionuclide ventriculogram)
RO (reverse osmosis)
R/O (rule out)
Ro antigen
r/o CA (carcinoma to be ruled out)
ROA (right occipitoanterior)
Roach (marijuana cigarette)
road
r. mapping, coronary
r. rage disorder
r. rage ▸ exhibits
roaring, ears
roaring unilateral tinnitus
Robert vascular dilation system ▸
Simpson-
Robert's pelvis
Robertson('s)
R. operation, Argyll
R. pupil, Argyll
R. sign
robin classification ▸ round-
Robin syndrome, Pierre
Robinia pseudacacia
robot, surgical
robot ▸ voice controlled surgical
robotic
r. assistance
r. knee
r. partial bypass procedure
r. patterns of speech
r. surgery
r. telesurgery
Rocha-Lima inclusion
Rochalimaea henselae
Rock(s) (rock)
R. (cocaine)
r. or crack cocaine
r., pelvic
r., pure cocaine
rocker, hematology
rocker-bottom foot
Rocket Fuel (phencyclidine analog)
rocking
r. and crying ▸ head rolling,
r. impulse ▸ paradoxical
r. motion, gentle
Rocky Mountain spotted fever
Rocky-Davis incision
rod(s)
r., aerobic gram-negative
r., anaerobic gram-negative

r. and cocci ▸ gram-negative
r. and cocci ▸ gram-positive
r., Auer
r. bacteria
r. cells
r., cluster of short gram-negative
r., Corti's
r. electrode
r., enamel
r., encapsulated gram-negative
r., flexible round silicone
r., fracture
r., germinal
r., gram-negative
r., gram-negative cigar-shaped
r., gram-positive
r. granules
r., Harrington
r., Heidenhain's
r. implant, silicone
r., inner
r. insertion, Rush
r., intramedullary
r., König's
r., large darkly staining gram-
positive
r. -like cells
r. -like forms
r. -like structures
r., long
r., Maddox
r., Meckel's
r., muscle
r., outer
r., pleomorphic gram-negative
r. prosthesis, Stenzel
r., radioactive
r., Reichmann's
r., retinal
r., Rush
r., Sage
r., Schneider
r. segment
r. -shaped bacteria
r. -shaped cells, pleomorphic
r. -shaped forms
r. -shaped organism in sputum
r. sheath, enamel
r., short
r. test, Maddox
r. vision
rodent cancer
rodent ulcer
Rodrigues' aneurysm
Roederer's obliquity

roentgen(s)
- r. delivered in air
- r. delivered to skin
- r. diagnosis
- r. dosage
- r. equivalent
- r. equivalent-man (REM)
- r. -equivalent-man period (REMP)
- r. equivalent physical (REP)
- r., gamma
- r. intoxication
- r. keratosis
- r. kymographic examination
- r. kymographic study
- r. kymography study
- r. per hour at one meter (rhm)
- r. per millimeter (r/mm)
- r. ray
- r. ray dosage, unit of
- r. ray therapy, deep
- r. rays ▸ intensity of
- r. studies, pyelographic
- r. therapy
- r. treatment
- r. unit (RU)

roentgenogram
- r., apical lordotic
- r., cephalometric
- r., chest
- r., lateral oblique jaw
- r., lateral ramus
- r., lateral skull
- r., maxillary sinus
- r., photo-
- r., skull
- r., submental vertex
- r., thoracic
- r., Towne projection

roentgenographic
- r. assessment
- r. differentiation
- r. examination
- r. examination, barium
- r. presentation
- r. study

roentgenography
- r., barium
- r., body section
- r., cardiac
- r., chest
- r., double contrast
- r., mass
- r., miniature
- r., mucosal relief
- r., selective

- r., serial
- r., soft tissue
- r., spot-film

roentgenologist's cancer
Roesler-Dressler infarction
Rogaine, minoxidil-based
Rogaine treatment
Roger('s) (s')
- R. bruit
- R., bruit de
- R. disease
- R. disease, Maladie-de-
- R. murmur
- R. reflex
- R. type spinal fusion

Rohr's stria
Rojo (barbiturates), Pajao
Rokitansky('s)
- R. cyst, Aschoff-
- R. disease
- R. disease, von
- R. diverticulum
- R. hernia
- R. kidney
- R. tumor

rolandic
- r. artery
- r. cortex
- r. epilepsy
- r. region

Rolando('s)
- R., fasciculus of
- R. fracture
- R. gelatinous substance

role(s) (Role)
- r. assignment
- r., causal
- r., causative
- r. change
- r. conflict ▸ parental
- r. counseling ▸ identity and
- r., counselor's
- r., family
- r. functioning ▸ social
- R. Inventory (BSRI), Bem Sex
- r. learning, behavior
- r. models
- r. of proprioception in control of behavior
- r. performance
- r. performance, altered
- r. play and interactional dynamics
- r. playing and response
- r. playing, systematic
- r., quasi-parental

- r. reversal, sudden
- r. transitions

Rolf's lance
roll(s)
- r. foot exercise ▸ golf ball
- r. independently, patient
- r., Kerlix gauze
- r. test, eye-
- r. tube
- r. upward, eyes

rolled back, eyes
rolled border, elevated
roller
- r. bandage
- r. coaster emotions
- r. dressing
- r. pump

Rollet's secondary substance
Rollet's stroma
rolling
- r. crutch
- r. hernia
- r. motion, pill
- r. movement
- r. papers
- r., patient independent in boosting and
- r., rocking and crying ▸ head

ROM (range of motion)
- ROM, active
- ROM, functional
- ROM, left ankle full
- ROM, left elbow full
- ROM, left femur full
- ROM, left knee full
- ROM, left lower extremity full
- ROM, left shoulder full
- ROM, left upper extremity full
- ROM, left wrist full
- ROM, limited
- ROM, neck full
- ROM, normal
- ROM, restricted
- ROM, right ankle full
- ROM, right elbow full
- ROM, right femur full
- ROM, right knee full
- ROM, right lower extremity full
- ROM, right shoulder
- ROM, right upper extremity full
- ROM, right wrist full

Romaña's sign
Romano-Ward syndrome
Romberg('s)
- R. disease

R. -Paessler syndrome
R. reflex
R. sign
R. station
R. unsteady
Rommel-Hildreth cautery
Rommel's cautery
Rönne's nasal step
R-on-T phenomenon
R-on-T premature ventricular complex
roof
 r. of mouth
 r. of sinus tarsi
 r., tegmental wall
room (Room)
 r. air, capillary blood gas at
 r., birthing
 r. care, emergency
 r., delivery
 r. deodorant
 R., Director of Operating
 r. episodes ▸ heroin-related emergency
 r., exercise
 r., footprint taken of infant in delivery
 r. (LAFR) ▸ laminar air flow
 r., laminar air flow (LAF) isolation
 r., mother thumbprinted in delivery
 r., newborn footprinted in delivery
 r. odor of body, locker
 R., Operating
 r., patient returned to
 R., patient sent to Recovery
 r., postanesthesia
 R., Recovery
 r., sanitized
 r. search
 r., seclusion
 r., slow rotation
 r. syndrome, locker
 r. temperature
rooming-in, infant
rooming-in, patient
Roos test
root(s) [*route*]
 r. amputation
 r. anomaly, conjoined nerve
 r., anterior nerve
 r., aortic
 r., apical portion of
 r. avulsion ▸ lumbar
 r. canal
 r. canal broach

r. canal filling
r. canal, fine
r. canal silver pinning
r. canal therapy
r. canal, tortuous
r. canal treatment
r. canal work
r. cap
r. cells
r. ▸ compressed nerve
r. compression, nerve
r. damage
r. dehiscence
r., demyelinated nerve
r. ▸ demyelinization of nerve
r. dimension, aortic
r., dorsal
r., dorsal nerve
r. elevator, Campbell's nerve
r. entry zone (DREZ) lesion, dorsal
r., excision of apex of tooth
r. ganglion, dorsal
r. hernia
r. injection
r. irritation, nerve
r. -mean-square (RMS)
r. -mean-square (RMS) voltage
r., motor nerve
r., nerve
r. of lung
r. of tongue
r. origin, lumbar spinal
r. pain
r. perforation
r. perfusion
r. planing
r. pliers, Allen's
r., posterior nerve
r. ratio, aortic
r., residual
r., retained
r. retractor ▸ Love nerve
r. rhizotomy, dorsal nerve
r. rhizotomy, ventral nerve
r., sacral nerve
r., sensory nerve
r. sign ▸ square
r. sleeves
r., spinal nerve
r. tip, retained
r., ventral
r., ventral nerve
rooting reflex
rootlet, nerve
ROP (right occipitoposterior)

rope flap
rope graft
ropy
 r. mass
 r. or granular, breasts
 r. saliva
 r. tumor
Rorschach ink blot test
Rorschach test
Rosa scleral implant ▸ Berens-
rosacea
 r., acne
 r. conjunctivitis, acne
 r., facial
 r. keratitis
 r. keratitis, acne
 r., ocular
rosaceum, Trichophyton
Rosas (amphetamines)
Rose('s) (rose)(s)
 R. (amphetamines)
 r. bengal antigen
 r. bengal dye
 r. bengal I 131, sodium
 r. bengal liver scan
 r. bengal scan
 r. bengal test
 R. -Bradford kidney
 R., lateral mammillary nucleus of
 R. position
 R. questionnaire
 R. skin test, Hanger-
 r. spot
 R. tamponade
 R. test
 R. -Thompson repair
 R. -Waaler test
Rose L-type nose bridge prosthesis
rosea, pityriasis
Rosenbach's syndrome
Rosenmüller's gland
Rosenthal('s)
 R., ascending vein of
 R. disease
 R. syndrome, Melkersson-
 R. vein
roseola
 r. infantilis
 r. infantum
 r. infantum incubation period
 r., syphilitic
 r. typhosa
roseopersicina, Lamprocystis
Roser-Braun sign

rosette(s)
r. cataract
r., cell
r. of hemorrhoids
roseum, Trichothecium
roseus
r., Acetobacter
r., Amoebobacter
r., Catharanthus
Roske syndrome, Caffey-Smyth-
Ross time frame of death, Kübler-
Rossetti modification of Nissen fundoplication
Rössle syndrome, Hanot-
Rossolimo's reflex
Rostan shunt
Rostan's asthma
rostral aspect
rostrate pelvis
rostrum of sinus
rostrum of sphenoid
ROT (right occipitotransverse)
rot, foot
Rot-Bielschowsky syndrome
rotary
r. atherectomy device
r. chorea
r. joint
r. microtome
r. nystagmus
r. prism, Risley's
r. vertigo
rotate fetal head
rotate scope
rotated
r. down, eye
r., externally
r., fetus
r., infant
r. kidney
r. to left
r. to right
r. upward, eyes
rotating
r. aid mattress
r. anode
r. disk oxygenation
r. forearm
r. hinge knee prosthesis, Kinematic
r. tourniquet, automatic
r. ultrasound beam
rotation
r., abduction, stress test ▸ external
r. advancement flap
r. and reduction of fracture

r. approach, arc
r. atherectomy extrusion angioplasty ▸ Kinsey
r. center
r., clockwise
r., counterclockwise
r. exercise
r. exercise ▸ shoulder external
r. exercise ▸ shoulder internal
r., external
r. flap
r. flap, Indian
r., internal
r., inward
r., limitation of
r., mediastinal volume
r., monocular
r. of eye around optical axis
r. of flap
r. of pelvis
r. operative delivery
r., outward
r. room, slow
r., shoulder
r. technique for dose calculation
r. test, fabere external
r. therapy
r. therapy, mediastinum volume
r. therapy, small volume
rotational
r. ablation
r. ablation, coronary
r. ablation laser
r. angioplasty ▸ low speed
r. angioplasty ▸ Osypka
r. angioplasty (PCRA) ▸ percutaneous coronary
r. atherectomy
r. atherectomy, coronary
r. atherectomy device
r. atherectomy ▸ high-speed
r. atherectomy ▸ percutaneous coronary
r. atherectomy system
r. coronary atherectomy
r. defect ▸ nonuniform
r. electron beam dosimetry
r. exercise
r. force
r. irradiation therapy ▸ supervoltage
r. movement, complex
r. thrombectomy ▸ percutaneous
r. x-ray beam dosimetry
rotator
r. cuff

r. cuff abnormality
r. cuff arthropathy
r. cuff injury
r. cuff lesion
r. cuff ▸ misalignment of
r. cuff muscles
r. cuff pathology
r. cuff repair
r. cuff rupture
r. cuff surgery
r. cuff tear
r. cuff tendon
r. cuff tendonitis
r. cuff, torn
r. muscles
r. muscles, long
r. muscles of neck
r. muscles of thorax
r. muscles, short
rotatory
r. chair, computer-driven
r. motion
r. nystagmus
r. spasm
r. tic
r. vertigo
rotavirus
r. gastroenteritis
r. vaccine
r. vaccine ▸ oral, tetravalent
Rotch's sign
rote memory ▸ superior
Roth('s)
R. -Bernhardt disease
R. disease
R. spots
R. ▸ vas aberrans of
Rothera's test
Rothmund's syndrome
Rothschild sign
rotifer compound
rotlauf bacillus, swine
rotoblator procedure
Rotor's syndrome
rotten stone
Rotter Incomplete Sentence Blank
rotund, abdomen
rotunda, fenestra
Rotunda treatment
rotundum ossis sphenoidalis, foramen
rotundus, Desmodus
rotundus, sacculus
roue de moulin, bruit de la
rouge, homme

Rouget's muscle
rough
   r. (R) cells
   r. (R.) colony
   r. endoplasmic reticulum
   r., scaly skin spots
roughness of photoaging
rouleaux formation
round(s)
   r. and regular (PRR) ▸ pupils
   r. atelectasis
   r., bedside
   r. bur
   r. cell
   r. cell accumulation ▸
     endobronchial
   r. cell carcinoma, small
   r. heart
   r. -house kicks
   r. ligament
   r., medical
   r. nucleus
   r., pharmaceutical
   r., prevalence
   r. pronator muscle
   r., react to light and accommodation
     (PERRLA) ▸ pupils equal,
   r., regular and equal (RRE)
   r. -robin classification
   r. silicone rod, flexible
   r. wheezes, year-
   r. window
   r. window ▸ intact
   r. window niche
   r. window reflex
rounded atelectasis
rounded edge
Rourke-Ernstein sedimentation rate
   (SR)
Rous sarcoma virus
Rous-associated virus (RAV)
roused, patient cannot be
roused, patient fully
Roussel's sign
Roussy
   R. -Carnil syndrome
   R. -Lévy disease
   R. -Lévy polyneuropathy
   R. -Lévy syndrome
   R. sarcoid, Darier-
   R. syndrome, Déjerine-
route [*root*]
   r., abdominal
   r., airborne

r. and method of administering
   medication ▸ action, dose,
r., fecal-oral
r., femoral
r. of administration
r. of infection
r. of infection, fecal-oral
r. of insertion
r. of transmission
r. of transmission, airborne
r., oral
r., percutaneous
Routier's operation
routine(s)
   r. admission, standing orders on
   r. aggressive management
   r. angiography
   r. cancer screenings
   r. care
   r. check
   r. chemistries
   r. culture
   r., daily
   r. ▸ detailed rituals and
   r. digitalization
   r. examination
   r. exercise
   r. fashion ▸ appendectomy
     performed in
   r. fashion, prepped in
   r. foot care
   r. general practitioner care
   r. gynecological examination
   r. home care
   r. mammogram
   r. mammography
   r. manner ▸ area prepped and
     draped in
   r. manner, patient prepared and
     draped in
   r. manner ▸ patient prepped and
     draped in
   r. medication
   r. method
   r. pelvic examination
   r. physical examination
   r. prenatal care
   r. preoperative screening
   r. preventive measures
   r. prophylaxis
   r. sampling
   r. screening
   r. skin transplant
   r. stick test
   r. stress test

r., stretch
r., strict exercise
r. studies
r. surveillance
r. tasks, decline in ability to perform
r. test dilution
r. treatment
r. warm-up
r. workup
routinely
   r. drawn blood specimen
   r. fatigued, patient
   r. monitored
Roux-en-Y
   R. anastomosis
   R. bypass
   R. cystojejunostomy
   R. gastrectomy
   R. gastrojejunostomy
   R., pancreaticojejunostomy with
   R. ▸ proximal loop of
Roux-Goldthwait operation
Rovsing('s)
   R. and Blumberg signs
   R. operation
   R. sign
row of sutures, transverse
rowing
   r. exercise ▸ seated
   r. machine
   r. motion
Rowinski's operation
Rowntree and Geraghty's test
Royalite body jacket
RP (resting pressure)
RP (retrograde pyelogram)
R-P interval
RPE (ratings of perceived exertion)
RPF (renal plasma flow)
RPM (rapid processing mode)
rpm (revolutions per minute)
RPO (right posterior oblique)
RPR (rapid plasma reagin)
RPR (rapid plasma reagin) test
R-prime complexes
RQ (respiratory quotient)
R-R
   R-R interval
   R-R prime
   R-R prime interval
RR cycle
RRE (round, regular and equal)
RRpm (respiratory rate per minute)
RRR (rate and rhythm regular)
RS (review of systems)

RS complexes
R/S ratio
RS (respiratory syncytial) virus
RSA (right sacroanterior)
RSB (right sternal border)
RScA (right scapuloanterior)
RScP (right scapuloposterior)
RSD (reflex sympathetic dystrophy)
   syndrome
RSI (rapid sequence induction)
RSI (repetitive strain injury)
RSI (repetitive stress injury)
RSI (rapid sequence induction)
   orotracheal intubation
RSP (right sacroposterior)
RSR (regular sinus rhythm)
RSR prime
RST (right sacrotransverse)
RS-T interval
RS-T segment
RSTL (relaxed skin tension lines)
RSV (right subclavian vein)
RT (repetition time)
RTF (Resistance Transfer Factor)
RTF (respiratory tract fluid)
RTV implant, Biocell
RTV total artificial heart
RU (rat unit)
RU (roentgen unit)
rub(s)
   r., absence of friction
   r., audible
   r., bilateral pleural
   r., friction
   r., pericardial
   r., pericardial friction
   r., pleural
   r., pleural friction
   r., pleuritic
   r., pleuropericardial
   r., right pleural
   r., saddle leather friction
   r. ▸ systolic pericardial friction
rubber
   r. band effect
   r. band ligation
   r. band ligation of hemorrhoids
   r. contact dermatitis
   r. dam
   r. dam drain
   r. drain
   r. endoscopic tube, flexible
   r., foam
   r. shoes, sutures tied over
   r. tissue

r. vaginal graft, foam
r. vaginal stent, foam
rubbing
   r. ▸ constant skin irritation and
   r. ▸ habitual eye
   r. heart sound
   r. on bone ▸ bone
Rubbrecht's operation
rubella
   r. immunity
   r. immunization
   r. incubation period
   r. scarlatinosa
   r. syndrome
   r. syndrome, congenital
   r. titer
   r. virus
rubellar titer
rubeola scarlatinosa
rubeosis iridis
rubeosis retinae
ruber, lichen
rubescens, Amanita
rubicornis, Sarcophaga
rubicundus, Cacajao
rubicundus, Ixodes
rubida, Trypanosoma
rubidium-82 imaging
Rubin('s)
   R. operation
   R. test
   R. tube
Rubinstein-Taybi syndrome
rubor, dependent
rubra
   r., lochia
   r., miliaria
   r., pityriasis
   r., polycythemia
   r., Rhodotorula
   r., trichomycosis
   r. vera, polycythemia
rubrum
   r., eczema
   r., Epidermophyton
   r., Saccharomyces
   r., Trichophyton
rubs or murmurs
ruby
   r. laser
   r. laser ▸ high energy pulsed
   r., solid state laser utilizing
rude respiration
rudimentary disc space
rudimentary white pulp

rudiments of pancreas
Rud's syndrome
RUE (right upper extremity)
RUE (right upper extremity)
   amputated
RUE (right upper extremity) flexed
rufescens, Protostrongylus
Rufus (Iranian heroin)
RUG (retrograde ureterogram)
rugae of vagina
rugae vaginales
rugal
   r. coarsening
   r. folds
   r. folds, congested
   r. folds, gastric
   r. folds of stomach
   r. pattern of stomach
   r. prominence, gastric
rugby knee
Ruggeri's reflex
Ruggieri stigma, Guiffrida-
Ruiz-Morgan procedure
RUL
   RUL (right upper lobe)
   RUL (right upper lobe) bronchial
     orifice
   RUL (right upper lobe) lesion
   RUL (right upper lobe) of lung
   RUL (right upper lobe) pneumonia
rule (Rule)
   r., Arey's
   R. ethics, Golden
   r., family
   r., Gibson's
   r. -governed behavior
   r., Hasse's
   r., His'
   r., Jackson's
   r., Liebermeister
   r., Luedde's transparent
   r., Nagele's
   r. of bigeminy
   r. out (r/o)
   r. out (r/o) appendicitis
   r. out myocardial infarction (MI)
   r., Simpson's
ruled out (r/o CA) ▸ carcinoma to be
ruling influence
rumble(s)
   r., Austin Flint
   r., bony
   r., booming
   r., filling
   r. ▸ mid-diastolic

r., protodiastolic
rumbling(s)
  r. diastolic murmur
  r. in abdomen
  r. murmur, atrioventricular (AV) flow
Rumel technique
Rumel tourniquet
ruminantium, Cowdria
rumination
  r. disorder of infancy
  r., endless
  r., guilty
  r., obsessive
  r., pessimistic
  r., psychogenic
ruminative activity
ruminative expression
rump
  r., crown-to-
  r. heel length (RHL)
  r. length (CRL) ▸ crown
  r. length ▸ head to
  r. measurement, crown
  r. to heel length
Rumpel-Leede capillary fragility
Rumpel-Leede phenomenon
Rumpf's sign
run, meter
run, quarter
runaway(s)
  r. adolescents
  r., halfway house for
  r. pacemaker
  r. pulse
rundown/run-down
Runeberg's type
Runge syndrome, Ballantyne
Runge test
runner('s)
  r. high
  r. knee
  r., knee pain in
  r., long distance
  r., marathon
running
  r. chromic suture
  r., downhill
  r. fits
  r. frequency and intensity
  r. imbricating suture
  r. injuries
  r. length of bone ▸ fracture
  r. lock stitch
  r. lock suture
  r. lock suture, continuous

r. nose, constantly
r. pneumonia
r. pulse
r. subcuticular suture of nylon ▸
  skin closed with
r. suture, continuous
r. suture, locking
r. technique
r. technique ▸ end-over-end
runny
  r., itchy nose
  r. nose
  r. nose and eyes ▸ itchy,
  r. nose ▸ body pain with
  r. nostril ▸ stuffed or
runoff
  r. angiography ▸ femoral
  r., aortofemoral arterial
  r., aortogram with distal
  r., arterial
  r. arteriogram
  r. arteriography ▸ femoral
  r., digital
  r., distal
  r., venous
runs
  r., longer
  r. of slow activity
  r., triangulation
  r., vertex
Runström projection
rupture
  r., Achilles tendon
  r., adventitial
  r., alveolar
  r., aortic
  r., aortic aneurysm
  r., artificial
  r., atherosclerotic plaque
  r., balloon
  r., cardiac
  r., chamber
  r., chordae tendineae
  r., chordal
  r., esophageal
  r. event scanning
  r., inflamed diverticulum
  r. ▸ interventricular septal
  r., intraperitoneal
  r., intrapleural
  r., liver
  r., membrane
  r., myocardial
  r., nonpenetrating

r. of anterior and posterior
  longitudinal ligaments
r. of cesarean section scar
r. of congenital aneurysm
r. of esophagus, spontaneous
r. of heart
r. of implant
r. of membranes
r. of membranes, artificial
r. of membranes (PROM),
  premature
r. of membranes, prolonged
r. of membranes ▸ spontaneous
r. of myocardium
r. of myocardium following
  infarction
r. of spleen ▸ traumatic
r. of tendon
r. of tibial tendon
r., oxytocic
r. ▸ papillary muscle
r., penetrating
r., pericardial
r., plaque
r., risk of cardiac
r. ▸ rotator cuff
r., spleen
r., splenic
r., spontaneous
r., tendon
r., traumatic
r., uterine
r., valve
r., ventricular
r. ▸ ventricular septal
ruptured
  r. abdominal aortic aneurysm
  r. aneurysm
  r. aneurysm mortality
  r. aortic aneurysm
  r. aortic artery
  r. appendix
  r. bag of waters
  r. Baker's cyst
  r. biceps tendon
  r. bladder
  r. blood vessels
  r. brain aneurysm
  r. brain blood vessel
  r. bronchus
  r. cerebral aneurysm
  r. cervical disc
  r. cuff
  r. diaphragm
  r. disc

ruptured—*continued*
- r. disc ▸ pain in back from slipped or
- r. eardrum
- r. eye
- r. follicle
- r. iliac aneurysm
- r. intervertebral disc
- r. ligament
- r. membranes
- r. membranes, premature
- r. muscle
- r. peritonitis from appendix
- r. peritonsillar abscess
- r. scar of uterus
- r. sclera
- r. sinus of Valsalva
- r. spinal disc
- r. spleen
- r. spontaneously
- r. spontaneously, membranes
- r. syphilitic aortic aneurysm
- r. traumatically
- r. tubal ectopic pregnancy
- r. tympanic membrane
- r. uterus

RUQ (right upper quadrant)
RUQ (right upper quadrant) of abdomen
rush (Rush)('s)
- r., adrenaline
- r., euphoric
- R. intramedullary nail
- R. intramedullary pin
- R. rod
- R. rod insertion

rushes, obstructive
rushes, peristaltic
Russell('s)
- R. Brain disease
- R. Brain reflex
- R. dwarf
- R. syndrome
- R. traction
- R. unit

Russe's bone graft
Russian influenza
Russian spring-summer encephalitis
rust ring
rusty sputum
Rutherford's syndrome
Ruysch's
- R. muscle
- R. tube
- R. veins

RV
- RV (respiratory volume)
- RV (right ventricle)
- RV (right ventricular) apex
- RV (right ventricular) apex electrogram
- RV (right ventricular) assist-device
- RV (right ventricular) cardiomyopathy
- RV (right ventricular) diastolic collapse
- RV (right ventricular) diastolic pressure
- RV (right ventricular) dimension
- RV (right ventricular) dysplasia
- RV (right ventricular) failure
- RV (right ventricular) function
- RV (right ventricular) heave
- RV (right ventricular) hypoplasia
- RV (right ventricular) inflow obstruction
- RV (right ventricular) myxoma
- RV (right ventricle) of heart
- RV (right ventricular) outflow obstruction
- RV (right ventricular) outflow tract
- RV (right ventricular) outflow tract tachycardia
- RV (right ventricular) study
- RV (right ventricular) systolic pressure
- RV (right ventricular) systolic time interval

RVE (right ventricular enlargement)
RVEDP (right ventricular end-diastolic pressure)
RVEDV (right ventricular end-diastolic volume)
RVET (right ventricular ejection time)
RVH (right ventricular hypertrophy)
RVI (relative value index)
RVM (right ventricular mean)
RV/TLC (residual volume to total lung capacity) ratio
Rx
- Rx (take)
- Rx (therapy)
- Rx (treatment)

ryanodine receptor
Ryle tube

S

s (without)
S and C (sclerae and conjunctivae)
S (smooth) cells
S. (smooth) colony
S deficiency ▸ protein
S, hemoglobin
S incision, lazy
S. (Streptococcus) pneumoniae
S, protein
s rays
S (Sarcoptes) scabiei mites
S, streptolysin
S virus, Uganda
S wave
S-A (sinoatrial)
    S-A arrest
    S-A cell analysis
    S-A conduction time
    S-A exit block
    S-A nodal reentrant tachycardia
    S-A node
    S-A node artery
    S-A node ▸ rhythmic pattern
    S-A pacemaker complex
    S-A recovery time
SA (Smokers Anonymous)
SA virus
SAA (Sex Addicts Anonymous)
Saal medullary pin, von
saber tibia
Sabia virus
Sabin('s)
    S. dye test
    S. -Feldman test
    S. vaccine
sabot, coeur en
sabot heart
sabouraudi, Trichophyton
Sabouraud's medium
saburral amaurosis
saburral colic
sac(s)
    s. ▸ abdominal aneurysm
    s., air
    s., alveolar
    s., amniotic
    s., aneurysmal

s., aortic
s., caudal
s., colostomy
s., congested air
s., conjunctival cul-de-
s. containing fluid, abnormal
s. containing gas, abnormal
s. containing semisolid material ▸ abnormal
s., cul-de-
s. cushions
s. discolored, pericardial
s. distended, pericardial
s., Douglas' cul-de-
s., drainage (dr'ge) of lacrimal
s., dural
s., dural cul-de-
s. ▸ elasticity of air
s. empty, scrotal
s., endolymphatic
s., enlarged air
s. entoderm, yolk-
s., excision of lacrimal
s., FB (foreign body) in lacrimal
s., fibrous
s., fistula of lacrimal
s., fluid
s. fluid ▸ cul-de-
s. ▸ fluid in heart
s., fluid-filled
s., free fluid in cul-de-
s. free of fluid ▸ pleural
s., fullness of cul-de-
s. fungus
s., gestational
s., heart
s., hernial
s., Hilton
s., ileostomy
s. in breast, fluid-filled
s., intrauterine gestational
s., lacrimal
s. ▸ large inguinal hernia
s., lateral
s., left pleural
s. -like defect
s. -like formation

s. -like gallbladder
s. -like protrusion
s., obliteration of cul-de-
s. of aneurysm, surgical closure of
s. of eye, lacrimal
s. of fluid
s. of vagina, posterior cul-de-
s., pericardial
s. placenta, yolk
s., pleural
s., polyp in lacrimal
s., rhinoscleroma of lacrimal
s., right pleural
s., scrotal
s., sporotrichosis of lacrimal
s., streptotrichosis of lacrimal
s., subarachnoid
s., tear
s., truncoaortic
s. tumor, yolk-
s. ▸ vital microscopic air
s., yolk
saccadic eye movement
saccadic velocity study
saccharide group
saccharolyticus, Peptostreptococcus
Saccharomyces (saccharomyces)
    S. albicans
    S. anginae
    S. apiculatus
    S. bayanus
    s., Busse
    S. cantliei
    S. capillitii
    S. carlsbergensis
    s. cerebisiae antibody (ASCA) ▸ anti-
    S. cerevisiae
    S. coprogenus
    S. dairensis
    S. ellipsoideus
    S. epidermica
    S. exiguus
    S. galacticolus
    S. glutinis
    S. granulomatosus
    S. guttulatus

S

Saccharomyces—*continued*
- S. hansenii
- S. hominis
- S. lemonnieri
- S. lipsoideus
- S. lithogenes
- S. mellis
- S. mesentericus
- S. mycoderma
- S. neoformans
- S. pastorianus
- S. rubrum
- S. subcutaneus tumefaciens
- S. tumefaciens albus

Saccharomycopsis guttulatus
Saccharum officinarum
sacciform kidney
saccular
- s. aneurysm
- s. aneurysm of abdominal aorta
- s. bronchiectasis
- s. herniation
- s. nerve
- s. outpouchings
- s. posterior pharyngeal diverticulum ▸ small

sacculated
- s. aneurysm
- s. bladder
- s. empyema
- s. pleurisy

sacculation, localized
saccule
- s., air
- s., alveolar
- s., laryngeal
- s. of larynx
- s., vestibular

sacculi, macula
sacculi, macula acustica
sacculus
- s. communis
- s. lacrimalis
- s. laryngis
- s. proprius
- s. rotundus
- s. ventricularis
- s. vestibularis

SACH heels
Sachs(')
- S. bacillus, Ghon-
- S. disease, Tay-
- S. infant, Tay-
- S. lesion, Hill-

Sacks
- S. endocarditis, Libman-
- S. lesion, Libman-
- S. syndrome, Libman-

sacral
- s. agenesis
- s. ala
- s. anesthesia
- s. aneurysm
- s. block
- s. block anesthesia
- s. bone
- s. cul-de-sac
- s. decubitus ulcer ▸ large
- s. edema
- s. flexure
- s. flexure of rectum
- s. ganglia
- s. nerves
- s. plexus
- s. prominence
- s. reflexes
- s. region
- s. region, mid-
- s. segment
- s. spine
- s. splanchnic nerves
- s. tuberosity
- s. vein, lateral
- s. vein, middle
- s. vertebra
- s. vertebrae bones

sacralization, lumbar pseudo◊
sacred mushroom (hallucinogen)
sacred mushrooms (psilocybin)
sacroanterior
- s., left
- s. position
- s., right

sacrococcygea, aorta
sacrococcygeal
- s. articulation
- s. cyst
- s. joint
- s. muscle, anterior
- s. muscle, dorsal
- s. muscle, posterior
- s. muscle, ventral

sacrodextra anterior
sacrodextra posterior
sacrofetal pregnancy
sacrogenital fold
sacrogenital ligament
sacrohysteric pregnancy

sacroiliac
- s. articulation
- s. belt, Mayo
- s. joint
- s. joint pain
- s. notch
- s. strain

sacrolaeva
- s. anterior
- s. posterior
- s. transverse

sacroposterior
- s., left
- s. position
- s., right

sacropubic diameter
sacrosciatic, notch, greater
sacrosciatic notch, lesser
sacrospinal muscle
sacrospinous ligament
sacrotransverse
- s., left
- s. position
- s., right

sacrouterine ligament
sacrum, lateral mass of
sacular (see saccular)
SAD (sad)
- S. (seasonal affective disorder)
- s., feeling
- s. or tearful appearance
- s., persistently

SADD (Students Against Drunk Driving)
saddle
- s. -back nose
- s. block
- s. block anesthesia
- s. deformity of nose
- s. embolism
- s. embolus
- s. embolus, aortic
- s. joint
- s. leather friction rub
- s. nose
- s. nose deformity
- s. sensation
- s. thrombus

sadism, sexual
sadistic (Sadistic)
- s. personality
- S. Ritual Abuse (SRA)
- s. tendencies

sadness
  s. and grief ▸ overwhelming feelings of
  s. and irritability
  s., extreme
  s., increased
  s. ▸ persistent feelings of
  s. ▸ pining, yearning and
SADS (seasonal affective disorder syndrome)
Saemisch's operation
Saemisch's ulcer
Saenger's
  S. macula
  S. operation
  S. reflex
  S. sign
Saethre-Chotzen syndrome
saevissima richteri, Solenopsis
SAF (self-articulating femoral) hip replacement
safe (Safe)
  s. and effective dosages
  s. and effective ▸ proven
  s. blood
  s. expression of anger ▸ permitting
  s. period
  S. Response manual resuscitator
  s. sex
  s. standing balance
  s. transfer
safety
  s. and stability at home ▸ evaluate
  s. awareness
  s. awareness, patient
  s., blood supply
  s. devices, bathroom
  s. guidewire
  s. of others ▸ reckless disregard for
  s. of self ▸ reckless disregard for
  s., patient
  s. precautions
  s. profile, drug
  s., quality assurance in radiation
  s., radiation
  s. ribbon
  s. studies ▸ long-term
  s. technique goals
  s. techniques, demonstration of
  s. test data
  s. tube
Saf-T-Coil
sag(s)
  s. and bags ▸ wrinkles,
  s. foot

  s., ST
Sage rod
sagging
  s. abdominal wall
  s. bladder
  s. breasts
  s. eyebrows
  s. eyebrows ▸ lift
  s. eyelids
  s. facial skin
  s. skin
  s. vitreous
saginata, Taenia
sagittal
  s. area
  s. cuts
  s. diameter
  s. fontanelle
  s. plane
  s. plane dose of rads in fractions, mid-
  s. plane, median-
  s. sections of brain
  s. sinus
  s. sinus, superior
  s. splitting of mandible
  s. suture
  s. suture lines
  s. suture synostosis
  s. view
sagittalis inferior, sinus
sagittalis superior, sinus
Sagnac rays
sago grains
sago-grain stool
Sahli's test
sail sound
Sainton syndrome, Scheuthauer-Marie-
sakazakii, Enterobacter
SAL (sensory acuity level)
SAL (sensory acuity level) test
Sala cells
salaam activity
salaam convulsion
salad, word
Salem sump tube, Argyle-
salicylate
  s., blood
  s., phenol
  s. poisoning
  s., serum
salicylic acid
salient
  s. features

  s. symptom
  s., ventricular
salinarium, Halobacterium
saline
  s. and dopamine infusion
  s., anterior chamber irrigated with
  s., area lavaged with sterile
  s. basin, sterile
  s., catheter aspirated and flushed with
  s. diuresis
  s. (N/S) enema, normal
  s. filled breast implant
  s., flushed with
  s., frozen
  s., glucose and
  s., heparinized
  s., iced
  s. implant
  s. implant, leaky
  s. infusion, intra-amniotic
  s., irrigated with
  s. loading
  s. mouthwash
  s. (N/S) ▸ normal
  s., operative area irrigated with
  s., phosphate-buffered
  s., physiological
  s. slush
  s. soaked cotton, bolus of
  s. solution
  s. solution, aerosol
  s. solution, buffered
  s. solution, cells suspended in
  s. (N/S) solution, normal
  s. solution, physiological
  s. solution, sterile
  s. solution, wound irrigated with
  s., sterile physiological
  s., wound irrigated with normal
saliva
  s., artificial
  s. bubbling from mouth
  s., chorda
  s., decreased flow of
  s., diminished secretion of
  s., excess
  s. ▸ excessive flow of
  s. ▸ flow of
  s., ganglionic
  s., leech
  s., lingual
  s., oral-oral transmission by
  s. output
  s., overproduction of

saliva—*continued*
s., parotid
s. ▸ reduced flow of
s., ropy
s., sublingual
s., submaxillary
s., sympathetic
s. test
s., whole
salivarius, gram-positive
Streptococcus
salivarius, Streptococcus
salivary
s. adenitis, acute
s. and lacrimal secretions
s. amylase
s. calculus
s. duct
s. dyspepsia
s. flow study
s. gland
s. gland ▸ atrophy of
s. gland carcinoma
s. gland disease
s. gland disorder
s. gland dysfunction
s. gland function
s. gland lesions
s. gland ▸ right submaxillary
s. gland, submandibular
s. gland tumor
s. gland virus
s. glands, overstimulation of
s. scintiscan
s. stone
s. tubes
salivatorius, nucleus
sallow complexion
sallow skin
salmincola, Troglotrema
salmon skin
Salmonella
S. abortus equi
S. aertrycke, gram-negative
S. anatum
S. bacteria
S. choleraesuis
S. derby
S. durazzo
S. enteritidis
S. enteritidis, gram-negative
S. enteritis
S. gallinarum
S. group
S. illness

S. montevideo
S. muenchen
S. organisms
S. paratyphi A
S. paratyphi B
S. paratyphi C
S. poisoning
S. pullorum
S. schottmülleri
S. schottmülleri, gram-negative
S. sendai
S. species
S. suipestifer, gram-negative
S. tyeora
S. typhi
S. typhimurium
S. typhisuis
S. typhosa
salmonicida, Aeromonas
Salmon's sign
Salomon test, Porges-
Salomon's test
salpingectomy, bilateral partial
salpingitis
s., chronic
s., chronic interstitial
s., chronic vegetating
s., hemorrhagic
s., hypertrophic
s. isthmica nodosa
s., mural
s., nodular
s., parenchymatous
s. profluens
s., pseudofollicular
s., purulent
s., recurrent
s., tuberculous
salpingo-oophorectomy (s-o)
s-o ▸ bilateral
s-o ▸ laparoscopic
s-o ▸ unilateral
salpingo-ovarian salpingolysis
salpingopalatine fold
salpingopharyngea, plica
salpingopharyngeal muscle
salpingostomy, cuff
Salpix contrast medium
salt(s)
s. agglutination
s. and water balance of body
s. and water imbalance
s. and water retention
s. antagonism
s. consumption

s. craving
s. depletion syndrome
s. deposits, uric
s. diet, low
s. (NAS) diet, no added
s., excesses of
s. excreted through urination
s. -free diet
s., gold
s. intake
s. intake, diminished
s. intake, limit
s. intake, reduce
s. intake ▸ reduction of
s. reduction, moderate
s. resistant
s. restriction diet
s. retention
s. sickness
s. solution, balanced
s. solution, Epsom
s. syndrome ▸ low
s., urinary
s. -losing nephritis
s. wasting
s. water implant
s. water solution
saltam, extension per
saltans, Bodo
saltatory
s. chorea
s. conduction
s. tic
saltatrix, Anthomyia
salted starches
Salter('s)
S. fracture
S. incremental lines
S. operation
S. osteotomy
saluretic agent
Salus' arch
Salus-Elschnig syndrome, Koerber-
salute, allergic
salvage
s. balloon angioplasty
s., intraoperative
s., limb
s., myocardial
salvarsan throat irrigation tubes
salvatella vein
salves ▸ tachycardia en
salvo of beats
salvo of ventricular tachycardia
Salzer's test meals

Salzmann's dystrophy
Salzmann's nodular corneal
    dystrophy
SAM (systolic anterior motion)
Samaritan Act, Good
Samaritan donation
same (Same)
    s. (COWS) ▸ cold to the opposite,
      warm to the
    S. Day Care Center
    S. Day Surgery Center
Sameness, insistence on
Samoan conjunctivitis
sample(s)
    s., arterial blood
    s., blood
    s., capillary
    s., DNA (deoxyribonucleic acid)
    s., drawing of blood
    s., filtered and cultured
    s. of tissue, removal of
    s., serum
    s., tissue
    s., umbilical arterial
    s., urine
    s., venous blood
sampling(s)
    s., arterial gas
    s., bioptic
    s., blood
    s. (CVS) ▸ chorionic villus
    s., fetal scalp
    s., mass
    s., microbiologic
    s., pelvic node
    s. (PUBS) ▸ percutaneous umbilical
      blood
    s., periaortic node
    s. rate
    s., routine
Sampson's cyst
San Joaquin fever
San Joaquin Valley disease
Sanchez-Cascos cardioauditory
    syndrome
Sanchez-Perez cassette
Sanctis-Cacchione syndrome, De
sanctuary irradiation, cranial
sand
    s. bath
    s. bodies
    s. walking foot exercise
sandbag placed for support
Sanders bed
sandpaper disc

sandwich
    s. appearance
    s. assay
    s. enzyme linked immunosorbent
      assay
    s. generation
    s. patch
    s. patch technique, anterior
    s. therapy
Sandwith's bald tongue
sane and sober
sane, patient legally
Sanfilippo's syndrome
Sanger-Brown syndrome
Sanger-Brown's ataxia
sanguinea integumenti communis ▸
    vasa
sanguinea retinae, vasa
sanguineous (*same as* sanguinous)
    s. cataract
    s. material
sanguinis, fragilitas
sanguinis, ictus
sanguinolenta, lochia
sanguinolentis, fetus
sanguinous (*see* sanguineous)
sanguis, streptococcus
sanguisorba, Hirudo
sanguisuga, Haemopis
sanguisuga, Trypanosoma
sanitized room
sanitizing, carpet
sanity ▸ periods of sobriety and
Sansom's sign
Sanson mirror images, Purkinje-
Santorini('s)
    S. cartilage
    S., concha of
    S. muscle
    S. muscles, circular
    S., parietal vein of
    S. plexus
Sanyal's conjunctivitis
SaO$_2$ (arterial oxygen saturation)
SaO$_2$ ▸ blood (arterial oxygen
    saturation)
SAP (systemic arterial pressure)
saphenofemoral junction
saphenofemoral system
saphenous
    s. artery
    s. graft
    s. nerve
    s. pulse
    s. system, greater

    s. system, lesser
    s. vein
    s. vein, accessory
    s. vein allograft, CryoVein
    s. vein bypass, aortocoronary
    s. vein bypass graft angiography
    s. vein bypass ▸ renal artery
      reverse
    s. vein graft
    s. vein graft ▸ reversed
    s. vein graft stenosis
    s. vein, greater
    s. vein ligation, high
    s. vein obstruction
    s. vein ▸ reverse
    s. vein, small
    s. vein varicosity
sapophore group
Sappey's fibers
Sappey's veins
Sappinia diploidea
saprophyte, nonpathogenic
saprophytic leptospirosis species
saprophyticus, Staphylococcus
Sarbo's sign
sarcasm ▸ displays extreme
sarcastic, patient
sarcogenic cells
sarcoid
    s., Boeck's
    s., Darier-Roussy
    s., equine
    s. granuloma
    s., Schaumann's
    s., Spiegler-Fendt
sarcoidosis
    s., Boeck's
    s., chronic
    s. cordis
    s., fibrocystic
    s., muscular
    s. myocarditis ▸ cardiac
    s., pulmonary
sarcolemma lipid
sarcolemmal level
sarcolemmal membrane
sarcoma
    s., advanced uterine
    s., alveolar soft part
    s., anaplastic
    s., bone forming
    s. botryoides of vagina
    s., carcino◊
    s., cardiac
    s., chondro◊

sarcoma—*continued*
- s., embryonal
- s., embryonal carcino◊
- s., Ewing's
- s., granulocytic
- s. herpes virus (KSHV) ▸ Kaposi's
- s., Hodgkin's
- s., Kaposi's
- s., lympho◊
- s., lymphosarcoma reticulum cell
- s., meningeal
- s., metastatic
- s., metastatic endometrial stromal
- s., mixed mesodermal
- s., myxo◊
- s. of brain, reticulum cell
- s. of the knee ▸ synovial cell
- s., osteo◊
- s., osteogenic
- s., periosteal
- s., primary bone
- s. ▸ pseudo-Kaposi
- s., reticulo◊
- s., reticulum cell
- s., rhabdomyo◊
- s., soft tissue
- s., somatic
- s., Sternberg's
- s., synovial
- s., tendosynovial tissue
- s., uterine
- s. virus, Moloney
- s. virus, murine
- s. virus, Rous

sarcomatodes, carcinoma
sarcomatodes, granuloma
sarcomatoid form
sarcomatosum
- s., ectropion
- s., glioma
- s., osteoma

sarcomatous
- s. changes
- s. leptomeningitis
- s. tumor

sarcopenia ▸ diagnosis of
Sarcophaga
- S. carnaria
- S. dux
- S. fuscicauda
- S. haemorrhoidalis
- S. nificornis
- S. rubicornis

sarcoplasmic reticulum
Sarcopsylla penetrans

Sarcoptes scabiei
Sarcoptes (S) scabiei mites
sarcoptic mange
sarcosporidian cysts
sarcotubular system
sarcous, substance
sardonicus, risus
sarmentosus, Strophanthus
Sarmiento cast
satanic alters, managing
satanic cult
satellite
- s., bacterial
- s. cells
- s., chromosomal
- s. colony
- s. lesion
- s. nodules
- s., nucleolar
- s. tumor nodules

satiety, early
satisfaction
- s. assessment, outpatient
- s., patient
- s., periods of

satisfactorily
- s., bowel fills and evacuates
- s., colon emptied
- s., colon fills and evacuates
- s., patient progressing
- s., wound healing

satisfactory
- s. akinesia of lids
- s. general anesthesia
- s. positioning of patient
- s., postreduction position
- s. recovery

satisfied, emotionally
satisfying relationships established
Sativa (marijuana)
sativus, Cucumis
Sattler's veil
saturated
- s. fat
- s. fat diet, low
- s. fat index, cholesterol
- s. fat intake
- s. fat, reducing
- s. for intake
- s. solution
- s. solution of potassium iodide (SSKI)

saturation [*maturation*]
- s. analysis
- s., arterial

- s. (SaO_2), arterial oxygen
- s. (SaO_2) ▸ blood arterial oxygen
- s. current
- s., fat
- s. index (SI)
- s. level ▸ iron
- s. level ▸ oxygen (O_2)
- s. meter (OSM) ▸ oxygen
- s. ▸ mixed venous oxygen (O_2)
- s., oxygen (O_2)
- s., peripheral
- s. point, tissue
- s. ▸ step-up in oxygen (O_2)
- s. test ▸ transferrin
- s. testing, oxygen (O_2)
- s. time
- s., venous

saturnine
- s. cachexia
- s. cerebritis
- s. gout
- s. nephritis

saturninus, halo
satyr ear
satyri, Bertiella
sauce appearance, apple
saucer, auditory
saucerization and biopsy
saucerize cyst
saucers (morning glory seeds) ▸ flying
Sauerbruch('s)
- S. -Herrmannsdorfer-Gerson diet
- S. rib guillotine
- S. prosthesis

Sauflon PW contact lens
sausaging of vein
Sauvage Dacron graft
Sauvage filamentous prosthesis
Sauvant syndrome
Sauvineau's ophthalmoplegia
savant, idiot-
saver, cell
saving
- s. antiviral drug ▸ life-
- s. assistance, life-
- s. decision, life-
- s. measures, life-
- s. medical care, life-
- s. organ, life-
- s. skills, life-
- s. treatment, life-
- s. treatment ▸ withdrawal of life-
- s. treatment ▸ withholding of life-

saw, sternum

saw-effect, band
sawtooth pattern
sawtooth wave
Saxtorph's maneuver
Sayre('s)
- S. apparatus
- S. bandage
- S. jacket
- S. operation
- S. Syndrome, Kearns-
- S. traction

SBE (subacute bacterial endocarditis)
SBE (subacute bacterial endocarditis) prophylaxis
SBE (supine bicycle echocardiogram)
SBFT (small bowel follow-through)
SBP
- SBP (spontaneous bacterial peritonitis)
- SBP (systemic blood pressure)
- SBP (systolic blood pressure)
- SBP (systolic blood pressure) ▸ decreased

SBS (shaken baby syndrome)
scab
- s., foot
- s., head
- s., sheep
- s., skin

scabbard trachea
scabbing, lesion
scabetic distribution
scabetic infection
scabiei
- s., Acarus
- s. mites, Sarcoptes (S)
- s., Sarcoptes

scabies
- s., bovine
- s. mite
- s., Norwegian
- s., nosocomial

SCAD (spontaneous coronary artery dissection)
Scag (heroin)
scala
- s. media
- s. tympani
- s. vestibuli of cochlea

scalar
- s. electrocardiogram (ECG)
- s. leads
- s. time

scalaris, Anthomyia
scalded skin syndrome
scale(s) (Scale)
- s., absolute
- s., activity
- s., Aldrich
- s., Apgar
- s., attitude
- s., Baumé's
- s., Benoist's
- s., Bloch's
- s., Borg numerical
- S. (BPES), Borg Perceived Exertion
- S. (BTES), Borg Treadmill Exertion
- s., Brazelton behavioral
- s., cardiac adjustment
- S., Cattell Infant Intelligence
- s., Celsius
- s., centigrade
- s., chair
- s., Charrière
- s., Clark's
- S., Clyde Mood
- S., Columbia Mental Maturity
- s. delusion ▸ full
- s., depression
- s., disability status
- s., double
- s., Dukes
- s., Dunfermline
- s., dyspnea
- s., Fahrenheit
- S. for Children (WISC) Test, Wechsler Intelligence
- S. for Children, Wechsler Intelligence
- s., French
- s., full
- s., Gaffky
- S. ▸ Geriatric Depression
- S. ▸ Glasgow Coma
- s., gray
- s., Grossman
- S., Hamilton rating
- s., Himmelsbach rating
- S. ▸ Holmes-Rahe
- s., Holzknecht's
- s., hydrometer
- s. imaging, gray-
- s., in-bed
- s. insulin therapy, sliding
- s. IQ (Intelligence Quotient) Test, full
- s., Karnofsky rating

s., Kelvin
S., Kent Emergency
s. lesion ▸ onion
S. (MSAS) ▸ Mandel Social Adjustment
s. method ▸ sliding
s. ▸ narcotic withdrawal
s. on elbows ▸ silvery
s. on knees ▸ silvery
s. on legs ▸ silvery
s. on scalp ▸ silvery
s., Outerbridge
s. ▸ over controlled hostility
s., Paykel
S. (PES) ▸ Perceived Exertion
s., performance
s., performing
s., prognostic
S. ▸ Psychosocial Adjustment to Illness
s., Rankine
s., Réaumur
s., Reisberg's
s., Schiotz's
s. screening, large
s., sliding
s., sliding fee
s., supplementary
s., Tallqvist's
S., Tanner Developmental
s., temperature
s. ▸ Tennant distress
S., Tennessee Self-Concept
S. (WAIS) Test, Wechsler Adult Intelligence
S. Test, Wittenborn Psychiatric Rating
s. testing, large
S. ▸ Thayer Clinical Anxiety
S. ▸ Toronto Alexithymia
s. ultrasonography, gray-
s. ultrasound, gray-
s. (VS) ▸ verbal
S. (VDRS) ▸ Verdun Depression Rating
S. (VTSRS) ▸ Verdun Target Symptom Rating
s. ▸ visual analogue
s. ▸ voxel gray
S. (WAIS) ▸ Wechsler Adult Intelligence
S. (WMS) ▸ Wechsler Memory
s., Wigle
S. (WPRS) ▸ Wittenborn Psychiatric Rating

scale(s)—*continued*
s., Ziegler's
S., Zung Depression
scalene
s. adenopathy
s. biopsy
s. fat pad biopsy
s. lesion
s. lymph node
s. lymph node biopsy
s. muscle
s. muscle, anterior
s. muscle, middle
s. muscle, posterior
s. muscle, smallest
s. node
s. node biopsy
s. triangle, Burger
s. tubercle
scalenotomy, Adson-Coffey
scalenus
s. anterior syndrome
s. anticus muscle
s. anticus syndrome
s. muscle
s. posterior, musculus
scaler
s., chisel
s., decade
s., deep
s., hoe
s., sickle
s., superficial
s., wing
scaliness of nipple
scaling
s., degree of
s. ▸ goal attainment
s., motion
s. of skin ▸ heavy
scalp
s. abrasions
s. abscess
s. and facial massage
s. ▸ blood flow to
s., centroparietal regions of
s., dandruff of
s. dermatitis
s. ▸ dermatophyte infections of
s. EEG (electroencephalogram)
s. electrode
s. electrode attachment
s. electrode mark
s., electrodes placed on
s., fetal

s. flap
s. flap surgery
s. hair, coarse
s. hematoma
s. implant
s. infection, fungal
s., interface between electrode and
s. irradiation, electron beam
s. itching from dermatitis
s. itching from eczema
s., local tenderness over
s. montage, posterior scalp to
s. muscle activity
s. muscle electrical interference ▸ extraneous
s. oils
s. pH
s. psoriasis
s. recording electrodes
s. reflected
s. sampling, fetal
s. ▸ seborrhea of
s. ▸ silvery scales on
s. site
s. stimulation test ▸ internal
s., subdermal layer of
s., temporal areas of
s., tender
s., tenderness of
s. to scalp montage, posterior
s. tourniquet
s. vertex
s. without palpable lesion
scalpel biopsy
scalpel vulvectomy
scaly
s. and itchy ▸ blister red,
s., disc-shaped rash
s. feet
s. patch ▸ red,
s. ▸ skin dry and
s. skin spots ▸ rough
s. surface
s. suture
scamping speech
SCAN (Stop Child Abuse and Neglect)
SCAN antitachycardia pacing protocol
scan (Scan)
s., A-
s. ▸ advanced imaging
s., alpha
s., angiography
s., B-

s., blood pool
s., bone
s., bone density
s., bone-mineral density
s., brain
s. ▸ brain imaging
s., cardiac
s., Cardiolite
s., CardioTec
s., carotid duplex
s., CAT (computerized axial tomography)
s., clear
s. ▸ computer enhancement
S. Computerized Tomography (CT) ▸ Fast-
s. converter, digital
s., coronary atherosclerosis
s. data
s. ▸ digital holographic CAT (computerized axial tomography)
s. ▸ Doppler ultrasound
s., dot
s., echo
s. echocardiography ▸ sector
s., enhanced
s., enhanced magnetic resonance imaging (MRI)
s., fluorescent
s. frame, B-
s. ▸ full body CT (computerized tomography)
s., gallbladder and liver
s., Gallium (Ga) 67
s. ▸ gated cardiac
s., heart
s. ▸ heel bone density
s., hepatic
s., hepatobiliary
s. ▸ hepato-iminodiacetic acid (HIDA)
s. ▸ hot spots on
s., indiam
s. interpretation
s., isotope bone
s., kidney
s., liver
s., lung
s. ▸ magnetic resonance imaging
s., milk
s., MR (magnetic resonance) brain
s. ▸ multigated acquisition (MUGA) blood pool radionuclide
s. ▸ multiple gated acquisition (MUGA) blood pool radionuclide

s. ▸ multiple-gated angiography (MUGA)
s., myocardial
s. negative, bone
s. negative, brain
s., normal bone
s., nuclear
s., nuclear heart
s., pancreatic
s., pancreatic liver
S., Pipida
s., perfusion
s., phosphate
s., placenta
s., positive bone
s., positive brain
s., postoperative
s., PYP
s., radioactive
s., radioactive brain
s. ▸ radioisotope bone
s., radionuclear bone
s., rapid flow brain
s., renal
s. reveals increased activity ▸ bone
s., RISA (radioiodinized serum albumin)
s., rose bengal
s., scintillation
s., sector
s., sestamibi
s., side-view MRI (magnetic resonance imaging)
s. ▸ single photon emission computed tomography (SPECT)
s., spleen
s., Tc (technetium) 99m
s., tebo
s., teboroxime
s., thallium
s. ▸ thallium exercise heart
s. thermograph, continuous
s. ▸ thin slice CT (computerized tomography)
s., thyroid
s., thyroid uptake
s., transabdominal
s., transvaginal
s. ▸ ultrafast computerized axial tomography (CAT)
s. ultrasonogram, B
s., ultrasound
s., unenhanced
s., ventilation
s. ▸ ventilation defect on lung

s. ▸ ventilation/perfusion
s., ventilation-perfusion lung

scanner (Scanner)
s. ▸ Biosound wide-angle monoplane ultrasound
s. ▸ computerized tomography (CT) body
s., Corometrics Doppler
s., Delmar Avionics
s., ECT (emission computerized tomographic) body
s., Electric and Musical Industries (EMI) brain
s., EMI
s. ▸ Imatron Ultrafast CT
s., laser
s., magnetic resonance
s., magnetic resonance imaging (MRI)
s., MedX
s., neurodiagnostic
s., nuclear
S. (NMRS), Nuclear Magnetic Resonance
s., optical
s. ▸ phased array sector
s., radioisotope
s., rectilinear
s., scintillation
s., supercam scintillation
s., tomographic multiplane
s., total body
s. ▸ ultrafast computed tomographic
s., ultrasonic
s., whole body

scanning (Scanning)
s., A-mode (amplitude modulation)
S. Beam Digital x-ray
s., bone
s., bone marrow
s., brain
s., brightness modulation (B-mode)
s., compound
s., computed tomography (CT)
s., coronary artery
S., Densitometer
s., depth dose in
s. device ▸ wavefront
s., diagnostic
s., duplex
s. electron microscope
s., electron microscopy
s., electronic
s., electrophoresis
s. equipment, computerized

s. equipment, electronic
s. ▸ exercise perfusion
s. format
s. ▸ fluorodopamine positron emission tomographic
s., Ga (gallium)
s. ▸ gated blood pool
s., interlaced
s., laser
s. laser ophthalmoscope (SLO)
s. laser tomograph
s., light
s., lung
s., motion modulation (M-mode)
s., nuclear cardiac
s., nuclear medicine
s. ophthalmoscope
s. probe microscopes
s. process
s., progressive
s., pulmonary perfusion
s., radioisotope
s., radionuclide
s., rapid sequential CT (computerized tomography)
s., renal
s. ▸ rupture event
s. speech
s. speech, patient has
s. ▸ stress thallium
s. studies
s. studies, isotope
s. studies of brain ▸ isotope
s. studies, radioisotope
s. technique, body
s. technique, echo
s. technique, nuclear
s. technique, positron
s., thallium
s. tunneling microscope (STM)
s. ▸ ventilation perfusion lung
s., visual

scanography
s., pelvic
s., slit
s., spot

scant infiltration

scanty
s. menstrual flow
s. menstrual periods
s. menstruation
s. pale cytoplasm

Scanzoni's maneuver
Scanzoni's operation
scaphocephalic idiocy

scaphoconchal angle
scaphoid
    s., abdomen
    s. bone
    s. fossa
    s. fracture, carpal
    s. implant, Swanson carpal
    s. projection
    s. scapula
scaphoiditis, tarsal
Scaptocosa raptoria
scapula
    s., alar
    s. alata
    s., coracoid process of
    s., dorsal nerve of
    s., elevated
    s., Graves'
    s., levator muscle of
    s., lower angle of
    s., lunula of
    s., neck of
    s., scaphoid
    s., semilunar notch of
    s., spine of
    s., wing of
    s., winged
scapulae, acromion
scapular
    s. area
    s. bone
    s. metastases
    s. notch
    s. reflex
    s. region
scapularis, Aedes
scapularis, Ixodes
scapuloanterior
    s., left
    s. position
    s., right
scapuloclavicular joint
scapulodextra anterior
scapulodextra posterior
scapulohumeral reflex
scapulohumeral type
scapulolaeva anterior
scapulolaeva posterior
scapuloposterior
    s., left
    s. position
    s., right
scapulothoracic motion
scar(s) [eschar]
    s., acne

    s., appendectomy
    s., bilateral mastectomy
    s., broad based
    s. camouflage
    s., chickenpox
    s. contracture, burn
    s. deformity
    s., dehiscence of cesarean section
    s., emotional
    s. emphysema
    s., excessive
    s. excision
    s., excisional
    s. formation
    s. from laceration
    s. from midepigastrium to pubis
    s., hypertrophic
    s., hypertrophic burn
    s., hypertrophied
    s., infarct
    s., interstitial
    s., keloid
    s. -like area
    s. -like growth
    s. lower pole left kidney
    s. lower pole right kidney
    s., midline
    s., multiple abdominal
    s. of ovary, white
    s. of uterus, ruptured
    s., old burn
    s., operative
    s., pathological
    s., pop
    s., psychological
    s., Reichert's
    s. removal
    s. retraction
    s. revision
    s. ▸ rupture of cesarean section
    s., S-shaped
    s., sternal splitting
    s. strands
    s., surgical
    s. tissue
    s. tissue ▸ abnormal development of
    s. tissue ▸ arthroscopic release of
    s. tissue, band of
    s. tissue, build up of
    s. tissue ▸ constricted by
    s. tissue detachment
    s. tissue ▸ diffuse
    s. tissue, fibrous
    s. tissue ▸ flexible

    s. tissue formation
    s. tissue ▸ formation of fibrous
    s. tissue, impassable
    s. tissue, internal
    s. tissue, massive
    s. tissue ▸ nonpumping
    s. tissue, revision of
    s., transverse mastectomy
    s., T-shaped
    s., U-shaped
    s., vaccination
    s., V-shaped
    s., well healed
    s., well healed previous excisional
    s. ▸ wide broad based
    s., wrist
    s., Y-shaped
    s., zipper
    s., Z-plasty
    s., Z-shaped
Scardino's ureteropelvioplasty
scarf sign
scarifier, Desmarres'
scarlatina, stomatitis
scarlatinal nephritis
scarlatinosa
    s., angina
    s., myocarditis
    s., rubella
    s., rubeola
scarlet fever
Scarpa('s) [dartos]
    S. fascia
    S. fluid
    S. foramen
    S. foramina
    S. ganglion
    S. ligament
    S. membrane
    S. method
    S. nerve
    S. operation
    S. sheath
    S. shoe
    S. staphyloma
    S. triangle
scarred
    s., antrum
    s. arm, needle
    s. connective tissue
    s. cornea
    s. fallopian tubes
    s. foci, hyaline
    s. heart
    s. kidney

s. lips
s. vessels
scarring
s. and narrowing of esophagus
s., apical
s. ▸ areas of focal
s., basilar
s., corneal
s., cortical
s., duodenal bulb
s., extensive
s., fibrocalcareous
s., fibrotic
s., focal
s., focal interstitial
s. from chemical burn ▸ corneal
s., hilar
s. in interstitium ▸ subcapsular
s., interstitial
s., linear
s., lung
s. lung destruction
s. ▸ mild focal interstitial
s., nodular
s. of anteroseptal wall
s. of aortic valve
s. of asbestosis
s. of breast tissue
s. of eardrum, residual
s. of heart muscle
s. of heart valve
s. of interstitium ▸ focal
s. of kidneys, cortical
s. of lung tissue
s., old
s. or cirrhosis ▸ tissue
s., parenchymal
s., perihilar
s., pleural
s., pulmonary fibrotic
s., pulmonic
s., renal
s., residual
s., retinal
s., subcapsular
s., tissue
scatoma (*same as* **scotoma**)
scatter
s. air ratio
s. factor, back
s. fraction
s. maximum ratio
s. photocoagulation
scattered
s. chronic inflammatory infiltrates

s. coarse rhonchi
s. degenerative changes
s. diverticula
s. echo
s. fibroglandular densities
s. fibrosis without pigmentation
s. hematopoietic elements
s. histiocytes
s. lymphocytic infiltrates
s. lymphocytic nodules
s. radiation
s. radiation within body
s. rales
s. rays
s. rhonchi
s. sclerotic tubules
s. slow waves
s. spikes
scattering
s., broad-beam
s., classical
s. coherent
s., Compton
s. foils in electron beam therapy
s. in brachytherapy
s. law, Rayleigh
s., self-
s., Thomson
s., tissue attenuation and
scatterplot smoothing technique
scavenger cell
scavenger cell pathway
scavenging tube
SCD (service-connected disability)
ScDA (scapulodextra anterior)
SCDK prosthesis, Cutter
ScDP (scapulodextra posterior)
SCDT heart valve prosthesis
scene, primal
scenes ▸ exploration of traumatic
scent ▸ loss of sensitivity to
SCG (serum chemistry graph)
Schachar's implant cataract lens
Schafer method of artificial respiration
Schafer's syndrome
Schäffer's reflex
Schamberg's disease
Schanz('s)
S. collar brace
S. disease
S. operation
S. syndrome
Schapiro sign
Scharf's implant cataract lens

Schatz('s)
S. maneuver
S. -Palmaz intravascular stent
S. -Palmaz tubular mesh stent
S. stent ▸ Palmaz-
Schatzki esophageal ring
Schaudinn's fluid
Schauffler's operation
Schaumann's
S. benign lymphogranuloma
S. disease
S. sarcoid
S. sarcoidosis
S. syndrome
Schauta('s)
S. operation
S. operation, Wertheim-
S. radical vaginal hysterectomy
S. -Wertheim operation
Schede thoracoplasty
Schede's operation
schedule (Schedule)
s. disturbance, chronic sleep
s., dosage
s., exercise
S., Gradual Dosage
s. of medication, daily
s. of medication, tapering
s., patient
s., strict catheterization
s., strict voiding
s., tapering
s., therapy
scheduled, patient tentatively
Scheie('s)
S. operation
S. ophthalmic cautery
S. syndrome
S. technique
schematic eye
schematic representation
scheme, decay
schemes, medical
schenckii, Sporothrix
schenckii, Sporotrichum
Schepelmann sign
Schepens-Okamura-Brockhurst technique
Scheuermann's disease
Scheuermann's kyphosis
Scheuthauer-Marie-Sainton syndrome
Schick's sign
Schick's test
Schiefferdecker's discs

Schiff's stain
Schiff's test
Schilder's disease
Schilder's encephalitis
Schiller('s)
   S. method
   S. stain
   S. test
Schilling('s)
   S. blood count
   S. leukemia
   S. test
   S. test for urine excretion
   S. -type monocytic leukemia
Schiøtz('s)
   S. scale
   S. tonometer
   S. tonometer, Sklar-
   S. tonometry
Schirmer's test
Schistosoma
   S. haematobium
   S. intercalatum
   S. japonicum
   S. mansoni
   S., Trematoda
schistosomal dysentery
schistosomiasis
   s., cutaneous
   s., hepatic
   s., pulmonary
   s., urinary
   s., vesical
schizoaffective
   s. disorder
   s. psychosis
   s. type schizophrenia
schizoid
   s. personality
   s. personality disorder
   s. type
   s. withdrawal
schizophrenia
   s., ambulatory
   s. and substance abuse,
      comorbidity of
   s., catatonic
   s., catatonic type
   s., catatonic type, chronic
   s., catatonic type, chronic with
      acute exacerbation
   s., catatonic type, subchronic
   s., catatonic type, subchronic with
      acute exacerbation
   s., catatonic type, unspecified

s., childhood
s., chronic
s., ▸ chronic paranoid
s., chronic undifferentiated
s., degeneration of
s., disorganized
s., disorganized type, chronic
s., disorganized type, chronic with
   acute exacerbation
s., disorganized type, subchronic
s., disorganized type, subchronic
   with acute exacerbation
s., disorganized type, unspecified
s., drug-resistant
s., hebephrenic-type
s., introvert-type
s., latent
s. -like behavior
s. -like psychosis
s. -like state ▸ chronic
s., paranoid
s., paranoid type, chronic
s., paranoid type, chronic with acute
   exacerbation
s., paranoid type, subchronic
s., paranoid type, subchronic with
   acute exacerbation
s., paranoid type, unspecified
s., prepubescent
s., process
s., pseudoneurotic-type
s., reactive
s. ▸ relapse in
s., residual
s., residual type
s., residual type, chronic
s., residual type, chronic with acute
   exacerbation
s., residual type, subchronic
s., residual type, subchronic with
   acute exacerbation
s., residual type, unspecified
s., schizoaffective-type
s., simple
s., undifferentiated
s., undifferentiated type
s., undifferentiated type, chronic
s., undifferentiated type, chronic
   with acute exacerbation
s., undifferentiated type, subchronic
s., undifferentiated type, subchronic
   with acute exacerbation
s., undifferentiated type, unspecified
s., unspecified
s. with prominent delusions

schizophrenic
   s. behavior, violent
   s. behavior with residual disability
   s. brain abnormalities
   s. cocaine abuser
   s. delusions
   s. disorder
   s. disorder, catatonic
   s. disorder, disorganized
   s. episode, acute
   s. hallucinations
   s. hallucinations and delusions
   s. -like psychotic state
   s. patient
   s. patient, chronic relapsing
   s. patient perseverating
   s. reaction
   s. spectrum disorders
   s. symptoms
   s. thought disorder
schizophreniform disorder
schizophrenoides, delirium
schizotypal personality
schizotypal personality disorder
Schlatter('s)
   S. disease
   S. disease, Osgood-
   S. syndrome, Osgood-
Schlein-type elbow arthroplasty
Schlemm's canal
Schlesinger's sign
Schlichting posterior polymorphous
   dystrophy
Schlichting's dystrophy
schlieren microscope
Schlossman syndrome, Posner-
Schmalz's operation
Schmidt's keratitis
Schmidt's syndrome
Schmiedel's ganglion
Schmincke tumor
Schmitt-Erlanger model of reentry
schmitzii, Shigella
Schmitz's bacillus
Schmorl's
   S. bacillus
   S. body
   S. disease
   S. furrow
   S. node
   S. nodule
Schmutz pyorrhea
Schnabel's atrophy
Schneider('s)
   S. catheter

S. hip fusion
S. index
S. intramedullary nail
S. medullary nail
S. rod
S. stent
schneiderian carcinoma
schneiderian respiratory membrane
Schnöbl's scleritis
Schnyder's dystrophy
Schoenander equipment
schoenleini, Trichophyton
Schöler's treatment
Scholz's disease
Schonander
S. cassette
S. procedure
S. technique
Schönberg
S. bone, Albers-
S. disease, Albers-
S. position, Albers-
S. syndrome, Albers-
Schönlein
S. -Henoch purpura
S. syndrome ► Henoch-
S. vasculitis ► Henoch-
Schön's theory
school
s. activities ► withdrawal from family, friends or
s. adjustment
s. adjustment, poor
s. avoidance syndrome
s. -based intervention
s. behavioral problems
s. examination
s. -made chorea
s. performance, altered
s. phobia
s. phobia in children
s. -related activities ► abnormal dread of
Schott treatment
schottmülleri, gram-negative Salmonella
schottmülleri, Salmonella
Schreger's striae
Schreiber's maneuver
Schridde's granules
Schrötter's chorea
Schuchardt's incision
Schuchardt's operation
Schüffner's granules
Schüffner's stippling

Schuknecht('s)
S. stapedectomy
S. stapedectomy technique
S. Teflon wire piston prosthesis
Schüle's sign
Schuletz pacemaker
Schüller('s)
S. -Christian syndrome, Hand-
S. method
S. position
S. stain
S. view
Schulte breast implant, Heyer-
Schultze's
S. bundle
S. fold
S. granular masses
S. mechanism
S. method
S. placenta
Schultz's angina
Schultz's syndrome
Schuman operation, McCall-
Schumann rays
Schuman's method
Schutz (*same as* Schultz)
Schutz's bundle
Schwabach's test
Schwachman's syndrome
Schwalbe('s)
S. corpuscles
S. fissure
S. foramen
S. line
S., nucleus of
S., olivary peduncle of
S. sheath
S. space
Schwann('s)
S. cell transplants
S. cells
S. cells, enlarged
S. sheath
S., white substance of
schwannoma, malignant
schwannoma, vestibular
Schwartz test, Watson-
Schwartze's sign
Schwartz's leukemia virus
Schweigger's capsule
Schweigger's perimeter
sciatic
s. component
s. hernia
s. nerve

s. nerve block
s. nerve distribution
s. nerve ► irritation of
s. nerve, pinched
s. nerve radiation
s. nerve, small
s. neuritis
s. notch
s. notch, greater
s. notch, lesser
s. pain
s. radiation, left
s. radiation, right
s. scoliosis
SCID (severe combined immunodeficiency)
SCIDS (severe combined immunodeficiency syndrome)
scie, bruit de
scie ou de rape, bruit
science
s., behavioral
s., brain
s., medical
s., molecular
s., social
s., sports
scientific
s. hydrotherapy
s. innovation
s. investigation, intensive
s. medicine
s. methodology
s. research ► authorization form for body to be donated for
s. research ► consent form for body to be donated for
s. understanding
scimitar
s. sign
s. syndrome
s. syndrome ► radiologic
scintigram, pyrophosphate
scintigraphic
s. angiography
s. perfusion defect
s. perfusion defection
scintigraphy
s., acute infarct
s., antimyosin infarct avid
s. ► dipyridamole thallium 201
s. ► exercise thallium 201
s. ► FFA labeled
s. ► gallium 67
s. ► gated blood pool

scintigraphy—*continued*
- s. ▸ indium 111
- s. ▸ infarct avid
- s. ▸ infarct avid hot spot
- s. ▸ infarct avid myocardial
- s. ▸ iodine 131 MIBG
- s. ▸ labeled FFA
- s. ▸ microsphere perfusion
- s. ▸ myocardial cold spot perfusion
- s. ▸ myocardial perfusion
- s. ▸ myocardial viability
- s., NEFA
- s., perfusion
- s. ▸ planar thallium
- s., pulmonary
- s., pyrophosphate
- s. ▸ single photon gamma
- s., SPECT
- s. ▸ stress thallium
- s. ▸ Tc-99 sestamibi
- s., thallium
- s. ▸ thallium-201 myocardial perfusion
- s. ▸ thallium-201 perfusion
- s. ▸ thallium-201 planar
- s. ▸ thallium-201 SPECT
- s. ▸ thyroidal lymph node
- s., ventilation

scintillans, synchysis
scintillating
- s. camera
- s. scotoma
- s. speckle pattern

scintillation
- s. camera
- s. camera ▸ gamma
- s. camera, positron
- s. cocktail
- s. counter
- s. counting technique
- s. probe
- s. scan
- s. scanner
- s. scanner, supercam

scintiphoto, combined transmission-emission
scintiphoto, liver
scintiscan, salivary
scirrhous/scirrhus [*serous, cirrus*]
- s. cancer
- s. carcinoma

scissors
- s. bite
- s. gait
- s. movement

- s. walking

ScLA (scapulolaeva anterior)
sclera
- s., blue
- s., buckling of
- s. cryotherapy
- s., ectasia of
- s., fibroma of
- s., fistula of
- s. marker
- s., optic foramen of
- s., preserved
- s. ▸ proper substance of
- s., ruptured
- s., superficial
- s., suture of
- s., thinning of
- s., venous sinus of

sclerae
- s. and conjunctivae (S and C)
- s. and conjunctivae (S and C) clear
- s., icteric
- s., jaundiced
- s., melanosis
- s., nonicteric
- s., sinus venosus

scleral
- s. bed
- s. buckle
- s. buckle ▸ vitrectomy and
- s. buckler implant, Silastic
- s. buckling
- s. buckling procedure
- s. crescent
- s. ectasia
- s. fistula operation
- s. flap
- s. hemorrhage
- s. icterus
- s. implant
- s. implant, Berens-Rosa
- s. insertion
- s. pigmentation
- s. resection
- s. rim
- s. ring, Bonaccolto's
- s. ring, Flieringa
- s. shortening
- s. staphyloma

sclerectomy
- s. with punch
- s. with scissors
- s. with trephine

scleredema
- s. adultorum
- s. neonatorum
- s. of Buschke

sclerema neonatorum
scleritis
- s., annular
- s., diffuse anterior
- s., necrotizing
- s., Schnöbl's

sclerocarpa, Acrocomia
sclerocorneal junction
scleroderma
- s., bullous
- s., localized
- s. lung
- s., pulmonary
- s. ▸ severe systemic
- s., systemic
- s., telangiectasia (CRST) syndrome ▸ calcification, Raynaud's phenomenon,

sclerolaser treatment
scleronyxis (*same as* scleroticonyxis)
sclerosed, glomeruli
sclerosed leiomyoma
sclerosing
- s. adenitis
- s. adenosis
- s. agent
- s. alveolitis, diffuse
- s. cholangitis, primary
- s. hemangioma
- s. keratitis
- s. leukoencephalitis ▸ subacute
- s. mastoiditis
- s. of bleeding esophageal varices ▸ endoscopic
- s. of esophageal varices
- s. panencephalitis (SSPE) ▸ subacute
- s. phlebitis
- s., variceal

sclerosis [*cirrhosis*]
- s., acute multiple
- s., Alzheimer's
- s. (ALS) ▸ amyotrophic lateral
- s., annular
- s., anterolateral
- s., aortic
- s., arterial
- s., arteriocapillary
- s., arteriolar
- s., benign
- s., benign multiple

s., bony
s., bulbar
s., cerebellar
s., cerebral
s., cerebrospinal
s., cervical
s., chronic esophageal
s. (MS) ▸ chronic progressive multiple
s. circle of Willis
s., combined
s., coronary
s., cutaneus systemic
s., dentinal
s., diffuse
s., diffuse systemic
s., disseminated
s., dorsal
s., endocardial
s., endoscopic
s., Erb's
s., esophageal variceal
s. (FALS) ▸ familial amyotrophic lateral
s., familial cerebral
s., focal
s., gastric
s., hereditary
s., hyaline
s., hyperplastic
s., insular
s., Krabbe's
s., labyrinthine
s., lateral
s., lichen
s., lobar
s., Marie's
s., miliary
s., Mönckeberg's
s. (MS) ▸ multiple
s. (MS) ▸ nerve degeneration in multiple
s., nodular
s., nuclear
s. of breast
s. of islets of Langerhans
s., plaques of multiple
s., posterior
s., posterolateral
s., presenile
s., primary lateral
s. (MS) ▸ primary progressive multiple
s., progressive multiple

s. (MS) ▸ progressive relapsing multiple
s. (PSS), progressive systemic
s. ▸ relapsing-remitting multiple
s., renal arteriolar
s., systemic
s. ▸ systemic progressive
s., tuberous
s. tubular lining
s., unicellular
s., valvular
s., vascular
s., vascular renal
s., venous
s., ventrolateral
s. virus ▸ multiple
s. (MS) ▸ worsening, relapsing-remitting multiple
sclerosus et atrophicus, lichen
sclerotherapy
s., acute endoscopic
s. ▸ long-term injection
s., painless
s. ▸ patient had
s., variceal
s., vein
sclerotic
s. aorta
s. aortic valve
s. glomeruli
s. keratitis
s. kidney
s. leiomyoma
s. ovary
s. patches
s. stomach
s. teeth
s. thickening
s. tubules, scattered
s. tumor
scleroticonyxis (*see* **scleronyxis**)
sclerotomy
s. with drainage (dr'ge)
s. with exploration
s. with removal foreign body (FB)
sclerous tissues
ScLP (scapulolaeva posterior)
SCM (sternocleidomastoid) muscle
SCN (Special Care Nursery)
scoleces ▸ hooklets and
scoliosis
s. and kyphosis ▸ lordosis,
s., artificial
s., Brissaud's
s., cicatricial

s., coxitic
s., dancer's
s., dextrorotatory
s., empyematic
s., ischiatic
s. ▸ juvenile idiopathic
s., list or
s., lumbar
s., myopathic
s., ocular
s. of spine
s., ophthalmic
s., osteopathic
s., paralytic
s., prominent
s., rachitic
s., rheumatic
s., sciatic
s., spinal
s., S-shaped
s., static
s. with concavity to left
s. with concavity to right
s. with convexity to left
s. with convexity to right
scolopendrium, Phymatosorus
scombroid poisoning
scooter, portable
scope
s. advanced directly into duodenum
s. advanced to cardia of stomach
s., fenestration
s., icono◊
s. inserted into trachea with ease
s. introduced
s., kineto◊
s., nonfade
s. passed
s. passed per ora
s. reverted to normal position
s., reverting
s., rotate
s., Welch-Allyn
s. withdrawn
scopolamine poisoning
Scopulariopsis
S. americana
S. aureus
S. blochi
S. brevicaulis
S. cinereus
S. koningi
S. minimus

scorbutic
- s. anemia
- s. dysentery
- s. gingivitis
- s. position

scorbutica, stomatitis

score (Score)
- s., age-equivalent
- s., Apgar
- s., Bishop's
- s., calcium
- s., clinical performance
- s. ▸ Duke treadmill prognostic
- s., echo
- s., electrocardiographic (ECG/EKG) Brush
- S., Expectation
- s., Gleason
- s. ▸ Goldman cardiac risk index
- s. ▸ Hollenberg treadmill
- s. index ▸ wall motion
- s., initial Apgar
- s., initial prognostic
- s., jeopardy
- s., Kurtzke
- s. ▸ lung injury
- s., Silverman's
- s., tender point
- s., trauma
- s. ▸ VAMC prognostic

scored tablets

scoring system, echocardiographic

scorpion venom

Scotch douche

scoterythrous vision

scotoma (*same as* scatoma)
- s., absolute
- s., annular
- s., arcuate
- s., aural
- s., Bjerrum's
- s., central
- s., centrocecal
- s., color
- s., filtering
- s., insular
- s., negative
- s., paracentral
- s., peripapillary
- s., physiologic
- s., relative
- s., ring
- s., scintillating
- s., Seidel's

scotometer, Bjerrum's

scotopic vision

Scott syndrome, Strachan-

scout
- s. film
- s. negative
- s. positive
- s. view

SCR (skin conductance response)

scraped free, iris

scraped vigorously, area

scrapings, skin

scrapings, uterine

scratch
- s. cycle ▸ itch
- s. disease, cat
- s. fever, cat-
- s. ▸ itch-
- s. ▸ Lerman-Means
- s. reflex
- s. tests
- s. -type incision

scratcher, Kratz

scratchy
- s., eye
- s. murmur
- s. sore throat ▸ itchy,

screaming, inconsolable

screen (Screen)
- s., antibody
- s., antigen
- s., Bjerrum's
- s. chart, computer
- s. colposcopic examination
- s. colposcopy
- s., detailed image on
- s., drug
- s. filtration pressure
- s., fluorescent
- s. for amphetamine, urine
- s. for cocaine, urine
- s. for drug use, blood
- s. format ▸ quad
- s. glare ▸ video display terminal (VDT)
- s., Hess diplopia
- s., intensifying
- s. mammography, film
- s. memory
- s., nonreflective glass
- s. ▸ normal pulmonary function
- s. oxygenation
- s. ▸ positive urine drug
- s., prepulmonary
- s., tangent
- s. test, coagulation

S. Testing (CAST) ▸ Children of Alcoholics
- s., toxicology
- s., type and
- s., urine
- s., urine drug
- s., vestibular
- s. ▸ viewer self-imaging

screening (Screening)
- s. and diagnosis ▸ eye
- s. and diagnostic technique
- s., antibody
- s., automated multiphasic
- s., blood
- s., blood cholesterol
- s. ▸ blood donor
- s., blood pressure (BP)
- s., body fat
- s., bone density
- s., cancer
- s. ▸ cancer detection, prevention and
- s. cancer of the cervix
- s. ▸ carotid artery
- S. Center, Cancer
- s., cervical cancer
- s., chemical
- s., cholesterol
- s., colon cancer
- s. ▸ colon cancer gene
- s., colorectal
- s., colorectal cancer
- s. criteria, medical generic
- s. criteria, nurse
- s., Denver
- s., depression
- s. device for drug abuse ▸ cutaneous signs as a
- s. device for drug abuse, diagnostic tests as a
- s. device for drug abuse, medical history as a
- s. device for drug abuse, patient behavior as a
- s. device for drug abuse, patient interview as a
- s. device for drug abuse, patient questionnaire as a
- s. device for drug abuse ▸ physical examination as a
- s. device for drug abuse, psychological history as a
- s. device for drug abuse, social history as a

s. device for drug abuse, symptoms as a
s. device, patient behavior as a
s. device, patient interview as a
s. device, patient questionnaire as a
s. device, psychological history as a
s., donor
s., drug
s. examination ▸ initial
s., foot
s. for drug abuse
s. for drug use ▸ urine
s., free blood sugar
s., free BP (blood pressure)
s., free glaucoma
s., free health
s., free medical
s., free posture
s., glaucoma
s., health
s., hearing
s., hearing acuity
s., heart
s. ▸ heart disease
s., Hemantigen
s., hemocult
s. ▸ hepatitis C
s., initial
s. initiative, nutrition
s., laboratory
s., large scale
s., lipid
s. mammography
s. ▸ mandated metabolic
s., mass
s., medical
s., method
s., multiphasic
s., multiple
s., noninvasive
s., oral cancer
s., osteoporosis
s. panel, drug
s. ▸ peripheral arterial disease
s. physical examination
s. physical examination, preoperative
s., porphyrin
s. potentially infectious blood
s., premarital
s., prenatal
s., preschool vision
s. procedure ▸ prostate cancer

s. program
S. Program, Breast
s. program, drug
s. program, hypertension
s. program, newborn
s., prostate
s., psychological
s., pulmonary function
s., routine
s., routine cancer
s. ▸ routine preoperative
s., Selectogen
s., sickle cell anemia
s., skin cancer
s., spirometric
s. study, genetic
s. summary, preadmission
s. system, automated cervical cell
s., stroke
s. test
s. test ▸ diagnostic
s. test, drug
s. test ▸ false-positive
S. Test ▸ Halstead-Wepman Aphasia
s. test ▸ initial drug
s. test, prenatal
s. test, Reitan-Indiana aphasia
s., thermographic
s., thyroid
s., TMJ (temporomandibular joint)
s. tool
s., ultrasound
s., universal blood
s., vascular
s., virus
s., vision
s., visual
s., visual acuity
s., vocational
s., wellness
screwdriver teeth
Scribner arteriovenous (AV) shunt
Scribner shunt ▸ Quinton-
script docs
scriptorius, calamus
scriptorum, chorea
scrofula, tubercular
scrofulaceum, Mycobacterium
scrofular conjunctivitis
scrofulous
s. gumma
s. keratitis
s. ophthalmia
s. rhinitis

scroll ear
scrotal
s. abscess
s. area
s. area, fluid in
s. hematocele
s. hernia
s. hydrocele
s. mass
s. nerves, anterior
s. nerves, posterior
s. reflex
s. sac
s. sac empty
s. swelling
s. tenderness
s. tongue
s. vein, anterior
s. vein, posterior
scroti
s. carcinoma
s., raphe
s., septum
scrotum
s. and pain ▸ chills with swollen
s. and testes ▸ trauma to
s., dartos muscle of
s., lapillosum
s., lymph
s., raphe of
s., septum of
s., shawl
s., testes in
s., watering-can
scrub
s., Betadine
s., hexachlorophene
s. nurse
s., pHisoHex
s., surgical hand
s. typhus
scrubbed, prepped and draped ▸ abdomen
SCT (Sentence Completion Test)
SCU (Self-Care Unit)
Scuffle (phencyclidine)
Scully's tumor
sculpt tissue
sculpting, body
sculpturing, body
scultetus (Scultetus')
s. bandage
s. binder
s. dressing
S. position

scurvy
- s. grass
- s., hemorrhagic
- s., infantile
- s., sea

scutatum, Gongylonema
scute, tympanic
scutellaris ▸ Aedes scutellaris pseudo◇
scutularis, parakeratosis
scybalous feces
scybalous stool
SD
- SD (septal defect)
- SD (speech discrimination)
- SD (speech discrimination) test

S/D (systolic to diastolic)
SDA (sacrodextra anterior)
SDAT (senile dementia, Alzheimer's type)
SDEEG (stereotactic/stereotaxic depth electroencephalogram)
SDM (standard deviation of the mean)
SDP (sacrodextra posterior)
se, felo-de-
se, per
Se 75 (selenomethionine)
sea
- s. -blue histiocyte
- s. fronds
- s. scurvy
- s. sickness
- s. swimmers eruption

seafood contamination
seafood poisoning
seagull bruit
seagull murmur
seal [feel]
- s. anterior chamber
- s., Asherman chest
- s. -bark cough
- s. bleeding blood vessels
- s., border
- s. chest tube ▸ water
- s., double
- s. drainage (dr'ge) bottle ▸ water
- s. drainage, closed chest water
- s. drainage system, closed water
- s. drainage (dr'ge) ▸ underwater
- s. fin deformity
- s. over victim's mouth, tight
- s., posterior palatal
- s., temporary
- s., velopharyngeal

- s., watertight

sealed
- s., aneurysm surgically
- s. applicator
- s. drainage unit ▸ intrapleural
- s. off, blood vessel
- s. over
- s. over, perforation
- s. vacuum bottle

sealing breast implant, self-
seam incision ▸ stocking
seam, pigment
seamless
- s. arterial graft
- s. prosthesis, bifurcated
- s. prosthesis, Edwards
- s. tube prosthesis, Helanca

sear [seer]
search, room
searcher, mastoid
searcher, stone-
searing facial pain ▸ severe,
searing pain
seasonal
- s. affective disorder (SAD)
- s. affective disorder syndrome (SADS)
- s. allergic conjunctivitis
- s. allergic rhinitis
- s. allergic rhinitis, congestive
- s. allergy
- s. allergy sufferer
- s. depression
- s. disorder
- s. exposure
- s. mood disorder
- s. mood swings
- s. rhinitis
- s. sneezes
- s. studies

seat
- s. angina ▸ toilet-
- s., basal
- s., infant car
- s., lumbar car
- s., rest
- s., shower
- s. syncope ▸ toilet

seated
- s. benign tumors ▸ deep-
- s. cancer, deep-
- s. cold, muscle
- s. guilt, deep-
- s. lesion, deep-
- s. pain, deep-

- s. psychopathology, deep-
- s. rowing exercise

Seattle angina questionnaire
Seattle, hemoglobin
sebacea, acne
sebaceous
- s. cyst
- s. cyst ▸ dermoid versus
- s. cyst, infected
- s. gland
- s. gland adenoma
- s. gland carcinoma
- s. gland neoplasm
- s. hyperplasia
- s. material

sebaceum, adenoma
seborrhea
- s., macular
- s. of face
- s. of scalp
- s. sicca

seborrheic
- s. dermatitis
- s. eczema
- s. keratosis
- s. keratosis, multiple
- s. wart

seborrheica, alopecia
seborrheica, keratosis
seborrhoeicum, eczema
sec (second)
secandi, mania
secant integral
Sechenoff's center
Seckel, bird-headed dwarf of
seclusion
- s. or restraints
- s. process
- s. /restraint observation form
- s. room

seclusive personality
seclusive type
2nd° (second degree) atrioventricular (AV) block
second(s) (sec)
- s. aortic sound (A2)
- s. areola
- s. atrioventricular (AV) node
- s. cartilaginous ring
- s. (cmps) ▸ centimeters per
- s. cranial nerve
- s. (cps or c/sec) ▸ cycles per
- s. degree (2nd°) atrioventricular (AV) block
- s. degree burn

s. degree burns ▸ patient sustained
s. degree heart block
s. degree uterine prolapse
s. digit of foot
s. digit of hand
s., dyne
s. echelon lymph nodes ▸ first or
s. filial generation
s. ▸ forced expiratory volume in one
s. (fps) ▸ frames per
s. -hand smoke
s. -hand smoking
s. -hand tobacco smoke
s. heart sound (A2)
s. incisor
s. intention, healing by
s. intention ▸ wound healed by
s. (kcps) ▸ kilocycles per
s. left interspace
s. (lps) ▸ liters per
s. look operation
s. look surgical management
s. (Mc.p.s.) ▸ megacycles per
s. messenger
s. (m/sec) ▸ meters per
s. (mas) ▸ milliampere-
s. mitral (M2) sound
s. nerve
s. obtuse margin
s. obtuse marginal artery
s. (mcs) of beta radiation ▸
    millicurie
s. opinion
s. or third degree sprain ▸ first,
s., per
s. portion of duodenum
s. positive spikes ▸ fourteen and six
    per
s. pulmonic (P2) sound
s. renal transplant
s. sight
s. signaling system
s. sound
s. sound (A2) accentuated ▸ aortic
s. sound (A2) ▸ aortic
s. sound (M2) ▸ mitral
s. sound (P2) ▸ pulmonic
s. sound (M2) split ▸ mitral
s. spike-and-wave discharge ▸ six
    per
s. spindle, per
s. spindle ▸ six to twelve per
s. (m/sec) squared, meters per
s. stage
s. stage of labor

s. station lymph nodes ▸ first or
s. strength
s. strength tuberculin test
s. through fifth shock count
s. toe
s. toe ▸ dorsal digital nerves of
    medial surface of
s. transplant
s. transplant, removal of
s. trimester abortion
s. trimester of pregnancy
s. ventricle of cerebrum
s., vibration
s. (ws) ▸ watt

secondary
s. adenoidectomy
s. adhesion formation
s. adrenocortical insufficiency
s. amenorrhea
s. amine
s. amputation
s. amyloidosis
s. anemia
s. aortic area
s. aplastic anemia
s. arrest of dilation
s. asphyxia
s. atelectasis
s. axillary adenopathy
s. bacterial infection
s. barium stasis
s. bilateral synchrony
s. biliary cirrhosis
s. bleeding
s. branch
s. bronchitis
s. bronchus
s. buffering
s. calcification
s. cardiomyopathy
s. carina
s. cataract
s. cataract membrane adjustments
s. cause
s. chemoprophylaxis
s. choana
s. closure
s. connective tissue diseases
s. constriction
s. delay in gastric emptying
s. dementia
s. deviation
s. dextrocardia
s. diagnosis
s. diaphragm

s. disabilities
s. disorder
s. disturbance
s. dysmenorrhea
s. effects of treatment
s. electron
s. encephalitis
s. fibrinolysis
s. follicle formation
s. fracture
s. gain
s. generalized seizure
s. glaucoma
s. growth
s. hemorrhage
s. high blood pressure (BP)
s. hydrocephalus
s. hyperparathyroidism
s. hypertension
s. hypertrophic arthropathy
s. hypertrophic osteoarthropathy
s. immune response
s. infection
s. infertility
s. integration
s. interpretation
s. intervention
s. lobule of lung
s. morphogenesis of heart
s. nodules
s. optic atrophy
s. organizer
s. pacemaker
s. palate
s. pancytopenia
s. partial paralysis
s. pleurisy
s. pneumonia
s. polycythemia
s. prevention
s. process
s. progressive multiple sclerosis
    (MS)
s. pulmonary hemosiderosis
s. pulmonary hypertension
s. pulmonary hypoplasia
s. puncture
s. puncture wounds endocervical
    canal
s. radiation
s. ray
s. repair
s. repression
s. response
s. sex characteristics

secondary—*continued*
s. shaping blocks for radiation
 beam
s. shock
s. side-effects
s. site
s. Sjögren's syndrome
s. stage
s. sterility
s. substance, Rollett's
s. sutures
s. syphilis
s. tachycardia
s. thrombosis
s. thrombus
s. to blood loss ▸ anemia
s. to carcinoma ▸ extrahepatic
 biliary obstruction
s. to cardiomyopathy ▸
 tachyarrhythmias
s. to cervical spine disease,
 headache
s. to endocrine disease, diabetes
 mellitus (DM)
s. to gallstones ▸ pancreatitis
s. to head trauma, coma
s. to heavy smoking ▸ emphysema
s. to hemorrhoids ▸ rectal bleeding
s. to hepatic failure ▸ hemorrhagic
 diathesis
s. to pancreatic disease, diabetes
 mellitus (DM)
s. to radiation therapy
s. to severe maturity
s. transformer coil, implanted
s. tumor
s. tympanic membrane
s. varicose veins
s. vitreous
s. vulvitis
secondhand smoke
secreta and excrements
secretase, gamma
secretase inhibitors
secrete(s)
s. excess mucus
s. fluid
s. gastric juice
s. insulin, pancreas
s. prolactin
secreted in kidneys, urine
secreted insulin
secretin test
secreting
s. alveoli, clusters of milk-

s. capacity ▸ enzyme-
s. cell ▸ metaplastic mucus-
s. glands ▸ milk-
s. granulosa cells ▸ estrogen-
s. pituitary tumor ▸ prolactin-
s. thecal cells ▸ androgen-
secretion(s)
s., acid
s. and excretions
s., apocrine
s., aspiration of
s., basal gastric
s., blood and
s., blood and body fluid
s., body
s., body fluids and
s., breast
s., bronchial
s. ▸ caustic gastric
s. collected
s., control gastric
s. defect, aldosterone
s., direct contact with body
s., direct contact with contaminated
 oral
s., enteric
s. ▸ excess mucus
s., excessive
s., exudates and fluids ▸ body
s., gastric acid
s., genital
s. gland ▸ internal
s., glandular
s. in the stomach ▸ retained
s. ▸ insufficiency of thyroid
s., insulin
s., internal
s., intestinal
s., lung
s., melatonin
s. ▸ microscopic analysis of
s., mouth
s., mucoid
s., mucosal
s., mucous
s., mucus
s., nasal
s. of body, internal
s. of hormones
s. of pancreas, external
s. of parathyroid ▸ increased
s. of saliva, diminished
s., oral
s., pancreatic
s., pancreatic exocrine

s., pituitary
s., pulmonary
s. rate
s. rate, aldosterone
s. rate, cortisol
s. rate, parathyroid hormone
s., respiratory
s., retained
s. ▸ salivary and lacrimal
s. spill
s. spill, blood or
s. spill, decontamination of
s. spills from AIDS (acquired
 immune deficiency syndrome)
 patients
s. spills from hepatitis patients
s. ▸ syndrome of inappropriate
 antidiuretic hormone (SIADH)
s., tenacious mucoid
s. tests ▸ pancreatic exocrine
s., thick bronchial
s., tracheal
s., tracheopulmonary
s., vaginal
s. ▸ virus contaminated nasal
s., wax-like
s., wound
secretory
s. activity
s. activity of pancreas, external
s. adenocarcinoma
s. adenocarcinoma ▸ endometrial
s. cell
s. diarrhea
s. diarrhea, chronic
s. endometritis
s. endometrium, early
s. function test ▸ pancreatic
s. granules
s. leukoprotease inhibitor protein
s. leukoproteinase inhibitor
s. nerve
s. otitis media
s. phase endometrium
s. testing ▸ gastric
s. vacuoles
s. vesicles
section(s)
s., abscess formation postcesarean
s., biopsy submitted for frozen
s., C- (cesarean)
s., capture cross
s., cervical cesarean (C-)
s. (CS or C-section) ▸ cesarean
s., classic cesarean (C-)

s., corneal
s., coronal
s. (CS), corporeal cesarean
s., cross
s. CT (computerized tomography) ▸ thin
s., cut
s. (cesarean) delivery, C-
s. done, frozen
s., emergency cesarean (C-)
s. examination, frozen
s., extraperitoneal cesarean (C-)
s., frozen
s., histologic
s., Kerr's cesarean (C-)
s. (CS), Krönig's cesarean
s. (CS), Latzko's cesarean
s. ▸ liver congested on cross
s., low cervical cesarean (C-)
s., low cesarean (C-)
s., lower segment cesarean
s. ▸ maternal death after cesarean
s., meridional
s., microscopic
s. ▸ multiple coronal
s. ▸ nail wedge
s., nonsmoking
s. of aorta ▸ multiple
s. of basal ganglia ▸ histologic
s. of bladder ▸ histologic
s. of brain ▸ histologic
s. of brain ▸ sagittal
s. of brain ▸ serial coronal
s. of brain ▸ transverse
s. of cerebellum ▸ histologic
s. of cortex ▸ histologic
s. of esophagus ▸ histologic
s. of heart ▸ transverse
s. of hippocampus ▸ histologic
s. of kidney ▸ histologic
s. of liver ▸ histologic
s. of liver parenchyma ▸ cut
s. of lungs ▸ histologic
s. of pancreas ▸ histologic
s. of pons ▸ histologic
s. of prostate, histologic
s. of spleen ▸ histologic
s. of stomach, cardiac
s. of vertebral bodies ▸ decalcified
s., pain postcesarean (PPC)
s., paraffin
s. ▸ paravesical extraperitoneal cesarean
s., patient delivered by cesarean (C-)

s. pattern on breast self-exam ▸ wedge
s., permanent
s., Porro's cesarean (C-)
s., post C-
s., postcesarean
s., primary cesarean (C-)
s., quadrant
s., radiography, body
s., recurrent nerve
s. (CS) ▸ repeat cesarean
s. roentgenography, body
s. scar, dehiscence of cesarean
s. scar ▸ rupture of cesarean
s., serial coronal
s., serial transverse
s., specimen submitted for frozen
s. ▸ supravesical extraperitoneal cesarean
s., tissue submitted for frozen
s. ▸ translabyrinthine vestibular nerve
s. (CS), transperitoneal cesarean
s., transverse
s., transverse cesarean (C-)
s. (CS), transverse cesarean
s., vaginal cesarean (C-)
s. view, cross-
s. (CS), Water's cesarean
sectional
s. echocardiography, cross-
s. electrocardiogram (EKG), cross
s. impression
s. plane, cross-
s. transverse projection, cross-
s. two-dimensional echocardiogram, cross-
s. views, cross-
sectioned, doubly ligated and
sectioning of brain ▸ fixation and
sectioning technique, Gregory Pell
sector
s. addiction programs ▸ private
s. iridectomy
s. program, private
s. scan
s. scan echocardiography
s. scanner ▸ phased array
secular equilibrium
secundines, retained
secundines, uterine
secundum
s. atrial septal defect
s. defect, ostium
s. foramen

s. healing, per
s. intentionem, per
s., ostium
s., septum
secured
s., airway
s., bleeding points
s., hemostasis
s. with tape, tubing
s. with ties, hemostasis
security (Security)
s., emotional
s., false
s. hospital treatment assistant (SHTA)
S., Social
S. Unit (MSU) ▸ Maximum
sed (sedimentation) rate elevated
sedated, patient
sedation
s., heavy
s., intravenous (IV)
s., patient under
s., pre◊
s., preoperative
s., sleep
sedative
s. abuse
s. action of drugs
s. amnestic disorder
s. effect
s. hypnotic drug
s., hypnotic or anxiolytic abuse
s., hypnotic or anxiolytic dependence
s., hypnotic or anxiolytic intoxication
s., intravenous
s. -like effects
s. narcotic
s., nerve
s., oral
s. similarly acting dependence
s. -stimulant
s. withdrawal delirium
Seddon's nerve graft
sedentary
s. culture
s. death syndrome (SEDS)
s. habits
s. inertia
s. patient
sediment, centrifuged
sediment, stained urinary
sedimentary cataract

sedimentation
- s. coefficient
- s., erythrocyte
- s. index
- s. rate (SR)
- s. rate (SR) ▸ blood
- s. rate (SR) ▸ corrected
- s. rate (SR) ▸ elevated
- s. rate (ESR) ▸ erythrocyte
- s. rate (SR) ▸ Rourke-Ernstein
- s. rate test, erythrocyte
- s. rate (SR) ▸ Westergren's
- s. rate (SR) ▸ Wintrobe's
- s. reaction
- s. reaction (ESR) ▸ erythrocyte

sedimented red cells
SEDS (sedentary death syndrome)
seductive
- s. appearance, sexually
- s., patient
- s. sexual behavior

seeberi, Rhinosporidium
Seecor pacemaker
seed(s)
- s. calculus, hemp
- s. cell carcinoma, oat
- s. cells, oat
- s. graft
- s. implant ▸ radioactive
- s. implant, radon
- s. implantation, radon
- s. injected ▸ morning glory
- s., iridium
- s. (flying saucers) ▸ morning glory
- s. (hallucinogens), Morning glory
- s. (heavenly blue) ▸ morning glory
- s. (licorice drops) ▸ morning glory
- s. (pearly gates) ▸ morning glory
- s., radioactive
- s., radium
- s. technique ▸ permanent
- s. treatment

seeded peritoneum, tumor
seeding
- s. in endometrial carcinoma, peritoneal
- s. of prostate ▸ radioactive
- s., pumpkin

SEEG (scalp electroencephalogram)
seeing ▸ sudden trouble
seek medical advice
seeker, bone
seeking
- s. behavior, attention-
- s. behavior, cocaine-
- s. behavior ▸ help-
- s. behavior ▸ unrecognized fluid-
- s. behavior ▸ water-
- s. catheter, coronary
- s. client, treatment-
- s., drug-
- s. environment, drug-
- s. excitement
- s. information, individual
- s. manipulative behavior, attention-
- s. praise or admiration ▸ constantly
- s. social support

seen in consultation, patient
seen on x-ray ▸ FB (foreign body)
seepage of gel ▸ leakage or
seeping silicone
seer [*sear*]
sees numerous physicians ▸ patient
sees visions ▸ patient
seesaw murmur
SEG (segmented) cell
segment(s)
- s., abnormal
- s. alternans ▸ ST
- s., antero-apical
- s., basal
- s., basilar
- s., bronchopulmonary
- s., bypass occluded
- s. cesarean (C-) section ▸ lower
- s. changes, ST
- s., coving of ST
- s., cranial
- s. depression ▸ downhill ST
- s. depression ▸ downsloping ST
- s. depression ▸ PQ
- s. depression ▸ ST
- s., discrete
- s., dyssynergic myocardial
- s. elevation, persistent ST
- s. elevation, ST
- s., flail
- s., frontal
- s., hepatic
- s., interannular
- s., lingular
- s., lower
- s., lower uterine
- s., medullary
- s., mesoblastic
- s., mesodermal
- s., occipital
- s. of artery, excision
- s. of bowel
- s. of bowel ▸ diseased
- s. of chromosome
- s. of colon, aganglionic
- s. of kidney
- s. of liver
- s. of lung
- s. of lung, anterior
- s. of lung, apical
- s. of lung, apicoposterior
- s. of lung, posterior
- s. of lung, superior
- s. of pelvis, pubic
- s. of Rivinus
- s., parietal
- s., postapical
- s., PQ
- s., PR
- s., primitive
- s., protovertebral
- s., pulmonary
- s., Ranvier's
- s., renal
- s., rivinian
- s., Rivinus'
- s., rod
- s., RST
- s., sacral
- s., skin
- s., spinal
- s., ST
- s., stenotic
- s., Ta
- s., TP
- s., TPQ
- s., TQ
- s., upper
- s., uterine
- s., ventricular

segmental
- s. analysis of hair follicles
- s. arterial disorganization
- s. artery
- s. atelectasis
- s. atelectasis ▸ lower lobe
- s. bronchi
- s. bronchi, upper lobe
- s. bronchus
- s. bronchus, basal
- s. colitis
- s. colon resection
- s. enteritis
- s. fracture
- s. fracture, closed
- s. lung resection
- s. mastectomy
- s. orifice

s. pressure index
s. pulmonary resection
s. reflex
s. resection
s. stenosis
s. stripping
s. wall motion
s. washings

segmentary syndrome
segmentation
s. anomaly
s. contraction
s., haustral
s. ▸ k-space
s. movement

segmented
s. (SEG) cell
s. forms
s. fracture
s. hyalinizing vasculitis
s. neutrophil(s)
s. ring tripolar lead

segnis, Ctenopsyllus
segnis, Leptopsylla
Segond's fracture
segregation, chromosomal
segregation, ecto/endocervical cell
SEGs (segmented cells)
Séguin's signal symptom
Seidelin bodies
Seidel's scotoma
Seidel's sign
Seiditz powder test
seismic wave
Seitz sign
Seitz's metamorphosing respiration
seize [*cease*]
seizure(s)
s. ▸ abnormalities characteristic of
s., absence of
s., active
s. activity
s. activity, build-up of
s. activity, continuous
s. activity indicative of brain
   metastases
s. activity, occasional
s. activity, questionable
s. activity, spike
s., acute traumatic
s., alcohol withdrawal
s. and paralysis ▸ uncontrollable
s. associated with drug withdrawal
s., atypical
s., audiogenic

s. ▸ brief recurrent
s., centrencephalic
s., cerebral
s., clinical
s., clinically diagnosable
s., clonic
s. cocaine
s., complex partial
s., continuous epileptic
s., continuous focal
s., convulsive
s., cortical
s., destructive
s. diathesis
s. discharges
s. disorder
s. disorder, idiopathic
s. disorder, mixed
s. disorder patients
s. disorder, previous
s. disorder ▸ primary generalized
s. disorders, epilepsy and
s. duration
s. dysrhythmia
s., epileptic
s. episode
s., fatal
s., febrile
s., focal
s., focal convulsive
s. focus
s. -free
s., frequent
s. from alcohol
s. from brain
s., generalized
s., grand mal
s., illusional
s., impending
s. impulses
s. in intracranial neoplasm
s. induction
s., infant with
s., isolated grand mal
s., jacksonian
s. ▸ Laennec's Gasteva
s., larval
s. ▸ little clusters of
s., localized clonic
s. medication, anti-
s., motor
s., myoclonic
s., neonatal
s., nocturnal
s. ▸ nonfever-related

s. or convulsions
s., partial
s. ▸ partial epileptic
s., patient had
s. pattern
s. pattern ▸ electroencephalogram
   (EEG)
s. pattern, pre◊
s., photogenic
s. ▸ postoperative neurological
s., post-traumatic
s. -producing areas of brain
s. prone
s., provoked
s., psychic
s., psychomotor
s. reaction
s., reducing frequency of
s., reduction in
s. ▸ secondary generalized
s., sensory
s., simple partial
s. specific brain waves ▸
   suppression of
s., spontaneous
s., subliminal
s. threshold
s., tonic
s., tonic-clonic
s. -triggering lesion
s., uncontrollable
s. ▸ uncontrolled generalized grand
   mal
s. ▸ uncontrolled generalized tonic
   clonic
s., unprovoked
s. variant
s. wave electroencephalogram
   (EEG) activity ▸ suppress
   specific
s., withdrawal

Seldinger technique
select diet
selected
s. frequency bands
s. insertion site
s. physiologic activity
s. population of patients
s. retroperitoneal lymph node
   biopsies

selecting treatment method
selecting treatment setting
selection
s., baby gender
s. bias

selection—*continued*
- s. of abused drug
- s., optimal dose
- s., patient
- s., recipient

selective
- s. ablation
- s. angiocardiography
- s. angiography
- s. aortography
- s. arterial magnetic resonance (MR) angiography
- s. arteriography
- s. blindness and paralysis
- s. chemotherapy
- s. coronary arteriography
- s. decontamination of digestive tract
- s. degeneration of nerve cells
- s. electrode ▸ ion
- s. estrogen receptor modulators (SERM)
- s. exertion
- s. hearing
- s. hearing loss (SHL)
- s. intracoronary thrombolysis
- s. memory
- s. past pathway
- s. photothermolysis
- s. prevention
- s. recall
- s. referral
- s. renal arteriography
- s. roentgenography
- s. serotonin re-uptake inhibitors (SSRI)
- s. stain
- s. studies
- s. surveillance
- s. targeting
- s. venography
- s. venous magnetic resonance (MR) angiography
- s. visceral aortography

Selectogen screening
selectors, electrode
Selig prosthesis
selenium
- s. deficiency
- s. poisoning
- s. sulfide

selenomethionine (Se 75)
self (Self)
- s. -absorbed ▸ patient
- s. -absorption

- s. -abuse ▸ agitation, delusions and tendency to
- s. -abusive patient ▸ severely
- s. -acceptance
- s. -actuated learning process
- s. -administered, drug
- s. -administered injection
- s. -administered systematic desensitization
- s. -administration of medication
- s. -administration of opioids ▸ long-term
- s., anticipation of misfortune to
- s. -appraisal, arrogant
- s. -appraisal ▸ inflated
- s. -articulating femoral (SAF) hip replacement
- s. -assertion
- s. -assertion ▸ healthy
- s. -assertive ▸ patient
- s. -assessment
- s. -assured manner
- s. -assured ▸ patient
- s. -attenuation, source
- s. -awareness
- s. -awareness in illness
- s. -awareness ▸ reflective
- s. -blame ▸ symptoms of recantation and
- s. -care
- s. -care activities
- s. -care deficit
- s. -care deficit, bathing
- s. -care deficit, dressing
- s. -care deficit ▸ feeding
- s. -care deficit ▸ grooming
- s. -care deficit ▸ hygiene
- s. -care deficit ▸ toileting
- s. -care function
- s. -care ▸ independent
- s. -care management
- s. -care measures
- s. -care, medical
- s. -care skills
- s. -care techniques
- s. -care ▸ understanding, insight and
- S. -Care Unit (SCU)
- s. -catheterization, intermittent
- s. -centered, excessively
- s. -centeredness and suspicion
- s. -centeredness, destructive
- s. -concept, improved
- s. -concept, realistic
- S. -Concept Scale, Tennessee

- s. -confidence
- s. -confidence, develop
- s. -confidence, increased
- s. -confidence, low
- s. -confidence ▸ severe loss of
- s. -confident
- s. -conscious ▸ patient
- s. -contained, transportable medical unit
- s. -contained underwater breathing apparatus
- s. -contradictory
- s. -control
- s. -control, loss of
- s. -control of heart rate
- s. -control skills
- s. -controlled intravenous system
- s. -created problems
- s. -critical patient
- s. -criticism, attendant
- s. -damaging behavior
- s. -defeating behavior
- s. -defeating behavior pattern
- s. -defeating personality
- s. -defeating personality disorder
- s. -defeating way ▸ patient a perfectionist in
- s. -denial
- s. -deprecating ▸ patient
- s. -deprecation
- s. -deprecation ▸ displays
- s. -depreciation
- s. -destruction
- s. -destruction, means of
- s. -destructive acts
- s. -destructive alcohol abuse
- s. -destructive behavior
- s. -destructive disease
- s. -destructive patient
- s. -destructiveness ▸ lack of
- S. -Determination Act (PSDA) ▸ Patient
- s. -determination, medical
- s. -diagnose
- s. -diagnose, patient tends to
- s. -differentiation
- s. -digestion
- s. -directed potential for violence
- s. -directed violence
- s. -discipline
- s. -disciplined, patient
- s. -dramatization
- s. -dramatizes ▸ patient
- s. -effacement
- s. -efficacy ▸ enhancing

s. -efficacy, low
s. -endangerment ▸ physical
s. -esteem
s. -esteem, building
s. -esteem child ▸ low
s. -esteem, chronic low
s. -esteem, diminished
s. -esteem disturbance
s. -esteem ▸ enhance
s. -esteem, enhancing
s. -esteem ▸ improve health
s. -esteem, inflated
s. -esteem is fragile ▸ patient
s. -esteem ▸ loss of
s. -esteem, low
s. -esteem of patient
s. -esteem or guilt ▸ low
s. -esteem ▸ poor
s. -esteem ▸ shame and
s. -esteem ▸ situational low
s. -esteem skills
s. -esteem ▸ vulnerability in
s. -evaluation
s. -evaluation and correction
s. -examination (BSE), breast
s. -examination, concentric circle pattern on breast
s. -examination (BSE) ▸ monthly breast
s. -examination of testicle
s. -examination ▸ skin
s. -examination (TSE) ▸ testicular
s. -examination ▸ vertical pattern on breast
s. -examination ▸ wedge section pattern on breast
s. -expanding stent
s. -expectation ▸ high
s. -exploration, psychologic
s. -fermentation
s. -fertilization
s. ▸ focus on
s. -fulfilling prophesies
s. -generation, affect
s. -harm
s. -harm ▸ potential for
s. -harming behavior
s. healing
s. -healing personality
s. -help
s. -help abortion
s. -help course
s. -help course, mutual
s. -help groups
S. -Help Groups, Community

s. -help, medical
s. -help program
s. -help skill
s. -help support group
s. -help techniques
s. -hypnosis
s. -hypnosis ▸ patient under
s. -image
s. -image, comfortable
s. -image, disturbance in
s. -image ▸ good
s. -image ▸ improve
s. -image ▸ patient
s. -image ▸ persistently unstable
s. -image ▸ poor
s. -image, positive
s. -image ▸ profound change in
s. -image, negative
s. -image ▸ stability of
s. -image ▸ unstable
s. -imaging screen ▸ viewer
s. -importance
s. -importance ▸ exaggerated sense of
s. -importance ▸ grandiose sense of
s. -imposed abstinence
s. -imposed starvation
s. -improvement groups
s. -improvement program
s. -improvement skills
s. -induced illness
s. -induced purging
s. -induced tattoos
s. -induced vomiting
s. -inductance
s. -infection
s. -inflicted abuse behavior
s. -inflicted injury
s. -inflicted wound
s. -inhibiting behavioral injury device (SIBID)
s. -injuring behaviors
s. -injurious habits
s. -inspections, regular
s. -introspection, positive
s. -knowledge ▸ loss of
s. -limited
s. -limited examination
s. -limiting illness
s. -limiting pain
s. -locking prosthesis ▸ Vitallium Moore
s. -locking stitch
s. -management

s. -management ▸ diabetes
s. -management ▸ instruction in
s. -management skills
s. -managing arthritis
s. -medicating ▸ patient
s. -monitoring blood pressure
s. -monitoring, glucose
s. -monitoring skills
s. -motivated, patient
s. -mutilating behavior
s. -mutilation, act of
s. -mutilation ▸ thoughts of
s. -mutilative acts
s. -mutilative behavior
s. -neglect, apathy and disorientation
s. -nurturing activities
s. -object experiences
s. -object transferences
s. -observation
s. or others ▸ threat to
s. ▸ patient blames
s., patient incapable of caring for
s. ▸ patient mutilates
s. -perceived worthlessness
s. -perception of
s. -perceptions, negative
s. -pity
s. -pity ▸ full of
s. -pity ▸ patient filled with
s. -powered treadmill
s. ▸ preoccupation with
s. -preoccupied
s. -preoccupied ▸ patient
s. -preservation
s. -psychological approach
s. -psychology
s. -psychology of dreaming
s. ▸ reckless disregard for safety of
s. -recriminatory
s. -referral
s. -regulates, patient
s. -regulating suggestion
s. -regulation, cardiac
s. -reliance, maximum
s. -reliant
s. -replication
s. -report measures
s. -reported history
s. -rescue method
s. -respect
s. -righteous ▸ patient
s. -righteousness
s. -scattering

self—*continued*

s. -sealing breast implant
s. ▸ sense of
s. -sensitization
s. -starvation
s. -starvation, voluntary
s. -sufficient
s. -sufficient, patient
s. -suspension
s. -talk, bad
s. -talk ▸ good
s. -talk ▸ realistic
s. -terminating tachycardia
s. -testing devices
s. -testing for alcoholism
s. -tolerance
s. ▸ totally incapable of caring for
s. -transmissibility region
s. -treatment
s. ▸ unstable sense of
s. -worth
s. -worth, augment individual's sense of
s. -worth, diminished
s. -worth ▸ rediscovering a sense of
s. -worth ▸ sense of
selfish dependency
Selivanoff's reaction
Selivanoff's test
Seliwanow's reaction
Seliwanow's test
sella
s., dorsum
s. syndrome, empty
s. turcica
s. turcica, diaphragm of
s. turcica, enlargement of
s. turcica normal
sellae, diaphragma
Sellards' test
Sellick maneuver
Selter's disease
SEM (scanning electron microscopy)
SEM (standard error of the mean)
SEM (systolic ejection murmur)
semantic
s. aphasia
s. dementia
s. memory
Semb's operation
semen
s. analysis test
s., blood in
s. ▸ chill with bloody

s. flows backward into bladder
s. from cancer ▸ bloody
s., hair and blood
semiambulatory patient
semiapochromatic objective
semiaxial
s. anteroposterior (AP) projection
s. projection
s. transcranial projection
semicanal of auditory tube
semicanal of tensor tympani
semichronic hypersomnia
semicircular
s. canal
s. canal, fenestration of
s. canal ▸ inflammation of
s. canal ▸ stimulation of
s. duct
s. rings
semicircularis corporis striati, taenia
semicircumferential fibrous thickening ▸ indistinct
semicomatose, patient
semiconductor detector
semiconscious level
semidirect leads
semierect position
semihorizontal heart
semi-invasive aspergillosis
semi-liquid tissue ▸ soft, spongy,
semilunar
s. bone
s. cartilage
s. fold
s. fold of colon
s. fold of conjunctiva
s. fold of fascia transversalis
s. ganglion
s. incision
s. line
s. lobule, inferior
s. lobule, superior
s. notch
s. notch of mandible
s. notch of scapula
s. space ▸ Traube's
s. valve regurgitation
s. valves
s. valves, aortic
s. valves, closure of
s. valves, lunulae of
s. valves of aorta, lunulae of
semilunaris, hiatus
semilunarium
s. aortae, lunulae valvularum

s. arteriae pulmonalis ▸ lunulae valvularum
s. trunci pulmonalis ▸ lunulae valvularum
semimembranous muscle
seminal
s. cells
s. duct
s. fibrinolysin
s. fluid
s. fluid, blood in
s. granules
s. vesicle, inflammation of
s. vesicles
s. vesiculitis
s. vesiculogram
seminis, liquor
seminoma
s., mediastinal
s. ovarian
s., retroperitoneal
s. testicular
semi-oval center
semipermeable membrane
semiprone position
semiquantitative measurement
semireclining position
semirecumbent position
semishell implant
semishelving incision
semisolid material ▸ abnormal sac containing
semispinal
s. muscle of head
s. muscle of neck
s. muscle of thorax
semistructured environment
semistuporous, patient
semisynthetic penicillin
semitendinous muscle
semiupright film of chest, portable
semivegetarian diet
semivertical heart
Semliki Forest virus
Semon sign
sendai, Salmonella
Sendai virus
Senear-Usher syndrome
senescence
s., cellular
s., dental
s., replicative
senescent
s. aortic stenosis
s. heart

s. myocardium
Sengstaken's tube
SENIC (Study on the Efficacy of Nosocomial Infection Control)
senile
s. amyloidosis
s. arrhythmia
s. arteriosclerosis
s. atrophic gingivitis
s. atrophy
s. atrophy of lung
s. atrophy of pigmented epithelium
s. bowing of vocal cords
s. cataract
s. chorea
s. chorioretinitis
s. cortical devastation
s. coxitis
s. delirium
s. dementia
s. dementia, Alzheimer's type (SDAT)
s. elastosis
s. emphysema
s. eversion of punctum
s. halo
s. insanity
s. keratosis
s. lentigines
s. macular degeneration
s. melanoderma
s. nephrosclerosis
s. onset, uncomplicated ▸ primary degenerative dementia of Alzheimer type,
s. onset, with delirium ▸ primary degenerative dementia of Alzheimer type,
s. onset, with delusions ▸ primary degenerative dementia of Alzheimer type,
s. onset, with depression ▸ primary degenerative dementia of Alzheimer type,
s. organic psychotic condition
s. paraplegia
s., patient
s. plaques
s. plaques ▸ neuritic
s. psychosis
s. purpura
s. reflex
s. tremor
s. tremor, benign
s. vaginitis

s. wart
senilis
s., arcus
s., choroiditis guttata
s., circus
s., ectropion
s., keratosis
s., linea corneae
s., malum articulorum
s., malum coxae
senility
s., Alzheimer's
s. and disorientation
s., comatose
s. ▸ early onset of
senior
s. assistance centers
s. day care
s. stress
Senning
S. operation
S. procedure
S. transposition procedure
sensation(s)
s., altered
s., altered somatic
s. and function ▸ return of
s. and motor function
s. and reflex testing ▸ strength,
s., anxiety-related
s., articular
s., atypical
s., auditory
s., basic
s., bearing-down
s., biting
s., bloated
s., burning
s., burning foot
s., chilly
s., choking
s., cincture
s., clicking
s., common
s., complete loss of
s., concomitant
s., controllable
s., cramp-like
s., cutaneous
s., defective cortical
s., delayed
s., dermal
s., deterioration in
s., diminution of pain
s., disorders of

s., distorted
s., disturbance of
s., dysesthetic
s. ▸ elephant-on-the-chest
s., epigastric
s., external
s., general
s., girdle
s., gnawing
s., gnostic
s., grating
s., heat
s. ▸ hot and cold
s., impaired
s. ▸ impaired discriminatory, vibratory and position
s. in chest, burning
s. in chest, crushing
s. in chest, fluttering
s. in chest ▸ painful, burning
s. in chest ▸ pressure
s. in chest ▸ squeezing
s. in chest, tight
s. in extremity, creeping
s. in extremity ▸ tingling
s. in eye ▸ burning
s. in eye ▸ stabbing
s. in feet, tingling
s. in fingertips, tingling
s. in hands, tingling
s. in mouth, tingling
s. in stomach, burning
s. in upper chest, burning
s., internal
s., itching
s. ▸ itching or burning
s., joint position
s. level
s., light
s. ▸ loaded breathing
s., loss of
s., loss of postural
s. magnitude
s. ▸ median nerve transmits
s., modalities of
s., needles-and-pins
s., negative
s., nerve
s., new
s., objective
s. of altered orientation in space
s. of facial fullness
s. of fullness in chest
s. of heaviness
s. of heaviness ▸ flushing

sensation(s)—*continued*
s. of intense dread
s. of pain
s. of pain ▸ loss of
s. of warmth
s. or function ▸ loss of
s., painful
s. ▸ painful, tingling
s., palmesthetic
s. ▸ perception of physical
s., persistent aching
s., physical
s., pins-and-needles
s., popping
s., premonitory subjective
s., pressure
s., primary
s., pulsating
s., reduction in pain
s., referred
s., reflex
s., respiratory
s., retrosternal burning
s., saddle
s. ▸ sharp prickly
s., skin
s. ▸ skin crawling
s., smothering
s., spontaneous
s., stinging
s., strain
s., subjective
s., substernal burning
s., suffocation
s., tactile
s., threshold of
s., tingling
s. ▸ tingling and burning
s. ▸ tingling or prickling
s. to pinprick, diminished
s., touch-and-pin
s., transferred
s., triggering
s. under kneecap ▸ grating
s. unit
s., vascular
s. ▸ vibratory, discriminatory and
    postural
s. ▸ violent spinning
s. while urinating ▸ burning
sense(s)
s. alteration
s. approach, common
s., chemical
s., color

s., decreased position
s. ▸ distortion of
s., equilibrium
s. factor, common
s., five
s., form
s. ▸ intensive stimulation of
s., internal
s. (JPS), joint position
s. judgment, common
s., kinesthetic
s., labyrinthine
s., light
s., muscle
s., muscular
s. of awareness, heightened
s. of balance
s. of balance, deteriorating
s. of betrayal
s. of confidence
s. of déjà vu
s. of depression
s. of disbelief, shock, numbness
s. of euphoria
s. of familiarity
s. of fatigue in leg muscles
s. of guilt
s. of hearing
s. of helplessness
s. of hopelessness
s. of impending doom
s. of increasing helplessness
s. of loss
s. of loss, recurring
s. of pain
s. of pain dulled
s. of panic
s. of panic ▸ overwhelming
s. of release
s. of responsibility, encourage
s. of self
s. of self ▸ unstable
s. of self-importance ▸ exaggerated
s. of self-importance ▸ grandiose
s. of self-worth
s. of self-worth, augment
    individual's
s. of self-worth ▸ rediscovering a
s. of sight
s. of smell
s. of smell, absence of
s. of smell, decrease in
s. of smell, diminished
s. of taste
s. of taste and smell

s. of taste, decreased
s. of taste ▸ lessening
s. of time and perception ▸
    distorted
s. of time ▸ disturbed
s. of time ▸ loss of
s. of touch
s. of touch, absence of
s. of touch and pain
s. of well-being
s. of well-being ▸ euphoric
s., organs of special
s. organs, peripheral
s., pain
s. perception
s., position
s., posture
s., proprioceptive
s., restricted
s., seventh
s., sixth
s., space
s., spatial
s., special
s., stereognostic
s., temperature
s., time
s., tone
s., vibratory
s., visceral
senseless
s. laughter
s. laughter, weeping or rage
s. rage
s., ritualistic acts
s. weeping
sensibilis' atrice, substance
sensibility
s., bone
s., common
s., cortical
s., deep
s., electromuscular
s., epicritic
s., joint
s., mesoblastic
s., pallesthetic
s., palmesthetic
s., proprioceptive
s., protopathic
s., recurrent
s., somesthetic
s., splanchnesthetic
s. to pain, absence of
s., vibratory

sensibilizing substance
sensible
   s. diet ▸ heart
   s. heat
   s. nutrition
Sensibly (TOPS) diet ▸ Take Off Pounds
sensing
   s., atrial
   s. capabilities
   s. cells ▸ light-
   s. conduction ▸ ventricular
   s. configuration, atrial
   s. device ▸ displacement
   s. (DDD) ▸ dual mode, dual pacing, dual
   s. function
   s. ▸ integrated bipolar
   s. pacemaker, activity
   s. pacemaker ▸ Q-T interval
   s. pacemaker ▸ temperature-
   s. spike
   s. thresholds ▸ pacing and
sensitive
   s., abnormally
   s. bronchial tree
   s. cells ▸ light
   s. cells, pressure
   s. chemicals, light-
   s. coccus, gram-positive penicillin
   s. drug, light-
   s., leucine
   s., pan-
   s. patient ▸ aspirin-
   s. receptor, temperature-
   s. to alcohol consumption
   s. to environmental circumstances
   s. to pain
   s. to _____ ▸ patient
   s. tumor, estrogen-
sensitivity(-ies) (Sensitivity)
   s. analysis
   s. and vulnerability ▸ extreme narcissistic
   s., antibiotic
   s., anxiety
   s., aspirin
   s., asthma-aspirin
   s., atrial
   s., carotid sinus
   s., chemical
   s. ▸ circulatory problem with cold
   s., cold
   s. ▸ confusion with light
   s. contaminated, urine culture and

   s. controls, operation of
   s. C-reactive protein (hs-CRP) ▸ high
   s., culture and
   s., decreased
   s., diagnostic
   s., digitalis
   s. ▸ disdain for others'
   s. ▸ drowsiness with light
   s., drug
   s., enhanced
   s. enteropathy, gluten
   s., ethanol
   s. from coldness ▸ light
   s., heat
   s., hidden
   s. ▸ high anxiety
   s., increased
   s. index (SISI) ▸ short increment
S. Index (SISI) Test, Short Increment
   s., instrumental
   s., insulin
   s., iodine
   s., light
   s. measured and recorded ▸ thresholds and
   s., milk
   s., minor light
   s. of electroencephalogram (EEG) channel
   s. of electroencephalogram (EEG) channel ▸ reduction of
   s. of eyes to light
   s. of others ▸ relative disregard for
   s., pacemaker
   s. pattern, antibiotic
   s. pattern, antimicrobial
   s., plane
   s., point
   s. ▸ postsynaptic receptor
   s., potential latex
   s., proportional
   s., reaction
   s., relative reduction of
   s., shock
   s., shyness, and social withdrawal disorder
   s., sodium
   s. studies
   s. studies, antibody
   s., sulfite
   s., sun
   s., sunburn
   s. syndrome ▸ chemical

   s. test
   s. test, insulin
   s. testing, antibiotic
   s. testing ▸ in vitro
   s. threshold
   s. to bright light
   s. to coldness
   s. to hyperthermia
   s. to light
   s. to light, acute
   s. to light and glare
   s. to light and noise
   s. to light and sound
   s. to odors, heightened
   s. to pain
   s. to painful stimuli ▸ excessive
   s. to scent ▸ loss of
   s. to sound, acute
   s. to sounds, heightened
   s. to stress ▸ enhanced
   s. to sunlight
   s. to sunlight, extreme
   s. to temperature
   s. to touch ▸ extreme
   s. to weather changes
   s., urine culture and
   s., ventricular
sensitization
   s., baroreceptor
   s., convert
   s., cross-
   s., cutaneous
   s., neurochemical
   s. response
   s., Rh (Rhesus)
   s., self-
sensitize heart muscle to digitalis toxicity
sensitized
   s. cell ▸ IgE
   s. cells
   s. culture
   s. material
sensitizer, cell
sensitizer enhancement ratio
sensitizing
   s. antibody, skin
   s. effects
   s. substance
   s. substance, erythrocyte
sensitometer, electroluminescent
sensitometric curve
sensor(s) (Sensor)
   s., alco
   S., Cosman ICM Tele-

sensor(s)—*continued*
s. -driven pacemaker
s., electronic
s., implantable glucose
s. ▸ light touch
s., microscopic
s. net ▸ geodesic
s., optical
s. pad, breast
s., photoelectric
s., pressure
s., skin contact of
s., telemetric pressure

sensorial
s. change
s. disturbance
s. idiocy

sensorimotor
s. cortex
s. polyneuropathy
s. rhythm (SMR)

sensorineural
s. deafness
s. hearing loss
s. hearing loss ▸ fluctuating
s. hearing loss ▸ high frequency
s. hearing loss ▸ low frequency

sensorium
s., clearing of
s., clouded
s., disturbance in thinking and
s. is clear

sensory
s. ability
s. abnormality
s. acuity level (SAL)
s. acuity level (SAL) test
s. alteration
s. amusia
s. aphasia
s. apraxia
s. area
s. area, primary
s. aspect of neurologic function
s. ataxia
s. awareness ▸ enhanced
s. belt
s. cell
s. center
s. change in extremities
s. changes
s. changes, motor and
s. component, somatic
s. component, splanchnic
s. conduction, median

s. control
s. cortex
s. cortex, somatic
s. defect
s. deficit
s. deficits ▸ motor and
s. deprivation
s. deprivation syndrome
s. -deprived state
s. dermatome level
s. disability
s. discrimination
s. disorder
s. distortions
s. disturbance
s. dysfunction
s. endings
s. epilepsy
s. epithelial cells
s. evoked potential
s. examination
s. feedback
s. feedback therapy
s. function, motor and
s. functions
s. hair cells
s. hairs
s. impaired support
s. impairment
s. impressions
s. influence
s. innervation, autonomic
s. input
s. input from spinal cord
s. integration
s. integration training
s. integrative problem
s. involvement
s. isolation
s. level
s. loss
s. mechanism ▸ pulmonary
s. memories ▸ fragmentary
s. modality
s. modality, individual
s. motor disease
s. motor syndrome
s. nerve
s. nerve action potential (SNAP)
s. nerve, cardiac
s. nerve cells
s. nerve conduction
s. nerve conduction study ▸ motor and
s. nerve deflection

s. nerve endings
s. nerve fibers
s. nerve in foot
s. nerve, peripheral
s. nerve roots
s. nerves of lung
s. nervous system
s. neural hearing loss
s. neuroanatomy
s. neurologic function
s. neuron
s. neuron, peripheral
s. paralysis
s. paralytic bladder
s. pathways
s. pathways, main
s. pathways ▸ referred pain
s. perception ▸ distortion of
s. perception, false
s. perceptions, blurred
s. perceptual alteration
s. phenomenon
s. physiology
s. psychophysics
s. receptor
s. receptor or nerve
s. receptors of ear
s. region
s. restriction
s. seizure
s. sound stimuli
s. stimulation
s. stimulation ▸ external
s. stimuli
s. stimuli, competing
s. stimuli, sudden
s. system
s. trace recall, immediate
s. tract, ascending
s. tract intact
s. variability

sensual pleasure
sent to Admitting Office ▸ admission orders
sent to Recovery Room ▸ patient
Sentence (sentence)
S. Blank, Rotter Incomplete
S. Completion Test
s. construction, verbal

sentinel
s. cells
s. node
s. node biopsy
s. pile
s. polyp

SEP or SSEP (somatosensory evoked potentials)
separate
- s. pockets of pus
- s. stab wound
- s. white blood cells

separated
- s. acromioclavicular (AC) joint
- s., ends divided and
- s. foci, spatially

separating medium
separation(s)
- s., acromioclavicular (AC)
- s. anxiety
- s. anxiety disorder (SAD)
- s. anxiety of children
- s., aortic cusp
- s. at fracture site
- s. counseling
- s., cranial
- s. ▸ E point to septal
- s., early parental
- s., epiphyseal
- s. from mother, short-term
- s., grief and
- s., incomplete
- s., marginal
- s., marital
- s. of fragments
- s. of leaves
- s. of placenta, premature
- s. of transudates and exudates ▸ diagnostic
- s. or loss ▸ abandonment,
- s. ▸ perception of impending
- s. ▸ realistic time-limited
- s., septal
- s., shoulder
- s., tissue
- s., traumatic
- s. ▸ vitreous pulling and
- s., wound

sepsis
- s., bacterial
- s., catheter
- s., E. (Escherichial)
- s., fungal
- s., gram-negative
- s., infant with
- s. ▸ jaundice associated with
- s. lenta
- s., localized
- s., neonatal
- s. peritonitis ▸ E. (Escherichia) coli
- s., postcesarean

- s. pseudomonas aeruginosa
- s., puerperal
- s. syndrome, meningitis
- s., systemic
- s., uremia and
- s., viral

septa
- s. collimator, thick-
- s. collimator, thin-
- s. interalveolaria maxillae

septal
- s. ablation ▸ alcohol
- s. amplitude ▸ apical interventricular
- s. amyloidosis, alveolar
- s. aneurysm, atrial
- s. apposition ▸ mitral-
- s. arcade
- s. atrium ▸ low
- s. cartilage
- s. cartilage deflection
- s. cell
- s. connective tissue
- s. defect (SD)
- s. defect, aortic
- s. defect, aorticopulmonary
- s. defect (ASD), atrial
- s. defect, atrioventricular (AV)
- s. defect, clamshell closure of atrial
- s. defect ▸ iatrogenic atrial
- s. defect ▸ infundibular
- s. defect, interatrial
- s. defect (IASD), interatrial
- s. defect (IVSD), interventricular
- s. defect ▸ perimembranous ventricular
- s. defect ▸ primum atrial
- s. defect ▸ secundum atrial
- s. defect shunt ▸ ventricular
- s. defect ▸ sinus venosus atrial
- s. defect ▸ subcristal ventricular
- s. defect umbrella, atrial
- s. defect vegetation ▸ ventricular
- s. defect, ventral
- s. defect (VSD) ▸ ventricular
- s. deviation
- s. dip
- s. dropout
- s. fracture
- s. gingiva
- s. hemiblock ▸ left
- s. hypertrophy
- s. hypertrophy (ASH), asymmetrical
- s. hypertrophy, basal

- s. hypertrophy ▸ borderline
- s. hypertrophy ▸ isolated
- s. impaction
- s. infarction
- s. lesion, posterior vaginal
- s. motion ▸ interventricular
- s. myectomy
- s. myotomy
- s. papillary muscles of right ventricle
- s. pathway
- s. perforating arteries
- s. perforation
- s. perforator
- s. process
- s. raphe
- s. resection
- s. resection ▸ myotomy-myectomy-
- s. right atrial electrogram ▸ low
- s. rupture ▸ interventricular
- s. rupture ▸ ventricular
- s. separation
- s. separation ▸ E point to
- s. spur
- s. structures, atrioventricular (AV)
- s. umbrella, Bard Clamshell
- s. umbrella, Clamshell
- s. wall motion
- s. wall ▸ posterior ventricle
- s. walls, thin

septate hymen
septate hyphae, broad
septation
- s., deficient atrioventricular (AV)
- s. ▸ normal atrioventricular (AV)
- s. of heart
- s. procedure

septi nasi muscle, depressor
septi pellucidi, cavum
septic
- s. abortion
- s. arthritis
- s. bursitis
- s. complications of drug abuse
- s. emboli
- s. embolization
- s. endocarditis
- s. factor, Simon's
- s. fever
- s. granuloma
- s. inflammation
- s. joint
- s. knee
- s. morbidity
- s. ▸ patient pancytopenic and

septic—*continued*
- s. pelvic thrombophlebitis
- s. peritonitis
- s. phlebitis
- s. phlebitis of cranial sinus
- s. pneumonia
- s. problems related to drug abuse
- s. process
- s. shock
- s. shock, clinical
- s. shock ▸ severe
- s. sore throat
- s. thrombophlebitis
- s. wound

septica, Pseudomonas

septicemia
- s., acute
- s., catheter-associated
- s., E. coli
- s., fungal
- s., gram-negative
- s. group, hemorrhagic-
- s. sputum
- s., transient

septicemic meningitis

septicemic plague

septicum, Clostridium

septicum, gram-positive Clostridium

septicus, Vibrio

septique, vibrion

Septisol, area prepared with

septotomy, balloon atrial

septum (septa)
- s. aneurysm ▸ interventricular
- s., aorticopulmonary
- s., apex ▸ posterior
- s., atrial
- s. bronchiale
- s. bulbi urethrae
- s., cartilaginous
- s., caudal
- s., conal
- s. corporum cavernosorum clitoridis
- s., deflection of
- s., deflection of nasal
- s., deviated
- s., deviated nasal
- s., enlarged
- s., fenestrated
- s. ▸ focal thickening of alveolar
- s. glandis penis
- s., high membranous interventricular
- s., hypokinetic
- s. in midline

- s. intact
- s., interarterial
- s. (IAS), interatrial
- s., interauricular
- s., interlobular
- s. interradiculare
- s., interventricular
- s., irregular
- s. mediastinale
- s., membranous
- s. mobile nasi
- s., nasal
- s. of Bertin ▸ large
- s. of glans penis
- s. of heart
- s. of heart, congenital defect interventricular
- s. of nose ▸ depressor muscle of
- s. of scrotum
- s., orbital
- s. pectiniforme
- s. pellucidum, vein of
- s. penis
- s., perforated
- s., placental
- s. primum
- s., quadrilateral
- s. rectovesicale
- s. renis
- s., retrovaginal
- s. scroti
- s. secundum
- s., sigmoid
- s. spurium
- s., subarachnoid
- s. subluxation ▸ nasal
- s. ▸ Swiss cheese interventricular
- s., tarsus orbital
- s., thickened
- s. tumors, rectovaginal
- s. ulceration, nasal
- s., ventricular

septus, uterus

Séquard lesion, Brown-

Séquard syndrome, Brown-

sequela (-ae)
- s., central nervous system (CNS)
- s., direct
- s., hypovolemic
- s., indirect
- s., long-term
- s. of radiation therapy
- s. of therapy
- s., treatment

sequence(s)
- s., amino acid
- s., anaplerotic
- s., degraded DNA (deoxyribonucleic acid)
- s., direct mapping
- s. excretory urography ▸ rapid
- s. filming, rapid
- s., genetic
- s. induction (RSI) orotracheal intubation ▸ rapid
- s. induction (RSI) ▸ rapid
- s. ▸ intra-atrial activation
- s. ▸ intracardiac atrial activation
- s. intravenous pyelogram (IVP) ▸ rapid
- s., long-short
- s. mapping, activation
- s., molecular
- s. of a gene, nucleotide
- s. of potential change
- s. of spike-and-slow wave complexes
- s. of waves
- s. of waves of inconstant period
- s. posture, developmental
- s. pyelogram, rapid
- s. ▸ spin-echo imaging
- s. tags, expressed

sequencing
- s. ▸ deoxyribonucleic acid (DNA)
- s. genes
- s. the genome ▸ mapping and

sequential (Sequential)
- s. approach, logical
- s. cephalometry
- s. CT (computerized tomography) scanning ▸ rapid
- s. film
- s. flow
- S. Multiple Analyzer Computer (SMAC)
- s. multiple analyzer (SMA-6) test
- s. multiple analyzer (SMA-12) test
- s. oppositional movements
- s. pacemaker, atrioventricular (AV)
- s. pacemaker, Avius
- s. pacing, atrioventricular
- s. quantitative evaluation
- s. steps
- s. type oral contraceptive

sequestered antigen

sequestrans, hepatitis

sequestrants, bile acid

sequestration(s)
s. bronchopneumonia
s., estimated fluid
s. of polymorphonuclear leukocytes
s., pulmonary
sequestrum formation
sequitur, non
SER (somatosensory evoked
response), short latency
Serafini's hernia
serenity, emotional
Serenity-Tranquility-Peace (STP) pill
sergenti, Phlebotomus
Sergent's white line
serial
s. angiogram
s. bilirubin
s. blood sugars
s. cephalometry
s. chest x-rays
s. coronal section of brain
s. cut films
s. dilatations
s. ECGs/EKGs
(electrocardiograms)
s. EEGs (electroencephalograms)
s. electrophysiologic testing
s. epilepsy
s. examinations
s. extraction
s. fashion ▸ incision closed in
s. films
s. lymph node involvement
s. rapist
s. roentgenography
s. sexual psychopath
s. sonography
s. stage
s. thrombin time
s. tracing
s. transverse sections
s. urinalyses
serially clamped
serially clamped, cut and ligated ▸
mesoappendix
serialographic filming
sericata, Phaenicia
series (Series)
s., decay
S., Doppler
s. elastic element
s., full mouth
s., GB (gallbladder)
s. GI (gastrointestinal)
s. of stimuli

s., oximetry
s., radioactive
s., small bowel
s., upper GI (gastrointestinal)
serine dehydrase
serine glycerophosphatide
serious
s. affective dyscontrol
s. ascites ▸ yellow-brown
s. brain disorder
s. depression
s. gum disease
s. health risks
s. hepatotoxicity
s. illness ▸ warning signs of
s. impulsive dyscontrol
s. muscle weakness
s. psychological disorder ▸
potentially
s. respiratory distress
s. side effects
seriously
s. ill (SI)
s. ill ▸ patient
s. retarded ▸ patient
SERM (selective estrogen receptor
modulators)
serocystadenoma of ovary
serodefined antigen
serodiagnosis, hepatitis
seroenzyme reaction
serofibrinous pericarditis
serofibrinous pleurisy
serologic
s. parameter
s. test
s. test ▸ Youman-Parlett
serological
s. indication
s. markers of disease
s. test for syphilis
serology
s., false positive
s. false positive syphilis
s., fungal
s., Laennec's
s., nonreactive
s. test
seromuscular
s. layer
s. stitch
s. sutures
seronegative arthropathy
seronegative spondyloarthropathy

seropositive
s. nonsyphilitic pneumopathy
s. reaction
s. recipient
seroprevalence rate, overall
seropurulent discharge
seropurulent sputum cultured
serosa
s., choroiditis
s. circumscripta cystica, meningitis
s., fibrotic
s., intestinal
s., meningitis
s., myositis
s., polyemia
s. ▸ smooth, glistening
s. ▸ tumor metastases throughout
s., tunica
serosal
s. abscess formation, focal
s. cell
s. deformity
s. fibroids
s. fold
s. hemorrhages
s. layer
s. peritoneal surfaces ▸ dry
s. petechiae
s. reflection
s. surface
serosanguineous (serosanguinous)
s. fluid
s. pleural effusion
s. pleural effusion ▸ bilateral and
right
s. turbid fluid
seroserous suture
serosum, pericardium
serosum simplex, cystoma
serosurvey, blinded
serotina, decidua
serotinergic nerve terminal ▸ central
dopaminergic and
serotonin
s. antagonist
s. deficiency
s. molecules
s. nerve receptors
s. syndrome
serotype A, B and C viruses
serotype ▸ M protein
serous [*cirrus, scirrhous, scirrhus*]
s. adenocarcinoma
s. atrophy
s. cavity

serous—*continued*
 s. cell
 s. chorioretinopathy, central
 s. cyclitis
 s. cystadenocarcinoma ▸ ovarian
 s. cystadenocarcinoma ovary ▸ papillary
 s. cystadenocarcinoma ▸ papillary
 s. cystadenoma
 s. diarrhea
 s. effusion
 s. exudation
 s. fat atrophy ▸ focal
 s. fluid
 s. fluid ▸ straw-colored
 s. fluid, yellow
 s. fold
 s. iritis
 s. labyrinthitis
 s. leptomeningitis
 s. membrane
 s. meningitis
 s. meningitis, chronic
 s. otitis
 s. otitis media
 s. otitis media ▸ acute
 s. pericarditis
 s. pericardium
 s. peritonitis
 s. pleural effusions
 s. pleurisy
 s. retinitis
 s. retinitis, central
 s. retinopathy, central
 s. straw-colored fluid
 s. tumor
serpens corneas, ulcus
serpent worm
serpentina, Rauwolfia
serpentine
 s. aneurysm
 s. incision
 s. plate
serpiginous
 s. border
 s. chancroid
 s. keratitis
serrata
 s., Linguatula
 s., ora
 s. retinas, ora
serrated appearance
serrated suture
Serratia
 S. indica

 S. kiliensis
 S. liquefaciens
 S. marcescens
 S. marcescens infection
 S. piscatorum
 S. plymuthica
 S. pneumonia
 S. species
serraticus, stridor
serratus
 s. anterior
 s. muscle
 s. muscle, anterior
 s. muscle, inferior posterior
 s. muscle, superior posterior
Sertoli('s)
 S. cell tumor
 S. cells
 S. column
 S. -Leydig cell tumor
serum (sera) [*cerumen*]
 s. acetate
 s. albumin
 s. albumin (HSA), human
 s. albumin, iodinated
 s. albumin, iodinated human
 s. albumin (human), iodinated I^{131}
 s. albumin, iodinated I^{125}
 s. albumin kit, Tc (technetium) 99m
 s. albumin, low
 s. albumin, normal human
 s. albumin, radioactive iodinated human
 s. albumin, radioiodinated
 s. albumin, radioiodine
 s. albumin, radioiodinized
 s. albumin (RISA) scan, radioiodinized
 s. albumin (RISA) study, radioactive iodinated
 s. alcohol level
 s. alkaline phosphatase
 s. ▸ alpha-l-antitrypsin
 s. amylase
 s. amylase ▸ decrease in
 s. amylase elevation
 s. and tissue, antibiotic concentration in
 s. antibiotic levels
 s. antigen ▸ mammary
 s., antihuman-lymphocyte
 s., antilymphatic
 s. (ALS) ▸ antilymphocyte
 s., antimacrophage
 s., antineutrophilic

 s., antirabies
 s., antireticular cytotoxic
 s., antitetanic
 s., antithymocyte
 s., anti-tissue
 s. bactericidal tissue
 s. bactericidal titer
 s. bilirubin
 s., blood
 s. -bound iodine
 s. -bound iron
 s. -bound iron, high
 s. -bound iron, low
 s. calcium
 s. calcium concentration
 s. calcium, low ionized
 s. calcium, lower
 s. calcium test
 s. catecholamines
 s. chemistry graph (SCG)
 s. chloride
 s. cholesterol
 s. cholesterol fluctuated
 s. complement
 s. complement level
 s. concentration, peak
 s. copper
 s. creatine kinase test
 s. creatine phosphokinase
 s. creatinine
 s. creatinine test
 s. defect
 s. diagnosis
 s., direct contact with contaminated
 s. electrolytes
 s. enzyme level
 s. enzyme study
 s. enzyme test
 s., Flexner's
 s. globulin
 s. globulin, immune
 s. glutamic-oxalic transaminase (SGOT)
 s. glutamic-oxaloacetic transaminase (SGOT)
 s. glutamic-pyruvic transaminase (SGPT)
 s. half-life
 s., haptoglobin
 s., hemolyzed
 s. hepatitis
 s. hepatitis antigen
 s. hepatitis, homologous
 s. hepatitis, icteric
 s. hyperviscosity

s. IgE
s., immune
s. intoxication
s. iron
s. isocitric dehydrogenase
s. jaundice, homologous
s. lactic dehydrogenase
s. level
s. level, peak
s. lipase
s., lipemic
s. lipid profile
s. magnesium, patient's
s. Mgb assay
s. myoglobin
s. neopterin
s., normal human
s., normal reference
s. opsonins
s. osmolality
s. osmolality, decreased
s. osmolarity
s. phosphatase
s. phosphorus
s. phosphorus test
s. potassium
s. precipitable iodine
s. prostatic acid phosphatase
   (TSPAP) ▸ total
s. protein
s. protein levels
s. protein (TSP) ▸ total
s. protein-bound iodine (SPBI)
s. prothrombin-conversion
   accelerator (SPCA)
s., radioiodinated
s. ratio, thyroid to
s. renin level
s. salicylate
s. sample
s. shock
s. sickness
s. sodium
s. testosterone
s. therapy
s. 3-hydroxybutyrate
   dehydrogenase
s. thrombotic accelerator
s. thyroxin level
s. triglyceride level
s. triglycerides
s. urea nitrogen (SUN)
s. uric acid
s. urine amylase
s. viscosity

s., Yersin's
Servat operation, Fasanella-
serve as baselines for future
   problems, studies to
service(s) (Service)
   s., air ambulance
   s., Alzheimer's diagnostic
      assessment
   s., Antabuse
   s., assessment
   s., better prevention
   s. ▸ cancer-related diagnostic
   S., Chief of
   s. -connected disability (SCD)
   s., consultation
   s., core
   s., crisis intervention
   s., diagnostic
   S., Dietary
   S. Director, Central
   s., discounted clinical
   s., emergency
   s. (EMS) ▸ emergency medical
   s., evaluation
   s., evaluative
   S., Family
   s., food
   s., general clinical
   s., geriatric
   S., Gerontology
   s., health care
   s. ▸ home health
   s., homemaker
   s. ▸ hospital's addiction medicine
   s., in vitro fertilization
   S., Infectious Disease
   s. intake process ▸ family
   s., intensity of
   s. intervention, social
   s., language pathology
   s. ▸ long-term care
   s. ▸ loss of desire to attend religious
   s. ▸ low vision
   s. ▸ management of psychiatric
   s., medical social
   s., mental health
   s., mini-nursing
   s., neurotrauma
   s., nonclinical
   s., nonemergency transportation
   s., nursing
   s., nutritional
   S., Obstetrical
   S., Oncology
   S., Outpatient

s. ▸ outpatient mental health
s., palliative
s. (PFS), patient financial
s., physical therapy
s., physician
s., physician referral
s., prevention
s., psychiatric
s. ▸ psychiatric and substance
   abuse
s., psychiatric emergency
s., psychiatric nursing
s., psychological
S. (PHS) ▸ Public Health
s., pulmonary
s., quality of
S., Radiotherapy
s., referral
s., referral resource
s., rehabilitation
s. -related disability (SRD)
s., respite
s., specialty
s., specialty inpatient
s., speech pathology
s. ▸ supervision of detox
s., support
s., support group
s., supportive
s., therapeutic
s., treatment
s., uncompensated clinical
S. ▸ Urgent Care
s., utilization management
s., visiting nurse
s. work, community
Servo-Driven Orthosis
sesamoid bone
sesamoid cartilage
sessile
   s. adenoma
   s. hydatid
   s. lesion
   s. polyp
session(s)
   s., alpha conditioning
   s., auditory training
   s., biofeedback training
   s., counseling
   s., family
   s., family outreach
   s., family-focused
   s. ▸ family-origin empowerment
   s., feedback
   s., group

session(s)—*continued*
- s., group support
- s., group therapy
- s., outpatient
- s., practice
- s., prenatal counseling
- s., rap
- s., relaxation training
- s., support
- s., therapy
- s., training
- s., transitional counseling

sestamibi
- s. imaging
- s. scan
- s. scintigraphy ▸ Tc-99
- s. stress test

set
- s. -back, emotional
- s., disposable cleansing
- s. ears, low
- s. of dentures, full
- s., recombined
- s., replicated
- s. -up and cueing ▸ assistance,

Setaria equina
Setchenow's centers
seton wound
Settegast's position
setting
- s., clinical
- s. detoxification, social
- s., emergency
- s. exercise, muscle-
- s., hospital
- s., inpatient
- s., outpatient
- s. potential ▸ fire-
- s. ▸ primary care
- s., residential
- s., selecting treatment
- s., treatment

settling culture, gravity
7 (#7) (seven)
- 7 artificial heart, Jarvik-
- 7 (HHV-7) ▸ Human Herpes Virus-
- 7 intrauterine device (IUD) inserted, Copper
- 7 mechanical pump, Jarvik-
- #7 NIH angiographic catheter
- s. pinhole tomography
- 7 -70 artificial heart ▸ Jarvik-
- 7 syndrome, monosomy

VII antigen, factor
714's (depressants)

733 CO$_2$ (carbon dioxide) laser, Sharplan
17
- 17 -hydroxycorticosteroid test
- 17 -hydroxylase deficiency syndrome
- 17 -ketosteroid test
- 17 -ketosteroids

seventh
- s. cranial nerve
- s. nerve
- s. sense

75%, hypaque-M
76 contrast material, Renograffin-
72 hours, organism isolated after
severance, partial
severe
- s. acidosis
- s. acute passive congestion
- s., acute respiratory syndrome
- s. addiction to alcohol
- s. addiction to drugs
- s. alcohol withdrawal syndrome
- s. alcoholic liver disease
- s. allergic reaction
- s. and persistent mental illness
- s. and relentless child abuse
- s. anoxic encephalopathy
- s. anxiety
- s. articulation delays
- s. articulation disorder
- s. atheromatous change of aorta
- s. atrophy of neocortex
- s. autonomic insufficiency
- s. back muscle spasms
- s. back pain
- s. behavior disorder
- s. bone loss
- s. bout of coughing
- s. brain damage
- s. brain stem disease
- s. bronchiectasis
- s. calcified atheroma
- s. cerebellar ataxia
- s. cerebral anoxia
- s. cerebrovascular occlusion
- s. characteristic disorders
- s. chest pain
- s. chest trauma
- s. chronic disease
- s. chronic tinnitus
- s. colonic dilation
- s. combined immune deficiency syndrome
- s. combined immunodeficiency

- s. combined immunodeficiency syndrome (SCIDS)
- s. concussion
- s. confluent bilateral bronchopneumonia
- s. constricting pain
- s. coronary arteriosclerosis
- s. cortical damage
- s. cramping pain
- s. cramps, sudden
- s. cystica
- s. daytime sleepiness
- s. debilitating symptoms
- s. dehydration
- s. dementia
- s. depression
- s. depression, episode of
- s. depressive illness
- s. depressive reaction
- s. diarrhea
- s. disabling handicap
- s. disorder of psychotic depth
- s. disordered water balance
- s. disuse atrophy
- s. dyskinesia
- s. dyslexia
- s. dysplasia
- s. dysplasia, cells indicative of
- s. emotional anguish
- s. emotional stress
- s. epileptic disorder
- s. eye dryness
- s. family dysfunction
- s. fatigue
- s. fetal distress
- s. fibrinous pleuritis
- s. functional insufficiency
- s. functional test
- s. head injury
- s. head trauma
- s. headache
- s. headache ▸ sudden,
- s. hearing loss
- s. heart valve narrowing
- s. heartburn
- s. hemophilia
- s. hemorrhagic pancreatitis
- s. hypertension
- s. hypochondriasis
- s. hypotension, acute
- s. illness
- s. impairment in interpretation of reality
- s. impairment in thinking
- s. impairment of hearing

s. impairment of ventricle
s. incapacitating vertigo
s. infection
s. inflammation
s. inherited disorder
s. insomnia
s. insulin resistance
s. intestinal infection
s. intracranial lesion
s., jabbing facial pain
s. joint pain
s. joint pain and fatigue
s. latex allergy
s. long-term depression
s. loss of self-confidence
s. low blood sugar
s. lung disorder
s. lymphocytic depletion
s. macromastia
s. malnourishment
s. mania ▸ symptoms of
s. maturity, secondary to
s. melancholia
s. memory loss
s. menstrual pain
s. mental anguish
s. mental deterioration
s. mental illness
s. mental retardation
s. mental subnormality
s. metabolic acidosis and coma
s. micronodular cirrhosis
s. midepigastric pain
s. mitral valve disease
s. mouth dryness
s. movement abnormality
s. multiple disabilities
s. muscle spasm
s. muscle wastage
s. muscular resistance
s. muscular weakness
s. myelofibrosis and myelosclerosis
s. myonecrosis
s. nail-biting habit
s. narrowing of artery
s. narrowing of ostia of coronary
    arteries
s. neurological deficits
s. neurological impairment
s. neurotic syndrome
s. neutropenia
s. obesity
s. occlusive disease
s. onset
s. or persistent vomiting

s. oxygen (O_2) deficiency
s. pain
s. pain and debility
s. pain and disability
s., painful skin rash
s. pancreatic insufficiency
s. paralytic illness
s. persistent dizziness
s. personality disorder
s. physical reaction
s. pitting edema
s. pitting edema all extremities
s. postchemotherapy nausea
s. postchemotherapy vomiting
s. postmortem rigidity
s. premenstrual changes in mood
s. psychiatric symptoms
s. psychosis
s. pulmonic stenosis
s. reaction
s., refractory angina
s. renal vascular disease
s. respiratory insufficiency
s. respiratory problem
s., retardation mental
s. rhythm disorder
s., searing facial pain
s. septic shock
s. side-effects
s. skin infection
s. sleep deprivation
s. spasm of blood vessel
s. spasms
s. stabbing pain
s. steatorrhea
s. stenosis left coronary artery
s. stenosis right coronary artery
s. structural damage
s. sunburn
s. swayback
s. symptoms
s. systemic reaction
s. systemic scleroderma
s. throbbing headache
s. throbbing pain
s. thyroidization
s. tinnitus
s. trauma and abuse
s. underlying esophagitis
s. unstable angina
s. valvular disease
s. vertigo ▸ intermittent attacks of
s. vision loss
s. visual loss
s. weakness

s. withdrawal reaction
s. withdrawal symptoms
s., without psychotic features ▸
    bipolar disorder, depressed,
s., without psychotic features ▸
    bipolar disorder, manic
s., without psychotic features ▸
    bipolar disorder, mixed
s., without psychotic features ▸
    major depression
s., without psychotic features ▸
    major depression, recurrent
s., without psychotic features ▸
    major depression, single episode
severed
s. digit reattached surgically
s. extremity reattached surgically
s. jugular vein
s. limb
s. limb reattached surgically
s. limb, reattaching
s. limb salvage technique
s. nerve endings
s. nerve ends
s. nerve ▸ surgical treatment for
s., spinal cord
s. surface of bone
s. tendon
severely
s. affected individual
s. affected patient
s. atherosclerotic
s. cachectic, patient
s. contaminated environment
s. debilitated patient
s. dehydrated, patient
s. demented
s. depressed
s. deteriorated
s. incapacitated
s. malnourished
s. restricted ▸ motion
s. retarded
s. self-abusive patient
s. swollen ankles
s. weakened heart
severity
s. and duration ▸ syndrome,
s. index (ASI), addiction
s. of attack
s. of cardiovascular disease
s. of duration ▸ insufficient
s. of injury
s. of medical problem ▸
    underestimate

severity—*continued*
- s., pain increasing in
- s., symptoms increased in

Sever-L'Episcopo repair of shoulder

Sever's disease

Sewell-Boyden flap

sewing
- s. ring
- s. ring ▸ knitted
- s. ring loop
- s. ring ▸ metal
- s. ring ▸ plastic
- s. ring ▸ prosthetic valve

Sex (sex)
- S. Addicts Anonymous (SAA)
- s. -behavior center
- s. characteristics, primary
- s. characteristics, secondary
- s. chromatin test
- s. chromosomes
- s. -conditioned character
- s., decline in interest of opposite
- s. determinant
- s. drive
- s. drive, decreased
- s. drive, low
- s. education
- s. estrogen hormone ▸ stimulate production of female
- s., extramarital
- s. for crack exchange
- s. headache
- s. hormone
- s. hormone, female
- s. hormone, male
- s. hormone, production of
- s. -influenced character
- s. -limited character
- s. -linked agammaglobulinemia, Bruton
- s. -linked character
- s. -linked defect
- s. -linked disease
- s. -linked disorders
- s. -linked genetic defect
- s. -linked heredity
- s. -linked traits
- s. offender
- s. partners, multiple
- s. pilus
- s. ratio
- S. Role Inventory (BSRI), Bem
- s., safe
- s. steroid
- s. therapy

sexalatus, Physocephalus

sexual
- s. aberration
- s. ability
- s. abuse
- s. abuse, childhood
- s. abuse ▸ dissociation and
- s. abuse group
- s. abuse of children
- s. abuse, preschool
- s. abuse ▸ survivors of
- s. abuse ▸ sustained
- s. abuse treatment, family
- s. abuse victims
- s. acting out
- s. activity
- s. activity ▸ forcible
- s. activity ▸ high-risk
- s. activity ▸ increase in
- s. activity ▸ increase in social, occupational,
- s. activity, teenage
- s. addiction
- s. addiction treatment
- s. adjustment therapy
- s. aggression
- s. angina
- s. appetite ▸ increased
- s. arousal
- s. arousal, decreased
- s. arousal disorder ▸ female
- s. arousal in infants
- s. assault
- s. assault nurse examiner (SANE)
- s. assault treatment center
- s. assault victim
- s. asthma
- s. aversion disorder
- s. battering
- s. behavior
- s. behavior, aberrant
- s. behavior, adolescent
- s. behavior, compulsive
- s. behavior, destructive
- s. behavior, deviant
- s. behavior ▸ high-risk
- s. behavior ▸ inappropriate
- s. behavior ▸ seductive
- s. cells
- s. cohabitation
- s. complications of drug abuse
- s. conduct
- s. contact
- s. cycle
- s. desire

- s. desire disorder ▸ hypoactive
- s. desire from anxiety ▸ loss of
- s. desire ▸ increased
- s. desire ▸ loss of
- s. desire psychosexual dysfunction ▸ inhibited
- s. development, deficient
- s. development, delayed
- s. development ▸ impaired
- s. development, normal
- s. deviant
- s. deviation
- s. differentiation ▸ process of neurobehavioral
- s. disorder
- s. disorders of drug abusers
- s. drive
- s. drive from diabetes ▸ loss of
- s. drive, heightened
- s. dwarf
- s. dysfunction
- s. dysfunction after heart attack
- s. dysfunction ▸ male
- s. excitement, inhibited
- s. experiences
- s. fixation
- s. freedom
- s. function
- s. function, decline in
- s. function, inadequate
- s. habits, changes in
- s. impairment
- s. impotence
- s. impulsiveness
- s. inadequacy
- s. instincts
- s. intercourse
- s. intercourse ▸ involuntary deviate
- s. interest
- s. interest, decreased
- s. interest ▸ loss of
- s. inversion
- s. issues
- s. malfunctioning
- s. masochism
- s. maturation in humans
- s. maturity
- s. maturity ▸ premature
- s. neurosis
- s. offense
- s. orientation
- s. orientation conflict
- s. partners
- s. partners, multiple
- s. performance problem

s. perversion
s. potency
s. practices
s. preoccupation
s. promiscuity
s. psychopath ▸ serial
s. reflex
s. relationship
s. reproductive system impairment
s. response
s. response, abnormal
s. response, heighten
s. sadism
s. stage, adult
s. stimulant
s. suicide
s. syncope
s. transmission
s. transmission of viral hepatitis
s. trauma
s. violence

sexuality
s., adolescent
s., alcohol and
s., built-in
s. issues
s., midlife
s. patterns, altered

sexually
s. abused children
s. abusive experience
s. active
s. active bisexual men
s. active homosexual men
s. active lesbian women
s. active person
s. disordered
s. maladjusted
s. provocative behavior
s. provocative behavior ▸ inappropriate
s. seductive appearance
s. transmitted disease (STD)
s. transmitted disease ▸ warning signs of
s. transmitted infection
s. transmitted pelvic inflammatory disease (PID)

Sézary cell
Sézary syndrome
SF (scarlet fever)
SF wave of cardiac apex pulse
SFP (spinal fluid pressure)
SG (specific gravity)
SGA (small for gestational age)

Sgambati's reaction
Sgambati's test
SGOT (serum glutamic-oxalic transaminase)
SGOT (serum glutamic-oxaloacetic transaminase)
SGPT (serum glutamic-pyruvic transaminase)
SH (sharp)
SH, hepatitis virus
shadow(s)
s., acoustic
s., adrenal
s., aortic
s., bat wing
s., bladder
s., breast
s., butterfly
s., calcific
s., cardiac
s. cell
s., confluent
s., diaphragmatic
s., gallbladder (GB)
s., heart
s., hilar
s. in urinary bladder
s., kidney
s., liver
s., mass
s., mediastinal
s., mottled
s., nipple
s., opaque
s., overlap
s., overlying gas
s., paramediastinal
s., psoas
s., renal
s., ring
s., snowstorm
s., soft tissue
s., splenic
s., summation
s., superimposition of bowel
s. test
s., uterine
shadowing, acoustic
shaft
s., distal fibular
s., femoral
s., fibular
s., fracture of ulnar
s., hair
s., humeral

s. of bone
s. of femur
s. of fibula
s. of humerus
s. of proximal phalanx
s., penile
s., proximal
s., radial
s., tibial
s., ulnar
s., verrucous penile
s. vision

shaggy pericardium
shagreen lesions of lens
shagreen of the lens
shake(s)
s. culture
s., jerks and falling ▸ tremors,
s., patient has the
s. test
s., tremors and
shaken baby syndrome (SBS)
shakiness
s. and jitteriness
s. in legs ▸ uncontrollable
s. ▸ trembling and
shaking
s. ague
s. and trembling ▸ disabling
s. ▸ body stiffening and
s. chill
s. chills and night sweats
s. chills, dyspnea ▸ fever,
s. chills ▸ fever
s. disorder
s. ▸ hyperventilating, sweating and
s. of limb ▸ uncontrolled
s. of part of body ▸ rhythmic
s. palsy
s. sound
s., uncontrollable
s., uncontrolled
s., violent
shaky, handwriting progressively
Shaldach pacemaker
shallow
s. accelerated breathing
s. accelerated-decelerated breathing
s. affect
s. breathing
s. breathing ▸ rapid
s. breathing, slow and
s. breathing with forced blowing out
s. chamber

shallow—*continued*
- s. erosion of skin
- s. expression of emotions
- s., rapid breathing
- s., respirations
- s. respirations ▸ rapid,
- s., respirations slow and
- s. subpleural, focal
- s. subpleural hemorrhage ▸ focal
- s. ulcer
- s., unrestful sleep
- s. water blackout

sham feeding
Shambaugh's endaural incision
Shambaugh's operating microscope
shambling gait
shame
- s. and addiction
- s. and codependency
- s. and guilt
- s. and self-esteem
- s. ▸ sustained feelings of

shampoo, Kwell lotion
shampoo vaccine
shape
- s. and consistency ▸ size,
- s. and motility ▸ size,
- s. and position ▸ size,
- s., body
- s. density, wedge-
- s. discrimination
- s., echo signal
- s., heart size and
- s. implant, reverse-
- s., normal size and
- s., spherical
- s., uterus normal in size and

shaped
- s. amputation stump ▸ cone-
- s. appearance, wedge-
- s. arch ▸ V-
- s. area, wedge-
- s. bacteria, rod-
- s. bacteria, spiral-
- s. body ▸ apple-
- s. body, irregularly
- s. body ▸ pear-
- s. bone, irregularly
- s. cataract, spindle-
- s. cells, oat-
- s. cells ▸ pleomorphic rod-
- s. cells, spindle-
- s. cells ▸ whorls of spindle-
- s. chest, barrel-
- s. continuous suture ▸ U-

- s. cut into bone, wedge-
- s. diplococci ▸ gram-negative bean-
- s. diplococci ▸ gram-negative extracellular bean-
- s. diplococci ▸ gram-negative extracellular kidney-
- s. diplococci ▸ gram-negative intracellular bean-
- s. diplococci ▸ gram-negative intracellular kidney-
- s., dome-
- s. face, moon-
- s. flap of tissue, crescent-
- s. forms, polyhedral-
- s. forms, rod-
- s. forms, spherical-
- s. fracture, T-
- s. graft, arrow-
- s. gram-positive diplococci, helmet-
- s. gram-positive diplococci, lancet-
- s. heart, balloon-
- s. heart, boat-
- s. heart, boot-
- s. heart ▸ egg-
- s. heart, flask-
- s. heart, pear-
- s. hemorrhage, flame-
- s. hemorrhage ▸ linear-
- s. implant, acorn-
- s. incision, crescent-
- s. incision, cross-
- s. incisions ▸ S-, T-, U-, V-, W-, Y-, and Z-
- s. incisor, shovel-
- s. murmur, diamond-
- s. node, spindle-
- s. nuclei ▸ basophilic pleomorphic irregularly
- s. opening, oval-
- s. organisms in sputum ▸ rod-
- s. pattern ▸ torpedo-
- s. pelvis, funnel-
- s. piece of tissue, wedge-
- s. polyp, mushroom-
- s. rash on face ▸ red butterfly-
- s. rash ▸ red, ring-
- s. rash ▸ scaly, disc-
- s. retinal hemorrhages
- s. retinopathy, central disk-
- s. rods, gram-negative cigar-
- s. scars ▸ S-, T-, U-, V-, W-, Y-, and Z-
- s. scoliosis, S-
- s. skin flap, horseshoe-
- s. stereotactic frame, arc-

- s. stools, pencil-
- s. stools, ribbon-
- s. thorax, barrel-
- s. tracing, diamond-
- s. ▸ unequal pupil size or
- s. waves, burst of arch-
- s., wedge-

shaping blocks for radiation beam, secondary
Shapiro sign
shared
- s. needles
- s. paranoid disorder
- s. psychotic disorder

sharing (Sharing)
- s. behaviors ▸ universality of needle
- s. drug needles
- s., history of needle
- s. infected intravenous drug needles
- s., intravenous (IV) needle
- s. needles
- S. Network, Organ
- s., organ
- S., United Network for Organ

Sharley tracheostomy tube
sharp (SH)
- s. and mobile, carina midline
- s. -and-slow wave
- s. -and-slow wave complex
- s. -and-slow waves, repetitive
- s. blow to region
- s. Bragg peak
- s., carina
- s. curettage
- s. cutting pain
- s. disc
- s. dissection
- s. dissection, blunt and
- s. dissection, freed by
- s. dose fall-off
- s. electroencephalogram (EEG) transients
- s., jabbing or electric pain
- s., jabbing pain
- s., localized pain
- s. margin
- s. osteotome dissection
- s. pain
- s. peaks of component waves
- s. prickly sensation
- s. pulse
- s. retrosternal pain

s., spike or delta waves (SSSDW) ▸ significant
s. spike transients
s. spikes, small
s. stabbing pain
s. stimuli
s. substernal pain
s. -toothed tenaculum
s. transient
s. transient, vertex
s. transient wave form
s. transients, central
s. transients of sleep, positive occipital
s. transients, positive occipital
s. wave
s. wave, positive
s. wave transient, central
s. waves, spikes and
s. wave-spike ▸ parietal area
sharpened reactions
sharper hearing
Sharpey's fibers
Sharplan 733 CO₂ (carbon dioxide) laser
sharply demarcated circumferential lesion
Sharrard-type kyphectomy
shave excision
shaved biopsy
shaved plaque
Shaver's disease
shawl scrotum
Shea
S. polyethylene drainage (dr'ge) tube
S. stapedectomy
S. stapedectomy technique
shear
s., atrial
s. force
s. rate of blood
s. stress
s. thinning
sheath(s) [*sheaf, chief*]
s. adenoma, carotid
s., adventitial
s. and dilator system
s., arterial
s. bronchial brushings ▸ double
s., carotid
s., check-valve
s., connective tissue
s., cystoscope
s., dermal

s., enamel rod
s., fascial
s., fatty
s., fibrous
s., glial
s., injected tendon
s., medullated fibers and
s., myelin
s. of optic nerve
s. of rectus muscle, anterior
s. of rectus muscle, posterior
s. of tendon
s. opening
s., panendoscope
s., peroneal
s., polyurethane
s., probing of tendon
s., rectus
s. reflected over periosteum
s., Scarpa's
s., Schwalbe's
s., Schwann's
s. syndrome, Brown's tendon
s., synovial
s., tendon
s., vascular
s., venous
shedding
s., asymptomatic viral
s. carrier
s., chronic fecal
s., excessive hair
s. phase
s. time ▸ viral
Sheehan's disease
Sheehy syndrome
Sheehy-House incus replacement prosthesis
Sheen airway reconstruction
sheen, skin
sheep scab
sheepskin boot
sheet(s)
s., discharge instruction
s., disposable examination
s., flow
s., medication flow
s., mucous
s. of skin ▸ multiple
s. ▸ patient education instruction
s., restraint
s. sign
s., tantalum
s., treatment flow
s. wadding, sterile

sheeting prosthesis, Teflon
Sheffield exercise stress test
Sheffield treadmill protocol
Shekelton's aneurysm
Sheldon-Pudenz's tube
Sheldon-Pudenz's valve
shelf
s., Blumer's
s., dental
s. life
s. of plaque
s. operation
s. procedure
s., rectal
s. -type implant
shell
s. cap
s. crown
s. fragment
s. image, ejection
s. implant
s. implant, corrected cosmetic contact
s. -K
s. -like demarcation
s., protein
s. shock
s. type implant, conventional
shelled cataract, dry-
shelled out from gallbladder bed ▸ gallbladder
shellfish allergy
sheltered environment
sheltered housing
shelving
s. border of inguinal ligament
s. incision
s. operation
s. portion of ligament
Shenstone's tourniquet
Shenton's arch
Shenton's line
shepherd's crook deformity
Shepherd's fracture
Sherman('s)
S. (phencyclidine)
S. cigarette
S. plate
S. plate and screws
S. screw
Sherrington reflex, Liddel and
Sherrington's law
Shiatsu massage
Shiatsu technique
Shibley's sign

shield
- s. applied, eye pad and
- s., barrier
- s., binocular
- s., bronchoscopic face
- s., Buller's
- s., chest
- s., Dacron
- s., Dalkon
- s., eye
- s., face
- s. for electron beam therapy, eye
- s., Fox
- s., Fox eye
- s., Fuller
- s., lead gonad
- s., metal
- s., perforated eye
- s., probe
- s., protective eye

shielding
- s. blocks, critical organ
- s. blocks, organ
- s. in electron beam therapy
- s. in radiation, lead
- s. of organ

Shier's total knee prosthesis

shift(s) [*drift*]
- s. artifact, chemical
- s. artifact ▸ phase
- s. assay ▸ mobility
- s., axis
- s., brain states
- s., cost-
- s. disruption of 24-hour sleep-wake cycle ▸ phase-
- s., Doppler
- s. from normal position ▸ uterus
- s. in attention
- s. in direction and pattern of brain electrical activity
- s. in frequency of sound waves
- s. in position
- s. in position of eyeball
- s., marked mood
- s. ▸ massive transference
- s., mediastinal
- s., mental-emotional
- s. method for air gap correction, isodose
- s. method, isodose
- s., midline
- s. of midline structures
- s. of pain
- s. of total pattern
- s., paradigm
- s., sleep-wake
- s., temporary threshold
- s. test in lateral position, pivot
- s. test of MacIntosh, pivot
- s. test, pivot
- s. to left
- s. to left, mediastinal
- s. to left, moderate
- s. to right
- s. to right, mediastinal
- s. to right, moderate

shifted to right, trachea
shifter, frequency
shifting
- s. border
- s., brain electrical activity toward sleep activity
- s. dullness
- s. emotions ▸ rapidly
- s. goals
- s. pacemaker
- s. values
- s. vocational aspirations
- s., weight

Shiga's bacillus
Shigella
- S. alkalescens
- S. ambigua
- S. arabinotarda Type A
- S. arabinotarda Type B
- S. boydii
- S. ceylonensis
- S. dispar
- S. dysenteriae
- S. dysentery
- S. enteritis
- S. etousae
- S. flexneri
- S. genus
- S., isolated
- S. madampensis
- S. newcastle
- S. organism
- S. paradysenteriae, gram-negative
- S. parashigae
- S. schmitzii
- S. shigae
- S. sonnei
- S. species
- S. wakefield

Shiley
- S. aortic valve prosthesis, Bjork-
- S. aortic valve prosthesis, Ionescu-
- S. cardiac jacket, Bonchek-
- S. cardiotomy reservoir
- S. convexoconcave heart valve
- S. heart valve
- S. mitral valve prosthesis ▸ Bjork-
- S. pericardial patch ▸ Ionescu-
- S. pericardial xenograft, Ionescu-
- S. Phonate speaking valve
- S. prosthesis, Ionescu-
- S. shunt
- S. Tetraflex vascular graft
- S. tracheostomy tube
- S. valve, Bjork-
- S. valve, Ionescu-
- S. valve prosthesis ▸ Kay-
- S. vascular graft ▸ Ionescu-

shill, protrusio
Shimadzu cardiac ultrasound
shimmering zigzag lines
shin [*skin, chin*]
- s. bone
- s. bone fracture
- s. splints
- s. test ▸ heel-to-

shiners, allergic
shingles
- s. (herpes zoster)
- s., chills from
- s. infection
- s., pain from
- s. pain ▸ persistent

Shinowara-Jones-Reinhard unit
shiny
- s. material
- s. nodule
- s. skin ▸ taut,

ship, hospital
Shipley-Hartford Test
Shirley drain
Shirodkar
- S. cerclage
- S. needle
- S. operation
- S. procedure

shivering, inhibition of
shivering, uncontrollable
SHL (selective hearing loss)
Shobert's maneuver
shock (Shock)
- s. absorber
- s. -absorbing and stabilizing
- s. absorption
- s. ▸ advanced stages of bacterial
- s., allergic
- s., anaphylactic
- s. and unconsciousness

s., anesthesia
s., apoplectic
s., asthmatic
s. aversion
s., bacteremic
s., bacterial
s., biphasic
s. blocks
s., break
s., burn
s. burst
s., cardiac
s., cardiogenic
s., cerebral
s., chronic
s., clinical septic
s., colloid
s., colloidoclastic
s., compensated
s. ▸ complementary therapy of
    bacterial
s. ▸ confusion from insulin
s. count
s. count ▸ first
s. count ▸ second through fifth
s. count ▸ total patient
s. count ▸ touch
s., culture
s., decompensated
s., deferred
s., defibrillation
s., defibrillatory
s., delayed
s., diabetic
s., diastolic
s., distributive
s. due to obstruction
s., electric
s., electrical
s. (ECS), electroconvulsive
s., emotional
s., endotoxic
s., epigastric
s., erethismic
s., faradic
s., gravitation
s., heart
s. heart into normal rhythm
s., hematogenic
s., hemoclastic
s., hemorrhagic
s. ▸ high energy transthoracic
s., histamine
s., hypnoclastic
s., hypoglycemic

s., hypovolemic
s. index
s., insulin
s. intensity ▸ levels of
s., internal
s., intractable
s., irreversible
s. -like complications
s. -like symptoms
s., liver
s. lung
s. ▸ management of bacterial
s., neurogenic
s., numbness and disbelief
s., numbness ▸ sense of disbelief,
s., obstructive
s. of _____ joules, heart
    defibrillated with single
s., oligemic
s., osmotic
s., paralytic
s. patient ▸ fluid retention of
s. ▸ patient in
s. ▸ patient in cardiogenic
s., patient in insulin
s., peptone
s., pleural
s. position
s. ▸ postheart attack
s., postoperative
s., postpartum
s., protein
s. protein, heat
s., psychic
s. ▸ QRS synchronous atrial
    defibrillation
s. reaction
s., respiratory
s., respiratory system
s., secondary
s., sensitivity
s., septic
s., serum
s. ▸ severe septic
s., shell
s., skin
s. sound, double
s., spinal
s., state of
s., static
s., sudden systemic
s., surgical
s. syndrome, declamping
s. syndrome ▸ dengue
s. syndrome ▸ diarrhea from toxic

s. syndrome ▸ dizziness from toxic
s. syndrome (TSS) ▸ menstrual
    toxic
s. syndrome (TSS), toxic
s., systolic
s., testicular
s. therapy
s. therapy (CST) ▸ convulsive
s. therapy, insulin
s. therapy, Metrazol
s., thyroxine
s. tissue
s., torpid
s., toxic
s. ▸ toxic factor in
s. trauma
S. Trauma Acute Resuscitation
    (MedSTAR), Medical
s., traumatic
s. treatment
s. treatment, insulin
s. ▸ treatment of circulatory
s., true convulsive
s., vasogenic
s. victims
s. wave
s. wave coupling
s. wave definition
s. wave ▸ electrically generated
s. wave, extracorporeal
s. wave focusing
s. wave lithotripsy (ESWL),
    extracorporeal
s. wave lithotripter
s. wave ▸ photo-acoustic
s. wave pressure measurement
s. wave reflection
s. wave treatment
shocked back into normal rhythm ▸
    patient
shocked during cardiac arrest, heart
shocky, pallid and
shocky, patient
shoddy (*same as* **shotty**)
shoddy fever
shoe(s) (Shoes)
s. adaptation, minor
S., Child Life Orthopedic
s., correction
s., exercise
s. heart, wooden-
s., ill-fitting
s., in-depth
s. insert
s., jogging

shoe(s)—*continued*
  s., orthotic
  s., out-flare
  s., Scarpa's
  s., soft soled
  s., sutures tied over rubber
  s., swing-out
  s., tarsomedial
  s., WACH (wedge adjustable cushioned heel)
  s., walking
Shone anomaly
Shone complex
shooting pains
shooting tattoos
shopper, compulsive
Shorr's stain
short (Short)
  s. abductor muscle of thumb
  s. -acting barbiturate
  s. -acting hallucinogen
  s. -acting insulin
  s. adductor muscle
  s. anconeus muscle
  s. arm cast
  s. attention span
  s. axis
  s. -axis parasternal view
  s. -axis plane
  s. axis view
  s. -axis view echocardiogram ▸ parasternal
  s. -axis view ▸ parasternal
  s. bone
  s. -bowel syndrome
  s. bursts
  s. -chain gram-positive cocci
  s. chains and tetrads
  s. ciliary nerves
  s. course
  s. crus of the incus
  s. cycle ▸ short-long-
  s. duration, deep sleep of
  s. esophagus
  s. extensor muscle of great toe
  s. extensor muscle of thumb
  s. extensor muscle of toes
  s. extensor tendon
  s. fibular muscle
  s. flexor muscle of great toe
  s. flexor muscle of little finger
  s. flexor muscle of little toe
  s. flexor muscle of thumb
  s. flexor muscles of toes
  s. gastric veins

  s. gram-negative rods ▸ cluster of
  s. -gut syndrome
  s. gyri of insula
  s. half-life
  s. in stature, patient
  s. increment sensitivity index (SISI)
  S. Increment Sensitivity Index (SISI) Test
  s. intense course
  s. inter-electrode distances
  s. latency somatosensory evoked response (SER)
  s. leg brace
  s. leg cast
  s. leg walking cast
  s. levator muscles of fibs
  s. limb dwarfism
  s. -lived
  s. -lived high
  s. -lived pain
  s. -long-short cycle
  s. neuron
  s. of breath, patient
  s. palmar muscle
  s. peroneal muscle
  s. posterior ciliary artery
  s. posterior ciliary axis
  s. P-R interval
  s. pulse
  s. pulse, periodic
  s. pulsed laser
  s. QRS complex
  s. rectangular flap
  s. rods
  s. rotator muscles
  s. sequences, long-
  s. sight
  s. stature
  s. stature, parents of
  s. -term amnesia
  s. -term anxiety ▸ intense
  s. -term care
  s. -term clinical trial
  s. -term detoxification
  s. -term dialysis
  s. -term follow-up
  s. -term goals
  s. -term improvements
  s. -term insomnia
  s. -term institutional respite care
  s. -term irritability ▸ intense,
  s. -term memory (STM)
  s. -term memory disruption
  s. -term memory ▸ impaired
  s. -term memory ▸ lapse in

  s. -term memory loss
  s. -term memory, patient's
  s. -term moodiness ▸ intense,
  s. -term mortality rates
  s. -term nursing care
  s. -term pain
  s. -term postsurgical use
  s. -term psychodynamic therapy
  s. -term psychotherapy
  s. -term recall
  s. -term relief
  s. -term separation from mother
  s. -term skilled nursing care
  s. -term smoking cessation
  s. -term stay
  s. -term steroid therapy
  s. -term stimulation
  s. -term stress
  s. -term therapeutic approach
  s. -term therapy
  s. -term verbal memory
  s. -term working relationship
  s. wave
  s. wave diathermy
  s. wave therapy
shortage of donor organs
shortened
  s. attention span from anxiety
  s. from anxiety ▸ attention span
  s. life expectancy
  s. uvula
shortening
  s., circumferential fiber
  s. fraction
  s. ▸ fractional myocardial
  s. indices, wall
  s. ▸ myocardial fiber
  s. osteotomy, femoral
  s., radial
  s. reaction
  s. relationship ▸ stress
  s., scleral
  s., tendon
  s. velocity
  s. ▸ velocity of circumferential fiber
  s. ▸ ventricular wall
shortness
  s. of breath ▸ acute
  s. of breath (SOB) ▸ chest discomfort with
  s. of breath (SOB) ▸ exercise induced
  s. of breath (SOB) from anxiety
  s. of breath ▸ increased
  s. of breath on exertion

s. of breath (SOB) ▸ palpitations and
s. of breath (SOB) ▸ progressive
s. of breath, recurrent
s. of breath (SOB) ▸ sudden
s. of breath (SOB) ▸ weakness, fatigue and

shortwinded, patient
Shoshin disease
shot
s. femoral sound ▸ pistol-
s., flu
s. -gun approach
s. -perforated
s. pulse, pistol-
s. -silk reflex
s. -silk retina
s., sinus
s., split
s., tetanus

shotted suture
shotty (*same as* **shoddy**)
shotty lymph nodes
shotty residual lymph nodes
shoulder(s)
s. abduction exercise
s. adduction exercise
s. area, atrophy in
s. arthrodesis
s. arthroplasty, Magnuson-Stack
s. arthroplasty, Stanmore
s. -blade
s. -blade bone
s. blade squeeze
s. blades ▸ prominent
s. bone
s., bursitis of
s. capsule
s. ▸ chest pain radiating to jaw and
s., contracted
s., dislocated
s. dislocation, Bankart procedure
s. dislocation, chronic
s., drooping
s., drop
s. dystocia
s. elevation exercises
s. external rotation exercise
s. fibromyalgia
s. flexed
s. flexibility
s. flexion exercise
s., frozen
s. full range of motion (ROM) ▸ left

s. full range of motion (ROM) ▸ right
s. girdle
s. -hand syndrome
s. holster
s. horizontal flexion
s. internal rotation exercise
s. joint
s. joint, anterior dislocation of
s. joint replacement
s., knocked-down
s., loose
s. motion
s. movement, spasticity with
s. muscle strength
s. pain
s., pain between
s. pain from disc ▸ neck and
s. ▸ pain spreading to
s., pillow inserted under
s. presentation
s. press
s. press exercise
s. prosthesis, Neer
s. reconstruction
s. repair, Mosely method anterior
s. replacement
s. rotation
s. separation
s., Sever-L'Episcopo repair of
s. shrug exercise
s. shrugging
s. shrugs
s. slip
s. spica cast
s. squeeze exercise
s. stiffness
s. strain
s. -strap incision
s. -strap resonance
s. stretch exercise
s. stretch ▸ knee-to-
s., stubbed
s. subluxation
s. subluxed
s. syndrome ▸ Milwaukee
s. ▸ tension in neck and

shouted voice (sv)
shouts, patient
shoveler fracture, clay-
Shoveller's fracture
shovel-shaped incisor
show, bloody
show, patient had evidence of

showed
s. evidence of weight loss ▸ abdomen
s. normal pattern ▸ electrocardiogram (ECG/EKG)
s. subjective improvement ▸ patient

shower
s., embolic
s. seat
s. transfer, bathtub and
s. trolley

shrapnel fragment
Shrapnell's membrane
shreds of mucus
shreds of tissue
shrink(s)
s. cancer
s., cysts
s. enlarged prostate gland
s. inoperable tumor
s. nasal blood
s. prostate with microwave
s. tumor

shrinkage
s. ▸ age-related tissue
s., bone
s., gum
s. of hemorrhoids
s. of tissue
s. of vitreous fluid
s., tumor

shrinking
s. cornea
s. field technique
s. gums
s. medication, brain
s. of testicles

shroom (psilocybin)
shrug exercise ▸ shoulder
shrugging, shoulder
shrugs, shoulder
shrunken
s. adrenal glands
s. atrophied neurons
s. brain
s. eyeball
s. kidney
s. torso ▸ pale

SHTA (security hospital treatment assistant)
shuckers' keratitis, oyster
shudder, carotid
shuffling, foot
shuffling gait
Shukuris operation, Falk-

Shultze test

shunt
- s., Allen-Brown
- s., Ames
- s., aortofemoral artery
- s., aortopulmonary
- s., arteriovenous (AV)
- s. ▸ ascending aorta-to-pulmonary artery
- s., atrial ventricular
- s., atrioventricular (AV)
- s., balloon
- s., bidirectional
- s., bladder
- s., Blalock-Taussig
- s., Brenner carotid bypass
- s., cardiac
- s., cardiac pulmonary
- s., cardiovascular
- s., carotid artery
- s., cavamesenteric
- s., Cavin
- s., cavocaval
- s., central nervous system (CNS)
- s., Cimino arteriovenous (AV)
- s., clogged
- s., Cordis-Hakim
- s. cyanosis
- s., Denver
- s., Denver peritoneal venous
- s., Denver pleuroperitoneal
- s. detection
- s. detection, cardiac
- s., dialysis
- s. ▸ distal splenorenal
- s., Dow Corning
- s., Drapanas mesocaval
- s., emergency ventriculoperitoneal
- s., endolymphatic-subarachnoid
- s., extracardiac
- s. function
- s. functioning optimally
- s., Glenn
- s., Gott
- s., hexose monophosphate
- s., Holter's
- s., hydrocephalus
- s. incapacitance, input
- s. infection
- s., initial venous
- s., interarterial
- s., intracardiac
- s., Javid's
- s., left-to-right
- s., LeVeen dialysis

- s., LeVeen peritoneal
- s., LeVeen peritoneovenous
- s. levels ▸ multiple
- s., Levine
- s., magnitude
- s. ▸ Marion-Clatworthy side-to-end vena caval
- s., mesocaval
- s. obstructed
- s. oozed blood
- s. operation
- s., parallel
- s., parietal
- s. pathway
- s., pentose
- s., peritoneal
- s., peritoneal insert of
- s., peritoneal venous
- s., peritoneovenous
- s., polystan
- s., portacaval
- s., portal
- s., portal systemic
- s., portal to systemic venous
- s., portarenal
- s., portopulmonary
- s., postcaval
- s., Potts
- s. procedure
- s. procedure, Torkildsen's
- s., proximal to
- s. ▸ Pruitt vascular
- s., Pruitt-Inahara carotid
- s., Pudenz's
- s., Pudenz's ventriculoatrial
- s. quantification
- s. ▸ Quinton-Scribner
- s., Ramirez
- s. ratio
- s., reversed
- s., right-to-left
- s. related
- s., Rostan
- s., Scribner arteriovenous (AV)
- s., Shiley
- s., Silastic ventriculoperitoneal
- s., silicone
- s. site, arteriovenous (AV)
- s. site, drainage (dr'ge) about
- s. site, leaking about
- s. site, oozing about
- s., Spetzler lumboperitoneal
- s., splenorenal
- s. ▸ Sundt carotid endarterectomy
- s. ▸ systemic to pulmonary

- s., Thomas
- s., Torkildsen's
- s. ▸ transjugular intrahepatic portosystemic
- s. tube
- s. tube, Teflon
- s. tube, Teflon endolymphatic
- s. ▸ Vascu Flo carotid
- s. ▸ vascular lung
- s., venous
- s., ventriculoatrial
- s., ventriculocaval
- s., ventriculocisternal
- s., ventriculojugular
- s., ventriculoperitoneal
- s. ▸ Vitagraft arteriovenous
- s., Warren's
- s., Waterston
- s., winged

shunted blood

shunting
- s., intrapulmonary
- s. urine
- s., venoarterial

shut ▸ eyes taped

shut, pinch nose

shutdown of kidneys

shutdown, renal

shut-in personality

shuttlemaker's disease

Shwachman syndrome, Riley-

Shwartzman's reaction, generalized

Shy-Drager syndrome

Shy-Magee syndrome

shyness
- s. and social withdrawal disorder ▸ sensitivity,
- s. ▸ anorexia, depression and
- s., behavioral
- s. disorder of childhood
- s. in adolescent

SI
- SI (saturation index)
- SI (seriously ill)
- SI (stroke index)

SIADH (syndrome of inappropriate antidiuretic hormone) secretion

sialadenitis/sialoadenitis

sialadenitis, chronic nonspecific

sialogram study

sialorrhea pancreatica

Siamese Cheddi

Siamese twins

SIBID (self-inhibiting behavioral injury device)

sibilant rale
sibilant rhonchi
sibling(s)
- s. adjustment
- s. classes
- s. deprivation
- s., difficulty with
- s. donor
- s. jealousy
- s. marrow
- s. rivalry
- s. stress
- s. transplants

Sibson's notch
Sibson's vestibule
Sicar sign
Sicard syndrome, Brissaud-
sicca
- s. bronchitis
- s. dolorosa, alveolitis
- s., hypophysis
- s., keratitis
- s., keratoconjunctivitis
- s., laryngitis
- s., Neisseria
- s., pericarditis
- s., pharyngitis
- s., rhinitis
- s., seborrhea
- s. syndrome
- s., tracheitis

siccatum, hepar
Sichel's disease
sick
- s. and dying
- s. cell
- s. headache
- s., healing the
- s. leave ‣ excessive use of
- s. sinus syndrome (SSS)
- s. syndrome, euthyroid
- s. to stomach ‣ feeling

sickhouse, sleeping
sickle
- s. cell
- s. cell abnormality
- s. cell anemia
- s. cell anemia screening
- s. cell crisis
- s. cell disease
- s. cell disorder
- s. cell gene
- s. cell test
- s. cell trait
- s. cell-hemoglobin C disease

- s. cell-hemoglobin D disease
- s. cell-thalassemia disease
- s. flap, New's
- s. scaler

sickling hemoglobins
sickling test
sickness
- s., acute mountain
- s., aerial
- s., African sleeping
- s., air
- s., altitude
- s., athletes'
- s., aviation
- s., balloon
- s., bay
- s., black
- s., Borna
- s., bush
- s., caisson
- s., car
- s., cave
- s., compressed-air
- s., chronic mountain
- s., decompression
- s., falling
- s. (gallsickness), gall
- s., green
- s., green tobacco
- s., high altitude
- s., lambing
- s., laughing
- s. ‣ layoff survivor
- s., milk
- s., morning
- s., motion
- s., mountain
- s., protein
- s., radiation
- s., railroad
- s., salt
- s., sea
- s., serum
- s. skin patch ‣ motion
- s., sleeping
- s., sweating
- s. syndrome ‣ motion
- s., talking
- s., veldt
- s., vomiting
- s., withdrawal
- s., x-ray

SICU (Surgical Intensive Care Unit)
SID (sudden infant death) syndrome

side(s)
- s., affected
- s. anastomosis, end-to-
- s. anastomosis, side-to-
- s., balancing
- s. bathing, sink
- s. bend exercises
- s. -biting clamp
- s. branch compromise
- s. branch occlusion
- s. colostomy, end-to-
- s. -effect, potential
- s. -effects
- s. -effects, adverse
- s. -effects, attendant
- s. -effects, clinical
- s. -effects, devastating
- s. -effects from medication
- s. -effects ‣ lethal
- s. -effects, long-term
- s. -effects, medical
- s. -effects, minor
- s. -effects, nervous system
- s. -effects of treatment
- s. -effects profile
- s. -effects ‣ secondary
- s. -effects, serious
- s. -effects, severe
- s. -effects, toxic
- s. -effects, tranquilizing
- s. -effects, unusual
- s., end-to-
- s. -entry access
- s. ileotransverse colostomy, end-to-
- s. immunization, side-to-
- s., impaired
- s. kicks
- s., left
- s. leg raise exercise
- s. lobe
- s. lobe artifact
- s., muscles of affected
- s. of baseline, alternate
- s. of body, left
- s. of body, muscular weakness one
- s. of body ‣ numbness one
- s. of body, paralysis one
- s. of body ‣ progressive weakness one
- s. of body, right
- s. of body ‣ sudden weakness one
- s. of body ‣ sudden weakness or numbness one

side(s)—*continued*
- s. of body ▸ temporary weakness one
- s. of brain, dominant
- s. of brain, left
- s. of brain, right
- s. of cerebellum, contralateral
- s. of face ▸ pain on affected
- s. of face ▸ sudden numbness one
- s. of face ▸ sudden paralysis one
- s. of face ▸ sudden weakness one
- s. of head, left
- s. of head, opposite
- s. of head, right
- s. of neck ▸ spasm one
- s., patient turned on
- s. port
- s., reposition patient on
- s., right
- s. splash lightning injury
- s. stitches
- s. stretching
- s. suture ▸ end-to-
- s. swinging of head ▸ pointless side-to-
- s. -to-end anastomosis
- s. -to-end vena caval shunt ▸ Marion-Clatworthy
- s. -to-side anastomosis
- s. -to-side immunization
- s. -to-side, patient turned from
- s. -to-side swinging of head ▸ pointless
- s. -to-side vein bypass
- s. transfer, cell-to-
- s. vein bypass, end-to-
- s. -view MRI (magnetic resonance imaging) scan
- s. vision
- s., working

sided
- s. appendicitis ▸ left-
- s. chorea, one-
- s. endocarditis, right-
- s. facial droop, left-
- s. facial droop, right-
- s. filling pressures, right-
- s. headaches, one-
- s. heart failure, left-
- s. heart failure, right-
- s., left-
- s., right-
- s. subclavian catheter, right-
- s. weakness, left-
- s. weakness, right-

sideline examination
siderans, encephalitis
siderans, pestis
Siderobacter [*Citrobacter*]
- S. brevis
- S. duplex
- S. gracilis
- S. latus
- S. linearis
- S. microorganism

sideroblastic anemia
Siderocapsa
- S. botryoides
- S. coronata
- S. eusphaera
- S. major
- S. monoaca
- S. treubii

siderochrestica hereditaria ▸ anemia hypochromica
Siderococcus communis
Siderococcus limoniticus
Sideromonas
- S. confervarum
- S. duplex
- S. major
- S. vulgaris

Sideronema globuliferum
sideropenic anemia
sideropenic dysphagia
Siderophacus corneolus
sideropous, Leptothrix
siderosis
- s. bulbi
- s. conjunctivae
- s., hematogenous
- s., hepatic
- s., nutritional
- s., pulmonary
- s., urinary
- s., xenogenous

siderosphaera conglomerata
siderotic nodules
siderotic splenomegaly
sidestream smoke
sidestream smoking
sideswipe fracture
Sidler-Huguenin's endothelioma
SIDS (Sudden Infant Death Syndrome)
Siegert's sign
Siegrist-Hutchinson syndrome
Siemens
- S. cyclographic tomogram
- S. open heart table

S. -Touraine syndrome, Christ-

sieve
- s. graft
- s. implanted surgically ▸ metal
- s. -like pores

Siever's disease
Sievert integral
sigh [*thigh*]
- s. function
- s., tendency to

sighing dyspnea
sighing respiration
sight (Sight) [*cite, site*]
- s., complete loss of
- s., day
- s. ▸ diminished hearing and
- s., far
- s., long
- s., loss of
- s., near
- s., night
- s., old
- S. Restoration, Eye Bank for
- s., restoration of
- s., second
- s., sense of
- s., short
- s. -threatening problems ▸ potentially

sighted, patient near◊
Sigma (sigma)
- S. method
- s. pattern
- s. reaction
- s. rhythm
- S. ▸ unipolar Pisces
- s. units

sigmoid
- s. colon
- s. colon, carcinoma of
- s. colon, diverticula of
- s. colon ▸ diverticulosis of
- s. colostomy
- s. diverticulosis
- s. flexure of colon
- s. folds of colon
- s. kidney
- s. loop colostomy
- s. mesocolon
- s. notch
- s., recto◊
- s. septum
- s. sinus
- s. sinus, drainage (dr'ge) of
- s. sinus, thrombosis of

s. sulcus
s. tender
s. veins
s. volvulus

sigmoidoscopy
s., flexible
s., ▸ postradiation flexible
s., rigid

sign(s)
s., Aaron's
s., Abadie's
s., abducens nerve
s., Abrahams'
s., accessory nerve
s., ace of spades
s., acoustic nerve
s., acute seaming
s., Adson's
s., Ahlfeld's
s., air bronchogram
s., air dome
s., Allis
s. and symptoms
s. and symptoms, clinical
s. and symptoms of anxiety, decreased
s. and symptoms of depression, decreased
s. and symptoms ▸ stages,
s., André-Thomas
s., Anghelescu's
s., anterior tibial
s., Apley's
s., applesauce
s., Arnoux's
s. as a screening device for drug abuse ▸ cutaneous
s., Aschner's
s., Auenbrugger's
s., Aufrecht's
s., auscultatory
s., Babinski
s., Baccelli's
s., bagpipe
s., Ballet's
s., Bamberger's
s., Barany's
s., Bard
s., Barre's pyramidal
s., Battle's
s., Beccaria's
s., Béclard's
s., Beevor's
s., Béhier-Hardy's
s., bent bronchus

s., Bespaloff's
s., Bethea's
s., Bezold's
s., Biederman's
s., Bieg's
s., Biot
s., Bird
s., Bjerrum's
s., black pleura
s., Bolt's
s., Bonnet's
s., Bouillaud's
s., bounce
s., Boyce
s., Bragard's
s., Branham's
s., Braun-Fernwald
s., Braunwald's
s., Braxton Hicks
s., bread and butter textbook
s., Broadbent's
s., Brockenbrough's
s., bronchial meniscus
s., Brudzinski's
s., Bryant's
s., calcium
s., Carabello
s., Cardarelli
s., Carvallo
s., Castellino
s., Cegka's
s., Chaddock's
s., Chadwick's
s., chandelier
s., Charcot
s. check, vital
s., Cheyne-Stokes
s., Chvostek's
s., Chvostek-Weiss
s., Claude's hyperkinesis
s., Cleeman's
s., clenched fist
s., clinical
s., Codman's
s., Comby's
s., Comolli's
s., contralateral
s., cooing
s., Coopernail
s., Corrigan's
s., cranial nerve
s., Cruveilhier
s., Cruveilhier-Baumgarten
s., cuff
s., Cullen's

s., Dalrymple's
s., D'Amato's
s., Danforth's
s., Davis
s., Dawbarn's
s., de la Camp's
s., de Musset's
s., Déjerine's
s., Delmege's
s., Demarquay's
s., Demianoff's
s., Desault's
s., Dew
s., DeWees'
s., Dieuaide's
s., doll's eye
s., Dorendorf
s., dorsiflexion
s., doughnut
s., drawer
s., Drummond's
s., Duchenne's
s., Dupuytren's
s., Duroziez's
s., early warning
s., Ebstein
s., Ellis'
s., Erb's
s., Erichsen's
s., Ewart's
s., Ewing's
s., fabere
s., facial nerve
s., failing lung
s., Fajersztajn's
s., fat pad
s., Fischer
s., focal and lateralizing neurologic
s., focal motor
s., focal neurologic
s., Fränkel's
s., Froment's
s., Gaenslen's
s., Galeazzi's
s., Gauss'
s., Gifford's
s., Glasgow
s., glossopharyngeal nerve
s., Golden's
s., Goldthwait's
s., Goodell's
s., Gowers'
s., Graefe's
s., Granger's
s., great toe

sign(s)—*continued*

s., Greene
s., Grossman
s., Guilland's
s. ▸ Gunn crossing
s., Halban's
s., Hamman's
s., Hefke-Turner
s., Hegar's
s., Heimlich
s., Hicks'
s. ▸ hilum convergence
s. ▸ hilum overlay
s., Hirschberg's
s., Hoehne's
s., Hoffmann's
s., Holmes'
s., Homans'
s., Hope's
s., Hueters
s., hypoglossal nerve
s. identification, warning
s., important warning
s. ▸ intravascular fetal air
s., Jaccoud
s., Jacquemier's
s., Jürgensen's
s., Kanavel's
s., Kanter's
s., Keen's
s., Kehr's
s., Kergaradec's
s., Kernig's
s., Kerr's
s., knuckle
s., Koplik's
s., Kussmaul's
s., Küstner's
s., Ladin's
s., Laennec's
s., Lafora's
s., Landou's
s., Langoria's
s. language (signing)
s. language alphabet
s., Lasègue's
s., Laugier's
s., Leichtenstern's
s., Leri's
s., Levine
s., Lhermitte's
s., Lichtheim's
s., Linder's
s. ▸ Litten diaphragm
s., Livierato

s., localized
s., localized neurological
s., localizing
s., localizing neurological
s., Lombardi's
s., long tract
s., Lorenz's
s. ▸ Löwenberg cuff
s., Ludloff's
s., Macewen's
s., Maisonneuve's
s. management, warning
s., Marie-Foix
s., Marie's
s., May
s., Mayor's
s., McBurney's
s., McGinn-White
s., McMurray
s. mechanism for ventilator
   breathing
s., Meltzer
s., meniscus
s., Mennell's
s., Mercedes Benz
s., Minor's
s., Möbius'
s., Morquio's
s., Murphy's
s., Munson's
s. ▸ mute toe
s., Myerson's
s., Naffziger
s., neck
s., neurological
s., neurovital
s. ▸ Nicoladoni-Branham
s., Nikolsky's
s. normal, vital
s., Nothnagel's
s., Ober's
s., objective
s. ▸ objective neurologic
s., obturator
s., oculomotor nerve
s. of alcoholism ▸ cardinal
s. of clearing
s. of drug abuse, cutaneous
s. of drug abuse, systemic
s. of drug abuse ▸ warning
s. of eye disease ▸ warning
s. of hearing loss ▸ warning
s. of heart attack ▸ warning
s. of hydronephrosis, calyceal
s. of hydronephrosis, crescent

s. of mental problems ▸ warning
s. of oral cancer ▸ warning
s. of rejection
s. of rejection, classical
s. of rejection, early
s. of relapse, early
s. of serious illness ▸ warning
s. of sexually transmitted disease ▸
   warning
s. of smoking-related problems ▸
   warning
s. of stress, warning
s. of suicide attempt ▸ warning
s. of transient ischemic attack (TIA)
   ▸ warning
s. of vulnerability
s. of weakness
s. of weakness, localized
s. of withdrawal
s., olfactory nerve
s., Oliver
s., Olshausen's
s. ▸ open bronchus
s., Oppenheim's
s. ▸ orthostatic vital
s., Ortolanti's
s., Osiander's
s., Osler's
s., pad
s., Parrot's
s., Pastia's
s. ▸ patent bronchus
s., Patrick's
s., Perez'
s., peroneal
s., Pfuhl-Jaffe
s., Pfuhl's
s., Phalen
s., physical
s., Pinard's
s., Piotrowski's
s., Piskacek's
s. ▸ pleural meniscus
s. ▸ plumb line
s., Pottenger's
s., pronation
s. ▸ Prussian helmet
s. ▸ pulmonary meniscus
s. ▸ pulmonary notch
s. ▸ pulmonary target
s., Queckenstedt's
s., Quénu-Muret
s., questionable Babinski
s., Quincke's
s., Quinquaud's

s. ▸ rabbit-ear
s., radialis
s. ▸ railroad track
s., Ramond's
s., Randall's
s., Rasch's
s., Raynaud's
s., Reusner's
s., Rifkind's
s., rim
s., ring
s., Rinman's
s., Rinne's
s., Riviera's
s., Robertson
s., Romaña's
s., Romberg's
s., Roser-Braun
s., Rotch's
s., Rothschild
s., Roussel's
s., Rovsing and Blumberg
s., Rovsing's
s., Rumpel-Leede
s., Rumpf's
s., Saenger's
s., Salmon's
s., Sansom's
s., Sarbo's
s., Schapiro
s., Schepelmann
s., Schick's
s., Schlesinger's
s., Schüle's
s., Schwartze's
s., scimitar
s., Seidel's
s., Seitz
s., Semon
s., Shapiro
s., sheet
s., Shibley's
s., Sicar
s., Siegert's
s., Signorelli's
s., silhouette
s., simian
s., Simon's
s., Skoda's
s., Smith
s. ▸ snake-tongue
s., Soto-Hall
s., Spalding's
s., Spurting's
s. ▸ square root

s., stable, vital
s., steeple
s. ▸ Steinberg thumb
s., Stellwag's
s., Sterles'
s., Sternberg's
s., Stiller's
s. ▸ stretched bronchus
s., string
s., stroke warning
s., Strümpell's
s., Strunsky's
s., T
s., tall
s., Tarnier's
s., tell-tale
s., tenting
s. test ▸ Phalen's
s., Thomas'
s. ▸ thumbprint bronchus
s., tibialis
s., Tinel's
s., toe
s. ▸ trapezius ridge
s., Traube's
s., trigeminal nerve
s., Trimadeau
s., trochlear nerve
s., Troisier's
s., Trousseau's
s., Turyn's
s., Unschuld's
s., vagus nerve
s., Vanzetti's
s. (VS), vital
s., von Fernwald's
s., von Graefe's
s. ▸ Walker-Murdoch wrist
s., warning
s., Wartenberg's
s., Warthin's
s., Weber's
s., Weill
s., Wenckebach's
s., Wernicke's
s., Westermark
s., Westphal's
s., Widowitz
s., Wilder's
s., Williams'
s., Williamson's
s., windsock
s., Wintrich
s., Wreden's
s., Zaufal's

s., Zugsmith's
signal(s)
s., amplitude of
s., analog
s., antiphase
s., artificial feedback
s. attenuation
s., audible
s., auditory and visual
s. -averaged echocardiogram
s. -averaged echocardiography
s. -averaged electrocardiogram (ECG)
s. -averaged electrocardiogram (ECG) ▸ time domain
s. -averaged electrocardiography (ECG)
s. averaging
s. averaging (EPSA), evoked potential
s., awareness of
s., background
s., biological
s., calibration
s., common mode
s., defective nerve
s. detectability, theory of
s., differential
s., digital
s., Doppler
s., electrical
s., electronic
s., gating
s., incoming
s., incoming pain
s., in-phase
s., isolate input
s., logic
s., low frequency alternating current (AC)
s. ▸ magnetic resonance
s., monitoring of
s. ▸ mosaic jet
s., myo-control
s., nerve
s. node
s., noise
s., nonbiological
s. of cancer, warning
s. or messages ▸ transmission of electric
s., out-of-phase
s., pain
s., primary
s. processing

signal(s)—*continued*
s., regularity of
s. shape, echo
s. symptom, Séguin's
s. -to-noise (S/N) ratio
s., visual
s. voltage, ratio of input
s. voltage, ratio of output

signalling
s., neuronal
s. system, second
s., transmembrane

signed
s., against medical advice (AMA) form
s., autopsy permit
s., operative permit
s., release slip
s., surgical permit

signet ring cells
signet-ring cell carcinoma
significance
s., behavior
s., clinical
s., controversial clinical
s., questionable

significant
s. abnormality
s. abnormality, no
s. calcification
s. change, no
s. changes
s. deformity
s. disabilities
s. dose (GSD), genetically
s. focal dysfunction
s. functional overlay
s. gain in weight
s. level of perceived pain
s. loss of weight
s. medical advances
s. others
s. pathology
s. risks ▸ free of
s. sharp, spike or delta waves (SSSDW)
s. stenosis ▸ hemodynamically
s. variation in pattern of excretion
s. weight gain
s. weight loss

signing (sign language)
Signorelli's sign
silacea, Chrysops
silantiewi, Ceratophyllus
silantiewi, Oropsylla

Silastic (silastic)
S. bead embolization
S. capping
S. catheter
S. corneal implant
S. corneal implant material
S. coronary artery cannula
S. Cronin implant
S. Cronin implant material
S. implant
S. implant material
S. injection
S. medical adhesive silicone implant
S. mushroom catheter
S. patch
S. penile prosthesis
S. prosthesis
S. prosthesis, Mulligan
S. scleral buckler implant
S. silo
S. sphere
S. subdermal implant
S. subdermal implant material
S. testicular prosthesis
S. trapezoid implant
S. tube, Guibor
S. valve ▸ Starr-Edwards
S. ventriculoperitoneal shunt

silence
s., EKG (electrocardiogram)
s., electrical
s. (ECS), electrocerebral
s. of apneic episode
s., record of electrocerebral
s. (ECS) recording, electrocerebral

silent
s. angina
s. area
s. attack
s. aura
s. carcinoma
s. coronary artery disease
s. counting
s. disease
s. electrode
s. epidemic
s. gallstones
s. gap
s. gene
s. heart attack
s. heart damage
s. heart muscle distress
s. infection
s. ischemia

s. ischemia, documented
s. ischemic heart disease
s. killer
s. mastoiditis
s. mitral stenosis
s. myocardial infarction
s. myocardial ischemia
s. myocardial ischemia ▸ exercise-induced
s. pericardial effusion
s. peritonitis
s. reaction ▸ rape trauma syndrome,
s. stroke

silhouette
s., cardiac
s., cardiomediastinal
s., cardiothymic
s., cardiovascular
s., diaphragmatic
s., heart
s. sign
s., supracardiac

silicate filling
silicon ion therapy
silicone
s. -based artificial joint
s. breast implant
s. chip
s., Dow Corning
s. -filled breast implant
s. -filled implant
s. gel breast implant
s. gel implant
s. gel, leaking
s. gel, viscous
s., gelatinous
s. gel-filled breast implant
s. gel-filled implants
s. grease
s. immersion
s. implant
s. implant, adhesive
s. implant material, adhesive
s. implant, Silastic medical adhesive
s. injection
s. into breast ▸ direct injection of
s. intraocular lens (IOL) ▸ foldable
s., liquid
s. orbital prosthesis, solid
s. prosthesis
s. rod, flexible round
s. rod implant
s., seeping

s. shunt
s. sponge implant
s. testicle
s. tube, encircling
s. tube, fil d'Arlon

silicosis
s., infective
s., nodular
s., simple

silicotic granuloma
silicotic pneumoconiosis
silicotuberculosis fibrosis
siliculose cataract
siliquose cataract
silk
s. braided suture
s. interrupted mattress sutures
s. keratitis, artificial
s., ligated with
s., pursestring of black
s. reflex, shot-
s. reflex, water-
s. retina, shot-
s. retina, watered-
s., skin closed with interrupted
s. stay suture
s. suture
s. suture, arterial
s. suture, black
s. suture, braided
s. suture, cardiovascular
s. suture, continuous
s. suture, Ethicon
s. suture, fine
s. suture, interrupted black
s. suture, interrupted fine
s. sutures, outer interrupted
s., temporal
s., virgin

silkworm gut
silkworm gut suture
Silly Putty (Psilocyn)
silo
s. filler's disease
s. filler's lung
s., Silastic

Silon tent
Silon test
Siltzbach test, Kveim-
Silva-Costa operation
silver('s) (Silver)
s. bead electrode
s. bunionectomy
s. cells
S. dwarf

s. -fork deformity
s. -fork fracture
s. nitrate (AgNO₃)
s. pinning, root canal
s. staining of tissue
s. stool
S. syndrome
s. wire effect
s. wiring of retinal arteries

Silverman syndrome, Caffey-
Silverman's score
Silverstein tube, Lindeman-
silvery
s. scales on elbows
s. scales on knees
s. scales on legs
s. scales on scalp

Simaruba amara
Simbu virus
simian
s. crease
s. crease of palm
s. immunodeficiency virus (SIV)
s. sign
s. T cell lymphotropic virus type
s. virus
s. virus 40 (SV40)

simii, Pinoyella
simii, Trichophyton
Similac feeding
similarity, behavioral
similarity, chemical
similarly
s. acting dependence ▸ barbiturate
s. acting dependence ▸ hypnotic
s. acting dependence ▸ sedative
s. acting sympathomimetic abuse ▸ amphetamine or
s. acting sympathomimetic delirium ▸ amphetamine or
s. acting sympathomimetic dependence ▸ amphetamine or
s. acting sympathomimetic intoxication ▸ amphetamine or
s. acting sympathomimetic withdrawal ▸ amphetamine or

Simkin analysis
Simmonds' disease
Simon('s)
S. foci
S. operation
S. septic factor
S. sign
S. test, Binet-
Simonelli's test

simple
s. atrophy
s. beam
s. bitter
s. blood test
s. bruising
s. comminuted fracture
s. dislocation
s. erythema
s. excision
s. fracture
s. fracture, complex
s. ganglion
s. glaucoma
s. glaucoma, chronic
s. goiter
s. hyperplasia
s. interrupted fashion
s. joint
s. marginal gingivitis
s. mastectomy
s. mastoidectomy
s. mastoidectomy, complete
s. meningitis
s. microscope
s. motor tic
s. obesity
s. operation
s. paranoid state
s. partial seizure
s. phobias
s. procedure
s. reflex
s. reflex arc
s. renal cyst
s. schizophrenia
s. silicosis
s. skull fracture
s. staining
s. sugar
s. suture
s. ureterocele

simplex (Simplex)
s., adiposis tuberosa
s., angina
s. antibody titers ▸ herpes
s., carcinoma
s. chronicus, lichen
s., cystoma serosum
s. encephalitis, herpes
s. gingivostomatitis, herpes
s., glaucoma
s., hemangioma
s., herpes
s., hydrosalpinx

simplex—*continued*
s., icterus
s., impetigo
s. infection, herpes
s., lobus
s., melancholia
S. P radiopaque bone cement,
Surgical
s., paranoia
s., pityriasis
s. pneumonitis ▸ herpes
s., purpura
s. Type 1, herpes
s. Type 2, herpes
s., uterus
s. virus, herpes
s., visceral herpes
simplification, work
Simpson('s)
S. lamp
S. light
S. -Robert vascular dilation system
S. rule
Sims
S. -Huhner test
S. position
S. suture
simulans, Staphylococcus
simulate [*stimulate*]
simulated, fields
simulated radiation arc
simulation
s., preliminary
s. study, altitude
s. test ▸ high altitude
s., treatment
s., treatment planning and
simulators, quality assurance in
Simulium
S. arcticum
S. columbaczense
S. damnosum
S. metallicum
S. pecuarium
S. venustum
simultaneous
s. activity
s. compression ventilation CPR
(cardiopulmonary resuscitation)
s. insanity
s. monitoring
s. pen deflections
Sindbis virus
sine
s. delirio, delirium

s. colors, angina
s. qua non, conditio
s. wave
s. wave carrier
s. -wave pattern
sinensis
s., caudamoeba
s., Clonorchis
s., Cordyceps
sinew, back
sinew, weeping
Singapore ear
singer's node
singers' nodule
single
s. ascertainment
s. atrium
s. atrium, congenital
s. balloon valvotomy
s. balloon valvuloplasty
s. breath diffusion
s. breath nitrogen curve
s. breath nitrogen washout test
s. breath test
s. breath test ▸ Fowler
s. causative genes
s. -celled organism
s. -celled protein
s. cells ▸ anaplastic infiltrating
s. chamber pacemaker
s. -chamber rate adaptic
pacemaker, Dash
s. -contrast study
s. crystal gamma camera
s. direct portal
s. dose, nominal
s. electron beam dosimetry
s. -ended amplifier
s. episode in full remission ▸ major
depression,
s. episode, in partial remission ▸
major depression,
s. episode ▸ major depression
s. episode ▸ major depressive
disorder,
s. episode ▸ manic disorder,
s. episode, mild ▸ major
depression,
s. episode, moderate ▸ major
depression
s. episode, severe without
psychotic features ▸ major
depression,
s. episode, unspecified ▸ major
depression,

s. episode, with psychotic features
▸ major depression,
s. family syndrome
s. focus lens
s. footling delivery
s. gene disease
s. gene disorder
s. gene inheritance
s. harelip
s. -hole collimator
s. intrauterine pregnancy
s. leaflet cardiac valve prosthesis ▸
Omniscience
s. leg raise
s. limb stance
s. lumen
s. lung reduction surgery
s. -lung transplant
s. motor unit
s. nucleotide polymorphisms
(SNPs)
s. object ▸ fixation on a
s. onlay cortical graft
s. pacemaker ▸ reprogram
s. papillary muscle syndrome
s. parent counseling
s. -parent status
s. pass lead
s. -pass pacemaker
s. -phase current
s. photon detection
s. photon emission
s. photon emission computed
tomography (SPECT)
s. photon emission computed
tomography (SPECT) scan
s. photon emission tomography
(SPET) imaging
s. photon gamma scintigraphy
s. plane aortography
s. pleurisy
s. premature extrastimulation
s. pressure transducer system
s. reference electrode
s. shock of _____ joules, heart
defibrillated with
s. -stage exercise stress test
s. strand conformational
polymorphism (SSCP)
s. symptom disorder
s. tooth tenaculum
s. tooth tenaculum, cervix grasped
with
s. umbilical artery
s. ventricle

s. ventricle malposition
s. vessel coronary stenosis
s. vessel disease
s. vision glasses
s. x-ray beam dosimetry
singultus gastricus nervosus
sinica, Ephedra
sinister, bronchus principalis
sinister cordis, ventriculus
sinistra (AS), auris
sinistrum, atrium
sinistrum, cor
sink side bathing
sinoaortic baroreflex activity
sinoatrial (S-A)
   s. arrest
   s. block
   s. bradycardia
   s. bundle
   s. cell analysis
   s. conduction time (SACT)
   s. exit block
   s. ganglion
   s. heart block
   s. node
   s. node artery
   s. node ▸ rhythmic pattern
   s. pacemaker complex
   s. recovery time (SART)
   s. rhythm
sinoauricular
   s. block
   s. heart block
   s. node
sinobronchial syndrome
Sinografin contrast medium
Sinomenium diversifolium
sinopulmonary disease
sinospiral muscle bundle
sinotubular junction
sinoventricular conduction
sinoventricular rhythm
Sinsemilla (marijuana)
Sinskey/Sinskey modified blue loop
   intraocular lenses (IOL)
sinuatrialis echo ▸ nodus
sinuotomy (*see* **sinusotomy)**
sinuous movements ▸ purposeless,
   uncontrolled
sinuous movements ▸ slow,
   repeated, involuntary
sinus(es)
   s., accessory
   s., actinomycosis of
   s., anal

s. aneurysm, cavernous
s., aortic
s., aperture of frontal
s., aperture of sphenoid
s. arrest
s. arrest, complete
s. arrhythmia
s. arrhythmia ▸ nonphasic
s. arrhythmia ▸ phasic
s. block
s., blood
s. blood flow, coronary
s. bradycardia
s. cancer, ethmoid
s. cancer, maxillary
s. cancer, paranasal
s. cancer, pyriform
s. cancer, sphenoid
s. cardiac rhythm
s. caroticus
s., carotid
s. catarrh
s. catheterization, coronary
s., cavernous
s. cavities
s., cerebral
s., clouding of
s., compression, carotid
s., congenital dermal
s., coronary
s., costophrenic
s., cribriform
s. cycle length
s. defect
s. disease
s. disease, nasal
s. drainage (dr'ge)
s., drainage (dr'ge) of cranial
s., drainage (dr'ge) of lateral
s., drainage (dr'ge) of sigmoid
s. durae matris
s. electrogram, coronary
s. endoscopy
s. epididymidis
s., ethmoidal
s., ethmoidal paranasal
s., exenteration of
s. exit block
s. exit pause
s. ▸ fistula of carotid cavernous
s., frontal
s., frontal paranasal
s. ganglion
s., granuloma of
s. groove

s. headache
s. headache from cold
s. heart rhythm ▸ normal
s. histiocytosis
s., Huguier's
s. hypersensitivity, carotid
s. infection
s. infection ▸ chronic
s. inflammation
s., inflammation of cerebral
s., laryngeal
s., lateral
s., lavage of
s., ligation superior longitudinal
s., lymphatic
s. massage, carotid
s., mastoid
s., maxillary
s., maxillary paranasal
s. mechanism
s., Meyer's
s., nasal
s. nerve
s. nerve, carotid
s. nodal automaticity
s. nodal dysfunction
s. nodal reentrant tachycardia
s. nodal reentry
s. node
s. node artery
s. node disease
s. node dysfunction
s. node function
s. node impulse
s. node ▸ pacemaking
s. node recovery time
s. node recovery time, corrected
s. node reentry
s., noncoronary
s., oblique
s., occipital
s. occlusion ▸ intermittent coronary
s. of epididymis
s. of Morgagni
s. of sclera, venous
s. of Valsalva
s. of Valsalva aneurysm
s. of Valsalva aortography
s. of Valsalva ▸ ruptured
s. opening
s. orifice electrogram, coronary
s. pacemaker
s. pain
s., paranasal
s. passage

sinus(es)—*continued*
- s. pause
- s. pericranii
- s., Petit's
- s. phlebitis
- s., phlebitis of cavernous
- s., phlebitis of cranial
- s., phlebitis of lateral
- s., pilonidal
- s., piriform
- s. polyp
- s., portal
- s. premature beats
- s. probe
- s. probe, frontal
- s., prostatic
- s. prostaticus
- s. ▸ proximal coronary
- s., pyriform
- s. rasp
- s. rasp, frontal
- s. reentrant tachycardia
- s. reflex
- s. reflex, carotid
- s. reflex, hyperactive carotid
- s., renal
- s. renalis
- s. retroperfusion, coronary
- s. rhythm
- s. rhythm, coronary
- s. rhythm (NSR) ▸ normal
- s. rhythm (RSR), regular
- s. rhythm (NSR) ▸ resumption of normal
- s., Ridley's
- s. roentgenogram, maxillary
- s. rostrum of
- s. sagittal
- s. sagittalis inferior
- s. sagittalis superior
- s. sensitivity, carotid
- s., septic phlebitis of cranial
- s. shot
- s., sigmoid
- s., sphenoidal
- s., sphenoidal paranasal
- s. standstill
- s. stimulation, carotid
- s., subarachnoidal
- s., subperiosteal abscess of frontal
- s., superior sagittal
- s. surgery
- s. surgery, endoscopic
- s. surgery (FESS) ▸ functional endoscopic

- s. syncope, carotid
- s. syndrome, carotid
- s. syndrome ▸ hypersensitive carotid
- s. syndrome (SSS), sick
- s. tachycardia (ST)
- s. tachycardia ▸ paroxysmal
- s., tarsal
- s. tarsi, roof of
- s. tenderness
- s. test, carotid
- s. thermodilution, coronary
- s. thrombosis
- s. thrombosis ▸ intracranial
- s., thrombosis of cavernous
- s., thrombosis of lateral
- s., thrombosis of sigmoid
- s. thrombosis ▸ venous
- s. tract
- s. transversus pericardii
- s. tumor, endodermal
- s. tumor, ovarian endodermal
- s. tympani
- s., Valsalva's
- s. valve of coronary
- s. venosus
- s. venosus atrial septal defect
- s. venosus defect
- s. venosus sclerae
- s. well aerated
- s. x-ray

sinusal aneurysm, aortic
sinusectomy, frontal
sinusitis
- s., acute
- s. ▸ acute bacterial
- s. ▸ acute exacerbation of
- s., allergic fungal
- s., chronic
- s. disorder
- s., recurrent

sinusography, cerebral
sinusoid(s)
- s. congested
- s. edematous
- s., myocardial
- s. of liver

sinusoidal
- s. biphasic wave form ▸ quasi-
- s. circulation
- s. delta activity, monorhythmic
- s. waves

sinusoideum, vas
sinusotomy (*same as* sinuotomy)
sinu-vertebral nerve

sip-and-puff mouthpiece
siphon(s)
- s., carotid
- s., Duquet
- s. ▸ Moniz carotid

Siphona irritans
siphonage, water test
Siphunculina funicola
Sippy diet
Sippy's dilator
sireniform fetus
siro, Tyroglyphus
SISI (Short Increment Sensitivity Index) Test
Sisyrinchium galaxioides
sit(s)
- s. still ▸ patient unable to
- s. -up exercise
- s. -up exercise, chair
- s. -up ▸ half
- s. up ▸ loss of ability to
- s. -ups ▸ straight leg

site(s) (Site) [*cite, sight*]
- s., active
- s., active oozing from
- s. affected
- s., allosteric
- s., amputation
- s., anastomotic
- s., anatomic
- s. antibody, combining
- s., antigenic
- s., antigenic determinate
- s., arterial entry
- s., arteriovenous (AV) shunt
- s. atrial pacing, dual-
- s., base of fracture
- s. -based physician
- s., binding
- s., biopsy
- s. ▸ bleeding from multiple
- s., body
- s., bone graft
- s., bony
- s., brain
- s. bruises, catheter
- s., cancer localized in ▸ original
- s. care
- s. care, intravenous (IV) needle
- s., catalytic
- s., catheter
- s., catheter insertion
- s. cauterized, bleeding
- s., colostomy
- s., combining

s., comminuted tibial fracture
s., crepitus at fracture
s., cut down
s., damaged
s. discomfort, infusion
s., donor
s., drain
s., drainage (dr'ge) about shunt
s., drainage at incision
s., draining, incisional
S. dressing, Dri-
s., electrode
s., entry
s., extrapulmonary
s., femoral neck fracture
s., fistula
s. for opioids, receptor
s., fracture
s. GC (gonococcus) cultures, four
s., greater curvature
s., healed cutdown
s., healed incision
s., healing incision
s., implant
s., incision
s., incision carried down to fracture
s., infected incision
s., infection
s. infection, IV (intravenous)
s. infection, operative
s. infection (SSI) ▸ surgical
s., infusion
s., initial
s., injection
s., injury
s., insertion
s. intervention, on-
s. ▸ intra-atrial
s., intraocular
s., intraventricular
s., involved
s. irrigated, operative
s., irritation of incision
s., joint
s., leaking about shunt
s., lesser curvature
s. lose function ▸ receptor
s., metastatic
s., motion at fracture
s. ▸ multiple body
s., needle
s., nipple
s., obstructive
s. occluded, fistula
s. of action

s. of bleeding
s. of blockage ▸ potential
s. of bone graft, donor
s. of electrode placement
s. of illness
s. of incision, tenderness at
s. of infection
s. of injection, bleeding at
s. of injection ▸ lump at
s. of nosocomial infection
s. of origin
s. of primary infection
s. of prophage
s., oozing about shunt
s., operative
s., opiate binding
s., optimal stimulation
s. ▸ original injection
s., original tumor
s., osteotomy
s., pain
s. ▸ pain at incision
s., placental
s., postsynaptic
s., presynaptic
s., primary
s., primary tumor
s., prime
s., procedure
s., puncture
s., pus at incision
s., radial fracture
s. reaction ▸ injection
s., receptor
s. ▸ receptor binding
s., recipient
s., recording
s., rectal
s., redness along incision
s. ▸ redness at incision
s., related
s., remottling fracture
s., repressor
s., residual tumor
s. ▸ residual tumor at primary
s., scalp
s., secondary
s. ▸ selected insertion
s., separation at fracture
s., smoke-free work
s., sterile
s., surgical
s. ▸ swelling at incision
s., swelling of
s., target

s. ▸ tender muscle
s., tibial fracture
s., tracheostomy
s., tracheotomy
s. unspecified ▸ psychogenic pain,
s., unsuspected disease
s., ureterotomy
s., venipuncture
s. ▸ warmth at incision
s., wound

sitology [*cytology*]
sitting
s. balance
s. blood pressure
s. height
s. position
s. posture
s. suprasternal height
s., transfer from supine to
s., unsupported
s. -up view
s. vertex height

situ
s., adenocarcinoma in
s. assay ▸ in-
s., cancer in
s. (CIS), carcinoma in
s. cells indicative of carcinoma in
s. disease, in
s. (DCIS) ▸ ductal carcinoma in
s. examination of abdomen ▸ in
s. hybridization ▸ in-
s., in
s. keratomileusis (LASIK)
 correction ▸ laser-assisted in
s. keratomileusis (LASIK) ▸ laser
 in
s. keratomileusis (LASIK) ▸ laser-
 assisted in
s. keratomileusis (LASIK) surgery ▸
 laser-assisted in
s. keratomileusis (LASIK) surgery ▸
 wavefront guided laser-assisted
 in
s., lobular carcinoma in
s. transitional bladder cell
 carcinoma, in
s., tumor in
s., vaginal carcinoma in

situation(s)
s., anxiety-producing
s., anxiety-provoking
s., catastrophic
s., competitive
s., crisis

situation(s)—*continued*

s., current family
s., depressed adult
s., emotional
s., external
s. ▸ extreme reticence in social
s. ▸ fear of social
s., group
s., high-risk
s., intolerable
s., knowledge
s., life-threatening
s., living
s., long-term living
s., monitoring
s. ▸ multiple victim
s., nonterminal
s., normal anatomic
s., perception of
s., reduced activity to emotional
s. ▸ relapse triggering
s. ▸ response to social
s., social or interpersonal
s., stress
s., stressful
s. ▸ stressful or anxious
s., stress-induced
s., terminal
s., traumatic
s., unbearable

situational

s. anxiety
s. demands
s. depression
s. disorder
s. disturbance, transient
s. low self-esteem
s. or stress reaction, acute
s. psychosis
s. reaction
s. reaction, acute
s. stress reaction, adult
s. syncope

situs

s. ambiguus
s. inversus, complete
s. inversus, dextrocardia with
s. inversus, incomplete
s. inversus ▸ levocardia with
s. inversus viscerum
s. solitus
s. transversus
s., visceroatrial

sitz bath
sitz baths ▸ daily warm

SIU (Stimulus Isolation Unit)
SIV (simian immunodeficiency virus)
Siwe

S. disease, Letterer-
S. syndrome, Abt-Letterer-
S. syndrome, Letterer-

six (6)

6 -amethopterin
s. and fourteen positive spikes
s. and fourteen spike rhythm
s. hertz (Hz) positive bursts ▸
   fourteen and
s. hertz (Hz) positive spikes ▸
   fourteen and
s. Hz spike-and-slow waves
6 -lead electrocardiogram (ECG)
6 -mercaptopurine/6-MP
   (Purinethol)
6 -mercaptopurine, and prednisone
   (VAMP) therapy ▸ vincristine,
   methotrexate,
6 -mercaptopurine and prednisone
   (VAMP) ▸ vincristine,
   amethopterin,
6 -mercaptopurine (POMP) ▸
   prednisone, Oncovin,
   methotrexate,
6 murmur, Grade 1 through
s. per second positive spikes ▸
   fourteen and
s. per second spike-and-wave
   discharge
6 -phosphate dehydrogenase
   deficiency anemia ▸ glucose-
6 -phosphate dehydrogenase
   deficiency, glucose-
s. to twelve per second spindle
6 ▸ V leads, 1 through

16-18 syndrome, trisomy
16-lead electrocardiogram (ECG)
sixth

s. cranial nerve
s. nerve
s. nerve palsy
s. sense
s. ventricle
s. -year molar

60

60 contrast medium, Reno-M-
60 (Co^{60}) eye plaques ▸ cobalt
60 (Co^{60}) teletherapy machine ▸
   cobalt
60 (Co^{60}) therapy ▸ cobalt

67

67 imaging ▸ gallium
67 scan, gallium (Ga)
67 scintigraphy ▸ gallium

size

s. and condition, normal
s. and configuration ▸ normal
s. and function ▸ cardiac
s. and outline, heart
s. and shape, heart
s. and shape, normal
s. and shape, uterus normal in
s. and/or configuration
s. ▸ breast
s. ▸ cardiac
s. ▸ configuration and
s. conformer, medium
s., decreased breast
s. discrepancy, tooth
s., field
s., gestational
s., gyri decreased in
s., heart
s., heart normal in
s., heart reduced to normal
s. in half body irradiation, field
s., increase in muscle
s., increased heart
s., liver generous in
s., normal
s., normal heart
s., normal in
s. of infarct
s. of tumor reduced
s. or shape ▸ unequal pupil
s., overall
s. per fraction, increased dose
s., pore
s., pupil
s., pupil reaction and
s., pupillary
s., reduce prostate
s., reduction of tumor
s., shape and consistency
s., shape and motility
s., shape and position
s., small head
s., suture
s., tumor
s., tumor increased in
s., uterus normal in

sizer ▸ Meadox graft
Sjögren('s)

S. disease
S. syndrome
S. syndrome, Marinesco-
S. syndrome, primary

S. syndrome, secondary
SK virus, Columbia
Skag (heroin)
skein cell
skein test, Holmgren's wool
skeletal
  s. abnormalities
  s. deformity
  s. disease
  s. disorder
  s., distorted chest
  s. dysplasia
  s. hyperostosis ▸ idiopathic
  s. maturation
  s. maturity
  s. metastases
  s. muscle
  s. muscle activity
  s. muscle, atrophy of
  s. muscle degeneration
  s. muscle disorder
  s. muscle fibers
  s. muscle ischemia
  s. muscle ▸ ischemic
  s. muscle plasticity
  s. muscle relaxant
  s. muscle reperfusion injury ▸
    postischemia
  s. muscle ▸ transplanted
  s. muscle wasting
  s. muscular defect
  s. muscular tone
  s. muscular tone, momentary loss
    of
  s. myoblasts
  s. pain
  s. structure
  s. survey
  s. system
  s. tissue
  s. traction
  s. traction, balanced
  s. traction, Crutchfield
skeletogenous cell
skeleton
  s., axial
  s., fetal
  s., fibrous
  s. hand
  s., infantile
Skene's
  S. duct
  S. glands
  S. (BUS) glands ▸ Bartholin's,
    urethral and

skew deviation
skew pupils
skewer technique
skiagram study
skid mat, no-
skids, bone
skier's thumb
skill(s)
  s., adaptive
  s., adequate literacy
  s., analytic
  s. and attention ▸ spatial
  s. and perception ▸ attention,
    orientation
  s., anger management
  s., anxiety management
  s. ▸ awkward motor
  s., balance
  s., basic mental
  s., basic physical
  s., bicultural communications
  s. building resources ▸ reproducible
  s. building ▸ social
  s., chemical dependency
  s., clinical
  s., codependency
  s., cognitive
  s., cognitive perceptual motor
  s., cognitive therapy
  s., communication
  s., compensatory
  s., comprehension
  s., conceptual
  s., conditioned reflex
  s., control motor
  s., conversational
  s., coping
  s., counseling
  s., crisis intervention
  s., culture centered
  s., daily living
  s., decision-making
  s., defensive behavior
  s. ▸ depression management
  s., develop coping
  s. development
  s. development ▸ social
  s., discipline
  s., driving
  s., effective
  s., effective communication
  s., effective parenting
  s., emotional
  s. ▸ evaluation of psychomotor
  s. ▸ functional memory

  s. ▸ group exercises for enhancing
    social
  s. group ▸ multiple
  s. ▸ impulse control
  s. ▸ inadequate literacy
  s. ▸ independent living
  s., insight
  s. ▸ intact motor
  s. ▸ intellectual and motor
  s., interpersonal
  s., intuitive
  s. ▸ journal writing
  s., language
  s. ▸ latency-based cognitive
  s., learning
  s. ▸ life changing
  s., lifesaving
  s. ▸ limited interpersonal
  s., loss of language
  s. ▸ loss of motor
  s. ▸ marginal literacy
  s., mobility
  s. modules
  s., motor
  s., obstructed airway
  s. of daily living ▸ relearn
  s. ▸ oral language
  s., oral motor
  s., perceptual and motor
  s. ▸ perfection of surgical
  s. ▸ poor management
  s., problem-solving
  s., procrastination
  s. ▸ progressive loss of mental
  s., psychological
  s., psychomotor
  s., pushing and pulling
  s. ▸ rational thinking
  s., reading
  s. ▸ recall and listening
  s. ▸ relapse prevention
  s., relaxation
  s. ▸ self-care
  s. ▸ self-control
  s. ▸ self-esteem
  s. ▸ self-help
  s., self-improvement
  s. ▸ self-management
  s. ▸ self-monitoring
  s. ▸ sleep management
  s. ▸ slow motor
  s. ▸ slowing down of motor
  s. ▸ sober leisure
  s., social

skill(s)—*continued*
s., social and leisure
s., social interpersonal
s., spatial
s., speech
s., stress
s. ▸ stress management
s., structured repetitive
s. support ▸ life
s., survival
s., therapeutic
s. therapy, coping
s. ▸ time management
s. training approach, cognitive
s. training for children
s. training ▸ problem-solving
s. training ▸ social
s. training ▸ special
s. ▸ transcendent coping
s., verbal
s., visitation
s. ▸ visual spatial
s., visual-motor
s., vocational

skilled
s. acts
s. facility
s. level of care criteria
s. movements
s. nursing care
s. nursing care ▸ intermittent
s. nursing care ▸ long-term
s. nursing care ▸ short-
s. nursing facility
s. nursing facility, certified
s. observation

Skillern's fracture
skim milk
skimming, plasma
skimming, platelet
skin (Skin) [*chin, shin*]
s., abraded
s. adhere, transplanted
s., age spots on
s. aging
s. anatomy
s. and hair, dry
s. and muscle, excess
s., anesthesia of
s., angioma of
s. anthrax
s. appendages
s. approximated
s. area ▸ central surface
s., artificial

s., ashen color
s. atriae
s. atrophy
s. bacteria, controlling
s., bacterial infection of
S. Bank
s. barrier
s. barrier, blood
s. biopsy
s. blanched
s. blemish
s. blistering
s. blisters
s., blotchy
s., blue
s., bluish colored
s., bluish tinge to
s. break in
s. breakdown
s. breakout
s., broken
s. bruises
s., bumpy
s., burning
s. ▸ burning, itching and redness of
s. burns
s. button
s. by contaminated instruments, puncturing of
s. by contaminated needle, puncturing of
s. cancer
s. cancer, basal cell
s. cancer ▸ eyelid
s. cancer ▸ nonmelanoma
s. cancer of lip
s. cancer screening
s. cancer ▸ squamous cell
s. cancer therapy, radiation necrosis in
s. carcinoma, squamous cell
s. care, clinical
s. care, decubitus
s. care teaching
s., cavernous hemangioma of
s. cells
s. cells, dead
s. cells layers of ▸ compacted dead
s. cells ▸ matured
s. changes
s. ▸ chronic ulcerations of
s., clamminess of
s., clammy
s. cleaning
s. cleansed

s. closed
s. closed with interrupted silk
s. closed with running subcuticular suture of nylon
s. closure, method of
s. closure, postoperative
s. cold and clammy
s., coldness of
s., color change of
s. condition, chronic
s. conductance response
s., congenital localized absence of
s., congested
s. contact of sensors
s. contamination
s. ▸ cool, clammy
s., cracked
s. cracking from athlete's foot
s. cracking from dermatitis
s. cracking from eczema
s. ▸ cracking, peeling or blistering of
s. crawling sensation
s. crease
s. crusting from dermatitis
s. crusting from eczema
s., crusting of
s. ▸ cyanotic discoloration of
s., darkening of the
s., dead
s., debridement infected
s. ▸ dermatophyte infections of
s. diaphoretic
s., diminution of breast
s., dimpling of
s. discoloration
s. disease, contagious
s. disease, exfoliative
s. disease ▸ facial
s. disinfection
s. disorder
s. disorder, alcohol-related
s. disorder from aspirin
s. disorder from birth control pill
s. disorder of cheek
s. disorder, rare
s. distance, focus to
s. distance (SSD), source to
s. distance (TSD) ▸ target
s. distance, tumor
s., donor
s. donor bank
s. dose
s. draped
s., dry
s. dry and itchy

s. dry and scaly
s., ▸ dry, cracked
s. ▸ dry, itching
s. ▸ dry, itchy, flaking
s. ▸ dry, mottled
s. ▸ dry, wrinkled
s. ▸ drying and wrinkling of
s. ▸ dryness and itching of
s. ▸ ear canal
s. edges, approximate
s. edges, attached to
s. edges, reapproximate
s. edges trimmed
s. edges undercut
s., elastic
s. elasticity
s. ▸ electrical response of
s. electrode attachment
s. electron beam therapy, total
s. emotional activity
s. equivalent, living
s. eruption
s. erythema dose
s., erythematous
s. evaluation
s., excess
s., exfoliative
s., facial
s. ▸ firm, elastic
s., flaccid
s., flaking
s. flap
s. flap, horseshoe-shaped
s. flap reflected
s. flaps raised
s. flora
s., flushed
s. flushing, alcohol
s., flushing of
s. fold
s. fold artifact
s. fold incision
s., fold of
s. fold thickness
s. fold ▸ wrinkled
s., fore▸
s. from blood clot ▸ blue
s. from dermatitis ▸ flaking
s. from dermatitis ▸ peeling
s. from eczema ▸ flaking
s. from eczema ▸ peeling
s. ▸ fungus infection of
s., gangrenous
s., glands of
s., good contact with

s. "goose bumps"
s. graft
s. graft, Blair-Brown
s. graft defatted
s. graft donor
s. graft donor site
s. graft, full-thickness
s. graft, intermediate
s. graft, intermediate split-thickness
s. graft, intermediate thickness
s. graft, partial thickness
s. graft slough
s. graft, split-
s. graft, split-thickness
s. graft, Thiersch's
s., grafted
s. grafting
s. grafting ▸ autologous cultured
s. grafting, repeated
s. growth
s. ▸ growth and maturation of new
s. growth and preserved ▸ generic
s. growth ▸ noncancerous
s. gun
s., hanging
s. hardening from dermatitis
s. heart
s. ▸ heavy scaling of
s. homograft
s., human
s. hydration
s., hypersensitive
s. impedance
s. incision
s. incision closed
s. incision, curvilinear
s. incision ▸ induration along
s. incision, midline
s. incision, wide
s. infection
s. infection, bacterial
s. infection ▸ chronic
s. infection, severe
s. infection ▸ spread of
s. infection, uncomplicated
s. infestation
s. inflammation
s. injury
s. integrity
s. integrity, impaired
s. integrity ▸ impairment of
s. interface, electrode
s. irritation
s. irritation and rubbing, constant
s. irritation from Benadryl

s. irritation, mild
S. Isolation, Wound and
s., itching of
s., itching of jaundiced
s., itchy
s. ▸ itchy or chapped
s. jaundiced
s. laceration
s. layers
s. lesion
s. lesion artifact
s. lesion biopsy
s. lesion, gram stain of
s. lesion, linear
s. lesion ▸ proliferative
s. leukosis
s. -like cell lining
s. lines
s. lipid
s., lividity and coldness of
s., loose
s. loss
s. loss, extensive
s. maceration
s. management
s. margins
s. medication ▸ topical
s. melanoma
s., mesh
s. metastases
s. moist
s., moist cold
s., mottled
s. ▸ multiple ecchymoses on
s. ▸ multiple moles on
s. ▸ multiple sheets of
s. necrosis
s. nerve ending
s. numbness
s., oily
s., open wound of
s. opened transversely
s. ▸ outer layer of
s., outermost layer of
s., overlying
s. ▸ pacemaker implanted under
s. pale
s. ▸ pale and clammy
s. pale and diaphoretic
s., pallid
s. pallor
s. pallor, marked
s. parasite
s. patch
s. patch ▸ motion sickness

skin—*continued*

s. patch ▸ nicotine
s. patches ▸ small adhesive
s. ▸ patchy depigmentation of
s., patient has leathery
s. ▸ patient picks at
s. peeling from athlete's foot
s., peeling of
s. pencil
s. pencil, Blaisdell
s., penile
s., perianal
s. ▸ petechial hemorrhages of
s. photosensitivity ▸ extreme
s. picking
s., picking and excoriating of
s. pigment
s. pigmentation
s. ▸ pitting of the
s. pliable
s., poor contact with
s. popper, mainliner and/or
s. potential
s. potential, electrodispersive
s. potential level
s. potential response
s., prematurely aging
s. preparation
s. preparation, preoperative
s. prepped
s. prepped and draped
s. ▸ puckering of
s. puncture
s. pupillary reflex
s. ▸ purplish hemorrhagic spots on
s. rash
s. rash, contact
s. rash, intractable
s. rash, itchy
s. rash, recurring
s. rash ▸ relapsing
s. rash ▸ severe, painful
s. reaction
s. reaction, allergic
s. reaction, psychogenic
s. reaction to electron beam therapy
s. reaction ▸ widespread allergic
s. receptors
s., red
s., reddened areas of
s. ▸ reddened, flushed
s. redness
s., redraped
s., redundant

s. reflex
s. reflex, galvanic
s. rejuvenation
s. rejuvenation ▸ laser
s. replacement
s. resistance
s. resistance, basal
s. resistance response
s. response
s. response, galvanic
s. restoration ▸ laser facial
s., resurface
s. resurfacing
s. resurfacing, carbon dioxide (CO_2) laser
s. resurfacing ▸ face laser
s. revision (FSR), fusiform
s. revitalization
s., roentgens delivered to
s., sagging
s. ▸ sagging facial
s., sallow
s. scab
s., scaling
s. scrapings
s., segment of
s. self-examination
s. sensation
s. sensitizing antibody
s. ▸ shallow erosion of
s. sheen
s. shocks
S. Skribe pen
s. ▸ sloughed-off
s., sloughing of
s. sloughs off, frozen
s. sores
s. sores ▸ festering
s. sparing mastectomy
s. spots
s. spots, aging
s. spots ▸ precancerous
s. spots ▸ rough, scaly
s., stimulation of
s. stones
s., stretchable
s. structure infection
s. subjected to friction
s., sun-damaged
s. surface
s. surgery ▸ laser
s. surrounding nipple, dark
s. sutures
s. sutures intact
s., sweaty

s. swelling ▸ local
s., swollen
s. syndrome, scalded
s. tag
s. tags, hemorrhoidal
s. tags, perineal
s. tags, rectal
s., taped to
s. ▸ taut, shiny
s. temperature
s. temperature, increased
s. tenderness
s. tension lines (RSTL), relaxed
s. ▸ tenting of
s. test antigen ▸ mumps
s. test dose (STD)
s. test for fungus organisms
s. test for tuberculosis (TB)
s. test, Hanger-Rose
s. test, histoplasmin
s. test ▸ Kveim antigen
s. test, Mantoux
s. test, patch
s. test, prick
s. test ▸ tuberculosis (TB)
s. test, tumor
s. test unit (STU)
s. testing
s. testing ▸ PPD (Purified Protein Derivative)
s. testing, vive
s. texture
s. texture ▸ improving
s. ▸ thick, red, itchy patches of
s., thickening of
s., thickness of
s., thinning
s. -tightening face-lift
s. tissue
s. to tumor distance
s. tone
s. tone pink and warm
s. transformer, belt
s., translucent
s. transplant
s. transplant ▸ feasible emergency
s. transplant, routine
s. transplantation
s. transplantation, autologous
s. transplantation ▸ autologous cultured
s. transplantation ▸ immunological barrier to
s. treatment, collagen
s. treatment ▸ laser

s. triangle excised
s. tumor
s. tumors ▸ recurrent
s. turgor
s. ulcer ▸ vascular
s. ulcerations
s. ulcers
s., underlying
s., undermined
s., unpigmented
s. vaporizes
s. vulnerable to injury ▸ grafted
s., wavy
s., wedge of
s. window
s. window technique, Rebuck
s. wound cleanser
s. wound, closure of
s. wound, minor
s., wrinkled
s. ▸ wrinkled lid
s. wrinkles, premature
s. ▸ yellowing of
s., yellowness of
skinfold thickness ▸ subscapular
skinfolds caliper
skinline incision
skinned patient, dark-
skinned, patient fair
skinning
s. colpectomy
s. vaginectomy
s. vulvectomy
s. vulvovaginectomy, partial
skinny needle aspiration
Skiodan
S. Acacia contrast medium
S. contrast medium
S. solution
skip
s. area
s. graft
s. lesions
skipped beat
skipping, verbal
Sklar-Schiøtz tonometer
Skoda('s)
S. rale
S. sign
S. tympany
skodaic resonance
skodaic tympany
skodique, bruit
Skoog procedure
Skribe pen, Skin

SKSD (streptokinase-streptodornase)
skujae, Leptothrix
skull
s., adult
s. base lesion ▸ benign
s. base lesion ▸ malignant
s., base of
s., bleeding inside
s., bur holes drilled in
s. cap
s., conformation of
s. defect
s., exophthalmos due to tower
s., external
s. film
s. fracture
s. fracture, basal
s. fracture, basilar
s. fracture, closed
s. fracture, compound
s. fracture ▸ debridement of compound
s. fracture, depressed
s. fracture, diastatic
s. fracture, elevation of
s. fracture, expressed
s. fracture, linear
s. fracture ▸ open reduction of
s. fracture, simple
s. ▸ hologram of
s., inner table bones of
s., inner tables of
s. irradiation, whole
s., lacunar
s. of fetus ▸ crushing procedure
s., outer table bones of
s., outer tables of
s. plate, Hoen's
s. portals, opposing
s., post-traumatic osteomyelitis of
s. roentgenogram
s. roentgenogram, lateral
s. survey
s., suture line of
s., sutures of
s. traction apparatus
s. traction, Vinke tong
s., vault of
SKY epidural pain control system
skyline projection
skyline view
sl (slow)
SLA (sacrolaeva anterior)
slant
s. culture

s., downward eye
s. -hole tomography
slapped cheek appearance
slapping gait
slapping percussion
slaved programmed electrical stimulation
SLE (systemic lupus erythematosus)
sleep(s) (Sleep)
s., active
s. activity ▸ shifting brain electrical activity toward
s. aid ▸ therapeutic
s. aids
s. anesthesia, twilight
s. anxiety dreams
s. anxiety dreams ▸ rapid eye movement (REM)
s. apnea
s. apnea, central
s. apnea ▸ drowsiness from
s. apnea ▸ mixed
s. apnea (OSA), obstructive
s. apnea ▸ problem with central nervous system from
s. apnea syndrome
s. apnea victim
s. apnea/hypopnea syndrome
s. architecture
s., arousal from
s. (h.s.) ▸ at bedtime or hour of
s. attacks ▸ irrepressible
s. behavior
s. behavior disorder
s. center technology
s. clinic
s., crescendo
s. cycle
s. cycle position
s., D
s., decreased deep
s. ▸ decreased need for
s., deep
s., deeper stage of
s. deficit
s., delta
s. deprivation
s. deprivation ▸ chronic
s. deprivation ▸ severe
s. deprivation therapy
s. deprived, chronically
s. deprived patient
s., desynchronized
s. difficulty
s. disorder

sleep(s)—*continued*

s. disorder center
s. disorder ▸ circadian rhythm
s. disorder ▸ complex
s. disorder, debilitating
s. disorder facilities ▸ certified
s. disorder, nonorganic
s. disordered breathing
S. Disorders Association ▸ American
s. disruption
s. disturbance, episodic
s. (DIMS), disturbance in maintaining
s. disturbances
s. -dream study
s., dreaming
s. dreamless
s., drifts into normal
s., drug-induced
s., early phases of
s., early stages of
s. efficiency
s. efficiency index
s., electric
s., electrotherapeutic
s. enhancing and pain relieving
s. environment
s. epilepsy
s. episodes, daytime
s. evaluation, overnight
s., fast wave
s., frozen
s. habits, revising
s. history
s. hygiene
s. hypoxia
s., inability to
s. ▸ increased rapid eye movement (REM)
s., induced
s., inducing
s., induction of
s. inertia
s., initiating
s., interrupted
s. interruption
s. interruption ▸ duration of
s. interruption insomnia ▸ rapid eye movement (REM)
s., K complexes during
s. lab
s. laboratory
s. latency
S. Latency Test, Multiple

s., light
s., lighter stage of
s. -like condition
s. -like state
s. log
s., longer periods of
s. loss
s., maintaining
s. maintenance disorder
s. maintenance insomnia
s. management skills
s. mentation
s., narcoleptic
s., natural
s., nighttime
s., nocturnal
s. (NREMS), nonrapid eye movement
s., normal spindles of
s. of short duration ▸ deep
s. onset
s. onset insomnia
s. onset REM (rapid eye movement) period
s. onset (WASO), wake after
s., orthodox
s., paradoxical
s. paralysis
s. paralysis attacks
s., paroxysmal
s., patient died in
s., patient expired in
s., patient in deep
s. pattern
s. pattern, alteration in
s. pattern ▸ disruptive
s. pattern, neonatal
s. pattern, therapeutic
s. patterns, abnormal
s. patterns, disordered
s. patterns ▸ disturbance in
s. patterns ▸ disturbed
s. patterns ▸ electroencephalogram (EEG)
s. patterns, monitoring
s. patterns of insomniacs
s. patterns, symmetrical
s. (PLMS) ▸ periodic limb movements in
s. ▸ persistent disorder initiating
s. ▸ persistent disorder of maintaining
s. phase, delayed
s. phase syndrome (DSPS), delayed

s. phase syndrome (FASPS) ▸ familial advanced
s. ▸ physiology of
s., positive occipital sharp transients of
s. problem
s. problem, child has
s., prolonged
s. quality, subjective
s., quiet
s., rapid eye movements (REM)
s. recording
s. recording, all night
s. -related disorder
s. -related hypoxemia ▸ rapid eye movement (REM)
s., REM (rapid eye movement)
s. ▸ repetitive intrusions of
s. research
s. respiratory rate
s. response
s., restorative
s. restriction therapy
s. schedule disturbance, chronic
s. sedation
s. ▸ shallow, unrestful
s. (SWS), slow wave
s. spindles
s., spontaneous
s. stage, deep
s. stage, delta
s. stage demarcation
s. stage, intermediary
s. stage, light
s. stage period
s. stages
s. stages and waking ▸ score
s. stages, dysfunction of
s. state
s. state, active
s. structure
s. study
s. (S sleep) ▸ synchronized
s. talking
s. technician
s., temple
s. terror disorder
s. time, total
s. ▸ transient disorder of initiating
s. ▸ transient disorder of maintaining
s., transitional
s. ▸ unable to
s. -wake cycle
s. -wake cycle, biological
s. -wake cycle, daily

s. -wake cycle ▸ phase-shift disruption of 24-hour
s. -wake disorders
s. -wake pattern
s. -wake pattern change
s. -wake pattern ▸ erratic
s. -wake shift
s. -waking
s. walking
sleeper, stomach
sleepiness
s., daytime
s., excessive
s., excessive daytime
s., mid-day
s., severe daytime
sleeping (Sleeping)
s., difficulty
s. disorder
s., excessive
s. habits ▸ change in eating or
s. pattern, change in
s. pattern, normal
S. Pills (barbiturates)
s. posture
s. sickhouse
s. sickness
s. sickness, African
s., stomach
s. subject
s. tachycardia
sleeplessness
s. and irritability
s., fatigue and
s. ▸ stress-related
sleeptalking, patient
sleepwalker, patient
sleepwalking disorder
sleepy and uncoordinated
sleepy staggers
sleeve
s. graft
s. graft, Dacron
s. lobectomy
s. resection, bronchial
s., root
s., trocar
slew rate
SLI (splenic localization index)
slice(s)
s., coronal
s. CT (computerized tomography) scan ▸ thin
s. graft
s., image

s. of heart muscle removed
s., transaxial
slick-gut syndrome
slide (Slide)
s. agglutination test, latex
s. air-dried
s., concave microscopic
s., etched circled
s. examination
s. heat fixed
s., microscopic
s. specimen
s. technology, dry
S. Test, Monospot
sliding
s. esophageal hiatal hernia
s. fee scale
s. filament theory
s. flap
s. flap, French
s. graft, massive
s. hernia
s. hiatal hernia
s. inlay bone graft
s. inlay graft
s. microtome
s. plasty
s. scale
s. scale insulin therapy
s. scale method
s. scale treatment
s. technique
s. transfer
s. -type hiatal hernia
slight
s. deformity
s. intention tremor
s. nystagmus on upward gaze
s. obstruction of esophagus
slightly [*tightly*]
s. displaced
s., fracture displaced
s. lipid, adrenals
s. nodular, mucosa
s. slow activity, generalized
s. thickened, arteries
slim disease
slime fungus
sling
s. and swathe
s., basket
s., cardiac
s. -dressing, Velpeau
s. elevation of eyelid
s., Glisson's

s., levator
s. operation
s., pericardial
s., pressure
s. procedure, esophageal
s. procedure, Lawman's
s. ▸ pulmonary artery
s., Rauchfuss'
s. ring complex
s., strap
s., Supramid ptosis
s., suspension
s. syndrome ▸ pulmonary
s., Tear's
s. ▸ vaginal wall
s., vascular
s., Velpeau
slip
s. hernia
s., shoulder
s. signed, release
slipped
s. disc
s. disc pain
s. epiphysis
s. hernia
s. meniscus
s. or ruptured disc ▸ pain in back from
s. upper femoral epiphysis
slipping
s. dentures
s. patella
s. rib syndrome
s. rib therapy
s. ribs
s. sound
slit(s)
s., dorsal
s., filtration
s., gill
s. in cornea, multiple
s. -lamp
s. -lamp examination
s. -lamp, Gullstrand's
s. -lamp, Haag-Streit
s. -lamp microscope
s. scanography
s. ventricle syndrome
slitting of canaliculus of eye
SLO (scanning laser ophthalmoscope)
Slocum's operation
slope
s. computer, electromechanical

slope—*continued*
- s. culture
- s., D to E
- s., down
- s., E to F
- s. ▸ mitral E to F

sloping surface
slot-blot hybridization analysis
slots, treatment
slotted plate
slough (*same as* sluff)
slough, skin graft
sloughed
- s. area
- s. bronchial epithelium
- s. off skin

sloughing
- s. ▸ chronic inflammation with alveolar
- s., dead tissue
- s., endometrial
- s., epithelial
- s. infiltrates ▸ extensive bilateral
- s. of cells
- s. of skin

sloughs off, frozen skin
slow (sl) [*flow*]
- s. activity
- s. activity, anterior temporal
- s. activity, background of
- s. activity, focal
- s. activity, focal moderately
- s. activity, focus of
- s. activity, frontal
- s. activity, generalized
- s. activity, generalized exceedingly
- s. activity, generalized slightly
- s. activity, midtemporal focus of
- s. activity, paroxysmal
- s. activity, posterior temporal
- s. activity, posterotemporal
- s. activity, runs of
- s. alpha variant
- s. alpha variant rhythm
- s. and inhumane
- s. and shallow breathing
- s. and shallow, respirations
- s. and unsteady speech
- s. A-V node pathway
- s. blood clotting
- s. brain wave activity ▸ deficiency of
- s. brain wave frequencies
- s. brain waves
- s. breathing, deep

- s. bursts, periodic
- s. cell degeneration
- s. channel
- s. channel blocker
- s. component
- s. component, fast and
- s. comprehension
- s., controlled movements
- s. death, painfully
- s. development
- s. diminished movement of bradykinesia
- s. -dissolving fluoride pills
- s. down cancer growth
- s. escape rhythm
- s. -fast tachycardia
- s. fetal growth
- s. frontal spindle
- s. fusion
- s. -growing acoustic neuroma
- s. growing cortical neoplasm
- s. growing virus
- s. growth
- s. growth rate
- s. healing sores
- s., heart
- s. heart beat, abnormally
- s. heart rate
- s. heart rhythm
- s. heartbeat
- s. hemoglobins
- s., hesitant urinary system
- s., high voltage waves
- s. immune response
- s. infusion intravenous (IV) drip
- s. intravenous (IV) infusion
- s. learner
- s. mentation
- s. metabolism
- s. metabolizer
- s. mitten pattern
- s. motor skill
- s. movement
- s. number
- s. pathway ablation
- s. pathway potential ▸ purative
- s. progression
- s. pulse
- s. reacting substance
- s. -reacting substance of anaphylaxis
- s. release of hormones
- s. renewal and nonrenewal systems of cells

- s., repeated, involuntary sinuous movements
- s. resolution
- s. respiration
- s. response
- s. rhythm, abnormally
- s. rotation room
- s. spike
- s. spike-and-wave
- s. spike-and-wave complex
- s. spread of cancer
- s., steady rhythm
- s. stretching exercise
- s. thaw treatment ▸ rapid freeze-
- s. thought processes ▸ disoriented or
- s. tumor growth
- s. virus
- s. vital capacity
- s. waking activity
- s. zone

slow wave(s)
- s.w. activity
- s.w. activity ▸ high voltage
- s.w., atypical repetitive spike-and-
- s.w. complex
- s.w. complex ▸ multiple spike-and-
- s.w. complex ▸ polyspike-and-
- s.w. complex ▸ sharp-and-
- s.w. complex ▸ spike-and-
- s.w. complexes ▸ sequence of spike-and-
- s.w., focal
- s.w. foci
- s.w. foci, occipital
- s.w. focus
- s.w. focus, anterior temporal
- s.w. focus, central
- s.w. focus, frontal
- s.w. focus, midtemporal
- s.w. focus, occipital
- s.w. focus, parietal
- s.w. generator
- s.w., high voltage arrhythmic
- s.w., high voltage diphasic
- s.w., independent
- s.w. ▸ irregular, extremely
- s.w., larval spike-and-
- s.w., medium voltage
- s.w., millisecond (msec)
- s.w., millivoltage (mv)
- s.w. of drowsiness
- s.w. of youth
- s.w., paroxysmal
- s.w., paroxysmal high voltage

s.w. pattern
s.w. phenomenon ▸ spike-and-
s.w. ▸ polymorphic
s.w., posterotemporal
s.w., repetitive sharp-and-
s.w. rhythm ▸ spike-and-
s.w., scattered
s.w., sharp-and-
s.w., six Hz (hertz) spike-and-
s.w. sleep (SWS)
s.w., spike-and-
s.w., sporadic
s.w., three hertz (Hz) spike-and-
s.w. transients
s.w. transients and eye blinks

slowed
  s. coordination
  s. gait and tremor
  s. intellectual function
  s. memory recall
  s. movements
  s. pulse
  s. reaction time
  s. reflexes
  s. respiration
  s. speech
  s. thinking

slowing
  s., bi-amplitude
  s., bioccipital
  s., cognitive
  s., diffuse paroxysmal
  s. down of motor skills
  s., focal
  s., focal temporal
  s., medium voltage
  s., midtemporal
  s. of motor responses
  s. of movements ▸ general
  s. of physical reactions
  s. of psychological reactions
  s. of pulse
  s., paroxysmal
  s., periodic
  s., post-ictal
  s. spikes, right frontal
  s., voltage

slowly
  s. developing brain disease
  s. developing lesion
  s., disease progressed
  s. growing invasive
    adenocarcinoma
  s. growing tumor
  s., heals

s. metabolize certain drugs
s., patient verbalizes
s. progressing memory loss
s. progressive hereditary disorder
s. progressive weakness

slowness
  s. of movement
  s. ▸ primary obsessional
  s., stiffness and unsteadiness ▸
    tremor,

SLP (sacrolaeva posterior)
SLR (straight leg raising)
SLR (straight leg raising) test
SLRT (straight leg raising
  tenderness)
SLRT (straight leg raising test)
SLT (sacrolaeva transverse)
sludge ball
sludged blood
sluff (_same as_ **slough)**
sluggish
  s. blood flow
  s. bowel
  s. circulation
  s. gallbladder
  s. movements of eyes and eyelids
  s. reaction
  s., reflexes
  s. to light, pupils
sluggishly, pupils react
sluggishness, mental
slumping, spinal
slurred
  s., indistinct speech
  s. speech
  s. speech, chronic
  s. speech ▸ sudden
slurring of QRS
slurring of ST
slurry, talc
slush, saline
slushed ice
slushing sound
Slyke test, Van
SM (systolic mean)
SM (syringomyelia) disorder
SMA (superior mesenteric artery)
SMAC (Sequential Multiple Analyzer
  Computer)
Smack (heroin)
smacking and licking of lips
smacking movements of tongue and
  lips
small (Small)
  s. adhesive skin patches

s. airway disease
s. arteries, embolized
s. based quad cane, patient
  independent with
s. blood vessel
s. blood vessel bleeding
s. blood vessel of the brain cover
s. bone density
s. bone structure
s. boost dose of radiation
s. bowel
s. bowel atresia
s. bowel biopsy
s. bowel, distal
s. bowel follow-through (SBFT)
s. bowel, gangrenous
s. bowel ischemia
s. bowel malabsorption
s. bowel mucosa
s. bowel, multiple loops of
s. bowel obstruction
s. bowel obstruction ▸ intermittent
s. bowel obstruction with ascites
s. bowel, proximal
s. bowel resection
s. bowel series
s. bowel, strangulated
s. brain hemorrhage
s. button of vein tissue
s. calcified leiomyomas ▸ multiple
s. caliber vessel
s. cardiac vein
S. -Carrion penile prosthesis
s. cell bronchogenic tumor
s. cell carcinoma
s. cell carcinoma of lung
s. cell carcinoma ▸ undifferentiated
s. cell lung cancer
s. cell ▸ typical
s. cell undifferentiated carcinoma
s. cell variety
s. cell variety ▸ bronchogenic
  carcinoma,
s. circumflex system
s. cystic infarct
s. duct disease
s. firm circumscribed nodule
s., flat, white patches on mucosa of
  stomach
s. focal hemorrhage
s. focus of hepatic necrosis
s. for gestational age (SGA)
s. fungating mucosal masses
s. gram-negative coccobacilli
s. group therapy

small—*continued*
s. growth
s. handwriting
s. head size
s. in stature
s. incision cataract surgery
s. infarct ▸ pulmonary emboli with
s. inflatable balloon
s., intact blister ▸ painless
s. interelectrode distances
s. intestinal submucosa
s. intestinal submucosa ▸ porcine
s. intestinal wall
s. intestine
s. intestine absorption
s. intestine as defense barrier
s. intestine cancer
s. intestine, distal portion of
s. intestine meridian
s. intestine ▸ mucosal surfaces of
s. intestine, solitary lymphatic
   nodules of
s. intestine transplant
s. joint replacement
s. left colon syndrome
s. -lunged emphysema
s. muscle coordination
s. nerve fibers
s. pedunculated adenomatous
   polyps
s. pelvis
s. prominent nucleolus
s. round cell carcinoma
s. saccular posterior pharyngeal
   diverticulum
s. saphenous vein
s. sciatic nerve
s. sharp spikes
s. stature, patient is of
s., tender lymph nodes
s. uterus
s. vein of heart
s. vessel circulation
s. vessel disease
s. vessel inadequate blood flow
s. vessel vasculitis
s. volume rotational therapy
s. white centers, oval lesions with
smaller
s. coronary vessels
s. pectoral muscle
s. psoas muscle
s. rib incision
smallest
s. adductor muscle

s. cardiac veins
s. scalene muscle
smallpox
s. vaccination
s. vaccine
s. vaccine reaction
s. virus
smart defibrillator
**SMAS (superficial
   musculoaponeurotic system)**
Smash (acetone extract of cannabis)
smasher, atom
**SMA-6 (sequential multiple analyzer)
   test**
SMA-12 profile test
**SMA-12 (sequential multiple
   analyzer) test**
smear(s)
s., abnormal Pap (Papanicolaou)
s. and culture
s. and cultures, stained
s., atypical Pap (Papanicolaou)
s., blood
s., bone marrow
s., buccal
s., buffy coat
s., cancer
s., cervical
s., cervical Pap (Papanicolaou)
s., concentrated
s., conjunctival
s. culture
s., differential
s., direct
s., fecal
s., fungi
s., lung Pap
s., nasal
s., nasopharyngeal
s., negative ▸ Pap (Papanicolaou)
s., Nickerson's medium
s. of clinical material ▸ stained
s. of stool, stained
s. overheated
s., Pagano-Levin medium
s., Pap (Papanicolaou)
s., peripheral blood
s., repeat
s. ▸ Richart and VCE (vaginal,
   cervical, endocervical) Pap
   (Papanicolaou)
s., sputum
s., stained
s., TB (tuberculosis)
s., throat

s., Tzanck
s., vaginal
s. ▸ vaginal, cervical, endocervical
   (VCE)
s., vaginal cuff Pap (Papanicolaou)
s., vaginal irrigation
s., wet
Smee cell
smegma
s. bacillus
s. clitoridis
s. embryonum
smegmatis, Mycobacterium
smell
s., absence of sense of
s. brain
s. ▸ decrease in sense of
s., diminished sense of
s. disorder
s. ▸ distortion in taste and
s., disturbance in
s. from aging ▸ loss of
s. ▸ impaired ability to
s., loss of memory for
s. of alcohol
s., sense of
s. ▸ sense of taste and
Smellie('s)
S. maneuver, Mauriceau-
S. method
S. -Veit maneuver, Mauriceau-
S. -Veit method
smelling
s. amniotic fluid ▸ foul-
s. phlegm ▸ foul-
s., sputum foul
s. ▸ sputum purulent and foul
s. urine ▸ foul-
s. urine from diabetes ▸ sweet
Smeloff
S. cardiac valve prosthesis ▸
   Cutter-
S. -Cutter valve prosthesis
S. heart valve
smile
s., disfigured
s. incision
s. ▸ loss of ability to
Smillie nail
Smith('s)
S. anastomosis ▸ Potts-
S. and Smith regime
S. brace, Lyman-
S. dislocation
S. fracture

S. -Gibson operation, Potts-
S. -Hodge pessary
S., Klein and French (SKF) culture
S. -Kuhnt-Szymanowski operation
S. -Lemli-Opitz syndrome
S. murmur, Eustace
S. operation
S. pessary
S. -Petersen approach
S. -Petersen hip cup prosthesis
S. -Petersen nail
S. -Petersen operation
S. -Petersen osteotomy
S. -Petersen prosthesis
S. sign

Smithwick's operation
SMO prosthesis, Lorenzo
Smoke (smoke)('s)
S. (hashish)
S. (marijuana cigarette)
s. asthma, cigarette
s. ► breathing in tobacco
s. ► environmental cigarette
s. (ETS), environmental tobacco
s. exposure, passive
s. -free environment
s. -free lifestyle
s. -free program
s. -free work site
s. -induced lung injury
s. inhalation
s. inhalation ► patient treated for
s., mainstream
s., passive
s. ► passive tobacco
s., patient
s., pot
s. ► puff of
s., second-hand
s., second-hand tobacco
s., sidestream

smokeable
s. cocaine
s. form
s. form of methamphetamine
s. methamphetamine

smoked
s. cannabis
s. cocaine
s., hashish
s., LSD
s., marijuana
s., mescaline
s., PCP (phencyclidine)
s., peyote

smokeless cigarette
smokeless tobacco
Smoker(s) ('s) (s') (smoker)
S. Anonymous (SA)
s. bronchitis
s., chain
s., chronic
s., cigarette
s., cocaine
s. cough
s. hack
s. heart
s., heavy
s., hypertensive
s., long-term
s. palate
s. patches
s., patient heavy
s. tongue

smoking
s. addiction
s., boozing and sniffing
s. cessation
s. cessation ► short-term
s. cessation therapy
s., cigarette
s. clinic, no
s. clinic, quit
s., cocaine
s., compensatory
s. death
s. during pregnancy ► maternal
s., emphysema secondary to heavy
s. free-base cocaine
s. habit
s. habit, kicking
s., hazards of
s., heroin
s. history
s. history, long
s. -induced angina
s., involuntary
s. of crystal methamphetamine
s. opium
s., passive
s. policy
s. pot
s. ► prenatal effects of
s. redistribution
s. reduction
s. -related disease
s. -related disorders
s. -related problems ► warning signs of
s. restrictions

s., second-hand
s., sidestream
smoldering myeloma
smoldering pneumonia
smooth
s. and glistening ► capsular surface
s. and glistening ► peritoneal surfaces
s. and glistening ► peritoneum
s. and repetitive stroke during massage
s. broach
s. (S) cells
s. (S.) colony
s. contour
s. cortical surfaces
s. endoplasmic reticulum
s., glistening serosa
s. liver edges
s. margin
s., mural endocardium
s. muscle
s. muscle cells
s. muscle cells ► vascular
s. muscle contraction ► vascular
s. muscle layer ► hypertrophic
s. muscle relaxation
s. muscle tone, bronchial
s. muscle ► venous
s. pursuit eye movement (SPEM)
s. tongue
s. walled uterus
smoothing, digital
smoothing technique ► scatterplot
smothering sensation
SMR (sensorimotor rhythm)
SMR (submucous resection)
SMR (submucous resection and rhinoplasty)
smudge cells
Smyth-Roske syndrome, Caffey-
S/N (signal-to-noise) ratio
snaggle tooth
snake
s. graft
s. -tongue sign
s. venom
SNAP (sensory nerve action potential)
snap
s., closing
s. (MOS) ► mitral opening
s., opening
s. packs, chemical
s. ► tricuspid opening

snapping finger
snapping hip
snare(s)
  s., cautery
  s., dissection and
  s. technique
  s. tonsillectomy ▸ dissection and
sneeze(s) [*wheeze, squeeze*]
  s. effect
  s. reflex
  s. reflex ▸ photic
  s., seasonal
  s. syncope
sneezed sputum
sneezing
  s., control itching and
  s. from allergy
  s. from cold
  s., recurrent
Snellen('s)
  S. chart
  S. conventional reform implant
  S. eye
  S. operation
  S. reflex
  S. reform eye
  S. test
Snell's law
sniff test
sniffed
  s. cocaine
  s. glue
  s. ▸ mescaline (Nutmeg)
sniffing
  s. cocaine
  s. death (SSD), sudden
  s., drug
  s., smoking and boozing
sniffling bronchophony
snobbish attitude
snoring, persistent
snoring rales
snorted
  s., cocaine
  s., Ketamine
  s., LSD
  s., mescaline
  s. phencyclidine (PCP)
snorting
  s. cocaine
  s. heroin
  s. lines of cocaine
  s. powder
  s., swallowing, or smoking ▸ drug

Snow (snow)
  S. (cocaine)
  s. ▸ anesthetizing effect of ice and
  s. blindness
  s. glasses
snowflake cataract
snowman abnormality
snowman heart
snowplow effect
snowstorm cataract
snowstorm shadow
SNPs (single nucleotide
  polymorphisms)
snuff box, anatomical
s-o (salpingo-oophorectomy)
s-o (salpingo-oophorectomy),
  bilateral
SO (Surveillance Officer)
soaked
  s. applicator, cocaine
  s. cotton, bolus of saline-
  s. Gelfoam ▸ thrombin
soaks, warm
SOAP (Subjective Objective
  Assessment Plan)
soap
  s., bacteriostatic
  s., Betadine
  s., coal tar
  s., hexachlorophene
Soapers (barbiturates)
soapsuds enema (SSE)
soapy kidney
Soave abdominal pull-through
  procedure
SOB (shortness of breath)
  SOB ▸ exercise induced
  SOB from anxiety
  SOB ▸ palpitations and
  SOB ▸ progressive
sober
  s. leisure skills
  s. patient
  s., sane and
sobria, Aeromonas
sobriety
  s., adjustment to
  s. and abstinence ▸ maintain
  s. and sanity ▸ periods of
  s., coping with
  s., detoxification and
  s., emerging
  s., enable
  s., fluid
  s., maintaining

  s. ▸ values of
  s., white knuckle
sociability, enhanced
social (Social)
  s. abilities ▸ decline in
  s. ability
  s. acceptance
  s. activities ▸ loss of interest in
    peer
  s. activity
  s. activity ▸ increase in
  s. adaptability
  s. adjustment
  S. Adjustment Scale (MSAS) ▸
    Mandel
  s. affliction
  s. aloofness
  S. and Addiction History form ▸
    Diagnostic
  s. and behavioral difficulties
  s. and emotional development
  s. and leisure skills
  s. anxiety
  s. behavior
  s. behavior and drug abuse, anti-
  s. behavior, anti-
  s. behavior, deviant
  s. behavior ▸ inappropriate
  s. beliefs
  s. betrayal
  s. breakdown syndrome
  s. class
  s. complications
  s. comprehension, nonverbal
  s. consciousness, changing
  s. considerations
  s. contact
  s. cues ▸ nonverbal
  s. disapproval
  s. dislocation
  s. drinkers, heavy
  s. drinking, casual
  s. drug
  s. dysfunction
  s. environment
  s. environment, patient's
  s. factors
  s. function ▸ impairment of
  s. functioning
  s. growth
  s. handicap
  s. history
  s. history as a screening device for
    drug abuse
  s. impairment ▸ occupational and

s. inadequacy, feelings of
s. interaction
s. interaction ▸ impaired
s. interpersonal skills
s. intervention
s. isolation
s. issue
s. learning
s. maladjustment
s. medicine
s. norms
s. norms, conforms to
s., occupational, sexual activity ▸ increase in
s. or interpersonal situation
s. pattern
s. personality and drug abuse, anti-
s. phobia
s. play, abnormal
s. play, absent
s. play ▸ absent or abnormal
s. potency
s. pressure
s. problems
s. psychiatry
s. psychology
s. psychology, experimental
s. pursuits
s. -recreational use
s. relationship
s. relationships, decline
s. resources
s. role functioning
s. science
S. Security
s. service intervention
s. services, medical
s. setting detoxification
s. situations ▸ extreme reticence in
s. situations ▸ fear of
s. situations ▸ response to
s. skills
s. skills building
s. skills development
s. skills ▸ group exercises for enhancing
s. skills training
s. stigma
s. stigmatization
s. stress
s. stressors
s. structure, supportive
s. support
s. support ▸ lack of
s. support ▸ low level of

s. support network structure
s. support ▸ seeking
s. tendencies, anti-
s. therapy ▸ psychological, educational and
s. withdrawal
s. withdrawal disorder ▸ sensitivity, shyness,
s. work
s. work, clinical
s. worker
s. worker, clinical
s. worker, psychiatric
socialized medicine
socializing, indiscriminate
socially
s. acceptable channels
s. debilitated
s. defined behavioral normalcy
s. disabled
s. disturbed
s. inappropriate behavior
s. incompetent
s. inept
s. isolated
s. maladroit
s. withdrawn
s. withdrawn ▸ patient
societal barrier
society (Society)
s. ▸ apathy and lack of interest in
S. of Addiction Medicine ▸ American
S. for Laser Medicine and Surgery (ASLMS) ▸ American
s. toward drug abusers ▸ attitudes of
sociocultural considerations
sociocultural environment
socioeconomic
s. status
s. stress
s. subcultures
socioemotional development
sociological phenomenon (ISP) ▸ interesting
sociopathic personality
sock(s)
s. array
s., knee high
s., TED (thromboembolic disease)
s., thigh high
socket
s., alveolar
s., bony
s., dry

s., eye
s., inflamed
s. inflammation ▸ eye
s. ▸ inflammation of tooth
s., joint
s. joint ▸ ball-and-
s., molar
s. prosthesis ▸ ball-and-
s., tooth
s. ▸ tooth extraction dry
s. ▸ tooth reimplanted in
SOD (superoxide dismutase)
soda
s., bicarbonate of
s., chlorinated
s. cum calce
s. headache
s. lime
s., washing
sodium (Na)
s., aminosalicylate
s. and water content, total
s. (Na) atom
s. bicarbonate
s., brequinar
s., cefazolin
s., cefmetazole
s., cefoxitin
s., cephalothin
s. channel
s. chloride
s. concentration, plasma
s. content, natural
s. contrast medium, acetrizoate
s. contrast medium, diatrizoate
s. contrast medium, Hypaque
s. contrast medium, iodophthalein
s. contrast medium, metrizoate
s. contrast medium, oragrafin
s. controlled diet
s. current, fast
s. diatrizoate contrast medium
s., dicloxacillin
s. diet, low
s., dietary
s. excretion, urinary
s., high potassium diet ▸ low
s. in urine, over-excretion of
s. intake
s. intake, low
s. intake, reduce
s. iodide (I_{123}, I_{125}, I_{131})
s. iodipamide
s. iodipamide contrast medium
s. iodohippurate (I_{131})

sodium (Na)—*continued*
s. iodohippurate contrast medium
s. iodomethamate
s. iodomethamate contrast medium
s. ion
s. iothalamate (I_{125})
s. iothalamate contrast medium
s. ipodate
s. ipodate contrast medium
s. kit, Tc (technetium) 99m etidronate
s. kit, Tc (technetium) 99m medronate
s. kit, Tc (technetium) 99m penetate
s., limit
s. load
s., mercaptomerin
s., methicillin
s. methiodal
s. methiodal contrast medium
s. morrhuate
s., nafcillin
s. nitrite
s. nitroprusside
s., Oragrafin
s., oxacillin
s. oxalate
s. penicillin G
s. pentobarbital
s. Pentothal
s. Pentothal anesthesia
s., pertechnetate
s. pertechnetate Tc 99m
s. phosphate P 32
s. polyanethole sulfonate (SPS)
s. potassium exchange
s. powder and liquid ▸ Hypaque
s., pravastatin
s. radioiodide
s. restricted diet
s. restricted diet, mild
s. restricted diet, moderate
s. restricted diet, strict
s. restriction
s. retention
s. rose bengal (I_{131})
s. sensitivity
s., serum
s. succinate ▸ methylprednisolone
s. syndrome ▸ low
s. test
s., thiamylal
s. thiopental
s., thiopentone

s. thorium tartrate contrast medium
s. tyropanoate contrast medium
s., warfarin
s., Yb (ytterbium) penetate
Soemmering('s)
S. area
S., arterial vein of
S. crystalline swelling
S., external radial vein of
S. gray substance
S. ring
S. ring cataract
S. spot
Soens approach
Sofield's operation
Soflens contact lens
soft
s., abdomen
s. and pliable, vagina
s. and ribbon-like stools
s. blowing diastolic murmur
s. cancer
s. cartilage
s. cataract
s. cervical collar
s. connective tissue, myxomatous
s. contact lenses
s. dental diet
s. diet
s. diet, mechanical
s. diet, surgical
s. disposable contact lenses
s. drugs
s. event
s. exudates
s. fleshy lesion
s. fleshy nodule
s. fluctuant nodular lesions
s. fold
s. foldable artificial lens
s. lens
s. lens ▸ daily-wear
s. lens, extended wear
s. mechanical diet
s., neck
s., nonmovable node ▸ tender,
s. oral tissues
s. palate
s. palate, pillars of
s. palates ▸ hard and
s. part sarcoma, alveolar
s. pulse
s. rays
s. soled shoe
s., spongy, semi-liquid tissue

s. spots
s. strategy
s. structure injury
s. tail of pancreas
s. ticks
s. tissue cancer
soft tissue
s.t. abscess
s.t. aging ▸ musculoskeletal
s.t. augmentation
s.t., benign lesion of
s.t. calcification
s.t. carcinoma
s.t. compression injury
s.t. damage
s.t. density, abdominal
s.t. ecchymosis
s.t., elastic
s.t. FB (foreign body)
s.t., fibrosarcoma of
s.t. hematoma
s.t. hemorrhage
s.t. hemorrhage into mesentery
s.t. hemorrhage ▸ recent
s.t., histiocytoma of
s.t. infection
s.t. injury
s.t. invasion
s.t. involvement
s.t. laceration
s.t. layers
s.t., leiomyosarcoma of
s.t., liposarcoma of
s.t. loss
s.t. mass
s.t. massage
s.t. metastases
s.t. muscle pain
s.t. of face
s.t., periarticular
s.t., periorbital
s.t., rhabdomyosarcoma of
s.t. rheumatism
s.t. roentgenography
s.t. sarcoma
s.t. shadow
s.t. swelling
s.t. tumor
softener, stool
softening
s. and swelling of cartilage
s., anemic
s., colliquative
s., diffuse hepatic
s., diffuse parenchymal

s., gray
s., green
s., hemorrhagic
s., inflammatory
s., mucoid
s. of brain
s. of the stomach
s., pyriform
s., red
s., white
s., yellow
Softgut suture
soilage, fecal
solanoid cancer
solanoid carcinoma
Solanum carolinense
Solanum tuberosum
solar
s. cautery
s. cheilitis
s. cheilitis, acute
s. elastosis
s. keratosis
s. plexus
s. radiation
s. retinitis
solaris, urticaria
Solcotrans autotransfusion unit
soldering flux
soldering fumes
soldier's heart
soldiers' patches
Sole(s) (sole)
S. (hashish)
s., convex
s., dropped
s., erythematous macules of palms and
s. ▸ hyperkeratosis of
s. ▸ hyperpigmented macules on heel and
s., quadrate muscle of
s. reflex
s. stroking
s. wedge
soled shoe, soft
Solenopsis geminata
Solenopsis saevissima richteri
soleus muscle
Solid(s) (solid)
S. (hashish)
s. angle concept
s. appearing mass
s. bone mass
s. bony union

s. chromatography, gas-
s. cysts
s. ▸ gastric emptying of
s. material ▸ abnormal sac containing semi◊
s. organ donation
s. organ graft
s. organ transplant
s. organs
s. silicone orbital prosthesis
s. state electronic behavior
s. state laser utilizing ruby
s. state physics
s. stool
s. (TS) ▸ total
s. tumor
s. tumor cancer
s. vision
s. waste
Solidago virgaurea
solis, ictus
solitary
s. aggressive type ▸ conduct disorder,
s. coronary ostium
s. focus
s. lesion
s. lymphatic nodules of large intestine
s. lymphatic nodules of small intestine
s. nodule
s. pulmonary arteriovenous fistula
s. pulmonary metastasis
s. pulmonary nodule
s. pyramidal cells
solitus, situs
solium larvae ▸ Taenia
solium, Taenia
sollicitans, Aedes
solubility, fat
solubility test, bile
soluble
s. dietary fiber
s. drugs, fat
s. dye, water
s. insulin
s. ligature
s. nitrogen, alkali-
s. ribonucleic acid (RNA)
s. substance, specific
s. vitamin, fat
s. vitamin, water
s., water-
solute, total body

solution(s)
s., aerosol saline
s., antiseptic
s., balanced salt
s. based therapy ▸ individual
s., bath
s. behavior change
s., Bouin's
s., Brompton's
s., buffered saline
s., Burow's
s., cardioplegic
s., collodion
s., colloid replacement
s., contamination from irrigating
s., crystalloid cardioplegic
s., Dakin's
s., disinfecting
s., enzyme
s., Epsom salt
s. focused group therapy
s., Fowler's
s., Harrington's
s., Holland's
s., hundredth-normal
s., hyperalimentation
s., hypertonic
s., infusing
s. infusion, heparinized
s., inhalation
s., iodophor
s., lactated Ringer's
s. line, main
s., Lugol's
s., Magendie's
s. mixture, dextrose
s., molal
s., Monzel
s., nebulized
s., normal dialysis
s., normal saline (N/S)
s., Nylmerate douche
s. of potassium iodide (SSKI), saturated
s., peritoneal dialysis
s., physiological saline
s., Plasmolyte
s., povidone-iodine
s., prepackaged irrigating
s., priming
s., priming of infusing
s., quaternary-amine type product/
s., rehydration
s., Ringer's lactate
s., saline

solution(s)—*continued*
- s., salt water
- s., saturated
- s., Skiodan
- s., sterile ophthalmic
- s., sterile saline
- s., stroma-free hemoglobin
- s., test
- s., volumetric
- s., white cells taken off top of
- s., wound irrigated with saline
- s., Zenker's
- s., Zephiran

Solvang graft

solving
- s. ability ‣ problem-
- s. capacity ‣ problem-
- s., critical problem
- s., daily problem
- s. devices, problem-
- s. mentality ‣ problem-
- s. skills, problem-
- s. skills training ‣ problem-
- s. therapy ‣ problem-

SOM (serrous otitis media)
Somagyi's reflex
somaliensis, Streptomyces
somatic
- s. aberration theory
- s. agglutinin
- s. alteration, psychotherapy by
- s. cells
- s. center
- s. coil
- s. complaints
- s. conversion
- s. correlates
- s. death
- s. delusion
- s. disturbance
- s. effect ‣ peripheral
- s. induction
- s. mechanism
- s. medicine
- s. motor component
- s. muscles
- s. mutations
- s. nerves
- s. nervous system
- s. reaction
- s. sarcoma
- s. sensation, altered
- s. sensory component
- s. sensory cortex
- s. stigma

- s. support ‣ psychologic, emotional,
- s. therapy
- s. treatment

somatization disorder
somatization reactions
somatoform
- s. disorder
- s. disorder, undifferentiated
- s. pain
- s. pain disorder

somatointestinal reflex
somatomammotropin, human
somatomammotropin, human chorionic
somatomedin levels
somatosensory
- s. area
- s. cortex
- s. evoked potentials (SEP or SSEP)
- s. evoked response (SER)
- s. evoked response (SER), short latency
- s. perceptions, enhanced
- s. receptor
- s. symptoms
- s. system

somatotropic hormone
somatotropin deficiency
somatotropin releasing factor
somatrophic adenoma
some appreciable change
somesthetic sensibility
somite embryo
sommeil, tic de
Sommer-Foegella method
somnambulism disorder
somnambulism or night terrors
somnolence, episodes of
somnolence, excessive daytime
somnolent
- s. and lethargic
- s., lethargic and weak
- s. metabolic rate

somnolentium, coma
Somogyi
- S. effect
- S. test
- S. unit

son of alcoholic parents
sonar, abdominal
sonarography, pelvic ultrasound
Sondergaard procedure
Sondergaard's cleft

S1 heart sound
S1 projection, L5
Sones catheter
sonic
- s. appearance, abnormal
- s. applicator
- s. imaging techniques
- s., ultra◊
- s. waves

sonication technique
Sonne dysentery
Sonneberg's operation
Sonne-Duval bacillus
sonnei, Bacterium
sonnei, Shigella
sonoencephalogram study
sonogram, cardiac
sonogram of heart
sonographic
- s. assessment
- s. criteria
- s. findings

sonography
- s., endovaginal
- s. of subfascial hematoma
- s. of uterus
- s., serial
- s. technique
- s., transabdominal
- s., transvaginal
- s., ultra◊

sonolucent area
sonolucent mass
sonometer, bone
sonorous
- s. breathing
- s. noise
- s. rales
- s. respiration
- s. rhonchi

sonotomy, ultra◊
Sonulator, Medical
soot cancer
Sopes (barbiturates)
sophistication, psychological
sopor (depressant)
soporific drug
sorbens, Musca
sorbitol dehydrogenase
sordellii, Clostridium
sordellii, gram-positive Clostridium
sordida, Trypanosoma
sore(s)
- s., bed
- s., bleeding

s. ▸ blister from cold
s. ▸ burning mouth from cold
s. calf muscle
s., canker
s., chancre
s., cold
s., denture
s. elbows
s., eyelid
s. ▸ festering skin
s. from anxiety ▸ canker
s. from chocolate ▸ cold
s., gaping
s. ▸ gaping, draining
s., genital
s. joint
s. lesion
s., mouth
s. mouth, Ceylon
s. on ear
s., open
s., open genital
s., persistent nonhealing open
s., pressure
s. ▸ recurring mouth
s., skin
s. ▸ slow healing
s. throat
s. throat from cancer
s. throat from chlamydia
s. throat ▸ itchy, scratchy
s. throat ▸ pain in ear from
s. throat, septic
s. throat, streptococcal
s., tongue
s., tropical
s., weeping
soreness
s., breast
s., delayed onset muscle
s. level
s., muscle
s. of tongue
s. ▸ rectal pain and
s. ▸ stiffness and
Soria's operation
Sorin mitral valve prosthesis
sorter, cell
sorter, dish
Sorting Test, Color-Form
sorting test, object
Soto-Hall sign
Sottas atrophy, Déjerine-
souffle
s., cardiac

s., fetal
s., funic
s., funicular
s. murmur ▸ mammary
s., placental
s. sound ▸ mammary
s., splenic
s., umbilical
s., uterine
soufflet, bruit de
soul pain
Soulier disease, Bernard-
sound(s)
s., abnormal
s., abnormal lung
s., absent breath
s. (A2) accentuated ▸ aortic second
s., active bowel
s., acute sensitivity to
s., adventitious
s., adventitious breath
s., amplification
s., aortic
s., aortic closure
s. (A2) ▸ aortic second
s., atrial
s., audible
s., auditory perception of speech
s., auscultatory
s., bandbox
s., Beatty-Bright friction
s., bell
s., bellows
s., blowing
s., bowel
s., breath
s., bronchovesicular
s., bronchovesicular breath
s., Cannon's
s., cardiac
s., characteristic wheezing
s., clicking
s., coarse breath
s., coin
s. -conducting
s., cracked-pot
s., crowing breath
s., crunching
s., decreased bowel
s., decreased breath
s. device, Doppler
s., diminished breath
s. ▸ distant breath
s., distant heart
s., double shock

s., dry crackling
s., eddy
s., ejection
s., enhance
s., esophageal
s., expiratory
s., extra
s., extra heart
s. (FHS), fetal heart
s., first heart
s. (M1) ▸ first mitral
s., flapping
s., fourth heart
s., friction
s., gallop
s., Gerhardt's change of
s., good breath
s. ▸ gradual distortion of
s., grating
s. guided into bladder
s., guttural
s., heart
s., heightened sensitivity to
s. ▸ high pitched
s., hippocratic
s., homogenous
s., hyperactive bowel
s., hypoactive bowel
s. in ears, ringing
s. in lungs, crackling
s. in lungs ▸ rattling
s., inspiratory
s. keying
s., Korotkoff's
s., lacrimal
s., LeFort urethral
s. level
s. ▸ mammary souffle
s., measure
s. medical practice
s., metallic
s. ▸ metallic breath
s., mitral
s. (M1) ▸ mitral first
s. (M2) ▸ mitral second
s. ▸ muffled heart
s., muscle
s., normal bowel
s. normal, cardiac
s., pacemaker
s. ▸ paradoxically split (S2)
s., passage of
s., percussion
s. ▸ pericardial friction
s., peristaltic

sound(s)—*continued*
s., physiological
s. ▸ physiological third heart
s. ▸ pistol-shot femoral
s., positive bowel
s. pressure level (SPL)
s. -proof tank
s., puffing
s., pulmonic
s. ▸ pulmonic closure
s. (P2) ▸ pulmonic second
s. ▸ pulmonic valve closure
s. ▸ quiet breath
s. ▸ quiet heart
s. receptor
s., respiratory
s. ▸ response to
s., ringing
s. ▸ rubbing heart
s., sail
s., second
s. (A2) ▸ second aortic
s., second heart
s. (M2) ▸ second mitral
s., second pulmonic (P2)
s. -sensing cells
s., sensitivity to light and
s., shaking
s., slipping
s., slushing
s. (M2) split ▸ mitral second
s. (P2) split ▸ pulmonic second
s., splitting of heart
s. ▸ squeaky leather
s. stimulation, repetitive
s. stimuli
s. stimuli, sensory
s., subjective
s., succussion
s., tambour
s., third heart
s., tick-tack
s., to-and-fro
s., to-and-fro friction
s., tracheal
s. training
s. ▸ tricuspid valve closure
s. ▸ tubular breath
s. ▸ tumor plop
s., tympanitic
s., ultra◊
s., urethral
s., uterine
s. vacuum
s., vesicular breath

s., waterwheel
s. wave cycle
s. wave techniques
s. wave technology
s. wave vibrations
s. waves
s. waves, high frequency
s. waves ▸ inaudible
s. waves, reflection of
s. waves, shift in frequency of
s. waves, transmit
s., whooshing
s. ▸ xiphisternal crunching
sounded
s., endometrial cavity
s. to depth of _____
s. to depth of _____ ▸ uterine cavity
s., uterine cavity
s., uterus
sounding, urethral
soup lines
soup stool, pea
soupy cytoplasm, cell's
soupy material
sour taste in mouth, bitter
source(s)
s. amnesia
s., applicator and
s., artificial
s., cesium
s., collateral
s. confusion
s., contamination of exogenous
s. distance
s., donor
s., extracerebral
s., fiberoptic cold light
s., fiberoptic light
s., high intensity light
s. imaging (MSI) ▸ magnetic
s., implanting radioactive
s., intracavitary radiation
s., linear
s. localization
s. of acquired torsades de pointes
s. of anxiety
s. of anxiety ▸ confront
s. of bacterial infection
s. of bleeding ▸ possible
s. of contamination
s. of contamination, eliminate
s. of infection, determine
s. of infection, exogenous
s. of infection, potential

s. of intraperitoneal bleeding
s. of potential change
s. of spread
s. of transmission
s., organ
s. penetrability
s. physics
s., primary
s., primary power
s., radiation
s., referral
s. self-attenuation
s. specifications
s. to skin distance (SSD)
s. unknown, primary
Sourdille's operation
South African tick fever
South African tick typhus
South American
S.A. blastomycosis
S.A. hemorrhagic fever
S.A. Junin virus
Southeast Asian mosquito-borne
Southern blot analysis
Southern transfer analysis
Southwick osteotomy
Souttar's cautery
Soviet gramicidin
soy milk
soy milk, corn-
soybean agglutinin
sp (spike)
SP (systolic pressure)
Sp gr (specific gravity)
spa ▸ holistic health
space(s) [*base*]
s. abscess ▸ premasseteric
s., air
s., alveolar
s., alveolar air
s., alveolar dead
s., anatomical dead
s., antecubital
s., arachnoid
s., basal subarachnoid
s., Broca's
s., chest
s. consolidation, air
s., corneal
s., costoclavicular
s., Czermak's
s., dead
s., disc
s. disease, air-
s. disease, diffuse air

s. ▸ disorientation of time and
s. ▸ distortion of time and
s., drainage (dr'ge) of cerebral epidural
s., drainage (dr'ge) of subarachnoid
s., drainage (dr'ge) of subdural
s. ▸ echo-free
s., enlarged subarachnoid
s. entered, retroperitoneal
s., epidural
s., extracellular
s., extrapleural
s. (ICS) ▸ fifth intercostal
s., Fontana's
s., Forel's
s., H
s. ▸ His perivascular
s., Holzknecht's
s. ▸ hyaline membranes lining alveolar
s., intercellular
s., intercellular tissue
s. (ICS) ▸ intercostal
s., interpedicular
s., interpedicular joint
s., interpleural
s., interproximal
s., interstitial
s., intervertebral disc
s., intraparenchymal air
s., intrathecal
s., intravascular
s., intravesical
s., joint
s., Larrey
s., lumbar
s., lumbar subarachnoid
s., Magendie's
s., marrow
s., masseteric
s., mediastinal
s. medicine
s. ▸ narrowed disc
s., narrowing of disc
s., narrowing of intervertebral disc
s., narrowing of joint
s. occupying change
s. occupying lesion
s. of Burns
s. of His
s. of Retzius abscess
s., palmar
s., Paron's
s. perceptual disturbances, color and

s., pericardial
s., peripheral air
s., perirenal
s., periscleral
s., peritoneal
s., perivascular
s., perivascular lymph
s. ▸ physiological dead
s., pleural
s., pneumatic
s. (PMI 5th ICS) ▸ point of maximum impulse fifth intercostal
s., popliteal
s., poststyloid
s., preperitoneal
s., prestyloid
s., prevertebral
s., prevesical
s., proximal
s., Prussak's
s., puncture of subarachnoid
s., retrocardiac
s., retrolental
s., retroperitoneal
s., retropharyngeal
s., retrosternal free
s., retrotracheal
s., rudimentary disc
s., Schwalb's
s. segmentation ▸ k-
s. ▸ sensation of altered orientation in
s. sense
s., subarachnoid
s., subdural
s., subphrenic
s., subpleural air
s. syndrome, retroparotid
s., Tenon's
s., thenar
s., time and persons ▸ patient alert to
s., tissue
s., translucent
s., Traube's semilunar
s. ventilation, dead
s., vitreous
s., web
s., Westberg
s., wide intervertebral
s., Zang's
s., zonular

spaced
s. electrodes, closely

s. out ▸ feeling
s. out, patient
SpaceLabs
S. Event Master
S. Holter monitor
S. pulse oximeter
spacial
s. orientation or perception
s. -perceptual data
s. relation
s. relationship
spacing between pairs of electrodes
spade(s)
s. hand
s. -like configuration
s. sign, ace of
Spaeth's operation
spagyric medicine
SPAI (steroid protein activity index)
Spalding-Richardson operation
Spalding's sign
span (Span)
s., attention
S., Digit
s., expected life
s. from anxiety ▸ shortened attention
s. in grief, attention
s. ▸ increased attention
s., life
s., limited attention
s., long attention
s. ▸ low attention
s. (MLS) ▸ mean life
s. ▸ poor attention
s., short attention
s., shortened from anxiety ▸ attention
Spanish
S. flu
S. patient
S. trots
Spanlang-Tappeiner syndrome
spared area, echo
sparing
s. agent ▸ steroid
s. diuretic ▸ potassium-
s. mastectomy ▸ skin
s., myocardial
s. stress test ▸ leg
s. surgery ▸ nerve
spark
s. chamber
s. erosion
s. x-rays

sparse infiltration of extramedullary hematopoietic cells
sparsity of bone formation
spasm(s)
s. ▸ abnormal uterine
s. and cramps ▸ muscle
s. and prolapse ▸ coronary
s. and twitches ▸ muscle
s., arterial
s., athetoid
s., back
s., Bell's
s., bladder
s., bronchial
s. ▸ bronchial constriction and
s., bronchopulmonary
s., cadaveric
s., cardiac
s., carpal
s., carpopedal
s., catheter induced
s., catheter-related peripheral
   vessel
s., catheter-tip
s., cecal
s., cerebral
s., cervical muscle
s., chest wall
s., choke
s., chronic
s., chronic muscular
s., clonic
s., colon
s., compulsive
s., coronary artery
s., coughing
s., diffuse esophageal
s., dystonic
s. ▸ ergonovine-induced
s., esophageal
s., facial
s., fatal cardiac
s., fixed
s., frequent
s., functional
s., gastrointestinal (GI)
s., glottic
s., hemifacial
s. in walls of intestines
s. induction, coronary
s., infantile
s., inspiratory
s., intention
s. ▸ intermittent continuous
s., intestinal

s. ▸ involuntary muscle
s. ▸ irregular esophageal
s., laryngeal
s., laryngo◊
s., leg
s., massive
s., mixed
s., muscle
s. ▸ muscle cramps and
s., muscular
s., nodding
s., nosecone
s., occupational muscle
s. of airway muscles ▸
   spontaneous
s. of anxiety
s. of arteries of brain
s. of artery ▸ angina from
s. of bladder
s. of blood vessel ▸ severe
s. of blood vessels
s. of blood vessels ▸ constriction or
s. of bronchial tubes
s. of coronary arteries
s. of diaphragm, involuntary
s. of esophagus
s. of external sphincter
s. of eyelid
s. of eyes ▸ muscle
s. of intestinal wall
s. of muscles, pain and
s. of voluntary muscles, clonic
s. of voluntary muscles, tonic
s. one side of neck
s. or rigidity ▸ tenderness,
s., painful
s., painful contractive
s., painful muscle
s., painless
s., paraspinal muscle
s., paroxysmal coughing
s., progressive torsion
s., protective
s., rectal sphincter muscle
s., relieve muscle
s., respiratory
s., rigidity or tenderness
s., rotatory
s., severe
s. ▸ severe back muscle
s., severe muscle
s., sphincter of Oddi
s., stomach
s., sudden torsion
s., synclonic

s., terminal laryngeal
s., tetanic
s., tonic
s., tonoclonic
s., torsion
s., toxic
s. ▸ twitching, grimacing, and
s. ▸ uncontrollable muscle
s., vascular
s., vasovagal
s., venous
s., vessel
s., winking
s., writers'
spasmodic
s. asthma
s. athetoid movements, periodic
s. blinking or squinting ▸
   involuntary
s. contractions
s. croup
s. diathesis
s. dysmenorrhea
s. dysphonia
s. dysphonia, abductor
s. dysphonia, adductor
s., involuntary movements ▸
   irregular,
s. movements
s. muscular contraction
s. rigidity
s. strabismus
s. stricture
s. synkinesis
s. tabes
s. talipes
s. tic
s. torticollis
spasmodica ▸ dysarthria syllabaris
spasmophilic diathesis
spastic
s. abasia
s. amaurotic axonal idiocy
s. angina, coronary
s. aphonia
s. bladder
s. blood vessel
s. bowel syndrome
s. colon
s. colon syndrome
s. constipation
s. contraction
s. diplegia
s. dysphonia
s. dysuria

s. ectropion lower lid
s. entropion
s. flatfoot
s. gait
s. hemiplegia
s. ileus
s. limbs
s. miosis
s. mucosal pattern
s. muscle activity
s. muscles
s. musculature
s. paralysis
s. paraparesis (TSP) ▸ tropical
s. paraplegia
s. quadriplegia
s. rigidity
s. stricture
s. subjects, neuromuscular firing in
s. torticollis
spastica, cholepathia
spastica, dysphagia
spasticity
s., colon
s., counteract
s., effect of emotional stress on
s., inhibit flexor
s., intestinal
s., muscle
s. of arm
s. of extremity
s. of hips, adductor
s. of leg
s., patient exhibits
s., reduced
s., relax
s., treatment of
s. treatment ▸ tone and
s. with shoulder movement
spasticum, ectropion
spatial
s. ability
s. ability test ▸ visual
s. cooperation in combined
    modality therapy
s. deficits
s. dimension
s. disorientation
s. dose distribution
s. dyslexia
s. intensity
s. memory
s. orientation
s. perception
s. sense

s. skills and attention
s. skills ▸ visual
s. relation
s. relationships
s. resolution
s. skills
s. tracking
s. vector
s. vectorcardiogram
s. vectorcardiogram study
s. vectorcardiography
s. vision system
s. -visual constructional task
s. words
spatially oriented behavior
spatially separated foci
Spatz syndrome, Hallervorden-
Spaulding-Richardson hysterectomy
SPBI (serum protein-bound iodine)
SPCA (serum prothrombin
    conversion accelerator)
speak(s)
s. ▸ difficulty or inability to
s. in rapid monotone
s. in staccato rhythm
s., inability to
s., loss of ability to
s., refusal to
speaking
s. ▸ pain on
s. valve ▸ Provox
s. valve ▸ Shiley Phonate
Speas' operation
Special (special)
S. Care Nursery (SCN)
S. Care Unit (ISCU) ▸ Infant
s. cushions
s. education
s. effects of drugs
s. electrode
s. handicaps
s. hosiery
S. K (Ketamine)
s. living arrangements
s. needs
s. purpose lens
s. rehabilitation products
s. sense
s. sense, organs of
s. skills training
s. teaching issues
s. wound care
specialist
s., cancer
s., clinical

s., clinical nurse
s., colorectal
s., drug treatment
s., exercise
s., fertility
s., health care
s., motivational
s., nurse
s., oral biology
s., pain
s., pain management
s. ▸ pediatric emergency medicine
s. preventive medicine
specialized
s. AIDS (acquired immune
    deficiency syndrome) home care
    programs
s. cells of retina
s. counseling
s. equipment
s. exercise program
s. nursing care
s. technique
s. ward
specially gifted child
specialties, treatment
specialty(-ies)
s. care nurse
s. hospital
s. inpatient service
s. mental health care
s. services
species
s., Acinetobacter
s., bacterial
s., Capnophagia
s., Citrobacter
s., clostridial
s., Clostridium
s., Enterobacter
s., gram-negative
s., gram-positive
s. immunity
s., Klebsiella
s., Mycobacterium
s., Neisserian
s., nontuberculous
s., pathogenic
s., Plasmodium
s., Proteus
s., Salmonella
s. ▸ saprophytic leptospirosis
s., Serratia
s., Shigella
s. specificity

specific
- s. activity
- s. activity, blood granulocyte
- s. activity, relative
- s. activity, thyroxine
- s. antigen ▸ organ
- s. antigen (PSA) ▸ prostate
- s. antigen ▸ tissue
- s. areas of body ▸ tender points
- s. arrhythmias
- s. behavior
- s. brain waves, suppression of seizure
- s. capsular substance
- s. cause
- s. compensatory mechanism ▸ activating
- s. component, group-
- s. delay
- s. delays in development
- s. developmental disorder
- s. drug analysis
- s. drugs, intolerance to
- s. endarteritis, Heubner's
- s. etiologic diagnosis
- s. febrile delirium
- s. findings
- s. foods, intolerance to
- s. function
- s. gamma ray constant
- s. gravity
- s. gravity, decreased
- s. gravity test
- s., group-
- s. heat
- s. immunity
- s. isolation precautions
- s. lag
- s. loss of consciousness
- s. lymphocyte transformation ▸ antigen
- s. membrane antigen (PSMA) ▸ prostate
- s. modalities
- s. parasite
- s. pathogen free (SPF)
- s. seizure wave electroencephalogram (EEG) activity ▸ suppress
- s. soluble substance
- s., strain-
- s. strain of bacteria
- s. strategies, relapse-
- s. substances ▸ blood grouping
- s. symptoms, list

- s. tenderness
- s. therapy
- s. to adolescence ▸ disturbance of emotions
- s. to childhood ▸ disturbance of emotions
- s. to childhood ▸ psychoses with origin
- s. transfusion (DST) ▸ donor
- s. transplantation antigen, tumor
- s. treatment programs ▸ gender-
- s. urethritis specifications, source

specificity(-ies)
- s., analytic
- s., relative
- s., species

specified family circumstances ▸ other

specimen(s)
- s. acellular
- s., biohazard
- s., biopsy
- s., catheterized
- s., clean-voided
- s., clinical
- s. collection
- s., concentrated
- s., cone
- s., culture of
- s., diseased tissue
- s., formalin fixed
- s., gram stain of stool
- s., initial urine
- s., nasopharyngeal
- s. of urine, catheterized
- s., pathological
- s., potentially infectious blood
- s., random
- s. ▸ routinely drawn blood
- s. sent to lab, tissue
- s., slide
- s., sputum
- s., sterile
- s., stool
- s. submitted for biopsy
- s. submitted for frozen section
- s. submitted for microsection
- s., test
- s., tissue
- s., urine
- s., voided

speciosa, Macaca
specked phlegm, blood
speckle, laser
speckled breast calcifications

speckled pattern, scintillating
specks in vision
SPECT (single photon emission computed tomography)
- SPECT scan
- SPECT scintigraphy
- SPECT scintigraphy ▸ thallium-201

spectacles, Masselon's
spectography ▸ magnetic resonance
spectography, Raman
spectral
- s. analysis
- s. analysis, Doppler
- s. array, compressed
- s. distribution curve for radiation
- s. envelope
- s. flow velocity ▸ translesional
- s. leakage
- s. peak velocity ▸ instantaneous
- s. phonocardiograph
- s. phonocardiography
- s. power
- s. temporal mapping
- s. turbulence mapping
- s. waveform

SpecTrax programmable Medtronic pacemaker
spectrometer
- s., beta-ray
- s., gamma-ray
- s., mass
- s., MRI (magnetic resonance imaging)

spectrometry, pulse height
spectrophotometer, absorption
spectrophotometry, infrared
spectroscopy
- s. -directed laser
- s. ▸ electron paramagnetic resonance
- s. ▸ flame emission
- s., fluorescence
- s. imaging (MRSI) ▸ magnetic resonance
- s., magnetic resonance
- s. ▸ near-infrared
- s., proton
- s., Raman

spectrum (spectra)
- s., absorption
- s., antibiotic, broad
- s., atomic
- s., bacterial
- s. behavioral treatment, broad
- s., broad

s., chromatic
s. disorder, autistic
s. disorder ▸ obsessive-compulsive
s. disorders ▸ schizophrenic
s., electroencephalogram (EEG) frequency
s., electromagnetic
s., frequency
s., gamma-ray
s., histological
s., microbicidal
s., normal
s. of cancer, clinical
s. of color
s. penicillins, extended-
s., pulse-height
s., thermal
s. thesis
s., x-ray

specular
s. echo
s. microscopy
s. writing

Spee, curve of

speech
s., absence of
s., alaryngeal
s., altered
s. and hearing impairment
s. and language disorders
s. and language impaired
s. and language pathologist
s. and language within normal limits
s. and swallowing ▸ difficulty with
s., appropriateness of
s. area
s. arrest
s. audiometry
s. center
s. center, auditory
s. center in brain
s. center, motor
s., chronic slurred
s., clipped
s., confused or impoverished thought and
s. defect
s. delay
s., delayed
s., delayed development of
s., delayed or impaired
s., deterioration in
s. ▸ deterioration of coordination, gait and

s. development
s. difficulties, emotional
s. difficulty
s. disabilities
s. discrimination (SD)
s. discrimination (SD) test
s. disorder
s. disorder, developmental
s., disturbance of
s., echo
s. echolalic
s., esophageal
s. evaluation
s. excessively impressionistic
s. ▸ exhibits nonsensical
s., explosive
s., eyes open to
s. frequencies
s., garbled
s., halting
s., impaired
s., impaired and difficult
s. impaired, child
s. impaired individual
s. impairment
s. impediment
s., impressionistic
s., incoherent
s., incomprehensible
s., intelligible
s., jargon
s., jumbled
s. lacking in detail
s., loss of
s. ▸ mechanical patterns of
s., mirror
s., motor
s. muscle activity, feedback of
s., nasal
s. ▸ neuromuscular development of
s., obsessional
s. oriented
s., overly impressionistic
s., palialic
s. pathologist
s. pathology
s. pathology service
s. patient has scanning
s. patient perseverates in
s. pattern, tangential
s., patterns
s., perception of
s. perseverative
s. phrase length
s., plateau

s., postlaryngectomy
s., pressured
s. problem ▸ stroke produces
s. processor
s. range
s., rapid
s. ▸ rapid and chaotic thinking and
s. reading
s. reception
s. reception test
s. reception threshold (SRT)
s. rehabilitation
s., repetitive
s. ▸ robotic patterns of
s., scamping
s., scanning
s. skills
s. ▸ slow and unsteady
s., slowed
s., slurred
s. ▸ slurred, indistinct
s. sounds, auditory perception of
s., spontaneous
s., staccato
s. ▸ sudden slurred
s. testing
s. therapist
s. therapy
s., thickening of
s. understanding
s. understanding assessment
s. vague
s. well articulated

Speed (speed)
S. (amphetamines)
s. (Crank) (methamphetamine)
s. (Crystal) (methamphetamine)
s. addiction
S. and Boyd reduction technique
S. -Boyd operation
s. drill, high-
s. engine, high-
S. (amphetamines) ingested
S. (amphetamines) injected
s. mechanism ▸ wave
S. operation, Kellog-
s., paper
S. radius cap prosthesis
s. rotational angioplasty ▸ low
s. rotational atherectomy ▸ high-
s. test ▸ motor
s. volumetric imaging ▸ high

Spee's embryo

spell(s)
s., blackout

spell(s)—*continued*
s., brief quivering
s., crying
s., dizzy
s., episodic coughing
s., fainting
s. ▸ near-fainting
s. of decreased consciousness
s. of Tumarkin, falling
s., presyncopal
s. ▸ repeated fainting
s., syncopal
s., tetrad
Spelunker's Crisis
SPEM (smooth pursuit eye movement)
Spemann's induction
Spence, tail of
spencerii, Aedes
Spencer-Watson operation
Spenco R analysis
spending sprees ▸ extravagant
sperm
s., abnormal
s. agglutinating antibodies
s. allergy problems
s. cell
s. count
s. -count evaluation
s. -count, low
s., deficient
s. duct, blocked
s., flow of
s., healthy motile
s., herring
s., incubated
s., live
s. motility
s., muzzled
s. output
s., pinheaded
s. production, enhance
s. production, normal
s., transport
s. washing
spermatic
s. artery
s. calculus
s. cord
s. fascia, external
s. fascia, internal
s. nerve, external
s. plexus
s. vein
s. vesicle

s. vessel, internal
spermatogenesis, active
spermatogenesis, ovulation and
spermatogenic
s. cells
s. epididymitis
s. granulomatous orchitis
spermicidal cream
spes phthisica
SPET (single photon emission tomography) imaging
Spetzler lumboperitoneal shunt
spewing obscenities
SPF (specific pathogen free)
SPF (sun protection factor)
sphaerocephalus, Trichodectes
sphenoethmoidal recess
sphenoethmoidal suture
sphenofrontal suture
sphenofrontal suture lines
sphenoid
s. angle
s. bone
s. bone, inferior lamina of
s. bone, tongue of
s. cells
s. fontanelle
s. ridge
s., rostrum of
s. sinus
s. sinus, aperture of
s. sinus cancer
s. turbinate
s. wing
sphenoidal
s. concha
s. electrode
s. paranasal sinus
s. process
s. yoke
sphenoidale, os
sphenoidale, planum
sphenoidalis, concha
sphenoidalis, foramen ovale ossis
sphenoidectomy, frontoethmoid
sphenoides, Amoebotaenia
sphenomalar suture
sphenomaxillary ganglion
sphenomaxillary suture
spheno-occipital suture
spheno-orbital suture
sphenopalatine
s. artery
s. block
s. ganglion

s. ganglionectomy
s. neuralgia
s. notch of palatine bone
sphenopalatinum, foramen
sphenoparietal suture
sphenoparietal suture lines
sphenopetrosal suture
sphenosquamous suture
sphenotemporal suture
sphenotic center
sphenozygomatic suture
sphere(s)
s., attraction
s. granule
s., hydroxyapatite
s. implant
s. implant, Berens
s. implant, Doherty
s. implant, Glass
s. implant, Gold
s. implant, Guist
s. implant, hollow
s. implant material, hollow
s. implant, plastic
s. of ideas
s., oriented in all
s. prosthesis, hollow
s., psychosexual
s., Silastic
spherical
s. aberration
s. aberration, negative
s. aberration, positive
s. bacterium
s. cell
s. equivalent
s. form of occlusion
s. implant
s. lens
s. lesion
s. mass
s. shape
s. -shaped forms
sphericity index
spherocytic anemia
spherocytosis anemia
spherocytosis, hereditary
spheroid joint
spheroidal cell carcinoma
spheron theory
spherons, bursting
sphincter
s., anal
s. ani
s. ani muscle

s., artificial urinary
s., cardiac
s., cardioesophageal
s., contract anal
s. contraction ▸ external
s. disorder, esophageal
s. disorder ▸ upper esophageal
s. dysfunction
s. dyssynergia, detrusor-
s., esophageal
s., esophagogastric
s. function ▸ loss of
s., gastroesophageal
s., Henle's
s., hypertonic
s., Hyrtl's
s. implant ▸ artificial
s., incompetent esophageal
s., inguinal
s., internal
s. iridis
s. ▸ lax anal
s. ▸ lower esophageal
s. malfunctioning
s. muscle
s. muscle ▸ anal
s. muscle ▸ external
s. muscle ▸ internal
s. muscle of anus, external
s. muscle of anus, internal
s. muscle of bile duct
s. muscle of hepatopancreatic
    ampulla
s. muscle of membranous urethra
s. muscle of pupil
s. muscle of pylorus
s. muscle of urethra
s. muscle of urinary bladder
s. muscle spasm, rectal
s., Nélaton's
s. oculi
s. of Oddi
s. of Oddi dysmotility disorder
s. of Oddi manometry
s. of Oddi spasm
s. of pupil
s. oris
s., precapillary
s. pressure
s. pressure, lower esophageal
s. pupillae
s., pyloric
s., rectal
s. ▸ relaxation internal
s. ▸ relaxed lower esophageal

s. ▸ spasm of external
s. stenosis
s., tight
s. tone
s. tone, rectal
s. ultrasound
s. urethras
s., urinary
s. vaginae
s. vesicae
sphincteral achalasia
sphincterotomy
s., anal
s., endoscopic
s., external urethral
s. ▸ lateral internal
s., rectal
sphingomyelin (LS) ratio, lecithin-
sphygmic interval
sphygmography study
spica
s. bandage
s. cast
s. cast, hip
s. cast, shoulder
s., double
s. dressing
s., hip
s., thumb
spicata, Actaea
spiculated calcification
spiculed mature red blood cells
spicules, bone
spicules evaluated
spicy foods (CAPS)-free diet ▸
    caffeine, alcohol, pepper,
spider
s. angioma
s. angiomata
s. bites, brown
s. burst veins
s. cancer
s. cell
s. finger
s. mark on arm
s. marks from cirrhosis
s. nevi
s. projection
s. vein treatment
s. veins
s. veins, red
s. venom
s. venom, black widow
Spiegler-Fendt sarcoid
Spielmeyer disease, Vogt-

Spielmeyer-Vogt syndrome, Stock-
Spigelia marilandica
spigelian hernia
spike(s) (sp)
s. -and-dome complex
s. -and-dome configuration
s. -and-dome pulse
s. -and-sharp waves
s. -and-slow wave
s. -and-slow wave ▸ atypical
    repetitive
s. -and-slow wave complex
s. -and-slow wave complex ▸
    multiple
s. -and-slow wave complexes ▸
    sequence of
s. -and-slow wave ▸ larval
s. -and-slow wave phenomenon
s. -and-slow wave rhythm
s. -and-slow waves ▸ six hertz (Hz)
s. -and-slow waves ▸ three hertz
    (Hz)
s. -and-wave
s. -and-wave bursts
s. -and-wave complex
s. -and-wave complex ▸ multiple
s. -and-wave complex ▸ slow
s. -and-wave discharge
s. -and-wave discharge ▸
    frontoparietal
s. -and-wave discharge ▸ six per
    second
s. -and-wave pattern
s. -and-wave ▸ slow
s. -and-waves ▸ phantom
s. artifact ▸ noise
s., biphasic
s. complex, multiple
s. detection error artifact, data
s., diffuse
s. discharges
s. discharges, nonspecific diffuse
s. ▸ double count of pacer
s. ▸ double counting of pacer
s., fever
s., focal
s., focal anterior temporal
s. foci, multiple
s. focus
s. focus, anterior temporal
s. focus, central
s. focus, frontal
s. focus, midtemporal
s. focus, occipital
s. focus, parietal

spike(s)—*continued*
s., fourteen and six hertz (Hz)
  positive
s., fourteen and six per second
  positive
s., generalized
s., hemagglutinin
s., hemisphere
s., isolated
s. -like emanations
s. -like formations
s., neuraminidase
s. or delta waves (SSSDW) ▸
  significant sharp,
s., pacemaker
s., pacer
s., parietal
s., parietal area left wave-
s., parietal area sharp wave-
s. pattern
s. pattern, positive
s. phenomenon
s., poorly developed
s. rhythm, six and fourteen
s., right frontal slowing
s., scattered
s. seizure activity
s., sensing
s., six and fourteen positive
s., slow
s., small sharp
s., temperature
s. transient
s. transients, isolated
s. transients, sharp
s., visual
s. wave abnormality
s., wave-and-
s. waves
s. waves, atypical
s. waves, multiple
spiked fever, patient
spiked temperature, patient
spikey dysrhythmic activity
spiking
s., anterior temporal
s., discharges
s. dysrhythmia
s. dysrhythmia, negative
s. fever
s., midtemporal
s., negative
s. phenomenon
s., sporadic negative
s., sporadic positive

s. temperature
spill(s)
s. area
s., blood
s., blood or secretion
s., contact with blood
s., contaminated blood
s., decontamination of blood
s., decontamination of secretion
s. from AIDS (acquired immune
  deficiency syndrome) patients ▸
  secretion
s. from hepatitis patients ▸
  secretion
s. into duodenum, prompt
s. of fluid ▸ hazardous
s., patency and
s., secretion
s. stomach, cup-and-
spilled
s. protein, patient
s., sugar
s. sugar, patient
Spiller operation, Frazier-
spilling into upper abdomen ▸ fluid
spillover ▸ jugular venous catechol
spilus, nevus
spin
s. density
s. -echo imaging
s. -echo imaging sequence
s. -echo MRI (magnetic resonance
  imaging)
s. -lattice time
s. -spin time
s. technique
s. -time ▸ spin
spina bifida
s.b. anterior
s.b. aperta
s.b. cystica
s.b. manifesta
s.b. occulta
s.b. posterior
s.b., repair of
s.b. with meningocele ▸ repair of
s.b. with meningomyelocele ▸
  repair of
s.b. with myelodysplasia
spinach stool
spinae reflex, erector
spinal [*final*]
s. accessory chain lymph nodes
s. accessory nerve

s. accessory-facial
  neuroanastomosis
s. accessory-hypoglossal
  neuroanastomosis
s. adjustment
s. alignment
s. analgesia
s. anatomy
s. anesthesia
s. anesthesia ▸ low
s. anomaly
s. arachnoid
s. artery
s. artery, anterior
s. arthritis
s. ataxia
s. atrophy, corticostriatal-
s. block
s. bone density
s. bone loss
s. bone mass
s. canal
s. canal ▸ narrowing of
s. canal tumor
s. canal vessels
s. channel, narrow
s. column
s. column, stabilize
s. compression
s. compression fracture
s. cord
s. cord abscess
s. cord, acute inflammation of
s. cord, anterior horns of
s. cord, arachnoid of
s. cord biopsy
s. cord birth defect
s. cord block
s. cord block in radiation therapy
s. cord, central canal of
s. cord, central ▸ intermediate
  substance of
s. cord compression
s. cord concussion
s. cord, contusion of
s. cord cyst
s. cord damage
s. cord, decompression of
s. cord, degeneration of
s. cord disease
s. cord disorder
s. cord, dorsal aspect
s. cord, dorsal horns of
s. cord, drainage (dr'ge) of
s. cord, dura mater of

s. cord dysfunction, transient
s. cord, electrical stimulation of
s. cord, excision lesion of
s. cord exploration
s. cord ▸ focal disorders of brain and
s. cord functions
s. cord ▸ gelatinous substance of
s. cord, gray matter in
s. cord, gray matter of
s. cord, gray substance of
s. cord, hemisection of
s. cord hemorrhage ▸ agonal
s. cord, horns of
s. cord ▸ impingement on
s. cord, inflammation of
s. cord injury
s. cord injury paralysis
s. cord ▸ intact
s. cord, lateral horns of
s. cord, lateral ▸ intermediate substance of
s. cord, lateral region of
s. cord lesion
s. cord, lining of
s. cord necrosis
s. cord ▸ neurons in
s. cord, outermost covering of
s. cord, pressure on
s. cord, protective layer of
s. cord ▸ proximal cervical
s. cord ▸ regenerate
s. cord ▸ regenerating nerves in
s. cord ▸ sensory input from
s. cord severed
s. cord stimulation ▸ electrical
s. cord stimulator
s. cord stroke
s. cord, terminal ventricle of
s. cord, thoracolumbar
s. cord tissue
s. cord tolerances in radiation therapy
s. cord tracts
s. cord ▸ transection of
s. cord tumor
s. cord tumor, metastatic
s. cord tumor, paraplegia in
s. cord, ventral gray columns of
s. cord ▸ ventral horns of
s. cord, white commissure of
s. cord ▸ white substance of
s. curvature
s. degeneration, corticostriatal-
s. deterioration due to radiation

s. disc degeneration
s. disc disease
s. disc ▸ ruptured
s. disease (DSD) ▸ degenerative
s. embolism
s. epidural abscess
s. epidural angiolipoma
s. epidural metastases
s. epilepsy
s. examination
s. fluid
s. fluid cell count
s. fluid circulation
s. fluid clear
s. fluid gram stains
s. fluid ▸ human
s. fluid level
s. fluid, normal
s. fluid pressure (SFP)
s. fluid rhinorrhea
s. fluid tap
s. fusion
s. fusion, Albee
s. fusion, Hibbs'
s. fusion, multilevel
s. fusion, Rogers' type
s. fusion surgery
s. ganglion
s. gliosis
s. headache
s. hemianesthesia
s. hemiplegia
s. immobilization
s. induction
s. injuries
s. injury ▸ immobilization of
s. instrumentation, Harrington
s. irritation
s. lesion, cervical
s. manipulation
s. marrow
s. meningitis
s. micturition reflex center
s. misalignment
s. motion, decrease
s. muscle
s. muscular atrophy
s. muscular atrophy, familial
s. muscular atrophy, progressive
s. mydriasis
s. myoclonus
s. nerve ▸ compression of
s. nerve cord
s. nerve fibers, afferent
s. nerve ▸ impingement on

s. nerve, inflamed
s. nerve neurotomy
s. nerve regeneration
s. nerve roots
s. nerves
s. nerves, filaments of
s. nerves, loops of
s. nerves, major
s. osteoporosis
s. paralysis
s. paralytic poliomyelitis
s. pathways
s. poliomyelitis
s. puncture
s. reflex
s. reflex, local
s. root origin, lumbar
s. scoliosis
s. segment
s. shock
s. slumping
s. spurs, treatment
s. stenosis
s. stenosis, cervical
s. stenosis ▸ congenital
s. stenosis ▸ lumbar
s. stiffness
s. stimulant
s. subarachnoid block
s. surgery, invasive
s. tap
s. tap, diagnostic
s. tap, headache after
s. tap ▸ traumatic
s. tissue
s. veins

spinale, tache
spinalis
s., arachnoidea
s., commotio
s., dura mater
s., medulla
s., pia mater
s. progressive, amyotrophia
s., tabes

spindle(s)
s. cataract
s. cell
s. cell cancer
s. cell carcinoma
s. cell nevus
s. cell stroma
s. cell thymoma
s., extreme
s., frontal

spindle(s)—continued
- s., His
- s., Krukenberg's
- s. of sleep, normal
- s., per second
- s. REMS (rapid eye movements)
- s. -shaped cataract
- s. -shaped cells
- s. -shaped cells ▸ whorls of
- s. -shaped node
- s., six to twelve per second
- s., sleep
- s., slow frontal

spindliform activity

spindling activity

spindling patterns

spine
- s. ▸ abnormal bone growth of
- s., anterior superior
- s. (ASIS), anterior superior iliac
- s., arachnoiditis of
- s., arthritis, inflammatory
- s., arthritis of
- s., bamboo
- s., cervical
- s., collapsed vertebrae of
- s., compensatory curvature of
- s., compression fracture of
- s. ▸ compressive force on
- s., concavity of
- s., convexity of
- s., curvature of
- s. deformity, cervical
- s., degenerative changes of
- s., dens view of cervical
- s. disease, headache secondary to cervical
- s., divisions of
- s., dorsal
- s. ▸ dysfunction of cervical
- s., erect
- s., erector muscle of
- s. ▸ excessive curvature of
- s., fetal
- s., flexion of
- s., fracture vertebrae of
- s. fractures, osteoporosis-related
- s., Henle's
- s., iliac
- s. in flexed position
- s., inflexible
- s. injury, cervical
- s., ischial
- s., lateral curvature of
- s., lumbar

- s., lumbosacral
- s. misalignment
- s. mobility
- s. motion, lumbar
- s., motion of
- s., nasal
- s. of Henle
- s. of maxilla, palatine
- s. of scapula
- s., open
- s., osteoarthritis of
- s., parallel to the
- s., poker
- s., protruding
- s. ▸ restricted excess motion in
- s., sacral
- s., scoliosis of
- s. spot films
- s., spurring of lumbar
- s., spurring of thoracic
- s., suprameatal
- s., thoracic
- s., thoracolumbar
- s., tibial
- s. ▸ twisting force on
- s., vertebral

Spinelli's operation

spinifera, Fasciolopsis

spinigera, Haemaphysalis

spinipalpus, Ixodes

spinnbarkeit testing

spinners' cancer, mule-

spinning sensation ▸ violent

spinocerebellar

spinocerebellar degeneration

spinoneural artery

spinosum, foramen

spinothalamic tract

spinothalamic tract cauterized

spinous cell layer

spinous process

spinulosa, trichostasis

spinulosum, Penicillium

spinulosus, lichen

spiny projections

spinyheaded worm

spiral(s)
- s. arterioles
- s., Curschmann's
- s. dissection
- s. flap, Hueston
- s. fold of cystic duct
- s. fracture
- s. ganglion
- s. ganglion of cochlea

- s. ganglion of cochlear nerve
- s., Herxheimer's
- s. incision
- s. joint
- s. -shaped bacteria
- s. tip catheter
- s. vein of modiolus
- s. wound

spirale, vas

spiraling death rate

spiralis, Aceraria

spiralis, Trichinella

Spira's disease

spirilla, gram-negative

spirillar dysentery

Spirillum genus

Spirillum minus

spiritual
- s. aspect of health
- s. assessment
- s. beliefs
- s. comfort
- s. concerns, human
- s. condition
- s. dimension of grief
- s. distress
- s. energy
- s. enrichment
- s. healing
- s. needs
- s. orientation
- s. pain
- s., physical and nutritional component ▸ medical, psychological,
- s. practices
- s. regeneration
- s. state
- s. support
- s. values, altered
- s. vitality

Spirochaeta
- S. daxensis
- S. eurystrepta
- S. genus
- S. marina
- S. pallida
- S. plicatilis
- S. pseudoicterogenes
- S. stenostrepta
- S. vincenti

spirochetal
- s. disease
- s. icterus
- s. infection

s. myocarditis
spirochetes, syphilitic
spirochetosis, bronchopulmonary
spirogram (FES) ▸ forced expiratory
spirometric screening
spirometry
s., bronchoscopic
s., incentive
s. test
s. ▸ Tri-flow incentive
spitting up blood
Spitz nevus
Spivack valve
SPL (skin potential level)
SPL (sound pressure level)
splanchnesthetic sensibility
splanchnic
s. aneurysm
s. bed perfusion
s. block
s. blood
s. blood flow
s. ganglion
s. mechanism
s. motor component
s. nerve
s. nerve, greater
s. nerve, inferior
s. nerve, lesser
s. nerve, lowest
s. nerves, lumbar
s. nerves, pelvic
s. nerves, sacral
s. sensory component
s. steal ▸ renal
s. venous thrombosis, central
s. vessel
Splash (splash)
S. (amphetamines)
s. lightning injury ▸ side
s., succussion
splashing body secretions
splaying open rib cage
spleen
s., accessory
s. colony assay
s. colony forming units
s., congestion of
s. does appear enlarged
s. does not appear enlarged
s., ellipsoid of
s. enlarged and congested
s. enlargement
s. enlargement ▸ acute
s. ▸ focal metastases to

s., Gandy-Gamna
s. grossly congested
s. had mottled appearance
s., hilus of
s. ▸ histologic sections of
s. injury
s., kidneys (LSK) not palpable ▸ liver,
s., lardaceous
s. ▸ leukemic infiltration of the
s. meridian
s. microscopically congested
s. not palpable
s. not palpably enlarged
s. palpated
s. pedicle, inverted Y and
s. ▸ red substance of
s. rupture
s., ruptured
s. scan
s., swollen
s., thromboembolism in
s. tip
s. ▸ traumatic rupture of
splendens, Eutrombicula
Splendore-de Almeida syndrome, Lutz-
splenial center
splenic
s. abscess
s. agenesis syndrome
s. anemia
s. aneurysm
s. angle
s. arteriography
s. arterioles
s. artery
s. capsule
s. cell cords
s. fever
s. flexure
s. flexure, carcinoma
s. flexure of colon
s. flexure syndrome
s. infarcts
s. localization index (SLI)
s. morphology
s. mycosis
s. panhematopenia, primary
s. phagocytosis
s. portogram
s. portography
s. puncture
s. red pulp
s. retinitis

s. rupture
s. shadow
s. souffle
s. system angiogram
s. tissue
s. vascular supply
s. vein
s. venogram
splenitis, patchy peri-
splenitis, spodogenous
splenius
s. muscle
s. muscle of head
s. muscle of neck
splenization, hypostatic
splenogastric omentum
splenogranulomatosis siderotica
splenomedullary leukemia
splenomegalic polycythemia
splenomegaly
s., congestive
s., dim use
s., febrile tropical
s., Gaucher's
s., hemolytic
s., hypercholesterolemic
s., myelophthisis
s., Niemann's
s., siderotic
s., spodogenous
s. syndrome, tropical
splenomyelogenous leukemia
splenoportal hypertension
splenoportal venography
splenoportography study
splenorenal shunt, distal
splenosis, pericardial
splice, breakaway
splice junction
splicing
s. defects
s. efficiency
s., gene
s., in vitro
splint [*squint*]
s. boots
s., molded plastic
s., muscle-relaxation
s., shin
splinted in flexion, hand
splinter hemorrhages
splintered fracture
splintered to pieces, fragments
splinting [*splitting*]
s., ankle

splinting [*splitting*]—*continued*
- s., arm
- s., dynamic
- s., hand
- s., kneecap
- s. leg ▸ immobilizing and
- s. limb ▸ bandaging and
- s., traction

split
- s. -brain patient
- s. -brain surgery
- s. -brain syndrome
- s. course dose fractionation
- s. course regimen
- s. course technique
- s. course treatment
- s. function lung test
- s. function study
- s. graft
- s. graft, thick-
- s. graft, thin-
- s. hand
- s. image artifact
- s. in line of fibers, muscles
- s. longitudinally, muscles
- s. lung ventilation
- s., mitral second sound (M2)
- s. personality
- s. products, fibrinogen-
- s. products, fibrinolytic-
- s. products of fibrin
- s. psychotherapy
- s., pulmonic second sound (P2)
- s., rectus muscle
- s. renal function study
- s. shot
- s. -skin graft
- s. (S2) sound ▸ paradoxically
- s., sternum
- s. -thickness graft
- s. thickness graft of pigskin
- s. -thickness skin graft
- s. -thickness skin graft, intermediate
- s. tongue
- s. urine
- s. virus vaccine

splitter, beam

splitting [*splinting*]
- s. breast bone
- s., cellulose
- s., commissural
- s. fingernails
- s. incision, muscle
- s. incision, rectus muscle
- s. incision, sternal
- s. of heart sounds
- s. of lacrimal papilla
- s. of mandible, sagittal
- s. procedure, sternal
- s. scar, sternal
- s. technique, muscle

SPO pacemaker ▸ Medtronic
spodogenous splenitis
spodogenous splenomegaly
spoken
- s., language
- s. language, normal comprehension of
- s. voice
- s. words, inability to remember

Spondee Word test, Harvard
spondylitis
- s., ankylosing
- s., Bekhterev's
- s. deformans
- s., hypertrophic
- s. infectiosa
- s., Kümmell's
- s., Marie-Strümpell
- s., rheumatoid
- s., tuberculosis
- s., von Bekhterev-Strümpell

spondyloarthropathy, seronegative
spondyloepiphyseal dysplasia
spondylolysis, cervical
spondylomalacia traumatica
spondylopathy, traumatic
spondylophyte impactor
spondylosis
- s., cervical
- s. chronica ankylopoietica
- s., rhizomelic
- s., uncovertebralis

sponge
- s., absorbable gelatin
- s., alcohol
- s. and lap count
- s. and needle count correct
- s. bath
- s., Bernay's
- s., biopsy
- s., contraceptive
- s. count correct
- s., ear
- s., fibrin
- s. forceps
- s., gelatin
- s., Gelfoam
- s. graft

- s. implant
- s. implant, Ivalon
- s. implant material, Ivalon
- s. implant, polyvinyl
- s. implant, silicone
- s., Ivalon
- s. kidney
- s. kidney, medullary
- s., lap
- s. -like holes in brain
- s., phantom
- s., RayTec
- s. stick
- s., surgical
- s. tent
- s. test
- s., vaginal

spongiform
- s. encephalopathy
- s. encephalopathy, bovine
- s. encephalopathy, subacute
- s. encephalopathy, transmissible
- s. leukodystrophy
- s. virus encephalopathy, transmissible

spongioblastoma multiforme
spongioblastoma unipolare
spongiosa graft, intramedullary and
spongy
- s. bone
- s., bone porous and
- s. iritis
- s. part of bone
- s., semi-liquid tissue ▸ soft,
- s. substance of bones
- s. tissue

sponsor, accredited
spontaneity
- s., creativity, and flexibility
- s., curiosity, and initiative ▸ reduced
- s., lack of initiative and

spontaneous
- s. abortion
- s. abortions, repeated
- s. activity
- s. activity, low level of
- s. amputation
- s. attack of unconsciousness
- s. bacterial peritonitis (SBP)
- s. bleeding
- s. breathing
- s. breathing, minimal
- s. breathing, stimulate adequate
- s. coronary artery dissection (SCAD)

s. delivery
s. delivery (NSD) ▸ normal
s. ecchymosis
s. echo contrast
s. echo contrast ▸ left atrial (LA)
s. fracture
s. hemorrhage
s. hypoglycemia
s. ischemia
s. labor
s. left hemothorax
s. lesion
s. miscarriage
s. movement
s. movement of limbs ▸ no
s. myoglobinuria
s. nystagmus
s. occurrences ▸ transient
s. onset of labor
s. onset of pain
s. panic attacks
s. passage of tissue
s. pneumothorax
s. premature labor
s. recall
s. reentrant sustained ventricular
  tachycardia
s. regression
s. remission
s. respiration
s. respiration, absent
s. retinal arterial pulsations
s. right hemothorax
s. rupture
s. rupture of esophagus
s. rupture of membranes
s. seizure
s. sensation
s. sleep
s. spasm of airway muscles
s. speech
s. vaginal delivery
s. vaginal delivery (NSVD) ▸ normal
s. vertex delivery
s. voiding
spontaneously
s. aborted human fetus
s., eyes open
s., fever subsided
s., heal
s., membranes ruptured
spooned nail from chemical
sporadic
s. arrhythmias
s. attack

s. bovine encephalomyelitis
s. colon cancer
s. dysentery
s. negative spiking
s. positive spiking
s. slow wave
sporadically occurring
spore(s)
s., anthrax
s., bacterial
s. containing dust
s. formation
s., fungi
s., inhaling
s., mold
s., swarm
s., washed
s., yeast
sporogenes, Clostridium
Sporothrix carnis
Sporothrix schenckii
sporotrichosis of canaliculus
sporotrichosis of lacrimal sac
Sporotrichum schenckii
Sporozoa Coccidia
Sporozoa Haemosporidia
sporozoan parasites
sports
s. injury
s. injury treatment
s. massage
s. medicine
s. medicine clinics
s. medicine programs
s., nonstrenuous contact
s. rage
s. -related injury
s. science
s., strenuous contact
s. vision
sporulation, endogenous
sporulation, exogenous
spot(s)
s., age
s., aging skin
s. and distortion of lines ▸ blank
s. and hot spots with electron beam
  dosimetry ▸ cold
s. artifact, black
s., bald
s. before eyes
s. before eyes from anemia
s. before eyes ▸ moving
s., Bitot
s., blind

s., Brushfield's
s., café au lait
s., Carleton's
s., cherry red
s. cholecystography
s., cold
s., DeMorgan's
s., Elschnig's
s. film
s. film device
s. film fluorography
s. film radiography
s. -film roentgenography
s. film study
s. films, pressure
s. films, spine
s., flame
s., focal
s., Förster-Fuchs' black
s., Fuchs'
s., Gaule's
s., Horner-Trantas
s., hot
s. imaging ▸ hot
s. in eye, ash leaf
s., Janeway's
s., Koplik's
s., laser
s., liver
s., Mariotte's
s., Mariotte's blind
s., Maxwell's
s., milk
s., multicolored
s. (YS) of retina, yellow
s. on breast ▸ red
s. on scan ▸ hot
s. on skin, age
s. on skin ▸ purplish hemorrhagic
s. pains
s. perfusion scintigraphy ▸
  myocardial cold
s., precancerous
s. ▸ precancerous skin
s. projection, erect fluoro
s. radiation
s., rose
s., Roth's
s. ▸ rough, scaly skin
s. scanography
s. scintigraphy ▸ infarct avid hot
s., skin
s., Soemmering's
s., soft
s., Tay's

spot(s)—*continued*
- s., tender trigger
- s., tendinous
- s., trigger
- s., Trousseau's
- s., unossified
- s. ▸ ventricular milk
- s. view
- s. view, oblique
- s. ▸ visual blind
- s., white
- s. with electron beam dosimetry ▸ cold spots and hot

spotted
- s. fever
- s. fever, Brazilian
- s. fever, Rocky Mountain
- s. tongue

spotting
- s. and cramping, intermittent
- s., first trimester
- s., IM (intermenstrual)
- s., intermittent
- s., intrauterine device (IUD)
- s. of blood
- s., postcoital
- s., vaginal

spotty loss of vision

spousal
- s. abuse
- s. impoverishment
- s. kidney
- s. kidney transplant

spouse
- s. abuse
- s., adjustment to death of
- s. beating
- s., substance-using
- s. syndrome (BSS), battered

SPR (skin potential response)

sprain [*strain*]
- s., ankle
- s., cervical
- s. ▸ first, second or third degree
- s., foot
- s. fracture
- s., inversion
- s. ▸ lateral ankle
- s., lumbosacral
- s. ▸ medial ankle
- s., rider's
- s., stable
- s., unstable

sprained joint

spray
- s., Dermoplast
- s. flu vaccine ▸ nasal
- s. inhaler, steam
- s., insulin nasal
- s., lysine pitressin
- s. ▸ metered-dose
- s., nasal
- s. ▸ nasal nicotine
- s. ▸ nicotine nasal
- s. ▸ steroid nasal

spread
- s. bacterial infection
- s. Bragg peak
- s., epithelial
- s. glomerulosclerosis and arteriosclerosis ▸ wide◊
- s. in cancer, pattern of local
- s. ▸ loco-regional
- s., lymphangitic
- s., lymphangitic pattern of cancer
- s., lymphatic
- s., metastatic
- s., middle-age
- s. of abnormal cells
- s. of cancer ▸ slow
- s. of infection
- s. of infection, mode of
- s. of infection, prevent
- s. of nasopharyngeal carcinoma, lymphatic
- s. of prostatic adenocarcinoma ▸ lymphangitic
- s. of skin infection
- s., patient-to-patient
- s. pattern of lung carcinoma, extrathoracic
- s. pattern of lung carcinoma, local
- s. pattern of lung carcinoma, lymphatic
- s., regional
- s. ribs apart
- s., source of
- s., tumor
- s., vehicular
- s., venous

spreading
- s. depression (CSD) ▸ cortical
- s. to arms ▸ pain
- s. to neck ▸ pain
- s. to shoulder ▸ pain

sprees ▸ extravagant spending

Sprengel's deformity

Spring(s) (spring)
- S. anemia, Bagdad

- s. appearance, coiled-
- s., arcing #80
- S. brace ▸ Warm
- s. diaphragm, coil
- s., disc
- s. finger
- s. lancet
- s. -loaded feet
- s. -loaded stent
- s., Mazlin
- s. -summer encephalitis, Russian
- s. water cyst

sprinter's fracture

sprue
- s., celiac
- s., nontropical
- s., tropical

sprung knee

spun in centrifuge, blood

spur(s)
- s., arthritic
- s., bone
- s., bony
- s., calcaneal
- s., cell
- s. cell anemia
- s. ▸ detection of bone
- s. excision ▸ heel
- s. formation
- s. formation, osteoarthritic hypertrophic
- s., heel
- s., hypertrophic
- s., Morand's
- s., nasal
- s., occipital
- s. of malleus
- s., olecranon
- s. ▸ painful heel
- s., plantar calcaneal
- s., scleral
- s., septal
- s. syndrome ▸ heel
- s., treatment spinal
- s., vomerine

spuria
- s., angina
- s., placenta
- s., polycoria

spurious
- s. aneurysm
- s. ejection fraction
- s. frequency
- s. hyperkalemia
- s. labor pains

s. parasite
s. polycythemia
s. pregnancy
spurium, septum
spurius, hydrops
Spurling's sign
Spurling's test
spurring
s., advanced
s., bony
s., degenerative
s., degenerative anterior
s., degenerative lateral
s., degenerative lumbar
s., hypertrophic
s., lumbar
s. of lumbar spine
s. of thoracic spine
spurter, arterial
spurts, growth
sputum
s., acid-fast stain of
s. aeroginosum
s., albuminoid
s. analysis
s., black stained
s., blood in
s., blood tinged
s., bloody
s., brown
s. coctum
s. collection
s., copious
s., cough and
s., cough productive of
s., cough productive of bloody
s. crudum
s. cruentum
s. culture
s. culture, premortem
s., cultured, seropurulent
s., currant jelly
s. cytology
s. cytology in lung cancer
s., early morning
s., egg yolk
s. ▸ elastic fibers in
s. examination
s., expectorated
s. ▸ fever, night sweats, cough, foul
s. foul smelling
s., frothy
s., globular
s. gram stain
s., green

s. grossly purulent
s., hemorrhagic
s., icteric
s. induction
s. ▸ malnourished, multiple caries, foul
s., moss-agate
s., mucopurulent
s., normal
s., nummular
s., pink
s. ▸ pinkish blood-tinged
s. -producing cough
s. production
s. production, excessive
s., productive
s., prune juice
s., purulent
s. purulent and foul smelling
s. ▸ rod-shaped organisms in
s., rusty
s., septicemia
s. smear
s., sneezed
s. specimen
s. stains
s. studies
s. studies, expectorated
s., tenacious
s. test
s. ▸ thick, tenacious
s. tube
s. viscosity and elasticity
s., white
s., yellow
s., yellowish
S-QRS interval
squamocolumnar junction
squamocolumnar junction, sharp
squamoid features
squamosa, blepharitis
squamosal bone
squamosal suture
squamosomastoid suture
squamosoparietal suture
squamososphenoid suture
squamous
s. alveolar cell
s. atypia, esophageal
s. carcinoma
s. cell
s. cell cancer
s. cell carcinoma
s. cell carcinoma base of tongue
s. cell carcinoma, bronchogenic

s. cell carcinoma, bronchogenic poorly differentiated
s. cell carcinoma buccal mucosa
s. cell carcinoma, cervical lymph node classification in
s. cell carcinoma dorsum of hand
s. cell carcinoma ear and nose
s. cell carcinoma ▸ electrodesiccation and curettage in
s. cell carcinoma eyelid
s. cell carcinoma gingiva
s. cell carcinoma ▸ infiltrating
s. cell carcinoma lip
s. cell carcinoma, locally advanced
s. cell carcinoma of cervix
s. cell carcinoma of lung
s. cell carcinoma of vocal cord
s. cell carcinoma ▸ perianal
s. cell carcinoma, poorly differentiated
s. cell carcinoma ▸ superficial
s. cell carcinoma tongue
s. cell in alveoli
s. cell, nonphagocytic
s. cell papilloma
s. cell skin cancer
s. cell skin carcinoma
s. cell tumor
s. cell tumor ▸ well differentiated
s. differentiation, adenocarcinoma with
s. epithelial cells
s. epithelial fragments
s. epithelium
s. epithelium, nonkeratinizing stratified
s. epithelium, stratified
s. -like polygonal cells
s. metaplasia
s. metaplasia ▸ focal areas of
s. metaplasia, marked
s. metaplasia of mucosa
s. suture
s. suture lines
s. suture of cranium
squandering of money ▸ repeated
square(s)
s. analysis, least-
s., blotter
s., chi-
s. deviations (SSD), sum of
s. inch (psi) ▸ pounds per
s. law, inverse-
s., mean

square(s)—*continued*
  s. regression ▸ least
  s. (RMS) ▸ root-mean-
  s. root sign
  s. test, chi
  s. voltage ▸ root-mean-
  s. wave pulse
  s. wave response
  s. wave stimulation
  s. wave stimulus
  s. waves of high frequency
squared
  s. (kg/m^2) ▸ kilogram per meter
  s. ▸ liters per minute per meter
  s. ▸ meters per second
squat(s)
  s. and lunge exercise
  s. exercise ▸ heel
  s. exercise ▸ knee lift
  s. exercise ▸ weighted
squatting exercise
squeaky leather sound
squeals ▸ grunts and
squeals ▸ patient grunts and
squeeze [*sneeze, wheeze*]
  s. dynamometer
  s. effect
  s. exercise ▸ shoulder
  s. exercise ▸ toe
  s. ▸ shoulder blade
  s., thoracic
  s., tussive
squeezing pain in chest
squeezing sensation in chest
SQUID (superconducting quantum
  interference device)
squint [*splint*]
  s., accommodative
  s., comitant
  s., concomitant
  s., convergent
  s., deviation
  s., divergent
  s., latent
  s. lines ▸ laugh and
  s., noncomitant
  s. of eyes
  s., upward and downward
squinting
  s. eye
  s. ▸ involuntary spasmodic blinking
    or
  s. of eyes ▸ increased winking,
    blinking or
squirrel plaque conjunctivitis

SR (sedimentation rate)
Sr (strontium)
  Sr 85, strontium nitrate
  Sr 87m, strontium
  Sr^{90} (strontium 90)
S-R interval
SRA (Sadistic Ritual Abuse)
SRD (service-related disability)
SRR (skin resistance response)
SRT (speech reception threshold)
ss (one-half)
SS (stainless steel)
SS (stainless steel) screw
Ssabanejew-Frank gastrostomy
SSCP (single strand conformational
  polymorphism)
SSD (source to skin distance)
SSD (sum of square deviations)
SSE (soapsuds enema)
SSEP or SEP (somatosensory
  evoked potentials)
S-shaped
  S-shaped incision
  S-shaped retractor, French
  S-shaped scar
  S-shaped scoliosis
SSI (surgical site infection)
SSKI (saturated solution of
  potassium iodide)
S-sleep (synchronized sleep)
SSPE (subacute sclerosing
  panencephalitis)
SSSDW (significant sharp, spike or
  delta waves)
ST
  ST alterations
  ST depression
  ST depression ▸ reciprocal
  ST elevation
  ST interval
  ST junction
  ST sag
  ST segment
  ST segment changes
  ST segment depression
  ST segment depression ▸ downhill
  ST segment depression ▸
    downsloping
  ST segment elevation
  ST segment elevation, persistent
  ST segments, coving of
  ST ▸ slurring of
  ST vector
  ST wave
ST

St. Jude('s)
  S.J. annuloplasty ring
  S.J. heart valve prosthesis
  S.J. Medical aortic valve prosthesis
  S.J. valve
St. Louis encephalitis
St. Louis encephalitis virus
St. Vitus' dance
stab
  s. cell
  s. culture
  s. form
  s. -in epicardial electrode
  s. incision
stab wound
  s.w. drain
  s.w., drain brought out through
  s.w. incision
  s.w., separate
stabbing
  s. chest pain
  s. joint pain
  s. pain
  s. pain, acute
  s. pain ▸ intense
  s. pain, severe
  s. pain, sharp
  s. sensation in eye
stability
  s. and optimal function
  s. at home ▸ evaluate safety and
  s., electrode
  s., joint
  s., medical
  s., mental
  s. of lesion
  s. of lesion, radiographic
  s. of self-image
  s. of subject differences
  s., personal
  s., postural
  s. test ▸ foam
  s. test, ligament
stabilization
  s. bar
  s., Grice
  s., medical
  s., neonatal
  s. of asthma
  s. of feelings
  s. of fracture
  s. of moods
  s. phase of treatment ▸ initial
  s., retentive
  s. test, clot

stabilize(s)
s., blood sugar
s. brain
s. cancer
s. heart function
s. injured knees ▸ protect and
s. knee
s. kneecap
s. patient
s. spinal column
s. weight
stabilized
s., blood pressure (BP)
s., condition
s., course
s., fracture
s. functional level
s., joint
s., patient
s., patient's condition
s. psychiatric condition
s., pulse
stabilizer, blood sugar
stabilizer, mood
stabilizing
s. activity ▸ membrane
s. blood coagulation factor ▸ fibrin-
s. drugs ▸ mood-
s. factor ▸ fibrin
s. fractures
s. prosthesis
s. ▸ shock-absorbing and
s. the backbone
stable
s., acid
s. alkaline phosphatase, heat
s. angina
s. angina, chronic
s., BP (blood pressure)
s., clinically
s. condition ▸ patient in
s., controlled heart failure
s. eating habits
s. family
s., fetal heart tones (FHT)
s. financial status
s. fracture
s. health status
s. heat
s. isotope
s. joint
s. medical condition
s. patient
s., patient clinically
s., patient emotionally

s., patient's condition
s. plaque
s., psychologically
s. sprain
s. teeth, adjacent
s., vital signs
s., weight
s. weight ▸ maintain
stabnuclear neutrophil
stabnuclear neutrophil steroid
staccato
s. pain
s. rhythm ▸ speaks in
s. speech
Stack operation, Magnuson-
Stack shoulder arthroplasty,
Magnuson-
staff
s. behavior, authoritarian
s. behavior, dysfunctional
s. cell
s., counseling
s. count
s. education, formal
s., hospital medical
s., in-service
s., intake assessment
s., medical
s. member, clinical
s. member, house
s. nurse
s., nursing
s. orientation
s. ▸ patient assault on
s. -patient interaction
s., professional
s. relationship, patient-
s. -to-patient transmission
s. training
s. training and interactions
s. transmission ▸ patient-to-
s., unit
staffing, continuing care
staffing, diagnostic
stage(s) (Stage) [phage]
s., acute
s., adolescent
s., adult sexual
s., advanced
s., algid
s., amphibolic
s. and waking, score sleep
s., asphyxial
s. breast cancer ▸ early
s. cancer, early

s. cancer ▸ end
s. cardiac disease, end-
s. cardiomyopathy, end-
s. cardiopulmonary disease, end-
s., chronic
s., clinical
s., clinically active
s., cold
s., curable
s., deep sleep
s., defervescent
s., delta sleep
s. demarcation, sleep
s., drowsing
s., dysfunction of sleep
s., early prodromal
s., end-
s., eruptive
s. esophagectomy in benign
    disease ▸ one-
s. esophagogastrostomy ▸ two-
s. exercise stress test ▸ single-
s., experimental
s., expulsive
s. failure, end-
s., fetal
s., genital
s. heart and liver disease, end-
s. heart factor ▸ end-
s. heart failure ▸ late-
s., hot
s., incubative
s., input
s., intermediary sleep
s., knäuel
s., light sleep
s. liver disease ▸ end-
s. liver failure, end-
s., localized
s., mechanical
s. melanoma, terminal-
s., menstrual
s., minimum
s. of alcoholism ▸ acute
s. of bacterial endocarditis,
    bacteria-free
s. of bacterial shock ▸ advanced
s. of cancer, advanced
s. of chemical dependency
s. of codependency
s. of congestive heart failure (CHF)
    ▸ advanced
s. of disease ▸ end-
s. of fervescence
s. of illness ▸ terminal

stage(s)—*continued*
- s. of infection ▸ incubative
- s. of labor, final
- s. of labor, first
- s. of labor, fourth
- s. of labor, second
- s. of labor, third
- s. of latency
- s. of recovery
- s. of sleep
- s. of sleep, deeper
- s. of sleep, lighter
- S. 1 hypertension
- s., oral
- s. period, sleep
- s., phallic
- s., placental
- s., precystic
- s., pre-epidemic
- s., pre-eruptive
- s. problem drinker ▸ early-
- s., prodromal
- s., progestational
- s., proliferative
- s. prostate cancer ▸ early
- s., psychosexual
- s., pyretogenic
- s., pyrogenetic
- s. radiograph ▸ 24-hour delayed lymph nodal
- s., Ranke's
- s., recovery
- s. renal disease (ESRD), end-
- S. Renal Disease (ESRD) Program, End
- s., resting
- s. retrosternal bypass coloplasty ▸ one-
- s., ring
- s., second
- s., secondary
- s., serial
- s., signs and symptoms
- s., stepladder
- s., stress injury
- s., successive
- s., sweating
- s., Tanner's
- s. terminal cancer, advanced
- s., transitional pulp
- s., treatable
- s., tumor
- s., ugly duckling
- s., vegetative
- s., zooglea

staged ulcer diet
staggering
- s. and falls ▸ frequent
- s. gait
- s. gait ▸ reeling,

staggers
- s., blind
- s., patient
- s., sleepy
- s., stomach

staghorn calculus
staghorn stone
staging
- s., clinical
- s., clinical diagnostic
- s., diagnostic workup and
- s. laparotomy
- s., lymphadenectomy
- s. of adenocarcinoma
- s., pathology and
- s., preoperative
- s. process and imaging
- s., surgical
- s., surgical evaluative
- s. system, Kirklin
- s. system ▸ tumor, nodes, metastases (TNM)
- s. systems in radiation therapy
- s. the disease

stagnant
- s. anoxia
- s. hypoxia
- s. urine

stagnation
- s., blood
- s. mastitis
- s. of urine

Stähli's line
Stahl's
- S. ear
- S. ear, No. 1
- S. ear, No. 2

stain [*gain, pain*]
- s., acid
- s., acid-fast
- s., after
- s., alcian blue
- s., Alzheimer's
- s., amyloid
- s., argentaffin
- s., argyrophil
- s., basic
- s., Bowie's
- s., Congo red
- s., connective tissue

- s., contrast
- s., counter
- s., differential
- s., elastic
- s., elastic fibers
- s., electron
- s., endocardial
- s., fat
- s., Feulgen
- s., fluorescent antibody
- s., Giemsa's
- s., gram
- s., heavy metal
- s., Heidenhain's
- s., Heidenhain's iron hematoxylin
- s., Heinz
- s., iron
- s., Jenner-Giemsa
- s., Kinyoun
- s., Leishman's
- s., lipoid
- s., Lugol's
- s., Mallory
- s., May-Grunwald-Giemsa
- s., metachromatic
- s. method, gram
- s., mucicarmine
- s. negative bacteremias ▸ gram's
- s. negative enteric bacilli ▸ gram's
- s., neutral
- s., nuclear
- s. of body fluid, gram
- s. of cervix, gram
- s. of exudate, gram
- s. of facial abscess, gram
- s. of pelvic abscess, gram
- s. of peritoneal fluid, gram
- s. of purulent discharge, gram
- s. of skin lesion, gram
- s. of sputum, acid-fast
- s. of stool specimen, gram
- s. of throat, gram
- s. of unspun urine, gram
- s. of urethra, gram
- s., Pap (Papanicolaou)
- s., Pappenheim's
- s., plasmatic
- s., plasmic
- s., port-wine
- s. procedure, gram
- s., protoplasmic
- s., Ringer's lactate
- s., Schiff's
- s., Schiller's
- s., Schuller's

s., selective
s., Shorr's
s., spinal fluid gram
s., sputum
s., sputum gram
s., Sudan
s., trichrome
s., tricose
s., tumor
s., van Gieson
s., Wade-Fite-Faraco
s., Weigert's
s., Weigert's hematoxylin
s., Wright's
s., Ziehl-Neelsen
stainable iron
stained
s. amniotic fluid, meconium
s. discharge, blood
s. fluid, dark blood
s. fluid, meconium
s., healthy tissue
s., meconium
s. mucus, blood
s. smear
s. smear and cultures
s. smear of clinical material
s. smear of stool
s. sputum, black
s. teeth
s. urinary sediment
staining
s., bipolar
s., chronic
s. coiled bacteria, lightly
s. cytoplasm, blue-
s., differential
s., double
s., fluorescent
s. gram-negative coccobacilli ▸ lightly
s. gram-positive rods ▸ large darkly
s., intravital
s., meconium
s. method, Harris
s., multiple
s., negative
s. nuclei, dark
s. nuclei, pale-
s. nucleus, deeply
s. of cornea, blood
s. of tissue ▸ silver
s., polar
s. polyhedral cells, pale-
s., postvital

s., preagonal
s. quality
s. reaction
s. simple
s., supravital
s. technique, gram
s., triple
s., vital
s., von Kossa
stainless steel
s.s. implant
s.s. mesh prosthesis, House
s.s. mesh stent
s.s. screw
s.s. strut
s.s. suture
s.s. wire, monofilament
stair(s)
s. claudication ▸ two flights of
s. climbing ▸ excessive
s., graduated
staircase phenomenon
stairclimbing exercise
stairway lift
stalk
s., abdominal
s., allantoic
s., basal
s., belly
s., body
s., cerebellar
s., connecting
s., connective tissue
s., degenerating yolk
s., hypophyseal
s., infundibular
s., neural
s., optic
s., pituitary
s., yolk
stalked hydatid
stall bars
stall the healing process
Stallard's operation
stamina
s. and endurance
s. and flexibility ▸ strength,
s., decreased
s., diminished
s., improved
stammering and stuttering
stammering bladder
Stamm's gastrostomy
Stamm's operation
Stamnosoma formosanum

stamp, muscle
stamper, optical disk
stance
s., disturbance of gait and
s., gait and
s., normal
s., single limb
s. time
stand
s. -alone laser treatment
s. crutch, jocked
s. exercise ▸ chair
s., inability to
s. -off, emotional
s. -off, verbal
s. transfer, sit-to-
standard(s)
s. antibody tests
s. Bruce protocol
s. cognitive technique
s. coil
s. configuration
s. dentures
s. deviation
s. deviation of the mean (SDM)
s. dose (NSD), nominal
s. electrode placement
s. error of the mean (SEM)
s., ethical
s., exposure
s. eye tests
s. gait
s. hospital treatment
s. hygienic practices
s. inpatient care
s. international system
s. isolation technique
s. limb lead
s. medical treatment
s. mortality ratio
s. of care
s. of clinical practice
s. of normality ▸ traditional
s. of practice, current
s. orders
s., Pignet's
s. procedure
s. procedure of rigorous analysis
s. psychological tests
s., quality control
s. radiation treatment
s. radical neck dissection
s. radiopharmaceutical
s. reduction rhinoplasty
s. rehabilitation technique

standard(s)—*continued*
- s. temperature and pressure (STP)
- s. 10-20 (ten-twenty) system
- s. test for syphilis
- s. therapy
- s. "Y" incision

standardized psychiatric evaluation
standardized treatment protocols
standby
- s. anesthesia
- s. assist, contact-
- s. assist with ambulation
- s. assistance
- s. assistance in transfers and ambulation
- s. assistance, patient transfers with
- s. pulse generator

standing (Standing)
- s. ambulation
- s. balance
- s. balance, safe
- s. clinic, free-
- S. Frame, Mobile
- s. frame, quadriplegic
- s. heart rate
- s. height
- s. ▸ lightheaded on
- s., long-
- s. orders
- s. orders on routine admission
- s. private psychiatric facility ▸ free-
- s., prolonged
- s., rapid
- s. symptomatology, long-

standpoint, clinical
standpoint, physical
standstill
- s., atrial
- s., auricular
- s., cardiac
- s., expiratory
- s., inspiratory
- s., respiratory
- s., sinus
- s., ventricular

Stanford
- S. -Binet test
- S. biopsy method
- S. -type aortic dissection

Stanicor pacemaker
Stanicor pacemaker, Omni-
Stanley Kent, bundle of
Stanmore shoulder arthroplasty

stannous pyrophosphate/polyphosphate, Tc (technetium) 99m
stapedectomy
- s., Guilford's
- s., Hough's
- s., House
- s., Schuknecht
- s., Shea
- s. technique, Guilford
- s. technique, Hough
- s. technique, House
- s. technique, Schuknecht
- s. technique, Shea

stapedial
- s. artery
- s. crus
- s. fold
- s. nerve
- s. tendon
- s. tendon cut

stapedis, caput
stapedis, plica
stapedius
- s., crus anterius
- s., crus posterius
- s. muscle
- s. nerve
- s. tendon

stapes
- s., abnormal
- s., anterior crus of
- s., base of
- s. bone
- s., capitulum of
- s., congenital defect in footplate of
- s., fixation of
- s., fixator muscle of base of
- s. fixed
- s. footplate
- s. hook
- s. mobilization
- s., posterior crus of

staph aureus prosthetic joint infection
staphylococcal (staphylococci) (Staph)
- s. abscess
- s., anaerobic
- s. bacteremia
- s. bronchitis
- s. carrier
- s. cellulitis
- s. clumping test
- s. contamination, environmental
- s. endocarditis
- s. enteritis
- s. enterocolitis
- s. impetigo
- s. infection
- s. infection of heart valve
- s. meningitis
- s. osteomyelitis
- s. pneumonia

Staphylococci, coagulase-negative
Staphylococcus/staphylococcus (Staph/staph)
- S. albus
- S. aureus
- S. aureus bacteremia
- S. aureus coagulase positive
- S. aureus, gram-positive
- S. aureus, hemolytic
- S. aureus (MRSA) ▸ methicillin-resistant
- S. aureus penicillinase
- s. bacterium
- s. bronchitis
- s. carrier, chronic
- S. citreus
- S. epidermidis
- S. genus
- S. haemolyticus
- S. hominis
- s. infection
- s., nonpenicillinase producing
- s. organism
- s. outbreak
- S. pyogenes
- S. saprophyticus
- S. simulans

staphylolysin
- s., alpha
- s., beta
- s., delta
- s., epsilon
- s., gamma

staphyloma
- s., annular
- s., anterior
- s., ciliary
- s. corneae
- s. corneae racemosum
- s., corneal
- s., equatorial
- s., intercalary
- s., posterior
- s. posticum
- s., projecting
- s., retinal

s., Scarpa's
s., scleral
s., uveal
Staple (staple)
S. implant cataract lens, Anis
s. lung reduction
s. procedure, Blount's
s. suture
stapler, EEA
stapler, TA-55
stapling
s., bleb
s. procedure, gastric
s., stomach
s. technique, stomach
star(s)
s. cells
s., daughter
s., lens
s., Winslow's
Starbardt's disease
starbursts of light
starch(es)
s. cone
s. equivalent
s., lichen
s., salted
s. sugar
stare(s)
s., blank
s., blank or downcast
s., fixed
s., patient
s. ▸ peculiar unblinking
s., wide
Starfish heart positioner
Stargardt's syndrome
staring and/or blinking
staring expression ▸ fixed
Starling('s)
S. curve
S. curve ▸ Frank-
S. equation
S. force
S. law
S. mechanism
S. mechanism ▸ Frank-
S. principle ▸ Frank-Straub-
Wiggers-
S. reserve ▸ Frank-
Starr-Edwards
S.E. aortic valve prosthesis
S.E. ball and cage valve
S.E. ball valve prosthesis
S.E. cardiac valve prosthesis

S.E. disk valve prosthesis
S.E. heart valve prosthesis
S.E. mitral prosthesis
S.E. mitral valve
S.E. pacemaker
S.E. prosthesis
S.E. prosthetic ball valve
S.E. Silastic valve
S.E. valve
S.E. valve prosthesis
start(s)
s. exercise ▸ stop-and-
s. heart ▸ jump-
s., hypnagogic
started ▸ heart jump-
started ▸ intravenous (IV) fluids
starting
s. and stopping of urinary stream
s. food and fluid ▸ stopping or
never
s. pains
s. urinary stream ▸ difficulty in
startle
s., hypnagogic
s. pattern
s. reaction ▸ heightened
s. reflex
s. response
startled, easily
startled reaction
starvation
s. acidosis
s. and dehydration ▸ death by
s. and purging (bulimarexia)
s. ketosis
s., self-
s. ▸ self-imposed
s., voluntary
s., voluntary self-
starved
s. brain ▸ oxygen (O_2)-
s. child, affect-
s. for oxygen-rich blood
s. heart muscle ▸ oxygen (O_2)-
s. heart muscle tissue, blood-
s. tissue, oxygen (O_2)-
starving behavior of anorexic
starving behavior of bulimic
stasis [*bases, basis*]
s., atrial
s., axoplasmic
s., bile
s. changes
s. changes, venous
s. cirrhosis

s. dermatitis
s. eczema
s. edema
s., extensive bile
s., focal bile
s., ileal
s., intestinal
s. ▸ massive centrilobular bile
s., papillary
s. pigmentation
s., pressure
s. retinopathy ▸ venous
s., secondary barium
s. ulcer ▸ venous
s. ulcers
s., urinary
s., venous
STAT (immediately)
STAT dialysis
STAT orders
state(s) (State) [*plate*]
s., active sleep
s., acute anxiety
s., acute pain
s., acute psychotic
s., alpha
s., altered mental
s. ▸ amphetamine-induced paranoid
psychotic
s. -and-trait anxiety
s., anxiety
s. (ATS) ▸ anxiety tension
s., anxious
s., awake
s., behavioral
s., borderline
s., cardiovascular steady
s., carrier
s., catatonic
s., central excitatory
s., central inhibitory
s., chronic anxiety
s. ▸ chronic schizophrenia-like
s. code
s., constitutional psychopathic
s. contraction, rested
s., correlated
s., cry
s., curarized
s., disease
s., disorganized
s. ▸ disorganized, dissociative
s., dissociative
s., dream
s., drowsing

state(s)—*continued*
s. during withdrawal, psychological
s. electronic behavior, solid
s., emotional
s., epileptic
s., euphoric
s., excited
s., febrile
s. -funded programs
s., ground
s., hyperadrenergic
s., hypercoagulable
s., hyperdynamic
s., hyperkinetic
s., hypnagogic
s., hypnoidal
s., hypnoleptic
s., hypnopompic
s., hypnotic
s., hysterical
s., immunity deficiency
s. in acute drug intoxication, psychological
s. in brain ▸ disordered
s. in flashback reactions, psychological
s. in panic reactions, psychological
s. induced by drugs ▸ hallucinatory
s. induced by drugs ▸ paranoid
s. induced, hyperdopaminergic
s., infantile
s., inotropic
s. laser utilizing ruby, solid
s., lethargic
s., local excitatory
s., lytic
s., marble
s. medicine
s., mental
s., metastable
s. ▸ near vegetative
s., noncurarized
s., noninfective
s. of conscious awareness, altered
s. of consciousness
s. of consciousness, alert
s. of consciousness, altered
s. of disease, advanced
s. of mental obtundity
s. of physical decay, patient in
s. of relaxation, induced
s. of shock
s. of unconsciousness
s. of untroubled calmness
s. -of-the-art medical care

s. -of-the-art techniques
s., overdose
s. ▸ pain-free
s., paranoid
s., patient in catatonic
s., patient in dazed
s., patient in vegetative
s. ▸ permanent vegetative
s., persistent vegetative
s. physics, solid
s., plastic
s., pluripotent
s., postabsorptive
s., postictal
s., postpartum
s., postsurgical
s., psychosis-like
s., psychotic
s., quiet-alert
s., refractory
s. ▸ relapse of paranoid psychotic
s., resting
s. ▸ schizophrenic-like psychotic
s., sensory-deprived
s., shift brain
s., simple paranoid
s., sleep
s., sleep-like
s., spiritual
s., steady
s., subjective
s., terminal
s., tolerate immune
S. total artificial heart ▸ Penn
s., toxic
S. -Trait Anxiety Inventory
s., trance-like
s., transitional
s., traumatic
s., twilight
s., typhoid
s., uncommunicative
s., voluntary control of internal
s., voluntary control of physiological
s., voluntary control of psychological
s., wakeful
s., waking
s. with overdosing, psychological

statement(s)
s., anatomical gift
s. ▸ makes abuse
s. ▸ makes obscene

Statham
S. electromagnetic flow meter

S. pressure transducer
S. strain gauge

static
s. activity, bacterio◇
s. ataxia
s. convulsion
s. dilation technique
s. disorder
s. exercise
s. reflex
s. refraction
s. scoliosis
s. shock
s. tremor

station
s., abnormal gait and
s. adequate, gait and
s. disturbance
s., gait and
s. lymph nodes ▸ first or second
s., proper
s. pull-through
s., Romberg

stationary
s. anode
s. bike
s. bridge
s. cataract
s. grid
s. lingual arch
s. paresis

statistics ▸ alcohol-related mortality
statistics, vital
statoconia ▸ traumatically detached
statotomic reflexes
stature
s., parents of short
s., patient is of small
s., patient short in
s., short
s. ▸ small in

status (Status)
s. ▸ alteration in mental
s. ▸ altered mentation or physical
s. anginosus
s., assessment of health
s., asthmaticus
s., bail
s., cardiac
s. changes ▸ mental
s. choreicus
s., cognitive
s., compensated cardiac
s. convulsivus
s., declining respiratory

s. degenerativus
s. dysmyelinatus
s. epilepticus
s. epilepticus electroencephalogram (EEG)
s. evaluation ▸ mental
S. Examination (BNMSE), Brief Neuropsychological Mental
s. examination, mental
s. examination ▸ psychiatric mental
s. ▸ fluctuating mental
s., functional
s. gastricus
s., grand mal
s., health
s., inpatient
s., intra-articular
s., Kamofsky
s. lymphaticus
s., marital
s., mental
s., mental health
s., muscle
s., neurologic
s., nutritional
s. of nodes, clinical
s. of patients, performance
s. offenders, delinquent
s. ▸ outpatient therapeutic suspension
s. parathyreoprivus
s., patient
s., patient performance
s., patient regained active
s., patient's emotional
s., perceptual
s. petit mal
s., physical
s. ▸ poor functional
s. postcholecystogastrostomy
s. postfistula placement
s., postmenopausal hormonal
s., postoperative
s., postreduction
s. praesens
s., preoperative
s. ▸ psychiatric mental
s., psychological
s. ▸ rapid change in mental
s., recovery
s. report, daily
s. scale, disability
s., single-parent
s., socioeconomic
s., stable financial

s., stable health
s., system parameter
s. test, mental
s. test, mini-mental
s. thymicolymphaticus
s. waxed and waned ▸ mental
s., work

Staunig's position
stay
s., appropriate lengths of
s. awake ▸ struggling to
s., hospital
s. (LOS), length of
s., length of hospital
s. ▸ short-term
s. suture, silk
s. sutures
s. unremarkable, hospital

STD (sexually transmitted disease)
STD (skin test dose)
steadily advancing tumor
steadily deteriorated, patient
steadiness, hand
steady
s. alpha rhythm
s. downhill course, patient had
s. potential
s. rhythm, slow
s. state
s. state, cardiovascular

steal [steel]
s., coronary
s., endoperoxide
s., iliac
s. mechanism
s. mechanism, coronary
s. phenomenon
s. phenomenon, coronary
s. ▸ pulmonary artery
s. ▸ renal splanchnic
s., subclavian
s. syndrome, carotid
s. syndrome, coronary
s. syndrome ▸ radial
s. syndrome, subclavian
s., transmural

steam
s. autoclaving
s. cautery
s. -fitters' asthma
s. inhalation
s. inhalation therapy
s. spray inhaler
s. sterilization
s. -sterilized gowns and masks

s. tent
s. vaporizer
Stearn's alcoholic
Stearn's alcoholic amentia
stearothermophilus, Bacillus
steatohepatitis (NASH) ▸ nonalcoholic
steatorrhea
s., idiopathic
s., mild
s., moderate
s., painless
s., severe
steatosis cardiaca
steatosis cordis
Stecher's position
steel [steal]
s. (SS) implant, stainless
s. (SS) mesh prosthesis ▸ House stainless
s. mesh stent ▸ stainless
s. (SS) screw, stainless
s. (SS) strut, stainless
s. (SS) suture, stainless
s. (SS) wire ▸ monofilament stainless
Steell murmur of heart, Graham-Steell's murmur
Steenbock unit
steepening of cornea, abnormal
steeple sign
steepling of trachea
steering-wheel injury
Steffanoff's ear reconstruction
Steidele complex
Stein
S. -Abbé lip flap
S. -Kazanjian lower lip flap
S. -Leventhal syndrome
Steinberg thumb sign
Steindler's
S. arthrodesis
S. flexorplasty
S. operation
Steinert's disease
Steinmann's extension
Steinmann's pin
Stella phenomenon, Arias-
stellata, Hemispora
stellata, rhinitis
stellate
s. block
s. block anesthesia
s. cataract
s. cell

stellate—*continued*
- s. cells of liver
- s. corpuscles, Langerhans'
- s. fracture
- s. ganglion
- s. ganglion block
- s. ganglion nerve block
- s. ganglion stimulation
- s. hair
- s. incision
- s. nerve block
- s. veins of kidney

stellatoidea, Candida
Stellwag's brawny edema
Stellwag's sign
stem(s)
- s. auditory evoked potentials (BAEP), brain
- s. auditory evoked response (BAER), brain
- s., blood effusion brain
- s., blood supply to brain
- s., brain
- s. bronchus
- s. bronchus ▸ distortion left main
- s. bronchus, left
- s. bronchus, main
- s. bronchus ▸ occlusion of main
- s. bronchus, right
- s. bronchus, right main
- s., cancer of brain
- s. cell
- s. cell autograft
- s. cell, committed
- s. cell engineering
- s. cell, hematopoietic
- s. cell leukemia
- s. cell lymphoma
- s. cell ▸ pleuripotential
- s. cell replacement
- s. cell transplant, autologous
- s. cell transplant ▸ fetus-to-fetus
- s. cell transplant ▸ limbal
- s. cell transplantation
- s. cells ▸ adult
- s. cells, bone marrow
- s. cells, donor
- s. cells ▸ harvested
- s. cells ▸ mesenchymal
- s. cells ▸ peripheral
- s. ▸ chemoreceptors in brain
- s. cirrhosis, pipe
- s. control, brain
- s., descending brain
- s. disease ▸ severe brain

- s., dorsal surface of brain
- s. evoked response (BSER), brain
- s. finger prosthesis, two-prong
- s. functions, brain
- s. glioma, brain
- s. hemorrhage, brain
- s., impairment of functions of brain
- s., irreversible cessation of all functions of entire brain including brain
- s., lesion of brain
- s., lower brain
- s., main
- s., massive infarct of brain
- s. nuclei, brain
- s. pessary
- s. reflexes, brain
- s. ▸ reticular formation of brain
- s. stool, pipe-
- s. stroke, brain
- s. stroke syndrome, post-brain
- s., tectum of brain
- s. ▸ transposition of arterial
- s. tumor, brain
- s., upper brain
- s. vascular disease, brain

Stenger hearing test
stenopeic disc
stenopeic iridectomy
stenosal murmur
stenosed aortic valve
stenosing
- s. tendinitis
- s. tendovaginitis
- s. tenosynovitis
- s. tenosynovitis, digital

stenosis(-es)
- s., airway
- s., anal
- s. and regurgitation, combined mitral
- s., anorectal
- s., antral
- s. (AS), aortic
- s., aortic valvular
- s., aortoiliac
- s., biliary
- s., bottle neck
- s., branch pulmonary artery
- s., bronchial
- s., buttonhole mitral
- s., calcific
- s., calcific aortic
- s., calcific mitral
- s., calcific nodular aortic

- s. (CAVS), calcific valve
- s., capillary
- s., caroticovertebral
- s., carotid artery
- s., cervical
- s., cervical spinal
- s., chronic aortic
- s., cicatricial
- s., circumflex artery
- s., congenital aortic
- s., congenital mitral
- s., congenital pyloric
- s. ▸ congenital spinal
- s., coronary
- s., coronary artery
- s., coronary ostial
- s. ▸ discrete subvalvular aortic
- s., distal
- s., Dittrich's
- s., double aortic
- s., eccentric
- s. ▸ enucleation of subaortic
- s., esophageal
- s. ▸ fibrous subaortic
- s. ▸ fish mouth-mitral
- s. ▸ flow limiting
- s. ▸ focal eccentric
- s., functional
- s., geometric
- s. ▸ geometry of
- s., granulation
- s. ▸ hemodynamically significant
- s. ▸ high grade
- s., hourglass
- s., hypertrophic muscular subaortic
- s., hypertrophic pyloric
- s., hypertrophic subaortic
- s. (IHSS), idiopathic hypertrophic subaortic
- s. in pulmonary valve
- s. infantile hypercalcemia syndrome ▸ supravalvular aortic
- s. jet, aortic
- s. left coronary artery, severe
- s. ▸ left main coronary
- s. ▸ lumbar spinal
- s. ▸ malignant esophageal
- s., meatal
- s. (MS), mitral
- s. ▸ mitral valve
- s. murmur, aortic
- s. murmur ▸ mitral
- s. ▸ myocardial infundibular
- s. ▸ napkin ring
- s., occult aortic

s. of aorta
s. of aortic valve
s. of bronchus
s. of canaliculus, cicatricial
s. of lacrimal passage
s. of lacrimonasal duct
s. of lacrimonasal duct, cicatricial
s. of mitral valve
s. of sphincter
s. of trachea
s. of vein
s., orificial
s. ▸ palliation of malignant
  esophageal
s., papillary
s. ▸ pathogenesis of pulmonary
  artery
s. ▸ peripheral pulmonic
s. ▸ point of critical
s., postdiphtheritic
s., postischemic
s., preventricular
s., pulmonary
s., pulmonary artery
s., pulmonary branch
s. ▸ pulmonary valve
s., pulmonic
s., pulmonic valvular
s., pyloric
s., renal artery
s., residual
s. ▸ rheumatic mitral valve
s. right coronary artery ▸ severe
s. ▸ saphenous vein graft
s., segmental
s. ▸ senescent aortic
s. ▸ severe pulmonic
s. ▸ silent mitral
s. ▸ single vessel coronary
s., spinal
s. ▸ stratified by carotid
s., subaortic
s., subglottic
s., subpulmonary
s., subpulmonic
s., subvalvular
s., subvalvular aortic
s. ▸ subvalvular mitral
s. ▸ symptomatic intracranial arterial
s. syndrome ▸ supravalvular aortic
s., tight
s., tracheal
s., tricuspid
s., urethral meatal
s., vaginal

s., valvular
s. ▸ valvular aortic
s., valvular pulmonic
s., vascular

stenostrepta, Spirochaeta
stenotic
s. area, fixed
s. esophagogastric anastomosis
s. femoral artery
s. lesion
s. process
s. segment
s. valve

stenotrophic parasite
Stenotrophomonas multiphilia
Stensen's
S. canal
S. duct
S. foramen
S. veins

Stenstrom foot flap
stent (Stent)('s)
s. apposition
s., balloon expandable intravascular
s., biodegradable
s., CardioCoil coronary
s., carotid
s., Carpentier's
s., chemically coated
s., coil
s., Cordis radiopaque tantalum
s., coronary
s. deployment
s. dressing
s. ▸ drug coated
s., eluting
s. expansion
s., foam rubber vaginal
S. graft
s. ▸ heat expandable
s. implantation
s. implantation, coronary
s., implanting
s., insertion of
s., intraoral
s., intravascular
s., keel
S. mass
s. ▸ Medtronic interventional
  vascular
s., mesh
s., metal
s. -mounted allograft valve
s. -mounted heterograft valve
s., occluded common bile duct

s. ▸ Palmaz-Schatz
s., percutaneous
s. ▸ physically coated
s. placement
s. placement ▸ coronary
s. plugging
s., polyethylene
s. ▸ polymeric endoluminal paving
s. procedure
s., radioactive
s. ▸ radiopaque tantalum
s. ▸ Schatz-Palmaz intravascular
s. ▸ Schatz-Palmaz tubular mesh
s., Schneider
s. ▸ self-expanding
s. ▸ spring-loaded
s. ▸ stainless steel mesh
s. strut
s., tantalum
s. technology
s. ▸ thermal memory
s., tie-over-
s. tube
s. tube with pigtail curl
s., ureteral
s., wall
s., Wiktor
s. ▸ zig-zag

stented coronary vessel
stenting
s., bailout
s., coronary
s., endoluminal
stentless
s. porcine aortic valve
s. porcine aortic valve prosthesis
s. porcine xenograft
Stenver x-ray view
Stenver's position
Stenzel rod prosthesis
step(s)
s. aerobics
s. -down therapy
s. exercise stress test ▸
  Gradational
s. exercise test ▸ two-
s. -families, blending of
s. -family couples
s. gait, double-
s. gait, intermittent double-
s., halting
s., Krönig's
s. program ▸ 12-
s., Rönne's nasal
s., sequential

step(s)—*continued*
- s., 12-
- s. -up in oxygen saturation
- s. -up transformer
- s. -wise movement ▸ jerky

stepladder appearance
stepladder stage
Step-One Diet
steppage gait
stepped contour
stepped-care antihypertensive regimen
stepping reflex
stercoraceous vomiting
stercoral colic
stercoral diarrhea
stercoralis, Strongyloides
stercorea, Chlamydophrys
stereognostic sense
stereologic assessment ▸ in vivo
stereopsis test, Worth
stereoroentgenography study
stereoscopic
- s. chest films
- s. interrogation
- s. microscope
- s. radiography
- s. vision
- s. zonography

stereotactic
- s. biopsy
- s. breast biopsy
- s. data
- s. /stereotaxic depth electroencephalogram (EEG)
- s. device
- s. frame, arc-shaped
- s. frame, Leksell's
- s. laser microsurgery, computer assisted
- s. localization
- s. measurements
- s. needle biopsy
- s. pallidotomy
- s. radiofrequency lesioning
- s. radiosurgery
- s. radiosurgery ▸ gamma knife
- s. surgery
- s. targeting

stereotaxic
- s. device, Leksell's
- s. neurosurgery
- s. surgery

stereotype/habit disorder

stereotyped
- s. behavior
- s. behavior of autistic children
- s. behavior ▸ repetitive
- s. repetitive movements

stereotypic behavior
stereotypical behavior ▸ increased
Sterges' carditis
sterile
- s. connecting tube
- s. drapes
- s. drapes applied
- s. draping of field
- s. dressing
- s. dressing applied
- s. dressing (DSD) applied ▸ dry
- s. dressing (DSD) ▸ dry
- s. drug
- s. environment
- s. field
- s. fluid
- s. immunity
- s. inflammation
- s. irrigation
- s. liquid cement, inject
- s. meningitis
- s. on culture, urine
- s. operative field
- s. ophthalmic solution
- s., patient
- s. pelvic examination
- s. physiological saline
- s. preparation and draping of field
- s. procedure
- s. redressing
- s. saline, area lavaged with
- s. saline basin
- s. saline solution
- s. sheet wadding
- s. site
- s. specimen
- s. technique
- s. thermometer
- s. towels, absorbent
- s. vacuum collection tube
- s. vaginal examination
- s. whirlpool therapy
- s. whirlpool treatment

sterilely, area prepared
sterilely prepped and draped
sterility
- s., absolute
- s. culture
- s., exercise induced
- s., female

- s., male
- s., one-child
- s., permanent
- s., primary
- s., relative
- s., secondary
- s., two-child
- s. workup

sterilization
- s., autoclaving
- s., chemical
- s., disinfection and antisepsis
- s., effective
- s., eugenic
- s., fractional
- s., gas
- s., heat
- s., intermittent
- s., involuntary
- s., irradiation
- s., laparoscopic
- s., mechanical
- s. procedure
- s. procedure evaluated
- s. procedure, proper
- s., steam
- s., tubal
- s. vasectomy

sterilized
- s. gowns and masks ▸ steam-
- s. instruments, gas
- s. instruments, inadequately
- s. membrane
- s. needles, inadequately
- s. syringes, inadequately

sterilizers, biological monitoring
sterilizers, monitoring of
sterilizing chamber
Steri-strips
Sterles' sign
sternal
- s. abscess
- s. angle
- s. biopsy
- s. border
- s. border (LSB) ▸ left
- s. border (RSB) ▸ right
- s. dehiscence
- s. depression
- s. infection
- s. intercostal retraction
- s. lead
- s. margin of left lung
- s. margin of right lung
- s. muscle

s. notch
s. plane
s. puncture
s. ribs
s. splitting incision
s. splitting procedure
s. splitting scar
s. synchondrosis
s. traction
s. wire sutures
s. wiring
s. wound infection

Sternberg('s)
S. cells ▸ Reed-
S. disease
S. myocardial insufficiency
S. pericarditis
S. sarcoma
S. sign

sternochondral junction
sternoclavicular
s. angle
s. articulation
s. joint
s. junction
s. ligament

sternocleidomastoid (SCM)
s. artery
s. hemorrhage
s. muscle
s. region
s. vein

sternocostal ligament
sternocostal triangle
sternohyoid muscle
sternomastoid muscle
sternospinal reference electrode
sternothyroid muscle
sternotomy
s., horizontal
s. incision ▸ median
s., median
s., vertical

sternoxiphoid plane
sternum
s. bone
s., clavicular notch of
s., costal notches of
s. depressed
s., jugular notch of
s., reflection of
s. saw
s., split
s. ▸ wiring of

steroid(s)
s. abuse, anabolic
s. administration, exogenous
s., anabolic
s., anti-inflammatory
s., cortisone
s. dependence
s. -dependent asthma
s. -dependent asthmatic
s. depletion
s. depletion of cortex
s. drug ▸ oral
s. eluting pacemaker lead
s. hormones
s. hormones, adrenal
s. implantation
s. -induced osteoporosis
s., inhaled
s., injected
s. injection
s., ketogenic
s. ▸ long-term
s. ▸ massive doses of
s. medication
s. myopathy
s. nasal spray
s. ointment
s., oral
s., oxogenic
s. pancreatitis
s., progestational
s. protein activity index (SPAI)
s., sex
s. sparing agent
s., stabnuclear neutrophil
s., synthetic
s., systemic
s. therapy
s. therapy in radiation therapy
s. therapy ▸ intermittent
s. therapy ▸ long-term
s. therapy ▸ prolonged
s. therapy, short-term
s., topical
s. treatment

steroidogenesis ▸ suppressing adrenal
steroidogenic potency
Steroli-Leydig cell tumor
stertorous breathing
stertorous respiration
stethoscope
s., binaural
s., Cammann's
s., decontaminate

s. ▸ DeLee-Hillis obstetric
s., differential
s., electronic
s., esophageal
s., Leff
s., obstetrical

stethoscopic phonocardiograph
Stevens-Johnson syndrome
Stevenson's test
sthenic [*asthenic*]
s. fever
s. type

STI (structured treatment interruptions)
Stick(s) (stick)
S. (marijuana cigarette)
s. ▸ accidental needle
s., arterial
s., blood gas
s., contaminated needle
s. deformity ▸ hockey
s. exposure, needle
s. fracture, hickory-
s. incision, hockey
s. incision, Meyer's hockey
s. injury, needle
s. ▸ intravenous needle
s. medicine ▸ finger-
s. -on electrode
s. -on nicotine patch
s. pain ▸ heel
s., sponge
s., swab
s. test ▸ routine
s. -tie suture
s. transmission ▸ needle

stickers, donor
stickiness of platelets
sticklandii, Clostridium
sticky
s. mucus ▸ thick,
s. plaques
s. proteins
s. stools

Stieda('s)
S. calcification, Pellegrini-
S. disease, Pellegrini-
S. fracture

stiff
s. -heart
s. -heart syndrome
s., inflamed joints ▸ swollen,
s. lung
s. neck
s. pupil

stiffening
- s. and deformity of legs
- s. and shaking ▸ body
- s., arthritic
- s. of body
- s. of joint
- s. of lens

stiffneck fever

stiffness
- s. ▸ aches, pains and
- s., aching and
- s., aching and burning pain
- s., active dynamic
- s. and discomfort in ligaments
- s. and discomfort in muscles
- s. and discomfort in tendons
- s. and pain ▸ edema,
- s. and restriction of movement
- s. and soreness ▸ muscle
- s. and unsteadiness ▸ tremor, slowness,
- s., arterial
- s., chamber
- s., diastolic
- s., disabling
- s., elastic
- s. ▸ feeling of tingling and
- s. from arthritis
- s. from disease of artery
- s., hip
- s. in back
- s., index
- s. ▸ joint pain and
- s., leg
- s., morning
- s., muscle
- s. ▸ muscle tension, aching, pain and
- s., myocardial
- s. of extremities
- s. of glands, goiter or
- s. of joints
- s. of neck
- s. or heaviness of limbs
- s., pain and
- s., pain and lack of mobility
- s., progressive
- s., shoulder
- s., spinal
- s., tremors and immobility
- s., vascular
- s., volume
- s. ▸ widespread muscle aching and

stifle joint

stigma
- s., costal
- s., follicular
- s., Giuffrida-Ruggieri
- s., hysteric
- s., malpighian
- s. of degeneracy
- s., psychic
- s., psychosocial
- s., social
- s., somatic

stigmata ▸ patent ductus renal agenesis with associated

stigmata, peripheral

stigmatic electrode

stigmatization, social

stilet/stilette (see stylet)

Still('s) (still)
- S. disease
- S. murmur
- s. ▸ patient unable to sit

stillbirth, patient had
- s. infant
- s., macerated
- s., patient delivered

stillborn, patient had

Stille('s)

Stiller's sign

Stilling('s)
- S. canal
- S. chart
- S. column
- S. fibers
- S. fleece
- S. nucleus
- S. -Türk-Duane syndrome

Stim apparatus, Osteo-

Stim-U-Dents

stimulans, Aedes

stimulant
- s. abuse, pattern of
- s. abuse, physical effects of
- s., abuse potential of
- s. abuse, prevalence of
- s. abusers, assessing needs of
- s., acute intoxication with
- s., adrenergic
- s., alcoholic
- s., cardiac
- s., central
- s., cerebral
- s., chronic
- s., CNS (central nervous system)
- s., dependence on
- s., detoxification from

- s., diffusible
- s. drug
- s., effects of
- s. expectorant
- s., flashback reactions with
- s., general
- s., genital
- s., heart
- s., hepatic
- s., intestinal
- s., kidney
- s., local
- s., long-acting thyroid
- s. medication
- s., mode of administration with
- s., nerve
- s., nervous
- s., organic brain syndrome with
- s., panic reactions with
- s., patient OD (overdosed) with
- s., psychoactive doses of
- s., psychoactive properties of
- s., psychological effects of
- s., psychotic reactions with
- s., respiratory
- s., sedative-
- s., sexual
- s., spinal
- s., stomachic
- s., sympathomimetic
- s., tolerance to
- s., topical
- s., toxicity of
- s., treatment of acute drug reactions to
- s., uterine
- s., vascular
- s., vasomotor
- s., withdrawal from

stimulate(s) [simulate]
- s. adequate spontaneous breathing
- s. appetite
- s. bone formation
- s. bone growth
- s. breathing
- s. calcium receptors in heart
- s. formation and increase mass in bone
- s. growth of prostate
- s. growth, protein
- s. heart muscle
- s. immune system ▸ vaccine
- s. mental function
- s. nerve impulse
- s. new vessel growth

s. pituitary gland
s. production of female sex estrogen hormone
s. production of progesterone
s. prolactin production
s. respiration
s. the immune system
s. viral replication

stimulated

s. analysis, pentagastrin
s. appetite
s. by injury, receptor
s. dopamine transmission
s. echo artifact
s. emission of radiation (laser) beam, light amplification by
s. emission of radiation (laser) ▸ light amplification by
s. emission of radiation (MASER) ▸ microwave amplification by
s., intellectually

stimulatic circulation

stimulatic dopamine production in brain

stimulating

s. activity ▸ intellectually
s. activity ▸ mentally
s. blood flow
s. cornea
s. electrode pair
s. electrodes
s. environment
s. factor, colony
s. factor, erythropoietic
s. factor (GM-CSF), human granulocytic-macrophage colony
s. fetus into activity
s. hobbies
s. hormone (FSH) ▸ follicle-
s. hormone, glomerular-
s. hormone, growth-
s. hormone inhibiting factor (MSHIF) ▸ melanocyte-
s. hormone, interstitial cell
s. (LATS) hormone, long-acting thyroid-
s. hormone (MSH) ▸ melanocyte-
s. hormone (MSH) ▸ melanophore-
s. hormone (TSH), thyroid
s. insulin release

stimulation (Stimulation)

s., alpha adrenergic
s., anti-gravity
s. ▸ audio-visual-tactile
s., beta adrenergic

s., beta adrenoceptor
s., block nervous system
s., brain
s., breast
s., caloric
s., cardiovascular
s., carotid sinus
s., chemical
s., deep brain
s., device, electrical
s., digital
s., electrical
s. (EMS) ▸ electrical muscle
s., electrical nerve
s. ▸ electrical spinal cord
s., electromagnetic
s., electronic
s., estrogenic
s., external
s. ▸ external sensory
s., faradic
s. (FAS) ▸ fetal acoustic
s., flash
s., forebrain
s., full field
s. (FES), functional electrical
s., galvanic
s., gentle
s. ▸ high frequency
s., hormonal
s. in pacing ▸ myocardial
s., insulin
s., intellectual
s., intermittent photic
s., levels of
s., light
s., locomotor
s., low intensity
s., marked respiratory
s., mechanical
s., mental
s., monotonous
s., muscle
s., nerve
s., neurohormonal
s., neurologically over-responsive
s., neuromuscular electrical
s., noninvasive programmed
s., nonspecific
s. of atria ▸ electrical
s. of auditory nerve ▸ electrical
s. of beta receptors
s. of brain, electrical
s. of hand ▸ electrical
s. of heart ▸ electrical

s. of leg ▸ electrical
s. of lower bowel
s. of lymphocytes, mitogenic
s. of muscle contraction
s. of nerve endings
s. of peripheral nerves
s. of pressure points
s. of receptors
s. of right atrium ▸ catheter
s. of semicircular canal
s. of senses ▸ intensive
s. of skin
s. of trigger areas
s. of urinary bladder
s. of ventricles ▸ electrical
s., outside
s. ▸ paired electrical
s., paradoxical
s., paraspecific
s., parasympathetic
s., pattern reversal
s., patterned visual
s. ▸ persistent inflammatory
s., photic
s., physical
s., pituitary
s., point of
s. procedure, photic
s., program
s., program, infant
s., programmed electrical
s. ▸ pulmonary hypothalamic
s., punctual
s., reaction to aversive
s., reduced
s., reflex
s., repeated electrical
s., repetitive electrical
s., repetitive photic
s., repetitive sound
s. response, Hallpike caloric
s., response of brain to electrical
s., response to light
s., restricted environmental
s., sensory
s. ▸ short-term
s. sites, optimal
s., skin
s. ▸ slaved programmed electrical
s., square wave
s. ▸ stellate ganglion
s. study
s., submaximal
s., subthreshold
s. ▸ supramaximal tetanic

stimulation—*continued*
s., sympathetic
s., synthesis
s., tactile
s., temporal bone
s. test, Hallpike caloric
s. test, histamine
s. test ▸ internal scalp
s. test, meal
s. test, penagastric
s., thalamic deep brain
s. therapy
S. Therapy (REST) ▸ Reduced
   Environmental
s. threshold
s. to brain, periodic electrical
s. to nerve, electrical
s. to spinal cord, electrical
s. ▸ transcranial magnetic
s. (TES), transcutaneous electrical
s. (TENS), transcutaneous
   electrical nerve
s., transcutaneous nerve
s. ▸ transesophageal atrial
s., tumor
s. ▸ ultrarapid subthreshold
s., unvarying
s., vagal
s., vagus
s. ▸ vagus nerve
s. ▸ ventricular programmed
s., virtual
s., visual
s., visual or auditory

stimulator
s., alpha
s., cardiac
s., deep brain
s. (DCS) ▸ dorsal column
s., electronic
s., external electronic
s. for pain relief, electrical
s., Hilger facial nerve
s., implantable bone growth
s. ▸ implantable gastric
s., impulse
s. ▸ long-acting thyroid
s., muscle
s., photic
s., receiver-
s., Reese's
s. ▸ spinal cord
s., thalamic
s., transcutaneous

s. (TENS), transcutaneous
   electronic nerve
s. ▸ 22 channel receiver
s. (VNS) ▸ vagus nerve
stimulus(-i) (Stimulus)
s., abdominal
s., abnormal electrical
s., acoustic
s. -action hunger
s., adequate
s., auditory
s., autonomic response to anxiety-
   evoking
s., aversive
s., binaural
s., chemical
s., conditioned
s. conditioning
s. control
s. control methods
s. control therapy
s., discriminative
s., double extra
s. ▸ double ventricular extra
s., electric
s., electrical
s., eliciting
s. environment, low
s. environment, normal
s., environmental
s., excessive sensitivity to painful
s., external
s., fat
s. frequency
s., gustatory
s., heterologous
s., heterotopic
s., homologous
s. hunger
s. ▸ hyperreactivity to
s., identical
s. -induced pain
s., intellectual
s. intensity
s. isolation
S. Isolation Unit (SIU)
s., liminal
s. magnitude
s., mechanical
s., neural
s., neurohumoral
s., nociceptive
s., nomotopic
s., noxious
s. of trauma

s., onset of
s., pacemaker
s., pacing
s., pain
s., painful
s., patient combative to
s. pattern
s., perception of noxious
s., phobic
s., physical
s., physiological
s., primary
s., proprioceptive
s., provocative
s., psychological
s. pulse
s., reinforcing
s., remote external
s., repetitive
s., resistant to
s. response mechanism
s. ▸ responsiveness to external
s., rhythmic
s., sensory
s., sensory sound
s., series of
s., sharp
s., sound
s. ▸ square wave
s., stressful
s., subliminal
s., sudden sensory
s., supraliminal
s., thermal
s. ▸ threatening external
s. threshold
s., tracewriting
s., triple
s., unconditioned
s., unknown
s., unstructured
s., various
s., verbal
s., vestibular
s., warning
s. wave
s. wave form
sting
s. ▸ allergic reaction to
s. allergy ▸ bee
s. allergy, insect
s. anaphylaxis ▸ insect
s., bee
s. ▸ blister from insect
s. ▸ dizziness from insect

s. hypersensitivity, bee
s., marine-life
s. ▸ pain in abdomen from insect
s., sunscreen
s. treatment ▸ emergency insect
s. treatment, insect
stinginess, emotional
stinging insect bite
Stipa viridula
stipple cell
stippled
s. appearance
s. epiphyses
s. tongue
stippling
s., basophilic
s., malarial
s., Maurer's
s., Schüffner's
stirrup(s)
s. anastomosis
s. bone
s. brace
s., Finochietto's
s., legs positioned in
stitch(es)
s. abscess
s. and no patch cataract removal ▸ no
s. cataract procedure ▸ one-
s. cataract surgery ▸ no
s., cosmetic
s., episiotomy
s., imbricating
s. ▸ inverting
s., no-patch cataract surgery ▸ no-
s., perineal support
s., running lock-
s., self-locking
s., seromuscular
s., side
s., subcuticular
s., supporting
s. suture, lock-
s. technique, one-
stitched together ▸ tongue-and-groove
stitching, peritoneal
stix, Dextro◊
STM (scanning tunneling microscope)
STM (short term memory)
stock (Stock)('s)
s. culture
s. operation

S. -Spielmeyer-Vogt syndrome
Stocker's needle
Stockert cardiac pacing electrode
Stockholm box
Stockholm syndrome
stockinette
s. amputation bandage
s. applied, dressings and
s. dressing
stocking(s)
s. -and-glove type hypesthesia
s., antiembolism
s., compression
s., elastic compression
s. glove distribution
s. ▸ graduated compression
s., Jobst's
s. ▸ pneumatic compression
s. seam incision
s., support
s., surgical support
s., TED (thromboembolic disease)
s. ▸ thigh-high antiembolic
s. ▸ venous pressure gradient support
Stoeckel operation ▸ Frangenheim-Goebell-
Stoeckel operation, Goebel-
Stoerck's loop
Stofa (heroin)
stoichiometric fashion
stoker's cramp
Stokes(')
S. -Adams syndrome
S. amputation
S. amputation, Gritti-
S. asthma, Cheyne-
S. attack, Adams-
S. breathing, Cheyne-
S., collar of
S. expectorant
S. lens
S. psychosis, Cheyne-
S. respiration, Cheyne-
S. sign, Cheyne-
S. syncope, Adams-
S. syndrome
S. syndrome, Adams-
S. syndrome ▸ Morgagni-Adams-
Stoll's pneumonia
stoma [*stroma, struma*]
s., abdominal
s., abdominal wall
s., artificial
s., formation of

s., gastric
s., gastroenterostomy
s., ileal loop
s. irrigated
s., tracheostomy
stomach
s., aberrant umbilical
s. acid
s., acid content of
s. acid into esophagus ▸ backwash of
s. acidity
s. acidity, neutralize
s. adenocarcinoma
s., anastomosis end of
s. and bowel functions ▸ normal
s. and duodenum ▸ closure open ends of
s. aspirate
s., aviator's
s., barium passed through esophagus into
s., bilocular
s. bleeding
s. bloating
s., burning sensation in
s. cancer of
s. capacity
s. carcinoma
s., cardia of
s. cardiac
s., cardiac notch of
s., cardiac section of
s. cascade
s. cirrhosis of
s. ▸ congestion of mucosa of
s. contents
s. contractions
s. cough
s. cramps
s., cup-and-spill
s. decompressed
s., diabetic
s., diffuse histiocytic lymphoma of
s. digestion
s., dilatation of
s. disorder
s. distended
s. distended with fluid
s., dumping
s. empties promptly
s. enzymes
s. epithelial lining of
s. erosions in
s. ▸ feeling sick to

stomach—*continued*
- s. filled
- s. flu
- s. fluid
- s. formation
- s. ▸ freshly clotted blood in
- s., fundus of
- s., gas in
- s., greater curvature of
- s., growling
- s., Holzknecht's
- s., hourglass
- s., inflammation of
- s., intrathoracic
- s., irritable
- s. irritation
- s., leather bottle
- s., lesser curvature of
- s. lining
- s. lining, aspirin irritates
- s. lining, irritation of
- s., lymphatic nodules of
- s. meridian
- s., miniature
- s. ▸ mucosal surfaces of
- s. ▸ multiple ulcers of
- s. ▸ muscular wall of
- s., nasogastric (NG) tube in
- s. nerves
- s. ▸ neutralizing acid in
- s. ▸ non-Hodgkin's lymphoma of
- s., normal appearing
- s. pain
- s. pain and vomiting
- s., partial emptying of
- s., partial resection of
- s., Pavlov's
- s. ▸ persistent inflammation of
- s. polyps
- s., powdered
- s. protective lining of mucous
- s., pumping
- s., pylorus of
- s., reflux from
- s., retained secretions in
- s., rugal folds of
- s., rugal pattern of
- s., sclerotic
- s., scope advanced to cardia of
- s. sleeper
- s. sleeping
- s. ▸ small, flat, white patches on mucosa of
- s., softening of the
- s. spasms
- s. staggers
- s. stapling
- s. stapling technique
- s., suction
- s., thoracic
- s. tooth
- s., trifid
- s. tube
- s. ulcer
- s. ulcer, bleeding
- s., upside-down
- s., villous folds of
- s. wall
- s. waterfall
- s. water-trap
- s. worm

stomachal vertigo
stomachic stimulant
stomachic tonic
stomal ulcer
stomatitis
- s., allergic
- s., angular
- s., annular
- s., aphthobullous
- s. aphthosa
- s., aphthous
- s., arsenicalis
- s., catarrhal
- s., contact
- s., epidemic
- s., epizootic
- s., erythematopultaceous
- s. exanthematica
- s., fusospirochetal
- s., gangrenous
- s., gonococcal
- s., herpetic
- s. herpetica
- s., hyphomycetica
- s., infectious
- s. intertropica
- s. intertropica, psilosis
- s., medicamentosa
- s., membranous
- s., mercurial
- s. mycetogenetica
- s., necrotizing ulcerative
- s. nicotina
- s., nonspecific
- s., oral
- s., residual
- s. scarlatina
- s. scorbutica
- s., syphilitic
- s. traumatica
- s., tropical
- s., ulcerative
- s., ulceromembranous
- s., uremic
- s. venenata
- s., vesicular
- s., Vincent's
- s. virus, vesicular
- s., vulcanite
- s. with bleeding

stomatology, forensic
stomatorrhagia gingivarum
stone(s) (Stone)('s)
- s., artificial
- s. asthma
- s., autochthonous
- s. basket
- s. basket, Dormia
- s. basket, Ellik kidney
- s., bile duct
- s., biliary
- s., bladder
- s., blue
- s., calcium
- s., calcium oxalate
- s., calyceal
- s., chalk
- s., cholesterol
- s., chronically inflamed gallbladder with
- s. ▸ common bile duct
- s., common duct
- s., crush large
- s. cutters' phthisis
- s., cystine
- s. degeneration, paving
- s. density classification
- s., dental
- s., disintegrating kidney
- s., disintegration, monitor
- s. dislodger
- s., dissolve common bile duct
- s., dissolve kidney
- s., eye
- s. formation
- s., fragment
- s. fragmentation ▸ kidney
- s. fragmentation ▸ renal
- s., gall◊
- s. heart
- s. imaging and localization
- s., impacted
- S. implant
- s. in gallbladder ▸ palpable

s., infection
s., kidney
s. ▸ kidney calcium
s. localization
s., lung
s. management
s. manipulation, percutaneous
s., metabolic
s., mixed
s., multiple facetted
s., palpable
s., passage of
s., passing of kidney
s., pigment
s. placenta
s. present in pancreatic duct
s., pulp
s., pulverize
s., puncta calcific
s., radiant
s., radio nonopaque
s., radiolucent
s. removal ▸ ureteroscopic
s., rotten
s., salivary
s. searcher
s., skin
s., staghorn
s., strain stools for
s. -strippers asthma
s., struvite
s., tear
s. tongue, cobble-
s., ureteral
s., urinary
s., vein
s., visible
s., womb
Stookey operation, Guleke-
Stookey reflex
stool(s)
  s., bilious
  s., black tarry
  s., blood coating
  s., blood in
  s. blood test
  s., blood tinged
  s., bloody
  s., bulky
  s., caddy
  s. card test
  s., change in color and consistency
    of
  s., clay-colored
  s., coke-colored

s. colonization
s. culture
s. culture negative for pathogens
s. ▸ dark, bloody
s., digital removal of
s. evaluation
s., explosive
s., fatty
s. for ova and parasites
s. for stones, strain
s., frequent
s., guaiac negative
s., guaiac positive
s., guaiac test of
s., hemocult positive
s., hemorrhagic
s., impacted
s., in rectum
s., inability to control
s. incontinence
s., lienteric
s., light-colored
s., loose
s., loose black
s., loose watery
s., meconium
s., melanotic
s., melenic
s., mucous
s. ▸ mucus in
s., occult blood in
s., oily
s. ▸ pale and malodorous
s. passage ▸ hard
s., pathological
s., patient incontinent of
s., pea soup
s., pencil-shaped
s., pencil-thin
s., pipe-stem
s. positive for occult blood
s., pus coating
s., residual
s., retained
s., ribbon-shaped
s., rice water
s., sago-grain
s., scybalous
s. showed normal flora
s., silver
s. ▸ soft and ribbon-like
s. softener
s., solid
s. specimen
s. specimen, gram stain of

s., spinach
s., stained smear of
s., sticky
s., tarry
s. ▸ tarry black
s., unable to control
s., watery
s. with Crohn's disease ▸ pale
stooped
  s. over posture
  s. posture
  s., rigid and
stop (Stop)
  s. and rest syndrome
  s. -and-start exercise
  S. Child Abuse and Neglect (SCAN)
  s. -cock
  s. hurting (MASH) ▸ make arthritis
  s. or reverse complication of
    diabetes ▸ prevent,
  s. -valve airway obstruction
stoppage, heart
stopping
  s. of urinary stream, starting and
  s. or never starting food and fluid
  s. power, total mass
  s., thought
storage
  s. and transportation ▸ tooth
  s. cells
  s. device
  s. disease, cholesterol ester
  s. disease, glycogen
  s. disease ▸ inherited iron
  s. disease ▸ iron
  s. disease ▸ polysaccharide
  s., intermediate
  s. location, memory
  s., memory
  s. of blood
  s. technique ▸ refine bone
  s. test, glycogen
stored
  s., bone marrow removed and
  s., excised cornea
  s. fat
  s. marrow ▸ reinfusion of
storiform pattern
storing medication
stork bite
storkleg deformity
storm, thyroid
Stormer viscosimeter
stormy course, patient had
stormy course postoperatively

story preference
Story Test ▸ Make-A-Picture-
Storz' magnet
STP (standard temperature and
    pressure)
STP (Serenity-Tranquility-Peace) pill
strabismic deviation
strabismus
    s., absolute
    s., accommodative
    s., acute paralytic
    s., alternating
    s., A-pattern
    s., bilateral
    s., binocular
    s., Braid's
    s., comitant
    s., concomitant
    s., constant
    s., convergent
    s. corrected
    s. deorsum vergens
    s., divergent
    s., dynamic
    s., external
    s. hook
    s., horizontal
    s., incomitant
    s., intermittent
    s., internal
    s., kinetic
    s., latent
    s., manifest
    s., mechanical
    s., monocular
    s., monolateral
    s., muscular
    s., nonconcomitant
    s., nonparalytic
    s. of eye
    s., paralytic
    s., periodic
    s., relative
    s., spasmodic
    s., suppressed
    s. sursum vergens
    s., unilateral
    s., uniocular
    s., vertical
Strachan-Scott syndrome
straddling
    s. aorta
    s. atrioventricular (AV) valve
    s. embolism
    s. embolus

    s. thrombus
    s. tricuspid valve
straight
    s. arm lifts
    s. back syndrome
    s. beam linear accelerator, low
    energy
    s. enamel
    s. flush percutaneous catheter
    s. front punches
    s. leg raising (SLR)
    s. leg raising (SLR) limited
    s. leg raising (SLR) ▸ negative
    s. leg raising tenderness (SLRT)
    s. leg raising (SLR) test
    s. leg raising test (SLRT)
    s. leg sit-ups
    s. -line EKG (electrocardiogram)
    s. line, patient walks
    s. -pin teeth
    s. protrusive occlusion
straighten back ▸ inability to
straighten ▸ pain in back with
    instability to
straightening, tooth
strain(s) [*sprain*]
    s. ▸ acute muscle
    s., back
    s., beta hemolytic
    s., blood-borne
    s., cardiovascular
    s., cell
    s., chronic low back
    s., drug-resistant
    s., emotional
    s. ▸ enterococcus faecalis
    s., epidemic
    s., eye
    s., family
    s. film
    s., flu
    s. fracture
    s. gauge
    s. gauge plethysmography
    s. gauge, Statham
    s., heterologous
    s., high-jumper's
    s., homologous
    s. in exercise ▸ avoid
    s., ingrown positive
    s. injuries, repetitive
    s. injury ▸ overuse
    s. injury (RSI), repetitive
    s., inversion
    s., jaw

    s., left ventricular
    s., ligamentous
    s. ▸ Listeria monocytogenes
    s., low back
    s., lumbosacral
    s., major viral
    s. ▸ minimize stress and
    s., muscle
    s., muscular
    s., musculoskeletal stress and
    s., myocardial injury
    s. of bacteria ▸ resistant
    s. of bacteria, specific
    s. of pneumococcus ▸ resistant
    s. or exhaustion
    s. or wrenching
    s. pattern
    s. pattern, ventricular
    s., physical
    s., predominant
    s., prototype
    s., psychological
    s. ▸ reduce stress and muscle
    s., relieve muscle
    s., resistance
    s., resistant
    s., right heart
    s., sacroiliac
    s. sensation
    s., shoulder
    s. -specific
    s. stools for stones
    s., stress and physical
    s., susceptible
    s., swine influenza
    s., thymidine dependent
    s., valgus
    s., varus
    s., Vi
    s., virulent
    s., virus
    s. x-ray, inversion
    s. x-rays
strained muscles
straining
    s., abdominal
    s. and coughing
    s., flexing, lifting
    s., lifting and/or
    s. on bowel movement
strait ▸ entrance of fetal head into
    superior pelvic
strait, pelvic
straitjacket, chemical
Strampelli implant cataract lens

strand(s) (Strand)
- s., Billroth's
- s. conformational polymorphism (SSCP) ‣ single
- s. crutches, Loft◊
- s., cut fibrous
- s., DNA (deoxyribonucleic acid)
- s., fibrotic
- s., fibrous
- s., genetic
- s., iridium
- s., lateral enamel
- s., linear
- s., muscle
- s. of tissue
- s. pulled taut
- s., scar
- s., visual
- s., vitreous

strandy infiltrate

strange environments

stranger anxiety

stranger donor

strangulated
- s. hemorrhoid
- s. hernia
- s. small bowel

strangulation
- s., death due to
- s., external
- s., intestinal
- s. of bladder

strangury/stranguria

strap (Strap)
- s., chin
- s. incision, shoulder-
- s., Montgomery
- s. muscles
- s. -on pump
- S. operation
- S. procedure
- s. resonance, shoulder-
- s. sling

strapping, eversion tape

Strassman-Jones operation

Strassmann's phenomenon

strategic
- s., experiential, and ego-analytic approach
- s. family therapy
- s. therapy

strategy(-ies) (Strategy)
- s., aggressive
- s., alcohol prevention
- s., apply coping

- s., attack
- s., bathroom
- s., cognitive
- s., coping
- s. ‣ effective treatment
- S. Enhancement (CSE), Coping
- s. ‣ expected intervention
- s., Gandhi
- s. ‣ hard-nose
- s., healthy coping
- s. ‣ innovative psychiatric nursing intervention
- s., intervention
- s. ‣ invasive management
- s., management
- s., pacemaker
- s. ‣ pain management
- s. ‣ perseveration of
- s., pharmacological
- s. procedure
- s. ‣ protective survival
- s., psychosocial
- s., psychotherapeutic
- S. questionnaire, Coping
- s., relapse-specific
- s., soft
- s., therapeutic
- s. ‣ therapeutic milieu management
- s., treatment
- s., vaccine

stratification, ring

stratification, risk

stratified
- s. by carotid stenosis
- s. squamous epithelium
- s. squamous epithelium, nonkeratinizing
- s. thrombus

stratum corneum

stratum granulosum

Straub-Wiggers-Starling principle ‣ Frank-

Strauss angiitis, Churg-

Strauss syndrome, Churg-

straw
- s. -colored fluid
- s. -colored fluid ‣ serous
- s. -colored pericardial fluid
- s. -colored serous fluid
- s. -colored urine

strawberry
- s. hemangioma
- s. mark
- s. tongue
- s. tongue, red

stray cancer cells

Strayer procedure

streak
- s., angioid
- s. culture
- s., fatty
- s., germinal
- s., Knapp's
- s., medullary
- s., meningeal
- s., primitive

streaked
- s. discharge, blood
- s. ovaries
- s. with blood
- s. with blood, mucous fluid

streaking, fibrous

streaky infiltrate

stream
- s., axial
- s., blood
- s. ‣ difficulty in starting urinary
- s., flow of urinary
- s. of thought
- s. ‣ slow, hesitant urinary
- s., starting and stopping of urinary
- s., urinary
- s. ‣ weak or interrupted urine
- s. ‣ weak urinary

street (Street)
- s. drugs
- s. impurities
- S. intramedullary nail, Hansen-
- S. nail, Hansen-
- S. nail, Vesely-
- s. names for drugs
- s. people
- S. pin, Hansen-
- S. -type medullary pin
- s. virus

Streiff syndrome, Hallermann-

Streit slit lamp, Haag-

strength(s)
- s., abdominal
- s., abdominal muscle
- s. and balance ‣ muscle mass,
- s. and coordination
- s. and endurance, muscle
- s. and endurance ‣ physical
- s. and flexibility
- s. and flexibility ‣ regain muscle
- s. and mobility
- s. and walking ‣ mobility, muscle
- s. and weakness, areas of

strength(s)—*continued*
s., balance and flexibility ▸ endurance,
s., bolster muscle
s., bone
s. -building experience ▸ aerobic and
s. conditioning
s., current
s., decreased
s., decreased muscle
s. duration curve
s., edge-
s., endurance and flexibility
s., first
s., gifts and creativity
s., grasp
s., greatest
s., grip
s. ▸ hand grip
s. ▸ increased muscle
s., leg
s. levels
s. ▸ long-term restoration of muscle
s. ▸ loss of
s. ▸ loss of bone
s., loss of muscle
s. ▸ lower body
s., lower extremity
s., maintain muscle
s., momentary loss of
s., muscle
s. ▸ muscle testing for
s., muscular
s. of bone mass ▸ density and
s. of myocardial contraction ▸ inherent
s. or fainting ▸ sudden loss of
s. ▸ overall body
s., patient lower extremity
s., patient upper extremity
s. rating
s. relation ▸ interval
s., second
s., sensation and reflex testing
s. ▸ shoulder muscle
s., stamina and flexibility
s. ▸ sudden loss of
s., tensile
s. test, hand
s. test ▸ muscle
s. training
s. training exercise
s. -training program
s., triple

s. tuberculin test, first
s. tuberculin test, second
s. ▸ upper body
s., upper extremity
s., voluntary control and

strengthen
s. and tone muscle groups
s. back muscles
s. muscles of evacuation
s. reality focus

strengthening
s. and flexibility exercises
s. bone mass
s., ego
s. exercise
s. exercise, back
s. exercise ▸ muscle
s. exercise ▸ neck
s. exercise ▸ toe
s. exercises, active quad
s. exercises, isometric quad
s. exercises, quad
s., muscle
s. technique, ego-

strenuous
s. activity
s. activity ▸ repetitive weight bearing,
s. contact sports
s. exercise
s. physical activity

strep (*see*** Streptococcus)**
strep endocarditis ▸ green
streptobacillary fever
Streptobacillus moniliformis
streptocerca, microfilaria
streptococcal (Streptococcal)
s. antibody
S. antibody titer
s. bacteria
s. bacteria, microscopic
s. bacterium
s. bronchitis
s. carditis
s. carrier
s. empyema
s. endocarditis
s. gingivitis
s. infection
s. meningitis
s. meningitis, neonatal
s. pharyngitis
s. pharyngitis ▸ Group A beta
s. pneumonia

s. throat and problem with central nervous system
s. tonsillitis

streptococci
s., aerobic
s. ▸ Group A beta hemolytic
s., hemolytic

Streptococcus/streptococcus (Strep/strep)
S. agalactiae
s., alpha
s., alpha hemolytic
s. angina
S. anginosus
s., anhemolytic
S., autopsy-acquired group A
s. bacterium
s., Bargen's
s., beta
s., beta hemolytic
S. bovis
s. bronchitis
S. cremoris
S. durans
s. enteritis
S. equi
S. equisimilis
S. fecalis
S. faecalis
S. faecalis, gram-positive
S. faecium
s., Fehleisen's
s., gamma
S. genus
s., hemolytic
S. hemolyticus
S. hemolyticus, gram-positive
s. infection
S. lactis
S. lactis, gram-positive
S. lanceolatus
S. laurentii
S. liquefaciens
s. MG
S. milleri
S. mitis
S. mucosus
s. mutans
s., nonhemolytic
s. of Ostertag
S. pneumoniae
S. pneumoniae ▸ drug-resistant
S. pyogenes
S. pyogenes infection
S. salivarius

S. salivarius, gram-positive
s. sanguis
s. sore throat
s. throat
S. uberis
S. viridans
s., viridans
S. viridans, gram-positive
S. zooepidemicus
S. zymogenes
streptodornase (SKSD) ▸ streptokinase-
streptogenes, erythema
streptogenes, impetigo
streptokinase
s. antibody
s. clot lysis time
s. complex ▸ plasminogen-
s. infusion, intracoronary
s., intracoronary
s. plasminogen complex
s. therapy
streptolysin O
streptolysin S
Streptomyces
S. albus
S. ambofaciens
S. antibioticus
S. lincolnensis
S. madurae
S. nodosus
S. pelletieri
S. pimprina
S. somaliensis
streptothrica, pseudotuberculosis hominis
Streptothrix genus
Streptothrix organism
streptotrichosis of canaliculus
streptotrichosis of lacrimal sac
stress(es) (Stress)
s. action
s. action pain
s. ▸ acute reaction to
s. -amplifying factors
s. and aging
s. and angina
s. and anxiety
s. and apprehension
s. and fatigue ▸ excessive
s. and motivation
s. and muscle strain ▸ reduce
s. and physical strain
s. and strain ▸ minimize
s. and strain, musculoskeletal

s. and tension
s. and tension ▸ excessive
s., anger and hopelessness
s. angioplasty ▸ percutaneous low
s. angioplasty (PLSA) ▸ physiologic low
s., angular
s. -attenuating factor
s., behavior adaption and
s., blood bank
s., brief exposure to heat
s., cardiac
s., cardiac rehabilitation mental
s. cascade
s. caused health problems
s., childhood
s., circumferential wall
s. component
s., condition related to
s., contraction
s. control and timing
s. control mechanism
s. control therapy
s., cope with daily
s., coping with
s., decreased
s., defuse
s., depression triggered by
s., dieting
s. dimension relation ▸ end-systolic
s., diminished
s. disorder
s. disorder patient
s. disorder, physical
s. disorder (PTSD) ▸ post-traumatic
s. disorder ▸ prolonged post-traumatic
s. disorder ▸ psychotherapy of post-traumatic
s. disorder ▸ repetitive
s. divider
s. ECG/EKG (electrocardiogram)
S. Echo bed
s. echocardiograph ▸ transesophageal dobutamine
s. echocardiography
s. echocardiography, dobutamine
s. echocardiography ▸ dobutamine-atropine
s. echocardiography ▸ exercise
s. echocardiography ▸ pharmacologic
s. echocardiography ▸ supine bicycle
s. education

s., emotional
s. ▸ emotional cues of
s. ▸ enhanced sensitivity to
s., environmental
s. equalizer
s. erythrocytosis
s. evoking event ▸ major
s., excess
s. exercise, low
s., extreme
s. ▸ extreme reactivity to interpersonal
s. factor
s., family
s. films
s. fracture
s. fracture ▸ pelvic
s. -free environment
s. -generating thesis
s., hazardous
s. headache
s., heart response to
s., heat
s., heightened
s. hormone
s. in hypertensive patient
s. incontinence
s. incontinence, increased
s. incontinence, urinary
s., increased
s., individual
s. -induced aggression
s. -induced chest pain
s. -induced reaction
s. -induced situation
s. inducer
s. injury (RSI) ▸ repetitive
s. injury stages
s. inoculation
s. inoculation training
s., intolerable emotional
s., inversion
s., job
s. job, high
s., job-related
s., knee
s. ▸ left ventricular (LV) end-systolic
s. ▸ left ventricular (LV) wall
s. level
s. level, natural
s., living under
s. management
s. management and imagery
s. management, critical incident
s. management ▸ hospital-based

stress(es)—*continued*

s. management, personal
s. management program
s. management relaxation training
s. management skills
s. management techniques
s. management therapy
s. management training
s., managing
s. ▸ maternal
s., measuring
s. ▸ medication-induced
s. menopause
s. ▸ meridional wall
s. ▸ mixed disorders as reaction to
s. moderating factors
s., modify
s. MUGA (multiple gated acquisition) electrocardiogram
s. -muscular headache
s., negative
s. of altitude
s. of birth
s. of daily living
s. of heart disease
s. of hospitalization ▸ psychological
s. of overlapping visits
s. of work
s. on cannula
s. on needle
s. on rigidity, effect of emotional
s. on spasticity, effect of emotional
s. on tendon ▸ repeated
s., ongoing
s. overload
s., oxidating
s., parental
s., pathologic
s., patient under constant
s. perfusion imaging ▸ pharmacologic
s. perfusion protocol ▸ rest metabolism/
s. ▸ periods of extreme
s. ▸ personality dysfunction and
s., pharmacologic
s., physical
s., physical cues of
s., physiological
s. physiology, pattern of
s., polycythemia
s., precipitating
s. producing factor
s., prolonged
s., prolonged emotional

s., psychogenic
s., psychological
s., psychopathological reaction to
s., psychosocial
S., Q-
s. reaction
s. reaction, acute
s. reaction, acute situational
s. reaction, adult situational
s. reaction, gross
s. reaction, tibial
s. reactions in dental patients
s. reducer, natural
s. reducing effects
s. reducing meditation
s. reducing techniques
s. reduction
s. reduction program
s. reduction ▸ relaxation and
s. -related aging of brain
s. -related arrhythmia
s. -related disease
s. -related disorder
s. -related factor
s. -related headache
s. -related heart condition
s. -related hormones
s. -related hypertension
s. -related problem
s. -related problems ▸ autogenic training and
s. -related sleeplessness
s. -related symptoms
s. -related tension
s. -related tremulousness
s. relaxation
s. release, temporary
s. -released hormones
s. relief methods
s., relieve
s., repetitive
s. response, inhibiting
s. responses
s. responses of cardiovascular system
s., senior
s., severe emotional
s., shear
s. shortening relationship
s., short-term
s., sibling
s. situation
s. skills
s., social
s., socioeconomic

s. ▸ sudden psychological
s. syndrome (ACSS) ▸ acute caretaker's
s. syndrome ▸ clutter
s. syndrome, delayed
s. syndrome ▸ repetitive
s., tensile
s., tension and
s. test
s. test, aerobic exercise
s. test, arm exercise
s. test ▸ Astrand bicycle exercise
s. test, atrial pacing
s. test, Balke exercise
s. test, bicycle ergometer exercise
s. test, Blake exercise
s. test, Bruce exercise
s. test, cardiac
s. test, dobutamine
s. test ▸ EKG (electrocardiogram) exercise
s. test ▸ electrocardiogram (ECG/EKG)
s. test ▸ elevated arm
s. test ▸ Ellestad exercise
s. test ▸ external rotation, abduction,
s. test ▸ Gradational Step exercise
s. test, inversion
s. test ▸ isoproterenol
s. test ▸ Kattus exercise
s. test ▸ leg sparing
s. test ▸ Master exercise
s. test ▸ mental
s. test, nuclear
s. test ▸ online
s. test ▸ Physical Work Capacity exercise
s. test ▸ routine
s. test ▸ sestamibi
s. test ▸ Sheffield exercise
s. test ▸ single-stage exercise
s. test ▸ Technetium Cardiolite
s. test, thallium-201
s. test, treadmill
s. test, treadmill exercise
s. test, valgus
s. test ▸ valgus-varus
s. test, varus
s. testing
s. testing, perinatal non-
s. thallium scanning
s. thallium scintigraphy
s. thallium study
s., thallium treadmill

s. thallium-201 myocardial perfusion imaging
s. to tissue lining ▸ repeated
s. ▸ tolerance for
s., tolerate heat
s., traumatic
s. treadmill ▸ electrocardiogram (ECG/EKG)
S. treadmill ▸ Q-
s. treatment group ▸ low
s. -type leukemoid reaction
s. ulcer
s. ▸ unduly vulnerable to
s., unmanaged
s. ▸ ventricular wall
s., wall
s., warning signs of
s. washout myocardial perfusion image
s. workout, high
s., work-related emotional
s., work-related physical

stressed
s., fatigued and
s. hypertensive
s. out, patient
s., patient feeling

stressful
s. activity
s. emotions
s. environments
s. exercise
s. experience
s. imagery
s. lifestyle
s. living habits, modify
s. or anxious situation
s., physically
s. ▸ physically and emotionally
s. situation
s. stimuli

stressor(s)
s., assessing life
s., current
s., daily
s., different
s., family
s., financial
s., legal
s., life
s., medical
s., negative
s., occupational
s. or impediment
s., peer

s., positive
s., psychosocial
s., social
s., traumatic

stretch(es)
s. and elongates
s. -and-reach test
s., calf muscle
s., chair
s. exercise, calf
s. exercise, calf-heel
s. exercise, chest
s. exercise ▸ elongation
s. exercise, hamstring
s. exercise, hip adductor
s. exercise ▸ low back
s. exercise, quadricep
s. exercise, shoulder
s. exercise ▸ thigh
s. exercise, upper thigh
s. ▸ knee-to-shoulder
s. ligaments
s. marks from pregnancy ▸ abdominal
s. marks from pregnancy ▸ breast
s. marks ▸ patient has
s. muscles
s. ▸ physical touch
s. ▸ post-exercise flexibility
s. receptor
s. reflex
s. reflexes, muscle
s. routines
s. stricture
s. tendons
s., yoga

stretchable skin
stretched
s. bronchi
s. bronchus sign
s. diameter
s. muscle
s. position, neutral or

stretching
s. and breathing exercises
s. and neck isometrics
s. and releasing exercises
s., birth canal
s. calves, thighs and hamstrings
s. esophagus
s. exercise, neck
s. exercise ▸ slow
s. exercises
s. exercises and meditating
s. exercises ▸ gentle

s. key muscles
s. massage ▸ deep and
s. of muscles
s. of nerves
s. of supratrochlear nerve
s. of ventricular muscle ▸ excessive
s. operation, iris
s. or damage to deep veins
s., passive
s. ▸ resistance to passive
s., side
s. syncope
s., tissue

stria(-ae)
s., acoustic
s., Amici's
s., auditory
s. ciliares
s., cutaneous
s., Francke's
s. from obesity
s. gravidarum
s., Knapp's
s., Langhans'
s., meningitic
s. of abdomen
s. of breasts
s. of pregnancy
s. of pregnancy, abdominal
s. of thighs
s., olfactory
s., Retzius' parallel
s., Rohr's
s., Schreger's

striatal nigral degeneration
striatal syndrome, Hunt's
striate
s. keratitis
s. retinitis
s. vein

striated
s. muscle
s. muscle fibers
s. muscular tissue of myocardium
s. reticulum

striati, taenia semicircularis corporis
striation
s. of myocardial fibers
s., tabby cat
s., tigroid

striatum, corpus
striatum palmare, xanthoma
striatus, lichen
strict (Strict)
s. bedrest ▸ patient at

strict (Strict)—*continued*
s. catheterization schedule
s. exercise routine
S. Isolation
s. limitations
s. medical criteria
s. sodium restricted diet
s. voiding schedule
stricture(s) [*structure*]
s., anal
s., anastomotic
s., annular
s., area of
s., bridle
s., cicatricial
s., contractile
s., dilated
s., dilation of
s., esophageal
s. ▸ esophageal lye
s., false
s. formation
s. formation, esophageal fibrous
s., fracturing the
s., functional
s., Hunner's
s., hysterical
s., impassable
s., impermeable
s., irritable
s., malignant
s. of bile duct
s. of cervical esophagus, caustic
s. of esophagus
s. of hypopharynx, caustic
s. of urethra
s. of urethra, granular
s., organic
s., peptic
s., permanent
s. ▸ pharyngoesophageal (PE) postcorrosive
s., recurrent
s. ▸ reflux-induced esophageal
s., spasmodic
s., spastic
s., stress
s., temporary
s., UP (ureteropelvic) juncture
s., urethral
s. ▸ Wickwitz esophageal
Stride cardiac pacemaker
striding ▸ fitness pole
stridor
s., biphasic

s., congenital laryngeal
s., inspiratory
s., laryngeal
s., respiratory
s., serraticus
stridulosa, laryngitis
stridulous respiration
strike, heel
strike, palm-heel
string
s. adhesions, banjo-
s. bladder
s. carcinoma
s., IUD (intrauterine device)
s. of pearls fashion
s. sign
s. test
s. test, duodenal
stringent technical precautions
stringy
s. density, minimal
s. infiltration
s. opacification
s. tangles
s. vitreous floaters
striocerebellar tremor
strip(s) (Strip)
s., bovine pericardium
s., collodion
s. easily, capsules
s., ECG (electrocardiogram)
s., gauze
s., Gelfoam
s., glucose
s., lead
s., motor
s. of gauze
s. percussion
s., rayon
s., rhythm
S., Steri-
stripe, flank
stripe ▸ subepicardial fat
striped muscle
stripped
s. and ligated, varicose veins
s. away, periosteum
s. capsule
s. cervix
s. easily, capsules
s. easily ▸ renal capsules
stripper(s)
s. asthma, stone-
s., Dunlop thrombus
s., intraluminal

s., vein
stripping
s. and dissection
s. and ligation
s. and ligation ▸ varicose vein
s. autoradiography, film-
s. bladder
s., cord
s. dissection and
s. ▸ erasing, ligation and
s., high ligation and
s., ligation and
s., multiple
s. of cord
s., peritoneal
s., segmental
s., vein
s., vocal cord
stroboscopic disk
stroboscopic microscope
stroboscopy, video
Stroganoff's (Stroganov's) treatment
stroke
s. and aging
s. and atherosclerosis
s., back
s., biofeedback treatment of footdrop after
s., brain stem
s., cardioembolic
s., cerebrovascular
s., confusion from
s. ▸ cooling therapy for
s., cryptogenic
s. culture
s. depression, post
s. diagnosis
s., disabling
s., dizziness from
s. due to cerebral hemorrhage
s. during massage ▸ smooth and repetitive
s. education classes
s., effective
s. ejection rate
s., embolic
s., evolving right parietal
s., fatal
s., footdrop after
s., full blown
s., heart
s., heat
s. hemorrhage and
s., hemorrhagic
s., history of

s., impending
s. ▸ increased risk of
s. index (SI)
s., initial
s. injury, butterfly
s. injury, freestyle
s., ipsilateral
s., ischemic
s., lacunar
s., light
s., lightning
s. -like syndrome of aphasia
s., major
s., minor
s., motor
s., nondisabling
s., nonfatal
s. onset ▸ symptoms of
s., optic
s. output
s. pain syndrome ▸ post-thalamic
s., paralytic
s., patient had mini-
s. patient ▸ recovering
s. patients ▸ increase of active
    extension in
s. prevention
s. produces speech problem
s. prophylaxis
s., recovery
s., recurrent
s., rehabilitation after
s., rehabilitation of disabilities as
    result of
s. -related disorder
s., repeated
s. risk ▸ ischemic
s., risk of
s., risk of recurrent
s. screening
s., silent
s. ▸ spinal cord
s., sun◊
s. ▸ surgical prevention of
s., surgical treatment for
s. survivor
s. symptoms
s. syndrome
s. syndrome, post-brain stem
s., temporary
s., thalamic
s., threatening
s., thromboembolic
s., thrombotic
s. treatment

s. victim ▸ nerve death in
s. victim, potential
s. volume
s. volume, conductance
s. volume, decreased
s. volume index (SVI)
s. volume (LVSV) ▸ left ventricular
s. volume of heart
s. warning signs
s. work
s. work index (SWI)
s. work (LVSW) ▸ left ventricular
s. work (VSW) ▸ ventricular
s. work-up

stroking
s. maneuver during massage ▸ cat
s. maneuver during massage ▸ fan
s. maneuver during massage ▸
    thumb

stroma [*stoma, struma*]
s., edematous
s. -free hemoglobin ▸ pyridoxilated
s. -free hemoglobin solution
s. iridis
s., loose fibromyomatous
s., loose fibrovascular
s., middle portion of
s. of cornea
s. of ovary
s., ovarian
s. ovarii
s., portio and
s., spindle cell
s. ▸ valvular myxoid
s., vitreous
s. vitreum

stromal
s. cell tumors
s. cells
s. cells ▸ marrow
s. herpetic keratitis
s. hyperplasia
s. hyperplasia, cortical
s. hyperplasia of ovary ▸ nodular
s. hyperplasia, ovarian
s. hypertrophy
s. mitosis
s. opacity
s. sarcoma, metastatic endometrial
s. tissue, cervical
s. tumor (GIST) ▸ gastrointestinal

Stromeyer's cephalohematocele
strong (Strong)('s)
s. and equal bilaterally ▸ reflexes
s. and regular, pulse

S. bacilli, Flexner-
S. bacillus
s. bones
s. depressive drive
s. educational component
s., pedal pulses
s. pulse
s. pulse ▸ full,

strongylina, Ascarops
Strongyloides stercoralis
Strongylus subtilis
strontium
s. 90 (Sr^{90})
s. nitrate Sr 85
s. Sr 87m

Stroop Color and Word Test
Strophanthus sarmentosus
structural
s. abnormality
s. alignment
s. anomaly
s. change
s. change in heart
s. changes in joints
s. changes, irreversible
s. chemistry
s. congenital anomaly
s. damage
s. damage, severe
s. defect
s. demarcations
s. disorder
s. elements
s. grouping, antigenic
s. heart defect
s. lesion
s. pathology
s. relationship, normal
s. therapy
s. unit
s. uterine defect

structure(s) [*stricture*]
s., abnormal bone
s., anatomic
s. and function of mitochondria ▸
    abnormalities
s. and function of valve
s., anterior commissure
s., antigenic
s., atomic and nuclear
s., atrioventricular (AV) septal
s., basic leukemia cell
s., biomolecular
s., Bohr model of atomic
s., bone

structure(s) [*stricture*]—*continued*
s., brain
s., cardiovascular
s., cell
s., cell-like
s., central
s., chordal
s., chromatic
s., coiled bony
s., collecting
s., congested vascular
s., cord
s., crystalline
s., deep
s., deep cerebral
s., delicate
s. demineralized, bony
s., denture-supporting
s., differentiated internal
s., dose-limiting
s., drainage (dr'ge)
s. drug-free environment
s., echodense
s., ego
s., facial
s., fine
s., genetic
s., glandular
s., hilar
s. infection ▸ skin
s., injury, soft
s., inner ear
s., intact bone
s., islet
s., ligamentous
s. ▸ loss of external
s., mediastinal
s., mesodermal
s., microfilament
s., microscopic
s., midline
s. ▸ minute embryonic
s., molecular
s., muscle
s., muscular
s., musculocartilaginous
s., nerve
s., neural
s., neurovascular
s., normal breast
s. of bone, dense
s. of nerve cells
s. of neurofilament subunits
s. of the ear ▸ inner
s. of the support system

s., orbital
s., organizational
s., osseous
s. ▸ periapical bone
s., phonating
s., polypoid cystic
s., rod-like
s., shift of midline
s., skeletal
s., sleep
s., small bone
s. ▸ social support network
s., subcortical
s., subintimal
s., subtentorial
s., superficial
s., supporting
s., supportive social
s., supraglottic
s., surrounding
s., thick
s., tree-like
s., underlying
s., urinary tract
s., urogenital
s., valve
s., vascular
s., venous
s., villous
s., viral antigenic
s., wall
s. weaken, supportive
s., yellow cortical
structured
s. adolescent psychotherapy group
s. elements
s. environment
s. environment, semi-
s. hospitalization, intensive
s. recreation
s. repetitive skills
s. responsibilities
s. treatment interruptions (STI)
struggle, life and death
struggling to stay awake
struma [*stoma, stroma*]
s. basedowificata
s., Hashimoto's
s. lymphomatosa
s., Riedel's
strumectomy, median
strumipriva, cachexia
strumosa exophthalmica ▸ tachycardia
strumous ophthalmia

Strümpell('s)
S. arthritis, Marie-
S. disease, Marie-
S. disease, Westphal-
S. -Leichtenstern encephalitis
S. reflex
S. sign
S. spondylitis, Marie-
S. spondylitis ▸ von Bekhterev-
strung-out, patient
Strunsky's sign
strut
s. fracture
s. fracture ▸ outlet
s. ▸ George Washington
s., piston
s., polyethylene
s., stainless steel (SS)
s., stent
s., tantalum
s., wire-loop
strutting, plaque
struvite calculus
struvite stone
strychnine poisoning
Stryker-Halbeisen syndrome
ST-T
ST-T deviations
ST-T wave
ST-T wave abnormalities
ST-T wave changes compatible with ischemia
ST-T wave changes, nonspecific
STU (skin test unit)
stubbed shoulder
stubborn, patient
stucco keratoses
Stuck nail, Venable-
stuckertianum, Chlorostigma
studded with numerous tumor nodules
studded with tumor nodules ▸ peritoneum
Studdiford perineorrhaphy ▸ Emmet-
Student (student)(s)
S. Against Drunken Driving (SADD)
s. disease ▸ medical
s., instructing nursing
studeri, Bertiella
study(-ies) (Study)
s., absorption
s., acoustogram
s., adjuvant
s., agglutination
s., air

s., air contrast
s., altitude simulation
s., angiocardiogram
s., angiocardiography
s., angiogram
s., angiographic
s., angiopneumogram
s., antibody sensitivity
s., aortic arch
s., aortogram
s., aortography
s., AP (anteroposterior)
s., apex cardiogram
s., arteriogram
s. ‣ arteriographical imaging
s., arteriography
s., arthrogram
s., ataxiagram
s., atrial
s., autopsy
s., ballistocardiogram
s., ballistocardiography
s., barium meal
s., baseline
s., behavioral genetic
s., biochemical
s., biofeedback pain
s. ‣ blinded, placebo-controlled, randomized
s., blood flow
s., blood gas
s., blood volume
s., brain imaging
s., bronchography
s., bronchoscopic
s., Bucky
s., cadaver preserved for anatomical
s., carcinogenicity
s., cardiac
s., cardiac-pulmonary angio-aortic arch
s., cardiography
s., cardiovascular diagnostic
s., case
s., case control
s., cell
s., cerebral blood flow
s., chemistry
s., cholangiogram
s., cholecystogram
s., choledochogram
s., chromoretinography
s., chronic electrophysiological
s., cine

s., cineangiocardiogram
s., cineangiocardiography
s., cineangiography
s., cinebronchogram
s., cinefluorography
s., cinephonation
s., cineradiography
s., clinical
s., clinical psychological
s., cohort
s., collaborative research
s., comparative
s., compared with previous
s., competitive binding
s., contrast
s., controlled
s., controlled outcome
s., crossover placebo controlled
s., current
s., cystometric
s., cytogenetic
s., cytologic
s., delayed
s. design, medical
s., diagnostic
s., double contrast
s., double-blind
s. ‣ double-blind controlled
s. ‣ double-blind placebo control
s. ‣ double-blind placebo control prophylactic
s., dual-contrast
s., ECG/EKG (electrocardiogram)
s., echocardiographic
s., EEG (electro-encephalogram)
s., EKY (electrokymogram/electrokymography)
s., electrocorticogram
s., electrocorticography
s., electromyogram
s., electromyography
s., electronystagmograph
s. (EPS), electrophysiologic
s., electroretinogram
s., embryolethality
s., empirical
s., encephaloarteriogram
s., endoscopic
s., enzyme
s., epidemiologic
s. ‣ equilibrium-gated blood pool
s., erythrokinetic
s., esophageal motility
s., esophageal pressure

s., estrogen receptor
s., ethnographic
s., exercise
s., expectorated sputum
s., experimental
s., fasciogram
s., fat absorption
s., fetogram
s., film
s. ‣ floating wall motion
s., fluoroscopic
s., follow-up
s., fracture/ultrasound
S. ‣ Framingham Heart
s., function
s., functional
s. ‣ gated blood pool
s., genetic screening
s., goniophotography
s., heart
S. ‣ Helsinki Heart
s., hemodynamic
s. ‣ hemodynamic angiographic
s., hepatic enzyme
s. ‣ hepatitis surface antigen
s., horizontal beam
s., hormone binding
s., hospital
s. ‣ hypertension optimal treatment
s., hypnosis
s. ‣ hypoxic response
s., hysterogram
s., hysterosalpingogram
s., imaging
s. in clinical trials, matched control
s. in clinical trials, pilot
s., in vitro
s. ‣ in vivo microdialysis
s., in-depth
s., infertility
s., infusion pyelographic
s., initial
s., interventional
s. ‣ intracardiac electrophysiologic
s., iodized oil
s., ionometric
s., isotope
s., isotope scanning
s., kinetocardiogram
s., kinetocardiography
s., laboratory
S. Laboratory, Motion
s., left ventricular
s., liver function
s. ‣ long-term safety

study(-ies)—*continued*

s., lumbar flexion and extension
s., lung function
s., lymphangiogram
s., manometry
s., matched control
s., medical
s., medical treatment
s., microscopic
s. ▸ mini-invasive vascular
s., minute
s., mortality
s., motility
s. ▸ motor and sensory nerve conduction
s., multigenerational
s. ▸ muscle immunocytochemical
s. ▸ myocardial perfusion
S. (NNIS) ▸ National Nosocomial Infection
s., naturalistic evaluation
s., nerve conduction
s. ▸ nerve conduction velocity
s., neuroimaging
s., normal exercise
s., normative
s. ▸ nuclear ventricular function
s., oblique
s., observational
s. of brain, isotope scanning
s. of cells ▸ Papanicolaou (Pap)
S. on the Efficacy of Nosocomial Infection Control (SENIC)
s., opacification
s. ▸ open label
s., PA (posteroanterior)
s., pain
s., paternity
s. ▸ pelvic radiation imaging
s., pelvimetry
s., pelviradiography
s., perfusion
s., peripheral blood
s., perirenal air
s. ▸ phased array
s., phonation
s., phonocardiogram
s., phonocardiographic
s., phonocardiography
s., photofluorographic
S. (PAS) ▸ Physicians Activities
s., placebo-controlled
s., pilot
s., pneumoarthrogram
s., pneumoencephalogram

s., pneumoencephalomyelogram
s., polysomnographic
s., posteroanterior (PA)
s., postmortem
s., precatheterization laboratory
s., preclinical
s., preliminary
s., previous
S. (PAS), Professional Activities
s., progress
s., prospective
s., prospective randomized
s. protocol
s., psychological
s., pulmonary blood flow
s., pulmonary diffusion
s., pulmonary function
s., pulmonary function ventilation
s., pyelographic roentgen
s., quantitative
s., quantitative regional function
s., radioactive iodinated serum albumin (RISA)
s., radioencephalogram
s., radiographic
s., radioisotope scanning
s., radioisotope uptake
s., radiologic magnification
s., radiological
s., radionuclide
s. ▸ radionuclide esophageal transit
s., randomized
s. ▸ randomized, blinded, controlled
s., recruitment
s., related
s., renal function
s., renogram
s., repeat
s., repeat water
s. ▸ reproductive toxicity
s., research
s. ▸ rest and exercise
s., retrococcygeal air
s., retrograde pyelographic
s., retrograde urogram
s., retroperitoneal air
s., retrospective
s., rheologic
s., right ventricular
s., roentgenkymographic
s., roentgenkymography
s., roentgenographic
s., routine
s., saccadic velocity
s. ▸ salivary flow

s., scanning
s., scintigraphic
s., seasonal
s., selective
s., sensitivity
s. ▸ serum enzyme
s., sialogram
s., single-contrast
s., skiagram
s., sleep
s., sleep-dream
s., sonoencephalogram
s., spatial vectorcardiogram
s., sphygmography
s., splenoportography
s., split function
s., split renal function
s., spot film
s., sputum
s., stereoroentgenography
s., stimulation
s. ▸ stress thallium
s., tachography
s., teleroentgenogram
s., teratogenicity
s., thermography
s., thyroid
s., thyroid function
s., tissue culture
s. ▸ tissue donation
s. to serve as baselines for future problems
s., tokodynagraph
s., tomography
s., tonography
s., toxicity
s., tracer
s., transient time
s., treatment effectiveness
S. (TOPS) ▸ Treatment Outcome Prospective
s., triolein fat absorption
s. ▸ triple-blind
s., tube dilution
s., tumorigenicity
s., unenhanced
s., uptake
s., ureterogram
s., ureteropyelogram
s., urological
s., vascular
s. (VPS) ▸ vasovagal pacemaker
s., vectorcardiogram
s., venogram
s. ▸ venous Doppler

s., ventilation
s., ventriculogram
s., vibrocardiography
s., videotape
s., virality
s. ▸ wall motion
s., washout
s., water
s. with nodules ▸ liver
s., xerography
s., xeromammogram
s., x-ray
s., x-ray diagnostic

Stuff (heroin)
stuffed
s. nostril
s. or runny nostril
s. -up feeling

stuffiness
s. from Actifed ▸ nose
s. from allergy ▸ altitude change, ear
s. from birth control pill ▸ nose
s., nasal
s. of ears

stuffy
s. head
s. nose
s. nose ▸ chronic

Stühmer's disease
Stumblers (barbiturates)
stump
s., amputated
s., amputation
s., appendiceal
s., Baylor's
s., bronchial
s., burying the
s., carbolized
s., carcinoma
s., carcinoma uterine cervical
s., cardiac
s., cervical
s., cone-shaped amputation
s., conical
s., cystic duct
s. doubly ligated, proximal
s., forklike
s., hallucination
s., healed
s., inverted
s., inverted, appendiceal
s., inverted, cardiac
s., lower end of
s., mature

s., mucosal
s. of appendix
s. of appendix, bury
s. of bronchus
s. of esophagus
s. of limb
s. of pedicle
s. phenolized
s. pregnancy
s. pressure
s. removed, cervical
s. shrinking
s., tracheal

stunned
s. atrium
s. feelings
s. myocardium
s., temporarily

stunning, myocardial
stunt virus, bushy
stunted growth
stupes, hot
stupor
s., anergic
s., benign
s., catatonic
s., delusion
s., dreamy
s., epileptic
s., lethargic
s., localized postseizure
s. ▸ muscular weakness and
s. ▸ patient in
s., postconvulsive
s., postictal
s., postseizure

stuporous
s. melancholia
s., patient
s., patient semi-

Sturge('s)
S. disease
S. -Weber syndrome
S. -Weber-Dimitri disease

Sturmdorf's operation
Sturmdorf's suture
Sturm's conoid
stuttering
s. and stammering
s., labiochoreic
s. myocardial infarction
s. of perfusion
s., urinary
s. urination

stutzeri, Pseudallescheria

stutzeri, Pseudomonas
S2 heart sound
S2 sound ▸ paradoxically split
stye/sty
s., meibomian
s., zeisian

style(s)
s., cognitive
s. of behaving ▸ negative
s. of breathing ▸ pursed lip
s. of thinking ▸ negative

stylet (*same as* stilet, stilette)
stylet, heart catheterization
styloglossus muscle
stylohyoid muscle
stylohyoid nerve
styloid
s. bone, ulnar
s. process
s. process of radius
s. process of ulna

stylomastoid vein
stylomastoideum, foramen
stylopharyngeal nerve
stylopharyngeus muscle
styptic
s., Binelli's
s. bitter
s., chemical
s., mechanical
s., vascular

Suarez-Villafranca operation
subacromial bursitis
subacute
s. bacterial endocarditis (SBE)
s. bacterial endocarditis (SBE) prophylaxis
s. bronchitis, chronic
s. bronchopneumonia
s. closure
s. combined degeneration
s. delirium
s. diffuse thyroiditis
s. inclusion body encephalitis
s. infective endocarditis
s. leukoencephalitis, chronic
s. myelomonocytic leukemia
s. myelo-opticoneuropathy
s. myocardial infarction
s. nephritis
s. pericarditis
s. sclerosing leukoencephalitis
s. sclerosing panencephalitis (SSPE)
s. spongiform encephalopathy

subacute—*continued*
- s. tamponade
- s. thyroiditis
- s. treatment for organic brain syndrome
- s. treatment for overdosing
- s. treatment of acute drug intoxication
- s. treatment of flashback reactions
- s. treatment of panic reactions
- s. treatment of psychotic reactions
- s. treatment on withdrawal
- s. yellow atrophy

subannular mattress suture

subaortic
- s. hypertension ▸ idiopathic hypertrophic
- s. stenosis
- s. stenosis ▸ enucleation of
- s. stenosis ▸ fibrous
- s. stenosis, hypertrophic
- s. stenosis, hypertrophic muscular
- s. stenosis ▸ idiopathic
- s. stenosis (IHSS), idiopathic hypertrophic

subarachnoid
- s. bleeding
- s. block
- s. block, spinal
- s. catheter, lumbar
- s. cavity
- s. cisterna
- s. hemorrhage
- s. hemorrhage in cranium
- s. hemorrhage ▸ intracerebral and
- s. hemorrhage ▸ surgical procedure for
- s. pathways
- s. sac
- s. septum
- s. shunt, endolymphatic
- s. space
- s. space, basal
- s. space, drainage (dr'ge) of
- s. space, enlarged
- s. space, lumbar
- s. space, puncture of

subarachnoidal cisterns
subarachnoidal sinus
subarachnoideale, cavum
subareolar duct papillomatosis
subareolar region
subastragalar amputation
subastragalar dislocation
subatomic particles

subauricular region
subcallosal gyrus
subcallosus, gyrus
subcapital fracture
subcapsular
- s. cataract
- s. cataract (PSC), posterior
- s. cortex
- s. hematoma
- s. hematoma of liver
- s. opacity
- s. scarring
- s. scarring in interstitium

subcardinal veins
subcarinal angle
subcarinal lymphadenopathy
subchondral bony reabsorption
subchorionic bleed
subchorionic hemorrhage
subchronic
- s. ▸ schizophrenia, catatonic type,
- s. ▸ schizophrenia, disorganized type,
- s. ▸ schizophrenia, paranoid type,
- s. ▸ schizophrenia, residual type,
- s. ▸ schizophrenia, undifferentiated type,
- s. with acute exacerbation ▸ schizophrenia, catatonic type,
- s. with acute exacerbation ▸ schizophrenia, disorganized type,
- s. with acute exacerbation ▸ schizophrenia, paranoid type,
- s. with acute exacerbation ▸ schizophrenia, residual type,
- s. with acute exacerbation ▸ schizophrenia, undifferentiated type

subclavian
- s. arteriogram
- s. arteriovenous fistula
- s. artery
- s. artery, aberrant right
- s. artery bypass graft
- s. artery, left
- s. artery, right
- s. artery, sulcus of
- s. bypass, carotid
- s. bypass ▸ subclavian-
- s. -carotid axilloaxillary bypass, aorto-
- s. carotid bypass
- s. catheter
- s. catheter, right-sided

- s. dialysis catheter
- s., double lumen
- s. flap technique, Waldhausen
- s. intravenous line
- s. line
- s. line in place
- s. loop
- s. lymphatic
- s. murmur
- s. nerve
- s. steal
- s. steal syndrome
- s. -subclavian bypass
- s. sulcus of lung
- s. Tegaderm dressing
- s. thrombosis
- s. transposition
- s. triangle
- s. vein
- s. vein cannulation
- s. vein dialysis catheter, right
- s. vein (LSV), left
- s. vein (RSV), right
- s. venous catheter

subclavicular murmur
subclavius muscle
subclinical
- s. asthma
- s. diabetes
- s. disease
- s. epilepsy
- s. form
- s. infection

subcollateral gyrus
subcoma insulin treatment
subconjunctival
- s. hemorrhage
- s. hemorrhage of eye
- s. injection

subconscious life
subconscious relationships, conscious-
subcoracoid dislocation
subcoracoid type displacement
subcortical
- s. aphasia
- s. area, left
- s. area, right
- s. dysfunction, diffuse
- s. encephalitis, chronic
- s. encephalopathy
- s. encephalopathy, progressive
- s. infarction ▸ old
- s. nuclei
- s. structures subcostal

s. flank incision
s. incision
s. muscles
s. nerve
s. retractions
s. vein
subcostal
s. retractions, mild
s. view
s. zone
subcrepitant, lungs
subcrepitant rale
subcristal ventricular septal defect
subcultures, socioeconomic
subcutaneous
s. adipose tissue
s. bleeders
s. connective tissues
s. electrode, implantation
s. emphysema
s. extravasation of blood
s. fat
s. fat layer
s. fracture
s. implantation, Oreton pellets for
s. injection
s. intraocular node
s. junction, dermal
s. mass
s. mastectomy
s. metastasis
s. nodule
s. nodule, hard
s. nodule, movable
s. perineal mass
s. plane
s. saw
s. suture
s. swelling
s. temporal nerves
s. tissue
s. tissues approximated
s. tissues closed
s. tissues reapproximated
s. tumor
s. tunneling device
s. veins of abdomen
s. wound
subcutaneously, adrenaline
subcutaneously, tunnel created
subcutaneum, condyloma
subcutaneus tumefaciens,
   Saccharomyces
subcuticular
s. fat

s. level
s. stitch
s. suture
s. suture of nylon ▸ skin closed with
   running
s. wire
subdeltoid bursitis
subdermal
s. implant
s. implant material
s. implant material, Silastic
s. implant, Silastic
s. layer of scalp
subdiaphragmatic
s. abscess
s. fields in radiation therapy
s. hernia
s. involvement
s. radiation therapy
s. sympathectomy
subdigastric lymph nodes
subdued personality
subdural
s. abscess
s. electrode
s. fluid
s. hematoma
s. hematoma, chronic
s. hematoma ▸ liquefaction of
s. hemorrhage
s. hemorrhage in cranium
s. hygroma
s. puncture
s. space
s. space, drainage (dr'ge) of
subdurale, cavum
subendocardial
s., anterior
s. blood flow ▸ impairment of
s. fibroelastosis
s. fibrosis
s. fibrosis, focal
s., focal
s. focal hemorrhages ▸ superficial
s. hemorrhage
s. hemorrhages, atrial
s. hemorrhages, focal
s. infarct, myocardial
s. infarction
s. injury
s. ischemia
s. layer
s. myocardial infarct ▸ acute
s. myocardial infarction
s. necrosis

s. petechial hemorrhages
s. region
s. sclerosis
s. zone
subependymal
s. germinal plate hemorrhage
s. giant cell astrocytoma
s. glial matrix
subepicardial
s. fat
s. fat stripe
s. injury
subepithelial
s. corneal edema
s. keratectomy (LASEK) procedure,
   laser-assisted
s. plexus
subepithelialis, keratitis punctata
subfascial emphysema
subfascial hematoma ▸ sonography
of
subgaleal hemorrhage in cranium
subgingival curettage
subglenoid dislocation
subglottic
s. area
s. carcinoma
s. laryngitis
s. stenosis
subgroups, patient
subhepatic abscess
subhyaloid hemorrhage
subhyoid laryngotomy
subhyoid region
subintimal plaques
subintimal structure
subinvolution of uterus
subinvolution of uterus, chronic
subitum, exanthema
subject(s)
s., alert awake
s., clinical research
s., control
s. differences, stability of
s. engaged in mental activity
s., escape and avoidance
   conditioning in human
s., human
s., individual
s. mobility
s., neuromuscular firing in normal
s., neuromuscular firing in spastic
s., normal control
s., patient normal
s., research

subject(s)—*continued*
s., sleeping
s., test
s., waking
subjected to friction ▸ skin
subjective (Subjective)
s. activity
s. awareness
s. behavior
s. change
s. decision
s. defect
s. difficulty
s. effect
s. evidence
s. experience
s. feeling
s. improvement
s. improvement, patient showed
s. material
S. Objective Assessment Plan
  (SOAP)
s. pain
s. relief
s. response
s. sensation
s. sensation, premonitory
s. sleep quality
s. sound
s. state
s. symptoms
s. tinnitus
s. weakness
subjunctional heart block
sublatio retinas
sublethal damage repair
sublethal doses
subleukemic leukemia
sublimate, corrosive
sublimation ▸ latency and adult
subliminal
s. angioplasty
s. cognition
s. seizures
s. stimulus
s. thirst
sublimis
s. muscle, flexor digitorum
s., tendinous chiasm of flexor
s., tendinous chiasm of musculus
  flexor digitorum
s. tendon
s. tendon, flexor digitorum
sublingual
s. caruncle

s. duct
s. fold
s. gland
s. hematoma
s. nerve
s. nitroglycerin
s. saliva
s. tablet
s. vein
sublobular veins
subluxation
s. and/or fracture
s. ▸ chronic patellar
s., forward
s., fracture and/or
s., joint
s., lateral
s. ▸ nasal septum
s. of knees ▸ congenital
s. of lens
s. ▸ radial head
s., shoulder
s., vertebral
s., Volkmann's
s., voluntary
subluxed, shoulder
submammary mastitis
submandibular
s. duct
s. ganglion
s. gland
s. gland, carcinoma
s. lymph nodes
s. salivary gland
submassive necrosis of liver
submassive pulmonary embolism
submaxillary
s. duct
s. ganglion
s. gland
s. gland tumor
s. nerves
s. region
s. saliva
s. salivary gland ▸ right
s. tumor
submaximal stimulation
submental
s. electromyogram (EMG)
s. glands
s. hematoma
s. lipectomy
s. lymph nodes
s. region
s. vein

s. vertex roentgenogram
submentovertical axial projection
submerged tonsil
submerged tooth
**submit to treatment, form for refusal
  to**
submitral area
submitral calcification
submitted
s. for biopsy, specimen
s. for frozen section, biopsy
s. for frozen section, specimen
s. for frozen section, tissue
s. for microsection, specimen
s. to pathologist, tissue
submucosa ▸ porcine small intestinal
submucosa ▸ small intestinal
submucosal
s. air
s. bacterial colonies
s. connective tissue
s. fibroid
s. gland hypertrophy
s. hemorrhage
s. implant
s. plaque
s. vascular pattern
submucous
s. leiomyoma
s. myomata
s. resection (SMR)
s. resection and rhinoplasty
  (SMRR)
subnormal
s. accommodation
s. excitability
s. temperature
subnormality
s., mental
s., profound mental
s., severe mental
suboccipital
s. decompression
s. incision
s. nerve
suboccipitobregmatic diameter
suboccluding ligature
suboxydans, Acetobacter
subpapillary zone
**subpectoral implantation of
  cardioverter-defibrillator**
subperiosteal
s. abscess of frontal sinus
s. amputation
s. bone

s. cortical abrasion
s. dissection
s. fracture
s. implant
s. implant material
subperiosteally resected, rib
subphrenic
s. abscess
s. collection
s. metastasis, retroperitoneal
s. space
subpial transection ‣ multiple
subpleural
s. air pockets
s. air space
s. bleb
s. blebs ‣ pinpoint
s. bullae
s. edema
s. emphysema
s., focal shallow
s. hemorrhage
s. hemorrhage ‣ focal shallow
s. interstitial fibrosis ‣ focal
s. mass
s. mediastinal plexus
s. reticulated carbon deposition
subpubic arch
subpubic hernia
subpulmonary obstruction
subpulmonary stenosis
subpulmonic stenosis
subretinal fluid
subsarcolemma cisterna
subsartorial tunnel
subscapular
s. muscle
s. nerves
s. skinfold thickness
subsegmental
s. area
s. atelectasis
s. bronchus
subseptus, hymen
subsequent treatment
subsequent weight gain
subserosal fibroids
subserous fascia
subshock insulin treatment
subsided spontaneously, fever
subsided, temperature
subsidiary atrial pacemaker
subsiding
s. asthmatic attack
s., swelling

s. with rest
subsidized funding
subsonic frequency
subspecialty, medical
subspinous dislocation
substance(s) (Substance)
s. abuse
s. abuse, alcohol
s. abuse benefits
s. abuse, chronic
s. abuse, cognitive therapy of
s. abuse, comorbidity of
    schizophrenia and
s. abuse counselor
s. abuse disorder
s. abuse disorder ‣ psychoactive
s. abuse during pregnancy
s. abuse ‣ perinatal
s. abuse ‣ pharmacotherapy
s. abuse, psychoactive
s. abuse rehabilitation
s. abuse services ‣ psychiatric and
s. abuse treatment
s. abuse treatment field
S. Abuse Treatment (JSAT) ‣
    Journal of
s. abuse treatment outcome
s. abuse treatment professionals ‣
    alcohol and
s., abused
s. abuser
s. abusing mothers
s. abusing patients
s., accessory food
s., active
s., addictive
s., agglutinable
s., agglutinating
s., alpha
s. amnestic disorder ‣
    psychoactive
s., anterior ‣ perforated
s., antidiuretic
s., anti-immune
s., antipetit mal
s. anxiety disorder ‣ psychoactive
s., autacoid
s., beta
s., black
s., blood
s., blood group
s. ‣ blood grouping specific
s., Blum
s. book, controlled
s., brain

s., carcinogenic
s., cement
s., cementing
s., chromidial
s., chromophil
s., colloid
s., comorbid
s., contact
s., controlled
s., coronal
s., cytotoxin
s. delirium, psychoactive
s. delusional disorder ‣ other or
    unspecified psychoactive
s. dependence
s. dependence disorder
s. dependence, psychoactive
s., dependence-producing
s. dependency
s. -dependent patient ‣
    psychoactive
s., depressor
s., electrode implanted within brain
s., erythrocyte sensitizing
s., estrogenic
s., exophthalmos producing
s., exposure to industrial
s. ‣ exposure to toxic
s. Fa, Reichstein's
s., fat mobilizing
s., fatty
s., foreign
s., gelatinous
s., hemolytic
s., I (iodine)
s., illegal controlled
s. -induced disorder
s. induced organic mental disorder
s. -induced organic mental disorder
    ‣ psychoactive
s., ingestion of poisonous
s., ingestion of potentially
    poisonous
s., inhalation of foreign
s., injection of contrast
s., injection of radiopaque
s., interfilar
s., interprismatic
s., interstitial
s. intoxication ‣ other or
    unspecified psychoactive
s. ‣ invasion of foreign
s., lethal
s., lung
s. M., Reichstein's

substance(s)—*continued*
s., medullary
s., metachromatic
s., methylene blue active
s. misuse
s., molecular
s. mood disorder ▸ psychoactive
s., mood-altering
s. ▸ mood-modifying
s. ▸ myocardial depressant
s., neurosecretory
s., neurotransmitter
s., no-threshold
s., noxious
s. of anaphylaxis ▸ slow-reacting
s. of bones ▸ compact
s. of bones ▸ cortical
s. of bones ▸ medullary
s. of bones, red ▸ medullary
s. of bones ▸ spongy
s. of cerebellum ▸ arborescent white
s. of cerebrum, central ▸ gray
s. of cornea ▸ proper
s. of Flemming ▸ interfibrillar
s. of gray substance ▸ gelatinous
s. of kidney ▸ cortical
s. of kidney ▸ medullary
s. of lens
s. of lens ▸ cortical
s. of lung ▸ hilar
s. of lymph nodes ▸ cortical
s. of Nissl
s. of prostate ▸ muscular
s. of Schwann, white
s. of sclera ▸ proper
s. of spinal cord, central ▸ intermediate
s. of spinal cord ▸ gelatinous
s. of spinal cord ▸ gray
s. of spinal cord, lateral ▸ intermediate
s. of spinal cord ▸ white
s. of spleen ▸ red
s. of suprarenal gland ▸ cortical
s. of suprarenal gland ▸ external
s. of suprarenal gland ▸ intermediate
s. of suprarenal gland ▸ internal
s. of suprarenal gland ▸ medullary
s. of tooth ▸ adamantine
s. of tooth ▸ bony
s. of tooth ▸ intertubular
s. of tooth ▸ ivory

s. of tooth ▸ proper
s., onychogenic
s. organic mental disorder ▸ psychoactive
s. P
s., paramagnetic
s. ▸ patient injected with lethal
s. ▸ pellagra-preventing (P-P)
s., periventricular gray
s. personality disorder ▸ psychoactive
s., poisonous
s., polysaccharide
s., posterior ▸ perforated
s. ▸ potentially hazardous
s., prelipid
s., pressor
s., preventive
s., proinflammatory
s., psychoactive
s., radioactive
s., radiopaque
s., receptive
s., Reichert's
s. -related disorder
s., renal pressor
s., reticular
s., Rolando's gelatinous
s., Rollett's secondary
s., sarcous
s. sensibilis' atrice
s., sensibilizing
s., sensitizing
s., slow reacting
s., Soemmering's gray
s., specific capsular
s., specific soluble
s., temperature elevating
s., threshold
s., thromboplastic
s., tigroid
s., toxic
s., transmitter
s., tumor polysaccharide
s. use, control
s. use disorders ▸ psychoactive
s. use, illicit
s. use ▸ psychoactive
s. user
s. -using spouse
s., vasodepressor
s., volatile
s., white
s. withdrawal, psychoactive
s., zymoplastic

substantia
s. nigra
s. nigra cells, loss of
s. ossea dentis
s. propria corneae
substantial arch support
substantial effect
substernal
s. burning sensation
s. discomfort
s. gastric bypass
s. goiter
s. pain ▸ sharp
s. pressing pain
s. thyroid
substitute
s. ▸ Hemopure blood
s., heroin
s. ▸ recycled human blood
s., sugar
substitution
s., enzymes inactivating by
s., freeze-
s. of bone ▸ creeping
s. transfusion
substitutional cardiac surgery
substrate
s., arrhythmogenic
s. of enzyme, normal
s., renin
s., tachyarrhythmic
subsynaptic web
subtalar joint
subtalar motion
subtemporal decompression
subtentorial structures
subtentorial tumor
subthalamic
s. nuclei
s. nucleus
s. nucleus implant
subthreshold stimulation
subthreshold stimulation ▸ ultrarapid
subtilis
s., Bacillus
s., Copromonas
s., Strongylus
subtle
s. and nonspecific symptoms
s. difficulties
s. microcalcifications
s. personality change
subtotal
s. cystectomy

s. esophagectomy ▸ emergency
s. gastrectomy
s. hysterectomy
s. removal of tumor
s. villose atrophy

subtraction
s. angiogram ▸ electrocardiogram (ECG) synchronized digital
s. angiography
s. angiography (DSA) ▸ digital
s. angiography ▸ intra-arterial digital
s. angiography (IDSA) ▸ intraoperative digital
s. angiography (IVDSA) ▸ intravenous digital
s. arteriography, digital
s., digital
s. echocardiography, digital
s. films
s., functional
s. imaging, digital
s. imaging system, radial
s. ▸ intraoperative digital
s. ▸ mask-mode
s. technique, background
s. technique, digital
s. ventriculography, digital
s. ventriculography ▸ exercise digital

subtrochanteric fracture
subtrochanteric osteotomy
subungual
s. hematoma
s. melanoma
s. onychomycosis ▸ distal

subunit(s)
s., functional
s., neurofilament
s. of hair, functional
s. radioimmunoassay, beta
s., ribosomal
s. ▸ structure of neurofilament
s. tissue, functional

suburban cirrhosis
suburethral melanoma
subvalvular
s. aortic stenosis ▸ discrete
s. mitral stenosis
s. obstruction
s. stenosis

subverterbral muscles
subvesical fascia
subwakefulness syndrome

subxiphoid
s. area
s. limited pericardiotomy
s. pain

sub-zero cryogenic fluid
succedaneous teeth
succedaneum, caput
succenturiata, placenta
succenturiate placenta
success
s. and failure rate
s. depression
s. -obsessed culture
s. rate
s., treatment

successful
s. passage of instrument
s. treatment
s. treatment outcomes

successfully resuscitated, patient
successional teeth
successive responses, amplitude of
successive stages
succinate, methylprednisolone sodium
succinic dehydrogenase
succinylcholine drip
succinylcholine poisoning
succirubra, Cinchona
succulent hand, Marinesco's
succus entericus
succussion
s., hippocratic
s. sounds
s. splash

suck is poor, infant
suck reflex
sucking
s. and swallowing difficulties
s. appliance, thumb-
s. chest wound
s., finger-
s. lice
s. louse
s. or chewing movements
s. pattern, monitoring
s. reflex
s. response
s., thumb-
s. wound
s. wounds of the chest

suckle ▸ inability to
Sucquet-Hoyer anastomosis
sucrose intolerance

suction
s. airway
s. and intubation
s. aspiration abortion
s. assisted lipectomy
s. biopsy instrument, Quinton
s. bulb
s. catheter
s. cup
s. curettage
s. curette
s. cutter (VISC), vitreous infusion
s. D and C (dilatation and curettage)
s., diastolic
s. drainage (dr'ge)
s. drainage (dr'ge) ▸ continuous
s. drainage system, continuous
s. drainage system, Surgivac
s., gastric
s., Gomco
s., Hemovac
s., intubation and
s. lipectomy
s. machine
s. method
s., nasogastric
s., nasotracheal
s., post-tussive
s. stomach
s. tube, Adson
s. tube, Baron
s. tube, Frazier
s. tube, Gomco
s. tube inserted
s. tube, Sachs
s. unit ▸ explosion-proof
s., Wangensteen

suctioned, patient
suctioning
s., endotracheal-bronchial
s., fat
s., nasogastric tube
s., nasotracheal
s. ▸ ultrasonic fat

Sudan stain
sudanophilic leukodystrophy
sudden (Sudden)
s. attack
s. blindness
s. body jerk
s. cardiac arrest
s. cardiac death
s. cardiopulmonary arrest

sudden (Sudden)—*continued*
- s. change in vision
- s. confusion
- s. congestive heart failure (CHF)
- s. death
- s. death, chronic
- s. death due to alcohol abuse
- s. death due to cocaine ingestion
- s. death during exercise
- s. death during jogging
- s. death ▸ ischemic
- s. death, risk of
- s. death situation
- s. despair
- s. dilation of pupil
- s. dimness
- s. dimness of vision
- s. dimness or loss of vision
- s. dizziness ▸ unexplained
- s. dizziness, weakness or change in vision
- s. fall ▸ unsteadiness or
- s. falls
- s. fatal heart attack
- s. headache
- s. hearing loss
- s. heart attack death
- s. heart failure
- s. illness
- s. impulse
- s. increase in temperature
- s. infant death (SID)
- S. Infant Death Syndrome (SIDS)
- s. insight
- s., involuntary contraction of muscle
- s. lassitude
- s. loss of balance
- s. loss of coordination
- s. loss of strength
- s. loss of strength or fainting
- s. loss of vision
- s. mood swings
- s. movement
- s. numbness
- s. numbness of arm
- s. numbness of leg
- s. numbness one side of face
- s. onset
- s. onset of fever
- s. onset of unconsciousness
- s. outbursts
- s. pain
- s. paralysis
- s. paralysis and coma
- s. paralysis of arm

- s. paralysis of leg
- s. paralysis one side of face
- s. psychological stress
- s. rhythm change
- s. role reversal
- s. sensory stimuli
- s. severe cramps
- s. severe headache
- s. shortness of breath
- s. slurred speech
- S. Sniffing Death (SSD)
- s. systemic shock
- s. torsion spasms
- s. trauma
- s. trouble seeing
- s. trouble talking
- s. trouble walking
- s. unexpected death
- s. unexplained death
- s., unexplainable fall
- s. unexplainable feeling of terror
- s. vertigo attack
- s. vision loss
- s. vision problem
- s. weakness
- s. weakness, numbness or paralysis
- s. weakness of arm
- s. weakness of face
- s. weakness of leg
- s. weakness of limb
- s. weakness of one side of body
- s. weakness one side of face
- s. weakness or numbness of arm
- s. weakness or numbness of extremity
- s. weakness or numbness of face
- s. weakness or numbness of one side of body
- s. weight gain
- s. weight loss

suddenly, patient died
suddenly, patient expired
Sudeck('s)
- S. atrophy
- S. disease
- S. -Leriche syndrome
- S. point

sudomotor nerves
sudorific centers
suffered respiratory arrest ▸ patient
sufferer(s)
- s., pain
- s., seasonal allergy
- s., ulcer

suffering
- s. alcoholic
- s., alleviate
- s., chronic emotional
- s., emotional
- s. from depression
- s. from malnutrition, patient
- s., mental
- s., patient perceived
- s., physical
- s., psychological

sufficient
- s. cognitive functioning
- s. diet, calcium
- s. impairments
- s. intrinsic factor
- s., patient self-
- s. quantity
- s. quantity (NSQ) ▸ not
- s., self-
- s. symptoms of depression
- s. tears ▸ lack of

suffocating sensation
suffocation, death due to
suffocation ▸ fear of
suffocative
- s. bronchitis
- s. catarrh
- s. goiter

sugar(s)
- s., actual
- s., anhydrous
- s., barley
- s., beechwood
- s., beet
- s., blood
- s., brain
- s. (heroin), Brown
- s., cane
- s. (CBS), capillary blood
- s., collagen
- s., compressible
- s., confectioner's
- s., control blood
- s. (FBS) ▸ daily fasting blood
- s., diabetic
- s., elevated blood
- s. (FBS) ▸ fasting blood
- s., fruit
- s., gelatin
- s., grape
- s., heart
- s., high blood
- s., increased blood
- s. ▸ increased level of blood

s. intake
s., invert
s., larch
s. level
s. level, blood
s., liver
s., low blood
s., malt
s., maple
s., milk
s., molecule
s. monitoring ▸ home blood
s., muscle
s. of lead
s. oil
s., palm
s., patient spilled
s., postprandial blood
s., qualitative
s., quantitative
s., reducing
s. screening, free blood
s., serial blood
s., severe low blood
s., simple
s. spilled
s. stabilizer, blood
s. stabilizes, blood
s., starch
s. substitute
s., sulfur
s. surge ▸ postmeal blood
s. test, blood
s., threshold
s. tumor
suggested relaxation, hypnotically
suggestion
s. and direction ▸ receptivity to
s., autogenic
s., hypnotic
s., mental
s., pain determined by
s., posthypnotic
s., power of
s., psychological effects of hypnotic
s., self-regulating
s. ▸ undisciplined interpretation and
suggestive findings
suggestive medicine
Sugiura operation
suicidal
s. behavior
s. behavior ▸ prior
s. behavior ▸ recurrent
s. child

s. contract, anti-
s. death
s. depression
s. gestures
s. ideation
s. impulses
s. individual
s. or homicidal feeling
s. overtures
s. patient
s. patients, treatment of
s. plan
s. tendencies
s. tendencies, hidden
s. tendencies in children
s. tendencies, patient has
s. tendencies, patient manifests
s. thoughts
suicide
s., adolescent
s., apparent
s. assessment
s., assisted
s. attempt
s. attempt, actual
s. attempt, failed
s. attempt ▸ warning signs of
s. -by-cop
s., cluster
s., death by
s. ▸ depression, anxiety, and
s., elderly
s. ▸ ethical validity of assisted
s. evaluation
s., high risk of
s. hotline
s. ideation
s., mass
s. motivation
s., nonfatal attempt at
s. pact
s., patient
s., patient contemplated
s., physician-assisted
s. plan
s. ▸ police-assisted
s., postvention of
s. precautions
s. prevention
s. -prone patient
s. rate
s. ▸ recurring thoughts of death
    or
s. risk
s., sexual

s. survivor
s. syndrome, contagious
s. ▸ talking of death or
s., teen
s., teenage
s., threatening
s. threats
s. ventricle
s. victim
suilla, Ascaris
suipestifer, Bacillus
suipestifer, gram-negative
    Salmonella
suis
s., Actinobacillus
s., Ascaris
s., Brucella
s., gram-negative Brucella
s., Haemophilus
suit(s) (Suit)
s., anti-G
S., Life
s. ▸ medical antishock
s. ▸ military antishock
suitable beam film localization
suitable donor, potentially
suitcase kidney
suite
s., operative
s., outpatient surgical
s., surgical
sulcated tongue
sulcus (sulci)
s., alveolabial
s., alveolingual
s., anterior
s., anterolateral
s. anthelicis ▸ transversus
s. aorticus
s., atrioventricular
s. basilaris
s. blunted, costophrenic
s., blunting of
s., buccal
s., bulboventricular
s. calcarine
s., callosal
s., cardiohepatic
s., central
s. centralis cerebri
s., cingulate
s. cinguli
s. cinguli, pars
s. circularis
s. coronarius cordis

sulcus (sulci)—*continued*
- s., coronary
- s., costophrenic
- s. for optic chiasm
- s. frontalis
- s., gingival
- s., gingivolabial
- s., gyri and/or
- s. hippocampi
- s. hypothalamicus
- s. in brain
- s. intermedius
- s., interparietal
- s., intraparietal
- s., labiodental
- s., lateral
- s. limitans
- s., lingual
- s., longitudinal
- s. lunatus
- s., median
- s. nasolabialis
- s., oculomotor
- s. of heart, interventricular
- s. of heart, longitudinal
- s. of heart, transverse
- s. of lung, subclavian
- s. of occipital lobes
- s. of subclavian artery
- s. of Turner, intraparietal
- s., paramedial
- s., postauricular
- s., posterior
- s., posterior median
- s., posterointermediate
- s., posterolateral
- s., retroauricular
- s., retrocentral
- s., sigmoid
- s., terminal
- s. terminalis
- s. tumor
- s. tumor syndrome, superior
- s., tympanic
- s., Waldeyer's

sulfa level

sulfate
- s., amphetamine
- s., androsterone
- s., barium
- s. contrast medium, barium
- s., copper
- s., creatinine
- s., morphine
- s. turbidity, zinc

sulfide, selenium
sulfite allergy
sulfite sensitivity
sulfonate (SPS) ▸ sodium polyanethole
sulfonic group
sulfoxide (DMSO), Dimethyl
sulfur
- s. colloid (TSC) ▸ technetium
- s. granules
- s. ▸ milk of
- s. sugar

sulfureum, Trichophyton
sulfuris, hepar
Sulkowitch's calcium
Sulkowitch's test
sulphate (Freebase), cocaine
Sulzberger syndrome, Bloch-
sum
- s. of square deviations (SSD)
- s. peak, coincidence
- s., ray

summary
- s., clinical trial
- s., diagnostic
- s. notation
- s., preadmission screening

summating potential
summation
- s. beat
- s., central
- s. device, electronic
- s. gallop
- s., impulse
- s. shadow
- s. techniques, computer

summer
- s. burns
- s. diarrhea
- s. doldrums
- s. encephalitis, Russian spring-
- s. wounds

summit
- s. of bladder
- s. of nose

sump
- s. catheter
- s. drainage system
- s. filter ▸ mediastinal
- s. pump
- s. syndrome
- s. tube, Argyle-Salem
- s. tube, Axiom double

Sun (sun)
- S. (serum urea nitrogen)

- s. block
- s. cautery
- s. damage
- s. damage, cumulative
- s. -damaged skin
- s. ▸ excessive exposure to
- s. exposure
- s. exposure, chronic
- s. exposure ▸ cumulative effects of unprotected
- s. exposure, excessive
- s. –induced keratosis ▸ noncancerous
- s., overexposure to
- s. protection
- s. protection factor (SPF)
- s. sensitivity
- s. texture
- s. ultraviolet radiation

sunburn sensitivity
sunburn, severe
sunburst appearance
sunburst lesion, black
sundown effect
sundown syndrome
sundowner's syndrome
sundowning, patient
Sundt carotid endarterectomy shunt
sunflower cataract
sunken
- s. acetabulum
- s. in appearance, eyes
- s. veins

sunlight
- s., exposure to
- s., extreme sensitivity to
- s., overexposure to

sunrise projection
sunscreen
- s. protection
- s. sting
- s., waterproof
- s., water-resistant
- s., waxy

Sunshine (LSD)
Sunshine (LSD), California
supercam scintillation scanner
superciliaris, arcus
superciliary arch
superciliary depressor muscle
superconducting quantum interference device (SQUID)
superego ▸ maturational vicissitudes of

superficial
- s. abdominal reflexes
- s. abrasion
- s. affect
- s. and deep parotid lymph nodes
- s. angioma
- s. basal cell carcinoma
- s. bites of tissue
- s. bladder cancer
- s. bleeders
- s. blood vessels
- s. branch of radial nerve
- s. branch of ulnar nerve
- s. bullae
- s. cancer
- s. cell
- s. cells, cornified
- s. cells, precornified
- s. cervical lymph nodes
- s. charm
- s. circumflex iliac vein
- s. cortical hemorrhage
- s. desquamation
- s. dorsal veins of clitoris
- s. dorsal veins of penis
- s. duodenitis
- s. epigastric vein
- s. erosion
- s. fascia
- s. femoral artery
- s. femoral artery contusion
- s. fibular nerve
- s. flexor muscle of fingers
- s. focal ulceration
- s. frostbite
- s. gastric ulcer
- s. gastritis
- s. hemorrhage distal esophagus
- s. idiot
- s. implant
- s. implantation
- s. incision
- s. infection
- s. inguinal lymph nodes
- s. irritation
- s. laceration
- s. laceration, healed
- s. layer of cervix
- s. layers of cornea
- s. middle cerebral vein
- s. middle petrosal nerve
- s. musculo-aponeurotic system (SMAS)
- s. myocardial layer
- s. nerve, greater

- s. nonhealing ulceration
- s., patient
- s. peroneal nerve
- s. phlebitis
- s. pneumonia
- s. radial nerve
- s. rationalization
- s. reflex
- s. scaler
- s. sclera
- s. squamous cell carcinoma
- s. structures
- s. subendocardial focal hemorrhages
- s. suture
- s. temporal artery
- s. temporal artery pressure points
- s. temporal vein
- s. thrombophlebitis
- s. tonsillitis
- s. transverse muscle of perineum
- s. treatments
- s. ulceration
- s. units
- s. varicosities
- s. vein
- s. venous markings
- s. vertebral veins
- s. wound

superficiale ▸ vas lymphaticum
superficialis
- s., colitis cystica
- s., esophagitis dissecans
- s., flexor digitorum
- s., keratitis ramificata
- s. muscle, flexor digitorum
- s., xerosis

superficially applied microwaves
superficially explored, wound
superfluous hair
Supergrass (hallucinogen)
Supergrass (phencyclidine)
superimposed
- s. acute inflammatory episodes
- s. bowel gas
- s. depression
- s. echodensity
- s. thrombus
- s. upper motor neuron dysfunction

superimposition of bowel shadows
superior
- s. alveolar nerve
- s. ampullar nerve
- s. anastomotic vein
- s., ankyloglossia

- s. annulus, posterior
- s., arcus palpebralis
- s. articular facet
- s. articulating process
- s. aspect
- s. auricular muscle
- s. azygos vein, lesser
- s. border
- s. cardiac nerve
- s. carotid artery
- s. carotid ganglion
- s. cavopulmonary anastomosis (BSCA) ▸ bidirectional
- s. cerebellar peduncle
- s. cerebellar vein
- s. cerebral veins
- s. cervical cardiac nerve
- s. cervical chain
- s. cervical ganglion
- s. clunial nerves
- s. colliculi
- s. commissure
- s. corner
- s. cul-de-sac
- s. duodenal fold
- s. epigastric veins
- s. flexure of duodenum
- s. fovea
- s. frontal gyrus
- s. ganglion of glossopharyngeal nerve
- s. ganglion of vagus nerve
- s. gemellus muscle
- s. gluteal nerve
- s. gluteal veins
- s., gyrus frontalis
- s., gyrus temporalis
- s. hemorrhagic polioencephalitis
- s. hemorrhoidal vein
- s. iliac spine (ASIS), anterior
- s. insular gyrus of brain
- s. intercostal vein, left
- s. intercostal vein, right
- s. internal laryngeal nerve
- s. labial region
- s. labial veins
- s. lacrimal gland
- s. laryngeal nerve
- s. laryngeal vein
- s. lateral cutaneous nerve of arm
- s. ligament
- s. ligament of the incus
- s. limbic keratoconjunctivitis
- s. lip, incisive muscles of
- s. lobe

superior—*continued*

- s. longitudinal muscle of tongue
- s. longitudinal sinus, ligation
- s. meatus
- s. mediastinum
- s. mediastinum, widening of
- s. mesenteric angiogram
- s. mesenteric artery (SMA)
- s. mesenteric artery bypass
- s. mesenteric artery syndrome
- s. mesenteric ganglion
- s. mesenteric lymph nodes
- s. mesenteric vascular occlusion
- s. mesenteric vein
- s. muscle, levator palpebrae
- s. muscle, obliquus
- s. muscle, rectus
- s., musculus obliquus
- s. nasal venule of retina
- s. oblique muscle
- s. oblique muscle, advancement
- s. oblique muscle of eyeball
- s. oblique tendon
- s. occipital gyrus
- s. ophthalmic vein
- s. ossea, concha nasalis
- s. ossicular chain
- s. palpebrae, tarsus
- s. palpebral region
- s. palpebral vein
- s. parietal lobule
- s. pedicle
- s. pelvic strait ▸ entrance of fetal head into
- s. perihilar mass
- s. phrenic vein
- s. pole of calyces
- s. portion of mesencephalon
- s. posterior serratus muscle
- s. projection, inferior-
- s. protoplasm
- s. pulmonary vein isolated
- s. pulmonary vein, left
- s. pulmonary vein, right
- s. QRS axis
- s. ramus
- s. rectal branch
- s. rectal vein
- s. rectus
- s. rectus bridle suture
- s. rectus muscle
- s. rectus muscle, advancement of
- s. rectus traction suture
- s. rote memory
- s. sagittal sinus

- s. segment of lung
- s. semilunar lobule
- s., sinus sagittalis
- s. spine, anterior
- s. sulcus tumor syndrome
- s. tangential projection, inferior-
- s. tarsal muscle
- s. temporal gyrus
- s. temporal venule of retina
- s. thyroid artery
- s. thyroid gland
- s. thyroid notch
- s. thyroid vein
- s. tracheobronchial lymph nodes
- s. turbinate
- s. vagal ganglion
- s. vena cava (SVC)
- s. vena cava (SVC) syndrome
- s., venula macularis
- s., venula nasalis retinae
- s., venula temporalis retinae
- s., vertebral notch

superioris, ankyloglossia

superioris, musculus levator palpebrae

superiority complex

superiorly, milked

Superjoint (hallucinogen)

supernormal artery

supernormal recovery phase

supernumerary
- s. bone
- s. cervical ribs
- s. digits
- s. kidney
- s. lacrimal gland
- s. lacrimonasal duct
- s. ribs
- s. teeth

superoinferior heart

superoinferior projection

superolateral aspect

superoxide dimutase gene

superoxide dismutase (SOD)

superparamagnetic contrast agent

supersonic
- s. frequency
- s. rays
- s. waves

superstitious false idea

supervised
- s. exercise program
- s. exercise training
- s. fasting protocol, medically
- s. urinalysis

- s. withdrawal, medically

supervising psychiatrist

supervision
- s., dietary
- s., general nursing
- s., medical/nursing
- s. of detoxification services
- s., patient does activities of daily living (ADL) with

Supervisor, Nursing

supervoltage
- s. generator
- s. rotational irradiation therapy
- s. technique
- s. therapy
- s. x-ray therapy

supination
- s., abnormal
- s. exercise, elbow
- s., pronation and

supinator longus reflex

supinator muscle

supinatus, pes

supinatus, talipes

supine
- s. bicycle echocardiogram (SBE)
- s. bicycle stress echocardiography
- s. exercise
- s. film
- s. hypotensive syndrome
- s. mediolateral view
- s. oblique approach
- s. position
- s. rest gated equilibrium image
- s. to sit transfer
- s. to sitting, transfer from

supinely, float

supple joints

supple, neck

supplement
- s., beta carotene
- s., calcium
- s., daily high fiber
- s., diet
- s., dietary
- s., enzyme
- s., favorite
- s., fish oil
- s., food
- s., herbal
- s., hormone
- s., iron
- s., melatonin
- s., mineral
- s., multivitamin

s., nourishing oral
s., nutritional
s., potassium
s. to diet ▸ liquid
s. ▸ unregulated dietary
s., vitamin

supplemental
s. dose
s. dose, daily
s. growth hormone therapy
s. inspired oxygen (O_2)
s. insurance
s. nutrition
s. oxygen (O_2)
s. oxygen (O_2), portable
s. oxygen (O_2) therapy
s. testosterone
s. therapy
s. treatment

supplementary
s. menstruation
s. motor area
s. respiration
s. scale

supplementation, nutritional
supplementation, vitamin
suppleness ▸ adequate range of
motion
supply(-ies) (Supply)
s., adequate blood
s., air
s. and matures ▸ develops new
blood
s., arterial
s., blood
S., Central
s. critical, oxygen
s., decreased blood
s., deficiency of blood
s., energy
s., inadequate blood
s., insufficient blood
s., interruption of blood
s., local diminution in blood
s. ▸ loss of blood
s., medical
s. ▸ myocardial oxygen (O_2)
s., nation's blood
s., occlusion of arterial
s. of brain, blood
s. ▸ oxygen (O_2)
s. ▸ oxygenated blood
s., renal vascular
s. safety, blood
s., splenic vascular

s. to brain stem, blood
s. to heart, blood
s. to heart ▸ reduced blood
s. to tissues, blood
s. ▸ tumor's blood
s., uncontaminated surgical
s., unimpaired nerve

support (Support)
s., Abée's
s., above knee (AK)
s. (ACLS) ▸ advanced cardiac life
s. (ALS), advanced life
s. (ATLS), advanced trauma life
s., airway
s., Antabuse
s., arch
s., artificial life
s., augmented psychological
s., basic cardiac life
s., basic life
s., behavioral
s., bereavement
s., biventricular
s., brain
s., cardiopulmonary
s., cardiovascular
s., clergy
s., clinical
s., constructive
s. defect, pelvic
s. device ▸ Medtronic defibrillator
implant
s. dressing, Jobst mammary
s. during labor, emotional
s., effective chemotherapeutic
s., emotional
s. environment, home care
s. ▸ extracorporeal life
s., family
s., financial
s., forego life
s. garment, Frederick foundation
s., good pelvic
s. group
s. group, anorexia
s. group, bereavement
s. group, community
s. group, divorce
s. group, family
s. group for Alzheimer's disease
s. group for epilepsy
s. group for paraplegics
s. group for quadriplegics
s. group, grief
s. group junkie

s. group, long-term
s. group, open ended
s. group ▸ pacemaker
s. group, pain
s. group, referral to
s. group, self-help
s. group services
S. Group ▸ Tough Love Parents
s. group ▸ youth/parent
s., hemodynamic
s., home care
s. hose ▸ elastic
s., hospice
s. hospital (CSH) ▸ combat
s. ▸ hypotensive and ventilatory
s., hysterectomy
s. in respiratory distress ▸
ventilatory
s., informal
s., inotropic
s., introitus with good
s., jaw
s. ▸ lack of
s. ▸ lack of social
s., learning
s. ▸ life skills
s., longitudinal
s. long-term recovery
s. ▸ low level of social
s., lumbosacral
s., mastectomy
s. measures, life
s., multihandicapped
s., network of
s. network structure ▸ social
s., nonmedical
s., nutritional
s., organ
s., peer
s., pelvic
s. ▸ percutaneous cardiopulmonary
s. ▸ percutaneous cardiopulmonary
bypass
s., perineal
s., physical
s. ▸ physical and emotional
s., prenatal
s. problem, pelvic
s. (ACLS) protocol ▸ advanced
cardiac life
s. provide appropriate nonverbal
s. ▸ psychologic, emotional, somatic
s., psychological
s. relaxed
s., religious

support—*continued*
s., removal of life
s., respiratory
s., sandbag placed for
s. ▸ seeking social
s. ▸ sensory impaired
s. services
s. session
s. sessions, group
s., social
s., spiritual
s. stitches, perineal
s. stockings
s. stockings, surgical
s. stockings ▸ venous pressure gradient
s., substantial arch
s. suture
s. sutures, perineal
s. system
s. system, circulatory
s. system, life-
s. system, positive
s. system ▸ structure of the
s. system ▸ withdrawing life
s. technique
s. technology, life
s., therapeutic
s. to family, emotional
s. to patient, emotional
s., uterus has good
s. ventilation ▸ pressure
s., ventilatory
s. ▸ volume-assured pressure
s., walking without
supported by mechanical respirator ▸ breathing
supported denture ▸ implant
supporting
s. cells
s. stitches
s. structures
s. structures, denture-
s. tissue of brain
s. tissue, vesicular
s. treatment, life-
supportive
s. care
s. care ▸ emotional aspects of
s. care environment
s. care of patient
s. care, patient transfused and treated with
s. care, patient treated with
s. care, potential benefits of

s. care withdrawn
s., church community
s. counseling
s. device to restrain hernia
s. environment
s. expressive therapy
s. halo cast
s. home care
s. intervention
s. measures
s. measures, general
s. medical/nursing care
s. nursing care
s. programs, intensive
s. psychiatric treatment
s. psychological treatment
s. psychotherapy
s. services
s. social structure
s. structures weaken
s. therapeutic contact
s. therapeutic recovery
s. therapy
s. therapy, minimal
s. therapy technique
s. tissue(s)
s. tissue ▸ overgrowth of non-nervous
s. treatment
suppository
s., glycerin
s. inserted, glycerin
s., rectal
s., vaginal
suppress
s. abnormal genes
s. drinking behavior
s. emotional responses
s. estrogen receptors in cancer cells
s. immune reaction
s. inhibitions
s. reflex contractions
s. specific seizure wave electroencephalogram (EEG) activity
suppressant
s., appetite
s. ▸ confusion from appetite
s., cough
s. therapy, chronic
s., vestibular
suppressed
s. immune response
s. memories

s. menstruation
s. pacemaker, ventricular
s. respiration
s. strabismus
suppressing
s. adrenal steroidogenesis
s. drug, fungus-
s. drug, pain-
s. drugs ▸ immune
s. symptoms
suppression (Suppression)
s., adrenal
s., auditory
s., bone marrow
s., burst-
s., chest
s., conscious
s. genes, tumor
s., immune
s., immuno◊
s., immunologic tumor
s., immunological
s., inducing
s., inflammatory
s. of bone marrow
s. of electroencephalogram (EEG) activity
s. of emotion
s. of immune system
s. of milk production
s. of seizure specific brain waves
s. of tumor growth
s. of voltage
s., overdrive
s. pattern, burst-
s. test (DST) ▸ dexamethasone
S. Trial (CAST), Cardiac Arrhythmia
s. ▸ white blood count
suppressive
s. activities of antibodies, tumor
s. antibiotics
s. anuria
s. medication
s. medication, immune-
s. or disease modifying drugs
s. therapy
suppressor
s. cells
s. gene
s. genes, tumor
s. lymphocytes
s., tumor
suppurating gastritis
suppuration, alveodental
suppuration, period of

suppurativa, hidradenitis
suppurativa, hidrosadenitis
   destruens
suppurative
  s. adenitis
  s. appendicitis
  s. appendix
  s. arthritis
  s. encephalitis
  s. hepatitis
  s. hidradenitis
  s. infection
  s. keratitis
  s. labyrinthitis
  s. labyrinthitis, acute
  s. marginal gingivitis
  s. mastitis
  s. myositis
  s. nephritis
  s. oropharyngeal disease
  s. otitis media, chronic
  s. pericarditis
  s. pericementitis, chronic
  s. phlebitis
  s. pleurisy
  s. pneumonia
  s. pyelitis
  s. retinitis
  s. thrombophlebitis
  s. tonsillitis
supra-annular mitral valve
  replacement
supra-annular prosthesis
supra-aortic angiography
supracallosal gyrus
supracallosus, gyrus
supracardiac silhouette
supracardinal veins
supracervical hysterectomy
supracervical incision
suprachoroid lamina
supraclavicular
  s. adenopathy
  s. and tangential fields, matching
  s. area
  s. bruit
  s. examination
  s. fascia
  s. fossa
  s. lymph node biopsy
  s. lymph nodes
  s. nerve block
  s. nerves
  s. nerves, anterior
  s. nerves, lateral

  s. nerves, medial
  s. nerves, middle
  s. nerves, posterior
  s. node
  s. node biopsy
  s. node masses
  s. node metastasis in lung
    carcinoma
  s. port
  s. region
supraclinoid carotid aneurysm
supracondylar fracture
supracondylar fracture of femur
supradiaphragmatic diverticulum
supradiaphragmatic sympathectomy
supraglottic carcinoma
supraglottic structures
supraglottitis, acute
suprahepatic venous obstruction
suprahilar mass
supra-Hisian block
suprahyoid muscles
suprahyoid musculature
supralevator abscess
supraliminal stimulus
supramarginal gyrus
supramarginalis, gyrus
supramaximal tetanic stimulation
suprameatal spine
supramediastinal mantle in radiation
  therapy
Supramid
  S. implant
  S. implant material
  S. ptosis sling
  S. suture
supranormal
  s. conduction
  s. excitability
  s. excitation
supranuclear palsy, progressive
supraomohyoid neck dissection
supraoptic commissures
supraorbital
  s. area
  s. artery
  s. nerve
  s. notch
  s. reflex
  s. region
  s. vein
suprapatellar
  s. effusion
  s. pouch
  s. reflex

suprapubic
  s. area ▸ manual percussion of
  s. aspiration
  s. catheter
  s. cystostomy
  s. cystotomy
  s. incision
  s. pressure
  s. prostatectomy
  s. rami
  s. reflex
  s. region
  s. tenderness
  s. transvesical prostatectomy
  s. tubes
suprarenal
  s. aortic aneurysm
  s. capsule
  s. epithelioma
  s. ganglion
  s. gland
  s. gland ▸ central vein of
  s. gland ▸ cortical substance of
  s. gland ▸ external substance of
  s. gland, fetal
  s. gland, hilus of
  s. gland ▸ intermediate substance
    of
  s. gland ▸ internal substance of
  s. gland ▸ medullary substance of
  s. medulla
  s. plexus
  s. vein, left
  s. vein, right
suprarenale, melasma
suprarenalis cachexia
suprarenalis, hilus glandulae
suprarenogenic syndrome
suprascapular
  s. nerve
  s. notch
  s. vein
suprasellar aneurysm
suprasellar tumor
supraspinous muscle
suprasternal
  s. examination
  s. height, sitting
  s. notch
  s. pulsation
  s. region
  s. retraction
  s. view
supratentorial astrocytoma

supratentorial parts of central nervous system
supratonsillaris, plica
supratrochlear
- s. artery
- s. depression
- s. foraminal bone
- s. nerve
- s. nerve, stretching of
- s. veins

supraumbilical reflex
supravaginal hysterectomy
supravalvular
- s. aortic stenosis
- s. aortic stenosis infantile hypercalcemia syndrome
- s. aortic stenosis syndrome

supraventricular
- s. arrhythmia
- s. arrhythmia ▸ paroxysmal
- s. arrhythmias ▸ refractory
- s. crest
- s. ectopy
- s. extrasystole
- s. premature contraction
- s. rhythm
- s. tachyarrhythmia ▸ sustained
- s. tachyarrhythmias
- s. tachycardia (SVT)
- s. tachycardia ablation
- s. tachycardia (PSVT) ▸ paroxysmal
- s. tachycardia ▸ paroxysmal reentrant
- s. tachycardia ▸ reentrant

supravesical extraperitoneal cesarean section
supravital staining
suprema ossea, concha nasalis
supreme cardiac nerves
surae
- s. jerk, triceps
- s. muscle, triceps
- s. reflex, triceps

sural nerve
surdocardiac syndrome
surf (surfactant) test
surface(s)
- s., abdominal wall
- s. anatomy
- s. anesthesia
- s., anterior
- s. antibody (HBsAb) ▸ hepatitis B
- s. antigen
- s. antigen (Anti-HBs) ▸ antibody to hepatitis B
- s. antigen, cell
- s. antigen (HBsAg) ▸ hepatitis B
- s. antigen (HBsAg) reactivity ▸ hepatitis B
- s. antigen studies ▸ hepatitis
- s. area
- s. area, body
- s. area ▸ proximal isovelocity
- s., articular
- s., assistive device on level
- s., atrophic mucosal
- s., back
- s. biopsy
- s. blood vessels
- s., body
- s., bosselated
- s., brain
- s. burned, body
- s. cancers
- s., capsular
- s., cell
- s. chemistry
- s., concave anterior
- s., concave posterior
- s., congested cortical
- s., conjunctivotarsal
- s. contaminant
- s., corneal
- s., cortical
- s., culturing of environmental
- s. curvature
- s., cut
- s. damage, articular
- s., debrided bone
- s. denuded, epithelial
- s., deperitonealized
- s., diaphragmatic
- s., dorsal
- s. dose, biological
- s. ▸ dry serosal peritoneal
- s. electrode
- s., epicardial
- s., exposed
- s. ▸ fibrinolytic activity of mesothelial
- s. film of liquid
- s., fissures on brain
- s., flexor
- s., friction of pericardial
- s., granular
- s. implant
- s. infiltration by hemorrhage
- s., inflamed

- s., joint
- s. lamellar transplant
- s. large intestine ▸ mucosal
- s., lateral
- s., lateral plateau joint
- s. layer of cervix
- s., level
- s., masticating
- s. membrane antigen
- s., mesial
- s., mucosal
- s., myometrial
- s., nonsterile
- s., nonsterile environmental
- s. occipital lobe, medial
- s., occlusal
- s. of abdominal wall ▸ inner
- s. of body, vertebral
- s. of bone, severed
- s. of brain
- s. of brain, elevated
- s. of brain stem, dorsal
- s. of cerebral hemisphere, medial
- s. of contact
- s. of cornea
- s. of duodenum ▸ mucosal
- s. of epithelial cells
- s. of esophagus ▸ mucosal
- s. of eye, outer
- s. of eye, protective outer
- s. of great toe ▸ dorsal digital nerves of lateral
- s. of great toe, lateral
- s. of head
- s. of head, electrodes placed on
- s. of knee, dorsolateral
- s. of knee, lateral
- s. of left lung ▸ diaphragmatic
- s. of lesion
- s. of lip, vermilion
- s. of occipital lobe of brain, mesial
- s. of ribs, inner
- s. of right lung ▸ diaphragmatic
- s. of second toe ▸ dorsal digital nerves of medial
- s. of small intestine ▸ mucosal
- s. of stomach ▸ mucosal
- s. of tongue
- s. of tooth
- s. of tooth, axial
- s. of tooth, buccal
- s. of tooth, cervical
- s. of tooth, distal
- s. of tooth, facial
- s. of tooth, gingival

s. of tooth, incisal
s. of tooth, lingual
s. of tooth, mesial
s. of tooth, occlusal
s. of wrist, ventral
s., palmar
s., peritoneal
s., plantar
s., pleural
s., posterior
s. reconstruction ▸ polyhedral
s. ▸ remesothelialization of
  peritoneal
s., scaly
s., serosal
s., skin
s. skin area ▸ central
s., sloping
s. smooth and glistening ▸ capsular
s. smooth and glistening ▸
  peritoneal
s., smooth cortical
s. tension
s. tension ▸ altered pulmonary
s. tension, interfacial
s. tissues
s. trauma
s., ventral
s. vertebral body disc
s. vessels
s., volar

**surfaced lesion, hyperkeratotic
  verrucoid**
surfactant
s., bovine lavage extract
s. deficiency
s. ▸ hydrolysis of
s., pulmonary
Surfer (hallucinogen)
surfers' nodules
surge ▸ postmeal blood sugar
surgeon
s., assistant
s., barber
s., oral
s., orthopedic
s., plastic reconstructive
s., transplant
surgery(-ies) (Surgery)
s., abdominal
s., ablative cardiac
s., additional
s., ambulatory
S. (ASLMS) ▸ American Society for
  Laser Medicine and

s. and irradiation, conservative
s., anesthetic
s., argon laser
s., arthroscopic
s., arthroscopic knee
s., asthetic plastic
s. authorization form, cosmetic
s., balloon videoscope
s., Band-Aid
s., bariatric
s. ▸ beating heart
s., belly button
s., bloodless
s., Botulinum Toxin (Botox)
  cosmetic
s., brain
s., brain graft
s., brain implant
s., breast augmentation
s., breast conservation
s., breast enhancement
s., breast reconstruction
s., breast reduction
s. ▸ brow lift
s., bypass
s., cardiac
s., cardiac bypass
s., cardiothoracic
s. (CVS), cardiovascular
s., cataract
s., cervical
s., closed heart
s., computer assisted laser
s. consent form, cosmetic
s., conventional
s., corneal transplant
s., coronary artery
s., coronary artery bypass (CAB)
s., coronary artery bypass grafting
s., corrective
s., cosmetic
s., cosmetic breast
s., cosmetic eyelid
s., cosmetic facial
s. ▸ cosmetic laser
s., cosmetic nasal
s., curative
s., decompression
s., definitive
s., deforming
s., denervation
s., detoxification before
s., diagnostic
s. ▸ double lung reduction
s., elective

s. ▸ elective abdominal
s., emergency
s., endoscopic
s., endoscopic plastic
s., endoscopic sinus
s. ▸ endoscopic vein
s., endovascular
s., epilepsy
s., excimer laser
s., excisional
s. ▸ excisional cardiac
s., experimental
s., experimental laser
s., exploratory
s., extracapsular
s. ▸ extracorporeal renal
s., eye
s., eyelid
s., eyesight
s. ▸ face lift
s., facial
s. ▸ facial cosmetic
s. ▸ facial implant
s. ▸ facial plastic
s. ▸ facial rejuvenation cosmetic
s., femoral popliteal bypass
s., fetal
s., flap
s. ▸ flap and zap
s. for cataracts
s. (FESS) ▸ functional endoscopic
  sinus
s., gallstone
s., gamma ray
s. ▸ gastric bypass
s., general
s. ▸ general reconstructive
s., gynecomastia
s. ▸ hair replacement
s. ▸ hair restoration
s., hand
s., hangman's
s., heart
s., heart bypass
s. ▸ heart port
s. ▸ heart reduction
s. ▸ heart valve
s. ▸ hip replacement
s. ▸ hologram-assisted
s., hypothermic
s. ▸ hypothermic cardiac arrest
s., ileus following abdominal
s., impatient
s., implant
s., in utero

surgery(-ies)—*continued*

s. ▸ injectable fillers in plastic
s., intestinal bypass
s., in-the-womb
s., intracranial
s., intraoperative radiation
s., intrusive
s., invasive
s. ▸ invasive brain
s., invasive spinal
s., irradiation and
s. ▸ irreversible laser
s., joint replacement
s. ▸ junctional rhythm after cardiac
s., keyhole
s. ▸ keyhole bypass
s. ▸ knee replacement
s., laparoscopic
s., laparoscopic gallbladder
s., laser
s., laser beam
s., laser eye
s. ▸ laser glaucoma
s. ▸ laser heart
s. ▸ laser refractive
s. ▸ laser skin
s. ▸ laser-assisted in situ
keratomileusis (LASIK)
s., left cataract
s. ▸ left ventricular (LV) reduction
s., lid
s., life-threatening
s., limitations of
s., limited
s., liposuction
s. ▸ liposuction cosmetic
s. ▸ lung reduction
s. ▸ lung volume reduction
s., major contraindication to
s., major intra-abdominal
s., major thoracic
s., micro◇
s., microvascular
s. ▸ microvascular decompression
s., minimally invasive brain
s. ▸ minimally invasive laparoscopy
s. ▸ minimally invasive valve
replacement
s., Mohs
s. ▸ Mohs micrographic
s. ▸ neck lift
s. ▸ nerve sparing
s. ▸ no stitch cataract
s., noncardiac
s., noninvasive

s., obesity
s., oculoplastic
s., open heart
s., open womb
s., oral
s., orbital
s., organ transplantation
s., orthopedic
s., otologic
s., outpatient
s., pain-free
s., palliative
s., patient candidate for
s., patient given enema prior to
s., patient prepped for
s., phacoemulsification
s., plastic
s., plastic and reconstructive
s., postmastectomy reconstructive
s., potential for
s., preoperative contraindication to
s., pretransplant
s. ▸ primary hip replacement
s. ▸ prophylactic breast
s. ▸ prosthetic heart valve
s. ▸ quintuple bypass
s. ▸ radial artery bypass
s., radical
s., radical brain
s. ▸ radical cancer
s. ▸ radical prostate
s., recent
s., reconstructive
s., reconstructive breast
s. ▸ reconstructive cosmetic
s. ▸ reconstructive eyelid
s., reconstructive hip
s., recovering from
s. ▸ re-excision
s., refractive
s., refractive eye
s., reparative
s. ▸ reparative cardiac
s. ▸ repeat hip replacement
s. ▸ rescue coronary bypass
s., retropubic
s. ▸ revision hip replacement
s., right cataract
s., risk of major
s., risk-free
s., robotic
s., rotator cuff
S., Same Day
s. ▸ scalp flap
s. ▸ single lung reduction

s., sinus
s. ▸ small incision cataract
s., spinal fusion
s. ▸ split brain
s., stereotactic
s., stereotaxic
s. ▸ substitutional cardiac
s., sutureless cataract
s., sweat
s., tattoo
s., thoracic
s., thyroplasty
s., traditional
s., transplant
s. treatment, laser
s., triple bypass heart
s. ▸ unilateral lung reduction
s., valve replacement
s. via laparoscope, laser
s. ▸ video-assisted thoracic
s., videoscopic
s. ▸ vision correction
s., vitrectomy
s. ▸ wavefront-guided LASIK (laser-
assisted in situ keratomileusis)
s. ▸ weight loss
s. ▸ weight reduction
s. with implant, cataract
s. ▸ wrap-around
s., written consent for

surgical (Surgical) [*Surgicel*]

s. abdomen
s. ablation
s. abortion
s. abscess
s. absence of breast
s. absence of fallopian tubes
s. absence of limb
s. absence of ovaries
s. absence of uterus
s. adjuvant therapy
s. alternative, non-
s. amputation
s. anastomosis of pancreatic duct
s. anatomy
s. and dental procedures
s. anesthesia
s. antibiotic utilization
s. approach
s. assistant
s. biopsy
s. biopsy, excisional
s. biopsy ▸ open
s. birth
s. cancer treatment

s. candidate
s. care, definitive
s. chromic suture
S. Clerk
s. clipping
s. closure of sac of aneurysm
s. closure, prompt
s. complications of drug abuse
s. consultation
s. contraception
s. correction
s. corset
s. course
s. criteria
s. debridement
s. decompression
s. defect
s. defects, irradiated
s. deliveries
s. diet, clear
s. discharge indicators
s. disease
s. dome
s. drainage
s. drapes
s. emphysema
s. engine
s. evaluative staging
s. excision
s. excision of organ
s. excisions, multiple
s. exploration
s. field
s. fixation
s. flap
s. gauze
s., general medical and
s. hand scrubs
s. hazard
s. histopathology
s. history
s. history (PSH) ▸ past
s. immobilization of joint
s. implant
s. implantation
s. incision
s. incision ▸ appendix brought into
s. incision, healed
s. incision, healing
s. infection
s. infection, post◊
s. infection prevention
s. inpatient care
S. Intensive Care Unit (SICU)
s. intervention

s. iridectomy
s. isolator
s. laser
s. lesion
s. liaison
s. limbus
S. Lint Pic-Ups
s. lung biopsy
s. management
s. management, cytoreductive
s. management, exploratory
s. management of drug abusers
s. management of metastatic
   disease
s. management, second look
s. menopause
s. mortality
s. navigation (ISN) ▸ interaction
s. neck
s. neck of humerus
s. neck of tooth
s. nurse
s. nurse-on-call
s. oncologist
s. option
s. packing
s. pain ▸ moderate post-
s. pain, post-
s. patch ▸ Gore-Tex
s. pathogens, gram-negative
s. pathogens, gram-positive
s. permit signed
s. prep
s. prevention of stroke
s. procedure
s. procedure for subarachnoid
   hemorrhage
s. procedure, modified
s. procedure, radical
s. procedure, reconstructive
s. prophylaxis
s. radiation therapy ▸ post-
s. recovery of donated organs and
   tissues
s. release and repair
s. removal
s. removal of donated organs
s. removal of organ
s. removal of tumor
s. repair
s. repair ▸ anal
s. replantation
s. resection
s. resection, activation map-
   guided

s. resection, failure patterns after
s. resident
s. revascularization procedure
s. revision
s. risk
s. risk, patient poor
s. robot
s. robot ▸ voice controlled
s. scar
s. shock
S. Simplex P radiopaque bone
   cement
s. site
s. site infection (SSI)
s. skills ▸ perfection of
s. soft diet
s. sponge
s. staging
s. suite
s. suite, outpatient
s. supplies, contaminated
s. supplies, uncontaminated
s. support stockings
s. suture, absorbable
s. suture, nonabsorbable
s. swelling
s. sympathectomy
s. team
s. technique
s. technique, image-guided
s. technique ▸ invasive
s. technique ▸ keyhole
s. template
s. testing, pre-
s. therapy
s. therapy, adjuvant
s. tissue, analyzing
s. trauma
s. treatment
s. treatment for aneurysm
s. treatment for brain tumor
s. treatment for epidural
   hemorrhage
s. treatment for epilepsy
s. treatment for Parkinson's
   disease
s. treatment for severed nerve
s. treatment for stroke
s. tuberculosis
s. urachus
s. use ▸ short-term post-
s. wound
s. wound, appendix brought into
s. wound classification
s. wound covered with collodion

surgical—*continued*
s. wound infection
s. wound surveillance
surgically
s. absent, breast
s. absent, uterus
s. created opening
s. implanted device
s. implanted electrode
s. implanted feeding tube
s. implanted medication tube
s. implanted neurostimulator
s. implanted pumps
s. implanted tube
s. ▸ metal sieve implanted
s. placed graft
s., repair
s. sealed, aneurysm
s., severed digit reattached
s., severed extremity reattached
s., severed limb reattached
Surgicel [*surgical*]
S. gauze
S. gauze implant placement
S. implant placement
S. implantation
Surgidev intraocular lens (IOL)
Surgitek mammary implant
Surgitek penile prosthesis
Surgivac suction drainage system
surrogate
s. decision-maker
s. mother
s. parenthood
s. parenting
surrounded by hematoma ▸ pelvic viscera
surrounding(s)
s. brain, alterations of media
s. breast tissue
s. erythema
s. graft material
s. lung parenchyma
s. myocardial fibers
s. nipple, dark skin
s., patient aware of
s., patient has interest in
s., patient has no interest in
s. structures
s. tissues
s. tissues, isodense with
surrounds carotid artery ▸ tumor
sursum vergens, strabismus
sursumduction
s. hyperphoria, alternating

s. of left eye
s. of right eye
surveillance (Surveillance)
s. angiography
s. artifacts
s., cardiovascular
s. data
s. data on infection, compiling
s., environmental
s., infection control
S. Nurse (ESN) ▸ Environmental
s. of infections
S. Officer (SO)
S. Officer (ESO) ▸ Environmental
s., ongoing
s. practices, effective
s. procedure
s. procedures, coordination of
S. Program
s., prospective
s., random
s., retrospective
s., routine
s., selective
s., surgical wound
s. system
survey (Survey)
s., bone
s., environmental
s., epidemiological
s., incidence
s., long bone
S. (NHDS) ▸ National Health Discharge
s., neurologic
s., prevalence
s., prospective
s., retrospective
s., skeletal
s., skull
survival
s., allograft
s. changes
s. curve, actuarial
s. curve, initial linear
s. curves, multifraction
s. data ▸ long-term
s. enhancement, allograft
s. factor
s., high probability of
s., intervener
s., linear quadratic formula for dose
s., management and
s., mean

s. period, long-term
s. probability
s. rate
s. rate, disease-free
s. rate, five-year
s. rate, long-term
s. rate, one-year
s. rate, patient
s. rates with combined modality therapy
s., red blood cell
s. relationship, linear quadratic
s. relative to nodal involvement in breast carcinoma
s. skills
s. strategy ▸ protective
s. ▸ surviving guilt and
s. time
s. time, erythrocyte
s. time, mean
s. time, median
s., total lymphoid irradiation for allograft
s., treatment and
SurVivaLink automated external defibrillator (AED)
surviving guilt and survival
survivor(s)
s., cancer
s., crash
s., depressed heart attack
s. guilt
s. ▸ heart attack
s. of abuse
s. of heart transplant, long-term
s. of sexual abuse
s. sickness ▸ layoff
s., stroke
s. ▸ psychopathology of Holocaust
s., trauma
susceptibility
s., alcoholism
s., antimicrobial
s. artifact ▸ magnetic
s., ethnic
s. genes
s., genetic
s., host
s., hypnotic
s., patient
s. patterns, antibiotic
s. testing
s. to alcohol ▸ ethnic
s. to cancer ▸ person's
s. to infection ▸ increased

s. to pneumonia

susceptible
s. group
s. hosts
s. microorganisms
s. patient
s. strain
s. to fractures
s. to radiation damage

suspect, glaucoma
suspected
s. child abuse
s. heart attack
s. infectious disease
s. transfusion reaction
s. trauma

suspects, brain tumor
suspended
s., bodily functions partially
s. heart
s. heart syndrome
s. in saline solution, cells
s. vaginal cuff, well

suspension
s., Abell-Gilliam
s., cystourethral
s. holder, Lewy's
s. laryngoscopy
s., Lynch's
s. of kidney
s. of uterus
s. of uterus, Gilliam
s. procedure, vaginal
s., self-
s. sling
s. status ▸ outpatient therapeutic
s. traction
s. traction, Jones
s., uterine

suspensory
s. ligament
s. ligament of lens
s. muscle of duodenum

suspicion
s. and paranoia
s. ▸ nervousness, confusion and
s. ▸ self-centeredness and

suspicious
s. area on xerogram
s. cells
s. lesion
s. lumps
s. mammogram
s. mammogram lesion
s. mass

s. mole
s. of others
s., patient
s. tissue
s. type

Sussman method, Colcher-
sustain consistent work behavior ▸
inability to
sustainable ventilatory capacity
(MSVC) ▸ **maximal**
sustained
s. action
s. activity
s. adrenal function
s. apical impulse
s. cardiac arrest
s. clonus
s. eye closure ▸ forceful
s. feelings of humiliation
s. feelings of shame
s. first, second or third degree burn
▸ patient
s. horizontal nystagmus
s. hypertension
s. monomorphic ventricular
tachycardia
s. odd play
s. periods of grandiosity
s. recovery
s. release
s. release medication
s. respiration
s. respiration ▸ prolonged time to
s. response rate
s. sexual abuse
s. supraventricular tachyarrhythmia
s. ventricular tachycardia
s. ventricular tachycardia ▸
spontaneous reentrant

sustaining
s. measures, life-
s. procedure, life-
s. procedures, withdraw life
s. procedures, withhold life
s. treatment, life-

sustentacular
s. cell tumor
s. cells
s. tissue

Sutton-Rendu-Osler-Weber
syndrome
sutural cataract
suture(s)
s., absorbable
s., angle

s., anterior palatine
s., apposition
s., approximation
s., arterial silk
s., atraumatic
s., atraumatic chronic
s. attached to arterial wall
s., baseball
s., basilar
s., biparietal
s., black silk
s., blanket
s., bolster
s., bony
s., braided silk
s., bridle
s., bronchial
s., bunching
s., Bunnell
s., buried
s., button
s. buttress ▸ Teflon pledget
s., cardiovascular silk
s., catgut
s., cervical
s., chain
s., chromic catgut (ccg)
s., chromic catgut mattress
s., chromic gut
s., circular
s., coaptation
s., coated polyester
s., cobbler's
s., collagen
s., Connell
s., continuous
s., continuous catgut
s., continuous circular inverting
s., continuous cuticular
s., continuous hemostatic
s., continuous inverting
s., continuous mattress
s., continuous running lock
s., corneal
s., corneoscleral
s., coronal
s., cranial
s., Cushing's
s., cushioning
s., cutaneous
s., cuticular
s., Czerny
s., Czerny-Lembert
s., Dacron
s., Dacron traction

suture(s)—*continued*

s., defect closed with
s., delayed
s., dentate
s., Dermalon
s., Dermalon cuticular
s., Dexon
s., direct radial
s., dissolving
s., double-armed mattress
s., double-button
s., doubly ligated with transfixion
s., Dupuytren's
s., edge-to-edge
s. ▸ end-to-side
s., Ethibond polyester
s., Ethicon silk
s., Ethilon
s., ethmoidomaxillary
s., evening
s., evening interrupted
s., everting mattress
s., false
s., far
s., figure-of-eight
s., fine silk
s., fixation
s., flat
s., frontal
s., frontoethmoidal
s., frontolacrimal
s., frontomalar
s., frontomaxillary
s., frontonasal
s., frontoparietal
s., frontosphenoid
s., frontozygomatic
s., Frost
s., furrier's
s., Gambee
s., Gély's
s., glover's
s., guide
s., Guyton-Friedenwald
s., Halsted
s., harelip
s., heavy retention
s., hemostatic
s., Herculon
s., horizontal mattress
s., implanted
s. incised, central
s., incisive
s., infraorbital
s., insert mattress

s., intact, skin
s., interdermal buried
s., interlocking
s., intermaxillary
s., internasal
s., interparietal
s., interrupted
s., interrupted black silk
s., interrupted chromic
s., interrupted chromic catgut
s., interrupted cotton
s., interrupted fine silk
s., interrupted mattress
s., intestinal
s., intracuticular nylon
s., intradermal mattress
s., intradermic
s., inverting
s., jugal
s., Kirby's
s., lacrimoconchal
s., lacrimoethmoidal
s., lacrimomaxillary
s., lacrimoturbinal
s., lambdoid
s., Le Fort's
s., Lembert
s. ligation
s., ligatures, anchor with
s., limbal
s. line, frontal zygomatic
s. line of skull
s. line, primary
s. line ▸ relieve pressure on primary
s. lines, coronal
s. lines, lambdoid
s. lines, occipitomastoid
s. lines, parietomastoid
s. lines, sagittal
s. lines, sphenofrontal
s. lines, sphenoparietal
s. lines, squamous
s. lines, widening of
s. lines, zygomaticofrontal
s., locking running
s., lock-stitch
s., longitudinal
s., loop
s., malomaxillary
s., mamillary
s., Marlex
s., mastoid
s. material
s. material, Ethibond synthetic
s. material, loop of

s. material, synthetic
s. material, Tycron
s. material, Vicryl
s., mattress
s., McLean
s., median palatine
s., Mersilene
s., metopic
s., middle palatine
s., monofilament
s. ▸ monofilament absorbable
s. ▸ monofilament polypropylene
s., nasal
s., nasofrontal
s., nasomaxillary
s., nerve
s., Neurolon
s., nonabsorbable
s., nonabsorbable surgical
s., nylon
s., nylon retention
s., occipital
s., occipitomastoid
s., occipitoparietal
s., occipitosphenoidal
s. of blood vessel
s. of cornea
s. of cranium, squamous
s. of eyeball
s. of Gruber, petrosphenooccipital
s. of iris
s. of Krause, transverse
s. of meninges
s. of nylon ▸ skin closed with
  running subcuticular
s. of palate, cutaneous
s. of palate, longitudinal
s. of sclera
s. of skull
s., outer interrupted silk
s., over-and-over
s., overlapping
s., palatoethmoidal
s., palatomaxillary
s., Pancoast's
s., parietal
s., parietomastoid
s., parietooccipital
s., perineal support
s., Perma-Hand
s., petrobasilar
s., petrosphenobasilar
s., petrosquamous
s., plain catgut
s., plain gut

s., plastic
s., ▸ pledgeted mattress
s., plication
s., Polydek
s., polyester fiber
s., polyethylene
s., posterior palatine
s., postplaced
s., premaxillary
s., preplaced
s., presection
s., primary
s., Prolene
s., pull-out wire
s., pursestring
s., quilt
s., reabsorbable
s., reinforcing
s., relaxation
s. removal, return for
s. removed
s., retained
s., retention
s., rhabdoid
s., right-angle mattress
s., running chromic
s., running imbricating
s., running lock
s., sagittal
s., scalp
s., secondary
s., seromuscular
s., seroserous
s., serrated
s., shotted
s., silk
s., silk braided
s., silk interrupted mattress
s., silk stay
s., silkworm gut
s., simple
s., Sims'
s. size
s., skin
s., Softgut
s., sphenoethmoidal
s., sphenofrontal
s., sphenomalar
s., sphenomaxillary
s., sphenooccipital
s., sphenoorbital
s., sphenoparietal
s., sphenopetrosal
s., sphenosquamous
s., sphenotemporal

s., sphenozygomatic
s., squamosal
s., squamosomastoid
s. squamosoparietal
s., squamosophenoid
s., squamous
s., stainless steel (SS)
s., staple
s., stay
s., sternal wire
s., stick-tie
s., Sturmdorf's
s. ▸ subannular mattress
s., subcutaneous
s., subcuticular
s., superficial
s., superior rectus bridle
s., superior rectus traction
s., support
s., Supramid
s., surgical chromic
s., swaged-on
s. synostosis, sagittal
s., tacking
s., temporal
s., temporomalar
s., temporozygomatic
s., tension
s., Tevdek
s., through-and-through
s. ▸ through-the-wall mattress
s., Ti-Cron
s. tied
s. tied down over cotton
s. tied over rubber shoes
s., tongue-and-groove
s., track
s., traction
s., transfixing
s., transverse row of
s., traumatic
s., true
s., uninterrupted
s., U-shaped continuous
s., uteroparietal
s., Verhoeff's
s., vertical mattress
s., Vicryl
s., wing
s., wire
s., wound closed with
s., Y-
s., zygomaticofrontal
s., zygomaticomaxillary
s., zygomaticotemporal

sutured
s., flap fashioned and
s. in place, graft
s., lacerations
s. parallel with edges of wound
s. wound
sutureless cataract surgery
suturing
s., coupled
s. cyst inside-out
s. of eyelid
suum, Ascaris
Suzuki disc valve prosthesis ▸ Kay-sv (shouted voice)
SVC (superior vena cava)
Svedberg flotation units
Svedberg unit
SV40 (simian virus 40)
SVI (stroke volume index)
SVT (supraventricular tachycardia)
swab(s)
s., alcohol
s., cervical
s., laryngeal
s., nasopharyngeal
s., rectal
s. stick
s., throat
s., vaginal
swabbed with gentian violet ▸ area
swabbing, concentric
swallow
s., barium
s., dry
s., impaired ability to
s., inability to
s., inability to chew or
s. ▸ lose ability to
s. response
s. syncope
s., wet
swallowed
s. blood syndrome
s. foreign body, accidentally
s. foreign object, patient
s. ▸ peyote chewed and
swallower, air
swallowing
s., act of
s., air
s. center
s. difficulties, sucking and
s., difficulty
s. ▸ difficulty with speech and
s. disorders

swallowing—*continued*
- s. function
- s., impaired
- s. ▸ impaired breathing and
- s. mechanism
- s. moderately impaired
- s. or smoking ▸ drug snorting,
- s. ▸ pain on
- s., painful
- s., patient has difficulty
- s. reflex
- s. therapy
- s., tongue

Swanson('s)
- S. carpal lunate implant
- S. carpal scaphoid implant
- S. finger joint implant
- S. great toe implant
- S. implant
- S. operation
- S. radial head implant
- S. radiocarpal implant
- S. trapezium implant
- S. ulnar head implant
- S. wrist joint implant

swarm spore
swathe, sling and
sway, baseline
sway ▸ sweep and glide, reach and
swayback
- s. deformity
- s. nose
- s., severe
- s. treatment

swaying gait
swaying of body
sweat(s)
- s., bloody
- s., blue
- s. centers
- s. ▸ chills, fever and night
- s. chloride determination
- s. chloride test
- s., cold
- s., cough, foul sputum ▸ fever, night
- s. crying test
- s., drenching night
- s. electrolyte test
- s., fetid
- s. gland
- s. gland adenoma
- s. gland, apocrine
- s. gland carcinoma
- s. gland, duct of
- s. gland, eccrine

- s., green
- s., malodorous
- s., night
- s., phosphorescent
- s. pores
- s. production
- s. retention
- s. ▸ shaking chills and night
- s. surgery
- s. test ▸ quantitative pilocarpine iontophoresis

sweating
- s. and disoriented ▸ patient
- s. and lacrimation ▸ yawning,
- s. and palpitation ▸ weakness,
- s. and shaking ▸ hyperventilating,
- s. and trembling
- s., chest discomfort with
- s. ▸ chest pain with
- s., decreased
- s., episodic
- s., excessive
- s. forehead, armpits, palms
- s., increased
- s., intense
- s. over eyebrow
- s., profuse
- s. profusely
- s. sickness
- s. stage

sweaty
- s. feet
- s. palms
- s. skin

Swediaur's disease
Swedish bitter
Swedish massage
sweep(s')
- s. and glide, reach and sway
- s. cancer, chimney-
- s., duodenal
- s., duodenal bulb and
- s. magnetic resonance imaging (MRI) ▸ gated

sweet(s) (Sweet)('s)
- s. clover disease
- s., craving for
- s. ▸ increased craving for
- S. localization
- S. method
- s. -smelling urine from diabetes
- S. syndrome

sweetener
- s., artificial
- s., diet

- s., nutritive
swell, cysts
swell with fluid
swelling
- s., abdominal
- s., abnormal tissue
- s., albuminous
- s. and breathing ▸ relieve
- s. and bruising
- s. and/or ecchymosis
- s. and pain
- s. and pain, abdominal
- s. and tenderness ▸ joint
- s. and tenderness of transplant ▸ fever,
- s. and tissue destruction ▸ fever,
- s., ankle
- s., arytenoid
- s. at incision site
- s., blennorrhagic
- s., bony
- s., brain
- s., breast
- s. ▸ breathing with abdominal
- s. ▸ breathing with neck
- s., Calabar
- s., capsular
- s., cerebral
- s., cloudy
- s. ▸ clubbing, edema or
- s., corneal
- s. deformity of affected bones
- s., dependent
- s. ▸ diarrhea with abdominal pain and
- s., diffuse
- s., diminish
- s., ecchymosis and
- s., eyelid
- s., facial
- s. ▸ fluid accumulation and
- s. ▸ fluid retention and
- s. from alcohol
- s. from birth control pill
- s., fugitive
- s. ▸ generalized lymph node
- s., genital
- s., giant
- s., glandular
- s., glassy
- s. hunger
- s. in armpit
- s. in brain ▸ reduce
- s. in colon
- s. in hemodialysis ▸ joint

s. in legs ‣ reduce
s., inflammation and/or
s., joint
s., joint contracture and
s., joint pain and
s., Kamerun's
s., labial
s., labioscrotal
s., leg
s., limb
s., limit
s., local
s. ‣ local skin
s. ‣ loss of appetite with joint
s., nasal
s. nasal mucosa
s. of abdomen
s. of airway walls
s. of ankle
s. of body tissues
s. of breast
s. of breast, painful
s. of cartilage, softening and
s. of ears
s. of face
s. of feet
s. of feet ‣ persistent
s. of finger
s. of forefoot
s. of genitalia
s. of gums
s. of hands
s. of hands or feet
s. of joint
s. of knee
s. of leg, pain and
s. of legs
s. of lining or airways
s. of lips
s. of lips, tongue and face
s. of liver
s. of lower extremities
s. of ovaries
s. of pancreas
s. of site
s. of throat
s. of toe
s. of tongue
s. of tongue ‣ itchy
s. of upper arm ‣ patient has
s. of upper extremities
s. of wall tissues
s. of wrist
s., pain and
s., painless

s., periodic
s., periorbital
s., reduce tissue
s., reduced by massage
s., scrotal
s., Soemerring's crystalline
s., soft tissue
s., subcutaneous
s., subsiding
s., surgical
s., testicular
s., tongue
s., tropical
s., tympanic
s. under chin ‣ lump or
s., vascular
s., white

Swenson pull-through procedure
SWI (stroke work index)
swimmer(s)('s)
    s. ear
    s. eruption ‣ sea
    s. view
swimming
    s. ‣ hypoxic lap
    s. injury
    s. pool granuloma
    s. -related illness
swine
    s. dysentery
    s. flu vaccine
    s. influenza
    s. influenza strain
    s. influenza vaccine
    s. orphan (ECSO) virus ‣ enteric
        cytopathic
    s. rotlauf bacillus
    s. (TGS) ‣ transmissible
        gastroenteritis of
swing(s)
    s. and depression, mood
    s., baseline
    s., disruptive mood
    s. ‣ dizzying mood
    s., emotional
    s., extreme mood
    s. ‣ frequent mood
    s. ‣ irritability and mood
    s., mood
    s., mood and energy
    s. -out shoe
    s. ‣ rapid mood
    s., respiratory
    s. ‣ seasonal mood
    s. ‣ sudden mood

s. -through gait
s. -to gait
s. ‣ volatile mood
s. ‣ wide-ranging mood
swinging
    s. flashlight test
    s. heart
    s. of head ‣ pointless side-to-side
Swiss
    S. cheese defect
    S. cheese endometrium
    S. cheese hyperplasia
    S. cheese interventricular septum
    S. -type agammaglobulinemia
switch(es)
    s. ‣ deoxyribonucleic acid (DNA)
    s., isoactin
    s., isomyosin
    s., mode
    s. operation
    s. operation, arterial
    s. probe ‣ Jatene arterial
    s. procedure
    s. procedure, arterial
switching (AMS), automatic mode
swollen
    s. and inflamed ‣ thumb joint
    s. and painful joints
    s. and tender
    s. and tender gums
    s. and tender ‣ hot,
    s. ankles
    s. ankles ‣ severely
    s. appendix
    s. artery
    s. blood vessel
    s. breasts ‣ tender,
    s., bulbous nose
    s. eyelid
    s. eyelids ‣ puffy,
    s. eyelids ‣ red and
    s. eyes
    s. feet
    s. fingers
    s. gland ‣ painful
    s. glands
    s. glands ‣ painfully
    s. ‣ irritated, red and
    s. ‣ itchy, red and
    s. joint ‣ inflamed
    s. joint ‣ red
    s. joints
    s. joints, painful
    s. ‣ kidneys pale and
    s. legs

swollen—*continued*
  s. lymph glands
  s. lymph nodes
  s. lymphoma glands
  s. nasal membranes
  s. nasal mucosa
  s. neck vein
  s. nerve
  s. scrotum and pain ▸ chills with
  s. skin
  s. spleen
  s., stiff, inflamed joints
  s., tender and
  s., tender gums ▸ red,
  s. tissue
  s. tissue lining
  s., tube edematous and
  s. underlying veins
SWS (slow wave sleep)
Sydenham's chorea
Sydenham's cough
Sydney virus
sydowi, Aspergillus
syllabaris spasmodica ▸ dysarthria
sylvian
  s. aqueduct
  s. area
  s. artery
  s. fissure
  s. fossa
  s. fossa, vein of
  s. line
  s. point
  s. vein
  s. waves, ischemic
sylvii, vallecula
Sylvius
  S., angle of
  S., aqueduct of
  S., cistern of
  S., cistern of fossa of
  S., fissure of
  S., valve of
  S., ventricle of
symbiosis
  s., antagonistic
  s., antipathetic
  s., conjunctive
  s., disjunctive
symbiotic psychosis
symbioticum, Chlorobacterium
symblepharon
  s., anterior
  s., posterior
  s., total

symbol, phallic
symbolic moralism
Syme's amputation
Symmers disease, Brill-
symmetric
  s. asphyxia
  s. polyneuropathy ▸ distal
  s. vitiligo
symmetrical
  s. and equal, extremities
  s., bilaterally
  s. brain
  s. brain, grossly
  s., breast
  s., chest
  s., chest bilaterally
  s. ▸ deep tendon reflexes (DTR)
  s., extremities equal and
  s., face
  s. in contour
  s. in contour, uterus
  s. lipomatosis
  s. patches of pigmentation
  s. phased array
  s. sleep patterns
  s., thorax
  s. uterine enlargement ▸ diffuse,
symmetrically reduced voltage
symmetry
  s. bilateral
  s., inverse
  s., radial
sympathectomy
  s., cervical
  s., cervicothoracic
  s., chemical
  s., dorsal
  s., lumbar
  s., periarterial
  s., regional
  s., subdiaphragmatic
  s., supradiaphragmatic
  s., surgical
  s., thoracic
  s., thoracolumbar
sympathetic
  s. activity
  s. block
  s. block anesthesia
  s. blockade ▸ regional
  s. cells
  s. chain
  s. dystrophy (RSD) ▸ reflux
  s. dystrophy (RSD) syndrome ▸
    reflex

  s. ganglia
  s. inhibitor
  s. innervation of lung
  s. iritis
  s. manifestation
  s. medicine
  s. nerve
  s. nerve activity
  s. nerve activity ▸ muscle
  s. nerve block
  s. nerve, cervical
  s. nerve fibers
  s. nerve trunks
  s. nervous pathways
  s. nervous system
  s. nervous system ▸ function of
  s. ophthalmia
  s. plexuses ▸ ganglia of
  s. reaction
  s. saliva
  s. stimulation
  s. system, peripheral
  s. trunk ▸ ganglia of
  s. uveitis
  s. vasoconstrictor tone
sympatheticotonic type
sympathica, meningitis
sympathica, ptosis
sympathicum, neuroblastoma
sympathizing eye
sympathoadrenal system
sympathoexcitation, reflex
sympatholytic agent
sympathomimetic
  s. abuse
  s. abuse ▸ amphetamine or
    similarly acting
  s. activity ▸ intrinsic
  s. amine
  s. delirium ▸ amphetamine or
    similarly acting
  s. delusional disorder
  s. dependence ▸ amphetamine or
    similarly acting
  s. drug
  s. intoxication ▸ amphetamine or
    similarly acting
  s. overdose
  s. stimulants
  s. syndrome
  s. withdrawal ▸ amphetamine or
    similarly acting
sympathovagal
  s. balance
  s. imbalance

s. transition
symphysis
s., cardiac
s., pleural
s., pubic
s. pubica
s., pubis
s. to umbilicus
symplastic tissue
symptom(s) (Symptom) [*system*]
s. abate
s. ▸ absence of premonitory
s., acute menopausal
s. ▸ adjustment react with physical
s., acute withdrawal
s., agoraphobia
s., allergic
s., alleviating psychiatric
s., alleviation of
s., ameliorate
s., anaphylactic
s., anxiety
s., arthritis-type
s. as a screening device for drug
abuse
s., associated
s., asthma-like
s., Bárány
s., behavioral
s., Bonhoeffer's
s., burnout
s., cardiac
s., cardinal
s., cause and treatment
s., chronic
s. ▸ chronic factitious illness with
physical
s., Chvostek's
s., cigarette withdrawal
s., clearing of mental
s., clinical
s., clinical signs and
s. clusters ▸ multiple
s., cognitive
s., cold
s., common dissociative
s. complex
s., compulsive
s., congestion
s. control
s. control, physical
s., control withdrawal
s., controlling
s., cosmetic
s., debilitating

s., depressive
s. diary
s., differential diagnosis of alcohol
withdrawal
s., disabling
s. disorder ▸ single
s., dissociative
s., diverse
s., dramatic relief of
s., dry eye
s. ▸ duration of
s. ▸ early identification of
s., eating disorder
s., elusive
s., emotional
s., endocrine
s., episodic
s., esophagosalivary
s. evaluation (ASE) ▸ abstinence
s., exacerbation of
s., experience
s., experiencing withdrawal
s. ▸ factitious disorder with physical
s. ▸ factitious disorder with
psychological
s. ▸ factitious illness with
psychological
s., feigning
s. fluctuate in duration
s., fluctuations
s., flu-like
s. formation
s. -free
s. -free interval
s. -free, patient
s., full-blown
s., full range of
s., functional
s., Ganser's
s., gastrointestinal
s., Haenel's
s., hay fever
s., heart attack
s. increased in severity
s., initial
s., labyrinthine
s. -limited treadmill exercise test
s., list specific
s. management
s. management, acute
s. management, pain and
s., Manchurian
s., manic
s. manifestation
s., medical

s., menopausal
s. ▸ minimization of alcohol
s., motor premonitory
s., multiple
s. ▸ multiple rheumatic
s. ▸ multiple vague
s., neurological
s., normative
s., objective
s., obsessional
s. ▸ obsessional and compulsive
s., obsessive
s., obstructive
s., Oehler's
s. of acute drug intoxication
s. of acute drug reactions
s. of anxiety, decreased signs and
s. of apnea
s. of clinical depression ▸ develop
s. of dementia ▸ mild
s. of depression
s. of depression, decreased signs
and
s. of drug abuse
s. of emergency cardiac care ▸
history and
s. of heart disease, overt
s. of heart failure
s. of heartburn
s. of hesitation and retreat
s. of menopause
s. of mittelschmerz
s. of neurological disorders
s. of nicotine withdrawal ▸ alleviate
s. of overdosing
s. of panic reactions
s. of proctitis
s. of psychotic reactions
s. of recantation and self-blame
s. of severe mania
s. of stroke onset
s. of toxicity
s., onset of
s. ▸ opiate withdrawal
s., other characteristic
s., painful
s. ▸ panic-like
s. ▸ perception of
s., perimenopausal
s., persistent
s. ▸ persistent chest pain
s., physical
s., physical withdrawal
s. ▸ post-traumatic
s. ▸ post-treatment

symptom(s)—*continued*
- s., postural reflux
- s., premenstrual
- s. ▸ presence of distinctive
- s., presenting
- s. ▸ prevent withdrawal
- s., prodromal
- s., progression of
- s., progressive
- s. ▸ prolonged psychotic
- s., psychiatric
- s., psychosomatic
- s., psychotic
- s. ▸ psychotic-like
- S. Rating Scale (VTSRS) ▸ Verdun Target
- s., Raynaud's
- s., recurrent
- s. ▸ recurrent psychotic
- s. reduction
- s. ▸ re-emergent
- s., regression of
- s., relief from
- s. relief ▸ improved
- s. relief, physical
- s., relieve fibromyalgia
- s., remission of
- s., respiratory
- s., reversible
- s., salient
- s., schizophrenic
- s., Séguin's signal
- s., severe
- s. ▸ severe debilitating
- s. ▸ severe psychiatric
- s. ▸ severe withdrawal
- s. ▸ shock-like
- s., signs and
- s. ▸ stages, signs and
- s., somatosensory
- s. ▸ stress-related
- s., stroke
- s., subjective
- s. ▸ subtle and nonspecific
- s., suppressing
- s., temporarily relieve
- s., total relief of
- s. transient
- s., transient visual
- s., Trendelenburg's
- s., triad of
- s., uncontrolled physical
- s., unpleasant withdrawal
- s., urinary
- s., vague

- s. ▸ vague and ambiguous
- s., varied nervous
- s., vasomotor
- s., vegetative
- s. ▸ vivid acute
- s. wax and wane
- s., Wernicke's encephalopathy
- s., whole body
- s. with back ▸ urgent
- s. with bone ▸ urgent
- s., withdrawal

symptomatic [*asymptomatic*]
- s. alcohol heart muscle disease
- s. asthma
- s. bradycardia
- s. disease
- s. disease, chronic
- s. enlargement
- s. epilepsy
- s. erythema
- s. fibroid
- s. fistula
- s. gallbladder disease
- s. gallstones
- s. headache
- s. hearing loss
- s. HIV (human immunodeficiency virus) infection
- s. hypertension
- s. illness, prolonged
- s. impotence
- s. infection
- s. intracranial arterial stensosis
- s. magnesium deficiency
- s. management
- s. medication
- s., overtly
- s. pain relief
- s., patient
- s. peritonitis
- s. progression of disease
- s. purpura
- s. relief
- s. treatment
- s. urinary tract infection
- s. vertigo

symptomatica ▸ porphyria cutanea tarda

symptomatically
- s. improved ▸ patient
- s., managed
- s. treated

symptomatologic factors

symptomatology
- s., abstinence

- s., cardiovascular
- s., cutaneous
- s., GI (gastrointestinal)
- s., increasing
- s., long-standing
- s., neurologic
- s. ▸ opiate withdrawal
- s., patient control of

synapse(s)
- s., autonomic ganglionic
- s., axodendritic
- s., excitatory
- s. in brain

synaptic
- s. branching of neurons
- s. cleft
- s. connections
- s. knobs
- s. level
- s. transmission

synarthrodial joint

sync ▸ patient out of

synchesis (*see* synchysis)

synchondrosis, sternal

SynchroMed pump ▸ Medtronic

synchronized
- s. cardioversion ▸ low energy
- s. digital subtraction angiogram ▸ electrocardiogram (ECG)
- s. intermittent mandatory ventilation
- s. sleep

synchronous
- s. activity
- s. airway lesions
- s. amputation
- s. atrial defibrillation shocks ▸ QRS
- s., bilaterally
- s. control
- s. forceful contraction
- s. pacemaker
- s. pacemaker, AV
- s. pacing, atrial
- s. pulse generator, atrial
- s. pulse generator ▸ ventricular
- s. rectification
- s. ventricular inhibited pacemaker atrial
- s. with heartbeat

synchronously, contract

synchronously ▸ occur bilaterally

synchrony
- s., atrial
- s., atrioventricular (AV)
- s., bilateral

s. biofeedback, hemispheric
s. biofeedback ▸ hemispheric alpha
s., consistent
s. ▸ normal atrioventricular
s., secondary bilateral
s. ▸ thalamus and cortex fire in
**synchroton-based transvenous
angiography**
synchysis (*same as* **synchesis**)
synchysis scintillans
synclonic spasm
syncopal
s. attack
s. episode
s. migraine headache
s. spell
syncope
s., Adams-Stokes
s., and hypotension ▸ vertigo,
s. anginosa
s. ▸ beauty parlor
s., cardiac
s., cardiac obstruction in
s., cardiogenic
s., cardioinhibitory
s., carotid
s., carotid sinus
s., cerebrovascular
s. clinic
s., convulsive
s., cough
s., defecation
s., deglutition
s., digital
s., diver's
s., exertional
s., heat
s., hypoglycemic
s., hypoxic
s., hysterical
s., laryngeal
s., local
s., micturition
s., migraine
s. ▸ mixed neurally mediated
s., near-
s. ▸ neurally mediated
s., neurocardiogenic
s., neuromediated
s., noncardiac
s., orthostatic
s., postmicturition
s. ▸ post-tussive
s., postural
s., sexual

s., situational
s., sneeze
s., stretching
s., swallow
s. ▸ toilet seat
s., transient
s., tussive
s. undetermined etiology
s. ▸ varying degrees of
s., vasodepressor
s. ▸ vasodepressor cardioinhibitory
s., vasomotor
s., vasovagal
s., vertigo and
s. with convulsions
**synctial cells, abnormal proliferation
of**
syncyanea, Pseudomonas
syncytial
s. cell
s. endometritis
s. knot formation
s. virus conduit ▸ respiratory
s. virus IV immune globulin ▸
respiratory
s. virus ▸ respiratory
syncytioma malignum
syncytiovascular membrane
syndactylism release
syndactyly deformity
syndesmochorial placenta
syndesmo-odontoid
syndesmosis, tibiofibular
syndromal episode
syndrome
s., Aarskog
s., Abderhalden-Fanconi
s., abstinence
s., Abt-Letterer-Siwe
s., Achard-Thiers
s. (AIDS), acquired immune
deficiency
s. (AVIDS), acquired violence
immune deficiency
s., acute
s., acute abstinence
s., acute brain
s. (ACSS) ▸ acute caretaker's
stress
s., acute chest
s., acute coronary
s., acute febrile
s., acute mononucleosis
s., acute organic brain
s., acute pharyngitis

s. (ARDS), acute respiratory
distress
s., acute retroviral
s., acute treatment for organic brain
s., acute urethral
s., acute withdrawal
s., Adams-Stokes
s., addictive relationships
s., addisonian
s., Adie's
s., adrenogenital
s. (ARDS), adult respiratory
distress
s., Agent Orange
s., Ahumada-del Castillo
s., Albers-Schönberg
s., Albright's
s., alcohol dependence
s. (AWS) ▸ alcohol withdrawal
s., alcoholic brain
s., Aldrich's
s., Alibert-Bazin
s., "Alice in Wonderland"
s., Allen-Masters
s. ▸ alpha thalassemia X-linked
retardation
s., Alport's
s., Alström-Olsen
s., Alzheimer's
s., amnestic
s., amniotic fluid
s., amniotic infection
s., amotivational
s., Andogsky's
s., Angelman's
s., Angelucci's
s., anginal
s., anomalous first rib thoracic
s., anterior chest wall
s., anterior compartment
compression
s., anterior tibial compartment
s. (AIDS) antibodies, acquired
immune deficiency
s., antibody deficiency
s. (AIDS) antibody test, acquired
immune deficiency
s., antiphospholipid
s., Anton-Babinski
s., aortic arch
s., aortic arteritis
s., aqueductal
s., Arakawa-Higashi
s., argentaffinoma
s., Arias'

syndrome—*continued*

s., Arneth's
s., Arnold-Chiari
s., arteriohepatic dysplasia
s., Asherman's
s., Asian flush
s., Asperger's
s., aspiration
s., asplenia
s. (AIDS) associated transfusion, acquired immune deficiency
s. ▸ athletic heart
s., atypical pneumonia
s., Austrian
s., autoexacerbating
s., Avellis'
s., Axenfeld
s., Ayerza's
s., Baastrup's
s., Babinski's
s., Baelz's
s., Bakwin-Eiger
s., Balint's
s., Ballantyne-Runge
s., ballooning mitral cusp
s., Bamatter's
s., Banti's
s., Bar
s., Bárány's
s., Bard-Pic
s., Bard's
s., Barlow's
s., Barrett's
s., Bársony-Polgár
s., Bartter's
s., basal cell nevus
s., Bassen-Kornzweig
s., battered child
s., battered husband
s., battered parent
s. (BSS), battered spouse
s., battered wife
s., Bauer
s., Beal's
s., Beard's
s., Bearn-Kunkel
s., Beau's
s., Beck's
s., Beckwith's
s., beer and cobalt
s., behavior
s., Behçet's
s., Behr's
s., Benedikt
s., Bernard

s., Bernheim's
s., Beuren
s., Bielschowsky-Lutz-Cogan
s., Bietti's
s., bilateral distress
s., Bilgert-Dreyfus'
s., billfold
s., billowing mitral valve
s., binge and purge
s., binge eating
s., Blackfan-Diamond
s., Bland-Garland-White
s., blind loop
s., bloating and irritable bowel
s., bloating from premenstrual
s., Bloch-Sulzberger
s., Bloom's
s., blue baby
s., blue finger
s., blue toe
s., blue velvet
s., Boerhaave
s., Bonnet
s., Bonnet-Dechaume-Blanc
s., Bonnevie-Ullrich
s., Bouillaud's
s., Bourneville's
s., Bouveret's
s., brachial
s., Brachmann-de Lange
s., brachy-tachy
s., bradycardia-tachycardia
s., bradytachycardia
s., brain
s., Brandt's
s., Brentano's
s., Briquet's
s., Brissaud-Sicard
s., Bristowe's
s., Brock
s., Brown's
s., Brown's tendon sheath
s., Brown-Séquard
s., Brueghel's
s., bubbly lung
s., Budd-Chiari
s., Burnett's
s., burning
s., burning foot
s., Buschke-Ollendorff
s., busulfan lung
s., Bywaters'
s., Caffey-Silverman
s., Caffey-Smyth-Roske

s. ▸ calcification, Raynaud's phenomenon, scleroderma, telangiectasia (CRST)
s., callosal
s., Calvé-Legg-Perthes
s., Camurati-Engelmann
s., cancer family
s., Capgras
s., capillary leak
s., Caplan's
s., capsular thrombosis
s., capsulothalamic
s., carbonless paper
s., carcinoid
s., cardio-auditory
s., cardiofacial
s., carotid steal
s. (CTS) ▸ carpal tunnel
s. (AIDS) carrier, patient acquired immune deficiency
s. (AIDS) carrier, patient unknown acquired immune deficiency
s., cauda equina
s., cave
s. cells ▸ Down's
s., cellular immunity deficiency
s., central cord
s., cerebellar
s., cervical anginal
s., cervical disc
s., cervical rib
s., Céstan-Chenais
s., Chapples
s., Charcot-Marie-Tooth-Hoffmann
s., Chédiak-Higashi
s. ▸ chemical sensitivity
s., Chiari
s., Chiari-Frommel
s., chiasma
s., Chilaiditi's
s., child abuse accommodation
s., child battering
s., childhood hyperkinetic
S. (CRS) ▸ Chinese Restaurant
s., Christ-Siemens-Touraine
s., chronic
s., chronic alcoholic brain
s., chronic brain
s. (CFS) ▸ chronic fatigue
s. (HVS) ▸ chronic hyperventilation
s., chronic itch and scratch
s., chronic itching
s., chronic muscle pain
s., chronic organic brain
s., chronic pain

s. ▸ chronic reflex pain
s., Churg-Strauss
s., Chvostek's
s., Cinderella
s. ▸ circadian rhythm disturbance
s., Clarke-Hadefield
s., classic
s., Claude's
s., click
s., click-murmur
s., clinical
s., clinical infection
s., clinical manifestations of chronic brain
s. ▸ clutter stress
s., cocaine addiction
s., Cockayne's
s., Cogan's
s., colon coagulation
s., compartment
s., compartmental
s. ▸ complex regional pain
s., compound reaction ▸ rape trauma
s., computer
s., computer vision
s., concussion
s., congenital central hypoventilation
s. ▸ congenital long QT
s., congenital rubella
s., congenital vs acquired
s., Conn's
s., contagious suicide
s., cord compression
s., Cornelia de Lange's
s., coronary insufficiency
s., coronary steal
s., Costen's
s., costochondral
s., costoclavicular rib
s., costosternal
s., Cotard's
s., Courvoisier-Terrier
s., crack baby
s., Creutzfeldt-Jakob
s., cricopharyngeal achalasia
s., cri-du-chat
s., Crigler-Najjar
s. (AIDS) crisis, acquired immune deficiency
s., Crouzon's
s., crush
s., crush injury
s., Cruveilhier-Baumgarten

s., cryptophthalmos
s., cubital tunnel
s., Curtius'
s., Cushing's
s., cutis laxa
s. (CVS) ▸ cyclic vomiting
s., Cyriax's
s., Dandy-Walker
s., Danlos'
s., Darrow-Gamble
s., de Clerembault's
s., debilitating
s., declamping shock
s., defibrination
s., Degos-Delort-Tricot
s., Dejean's
s., Déjerine-Roussy
s., Déjerine's
s., de Lange's
s., de Morsier-Gauthier
s., De Sanctis-Cacchione
s., de Toni-Fanconi-Debre
s. (DSPS) ▸ delayed sleep phase
s., delayed stress
s. (AIDS) dementia complex, acquired immune deficiency
s. ▸ Dengue shock
s., Dennie-Marfan
s. ▸ dental enamel dysplasia
s., depersonalization
s. ▸ depression from premenstrual
s., depressive
s. (DLS) ▸ depressive living
s., DeQuervain's
s., Devic's
s. ▸ diabetic hyperosmolar
s., dialysis equilibrium
s., Diamond-Blackfan
s. ▸ diarrhea from toxic shock
s., diencephalic
s., differential diagnosis in acute
s., DiGeorge's
s., DiGuglielmo's
s., disability
s. disorder ▸ organic mental
s. ▸ distal intestinal obstruction
s., disuse
s. ▸ dizziness from toxic shock
s., Down's
s., Dresbach's
s., Dressler's
s., drowned newborn
s., drug reactions in organic brain
s., drug withdrawal
s., drug-induced amnestic

s. ▸ drug-induced lupus
s., drug-induced organic affective
s., drug-induced organic delusional
s., drug-induced Parkinson's
s., dry eye
s., Duane
s., Duane retraction
s., Dubin-Johnson
s., Dubovitz's
s., dumping
s., dysglandular
s., dysmaturity
s., dysmetabolic
s., dysmorphic
s., dysplastic nevus
s., dystrophy-dystocia
s., Eagle
s., Eagle-Barrett
s., early respiratory distress
s., economy class
s., ectodermal dysplasia
s., ectopic ACTH (adreno-corticotropic hormone)
s., ectopic Cushing's
s., Edwards
s., effort
s., Ehlers-Danlos
s., Eisenmenger's
s., Ekbom
s. ▸ elfin facies
s., Ellis-van Creveld
s., Elschnig's
s. (AIDS) ▸ emotional effects of acquired immune deficiency
s., empty nest
s., empty sella
s., endocrine neoplasia
s. (EMS) ▸ eosinophilia myalgia
s., eosinophilic pulmonary
s. ▸ epibronchial right pulmonary artery
s. (AIDS) epidemic, acquired immune deficiency
s., epiphyseal
s., Epstein-Barr (EB)
s., Epstein-Barr (EB) virus
s., Erb's
s., Erlacher-Blount
s., euthyroid sick
s., extrapyramidal
s., Faber's
s., false memory
s. ▸ (FASPS) familial advanced sleep phase
s. ▸ familial cholestasis

syndrome—*continued*

s. ▸ family cancer
s., Fanconi
s., Fanconi-Albertini-Zellweger
s., Fanconi-Petrassi
s. ▸ fat emboli
s., fat embolism
s., Felty's
s. (AIDS) ▸ fetal acquired immune deficiency
s. (FAS) ▸ fetal alcohol
s. ▸ fibrinogen fibrin conversion
s., fibromyalgia
s., fidgety leg
s. ▸ fight-or-flight
s., Fitz-Hugh-Curtis
s., Fitz-Hugh's
s., Fitz's
s. ▸ flapping valve
s., Fleischner
s., floppy infant
s., floppy valve
s., flu-like
s., focal dermal hypoplasia
s., Foix's
s. ▸ Forbes-Albright
s. ▸ foreign accent
s., Forrester
s., Foster Kennedy
s., Foville's
s., Foville-Wilson
s. ▸ fragile child
s., Fragile X
s., Franceschetti's
s., Friedenwald's
s., Friedmann's vasomotor
s., Fritz-Asherman
s., Froin's
s. from aspirin, Reye's
s., frontal lobe
s., Fuchs'
s., Fuchs-Kraupa
s., full alcohol
s., functional bowel
s., Gaisböck's
s., Ganser's
s., Garcin's
s., Gardner's
s., Gasser's
s., Gastaut
s., Gastaut-Lennox
s., gastrocardiac
s., gay bowel
s., gay immunocompromise
s., Gélineau's

s., general adaptation
s., Gerstmann's
s., Gianotti-Crosti
s., Gilbert-Lereboullet
s., Gilbert's
s., Gilles de la Tourette's
s., Glanzmann's
s., Glénard's
s., Goltz
s., Goltz-Gorlin
s., Goodpasture's
s., Gordan-Overstreet
s., Gougerot's
s., Gower's
s., Gradenigo's
s., Graefe's
s., gray baby
s., Gregg
s., Greig
s., Guillain-Barré
s. ▸ Gulf War
s., Gunn's
s., Günther's
s., Halbrecht's
s., Hallermann-Streiff
s., Hallervorden-Spatz
s., Hamman-Rich
s., Hand-Schüller-Christian
s., Hanhart's
s., Hanot-Rössle
s. ▸ Hantavirus pulmonary
s., happy puppet
s., Harada's
s., Harris'
s., Hartnup's
s., Hart's
s. ▸ haunted womb
s., Hayem-Widal
s., heart-hand
s., heat illness
s. ▸ heel spur
s., Heerfordt's
s. ▸ hemangioma thrombocytopenia
s. ▸ hemiconvulsion, hemiplegia, epilepsy (HHE)
s. (HUS) ▸ hemolytic uremic
s., hemopleuropneumonic
s., hemorrhagic fever with renal
s. ▸ Henoch-Schönlein
s., hepatorenal
s., hereditary benign intraepithelial dyskeratosis
s. ▸ hereditary breast-ovarian cancer
s., herniated disc

s., Hertwig-Magendie
s. (AIDS) ▸ heterosexual contact with male carriers of acquired immune deficiency
s., heterotaxy
s., Hippel-Lindau
s. ▸ holiday heart
s., Holt-Oram
s., Homén's
s., homocystinuria
s., Horner-Bernard
s., Horner's
s., Horton's
s. ▸ hot reactor
s., Hunter's
s., Hunt's
s., Hunt's striatal
s., Hurler's
s., Hutchinson-Gilford
s., Hutchinson's
s., hydralizine lupus
s., hyperabduction
s., hypereosinophilia
s., hyperglycemic hypersmolar
s., hyperlucent lung
s., hyperkinetic
s., hyperkinetic heart
s., hypermetabolic
s., hyperosmolar
s. ▸ hypersensitive carotid sinus
s., hyperventilation
s., hyperviscosity
s., hypoplastic left heart
s., hypoplastic lung
s. ▸ hypothenar hammer
s. ▸ identifiable psychiatric
s. ▸ idiopathic hypereosinophilic
s. ▸ idiopathic long Q-T interval
s., idiopathic nephrotic
s. (IRDS) ▸ idiopathic respiratory distress
s. (AIDS) illness ▸ acquired immune deficiency
s. ▸ immotile cilia
s., impingement
s. ▸ infant respiratory distress
s. (AIDS) infected child ▸ acquired immune deficiency
s. ▸ inherited cancer
s., inspissated milk
s. ▸ insulin resistance
s. ▸ intensive care unit (ICU)
s., intermediate
s., intimectomy for Leriche
s. (IBS) ▸ irritable bowel

s., irritable colon
s. (IMS) ▸ irritable male
s., Ivemark's
s., Jackson's
s. ▸ Jakob-Creutzfeldt
s., Jansen's
s., jaw-winking
s. ▸ Jervell and Lange-Nielsen
s., jet-lag
s., Joseph's
s., Josephs-Diamond-Blackfan
s., jugular foramen
s., Kallmann's
s., Kanner's
s., Kartagener's
s., Kasabach-Merritt
s., Kawasaki's
s., Kearns-Sayre
s., Kennedy's
s., Kiloh-Nevin
s., Kimmelstiel-Wilson
s., Kleine-Levin
s., Klinefelter's
s., Klippel-Feil
s., Klippel-Feldstein
s., Kloepfer's
s., Klüver-Bucy
s., Koerber-Salus-Elschnig
s., Korsakoff's
s., Krause's
s., Kurz's
s. ▸ Landouzy-Déjerine
s., Landry-Guillain-Barré
s., Larsen's
s., Launois
s., Laurence-Moon-Biedl
s. (LLS) ▸ lazy leukocyte
s., lazy-eye
s., Leitner's
s., Lennox's
s., leopard
s., Leredde's
s., Leriche
s., Lermoyez's
s., Letterer-Siwe
s., Libman-Sacks
s., Lieou-Barré
s., Lightwood-Albright
s., Lignac-Fanconi
s., lipogenesis
s., locked-in
s., locker room
s., Löffler's
s. ▸ long Q-T
s. ▸ long Q-TU

s., Long-Ganong-Levine (*see* s., Lown-Ganong-Levine)
s., Looser-Milkman
s., Louis-Bar
s., low back
s. ▸ low salt
s. ▸ low sodium
s., Lowe's
s., Lown-Ganong-Levine
s., Luft's
s., Lutembacher's
s., Lutz-Splendore-de Almeida
s., Lyell's
s., Lyle's
s. (LAS) ▸ lymphadenopathy
s., lymphoproliferative
s., Lynch
s., Maffucci's
s., malabsorption
s. ▸ malignant carcinoid
s., malignant neuroleptic
s., Mallory-Weiss
s. (AIDS) mandatory testing ▸ acquired immune deficiency
s., Marchiafava-Bignami
s., Marchiafava-Micheli
s., Marcus Gunn
s., Marfan's
s., Marie's
s., Marinesco-Sjögren
s., Maroteaux-Lamy
s., mastocytosis
s., Maugeri's
s., Mauriac's
s., McCune-Albright
s. ▸ meconium aspiration
s., meconium plug
s., medical
s., Meigs'
s., Melkersson-Rosenthal
s., Mendelson's
s., Meniere's
s., meningitis sepsis
s., menopausal
s., menstrual
s. (TSS) ▸ menstrual toxic shock
s., metabolic
s. ▸ metabolic renal
s., metameric
s. ▸ metastatic carcinoid
s., methionine malabsorption
s., micrognathia-glossoptosis
s., middle lobe
s. ▸ midsystolic click
s., Miege's

s., Milian's
s., Mikity-Wilson
s., Mikulicz's
s. ▸ milk-alkali
s., Milkman's
s., Millard-Gubler
s., Miller's
s. ▸ Milwaukee shoulder
s., Minkowski-Chauffard
s. ▸ mirror image lung
s. ▸ mitral valve prolapse
s., Möbius
s., monosomy 7
s., Morgagni-Adams-Stokes
s., Morquio's
s., Morquio-Ullrich
s. ▸ motion sickness
s., motivational
s. (MLNS) ▸ mucocutaneous lymph node
s., multifaceted
s., multiple clinical
s., multiple endocrine neoplasia
s., multiple lentigines
s., Munchausen's
s., myelodysplastic
s., myeloproliferative
s. ▸ myocardial ischemic
s., myofascial
s. ▸ myofascial pain
s. (MPD) ▸ myofascial pain dysfunction
s. ▸ myonephropathic metabolic
s. ▸ myonephropathic metabolism
s. ▸ myonephrotic metabolic
s., myositis
s., Naffziger's
s., narcolepsy
s., neonatal withdrawal
s., nephrotic
s., Nettleship's
s., neurocutaneous
s., neurological
s., nevoid basalioma
s., Nezelof's
s. ▸ nicotine withdrawal
s., Nonne's
s. ▸ nonthoracotomy defibrillation lead
s., Noonan's
s., Nothnagel's
s., nursing bottle
s. ▸ obesity hypoventilation
s., occipital condyle metastasis
s. ▸ ocular histoplasmosis

syndrome—*continued*

s. ▸ ocular ischemic
s., oculomucocutaneous
s. of aphasia ▸ stroke-like
s. of childhood ▸ hyperkinetic
s. of disordered water balance (DWB)
s. of hyperserotonemia ▸ vasculocardiac
s. of inappropriate anti-diuretic hormone (SIADH) secretion
s. of legs, creepy-crawly
s. of RAEB (refractory anemia with excess blasts) dysmyelopoietic
s., Ollier's
s. ▸ opiate withdrawal
s. or glossodynia ▸ burning tongue
s. ▸ oral allergy
s., orbital metastasis
s., organic affective
s., organic brain
s., organic delusional
s., organic hallucinosis
s., organic mental
s., organic personality
s., Osgood-Schlatter
s., Osler's
s. ▸ overactive bladder
s., overuse
s., pacemaker
s. ▸ pacemaker Twiddler's
s., pain
s. ▸ pain in abdomen from irritable bowel
s., painful
s., painful heel
s., Pancoast's
s., pancreatic insufficiency
s., pancreatic tumor
s., pancreaticohepatic
s. ▸ papillary muscle
s., paraneoplastic
s. ▸ parasellar and middle fossa metastasis
s., paratrigeminal
s., Parinaud's
s., Parkinsonian
s., Parkinson's
s., Patau's
s., Paterson-Brown-Kelly
s. (AIDS) patient ▸ acquired immune deficiency
s. (AIDS) ▸ patient at risk for acquired immune deficiency
s. ▸ pediatric heart

s., Pellizzi's
s., Penderluft
s., Pendred's
s. ▸ pericarditis-myocarditis
s., perineoplastic
s., periodic
s., petrosphenoidal
s., Petzetakis-Takos
s., Peutz-Jeghers
s. ▸ pharyngeal pouch
s., phase advance
s., phase delay
s., Pick's
s., pickwickian
s., Pierre Robin
s., piriformis
s., placental dysfunction
s. ▸ platelet dysfunction
s., Plummer-Vinson
s., polyglandular
s., polyposis coli
s., polysplenia
s. (PCOS) ▸ polycystic ovarian
s. (PCOS) ▸ polycystic ovary
s., Posner-Schlossman
s., postabortion
s., post-brain stem stroke
s., postcardiotomy
s., postcommissurotomy
s., postconcussion
s. ▸ postgastrectomy dumping
s., postinfarction
s. ▸ postmyocardial infarction
s., postperfusion
s., postpericardiotomy
s., postphlebitis
s., postpolio
s., postpump
s. ▸ post-thalamic stroke pain
s. ▸ post-transfusion
s. ▸ post-trauma response
s., post-traumatic
s. (POTS) ▸ postular orthostatic tachycardia
s., post-Vietnam
s., postviral
s., Potter's
s. ▸ precordial catch
s., preexcitation
s., preinfarction
s. (PMS) ▸ premenstrual
s., premonitory
s. (AIDS) prevention ▸ acquired immune deficiency
s., primary

s. (AIDS) primary pathogen ▸ acquired immune deficiency
s., primary Sjögren's
s. ▸ prolapsed mitral valve
s., prolonged Q-T
s. ▸ prolonged Q-T interval
s., protracted withdrawal
s., prune-belly
s., pseudoexfoliation
s. ▸ pseudoxanthoma elasticum
s., psychiatric
s., psychic
s., psychotic
s. ▸ pulmonary acid aspiration
s. ▸ pulmonary disease anemia
s. ▸ pulmonary dysmaturity
s. ▸ pulmonary infarction
s. ▸ pulmonary insufficiency revascularization
s. ▸ pulmonary sling
s., Q-T
s. ▸ Q-TU interval
s., rabbit
s. ▸ radial steal
s. ▸ radiologic scimitar
s., Raeder's
s. ▸ Ramsay Hunt
s. ▸ rape trauma
s., Rasmussen
s., Raynaud's
s. (RADS) ▸ reactive airways disease
s. ▸ recurrent thoracic outlet
s. ▸ redundant cusp
s., Reese's
s. ▸ reflex sympathetic dystrophy (RSD)
s., Refsum's
s., Reifenstein's
s., Reiter's
s. (AIDS) related complex (ARC) ▸ acquired immune deficiency
s. (AIDS) related pneumonia ▸ acquired immune deficiency
s. (AIDS)-related complex ▸ acquired immune deficiency
s. (AIDS)-related dementia ▸ acquired immune deficiency
s. (AIDS)-related macular degeneration ▸ acquired immune deficiency
s., Rénon-Delille
s., reperfusion
s. ▸ repetitive stress

s. (AIDS) residential treatment facility ▸ acquired immune deficiency

s., respiratory disease

s. (RDS) ▸ respiratory distress

s., respiratory failure

s., restless leg

s. ▸ retinitis pigmentosa

s., retraction

s., retroparotid space

s., Rett

s. ▸ reversible brain

s., Reye's

s., rhabdomyolytic

s., Riddoch's

s., Rieger's

s., right middle lobe (RML)

s., Riley-Day

s., Riley-Shwachman

s., Robin's

s., Rollet's

s. ▸ Romano-Ward

s., Romberg-Paessler

s., Rosenbach's

s., Rot-Bielschowsky

s., Rothmund's

s., Rotor's

s., Roussy-Cornil

s., Roussy-Levy

s., rubella

s., Rubinstein-Taybi

s., Rud's

s., Russell's

s., Rutherfurd's

s., Saethre-Chotzen

s. ▸ salt depletion

s. ▸ Sanchez-Cascos cardioauditory

s., Sanfilippo's

s., Sanger-Brown

s., sauvant

s., scalded skin

s. ▸ scalenus anterior

s., scalenus anticus

s., Schafer's

s., Schanz's

s., Schaumann's

s., Scheie's

s., Scheuthauer-Marie-Sainton

s., Schmidt's

s., school avoidance

s., Schultz's

s., Schwachman's

s., scimitar

s. ▸ scratch-like

s. (SADS) ▸ seasonal affective disorder

s., secondary Sjögren's

s. (SEDS) ▸ sedentary death

s., segmentary

s., Senear-Usher

s., sensory deprivation

s. ▸ sensory motor

s., serotonin

s., 17-hydroxylase deficiency

s. ▸ severe, acute respiratory

s., severe alcohol withdrawal

s. (SCIDS) ▸ severe combined immune deficiency

s., severe neurotic

s., severity and duration

s., Sézary

s. (SBS) ▸ shaken baby

s., Sheehy

s. ▸ short bowel

s. ▸ short gut

s., shoulder-hand

s. ▸ Shy-Drager

s. ▸ Shy-Magee

s., sicca

s. (SSS) ▸ sick sinus

s., Siegrist-Hutchinson

s., silent reaction ▸ rape trauma

s., Silver's

s., single family

s. ▸ single papillary muscle

s., sinobronchial

s., Sjögren's

s., sleep apnea

s. ▸ sleep apnea/hypopnea

s., slick-gut

s., slipping rib

s. ▸ slit ventricle

s., small left colon

s. ▸ Smith-Lemli-Opitz

s., social breakdown

s., Spanlang-Tappeiner

s., spastic bowel

s., spastic colon

s., splenic agenesis

s. ▸ splenic flexure

s., split-brain

s., Stargardt's

s., Stein-Leventhal

s., Stevens-Johnson

s., stiff-heart

s., Stilling-Türk-Duane

s., Stockholm

s., Stock-Spielmeyer-Vogt

s., Stokes

s., Stokes-Adams

s., stop and rest

s., Strachan-Scott

s., straight back

s., stroke

s., Stryker-Halbeisen

s., Sturge-Weber

s., subacute treatment for organic brain

s., subclavian steal

s., subwakefulness

s. (SIDS) ▸ sudden infant death

s. ▸ sudden sniffing death

s., Sudeck-Leriche

s., sump

s., sundown

s. ▸ sundowner's

s. ▸ superior mesenteric artery

s., superior sulcus tumor

s., superior vena cava (SVC)

s., supine hypotensive

s., suprarenogenic

s. ▸ supravalvular aortic stenosis

s. ▸ supravalvular aortic stenosis infantile hypercalcemia

s., surdocardiac

s. ▸ suspended heart

s. ▸ swallowed blood

s., Swan

s., Sweet's

s., sympathomimetic

s. ▸ systemic inflammatory response

s. ▸ systolic click murmur

s., tachybradycardia

s. ▸ tachycardia-bradycardia

s. ▸ tachycardia-polyuria

s. (AIDS)-tainted transfusion ▸ acquired immune deficiency

s., Takayasu's

s., Taussig-Bing

s., temporomandibular joint (TMJ)

s., Terry's

s., testicular feminizing

s. (AIDS) testing ▸ acquired immune deficiency

s. (AIDS) testing ▸ mandatory acquired immune deficiency

s., tetany

s., tethered cord

s., thalamic

s. ▸ thalamic pain

s., 13q deletion

s., Thompson's

s. ▸ thoracic endometriosis

syndrome—*continued*
s., thoracic outlet
s. ▸ thrombocytopenia-absent radius
s., thromboembolic
s., Tietze's
s., TMJ (temporomandibular joint)
s., Tolosa-Hunt
s., tonsillitis
s., total allergy
s., Touraine's
s., Tourette
s., toxic
s. (TSS) ▸ toxic shock
s., toxicologic-pharmacologic
s., translocation Down's
s. (AIDS) transmission ▸ acquired immune deficiency
s., trauma
s. ▸ traumatic disability
s., Treacher Collins
s. (AIDS) treatment ▸ acquired immune deficiency
s., treatment of organic brain
s. (AIDS) treatment trials ▸ federal acquired immune deficiency
s., Trenaunay
s., trisomy D
s., trisomy D₁
s., trisomy E
s., trisomy 13-15
s., trisomy 16-18
s., trisomy 18
s., trisomy 21
s., Troisier-Hanot-Chauffard
s., Troisier's
s., tropical splenomegaly
s., Trousseau
s., Turcot
s., Turner's
s., 20th century
s., Twiddler's
s., twin-twin transfusion
s., ulcerogenic tumor of pancreas
s. ▸ uneven limb
s. ▸ upper respiratory viral
s., urethral
s., Usher
s., Uyemura's
s. (AIDS) vaccine ▸ anti-acquired immune deficiency
s., vascular headache
s., vasovagal
s., velocardiofacial
s. ▸ vena cava

s., venolobar
s., vertigo
s. (AIDS) victim ▸ acquired immune deficiency
s., Vietnam
s. (AIDS) virus infection ▸ acquired immune deficiency
s. (AIDS) virus ▸ mother infected with acquired immune deficiency
s. (AIDS) virus testing ▸ acquired immune deficiency
s. ▸ visceroatrial heterotaxy
s., Vogt
s., Vogt-Koyanagi
s., Volkmann's
s., von Hippel-Lindau
s., Waardenburg's
s., Wallenberg's
s., Wartenberg's
s., wasting
s., Waterhouse-Friderichsen
s., Weber-Christian
s., Weber's
s., Weill-Marchesani
s., Weil's
s., Werdnig-Hoffmann
s., Wermer's
s., Werner's
s., Wernicke
s., Wernicke-Korsakoff
s. ▸ wet brain
s., wet lung
s. ▸ white clot
s. ▸ white coat
s., Wiedemann's
s., Willebrand-Jürgens
s., Wilson-Mikity
s., Wilson's
s., Wiskott-Aldrich
s., winter
s. with cannabinoids ▸ organic brain
s. with constipation ▸ irritable bowel
s. with depressants ▸ organic brain
s. with hallucinogens ▸ organic brain
s. with inhalants ▸ organic brain
s. with multiple drugs ▸ organic brain
s. with opioids ▸ organic brain
s. with phencyclidines ▸ organic brain
s. with stimulants ▸ organic brain
s., withdrawal
s., Wolff-Parkinson-White (WPW)

s., Wolf's
s. X
s. X ▸ cardiac
s. ▸ X-linked immunoglobulin M
s. ▸ X-linked lymphoproliferative (XLP)
s., XXY
s. ▸ yellow nail
s., yo-yo
s., Zollinger-Ellison
synechia(-ae)
s., anterior
s., cervical
s., dissolved
s. pericardii
s., vulvae
synergic muscles
synergism
s., antibiotic
s., in vitro
s., therapeutic additivity and
synergist, pituitary
synergistic
s. activity
s. bactericidal effect
s. effect
s. interaction
s. muscles
s. pressor effect
s. treatment
synergy, extensor
synergy, flexor
synesthesia algica
synesthesia, occasional
Syngamus trachea
syngeneic graft
syngenesioplastic transplant
synizesis pupillae
synkinesis/synkinesia
s., imitative
s., mouth-and-hand
s., spasmodic
synkinetic movements
synostoses, cranial
synostosis
s., congenital radioulnar
s., radioulnar
s., sagittal suture
s., tarsal
s., tribasilar
synovial
s. capsule
s. cavity
s. cell sarcoma
s. cell sarcoma of the knee

s. chondroma
s. chondromatosis
s. cyst
s. flap
s. fluid
s. fold
s. fold, infrapatellar
s. fold of hip
s. fold, patellar
s. ganglion
s. hernia
s. inflammation
s. joint
s. membrane
s. membrane, inflammation of
s. membrane of joint
s. membrane ▸ thickened
s. osteochondromatosis
s. plica
s. sarcoma
s. sheaths
s. tissue ▸ inflamed
s. villi
synovitis, hypertrophic
synovitis, rheumatoid
synovium, inflammation of
synpneumonic empyema
syntactical aphasia
synthesis
s., antibody
s., blocking testosterone
s., cell wall
s., cholesterol
s., collagen
s., decreased protein
s., diagnostic
s., disease
s., distributive analysis and
s., DNA (deoxyribonucleic acid)
s., enzymatic
s., folic acid
s., impair protein
s., inducible enzyme
s., inhibition, protein
s., molecular
s., morphologic
s. of continuity
s. of continuity of fracture
s. of immunoglobulins
s. of virus
s., prostaglandin
s., protein
s., stimulation
s., thromboxane
synthesize fatty acids

synthesize gamma globulin
synthesizing enzymes, testosterone-synthetase
s., amide
s., glycogen
s., pantothenate
synthetic
s. androgen
s. bone material
s. calcitrol
s. chemistry
s. colloid
s. DNA ▸ molecules of
s. drug
s. estrogen and progestin
s. graft
s. graft material
s. heart valve
s. hemoglobin
s. hormone
s. hormones ▸ natural or
s. human gastrin
s. human growth hormone
s. insulin
s. lecithin, cardiolipin
s. male hormones
s. opiate
s. penicillins, semi◊
s. progesterone
s. prostaglandins
s. protein
s. retinoids
s. steroid
s. suture material
s. suture material, Ethibond
s. suture material, Ethiflex
s. thyroid hormone
s. thyroid medication
s. tube ▸ insertion of
s. vaccine
s. virus
syntonic, ego-
syntonic type
Syphacia obvelata
syphilis (Syphilis)
s., Bejel
s., cardiovascular
s., cerebrospinal
s., congenital
s., incubating
s., latent
s., meningovascular
s., neonatal
s. of bone
s. of conjunctiva

s. of iris
s. of lacrimal gland
s., secondary
s. serology, false positive
s., standard test for
s., tertiary
S. Test (DST) ▸ Daya
s., treated
s. (VDS), venereal disease-
syphilitic
s. alopecia
s. aneurysm
s. aortic aneurysm, rupture of
s. aortic valvulitis
s. aortitis
s. arteritis
s. cataract
s., cerebrospinal
s. choroiditis
s. cirrhosis
s. dacryocystitis
s. endarteritis
s. endocarditis
s. infection, chronic
s. laryngitis
s. leptomeningitis
s. lesion, initial
s. meningitis
s. myocarditis
s. nephritis
s. node
s. pseudoparalysis
s. psychosis
s. rhinitis
s. roseola
s. spirochetes
s. stomatitis
syphilitica, lues
syphilitica, retinitis
syphiliticum, erythema nodosum
syphiliticus, pemphigus
syphiliticus, tophus
syringe(s)
s., contaminated needles and
s., disposable
s. exchange ▸ needle and
s., inadequately sterilized
s., laryngeal
s., Luer-Lok
s. pump
s. push
s. ▸ used needles, instruments or
syringomyelia (SM) disorder
syringomyelic clawhand
syrup of ipecac

**syrup urine disease (MSUD), maple
system(s) (System) [*symptom*]**
- s. abuse
- s., abusive family
- s., activate immune
- s. (CNS) activity ▸ central nervous
- s., adrenergic nervous
- s., after-loading
- s., air delivery
- s., alcohol family
- s., allergy/immune
- s. analyzer ▸ pacing
- s. anatomy ▸ immune
- s. and anxiety, autonomic nervous
- s., angiogram, splenic
- s., angled-vision lens
- s., annular phased array
- s. approach, family
- s., arterial
- s., atrioventricular conduction
- s. atrophy ▸ multiple
- s., augmentative communication
- s., automated cervical cell
  screening
- s., automatic exposure
- s., autonomic nervous
- s., autotransfusion
- s., background
- s., biliary
- s., biliary duct
- s. bleeding, digestive
- s., blood circulation
- s., blood clotting
- s., blood group
- s., body's defense
- s., body's infection-fighting immune
- s., brachiocephalic
- s., brain's limbic
- s., brain's motor control
- s. ▸ breathing difficulty with
  problems from central nervous
- s., calyceal
- s., canalicular
- s. cancer, immune
- s. cancer, nervous
- s. ▸ cancer of reproductive
- s., cardiac conduction
- s. ▸ cardiac-related vertebrate blood
- s. (CVS), cardiovascular
- s., carotid arterial
- s., catenary
- s., cell
- s. cells, immune
- s., cellular immune
- s. (CNS) ▸ central nervous

- s. check, body
- s., cine pulse
- s., circulatory
- s., circulatory support
- s., closed water seal drainage
- s., codominant
- s., collecting
- s., commercial dose computation
- s., complement
- s., complete pacemaker patient
  testing
- s., computer-imaging
- s., conceptual
- s., conduction
- s., connecting
- s., Conolly's
- s. ▸ constipation with problems of
  central nervous
- s., continuous drainage (dr'ge)
- s., continuous suction drainage
- s., control of hormonal
- s., controlled release
- s., coordinate
- s. (COEPS) ▸ cortically originating
  extrapyramidal
- s. damage, immune
- s. ▸ damage to central nervous
- s. (CNS) defect, central nervous
- s., degenerative disorder of nervous
- s. (CNS) depressant ▸ central
  nervous
- s. (CNS) depression ▸ central
  nervous
- s. (CNS) deterioration, organic
  central nervous
- s., didactic
- s., digestive
- s. ▸ digital cardiac imaging
- s., dilatation of ventricular
- s., dilated ventricular
- s. (CNS) disease ▸ central nervous
- s. disease ▸ peripheral nervous
- s. (CNS) disorder ▸ central nervous
- s. disorder, immune
- s. ▸ disorder of brain and nervous
- s., distention of ventricular
- s., drainage (dr'ge)
- s., drug delivery
- s., duplication of left collecting
- s., duplication of right collecting
- s. dysfunction ▸ autonomic nervous
- s. (CNS) dysfunction ▸ central
  nervous
- s. dysfunction ▸ immune
- s., dysfunctional family

- s., dysfunctional thermoregulatory
- s., dysplasia of nervous
- s. ▸ echocardiographic automated
  boundary detection
- s. ▸ echocardiographic scoring
- s. effect ▸ peripheral autonomic
  nervous
- s., electrode
- s., emission computerized
  tomographic (ECT)
- s., endocrine
- s., enteric nervous
- s., enzyme
- s., excretory
- s., expanding cellular
- s., extrahepatic
- s., extrahepatic biliary
- s., extrapyramidal
- s. failure of vital organs, total
- s., faulty warning
- s., fetal monitoring
- s. ▸ fiberoptic catheter delivery
- s., fibrinolytic
- s., flatworm ▸ nervous
- s., flexible fiberoptic
- s. for cancer ▸ classification
- s., foreground
- s. from AIDS ▸ problems with
  central nervous
- s. from alcoholism ▸ problem with
  central nervous
- s. from diet pills ▸ problem with
  central nervous
- s. from sleep apnea ▸ problem with
  central nervous
- s. from vomiting ▸ problem with
  central nervous
- s. function ▸ circulatory
- s. function ▸ immune
- s. function ▸ normal immune
- s. ▸ function of sympathetic nervous
- s. function ▸ perturbed autonomic
  nervous
- s., functional
- s., functional communication
- s. ▸ fungal infection of nervous
- s., gastrointestinal (GI)
- s. ▸ gastrointestinal therapeutic
- s., gated
- s., genitourinary (GU)
- s. ▸ Gleason grading
- s., Glover's drainage
- s., greater saphenous
- s., headwall
- s., health care

s., hearing
s., hematopoietic
s., hereditary disease of nervous
s. ▸ hexaxial reference
s. ▸ His-Purkinje
s. homeostatic
s., hospital
s., hot-cold
s., humoral
s. ▸ hyperactive immune
s. (CNS) hypersomnolence ▸ idiopathic central nervous
s., imaging
s., immune
s., immune defense
s. ▸ impair the immune
s. ▸ impaired reticuloendothelial
s. impairment ▸ sexual/reproductive
s. ▸ implantable left ventricular (LV) assist
s. in drug abuse, monitoring
s. in radiation therapy, staging
s. ▸ incomplete development of autonomic nervous
s. (CNS) infarction ▸ central nervous
s. (CNS) infection ▸ nosocomial central nervous
s. (CNS) ▸ infratentorial parts of central nervous
s., inhibit immune
s. ▸ integrated lead
s., intracranial nervous
s. (CNS) ▸ intracranial part of central nervous
s., inventory by
s., involuntary nervous
s., isocenter
s., Kardex
s., Kirklin staging
s., laboratory computer
s., lacrimal
s., laser alignment
s., lead
s., lens
s. (CNS) lesion ▸ macroscopic central nervous
s. (CNS) lesion ▸ microscopic central nervous
s., lesser saphenous
s., life support
s., limbic
s., linear
s., linear compartmental
s., lower collecting

s., lymph
s., lymph node
s., lymphatic
s. (CNS) lymphoma ▸ primary central nervous
s., magnetic induction coaxial electrode
s., maintenance of nervous
s., maldeveloped nervous
s., malformed reproductive
s., malfunction of permanent demand ventricular pacing
s., malfunctioning immune
s. malfunctions ▸ major organ
s., malignancy of lymphatic
s., mamillary
s. ▸ managed care
s., Manchester dose distribution
s., medical information
S. (MEDLARS) ▸ Medical Literature Analysis and Retrieval
s. ▸ Medtronic transvene endocardial lead
s., mental health delivery
s., mesolimbic
s., metric
s. ▸ microwave ablation
s., Monaldi's drainage
s., monitoring
s., mononuclear phagocyte
s., motor
s., multiaxial
s., multihospital
s., multiple pressure transducer
s., muscular
s., myocardium electrical
s., nasolacrimal
s., negative airflow
s. neoplasm ▸ nervous
s., nervous
s., nicotine transdermal
S., Nobelpharma Implant
s., nonrenewal cellular
s., object vision
s. of body ▸ circulatory
s. of body ▸ immune
s. of brain ▸ chemical
s. of brain ▸ vascular
s. of brain ▸ ventricular
s. of cancer patient ▸ immune
s. of cells ▸ slow renewal and nonrenewal
s. of neurotransmitters ▸ brain's
s. of refraction ▸ fogging
s. of the body ▸ circulatory

s. of tubules
s., on-line appointment
S. (OTS), Optical Tracking
s., organ
s. ▸ orthogonal lead
s., orthotic
s., outpatient drug treatment
s., overactive immune
s. ▸ pacemaker code
s. parameter status
s., parasympathetic
s., parasympathetic nervous
s., Paris dose distribution
s., patent, biliary
s., pediatric monitoring
s., peripheral
s. ▸ peripheral access
s. ▸ peripheral atherectomy
s., peripheral circulatory
s., peripheral nervous
s., peripheral sympathetic
s., permanent cardiac pacing
s., permanent demand ventricular pacing
s. (PERS) ▸ personal emergency response
s., perturbation in cardiovascular
s. ▸ phased array
s., Pinel's
s. ▸ plasma coagulation
s., pneumatic conveying
s., poisoning of nervous
s., portable insulin infusion
s., portal
s., positive support
s., postural drainage
s., preprogrammed insulin delivery
S. (PAIRS) program ▸ Psychiatric Alcohol Inpatient Review
s. (PIMS) ▸ programmable implantable medication
s. programmer
s., prospective payment
s., prosthetic
s., Purkinje
s., pyelocalyceal
s., quality information monitoring
s., Quimby dose distribution
s., radial subtraction imaging
s., radiation injury of vascular
s., radionuclide emission computerized tomographic (ECT)
s., rapid renewal cell
s. ▸ regulated perfusion

system(s)—*continued*

s. relaxation techniques ▸ autonomic nervous
s., remote metastases
s., renal collecting
s. ▸ renin angiotensin aldosterone
s. (RAS) ▸ renin-angiotensin
s., reproductive
s. ▸ reroute digestive
s., research
s., respiratory
s., reticular activating
s., reticuloendothelial
s. review
s. ▸ rotational atherectomy
s., saphenofemoral
s., sarcotubular
s., second signalling
s., self-controlled intravenous
s., sensory
s., sensory nervous
s. (CNS) sequelae ▸ central nervous
s. ▸ sheath and dilator
s. shock ▸ respiratory
s. (CNS) shunt ▸ central nervous
s. side-effects, nervous
s. ▸ Simpson-Robert vascular dilation
s., single pressure transducer
s., skeletal
s. ▸ SKY epidural pain control
s., small circumflex
s., somatic nervous
s., somatosensory
s., spatial vision
s., standard international
s., standard 10-20 (ten-twenty)
s. (CNS) stimulant ▸ central nervous
s., stimulate the immune
s., stimulation, block nervous
s. ▸ strep throat and problem with central nervous
s., stress responses of cardiovascular
s., structure of the support
s., sump drainage
s. (SMAS) ▸ superficial musculo-aponeurotic
s., support
s. ▸ suppression of immune
s., supratentorial parts of central nervous
s., Surgivac suction drainage

s., surveillance
s., sympathetic nervous
s., sympathoadrenal
s., T
s. ▸ tear drainage
s., ten-twenty (10-20)
s. (CNS) therapy ▸ central nervous
s., three-bottle drainage
s., three-compartment
s., three-dose distribution
s., three-phase
s., tidal drainage
s. tolerance to radiation therapy ▸ central nervous
s., transducer
s. ▸ transluminal lysing
s. ▸ transtelephonic ambulatory monitoring
s. (CNS) trauma ▸ central nervous
s. ▸ triaxial reference
s., trypanosomiasis of nervous
s. ▸ tumor, nodes, metastases (TNM) staging
s. tumors, lacrimal drainage
s., two-bottle drainage
s., two-compartment
s., ultraviolet purification
s. ▸ underactive immune
s., unstable vasomotor
s., upper collecting
s. ▸ urinary tract
s., urogenital
s., using
s., vaccine stimulates immune
s., vacuum drainage
s., vascular
s. vascular disease ▸ digestive
s., vegetative nervous
s., venous
s., ventricular conduction
s., vertebrobasilar
s. ▸ vessel occlusion
s., vestibular
s., video
s., visceral nervous
s., visual
s., vocal
s., water purification
s., waterseal drainage
s. ▸ weakened immune
s., withdrawing life support

systematic

s. anatomy
s. approach
s. desensitization

s. desensitization of pervasive anxiety
s. desensitization of phobic reactions
s. desensitization procedure
s. desensitization, relaxation in
s. desensitization, self-administered
s. follow-up procedures
s. monitoring
s. role playing
s. therapeutical friction

systematica, paraphrenia
systematized delusion
systemic

s. absorption
s. adjuvant therapy
s. allergic reaction
s. amyloidosis ▸ primary
s. antibiotics
s. arch
s. arterial pressure (SAP)
s. arteriolar resistance
s. atherosclerosis, mild
s. blood flow
s. blood flow ratio ▸ pulmonary
s. blood pressure (SBP)
s. body infection
s. cancer
s. cancer, neurologic complications of
s. Candida infection
s. candidemia
s. candidiasis
s. cardiac output
s. change
s. chemotherapy
s. chondromalacia
s. circulation
s. circulation, inadequacy of
s. collateral
s. corticosteroids
s. desensitization
s. disease
s. disease, control of local and
s. disorder
s. effect
s. emetic
s. encephalopathy, portal-
s. flow
s. hamartomatosis
s. heart
s. hemodynamic parameters
s. hemodynamics
s. hypertension

s. illness
s. infection
s. infection, fatal
s. inflammation
s. inflammatory response syndrome
s. injection
s. lesion
s. lupus erythematosus (SLE)
s. mastocytosis
s. mean arterial pressure
s. medication
s. myalgia
s. mycosis
s. mycotic infection
s. necrotizing vasculitis
s. oxygen (O₂) consumption
s. poison
s. pressure
s. progressive sclerosis
s. psychotherapy
s. radiation therapy
s. reaction, severe
s. resistance
s. scleroderma
s. scleroderma ▸ severe
s. sclerosis
s. sclerosis, cutaneous
s. sclerosis, dim use
s. sclerosis (PSS), progressive
s. sepsis
s. shock, sudden
s. shunt, portal
s. signs of drug abuse
s. steroids
s. to pulmonary artery anastomosis
s. to pulmonary shunt
s. toxicity
s. therapy
s. therapy ▸ adjuvant
s. therapy ▸ cancer responsive to
s. treatment
s. vascular disorder
s. vascular hypertension
s. vascular resistance index
s. venous hypertension
s. venous return
s. venous shunt, portal to
s. yeast infection

systole [*cystocele*]

s., aborted
s. alternans
s., anticipated
s., arterial
s., atrial

s., atrioventricular (AV) nodal
s., auricular
s., cardiac
s., catalectic
s., electrical
s., electromechanical
s., end-
s., extra◊
s., frustrate
s., hemic
s., internal dimension-
s., isovolumic
s., late
s., posterior wall thickness-
s., premature
s., premature junctional
s. (PVS) ▸ premature ventricular
s. ▸ total electromechanical
s., ventricular
s. ▸ ventricular ectopic

systolic

s. and diastolic performance ▸ impairment of
s. anterior motion (SAM)
s. aortic pressure (PSAP) ▸ peak
s. apical impulse
s. apical murmur
s. blood pressure (SBP)
s. blood pressure (SBP) ▸ decreased
s. bruit
s. click
s. click murmur syndrome
s. click ▸ nonejection
s. contraction
s. count ▸ end-
s. current of injury
s. depression
s. diameter ▸ total end-
s. dimension ▸ end-
s. dimension ▸ left ventricular (LV) end-
s. discharge
s. doming
s. dysfunction
s. ejection click
s. ejection murmur (SEM)
s. ejection period
s. ejection rate (SER)
s. ejection rate (MSER) ▸ mean
s. ejection rate ▸ mean normalized
s. ejection time
s. elastance ▸ end-
s. expansion
s. force velocity indices ▸ end-

s. function
s. function, impaired
s. gallop
s. gallop rhythm
s. gradient
s. gradient (PSG) ▸ peak
s. gradient, peak-to-peak
s. gradient pressure ▸ peak
s. heart failure
s. heart murmur, apical
s. heave
s. honk
s. hypertension
s. hypertension, borderline
s. hypertension in the elderly
s. hypertension ▸ isolated
s. hypotension
s. ▸ left ventricular (LV) end-
s. left ventricular (LV) pressure
s. left ventricular (LV) pressure ▸ mean
s. lift ▸ parasternal
s. mean (SM)
s. mitral prolapse
s. motion
s. murmur
s. murmur, blowing
s. murmur, blowing ejection
s. murmur, decrescendo early
s. murmur ▸ early peaking
s. murmur (ESM), ejection
s. murmur, end-
s. murmur, harsh
s. murmur (LSM), late
s. murmur ▸ late apical
s. murmur ▸ late peaking
s. murmur, loud
s. performance ▸ left ventricular (LV)
s., pericardial friction rub
s. pressure (SP)
s. pressure (ASP) ▸ area
s. pressure, depressed
s. pressure, end-
s. pressure ▸ high risk
s. pressure (LVSP) ▸ left ventricular
s. pressure, maintain
s. pressure ▸ right ventricular (RV)
s. pressure time index
s. pressure volume relation ▸ end-
s. pressure volume relation ▸ ventricular end-
s. reading
s. regurgitant murmur
s. reserve

systolic—*continued*
- s. shock
- s. stress dimension relation ▸ end-
- s. stress ▸ left ventricular (LV) end-
- s. tension, ventricular
- s. thrill
- s. thrill ▸ parasternal
- s. time interval
- s. time interval ▸ right ventricular (RV)
- s. to diastolic
- s. trough
- s. velocity ▸ peak
- s. velocity ratio
- s. volume ▸ end
- s. volume index ▸ end
- s. volume, ventricular end-
- s. whipping
- s. whoop

Sz (skin impedance)
Szabo's test
Szymanowski('s)
- S. -Kuhnt operation
- S. operation
- S. operation, Kuhnt-
- S. operation, Smith-Kuhnt-
- S. procedure, Kuhnt-

T

T (hallucinogen)
t (temporal)
T and A (tonsillectomy and
    adenoidectomy)
T appearance ▸ inverted-
T artifact
T categories in hollow organs
T cell
    T. cell antigen ▸ pan
    T. cell defect
    T. cell, disease fighting
    T. cell, helper
    T. cell ▸ infection fighting
    T. cell Lymphocytic Virus (HTLV),
        Human
    T. cell lymphoma
    T. cell lymphoma, cutaneous
    T. cell lymphoma ▸ erythrodermic
        cutaneous
    T. cell lymphotropic virus type ▸
        simian
T fashion, inverted
T incision, inverted
T lens contact lenses
T loop
T, peptide
T phenomenon ▸ R-on-
T premature ventricular complex ▸ R-
    on-
T sign
T system
T vector
T. water test
T wave(s)
    T w. abnormalities, ST and
    T w. alternans
    T w. changes
    T w. changes compatible with
        ischemia ▸ ST-
    T w., depressed
    T w., diphasic
    T w., flattening
    T w., flipped
    T w., inversion
    T w., isoelectric
    T w. ▸ postextrasystolic
    T w. ▸ pseudonormalization of

Ta (tantalum)
Ta segment
TAB (therapeutic abortion)
tabac, nodules
Tabanus
    T. atratus
    T. bovinus
    T. ditaeniatus
    T. fasciatus
    T. gratus
tabby cat heart
tabby cat striation
tabes
    t., cerebral
    t., cervical
    t., diabetic
    t. dorsalis
    t. ergotica
    t., Friedreich's
    t., hereditary
    t. infantum
    t., interstitial
    t. mesaraica
    t. mesenterica
    t., nerve
    t., spasmodic
    t. spinalis
tabetic
    t. cuirass
    t. dementia
    t. foot
    t. gait
    t. mast
    t. neurosis
    t. neurosyphilis
table(s)
    t., Albee fracture
    t., anterior
    t., Bell fracture
    t. bones of skull, inner
    t. bones of skull, outer
    t., bony
    t., conversion
    t. drugs, under the
    t., fracture
    t. frontal bone, inner
    t. frontal bone, outer
    t. graft, outer

    t., inadequately cleaned x-ray
    t. lateral position, cross-
    t. of skull, inner
    t. of skull, outer
    t., overbed
    t., periodic
    t., Reuss's
    t. ▸ Siemens open heart
    t. test ▸ head up tilt
    t. test ▸ isoproterenol tilt
    t. test ▸ tilt
    t., vitreous
tablet(s)
    t., buccal
    t., dispensing
    t., enteric-coated
    t., estrogen
    t. form
    t., hypodermic
    t., oral hormone
    t., scored
    t., sublingual
    t., vaginal
tabourka, bruit de
Tabs (LSD)
tabs [tags]
tac (Tac) (TAC)
tac rhythm ▸ tic-
tach (ventricular tachycardia) ▸ V
tache
    t. blanche
    t. cérébrale
    t. laiteuse
    t. méningéale
    t. spinale
tachography study
tachy syndrome, brachy-
tachyarrhythmia(s)
    t. ▸ life-threatening ventricular
    t. pacing
    t., resistant
    t., supraventricular
    t. ▸ sustained supraventricular
    t., ventricular
tachyarrhythmic substrate
tachy-brady arrhythmia
tachy-bradycardia syndrome

tachycardia
- t. ablation ▸ supraventricular
- t., aborted paroxysmal atrial
- t., accelerated idioventricular
- t., alternating bidirectional
- t., antidromic
- t. ▸ antidromic atrioventricular (AV) reciprocating
- t. ▸ antidromic circus movement
- t. ▸ arteriovenous (AV) junctional
- t., atrial
- t. ▸ atrial atrioventricular (AV) nodal reentrant
- t., atrial chaotic
- t. (AET), atrial ectopic
- t., atrial paroxysmal
- t., atrial reentry
- t. ▸ atrial ventricular (AV) nodal reentry
- t. ▸ atrial ventricular (AV) reciprocating
- t., atrioventricular (AV) junctional
- t., atrioventricular (AV) junctional reciprocating
- t., atrioventricular (AV) nodal
- t., atrioventricular (AV) nodal reentrant
- t., atrioventricular (AV) nodal reentrant paroxysmal
- t. (AVRT), atrioventricular reciprocating
- t., auricular
- t., automatic atrial
- t., automatic ectopic
- t., AV (arteriovenous) junctional
- t., AV (arteriovenous) reciprocating
- t., baseline
- t., bidirectional
- t., bidirectional ventricular
- t. -bradycardia syndrome
- t., bundle branch reentrant
- t. ▸ bursts of ventricular
- t., chaotic atrial
- t., chronic
- t., circus movement
- t. cycle length
- t. cycle length ▸ ventricular
- t. -dependent aberrancy
- t. detection rate
- t., differential diagnosis of
- t., double
- t., drug-refractory
- t., ectopic
- t. ▸ ectopic atrial
- t. en salves
- t. ▸ endless loop
- t., entrainment of
- t., essential
- t. ▸ exercise-induced ventricular
- t., fetal
- t. ▸ hypertension and
- t., hypotension and
- t. ▸ idiopathic ventricular
- t., idioventricular
- t., incessant
- t. -induced cardiomyopathy
- t. ▸ inducible polymorphic ventricular
- t. ▸ intra-atrial reentrant
- t. ▸ intractable junctional
- t., junctional
- t. ▸ junctional ectopic
- t. ▸ junctional reciprocating
- t. ▸ macroreentrant atrial
- t. ▸ malignant ventricular
- t., monoform
- t. ▸ monomorphic ventricular
- t. (MAT) ▸ multifocal atrial
- t., multiform
- t. ▸ narrow complex
- t., nodal
- t. ▸ nodal paroxysmal
- t. ▸ nodal reentrant
- t. ▸ nonparoxysmal atrioventricular junctional
- t. ▸ nonparoxysmal junctional
- t., nonparoxysmal nodal
- t. ▸ nonsustained ventricular
- t., normal
- t., orthodromic
- t. ▸ orthodromic atrioventricular (AV)
- t. ▸ orthodromic atrioventricular (AV) reciprocating
- t., orthostatic
- t. (PMT), pacemaker mediated
- t. ▸ parasystolic ventricular
- t., paroxysmal
- t. (PAT) ▸ paroxysmal atrial
- t. ▸ paroxysmal junctional
- t. ▸ paroxysmal nodal
- t. ▸ paroxysmal reentrant supraventricular
- t. ▸ paroxysmal sinus
- t. (PSVT) ▸ paroxysmal supraventricular
- t. (PVT) ▸ paroxysmal ventricular
- t. pathway mapping
- t. ▸ patient has
- t. (PJRT) ▸ permanent junctional reciprocating
- t., pleomorphic
- t. ▸ polymorphic ventricular
- t. ▸ polymorphous ventricular
- t. -polyuria syndrome
- t. ▸ primary ventricular
- t. ▸ rapid nonsustained ventricular
- t., reciprocating
- t. ▸ reciprocating macroreentry orthodromic
- t. ▸ recurrent paroxysmal
- t., recurring
- t., reentrant
- t. ▸ reentrant atrial
- t. ▸ reentrant supraventricular
- t., reflex
- t., refractory
- t. ▸ regular, wide QRS
- t. ▸ repetitive monomorphic ventricular
- t. ▸ repetitive paroxysmal ventricular
- t., resting
- t. reversion pacemaker, Pasar
- t. ▸ right ventricular (RV) outflow tract
- t. ▸ S-A nodal reentrant
- t. ▸ salvo of ventricular
- t., secondary
- t. ▸ self-terminating
- t., sinus
- t. ▸ sinus nodal reentrant
- t. ▸ sinus reentrant
- t., sleeping
- t. ▸ slow-fast
- t. ▸ spontaneous reentrant sustained ventricular
- t. strumosa exophthalmica
- t. (SVT) ▸ supraventricular
- t. ▸ sustained monomorphic ventricular
- t. ▸ sustained ventricular
- t. syndrome, bradycardia
- t. syndrome (POTS) ▸ postular orthostatic
- t. therapy
- t. (V tach) ▸ ventricular
- t. ▸ wide QRS
- t. window
- t. with aberrancy, paroxysmal atrial
- t. with high degree atrioventricular block ▸ atrial
- t. with torsades de pointes, ventricular

t. ▸ Wolff-Parkinson-White reentrant
Tachylog pacemaker
tachypnea
  t., nervous
  t. of newborn ▸ transient
  t., transient
tachypneic, patient
tachysystole, atrial
tachysystole, auricular
tack sounds, tick-
tacking suture
tactics, confrontational
tactics, diversionary
tactile
  t. amnesia
  t. aphasia
  t. astereognosis
  t. cell
  t. deficits
  t. delusions
  t. disc
  t. discs, Ranvier's
  t. fremitus
  t. hairs
  t. hallucination
  t. hallucinations ▸ occasional
  t. pressure ▸ light
  t. sensation
  t. stimulation
  t. stimulation ▸ audio-visual-
  t. tension
TActile CONverter (OPTACON),
  OPtical
TAD (thoracic asphyxiant dystrophy)
tadpole cells
Taenia (taenia)
  T. africana
  T. antarctica
  T. balaniceps
  T. brachysoma
  T. bremneri
  T. brunerri
  t. choroidea
  t. cinerea
  T. confusa
  T. crassiceps
  T. crassicollis
  T. cucurbitina
  T. demarariensis
  T. echinococcus
  T. elliptica
  t. fimbriae
  t. fornicis
  t. hippocampi
  T. hydatigena

T. krabbei
T. madagascariensis
T. marginata
T. mediocanellata
t. medullaris thalami optici
T. nana
t. organism
T. ovis
T. philippina
T. pisiformis
t. pontis
T. saginata
t. semicircularis corporis striati
T. solium larvae
T. taeniaeformis
t. tectae
t. terminalis
t. thalami
t. violacea
taenioides, Diphyllobothrium
taenioides, Pentastoma
taeniola cinerea
taeniola corporis callosi of Reil
taeniorhynchus, Aedes
TAF (trypsin, aldehyde-fuchsin)
tag(s) [*tabs*]
  t., auricular
  t., cutaneous
  t., epicardial fat
  t., expressed sequence
  t., hemorrhoidal skin
  t. on patient, toe
  t., perineal skin
  t., peritonsillar
  t., pleural
  t., radioactive
  t., rectal
  t., rectal skin
  t., skin
  t., toe
  t., tonsillar
tagged
  t. atom
  t., muscles isolated and
  t. with radioactive material, red
    cells
tagging, cardiac
T-agglutination
tagliacotian operation
tagliacotian rhinoplasty
Tagliacozzi's flap
Tagliacozzi's nasal reconstruction
TAH (total abdominal hysterectomy)
TAH (total artificial heart)

tai chi
  t.c. martial arts
  t.c. technique
  t.c. treatment
tail
  t., elongated cytoplasmic
  t. fold
  t. gut
  t. of pancreas
  t. of pancreas necrotic
  t. of pancreas, perfusion in
  t. of pancreas soft
  t. of Spence
  t. pulse, mouse
  t. sign
tailbone
  t. area
  t. pain
  t. pain from cyst ▸ pilonidal
tailed bandage, many-
tailed dressing, many-
tailoring of flaps
tailors' ankle
tainted
  t. blood ▸ hepatitis-
  t. blood, HIV-
  t. blood transfusion
  t. drugs
  t. restaurant food
  t. transfusion, AIDS-
Takayasu-Onishi disease
take(s) (Take)
  t. as directed
  T. Off Pounds Sensibly (TOPS) diet
  t. risk ▸ unwilling to
taken
  t., biopsies of area
  t., biopsies of tissue
  t., bites of ribs
  t. cells
  t., effective action
  t. for examination, multiple
    washings
  t., multiple biopsies
  t. off top of solution, white
taking
  t. and publication of photographs ▸
    authorization form for
  t. and publication of photographs ▸
    consent form for
  t. behavior, drug-
  t. behavior, risk-
  t. of motion pictures of operation ▸
    authorization form for

taking—*continued*
- t. of motion pictures of operation ▸ consent form for

Takos syndrome, Petzetakis-

talar tilt

talc
- t. insufflation ▸ thorascopic
- t. operation
- t. plaques
- t. pleurodesis
- t. pleurodesis ▸ thorascopic
- t. pneumoconiosis
- t. poudrage
- t. retinopathy
- t. slurry

tale signs, tell-

Talion law or principle

talipes
- t. calcaneovalgus
- t. calcaneovarus
- t. calcaneus
- t. cavus
- t. equinovalgus
- t. equinovarus
- t. equinus
- t. percavus
- t. planovalgus
- t. planus
- t., spasmodic
- t. supinatus
- t. valgus
- t. varus

talk(s)
- t. back
- t., bad self-
- t. constantly
- t. ▸ good self-
- t., inability to
- t. pacemaker, cross-
- t. ▸ realistic self-
- t. therapy

talkative, patient

talking
- t., compulsive
- t., difficulty
- t., increased
- t. of death or suicide
- t. or understanding ▸ trouble
- t., rapid
- t. sickness
- t., sleep
- t. ▸ sudden trouble
- t. tracheostomy tube, Pitt
- t., trouble

Tallqvist's scale

Talma's disease

talocalcaneal angle

talocalcaneal ligament

talocalcaneonavicular articulation

talofibular ligament

talonavicular
- t. articulation
- t. joint
- t. ligament

talpae, Grahamella

talus [*callous, callus*]
- t. foot deformity, congenital vertical
- t., head of

tambour, bruit de

tambour sound

tamoxifen, patient treated with

tampering, drug

tampon
- t., Corner
- t., Dührssen's
- t., Genupak
- t. injuries
- t., nasal
- t., tracheal
- t., Trendelenburg's
- t. tube

tamponade
- t. action
- t., acute
- t., atypical
- t., balloon
- t., cardiac
- t., chronic
- t., esophageal
- t., finger
- t., heart
- t. ▸ low pressure
- t., nontraumatic cardiac
- t., pericardiac
- t., pericardial
- t. ▸ pericardial effusion and
- t., Rose's
- t., subacute
- t., traumatic

tan parenchyma ▸ lobulated firm,

tandem
- t., Ernst radium
- t., Fletcher after-loading
- t. gait
- t. insertion
- t. lesion
- t. walking

tangent screen

tangential
- t. beam, alignment of

- t. breast, medial and lateral
- t. field with internal mammary field, matching
- t. fields, matching supraclavicular and
- t. fields, parallel opposing
- t. percussion
- t. plane, dose calculated in a
- t. projection
- t. projection, inferior-superior
- t. speech pattern
- t. thinking
- t. views
- t. wound

Tangier disease

tangled fibers ▸ clumps of

tangles
- t. in brain
- t. (NFT) ▸ neurofibrillary
- t., neuronal
- t. of Alzheimer's disease, brain plaques and
- t. of filaments ▸ abnormal
- t., plaques and

tank
- t. ear
- t., flotation
- t., Hubbard
- t., hyperbaric
- t. massage, Hubbard
- t., nitrous oxide (N_2O)
- t., portable oxygen (O_2)
- t., sound-proof
- t. suit, hydrotherapy
- t. therapy, Hubbard
- t. ventilator

tannate, albumin

tanned red cells (TRC)

tanned red cells (TRC) antibody titer, microsomal

Tanner
- T. Developmental Scale
- T. mesher
- T. operation
- T. stage
- T. -Vanderput graft

tannex, bisacodyl

tanning pills

tanning, postirradiation

Tansley's operation

tantalum
- t. bronchogram
- t. implant
- t. implant material
- t. mesh

t. mesh graft
t. mesh implant
t. mesh implant material
t. 182 (Ta^{182})
t. -132
t., powdered
t. ring
t. sheet
t. stent
t. stent, Cordis radiopaque
t. stent ▸ radiopaque
t. strut
t. wire
t. wire fixation
tantrum(s)
t., infantile
t., intense
t. ▸ patient has
t. ▸ repetitious behavior and
t., temper
Tanzer's auricle reconstruction
Ta^{182} (tantalum 182)
tap(s)
t., belly
t., bloody
t., bone marrow
t., cisternal
t., diagnostic spinal
t., headache after spinal
t., mitral
t., non-traumatic
t., pericardial
t., peritoneal
t., pleural
t. reflex, front-
t. reflex, heel-
t., spinal
t., spinal fluid
t. ▸ traumatic spinal
t., ventricular
t. water
t. water, contaminated
t. water, filtered
tape(s) (Tape)
t. closure of laceration
t. drain, umbilical
t., fiberglass casting
t., Mersilene
T., Micropore
t. prosthesis, collagen
t., relaxation
t., restraining
t. strapping, eversion
T., Tes-
t., tubing secured with

t., umbilical
taped shut ▸ eyes
taped to the skin
tapering
t. of therapy
t. off drugs
t. schedule
t. schedule of medication
tapetal light reflex
tapetum nigrum
tapetum oculi
tapeworm, pork
tapeworm, unarmed
tapir, bouche de
tapped daily ▸ ascitic fluid
Tappeiner syndrome, Spanlang-
tapping of chest for fluid
TAR (tar)
T. (thrombocytopenia with absent radii)
t. bath, coal
t., black
t. cancer
t. /nicotine (T/N) cigarettes, low
t., coal
t. soap, coal
TARA (Total Articular Replacement Arthroplasty)
tarda
t., dyskinesia
t., lues
t. (PCT) ▸ porphyria cutanea
t. symptomatica, porphyria cutanea
tardive
t. cyanosis
t. dyskinesia
t. dyskinesia ▸ antipsychotic-induced
t. dystonia
t., forme
t. muscular dystrophy, Becker-type
tardus pulse ▸ parvus et
tardy epilepsy
target (Target)
t. absorbed dose, average
t. absorbed dose, maximum
t., antigenic
t. appearance, ulcer crater with
t. brain tumors
t. cell
t. cells, radiation injury of
t. DNA (deoxyribonucleic acid)
t., dyspnea
t. enzyme
t. enzyme insensitive to inhibitor

t. enzyme, modification of
t. erythrocyte
t. heart rate
t. heart rate zone (THRZ)
t. lesion
t. of conspiracy
t. organ disease
t. region
t. sign ▸ pulmonary
t. site
t. skin distance (TSD)
T. Symptom Rating Scale (VTSRS) ▸ Verdun
t. tissue
t. -to-nontarget ratio
t. volume, initial
t. volume localization
targeted
t. cells
t. chemicals
t. contact tracing
t. radiation
t. tissue
t. treatment
targeting
t. ability ▸ tumor
t. agent
t. (BAT) ▸ B-mode acquisition and
t., selective
t., stereotactic
tarini, pons
Tarnier's sign
Tarrant's position
tarry
t. black bowel movement
t. black stool
t. stool
tarsal
t. arches
t. bones
t. cyst
t. glands
t. joint
t. muscle, inferior
t. muscle, superior
t. plate
t. scaphoiditis
t. sinus
t. synostosis
t. tunnel
tarsalis, Culex
tarsi, os trigonum
tarsi, roof of sinus
tarsoepiphyseal aclasis
tarsomedial shoes

tarsometatarsal articulations
tarsophalangeal reflex
tarsorrhaphy, internal
tarsus
    t. inferior palpebrae
    t. orbital septum
    t. superior palpebrae
tart cell
tartar emetic
tartrate
    t. contrast medium sodium thorium
    t., ergotamine
    t. nephritis
task(s)
    t. ▸ decline in ability to perform routine
    t. ▸ difficulty performing familiar
    t. ▸ efficient performance of
    t. ▸ goal oriented
    t., learning
    t. ▸ metabolic equivalents of
    t. -oriented activity ▸ prolonged
    t. -related motion
    t., repetitive
    t., spatial-visual constructural
    t., visual-motor
taste
    t. abnormalities from cranial nerve problem
    t. abnormalities from dentures
    t. abnormality
    t. and smell ▸ distortion in
    t. and smell ▸ sense of
    t., aura of peculiar
    t. aversion ▸ mechanism of
    t. buds
    t. cells
    t. center
    t. corpuscles
    t., decreased sense of
    t. disorder
    t. disturbance
    t. enhancers
    t. hairs
    t., heightened awareness of touch or
    t. in mouth, acid
    t. in mouth, bad
    t. in mouth ▸ bitter, sour
    t., lessening sense of
    t., loss of
    t., metallic
    t. of alcohol
    t., sense of
    t., unpleasant

taster's cough, tea
tasting discharge around tooth ▸ foul
TAT (Thematic Apperception Test)
TAT (toxin-antitoxin)
tatlock organism
Tatlockia micdadei
tattoo
    t. of cornea
    t. removal
    t., self-induced
    t., shooting
    t. surgery
tattooing instruments
tattooing needle, Agnew
tau
    t., human
    t. molecules
    t., nuclear
taught deep breathing, patient
taught leg exercises, patient
taurinum, cor
Taussig('s)
    T. -Bing anomaly
    T. -Bing disease
    T. -Bing heart
    T. -Bing syndrome
    T. -Morton operation
    T. operation
    T. operation, Blalock-
    T. procedure, Blalock-
    T. shunt, Blalock-
taut
    t. and distended ▸ abdomen
    t. band of muscles
    t. foot
    t., shiny skin
    t., strand pulled
Tawara
    T. node, Aschoff-
    T. node, His-
    T., node of
Tay('s)
    T. choroiditis
    T. -Sachs disease
    T. -Sachs infant
    T. spot
Taybi syndrome, Rubinstein-
Taylor('s)
    T. back brace
    T. position
    T. position, Wigby-
    T. procedure, Girdlestone-
TB (tuberculosis)
    TB ▸ extrapulmonary
    TB ▸ multi-drug resistant

    TB of lacrimal gland
    TB patch test
    TB reactivated
    TB skin test
    TB smear
TBG (thyroxine binding globulin)
TBI (thyroid binding index)
TBI (thyroxine binding index)
Tc (technetium) 99m
    Tc (technetium) 99m aggregated albumin kit
    Tc (technetium) 99m albumin microspheres kit
    Tc (technetium) 99m etidronate sodium kit
    Tc (technetium) 99m generator
    Tc (technetium) 99m medronate sodium kit
    Tc (technetium) 99m pentetate sodium kit
    Tc (technetium) 99m, radioactive
    Tc (technetium) 99m scan
    Tc (technetium) 99m serum albumin kit
    Tc (technetium) 99m sestamibi scintigraphy
    Tc (technetium) 99m, sodium pertechnetate
    Tc (technetium) 99m stannous pyrophosphate/polyphosphate
    Tc (technetium) 99m sulfur colloid
TCF (total coronary flow)
TCP/TPCP (phencyclidine analog)
TD (total discrimination)
TD (tumor dose)
TDD (Telecommunications Device for the Deaf)
TDF (time, dose, fractionation) factor
TDI (therapeutic donor insemination)
TDP (thoracic duct pressure)
Te Linde operation
Tea (tea)
    T. (hashish)
    T. (marijuana)
    T. Leaves (hallucinogens), Green
    t., pectoral
    t. taster's cough
teacher(s) ('s)
    t., conflict with
    t. node
    t. nodule
teaching
    t. alternatives
    t., discharge
    t. hospital, academic

t. issues, special
Teale's amputation
team (Team)
t. approach
t. approach ▸ interdisciplinary
t. approach ▸ multidisciplinary treatment
t. ▸ attending designated treatment
t., bioethical
t., cardiac rehabilitation
t. concept
t., emergency cardioresuscitation
t., field
t. goals, rehabilitation
t., health care
T., Home Care
t., hospice
t., hospital
T., Infection Control
t. leader ▸ treatment
t. (IDT) meeting, interdisciplinary
t. members, trauma
t., multidisciplinary
t., multidisciplinary treatment
t. ▸ organ recovery
T., Paramedic
t. recommendations, treatment
t., rehabilitation
t., surgical
t. technique, two-
t., trauma
tear(s)
t., anal
t., aortic
t. arthritis ▸ wear-and-
t., artificial
t. at 1 (2, 3, etc.) o'clock
t., Boerhaave
t., bucket-handle
t., cartilage
t., cauded
t., cruciate ligament
t., decreased flow of
t., deficient drainage of
t., degenerative
t., diminished flow of
t. drain
t. drainage
t. drainage system
t. duct
t. duct, blocked
t. ducts, plug
t., esophageal
t., excessive
t. film

t. from eyes ▸ drain
t. in mucosa at cardioesophageal junction
t., intimal
t. ▸ lack of sufficient
t., Mallory-Weiss
t., medial
t., muscle
t. of capsule
t. of ligament
t. of meniscus
t. of meniscus, bucket-handle
t. of muscle
t., overflow of
t., perineal
t. pipe
t. pipe ▸ artificial
t., pleural
t. -producing gland ▸ atrophy of
t. production ▸ decreasing
t., rectal
t. -related problem
t., retinal
t., rotator cuff
t. sac
t. stone
t., tendon
t., uterine
teardrop(s)
t. appearance
t. fracture
t. heart
Teare's sling
tearful appearance, sad or
tearful, patient
tearing
t., excess
t., excessive
t. of blood vessel
t. of eyes ▸ excessive
t. pain
t., reflex
teary eyes
teased open
tebo scan
teboroxime imaging
teboroxime scan
TECAB (total endoscopic coronary artery bypass)
Technetium Cardiolite stress test
technetium (Tc) 99m
t. (Tc) 99m aggregated albumin kit
t. (Tc) 99m albumin microspheres kit
t. (Tc) 99m etidronate sodium kit

t. (Tc) 99m generator
t. (Tc) 99m hexamibi
t. (Tc) 99m imaging
t. (Tc) 99m medronate sodium kit
t. (Tc) 99m MIBI imaging
t. (Tc) 99m pentetate sodium kit
t. (Tc) 99m pyrophosphate
t. (Tc) 99m pyrophospate scintigraphy
t. (Tc) 99m, radioactive
t. (Tc) 99m radioisotope
t. (Tc) 99m scan
t. (Tc) 99m serum albumin kit
t. (Tc) 99m stannous pyrophosphate/polyphosphate
t. (Tc) 99m sulfur colloid
technic (*see* technique)
technical precautions, stringent
Technician (technician)
T. (EMT), Emergency Medical
t., monitor
t. -on-call, laboratory
t. on-call, respiratory care
t. -on-call, x-ray
t., sleep
t., tissue typing
technique(s)
t., ablative
t., acupuncture
t., adaptive
t., adjunctive
t., adult CPR (cardiopulmonary resuscitation)
t., advanced
t., airway occlusion
t., Albee
t., Alexander's
t., algebraic reconstruction
t., Amplatz
t., amputation
t., AngioJet
t. ▸ anterior sandwich patch
t., anterograde transseptal
t., antiseptic
t., apex cardiography
t., aseptic
t., aseptic catheterization
t., assisted reproductive
t., atherectomy
t., Atkinson's
t., atrial well
t., autonomic nervous system relaxation
t., autoradiographic
t., awakening

technique(s)—*continued*
t., background subtraction
t., balance improvement
t., Baron
t., Bassini's
t., behavior modification
t., behavioral
t., behavioral management
t., behavioral psychological
t., Bentall inclusion
t., biofeedback
t. ▸ biofeedback, imagery and relaxation
t., biotelemetry
t., blind
t., Blitz
t., Bloodgood
t., body manipulation
t., body scanning
t., bootstrap two-vessel
t., brain imaging
t., branching
t., Brandt's
t., Braun pinch graft
t., breathing
t., breathing and relaxation
t., Bucky
t., button
t., cardiac catheterization
t., cardiac-imaging
t. ▸ child and infant CPR (cardiopulmonary resuscitation)
t., childbirth
t., chromatographic-fluorometric
t., classic
t., clearance
t., clonogenic
t., closed
t., closed womb
t., Coffey
t., cognitive
t., cognitive behavioral
t., compensatory communication
t., computer averaging
t., computer summation
t., computerized display
t., computerized imaging
t., confrontational
t., controlled double-blind
t., Conway
t., coping
t., coronary flow reserve
t., cough CPR (cardiopulmonary resuscitation)

t., CPR (cardiopulmonary resuscitation)
t., crash
t., Crawford graft inclusion
t., Crobin
t., Crutchfield reduction
t., cryosurgery
t., culture
t., cupula
t., cutdown
t., cytological
t., deep-breathing
t., defibrillation
t., demonstration of safety
t., desensitization
t., develop isolation
t., diagnostic
t., diffusible tracer
t., digital subtraction
t., dilution-filtration
t., direct insertion
t., diskectomy
t. ▸ Doppler auto correlation
t., dosimetry and
t., double dose
t., double dummy
t., drainage
t., drip infusion
t., echo scanning
t., effleurage
t., ego strengthening
t., electromyograph (EMG) feedback as relaxation
t. ▸ emotional freedom
t. ▸ en bloc no touch
t., end-over-end running
t., entangling
t., enzymatic debridement
t., Essex-Lopresti reduction
t., exchange
t. ▸ excimer laser
t., extinction
t. ▸ extractable tracer
t., Fick's
t., first aid
t. ▸ first pass
t. ▸ flap transplant
t. ▸ flow mapping
t. ▸ flush and bathe
t. for deep relaxation, feedback
t. for dose calculation, irregular field
t. for dose calculation, isocentric
t. for dose calculation, rotation
t. ▸ forced oscillation
t. ▸ forward triangle

t., four field
t., four field isocentric
t., four portal
t., ▸ freeze-thaw-freeze
t., G banding
t., gated
t. ▸ gene therapy
t., general relaxation training
t., genetic engineering
t., George Lewis
t., George Winter elevation torque
t. ▸ gloved fist
t. goals, safety
t., grabbing
t., gram staining
t., Gregory Pell sectioning
t., grid
t., Guilford stapedectomy
t., guillotine
t., hand washing
t., hanging-drop
t., Hartel's
t., heavy exposure
t. ▸ hot biopsy
t., Hough stapedectomy
t., House stapedectomy
t., hypnosis
t., hypothermic
t., image-guided surgical
t., imaging
t., immunofluorescent
t., implant
t., implantation
t. in radiation therapy, mantle
t. in radiation therapy, photon irradiation
t., in vitro
t., indocyanine green
t. ▸ indocyanine green indicator dilution
t. ▸ interventional radiologic
t., invasive
t. ▸ invasive surgical
t., irrigation
t., isolation
t., Johnson
t., Karman
t., Kerrison
t. ▸ keyhole surgical
t. ▸ kissing balloon
t., Kleinschmidt
t., Kristeller
t., Lamaze
t., laparoscopic
t., laser

t., Lash's
t. ▸ latissimus dorsi flap
t., lifting
t., Lottes' reduction
t., low dose x-ray
t., macro-Kjeldahl
t. ▸ magnetoencephalography
   (MEG)
t., Magnuson reduction
t., maladaptive
t., mantle
t., Maquet
t., Martin reduction
t., massive dose
t., Michel
t., microelectrode
t., microsphere
t., microsurgery
t., microsurgical
t., Millen
t. ▸ minimal leak
t. ▸ minimally invasive
t. ▸ minimally invasive biopsy
t. ▸ modified brachial
t., modified Hibbs'
t., modified Richardson
t., Mohs'
t., monitoring
t., motivational
t., multiplanar
t. ▸ multiple parameter
t., muscle splitting
t. ▸ natural holistic
t. ▸ nerve block
t. ▸ neuro-imaging
t. ▸ no-leak
t. ▸ nonablative laser
t., noninvasive
t., nonsterile catheterization
t., nonsterile irrigation
t., no-touch
t., nuclear scanning
t. of recording
t. of relaxation during childbirth ▸
   biofeedback
t., one-stitch
t., open
t., operational
t., Orr
t., Ouchterlony
t., pacing
t. ▸ pancreatic cell transplant
t., parapsychological
t., patch
t., patient care

t., percutaneous
t., perfusion
t. ▸ permanent seed
t., photosensitization
t., physical agents and
t. ▸ polymerase chain reaction
   (PCR)
t., positron scanning
t. ▸ pressure half-time
t., programmed behavior therapy
t., prolotherapy
t., proper exercise walking
t., psychological
t., psychophysical
t., psychosocial
t. ▸ radial keratotomy
t., radiation mantle
t., radiation therapy
t., radiographic
t., radioimmunometric
t., radionuclide
t. ▸ rage reduction
t. ▸ Rashkind balloon
t., Rebuck skin window
t., reconstructive
t., recovery
t. ▸ refine bone storage
t., relation
t., relaxation
t., relaxation and meditation
t., restricted environmental
t., revival
t., Richardson
t., Ritter-Oleson
t., Rumel
t., running
t. ▸ scatterplot smoothing
t., Scheie
t., Schepens-Okamura-Brockhurst
t., Schonander
t., Schuknecht stapedectomy
t., scintillation counting
t., screening and diagnostic
t., Seldinger
t., self-care
t., self-help
t., severed limb salvage
t., Shea stapedectomy
t., shiatsu
t., shrinking field
t., skewer
t., sliding
t., snare
t., sonic imaging
t., sonication

t., sonography
t., sound-wave
t., specialized
t., Speed and Boyd reduction
t., spin
t., split course
t. ▸ standard cognitive
t., standard rehabilitation
t. ▸ static dilation
t., sterile
t., stomach stapling
t., stress management
t., stress reducing
t., stress reduction
t., supervoltage
t., support
t. ▸ supportive therapy
t., surgical
t. ▸ tai-chi
t., telemetric
t., therapeutic
t., therapeutic endoscopic
t., therapy
t., thermodilution
t., Thomson reduction
t., time diffusion
t. ▸ time-out
t., tissue culture
t., treatment
t., Trueta
t., tumor infiltrating lymphocytes
   (TIL)
t. ▸ two-patch
t., two-team
t., ultrasound
t., vaccination
t., Van Lint
t., vascular invasive
t., vibrocardiography
t., Wagner reduction
t., Waldhausen subclavian flap
t. ▸ wax matrix
t., Welin's
t., Winter's
t. with drug abusers, confrontation
t., Yasargil
technological advancement
technological disaster
technologist, radiation
technologist, radiological
technologist, trauma
technology(-ies)
   t. ▸ adaptive phased array
     microwave
   t., adjunctive

technology(-ies)—*continued*
t., alternative
t. assessment
t., assistive
t., averaging
t., breast imaging
t., dental implant
t., dry slide
t., genetic
t., health care
t., hemapheresis
t., Holter
t., imaging
t., life support
t., micro chip
t. ▸ nucleic acid
t. ▸ phased array
t., pulmonary
t., recombinant
t., recombinant DNA
    (deoxyribonucleic acid)
t., reproductive
t., sleep center
t., sound-wave
t., stent
t., therapeutic
t., transplant
t., treatment
t., ultrasound
tectae, taenia
tectonic keratoplasty
tectorial membrane
tectospinal tract
tectum, Ochrobium
tectum of brain stem
TED
TED (threshold erythema dose)
TED (thromboembolic disease)
TED (thromboembolic disease)
    hose
TED (thromboembolic disease)
    socks
TED (thromboembolic disease)
    stockings
tedding device
**TEE (transesophageal echocardio-
    graphy)**
teen suicide
teen suicide prevention
teenage
t. addict
t. alcoholic
t. drinking
t. pregnancy
t. sexual activity

t. suicide
teenager, patient
teeth (*see also* **tooth**)
t., abutment
t., accessional
t., acrylic resin
t., adjacent stable
t., anatomic
t., anterior
t., artificial
t. ▸ artificial replacement
t., avulsed
t. avulsed, reimplant
t., baby
t., barred
t., bicuspid
t., brushing and flossing
t., buccal
t., canine
t., carious
t., chattering of
t., cheek
t., cheoplastic
t., chiaie
t., chipped
t. clenching and grinding
t., connate
t., crooked
t., cross-bite
t., cross-pin
t., cuspid
t., cuspless
t., cutting of
t., decayed
t., deciduous
t. descaling
t., diatoric
t., discolored
t., erupted
t., extraction of
t., eye
t., false
t., filled
t., flossing of
t., Fournier
t., front
t., fused
t., fusion of
t., geminate
t. ▸ gnashing and clenching of
t. grinding disorder
t., grinding ▸ nocturnal
t., grinding of
t., hag
t., hair

t., Horner's
t., Huschke's auditory
t., Hutchinson's
t., impacted
t., impacted molar
t., implanting
t. in good dental condition
t. in good dental repair
t. in poor dental repair
t., incisor
t., irregularities of
t., labial
t. ▸ loss of
t., lower
t., malacotic
t., malaligned
t., mandibular
t., maxillary
t., metal insert
t., milk
t. ▸ misalignment of
t., missing
t., molar
t., Moon's
t., morsal
t., mottled
t., multicuspid
t., natural
t., neonatal
t., night grinding of
t., patient grinds
t., peg
t., permanent
t., permanent prosthetic
t., posterior
t., premolar
t., primary
t. ▸ proper realignment of
t., pyorrhea around lower
t., pyorrhea around upper
t., rake
t. replacement ▸ permanent
t., sclerotic
t., screwdriver
t., stained
t., straight-pin
t., succedaneous
t., successional
t., supernumerary
t., temporary
t., transplanting
t., upper
t. whitening
t. wired together
t., wisdom

t., zero degree
Teflon
  T. button
  T. catheter
  T., cellular
  T. coating
  T. endolymphatic shunt tube
  T. felt
  T. felt pledget ▸ Meadox
  T. graft
  T. implant
  T. implant material
  T. intracardiac patch implant ▸ Edwards
  T. intracardiac patch prosthesis ▸ Edwards
  T. material
  T. mesh
  T. mesh implant
  T. mesh implant material
  T. mesh prosthesis
  T., molded
  T. patch
  T. pledget
  T. pledget suture buttress
  T. pledgets, prethreaded
  T. prosthesis
  T. prosthesis ▸ woven
  T. sheeting prosthesis
  T. shunt tube
  T. tri-leaflet prosthesis
  T. wire piston prosthesis ▸ Schuknecht
  T., woven
Tegaderm dressing
Tegaderm dressing, subclavian
tegmen tympani
tegmental
  t. cells
  t. part of pons
  t. region, medial
  t. wall
  t. wall roof
tegmentalis, paries
tegumentary amidine
teichoic acid titers, anti-
Teicholz ejection fraction
Tek cryostat, Ames Lab-
telangiectasia
  t. (AT), ataxia-
  t., hemorrhagic
  t., hereditary hemorrhagic
  t., oculocutaneous

t. (CRST) syndrome ▸ calcification, Raynaud's phenomenon, scleroderma,
telangiectatic
  t. angioma
  t. glioma
  t. wart
telangiectaticum, carcinoma
telangiectaticum, granuloma
telangiectodes, carcinoma
telecanthus deformity
telecanthus deformity, epicanthus with
Telecommunications Device for the Deaf (TDD)
Telectronics ATP implantable cardioverter defibrillator
Telectronics pacemaker
telemetric
  t. monitoring
  t. pressure sensor
  t. technique
telemetry
  t., cardiac
  t., cardiac stepdown unit and
  t., electrocardiogram (ECG/EKG)
  t. ▸ interrogation of
  t. monitor
telencephalic ventriculofugal artery
Telepaque contrast medium
telephone order (TO)
telephone tooth
teleroentgenogram study
telescope, fiberoptic
telescope-like instrument
telescopic glasses
Tele-Sensor, Cosman ICM
telesurgery, robotic
teletherapy
  t. machine, cesium 137
  t. machine, cobalt-60 (Co^{60})
  t. procedure
  t. unit
televising of operation ▸ authorization form for
televising of operation, consent form for
television
  t. microscope, ultraviolet color-translating
  t. microscopy
  t. monitor
Telfa dressing
tell-tale signs
Tellyesniczky's fluid

telogen effluvium
Telson hinged walking heel
temper
  t., explosive
  t., pathological
  t. tantrums
temperate virus
temperature
  t., absolute
  t., alteration of
  t., altered body
  t. and pressure (ATP) ▸ ambient
  t. and pressure (NTP), normal
  t. and pressure (STP) ▸ standard
  t. autoregulation, digital
  t., axillary
  t. (BBT) ▸ basal body
  t. biofeedback, autogenic training in
  t., body
  t., brain
  t. change
  t. chart
  t. compensation
  t. control
  t. control, autosuggestion
  t. cooled, patient's body
  t., core
  t. ▸ core body
  t. curve
  t. cycle
  t., digital
  t. ▸ diminished perception of pain and
  t., effective
  t. -elevating substances
  t. elevation
  t., elevation of body
  t. feedback and cognition
  t., fluctuation of
  t. graph
  t. graph, basal metabolic
  t., increased skin
  t., internal body
  t. inversion
  t., limb
  t. ▸ low body
  t., low grade
  t., mean
  t. melting out
  t., normal
  t. of extremity
  t. of limb elevated
  t., oral
  t., patient had elevated
  t., patient spiked

temperature—*continued*
- t., peak
- t. ▸ perception of
- t., postoperative rise in
- t. probe, esophageal
- t., pulse and respiration (TPR)
- t., rectal
- t., reduced blood
- t., reduced body
- t., regulate body
- t. regulation
- t., regulation of body
- t., retrocardiac
- t. reversals
- t., room
- t. scale
- t. sense
- t. -sensing pacemaker
- t. -sensitive receptor
- t., sensitivity to
- t., skin
- t. spike
- t., subnormal
- t. subsided
- t. ▸ treatment of contrasting
- t. ▸ tympanic membrane

tempestuous ▸ callous, cynical and

template
- t. bleeding time
- t. markings
- t., Moore's
- t. splint, clear acrylic
- t., surgical
- t., wire

Temple procedure

temple sleep

Templeton and Zim carpal tunnel projection

temporal
- t., anterior
- t. area
- t. areas of scalp
- t. arteriole of retina
- t. arteritis
- t. artery
- t. artery biopsy
- t. artery pressure point ▸ superficial
- t. artery ▸ superficial
- t. arthritis
- t. bone
- t. bone bank
- t. bone fracture
- t. bone fracture ▸ preexisting
- t. bone, interclavicular notch of
- t. bone, jugular notch of

- t. bone, parietal notch of
- t. bone, pneumatization of
- t. bone stimulation
- t. canthus
- t. consolidation in combined modality therapy
- t. cortex
- t. diameter
- t. diploic vein, anterior
- t. diploic vein, posterior
- t. dispersion
- t. electrode, anterior
- t. electrodes, true anterior
- t. facial nerve
- t. field
- t. field defect
- t. field loss
- t. field of vision
- t. fossa
- t. granulomatous arteritis
- t. gyri, transverse
- t. gyrus
- t. gyrus, anterior transverse
- t. gyrus, inferior
- t. gyrus, middle
- t. gyrus, superior
- t. headache
- t. hemianopia
- t. horn
- t. horn of lateral ventricle
- t. instability artifact
- t. line
- t. lobe
- t. lobe epilepsy
- t. lobe focus, right
- t. lobe lesion
- t. lobe of brain
- t. lobe of brain, excision
- t. mapping ▸ spectral
- t. muscle
- t. nerves, deep
- t. nerves, subcutaneous
- t. processing, cross-
- t. region
- t. resolution
- t. retina
- t. silk
- t. slow activity, anterior
- t. slow activity, posterior
- t. slow wave focus, anterior
- t. slowing, focal
- t. spike, focal anterior
- t. spike focus, anterior
- t. spiking, anterior
- t. suture

- t. theta burst of drowsiness ▸ rhythmic
- t. vein, deep
- t. vein, middle
- t. vein, superficial
- t. venule of retina, inferior
- t. venule of retina, superior

temporale, os

temporales transversi, gyri

temporalis
- t. fascia
- t. inferior, gyrus
- t. medius, gyrus
- t., musculus
- t., planum
- t. retinas inferior, venula
- t. superior, gyrus

temporarily relieve symptoms

temporarily stunned

temporary
- t. absence of breathing
- t. absence of consciousness
- t. alterations in mood
- t. atrial pacing electrode
- t. baldness
- t. Bell's palsy
- t. blindness
- t. breast implant
- t. breathing difficulty
- t. cardiac pacemaker
- t. cessation
- t. closure
- t. closure reopened
- t. colostomy
- t. coma
- t. confusion
- t. crisis
- t. delusions
- t. deprivation of maternal touch
- t. disability
- t. electrode ▸ monopolar
- t. epicardial pacing electrode
- t. facial weakness or drooping
- t. global amnesia
- t. hair loss
- t. hardness
- t. hearing loss
- t. heart transplant
- t. impairment
- t. impotence
- t. ischemia
- t. loss of memory
- t. memory loss
- t. menopause
- t. mental derangement

t. mild euphoria
t. numbness or weakness
t. obliteration
t. obstruction
t. opening
t. opening in joint
t. ostomy
t. pacemaker
t. pacemaker implant
t. pacemaker management
t. pacemaker ▸ Medtronic
t. pacemaker ▸ noninvasive
t. pacing
t. pacing ▸ noninvasive
t. paralysis
t. parasite
t. pervenous lead
t. plaster cast
t. recollection
t. relief
t. relief of headache pain
t. seal
t. stress release
t. stricture
t. stroke
t. teeth
t. threshold shift
t. tinnitus
t. transvenous pacemaker
t. transvenous pacemaker
   placement
t. unilateral pulmonary artery
   occlusion
t. unresponsiveness
t. urinary opening
t. vasodilatation
t. vision loss
t. weakness one side of body
temporofacial graft
temporomalar suture
temporomandibular (TM)
t. joint (TMJ)
t. joint (TMJ) dislocation
t. joint (TMJ) disorder
t. joint (TMJ) dysfunction
t. joint (TMJ) ▸ proper alignment of
t. joint (TMJ) screening
t. joint (TMJ) syndrome
t. joints (TMJ) ▸ osteoarthritis
temporomaxillary joint, meniscus
  of
temporo-occipital artery
temporoparietal aphasia
temporoparietal muscle
temporozygomatic suture

Ten (10)
T. Channel Instrument, Grass
#10 lens implant, Leiske
10 pacemaker, Vivalith-
10-20 (ten-twenty)
10-20 electrode system
10-20 system
10-20 system, standard
tenacious
t. mucoid secretion
t. sputum
t. sputum ▸ thick,
tenax, Eristalis
tenax, Trichomonas
tendency(-ies)
t., achieving
t., anti-social
t., bleeding
t., elastic recoil
t., epileptic
t., exhibitionistic
t., familial
t., genetic
t., hereditary
t., hidden suicidal
t. in children ▸ suicidal
t., inherited
t., introverted
t., invasive
t. ▸ long-term
t., patient has suicidal
t., patient manifests suicidal
t. ▸ rebellious, aggressive acting-out
t., sadistic
t., suicidal
t. to be distracted
t. to self-abuse ▸ agitation,
   delusions and
t. to sigh
t. toward bullying
t. toward cruelty
tender
t. and swollen
t. blisters on feet
t. gums ▸ red, swollen,
t. gums ▸ swollen and
t. ▸ hot, swollen and
t. joint
t. joint and muscle
t., liver
t. liver ▸ enlarged,
t. loving care (TLC)
t. lymph nodes ▸ small
t. mass
t. muscle sites

t. point score
t. points specific areas of body
t. scalp
t., soft, nonmovable node
t., swollen breasts
t. to motion, uterus
t. to palpation ▸ abdomen
t. trigger spots
t., tympanitic ▸ abdomen distended,
tenderness
t., abdominal
t., abdominal distention and
t. ▸ acute thyroiditis with
t., adnexal
t. and pain
t. and rigidity
t., anserine bursa
t., areas of
t. at site of incision
t., bony
t., breast
t., calf muscle
t. ▸ CVA (costovertebral angle)
t., deep abdominal
t., diffuse abdominal
t. elicited
t., epigastric
t., flank
t., focal
t. from appendicitis ▸ abdominal
t. ▸ gas, bloating and abdominal
t., generalized
t. in abdomen from appendicitis
t. in abdomen from diverticulosis
t. in abdomen from gastritis
t. in abdomen from hepatitis
t. in abdomen from pancreatitis
t. in abdomen from peritonitis
t. in both adnexa
t., intercostal
t., joint
t. ▸ joint swelling and
t., localized
t. ▸ lymph node
t. ▸ masses, induration or
t., midepigastric
t. of abdomen
t. of breasts
t. of jaw muscle
t. of scalp
t. of transplant ▸ fever, swelling and
t. of umbilical region
t. on palpation ▸ masses, organs or
t. on pressure
t. or rebound

tenderness—*continued*
- t. or weakness ▸ muscle pain,
- t. over scalp, local
- t., pain and
- t., parasternal intercostal
- t., point
- t., premenstrual breast
- t., punch
- t., rebound
- t. ▸ restoring nurturance and
- t., rib
- t., right upper quadrant (RUQ)
- t., scrotal
- t., sinus
- t., skin
- t., spasm or rigidity
- t., specific
- t. (SLRT), straight leg raising
- t., suprapubic
- t. to palpation or percussion
- t. to percussion
- t. to touch
- t., vertebral percussion
- t. without rebound
- t., wound

tendinea, macula
tendineus communis, anulus
tendinitis
- t., Achilles
- t., bicipital
- t., calcific
- t., hypertrophic infiltrative
- t. ossificans traumatica
- t., overuse
- t., peroneal
- t., radiation treatment of
- t., rotator cuff
- t., stenosing
- t., trochanteric

tendinosa, paronychia
tendinosum, xanthoma
tendinotrochanteric ligament
tendinous
- t. arch
- t. center
- t. chiasm of flexor sublimis
- t. chiasm of musculus flexor digitorum sublimis
- t. galea
- t. ring, common
- t. spot
- t. xanthoma
- t. zones of heart

tendinum digitorum manus, chiasma
tendinum, tremor

tendon(s)
- t., Achilles
- t. advancement
- t. advancement, patellar
- t., aspiration and injection of
- t. bearing, patellar
- t. blockage
- t. calcaneus
- t. cartilage
- t. cells
- t., common
- t., conjoined
- t. cut, stapedial
- t., divided
- t., extensor
- t., extensor pollicis brevis
- t., false
- t. ▸ fatigue and muscle
- t., flexor carpi radialis
- t., flexor digitorum profundus
- t., flexor digitorum sublimis
- t., flexor profundus
- t. graft
- t., Hibbs'
- t. identified, proximal ends of
- t. implant
- t., inflamed
- t., inflammation of
- t. injury
- t. insertion, medial transplantation of patellar
- t. insertion, patellar
- t. intact
- t. jerk
- t., lacerated
- t. lengthening
- t., Lockwood's
- t., long abductor
- t., muscle
- t. nerve deficit, functional
- t. nodule
- t., palmaris longus
- t., patellar
- t., percussion of
- t., peroneal
- t., popliteus
- t. ▸ posterior tibial
- t., primary bundles of
- t., pulley
- t., quadriceps
- t. reaction
- t., reattachment of
- t., rectus femoris
- t. reflex
- t. reflex, Achilles

- t. reflex (DTR) ▸ deep
- t. reflex, patellar
- t. reflex, timed Achilles
- t. reflexes
- t. reflexes (DTR) equal and active bilaterally ▸ deep
- t. reflexes, excessive reactivity to
- t. reflexes (DTR) ▸ hypoactive deep
- t. reflexes (DTR) ▸ increased deep
- t. reflexes (DTR) ▸ monitoring of deep
- t. reflexes (DTR) symmetrical ▸ deep
- t. release, adductor
- t. released
- t. ▸ repeated stress on
- t., rider's
- t. ▸ rotator cuff
- t. rupture, Achilles
- t., rupture of
- t. ▸ rupture of tibial
- t., ruptured biceps
- t., severed
- t. sheath
- t. sheath, injected
- t. sheath, probing of
- t. sheath syndrome, Brown's
- t., short extensor
- t. shortening
- t., stapedial
- t., stapedius
- t. ▸ stiffness and discomfort in
- t., stretch
- t., sublimis
- t., superior oblique
- t. tear
- t., tenotomy of ocular
- t. tightness
- t. transfer
- t. transfer, Bunnell
- t. transfer, patellar
- t. transfer, Velpeau's
- t. transplant
- t. transplant, patellar
- t., transplantation of
- t. transposition, patellar
- t., weak
- t., Zinn's

tendonitis (*see* tendinitis)
tendoplastic amputation
tendosynovial tissue sarcoma
tendovaginitis, stenosing
tends to self-diagnose, patient
tenella, Eimeria
tenellum, Coccidium

tenesmus, rectal
tenesmus, vesical
tenia/taenia (*see* Taenia)
tenia organism
Tennant distress scale
Tennessee Self-Concept Scale
tennis elbow
tennis thumb
Tennison-Randall repair
tenodesis, Jones
tenolysis, DeQuervain's
Tenon('s)
    T. capsule
    T. capsule dissected
    T. fascia
    T. membrane
    T. space
tenoplasty/tenontoplasty
tenorrhaphy, primary
tenosuspension, Jones'
tenosynovial chondrometaplasia
tenosynovitis
    t., biceps
    t., digital stenosing
    t., stenosing
tenotomy
    t., curb
    t., graduated
    t. of ocular tendon
TENS (transcutaneous electrical nerve stimulation)
TENS (transepidermal nerve stimulation)
tensa, pars
tense
    t., abdomen
    t. and apprehensive
    t., back
    t. edema
    t., patient
    t., patient irritable and
    t. pulse
tensed up, patient
tensile strengths
tensile stress
Tensilon
    T. implant
    T. implant material
    T. injection
    T. test
    T. test for myasthenia gravis
tensin converting enzyme (ACE), angio-

tension
    t., aching, pain and stiffness ▸ muscle
    t., acute anxiety
    t. ▸ altered pulmonary surface
    t., alveolar oxygen (O_2)
    t. and anxiety, chronic
    t. and anxiety, decrease
    t. and anxiety, muscle
    t. and distress, reduce
    t. and emotional problems
    t., and fatigue ▸ anger
    t. and frustration
    t. and headache ▸ anxiety,
    t. and relaxation
    t., arterial
    t., arterial carbon dioxide (CO_2)
    t. artifact
    t. artifact, muscle
    t., autogenic training for anxiety and
    t., body
    t., chronic muscle
    t. /concentration, oxygen
    t., continuous
    t. curve ▸ length active
    t. cycling, low-
    t., decreased
    t., decreased mental
    t. ▸ dysphoria and
    t., electric
    t., emotional
    t. ▸ excessive stress and
    t., extraocular
    t., eyeball under
    t., family
    t. ▸ fatigue and
    t., fear and
    t., feeling of inner
    t., frontalis muscle
    t. gradient, alveoloarterial oxygen (O_2)
    t. headache
    t. headache frequency, reduce
    t. headache, muscle
    t. headache, nervous
    t. headaches ▸ voluntary control of
    t. in feedback groups
    t. in neck and shoulders
    t., increased
    t., increased eye
    t., increased mental
    t. index (TTI) ▸ time-
    t., interfacial surface
    t., intraocular
    t., intravenous (IV)

    t. irritability
    t., jaw
    t. ▸ left ventricular
    t. -length relation
    t. line
    t. line, increased
    t. line, maximal
    t. line, minimal
    t. lines (RSTL), relaxed skin
    t., mental
    t., muscle
    t., muscular pain and
    t., myalgia
    t., myocardial
    t., myocardial wall
    t., neck
    t., nervous
    t., normal intraocular
    t., ocular
    t. of right eye (TOD)
    t. on wound
    t. overload, muscle
    t. ▸ oxygen (O_2)
    t. -pain cycle, fear-
    t. perception
    t., physical
    t. pneumopericardium
    t. pneumothorax
    t. (PMT), premenstrual
    t. pulse, high-
    t. pulse, low-
    t., reduce
    t., reduced oxygen
    t. relation ▸ length
    t. relation ▸ length resting
    t. relation ▸ resting length
    t., release
    t., release pent-up
    t., relieve
    t. relieving exercise
    t. relieving formula
    t. state (ATS) ▸ anxiety
    t., stress and
    t., stress-related
    t., surface
    t. suture
    t., tactile
    t. test
    t. -time index
    t., tissue
    t. variability, muscle
    t., ventricular systolic
    t., volume and
    t., wall

tensor
- t. fasciae latae muscle
- t. muscle of fascia lata
- t. muscle of tympanic membrane
- t. muscle of tympanum
- t. muscle of velum palatine
- t. test
- t. tympani, musculus
- t. tympani, nerve of
- t. tympani, semicanal of
- t. veli palatini muscle
- t. veli palatini ▸ nerve of

tent
- t., Cam
- t., croup
- t., Croupette child
- t., iridial
- t. isolator, plastic
- t., Laminaria
- t., mist
- t., mistifier
- t., oxygen
- t., pleural
- t., Silon
- t., sponge
- t., steam

tentative
- t. diagnosis
- t. dose
- t. etiologic diagnosis

tentatively scheduled, patient
tenth
- t. cranial nerve
- t. nerve
- t. value layer

tenting
- t. of diaphragm
- t. of hemidiaphragm
- t. of skin
- t. sign

tentorial
- t. herniation
- t. line
- t. nerve
- t. notch
- t. region

tentorium
- t. cerebelli
- t., cyst of
- t. of cerebellum
- t. of hypophysis

tenuicollis, Cysticercus
Tenz unit
tepid water
teratic implantation

teratogenesis ▸ oncogenesis and
teratogenic
- t. effect
- t. potential
- t. virus

teratogenicity study
teratoid
- t. parasite
- t. tumor
- t. tumor, atypical rhabdoid/

teratoma
- t., adult
- t., extragenital
- t., genital
- t., immature
- t., immature ovarian
- t., intermediate malignant
- t., malignant
- t., mature cystic
- t., pericardial
- t., trophoblastic malignant
- t. tumor

tercile value
terebrant pain
terebrating pain
teres
- t. cardiopexy ▸ ligamentum
- t. femoris, ligamenta
- t. major, musculus
- t. minor, musculus
- t. muscle
- t. muscle, pronator
- t., notch of ligamentum
- t., pronator

term(s)
- t. acupuncture treatment, long-
- t. adjustment, long-
- t. aftercare treatment, long-
- t. AGA (appropriate for gestational age) female neonate
- t. AGA (appropriate for gestational age) male neonate
- t. alcohol exposure ▸ long-
- t. amnesia, short-
- t., amniotic fluid at
- t. aspirin therapy ▸ long-
- t. behavior modification treatment, long-
- t. behavioral change, long-
- t. biofeedback relaxation therapy, long-
- t. birth, post-
- t. birth, pre-
- t. birth, reduced risk of pre-
- t., bland

- t. breast feeding, long-
- t. care facility, long-
- t. care, long-
- t. care services ▸ long-
- t. care, short-
- t. chronic pain ▸ long-
- t. clinical trial ▸ short-
- t. cohabitation, long-
- t. complications, long-
- t. contractions ▸ pre-
- t. counterconditioning treatment, long-
- t. damage, acute and long-
- t. delivery
- t. delivery, antepartum death
- t. delivery, intrapartum death
- t. delivery, neonatal death
- t. delivery, normal full
- t. depression ▸ long-
- t. depression ▸ severe, long-
- t. detoxification, short-
- t. detoxification treatment, long-
- t. dialysis, long-
- t. dialysis, short-
- t. drug therapy ▸ long-
- t. drug treatment, long-
- t. edema ▸ long-
- t. effectiveness, long-
- t. effects, long-
- t., engagement at
- t. exercise ▸ long-
- t. exposure, long-
- t. family therapy, long-
- t. fetus, full
- t. followup, short-
- t., full
- t. gestation, near-
- t. goals ▸ long-
- t. goals ▸ short-
- t. health care facilities, long-
- t. heavy drinking, long-
- t. heroin addicts, long-
- t. hospitalization, long-
- t. illness, chronic long
- t. illness, long-
- t. improvements, short-
- t. in labor
- t. individual counseling, long-
- t. infant
- t. infant, full-
- t. infant, post-
- t. inhalation, long-
- t. injection sclerotherapy ▸ long-
- t. insomnia, short-
- t. institutional respite care, short-

t., intrauterine pregnancy at
t. irritability ▸ intense, short-
t. living birth (FTLB), full
t. living situation, long-
t., long-
t. management ▸ long-
t. mechanical assistance, long-
t. mechanical ventilation, long-
t. memory disruption ▸ short-
t. memory function ▸ long-
t. memory, impaired short-
t. memory ▸ lapse in short
t. memory (LTM), long-
t. memory loss, long-
t. memory loss, short-
t. memory, patient's short
t. memory (STM), short
t. mood disorder ▸ long-
t. moodiness ▸ intense, short-
t. morbidity and mortality ▸ long-
t. mortality rates, short-
t. neurologic disease ▸ long-
t. normal delivery
t. normal delivery (FTND), full
t. nursing care, short-
t. outpatient treatment, long-
t. oxygen (O₂) therapy ▸ long-
t. pain ▸ long-
t. pain relief ▸ long-
t. pain, short-
t. paralysis, long-
t. post-surgical use ▸ short-
t., pregnancy at
t. pregnancy, full-
t. prognosis ▸ long-
t. psychodynamic therapy ▸ short-
t. psychological morbidity ▸ long-
t. psychotherapy, long-
t. psychotherapy, short-
t. reaction, long-
t. recall, short-
t. recovery ▸ long-
t. recovery, support long-
t. relief, long-
t. relief, short-
t. remission ▸ long-
t. restoration of muscle strength ▸ long-
t. safety studies ▸ long-
t. self-administration of opioids ▸ long-
t. separation from mother ▸ short-
t. sequelae, long-
t. side-effects, long-
t. skilled nursing care ▸ long-

t. skilled nursing care ▸ short-
t. smoker, long-
t. smoking cessation ▸ short-
t. stay ▸ short-
t. steroid ▸ long-
t. steroid therapy ▸ long-
t. steroid therapy, short-
t. stimulation ▸ short-
t. stress, short
t. support group, long-
t. survival data, long-
t. survival period, long-
t. survival rate, long-
t. survivor of heart transplant ▸ long-
t. tendency ▸ long-
t. therapeutic approach, short-
t. therapy ▸ short-
t. toxicity, long-
t. trauma, long-
t. treatment, indications for long-
t. ultraviolet exposure ▸ long-
t. unit, adult long-
t. use, long-
t. use of free-base cocaine ▸ long-
t. verbal memory ▸ short-
t. ward ▸ restrictive long-
t. weight control ▸ long-
t. working relationship, short-

terminal(s)

t. aorta
t. aspects
t. aspiration of gastric contents
t. assay, C-
t. bronchiole
t. cancer
t. cancer, advanced stage
t. cancer pain
t. carcinoma
t. care
t. care, patient admitted for
t. care program
t. ▸ central dopaminergic serotinergic nerve
t. cisterna
t. condition
t. death
t. dehydration
t. dementia
t. diagnosis
t. disease
t. disease, potentially
t. disinfection
t. edema

t. electrode, central
t. emphysema
t. endocarditis
t. event
t. flow (MTF) ▸ maximum
t. force ▸ P
t. frame, Deiters'
t. ganglion
t. genetic disorder
t. genetic illness
t. groove
t. hair
t. ileal loop
t. ileitis
t. ileum
t. ileum normal, reflux into
t. illness
t. infection
t., input
t. laryngeal spasm
t. ligature
t. line
t. lung ailment
t. lung cancer
t., negative output
t. nerves
t. occlusion
t. 1, input
t., patient
t. periodontosis
t. peritonitis
t. phalanx
t. pneumonia
t., postsynaptic
t., presynaptic
t. Purkinje fibers
t., respective input
t. respiratory acidosis
t. (VDT) screen glare ▸ video display
t. situation
t. -stage melanoma
t. stage of illness
t. state
t. sulcus
t. tuft fracture
t. tumor, mixed
t., two input
t. 2, input
t. use, video
t. vein
t. ventricle
t. ventricle of spinal cord
t. (VDT) ▸ video display
t. web

terminal(s)—*continued*
- t. ▸ Wilson central

terminale, filum
terminalis, crista
terminalis, sulcus
terminally ill children
terminally ill, patient
terminate [*turbinate*]
terminated
- t., investigation
- t. patient, actively
- t. pregnancy

terminating care
terminating tachycardia ▸ patient self-
termination [*determination*]
- t., genetic
- t., treatment
- t., underdrive

terminoterminal anastomosis
terpin hydrate elixir
Terrien's degeneration
Terrier syndrome, Courvoisier-
terror(s)
- t., attack of intense
- t. disorder, sleep
- t., night
- t. ▸ overwhelming episode of
- t., psychological
- t., somnambulism or night
- t., sudden unexplainable feeling of

Terry's syndrome
Terson's operation
tertian ague
tertian malaria, benign
tertiary
- t. amine
- t. amputation
- t. care center
- t. care facility
- t. carina
- t. contractions
- t. contractions of esophagus
- t. dehiscence
- t. organizer
- t. peristaltic activity
- t. syphilis
- t. transmission
- t. vitreous

tertium, Clostridium
tertius muscle, peroneus
tertius, palpebra
TES (transcutaneous electrical stimulation)
Teschen virus

tesquorum, Ceratophyllus
tessellated fundus
test(s) (Test)
- t., abdominal jugular
- t., acetic acid
- t., acetoacetic acid
- t., acetone
- t., acid phosphatase
- t., acidosis
- t., ACTH (adrenocorticotropic hormone)
- t., Adamkiewicz's
- t., Addis
- t., adenosine thallium
- t., Adler's
- t., adrenaline
- t., adrenocortical inhibition
- t., adrenocorticotropic hormone (ACTH)
- t., AD7C
- t., Adson's
- t., aerobic exercise stress
- T. ▸ AGC (Army General Classification)
- t., agglutination
- t., agglutination inhibition
- t., AIDS (acquired immune deficiency syndrome) antibody
- t., air calorics
- t., airway function
- t., albumin
- t., albumin/globulin (A/G) ratio
- t., aldolase
- t., aldosterone
- t., alkali
- t., alkali denaturation
- t., alkali tolerance
- t., alkaline phosphatase
- t., alkaloid
- t., Allen's
- t., Allen's vision
- t., alpha amino nitrogen
- t., alpha fetoprotein
- T., Amsler Grid
- t., amylase
- t. and procedures, diagnostic
- t., anoxemia
- t., anterior drawer
- t., antibody
- t. antigen ▸ mumps skin
- t., antiglobulin
- t., aortic jugular
- t., Apley's
- t. (ATT), arginine tolerance
- t., Arloing-Courmont

- t., arm exercise stress
- t., arm-tongue time
- T. ▸ Army General Classification (AGC)
- t. as a screening device for drug abuse, diagnostic
- t., Aschheim-Zondek (A-Z)
- t., ascorbic acid
- t., aspirin tolerance
- t. ▸ Astrand bicycle exercise stress
- t., atrial pacing stress
- t., atropine
- t., attention
- t., audiometry
- t., augmented histamine
- t., Australia antigen
- t., A-Z (Aschheim-Zondek)
- t., balance
- t., Balke exercise stress
- t., Balke-Ware
- t., Bárány
- t., Barony's pointing
- t. ▸ baseline exercise
- T. Battery for Adults or Children ▸ Halstead Neuropsychological
- t., behavioral
- t., behavioral avoidance
- t., Bekesy
- t., Bekhterev's
- t., Bence Jones protein
- T., Bender-Gestalt
- t., Benedict's
- T., Benton Visual Retention
- t., bentonite flocculation
- t., benzidine
- t., bicycle ergometer exercise stress
- t., Bielschowsky's
- t., bile acid
- t., bile pigment
- t., biliary function
- t., Binet's
- t., Bing
- t., Biocept-G
- t., Blacky pictures
- t., Blake exercise stress
- t., blanch
- t., blood
- t., blood pressure (BP)
- t., blood sugar
- t., blood urea nitrogen (BUN)
- t., blood volume
- t., Blumenau's
- t., Boas
- t., Bonanno's
- t., bone density

t., bone mineral
t., borderline glucose tolerance
t., BP (blood pressure)
t., breath
t., breath excretion
t., breath holding
t., breath pentane
t., breathalyzer
t., Bromsulphalein
t., bronchial challenge
t., bronchoprovocation
t., broth
t., Brouha's
t., Bruce exercise stress
t., Bruce protocol exercise
t., BUN (blood urea nitrogen)
t. -butyl ether (MTBE) ▸ methyl
t., calcium
t., Callaway's
t., caloric
t., capillary fragility
t., cardiac stress
t., cardiopulmonary exercise
t., carotid sinus
t., Casoni's
t., Casoni's intradermal
t., Castellani
t., catecholamine
t., cephalin flocculation
t., cephalin-cholesterol flocculation
t., cervical mucus
t., cervigram
t., chi square
t., Chiene's
T. ▸ Children's Apperception
t. (CAT), chlormerodrin
    accumulation
t., cholesterol
t., cholinesterase
t., chorionic gonadotropin
t., clivogram
t., clock-drawing
t., clot retraction
t., clot stabilization
t., coagulation
t., coagulation screen
t., coccidioidin
t., cognitive
t., coin
t., cold pressor
t., colloidal benzoin
t., colloidal gold
t., color vision
T., Color-A-Person
T. ▸ Color-Form Sorting

t., common electroencephalogram
    (EEG) input
t., complement fixation
t., concentration
t., confirmatory
t., conglutinating complement
    absorption
t., Congo red
t., Coombs'
t., Cooper's irritable
t., coproporphyrin
t., Core antibody
t., Corner-Allen
t., cortisone-glucose tolerance
t., cover
t., cover-uncover eye
t., Craig's
t., C-reactive protein
t., creatinine
t., creatinine clearance
t., critical flicker fusion
t., cross-matching
t., cross-modal
t., cuff
t., cytological diagnostic
t., daily urine
t. data, safety
t., Davidson protocol exercise
T. (DST) ▸ Daya Syphilis
t., decibel hearing
t., Dehio's
t. ▸ delayed word recall
t. (DST) ▸ dexamethasone
    suppression
t., dextrose
t., Dextrostix
t., Diagnex Blue
t., diagnostic
t. ▸ diagnostic screening
t., Dick
T., Dienst's
t. diet for papillotomy patient
t., digital rectal
t., dilution
t. dilution, routine
t., direct agglutination pregnancy
t., direct bilirubin
t., direct Coombs'
t., distance
t., dobutamine stress
t. donated blood
t. dose (STD) ▸ skin
t., dot pattern
t., double triangular
T. ▸ Draw Person, Tree, House

T., Draw-A-Man
T. ▸ Draw-A-Person
t., drug screen
t. ▸ dual energy x-ray
    absorptiometry (DEXA) bone
    density
t., duction eye
t., Dugas'
t. ▸ duodenal string
t., d-Xylose absorption
t., d-Xylose tolerance
t., dye
t., E
t., ear occlusion
t., early detection
t., Ebbinghaus'
t., ECG (electrocardiogram) stress
t., EEG (electroencephalogram)
t., Ehrlich
t. ▸ electrocardiogram (EKG)
    exercise stress
t., electrophysiological
t., electrophysiology
t. ▸ elevated arm stress
t. ▸ ELISA (enzyme-linked
    immunosorbent assay)
t. ▸ Ellestad exercise stress
t., Ely's
t., ER (estrogen receptor) assay
t. ▸ ergonovine provocation
t., Erhard's
t., erythrocyte sedimentation rate
t., Escherich's
t., esophageal motility
t., ether
t., evoked response
t. ▸ executive function
t., exercise stress
t. ▸ exercise thallium
t. (ETT) ▸ exercise tolerance
t. ▸ exercise treadmill
t., extensive
t. ▸ external rotation, abduction
    stress
t., extrastimulus
t., eye-roll
t., fabere
t., fabere abduction
t., fabere extension
t., fabere external rotation
t., fabere fixation
t., false negative
t. ▸ false positive
t. ▸ false-positive screening
t., Farber's

test(s)—*continued*

t., Farris'
t., fat absorption
t., fecal fat
t. (FOBT) ▸ fecal occult blood
t., fern
t., fetal ECG (electrocardiogram)
t., fetal hemoglobin
t., Fetaldex
t., F-F (finger-to-finger)
t., Fibrindex
t., fibrinogen
t., filter paper microscopic
t., finger prick
t., finger-nose (F-N)
t., fingerstick
t., finger-to-finger (F-F)
t., Finkelstein's
t., first strength tuberculin
t., Fishberg's concentration
t., fitness
t., flexibility
t., flicker
t., flocculation
t., fluorescent antibody
t., fluorescent treponemal antibody
   absorption
t., F-N (finger-nose)
t. ▸ foam stability
t. ▸ focal occult blood
t. for allergy, patch
t. for diplopia, Lancaster's red-
   green
t. for fungus organisms, skin
t. for glutaric aciduria
t. for hypertension, Regitine
t. for ketones, Ketostix
t. for myasthenia gravis, Tensilon
t. for syphilis, serological
t. for syphilis, standard
t. for tuberculosis (TB) ▸ skin
t. for tuberculosis, tine
t. for urine excretion ▸ Schilling
t., formol-gel
t., Fowler loudness balance
t. ▸ Fowler single breath
t., fragility
t., Frei's
t., Friedman-Lapham
t., Friedman's
t., frog
t., Fukuda
T., full scale Intelligence Quotient
   (IQ)
t., functional hearing

t. ▸ functional memory
t., Gaenslen
t., galactose tolerance
t. ▸ gallbladder function
t., Galli-Mainini
T. (GOAT) ▸ Galveston Orientation
   and Amnesia
t., gastrointestinal (GI) protein loss
t., Gault's
t., Gellé's
t., Gerhardt's
t., GI (gastrointestinal) blood loss
t., Gibbon-Landis
t., glucagon
t., glucose
t., glucose absorption
t., glucose tolerance
t., glucose-insulin tolerance
t., glycogen storage
t., Gmelin's
t., gonioscopy
t., Goodenough
t. ▸ Gradational Step exercise
   stress
t., graded exercise
t., Gravindex
t., guaiac stool
t., hair analysis
t., Hallpike caloric stimulation
T., Halstead Category
t., Halstead-Reitan
T. ▸ Halstead-Wepman Aphasia
   Screening
t., Hamburger's
t., Hamilton's
t., hand strength
t., Hanger-Rose skin
t., Hanger's
t., Harvard P.B.
t., Harvard Spondee Word
t. ▸ head down tilt
t. ▸ head up tilt table
t., head-tilt
t., Heaf
t., hearing
t., heat detection
t., heel-knee
t. ▸ heel-to-shin
t., hemagglutination-inhibition
t. ▸ hepatojugular reflux
t. ▸ hereditary hemolytic anemia
   (HHA)
t., Hering's
t., heterophil antibody
t., Hickey-Hare

t., Hicks-Pitney thromboplastin
   generation
t. ▸ high altitude simulation
t., hippuric acid
t., histamine
t., histamine stimulation
t., histoplasmin skin
t., Hitzenberg's
t., Hofmeister's
t., Hogben's
t., Holmgren's
t., Holmgren's wool skein
t., homocysteine
t., homogentisic acid
t. ▸ hormone receptor
t., Howard
t., Huhner's
t., human erythrocyte agglutination
t., Hunt's
t., hypoxemia
t., icterus index
t., immunofluorescence assay
t., immunologic
t., implantation
t. in drug abuse, diagnostic
t. in lateral position, pivot shift
t., in vitro
t., indican
t., indigo carmine
t., indirect bilirubin
t., indirect Coombs'
t., infertility
t., inhalation
t. ▸ initial drug screening
t., ink blot
t., insulin clearance
t., insulin sensitivity
t., insulin tolerance
t., intelligence quotient (IQ)
t. ▸ internal scalp stimulation
t., interpersonal reaction
t., intracellular magnesium
t., intradermal
t., intravenous (IV) glucose
   tolerance
t., intravenous (IV) tolbutamide
   tolerance
t., invasive
t., invasive activity
t., inversion stress
t., iodine-azide
t., I^{131} (radioactive iodine) uptake
T. ▸ Iowa
t., iron-binding capacity
t., irresistible impulse

t., Ishihara's
t., Isoiodeikon
t. ▸ isometric hand grip
t. ▸ isoproterenol stress
t. ▸ isoproterenol tilt table
t., IV (intravenous) glucose tolerance
t., IV (intravenous) tolbutamide tolerance
t. ▸ J point treadmill
t., Janet's
t., Jansen's
t., Kahn's
t., Kapeller-Adler
t. ▸ Kattus exercise stress
t., ketone body
t., kidney function
t. kits ▸ home medical
t., Kleihauer-Betke
t., Kline flocculation
t., knee-heel
t., Kolmer's
t., Korotkoff's
t., Kupperman's
t., Kveim
t. ▸ Kveim antigen skin
t., Kveim-Siltzbach
t., Lachman's
t., lactic acid
t., lactic dehydrogenase (LDH)
t., lactose tolerance
t., Landau
t., language
t., lantern
t., Lasegue
t., latex agglutination inhibition
t., latex fixation
t., latex flocculation
t., latex slide agglutination
t., Lautier's
t., LE (lupus erythematous) cell
t. ▸ leg sparing stress
t., leukocyte alkaline phosphatase (LAP)
t., Levinson
t., levulose tolerance
t., ligament stability
t., Lingieres
t., lipase
t., lipid
t. (LFT), liver function
t., Livierato's
t. ▸ log rank
t., Lombard's
t., lung functioning

T., Luria-Nebraska
t., Luscher-Zwislocki
t., lymphocyte transfer
t., Maddox rod
t., magnesium
T. ▸ Make-A-Picture-Story
t., malaria film
t., mallein
t., Mantoux skin
t., manual muscle
t., Marchetti
t., Marlow's
t., Marshall's
t., masking
t. ▸ Master exercise stress
t., Master "2-step" exercise
t., Master's exercise tolerance
t., mastic
t., Matas
t., Mauthner's
t., McMurray
t. meal, Boas
t. meal, Boyden's
t. meal, Dock's
t. meal, Ehrmann's alcohol
t. meal, Ewald's
t. meal, Fischer's
t. meal, Leube's
t. meal, motor
t. meal, Riegel's
t. meal, Salzer's
t., meal stimulation
t., mecalil provocation
t., Meigs'
t., Meinicke
t., melanin
t., memory
t. ▸ memory and concentration
t., meniscal
t., mental status
t. ▸ mental stress
t. method ▸ prick
t., methylene blue dye
t., Metopirone
t., milk ring
t., Mill's
t., mini-mental status
t., MMPI (Minnesota Multiphasic Personality Inventory)
t., moan
t., modified tone decay
T., Monospot Slide
t., Moro's
t. ▸ motor speed
t., Moynihan's

t., mucoprotein
t., Müller's
T., Multiple Sleep Latency
t., Murphy-Pattee
t. ▸ muscle strength
t. ▸ Myers-Briggs Type Indicator (MBTI)
t., Naffziger
t., Naloxone
t., Nathan's
t., near vision
t. ▸ negative exercise
t., neoprecipitin
t. ▸ nerve conduction velocity
t., neutralization
t., nitrazine
t., nitrogen retention
t., nonintrusive
t., noninvasive
t., noninvasive brain
t. ▸ noninvasive diagnostic
t., nonprotein nitrogen
t., nonstress
t. ▸ nonverbal memory
t., norethindrone
t., norethynodrel
t., normal lymphocyte transfer
t., nuclear stress
t., Obermayer's
t., Ober's
t., object sorting
t., occult blood
t., octopus
t. of blood, compatibility
t. of blood, fragility
t. of Hughston, jerk
t. of Macintosh, pivot shift
t. of vision, finger-counting
t. ▸ online stress
t., ophthalmodynamometry
t., ophthalmoscopy
t., oral glucose tolerance
t., Ortolani's
t., osazone
t., ovulation
t., ox cell hemolysin
t., pancreatic exocrine function
t., pancreatic exocrine secretion
t., pancreatic function
t., pancreatic secretory function
t., Pandy's
t., Papanicolaou (Pap)
t., partial thromboplastin time
t., past-pointing
t., patch

test(s)—*continued*

t., patch skin
t., pathological
t., Patrick's
t., Paul-Bunnell
t., Paul-Bunnell-Barrett
T., Peg
t., penagastric stimulation
t., peppermint
t., perceived exertion
t., personality
t., Petri
t., pH
t., Phalen
t. ▸ Phalen's sign
t., phenolphthalein
t., phenolsulfonphthalein
t., phenylketonuria
t., phosphatase
t., phospholipid
t., phosphoric acid
t. ▸ Physical Work Capacity
   exercise stress
t., Piazza's
t., pivot shift
t. ▸ planar thallium
t., plant protease
t. ▸ plantar ischemia
t., plasma glucose tolerance
t., Politzer's
t., polygraph
t., Porges-Meier
t., Porges-Salomon
t., porphobilinogen
t., porphyrin
t. positive for tuberculosis (TB) ▸
   patch
t., positive washout
t., postcoital
t., posterior drawer
t., potassium
t., precipitin
t., pregnancy
t., prenatal diagnostic
t., prenatal screening
t. ▸ pretransplant pulmonary
   function
t., prick skin
t. ▸ primed lymphocyte
t. (PCT) ▸ progesterone challenge
t., progesterone withdrawal
t., projective
T., Projective Human Figure
   Drawing
t., protein

t. ▸ protein level
t., proteinuria
t., prothrombin
T., Proverbs
t., provocation
t., pulmonary
t. (PFT), pulmonary function
t., pure tone
t., purine bodies
t., quadrivation
t. ▸ quantitative pilocarpine
   iontophoresis sweat
t., Queckenstedt's
t., Quick
t., RA (rheumatoid arthritis) latex
   fixation
t., radioactive fibrinogen uptake
t., radioactive Hippuran (RAH)
t., radioactive iodine (RAI) uptake
t. ▸ radioactive thallium exercise
t. ▸ radioactive treadmill
t. (RAST), radioallergo-absorbent
t., radiographic
t., radioimmunoprecipitation
t., radioiodine
t., radioisotope renogram
t., radiosensitivity
t., RAH (radioactive Hippuran)
t., RAI (radioactive iodine) uptake
t., Rainville
t., Raji cell assay
t., rapid plasma reagin (RPR)
T., Raven's Progressive Matrix
t., red glass
t., refraction
t., Regitine
t., Reitan-Indiana aphasic screening
t., Reiter protein complement
   fixation
t., respiratory drive
t. result ▸ true-negative
t. result ▸ true-positive
t. -retest consistency
t. -retest reliability
t. ▸ reverse transcriptase
   polymerase chain reaction
T., Rey Auditory Verbal Learning
t. ▸ rheumatoid arthritis (RA) latex
   fixation
t., rheumatoid factor
t., RhoGAM
t., Rinne's
t., Roos
t., Rorschach
t., rose bengal

t., Rose's
t., Rose-Waaler
t., Rothera's
t. ▸ routine stick
t. ▸ routine stress
t., Rowntree and Geraghty's
t., Rubin's
t., Sabin dye
t., Sabin-Feldman
t., Sahli's
t., SAL (sensory acuity level)
t., saliva
t., Salomon's
t., Schick's
t., Schiff's
t., Schiller's
t., Schilling
t., Schirmer's
t., Schwabach's
t., scratch
t., screening
t., SD (speech discrimination)
t., second strength tuberculin
t., secretin
t., Seiditz powder
t., Selivanoff's
t., Seliwanow's
t., Sellards'
t., semen analysis
t., sensitivity
t., sensory acuity level (SAL)
T. ▸ Sentence Completion
t., sequential multiple analyzer
   (SMA-6)
t., sequential multiple analyzer
   (SMA-12)
t., serologic
t., serology
t., serum calcium
t., serum creatine kinase
t., serum creatinine
t., serum enzyme
t., serum phosphorus
t. ▸ sestamibi stress
t., 17-hydroxycorticosteroid
t., 17-ketosteroid
t., severe functional
t., sex chromatin
t., Sgambati's
t., shadow
t., shake
t. ▸ Sheffield exercise stress
T., Shipley-Hartford
t., Shultze
t., sickle cell

t., sickling
t., sigmoidoscopy
t., Silon
t., Simonelli's
t., simple blood
t., Sims-Huhner
t., single breath
t. ▸ single breath nitrogen washout
t. ▸ single-stage exercise stress
T., SISI (Short Increment Sensitivity Index)
t., SLR (straight leg raising)
t., SMA-12 profile
t., Snellen's
t., sniff
t., sodium
t. solution
t., Somogyi
t., specific gravity
t. specimen
t., speech discrimination (SD)
t., speech reception
t., spirometry
t. ▸ split function lung
t., sponge
t., Spurling
t., sputum
t., standard antibody
t., standard eye
t., standard psychological
t., Stanford-Binet
t., staphylococcal clumping
t., Stenger hearing
t., Stevenson
t., stool blood
t. ▸ stool card
t. (SLRT), straight leg raising
t., stress
t. ▸ stretch-and-reach
t., string
T., Stroop Color and Word
t. subject
t., Sulkowitch's
t., surf (surfactant)
t. ▸ sweat chloride
t. ▸ sweat crying
t. ▸ sweat electrolyte
t., swinging-flashlight
t. ▸ symptom-limited treadmill exercise
t., Szabo's
t., T water
t., TB (tuberculosis) patch
t., TB (tuberculosis) skin
t., TBI (thyroxine binding index)

t., Tensilon
t., tension
t., tensor
t., thallium 201 stress
T. (TAT) ▸ Thematic Apperception
t., thermodilution
t., Thomas'
t., Thorn
t., thromboplastin generation
t., thumbnail
t., thymol turbidity
t., thyrocalcitonin
t., thyroid function
t. ▸ tilt table
t., tine tuberculin
t. (TTT) ▸ tolbutamide tolerance
t., tone decay
t., tonometry
t., Töpfer's
t., torsion
t., transaminase
t. ▸ transcranial Doppler
t. ▸ transferrin saturation
t., transillumination
t., treadmill exercise stress
t., treadmill stress
t., Trendelenburg's
t., triglyceride
t., triiodothyronine red cell uptake
t., triiodothyronine resin
t., triiodothyronine (T_3) uptake
t., trypsin
t., Tschiassny
t., T_3 (triiodothyronine) uptake
t., tubal potency
t. tube
t., tuberculosis (TB)
t., tuberculosis (TB) patch
t., tuberculosis (TB) skin
t., tumor skin
t., tuning
t., tuning fork
t. ▸ two-step exercise
t., tympanometry
t. type
t. types, Jaeger's
t., tyramine
t., tyrosine
t., tyrosine tolerance
t., ultrasound
t. ▸ ultrasound vascular
t. unit (STU) ▸ skin
t., urea clearance
t., urea nitrogen
t., uric acid

t., urinalysis
t. ▸ urinary flow
t., urine
t., urine chloride
t., urine concentration
t., urobilinogen
t., valgus stress
t. ▸ valgus-varus stress
t., Valsalva's
t., van den Bergh
t., Van Slyke
t., varus stress
t., vasography
T., Venereal Disease Research Laboratories (VDRL)
t. ▸ verbal memory
t., vestibular
t., Visscher-Bowman
t., visual acuity
t., visual field
t. ▸ visual spatial ability
t., Vollmer's
t. ▸ volume-challenge
t., von Poehl's
t., Wadas
T., WAIS (Wechsler Adult Intelligence Scale)
t. ▸ walking ventilation
t., Walter's bromide
t., Wampole's
t., washout
t., Wassermann
t., watch
t. ▸ water gurgle
t., water load
t., water siphonage
t., Watson
t., Watson-Schwartz
t., Weber's
T., Wechsler Adult Intelligence Scale (WAIS)
T., Wechsler Intelligence Scale for Children (WISC)
T. ▸ Wechsler-Bellevue
t., Weinberg's
t., Westcott's
T., Western Blot
t., WHIFF
t., whisper
t., whistle
T., Wide Range Achievement
t., Wills
t., Wilson's
t., Wintrobe
t., wire-loop

test(s)—*continued*
- T., WISC (Wechsler Intelligence Scale for Children)
- T., Wittenborn Psychiatric Rating Scale
- t., Worth stereopsis
- t., Xenopus laevis
- t., xylose concentration
- t., Yerkes-Bridges
- t., Youman-Parlett serologic
- t., Yvon's
- t., Ziehen's
- t., zinc flocculation
- t., zinc turbidity

testamentary capacity
testamentary competence
Tes-Tape
tested
- t. cognitively, patient
- t. for albumin, blood
- t. for albumin, urine
- t. with Clinitest, urine

testes
- t. atrophic
- t. in scrotum
- t. torsion of
- t. ▸ trauma to scrotum and
- t., undescended

testicle(s)
- t. cancer
- t., mobile
- t. self-examination
- t. ▸ shrinking of
- t., silicone
- t. transplant
- t., undescended

testicular
- t. abscess
- t. appendage
- t. artery
- t. atrophy
- t. biopsy
- t. cancer
- t. cancer, metastatic
- t. carcinoma
- t. choriocarcinoma
- t. failure
- t. feminization
- t. feminizing syndrome
- t. growth
- t. implant
- t. injuries
- t. injury, mechanisms of
- t. lymphoma
- t. parenchyma

- t. plexus
- t. prosthesis, Silastic
- t. self-examination (TSE)
- t. seminoma
- t. shock
- t. swelling
- t. torsion
- t. tubules
- t. vein, left
- t. vein, right

testiculare, adenoma ovarii
testiculare ovarii, adenoma tubulare
testiculoma ovarii
testing (Testing)
- t., acoustic reflex
- t., acquired immune deficiency syndrome (AIDS)
- t., acquired immune deficiency syndrome (AIDS) mandatory
- t., acquired immune deficiency syndrome (AIDS) virus
- t., alcohol and drug abuse
- t. and mapping ▸ electrophysiologic
- t., antepartum
- t., antibiotic sensitivity
- t., audiology
- t., breath alcohol
- T. (CAST) ▸ Children of Alcoholic Screen
- t., clinical
- t., cortical function
- t., cytotoxic
- t., daily urine
- t., defibrillation threshold
- t., definitive
- t. devices, self-
- t., diagnostic
- t., DNA (deoxyribonucleic acid)
- t., electrodiagnostic
- t., electrophysiologic
- t., electrophysiology
- t., exercise
- t., eye
- t. ▸ fecal occult blood
- t. for alcoholism, self-
- t. for strength ▸ muscle
- t., frequency of
- t. ▸ gastric secretory
- t., genetic
- t. ▸ genetic predisposition
- t. (GART) ▸ genotypic antiretroviral resistance
- t., gross
- t., hair
- t., human

- t. ▸ impaired reality
- t. ▸ in vitro sensitivity
- t. ▸ invasive electrophysiologic
- t., large scale
- t., magnet
- t., mandatory AIDS (acquired immune deficiency syndrome)
- t., mandatory blood
- t. maneuver, cold pressor
- t., manual muscle
- t., neurological
- t., neuropsychological
- t., noninvasive
- t., objective personality
- t. of newborn for galactosemia
- t. of vestibular function ▸ caloric
- t., oxygen (O₂) saturation
- t., patch
- t., paternity
- t., perinatal non-stress
- t., perinatal stress
- t., positive for drugs
- t., post-training
- t. potential donors
- t. ▸ preembryotic genetic
- t., prenatal
- t., pre-surgical
- t., pretransfusion
- T. Program ▸ Forensic Urine Drug
- t. program, voluntary
- t., psychological
- t., psychometric
- t., pulmonary function
- t., Purified Protein Derivative (PPD) skin
- t., random drug
- t., reality
- t., relapse
- t., result of
- t. ▸ serial electrophysiologic
- t., skin
- t., speech
- t., spinnbarkeit
- t. ▸ strength, sensation and reflex
- t., stress
- t., susceptibility
- t. system, complete pacemaker patient
- t., treadmill
- t., unit, mobile
- t., urodynamic
- t. ▸ viral lode
- t., vive skin

testis(-es)
- t., appendage of

t., carcinoma of
t., ectopia
t., ectopic
t., fungus
t., gubernaculum
t., inverted
t., lobules of
t., obstructed
t., parenchyma
t., pulpy
t., redux
t., retained
t., tumor
t., undescended

testosterone
t. binding affinity
t. level
t., male hormone
t. measurement, plasma
t. patch ▸ abdominal
t. production rate
t. production, trigger
t. receptors
t. replacement therapy
t., serum
t., supplemental
t. synthesis, blocking
t. -synthesizing enzymes
t. therapy

tetani, Bacillus
tetani, Clostridium
tetanic
t. contraction
t. convulsion
t. motor response
t. spasm
t. stimulation ▸ supramaximal

tetanoid chorea
tetanomorphum, Clostridium
tetanus
t. and diphtheria toxoid
immunization
t. and rabies control programs
t., anodal closure
t., anodal duration
t. (AOT), anodal opening
t. antitoxin
t. bacillus
t., bony
t. booster
t., cathodal closure
t., cathodal duration
t. (DPT) ▸ diphtheria, pertussis,
t. immune globulin
t. immunization

t., kopf
t. shot
t. toxoid
t. toxoid immunization
t. toxoids, and acellular pertussis
vaccine ▸ diphtheria,
t. toxoids, and whole cell pertussis
vaccine ▸ diphtheria,

tetany
t. cataract
t., contraction of hand in
t., duration
t., hyperventilation
t., latent
t., parathyroid
t., parathyroprival
t., rheumatic
t. syndrome
t. thyroprival

tether device, implanted
tethered cord syndrome
tetracaine, adrenaline and cocaine (TAC)
tetracycline antiulcer agent
tetrad(s)
t., Fallot
t., narcoleptic
t., short chains and
t. spell

tetraethyl pyrophosphate
Tetraflex vascular graft ▸ Shiley
tetragena, Entamoeba
tetragena, Gaffkya
tetrahedon chest
tetrahydrofolic acid
tetralogy
t., Eisenmenger
t. of Fallot
t. of Fallot ▸ pink

tetramethyl lead
tetraphasic action potentials
tetraptera, Aspicularis
tetravalent rotavirus vaccine ▸ oral
tetra-X chromosomal aberration
tetrazolium reduction
tetrazolium-reduction inhibition
Teulon law, Giraud-
Tevdek suture
Tex
T. baffle ▸ Gore-
T. cardiovascular patch ▸ Gore-
T. graft, Gore-
T. graft, PTFE (polytetra-
fluoroethylene) Gore-
T. jump graft ▸ Gore-

T. ligament, Gore-
T. surgical patch ▸ Gore-
T. vascular graft ▸ Gore-

Texas influenza
Texas mange
textbook
t. depression
t. norms
t. sign, bread and butter

texture
t., hair normal
t. ▸ improving skin
t., normal color and
t., skin

textured breast augmentation ▸ female
TF (total flow)
T-4 cells
T-4 lymphocytes
TGA (transient global amnesia)
TGAR (total graft area rejected)
TGF (Tumor Growth Factor)
TGS (transmissible gastroenteritis of swine)
TGT (thromboplastin generation test)
THA (tetrahydroaminoacridine)
THA (total hydroxyapatite)
Thal fundoplasty ▸ modified
thalami optici, taenia medullaris
thalami, taenia
thalamic
t. deep brain stimulation
t. electrode, VPL
(ventroposterolateral)
t. epilepsy
t. nuclei, anterior
t. pain
t. pain syndrome
t. radiation
t. stimulator
t. stroke
t. stroke pain syndrome ▸ post-
t. syndrome
t. tumor

thalamocortical dysrhythmia
thalamomamillary bundle
thalamoperforating artery
thalamostriate vein
thalamotomy
t., anterior
t., dorsomedial
t. procedure
t., radiofrequency

thalamus
t. and cortex fire in synchrony

thalamus—*continued*
- t., function of
- t., inferior peduncle of
- t., lateral
- t., left
- t., optic
- t., posterior
- t., right
- t., ventroposterolateral nucleus of

thalassemia
- t. disease, hemoglobin C-
- t. disease, hemoglobin E-
- t. disease, sickle cell
- t. gene
- t. intermedia, beta
- t. major
- t. major anemia
- t. major, beta
- t. minor
- t. trait
- t. X-linked retardation syndrome ▸ alpha

thalictroides, Caulophyllum

thalidomide-induced birth defects

thallium
- t. (Tl)
- t. electrocardiogram (ECG)
- t. exercise heart scan
- t. exercise test ▸ radioactive
- t. imaging ▸ dipyridamole
- t. perfusion imaging
- t. poisoning
- t. scan
- t. scanning
- t. scanning ▸ stress
- t. scintigraphy
- t. scintigraphy ▸ dipyridamole
- t. scintigraphy ▸ planar
- t. scintigraphy ▸ stress
- t. stress test
- t. study ▸ stress
- t. test, adenosine
- t. test ▸ exercise
- t. test ▸ planar
- t. toxicity
- t. treadmill stress test
- t. -201 imaging ▸ rest redistribution
- t. -201 myocardial perfusion imaging ▸ stress
- t. -201 perfusion scintigraphy
- t. -201 planar scintigraphy
- t. -201 scintigraphy ▸ dipyridamole
- t. -201 scintigraphy ▸ exercise
- t. -201 SPECT scintigraphy
- t. washout

thanatophoric dwarf

thaw
- t. cryotherapy, freeze-
- t. -freeze technique ▸ freeze-
- t. treatment ▸ rapid freeze-slow

Thayer Clinical Anxiety Scale

THC (depressant)

THE (transhepatic embolization)

The Force (LSD)

theatrical, patient

thebesian
- t. circulation
- t. foramina
- t. valve
- t. vein

Thebesius, vein of

theca
- t. cell
- t. cell carcinoma, granulosa
- t. cell tumor
- t. cordis
- t. folliculi
- t. -lutein cells
- t. -lutein cyst
- t. vertebralis

thecal [*cecal, fecal, fetal*]
- t. cells ▸ androgen-screening
- t. puncture
- t. whitlow

thecocellulare, xanthofibroma

Theiler's mouse encephalomyelitis

Theiler's virus

Theile's glands

thelarche, pubarche and

Thematic (thematic)
- T. Apperception Test (TAT)
- t. paralogia
- t. paralogism
- t. process group

thenar
- t. atrophy
- t. eminence
- t. muscle
- t. muscle contraction
- t. muscles, atrophy of
- t. space
- t. web

theorem, Bernoulli

theoretical
- t. data
- t. psychology
- t. renal phosphorus threshold

theorist, behavioral

theorist, learning

theory(-ies)
- t., Adler's
- t., Altmann's
- t., anatomical
- t., arousal
- t., attachment
- t., Bayliss
- t., Cannon
- t., cross-linkage
- t., dipole
- t. -driven treatment
- t., ethical
- t., free radical
- t., Freud's
- t., gate-control
- t., Gestalt
- t., Hering's
- t., immunological
- t., Jungian
- t., latency
- t., Meyer's
- t., myogenic
- t., neuroendocrine
- t., neurogenic
- t. ▸ object relations
- t. of anxiety ▸ learning
- t. of atherogenesis ▸ monoclonal
- t. of atherosclerosis ▸ encrustation
- t. of atherosclerosis ▸ lipogenic
- t. of development, biosocial
- t. of signal detectability
- t., Planck's quantum
- t., primary therapeutic
- t., psychodynamic
- t., psychotic
- t., quack
- t., quantum
- t., reentry
- t. ▸ response to injury
- t., Schön's
- t. ▸ sliding filament
- t., somatic aberration
- t., spheron
- t., translation
- t., viral oncogenesis
- t., Young-Helmholtz

therapeutic(s)
- t. abortion (TAB)
- t. action
- t. activity
- t. activity ▸ legitimate
- t. acupuncture
- t. additivity and synergism
- t. agent
- t. alliance

t. approach
t. approach, short-term
t. aspect
t. benefits of humor
t. blood level
t. chemistry
t. classification
t. community
t. contact, supportive
t. control
t. demands
t. device
t. diet
t. dilemmas, common
t. dissection
t. donor insemination (TDI)
t. dose
t. drug level
t. drugs
t. effect
t. effect ▸ positive
t. effectiveness
t. effects of medication
t. efficacy
t. electrode
t. encounter
t. endoscopic procedure
t. endoscopic technique
t. endoscopy
t. endpoint
t. environment
t. equivalent
t. exercise
t. exercise for reminiscence
t. exercise for remotivation
t. exercise for validation
t. exercise program
t., experimental
t. eye movement
t. factors
t. failures
t. formulation
t. friction, systematic
t. goals, overall
t. grieving process
t. hemapheresis
t. home pass
t., human
t. humor
t. humor movement
t. impact
t. impasses ▸ negotiate
t. incompatibility
t. instructions, intratreatment
t. instructions, pretreatment

t. intervention
t. ionizing radiation
t. iridectomy
t. limitations of delayed recall
t. maneuver
t. massage
t. measures
t., medical
t. milieu
t. milieu management strategy
t. modality
t. nature, beneficial
t. needle punctures
t. nutritional intake
t. options
t. outcome, diagnosis and
t. paracentesis
t. philosophy
t. phlebotomy
t. pneumothorax
t. poisoning
t. pool
t. potential
t. potential of cannabinoids
t. potential of delayed recall
t. procedure
t. process
t. products
t. qualities of ice
t. radiology
t. ratio
t. ratio in radiation therapy
t. reaction, negative
t. recovery, supportive
t. regimens
t. relationship
t. resistance
t. response
t. result
t. services
t. skills
t. sleep aid
t. sleep pattern
t. strategy
t. support
t. suspension status ▸ outpatient
t. system ▸ gastrointestinal (GI)
t. technique
t. technology
t. theories, primary
t. thoracentesis
t. touch
t. training
t. treatment
t. trial

t. usefulness of antibodies
t. vitamins
t. window
t. zeal
therapeutically, work
therapist
t., activity
t., behavior
t., chemo◇
t. confidentiality ▸ patient-
t. coordinator, family
t., deep tissue massage
t., dynamic
t., enterostomal
t., fetal
t., grief
t., home
t., humor
t., massage
t., neuropsychology
t., occupational
t., physical
t. ▸ recovered memory
t., rehabilitation nurse
t., respiratory
t., speech
t., vocational
t., water
therapy(-ies) (Therapy)
t., ablation
t., ablative
t., ablative hormonal
t., ablative pace
t., abnormal gene
t., acid base
t., ACTH (adrenocorticotropic
  hormone)
t., action
t., activity
t. ▸ activity based
t., acupuncture
t., acute migraine
t., acute reaction to radiation
t., adaptive
t., additive hormonal
t., adjunct
t., adjunctive
t., adjunctive glucocorticoid
t., adjuvant
t., adjuvant medical
t., adjuvant surgical
t. ▸ adjuvant systemic
t., adverse reaction to
t., adversive
t., aerosol

therapy(-ies)—*continued*

t., aggressive
t. ‣ aggressive intense
t., aggressive medical
t. aide
t., alternative
t. ‣ alternative empiric
t., anaclitic
t., anatomical considerations in radiation
t. ‣ androgen ablation
t., anemia
t., angina-guided
t., Antabuse
t., antacid
t., antagonist
t., anti-aging
t., antialdosterone
t., anti-anginal
t., antiarrhythmic
t. antiarrhythmic device ‣ tiered
t., antibiotic
t., antibiotic combination
t., antibiotic drug
t., anticholinergic
t., anticoagulant
t., anticonvulsive
t., antidepressant
t., antidiabetic
t., antiemetic
t., anti-fibrinolytic
t., antifungal
t., antihypertensive
t., antimicrobial
t., antineoplastic
t., antiplatelet
t., antirejection
t., antiretroviral
t., antitetanus
t., antituberculosis
t., antituberculous
t., antiviral
t., appropriate
t., aquatic
t., aroma
t., Artane
t., arterial infusion
t. ‣ arterial plaque
t., aspirin
t., attack
t., augmentation
t., auricular
t., aversion
t., aversive
t., barbiturate

t., beam direction
t., behavior
t., behavior modification
t., behavioral
t., best-chance experimental
t., beta blocker
t., bicarbonate
t., biofeedback
t., biofeedback relaxation
t., biologic
t., biologic basis of radiation
t., biologic cancer
t., biological
t., biological tumor dose
t., bleeding
t., block placement in radiation
t., blood component
t., blood component replacement
t., blood transfusion
t., Borox
t., breast
t. ‣ breast conservation
t., cancer
t., cancer radiation
t. ‣ cancer responsive to systemic
t., carbon dioxide
t., carbon ion
t., cardiac drug
t. ‣ cardiac gene
t. ‣ cardiac resynchronization
t., cardiovascular
t., cell
t., cellular breast cancer
t., central axis dose of electron beam
t., central nervous system (CNS)
t., central nervous system tolerance to radiation
t., cerebral protective
t., chelation
t., chemical
t., chemo◊
t., chemoprevention
t., chemotherapy and radiation
t. ‣ cholesterol-lowering drug
t., chronic
t. ‣ chronic aspirin
t., chronic maintenance
t., chronic suppressant
t., cimetidine
t., client-centered
t., clinical radiation
t. ‣ clot dissolving
t., coagulant
t., cobalt 60 (Co^{60})

t., codependency
t., cognitive
t., cognitive behavior
t. (CBT), cognitive behavioral
t., cold
t., collaborative
t., collagen
t., collapse
t., combination
t., combination drug
t., combination electron and photon
t., combination high and low energy x-ray
t., combined chemotherapy/radiation
t., combined modality
t., compassion
t., complementary
t. complications in radiation therapy
t., complications of radiation
t., composite cyclic
t., compression
t., concomitant
t., conditioned reflex (CR)
t. ‣ conformal radiation
t. ‣ congestive heart failure (CHF)
t., conservative
t. ‣ conservative nonpharmacologic
t. ‣ constraint-induced movement
t., contact
t. contamination ‣ gene
t., continuous combined
t., controversial
t., conventional
t. ‣ conventional physical
t. ‣ convulsive shock
t., cool
t., coping skills
t., COPP
t., COPP chemo◊
t., cord blood cell
t., coronary
t., coronary gene
t., corporate
t. ‣ corrective attachment
t., corticosteroid
t., cortisone
t., couples
t. (first, second, etc.) ‣ course of
t., craniosacral
t., cryosurgery and laser
t., cyclic
t., cyclosporine
t., daily
t., daily group

t., daily preventive
t., deep chest
t. ▸ deep muscle
t., deep roentgen ray
t., deep tissue massage
t., deep x-ray
t., definitive
t., delayed reaction to radiation
t., dendritic cell
T. (PT) Department, Physical
T. Department, Respiratory
t. dermagraphic ▸ macro
t., desensitization
t., detoxification
t. ▸ development of gene
t., device
t. devices, effluent gas from
   respiratory
t. devices, respiratory
t., diabetes
t., diagnostic
t. ▸ dialectical behavior
t., dialysis
t., diathermal
t., diathermy
t., diet
t., dietary
t., differential
t., digitalis
t., directive
t. ▸ directive group play
t. ▸ directly observed
t. discontinued
t., discontinuing drug
t., dissolution
t., diuretic
t., dosimetry in radiation
t., drug
t., dynamic
t., educational
t., effective
t., electrical
t., electrical aversive
t. (ECT) ▸ electroconvulsive
t., electrolyte
t., electron
t., electron beam
t. (EST) ▸ electroshock
t., embolization
t., emergency
t., emergency radiation
t., empiric
t. ▸ empiric antibiotic
t., endocavitary radiation
t., endocrine

t. ▸ endoluminal radiation
t., enterostomal
t., environmental
t., established
t., estrogen
t. (ERT) ▸ estrogen replacement
t., ethnomedical
t. evaluation, occupational
t., exercise
t. exercise ▸ relaxation
t., experimental
t., experimental cancer
t., exposure
t., expressive
t., external
t. ▸ external beam
t., external irradiation
t., external radiation
t. ▸ eye movement
t., eye shields for electron beam
t., eyebrow and eyelash loss in
   radiation
t., fallback
t., family
t., family group
t., fast neutron beam
t., fetal
t., fever unresponsive to antibiotic
t., fibrillation
t., fibrinolytic
t. field localization
T., Flexicair
T., Flexicair Low Airloss
t., flooding
t., fluid
t., fluid replacement
t., focal radiation
t. follow-up, radiation
t. for alcoholism
t. for bone pain, radiation
t. for breast cancer ▸ adjuvant
t. for carcinoma, radiation
t. for heart ▸ gene
t. for hyperactivity ▸ relaxation
t. for intact breast, radiation
t. for men ▸ estrogen
t. for stroke ▸ cooling
t., full brain radiation
t., full course radiation
t., furosemide
t., gamma ray
t., garlic
t., gene
t., genetic
t., glandular

t., glaucoma
t., greyhound
t., grief
t., group
t., group and family
t. group, cognitive
t. group, conventional
t. group ▸ intensive
t., headache
t. ▸ heart disease
t., heat
t., heat and massage
t., heavy charged particle beam
t., heavy particle
t., hemibody radiation
t., heparin
t., herbal
t., high dose aspirin
t. ▸ high dose fractional radiation
t., high dose radiation
t. (HAART) ▸ highly active
   antiretroviral
t., holistic
t., home oxygen (O_2)
t., homeopathic
t., hormonal
t., hormone
t. (HRT) ▸ hormone replacement
t., Hubbard tank
t., hug
t., human
t., humeral block in radiation
t., hyperalimentation
t., hyperbaric oxygen (O_2)
t., hypertensive
t. ▸ iatrogenic effects of behavior
t., ice
t., immunization
t., immuno◇
t., immunological
t., immunomodular
t., immunosuppressant
t., immunosuppression
t., immunosuppressive
t., immunosuppressive drug
t., implant
t., implosive
t. in acromegaly, conventional
   radiation
t. in endometrial carcinoma,
   hormonal
t. in eye tumors, heavy charged
   particle
t. in patient management,
   combination

therapy(-ies)—*continued*

t. in radiation therapy, steroid
t. in trauma, fluid and electrolyte
t. in tumors, electron beam
t., independent toxicity in combined modality
t., indications for
t., individual
t. ▸ individual solution based
t. ▸ individualized behavior
t., individualized transfusion
t., Indoklon
t., infrared light
t., infusion
t., inhalation
t., inhomogeneities in electron beam
t., initial
t., initiating
t., injection
t. injection ▸ gene
t., innovative
t. ▸ insight-oriented
t., institution of
t., insulin
t., insulin coma
t., insulin shock
t., integrated
t. (ICT) ▸ integrative couple
T. (IMRT) ▸ Intensity Modulated Radiation
t., intensive
t. ▸ intensive antimicrobial
t. ▸ intensive dietary
t., intensive insulin
t., intensive topical antibiotic
t., interferon
t. ▸ interferon alpha
t., interleukin II
t., intermittent
t., intermittent diuretic
t., intermittent radiation
t. ▸ intermittent steroid
t. ▸ internal antifungal
t., internal radiation
t., interpersonal
t., interstitial
t., intracavitary
t., intracavitary cesium
t. ▸ intracavitary radiation
t. (IDET), intradiskal electrothermal
t., intraluminal radiation
t., intraoperative radiation
t., intraoral cone for electron beam
t., intrathecal
t., intravaginal

t., intravenous (IV)
t. ▸ intravenous anticoagulant
t. ▸ intravenous antioxidant
t., intravenous (IV) nutritional
t., invasive
t., investigational
t., irradiation
t. ▸ ischemia-guided medial
t., isotope
t., language
t., laryngeal block in radiation
t., laser
t., laser light
t., last-chance experimental
t., late reactions to radiation
t., light
t., light-beam
t., limitations of radiation
t., lipid
t., lithium
t., local
t., local radiation
t., local recurrence after radiation
t. ▸ long-term anticoagulation
t., long-term biofeedback relaxation
t. ▸ long-term drug
t., long-term family
t. ▸ long-term oxygen (O_2)
t. ▸ long-term steroid
t., low dose
t., low dose aspirin
t., low dose intravenous (IV) insulin
t., low insulin
t. ▸ low vision
t., lumbosacral fields for radiation
t., lung radiation
t., lymphedema
t., macrobiotic
t., magnesium
t., magnet
t., maintenance
t. ▸ malaria fever
t. manager
t., manipulative
t., mantle
t., mantle field in radiation
t., mantle technique in radiation
t., marital
t., massage
t., maximal
t., mediastinum volume rotation
t., medical
t. ▸ medical nutrition
t., medication
t. ▸ megadose vitamin

t., megavitamin
t., megavolt
t., mental
t., mercaptopurine
t., metabolic
t., Metrazol shock
t., microinjection
t., microwave
t., milieu
t. ▸ mind-body
t., mineral
t. ▸ mineral replacement
t., minimal supportive
t., modify
t. ▸ molecular breast cancer
t., molybdenum radiation
t., monitor
t. ▸ monoclonal antibody
t. (MET) ▸ motivational enhancement
t., multimodal
t., multimodality
t., multiple drug
t., multiple drug chemo◊
t., multiple family
t., music
t., myoblast
t., myoblast transfer
t. ▸ myocardial infarction
t. ▸ naturopathic manipulative
t. ▸ negative ion
t., neon ion
t., network
t., neural
t., neuraxis irradiation in radiation
t., neurobehavioral
t., neuroleptic
t., neuromuscular
t., neuroprotective
t., new drug
t., niacin
t., nicotine replacement
t. ▸ nicotinic receptor blockade
t., nitrogen mustard
t., nitroglycerin
t., nonbarbiturate
t., nondirective
t., noninvasive
t. ▸ non-nicotine
t., nonsurgical
t., normal tissue considerations in radiation
t. nurse ▸ radiation
t., nutrition
t., nutritional

t. observation unit (ITOU) ▸ intensive
T. (OT) ▸ Occupational
t. of arrhythmias ▸ pharmacological
t. of bacterial shock ▸ complementary
t. of depression, cognitive
t. of diabetic retinopathy, laser
t. of hemorrhoids ▸ laser
t. of migraine, biofeedback
t. of personality, cognitive
t. of substance abuse, cognitive
t. on prophylactic basis, radiation
t., oncotic
t., one-on-one
t., operative
t. ▸ oral antiarrhythmic
t. ▸ oral anticoagulant
t. ▸ oral chelation
t. ▸ oral dissolution
t., oral drug
t., oral estrogen
t. ▸ organizing interstitial pneumonia
oxygen (O_2)
t., osteoporosis
t., outpatient
t., ovary protection in radiation
t., oxygen (O_2)
t., pacemaker
t., pain medication and
t., palliative
t., palliative radiation
t., pancreatic replacement
t., paraffin
t., parenteral
t., parenteral prophylactic
t., particle
t., passive
t., patch
t. ▸ patient intolerant to aspirin
t., patient tolerated
t., patient treated with radiation
t., pattern
t. ▸ percutaneous dissolution
t. perineal area, radiation
t. ▸ perioperative antimicrobial
t., permanent implant
t., personal
t., pharmacologic
t., pharmacological
t. (PDT) ▸ photodynamic
t. ▸ photodynamic tumor
t., photon
t., photon irradiation technique in
radiation

T. (PT) ▸ Physical
t., placebo
t., plasma component
t. ▸ plasma exchange
t., plastic mask for electron beam
t., play
t. pneumonitis, radiation
t., polarizing
t., postmantle radiation
t. ▸ postmenopausal estrogen
t. ▸ postmenopausal hormone
t., postoperative radiation
t., postradiation
t., postsurgical radiation
t., potential
t., preauricular radiation
t., preferred
t., preoperative
t., preoperative radiation
t., prescription drug
t., preventive
t., preventive aspirin
t., previous
t., primary
t., primary radiation
t. ▸ problem-solving
t. procedure, gene
t. program, computer
t. program ▸ coronary gene
t. progress
t., prolonged
t., prolonged antibiotic
t., prolonged drug
t. ▸ prolonged steroid
t., prophylactic
t. ▸ prostate hormone
t. ▸ protease inhibitor
t., protocol design in combined
modality
t. protocols, complex oncologic
t. ▸ proton beam
t., pseudomedical
t., psychedelic-peak
t., psychiatric
t., psychoanalysis
t., psychoanalytic
t., psychodynamic
t. ▸ psychodynamic play
t. ▸ psychodynamically oriented
t., psychoeducational group
t., psychological
t. ▸ psychological, educational and
social
t., psychosocial
t., psychosocial occupational

t., psychotropic
t. ▸ pulsed light
t. (RET) ▸ rad equivalent
t., radiation
t., radiation necrosis in skin cancer
t., radical radiation
t., radio◊
t., radioimmunoglobulin
t., radium
t. ▸ rage reduction
t., rational hypertensive
t. reaction, adverse
t., reality
t., recommend continued medical
t. ▸ recovered memory
t., recreational
t. ▸ red cell
t., red light
t., reduced active
T. (REST) ▸ Reduced
Environmental Stimulation
t. ▸ re-evaluation of existing drug
t., regenerative
t. ▸ regenerative heart
t., rehabilitation
t. ▸ rehabilitation occupational
t., rehabilitative
t. ▸ rehabilitative physical
t. ▸ relationship enhancement (RE)
t. ▸ relationship enhancement (RE)
family
t., relaxation
t., relaxation response in headache
t., replacement
t., research design in combined
modality
t. research ▸ gene
t., respiratory
t., response and combined modality
t., response to
t. ▸ response to relaxation
t., restorative
t. results
t. resumed in full course, radiation
t., retail
t., rheologic
t., roentgen
t., root canal
t., rotation
t., sandwich
t., scattering foils in electron beam
t. schedule
t. ▸ secondary to radiation
t., sensory feedback
t., sequelae of

therapy(-ies)—*continued*
t., sequelae of radiation
t., serum
t. services, physical
t. session
t. sessions, group
t., sex
t., sexual adjustment
t., shielding in electron beam
t., shock
t., short wave
t. ▸ short-term
t. ▸ short-term psychodynamic
t., short-term steroid
t., silicon ion
t. skills, cognitive
t., skin reactions to electron beam
t. ▸ sleep restriction
t., sleep-deprivation
t., slipping rib
t., small group
t., small volume rotational
t. ▸ smoking cessation
t. ▸ solution focused group
t., somatic
t., spatial cooperation in combined modality
t., specific
t., speech
t., spinal cord block in radiation
t., spinal cord tolerance in radiation
t., staging systems in radiation
t., standard
t. ▸ steam inhalation
t. ▸ step-down
t. ▸ sterile whirlpool
t., steroid
t., steroid therapy in radiation
t., stimulation
t. ▸ stimulus control
t., strategic
t. ▸ strategic family
t., streptokinase
t., stress control
t. ▸ stress management
t., structural
t., subdiaphragmatic fields in radiation
t., subdiaphragmatic radiation
t., supervoltage
t., supervoltage rotational irradiation
t., supervoltage x-ray
t., supplemental
t., supplemental growth hormone
t. ▸ supplemental oxygen (O_2)

t., supportive
t. ▸ supportive expressive
t., suppressive
t., supramediastinal mantle in radiation
t., surgical
t., surgical adjuvant
t., survival rates with combined modality
t., swallowing
t., systemic
t., systemic adjuvant
t., systemic radiation
t., tachycardia
t., talk
t. technique
t. technique ▸ gene
t. technique, radiation
t. technique ▸ supportive
t. techniques, programmed behavior
t., temporal consolidation in combined modality
t., testosterone
t. ▸ testosterone replacement
t., therapeutic ratio in radiation
t. ▸ therapy complications in radiation
t., thin liver block in radiation
t., thin lung blocks in radiation
t., thoracentesis
t. ▸ thought field
t. ▸ three-dimensional conformal radiation
t. ▸ three-dimensional radiation
t. ▸ three-drug
t., thrombolytic
t., thymic radiation
t., thyroid
t., tiered
t., topical
t., total body radiation
t., total parenteral nutrition (TPN)
t., total push
t., total skin electron beam
t., touch
t., traditional
t. ▸ traditional behavioral
t., transcatheter
t., transdermal estrogen
t., transfer factor
t., transfusion
t. ▸ treadmill walking
t., treatment

t. (PDT) treatment for cancer ▸ photodynamic
t. treatment, radiation
t., treatment volume in radiation
t. trials ▸ gene
t. ▸ trigger point
t., tumor
t. ▸ tumor photodynamic
t., ultrasonic
t., ultrasound
t. ▸ ultrasound-guided injection
t. ▸ ultraviolet (UV)
t., ultraviolet light
t., unconventional
t., underwater
t. unit (ITU) ▸ intensive
t. unit, Picker Vanguard deep
t., upper mantle
t., urokinase
t. ▸ uterine balloon
t., vaccine
t. ▸ vascular endothelial growth factor (VEGF)
t., vasodilating
t., vasodilator
t. ▸ vestibular and balance rehabilitation
t. ▸ vincristine, methotrexate, 6-mercaptopurine, and prednisone (VAMP)
t. ▸ virus injected
t., vision
t., visual
t., Visudyne
t., vitamin
t., voice
t., warfarin
t., water
t., whirlpool
t., whole abdomen radiation
t., whole abdominal treatment in radiation
t., whole brain radiation
t., whole brain vs local brain radiation
t., x-ray
THERM, Auto-MEDI-Therma Choice procedure
thermal
t. ablation
t. angiography
t. approach
t. ataxia
t. balloon
t. balloon ablation

t. burn
t. capacity
t. conductivity
t. destruction
t. dilution
t. dose
t. effect
t. energy
t. injury
t. keratoplasty ▸ laser
t. laser
t. memory stent
t. neutrons
t. number
t. /perfusion balloon angioplasty (TPBA)
t. shock
t. spectrum
t. stimulus
t. walks
t. wheel
thermalis, Leptothrix
thermally induced nystagmus
thermic fever
thermionic emission
thermistor plethysmography
thermodilution
    t. cardiac output
    t., coronary sinus
    t. measurement
    t. method
    t. technique
    t. test
thermodynamics, law of
thermodynamics, muscle
thermogenesis
    t., dietary
    t. (NEAT) ▸ nonexercise activity
    t. reaction, dietary
thermogenic effect
thermogenic effect exercises
thermogram, abnormal
thermogram (LCT), liquid crystal
thermograph, continuous scan
thermographic screening
thermography
    t., breast
    t., clinical application of
    t., heat pattern
    t., infrared
    t., liquid crystal
    t., neuromuscular
    t. study
thermoluminescent dosimeter (TLD)

thermometer(s)
    t., centigrade
    t., disposable
    t., electronic
    t., electronic digital
    t., Fahrenheit
    t., fiberoptic
    t., glass
    t. monitoring in hyperthermia
    t., oral
    t., rectal
    t., sterile
thermoneutral environment
thermonuclear reaction
thermophilia, Actinomyces
thermophilic actinomycetes
thermoregulation, ineffective
thermoregulation, neonatal
thermoregulatory
    t. center
    t. mechanism
    t. system, dysfunctional
thermoresistable, Mycobacterium
Therm-O-Rite blanket
Therm-O-Rite mattress
Thermos pacemaker
thermosaccarolyticum, Clostridium
thermosetting resin
thermotherapy
    t., patient treated with
    t., Prostatron
    t. (TUMT) ▸ transurethral microwave
thermotic drainage (dr'ge) unit
thermovision camera
thesis
    t., characterological predisposition
    t., characterological vulnerability
    t., co-effect
    t., complication
    t., etiologic
    t., orthogonal
    t., spectrum
    t. ▸ stress generating
theta [*beta*]
    t. activity
    t. activity, bursts of
    t. band
    t. biofeedback, alcoholism and alpha-
    t. biofeedback training ▸ electroencephalogram (EEG)
    t. bursts
    t. bursts of drowsiness ▸ rhythmic temporal

    t. electroencephalogram (EEG) frequency range ▸ alpha-
    t. frequencies
    t. frequency, burst of
    t. pattern
    t. rhythm
    t. wave
    t. waves, alpha-
thiamine deficiency
thiamine pyrophosphate
thiamylal sodium
thiazide diuretic
thiazole ring
thick
    t. and closed ▸ cervix long,
    t. bronchial secretions
    t. elastic tissue
    t. -layer autoradiography
    t. mucoid material
    t., red, itchy patches of skin
    t. -septa collimator
    t. -split graft
    t., sticky mucus
    t. structure
    t., tenacious sputum
    t. visceral peel
    t. walled
thicken and grow ▸ villus hairs to
thicken ▸ cause bones to
thickened
    t., aortic valve
    t. arterial wall
    t., arteries slightly
    t., bladder wall
    t. connective tissue
    t. folds
    t. heart muscle
    t. heart walls
    t. musculature
    t. pericardium
    t. plaque, fatty
    t. pleura
    t. septum
    t. synovial membrane
    t. toenail
    t. whitish plaques
thickening(s)
    t., alveolar capillary
    t., apical pleural
    t., arteriolar
    t., cardiac wall
    t., cortical
    t., diffuse intimal
    t., endocardial
    t., focal pleural

thickening(s)—*continued*
t. ▸ heart wall
t. in the breast
t. ▸ indistinct semicircumferential
  fibrous
t., intimal
t., leaflet
t., marked muscular
t., membrane
t. mitral valve ▸ fibrous
t., mucosal
t. of alveolar septum ▸ focal
t. of aortic valve
t. of breast
t. of capillary walls
t. of chordae ▸ fibrous
t. of colon muscle
t. of left ventricle ▸ apical
t. of muscle wall
t. of periosteum
t. of pleura
t. of skin
t. of speech
t. of tunica intima
t. of uterine lining
t., parametrial
t., pericardial
t., periosteal
t., pleural
t., sclerotic
t., tongue
t. ▸ valve
t., wall

thickly gnarled knuckles
thickness
t. (AET) ▸ absorption equivalent
t. bone
t. (CET) ▸ coefficient of equal
t., cortical
t. -diastole, posterior wall
t., diastolic
t. graft, full-
t. graft of pigskin, split
t. graft, split-
t., half-
t., half-value
t. index ▸ volume
t. ▸ intimal medial
t., left ventricular posterior wall
t. (MCT) ▸ mean corpuscular
t., myocardial wall
t., narrow beam half-
t. of skin
t. of ventricular wall
t. postauricular graft, full-

t. ratio (MDTR) ▸ mean diameter-
t. ▸ relative wall
t. skin graft, full-
t. skin graft, intermediate
t. skin graft, intermediate split-
t. skin graft, partial
t. skin graft, split-
t., skinfold
t. ▸ subscapular skinfold
t. -systole, posterior wall
t. transplant ▸ full
t. transplant ▸ partial
t., wall

Thiers syndrome, Achard-Thiersch('s)
T. cerclage
T. -Duplay urethroplasty
T. graft
T. graft, Ollier-
T. operation, Ollier-
T. skin graft
T. wire

thigh(s) [*sigh*]
t. and hamstrings ▸ stretching
  calves,
t., biceps muscle of
t. bone
t. bone ▸ upper
t., chafing of
t., deep vein of
t., flexion of
t. hair
t. high antiembolic stockings
t. high socks
t. injury
t., lateral cutaneous nerve of
t., left
t. on abdomen, flexion of
t., posterior cutaneous nerve of
t., quadrate muscle of
t., quadriceps muscle of
t., right
t. stretch exercise
t. stretch exercise ▸ upper
t., striae of

thimble valvotomy
thin
t. and trabeculated ▸ bladder wall
t. cancerous tumor
t. cornea
t. disc
t. edge
t. fibrous cap
t. layer chromatography
t. layer chromatography, instant

t. layer electrophoresis
t. liver block in radiation therapy
t. lung blocks in radiation therapy
t. panniculus
t. plastic membrane
t. section CT (computerized
  tomography)
t. -septa collimator
t. septal walls
t. slice CT (computerized
  tomography) scan
t. -split graft
t. stools, pencil-
t. -walled bleb
t. -walled blood vessels
t. -walled cyst of liver
t. walled veins

Thing (heroine)
things ▸ patient misplacing
think abstractly
think or concentrate ▸ ability to
thinking
t., ability of abstract
t., abstract
t., abstract operational
t. and sensorium disturbance
t. and speech ▸ rapid and chaotic
t., autistic
t., automatic
t., behavior and
t., bizarre incoherent
t., bizarre way of
t., circular
t., coherent
t., confused
t., constructive
t. cortex
t., creative
t., creative-associative
t., deficient cognitive
t., delusional
t., deranged
t. ▸ disordered
t., disorganized
t., distorted
t., distorted negative
t. distortion
t., disturbed
t., divergent
t., foggy
t. ▸ hallucinations and incoherent
t., impaired
t., impaired abstract
t., incoherent
t., inconsistent and inappropriate

t., irrational
t., logical
t., magical
t., muddled
t. ▸ negative style of
t. ▸ nonpsychotic distorted
t. or concentration ▸ impaired
t., paranoid
t., patient acts before
t., patient paranoic in
t. process ▸ negative
t., rational
t., referential
t. ▸ right in
t. ▸ severe impairment in
t. skills ▸ rational
t., slowed
t., tangential
t., unrealistic
t., visual
t., woolly
thinks about ending life ▸ patient
Thinlith II pacemaker, Intermedics
thinned, cortex
thinner, blood
thinning
    t. agents, blood
    t., blood
    t., bone
    t. drug, blood
    t. effects of estrogen loss, bone
    t. hair
    t. hair ▸ restore lost or
    t., infarct
    t. medication, blood
    t. of blood
    t. of cervix
    t. of sclera
    t. of vertebral column ▸
        osteoporotic
    t. process of bone
    t., retinal
    t., shear
    t. skin
    t. ▸ vaginal tissue
    t. ▸ ventricular wall
thiocyanate level
thiopental, sodium
thiopentone sodium
thiosulfatophilum, Chlorobium
third
    t. cartilaginous ring
    t. cranial nerve
    t. degree (3rd) atrioventricular (AV)
        block

t. degree burn
t. degree burns, patient sustained
t. degree heart block
t. degree sprain ▸ first, second or
t. degree uterine prolapse
t. digit of foot
t. digit of hand
t., distal
t. fibular muscle
t. filling fraction ▸ first-
t. heart sound
t. heart sound ▸ physiologic
t. intention, healing by
t., junction of distal
t., junction of middle
t., middle
t. molar
t. nerve
t. occipital nerve
t. of esophagus, carcinoma upper
t. -party payor
t. peroneal muscle
t., proximal
t. renal transplant
t. stage of labor
t. toe
t. tonsil
t. trimester bleeding
t. trimester of pregnancy
t. ventricle, floor of
t. ventricle of brain
t. ventricle of cerebrum
thirst
    t., abnormal
    t., chronic
    t. enema
    t., excessive
    t., extreme
    t. from diabetes
    t. from diuretics
    t., increased
    t., insensible
    t., real
    t., subliminal
    t., true
    t., twilight
thirsty and tired ▸ patient
thirsty, patient excessively
13 hertz (Hz), eight to
13q-deletion syndrome
13-15 syndrome, trisomy
30 contrast medium, Reno-M-
30-minute interval
32, chromic phosphate P
32^p (radioactive phosphorus)

Thixokon contrast medium
Thoma('s)
    T. ampulla
    T. fluid
    T. -Zeiss counting cell
    T. -Zeiss counting chamber
Thomas(')
    T. atrophy, Déjerine-
    T. collar
    T. cryoptor
    T. erysiphake, Dimitry-
    T. heel
    T. leg splint
    T. operation
    T. pessary
    T. shunt
    T. sign
    T. sign, André
    T. test
Thompson('s)
    T. catheter
    T. femoral head
    T. prosthesis
    T. reduction technique
    T. repair, Rose-
    T. syndrome
Thoms'
    T. flap
    T. method
    T. pelvimeter
Thomsen's disease
Thomson scattering
thoracalis, aorta
thoracenteses, multiple
thoracentesis
    t., aspirated
    t., blind
    t. chest film, post-
    t., emergency
    t., therapeutic
    t. therapy
thoracic
    t. adenopathy
    t. aneurysm
    t. angiography
    t. aorta
    t. aorta aneurysm
    t. aorta, arteriosclerotic elongation
    t. aorta, descending
    t. aorta, ectasia of
    t. aorta, elongation of
    t. aortic aneurysm, descending
    t. aortic dissection
    t. aortofemoral-femoral bypass,
        descending

thoracic—*continued*
- t. aortography
- t. arch aortography
- t. artery, internal
- t. asphyxiant dystrophy (TAD)
- t. axis
- t. cage
- t. cage, bony
- t. cancer ▸ extended dissection for
- t. cardiac nerves
- t. cavity
- t. choke
- t. cord lesion, high
- t. crisis
- t. curve
- t. diameter, anteroposterior
- t. disease
- t. drainage (dr'ge) tube
- t. duct
- t. duct, arch of
- t. duct fistula
- t. duct flow
- t. duct lymph
- t. duct pressure (TDP)
- t. dystrophy, asphyxiating
- t. dystrophy ▸ familial asphyxiant
- t. electrical bioimpedance
- t. empyema
- t. endometriosis syndrome
- t. esophageal cancer
- t. esophagus
- t. esophagus, cervical
- t. esophagus ▸ Torek resection of
- t. fine needle aspiration biopsy
- t. ganglia
- t. gas volume
- t. impedance
- t. incisure
- t. index
- t. inferior vena cava (TIVC)
- t. injury
- t. inlet
- t. laminectomy
- t. limb
- t. medical workup
- t. nerve, long
- t. nerves
- t. outlet decompression
- t. outlet syndrome
- t. outlet syndrome ▸ recurrent
- t. patch electrode, cutaneous
- t. -pelvic-phalangeal dystrophy
- t. region
- t. respiration
- t. respiratory movements

- t. roentgenogram
- t. spine
- t. spine, spurring of
- t. squeeze
- t. stomach
- t. surgery
- t. surgery, major
- t. surgery ▸ video-assisted
- t. sympathectomy
- t. syndrome, anomalous first rib
- t. vein, internal
- t. vein, lateral
- t. vertebrae (T1-T12 or D1-D12)
- t. vertebrae bones
- t. vertebral bodies
- t. vertebral column
- t. vessel
- t. viscera
- t. volume
- t. wall

thoracica, aorta
thoracicolumbar division
thoracis muscle, iliocostalis
thoracis, paracentesis
thoracoabdominal
- t. aortic aneurysm
- t. dyssynchrony
- t. paradox

thoracoacromial artery
thoracoacromial vein
thoracodorsal artery
thoracodorsal nerve
thoracoepigastric veins
thoracolumbar
- t. curve
- t. division
- t. spinal cord
- t. spine
- t. sympathectomy

thoracopagus twins
thoracoplasty
- t., complete
- t., costoversion
- t., partial
- t., Schede

thoracoscopic talc insufflation
thoracoscopy with biopsy
thoracoscopy with excision
Thoracoseal drainage
thoracostomy
- t., closed
- t., closed chest
- t., left
- t., right
- t. tube

thoracotomy
- t. changes, post-
- t., clamshell
- t., emergency
- t., exploratory
- t. incision
- t., left
- t., Lewis
- t., ▸ patient had a mini-
- t. procedure
- t., right
- t. tube in place
- t. with closed drainage (dr'ge)
- t. with exploration
- t. with open drainage (dr'ge)
- t. wound

thorascopic
- t. apical pleurectomy
- t. talc pleurodesis
- t. thymectomy ▸ video-assisted

thorax (thoraces)
- t., amazon
- t., barrel-shaped
- t., bony
- t., cholesterol
- t., frozen
- t., interspinal muscles of
- t., intertransverse muscles of
- t., left lateral
- t., longissimus muscle of
- t. paralyticus
- t., Peyrot's
- t., piriform
- t., pneumo◊
- t., pyriform
- t. resonant on percussion
- t., right lateral
- t., rotator muscles of
- t., semispinal muscle of
- t., symmetrical
- t., transverse muscle of

Thoreau's filter
Thorel pathway
Thorel's bundle
thorium
- t. dioxide (Th-O$_2$)
- t. dioxide (Th-O$_2$) contrast medium
- t. emanation
- t. tartrate contrast medium sodium

Thorn test
Thornton's nail
Thornwaldt's (*see* Tornwaldt's)
thorny-headed worm
Thorotrast contrast medium
thorough physical

Thorpe plastic lens
Th-O₂ (thorium dioxide)
thought(s)
    t. activity
    t. and compulsions ▸ persistent, intrusive
    t. and ideas ▸ senseless
    t. and recognition of information ▸ perception,
    t. and speech, confused or impoverished
    t., change in
    t., conscious
    t. content
    t., decreased capacity for abstract
    t. ▸ disconnected and racing
    t. disorder
    t. disorder, acute psychotic
    t. disorder, psychotic
    t. disorder ▸ schizophrenic
    t., distressing
    t., duplicitous
    t. field therapy
    t., flow of
    t., fragmentation of
    t., grandiose
    t., homicidal
    t., impoverished
    t., incoherent
    t., interfering
    t., intrusive
    t., irrational
    t., negative
    t., obsessional
    t. of death or suicide ▸ recurring
    t. of death ▸ recurrent
    t. of dying
    t. of self-mutilation
    t. of suicide ▸ recurrent
    t., omnipotence of
    t. pattern
    t. pattern, destructive
    t. patterns ▸ associative
    t., persistent
    t. process
    t. process, altered
    t. process, blocking of
    t. process ▸ disoriented or slow
    t. process, improved
    t. processes, alteration in
    t., racing
    t. -stopping
    t., stream of
    t., suicidal
    t., train of

    t., trend of
    t. ▸ vague obsessional
thoughtless hostility
THR (thyroid hormone replacement)
Thrassis francisi
thread(s)
    t. -elastic ligature
    t. fungus
    t. granules
    t., mucous
    t. protein level, neural
    t. protein (NTP) ▸ neural
threaded portion of nail
threading catheter into artery
thready pulse
thready ▸ pulse weak and
threat(s)
    t., drug abuse
    t., major health
    t. of physical harm
    t. of physical violence
    t. reflex
    t., suicide
    t. to self or others
threatened
    t. abortion
    t. labor
    t. miscarriage
    t. premature delivery
    t. rejection of transplant
threatening
    t. abnormal heartbeat ▸ life-
    t. allergic reaction ▸ life-
    t. and aggression ▸ physical
    t. angina ▸ life-
    t. arrhythmias, life-
    t. asthma attack ▸ life-
    t. behavior
    t. behavior ▸ problematic life-
    t. bleeding ▸ life-
    t. blood clots ▸ dissolve life-
    t. blood clots ▸ life-
    t. brain injury, life-
    t. cataracts, vision-
    t. circumstances, life-
    t. complications, life-
    t. conditions, life-
    t. crisis, life-
    t. disease, chronic life-
    t. disease, life-
    t. disease process, life-
    t. disorder, life-
    t. disorder ▸ nonlife-
    t. dose ▸ life-
    t. drug interaction ▸ life-

    t. dysrhythmias, life-
    t. emergency, life-
    t. event (ALTE), apparent life-
    t. event, life-
    t. external stimuli
    t. graft vs. host disease (GVHD) ▸ life-
    t. heart arrhythmias ▸ life-
    t. heart rhythm abnormality ▸ life-
    t. heart rhythm, life-
    t. heatstroke, life-
    t. hypertension ▸ heart
    t. illness, catastrophic life-
    t. illness, life-
    t. illness, potentially life-
    t. infection, life-
    t. infectious agent, life-
    t. injury, life-
    t. ischemia ▸ life-
    t. manifestation ▸ life-
    t. microbial contamination ▸ life-
    t., patient
    t. problem, extremity-
    t. problem, life-
    t. problem, limb-
    t. problem, potentially sight-
    t. reaction, life-
    t. respiratory complications, life-
    t. rhythm disorder, life-
    t. rhythm disturbance, life-
    t. situation, life-
    t. stroke
    t. suicide
    t. surgery, life-
    t. ventricular arrhythmia ▸ life-
    t. ventricular tachyarrhythmias ▸ life-
three (3) (III)
    3, adenovirus type
    t. -block claudication
    t. -bottle drainage system
    t. -chambered heart
    t. -channel electrocardiogram (ECG)
    3 channel Holter monitor
    t. -compartment system
    3 -D computer graphics
    t. -dimensional
    t. -dimensional analysis
    t. -dimensional computed tomographic (CT) colonography
    t. -dimensional conformal radiation therapy
    t. -dimensional echocardiography ▸ real time

three (3) (III)—*continued*
- t. -dimensional image
- t. -dimensional radiation therapy
- t. -dimensional view
- t. -dimensional x-ray images
- t. -dose distribution systems
- t. -drug combination of chemotherapy
- t. -drug protocol
- t. -drug therapy
- t. hertz (Hz) spike-and-slow waves
- 3 Holter scanner, CardioData MK
- 3 -lead electrocardiogram (ECG)
- t. -part breath
- t. -phase current
- t. -phase generator
- t. -phase system
- t. -pillow orthopnea
- t. -pillow orthopnea, two- or
- t. -point gait
- III pulse generator ‣ Programalith
- t. times a day (t.i.d.)
- t. times a week (t.i.w.)
- 3 :1 conduction, atrial flutter with
- 3 :1 heart block
- 3 :2 heart block
- t. -turn epicardial lead
- t. vein graft
- t. vessel disease
- t. -way irrigating catheter

thresher's lung

threshing fever

threshold(s)
- t., ablation
- t., activity
- t., aerobic
- t., alpha
- t. amount of asbestos exposure
- t., amplitude
- t., anaerobic
- t. and sensitivities measured and recorded
- t. angina ‣ variable
- t., anginal perceptual
- t., atrial capture
- t., atrial defibrillation
- t., capture
- t., cough
- t., energy
- t., epidemic
- t. erythema dose (TED)
- t., fibrillation
- t., flicker fusion
- t., fracture
- t. ‣ increased pain

- t., ischemic
- t., lactate
- t., lead
- t. limit value
- t., low
- t. ‣ low pain
- t., median detection
- t., median recognition
- t., nicotine
- t., nociceptive
- t. of consciousness
- t. of discomfort
- t. of sensation
- t., pacemaker
- t. ‣ pacing and sensing
- t., pain
- t. percussion
- t., risk-benefit
- t., seizure
- t., sensitivity
- t. shift, temporary
- t. (SRT) ‣ speech reception
- t., stimulation
- t., stimulus
- t. substances
- t. substances, no-
- t. sugar
- t. testing, defibrillation
- t., theoretical renal phosphorus
- t., ventilation
- t., ventilatory
- t. ‣ ventricular capture
- t., weeping
- t., work

threw an embolus ‣ patient

thrill(s)
- t. and/or friction rub
- t., aneurysmal
- t., aortic
- t., apical
- t., arterial
- t., coarse
- t., dense
- t., diastolic
- t., no palpable
- t. or murmur ‣ enlargement,
- t., palpable
- t. ‣ parasternal systolic
- t., precordial
- t., presystolic
- t., prominent
- t. purring
- t., systolic

thrive, failure to

thrive ‣ nonorganic failure to

throat
- t. abscess
- t. and problem with central nervous system ‣ strep
- t. clearing
- t. clearing from anxiety
- t., clears
- t., collapsed tissue in
- t. constriction
- t. culture
- t. discomfort, mouth and
- t., dry
- t. (ENT) ‣ ears, nose and
- t. (ENT) emergency ‣ ear, nose and
- t. flora
- t. from cancer ‣ sore
- t. from chlamydia ‣ sore
- t., gram stain of
- t. (HEENT) ‣ head, eyes, ears, nose and
- t. infection
- t. infection ‣ acute
- t. ‣ infection of mouth and
- t. inflammation
- t. injected
- t. injury
- t. irrigation tubes, salvarsan
- t. irritation
- t. irritation, acute
- t. ‣ itchy, scratchy sore
- t. lift
- t., lump in
- t. mucosa
- t., mucus in
- t. (HEENT) not remarkable ‣ head, eyes, ears, nose and
- t., obstructed
- t. ‣ pain in ear from sore
- t., patient has lump in
- t., quinsy
- t., septic sore
- t. smear
- t., sore
- t., strep
- t., streptococcal sore
- t. swab
- t. ‣ swelling of
- t., tightness in
- t. (ENT) trauma ‣ ear, nose and
- t., trench
- t., ulceration of
- t. washings

throbbing
- t. aorta

t. headache
t. headache ‣ severe
t. headache ‣ unilateral
t. neck pain
t. pain
t. pain in head
t. pain ‣ intense
t. pain ‣ severe
t., pulsating pain
Throckmorton's reflex
thrombectomy ‣ percutaneous rotational
thrombectomy, venous
thrombi, acute aortic
thrombi, intramural
thrombic thrombocytopenic purpura (TTP)
thrombin
t. clotting time
t. generation
t. soaked Gelfoam
t. time
t. time, serial
t., topical
thromboangiitis obliterans
thromboangiitis obliterans, cerebrospinal
thromboaortopathy, occlusive
thromboarteriosclerosis obliterans
thromboarteritis purulenta
thrombocytopenia
t. -absent radius
t. -absent radius syndrome
t., drug-induced
t., essential
t., heparin
t., idiopathic
t., malignant
t., precipitous
t. purpura (ATP) ‣ autoimmune
t. syndrome ‣ hemangioma
t. with absent radii (TAR)
thrombocytopenic
t. purpura
t. purpura (ITP), idiopathic
t. purpura (TTP), thrombic
t. purpura, thrombotic
thromboemboli
t., massive pulmonary
t., pulmonary
t., recurrent
thromboembolic
t. disease (TED)
t. disease, aortic
t. disease (TED) hose

t. disease, pulmonary
t. disease (TED) socks
t. disease (TED) stockings
t. disorder
t. pulmonary hypertension ‣ chronic
t. stroke
t. syndrome
thromboembolism
t., acute pulmonary
t. in liver
t. in pancreas
t. in pregnancy
t. in spleen
t., pulmonary
t., venous
thromboembolization, recent
thromboembolus, pulmonary
thromboendarterectomy, pulmonary
thromboglobulin, beta
thrombolysis
t., aortic
t. balloon valvuloplasty ‣ intracoronary
t., coronary
t. ‣ high frequency
t. ‣ selective intracoronary
thrombolytic
t. drug
t. drug, clot dissolving
t. enzymes
t. medication
thrombopenia, essential
thrombopenic anemia
thrombophlebitis
t., chronic
t., iliofemoral
t., local
t. migrans
t., migratory deep vein
t., puerperal
t., septic
t., septic pelvic
t., superficial
t., suppurative
thromboplastic substance
thromboplastin
t. antecedent (PTA) ‣ plasma
t. component (PTC) ‣ plasma
t. generation test
t. generation test, Hicks-Pitney
t. generation time
t. time (APTT), activated partial
t. time, kaolin partial
t. time ‣ partial
t. time test, partial

thrombosed
t. giant vertebral artery aneurysm
t. hemorrhoid
t. veins
thrombosis
t., acute
t. ‣ acute middle cerebral artery
t., agonal
t., aortoiliac
t., arterial
t., atrophic
t., brachial artery
t., cardiac valve
t., central splanchnic venous
t., cerebral
t., cerebral artery
t., cerebral vein
t., cerebrovascular
t., coaglation
t., compression
t., coronary
t., creeping
t., deep vein
t. (DVT) ‣ deep venous
t., dilatation
t., dilation
t., effort
t. ‣ effort-induced
t., embolic
t. ‣ femoral artery
t. ‣ femoral venous
t., graft
t. ‣ iliac vein
t., iliofemoral deep vein
t., incomplete
t., infarction of lung due to
t., infective
t. ‣ infrarenal aortic
t., intracranial
t. ‣ intracranial sinus
t., intramural
t., jumping
t., large artery
t. ‣ laser-induced
t., major arterial
t., marantic
t., marasmic
t., mesenteric arterial
t., mesenteric vein
t. ‣ mesenteric venous
t., mural
t. of artery
t. of cavernous sinus
t. of jugular bulb
t. of lateral sinus

thrombosis—*continued*
- t. of sigmoid sinus
- t. of vessels of brain
- t. ▸ ophthalmic artery
- t., peripheral
- t., placental
- t., plate
- t., platelet
- t. (PVT) ▸ portal vein
- t., propagating
- t. ▸ prosthetic valve
- t., puerperal
- t., pulmonary
- t., recanalizing
- t., renal
- t., renal vein
- t., secondary
- t., sinus
- t., subclavian
- t. syndrome, capsular
- t., transient cerebral vein
- t., traumatic
- t. traveler's
- t., vascular
- t., venous sinus

thrombotic
- t. accelerator, serum
- t. aneurysm, abdominal aorta
- t. aneurysm, acute
- t. apoplexy
- t. endocardial lesion ▸ nonbacterial
- t. endocarditis
- t. endocarditis, abacterial
- t. endocarditis, nonbacterial
- t. microangiopathy
- t. occlusion
- t. purpura
- t. stroke
- t. thrombocytopenic purpura (TTP)

thromboxane
- t. levels
- t. receptor antagonist
- t. synthesis

thrombus (thrombi)
- t., agglutinative
- t., agonal
- t., annular
- t., antemortem
- t., antemortem mural
- t., artery clogging
- t., atrial
- t., ball
- t., ball valve
- t., bile
- t., blood platelet

- t., calcified
- t., coral
- t., fibrin
- t. formation
- t., globular
- t. grade
- t., hyaline
- t. in vessels of heart ▸ multiple
- t., infective
- t., intracardiac
- t., intravascular
- t., Laennec's
- t., laminated
- t., lateral
- t., marantic
- t., marasmic
- t., migratory
- t., mixed
- t., mural
- t., obstructive
- t., occluding
- t., occlusive
- t. of basilar artery, organizing
- t., organized
- t., pale
- t., parietal
- t., pedunculated
- t., plate
- t., platelet
- t., postmortem
- t. precursor protein
- t., primary
- t., progressive
- t., propagated
- t., red
- t. ▸ right atrial (RA)
- t., saddle
- t., secondary
- t., straddling
- t., stratified
- t., superimposed
- t., traumatic
- t., valvular
- t., vascular
- t., ventricular
- t., white

through
- t. -and-through avulsion injury
- t. -and-through myocardial infarction
- t. -and-through sutures
- t. angina ▸ walk-
- t., break◊
- t., clinical follow-
- t. drainage (dr'ge)

- t. esophagus into stomach, barium passed
- t. fifth digits of hand ▸ first
- t. fifth shock count ▸ second
- t. gait, swing-
- t. illumination
- t. incision, forceps passed up
- t. mammography, early detection
- t. myocardial infarction ▸ through-and-
- t. procedure, Soave abdominal pull-
- t. procedure, Swenson pull-
- t. scar of uterus, rupture
- t. 6 murmur ▸ Grade 1
- t. (SBFT), small bowel follow-
- t. stab wound ▸ drain brought out
- t. -the-wall mattress suture
- t. vocal cords with ease ▸ bronchoscope inserted
- t. wall of cavity, incision
- t., working
- t. wound, tissue brought out

throughout serosa ▸ tumor metastases

**thrower fracture, grenade-
thrust**
- t., abdominal
- t. breast heart
- t., cardiac
- t. culture
- t. maneuver ▸ jaw
- t. of apex of heart
- t., quick upward

**Thrusters (amphetamines)
thrusting, tongue-
thumb(s)**
- t. abduction
- t., adductor muscle of
- t., basal joint of
- t., base of
- t., bifid
- t., broad
- t., cortical
- t. finger
- t. fracture
- t. fracture, gamekeeper's
- t. joint swollen and inflamed
- t., long abductor muscle of
- t., long extensor muscle of
- t., long flexor muscle of
- t. mobility
- t., opposing muscle of
- t. pad
- t. reflex, finger-
- t. release ▸ trigger

t., short abductor muscle of
t., short extensor muscle of
t., short flexor muscle of
t. sign ▸ Steinberg
t. spica
t. splint, Lewin-Stern
t. stroking maneuver during massage
t. sucking
t. -sucking appliance
t. sucking ▸ prolonged
t., tennis
t. transplant, toe-to-
t., trigger
t. twitch
thumbnail test
thumbprint bronchus sign
thumbprinted in delivery room, mother
thump, chest
thump, precordial
Thunberg tube
thunderclap headache
Thygeson's keratitis
thymectomy ▸ video-assisted thorascopic
thymectomy/thymusectomy
thymic
t. agenesis
t. aplasia
t. asthma
t. cyst
t. depletion
t. dysplasia
t. dysplasia, congenital
t. humoral factor
t. lymphocyte antigen
t. nodules, accessory
t. -parathyroid aplasia
t. radiation therapy
t. tumor
t. vein
thymicolymphaticus, status
thymidine
t. (AZT), azido-
t. dependent strain
t. monophosphate
t. triphosphate
t., tritiated
thymocyte depletion
thymocytes, human
thymol flocculation
thymol turbidity test
thymoma, invasive
thymoma, noninvasive

thymopriva, cachexia
thymus
t. and mediastinal fat
t. and mediastinal fat ▸ indentation for
t. antiserum, human
t. barrier, blood
t. -dependent
t. dependent antigen
t. dependent cells
t. gland
t. gland function
t. gland, removal of
t. independent antigen
t., lobules of
t., lymphoepithelioma of
t. retractor
thyroarytenoid muscle
thyroarytenoid muscle, internal
thyrocalcitonin test
thyrocardiac disease
thyroepiglottic ligament
thyroepiglottic muscle
thyroglossal
t. cyst
t. duct
t. duct cyst
thyrohyoid
t. arch
t. laryngotomy
t. ligament
t. membrane
t. muscle
thyroid [*fibroid, euthyroid*]
t., aberrant
t. abscess
t., accessory
t. acini
t. activity ▸ abnormal
t. activity, increased
t. adenoma
t. adenoma, calcified
t. antibodies
t. artery
t. artery ▸ superior
t., benign granuloma of
t. binding index (TBI)
t., blood
t. bruit
t. cachexia
t. cancer
t. carcinoma
t. carcinoma ▸ ossified papillary
t. carcinoma, papillary
t. cartilage

t. ▸ colloid nodules of
t. congested
t. deficiency
t. deficient dwarf
t., desiccated
t., diffusely enlarged
t. disease
t. disease, primary
t. disease ▸ undiagnosed
t. disorder
t. disorder, overactive
t. diverticulum
t. does not appear enlarged
t. drain
t. dysfunction
t. dyshormonogenesis
t., enlarged
t. extract
t. eye disease
t. failure ▸ mild
t. function
t. function ▸ low
t. function profile
t. function reaction
t. function study
t. function test
t. gland
t. gland activity
t. gland ▸ excessive activity of
t. gland, inferior
t. gland, levator muscle of
t. gland, lobules of
t. gland, multinodular
t. gland, overactive
t. gland, superior
t. gland, underactive
t. hormone
t. hormone production
t. hormone replacement (THR)
t. hormone resistance
t. hormone, synthetic
t. hormone treatment
t., hyperactive
t. imaging, fluorescent
t. imaging, radionuclide
t. insufficiency
t. intoxication
t., intrathoracic
t. isthmus
t., lingual
t., lobe of
t. malfunction
t. mass causing obstruction
t. medication ▸ synthetic
t. ▸ medullary carcinoma of

thyroid—*continued*
- t. ‣ metastases to the
- t., multinodular
- t. nodule
- t. nodule ablation
- t. nodule, cancerous
- t. nodule, malignant
- t., nonpalpable
- t. notch
- t. notch, inferior
- t. notch, superior
- t., overactive
- t. palpable
- t. panel
- t. profile
- t. ratio (ETR) ‣ estimated
- t. region
- t., residual nodular
- t., retrosternal
- t. scan
- t. screening
- t. secretion ‣ insufficiency of
- t. stimulant, long-acting
- t. -stimulating hormone (TSH)
- t. -stimulating (LATS) hormone, long-acting
- t. stimulator, long-acting
- t. storm
- t. studies
- t., substernal
- t. therapy
- t. tissue
- t. tissue, ectopic
- t. to serum ratio
- t. tumor
- t. tumor, anaplastic
- t. tumor, benign
- t. tumor, malignant
- t. tumor ‣ removal of benign
- t., underactive
- t. uptake scans
- t. vein, inferior
- t. vein, middle
- t. vein, superior

thyroidal hernia
thyroidal lymph node scintigraphy
thyroidectomy
- t., medical
- t., partial
- t., total

thyroiditis
- t., acute
- t., chronic
- t., chronic lymphocytic
- t., de Quervain's

- t., giant cell
- t., giant follicular
- t., granulomatous
- t., Hashimoto's
- t., invasive
- t., ligneous
- t., lymphocytic
- t., lymphoid
- t. ‣ nonspecific chronic lymphocytic
- t., Riedel's
- t., subacute diffuse
- t. with tenderness ‣ acute
- t., woody

thyroidization, severe
thyromegaly, palpable
thyroneural dystrophy
thyropharyngeal muscle
thyroplasty surgery
thyroprival tetany
thyrotoxic
- t. cardiopathy
- t. goiter
- t. heart disease

thyrotropic hormone
thyrotropin-releasing hormone response
thyroxin/thyroxine
- t. binding globulin
- t. binding globulin ‣ unbound
- t. binding index (TBI) test
- t. binding protein
- t., blood
- t., extrathyroidal
- t., free
- t. index (FTI) ‣ free
- t. level, normalize
- t. level, serum
- t. (PBT) ‣ protein-bound
- t. shock
- t. specific activity
- t. (TT) ‣ total

Ti (TI)
- Ti (titanium)
- TI (tricuspid incompetence)
- TI (tricuspid insufficiency)
- Ti -Cron suture

TIA (transient ischemic attack)
TIBC (total iron-binding capacity)
tibia
- t. bone
- t. enchondroma
- t., lengthening
- t. ‣ medial malleolus of
- t., medullary nailing of
- t., proximal

- t., saber
- t. valga
- t. vara

tibial
- t. artery
- t. artery, anterior
- t. artery, posterior
- t. bypass ‣ femoral
- t. bypass vein graft ‣ popliteal
- t. compartment, anterior
- t. compartment syndrome, anterior
- t. condyle
- t. crest palpated
- t. cuff, long leg brace with large
- t. dysfunction, posterior
- t. fracture, comminuted
- t. fracture site
- t. fracture site, comminuted
- t. graft
- t. lymph nodes, anterior
- t. malleolus
- t. muscle
- t. muscle, anterior
- t. muscle, posterior
- t. nerve
- t. perforator, mid◇
- t. -peroneal bypass ‣ femoral-
- t. plateau
- t. plateau fracture
- t. plateau, lateral
- t. plateau prosthesis, MacIntosh
- t. prosthesis
- t. pulse
- t. pulse, posterior
- t. shaft
- t. sign, anterior
- t. spine
- t. stress reaction
- t. tendon ‣ posterior
- t. tendon ‣ rupture of
- t. torsion
- t. tubercle
- t. vein, anterior
- t. vein, posterior

tibialis
- t., anterior
- t. muscle
- t. sign

tibiarum, anxietas
tibioadductor reflex
tibiofibular
- t. articulation
- t. joint
- t. mortise
- t. syndesmosis

tibioperoneal trunk angioma
tibioperoneal vessel angioplasty
tic(s) (Tic)
- t. and fasciculations ▸ tremors,
- t. and twitches
- t., bowing
- t. chorea
- t. ▸ chronic facial
- t., complex
- t., compulsive
- t., convulsive
- t. de Guinon
- t. de pensée
- t. de sommeil
- t., degenerative
- t., diaphragmatic
- t. disorder
- t. disorder, chronic motor
- t. disorder, chronic motor or vocal
- t. disorder of childhood, transient
- t. disorder, transient
- t. douloureux
- t. douloureux ▸ dizziness from
- t. douloureux, feigned
- t., facial
- t., generalized degenerative
- t., gesticulatory
- t. ▸ involuntary motor
- t. ▸ involuntary verbal
- t., laryngeal
- t., local
- t., localized degenerative
- t., mimic
- t., motor
- t., nervous
- t., nondouloureux
- t., occupation
- t., progressive choreic
- t., respiratory
- t., rotatory
- t., saltatory
- t. ▸ simple motor
- t., spasmodic
- T. Tac (hallucinogen)
- t. -tac rhythm
- t. ▸ transient motor
- t., verbal

tick
- t. bite
- t. -borne encephalitis
- t. -borne encephalitis virus
- t. -borne illness
- t. -borne viruses
- t. fever
- t. fever, Colombian
- t. fever, South African
- t. fever virus, Colorado
- t., hard
- t. paralysis
- t., soft
- t. -tack sounds
- t. typhus, African
- t. typhus, Indian
- t. typhus ▸ Queensland
- t. typhus, South African
- t., watch

t.i.d. [*b.i.d.*] (three times a day)
tidal
- t. air
- t. carbon dioxide (ETCO$_2$) ▸ end-
- t. drainage (dr'ge)
- t. drainage system
- t. ▸ end-
- t. inspiratory flow ▸ peak
- t. volume
- t. wave
- t. wave pulse

tie(s)
- t. at birth ▸ tongue-
- t., breast tissue approximated with
- t., hemostasis secured with
- t. of chromic catgut
- t. -over graft, bolus
- t. -over-stent
- t. suture, stick-
- t., tongue-

tied
- t., bleeders clamped and
- t. ▸ clamped, divided and
- t. down over cotton, sutures
- t. over rubber shoes, sutures
- t., perforators
- t., sutures

Tiedemann's nerve
tiered-therapy antiarrhythmic device
Tietze's syndrome
tiger heart
tiger lily heart
tight
- t. bladder neck
- t. calf muscles
- t. feeling in head
- t. junction
- t., knotted muscles
- t. muscles
- t. seal over victim's mouth
- t. sensation in chest
- t. sphincter
- t. stenosis

tightened fascia

tightened, tourniquet
tightening
- t. face-lift ▸ skin-
- t. of eyelid
- t., tummy

tightly [*slightly*]
tightness
- t. capsular
- t., chest
- t., chest pain and
- t. in chest ▸ feeling of
- t. in throat
- t., muscle
- t., muscular
- t. of hamstring
- t., tendon

tiglium, Croton
tigre, fundus
tigroid
- t. fundus
- t. masses
- t. retina
- t. striation
- t. substance

TIL (tumor infiltrating lymphocytes)
TIL (tumor infiltrating lymphocytes) ▸ genetically altered
TIL (tumor infiltrating lymphocytes) technique
Tillaux, fracture of
tilt
- t. and chin lift maneuver ▸ head
- t., chin
- t., dorsal
- t. exercise, pelvic
- t., head
- t., head tilt with chin
- t., lateral
- t. method ▸ head
- t. -table test
- t. -table test ▸ head up
- t. -table test ▸ isoproterenol
- t., talar
- t. test, head
- t. test ▸ head down
- t. with chin lift, head
- t. with neck lift, head

tilting
- t. disk aortic valve prosthesis
- t. disk prosthetic valve
- t. disk valve prosthesis ▸ Medtronic-Hall
- t. disk valve prosthesis ▸ Omniscience
- t., head

timber tongue
Timberlake obturator
time(s)
t. a day (q.i.d.) ▸ four
t. a day (t.i.d.) ▸ three
t. a day (b.i.d.) ▸ two
t. a week (t.i.w.) ▸ three
t., acceleration
t., access
t., acquisition
t., activated clotting
t., activated coagulation
t. (APTT), activated partial thromboplastin
t. activities ▸ leisure-
t. activity curve
t., analyzer
t. and distance, poor perception of
t. and perception ▸ distorted sense of
t. and persons ▸ patient alert to space,
t. and place, confusion about
t. and space ▸ disorientation of
t. and space ▸ distortion of
t., aspirin tolerance
t., atrioventricular (AV)
t. -averaged peak velocity
t. axis
t., bleeding
t., blood clot lysis
t., blood coagulation
t., bypass
t., carotid ejection
t., cell cycle
t., charge
t., cinedensitometric assessment of transit
t., cinedensitometric transit
t., circulation
t., clot lysis
t., clot retraction
t., clotting
t., coagulation
t. compensation gain
t. constant
t. constant control
t., contraction
t., corrected sinus node recovery
t., crest
t., cross-clamp
t., curve ▸ volume
t. -cycled ventilation
t., Dale-Laidlaw's clotting
t., dead

t., deceleration
t. delay
t. dependent
t., detect
t., dialysis
t. diffusion technique
t. ▸ disorientation in place and
t. distortion
t. ▸ disturbed sense of
t. domain
t. domain analysis
t. domain signal averaged electrocardiogram (ECG)
t. ▸ donor organ ischemic
t., dose, fractionation (TDF) factor
t., doubling
t., down
t. ▸ echo delay
t., ejection
t., emptying
t., erythrocyte survival
t., esophageal transit
t., euglobulin clot lysis
t., euglobulin lysis
t., exercise
t. ▸ exercise treadmill
t., external clock
t., fixing
t., flushing
t. (FET) ▸ forced expiratory
t. frame of death, Kübler-Ross
t. -gain compensation
t. -gain control
t., gastric emptying
t., gastric emptying half-
t., generation
t., generosity of
t., helium equilibration
t. in lung carcinoma, tumor doubling
t. index, diastolic pressure
t. index ▸ relaxation
t. index ▸ systolic pressure
t. index ▸ tension-
t. interval
t. interval between doses
t. interval (MTI) ▸ minimum
t. interval ▸ right ventricular (RV) systolic
t. interval ▸ systolic
t. ▸ intra-atrial conduction
t., ischemic
t., isovolumic contraction
t. ▸ isovolumic relaxation
t., Ivy's method bleeding

t., kaolin partial thromboplastin
t., lag
t. lapse
t. (LVET) ▸ left ventricular ejection
t. -limited separation ▸ realistic
t. ▸ loss of sense of
t., lysis
t. ▸ magnetic relaxation
t. management skills
t. marker
t. ▸ maximum walking
t. (MCT) ▸ mean circulation
t., mean survival
t., median survival
t. method ▸ half-
t. method, Lee-White clotting
t. motion (TM)
t., movement
t. ▸ myocardial transit
t., nondialysis
t., occlusion
t. of arrival (ETA), estimated
t. of barium, transient
t. of birth
t. of death
t. of death, family present at
t. of demise, family present at
t. of exchange, half-
t. of last food/fluids
t. -of-flight angiography
t. -out technique
t. ▸ pacemaker lag
t. ▸ pain-free walking
t. ▸ partial thromboplastin
t. particle transport
t. patient expired
t. ▸ patient oriented as to person, place and
t., percent
t. perception, alteration in
t. perception, altered
t. perception distorted
t., place and person ▸ oriented to
t., plasma iron disappearance
t., predetermined intervals of
t., pre-ejection
t. ▸ pressure half-
t., prothrombin (Pro)
t. ▸ quick prothrombin
t., reaction
t., read
t., recovery
t., recuperation
t., relaxation
t. -released

t. (RT), repetition
t., resolving
t., response
t., reversal
t. (RVET) ▸ right ventricular ejection
t., rise
t., saturation
t., scalar
t. sense
t., serial thrombin
t. ▸ sinoatrial (SA) conduction
t. ▸ sinoatrial (SA) recovery
t., sinus node recovery
t., slowed reaction
t. ▸ spin-lattice
t. ▸ spin-spin
t., stance
t. ▸ streptokinase clot lysis
t. studies ▸ transient
t., survival
t., systolic ejection
t. technique ▸ pressure half-
t., template bleeding
t. -tension index (TTI)
t. test, arm-tongue
t. test, partial thromboplastin
t. three-dimensional echocardiography ▸ real
t., thrombin
t., thrombin clotting
t., thromboplastin generation
t. (TOT) ▸ tincture of
t. to sustained respiration ▸ prolonged
t. -to-peak contrast
t. (TT) ▸ total
t., total labor
t., total sleep
t. -to-treatment bias
t., transit
t. ▸ transmitral E wave deceleration
t. ▸ T2 relaxation
t., tumor doubling
t. ultrasonography ▸ real-
t. ultrasound ▸ real-
t. urination ▸ frequent night-
t. varied gain
t. -varied gain control
t., ventilator
t. ▸ ventricular activation
t. ▸ viral shedding
t., wake
t., workout
t., write

timed
  t. Achilles tendon reflex
  t. contractions
  t. forced expiratory volume
  t. vital capacity (VC)
timely admissions
timing ▸ stress control and
timori, Brugia
timothy bacillus
tincture [*cincture*]
tincture of opium
tincture of time (TOT)
tine
  t. test
  t. test for tuberculosis
  t. tuberculin test
tinea [*tenia*]
  t. capitis
  t. corporis
  t. cruris
  t. pedis
  t. versicolor
Tinel's sign
tinge to lips and nailbeds, blue
tinge to skin, bluish
tinged
  t. fluid ▸ blood
  t., fluid content blood
  t. froth ▸ blood
  t. mucoid material ▸ blood
  t. sputum ▸ blood
  t. sputum ▸ pinkish blood
  t. stools ▸ blood
  t. urine ▸ blood
tingle, feet
tingling
  t. and burning ▸ numbness,
  t. and burning sensation
  t. and numbness in feet
  t. and pain ▸ numbness,
  t. around mouth ▸ numbness and
  t., blood
  t. in arm
  t. in fingers ▸ numbness and
  t. in hands and feet
  t., numbness and
  t., numbness and weakness
  t. of fingers
  t. of fingertips
  t. on percussion (DTP) ▸ distal
  t. or numbness in extremities
  t. or numbness in feet
  t. or numbness ▸ localized
  t. or prickling sensation
  t. or prickly feeling ▸ burning,

t. or stiffness ▸ feeling of
t. or weakness ▸ numbness,
t. pain
t., prickling, or numbness
t. sensation
t. sensation in extremity
t. sensation in feet
t. sensation in fingertips
t. sensation in hands
t. sensation in mouth
t. sensation ▸ painful,
t., transient
tinkle, Bouillaud's
tinkle, metallic
tinnitus
  t. and aging
  t. aurium
  t., bilateral
  t., chronic
  t. ▸ deafness, vertigo and
  t., deafness with
  t. from anxiety
  t. from aspirin
  t. from diabetes
  t. from diuretics
  t., mild
  t., objective
  t., persistent
  t., pulsatile
  t. ▸ roaring unilateral
  t., severe
  t. ▸ severe chronic
  t., subjective
  t., temporary
  t., tonal
Tinospora cordifolia
tiny bones
tiny bronchioles lack cartilage
tip(s)
  t. angle
  t., aspirating
  t., broken catheter
  t. catheter ▸ olive
  t. catheter ▸ spiral
  t. catheter ▸ whistle-
  t. cautery ▸ nasal
  t. culture ▸ catheter
  t., diathermy
  t. drain ▸ whistle-
  t. electrode ▸ ball
  t. electrode ▸ bayonet
  t. electrode ▸ conical
  t., laser
  t. laser ▸ cool
  t. laser probe ▸ hot

tip(s)—*continued*
- t. lead, barb-
- t. of acromion
- t. of cecum ‣ distal
- t. of coracoid process drilled
- t. of malleolus
- t. of tongue
- t. ‣ papillary muscle
- t., petrous
- t., retained root
- t. spasm, catheter-
- t., spleen

tipped
- t. bougie ‣ acorn-
- t. catheter ‣ acorn-
- t. uterus

tire implant

tired
- t., aching feet
- t. and irritated
- t. eyes
- t. feeling ‣ listless and
- t. ‣ patient thirsty and

tiredness
- t., excessive
- t., extreme
- t., limb
- t., physical

tissue(s) (Tissue)
- t. ‣ aberrant endometrial
- t. ablation
- t. ablation, incision, and excision
- t., abnormal
- t., abnormal brain
- t. ‣ abnormal development of scar
- t., abnormal fatty
- t., abnormal residual
- t. abnormality, liver
- t. abscess, soft
- t. absorption by radiation
- t., accidental
- t., active brain
- t., acute responding vs late responding
- t., adenoid
- t. adhesive
- t. adhesive ‣ polymerizing
- t., adipose
- t., adjacent
- t., adrenal
- t., adrenogenic
- t., adventitial
- t. aging ‣ musculoskeletal soft
- t. air ratio
- t., analogous

- t., analyzing surgical
- t. and bone disease
- t., antibiotic concentration in serum and
- t., aortic
- t., appendiceal
- t. appendix, lymph
- t. approximate, subcutaneous
- t. approximated with ties, breast
- t., areolar
- t., areolar connective
- t. arm ‣ dissected
- t. ‣ arthroscopic release of scar
- t. atelectatic, lung
- t., atrial
- t., atrioventricular (AV) conduction
- t., atrophy of acinar
- t., atrophy of glandular
- t., atrophy of muscular
- t. attenuation and scattering
- t. augmentation ‣ soft
- t., authorization form for operation and grafting of
- t., autodigestion of connective
- t., autodigestion of pancreatic
- t., autolysis of pancreatic
- t., avascular
- t., bacterial contamination of
- t. band
- t., band of scar
- T. Bank
- t. bank ‣ registry and
- t., banking, cryopreserved
- t., banking, ovarian
- t., basement
- t. bed
- t., benign lesion of soft
- t. ‣ biologically engineered
- t. biopsy
- t., bleeding into brain
- t., blood
- t., blood forming
- t., blood supply to
- t., blood-starved heart muscle
- t., body
- t., bone
- t., bony
- t., brain
- t. breakdown
- t. breakdown ‣ gum
- t., breast
- t., bronchial
- t. brought out through wound
- t., brown fat
- t., bruised

- t., bruised brain
- t., build up of scar
- t. burn
- t., burn healthy
- t., burn off
- t., bursal equivalent
- t. calcification, soft
- t., cancellous
- t. cancer ‣ soft
- t., cancerous
- t. carcinoma, soft
- t., cartilaginous
- t., caseated
- t., cauterized
- t., cavernous
- t. cell, connective
- t. cells
- t. cells, embryonal connective
- t. cells, fixed-
- t. cells, flattened
- t. cells ‣ invasive breast
- t. cells ‣ normal breast
- t., cervical stromal
- t. change
- t. changes ‣ pre-malignant
- t., charred
- t., chondroid
- t., chordal
- t., chorionic
- t., chromaffin
- t., cicatricial
- t. closed, subcutaneous
- t., coagulate
- t., coagulation of
- t. coding factor
- t., collar of
- t., compact
- t. compression injury, soft
- t. ‣ compression of pulmonary
- t. concentration ‣ prolonged
- t. congested, lung
- t., connective
- t., consent form for operation and grafting of
- t. considerations in radiation therapy, normal
- t. ‣ constricted by scar
- t. consultation
- t., corneal
- t., cortical
- t., crescent-shaped flap of
- t., cribriform
- t. culture
- t. culture cells
- t. culture dose

t. culture dose, median
t. culture, infected
t. culture infective dose, median
t. culture medium
t. culture studies
t. culture technique
t., cultured brain
t. damage
t. damage, actual
t. damage, potential
t. damage, soft
t. ▸ damage to healthy
t., damaged brain
t. ▸ damaged connective
t. damaging factor
t., dartoid
t., dead
t. death
t., death of brain
t., death of heart muscle
t., debridement of bruised
t., debridement of necrotic
t., decidual
t., deciduous
t., deep bites of
t., degenerated
t. degenerates ▸ brain
t., degenerating decidual
t. ▸ dense breast
t., dense collagenous
t., dense fibrous
t. density, abdominal soft
t., dermal
t., destroy
t., destroy healthy
t. ▸ destroyed brain
t., destroyed nasal
t. destruction ▸ fever, swelling and
t., destruction of
t. detachment ▸ scar
t. ▸ deterioration of bone
t., devitalized
t. diagnosis
t. ▸ diffuse scar
t. disease, connective
t. disease ▸ degenerated
t. disease (MCTD) ▸ mixed
    connective
t. disease ▸ secondary connective
t., diseased
t., diseased cardiac
t., disfigured
t. disintegration
t. disorder, chronic connective
t. disorder ▸ genetic connective

t. disorders, connective
t. ▸ distorted brain
t., distribution of donor organs and
t. donated
t. donation
t. donation study
t., donor
t. Doppler imaging
t. dose
t., dose limiting
t. -eating toxin
t. ecchymosis, soft
t., ectopic thyroid
t. effects of dose fractionation,
    normal
t., elastic
t., elastic connective
t., elastic soft
t., endometrial
t., endothelial
t. ▸ enlargement of lymphadenoid
t., envelope of
t., eosinophilic endometrial
t., episcleral
t., epithelial
t., epivaginal connective
t., equal bites of
t. equivalent
t. -equivalent detector
t., erectile
t. ▸ eroding gum
t. evacuated
t. examination
t. examination, pathological
t., excess fluid in
t., excess hemorrhoidal
t. ▸ excess prostate
t., exocrine
t. expander, breast
t. expanders
t. expansion
t. extenders
t., extracellular
t. extract, adipose
t. extruding at cervical os
t., eye
t., eyelid
t., facial
t. factor
t., fat
t., fatty
t. FB (foreign body) ▸ soft
t., fetal
t., fibrinous
t., fibroadipose

t., fibrofatty
t., fibrohyaline
t., fibrolipomatous
t., fibrosarcoma of soft
t., fibrous
t., fibrous connective
t. ▸ fibrous scar
t., firm
t., flap of
t., flap of abdominal
t. flap transplanted
t. ▸ flexible scar
t. fluid
t., fluid in body
t. for grafting ▸ authorization form
    for removal of
t. for grafting ▸ consent form for
    removal of
t., foreign
t. foreign body (FB) soft
t. formation, fibrous
t. ▸ formation of fibrous or scar
t. formation ▸ scar
t. ▸ fragments of endometrial
t. ▸ fragments of medial
t., fresh corneal
t., fresh granulation
t., friable necrotic
t., frozen corneal
t., functional subunit
t. ▸ functioning of normal epithelial
t., Gamgee
t., gelatiginous
t., gelatinous
t., glandular
t. ▸ gradual loss of bone
t. graft
t., granulated
t., granulation
t., grayish
t. growth
t. growth, abnormal mass of
t., gum
t. (GALT) ▸ gut-associated
    lymphoid
t., hardened
t., hardening of breast
t. harvest
t. health ▸ analyzes
t., healthy
t., heart
t. ▸ heart muscle
t. hematoma, soft
t., hematopoietic
t. hemorrhage into mesentery ▸ soft

tissue(s)—*continued*

t. hemorrhage, recent soft
t. hemorrhage, soft
t., heterologous
t., heterotopic
t. ▸ His-Purkinje
t. histidine
t., histiocytoma of soft
t., homologous
t., human
t., hyalin fibrotic
t., hyalinized fibrous
t., hylic
t., hypergranulation
t., hyperplastic
t. imaging, Doppler
t., immobile
t. immunity
t. impassable scar
t. implants ▸ brain
t. in os
t. in paraffin block ▸ embedded
t. in throat ▸ collapsed
t., indifferent
t., induration of
t., infected
t. ▸ infected lung
t. ▸ infection in leg
t. infection, soft
t. ▸ inflamed airway
t. ▸ inflamed synovial
t., inflammation of biopsy
t., inflammation of connective
t., inflammation of vaginal
t. inflammation ▸ persistent
t., inflammatory
t., injured
t. injury
t., injury, soft
t., innocent appearing
t., intact
t. integrity ▸ impaired
t. interaction ▸ laser
t. ▸ interfascicular fibrous
t., internal scar
t., interstitial
t., intertubular
t., intervening
t., intestinal
t., intracranial calcification benign
    glandular
t., intravesical prostatic
t. invasion
t. invasion ▸ soft
t. involvement, soft

t. irritant, lung
t. irritation, localized
t., ischemic
t., isodense with surrounding
t., joint
t., junctional
t., kidney
t., Kuhnt's intermediary
t., laceration, soft
t., lardaceous
t., laser destroyed
t., laser excess
t., laser vaporized
t. ▸ layer of connective
t. layers, soft
t., leiomyosarcoma of soft
t., lepidic
t. level
t. lining ▸ repeated stress to
t. lining ▸ swollen
t., liposarcoma of soft
t., liver
t., living mammalian
t. ▸ long fronds of connective
t., loose connective
t. loss
t. loss ▸ soft
t., lost muscle
t., lung
t., lymphadenoid
t., lymphatic
t., lymphoid
t. macrophages
t. maintenance ▸ inadequate
t., malignant
t., marrow
t. mass
t. mass ▸ abnormal
t. mass ▸ soft
t. massage ▸ deep
t. massage ▸ soft
t. massage therapist ▸ deep
t. massage therapy ▸ deep
t., massive scar
t. match
t. match, blood and
t. material
t. maximum ratio
t., mediastinal fatty
t., membranous
t., mesenchymal
t. ▸ metabolically active
t., metanephrogenic
t. metastases, soft
t. microcirculation, normal

t., mobile
t., mucous
t., multicellular
t., muscle
t. muscle pain ▸ soft
t., muscular
t., myeloid
t., myocardial
t., myxomatous
t., myxomatous soft connective
t., nasal
t., nasopharyngeal
t. necrosis
t. ▸ necrosis of brain
t. ▸ necrosis of pancreatic
t., necrotic
t., necrotic decidual
t., necrotic gangrenous
t., necrotic kidney
t. ▸ necrotic lung
t., necrotic pancreatic
t., necrotic placental
t. negative for malignancy
t., neighboring
t., nephrogenic
t., nerve
t., nervous
t., neural
t., nodal
t., nodular growth of
t., nonmalignant
t. ▸ nonpumping scar
t., nonviable
t., normal
t., normal brain
t., normal immature brain
t., ocular
t. of brain, supporting
t. of face, soft
t. of myocardium ▸ striated
    muscular
t. of prostatic origin
t., oral
t. ▸ organs, corneas and
t., osseous
t., osteogenic
t., osteoid
t., overgrowth of interacinar
    connective
t. ▸ overgrowth of non-nervous
    supportive
t. ▸ oxidative process in
t. oxygen
t. oxygenation
t. ▸ oxygen-starved

t., pancreatic
t., parasternal
t., parathyroid
t., parenchymatous
t., passage of
t. pedicle
t. perfusion, alteration
t. perfusion, altered cerebral
t. perfusion, altered renal
t., perfusion of
t., periarticular soft
t., peribronchiolar connective
t., perineal
t., perinodal
t., periodontal
t., periorbital soft
t., perirenal
t. phantom ratio
t., placental
t. plasminogen activation (TPA)
t. plasminogen activator (TPA) infusion
t., polypoid
t. ▸ porcine pericardial
t., portal connective
t., postirradiation necrotic
t., postmortem
t., postnecrotic
t. prepared for microsection
t. preservation
t. preservation of donor organs and
t., primitive pulp
t. procurement
t. procurement of donor organs and
t. procurement, organ-
t., progressive growth of
t., prostate
t., prostatic
t., radiation treatment of glandular
t. radiobiology
t. reapproximated, subcutaneous
t. reconnected
t. reconstruction of breast
t. recovery, organ-
t., recreating heart
t., redundant
t. regeneration
t. regeneration, accelerated
t., regrowth, excess
t., regrowth, nerve
t. rejection
t., rejection of transplanted
t. removal sample of
t. removed for pathological examination

t., renal
t. repair
t. repair ▸ gastrointestinal (GI) tract
t. repair ▸ inadequate
t. reperfusion ▸ ischemic
t., replacement
t. replacement of lung
t., replica of donor
t. reposition
t. research
t. resected, estimated
t., residual
t., residual lymphoid
t., residual necrotic
t. respiration
t., retained placental
t., reticular fibers of connective
t., reticulated
t., retinal
t., revision of scar
t. rhabdomyosarcoma of soft
t. rheumatism, soft
t. roentgenography, soft
t., rubber
t. samples
t. sarcoma, soft
t. sarcoma, tendosynovial
t. saturation point
t., scar
t., scarred connective
t. scarring
t., scarring of breast
t., scarring of lung
t. scarring or cirrhosis
t., sclerous
t., sculpt
t. separation
t., septal connective
t. sera, anti-
t. ▸ serum bactericidal
t., shadow, soft
t. sheath, connective
t., shock
t. shreds
t., shrinkage ▸ age-related
t., shrinkage of
t., silver staining of
t., skeletal
t., skin
t. sloughing, dead
t. small button of vein
t., soft
t., soft oral
t. ▸ soft, spongy, semi-liquid
t. spaces

t. spaces, intercellular
t. specific antigen
t. specimen, diseased
t. specimens
t. specimens sent to lab
t., spinal
t. ▸ spinal cord
t., splenic
t., spongy
t., spontaneous passage of
t. stained, healthy
t. stains, connective
t. stalk, connective
t. strands of
t. stretching
t., subcutaneous
t., subcutaneous adipose
t., subcutaneous connective
t. submitted for frozen section
t. submitted to pathologist
t., submucosal connective
t., superficial bites of
t., supportive
t., surface
t., surgical recovery of donated organs and
t., surrounding
t., surrounding breast
t., suspicious
t., sustentacular
t. swelling ▸ abnormal
t. ▸ swelling of body
t., swelling of wall
t. swelling, reduce
t. swelling ▸ soft
t., swollen
t., symplastic
t., taken, biopsies of
t., target
t., targeted
t. tension
t., thick elastic
t., thickened connective
t. thinning ▸ vaginal
t., thyroid
t. to affected area ▸ restore
t., tolerance dose (TTD)
t., tonsillar
t., transparent
t. transplant
t. transplant ▸ adrenal gland
t. transplant ▸ animal
t. transplant, corneal
t. transplant ▸ fetal
t. transplantation

tissue(s)—*continued*
- t., transplanted
- t., transplanting human fetal
- t. transport
- t. ▸ transurethral vaporization of prostate
- t. trauma
- t., trimmed torn
- t., trophoblastic
- t., tuberculosis granulation
- t. tumor
- t. tumor, placental
- t. tumor, soft
- t. tumors, mixed
- t. turgor
- t. turgor, good
- t. typing
- t. -typing laboratories, transplant
- T. Typing Laboratory
- t. typing technician
- t., underlying
- t. ▸ underlying connective
- t. ▸ underlying fatty
- t., uterine
- t., uterine lining
- t., vaginal
- t. ▸ vagrant endometrial
- t. valve
- t., vaporize
- t. ▸ vaporized hemorrhoidal
- t., vaporizing diseased
- t., vascular
- t., vascular granulation
- t. ▸ vascular intermediate
- t. ▸ vascular poor
- t. ▸ vascular rich
- t., vesicular supporting
- t. viability, muscle
- t., viable
- t. vibration
- t., vital
- t. wall ▸ weakened
- t. wasting
- t. water pressure
- t., waxy
- t. wedge
- t., wedge-shaped piece of
- t., white fibrous
- t., xenotransplant
- t., yellow elastic

titanium (Ti)
- t. cage
- t. fixture
- t. implant
- t. ray

titanyl phosphate laser ▸ potassium
titer(s)
- t., agglutination
- t., agglutination inhibition
- t., antiheart antibody
- t., antihyaluronidase
- t., antistreptolysin
- t., antistreptolysin O (ASO)
- t., anti-teichoic acid
- t., bactericidal
- t., complement fixation
- t. determination, antibody
- t., differential agglutination
- t. (GMT) ▸ geometric mean
- t., gonadotropin
- t., hemagglutination
- t. ▸ herpes simplex antibody
- t., heterophil antibody
- t., hormone
- t., Legionnaires'
- t., levels of antibody
- t., Lyme
- t., microsomal tanned red cells (TRC) antibody
- t., Rh (Rhesus) antibody
- t., rubella
- t., rubellar
- t. ▸ serum bactericidal
- t. ▸ streptococcal antibody
- t., toxoplasma
- t., viral

titrate dosage
titrated initial dose
Titterington's position
titubation
- t. and tremor, ataxia
- t., ataxia and
- t., lingual

TIVC (thoracic inferior vena cava)
Tivoli douche
t.i.w. (three times a week)
TKG (tokodynagraph)
Tl (thallium)
TL (total lipids)
TLC
- TLC (tender loving care)
- TLC (total L-chain concentration)
- TLC (total lung capacity)
- TLC (total lung compliance)

TLD (thermoluminescent dosimeter)
TLD (tumor lethal dose)
TLQ (total living quotient)
T-lymphocyte binding
TM
- TM (time motion)

- TM (transcendental meditation)
- TM (tympanic membrane)
- TM (tympanic membrane) ▸ perforation of

TMH (trainable mentally handicapped)
TMJ (temporomandibular joint)
- TMJ dislocation
- TMJ disorder
- TMJ disorder ▸ chest pain from
- TMJ disorder ▸ dizziness from
- TMJ disorder ▸ pain in back from
- TMJ disorder ▸ pain in ear from
- TMJ ▸ proper alignment of
- TMJ screening
- TMJ syndrome

TMP (transmembrane pressure)
TMR (transmyocardial revascularization)
TMV (tobacco mosaic virus)
TN (total negatives)
T/N (tar/nicotine) cigarette, low
TNF (tumor necrosis factor) gene-altered cells
TNI (total nodal irradiation)
TNM (tumor, nodes, metastases)
TNM (tumor, nodes, metastases) classification
TNM (tumor, nodes, metastases) staging system
TNTC (too numerous to count)
TO (telephone order)
tobacco
- t. abuse
- t. addiction
- t. and marijuana mix (Kiff)
- t., craving for
- t. dependence
- t. mosaic virus (TMV)
- t. -related cancer
- t. sickness, green
- t. smoke ▸ breathing in
- t. smoke (ETS), environmental
- t. smoke ▸ passive
- t. smoke, second-hand
- t., smokeless
- t. use disorder

tocodynamometer, external
TOD (tension of right eye)
Todd('s)
- T. bodies
- T. cautery, Wadsworth-
- T. cirrhosis
- T. gouge
- T. palsy

T. paralysis
T. process
T. units
toddler vision
toe(s)
   t., abductor muscle of great
   t., abductor muscle of little
   t., abscess of
   t., adductor muscle of great
   t. alignment
   t. and/or fingers ▸ numbness in
   t. bone
   t., cellulitis of
   t. ▸ change of color in
   t., claw
   t., clubbing of
   t. correction, hammer
   t. cramps
   t. curl exercise
   t., curly
   t. defect, hammer
   t., dorsal digital nerve of lateral
      surface of great
   t., dorsal digital nerve of medial
      surface of second
   t., dorsal regions of
   t. downgoing
   t. exercise ▸ marble pickup
   t. exercise ▸ towel curl
   t., extension of
   t., extension of great
   t. extensor
   t., fanning of
   t., fifth
   t., finger and
   t., first
   t. flexed
   t., flexion of
   t. flexor
   t., fourth
   t., frostbite
   t. gait, heel-to-
   t., great
   t., hammer
   t. -heel raise exercise
   t. implant, Swanson great
   t., infected
   t. injury
   t. joint ▸ pressure on
   t., lateral surface of great
   t., little
   t., long extensor muscle of
   t., long extensor muscle of great
   t., long flexor muscle of great
   t., long flexor muscles of

t., mallet
t., Morton's
t. motion ▸ heel-
t., necrotic
t., normal flexion of great
t. partially amputated
t., pigeon
t., plantar regions of
t. point exercise
t., poor circulation in
t. position, claw
t. prosthesis, Joplin
t. pull exercise
t. raise exercise
t. reflex
t. repair, DuVries hammer
t., second
t., short extensor muscle of
t., short extensor muscle of great
t., short flexor muscle of great
t., short flexor muscle of little
t., short flexor muscles of
t. sign
t. sign, great
t. signs ▸ mute
t. squeeze exercise
t. strengthening exercise
t., swelling of
t. syndrome, blue
t. tag on patient
t., third
t. -to-thumb transplant
t. touch
t. touch exercise
t. upgoing
t. walking ▸ heel-to-
t., weakness of great
t., webbed
toedrop brace
toeing, bilateral in-
toeing, out-
toenail(s)
   t., bluish
   t., curved
   t. excision, radical
   t., fungal
   t. fungus
   t. fungus ▸ chronic
   t., ingrown
   t. ▸ misshapen brittle
   t., thickened
Togaviridae virus
together, teeth wired
together, tongue-and-groove stitched
togoi, Aedes

toilet
   t., bronchial
   t. facilities, private
   t., joint
   t. plunger CPR (cardiopulmonary
      resuscitation)
   t., pulmonary
   t., respiratory
   t. -seat angina
   t. -seat syncope
   t., tracheal
   t., tracheobronchial
   t. training
   t. -training trauma
   t. transfer, patient completes
   t., vaginal
   t., vigorous pulmonary
toileting ▸ eating, grooming and
toileting self-care deficit
Toison's fluid
token economy
tokodynagraph study
tolbutamide tolerance test (TTT)
tolbutamide tolerance test ▸
   intravenous (IV)
Toldt, ligament of
Toldt, line of
tolerable levels
tolerance
   t., acquired
   t., alcohol
   t. and dependence ▸ morphine
   t. and endurance, patient's
   t., biliary duct
   t., cold
   t., cross-
   t., decreased
   t., dispositional
   t., distress
   t. dose
   t. dose, minimal
   t. dose (OTD), organ
   t. dose (TTD), tissue
   t., drug
   t., exercise
   t. for activity
   t. for physical activity ▸ reduced
   t. for stress
   t., frustration
   t., glucose
   t., heat
   t., hemodynamic
   t. (IGT) ▸ impaired glucose
   t. ▸ improved performance and
   t. in radiation therapy, spinal cord

tolerance—*continued*
- t. ▸ increased pain
- t. level for pain
- t. ▸ low frustration
- t., mechanism of
- t., medication
- t., normal fetal
- t. of pain, increased
- t., pain
- t. peak, work-
- t., potential for
- t., professional and public
- t., reverse
- t., self-
- t., smoker
- t. test, abnormal glucose
- t. test, alkali
- t. test (ATT), arginine
- t. test, aspirin
- t. test, borderline glucose
- t. test, cortisone-glucose
- t. test, d-Xylose
- t. test (ETT), exercise
- t. test, galactose
- t. test, glucose
- t. test, glucose-insulin
- t. test, insulin
- t. test, intravenous (IV) glucose
- t. test, intravenous (IV) tolbutamide
- t. test, lactose
- t. test, levulose
- t. test, Master's exercise
- t. test, oral glucose
- t. test, plasma glucose
- t. test (TTT) ▸ tolbutamide
- t. test, tyrosine
- t. to cannabinoids
- t. to cannabinoids, potential
- t. to depressants, potential
- t. to hallucinogens
- t. to hallucinogens, potential
- t. to inhalants, potential
- t. to opioids
- t. to opioids, potential
- t. to phencyclidines
- t. to phencyclidines, potential
- t. to radiation therapy, central nervous system
- t. to stimulants
- t. to stimulants, potential
- t. to treatment
- t. to treatment, lack of

tolerant infection, persistent
tolerate
- t. boredom ▸ inability to

- t. heat stress
- t. immune stress
- t. stress

tolerated
- t. diagnostic procedures well, patient
- t. dose
- t. dose (MTD) ▸ maximum
- t. full course of radiation, patient
- t. procedure well, patient
- t. therapy, patient
- t., weight bearing as

Tolosa-Hunt syndrome
toluene poisoning
toluidine blue O
Tom Jones closure
tomogram
- t., computed
- t., interauditory canal
- t., Siemen's cyclographic
- t., total chest

tomograph, mechanical
tomograph ▸ scanning laser
tomographic
- t. (ECT) body scanner ▸ emission computerized
- t. (CT) colonography ▸ three dimensional computed
- t. control console
- t. cut
- t. examination
- t. images of body
- t. images of head
- t. multiplane scanner
- t. radionuclide ventriculography
- t. scanner ▸ ultrafast computed
- t. scanning ▸ fluorodopamine positron emission
- t. study
- t. (ECT) system ▸ emission computerized
- t. (ECT) system ▸ radionuclide emission computerized

tomography (Tomography)
- t. angiographic portography, computed
- t., atrial bolus dynamic computer
- t. (ACAT) ▸ automated computerized axial
- t., automatic
- t. (ACT) ▸ axial computed
- t., axial transverse
- t., biplanar
- t. (CT) body scanner ▸ computerized

- t., cine computed
- t. (CT) ▸ computed
- t. (CAT) ▸ computed axial
- t. (CT) ▸ computerized
- t. (CAT) ▸ computerized axial
- t. ▸ dynamic computerized
- t. (EBCT) ▸ electron beam computed
- t. (EBCT) ▸ electron beam computerized
- T. (CT) ▸ Fast-Scan Computerized
- t. ▸ focal plane
- t. ▸ gated computed
- t. ▸ images produced by computerized
- t. (SPET) imaging ▸ single photon emission
- t. of both kidneys
- t. (CT) of chest ▸ computed
- t. of upper mediastinum
- t. ▸ optical coherence
- t. ▸ panoramic
- t. ▸ plesiosectional
- t. ▸ polycycloidal
- t. ▸ positron computed
- t. (PET) ▸ positron emission
- t. (PETT) ▸ positron emission transaxial
- t. (PETT) ▸ positron emission transverse
- T. (QCT) ▸ Quantitative Computed
- t. ▸ rapid acquisition computed axial
- t. (CAT) scan ▸ computerized axial
- t. (CAT) scan ▸ digital holographic computerized axial
- t. (HRCT) scan ▸ high resolution computed
- t. (SPECT) scan ▸ single photon emission computed
- t. (CT) scan ▸ thin slice computerized
- t. (CAT) scan ▸ ultrafast computerized axial
- t. (CAT) scanner ▸ helical computerized axial
- t. (CT) scanning ▸ computed
- t. (CT) scanning ▸ rapid sequential computerized
- t. ▸ seven pinhole
- t. (SPECT) ▸ single photon emission computed
- t. ▸ slant-hole
- t. (CT) ▸ thin section computerized
- t. ▸ transversal

t. (CT) ▸ ultrafast computed
t. ▸ ultrasonic
t. ▸ xenon-enhanced computed
tonal tinnitus
tone(s)
  t., abdominal muscle
  t., active bowel
  t., alteration of body
  t., alteration of muscle
  t., anal
  t. and collapse ▸ loss of muscle
  t. and elasticity, vascular
  t. and rhythm
  t. and spasticity treatment
  t. audiometric findings, pure
  t., bladder
  t., bowel
  t. burst
  t. contraction
  t. deafness
  t. decay
  t. decay test
  t. decay test, modified
  t. ▸ disordered muscle
  t. (FHT), Doptone monitoring of
    fetal heart
  t., emotional feeling
  t., enhance muscle
  t., feeling
  t. (FHT) ▸ fetal heart
  t., flexor
  t. hearing loss, high
  t. (HT) ▸ heart
  t., high
  t., hyperactive bowel
  t., hypoactive bowel
  t., improve muscle
  t., increased flexor
  t. ▸ increased muscle
  t., jecoral
  t. ▸ lack of muscle
  t., loss of muscle
  t., loss of postural
  t., low
  t., momentary loss of skeletal
    muscular
  t., muscle
  t. muscle groups ▸ strengthen and
  t., muscular
  t., normoactive bowel
  t. (FHT) obtained with Doptone,
    fetal heart
  t. ▸ persistent abnormal muscle
  t. pink and warm, skin
  t., plastic

t. ▸ poor muscle
t., postural
t., rectal sphincter
t. regular, heart
t., rhythm and
t. sense
t., skeletal muscular
t., skin
t., smooth bronchial muscle
t., sphincter
t., stable fetal heart
t., sympathetic vasoconstrictor
t. test, pure
t., Traube's double
t. -up, pelvic
t., uterine muscle
t., vagal
t., Williams' tracheal
T1-T2 or D1-D12 (thoracic vertebrae)
T1-T2 weighted image
tongs or halo, Crutchfield
tongue
  t. abnormalities from antibiotic
  t., adherent
  t., amyloid
  t. and face ▸ swelling of lips,
  t. and lips, smacking movements of
  t. -and-groove stitched together
  t. -and-groove suture
  t., antibiotic
  t., baked
  t., bald
  t. base carcinoma
  t., beefy
  t., bifid
  t. biting
  t., black
  t., black hairy
  t. blade
  t., blue
  t. buds
  t., burning
  t. cancer
  t. carcinoma
  t., cardinal
  t., cerebriform
  t., choreic
  t., cleft
  t. coated
  t. coating
  t., cobble-stone
  t., crocodile
  t., deep vein of
  t. depressor
  t. deviation

t. discomfort
t. disorder
t., dorsal vein of
t., dotted
t., double
t., earthy
t., encrusted
t., fern leaf
t., fibrillary twitchings of
t., filmy
t., fissured
t. flap, lingual
t., flat
t., furred
t., furrowed
t., geographic
t., grooved
t., hairy
t. ▸ inability to move
t., inferior longitudinal muscle of
t. inflammation from pernicious
  anemia
t. ▸ itchy swelling of
t., large
t., lazy
t., lesion
t., lobulated
t., magenta
t., mappy
t., mobile portion of
t., motor nerve of
t. ▸ numbness of
t. obstructing airway
t. of sphenoid bone
t. ▸ outstretched hand or
t. pain from dentures
t., parrot
t. ▸ petechiae of
t. piercing
t., plicated
t. problem ▸ pain in ear from
t. problems from anemia
t. protrudes in midline
t., protruding
t. protrusion
t., raspberry
t., red strawberry
t., rhabdomyoma of
t., root of
t., Sandwith's bald
t., scrotal
t. sign ▸ snake-
t., smoker's
t., smooth
t., soreness of

tongue—*continued*
- t. sores
- t., split
- t., spotted
- t., squamous cell carcinoma
- t., squamous cell carcinoma base of
- t., stippled
- t., strawberry
- t., sulcated
- t., superior longitudinal muscle of
- t., surface of
- t. swallowing
- t. ▸ swelling of
- t. syndrome or glossodynia ▸ burning
- t. thickening
- t. -thrusting
- t. -tie
- t. -tie at birth
- t., timber
- t. time test, arm-
- t. traction
- t., transverse muscle of
- t., trombone tremor of
- t., vallecula of
- t., vertical muscle of
- t., white
- t. ▸ whitish coating back of
- t., wooden
- t. worm
- t., wrinkled

tonic [*chronic, clonic*]
- t., bitter
- t., cardiac
- t., clonic-
- t. -clonic movement
- t. -clonic seizure
- t. clonic seizures ▸ uncontrolled generalized
- t. -clonic spasm
- t. contraction
- t. convulsion
- t., digestive
- t. EMG (electromyogram) activity, decreased
- t. EMG (electromyogram) activity, increased
- t. epilepsy
- t., general
- t. heart level
- t., intestinal
- t. muscular contractions, intermittent
- t. neck reflex
- t. perseveration

- t. phase
- t. postural epilepsy
- t. pupil
- t. purpura ▸ gin and
- t. reflex
- t. seizure
- t. spasm of voluntary muscles
- t. spasms
- t., stomachic
- t., vascular

tonicity, muscle
Toni-Fanconi-Debre syndrome, de
toning, body
toning muscles
tonoclonic spasm
tonofilaments, bundles of
tonofilaments ▸ desmosomes with bundles of
tonography study
tonometer
- t., air-puff
- t., Gartner

tonometered whole blood
tonometry, carotid applanation
tonometry test
tonsil(s)
- t. and adenoids ▸ hypertrophy of
- t. appear enlarged
- t., buried
- t. calculus
- t. calculus, palatine
- t. cerebellar
- t., chronically infected
- t., cryptic
- t., crypts of palatine
- t., crypts of pharyngeal
- t. dissector, Colver
- t. do not appear enlarged
- t., enlarged
- t., eustachian
- t., faucial
- t. fossa
- t. function
- t., Gerlach's
- t. grasped
- t., hypertrophied
- t. infected
- t. inflamed
- t., intact
- t., intestinal
- t., lingual
- t., Luschka's
- t. of cerebellum
- t., palatine
- t., pharyngeal

- t. problem ▸ pain in ear from
- t. puncture
- t., resected
- t., submerged
- t., third

tonsillar
- t. abscess
- t. crypts
- t. enlargement
- t. exudate
- t. fossa
- t. fossa carcinoma
- t. hernia
- t. herniation
- t. nerves
- t. pillar
- t. tag
- t. tissue

tonsillectomy
- t. and adenoidectomy (T and A)
- t. diet
- t., dissection and snare
- t. hemorrhage, post-
- t., LaForce

tonsillitis
- t., acute catarrhal
- t. ▸ acute exacerbation
- t., acute parenchymatous
- t., caseous
- t., catarrhal
- t., chronic
- t., chronic catarrhal
- t., diphtherial
- t., erythematous
- t., exudative
- t., follicular
- t., herpetic
- t., lacunar
- t. lenta
- t., lingual
- t., mycotic
- t., parenchymatous
- t., pharyngitis
- t., preglottic
- t., pustular
- t., streptococcal
- t., superficial
- t., suppurative
- t. syndrome
- t., Vincent's
- t., white

tonsurans, Trichophyton
tonus [*clonus, conus*]
- t. fracture
- t., muscle

t., neurogenic
t. of extrinsic laryngeal muscles
t., perception and
too numerous to count (TNTC)
Tooies (barbiturates)
tool, diagnostic
tool, screening
Toot (cocaine)
tooth (*see also* **teeth**) **(Tooth)**
t. abscess
t. ▸ adamantine substance of
T. atrophy, Charcot-Marie-
t. attachment
t. avulsion
t., axial surface of
t. ▸ bony substance of
t. -borne
t. brushing and flossing
t., buccal surface of
t., cervical surface of
t., dead nerve in
t. decay
t. decay ▸ pain in ear from
t. discolorization from calculus
T. disease, Charcot-Marie-
T. disease, Marie-
t., distal surface of
t. enamel
t., eruption of
t. extraction
t. extraction dry socket
t., facial surface of
t. ▸ foul tasting discharge around
t., gingival surface of
t., Goslee
T. -Hoffman syndrome, Charcot-
Marie-
t., impacted
t., incisal surface of
t., infected
t. ▸ intertubular substance of
t. ▸ ivory substance of
t. -like calcification
t., lingual surface of
t. malformation
t., malposed
t., mesial surface of
t., misaligned
t., molar
t., mulberry
t., multirooted
t., Mummery's pink
t., neck of
t., nonfunctional
t., nonvital

t., occlusal surface of
t. of malleus, cog-
t. pocket
t. ▸ proper substance of
t., pulpless
t., reimplanted
t. reimplanted in socket
t. reshaping
t., restoration of
t. root, excision of apex of
t. size discrepancy
t., snaggle
t. socket
t. socket ▸ inflammation of
t., stomach
t. storage and transportation
t. straightening
t., submerged
t. surface of
t., surgical neck of
t., telephone
t. tenaculum, cervix grasped with
single
t. tenaculum, single
t. treated
t., Turner's
t., unerupted
t. yellowing from aging
toothache, feigned
toothache, patient has
toothed tenaculum, sharp-
top
t. murmur, humming-
t. of container, red cells float to
t. of solution, white cells taken
off
Töpfer's test
tophaceous gout
tophus
t., auricular
t., dental
t. syphiliticus
topical
t., anesthesia
t. anesthetic
t. antibiotic
t. antibiotic therapy, intensive
t. antipruritic
t. application
t. bacteria ▸ Bartonella henselae
t. cannabinoid
t. cartilage
t. chemotherapy
t. cocaine anesthesia
t. cooling

t. coronary vasodilator
t. estrogen
t. eye medications
t. fluorides
t. hypothermia
t. mechlorethamine chemotherapy
t. medication
t. medicine
t. ointment
t. pain reliever
t. prescription medication
t. skin medication
t. steroid
t. stimulant
t. therapy
t. thrombin
t. treatment
topic-oriented process group
topogram (CET), computed EEG
(electroencephalogram)
topographer, corneal
topographic
t. anatomy
t. examination
t. location
topography
t. and anatomic measurements of
patient
t. and/or reactivity
t., corneal
t. ▸ frequency, form and
toppling gait
TOPS (Treatment Outcome
Prospective Study)
TOPS (Take Off Pounds Sensibly)
diet
Torek operation
Torek resection of thoracic
esophagus
toric lens
Torkildsen's operation
Torkildsen's shunt procedure
torn
t. anterior cruciate ligament
t. cartilage
t. knee cartilage
t. knee ligament
t. lateral meniscus
t. ligament
t. medial meniscus
t. muscle
t. retina
t. rotator cuff
t. tissue, trimmed

Tornwaldt's (*same as* **Thornwaldt's**)
  T. bursitis
  T. cyst
  T. disease
Toronto Alexithymia Scale
Toro's operation, Del
TORP (total ossicular replacement
  prosthesis)
TORP (total ossicular replacement
  prosthesis), Plastiport
torpedo-shaped pattern
torpid
  t. idiocy
  t. idiot
  t. shock
Torpin's operation
torpor retinae
torque
  t., clockwise
  t. control
  t. of femur
  t. technique, George Winter
    elevation
  t. -type prosthesis, Plasticor
  t. vise
torr
  t. pressure
  t. ▸ pressure kept at ___ torr,
    dropped to ___
  t. units
torse ▸ pale shrunken
torsion [*portion*]
  t. balance
  t. dystonia
  t., elongation and
  t. neurosis
  t. fracture
  t., gastric
  t., multiangular
  t. of testes
  t., ovarian cyst
  t., positive
  t. spasm
  t. spasm, progressive
  t. spasms, sudden
  t. test
  t., testicular
  t., tibial
torsional diplopia
torsional, upbeat nystagmus
torso presentation
tort, toxic
tortuosity
  t., arterial
  t. of glands

  t. of vessels
tortuous
  t. aorta
  t. aorta, wide
  t. aortic arch
  t. root canal
  t. uterine artery
  t. varicosities in lower extremities
  t. varicosity
  t. veins
  t. vessels
Torula (torula)
  T. capsulatus
  T. histolytica
  t. meningitis
Torulopsis glabrata
Torulopsis glabrata pneumonia
torus
  t. crush
  t. fracture
  t. frontalis
  t. levatorius
  t., mandibular
  t. mandibularis
  t., maxillary
  t. palatinus
  t. tubarius
TOS (tension of left eye)
TOT (tincture of time)
TOT (tip of tongue)
TOT (Tubal Ovum Transfer)
total (Total)
  t. abdominal hysterectomy (TAH)
  t. absence of circulation on four
    vessel angiography
  t. abstinence
  t. acidity
  t. activity
  t. admissions ▸ total infections vs.
  t. air
  t. air volume
  t. allergy syndrome
  t. alopecia
  t. alternans
  t. amnesia
  t. anomalous pulmonary venous
    connection
  t. anomalous pulmonary venous
    drainage (dr'ge)
  t. anomalous pulmonary venous
    return
  T. Antibody to Hepatitis B Core
    Antigen (Anti-HBc)
  t. aphasia

  T. Articular Replacement
    Arthroplasty (TARA)
  t. artificial heart (TAH)
  t. artificial heart, Baylor
  t. artificial heart, Berlin
  t. artificial heart, CardioWest
  t. artificial heart ▸ Hershey
  t. artificial heart ▸ Liotta
  t. artificial heart ▸ RTV
  t. artificial heart ▸ Utah
  t. artificial heart ▸ Vienna
  t. autopsy
  t. avulsion
  t. axial node irradiation
  t. baldness
  t. base
  t. bed capacity
  t. bilirubin
  t. biopsy
  t. blackout mentally
  t. bladder capacity
  t. bladder resection
  t. blindness
  t. blood cholesterol
  t. blood granulocyte pool
  t. blood loss
  t. blood volume
  t. body
  t. body density
  t. body fat
  t. body irradiation
  t. body potassium
  t. body radiation
  t. body radiation therapy
  t. body scanner
  t. body solute
  t. body treatment
  t. body water
  t. body weight
  t. breech extraction
  t. calorie expenditure
  t. capacity
  t. cardiopulmonary bypass
  t. cataract
  t. cavopulmonary connection
  t. chemical freedom
  t. chest tomogram
  t. cholesterol
  t. circulating hemoglobin
  t. collapse of lung
  t. color blindness
  t. coronary flow (TCF)
  t. cystectomy
  t. deafness
  t. disability

t. discrimination (TD)
t. dosage, maximum
t. dose
t. dose infusion
t. dose of rads in fractions
t. dullness
t. duodenal bypass
t. elasticity of muscle
t. elbow arthroplasty
t. electromechanical systole
t. end-diastolic diameter
t. endoscopic coronary artery
   bypass (TECAB)
t. end-systolic diameter
t. eradication
t. estrogen excretion
t. exhaustion
t. fat intake
t. fatty acids
t. fitness program
t. flow (TF)
t. gastrectomy
t. graft area rejected (TGAR)
t. health care
t. hemolytic complement (C'H$_{50}$)
t. hip arthroplasty
t. hip arthroplasty, McKee-Farrar
t. hip, ceramic
t. hip prosthesis, HD II
t. hip replacement
t. hip replacement ▸ dual lock
t. hip replacement operation
t. hip replacement procedure
t. hydroxyapatite (THA)
t. hydroxyproline
t. hypermetropia
t. hyphema
t. hysterectomy
t. immobility
t. inability to urinate
t. incontinence
t. infections vs. total admissions
t. infusion
t. infusion period
t. iron-binding capacity (TIBC)
t. joint arthroplasty
t. joint reconstruction
t. joint replacement
t. knee arthroplasty
t. knee prosthesis, Shier's
t. knee replacement
t. labor time
t. laryngectomy
t. L-chain concentration (TLC)
t. lesion

t. lipid profile
t. lipids (TL)
t. living quotient (TLQ)
t. loss of consciousness
t. loss of motor function
t. loss of vision
t. lung capacity (TLC)
t. lung capacity (RV/TLC) ratio ▸
   residual volume to
t. lung compliance (TLC)
t. lung volume
t. lymphoid irradiation
t. lymphoid irradiation for allograft
   survival
t. lymphoid irradiation in arthritis
t. lymphoid irradiation in organ
   transplantation
t. lymphoid irradiation in
   rheumatoid arthritis
t. mass stopping power
t. mastectomy
t. memory loss
t. meniscectomy
t. negatives (TN)
t. nerve deafness
t. nodal irradiation (TNI)
t. obstruction
t. occlusion basilar artery
T. Occlusion Device ▸ Prima
t. occlusion ▸ nonacute
t. ossicular replacement prosthesis
   (TORP)
t. ossicular replacement prosthesis
   (TORP), Plastiport
t. outlet occlusion
t. paralysis
t. parenteral nutrition
t. parenteral nutrition (TPN)
   catheter
t. parenteral nutrition (TPN)
   hyperalimentation
t. parenteral nutrition (TPN) line
t. parenteral nutrition (TPN) therapy
t. patient care
t. patient shock count
t. pattern of waves
t. pattern, shift of
t. pelvic exenteration
t. peripheral parenteral nutrition
   (TPPN)
t. peripheral resistance (TPR)
t. peripheral resistance index
t. placenta previa
t. pneumonectomy
t. proctocolectomy

t. protein (TP)
t. pulmonary blood flow (TPBF)
t. pulmonary resistance (TPR)
t. pulmonary vascular resistance
   (TPVR)
t. push therapy
t. quadriplegia
t. relief of pain
t. relief of symptoms
t. remission
t. renal blood flow (TRBF)
t. resistance (TR)
t. resistance (PTR) ▸ peripheral
t. response (TR)
t. ridge-count (TRC)
t. serum cholesterol
t. serum prostatic acid
   phosphatase (TSPAP)
t. serum protein (TSP)
t. shoulder arthroplasty
t. skin electron beam therapy
t. sleep time
t. sodium and water content
t. solids (TS)
t. symblepharon
t. system failure of vital organs
t. thyroidectomy
t. thyroxine (TT)
t. time (TT)
t. transverse fracture
t. treatment plan
t. urinary gonadotropin (TUG)
t. urine protein
t. vaginal hysterectomy (TVH)
t. ventilatory assistance
t. ventricular blood expelled
t. vital capacity (VC)
t. volume
t. volume capacity (TVC)

totalis
t., alopecia
t., hyperostosis
t., ophthalmoplegia

totally
t. abstinent
t. dependent individual
t. dependent, patient
t. disabled, patient
t. incapable of caring for self
t. inoperable, patient
t. nonfunctional

Toti('s)
T. -Mosher operation
T. operation
T. operation, Mosher-

totipotential cell
totipotential protoplasm
toto, in
toto, removed in
touch
- t., absence of sense of
- t. and pain, sense of
- t. -and-pin sensation
- t., bleeding on
- t., caring
- t. cell
- t. exercise ▸ toe
- t. ▸ extreme sensitivity to
- t., healing
- t., human
- t. ▸ importance of
- t., mother's
- t., need for
- t. or taste, heightened awareness of
- t. ▸ perception of
- t., sense of
- t. sensors ▸ light
- t. shock count
- t. stretch ▸ physical
- t. technique ▸ en bloc no
- t. technique, no-
- t., temporary deprivation maternal
- t., tenderness to
- t., therapeutic
- t. therapy
- t., toe

touching compulsions ▸ arranging and
Tough Love Parents Support Group
tough-minded ▸ patient
toughness, mental
tour de maitre
Touraine syndrome, Christ-Siemens-
Touraine's syndrome
Tourette('s)
- T. disease
- T. disease, Gilles de la
- T. disorder
- T. disorder, Gilles de la
- T. syndrome
- T. syndrome, Gilles de la

tourniquet
- t. applied
- t., automatic rotating
- t., Bethune's
- t. control
- t. control, pneumatic
- t. controlled bleeding, pneumatic
- t. deflated

- t. inflated
- t. ischemia
- t. pigmentation
- t., pneumatic
- t. released
- t. removed
- t., Rumel
- t., scalp
- t., Shenstone's
- t. tightened

Touton giant cells
toward
- t. bullying ▸ tendency
- t. cruelty ▸ tendency
- t. drug abusers, attitudes of society
- t. illness, predisposition
- t. sleep activity ▸ shifting brain electrical activity

towel(s) [*dowel*]
- t., absorbent sterile
- t. curl toe exercise
- t., Kaycel

tower skull, exophthalmos due to
Town prosthesis, Cape
Towne('s)
- T. position
- T. projection roentgenogram
- T. view
- T. x-ray view, Chamberlain-

Townley prosthesis
Townsend's avalanche
toxemia
- t., alimentary
- t., eclamptic
- t. of pregnancy
- t., preeclamptic

toxemic epilepsy
toxemic pneumonia
toxic
- t. agent, exogenous
- t. agents, ingestion of
- t. air pollutants
- t. amaurosis
- t. atrophy
- t. cardiomyopathy
- t. cardiopathy
- t. cataract
- t. chemicals
- t. cirrhosis
- t. deafness
- t. delirium
- t. dementia
- t. diabetes
- t. dilatation
- t. disorder, acute

- t. drug ▸ ingestion of
- t. drugs
- t. effects
- t. effects of copper
- t. effects of radiation
- t. effects, potential
- t. elements
- t. emotions
- t. environment
- t. epidermal necrolysis
- t. equivalent
- t. erythema
- t. factor
- t. factor in shock
- t. fumes
- t. gas
- t. gastritis
- t. goiter
- t. granules
- t. headache
- t. hepatitis
- t. hepatitis, acute
- t. injury
- t. insanity
- t. iron damage
- t. level
- t. level of drugs
- t. megacolon
- t. metabolic encephalopathy
- t. metabolic etiology
- t. mold
- t. molecules
- t. myocarditis
- t. nephropathy
- t. nephrosis
- t. neuropathy
- t. ocular effects
- t. optic nerve atrophy
- t. overdose
- t., patient
- t. poison
- t. poisoning
- t. psychosis
- t. purpura
- t. radiation
- t. reaction
- t. reaction to local anesthesia
- t. shock
- t. shock syndrome (TSS)
- t. shock syndrome (TSS) ▸ diarrhea from
- t. shock syndrome (TSS) ▸ dizziness from
- t. shock syndrome (TSS) ▸ menstrual

t. side-effects
t. spasm
t. state
t. substance
t. substance ▸ exposure to
t. syndrome
t. tort
t. treatment
t. tremor
t. unit (TU)
t. vasculitis, noninflammatory
t. wastes
t. wastes, body's
t. weight
toxicaria, Chailletia
toxicity
    t., aminoglycosides
    t., amphetamine
    t., antibiotic
    t., aspirin
    t., behavioral
    t., bone marrow
    t., cardiac
    t., cartilage
    t., cephalosporin
    t., clinical
    t., digitalis
    t., digoxin
    t., direct
    t., drug
    t. ▸ drug-induced liver
    t., eight nerve
    t., fatal liver
    t., gastrointestinal
    t., hematologic
    t., high
    t., histamine
    t., hydrocarbon
    t. in combined modality therapy, independent
    t. in immature lung ▸ oxygen (O_2)
    t., increased
    t., industrial
    t. information
    t., intraocular
    t., kidney
    t., lethal
    t., liver
    t., long-term
    t. ▸ newborn drug
    t. of cannabinoids
    t. of depressants
    t. of hallucinogens
    t. of inhalants
    t. of multiple drugs

t. of opioids
t. of phencyclidines
t. of stimulants
t. or drug interactions
t., oxygen (O_2)
t. ▸ peripheral autonomic
t., plant
t., potential
t., procaine
t., renal
t. retention
t. risk, antibiotic
t. ▸ sensitize heart muscle to
t. study
t. study reproductive
t., symptoms of
t., systemic
t., thallium
t., vitamin
toxicodendron, Rhus
toxicologic
    t. aspect
    t. -pharmacologic syndromes
    t. screens
toxicologist
    t., clinical
    t., forensic
    t., medical
toxicology
    t. laboratory
    t. screen
    t., trauma
toxicum, erythema
toxicum neonatorum, erythema
toxigenic diarrhea
toxigenic mycosis
toxin(s) (Toxin)
    t. -antitoxin immunity
    t. -antitoxin reaction
    t., bacterial
    t., botulism
    t., brain
    t., Clostridium difficile
    t. colitis
    T. (Bo-Tox) cosmetic surgery, Botulinum
    t., Dick
    t., endogenous
    t., environmental
    t., exposure to
    t. -filled environment
    t. from blood ▸ filtering
    T. (Bo-Tox) injection ▸ Botulinum
    t. insensitive current
    t. neutralization

t. panel
t., pertussis
t. -producing common organisms
t., radioactive
t., tetanus anti◇
t., tissue-eating
toxipathic hepatitis
Toxocara canis
Toxocara cati
toxoid(s)
    t., and acellular pertussis vaccine ▸ diphtheria, tetanus
    t., and whole cell pertussis vaccine ▸ diphtheria, tetanus
    t. -antitoxin floccule
    t. -antitoxoid
    t. immunization, tetanus
    t. immunization, tetanus and diphtheria
    t. ▸ inactive vaccines and
    t., tetanus
toxophore group
Toxoplasma
    T. antibodies, anti-
    T. gondii
    T. pyrogenes
    T. titer
toxoplasmic
    t. choroiditis
    t. encephalitis
    t. retinochoroiditis
toxoplasmosis
    t., congenital
    t. infection, acute
    t., neonatal
Toynbee maneuver
toys, adaptive
TP (total protein)
T-P interval
T-P segment
TPA (tissue plasminogen activation)
TPA (tissue plasminogen activator)
TPA (tissue plasminogen activator) infusion
TPBA (thermal/perfusion balloon angioplasty)
TPBF (total pulmonary blood flow)
TPCP (phencyclidine analog), TCP/
TPI (Treponema pallidum immobilization)
TPN
    TPN (Trained Practical Nurse)
    TPN (total parenteral nutrition) catheter

TPN—*continued*
    TPN (total parenteral nutrition)
      hyperalimentation
    TPN (total parenteral nutrition) line
    TPN (total parenteral nutrition)
      therapy
TPPN (total peripheral parenteral
  nutrition)
T-P-Q segment
TPR
    TPR (temperature, pulse and
      respiration)
    TPR (total peripheral resistance)
    TPR (total pulmonary resistance)
TPT (typhoid-paratyphoid) vaccine
TPVR (total pulmonary vascular
  resistance)
TQ segment
TR (total resistance)
TR (total response)
trabecula
    t. cerebri
    t. cinerea
    t. cranii
trabeculae of heart, flesh
trabecular
    t. bone
    t. degeneration
    t. hypertrophy
    t. meshwork
    t. pattern
    t. region
    t. vein
trabeculated, bladder wall
trabeculated ▸ bladder wall thin and
trabeculation
    t., coarse
    t., mild
    t., muscular
    t., vesical
trabeculoplasty (LTP), laser
trace
    t. degree
    t., EEG (electroencephalogram)
    t. elements
    t., memory
    t. metal
    t. recall, immediate sensory
    t. ▸ residual drug
tracé alternant
traceable element, magnetically
tracer
    t., frequency
    t., low level radioactive
    t., nuclear

    t., radioactive
    t. study
    t. technique, diffusible
    t. technique ▸ extractable
tracewriting stimulus
trach (tracheostomy) tube
  replacement
trachea (tracheae)
    t. anesthetized ▸ pharynx, larynx
      and
    t., annulus
    t., bifurcatio
    t., bifurcation of
    t., carcinoma of epidermoid
    t., carina of
    t., cervical
    t., deviation of
    t., deviation upper
    t., diverticulum of
    t., esophagus with
    t. exposed
    t., FB (foreign body) in
    t., food lodged in
    t., food trapped in
    t. forceps
    t., foreign body (FB) in
    t., fractured
    t. incised
    t., lining of
    t. ▸ lipoma of
    t. markedly inflamed
    t. midline
    t., paries membranaceous
    t., scabbard
    t. shifted to right
    t. ▸ steepling of
    t., stenosis of
    t., Syngamus
    t., varix of
    t. with ease ▸ scope inserted into
tracheal
    t. adenoma
    t. aspirate culture
    t. bifurcation angle
    t. biopsy
    t. bronchitis
    t. bronchus
    t. button
    t. button ▸ Kistner
    t. calcification
    t. cartilage
    t. catheterization
    t. compression
    t. deviation
    t. diverticulum

    t. erosion ▸ tracheotomy with
    t. FB (foreign body)
    t. fistula
    t. fistula, closure of
    t. foreign body (FB)
    t. fracture
    t. incision
    t. intubation
    t. lavage
    t. lipoma
    t. lymph nodes
    t. mucosa
    t. mucus velocity
    t. muscle
    t. obstruction
    t. papilloma
    t. prosthesis ▸ Neville
    t. rales
    t. reflex
    t. rings
    t. secretions
    t. sound
    t. stenosis
    t. stump
    t. tampon
    t. toilet
    t. tone, Williams'
    t. tree
    t. tube
    t. tug
    t. tumor
    t. ulceration
    t. vein
    t. wall
trachealis, angina
tracheitis (*same as* trachitis)
    t., acute laryngeal
    t., chronic
    t., erosive
    t. sicca
trachelomastoid muscle
tracheobronchial
    t. amyloidosis
    t. lavage
    t. lymph node
    t. lymph nodes, inferior
    t. lymph nodes, superior
    t. toilet
    t. tree
    t. tuberculosis
tracheobronchitis, acute
tracheoesophageal
    t. atresia ▸ gross
    t. fistula embryology
    t. fistula ▸ gross

t. fistula ▸ malignant
t. fistula ▸ trifurcation
t. junction
t. puncture

tracheopulmonary secretions

tracheoscopy
t. with biopsy
t. with dilatation
t. with excision
t. with irrigation
t. with removal

tracheostomy
t. button
t. button, Moore's
t. care
t., cricothyroidotomy and
t. cuff
t., flap
t. ▸ percutaneous dilational
t. site
t. stoma
t. tube
t. tube, cuffed
t. tube, fenestrated
t. tube in place
t. tube inserted
t. tube, Kistner
t. tube, Mörch
t. tube, Pitt talking
t. tube placed
t. tube, Portex
t. (trach) tube replacement
t. tube, Sharley
t. tube ▸ Shiley

tracheotomy
t., emergency
t., high
t., low
t., permanent
t. site
t. with biopsy
t. with excision
t. with tracheal erosion

trachitis (see tracheitis)

trachoma
t., Arlt's
t., brawny
t. inclusion conjunctivitis (TRIC)
t. virus

trachomatis, Chlamydia

trachomatous
t. conjunctivitis
t. dacryocystitis
t. keratitis

Trachybdella bistriata

tracing(s)
t. (CT), carotid
t., carotid pulse
t. ▸ complete, mandatory contact
t., computerized edge
t., contact
t. ▸ diamond-shaped
t. display, ECG (electrocardiogram)
t. display, EEG
   (electroencephalogram)
t., edge
t., electrocardiogram (ECG/EKG)
t., electroencephalogram (EEG)
t., electroencephalographic
t., fetal heart monitor
t., Gothic arch
t. ▸ jugular venous pulse
t., monitor
t. of electrocerebral inactivity
t., polygraph
t., pressure
t., previous
t., pulse
t., serial
t., targeted contact
t., venous pulse

track(s) [*tract*]
t. appearance ▸ railroad
t., blood pressure (BP)
t. detector, dielectric
t. ductus arteriosus ▸ railroad
t. movement, infant
t., patient has needle
t. sign ▸ railroad
t. suture
t., tram

tracked, eyes

tracking (Tracking)
t. device, A-mode echo-
t. pacemaker, atrial
t., spatial
T. System (OTS), Optical

tract(s)
t. ▸ acute inflammation of portal
t. adenocarcinoma ▸
   gastrointestinal
t., afferent
t., alimentary
t. anomaly ▸ urinary
t., ascending sensory
t., atrial internodal
t., atriodextrofascicular
t., atrio-Hisian bypass
t. ▸ bacterial balance in digestive
t., biliary

t., biliary outflow
t., blocked digestive
t., blocked urinary
t., Burdach's
t., bypass
t. calculi, urinary
t. cancer, biliary
t. cancer of male reproductive
t. cancer, urinary
t. carcinoid ▸ intestinal
t. carcinoma ▸ gastrointestinal (GI)
t. cauterized, spinothalamic
t., clogged urinary
t. concealed bypass
t., corticobulbar
t., corticospinal
t., descending
t., descending motor
t., digestive
t. discomfort, upper respiratory
t. disease, biliary
t. disease, hepatobiliary
t. disorder, digestive
t. disorder, gastric
t. disorder, urinary
t. drained, fistulous
t. dysfunction, urinary
t. ▸ extensive fibrosis of portal
t., female genital
t., female reproductive
t. fistula ▸ esophageal carcinoma
   with respiratory
t. fistula ▸ respiratory
t., fistulous
t., flow
t. fluid (RTF), respiratory
t., Foville's
t. from gases ▸ burns to respiratory
t. gas, intestinal
t., gastrointestinal (GI)
t., geniculocalcarine
t., genital
t., genitourinary (GU)
t., Goll's
t., Gudden's
t., Helweg's
t., iliotibial
t., incision and drainage (I and D) of
   fistulous
t. infection, acute respiratory
t. infection, asymptomatic urinary
t. infection, candida urinary
t. infection ▸ catheter-related
   urinary

tract(s)—*continued*

- t. infection ▸ Citrobacter freundii urinary
- t. infection cleared, urinary
- t. infection, concurrent upper respiratory
- t. infection (UTI), congenital urinary
- t. infection ▸ enterococcal urinary
- t. infection ▸ hospital-acquired urinary
- t. infection ▸ hospital-associated respiratory
- t. infection ▸ Klebsiella urinary
- t. infection ▸ nosocomial respiratory
- t. infection, pin
- t. infection ▸ recurrent upper respiratory
- t. infection ▸ recurrent urinary
- t. infection ▸ reproductive
- t. infection, respiratory
- t. infection ▸ symptomatic urinary
- t. infection (U.T.I.), urinary
- t. inflammation ▸ lower respiratory
- t., inflammation of urinary
- t. inflammation ▸ respiratory
- t., inflow
- t. injury, urinary
- t. intact, motor
- t. intact, sensory
- t., internodal
- t., intestinal
- t., left flow
- t. ▸ left ventricular outflow
- t. lesions, corticospinal
- t. lesions, genital
- t., Lissauer's
- t., lower respiratory
- t., Meynert's
- t. ▸ nodo-Hisian bypass
- t., nodoventricular
- t. ▸ normal functioning of GI
- t. obstruction, biliary
- t. obstruction ▸ left ventricular (LV) inflow
- t. obstruction ▸ left ventricular (LV) outflow
- t. obstruction ▸ outflow
- t. of liver ▸ portal
- t., olivocerebellar
- t., optic
- t., outflow
- t., pancreaticobiliary
- t., pin
- t., portal
- t., pulmonary outflow

- t., pyramidal
- t., reproductive
- t., respiratory
- t., right flow
- t. ▸ right ventricular (RV) outflow
- t. ▸ selective decontamination of digestive
- t. signs, long
- t., sinus
- t., spinal cord
- t., spinothalamic
- t. structures, urinary
- t. system ▸ urinary
- t. tachycardia ▸ right ventricular (RV) outflow
- t., tectospinal
- t. tissue repair ▸ gastrointestinal (GI)
- t., upper respiratory
- t., upper urinary
- t., urinary
- t., urogenital
- t., vaginal
- t. velocity ▸ left ventricular (LV) outflow
- t., ventricular outflow
- t. ▸ Wolff-Parkinson-White bypass

traction [*faction, fraction*]

- t. aneurysm
- t. apparatus, skull
- t. applied to extremity
- t., balanced
- t., balanced skeletal
- t., bed rest and
- t. bows
- t., bronchiectasis
- t., Bryant's
- t., Buck's
- t., Buck's extension
- t., cervical
- t., cord
- t., Crego
- t., Crile head
- t., Crutchfield skeletal
- t., Crutchfield tong
- t. diverticula
- t., diverticulum
- t., Dunlop
- t., elastic
- t., fiber
- t., Forrester-Brown head halter
- t., gentle
- t., halo
- t., halo-pelvic
- t., handle

- t., head halter
- t. headache
- t., intermittent
- t., intermittent cervical
- t., Jones suspension
- t., Kuhlmann cervical
- t., manual
- t., McBride tripod pin
- t., patient placed in
- t., pelvic
- t., ___ pounds of
- t., radial
- t. retinal detachment
- t., Russell
- t., Sayre
- t., skeletal
- t. splinting
- t., sternal
- t., suspension
- t. suture
- t. suture, Dacron
- t. suture, superior rectus
- t., tongue
- t. ▸ umbilical cord
- t., Vinke tong
- t., Vinke tong skull
- t., Zimfoam head halter

tractotomy, mesencephalic

Trade Center cough ▸ World

tradition, faith

traditional

- t. attitudes
- t. behavioral therapy
- t. care
- t. chemotherapy
- t. disease concept
- t. drug program
- t. enzyme measurements
- t. hearing aid
- t. home care
- t. metal braces
- t. programs
- t. psychotherapy
- t. standard of normality
- t. surgery
- t. therapy
- t. treatment

traffic, illegal drug

traffickers, drug

tragacanth, gum

tragal perichondrium

tragus, muscle of

train of thought

trainable mentally handicapped (TMH)

trainable mentally retarded patient
trained (Trained)
    t. adolescent psychologist
    t. clinician
    T. Practical Nurse (TPN)
    t. reflex
training
    t. and deprogramming ▸ unlearning
       the
    t. and electroencephalogram (EEG)
       patterns ▸ autogenic
    t. and interactions ▸ staff
    t. and stress-related problems ▸
       autogenic
    t. approach, cognitive skills
    t., assertiveness
    t., auditory
    t., autogenic
    t., autogenic feedback
    t., autosuggestion in autogenic
    t., balance
    t., biofeedback
    t., biofeedback-assisted muscular
       relaxation
    t., bladder
    t., bowel
    t., clinical
    t., cognitive
    t., counterproductive
    t., custom
    t., diagnostic
    t., educational
    t. effect
    t., electroencephalogram (EEG)
       theta biofeedback
    t., endurance
    t. exercise ▸ strength
    t. exercise ▸ weight
    t. for anxiety and tension ▸
       autogenic
    t. for children ▸ skills
    t. for drug abuse ▸ autogenic
    t. for headache, autogenic
    t. for hypertension, autogenic
    t. for insomnia, autogenic
    t. for migraine headache ▸
       autogenic
    t., gait
    t., gentle resistance
    t. heart rate
    t., hypnotic
    t. in temperature biofeedback ▸
       autogenic
    t., Lamaze
    t. ▸ low vision

    t., marathon
    t., medical
    t., neuromuscular feedback
    t. of cardiovascular control
    t. of parts of buccinator muscle ▸
       feedback
    t., orthoptic
    t., paramedic
    t., parent effectiveness
    t., physical
    t., physiological response to
       relaxation
    t. ▸ problem-solving skills
    t. program, bowel
    t. program, strength-
    t., progressive relaxation
    t., psychological effects of
       relaxation
    t. qualifications
    t., relaxation
    t. relaxation exercises, autogenic
    t., resistance
    t. ▸ respiratory muscle
    t. ▸ sensory integration
    t. sessions
    t. sessions, auditory
    t. sessions, biofeedback
    t. sessions, relaxation
    t. ▸ social skills
    t., sound
    t. ▸ special skills
    t., staff
    t., strength
    t. ▸ stress inoculation
    t., stress management
    t. ▸ stress management relaxation
    t. ▸ supervised exercise
    t. technique, general relaxation
    t. testing, post-
    t., therapeutic
    t., toilet
    t., transfer
    t., trauma ▸ toilet-
    t., treadmill
    t. ▸ upper extremity
    t., weight
trains of ventricular pacing
trainwheel rhythm
trait(s) (Trait)
    t., antisocial
    t., antisocial personality
    T. Anxiety Inventory ▸ State
    t. anxiety, state-and-
    t., autosomal (asexual)
    t., biological

    t., character
    t., compulsive
    t., gait
    t., genetic
    t. ▸ health enhancing
    t., hereditary
    t. ▸ histrionic personality
    t., human
    t. in alcoholics ▸ personality
    t., inflexible
    t. ▸ inflexible antisocial personality
    t., inherited
    t., maladaptive
    t. ▸ maladaptive antisocial
       personality
    t., narcissistic
    t. of patient, premorbid personality
    t. pattern
    t. ▸ persistent antisocial personality
    t., personality
    t., physical
    t., psychological
    t., sex-linked
    t., sickle cell
    t., thalassemia
    t., unattractive character
tram (TRAM)
    T. (Treatment Rating Assessment
       Matrix)
    T. (Treatment Response
       Assessment Matrix)
    T. (Treatment Response
       Assessment Method)
    t. lines
    t. tracks
trance
    t. capabilities
    t. capacity, natural
    t. coma
    t., hypnotic
    t. -like attack
    t. -like behavior
    t. -like state
    t. logic
Tranq (phencyclidine)
Tranquility-Peace (STP) pill, Serenity-
tranquilize feelings
tranquilized, patient
tranquilizer
    t. (phencyclidine), elephant
    t. (phencyclidine) ▸ horse
    t., major
    t., minor
tranquilizing side-effects

transabdominal
- t. cholangiography
- t. scan
- t. sonography

transaction, consent

transaminase
- t. enzymes
- t. (EGOT) ▸ erythrocyte glutamic-oxaloacetic
- t. (GOT) ▸ glutamic-oxaloacetic
- t. (GPT) ▸ glutamic-pyruvic
- t. (SGOT) ▸ serum glutamic-oxaloacetic
- t. (SGPT) ▸ serum glutamic-pyruvic
- t. test

transaortic valve gradient

transaortic valve gradient ▸ peak

transatrial mitral commissurotomy ▸ percutaneous

transatrial pacing

transaxial
- t. plane
- t. slice
- t. tomography (PETT) ▸ positron emission

transbrachial arch aortogram

transbronchial
- t. biopsy
- t. brush biopsy
- t. lung biopsy

transcapillary refill

transcatheter
- t. arterial embolization
- t. embolization
- t. therapy
- t. umbrella

transcellular fluid

transcellular redistribution

transcendent coping skills

transcendental meditation (TM)

transcervical fracture

transcondylar fracture

transconjunctival blepharoplasty

transcortical aphasia

transcortical apraxia

transcranial
- t. Doppler probe
- t. Doppler test
- t. magnetic stimulation

transcriptase
- t. inhibitors ▸ nucleoside reverse
- t. polymerase chain reaction test ▸ reverse
- t., reverse
- t. ▸ ribonucleic acid (RNA) reverse

transcription
- t. assay ▸ gene transfer
- t., gene
- t., parallel

transcubital approach

transcultural psychiatry

transcutaneous
- t. echo
- t. electrical nerve stimulation (TENS)
- t. electrical stimulation (TES)
- t. electronic nerve stimulator (TENS)
- t. nerve stimulation
- t. oximetry
- t. oxygen (O_2)
- t. oxygen (O_2) monitor
- t. stimulator

transdermal (Transdermal)
- t. estrogen therapy
- t. nicotine patch
- T. -NTG (nitroglycerin) Patch
- t. patches, nicotine
- t. system, nicotine

Transderm-Nitro 5

transdiaphragmatic sympathectomy

transducer
- t., annular array
- t., diaphragm
- t., echocardiographic
- t., electronic
- t., external
- t., linkages, cellular
- t., phonocardiographic
- t., pressure
- t., quartz
- t., Statham pressure
- t. system
- t. system, multiple pressure
- t. system, single pressure
- t., ultrasound

transduction
- t., generalized
- t., genetic
- t., restricted
- t., transferred by
- t. ▸ transformation, conjugation or

transduodenal fiberscopic duct injection

transdural approach

transected
- t. and closed, bronchus
- t. and stump ligated ▸ doubly clamped,
- t. pancreas

- t. spinal cord
- t., vein ligated and

transection
- t., cord
- t., cranial nerve
- t. ▸ multiple subpial
- t. of pancreas, traumatic
- t. of proximal duodenum, traumatic
- t. of spinal cord

transepidermal nerve stimulation (TENS)

transepidermal water loss

transesophageal
- t. atrial pacing
- t. atrial stimulation
- t. color flow imaging ▸ Doppler
- t. contrast echocardiography
- t. dobutamine stress echocardiograph
- t. echo probe
- t. echocardiogram
- t. echocardiography (TEE)
- t. echocardiography with pacing
- t. probe

transfacial projection, lateral

trans-fatty acids

transfer (Transfer)
- t., adenovirus mediated gene
- t., advanced
- t. agent, heat
- t. analysis ▸ Southern
- t. and ambulation, standby assistance in
- t., bathtub and shower
- t., blastocyst
- t., Bunnell tendon
- t., cell-to-side
- t., chordal
- t. diagnosis
- t. ▸ ex vivo gene
- t., facilitate
- t. factor
- t. factor, blood element
- T. Factor (RTF) ▸ Resistance
- t. factor therapy
- t. flap, delayed
- t. flap, direct
- t. flap, immediate
- t. from supine to sitting
- t. function analysis
- t. function (MTF), modulation
- t. (GIFT), gamete intrafallopian
- t., gas
- t., gene
- t., group-

t., heat
t. ▸ in vivo gene
t., inpatient to outpatient
t., intrafallopian
t. (LET), linear energy
t., maximum assisted
t., minimal assistance for
t., minimal assisted
t., nutrient
t. of disease
t., patellar tendon
t., patient completes basic
t., patient completes independent
t., patient completes toilet
t., patient independent in
t., pes anserine
t., pivot
t. radiation, high linear energy
t., replication and
t., safe
t., sit-to-stand
t., sliding
t., supine to sit
t., tendon
t. test, lymphocyte
t. therapy, myoblast
t. to blood ▸ nutrients
t. to nursing home
t. to wheelchair, pivot
t. training
t. transcription assay ▸ gene
T. (TOT), Tubal Ovum
t., two-chair tub
t., unplanned
t. ▸ vascular gene
t., Velpeau's tendon
t. with standby assistance, patient
t. with walker, patient
t. (ZIFT) ▸ zygote intrafallopian

transferase
t. (ALT), alanine amino
t., galactose phosphate uridyl
t., hypoxanthine guanine
   phosphoribosyl
t., uridine diphosphoglycyronyl

transference(s)
t. and counter-transference
t. neurosis
t. paradigms, unrecognized
t., self-object
t. shift ▸ massive

transferred
t. by transduction
t. cells
t. for custodial care ▸ patient

t. ophthalmia
t., patient
t. sensation
t. to morgue, body
t. to nursing home ▸ patient
t. to recipient, donor's chromosome
transferrin saturation test
transferring immature muscle cells
transfixing suture
transfixion
t. ligature
t. of iris
t. screws
t. suture, doubly ligated with
transformable bacteria
transformation
t. ▸ antigen specific lymphocyte
t., chemical
t., conjugation or transduction
t. constant
t., genetic
t. ▸ growth and
t., human lymphocyte
t. imaging ▸ direct Fourier
t., lymphoblastic
t., metabolic
t. ▸ multiple myeloma with leukemic
t. of cell ▸ malignant
t., photochemical
t. process, endothelial
t. zone
t. zone, benign
t. zone, mature
t. zone, prophylactic destruction of
transformed cancer cells
transformer(s)
t., belt skin
t., cell
t. coil ▸ implanted secondary
t. coil, primary
t., filament
t., high voltage
t., ratio
t., step-down
t., step-up
transforming growth factor
transfused
t. and treated with supportive care
   ▸ patient
t. back into donor ▸ red cells
t., patient
t. with fresh frozen plasma ▸ patient
   admitted and
t. with whole blood ▸ patient
   admitted and

transfusion(s)
t. ▸ AIDS (acquired immune
   deficiency syndrome) associated
t. ▸ AIDS (acquired immune
   deficiency syndrome) tainted
t. -associated AIDS (acquired
   immune deficiency syndrome)
t. associated disease
t. associated infection
t., autologous
t., autologous blood
t., blood
t., blood for
t., blood product
t., cell mass
t., contaminated
t., contaminated blood
t., delayed reaction to
t., direct
t., directed donor
t. disease ▸ incompatible hemolytic
   blood
t., donor specific
t., exchange
t. ▸ exchange blood
t. form refusing permission for
   blood
t., fresh frozen plasma
t., granulocyte
t. hepatitis
t. hepatitis, post-
t. ▸ heterologous blood
t., homologous
t., immediate
t., incompatible blood
t., indirect
t., intraperitoneal
t., intrauterine
t., intravenous (IV)
t., massive
t. medicine
t. (MET) ▸ minimal exposure
t. mononucleosis, post-
t., neonatal
t. nephritis
t. of cryoprecipitate
t. of leukocytes
t. of red blood cells (RBC)
t. of tainted blood
t., packed cell
t. ▸ packed red blood cell (RBC)
t., periodic blood
t. ▸ perioperative red cell
t., placental
t., plasma

transfusion(s)—*continued*
t., platelet
t. procedure
t. protocol
t. purpura ▸ post-
t. reaction
t. reaction, anaphylactic
t. reaction, fatal
t. reaction ▸ febrile
t. reaction, immediate
t. reaction, suspected
t. recipients, blood
t., reciprocal
t., red cell
t. refusal form, blood
t. -related disease
t. -related disease ▸ minimize risk of
t. -related infection
t., replacement
t., substitution
t. syndrome ▸ post-
t. syndrome ▸ twin-twin
t., tainted blood
t. therapy
t. therapy, blood
t. therapy, individualized
t. transmissable
t. transmission of viral hepatitis
t. -transmitted AIDS (acquired immune deficiency syndrome)
t. transmitted disease
t. ▸ twin-to-twin
t., untoward reaction to
t., white blood cell
t., whole blood
transfusional hemosiderosis
transgluteal approach
transhepatic
t. catheterization ▸ percutaneous
t. cholangiogram
t. cholangiogram (PTC), percutaneous
t. cholangiography
t. cholangiography, direct percutaneous
t. cholangiography (FNTC) ▸ fine needle
t. cholangiography (PTC), percutaneous
t. drainage ▸ percutaneous
t. embolization (THE)
t. portography, percutaneous
transient(s) (Transients)
t. abnormal behavior

t., abrupt
t. acantholytic dermatosis
t. and eye blinks ▸ slow wave
t. anesthesia
t. asystole
t. ataxia
t. bacteremia
t. capillary leak
t. cardiac arrest
t., central sharp
t., central sharp wave
t. cerebral ischemia
t. cerebral ischemic episode
t. cerebral vein thrombosis
t. clinical hepatitis
T. Computer of Average
t. confusion
t. contact
t. contact between donor and recipient
t. depolarization
t. depression white blood count (WBC)
t. disorder
t. disorder of initiating sleep
t. disorder of initiating wakefulness
t. disorder of maintaining sleep
t. disorder of maintaining wakefulness
t. dissection
t. dizziness
t. edema
t., electroencephalogram (EEG)
t. emotional distress
t. equilibrium
t. evoked potential
t. global amnesia (TGA)
t. heart block
t. hemispheric attack
t. hypogammaglobulinemia
t. ideas of reference
t. impairment
t. insomnia
t. inward current
t. ischemia
t. ischemic attack (TIA)
t. ischemic attack and aging
t. ischemic attack (TIA) ▸ warning signs of
t. ischemic episode
t., isolated spike
t. joint pain
t. leukocytosis
t. loss of consciousness
t. loss of function

t. loss of respiratory reflex
t. loss of vision
t. mesenteric ischemia
t. motor tics
t. neurologic disturbance
t. of sleep, positive occipital sharp
t. organic mental disorder
t. organic psychotic condition
t. pain
t. paralysis
t. paranoid ideation
t. pericarditis
t., positive occipital sharp
t. respiratory distress
t. response imaging
t. septicemia
t., sharp
t., sharp central
t., sharp electroencephalogram (EEG)
t., sharp spike
t. situational disturbance
t., slow wave
t., spike
t. spinal cord dysfunction
t. spontaneous occurrences
t. symptoms
t. syncope
t. tachypnea
t. tachypnea of newborn
t. tic disorder
t. tic disorder of childhood
t. time of barium
t. time studies
t. tingling
t., vertex
t., vertex sharp
t. vertigo
t. visual symptoms
t. wave form, sharp
t. weakness
transillumination
t. light
t. procedure
t. test
transit
t., radionuclide
t., rapid
t. study ▸ radionuclide esophageal
t. time
t. time, cinedensitometric
t. time, esophageal
t. time ▸ myocardial
t. times, cinedensitometric assessment of

transition (Transition)
- t., allowed beta
- t. and expulsion
- t. back into community
- t., beta
- t. breathing
- t. contraction
- t. douche
- T. Dyspnea Index
- t. ▸ effacement, dilatation and
- t. ▸ forced ischemia reperfusion
- t., isobaric
- t., isomeric
- t., isometric
- t., life
- t., midlife
- t. phase
- t. rays
- t., role
- t., sympathovagal

transitional
- t. bladder cell carcinoma, in situ
- t. care
- t. cell
- t. cell carcinoma
- t. cell carcinoma of bladder
- t. cell carcinoma of renal pelvis
- t. cell papilloma
- t. cell zone
- t. counseling session
- t. development
- t. epithelial cells
- t. lumbosacral joint
- t. object
- t. pulp stage
- t. respiration
- t. sleep
- t. state
- t. tumor

transitive cerebri, gyri
transitory
- t. fever
- t. hallucinations
- t. hypertension
- t. mania
- t. mental disorder
- t. rales

transjugular cholangiography
transjugular intrahepatic
  portosystemic shunt
transketolase activity
translabyrinthine vestibular nerve
  section
translateral films

translating television microscope ▸
  ultraviolet color-
translation theory
translesional spectral flow velocity
translocation Down's syndrome
translocation mongolism
translucent
- t. goggles
- t. skin
- t. space

translumbar aortogram
translumbar aortography
transluminal
- t. angioplasty
- t. angioplasty ▸ infrapopliteal
- t. angioscopy ▸ percutaneous
- t. balloon valvuloplasty ▸
    percutaneous
- t. coronary angioplasty
- t. coronary revascularization
    (PTCR) ▸ percutaneous
- t. extraction atherectomy
- t. extraction endarterectomy
- t. lysing system

transmandibular implant
transmastoid labyrinthectomy
transmeatal atticotomy
transmeatal labyrinthotomy
transmembrane
- t. calcium flux
- t. potential
- t. signalling
- t. voltage

transmesenteric hernia
transmetatarsal amputation
transmissable, transfusion
transmissibility region, self-
transmissible
- t. infection
- t. spongiform encephalopathy
- t. spongiform virus encephalopathy

transmission
- t. ▸ AIDS (acquired immune
    deficiency syndrome)
- t. ▸ AIDS (acquired immune
    deficiency syndrome) virus
- t., airborne route of
- t. ▸ autosomal dominant
- t., blockage of light
- t., blood
- t. by contact
- t. by saliva, oral-oral
- t. chemoreceptor, deficient
- t., disease
- t., efficient means of

- t. electron microscopy
- t. -emission scintiphoto, combined
- t., environmental vector
- t. factor
- t. from infected mother to infant
- t., genetic
- t., hand-to-hand
- t., hepatitis
- t., heterosexual
- t., homosexual
- t., human
- t., impulse
- t., internal
- t. ▸ irregular dopamine
- t., mode of
- t. ▸ needle stick
- t., nerve
- t., neural
- t. of AIDS (acquired immune
    deficiency syndrome)
- t. of bacteria
- t. of disease ▸ prevent
- t. of electric signals or messages
- t. of infection
- t. of microbe to host
- t. of murmur
- t. of nerve impulses
- t. of organisms, nosocomial
- t. of risk factors, genetic
- t. of viral hepatitis ▸ confirmed
- t. of viral hepatitis ▸ food-borne
- t. of viral hepatitis ▸ hemodialysis
- t. of viral hepatitis ▸ inoculation
- t. of viral hepatitis ▸ intrafamily
- t. of viral hepatitis ▸
    intrainstitutional
- t. of viral hepatitis ▸ maternal-
    neonatal
- t. of viral hepatitis ▸ oral
- t. of viral hepatitis ▸ sexual
- t. of viral hepatitis ▸ transfusion
- t. of viral hepatitis ▸ waterborne
- t., parenteral
- t., patient-to-patient
- t., patient-to-staff
- t., perinatal
- t., respiratory
- t., risk of
- t., route of
- t., sexual
- t., source of
- t., staff-to-patient
- t. ▸ stimulated dopamine
- t., synaptic
- t., tertiary

transmission—*continued*
- t., transplacental
- t., ultraviolet
- t., vector
- t., viral

transmitral
- t.   Doppler E:A ratio
- t.   E:A ratio
- t.   E-wave deceleration time

transmits
- t.   sensation ▸ median nerve
- t.   sound waves
- t.   virus to unborn child

transmitted
- t.   acquired immune deficiency syndrome (AIDS) ▸ transfusion-
- t.   carotid pulsation
- t.   disease (STD), sexually
- t.   disease, transfusion
- t.   disease ▸ warning signs of sexually
- t.   diseases
- t.   infection ▸ sexually
- t.   murmurs
- t., pain impulses
- t.   pelvic inflammatory disease (PID) ▸ sexually

transmitter(s)
- t.   action, inhibitory neuro-
- t., event
- t., excitatory
- t., false
- t.   in brain, chemical
- t., inhibitory
- t., mood altering chemical
- t., neural
- t.   -receiver
- t.   substance

transmitting electrochemical messages to brain
transmitting infection
transmural
- t.   colitis
- t.   hemorrhage
- t.   infarction
- t.   myocardial infarction
- t.   pressure
- t.   steal

transmyocardial
- t.   perfusion pressure
- t.   revascularization (TMR)
- t.   revascularization ▸ percutaneous

transnasal drain
transoral projection, Pirie
transorbital leukotomy

transorbital lobotomy
transosteal implant
transparency ▸ illusion of
transparent
- t.   dressing, Bioclusive
- t.   granules, pale
- t.   jelly-like mass
- t.   meninges, glistening
- t.   rule, Luedde's
- t.   tissue

transpeptidase, gamma-glutamyl
transpeptidase, glutamyl
transperitoneal cesarean section (CS)
transpersonal medicine
transpersonal treatment for addictions
transplacental
- t.   gradient
- t.   hemorrhage
- t.   transmission

transplant(s)
- t., adrenal
- t., adrenal gland tissue
- t., allogeneic
- t., animal tissue
- t., authorization form for recipient of organ
- t., authorization form for removal of organ for
- t., autogenous
- t., autologous
- t., autologous bone marrow
- t., autologous stem cell
- t., Baffes
- t.   bilateral lung
- t.   bilateral nephrectomy, pre◊
- t., blood cell
- t., bone
- t., bone marrow
- t., brain cell
- t., cadaveric
- t.   candidate
- t., cardiac
- t., cartilage
- t.   cell
- t.   center
- t.   center, organ
- t.   center, referral
- t., cochlear
- t., consent form for recipient of organ
- t., consent form for removal of organ for
- t.   coordinator

- t., cord blood
- t., cornea
- t., corneal
- t., corneal tissue
- t.   coronary artery disease
- t. ▸ deep lamellar
- t., domino
- t., double lung
- t. ▸ en bloc bilateral lung
- t., eyes donated for corneal
- t., fat
- t.   feasible ▸ emergency skin
- t. ▸ fetal nerve cell
- t. ▸ fetal pig cell
- t., fetal tissue
- t. ▸ fetus-to-fetus stem cell
- t. ▸ fever, swelling and tenderness of
- t., first renal
- t., free nipple
- t. ▸ full thickness
- t., gene
- t., genetic
- t.   graft, whole bone
- t., hair
- t., hand
- t., Hauser
- t., heart
- t., heart-lung
- t. ▸ heterologous cardiac
- t. ▸ heterotopic cardiac
- t., homogeneous
- t. ▸ homologous cardiac
- t. ▸ human fetal pancreas
- t., identical twin
- t., islet cell
- t.   isolation ▸ post-
- t., kidney
- t., kidney-pancreas
- t., kidneys donated for kidney
- t. ▸ limbal stem cell
- t. ▸ live donor
- t., liver
- t., local irradiation of
- t., long-term survivor of heart
- t., lung
- t., mammary artery
- t., marrow
- t., McReynolds' pterygium
- t., meniscus
- t., microhair
- t., multiple organ
- t., nerve
- t. ▸ nerve cell
- t., nonidentical twin

t. of human fetal cells
t. of pterygium
t., organ
t. ▸ orthotopic cardiac
t. ▸ orthotopic heart
t., orthotopic hepatic
t., pancreas
t., parental
t., partial pancreas
t. ▸ partial thickness
t., patellar tendon
t. patient
t. patient, heart
t. patient, kidney
t. patient, liver
t. patient ▸ post-
t. patient ▸ prospective
t., peroneus brevis
t. physician
t. pneumonia
t., prenatal
t. procedure ▸ islet cell
t. recipient
t. recipient, cardiac
t. recipient, corneal
t. recipient, heart
t. recipient, organ
t. recipient ▸ prospective
t. recipients ▸ matching organ
t. rejection
t. rejection, bone marrow
t. ▸ rejection cardiomyopathy
t. rejection, kidney
t., removal of first
t., removal of second
t., renal
t., right pulmonary vein
t., routine skin
t. ▸ Schwann cell
t., second
t., second renal
t., sibling
t., single-lung
t., skin
t., small intestine
t. ▸ solid organ
t. ▸ spousal kidney
t. ▸ surface lamellar
t. surgeon
t. surgery
t. surgery, corneal
t. surgery, pre◊
t., syngenesioplastic
t. technique ▸ flap
t. technique ▸ pancreatic cell

t. technology
t., temporary heart
t., tendon
t., testicle
t., third renal
t., threatened rejection of
t., tissue
t. tissue-typing laboratories
t., toe-to-thumb
t., unrelated donor
t., vascular organ
t., whole organ
transplantable cadaver organ
transplantation (Transplantation)
t., allogenic
t., allogenic marrow
t. antigen
t. antigen, tumor specific
t. ▸ autologous cultured skin
t. ▸ blood and marrow
t., bone marrow
t., brain
t., cadaveric donor
t., cardiopulmonary
t., cartilage
t., cell
t. center
t., corneal
t., cryopreserved venous
t., fat
t., hair
t., heart
t., human organ
t. ▸ immunological barrier to skin
t., intestinal
t., islet
t., kidney
t., lung
t. metastasis
T. Network, Organ Procurement
    and
t., neural
t. of ocular muscle
t. of patellar tendon insertion,
    medial
t. of tendon
t., organ
t., orthotopic
t., pancreas
t., periosteal
t. pneumonia
t., post-
t. procedure
t. ▸ procurement of cadaver organs
    of

t., renal
t., skin
t., stem cell
t. surgery, organ
t., tissue
t., total lymphoid irradiation in organ
t., venous
t., xenograft
transplanted
t. blood vessels
t. cells
t. cord blood cells
t. fetal cells
t. heart, immune rejection of
t. immunity
t. islets
t. marrow
t. nerve
t. organ
t. organ ▸ block rejection of
t. organ ▸ blood flow to
t. organ ▸ combat rejection of
t. organ ▸ rejection of
t. skeletal muscle
t. skin adheres
t. tissue
t. ▸ tissue flap
t. tissue ▸ rejection of
t. vein
transplanting
t. hair
t. human fetal tissue
t. teeth
transport
t., aeromedical
t., calcium
t., critical care air
t. ▸ deficit in oxygen
t. function, atrial
t., immediate
t. of patient ▸ air
t., oxygen (O_2)
t., patient
t., placental
t. protocol, organized
t. sperm
t. time, particle
t., tissue
t. tubes
t. vials
transportation services,
    nonemergency
transportation ▸ tooth storage and
transported on gurney, patient
transporter cart

transposed adnexa
transposition
- t. complex
- t., corrected
- t. of arterial stems
- t. of great arteries
- t. of great arteries, complete
- t. of great arteries, corrected
- t. of great vessels
- t. of great vessels, corrected
- t., ovarian
- t., patellar tendon
- t., portacaval
- t. procedure ▸ Senning
- t., subclavian

transpulmonary pressure
transrectal
- t. needle biopsy
- t. probe
- t. ultrasound

transsacral anesthesia
transsacral block
transsarcolemmal calcium current
transseptal
- t. angiocardiography
- t. commissurotomy, Brock
- t. commissurotomy, Brockenbrough
- t. left heart catheterization
- t. puncture
- t. technique, anterograde

transsphenoidal resection in acromegaly
transstenotic pressure gradient measurement
transsynaptic retrograde degeneration
transtabular AP/PA projection
transtelephonic
- t. ambulatory monitoring system
- t. arrhythmia monitoring
- t. ECG (electrocardiograph) monitor
- t. exercise monitor
- t. monitor ▸ electrocardiographic (ECG)
- t. pacemaker monitoring

transtentorial herniation
transtentorial herniation ▸ traumatic
transthoracic
- t. approach
- t. biopsy
- t. biopsy chest wall
- t. diameter
- t. echocardiography
- t. impedance

- t. needle aspiration biopsy
- t. pacemaker
- t. projection
- t. shock ▸ high energy

transtracheal
- t. anesthesia
- t. aspirate
- t. bronchography, percutaneous
- t. oxygen (O_2)

transtrochanteric osteotomy
transudate, peritoneal
transudates and exudates ▸ diagnostic separation of
transudation of fluid
transudative ascites
transudative pleural effusion
transureteroureteral anastomosis
transurethral
- t. incision of prostate (TUIP)
- t. microwave thermotherapy (TUMT)
- t. needle ablation (TUNA)
- t. prostatectomy
- t. resection (TUR)
- t. resection (TUR) of bladder
- t. resection of prostate (TURP)
- t. ultrasound-guided laser-induced prostatectomy (TULIP)
- t. vaporization of prostate tissue

transvaginal
- t. approach
- t. cone
- t. scan
- t. sonography
- t. ultrasound

transvalensis, Nocardia
transvalvular aortic gradient
transvalvular flow
Transvene endocardial lead system ▸ Medtronic
Transvene nonthoracotomy implantable cardioverter defibrillator
transvenous
- t. angiography ▸ synchroton-based
- t. aortovelography
- t. approach
- t. catheter pacemaker
- t. defibrillation lead ▸ nonintegrated
- t. defibrillator lead
- t. device
- t. electrodes
- t. implantation of cardioverter defibrillator

- t. mitral commissurotomy ▸ percutaneous
- t. pacemaker
- t. pacemaker line
- t. pacemaker, permanent
- t. pacemaker placement, temporary
- t. pacemaker, temporary
- t. pacer

transventricular
- t. mitral commissurotomy, closed
- t. mitral valve commissurotomy
- t. valvotomy

transversa
- t., frontodextra
- t., frontolaeva
- t., mentodextra
- t., mentolaeva
- t., occipitodextra
- t. pelvis, diameter
- t., plica vesicalis
- t., sacrolaeva

transversal tomography
transversalis
- t. divided, fascia
- t., fascia
- t. muscle
- t., musculus
- t., semilunar fold of fascia

transverse [*traverse*]
- t. abdominal incision, lower
- t. and descending colon ▸ diverticulosis of
- t. arch
- t. arrest, deep
- t. arytenoid muscle
- t. bipolar montage
- t. bundles of palmar aponeurosis
- t. cervical nerve
- t. cervical veins
- t. cesarean (C-) section
- t. cesarean section (CS)
- t. colon
- t. colon ▸ diverticula of
- t. colon, infarcted
- t. colon obstruction
- t. colostomy
- t. colostomy, normal functions ileal
- t. commissure
- t. commissure, great
- t. diameter
- t. diameter of heart
- t. diameter of pelvic outlet
- t. diameter of pelvis
- t. disc
- t. facial fracture

t. facial vein
t. fascia
t. fibers, deep
t. folds of rectum
t. fracture
t. fracture, total
t. fragmentation
t. incision
t. incision, linear
t. lie
t. lie presentation
t. ligament
t. mastectomy scar
t. maxillary fracture
t. mesocolon
t. muscle
t. muscle of abdomen
t. muscle of auricle
t. muscle of chin
t. muscle of nape
t. muscle of perineum, deep
t. muscle of perineum, superficial
t. muscle of thorax
t. muscle of tongue
t. myelitis
t. myelitis, acute
t. nerve of neck
t. occipital protuberance
t. palatine folds
t. palatine suture
t. perinei muscle
t. plane
t. presentation
t. process
t. projection, cross-sectional
t. ridge
t. row of sutures
t. section
t. section of brain
t. section of heart
t. sections, serial
t. sulcus of heart
t. suture of Krause
t. temporal gyri
t. temporal gyrus, anterior
t. tomography, axial
t. tomography (PETT), positron emission
t. tubule
t. vein of face
t. vein of neck
t. vesical fold
t. wave
transversely, fascia incised
transversely, skin opened

transversi, gyri temporales
transversospinal muscle
transversus
  t. pericardii, sinus
  t., situs
  t., sulcus anthelicis
transvesical prostatectomy, suprapubic
transvestic fetishism
Trantas(')
  T. dots
  T. operation
  T. spots, Horner-
trap(s)
  t., bubble
  t., mucus
  t., reinforcement
  t. stomach, water-
trapanicum, Halobacterium
trapeze bar
trapezium bone
trapezium implant, Swanson
trapezius muscle
trapezius ridge sign
trapezoid
  t. bone
  t. implant
  t. implant ▸ Silastic
  t. ligament
trapped
  t. blood, drain
  t. gas volume
  t. in trachea, food
trapping
  t. filters, clot
  t., lymphocyte
  t. of air
  t. of air, expiratory
trash foot
trash, isolation
Traube('s)
  T. bruit
  T. curves
  T. double tone
  T. dyspnea
  T. heart
  T. -Hering waves
  T. murmur
  T. semilunar space
  T. sign
  T. space
trauma (Trauma)
  t., abdominal
  t., acoustic
  t., acute neurological

T. Acute Resuscitation (MedSTAR), Medical Shock
t., adult
t., adult betrayal
t. and abuse ▸ severe
t., arterial
t. -associated anuria
t., attachment
t., barometric
t. -based mastery fantasy
t., battlefield
t., betrayal
t., birth
t., blunt
t. ▸ blunt force
t., bone
t., bony
t., brain
t., burn
t., cardiac arrest following
t. care, prehospital
t. case
t. center
t. center, pediatric
t. center, regional
t., central nervous system (CNS)
t., cerebral
t., chest
t., childhood
t., coma secondary to head
t., controlled
t., cranial
t., crime victim
t., cumulative effects of
t. deafness, acoustic
t. death
t., dentoalveolar
t., destabilizing impact of
t. disorder, cumulative
t. dyscontrol
t. ▸ ear, nose and throat (ENT)
t., emotional
t., exacerbate
t., facial
t., fluid and electrolyte therapy in
t. -focused approach to psychotherapy
t. framework, basic
t., functional decortication from
t., head
t., hidden
t. ▸ high impact
t., iatrogenic
t. incident reduction
t. index

trauma—*continued*

- t. -induced hysterical paralysis
- t. ▸ influence of
- t., initial
- t., joint
- t., laryngotracheal
- t. life support (ATLS), advanced
- t., localized
- t., long-term
- t. ▸ low impact
- t., major
- t., major physical
- t. management
- t., massive multiple
- t. medicine
- t. ▸ memory for
- t., multiple
- t., multisystem
- t. ▸ pain and
- t. patient
- t. patient, air evacuation of
- t., patient has multiple
- t., pediatric
- t., penetrating
- t., peritoneal
- t., pharmacology in
- t., physical
- t. ▸ physical evidence of
- t., postabortion
- t., psychic
- t., psychological
- t. recovery
- t. researcher
- t. response ▸ post-
- t. response syndrome ▸ post-
- t. score
- t., severe chest
- t., severe head
- t., sexual
- t., shock
- t., stimulus of
- t., sudden
- t., surface
- t., surgical
- t. survivor
- t., suspected
- t. syndrome
- t. syndrome, compound reaction ▸ rape
- t. syndrome ▸ rape
- t. syndrome, silent reaction ▸ rape
- t. team
- t. team members
- t. technologist
- t., tissue

- t. to chest, massive
- t. to eyeball
- t. to scrotum and testes
- t. to vein
- t. ▸ toilet-training
- t., toxic
- t. toxicology
- t. treatment
- t. unit
- t. units, pediatric
- t., vascular

traumatic

- t. abscess
- t. acute renal failure (PTARF) ▸ post-
- t. amaurosis
- t. amnesia
- t. amnesia, post-
- t. amputation
- t. aneurysm
- t. aortic disruption
- t. apnea
- t. arthritis
- t. arthritis ▸ post-
- t. asphyxia
- t. atrophy of bone, post-
- t. avulsion
- t. brain death
- t. brain injury
- t. cardiopulmonary arrest
- t. cataract
- t. cervicitis
- t. childhood
- t. childhood experiences
- t. deafness
- t. death
- t. delirium
- t. depression
- t. disability syndrome
- t. discopathy
- t. dislocation
- t. displacement
- t. effect
- t. emergency
- t. emphysema
- t. encephalopathy
- t. epilepsy
- t. epilepsy, post-
- t. event
- t. experience
- t. experience ▸ recall of
- t. fever
- t. fistula
- t. flashbacks ▸ post-
- t. forgetting

- t. glaucoma
- t. grief
- t. headache
- t. headache ▸ post-
- t. heart disease
- t. hemopericardium
- t. hemorrhage
- t. hemorrhagic bursitis
- t. hemothorax
- t. idiocy
- t. in origin
- t. influence
- t. injury
- t. lacerations
- t. memories
- t. multiple hemorrhage
- t. neurosis
- t. occlusion
- t. orchitis
- t. osteomyelitis of skull, post-
- t. pain
- t. pancreatitis
- t. pancreatitis, post-
- t. perforation of esophagus
- t. pericarditis
- t. pneumonia
- t. pneumothorax
- t. reaction, adult
- t. reenactments
- t. rhabdomyolysis
- t. rupture
- t. rupture of spleen
- t. scenes ▸ exploration of
- t. seizure, acute
- t. seizures, post-
- t. separation
- t. shock
- t. situation
- t. spinal tap
- t. spondylopathy
- t. state
- t. stress
- t. stress disorder (PTSD) ▸ post-
- t. stress disorder ▸ prolonged post-
- t. stress disorder ▸ psychotherapy of post-
- t. stressors
- t. sutures
- t. symptoms ▸ post-
- t. syndrome, post-
- t. syringomyelia
- t. tamponade
- t. tap, non-
- t. thrombosis
- t. thrombus

t. transection of pancreas
t. transection of proximal
    duodenum
t. transtentorial herniation
t. ureteral injury
t. vaginal delivery
t. vertigo
t. vertigo, chronic post-
t. vertigo ▸ post-
t. wet lung
t. wounds, open fresh
traumatica
   t., spondylomalacia
   t., stomatitis
   t., tendonitis ossificans
traumatically detached statoconia
traumaticum, erythema
traumatization, vicarious
traumatized child
traumatized zone
traumatogenic
   t. occlusion
   t. pulpal necrosis
   t. wound
Trautmann's triangle
traveler's
   t. diarrhea
   t. disease
   t. thrombosis
travel-related blood clot
traverse [*transverse*]
tray assembly, automated
TRBF (total renal blood flow)
TRC (total ridge-count)
TRC (tanned red cells) antibody titer,
    microsomal
Treacher-Collins syndrome
treadmill (Treadmill)
   t., arm ergometry
   t., Bruce
   t. echocardiography
   t., electrocardiogram (ECG/EKG)
   t., electrocardiogram (ECG/EKG)
      stress
   t. exercise
   t. exercise stress test
   t. exercise test ▸ symptom-limited
   T. Exertion Scale (BTES), Borg
   t. -induced angina
   t. prognostic score ▸ Duke
   t. protocol, Bruce
   t. protocol ▸ Naughton
   t. protocol ▸ Reeves
   t. protocol ▸ Sheffield
   t. score ▸ Hollenberg

t. ▸ self-powered
t. stress test
t. stress, thallium
t. test ▸ exercise
t. test ▸ J point
t. test ▸ radioactive
t. testing
t. time ▸ exercise
t. training
t. walking therapy
treat alcoholics
treat empirically
treatable
   t. arrhythmias
   t. blindness
   t. condition
   t. depression
   t. disease
   t. disorder
   t. illness
   t. lesion
   t. mental disease
   t. psychiatric disorder
   t. stage
   t. vascular occlusions
treated
   t. conservatively, patient
   t. for comfort only, patient
   t. for smoke inhalation, patient
   t. in external irradiation, volume
   t. in hospital, patient
   t. initially, patient
   t. initially with intravenous (IV)
      fluids ▸ patient
   t. lesions, antibiotic-
   t. marrow
   t. medically, patient
   t. milk, lactase-
   t. on an outpatient basis
   t. pain, incompletely
   t. ▸ patient diagnosed and
   t., patient empirically
   t., symptomatically
   t. syphilis
   t. with placebo ▸ patient
   t. with radiation and chemotherapy
      ▸ patient
   t. with radiation therapy ▸ patient
   t. with supportive care ▸ patient
   t. with supportive care ▸ patient
      transfused and
   t. with tamoxifen ▸ patient
   t. with thermotherapy ▸ patient
treatment(s) (Treatment)
   t. abstinence, post

t., abstinence-oriented
t., accelerated
t. ▸ accept or reject medical
t., acquired immune deficiency
    syndrome (AIDS)
t., active
t., active care
t., acupuncture
t. ▸ acute phase of
t., addiction
t. ▸ adequacy of
t., adequate
t., adjunct
t., adjuvant
t. ▸ adjuvant hormonal or
    chemotherapy
t., aerosolized
t., aggressive
t., aggressive laser
t., aggressive medical
t. agreement, family
t., alcohol
t., alcohol abuse
t., alcohol and drug abuse
t. alcohol use ▸ post-
t., alcoholism community
t., alternative
t., alternative method of
t., anaphylaxis emergency
t. and observation
t. and prevention programs
t. and recovery, diagnosis
t. and survival
t., angiogenesis
t., Antabuse
t., anti-aging
t., antianginal
t., antibiotic
t., antidepressant
t., antimicrobial
t., antiviral drug
t., application to
t., approaches
t., appropriate
t. as indicated
t. assistant (SHTA) ▸ security
    hospital
t., axiomatic
t. (AZT) ▸ azidothymidine
t., baldness
t. barriers
t., behavioral
t., behavioral health
t., beneficial
t. bias ▸ time-to-

treatment(s)—*continued*

t., biofeedback
t., biological
t., blanket
t. bleeding, post-
t., bloodletting
t., bogus
t., brachytherapy
t., brain cancer
t., brain tumor
t., Brandt's
t., breast cancer
t., broad spectrum behavioral
t. by manipulation of the body
t., cancer
t. ▸ cancer detection, prevention and
t., cataract
t., catheter administered
t., cellulite
T. Center, Drug
T. Center, Pain
t. center ▸ patient discharged to convalescent
t. center, sexual assault
t., chemical dependency
t., chemotherapy
t., childhood psychiatric
t., choice of
t., choice of medical
t. choices, factor in
t. chronic
t., chronic antidepressant
t., clinic, free drug
t., clinical
t., cocaine
t., cocaine abuse
t., cocaine addiction
t., cocaine dependence
t., coercive
t., cognitive behavioral
t. ▸ cold or ice whirlpool
t., collagen skin
t. ▸ combined hyperthermia and radiation
t. completion
t. compliance
t., compound-Q
t., comprehensive
t., compulsory
t., concurrent
t., conducting
t. ▸ conformed radiation
t., conjoint
t., conservative

t., conventional
t. ▸ conventional radiation
t., cornerstones of
t., cost-effective quality
t. costs
t., costs, direct
t., course of
t., court ordered medical
t. criteria, addiction
t., cross-fire
t., cryokinetic
t., cryopexy
t., cryotherapy
t., curative
t., current medication
t. decision
t., definitive
t. ▸ denial of lifesaving medical
t., depression-anxiety
T. (D/ART) ▸ Depression/Awareness Recognition and
t., description of
t., detoxification and brief
t., diabetic laser
t., diagnosis and
t. ▸ diagnosis, prevention and
t., diagnostic
t., diagnostic procedure and
t., dialysis
t. directive ▸ advanced
t., discharged to
t. discontinued
t., drug
t., drug abuse
t. drug, prostate
t. drug use ▸ post-
t., drug-free
t., dual approach to
t. duration, increased overall
t. during pregnancy, care and
t., early burn
t., effective
t. effectiveness studies
t., effects of
t., effects of behavioral
t. efficacy
t. (ECT), electroconvulsant
t. (ECT) ▸ electroconvulsive
t. (EST) ▸ electroshock
t., embolization
t., emergency
t. ▸ emergency insect-sting
t. ▸ emergency pain
t., empirical

t., endodontic
t., endovascular
t., enhance
t. environment ▸ post-
t., epilepsy laser
t. essentials
t., established
t., ethically extraordinary
t., evaluate
t., evaluation and
t., exercise
t. experience criteria ▸ previous
t. experience ▸ previous
t., experimental
t., experimental breast cancer
t., exploratory
t., extended medical
t. facilities, narcotic
t. facility ▸ acquired immune deficiency syndrome (AIDS) residential
t. facility ▸ residential
t. failure
t. failure pattern
t., family based
t., family sexual abuse
t., fibroid
t. field
t. field, alcoholism
t. field ▸ substance abuse
t. flow sheet
t., follow-up
t. for acute drug intoxication ▸ acute
t. for addictions ▸ transpersonal
t. for aneurysm ▸ surgical
t. for brain tumor ▸ surgical
t. for bursitis ▸ radiation
t. for cancer
t. for cancer ▸ photodynamic therapy (PDT)
t. for children ▸ group
t. for depression, cognitive
t. for drug abuse, behavioral
t. for drug dependence, behavioral
t. for epidural hemorrhage ▸ surgical
t. for epilepsy ▸ surgical
t. for flashback reactions, acute
t. for hair loss
t. for hypertension
t. for organic brain syndrome, acute
t. for organic brain syndrome, subacute
t. for overdosing, acute

t. for overdosing, subacute
t. for panic reactions, acute
t. for Parkinson's disease ▸ surgical
t. for psychotic reactions, acute
t. for severed nerve ▸ surgical
t. for stroke ▸ surgical
t. for withdrawal, acute
t. for wrinkles ▸ laser
t., Forlanini's
t., form for refusal to submit to
t., Fränkel's
t., functioning after
t., gastroenteritis
t., gentian violet
t., glaucoma
t. goal
t., grenz ray
t. group, combined
t. group, drug
t. group ▸ low stress
t., hair loss
t. ▸ hair removal
t., Hartel's
t. ▸ heart failure
t., herbal
t., high pressure
t. ▸ high-quality and effective
t., homeopathic
t., hormonal
t. ▸ hormonal cancer
t., hormone
T. ▸ Hydrotherapy
t. ▸ hyperbaric oxygen (O₂)
t., hypertension
T. (HOT), Hypertension Optimal
t., hypnotic
t., immunotherapy
t. implications
t. improvement
t., Imre
t. in advanced disease, combined
t. in cancer, preferred
t. in radiation therapy, whole abdominal
t., indications for long-term
t., ineffective
t., infertility
t., inhalation chemotherapy
t., initial
t., initial diagnosis and
t., initial evaluation and
t. ▸ initial stabilization phase of
t., initiate
t., injection
t., innovative

t., inpatient
t., inpatient psychiatric
t., insect sting
t., insulin
t., insulin coma
t., insulin shock
t., integrated
t., intensive
t. ▸ intensive chemotherapy
t., interferon
t. interruptions (STI) ▸ structured
t. intervention
t. ▸ intractable pain
t., invasive
t. issues ▸ impaired employees alcohol and drug
T. (JSAT) ▸ *Journal of Substance Abuse*
t., Karell's
t., kyphoplasty
t., lack of tolerance to
t., laser
t. ▸ laser hair removal
t. ▸ laser skin
t., laser surgery
t. ▸ leg vein
t. level
t., life-prolonging
t., life-saving
t., life-saving medical
t., life-supporting
t., life-sustaining
t. literature
t., lithium
t., local
t., long-term
t., long-term acupuncture
t., long-term aftercare
t., long-term counterconditioning
t., long-term detoxification
t., long-term drug
t., long-term outpatient
t., lymphoma
t. machines, quality assurance in
t. ▸ marijuana dependence
t., maternal
t., medical
t., medication
t., mental health
t., methadone
t. method, selecting
t. methods
t. methods ▸ moderation-oriented
t., microdermabrasion
t. modalities ▸ psychiatric

t. modality, major
t., modality of
t., modified upper mantle radiation
t., moist heat
t., monotherapy
t., moral
t., motivated for
t., multidisciplinary
t., multidisciplinary method of
t. necessary, no
t., nervous disorder
t. ▸ nicotine patch
t. ▸ noncompliance with medical
t., noninvasive
t. ▸ nonpharmacologic measure of
t., nonsurgical
t., nontoxic
t., nontraditional
t., nursing
t. objectives, establish
t., observation and
t., Ochsner's
t., Oertel's
t. of a minor ▸ authorization for
t. of accidents
t. of acute drug intoxication, subacute
t. of acute drug reaction withdrawal
t. of acute drug reactions
t. of acute drug reactions in violent patients
t. of acute drug reactions to cannabinoids
t. of acute drug reactions to depressants
t. of acute drug reactions to hallucinogens
t. of acute drug reactions to inhalants
t. of acute drug reactions to multiple drugs
t. of acute drug reactions to opioids
t. of acute drug reactions to phencyclidines
t. of acute drug reactions to stimulants
t. of acute intoxication
t. of addictive behaviors
t. of alcoholism ▸ diagnosis and
t. of cervical neoplasia, laser
t. of choice
t. of chronic anxiety
t. of chronic pain
t. of circulatory shock
t. of cocaine addiction

treatment(s)—*continued*

t. of contrasting temperatures
t. of delusions ▸ psychiatric
t. of diabetes
t. of digestive disease
t. of disease
t. of drug abuse and addiction
t. of eating disorders ▸ evaluation
t. of flashback reactions
t. of flashback reactions, subacute
t. of footdrop after stroke ▸ biofeedback
t. of gingiva
t. of glandular tissue, radiation
t. of heart disease
t. of infertility
t. of insomnia, group
t. of localized neurodermatitis
t. of mental illness
t. of opiate addict
t. of organic brain syndrome
t. of overdose
t. of panic reactions
t. of panic reactions, subacute
t. of patient, ongoing
t. of pericular infection
t. of physicians who abuse drugs
t. of poisoning of adolescents
t. of poisoning of children
t. of psychotic reactions
t. of psychotic reactions, subacute
t. of rheumatic fever
t. of spasticity
t. of suicidal patients
t. of tendinitis, radiation
t. of vaginal neoplasia, laser
t., off-trail
t. on withdrawal, subacute
t. options
t., oral
t., oral disulfiram
t., Orr
t., orthodontic
T. Outcome Prospective Study (TOPS)
t. outcome research
t. outcome ▸ substance abuse
t. outcomes, successful
t., outpatient
t., outpatient drug-free
t., outpatient psychiatric
t., overall
t., pain
t., palliative
t., parenteral

t., parenteral injection
t., passive
t., patient admitted for observation and
t., patient discharged to
t., patient responded to
t., Paul's
t. ▸ pelvic radiation
t., period, active
t., pharmacological
t., phases of
t. philosophy
t. ▸ physiology, disease and
t. placement
t. placement decisions
t. plan, developing
t. plan, individual
t. plan, initial
t. plan, initial psychiatric
T. Plan, Master
t. plan, process of
t. plan review
t. planning
t. planning and simulation
t. planning format
t. planning ▸ joint
t. planning, multidisciplinary
t. planning, quality assurance in
t., plasmapheresis
t., Politzer's
t. ▸ poly-antiviral
t. portals
t., postlaser
t., postsurgical
t. practice
t., preferred
t., preventive
t., primary
t., prior to
t. problems
t. process
t., Proetz's
t. professionals
t. professionals ▸ alcohol and substance abuse
t. program
t. program, drug
t. program, drug-free
t. program, experimental
t. program, extensive
t. program, gender-specific
t. program, intense outpatient
t. program, intensive outpatient
t. program, methadone maintenance

t. program ▸ pain
t. program, partial hospital
t. program, publicly assisted drug abuse
t. program, rigid
t., proposed
t., prostate cancer
t. protocol ▸ multinodal
t. protocols, inpatient
t. protocols, standardized
t. protocols, written
t., psora-lens plus ultraviolet light (PUVA)
t., psoriasis
t., psychedelic
t., psychiatric
t., psychodynamic
t., psychological
t., psychopharmacological
t., psychosocial
t., psychotherapeutic
t., quality of
t., radiation
t., radiation therapy
t., radical
t. ▸ radioactive iodine
t., radiotherapy
t. ▸ rapid-freeze, slow-thaw
T. Rating Assessment Matrix (TRAM)
t. record
t., recovery, and relapse prevention
t., reflexology
t., refractive to
t., refractory to
t. regimen
t., rehabilitative
t., residential
t. resistant alcoholism
t. -resistant depression
t. -resistant obsessive-compulsive disorder
t. resource, addiction
t. resource available
T. Response Assessment Matrix (TRAM)
T. Response Assessment Method (TRAM)
t., response to
t. restrictions
t., retroviral
t., rib field
t. ▸ right to reject medical
t. ▸ risks and benefits of
t., roentgen

t., Rogaine
t. ▸ root canal
t., Rotunda
t., routine
t., Schlösser's
t., Schott
t., sclerolaser
t., sclerotherapy
t., secondary effects of
t., seed
t. -seeking client
t., self-
t. sequelae
t. services
t. setting
t. setting, selecting
t., shock
t. ▸ shock wave
t., side-effects of
t. simulation
t. slots
t., somatic
t. specialist, drug
t. specialties
t. ▸ spider vein
t. spinal spurs
t., split course
t. ▸ sports injury
t. ▸ stand-alone laser
t., standard hospital
t. ▸ standard medical
t., standard radiation
t. ▸ sterile whirlpool
t., steroid
t. strategy
t. strategy ▸ effective
t., Stroganoff's (Stroganov's)
t., stroke
t. studies, medical
t. study ▸ hypertension optimal
t., subcoma insulin
t., subsequent
t., subshock insulin
t., substance abuse
t. success
t., successful
t., superficial
t., supplemental
t., supportive
t., supportive care
t., supportive psychological
t., surgical
t. ▸ surgical cancer
t., surgical removal
t., swayback

t., symptomatic
t. ▸ symptoms cause and
t. symptoms ▸ post-
t., synergistic
t. system ▸ outpatient drug
t., systemic
t. ▸ tai-chi
t. team
t. team approach ▸ multidisciplinary
t. team ▸ attending designated
t. team leader
t. team ▸ multidisciplinary
t. team recommendations
t. technique
t. technologies
t. termination
t. ▸ theory-driven
t., therapeutic
t. therapeutic instructions ▸ intra◊
t. therapeutic instructions ▸ pre◊
t. therapy
t. ▸ thyroid hormone
t., tolerance to
t. ▸ tone and spasticity
t., topical
t., total body
t., total eradication
t., toxic
t., traditional
t., trauma
t. trial, randomized
t. trials ▸ federal acquired immune
    deficiency syndrome (AIDS)
t., Trueta
t., tumor regeneration and
    protracted
T., Tuneable Dye Laser
t., types of
t., ultrasonic
t., ultrasound
t., unconventional
t., undergoing cancer
t. unit ▸ medically managed
    intensive addiction
t., units, methadone
t., unproven
t., vertebroplasty
t., viable
t., vibratory
t. volume
t. volume and dose
t. volume in radiation therapy
t., Weir Mitchell's
t. ▸ withdrawal of life-saving
t. ▸ withholding of life-saving

t., worthless
t., Yeo's
t., yoga
t., zyderm collagen

Tree (tree)(s)
T. (barbiturates)
t. appearance pruned
t. arteriogram, pruned-
t., biliary
t. branches of bronchial
t., bronchial
t. cannulated, biliary
t. carcinoma, biliary
T. (barbiturates), Christmas
t., distortion endobronchial
t., embryo bronchial
•t., endobronchial
•t. examined, bronchial
t., flexibility of bronchial
T., House Test ▸ Draw Person,
t. in patient management, decision
t., left bronchial
t., left endobronchial
t. -like structure
t. ▸ mucus plugging of bronchial
t. -person (HTP) ▸ house-
t., right bronchial
t., right endobronchial
t., sensitive bronchial
t., tracheal
t., tracheobronchial

Treitz('s)
T., arch of
T., fossa of
T. hernia
T., ligament of
T., muscle of

Trematoda
T. Clonorchis
T. Dicrocoelium
T. Echinostoma
T. Fasciola
T. Fasciolopsis
T. Gastrodiscoides
T. Heterophyes
T. Metagonimus
T. Opisthorchis
T. Paragonimus
T. Schistosoma

trematode parasite
trembling
t. abasia
t. and shakiness
t. convulsion
t. ▸ disabling, shaking and

trembling—*continued*
  t. from anxiety
  t. from atherosclerosis
  t. from caffeine
  t. from coldness
  t. in aging
  t., involuntary
  t. of arm
  t. of body, involuntary
  t. of hands
  t. of limbs, involuntary
  t., patient
  t. pulse
  t., rhythmic
  t. ▸ sweating and
  t. ▸ tremor or
  t. ▸ twitching and
tremendous fatigue
tremens (DTs) ▸ delirium
tremens, rigor
tremolo massage
tremor(s)
  t., abnormal
  t., action
  t. and chills
  t. and dyskinesia
  t. and immobility ▸ stiffness,
  t. and jerky movements
  t. and rigidity ▸ diminish
  t. and shakes
  t. artifact, ocular
  t., ataxia and intention
  t. ▸ ataxia titubation and
  t., benign essential
  t. ▸ benign hereditary
  t., benign senile
  t., bradykinesia and rigidity
  t., clubbing or
  t., coarse
  t., coarse hand
  t., continuous
  t., cordis
  t., darkness
  t., definite
  t., disabling essential
  t. disorder ▸ Parkinson's
  t., drug-induced
  t., epidemic
  t., epileptoid
  t., essential
  t., familial
  t., fibrillary
  t., fine
  t., flapping
  t., forced

  t., hand
  t., head
  t., hereditary essential
  t., heredofamilial
  t., Hunt's
  t., hysterical
  t. in hands
  t. in upper extremity
  t., incapacitating
  t., intention
  t., intermittent
  t., involuntary
  t. ▸ irritability and
  t., kinetic
  t. linguae
  t., marked observed
  t. mercurialis
  t., metallic
  t., mild
  t., mild observed
  t., motofacient
  t., muscle
  t. ▸ muscle rigidity and
  t., muscular
  t., normal
  t., ocular
  t. of extremities ▸ intention
  t. of eyelids
  t. of hand
  t. of head
  t. of legs, coarse
  t. of tongue, trombone
  t., opiophagorum
  t. or trembling
  t., Parkinson-like
  t., passive
  t. ▸ patient has
  t., perioral
  t., persistent
  t., physiologic
  t. potatorum
  t., purring
  t. reduction
  t., Rendu's
  t., resting
  t., rhythmic
  t., rhythmical
  t., senile
  t., shakes, jerks and falling
  t., slight intention
  t. ▸ slowed gait and
  t., slowness, stiffness and
    unsteadiness
  t., static
  t., striocerebellar

  t. tendinum
  t., tics and fasciculations
  t., toxic
  t., voice
  t., volitional
  t., voluntary
  t., weakness and rigidity ▸ poor
    balance,
tremulous
  t. cataract
  t. iris
  t., patient
  t. pulse
tremulousness ▸ stress-related
Trenaunay syndrome
trench
  t. fever
  t. foot
  t. hand
  t. lung
  t. mouth
  t. mouth from anxiety
  t. nephritis
  t., paranoid
  t. throat
trend(s)
  t. in drug abuse
  t. in drug abuse, international
  t., inversional
  t. of thought
Trendelenburg('s)
  T. gait
  T. operation
  T. position
  T. symptom
  T. tampon
  T. test
trepanation, corneal
trephination/trepanation
trephining, corneal
trepidans, abasia
trepidant abasia, paroxysmal
trepidatio cordis
Treponema
  T. calligyrum
  T. carateum
  T. genitalis
  T. macrodentium
  T. microdentium
  T. mucosum
  T. pallidum
  T. pallidum immobilization (TPI)
  T. pallidum ▸
    microhemagglutination
  T. pertenue

T. pintae
T. refringens
treponemal
    t. absorption fluorescent
    t. antibody absorption test ▸
       fluorescent
    t. antibody, fluorescent
treppe
    t., negative
    t. phenomenon
    t., positive
treubii, Siderocapsa
Treves' fold
TRF (thyrotropin-releasing factor)
triad
    t., acute compression
    t., adrenomedullary
    t. asthma
    t., Beck's
    t., Bezold's
    t., Cushing
    t., Fallot
    t., Falta's
    t., hepatic
    t., Hutchinson's
    t., Kartagener's
    t., Merseburg
    t. of city cultures
    t. of symptoms
    t., Osler
    t., portal
    t. ▸ Q fever, psittacosis, cocci
    t., Virchow
triadic junction
Triage (triage)
    T., Nursing
    t. patients
    t., prehospital
trial(s) (Trial)
    t., adequate clinical
    t., analysis at conclusion of clinical
    t. basis
    t., cancer
    T. (CAST), Cardiac Arrhythmia
       Suppression
    t., clinical
    t., clinical research
    t., continuous
    t., controlled
    t., controlled clinical
    t., crossover
    t., double-blind clinical
    t., double-blind placebo
    t., double-blinded
    t., drug

t. drug, on-
t., empiric
t., exclusion rate and clinical
t., false-negative results in clinical
t. ▸ federal acquired immune
    deficiency syndrome (AIDS)
    treatment
t. feedback, discrete post-
t. frame
t. ▸ gene therapy
t., international
t. ▸ Magnesium in Coronaries
    (MAGIC)
t., matched control studies in clinical
t., methodology clinical
t., multicenter
t., multi-institutional clinical
t., national clinical
t., nonrandomized
t. of labor
t. of labor ▸ mandatory
t., ongoing clinical
t. period
t., pilot study in clinical
t., placebo-controlled
t. ▸ placebo-controlled clinical
t., protocol for clinical
t. ▸ random control clinical
t., randomized
t., randomized clinical
t., randomized controlled
t. ▸ randomized controlled clinical
t. ▸ randomized double blinded
    placebo-controlled
t. ▸ randomized, placebo-controlled
t., randomized vs nonrandomized
    clinical
t. results
t. ▸ short-term clinical
t. summary, clinical
t., therapeutic
t. treatment, off-
t., vaccine
t. visit
triangle(s)
    t., aortic
    t., axillary
    t., Burger scalene
    t., Burger's
    t., cardiohepatic
    t., carotid
    t., clavipectoral
    t., Codman's
    t., Einthoven's
    t. excised, skin

t., femoral
t., Hesselbach's
t., infraclavicular
t., intraclavicular
t., Kiesselbach's
t., Middeldorpf's
t., Pawlik's
t., Rauchfuss
t., retentive
t., retromolar
t., Scarpa's
t., sternocostal
t., subclavian
t. technique ▸ forward
t., Trautmann's
triangular
    t. bandage
    t. bipolar montage
    t. bone
    t. defect
    t. dressing
    t. fold
    t. fossa
    t. infarct
    t. muscle
    t., plica
    t. ridge
    t. test, double
triangulation of drugs
triangulation runs
Triatoma infestans
triatrial heart
triatriatum cor
triatriatum dexter, cor
triaxial reference system
triazeno imidazole carboxamide
    (DTIC/DIC) ▸ dimethyl
tribasilar synostosis
tributaries and perforators
tributaries, renal vein
TRIC (trachoma inclusion
    conjunctivitis)
triceps
    t. brachii muscle
    t. extension
    t. extension exercise
    t. muscle of arm
    t. muscle of calf
    t. pushdown
    t. reflex
    t. surae jerk
    t. surae muscle
    t. surae reflex
trichiasis of eyelashes
trichina worm

Trichinella spiralis
trichinous embolism
trichiura, Trichuris
trichloroacetic acid
Trichobilharzia ocellata
Trichodectes
    T. canis
    T. climax
    T. equi
    T. hermsi
    T. pilosus
    T. retusis
    T. sphaerocephalus
trichoepithelioma papillosum
    multiplex
trichoides, Cladosporium
Trichomonas
    T. buccalis
    T. columbae
    T. columbarum
    T. elongata
    T. foetus
    T. gallinae
    T. gallinarum
    T. genus
    T. hominis
    T. infection
    T. infestation
    T. intestinalis
    T. muris
    T. pulmonalis
    T. resistance
    T. tenax
    T. vaginalis
    T. vaginitis
trichomycosis
    t. axillaris
    t. chromatica
    t. favosa
    t. nodosa
    t. palmellina
    t. pustulosa
    t. rubra
trichophytic granuloma
Trichophyton
    T. acuminatum
    T. album
    T. asteroides
    T. cerebriforme
    T. concentricum
    T. crateriforme
    T. discoides
    T. ectothrix
    T. endothrix
    T. epilans

    T. faviform
    T. ferrugineum
    T. gallinae
    T. gypseum
    T. mentagrophytes
    T. neoendothrix
    T. ochraceum
    T. radians
    T. rosaceum
    T. rubrum
    T. sabouraudi
    T. schoenleini
    T. simii
    T. sufureum
    T. verrucosum
    T. violaceum
trichorrhexis nodosa
trichosis carunculae
Trichosoma contortum
Trichosomoides crassicauda
Trichosporon
    T. beigelii
    T. cutaneum
    T. fungus
    T. giganteum
    T. pedrosianum
trichosporosis
    t. indica
    t. nodosa
    t. tropica
trichostasis spinulosa
Trichostrongylus
    T. capricola
    T. colubriformis
    T. instabilis
    T. orientalis
    T. probolurus
    T. vitrinus
Trichothecium roseum
trichrome stains
Trichuris trichiura
trick knee
tricose stain
Tricot syndrome, Degos-Delort-
tricrotic pulse
tricrotic wave
tricuspid
    t. atresia
    t. commissurotomy
    t. endocarditis in drug addict
    t. heart valve
    t. incompetence (TI)
    t. insufficiency (TI)
    t. murmur
    t. opening snap

    t. orifice
    t. position
    t. regurgitation
    t. restenosis
    t. stenosis
    t. valve
    t. valve closure sound
    t. valve disease
    t. valve disorder
    t. valve doming
    t. valve ‣ Ebstein's malformation of
    t. valve flow
    t. valve gradient
    t. valve prolapse
    t. valve ‣ straddling
    t. valve vegetation
    t. valvotomy
    t. valvotomy, balloon
    t. valvular leaflet
    t. valvuloplasty
    t. valvulotomy
tricuspidatus, Paragordius
tricyclic antidepressant
trident hand
trifascicular block
trifascicular heart block
trifid stomach
trifida, Ambrosia
Tri-flow incentive spirometry
trifocal glasses
trifocal lens
Trifolium hybridum
trifurcation tracheoesophageal fistula
trigeminal
    t. artery ‣ persistent primitive
    t. cough
    t. disorder
    t. ganglion
    t. gland
    t. nerve
    t. nerve, fifth
    t. nerve, gland of
    t. nerve irritation
    t. nerve signs
    t. neuralgia
    t. pulse
    t. rhizotomy
    t. rhythm
    t. zoster
trigeminus reflex
trigeminy, ventricular
trigeminy with aberrancy, atrial
trigger(s)
    t. action
    t., anxiety

t. area
t. areas, stimulation of
t., dietary
t., environmental
t. factors for epilepsy
t. factors for migraine
t. finger
t., food
t. gag reflex, hair-
t., headache
t. ▸ heart attack
t. ▸ hot flash
t. hypothesis ▸ premature
ventricular complex
t. of asthma
t., old
t. ovulation ▸ pituitary hormone
t. pain
t. paint
t., personal
t. ▸ personal asthma
t., physical
t. point injection
t. point ▸ massage
t. point therapy
t., potential
t. reaction
t. spots
t. spots, tender
t. testosterone production
t. thumb
t. thumb release

triggered
t. by physical illness ▸ depression
t. by stress ▸ depression
t., disease
t. pacemaker, atrial demand
t. pacemaker ▸ ventricular-
t. pacemaker ▸ ventricular demand
t. pacing
t. pulse generator, atrial
t. ventricular inhibited pacemaker ▸
atrial
t. ventricular pacemaker ▸ P wave

triggering
t. sensations
t. situations ▸ relapse
t. unit ▸ electrocardiogram (ECG)

triglyceride(s)
t., decreased
t. diet, medium chain
t. elevated
t., fasting plasma
t. fatty acid
t. level

t. level, blood
t. level, normal
t. level, serum
t. lipase
t., long chain
t., medium chain
t., plasma
t., serum
t. test

trigone
t. depressed
t. edematous and friable
t., fascia of urogenital
t., hypertrophy of
t., Müller's
t., retromolar
t., urogenital

trigonitis, chronic
trigonitis, urethral
trigonum tarsi, os
triiodothyronine
t. ▸ iodine 131 with
t. red cell uptake test
t. resin test
t. (T_3) uptake test

tri-leaflet aortic prosthesis
tri-leaflet prosthesis, Teflon
triloba, placenta
trilobar hyperplasia
trilobate placenta
trilocular heart
triloculare
t. biatriatum, cor
t. biventriculare, cor
t., cor

trilogy of Fallot
Trimadeau sign
trimalleolar fracture
trimalleolar fracture of ankle
trimester
t. abortion, second
t. bleeding ▸ third
t. of pregnancy ▸ first, second or
third
t. spotting ▸ first

trimethoxy
t. -amphetamine (Nutmeg)
t. -amphetamine (Nutmeg) ingested
t. -amphetamine (Nutmeg) sniffed

trimmed
t., callus
t., cast
t., edges
t., edges of cartilage
t., skin edges

t. torn tissue
trimming
t., improper nail
t., mucoperiosteal flap
t. procedure ▸ heart
trinitrate, glycerol
trinocular microscope
Triodontophorus diminutus
triolein fat absorption study
triolein I 131
triolet, bruit de
triorthocresyl phosphate
triose phosphate isomerase
tripartita, placenta
tripartite fracture of patella
tripartite placenta
tripetala, Magnolia
trip-hammer pulse
triphasic action potential
triphasic wave
triphenyl albumin
Triphleps insidiosus
triphosphate
t. (ATP) ▸ adenosine
t., guanosine
t., thymidine
t., uridine
triphosphopyridine nucleotide
Tripier's amputation
triple
t. -angle
t. arthrodesis, Lambrinudi
t. balloon valvuloplasty
t. bandpass filter
t. -blind study
t. burner meridian
t. bypass heart surgery
t. discharges
t. distance
t. drug chemotherapy
t. -humped pressure pulse
t. lumen catheter
t. phosphate crystals
t. rhythm
t. staining
t. stimulus
t. strength
t. vessel disease
t. vision
t. voiding cystogram
t. voiding cystography
t. -X chromosomal aberration
triplets, patient delivered
triplex, placenta

tripod (Tripod)
- t. cane
- t. fracture
- T. implant cataract lens, Azar
- T. implant cataract lens, Pearce
- t. pin traction, McBride

tripolar
- t. lead
- t. lead ▸ nonintegrated
- t. lead ▸ segmented ring

triquestropisiform articulation
triquetral bone
triquetrum, os
trisection, pulse
trisimilitubis, Isoparorchis
trismus
- t. nascentium
- t. neonatorum
- t. of masseter muscle

trisomy
- t. C, mosaic
- t. D syndrome
- t. D₁ syndrome
- t. E syndrome
- t. -G
- t., mongolism double-
- t. 13-15 syndrome
- t. 16-18 syndrome
- t. 18 syndrome
- t. 21 syndrome
- t. 22

tritaeniorhyncus, Culex
tritiated thymidine
tritiated water
triticeous node
triticeous nodule
tritium nuclei
trivalent oral poliovirus vaccine
trochanter
- t., greater
- t., lesser
- t. muscle, greater

trochanteric bursitis
trochanteric tendonitis
trochlear
- t. nerve
- t. nerve signs
- t. notch
- t. notch of ulna

trochoid joint
trochoidal articulation
troctina, Hirudo
Troglotrema salmincola
Troisier('s)
- T. ganglion

T. -Hanot-Chauffard syndrome
T. node
T. sign
T. syndrome
Trolard, vein of
trolley, shower
Trombicula
- T. akamushi
- T. autumnalis
- T. irritans
- T. tsalsahuatl
- T. vandersandi

trombone tremor of tongue
Troncoso gonioscope
Tropherem whippelii
Tropheryma whipplei
trophic
- t. changes
- t. cicatrix
- t. factor
- t. fracture
- t. keratitis
- t. lesion
- t. nerve
- t. ulcer

trophoblast cell
trophoblastic
- t. cells
- t. disease
- t. disease ▸ gestational
- t. malignant teratoma
- t. tissue
- t. tumor
- t. tumor, malignant

trophoneurotic atrophy
trophopathic hepatitis
tropica
- t., Leishmania
- t., Malassezia
- t., stomatitis
- t., trichosporosis

tropical [*topical*]
- t. amnesia
- t. cachexia
- t. cardiospasm
- t. diarrhea
- t. diseases
- t. dysphagia
- t. ear
- t. endomyocardial fibrosis
- t. macrocytic anemia
- t. medicine
- t. phagedenic ulcer
- t. pulmonary eosinophilia
- t. sore

- t. spastic paraparesis (TSP)
- t. splenomegaly, febrile
- t. splenomegaly syndrome
- t. sprue
- t. swelling

tropicalis, Candida
tropicalis, Entamoeba
tropicum, granuloma
tropicum, granuloma pudente
trots, Spanish
trouble
- t. breathing
- t. concentrating
- t. seeing ▸ sudden
- t. talking or understanding
- t. talking ▸ sudden
- t. walking ▸ sudden

trough
- t. -and-peak levels
- t. concentration
- t., gingival
- t. level
- t. levels ▸ peak and
- t., systolic
- t., vestibular
- t. ▸ X-descent
- t. ▸ Y-descent

troughing, venous
trousers, air
trousers (MAST) ▸ medical antishock
Trousseau('s)
- T. phenomenon
- T. sign
- T. spot
- T. syndrome
- T. twitching

Troutman's implant
Troutman's operation
TRU (turbidity reducing unit)
Truck Drivers (amphetamines)
true
- t. accusations ▸ retract
- t. aneurysm
- t. anterior temporal electrodes
- t. aphasia
- t. average
- t. conjugate diameter
- t. convulsive shock
- t. cords
- t. cyst
- t. dwarf
- t. epilepsy
- t. hemianopia
- t. hyperplasia
- t. hypertrophy

t. fungus
t. intersex
t. labor
t. lumen
t. memory
t. negative
t. -negative test result
t. -negative undetected disease
t. neurosis
t. pelvis
t. petit mal
t. phase reversal
t. positive
t. -positive test result
t. restenosis
t. ribs
t. suture
t. thirst
t. ventricular aneurysm
t. vocal cords
Trueta technique
Trueta treatment
truffée, placenta
truncal
t. abrasions
t. asynergy
t. ataxia
t. instability
t. obesity
truncata, Physaloptera
truncate ascertainment
truncated
t. cone
t. nerve endings
t. osteotomy
truncation artifact
truncatum, Pseudo-amphistomum
trunci pulmonalis, lunulae
valvularum semilunarium
truncoaortic sac
truncus
t. arteriosus
t. arteriosus, persistent
t. brachiocephalicus
t. fasciculi atrioventricularis
trunk
t. and hip flexibility
t. angiography ▸ digital celiac
t. angioma ▸ tibioperoneal
t. ▸ base of pulmonary
t., bifurcation of pulmonary
t., brachiocephalic
t. ▸ complete occlusion of right
coronary
t. curls exercise

t., forward flexion of
t., ganglia of sympathetic
t., jugular
t. movement
t. muscles
t. presentation
t., pulmonary
t. ▸ rhythmic instability of head and
t., sympathetic nerve
t. valves, lunulae of pulmonary
t. valves, nodules of pulmonary
trust, betrayal of
trust, mutual
trusting relationship
Trypanosoma
T. brucei
T. cruzi
T. dimidiata
T. equinum
T. escomili
T. evansi
T. gambiense
T. geniculata
T. gerstaeckeri
T. hippicum
T. infestans
T. megista
T. mexicana
T. nigrovarius
T. protracta
T. recurva
T. rhodesiense
T. rubida
T. sanguisuga
T. sordida
T. vitticeps
trypanosome protozoan
trypanosomiasis, American
trypanosomiasis of nervous system
trypsin
t., aldehyde-fuchsin
t. -inhibitory capacity
t. test
TS (total solids)
Ts and Blues (heroin substitute)
tsalsahuatl, Trombicula
TSC (technetium sulfur colloid)
Tschiassny recruitment
Tschiassny test
TSD (target skin distance)
TSE (testicular self-examination)
tsetse fly
TSH (thyroid stimulating hormone)
tsp (teaspoonful)
TSP (total serum protein)

TSP (tropical spastic paraparesis)
TSPAP (total serum prostatic acid
phosphatase)
TSS (toxic shock syndrome) ▸
menstrual
tsutsugamushi
t. disease
t. fever
t., Rickettsia
TT (total thyroxine)
TT (total time)
TTD (tissue tolerance dose)
T₃ (triiodothyronine)
T₃ (triiodothyronine) uptake test
TTI (time-tension index)
TTP (thrombic thrombocytopenic
purpura)
T-tube
T-tube cholangiogram
T-tube cholangiography
T2
T2 relaxation time
T2 weighted image
T2 weighted image ▸ T1-
TU
TU (toxic unit)
TU (tuberculin unit)
TU complex
TU wave
tub
t. bath
t. bench
t. dermatitis ▸ hot
t., Hubbard
t. lung ▸ hot
t. transfer ▸ two-chair
tubae
t. uterinae, infundibulum
t. uterinae, isthmus
t. uterinae, ostium abdominal
t. uterinae, ostium uterinum
t. uterinae, pars uterine
t. uterinae, plica isthmicae
t. uterinae, plicae ampullares
t. uterinae, plicae tubariae
tubal (Tubal)
t. abortion
t. air cells
t. block
t. blockage
t. dysmenorrhea
t. ectopic pregnancy ▸ ruptured
t. folds of uterine tube
t. fulguration
t. infertility

tubal—*continued*
- t. inflation
- t. insufflation
- t. ligation, Irving type
- t. ligation ▸ laparoscopic
- t. ligation/tuboligation
- t. mass
- t. nephritis
- t. obstruction
- t. occlusion
- T. Ovum Transfer (TOT)
- t. patency, postoperative
- t. potency test
- t. pregnancy/tubopregnancy
- t. protuberance
- t. reconstruction
- t. reversal
- t. ring
- t. sterilization

tubariae tubae uterinae, plicae
tubarius, torus
tube(s) [pubes]
- t., Abbott-Miller
- t., abdominal orifice of uterine
- t., Adson suction
- t., air
- t., air-filled
- t., Andrews-Pynchon
- t., angled pleural
- t., Argyle chest
- t., Argyle-Salem sump
- t., Atkins-Cannard
- t., auditory
- t., Axiom double sump
- t., Baker's
- t., Baron suction
- t., bilateral chest
- t., Blakemore's
- t. blockage, fallopian
- t. blocked by infection of ear ▸
  eustachian
- t., Bouchut's
- t. bound down, fallopian
- t. brachytherapy, cesium 137
  bougie
- t., breathing
- t., bronchial
- t., Broyles'
- t., buccal
- t., bulboventricular
- t. cancer, fallopian
- t., Cantor
- t., Carabelli's
- t. carcinoma, fallopian
- t., Carlen

- t. carrier
- t., cartilaginous
- t., Castelli's
- t., catheterization of eustachian
- t. (CRT), cathode ray
- t., Celestin's
- t., cerebromedullary
- t., cesium
- t., Chaussier's
- t., chest
- t., Chevalier-Jackson
- t., cholangiogram, T-
- t., cholangiography, T-
- t., collar button
- t., collecting
- t., colostomy
- t., column
- t., complex
- t. constrict, bronchial
- t. conveyor, pneumatic
- t., corneal
- t., cuffed endotracheal
- t., cuffed tracheostomy
- t. culture
- t., cultures, catheter
- t. defect (NTD) ▸ neural
- t., digestive
- t. dilate bronchial
- t., dilution studies
- t., discharge
- t. disorder ▸ neural
- t., Dobhoff feeding
- t., double cuffed
- t., double lumen endobronchial
- t., drainage (dr'ge)
- t. drainage, chest
- t., drainage (dr'ge) ▸ closed
- t., dressed
- t. ▸ drug coated
- t., duodenal
- t., Durham's
- t. dysfunction, eustachian
- t., edematous and swollen
- t., electron multiplier
- t., electronic vacuum
- t., embryonic neural
- t., empyema
- t., encircling silicone
- t., end
- t., endobronchial
- t., endocardial
- t. (ET), endotracheal
- t., enlarged bronchial
- t., esophageal
- t., eustachian

- t., fallopian
- t., feeding
- t. feeding, blenderized
- t. feeding, casein based
- t. feeding ▸ forced
- t. feeding, mild based
- t., fenestrated tracheostomy
- t., fermentation
- t., fiberoptic
- t., fil d'Arion silicone
- t., fimbriae of uterine
- t. flap
- t. ▸ flexible, lighted
- t., flexible rubber endoscopic
- t. ▸ fluffy cuffed
- t., Frazier suction
- t. free of obstruction
- t. function (ETF), eustachian
- t., fusion
- t., Gabriel-Tucker
- t., gas
- t., gastric
- t., gastrostomy
- t., gavage
- t., glow modular
- t., Gomco suction
- t. graft
- t. graft, aortic
- t. graft, Dacron
- t. graft ▸ woven Dacron
- t., granulation
- t., Guibor Silastic
- t., Guisez's
- t., Harris
- t., Hemovac
- t., Holinger
- t., Holter
- t., horizontal
- t., hot-cathode
- t. hydrosalpinx, both
- t. ▸ hyperreactive bronchial
- t. in esophagus ▸ flexible
- t. in place ▸ drainage (dr'ge)
- t. in place ▸ endotracheal
- t. in place ▸ patient has
  endotracheal
- t. in place, thoracotomy
- t. in place, tracheostomy
- t. in stomach nasogastric (NG)
- t., infant feeding
- t. ▸ inflammation of bronchial
- t. inflation, eustachian
- t., infundibulum of fallopian
- t., infundibulum of uterine
- t. inserted

t. inserted, suction
t. inserted, tracheostomy
t. ▸ insertion of synthetic
t. insertion ▸ tympanostomy
t. insufflator
t. intercostal
t., intraesophageal feeding
t., intratracheal
t., intubation
t., isthmus of fallopian
t., Jackson's
t., jejunal feeding
t., Jergesen
t., Kelly's
t., Keogh feeding
t., Killian's
t., Kistner tracheostomy
t., Kistner's
t., Lanz'
t., LaRocca's
t., laryngeal
t., Lennarson's
t., Lepley-Ernst
t., Levin
t., Lewis'
t., Lindeman-Silverstein
t., Linton
t., liposuction
t., Luer's
t., Mackenty's
t. malplacement ▸ endotracheal
t., Martin's
t., medullary
t., membranous
t., Miescher's
t., Miller-Abbott
t., Minnesota
t., Mörch tracheostomy
t., Mosher's esophagoscope
t., multiple lumen
t., nasoesophageal feeding
t., nasogastric (NG)
t., nasogastric feeding
t., nasotracheal
t., nephrostomy
t., neural
t., New's
t., NG (nasogastric)
t. obstructed
t. obstruction, eustachian
t., obstruction of fallopian
t. ▸ open blocked fallopian
t., oroendotracheal
t., orotracheal
t., otopharyngeal

t., ovarian
t. patent
t., patent fallopian
t., pharyngotympanic
t., photomultiplier
t., Pilling's
t., Pitt talking tracheostomy
t. placed, tracheostomy
t. placement
t., placement, chest
t., pleural
t., plugged
t., polyethylene
t., Portex tracheostomy
t. positioning controls
t., postnasal
t., precipitin
t. present in abdomen ▸ chest
t. ▸ pressure equalizing (PE)
t. pressure, eustachian
t. prosthesis, Helanca seamless
t. prosthesis, Mackler intraluminal
t., Pudenz's
t., pus
t., pyramidal
t. radiation, cesium
t., Rainey's
t. removal of chest
t. replacement ▸ trach
   (tracheostomy)
t., respiratory
t., retractable fiberoptic
t. ▸ right angle chest
t., roll
t., Rubin
t., Ruysch's
t., Ryle
t., Sachs' suction
t., safety
t., salivary
t., salvarsan throat irrigation
t., scarred fallopian
t., scavenging
t., semicanal of auditory
t., Sengstaken's
t., Sharley tracheostomy
t., shea polyethylene drainage
   (dr'ge)
t., Sheldon-Pudenz's
t. ▸ Shiley tracheostomy
t., shunt
t. ▸ spasm of bronchial
t., speaking
t., sputum
t., stent

t., sterile connecting
t., sterile vacuum collection
t., stomach
t. suctioning, nasogastric
t., suprapubic
t. ▸ surgical absence of fallopian
t., surgically implanted
t. ▸ surgically implanted feeding
t. ▸ surgically implanted medication
t., T
t., tampon
t., Teflon endolymphatic shunt
t., Teflon shunt
t., test
t., thoracic drainage (dr'ge)
t., thoracostomy
t., thoracotomy
t., Thunberg
t., tracheal
t., tracheostomy
t., transport
t., Tucker's
t., urinary
t., uterine
t., vacuum
t., valve
t., ventriculocisternostomy by
t., vertical
t., Wangensteen
t. ▸ water seal chest
t. with pigtail curl, stent
t. ▸ withdrawal feeding
t. ▸ withholding feeding
t., x-ray
t. ▸ Z-wave
tubed pedicle flap
tubeless cystostomy
tubercle(s)
   t., acoustic
   t. bacillus
   t., clusters of
   t., cuneate
   t., cuneiform
   t., Darwin's
   t., Farre's
   t., Ghon
   t., greater
   t. in knee, Gerdy's
   t., lesser
   t., pubic
   t., scalene
   t., tibial
tubercular
   t. diarrhea
   t. meningitis

tubercular—*continued*
t. scrofula
tuberculatum, Amblyomma
tuberculin
t., albumose-free
t., alkaline
t. -delayed hypersensitivity
t. filtrate
t., original
t. precipitation
t. reaction
t. test, first strength
t. test, second strength
t. test, tine
t. unit (TU)
t., vacuum
tuberculoid myocarditis
tuberculosa, gonitis
tuberculosis (TB)
t., active
t., active pulmonary
t., acute miliary
t., adrenal
t., adult
t., advanced
t., aerogenic
t., anthracotic
t., arrested
t., arthritic
t., atypical
t., autopsy-acquired
t., avian
t., Bacillus
t., basal
t., bilateral
t., calcified focus of
t., cavitary
t., cerebral
t., cestodic
t., childhood
t. culture
t. cutis
t., disseminated
t., dormant
t., drug-resistant
t., early
t. (TB) ▸ extrapulmonary
t., exudative
t., gram-positive Mycobacterium
t. granulation tissue
t., hematogenous
t., hilus
t., inactive
t., inhalation
t., intestinal

t. ▸ knee monarthritis caused by
t., late
t. lichenoides
t., lymphatic
t. miliaris disseminata
t., miliary
t. morbidity
t. ▸ multidrug-resistant
t., mycobacterial
t., Mycobacterium
t. of bone
t. of kidney and bladder
t. of lacrimal gland
t. of larynx
t. of lung
t., open
t., oral
t., orificial
t., papulonecrotic
t. patch test
t. patch test positive for
t., patient exposed to
t., postprimary
t., primary
t., productive
t., pulmonary
t., reactivation
t., reinfection
t., renal
t. skin test
t. smear
t., surgical
t., tine test for
t., tracheobronchial
tuberculous
t. adenitis
t. arthritis
t. caseation
t. chemotherapy
t. colitis
t. dacryocystitis
t. diaphysitis
t. empyema
t. empyema ▸ postpneumonectomy
t. empyesis
t. endocarditis
t. endometritis
t. gumma
t. infiltrate, Assmann
t. iritis
t. laryngitis
t. leptomeningitis
t. lesion
t. mediastinal adenopathy
t. meningitis

t. myocarditis
t. nephritis
t. pericarditis
t. peritonitis
t. pleurisy
t. pneumonia
t. prostatitis
t. rhinitis
t. salpingitis
t. spondylitis
tuberoeruptive xanthoma
tuberosa
t., chorditis
t. papulosa, endometritis
t. simplex, adiposis
tuberosity
t. deformities, maxillary
t., ischial
t., maxillary
t., radial
t. resectional ostectomies,
    maxillary
t., sacral
tuberosum
t., carcinoma
t. multiplex, xanthoma
t., Solanum
tuberous
t. carcinoma
t. sclerosis
t. xanthoma
tubifera, Stachys
tubing
t., flexible
t., hyperalimentation
t. ▸ medical equipment or
t. secured with tape
tubo
t. -insufflation
t. -ovarian abscess
t. -ovarian cyst
t. -ovarian pregnancy
tuboligation, Pomeroy's
tuboplasty, balloon
tubouterine pregnancy
tubular
t. acidosis, renal
t. adenoma
t. adenoma ▸ ovarian
t. adenoma ▸ proximal
t. aneurysm
t. breath sounds
t. cancer
t. defect, renal
t. degeneration, proximal

t. diuresis
t. dysfunction ▸ renal
t. ectasia
t. epithelial regeneration ▸ renal
t. excretory capacity
t. excretory capacity, maximal
t. fluid
t. graft
t. lining
t. mesh stent ▸ Schatz-Palmaz
t. narrowing
t. necrosis
t. necrosis (ATN), acute
t. necrosis, premortem
t. necrosis ▸ renal
t. reabsorption, altered
t. reabsorption of amylase ▸
    decreased
t. reabsorption of glucose
t. reabsorption of phosphate
t. respiration
t. tumor
t. visual fields
tubulare testiculare ovarii, adenoma
tubule(s)
t., atrophied
t., Bellini's
t., collecting
t., dilated kidney
t. ▸ distal convoluted
t. hypokalemia ▸ renal
t., Miescher's
t. ▸ proximal convoluted
t., renal
t., scattered sclerotic
t., system of
t., testicular
t., transverse
tubulointerstitial nephritis, allergic
tubulovillous adenoma
tucking, tummy
tucks, chin
tuft(s)
t., distal
t. fracture
t. fracture, terminal
t., malpighian
t. of bone
t., phalangeal
t., renal
t., ungual
TUG (total urinary gonadotropin)
tug, tracheal
TUIP (transurethral incision of
    prostate)

Tuksu tumble flap, Hodgson-
tularemia, oropharyngeal
tularemic pneumonia
tularense, Bacillus
tularense, Bacterium
tularensis
t., conjunctivitis
t., Francisella
t., gram-negative Pasteurella
t., Pasteurella
TULIP (tulip)
T. (transurethral ultrasound-guided
    laser-induced prostatectomy)
t. bulb aorta
t. fingers
Tumarkin, falling spells of
tumble flap, Hodgson-Tuksu
tumbling
t. fashion
t. fashion, lens extracted in
t. procedure
t. procedure, lens delivered by
tumefaciens albus, Saccharomyces
tumefaciens, Saccharomyces
    subcutaneous
tumefaction
t., area of
t., breast
t., cystic
tumescent fluid
tumescent liposuction
tummy
t. crunch exercise
t. tightening
t. tucking
tumor(s) (Tumor)
t., abdominal
t. ablation
t. ablation ▸ parathyroid
t. ablation ▸ percutaneous
t., Abrikosov's (Abrikossoff's)
t., acoustic
t., active
t. activity
t. activity, continuing
t. activity, renewed
t., adenocystic
t., adrenal
t., adrenal gland
t., adult Wilms'
t., advanced uterine mixed
    mesodermal
t. albus
t., alveolar cell
t., amyloid

t., anaplastic thyroid
t. and/or ulceration
t. angiogenesis factor
t. antibody
t. antigen
t. antigenicity
t. antigenicity ▸ lowered
t., aortic
t., aortic body
t. -associated antigens
t. at primary site ▸ residual
t., atypical rhabdoid
t., atypical rhabdoid/teratoid
t., benign
t., benign brain
t., benign breast
t. ▸ benign essential
t., benign myocardial
t., benign thyroid
t., bile duct
t. biology
t. biopsy
t., bladder
t., blasting
t. blood
t. blood flow
t. blood supply
t. blood vessel cells
t. blush
t., bone marrow invasion by
t. border extent
t., brain
t., brain stem
t., Brenner's
t., bronchogenic Pancoast-type
t., Burkitt's
t., Buschke-Loewenstein
t. cancer ▸ solid
t., cancer-causing
t., cancerous
t., canine transmissible
t. capsule
t., carcinoid
t., cardiac
t., carotid body
t., cartilaginous
t., cauda equina
t. -caused headaches
t. cell hypoxia
t. -cell kill
t. cell kinetics
t. cells
t. cells, cluster of
t. cells, extension of
t. cells ▸ genetically altered

tumor(s)—*continued*

t. cells ‣ infiltration by
t. cells ‣ microscopic
t. cells, primitive
t. cells ‣ virus infected
t., cerebellopontine angle
t., ceruminous gland
t., chiasmal
t., childhood brain
t., choroid
t., chromaffin cell
t., classification of malignant
t., clear cell
t. complement
t. concentration
t., conjunctival
t. control dose
t. control, local
t. control probability
t. control with dose fractionation
t., cord
t., cortical fatty
t., corticoadrenal
t., craniopharyngeal duct
t., curable breast
t., Cushing's
t., cystic
t. debulked
t. debulking, intra-abdominal
t. decompression
t., deep
t., deep cerebral
t., deep midline
t. ‣ deep seated benign
t. deposits, extensive
t. -derived cells
t. -derived immunosuppression
t., dermoid
t., destroy brain
t. destruction
t. development
t. ‣ direct extension of
t., distal common duct
t. distance, skin to
t., dormant
t. dose
t. dose in radiation therapy
t. dose therapy, biological
t. doubling time
t. doubling time in lung carcinoma
t. electron beam therapy in
t., embolism
t., embryonal
t., embryonal cell
t., encapsulated

t. encroachment
t., endobronchial
t., endocardial
t. ‣ endocrine inactive pituitary
t., endodermal sinus
t., endometrial
t., endotracheal
t., epidermoid
t., esophageal
t. estradiol receptor
t., estrogen sensitive
t. evaluation
t., Ewing's
t. excavated, interior of
t. excision
t. excision, local
t. excision, mediastinal
t. excision with irradiation, local
t., extensive residual
t. extent
t., extrathoracic
t., eye
t., familial bilateral giant cell
t. ‣ fast growing
t., fatty
t., fetal lung
t., fibrillatory
t. -fighting lymphocytes
t. ‣ focal nodules of residual
t. formation
t., fungating
t., gastric
t. (GIST) ‣ gastrointestinal stomal
t., germ cell
t., giant cell
t., glomus
t. grade
t., granular cell
t., granulosa cell
t., Grawitz's
t., gross
t., growing
t. growth
T. Growth Factor (TGF)
t. growth, Gompertzian
t. growth, inhibit
t. growth, suppression of
t., hard
t., heavy charged particle therapy in eye
t., hepatic
t. ‣ hormone receptor negative
t. ‣ hormone receptor positive
t., hot vs cold breast
t., Hürthle cell

t., hyperfunctional pituitary
t., hypernephroid
t. identified
t. impinging on cortex
t. implants
t. in children ‣ kidney
t. in situ
t. increased in size
t. -induced changes
t. infiltrating lymphocytes (TIL)
t. infiltrating lymphocytes (TIL) ‣ genetically altered
t. infiltrating lymphocytes (TIL) technique
t. infiltration
t., inhibit growth of
t., initial
t., innocuous
t. inoperable
t., inoperable brain
t., interstitial cell
t., intracranial
t., intraocular
t. invasion
t. involvement
t., islet cell
t. -killing ability ‣ body's
t., Krukenberg's
t., lacrimal drainage system
t., lacrimal gland
t., laryngeal
t., late responding
t. length
t., lethal childhood
t. lethal dose (TLD)
t., lip
t., liver
t. lobule
t. ‣ local recurrence of
t. ‣ local resection of rectal
t. localization
t. localization scan
t. localized
t. ‣ localized cancerous breast
t., lower brain
t., malignant
t. ‣ malignant brain
t., malignant germ cell mediastinal
t., malignant mediastinal
t., malignant parotid
t., malignant renal
t., malignant trophoblastic
t., malignant vascular
t. marker
t. mass

t. mass ▸ embedded in
t. mass ▸ excisional biopsy of
t. mass, friable
t. mass ▸ high dose radiation to
t. mass ▸ infiltrating irregular
t. mass, lobulated
t. mass ▸ resection of
t., massive
t., massive brain
t., mast cell
t., mediastinal
t., medullary
t., melanotic neuroectodermal
t., mesenchymal
t. ▸ mesenchymal-derived
t., mesodermal
t., metastases
t. metastases ▸ focal infiltrating
t. metastases, hemorrhagic
t. metastases ▸ membranes matted
   with
t. metastases, multiple
t. metastases, necrotic
t. metastases throughout serosa
t. metastasis, nodular
t., metastasizing
t., metastatic
t. ▸ metastatic brain
t., metastatic cardiac
t., metastatic orbital
t., metastatic pericardial
t., metastatic spinal cord
t. microcirculation
t., microscopic
t. ▸ microscopic granular cell
t., migrated
t., mixed
t., mixed mammary
t., mixed nodular
t., mixed terminal
t., mixed tissue
t. morphology
t., mucinous
t., mucosal
t., muscle
t., musculoskeletal
t., myasthenia gravis and
   mediastinal
t., myocardial
t., myxoma
t. necrosis factor (TNF)
t. necrosis factor (TNF) gene-
   altered cells
t., necrosis of
t., necrotic

t. ▸ neural crest
t., neuroendocrine
t., neurogenic
t., neurogenous
t., neuroma
t., nodes, metastases (TNM)
t., nodes, metastases (TNM)
   classification
t., nodes, metastases (TNM)
   staging system
t. nodule
t. nodules on liver
t. nodules, peritoneal
t. nodules ▸ peritoneum studded
   with
t. nodules, satellite
t. nodules ▸ studded with numerous
t., noncancerous
t., nonepithelial
t., nonoperable
t., nonresponsive
t., oat cell
t. of abdomen
t. of anus
t. of blood vessel
t. of bone
t. of brain, excision
t. of breast
t. of intestine, carcinoid
t. of kidney, malignant
t. of lacrimal gland, mixed
t. of lung
t. of pancreas
t. of pancreas syndrome,
   ulcerogenic
t. of urinary bladder, malignant
t. of uterus, fibroid
t., ophthalmic
t., orbital
t., original site of
t., ovarian
t., ovarian endodermal sinus
t., oxygen flow to
t., painting base of
t., Pancoast's
t., pancreatic
t., papillary
t., paraganglioma
t., paraplegia in spinal cord
t., parotid
t., pelvic
t., pericardial
t., peripheral nerve
t. ▸ peripheral primitive
   neuroectodermal

t., phantom
t. photodynamic therapy
t., pineal
t., pituitary
t., placental tissue
t., plasma cell
t., pleural based
t. plop sound
t., plug of
t. polycystic
t. polysaccharide substance
t., pontine
t., posterior fossa
t., postirradiation residual
t., Pott's puffy
t., preexisting breast
t., primary
t., primary brain
t., primary malignant cardiac
t. progression
t., prolactin secreting pituitary
t. proliferation, fibrous
t., prostate
t., pulmonary artery
t., Purkinje
t., radiation assaults on
t., radiation attack on
t., radical excision of
t., radiocurable
t., radioresistant
t., rapidly growing
t. ▸ rapidly growing brain
t., rapidly proliferating
t., Rathke's
t., rectal
t., rectovaginal septum
t. recurrence ▸ ipsilateral breast
t., recurrent
t., recurrent brain
t. ▸ recurrent skin
t. reduced, size of
t., reducing
t. re-excision
t. regeneration
t. regeneration and protracted
   treatment
t. ▸ regional recurrence of
T. Registry, Ovarian
t. regression
t. regrowth
t. ▸ removal of benign thyroid
t., renal
t. research, brain
t. resectable
t. ▸ resection of mediastinal

tumor(s)—*continued*
t., residual
t. response
t. response in antibodies, radiobiology and
t., responsive
t. retardant
t., retroperitoneal
t., rhabdomyosarcoma orbital
t., Rokitansky's
t., ropy
t., salivary gland
t., sarcomatous
t., Schmincke
t., sclerotic
t., Scully's
t., secondary
t. seeded peritoneum
t., serous
t., Sertoli cell
t., Sertoli-Leydig cell
t., shrink
t., shrink inoperable
t., shrinkage
t. site, original
t. site, primary
t. site, residual
t. size
t. size, reduction of
t., skin
t. skin distance
t. skin test
t., slowly growing
t., small cell bronchogenic
t., soft tissue
t., solid
t. specific transplantation antigen
t., spinal canal
t., spinal cord
t. spread
t., squamous cell
t. stage
t. stain
t., steadily advancing
t., stimulation
t., stromal cell
t., subcutaneous
t., submaxillary
t., submaxillary gland
t., subtentorial
t., subtotal removal of
t., sugar
t., sulcus
t. suppression genes
t. suppression, immunologic

t. suppressive activities of antibodies
t. suppressor
t. suppressor genes
t., suprasellar
t., surgical removal of
t. ▸ surgical treatment for brain
t. surrounds carotid artery
t. suspects, brain
t. sustentacular cell
t. syndrome, pancreatic
t. syndrome, superior sulcus
t., target brain
t. targeting ability
t., teratoid
t., teratoma
t., testis
t., thalamic
t., theca cell
t. therapy
t., therapy ▸ photodynamic
t., thin cancerous
t., thymic
t., thyroid
t. tissue
t., tracheal
t. transitional
t. treatment, brain
t., trophoblastic
t., tubular
t. ▸ ulcers, polyps or
t., unknown primary
t. unresectable
t., vaginal
t., vaporize cancerous
t., vaporize fibroid
t. ▸ vaporizing breast
t., vascular
t., vena caval
t., viable
t., villous
t., virilizing
t. virus
t. virus, mammary
t., Warthin's
t. ▸ well differentiated squamous cell
t., Wilms'
t. with microinvasion
t. xenograft, human
t., yolk-sac
tumorigenicity study
tumorous portion
TUMT (transurethral microwave thermotherapy)

tumultuous personal relationship
tumultus cordis
TUNA (transurethral needle ablation)
Tuneable Dye Laser Treatment
Tunga penetrans
tungsten arc lamp
tunic
t., fibrous
t., nervous
t., vascular pigmented
tunica
t. adnata oculi
t. adventitia
t. adventitia, aortic
t. albuginea
t. intima
t. intima, aortic
t. intima, thickening of
t. media
t. media, aortic
t. nervea of Brücke
t. propria
t. serosa
t. vaginalis
t. vasculosa lentis
t. vasculosa oculi
tunicary hernia
tuning
t. fork
t. fork, Hartmann
t. fork test
t. test
tunnel(s)
t., air
t., carpal
t. cells
t. created subcutaneously
t. decompression, carpal
t. endoscopy, carpal
t. flap
t. graft
t. ▸ Kawashima intraventricular
t. -like vision
t. murmur, aortic left ventricular (LV)
t. of Corti
t., percutaneous
t. projection
t. projection, Templeton and Zim carpal
t. release, carpal
t., subsartorial
t. syndrome (CTS) ▸ carpal
t. syndrome, cubital
t., tarsal

t. view
t. vision
tunneled implant
tunneling device ▸ **subcutaneous**
tunneling microscope (STM) ▸
scanning
**TUR (transurethral resection) of
bladder**
**TUR (transurethral resection) of
prostate**
turbid
t. fluid
t. fluid, serosanguineous
t. milky fluid
t. yellow urine
turbidity
t. reaction, Meinicke
t. -reducing unit (TRU)
t. test, thymol
t. test, zinc
t., zinc sulfate
turbinate(s) [*terminate*]
t. bone
t., bulbous
t., conchae nasal
t., crushing
t., enlarged
t., inferior
t., infracted
t., middle
t., nasal
t., sphenoid
t., superior
turbulence mapping ▸ **spectral**
turbulence of flow of blood
turbulent
t. blood flow
t. diastolic mitral inflow
t. jet
t., patient's hospital course
turcica
t., diaphragm of sella
t., enlargement of sella
t. normal, sella
t., sella
Türck line, Ehrlich-
Türck's bundle
Turcot syndrome
Turek's spreader
turgescence of neck veins
turgescent vessel
turgor
t., coronary vascular
t., good tissue
t., hydration and

t., skin
t., tissue
t. vitalis
turicatae, Borrelia
Türk-Duane syndrome, Stilling-
Turkel's needle
Turkel's trephine
turkey ▸ **quit cold**
Turko's operation
Turlock virus
turmoil, emotional
turmoil, psychological
turn
t. a flap
t. epicardial lead ▸ three-
t. epicardial lead ▸ two-
turned
t. from side to side
t. -in eyelid
t. mouth corners ▸ down-
t. on side, patient
t. -out eyelid
Turner('s)
T. acetabular cup, Aufranc-
T. arthroplasty, Aufranc-
T., intraparietal sulcus of
T., marginal gyrus of
T. mosaicism
T. pin
T. prosthesis, Aufranc-
T. sign, Hefke-
T. syndrome
T. tooth
T. -Warwick urethroplasty
turning in ▸ **conjunctivitis with
eyelashes**
turnover
t., bone
t., plasma
t. (PIT), plasma iron
t. rate, plasma iron
**TURP (transurethral resection of
prostate)**
turpentine enema
Turyn's sign
tussive
t. fremitus
t. squeeze
t. suction, post-
t. syncope
Tut (LSD), King
TV (tidal volume)
TV light camera
TVC (total volume capacity)
TVH (total vaginal hysterectomy)

'tween-brain
twelfth
t. cranial nerve
t. nerve
t. -year molar
12 (twelve) (Twelve)
12 deficiency, vitamin B-
12, Freon
12 -lead electrocardiogram
(ECG/EKG)
12 o'clock position
12 per second ▸ six to
12 profile test, SMA-
12 -step program
12 steps
20
20 (ten-twenty) electrode system ▸
10-
20 %, hypaque
20 (ten-twenty) system ▸ standard
10-
20 (ten-twenty) system ▸ 10-
20 /20 vision
20th century syndrome
28 virus ▸ **enteric cytopathic human
orphan (ECHO)**
25 virus, M-
24
24 -hour delayed lymph nodal
stage radiograph
24 -hour emergency care
24 -hour monitoring
24 -hour period of observation and
hydration
24 -hour sleep-wake cycle ▸ phase-
shift disruption of
24 -hour urines
21 Chromosome
21 syndrome, trisomy
2060 virus (ECHO 28 virus)
22 channel receiver/stimulator
22, trisomy
twice a day (b.i.d.)
twiddler's syndrome
twiddler's syndrome ▸ **pacemaker**
twilight
t. anesthesia
t. blindness
t. sleep
t. sleep anesthesia
t. state
t. thirst
t. vision
twin(s)
t., cephalopagus

twin(s)—*continued*
t., conjoined
t., craniopagus
t., dissimilar
t., dizygotic
t., false
t., fraternal
t. gestation
t., identical
t., impacted
t. intrauterine pregnancy
t., mirror
t., monozygotic
t., nonidentical
t., patient delivered
t. pregnancy
t., Siamese
t., thoracopagus
t. -to-twin transfusion
t. transfusion syndrome ▸ twin-
t. transfusion ▸ twin-to-
t. transplants, identical
t. transplants, nonidentical
t. -twin transfusion syndrome
t. wire appliance, Johnson
twinge of pain
Twining's position
twist of neck
twisted hair
twisted nerve cell fibers
twisting
t. and/or bending
t. force
t. force on spine
t. injury to joint
t. movement ▸ repetitive
t. of vas deferens
twitch(es)
t. and involuntary movements
t., body
t. contraction
t., eye
t., muscle
t. ▸ muscle spasms and
t. of extremities ▸ flicking of
t. ▸ recurrent eye
t., thumb
t. ▸ tics and
twitching(s)
t. and trembling
t. around eye
t. artifact, eye
t. ▸ blinking and
t., continuous muscular
t. episodes

t. eyeball
t., eyelid
t. ▸ facial pain and
t., fascicular
t., fibrillar
t. from caffeine ▸ eye
t., grimacing, and spasm
t., involuntary
t., irregular
t., muscle
t., muscular
t. of muscles
t. of tongue, fibrillary
t., Trousseau's
t., uncontrollable
twitchy eyelid
two (2) (II)
II, Accu-Chek
II alcoholic, Type
t. algorithm ▸ radix
t. block claudication
t. -bottle drainage system
t. cerebral hemispheres
t. -chair tub transfer
t. chamber view
t. chamber view echocardiogram ▸
  apical
t. -child sterility
t. -compartment system
2 -D echocardiogram
t. -dimensional echocardiogram,
  cross sectional
t. -dimensional echocardiograms
t. -dimensional echocardiography
t. -dimensional echocardiography ▸
  quantitative
t. -dimensional imaging ▸ Fourier
t. disorder, Axis
II dual chamber pacemaker
t. -emulsion autoradiography
2 fat cells, alpha
t. -flight exertional dyspnea
t. flights of stairs claudication
II, Gamma Med
II gastrostomy, Billroth
2, grid
2 hemadsorption virus (HA2) ▸ type
t. hours postprandial
2, input terminal
t. -light discrimination
II, Mobitz
II -NIDD (noninsulin dependent
  diabetes mellitus), Type
t. or three pillow orthopnea
II pacemaker, Autima

II pacemaker, Intermedics Thinlith
II pacemaker, Intermedics Thinlith
II pacemaker ▸ Medtronic Elite
II pacemaker ▸ Paragon
II pacer ▸ Intertach
t. parainfluenza virus
t. -patch technique
t. -pillow orthopnea
t. plane needle implant
t. plane radium implant
t. -point gait
t. -prong stem finger prosthesis
2. receptors, alpha
t. -rescuer CPR (cardiopulmonary
  resuscitation)
t. rescuer CPR (cardiopulmonary
  resuscitation), one and
t. -stage esophagogastrostomy
2 ▸ Stahl ear, No.
t. -step exercise test
2 -step exercise test, Master
t. -team technique
II therapy, interleukin
t. times a day (b.i.d.)
2 :1 block, Wenckebach with
2 :1 loading
II total hip prosthesis, HD
t. -turn epicardial lead
II vascular prosthesis, DeBakey
  Vasculour
t. -vessel angioplasty, bootstrap
t. -vessel technique, bootstrap
201
201 imaging ▸ rest redistribution
  thallium-
201 myocardial perfusion imaging ▸
  stress, thallium-
201 myocardial perfusion
  scintigraphy ▸ thallium-
201 perfusion scintigraphy ▸
  thallium-
201 planar scintigraphy ▸ thallium-
201 scintigraphy ▸ dipyridamole
  thallium-
201 scintigraphy ▸ exercise
  thallium-
201 SPECT (single photon
  emission computed tomography)
  scintigraphy ▸ thallium-
201 stress test ▸ thallium-
203, chlormerodrin Hg
2000 artificial heart ▸ Jarvik-
Twombly's operation
Twombly-Ulfelder's operation
twoness, limen of

Twort-d'Herelle phenomenon
Tycron suture material
Tyding snare
tying, knot
tympani
    t., canaliculus chordae
    t., canaliculus of chorda
    t., cavum
    t., cholesteatoma
    t., chorda
    t., fundus
    t., membrana
    t., musculus tensor
    t. nerve, chorda
    t., nerve of tensor
    t., scala
    t., semicanal of tensor
    t., sinus
    t., tegmen
tympanic
    t. annulus
    t. antrum
    t. aperture
    t. bone
    t. cavity
    t. cells
    t. ganglion
    t. lead
    t. nerve
    t. notch
    t. orifice
    t. percussion note
    t. plexus
    t. scute
    t. sinus
    t. sulcus
    t. swelling
    t. vein
tympanic membrane (TM)
    TM ▸ anterior mallear fold of
    TM ▸ bulging red
    TM ▸ bulging yellow
    TM gray
    TM inflammation
    TM injected
    TM perforation
    TM ▸ posterior mallear fold of
    TM ▸ rupture of
    TM ▸ secondary
    TM temperature
    TM ▸ tensor muscle of
    TM ▸ umbo of
tympanica, incisura
tympanicum, antrum
tympanicus, anulus

tympanicus, canaliculus
tympanites, false
tympanites, uterine
tympanitic ▸ abdomen distended tender,
tympanitic sound
tympanocentesis and myringotomy
tympanomastoid abscess
tympanomastoid cavity
tympanomeatal flap
tympanometry test
tympanoplasty (type I, II, III, IV, V)
tympanoplasty, Wullstein's type
Tympan-O-Scope, Madsen
tympanostomy tube insertion
tympanotomy
    t., bilateral
    t., exploratory
    t. flap
tympanum
    t., hypo◇
    t., mallear fold of mucous membrane of
    t., promontory of
    t., tensor muscle of
tympany
    t., bell
    t., skodaic
    t., Skoda's
type(s) (Type) [*like*]
    t. A, B, AB, O ▸ blood
    t. A behavior
    T. A personality
    t. A ▸ Shigella arabinotarda
    t. aberration, chromatid-
    t., ABO blood
    t. acute lymphocytic leukemia, Burkitt-
    t., allotropic
    t., amyostatic-kinetic
    t. and cross-match blood
    t. and screen
    t. aortic dissection, DeBakey-
    t. aortic dissection ▸ Stanford-
    t., apoplectic
    t., asthenic
    t., athletic
    t. B behavior
    t. B (HIB), Hemophilus influenza
    T. B personality
    t. B ▸ Shigella arabinotarda
    t. B (HIB) vaccine ▸ Hemophilus influenza
    t. ▸ Bence Jones light chain
    t., Blastomycoides

    t., blood
    t., body
    t. brace, chair-back
    t. carcinoma, colloid
    t., cardioinhibitory
    t., cell
    t., chronic ▸ schizophrenia, catatonic
    t., chronic ▸ schizophrenia, disorganized
    t., chronic ▸ schizophrenia, paranoid
    t., chronic ▸ schizophrenia, residual
    t., chronic ▸ schizophrenia, undifferentiated
    t., chronic with acute exacerbation ▸ schizophrenia, catatonic
    t., chronic with acute exacerbation ▸ schizophrenia, disorganized
    t., chronic with acute exacerbation ▸ schizophrenia, paranoid
    t., chronic with acute exacerbation ▸ schizophrenia, residual
    t., chronic with acute exacerbation ▸ schizophrenia, undifferentiated
    t. ▸ conduct disorder, group
    t. ▸ conduct disorder, solitary aggressive
    t. ▸ conduct disorder, undifferentiated
    t. culture
    t. deafness, conductive
    t. deafness, nerve-
    t. deformity, cloverleaf-
    t. deformity, compression-
    t. dependence, opioid
    t. diet, fasting-
    t. diseases, pneumoconiosis
    t. displacement, subcoracoid
    t., dysplastic
    t. epilepsy, mixed
    t. factor, blood
    t. ▸ gender identity disorder of adolescence or adulthood, nontranssexual
    t. growth, exophytic-
    t. head halter, Forrester-
    t. hiatal hernia, sliding-
    t. hypersensitivity reaction, delayed-
    t. ileus, reflex-
    t. implant, conventional shell
    t. incision, scratch-
    t. incision, Y-
    T. Indicator (MBTI) test ▸ Myers-Briggs

type(s)—*continued*

t., Jaeger's test
t. kidney, horseshoe-
t., koinotropic
t., Kretschmer
t. laceration, flap-
t., Langhans'
t., leg
t. lesion ▸ painful, blister-
t. leukemoid reaction, stress-
t. lid block, Atkinson-
t. medullary pin, Street-
t. monocytic leukemia ▸ Schilling-
t. non-Hodgkins lymphoma, null-
t. nose bridge prosthesis ▸ Rosi L-
t. nystagmus, fine
t. of activity, delusional
t. of adolescence, nontranssexual
t. of adulthood ▸ nontranssexual
t. of assertion
t. of assessment
t. of care
t. of depression ▸ reactive
t. of isolation, enteric
t. of treatments
T. I alcoholic
T. I and II alcoholism
t. I cells
t. 1 hemadsorption virus (HA1)
T. 1, herpes simplex
t. I, II, III Bondy mastoidectomy
T. I-IDDM (insulin dependent diabetes mellitus)
t. operation, McGavic
t., organic reaction
t. osteotomy, opening wedge-
t. papilloma, mulberry
t., paranoid
t. personality, obsessive-
t., phage
t., phthinoid
t., phthisic
t. plasminogen activator ▸ urokinase-
t., presenile onset, with delirium ▸ primary degenerative dementia of Alzheimer
t., presenile onset, with delusions ▸ primary degenerative dementia of Alzheimer
t., presenile onset, with depression ▸ primary degenerative dementia of Alzheimer
t. product/solution ▸ quaternary-amine

t. prosthesis, piston-
t. psychosis, depressive
t. psychosis, excitative
t., pyknic
t. reactions, allergic-
t. reflex, Bezold-
t. retroviral particle, human intracisternal A-
t., Runeberg's
t., scapulohumeral
t., schizoid
t. ▸ schizophrenia, catatonic
t. ▸ schizophrenia, residual
t. ▸ schizophrenia, undifferentiated
t., seclusive
t. (SDAT) senile dementia ▸ Alzheimer's
t., senile onset, uncomplicated ▸ primary degenerative dementia of Alzheimer
t., senile onset, with delirium ▸ primary degenerative dementia of Alzheimer
t., senile onset, with delusions ▸ primary degenerative dementia of Alzheimer
t., senile onset, with depression ▸ primary degenerative dementia of Alzheimer
t. ▸ simian T cell lymphotropic virus
t. spinal fusion, Rogers'
t., sthenic
t., subchronic ▸ schizophrenia, catatonic
t., subchronic ▸ schizophrenia, disorganized
t., subchronic ▸ schizophrenia, paranoid
t., subchronic ▸ schizophrenia, residual
t., subchronic ▸ schizophrenia, undifferentiated
t., subchronic with acute exacerbation ▸ schizophrenia, catatonic
t., subchronic with acute exacerbation ▸ schizophrenia, disorganized
t., subchronic with acute exacerbation ▸ schizophrenia, paranoid
t., subchronic with acute exacerbation ▸ schizophrenia, residual

t., subchronic with acute exacerbation ▸ schizophrenia, undifferentiated
t., suspicious
t., sympatheticotonic
t. symptom, arthritis-
t., syntonic
t. tardive muscular dystrophy, Becker-
t., test
t. 3, adenovirus
t., tissue
t. tubal ligation, Irving
T. II alcoholic
t. II cells
t. II heat exhaustion
t. 2 hemadsorption virus (HA2)
T. 2, herpes simplex
T. II-NIDDM (noninsulin dependent diabetes mellitus)
t. tympanoplasty, Wullstein's
t. ▸ undersocialized conduct disorder, aggressive
t., undifferentiated
t., unspecified ▸ schizophrenia, catatonic
t., unspecified ▸ schizophrenia, disorganized
t., unspecified ▸ schizophrenia, paranoid
t., unspecified ▸ schizophrenia, residual
t., unspecified ▸ schizophrenia, undifferentiated
t., unstable
t. ureteropelvioplasty, Foley Y-
t., vagotonic
t., visual
t., voyeur exhibitionist

typhi
t., Bacillus
t., Eberthella
t., gram-negative Eberthella
t., Rickettsia
t., Salmonella
typhimurium, Salmonella
typhisuis, Salmonella
typhoid
t. dysentery group, colon-
t. fever
t. nodule
t. -paratyphoid vaccine
t. pleurisy
t. pneumonia

typhosa
    t., Eberthella
    t., gastroenteritis
    t., roseola
    t., Salmonella
typhosum, Bacterium
typhosus, Bacillus
typhus
    t., African tick
    t., Indian tick
    t. nodules
    t. ▸ Queensland tick
    t., scrub
    t., South African tick
typical [*atypical*]
    t. alcoholic
    t. alveolar damage
    t. behavior and attitude
    t. cells
typing (Typing)
    t. ▸ human lymphocyte antigen
    t. laboratories, transplant tissue
    T. Laboratory, Tissue
    t., maternal blood
    t. of organisms, phage
    t., phage-
    t. technician, tissue
    t., tissue
typologies, behavioral
tyramine and MAO (monoamine
    oxidase) inhibitor diet ▸ restricted
tyramine test
tyrogenus, Vibrio
Tyroglyphus siro
tyropanoate contrast medium,
    sodium
tyrosine
    t. aminotransferase
    t. ethyl ester
    t. test
    t. tolerance test
tyrosinogenes, Clostridium
Tzanck preparation
Tzanck smear

U

U (unit)
U virus (Uppsala virus)
U wave alternans
U wave inversion
UA (urinalysis)
uberis, Streptococcus
UC (uterine contractions)
UCD (usual childhood diseases)
Uchida's operation
UCR (unconditioned reflex)
U-Dents, Stim-
Uganda S virus
UGI (upper gastrointestinal)
ugliness imagined
ugliness ▸ irrational obsession with
    imagined
ugly duckling stage
Uhl's anomaly
UIBC (unsaturated iron-binding
    capacity)
ulcer(s)
    u., acid
    u., active
    u., acute duodenal
    u., acute gastroduodenal
    u., acute nonperforated
    u., amebic
    u., antral
    u., aphthous
    u., atheromatous
    u., bacterial corneal
    u., benign gastric
    u. biopsy
    u., biopsy of
    u., bleeding
    u., bleeding gastrointestinal (GI)
    u., bleeding stomach
    u., chronic gastric
    u., chronic prepyloric
    u., colonic
    u., contact
    u., corneal
    u. crater
    u. crater, active
    u., crater with target appearance
    u., Crombie's
    u., Curling's

u., debridement
u., decubitus
u., dendritic
u., develop mouth
u., diabetic
u. diet, bland
u. diet, staged
u. disease (PUD), peptic
u., duodenal
u., duodenal bulbar
u. ▸ duodenum free of
u., esophageal
u., foot
u. from alcohol
u. from aspirin
u. from caffeine
u., full-blown
u. (GU), gastric
u., gastrointestinal (GI)
u., genital
u., healing duodenal
u., heel
u. in mouth
u., infected decubitus
u., ischemic
u., jejunal
u., kissing
u. ▸ large sacral decubitus
u., leg
u., local
u., low incidence of peptic
u. margin
u., marginal
u., Mooren's
u., mouth
u., necrotic
u. niche
u., noninfectious
u., nonperforated
u., nonspecific
u. of cornea, dendritic
u. of esophagus ▸ multiple
u. of stomach ▸ multiple
u., oral
u. pain
u. ▸ pain in abdomen from
u., painful

u., painless
u., Parrot's
u. patient, duodenal
u., penetrating
u. (PU), peptic
u., perforated
u., perforated corneal
u., perforated peptic
u., perforating
u., persistent foot
u., phagedenic
u., polyps or tumors
u., postbulbar
u., prepyloric
u., pressure
u. program
u., pyloric channel
u., refractory
u. regimen
u., rodent
u., Saemisch's
u., shallow
u., skin
u., stasis
u., stomach
u., stomal
u., stress
u. sufferer
u., superficial gastric
u., trophic
u., tropical phagedenic
u., varicose
u. ▸ vascular skin
u., venous
u., venous stasis
ulcerans, Corynebacterium
ulcerans, Mycobacterium
ulcerated
    u. area
    u. buccal mucosa
    u. eccentric lesion
    u. lesion
    u. neurofibroma
    u. nodule
    u. plaque
    u. wound

ulcerating
- u. area
- u. granuloma of the pudenda
- u. lesion
- u. plaque

ulceration(s)
- u. and/or tumor
- u., corneal
- u., deep
- u. ▸ erosive gastritis with
- u., esophageal
- u., focal
- u. ▸ foci of mucosal
- u. ▸ gastrointestinal irritation and
- u., herpetic
- u., mouth
- u., mucosal
- u., multiple
- u., nasal septum
- u., necrosis and
- u., nonhealing
- u. of bronchus
- u. of mouth
- u. of mucosa
- u. of pancreas
- u. of skin ▸ chronic
- u. of the globe
- u. of throat
- u. of trachea
- u. peptic
- u. ▸ perforating acute
- u., skin
- u., superficial
- u., superficial focal
- u., superficial nonhealing
- u., tracheal

ulcerative
- u. blepharitis
- u. blepharitis ▸ recurrent
- u. bowel disease
- u. colitis
- u. colitis, chronic
- u. colitis ▸ diarrhea from
- u. colitis with Crohn's disease
- u. endocarditis
- u. esophagitis
- u. gingivitis, necrotizing
- u. gingivostomatitis, necrotizing
- u. keratitis
- u. lesion
- u. proctitis
- u. stomatitis
- u. stomatitis, necrotizing
- u. vulvitis

ulcere, carcinoma ex

ulcerogenic medication
ulcerogenic tumor of pancreas syndrome
ulceromembranous gingivitis
ulceromembranous stomatitis
ulcerosa
- u., angina
- u., blepharitis
- u., pharyngitis

ulcus serpens corneae
Ulfelder's operation, Twombly-
Ullmann's line
Ullrich syndrome, Bonnevie-
Ullrich syndrome, Morquio-
ulna
- u. bone
- u., distal
- u., radial notch of
- u., styloid process of
- u., trochlear notch of

ulnar
- u. antebrachial region
- u. artery
- u. aspect
- u. compression neuropathy
- u. cutaneous vein
- u. deviation
- u. deviation, partial
- u. drift
- u. drift deformity
- u. head implant, Swanson
- u. ligament
- u. malleolus
- u. nerve
- u. nerve ▸ common palmar digital nerves of
- u. nerve compression
- u. nerve distribution
- u. nerve ▸ dorsal branch of
- u. nerve ▸ dorsal digital nerves of
- u. nerve entrapment
- u. nerve palsy
- u. nerve ▸ proper digital nerves of
- u. nerve ▸ superficial branch of
- u. notch
- u. notch of radius
- u. palsy
- u. pulse
- u. reflex
- u. resection
- u. shaft
- u. shaft, fracture of
- u. styloid bone
- u. synostosis, radio◊
- u. vein

ulnaris
- u., flexor carpi
- u. muscle, extensor carpi
- u. muscle, flexor carpi

ulnocarpal ligament
ultimate cause
ultimate goal
ultimobranchial body
ultra
- u. low profile
- u. low resistance voice prosthesis
- u. low risk category patient
- u. x-ray

ultradian rhythm
ultrafast
- u. CAT (computerized axial tomography) scan
- u. computed tomographic scanner
- u. computed tomography (CT)
- u. CT (computed tomography)
- u. CT scanner ▸ Imatron

ultrafiltration hemodialyzer
ultraflow coil
ultrahigh frequency ventilation
Ultralente insulin
ultrarapid subthreshold stimulation
ultrasensitive to noise
ultrashort wave
ultrashort wave diathermy
ultrasonic
- u. angioplasty
- u. attenuation
- u. cardiography
- u. cephalometry
- u. electrode
- u. fat suctioning
- u. fragmenter
- u. frequency
- u. heat
- u. humidifier
- u. imager
- u. liposuction
- u. liposuction ▸ external
- u. microscope
- u. mist
- u. nebulizer
- u. needle
- u. scanner
- u. therapy
- u. tomography
- u. treatment
- u. waves

ultrasonogram, B scan
ultrasonogram, renal
ultrasonographic echoes

ultrasonographic investigation
ultrasonography
    u., A-mode (amplitude modulation)
    u., B-mode
    u., cardiac
    u., compression
    u., Doppler
    u., duplex
    u. ▸ duplex pulsed Doppler
    u., endoscopic
    u. examination
    u., gray-scale
    u. ▸ high resolution B-mode
    u. ▸ intracaval endovascular
    u., prenatal
    u., real-time
ultrasound
    u., abdominal
    u. angiography
    u. assessment
    u. beam ▸ rotating
    u. blood flow detector
    u., B-mode
    u. breast biopsy
    u., cardiac
    u. cardiography
    u., carotid
    u., carotid artery
    u. catheter ▸ intravascular
    u., continuous wave Doppler
    u., diagnostic
    u., Doppler
    u. Doppler, color flow
    u., duplex
    u. ▸ echo guided
    u. (EUS) ▸ endoscopic
    u., endovaginal
    u. examination
    u. examination, abdominal
    u., fetal
    u., gallbladder
    u. gallstone detection
    u., gray-scale
    u. -guided bronchoscopy
    u. -guided injection therapy
    u. -guided laser-induced
        prostatectomy (TULIP) ▸
        transurethral
    u. hyperthermia
    u. image
    u. imaging
    u. imaging, Doppler
    u., intracoronary
    u., intraluminal
    u., intravascular

    u., Level 2
    u. liposuction
    u. of prostate
    u. of uterus
    u., ophthalmic
    u., pelvic
    u. ▸ power Doppler
    u. ▸ pre-exercise
    u. radiology
    u., real-time
    u., renal
    u. scan
    u. scan ▸ Doppler
    u. scanner ▸ Biosound wide-angle
        monoplane
    u. screening
    u. ▸ Shimadzu cardiac
    u. sonarography, pelvic
    u., sphincter
    u. study, fracture/
    u. technique
    u. technology
    u. test
    u. therapy
    u. transducer
    u., transrectal
    u., transvaginal
    u. treatment
    u. vascular test
    u. vibrations
    u. waves
ultraspeed engine
ultraviolet (UV)
    u. absorbing quality
    u. B (UVB) light
    u. B (UVB) radiation
    u. blood irradiation
    u. color-translating television
        microscope
    u. cytoscopy
    u. (UV) exposure
    u. exposure, chronic
    u. exposure ▸ long-term
    u. fluorescent dosimeter
    u. irradiation
    u. lamp
    u. (UV) laser
    u. light
    u. light, exposure to
    u. light (PUVA) regimen, psora-lens
        plus
    u. light therapy
    u. light (PUVA) treatment, psora-
        lens plus
    u. microscope

    u. protection, lack
    u. purification system
    u. (UV) radiation
    u. radiation, sun's
    u. ray
    u. ray ophthalmia
    u. (UV) therapy
    u. transmission
Ultravist contrast
umbilical
    u. areola
    u. arterial line
    u. arterial samples
    u. artery catheter
    u. artery catheterization
    u. artery, single
    u. blood sampling (PUBS) ▸
        percutaneous
    u. blood vessels
    u. catheter
    u. catheter, infant with
    u. cicatrix
    u. circulation
    u. cord
    u. cord blood
    u. cord blood banks
    u. cord, cleansing
    u. cord compression
    u. cord cut
    u. cord, cutting of
    u. cord fluid
    u. cord traction
    u. eventration
    u. fold, infra◇
    u. fold, lateral
    u. fold, medial
    u. fold, median
    u. fold, middle
    u. fungus
    u. graft
    u. granuloma
    u. hernia
    u. infection
    u. ligament, middle
    u. notch
    u., par◇
    u. region
    u. region of abdomen
    u. region, tenderness of
    u. souffle
    u. stomach, aberrant
    u. stump
    u. tape
    u. tape drain
    u. vein

umbilical—*continued*
 u. vein (HUV) bypass graft ▸
  human
 u. vein catheter
 u. vein ▸ human
 u. vein, left
umbilicalis, arteritis
umbilicated mass
umbilicus
 u., amniotic
 u., decidual
 u., rebound in region of
 u., symphysis to
umbo of tympanic membrane
umbrella
 u., atrial septal defect
 u., Bard clamshell septal
 u., clamshell septal
 u. closure
 u. closure, double
 u. device, double
 u., double
 u. filter
 u. ▸ patent ductus arteriosus
 u. ▸ Rashkind double
 u., transcatheter
unable to
 u.t. control stool
 u.t. control urine
 u.t. cope, patient
 u.t. perform basic activity ▸ patient
 u.t. relax, patient
 u.t. resuscitate patient
 u.t. sit still ▸ patient
 u.t. sleep
 u.t. understand language
 u.t. void, patient
 u.t. walk, patient
unaffected extremity
unaggressive type ▸ undersocialized
  conduct disorder,
unarmed tapeworm
unassigned claim
unassisted detox
unattached to chromosome, bacterial
  cell
unattractive character traits
unattractiveness ▸ delusions of
  physical
unavoidable changes in plans
unavoidable hemorrhage
unbearable situation
unblinking stare ▸ peculiar
unborn child ▸ transmit virus to
unborn offspring

unbound thyroxine binding globulin
uncal herniation
uncal herniation, bilateral
uncaring ▸ caregiver withholding and
uncemented joint
uncertainty principle
unciform bone
Uncinaria braziliense
uncinate
 u. bone
 u. epilepsy
 u. fasciculus
 u. gyrus
 u. process
uncinatus, Chilodon
uncinatus, gyrus
uncircumcised male
unclogged, artery
unclogging coronary artery
uncoiling aorta
uncommunicative state
uncompensated care
uncompensated clinical services
uncomplicated
 u. alcohol withdrawal
 u. ▸ arteriosclerotic dementia,
 u. bereavement
 u. birth
 u. cystitis ▸ acute
 u. delivery
 u. ▸ multi-infarct dementia,
 u. postoperative course
 u. ▸ primary degenerative dementia
  of the Alzheimer type, senile
  onset
 u. skin infections
unconditioned reflex (UCR)
unconditioned stimulus
unconscious
 u. activity
 u. airway obstruction
 u. cerebration
 u. choking victim
 u., collective
 u. conflicts
 u. ▸ immobilized and
 u. memory
 u., patient
 u., permanently
 u. person
 u., racial
 u., shock and
 u. victim
unconsciousness
 u., period of

 u., prolonged
 u., spontaneous attack of
 u., state of
 u., sudden onset of
uncontaminated blood
uncontaminated surgical supplies
uncontrollable
 u. behavior ▸ random
 u. bladder
 u. bleeding
 u. body movements
 u. diarrhea
 u. hemorrhaging
 u. manic behavior
 u. muscle spasm
 u. nosebleed
 u. pain
 u., patient
 u. seizures
 u. seizures and paralysis
 u. shakiness in legs
 u. shaking
 u. shivering
 u. twitching
 u. walking
uncontrolled
 u. atrial fibrillation
 u. bleeding
 u. cell division and growth
 u. cell growth of cancer
 u. diabetes
 u. generalized grand mal seizures
 u. generalized tonic clonic seizures
 u. high blood pressure
 u. hypertension
 u. intrusive reliving
 u. menometrorrhagia
 u. movement
 u. movement of limbs and face
 u. muscle contractions, bursts of
 u. physical symptoms
 u. rhythmic limb movements
 u. shaking
 u. shaking of limb
 u. sinuous movements ▸
  purposeless,
 u. urethral bleeding
unconventional therapy
unconventional treatment
uncoordinated
 u. arm movement
 u. atrial impulses
 u. esophageal peristalsis
 u., feeling
 u. leg movement

u. movements
u. ▸ sleepy and
uncorroborated memory
uncoupling of receptors
uncover eye test, cover-
uncovertebralis, spondylosis
undemanding responsibilities
under
u. anesthesia, examination
u. anesthesia, pelvic examination
u. Bili-Lites ▸ infant placed
u. chin ▸ lump or swelling
u. conjunctiva, medication injected
u. eyes, bags
u. eyes, dark circles
u. fingernail ▸ blood clot
u. high pressure, oxygen
u. kneecap ▸ grating sensation
u. self-hypnosis ▸ patient
u. skin ▸ pacemaker implanted
u. tension, eyeball
u. the influence ▸ working
u. the table drugs
u. x-ray control, biopsy
underachievement disorder, academic
underactive
u. glands
u. immune system
u. thyroid
u. thyroid gland
underarm lymph node
undercut, skin edges
underdeveloped lungs
underdeveloped thigh
underdrive pacing
underdrive termination
underestimate severity of medical
problem
undergoing cancer treatment
undergoing personality change, patient
undergraded insulin factor
underhung bite
underinsured ▸ uninsured and
underlay fascial graft
underline [undermine]
underlying
u. apprehension
u. blood disorder
u. cause
u. chest muscles
u. connective tissue
u. conus
u. defect
u. disease
u. disease, chronic

u. disease ▸ non-lethal
u. disease, patient's
u. disease process
u. disorder
u. esophagitis
u. esophagitis, severe
u. fascia
u. fatty tissue
u. illness
u. immune dysfunction
u. lesion
u. lipid abnormality ▸ genetic
u. malignancy
u. muscle
u. nodularity
u. obstructive coronary disease
u. physical illness
u. physiological problems
u. psychiatric disorder
u. skin
u. structures
u. tissue
u. undifferentiated large cell
carcinoma
u. veins ▸ swollen
undermedication for pain
undermine [underline]
undermined
u., edges
u., lacerations
u., pterygium
u., skin
u., wound margins
underpad, disposable
underperfused myocardium
undersensing, pacemaker
undersensing, ventricular
undersensitive nipple
undersensitivity to pain
underside of nose
undersized person, abnormally
undersocialized conduct disorder,
aggressive type
undersocialized conduct disorder,
unaggressive type
understand, ability to
understand language ▸ unable to
understanding
u. assessment ▸ speech
u., cognitive
u., experiential
u., insight and self-care
u. ▸ lack of
u., scientific
u., speech

u. ▸ trouble talking or
understood ▸ follow-up instructions
undertreatment of pain
underuse of shoulder
underwater
u. breathing apparatus, self-
contained
u. drainage (dr'ge)
u. exercise
u. seal drainage (dr'ge)
u. therapy
undescended testicle
undescended testis
undesirable hypnotic
undesired motor activity
undetected
u. aneurysm
u. disease ▸ true-negative
u. fungal infections ▸ clinically
u. infarcts
u. microscopic disease
undetermined
u. (CU) ▸ cause
u., diagnosis
u., etiology
u. etiology, syncope
u. etiology, urinary frequency
u. myocardial infarction, age-
u. origin
u. origin ▸ anemia of
u. origin (FUO) ▸ fever of
undiagnosed
u. diabetes
u. endometriosis
u. hepatitis
u. hydrocephalus
u. thyroid disease
undifferentiated
u. adenocarcinoma
u. adenocarcinoma of bladder
u. attention deficit disorder
u. body cells
u. bronchogenic carcinoma
u. carcinoma
u. carcinoma ▸ metastatic large
cells
u. cell adenoma
u. cell leukemia
u. cells
u. epidermoid carcinoma
u. large cell carcinoma
u. large cell carcinoma ▸ underlying
u. lesion
u. leukemia, acute
u. lymphoma

undifferentiated—*continued*
 u. malignant lymphoma
 u. mental retardation
 u. mesenchymal cell
 u. neoplasm
 u. protoplasm
 u. renal carcinoma
 u. schizophrenia
 u. schizophrenia, chronic
 u. small cell carcinoma
 u. somatoform disorder
 u. type
 u. type, chronic ▸ schizophrenia
 u. type, chronic with acute
  exacerbation ▸ schizophrenia
 u. type ▸ conduct disorder
 u. type ▸ schizophrenia
 u. type, subchronic ▸
  schizophrenia,
 u. type, subchronic with acute
  exacerbation ▸ schizophrenia,
 u. type, unspecified ▸
  schizophrenia,
undigested
 u. food
 u. food particles
 u. food particles, patient vomited
Undine's dropper
undirected behavior
undirectional block
**undisciplined interpretation and
 suggestion**
undisplaced fracture
Undritz' anomaly
undue physical discomfort
undue retraction of muscles
undulans, Entamoeba
undulant fever
undulating pulse
undulatory nystagmus
unduly vulnerable to stress
uneasiness, feeling of
unempathic, patient
unencapsulated, colloid follice
unengaged, head
unenhanced
 u. CAT (computerized axial
  tomography) scan
 u. scan
 u. study
unequal
 u. amplitude
 u. curvature of cornea
 u. development of electroencephalogram (EEG) waves

 u. pulse
 u. pupil size or shape
 u., pupils
unequivocal diagnosis
unerupted tooth
unesterified fatty acid
unethical practitioner
uneven contour
uneven limb syndrome
uneventful
 u., course of dialysis
 u., operation
 u. postoperative convalescence
 u., postoperative course
 u. postoperative course ▸ patient
  had
 u. prenatal course
unexpected breathlessness
unexpected death
unexpectedly
 u., crying
 u., patient died
 u., patient expired
unexplainable fall ▸ sudden
unexplainable feeling of terror, sudden
unexplained
 u. angina
 u. cough
 u. death, sudden
 u. depression and lethargy
 u. dizziness
 u. fatigue and breathlessness
 u. feeling
 u. generalized weakness
 u. hyperbilirubinemia, prolonged
 u. irritability
 u. pain
 u. personality changes
 u. protrusion
 u. sudden dizziness
 u. weight loss
unexpressed emotions
unfertilized ova
unfocused
 u. behavior
 u. behavior ▸ jittery,
 u. ▸ eyes distant and
unfolding ▸ normal maturational
ungual process
unguiculata, Linuche
unguis
 u. incarnatus
 u., lunula
 u., matrix
 u., os

 u., pterygium
unhappiness disorder, miser and
unhealthy eating patterns
uniaxial joint
unicellular organisms
unicellular sclerosis
unicompartmental knee prosthesis
unicornis, uterus
unidirectional current
unifocal contractions
**unifocal PVCs (premature ventricular
 contractions)**
Uniform (uniform)
 U. Anatomical Gift Act
 u. behavior
 u., colloid content
 u. consistency
 U. Donor Card
 u. frequency
uniformity determination, field
unilateral
 u. activities
 u. cerebellar ataxia
 u. disease
 u. EEG (electroencephalogram)
  activities
 u. emphysema
 u. facial atrophy
 u. facial atrophy, progressive
 u. gliosis
 u. head pain
 u. hearing loss
 u. hearing loss ▸ progressive
 u. hemianopia
 u. hyperlucency of lung
 u. hyperplasia
 u. hypertrophy
 u. lung reduction surgery
 u. mass
 u. nasal obstruction
 u. neglect
 u. nonfunctioning lung
 u. pain
 u. polyps
 u. ptosis of eyelid
 u. pulmonary agenesis
 u. pulmonary artery occlusion ▸
  temporary
 u. salpingo-oophorectomy (s-o)
 u. strabismus
 u. throbbing headache
 u. tinnitus ▸ roaring
 u. ureteral obstruction
unilobar emphysema, idiopathic
unilobular cirrhosis

unilocular cyst
unilocular joint
unimpaired
    u. function
    u. motor function
    u. nerve supply
    u., perception
unimpeded, blood flow
unimproved, condition
unimproved, patient
uninflamed, appendix
uninflamed diverticula, multiple
uninhibited
    u. behavior, brash and
    u. bladder
    u. neurogenic bladder
uninsured and underinsured
unintended pregnancy
unintentional movement
uninterrupted suture
union
    u., bony
    u., cross
    u., delayed
    u., fibrous
    u., fracture with cross
    u., fracture with delayed
    u. of fracture
    u. of fracture, advancing
    u. of fracture, delayed
    u. of fracture, partial
    u., solid bony
un-ionized hemoglobin
uniparental disomy, human
unipennate muscle
uniphasic reaction
unipolar
    u. depression
    u. depression with psychosis
    u. depressive disorder
    u. depth electrode
    u. derivation
    u. disorder
    u. electrocardiogram (ECG)
    u. endocardial electrode ▸
        implantable
    u. lead
    u. limb leads
    u. montage
    u. pacemaker
    u. pacemaker generator
    u. pacing
    u. Pisces Sigma
    u. precordial lead
    u. psychosis

u., spongioblastoma
u. ventricular pacemaker ▸
    Medtronic Activitrax rate
    responsive
unique recovery needs
unit(s) (Unit)
    u. action potential, motor
    u. action potentials, individual
        motor
    u., acute care medical
    u., acute detoxification
    u., adult long-term
    u., Aloe reading
    u., alveolar capillary
    U. (ACU) ▸ Ambulatory Care
    u., AMX 110 mobile x-ray
    u. and telemetry, cardiac stepdown
    u., Angstrom
    u., antitoxin
    u. area, cells per
    u., arithmetic
    u. (a.m.u.), atomic mass
    u., audio response
    u., bedside
    u., Behnken's
    u., Bessey-Lowry
    u., Bodansky
    u., Bovie
    U., Burn
    U. (CCU) ▸ Cardiac Care
    U. (CICU) ▸ Cardiology Intensive
        Care
    u., C-arm fluoroscopy
    u., cautery
    u. cell
    u. (CPU), central processing
    u. character
    u., Cherry-Crandall
    U., Chest Pain
    u. clerk
    u., clinical research
    u., colony forming
    U. (CCU) ▸ Community Care
    u., conscious control of motor
    u., contact
    u., convalescent
    u., Cordis pacemaker
    U. (CCU) ▸ Coronary Care
    U. (CICU) ▸ Coronary Intensive
        Care
    u. ▸ custom fit in ear
    u., death on
    u., digital fluoroscopic
    U. Director
    u. dose

u., Ehrlich
u. ▸ electrocardiogram (ECG)
    triggering
u., electrocautery
u., electrostatic
u. ▸ enhanced external
    counterpulsation
U. (ECU) ▸ Environmental Control
u., enzyme
u., explosion-proof suction
u. for fast neutrons
u. ▸ fungal infection of nail
u. germ-free isolation
u. graft ▸ follicular
u., Gutman
u., hair
u., hemagglutinating
u., hemodialysis
u., Hemovac
u., hertz (Hz)
u., Holzknecht's
u., Hounsfield
u., hybrid
u., hyperemia
u., immunizing
U. (ISCU) ▸ Infant Special Care
u., inpatient
u., institutional
U. (ICU) ▸ Intensive Care
U. (ICCU) ▸ Intensive Coronary
    Care
u. (ITU) ▸ intensive therapy
u. (ITOU) ▸ intensive therapy
    observation
U. (IMCU) ▸ Intermediate Medical
    Care
U. (IU) ▸ International
u. (IBU) ▸ international benzoate
u. ▸ intrapleural sealed drainage
u., isolated
u., Karman
u., Keeler cryophake
u., King-Armstrong
u., Kreiselman
u. (LAFU) ▸ laminar airflow
u., Leksell gamma
u. (LCU) ▸ life change
u., logarithmic
u., Mache
u. (mu) ▸ machine
U. (MSU) ▸ Maximum Security
U. (MICU) ▸ Medical Intensive Care
u. ▸ medically managed intensive
    addiction treatment
u., methadone treatment

unit(s)—*continued*

u., microcautery
u. (MIU) ▸ million international
U. (MCCU) ▸ Mobile Coronary Care
U. (MICU) ▸ Mobile Intensive Care
u., mobile mammography
u., mobile testing
u., Montevideo
u. (MU) ▸ mouse
u. (MUU), mouse uterine
u. ▸ myocardial oxygen (O₂)
u., myocardial research
U. (NICU) ▸ Neonatal Intensive Care
U., Obstetrical
u. of blood
u. of frequency
u. of heat capacity
u. of magnetic energy
u. of packed cells
u. of platelets
u. of radioactivity
u. of roentgen ray dosage
u. of x-ray dosage ▸ Kienböck's
u., orthovoltage
u., oxygen (O₂)
U., Paramedic
u., pediatric trauma
u. (PRU) ▸ peripheral resistance
u., photodisplay
u., Picker Vanguard deep therapy
u., pilosebaceous
u. (PFU) ▸ plaque-forming
u. ▸ portable biofeedback
u. ▸ portable defibrillator
u., portable dialysis
u. potentials, motor
U. (PICU), Prenatal Intensive Care
u. (PNU) ▸ protein nitrogen
u. (ICU) psychosis ▸ intensive care
U. (PICU) ▸ Pulmonary Intensive Care
u., pump/drive
u., R
u. (RU) ▸ rat
u. (RFU) ▸ Reitland-Franklin
U., Renal Dialysis
u., resistance
U., Respiratory
U. (RCU) ▸ Respiratory Care
u. (RU) ▸ roentgen
u., Russell
U. (SCU) ▸ Self-Care
u. ▸ self-contained, transportable medical

u., sensation
u., Shinowara-Jones-Reinhard
u., sigma
u., single motor
u. (STU) ▸ skin test
u. ▸ Solcotrans autotransfusion
u., Somogyi
u., spleen colony forming
u. staff
u., Steenbock
U. (SIU), Stimulus Isolation
u., structural
u., superficial
U. (SICU) ▸ Surgical Intensive Care
u., Svedberg
u., Svedberg flotation
u. (ICU) syndrome ▸ intensive care
u., Tenz
u., thermotic drainage (dr'ge)
u., Todd
u., torr
u. (TU) ▸ toxic
u., trauma
u. (TU) ▸ tuberculin
u. (TRU) ▸ turbidity reducing
u., voice activated
u., voltage
u. weight, per
u., Wohlgemuth
u., Wood

United Network for Organ Sharing (UNOS)
unity and continuity of consciousness
univariant analysis
univariate analysis
univentricular
  u. artificial heart ▸ orthotopic
  u. atrioventricular connection
  u. heart
  u. heart probe ▸ Norwood
universal
  u. appliance
  u. blood screening
  u. fantasies of loneliness
  u. pacemaker
  u. precautions
  u. proximal femur (UPF) prosthesis, Bateman
universalis, adiposis
universalis, calcinosis
universality of needle sharing behaviors
University of Akron artificial heart

unknown
  u. AIDS (acquired immune deficiency syndrome) carrier, patient
  u. cause ▸ impaired memory of
  u. cell type ▸ bronchogenic carcinoma,
  u. (E.U.) ▸ etiology
  u. etiology, pyrexia of
  u., exact nature
  u. origin
  u. origin (FUO) ▸ fever of
  u. origin ▸ myocardial disease of
  u. origin, pyrexia of
  u., primary carcinoma
  u., primary source
  u. primary tumor
  u. risk factor
  u. stimulus
unlearning the training and deprogramming
unlimited potential
unmanageable pain
unmanaged stress
unmyelinated nerve fibers
Unna's
  U. boot
  U. paste
  U. paste boot
  U. wrap
unnatural death, patient died
unobstructed, nasal airways
unorganized virus
unossified cartilage
unossified spot
unoxygenated blood
unpersuasive false idea
unpigmented malignant melanoma
unpigmented skin
unplanned transfer
unpleasant taste
unpleasant withdrawal symptoms
unpredictable
  u. behavior
  u. emotions
  u. moods
unproductive mania
unprofessional conduct
unprotected sun exposure ▸ cumulative effects of
unproven health claims
unproven treatment
unprovoked
  u. anger
  u. rage attacks

u. seizure
unreactive, pupils
unrealistic thinking
unreality ▸ feeling of
unreasonable anger
unreasonable expectations of others
unrecognized
u. disease
u. fluid-seeking behavior
u. mental illness ▸ previously
u. past experience
u. transference paradigms
unregulated dietary supplement
unrelated
u. donor ▸ genetically
u. donor (LURD) ▸ living,
u. donor transplant
u. kidney ▸ living
u. living donors
unrelieved fatigue
unrelieved pain
unremarkable
u., face
u., grossly
u., head
u., HEENT (head, eyes, ears, nose and throat)
u., patient stay
unremitting cough ▸ chronic
unresectable
u. adenocarcinoma
u. carcinoma
u. disease, localized
u. lesion
u., tumor
unresolved grief
unresolved pneumonia
unresponsive
u. cancer
u., emotionally
u., patient
u. ▸ patient weak, hypotensive and
u. to antibiotic therapy ▸ fever
unresponsiveness, emotional
unresponsiveness, temporary
unrest, peristaltic
unrestful sleep ▸ shallow,
unrestrained cell division
unripe cataract
unripe, cervix
unruptured
u. brain aneurysm
u. ectopic pregnancy
u. vascular anomalies

unsaturated
u. compounds
u. fat
u. iron-binding capacity (UIBC)
Unschuld's sign
unsealed radioisotopes
unsoundness of mind
unspecific
u. ▸ bipolar disorder, depressed,
u. ▸ bipolar disorder, mixed,
u. ▸ eating disorder,
u. ▸ major depression, recurrent,
u. ▸ major depression, single episode,
u. mental disorder (nonpsychotic)
u. psychoactive substance delusional disorder ▸ other or
u. psychoactive substance intoxication ▸ other or
u. ▸ psychogenic pain, site
u. schizophrenia
u. ▸ schizophrenia, catatonic type,
u. ▸ schizophrenia, disorganized type,
u. ▸ schizophrenia, paranoid type
u. ▸ schizophrenia, residual type
u. ▸ schizophrenia, undifferentiated type,
unspecified hypertension
unspun urine ▸ gram stain of
unstable
u. and intense relationships
u. angina
u. angina ▸ severe
u. blood pressure (BP)
u. colon
u., emotionally
u., heart electrically
u. interpersonal relationship
u. knee
u. mood
u. or erratic parenting
u. oxygen (O₂) molecules
u., patient emotionally
u. ▸ patient physiologically
u. plaque
u. self-image
u. self-image ▸ persistently
u. sense of self
u. sprain
u. type
u. vasomotor system
unstained ring, pale
unsteadiness
u., faintness and

u. or sudden fall
u. ▸ patient has vertigo and
u. ▸ tremor, slowness, stiffness and
u. while walking
unsteady
u. feelings
u. gait
u. in gait ▸ patient
u., Romberg
u. speech ▸ slow and
u. walk
unsterile needles, contamination from
unsterilized needle
unstimulating occupation ▸ mentally
unstressed heart
unstriated muscle
unstripped bladder
unstructured stimulus
unstructured work
unsuitable donor
unsupported balance
unsupported sitting
unsuspected disease site
unsuspected hydrocephalus
unsustained clonus
unsystematized delusion
untidy appearance
untimely death
untoward reaction
untoward reaction to transfusion
untrainable mentally retarded patient
untraining, bladder
untreatable
u. cardiomyopathy
u. condition, chronic
u. coronary disease
u. epilepsy
u., injury
untreated
u. addictions
u. controls
u. disease
u. mania
untroubled calmness, state of
ununited fracture
unusual
u. behavior
u. bleeding
u. risky behavior
u. side-effects
u. uterine bleeding
u. water drinking behavior

unusually hostile or aggressive
    behavior
unvarying stimulation
unverifiable memories of incest
Unverricht's disease
unwanted pregnancy
unwilling to make decisions
unwilling to take risk
unwitting exploitation of others
up(s) (Ups)
    u. and cool down ▸ warm
    u. and down flap, Gillies'
    u., annual check-
    u., appendix freed
    u. arm ▸ red line
    u. blood, spitting
    u., build-
    u. care, follow-
    u., classic push-
    u. ▸ developmental catch-
    u., drain fluid build-
    u. ▸ ear wax build-
    u. exercise, abdominal crunch/curl-
    u. exercise, chair sit-
    u. exercise ▸ sit-
    u. feeling ▸ stuffed-
    u. feelings, pent-
    u. ▸ fluid build-
    u., freed
    u. ▸ half sit-
    u. hostility ▸ pent-
    u. implant, build-
    u. in chair, patient
    u. in oxygenation saturation ▸ step-
    u. ▸ loss of ability to hold head
    u. ▸ loss of ability to sit
    u. ▸ modified push-
    u. ▸ neck push-
    u. of pressure ▸ rapid build
    u. of scar tissue, build
    u., patient discharged to follow-
    u., patient discharged to office
        follow-
    u., pelvic tone-
    u. phenomenon ▸ warm-
    u. position, brow-
    u., pull-
    u. region, build-
    u. response ▸ giving
    u. ▸ straight leg sit-
    U. ▸ Surgical Lint Pic-
    u. tilt table test ▸ head
    u. transformer, step-
    u. view ▸ sitting
UP (ureteropelvic) juncture stricture

U/P (urine/plasma) ratio
upbeat nystagmus ▸ torsional,
upbringing, chaotic
update isolation techniques
update, medical
updrawn pupil
UPF (universal proximal femur)
    prosthesis, Bateman
upgated technique
upgoing, toes
upheaval, emotional
UPJ (ureteropelvic junction)
upon itself, catheter coiled
Uppers (upper)
    U. (amphetamines)
    u. abdomen
    u. abdomen ▸ fluid spilling into
    u. abdominal area
    u. abdominal flap
    u. abdominal radiation
    u. airway disease
    u. airway ▸ froth in
    u. airway, obstructed
    u. airway receptor
    u. and lower
    u. and lower extremities ▸ mild
        edema
    u. arm ▸ patient has swelling of
    u. back and in neck ▸ pain in
    u. back ▸ hump in
    u. back, patient flexed
    u. body dressing
    u. body dressing, independent
    u. body dressing, maximum
        assistance for
    u. body dressing, minimal
        assistance for
    u. body dressing, patient
        independent in
    u. body exercise
    u. body, flushing of
    u. body strength
    u. border of pupil
    u. brain stem
    u. cervical region
    u. chamber of heart
    u. chest, burning sensation in
    u. collecting system
    u. denture
    u. denture, complete
    u. denture, partial
    u. ear cartilage
    u. edge of rib
    u. esophageal sphincter disorder
    u. esophagus

u. extremities atrophic ▸ muscles of
u. extremities bilaterally amputated
u. extremities ▸ clubbing and
    cyanosis
u. extremities ▸ marked atrophy of
u. extremities, swelling of
u. extremities, vasomotor changes
    in
u. extremity
u. extremity (LUE) amputated ▸ left
u. extremity (RUE) amputated ▸
    right
u. extremity ▸ edema of
u. extremity (LUE) flexed ▸ left
u. extremity (RUE) flexed ▸ right
u. extremity full range of motion
    (ROM) ▸ left
u. extremity full range of motion
    (ROM) ▸ right
u. extremity ▸ intramuscular
    arteries of
u. extremity (LUE) ▸ left
u. extremity (RUE) ▸ right
u. extremity strength
u. extremity strength, patient
u. extremity training
u. extremity ▸ tremor in
u. extremity vascular disorder
u. eyelid
u. eyelid crease
u. eyelid, drooping of
u. eyelid infiltrated
u. eyelid, levator muscle of
u. eyelid ptosis
u. femora
u. femoral epiphysis, slipped
u. ganglion
u. gastrointestinal (UGI)
u. gastrointestinal endoscopy
u. gastrointestinal (GI) series
u. GI (gastrointestinal) bleed ▸
    massive
u. gut
u. half
u. hemianopia
u. impression
u. inner quadrant
u. intestinal disorder
u. jawbone
u. left quadrant
u. lid
u. limb amputee, patient bilateral
u. limb cardiovascular disease ▸
    Lewis
u. limbus

u. limits of normal
u. lip
u. lip and ala of nose ▸ levator muscle of
u. lip, incisive muscles of
u. lip, levator muscle of
u. lip mucosa
u. lip ▸ quadrate muscle of
u. lobe
u. lobe (LUL) bronchial orifice ▸ left
u. lobe (RUL) bronchial orifice ▸ right
u. lobe bronchus
u. lobe (LUL) ▸ left
u. lobe (LUL) lesion ▸ left
u. lobe (RUL) lesion ▸ right
u. lobe of left lung
u. lobe (LUL) of lung ▸ left
u. lobe (RUL) of lung ▸ right
u. lobe of right lung
u. lobe (LUL) pneumonia ▸ left
u. lobe (RUL) pneumonia ▸ right
u. lobe (RUL) ▸ right
u. lobe segmental bronchi
u. mantle radiation
u. mantle radiation treatment ▸ modified
u. mantle therapy
u. mediastinum, tomography of
u. motoneurons/motor neurons
u. motor neuron dysfunction ▸ superimposed
u. nodal extrasystole
u. outer quadrant
u. peritoneal edge
u. peritoneal flap
u. plate
u. pole of uterine incision
u. portion of lung ▸ artificial collapse of
u. quadrant (LUQ) ▸ left
u. quadrant (LUQ) of abdomen ▸ left
u. quadrant (RUQ) of abdomen ▸ right
u. quadrant (RUQ) ▸ right
u. quadrant (RUQ) tenderness ▸ right
u. respiratory congestion
u. respiratory disease
u. respiratory infection (URI)
u. respiratory tract
u. respiratory tract discomfort
u. respiratory tract infection (URI), concurrent

u. respiratory tract infection ▸ recurrent
u. respiratory viral syndrome
u. retina
u. right quadrant (URQ)
u. segment
u. teeth
u. teeth, pyorrhea around
u. thigh bone
u. thigh stretch exercise
u. third of esophagus, carcinoma
u. trachea, deviation
u. urinary tract
u. uterine canal curettings
u. vagina ▸ force on uterus and
UPPP (uvulopalatopharyngoplasty)
Uppsala virus (U virus)
upright
u. film
u. film of abdomen
u. film of chest, portable semi-
u. position
u. posture
upset
u., emotional
u., emotionally
u., intestinal
upside-down stomach
upstairs-downstairs heart
upstroke
u., decreased carotid
u. pattern on apexcardiogram
u. velocity
uptake
u. (AIU) ▸ absolute iodine
u., areas of increased
u., fluorescein
u., glucose
u., lung
u., maximum oxygen (O_2)
u. mismatch pattern
u. ▸ myocardial oxygen (O_2)
u. of isotope, increased
u., radioactive iodine (I^{131}/RAI)
u. ratio, resin-
u., resin
u. scans, thyroid
u. studies
u. studies, radioisotope
u. test, radioactive fibrinogen
u. test ▸ radioactive iodine (I^{131}/RAI)
u. test, triiodothyronine (T_3)
u. test, triiodothyronine red cell
uptight, patient

upward
u. and downward
u. and downward squint
u., blunt dissection carried
u., displacement of larynx backward and
u., eyes roll
u., eyes rotated
u. gaze
u. gaze, paralysis of
u. gaze ▸ slight nystagmus on
u., knife advanced
u. movement
u. pen deflection
u., reflected
u. relaxation
u. thrust, quick
urachal abnormality
urachal cyst
urachus, patent
urachus, surgical
uracil mustard
urate(s)
u., amorphous
u. calculus
u. crystals
u. deposition
u., monosodium
uratic conjunctivitis
uratic iritis
urban legends
URD (upper respiratory disease)
urea
u., Blastomycoides
u., blood
u. clearance
u. clearance, blood
u. clearance test
u. concentration, blood
u. excretion ratio
u. nitrogen
u. nitrogen (BUN) ▸ blood
u. nitrogen (BUN) ▸ elevated blood
u. nitrogen (BUN) fluctuation ▸ blood
u. nitrogen (SUN) ▸ serum
u. nitrogen test
u. nitrogen (BUN) test ▸ blood
u. nitrogen (UUN) ▸ urine
u. production
ureae, Actinobacillus
Ureaplasma urealyticum
uremia
u. and sepsis

uremia—*continued*
 u., azotemic
 u., eclampsia due to
 u., extrarenal
 u. of pregnancy
 u., prerenal
 u., puerperal
 u., retention

uremic
 u. acidosis
 u. amaurosis
 u. amblyopia
 u. cachexia
 u. coma
 u. convulsion
 u. eclampsia
 u. frost
 u. pericarditis
 u. pneumonia
 u. poisoning
 u. pulmonary edema
 u. retinitis
 u. stomatitis
 u. syndrome (HUS), hemolytic

ureter(s)
 u., adenocarcinoma
 u. and bladder (KUB) film ▸ kidneys,
 u. and bladder (KUB) ▸ kidneys,
 u. cancer
 u., circumcaval
 u., congenital absence of
 u., course of
 u., dilatation of
 u., ectopic
 u. exposed
 u. freed
 u. into rectum, implantation of
 u., left
 u., obstruction of
 u., orifice of
 u. patent
 u. patent and not dilated
 u. ▸ pelves, calyces and
 u., postcaval
 u., proximal
 u., retrocaval
 u., retroiliac
 u., right

ureteral
 u. abnormality
 u. anastomosis, transuretero-
 u. calculus
 u. calculus, left
 u. calculus, right
 u. catheter

 u. colic
 u. electromyography
 u. fibrosis
 u. implant
 u. implant material
 u. implantation
 u. injury, iatrogenic
 u. injury, traumatic
 u. meatotomy electrode
 u. obstruction
 u. obstruction ▸ unilateral
 u. orifice
 u. pressure
 u. pyelocaliectasis
 u. pyelography, retrograde
 u. reflux of urine
 u. ridge
 u. stent
 u. stone

ureteric
 u. injury
 u. plexus
 u. ridge

ureterocele, simple
ureterogram (RUG), retrograde
ureterogram study
ureteroileal loop, Cordonnier
ureteroileocutaneous anastomosis
ureterolithiasis, proximal
ureterolithotomy, proximal
ureteropelvic (UP)
 u. junction (UPJ)
 u. junction obstruction
 u. juncture stricture
 u. obstruction

ureteropelvioplasty
 u., Culp's
 u., Foley Y-type
 u., Scardino's

ureteropyelogram study
ureteroscopic stone removal
ureterostomy, cutaneous
ureterotomy site
ureterotubal anastomosis
ureteroureteral anastomosis
ureterovesical junction (UVJ)
urethra
 u., adenocarcinoma
 u. and bladder, prolapse of
 u., blockage of
 u., bulbous
 u., calibration of
 u. carcinoma
 u., cervical colliculus of female
 u., closing force on

 u. completely obstructed
 u. constricted
 u. feminina
 u., gram stain of
 u., granular stricture of
 u. ▸ inflammation of
 u., inflammation of bladder and
 u., irritation of
 u. masculina
 u., membranous
 u. muliebris
 u., muscles constrict
 u., narrowed
 u., navicular fossa of male
 u., obstruction of
 u., orifice of male
 u., pendulous
 u., pressure on
 u., prostatic
 u., relieve pressure on
 u., sphincter muscle of
 u., sphincter muscle of membranous
 u. virilis
 u. ▸ walls of

urethrae
 u., bulbus
 u., fossa navicularis
 u. muliebris, corpus spongiosum
 u., septum bulbi
 u., sphincter

urethral
 u. and Skene's (BUS) glands ▸
  Bartholin's,
 u. bleeding, uncontrolled
 u. calculus
 u. calibration
 u. caruncles
 u. catheter, indwelling
 u. catheterization
 u. chill
 u. dilatation
 u. discharge
 u. fever
 u. gland
 u. hematuria
 u. incompetence
 u. instrumentation
 u. lesions, female
 u. lining
 u. meatal stenosis
 u. meatus
 u. melanoma, sub◊
 u. opening
 u. orifice, external
 u. orifice, internal

u. profile pressure
u. resistance, external
u. sound
u. sound, Le Fort
u. sounding
u. sphincterotomy, external
u. stricture
u. syndrome
u. syndrome, acute
u. trigonitis
u. utricle
u. wall
u. wall, patulous

urethralis
u., annulus
u. femininae, crista
u. muliebris, crista
u. vaginae, carina

urethritis
u. and cystitis cystica ▸ pyelitis,
u., Chlamydiae
u., chronic
u. cystica
u. glandularis
u., gonococcal
u., gonorrheal
u., gouty
u., granular
u., granulosa
u., nongonococcal
u. (NSU), nonspecific
u. orificii externi
u. petrificans
u., polypoid
u., prophylactic
u., specific
u. venerea

urethrogram, excretory
urethroplasty, Thiersch-Duplay
urethroplasty, Turner-Warwick
urethroscopic examination
urethrotomy (DVIU), direct vision
    internal
urethrovesical angle ▸ posterior
urethrovesiculo-differential reflux
urge(s)
u., compulsive
u. ▸ cravings and
u. incontinence
u. to defecate
u. to urinate
u. ▸ violent obsessional

urgency
u. and frequency
u. and frequency of urination

u., bladder
u., hypertensive
u., precipitate
u., pressure
u., urinary

urgent (Urgent)
u. admissions, elective
u. bowel movement
U. Care Center
U. Care Physician
u. care service
u. symptoms with back
u. symptoms with bone

Urginea maritima
URI (upper respiratory infection)
uric
u. acid
u. acid, blood
u. acid calculus
u. acid crystals
u. acid diathesis
u. acid diet, low
u. acid, excess
u. acid infarct
u. acid level
u. acid, serum
u. acid test
u. salt deposits

uricosuric agents
Uricult dipslides
uridine
u. diphosphate
u. diphosphoglucose
u. diphosphoglucuronic acid
u. diphosphoglycyronyl transferase
u. monophosphate
u. triphosphate

uridyl transferase, galactose phosphate
urinae granulata, Amoeba
urinae muscle, detrusor
urinal, assist with
urinalysis(-es) (UA)
u., admission
u., clean catch
u., initial
u., serial
u., supervised

urinaria, Bodo
urinary
u. abnormalities
u. acidifiers
u. amylase
u. amylase excretion
u. bladder
u. bladder, adenocarcinoma

u. bladder, atonia of
u. bladder calculi
u. bladder cancer
u. bladder, congenital absence of
u. bladder contracted
u. bladder ▸ distended
u. bladder, fundus of
u. bladder, inflammation of
u. bladder, infundibulum of
u. bladder ▸ irrigation of
u. bladder, level of
u. bladder, malignant tumor of
u. bladder, mucosa of
u. bladder, peak flow of
u. bladder, rhabdomyosarcoma of
u. bladder, shadows in
u. bladder, sphincter muscle of
u. bladder, stimulation of
u. bladder, vertex of
u. bladder, wall of
u. blockage
u. burning
u. cachexia
u. calcium level
u. calculus
u. catheter
u. catheter care kit
u. catheter, indwelling
u. catheterization
u. chorionic gonadotropin
u. concentration, maximum
u. continence
u. coproporphyrin
u. cramping
u. culture
u. diversion
u. drainage (dr'ge) bag with drip
    chamber ▸ closed
u. dribbling
u. elimination
u. elimination, alteration in pattern of
u. elimination, altered patterns of
u. estriol
u. estriol values
u. excretion
u. excretion ▸ disorder of
u. excretion, increasing
u. extravasation
u. fever
u. findings
u. fistula
u. flow
u. flow ▸ increased
u. flow ▸ reduced
u. flow test

urinary—*continued*
- u. frequency
- u. frequency of undetermined etiology
- u. function, normal
- u. gonadotropin (TUG) ▸ total
- u. hemorrhage
- u. hesitancy
- u. incontinence
- u. incontinence ▸ frequent
- u. incontinence ▸ minimize or delay
- u. infection
- u. infection, chronic
- u. infection, hospital-acquired
- u. infection in children
- u. meatus
- u. obstruction
- u. opening, permanent
- u. opening, temporary
- u. output
- u. output, decreased
- u. output, increased
- u. problems
- u. reflexes
- u. reflux
- u. retention
- u. retention, acute
- u. retention cysts
- u. retention, patient has
- u. salts
- u. schistosomiasis
- u. sediment, stained
- u. siderosis
- u. sodium excretion
- u. sphincter
- u. sphincter, artificial
- u. stasis
- u. stone
- u. stream
- u. stream ▸ difficulty in starting
- u. stream, flow of
- u. stream ▸ slow, hesitant
- u. stream, starting and stopping of
- u. stream ▸ weak
- u. stress incontinence
- u. stuttering
- u. symptoms
- u. tract
- u. tract anomaly
- u. tract, blocked
- u. tract calculi
- u. tract cancer
- u. tract, clogged
- u. tract disorder
- u. tract dysfunction

- u. tract infection (UTI)
- u. tract infection, asymptomatic
- u. tract infection, candida
- u. tract infection (UTI), catheter-related
- u. tract infection (UTI) ▸ Citrobacter freundii
- u. tract infection (UTI), congenital
- u. tract infection (UTI) ▸ enterococcal
- u. tract infection (UTI), hospital-acquired
- u. tract infection (UTI) ▸ Klebsiella
- u. tract infection (UTI), recurrent
- u. tract infection ▸ symptomatic
- u. tract, inflammation of
- u. tract injury
- u. tract structures
- u. tract system
- u. tract, upper
- u. tube
- u. urgency
- u. volume
- u. washings

urinate
- u. ▸ partial inability to
- u. ▸ total inability to
- u., urge to

urinating ▸ burning sensation while
urinating, difficulty in
urination
- u. at night ▸ excessive
- u. ▸ bladder burning during
- u. ▸ burning and frequent
- u., burning on
- u., decreased
- u. ▸ difficulty in initiating
- u., difficulty on
- u. ▸ disruption in normal
- u. ▸ dribbling at end of
- u., dribbling on
- u., excessive
- u., frequency and urgency of
- u., frequent
- u. ▸ frequent nighttime
- u. from alcohol
- u. from anxiety
- u. from caffeine
- u. from diabetes
- u., increased
- u. ▸ increased frequency of
- u., interruption of flow of
- u., pain during
- u., pain on
- u., painful

- u., patient has frequency of
- u., precipitant
- u., salt excreted through
- u., stuttering

urine(s) (Urine)
- u., abnormally high concentration of
- u. acetone
- u., amber-colored
- u. amylase
- u. amylase, serum
- u. analysis
- u. and plasma aldosterone
- u., anemic
- u., bacteria in
- u., Bence-Jones
- u. bilirubin
- u., black
- u., bladder
- u., blood in
- u., blood tinged
- u., calcium in
- u., catheterized specimen of
- u. chloride test
- u., cholesterol in
- u., chylous
- u., clean catch
- u., clear
- u. cloudy
- u. collections
- u. concentration
- u. concentration test
- u. copper
- u. creatinine clearance
- u., crude
- u. culture
- u. culture and sensitivity
- u. culture and sensitivity contaminated
- u. cultures, followup
- u., dark
- u., diabetic
- u. dilution
- u., diphtheroids isolated in
- u., discharge of
- u. discoloration
- u. disease (MSUD), maple syrup
- u. drug screen
- u. drug screen ▸ positive
- U. Drug Testing Program ▸ Forensic
- u., dyspeptic
- u., effluxed clear
- u., excessive discharge of
- u. excretion, decrease in
- u., excretion of
- u. excretion, Schilling test for

u., febrile
u., fetal
u., fibrin in
u. flow from constipation ▸ change in
u. flow, interrupted
u. flow, normal
u. ▸ flow of
u., foamy
u. ▸ foul-smelling
u. ▸ free passage of
u. from antidepressant ▸ green
u. from diabetes ▸ sweet smelling
u. glucose
u., gouty
u., gram stain of unspun
u. hazy
u. ▸ hypo-osmolarity of blood and
u., inability to control
u., inability to pass
u., incontinence of
u. ▸ involuntary discharge of
u. ▸ involuntary dribbling of
u. ▸ leakage or dribbling of
u. level
u. level of amphetamine
u. level of cocaine
u. level of depressant
u. level of opioids
u. midstream culture
u., milky
u. mucoid
u. myoglobin
u., nebulous
u., nervous
u. osmolality
u. osmolality, increased
u. output, normal
u., over-excretion of sodium in
u. ▸ passage of dark brown
u., patient incontinent of
u. /plasma (U/P) ratio
u., porphyrins in
u. (PU), pregnancy
u. protein ▸ rat
u. protein, total
u. ▸ pus in
u. radiography
u. reaction
u., residual
u., retained
u. samples
u. screen
u. screen for amphetamine
u. screen for cocaine
u. screening for drug use

u. secreted in kidneys
u., shunting
u. specimen
u. specimen, initial
u., split
u., stagnant
u., stagnation of
u. sterile on culture
u., straw-colored
u. stream ▸ weak or interrupted
u. tested for albumin
u. tested with Clinitest
u. testing, daily
u., turbid yellow
u., 24-hour
u., unable to control
u. urea nitrogen (UUN)
u., ureteral reflux of
u. urobilinogen (UU)
u., voided
u. volume ▸ low residual
urobilin icterus
urobilinogen
    u. (FU) ▸ fecal
    u. test
    u. (UU) ▸ urine
urodynamic testing
urogenital
    u. atrophy
    u. diaphragm
    u. fold
    u. region
    u. structures
    u. tract
    u. trigone
    u. trigone, fascia of
    u. vestibule
urogenitalis, Amoeba
urogenous pyelitis
urogram
    u., constant infusion excretory
    u., drip-infusion
    u. (XU), excretory
    u., IV (intravenous)
    u., retrograde
urographic contrast agent
urography
    u., ascending
    u., cystoscopy
    u., descending
    u., excretory
    u., intravenous (IV)
    u., oral
    u., percutaneous antegrade
    u. ▸ rapid sequence excretory

u., retrograde
urokinase therapy
urokinase-type plasminogen activator
urologic oncologist
urological
    u. evaluation
    u. medical evaluation
    u. studies
urology, gynecologic
Uronema caudatum
uropathy, obstructive
urophilus, Leptomitus
uroporphyrin isomerase
uroporphyrinogen decarboxylase
urostealith calculus
urostomy, patient has
urostomy procedure
urticans, purpura
urticaria
    u., aquagenic
    u., chronic
    u. ▸ cold-induced
    u., exercise-induced
    u., giant
    u. hemorrhagica
    u. maculosa
    u. multiformis endemica
    u. papulosa
    u. pigmentosa
    u., pressure
    u. solaris
urticarial
    u. rash
    u. reaction
    u. valiant
urticata, acne
urticatus, lichen
Uruma virus
U.S. Centers for Disease Control (CDC)
usage
    u., antibiotic
    u., cannabis
    u., hard drug
    u., heavy alcohol
    u., intravenous
    u. pattern, chemical
use(s) (Use)
    u., abstention versus moderation of
        drug
    u., active alcohol
    u., addictive
    u., adolescent drug
    u., adolescent polydrug
    u., alcohol and drug
    u. and abuse, antibiotic

use(s)—*continued*
u. and abuse, cyclic epidemics of
u. and abuse, polysubstance
u., blood screen for drug
u., chronic cocaine
u., chronic marijuana
u., clinical
u. cocaine, patient
u., continuous
u., crack cocaine
u. dependence
u. disorder ▸ psychoactive substance
u. disorder, tobacco
u. ▸ elderly alcohol
u., encouragement of drug
u., excessive
u. ▸ excessive alcohol
u., experimental drug
u. eyes (donor) ▸ authorization form to
u. eyes (next of kin) ▸ authorization form to
u. eyes (donor) ▸ consent form to
u. eyes (next of kin) ▸ consent form to
u., history of pathological
u., illegal drug
u., illegal IV (intravenous) drug
u., illicit drug
u., illicit substance
u. in brain ▸ energy
u. in detoxification, methadone
u. inappropriate words ▸ patient
u., intensive
u., intravenous (IV) drug
U. Inventory (AUI) ▸ Alcohol
u. kidneys (donor) ▸ authorization form to
u. kidneys (next of kin) ▸ authorization form to
u. kidneys (donor) ▸ consent form to
u. kidneys (next of kin) ▸ consent form to
u., long-term
u. ▸ multigenerational drug
u., occasional drug
u. of aliases
u. of cocaine ▸ addictive
u. of drugs
u. of drugs ▸ curb intravenous
u. of drugs ▸ off label
u. of free-base cocaine ▸ long-term
u. of involved muscle ▸ excessive
u. of medication ▸ off label
u. of prescription ▸ improper

u. of restraint
u. of sick leave ▸ excessive
u. ▸ opiate
u. ▸ pathological
u. ▸ pattern of
u. ▸ pattern pathological alcohol
u. ▸ polydrug
u. ▸ post-treatment alcohol
u. ▸ post-treatment drug
u. ▸ psychoactive substance
u. ▸ recent alcohol or drug
u. ▸ recovery of alcohol or drug
u. ▸ recreational
u. ▸ regular drug
u. ▸ resume drug
u. ▸ screening for drug
u. ▸ short-term post-surgical
u. ▸ social/recreational
u. ▸ video terminal
u. water cooler ▸ dual

used
u. needles, instruments or syringes
u. needles ▸ recapping
u. to prime coil, blood

useful beam
usefulness of antibodies, therapeutic
useless rhythm ▸ chaotic
user(s)
u., active drug
u., Big H (heroin)
u., casual drug
u., chronic drug
u., cocaine
u., dependent drug
u., drug
u., hallucinogen (LSD)
u., hard alcohol
u., heavy alcohol
u., heroin (Big H)
u., IV (intravenous) drug
u., LSD (lysergic acid diethylamide)
u., marijuana
u. needle sticks
u. ▸ opioid-dependent cocaine
u., patient occasional drug
u., substance

uses
u. cane, patient
u. quad cane with verbal cueing, patient
u. walker, patient

U-shaped
U-s. continuous suture
U-s. incision
U-s. scar

Usher('s)
U. Marlex mesh implant
U. Marlex mesh implant material
U. Marlex mesh prosthesis
U. syndrome

using
u. bolus adjacent to chest wall
u. peer groups ▸ drug-
u. population ▸ heroin-
u. spouse ▸ substance-
u. system

Uskow's pillars
usnic acid
Ustilago maydis
ustus, Aspergillus
usual
u. activities ▸ loss of interest in
u. anatomic locations
u. anatomic position
u. childhood diseases (UCD)
u. state of good health (USGH)

Utah total artificial heart
utensils, weighted
uteri
u., adenomyosis
u., adnexa
u., apoplexia
u., ascensus
u., cavum
u., cervix
u., corpus
u., descensus
u. ▸ dilatation of os
u., discission of cervix
u., fibromyomata
u., fundus
u., inertia
u., isthmus
u., leiomyoma
u., leiomyomata
u., lyra
u., myomata
u., os
u., ostium
u., partial excision mucous membrane of cervix
u. rigidity, cervix

uterina
u., endometriosis
u., lyra
u., placenta
u., placentae, pars

uterinae
u., ostium abdominal tubae
u., ostium uterinum tubae

u., plica isthmicae tubae
u., plicae ampullares tubae
u., plicae tubariae tubae

uterine
u. activity
u. adenocarcinoma
u. adenomyosis
u. agenesis
u. angiosarcoma
u. anomaly
u. aplasia
u. apoplexy
u. appendage
u. artery
u. artery embolization
u. artery ▸ tortuous
u. aspiration
u. atony
u. balloon therapy
u. bleeding
u. bleeding, abnormal
u. bleeding during pregnancy
u. bleeding (DUB), dysfunctional
u. bleeding, irregular
u. bleeding, prolonged
u. bleeding, unusual
u. blood flow
u. calculus
u. canal curettings, lower
u. canal curettings, upper
u. cancer
u. cancer risk
u. cavity
u. cavity curetted
u. cavity sounded
u. cavity sounded to depth of _____
u. cervical carcinoma
u. cervical stump, carcinoma
u. cervix
u. colic
u. configuration
u. contractions (UC)
u. corpus
u. cramping
u. curettement
u. curettings
u. cycle
u. defect ▸ structural
u. descensus
u. didelphia
u. dilatation
u. distress, intra-
u. dysfunction, hypertonic
u. dyskinesia
u. dysmenorrhea

u. elevator
u. endometrium ▸ normal
u. enlargement
u. enlargement, diffuse
  symmetrical
u. environment
u. evacuation
u. exploration
u. exteriorization ▸ extra-abdominal
u. fibroid
u. fibroid, calcified
u. fibroid embolization
u. fibroma
u. flap, bleeding
u. fundus
u. hemorrhage
u. hemorrhage, essential
u. hernia
u. hyperplasia
u. incision
u. incision ▸ horizontal
u. incision, upper pole of
u. incision, vertical
u. inertia
u. insufficiency
u. irritability
u. isodose, intra◇
u. laceration
u. leiomyosarcoma
u. life
u. lining
u. lining ▸ precancerous overgrowth of
u. lining ▸ thickening of
u. lining tissue
u. manipulation
u. mass ▸ palpable extra-
u. milk
u. mixed mesodermal tumor,
  advanced
u. mucosa
u. mucous
u. muscle, contraction of
u. musculature
u. myoma
u. myomata
u. myomectomy
u. nerve
u. orifice
u. overdistention
u. placenta
u. plexus
u. polyp
u. pregnancy
u. procidentia
u. prolapse

u. prolapse ▸ first, second or third
  degree
u. prolapse repair, Le Fort
u. reflection
u. rupture
u. sarcoma
u. sarcoma, advanced
u. scrapings
u. secundines
u. segment
u. segment, lower
u. shadow
u. souffle
u. sound
u. spasm ▸ abnormal
u. stimulant
u. suspension
u. tear
u. tissue
u. tubae uterinae, pars
u. tube
u. tube, abdominal orifice of
u. tube, fimbriae of
u. tube, infundibulum of
u. tube, tubal folds of
u. tympanites
u. units (MUU) ▸ mouse
u. veins
u. vessels
u. wall

uterinum, chloasma
uterinum tubae uterinae, ostium
uteris, mons
utero
u., dead fetus in
u. ▸ fetus in
u., in
u. -ovarian pregnancy
u. -ovarian varicocele
u. surgery, in
uteroabdominal pregnancy
uteroparietal suture
uteroplacental apoplexy
uteroplacental insufficiency
uterosacral ligaments
uterotubal pregnancy
uterovaginal fistula
uterovaginal plexus
uterovaginalis, plexus
uterovesical fold
uterus
u., abdominal removal of pregnant
u. acollis
u., adenocarcinoma of
u. and cervix, extirpation of

uterus—*continued*
- u. and upper vagina ▸ force on
- u. anteflexed
- u., anteflexion of
- u. anterior
- u., anteversion of
- u. appears enlarged
- u., arcuate
- u. arcuatus
- u., atonia of
- u. bicornis
- u., bicornuate
- u. biforis
- u. bilocularis
- u. bipartitus
- u., boggy
- u., bosselated
- u., calcified leiomyoma of
- u. cancer of
- u., carcinoma of body of
- u., cauterize lining of
- u., cervical ganglion of
- u., chronic subinvolution of
- u., cochleate
- u., contractions of
- u. cordiformis
- u., cornual portion of
- u., Couvelaire
- u., dehiscence of
- u., dextrorotation of
- u. didelphys
- u., dilatation and aspiration (D and A)
- u. does appear enlarged
- u. does appear enlarged ▸ fibroid of
- u. does not appear enlarged
- u., dropped
- u. duplex
- u., dysfunction of
- u., effleurage on
- u. enlarged
- u., exteriorizing
- u., fetal
- u. fibroid
- u., fibroid tumor of
- u. firm
- u. freely mobile
- u., freely movable
- u., fundal portion of
- u., fundus of
- u., Gilliam suspension of
- u., gravid
- u. has good support
- u., horn of
- u. incudiformis
- u., infection of the
- u., inversion of
- u., involution of
- u., isthmus of
- u., lining of
- u., lyre of
- u. masculinus
- u., massaged
- u. mobilized
- u., muscle tone of
- u. ▸ nonmalignant lesion of
- u. normal in anteroposterior (AP) diameter
- u. normal in length
- u. normal in size
- u. normal in size and shape
- u. packed
- u. packed with gauze
- u. parvicollis
- u., perforated
- u., Pituitrin injected into
- u., procidentia of
- u., prolapse of
- u., pubescent
- u., recurrent fibrosarcoma of
- u., rent in
- u., retrocession of
- u., retroflexed
- u., retroverted
- u., rupture of
- u., ruptured scar of
- u. septus
- u. shifts from normal position
- u. simplex
- u., small
- u., smooth walled
- u., sonography of
- u. sounded
- u., subinvolution of
- u., surgical absence of
- u. symmetrical in contour
- u. tender to motion
- u., tipped
- u., ultrasound of
- u. unicornis
- u., weeping of
- u., well differentiated adenocarcinoma of

UTI (urinary tract infection)
utility programmer
utilization
- u. and quality review mechanisms
- u., health care
- u. management services
- u., medical care
- u., net protein
- u., patient
- u. review
- u. review, antibiotic
- u. review program
- u. ▸ surgical antibiotic

utilize galactose in diet
utilizing ruby, solid state laser
utricle, prostatic
utricle, urethral
utricular crises
utricular nerve
utriculi, macula
utriculi, macula acustica
utriculoampullar nerve
utterance, phrase length
UU (urine urobilinogen)
UUN (urine urea nitrogen)
UV (ultraviolet)
- UV exposure
- UV laser
- UV radiation
- UV therapy

uvea, inflammation of
uveae, ectropion
uveal melanoma
uveal staphyloma
uveitis
- u., acute
- u., Förster's
- u., heterochromic
- u., prolonged
- u., sympathetic

uvivittatus, Culex
UVJ (ureterovesical junction)
uvula
- u., bifid
- u., birth disorder of
- u. edema
- u., elongated
- u., muscle of
- u. of bladder
- u., palatine
- u., shortened
- u. vesicae

uvulopalatopharyngoplasty (UPPP)
uvulopalatoplasty (LAUPP) ▸ laser-assisted
Uyemura's syndrome

V

V Leads, 1 through 6
V tach (ventricular tachycardia)
V (vertex) wave
v wave ▸ giant
VA (visual acuity)
vaccae, Mycobacterium
vaccinal areola
vaccinal fever
vaccination(s)
    v. ▸ anti-anthrax
    v., BCG (bacille Calmette-Guerin)
    v. booster ▸ pneumonia
    v. clinic
    v., influenza
    v., pneumococcal
    v., pneumonia
    v. program ▸ mandatory
    v. reaction
    v. scar
    v., smallpox
    v. technique
    v., varicella
vaccinatum, eczema
vaccine(s)
    v., active
    v. and toxoids ▸ inactive
    v., anti-AIDS (acquired immune
       deficiency syndrome)
    v., antiviral
    v. -associated paralytic polio
       (VAPP)
    v., BCG (bacille Calmette-Guerin)
    v., bivalent
    v. ▸ bivalent conjugate
    v., bivalent influenza
    v., cancer
    v., conjugate
    v. ▸ diphtheria, tetanus toxoids, and
       acellular pertussis
    v. ▸ diphtheria, tetanus toxoids, and
       whole cell pertussis
    v., experimental
    v., experimental cancer
    v. ▸ genetically engineered
    v., Haemophilus pertussis
    v., hepatitis
    v., hepatitis B

v., inactivated
v. ▸ inactivated influenza
v. (IPV) ▸ inactivated polio
v. ▸ inactivated poliovirus
v. -induced immunity
v., influenza
v. ▸ influenza virus
v. ▸ intranasal influenza
v., killed poliomyelitis
v., lipopolysaccharide
v., live
v., live poliomyelitis
v., live-virus
v. ▸ Lyme disease
v., melanoma
v., meningococcal
v., monovalent influenza
v. ▸ nasal spray flu
v., oral monovalent poliovirus
v. (OPV) ▸ oral polio
v., oral poliovirus
v. ▸ oral, tetravalent rotavirus
v., passive
v., pertussis
v., pneumococcal
v. ▸ pneumococcal conjugate
v., polio
v. preventable disease
v. reaction, cholera
v. reaction ▸ smallpox
v., retroviral
v., RhoGAM
v., rotavirus
v., Sabin's
v., shampoo
v., smallpox
v. ▸ split virus
v. stimulates immune system
v. strategy
v. ▸ swine flu
v. ▸ swine influenza
v., synthetic
v. therapy
v. trials
v., trivalent oral poliovirus
v., typhoid-paratyphoid
vaccinia gangrenosa

vaccinia virus
vaccinicum, virus
vaccinoid reflex
vacuo
    v. change ▸ hydrocephalus ex
    v. effect, ex
    v., hydrocephalus ex
vacuolar degeneration
vacuolar nephrosis
vacuolated
    v. basophil cells
    v. cells
    v. plasma cells
vacuolation/vacuolization
    v., cytoplasmic
    v., fatty
    v., glycogen
    v. of cerebral matrix
vacuolative virus
vacuole(s)
    v., autophagic
    v., coarse cytoplasmic
    v., contractile
    v., fatty
    v., food
    v., host cell
    v., plasmocrine
    v., rhagiocrine
    v., secretory
    v., water
vacuum
    v. aspiration
    v. bottle, sealed
    v. cap delivery
    v. collection tube, sterile
    v. culture bottle
    v. curettage
    v. drainage system
    v. extraction operative delivery
    v. formed drum
    v. headache
    v. phenomenon
    v. retraction
    v., sound
    v. tube
    v. tube, electronic
    v. tuberculin

vacuum—*continued*
   v. vaginal delivery
vacuuming needle, Charles
vacuus, pulsus
VAD (ventricular assist device)
VAD (ventricular assist device)
   permanently implanted
vag (vaginal) pad
vagal
   v. accessory nerve
   v. action
   v. afferent fibers, blocking
   v. attack
   v. block
   v. bradycardia
   v. efferent fibers, blocking
   v. escape
   v. ganglion, inferior
   v. ganglion, superior
   v. nerve
   v. nerve damage
   v. nerve damage ▸
      postfundoplication
   v. neural crest
   v. reaction
   v. reflex
   v. response
   v. stimulation
   v. tone
vagina
   v., acid balance
   v., apex of
   v. ▸ bladder descends into
   v., carcinoma of
   v., congenital absence of
   v. ▸ force on uterus and upper
   v., fossa of vestibule of
   v., lesion of
   v. ▸ lining of
   v., lyre of
   v. packed
   v., posterior cul-de-sac of
   v. prepped
   v. ▸ rectum prolapse into
   v., rhabdomyosarcoma of
   v., rugae of
   v., sarcoma botryoides of
   v. soft and pliable
   v., vestibule of
vaginae
   v., atrium
   v., carina urethralis
   v., fossa vestibule
   v., fundus
   v., introitus

v., Leptomitus
v., lyra
v., ostium
v., paries anterior
v., plicae
v., sphincter
vaginal
   v. acidity
   v. agenesis
   v. air
   v. atrophy
   v. birth
   v. birth after cesarean (VBAC)
   v. birth, normal
   v. bleeding
   v. bleeding, abnormal
   v. bleeding, active
   v. bleeding, dysfunctional
   v. bleeding, frequent
   v. bleeding from chlamydia
   v. bleeding in pregnancy
   v. bleeding, irregular
   v. bleeding, recurrent
   v. breech, complete
   v. breech delivery
   v. breech, frank
   v. cancer
   v. candidiasis
   v. carcinoma in situ
   v. celiotomy
   v., cervical, endocervical (VCE) Pap
      (Papanicolaou) smears
   v., cervical, endocervical (VCE)
      Papanicolaou (Pap) smears ▸
      Richart and
   v., cervical, endocervical (VCE)
      smear
   v. cervix
   v. cesarean (C-) section
   v. contraceptive film (VCF)
   v. cream
   v. cuff
   v. cuff abscess
   v. cuff Pap (Papanicolaou) smear
   v. cuff reefed
   v. cuff, well suspended
   v. culture
   v. cycle
   v. delivery
   v. delivery, difficult
   v. delivery (NSVD) ▸ normal
      spontaneous
   v. delivery, spontaneous
   v. delivery, traumatic
   v. delivery, vacuum

v. diaphragm
v. discharge
v. discharge, bloody
v. discharge ▸ chills with
v. discharge, heavy
v. discharge in children
v. discharge ▸ itchy, whitish
v. discharge, malodorous
v. discharge, mucopurulent
v. discharge ▸ pain in abdomen
   with
v. discharge, pinkish
v. dose
v. douche
v. dryness
v. dryness, estrogen-dependent
v. examination, sterile
v. flora
v. flora, normal
v. flow of blood
v. folds
v. fornix
v. gel
v. graft, foam rubber
v. hematocele
v. hemorrhage
v. hernia
v. hernia, posterior
v. hysterectomy
v. hysterectomy, Doyen's
v. hysterectomy, Heaney's
v. hysterectomy (LAVH) ▸
   laparoscopically assisted
v. hysterectomy, Mayo-Ward
v. hysterectomy (TVH) ▸ total
v. hysterectomy, Ward-Mayo
v. inclusion cyst
v. infection
v. inflammation
v. intercourse
v. intraepithelial neoplasia
v. irrigation smear
v. irritation
v. itch
v. itching
v. itching from diabetes
v. lubrication
v. lumen
v. metastasis
v. mucosa
v. muscles
v. myomectomy
v. narrowing
v. neoplasia, laser treatment of
v. nerves

v. orifice
v. outlet
v. outlet, relaxed
v. pack
v. packing
v. pad
v. pessary donut
v. plexus
v. portio
v. pouch
v. pressure
v. prolapse
v. repair
v. ring
v. secretion
v. septal lesion, posterior
v. smear
v. sponge
v. spotting
v. stenosis
v. stent, foam rubber
v. suppositories, Mycostatin
v. suppository
v. suspension procedure
v. swab
v. tablet
v. tissue
v. tissue thinning
v. tissues, inflammation of
v. toilet
v. tract
v. tumors
v. varicose vein
v. vault
v. vault repair, anteroposterior (AP)
v. vertex delivery
v. wall
v. wall, atrophic
v. wall lesion, posterior
v. wall, prolapsed
v. wall sling
v. yeast
v. yeast infection
v. yeast infection ▸ recurrent
vaginales, rugae
vaginalis
v., Haemophilus
v., Hemophilus
v., phimosis
v., plexus venosus
v., processus
v., Trichomonas
v., tunica
vaginectomy, skinning
vaginicola, Herellea

vaginismus, psychogenic
vaginitis
v., atrophic
v., bacterial
v., Candida
v., catarrhal
v., cervical
v. chronic
v. ▸ chronic yeast
v., diphtheritic
v., emphysematous
v., glandular
v., granular
v., mixed
v., Monilia
v., monilial
v., papulous
v. ▸ recurring yeast
v., senile
v., Trichomonas
v., yeast
vaginolabial hernia
vaginoperineal fistula
vaginorectal examination
vaginosis, bacterial
vagomimetic intervention
vagotomy
v., delayed
v., hemigastrectomy and
v., pyloroplasty and
vagotonic type
vagovagal spasm
vagrant endometrial tissue
vague
v. abdominal complaints
v. abdominal pain
v. aches and pains
v. and ambiguous symptoms
v. chest discomfort
v. confusion
v. conspiracy ▸ delusion with
v. increased density
v. obsessional thoughts
v., speech
v. symptoms
v. symptoms ▸ multiple
vagus
v. area
v. arrhythmia
v. nerve
v. nerve, auricular branch of
v. nerve, auricular nerve of
v. nerve, inferior ganglion of
v. nerve, jugular ganglion of
v. nerve, lower ganglion of

v. nerve signs
v. nerve stimulation
v. nerve stimulator (VNS)
v. nerve, superior ganglion of
v. pneumonia
v. pulse
v. reflex
v. stimulation
valency electron
valga, coxa
valga, tibia
valgum, genu
valgus [*varus*]
v., cubitus
v. deformity
v. deformity, hallux
v., hallux
v., pes
v. strain
v. stress test
v., talipes
v. -varus stress tests
valid consent
validate memory
validation
v., experimental
v., functional
v. ▸ therapeutic exercise for
validity
v., clinical
v., concurrent
v., construct
v., content
valise handle graft
vallecula
v. cerebelli
v. epiglottica
v. of tongue
v. sylvii
vallecular dysphagia
vallecular pouch
Vallet's mass
Valley (valley)
V. disease ▸ San Joaquin
V. encephalitis virus, Murray
V. fever
V. fever virus, Rift
V. virus, Cache
Valsalva('s)
V. aneurysm ▸ sinus of
V. aortography ▸ sinus of
V. experiment
V. maculopathy
V. maneuver
V. procedure

Valsalva('s)—*continued*
- V. ▸ ruptured sinus of
- V. sinus
- V. test

valsalviana, dysphagia
Valsuani's disease
value(s)
- v., alpha/beta
- v., altered spiritual
- v., Astrup blood gas
- v., biologic
- v., diagnostic
- v., fixed
- v., half-
- v. index (RVI) ▸ relative
- v. layer (HVL), half-
- v. layer, tenth
- v., mean
- v. (MCV) ▸ mean clinical
- v., normal
- v., observed
- v., ocular density (OD)
- v. of food, energy
- v. of sobriety ▸ positive
- v., optical density (OD)
- v., patient has religious
- v., peripheral circulatory
- v., QRS-T
- v. ▸ redefining family's
- v., reference
- v. thickness, half
- v., threshold limit
- v., urinary estriol

valve(s)
- v., abnormal cleavage of cardiac
- v., abnormal development of
- v. abnormality ▸ heart
- v. abnormality, mitral
- v. action, faulty
- v., age-related degeneration of
- v. airway obstruction ▸ stop-
- v. allograft, cryopreserved heart
- v. aneurysm ▸ mitral
- v. anomaly, cardiac
- v. anomaly ▸ pulmonary
- v. anterior leaflet, mitral
- v., aortic
- v., aortic semilunar
- v. area, aortic
- v. area, mitral
- v. area ▸ pulmonary
- v., artificial
- v., artificial cardiac
- v., artificial heart
- v. atresia, aortic

- v., atrial
- v., atrioventricular
- v., auriculoventricular
- v. autotransplantation
- v., ball
- v., Beall mitral
- v., bicommissural aortic
- v., bicuspid
- v., bicuspid aortic
- v., biological
- v. bioprosthesis ▸ porcine
- v., bioprosthetic
- v., bioprosthetic heart
- v., Bjork-Shiley
- v., Blom-Singer
- v., bovine heart
- v., bovine pericardial
- v., broken heart
- v., caged ball
- v., caged ball prosthetic
- v., calcified
- v., calcified aortic
- v., calcium deposits on heart
- v. ▸ carcinoid involving pulmonary
- v., cardiac
- v., caval
- v., check
- v., cleft mitral
- v., clicking of malfunctioning
- v., closed mitral
- v. closure index ▸ mitral
- v., closure of semilunar
- v. closure sound ▸ pulmonic
- v. closure sound ▸ tricuspid
- v. commissurotomy ▸ mitral
- v. commissurotomy ▸ transventricular mitral
- v., congenital anomaly of mitral
- v., convexo-concave (C-C)
- v., crisscross atrioventricular (AV)
- v., cryopreserved homograft
- v., cultural
- v. damage ▸ heart
- v., debris
- v., defect
- v. defect ▸ heart
- v., defective aortic
- v., defective artificial heart
- v., defective heart
- v. ▸ diastolic fluttering aortic
- v., disc
- v., disease, aortic
- v. disease, carcinoid
- v. disease, heart
- v. disease ▸ lupus-associated

- v. disease, mitral
- v. disease ▸ pulmonary
- v. disease ▸ severe mitral
- v. disease ▸ tricuspid
- v., diseased
- v., diseased heart
- v. ▸ diseased mitral
- v. ▸ disk cage
- v. disorder, aortic
- v. disorder, asymptomatic pulmonary
- v. disorder, cardiac
- v. disorder, congenital aortic
- v. disorder ▸ heart
- v. disorder ▸ mild pulmonary
- v. disorder ▸ mitral
- v. disorder ▸ pulmonary
- v. disorder ▸ pulmonary heart
- v. disorder ▸ tricuspid
- v. doming ▸ tricuspid
- v., drip infusion
- v. ▸ dysfunctional heart
- v. ▸ Ebstein's malformation of tricuspid
- v. echocardiography ▸ mitral
- v. echocardiography ▸ pulmonary
- v., ectatic aortic
- v. endocarditis ▸ mitral
- v. endocarditis, prosthetic
- v., eustachian
- v., expand narrowed
- v. failure, vein
- v., fenestrated
- v. ▸ fibrous thickening mitral
- v. ▸ flail mitral
- v., flair
- v., Foltz's
- v., floppy
- v., floppy mitral
- v. flow ▸ tricuspid
- v., fractured
- v. function, abnormal heart
- v. function ▸ heart
- v. function ▸ ineffective
- v. gradient, aortic
- v. gradient, mitral
- v. gradient ▸ peak transaortic
- v. gradient ▸ pulmonary
- v. gradient (PVG) ▸ pulmonic
- v. gradient ▸ transaortic
- v. gradient, tricuspid
- v. graft, Cryolife
- v. graft ▸ Hancock pericardial
- v., heart

v. ▸ Heimlich heart
v., Heister's
v., hemostasis
v., Holter
v., Huschke's
v. hypoplasia ▸ mitral
v., ileocecal
v. ▸ incompetence of the cardiac
v., incompetent
v., incompetent atrioventricular
v. infection
v. infection ▸ bacterial heart
v. infection ▸ heart
v. insufficiency, atrioventricular (AV)
v. insufficiency ▸ mitral
v., Ionescu-Shiley
v. leaflet
v. leaflet, aortic
v. leaflet, bowing of mitral
v. leaflet, cardiac
v. leaflet ▸ mitral
v. leaflet prolapse, aortic
v. leakage ▸ replacement
v., leaking
v. ▸ leaking aortic
v. ▸ leaking heart
v., leaky
v. ▸ leaky heart
v. ▸ leaky mitral
v. ▸ liver enzyme
v., lunulae of aortic
v., lunulae of pulmonary trunk
v., lunulae of semilunar
v. ▸ malformed heart or heart
v. malfunction
v. malfunction, vein-
v., mechanical
v. ▸ mechanical heart
v. ▸ metal heart
v. ▸ mild leaking of aortic
v. (MV), mitral
v. ▸ mitral balloon
v. ▸ moderate leaking of
v. ▸ moderate leaking of mitral
v., mucinous layer of
v. ▸ myxomatous degeneration of heart
v., myxomatous degeneration of mitral
v., narrowed
v., narrowed atrial ventricular
v., narrowed heart
v. ▸ narrowed pulmonary
v., narrowing of aortic

v., narrowing of heart
v. narrowing, severe heart
v., native
v. ▸ negative predictive
v., nodules of aortic
v., nodules of pulmonary trunk
v., noncalcified
v. obstruction, aortic
v. of aorta, lunulae of semilunar
v. of coronary sinus
v. of Kerckring
v. of Sylvius
v. of Vieussens
v. opening, aortic
v., opening of atrioventricular
v. orifice
v. ▸ parachute mitral
v. ▸ Passy-Muir
v. peak gradient ▸ aortic
v. ▸ plastic heart
v., porcine
v. ▸ porcine heart
v. ▸ porcine prosthetic
v. posterior leaflet, mitral
v., predictive
v. prolapse (MVP), mitral
v. prolapse syndrome ▸ mitral
v. prolapse ▸ tricuspid
v., prolapsed
v. prosthesis
v. prosthesis, Alvarez
v. prosthesis, aortic
v. prosthesis, ball
v. prosthesis, Barnard mitral
v. prosthesis, Beall disk
v. prosthesis, Beall mitral
v. prosthesis, Bjork-Shiley aortic
v. prosthesis, Bjork-Shiley mitral
v. prosthesis, Capetown aortic
v. prosthesis, cardiac
v. prosthesis, Carpentier-Edwards aortic
v. prosthesis, Cartwright
v. prosthesis, Cooley-Bloodwell mitral
v. prosthesis, Cross-Jones
v. prosthesis, Cutter-Smeloff cardiac
v. prosthesis, Dacron
v. prosthesis, DeBakey ball
v. prosthesis, disc
v. prosthesis, 4-A Magovern
v. prosthesis, Gott and Daggett
v. prosthesis, Hall-Kaster mitral
v. prosthesis ▸ Hancock mitral

v. prosthesis, Harkins
v. prosthesis ▸ heart
v. prosthesis, Hufnagel
v. prosthesis, Hufnagel low profile heart
v. prosthesis, Ionescu-Shiley aortic
v. prosthesis, Kastec mitral
v. prosthesis, Kay-Shiley
v. prosthesis, Kay-Suzuki disc
v. prosthesis ▸ Lillehei-Kaster cardiac
v. prosthesis, Magovern-Cromie
v. prosthesis ▸ Medtronic-Hall heart
v. prosthesis ▸ Medtronic-Hall tilting disk
v. prosthesis ▸ Omniscience single leaflet cardiac
v. prosthesis ▸ Omniscience tilting disk
v. prosthesis, Pemco
v. prosthesis, SCDT heart
v. prosthesis ▸ Smeloff cardiac
v. prosthesis, Smeloff-Cutter
v. prosthesis ▸ Sorin mitral
v. prosthesis ▸ St. Jude heart
v. prosthesis, St. Jude Medical aortic
v. prosthesis, Starr-Edwards aortic
v. prosthesis ▸ Starr-Edwards ball
v. prosthesis ▸ Starr-Edwards cardiac
v. prosthesis ▸ Starr-Edwards disk
v. prosthesis ▸ Starr-Edwards heart
v. prosthesis ▸ stentless porcine aortic
v. prosthesis ▸ tilting disk aortic
v. prosthesis, Wada
v. prosthesis, Wada hingeless heart
v. ▸ prosthetic aortic
v., prosthetic ball
v. ▸ prosthetic heart
v. ▸ Provox speaking
v., Pudenz's
v., pulmonary
v., pulmonic
v. ▸ quadricuspid pulmonic
v. regurgitation, aortic
v. ▸ regurgitation in mitral
v. regurgitation ▸ mitral
v. regurgitation ▸ semilunar
v. repair
v. repair ▸ mitral
v., repair or replace damaged
v. replacement

valve(s)—*continued*
v. replacement (AVR), aortic
v. replacement, Cosgrove mitral
v. replacement ▸ heart
v. replacement, mitral
v. replacement ▸ supra-annular mitral
v. replacement surgery
v. replacement surgery ▸ minimally invasive
v. resistance, aortic
v. restenosis, aortic
v. restenosis ▸ pulmonary
v., resting
v. ring
v. ring, mitral
v. rings and leaflets
v. rupture
v. ▸ scarring of aortic
v., scarring of heart
v. ▸ sclerotic aortic
v., semilunar
v. sewing ring ▸ prosthetic
v. sheath, check-
v., Sheldon-Pudenz's
v., shifting
v. ▸ Shiley convexo-concave heart
v. ▸ Shiley heart
v. ▸ Shiley Phonate speaking
v., Singer-Blom
v. ▸ Smeloff heart
v., Spivack
v. ▸ St. Jude's
v. ▸ staphylococcal infection of heart
v. ▸ Starr-Edwards
v. ▸ Starr-Edwards ball and cage
v. ▸ Starr-Edwards mitral
v., Starr-Edwards prosthetic ball
v. ▸ Starr-Edwards Silastic
v., stenosed aortic
v. stenosis (CAVS) ▸ calcific aortic
v. ▸ stenosis in pulmonary
v. stenosis ▸ mitral
v. stenosis ▸ pulmonary
v. stenosis ▸ rheumatic mitral
v., stenotic
v. ▸ stent-mounted allograft
v. ▸ stent-mounted heterograft
v. ▸ straddling atrioventricular (AV)
v. ▸ straddling tricuspid
v. structure
v., structure and function of
v. surgery ▸ heart

v. surgery, prosthetic heart
v. syndrome, billowing mitral
v. syndrome ▸ flapping
v. syndrome, floppy
v. syndrome ▸ prolapsed mitral
v. ▸ synthetic heart
v., tercile
v., thebesian
v. thickened, aortic
v. thickening
v. thrombosis, cardiac
v. thrombosis ▸ prosthetic
v. thrombus, ball
v. ▸ tilting disk prosthetic
v., tissue
v., tricuspid
v., tricuspid heart
v. tube
v. vegetation
v. vegetation, aortic
v. vegetation ▸ prosthetic
v. vegetation ▸ pulmonary
v. vegetation ▸ tricuspid
v. velocity profile, aortic
v. xenograft

valvotomy
v., aortic
v., balloon
v., balloon aortic
v., balloon mitral
v., balloon pulmonary
v., balloon tricuspid
v., bicuspid
v., double balloon
v., mitral
v. ▸ percutaneous mitral balloon
v., pulmonary
v. ▸ repeat balloon mitral
v. ▸ single balloon
v., thimble
v., transventricular
v., tricuspid

valvular
v. aortic stenosis
v. calcification
v. cardiopathy
v. defect
v. defect, congenital
v. deposits of calcium
v. disease
v. disease, mitral
v. disease of heart (VDH)
v. disease, rheumatic
v. disease ▸ severe
v. dysfunction

v. endocarditis
v. function, loss of
v. heart disease
v. incompetence
v. infection
v. insufficiency
v. insufficiency, aortic
v. insufficiency ▸ venous
v. leaflet ▸ tricuspid
v. myxoid stroma
v. orifice
v. pneumothorax
v. prolapse
v. pulmonic stenosis
v. regurgitation
v. regurgitation ▸ pulmonary
v. sclerosis
v. stenosis
v. stenosis, aortic
v. stenosis, pulmonic
v. thrombus

valvularum
v. semilunarium aortae, lunulae
v. semilunarium arteriae pulmonalis, lunulae
v. semilunarium trunci pulmonalis, lunulae

valvulitis
v., aortic
v., chronic
v., mitral
v., rheumatic
v. ▸ syphilitic aortic

valvuloplasty
v., aortic
v., bailout
v., balloon aortic
v., balloon mitral
v., balloon pulmonary
v. catheterization, balloon
v., double balloon
v. ▸ intracoronary thrombolysis balloon
v., mitral
v. ▸ multiple balloon
v. ▸ percutaneous balloon
v. ▸ percutaneous balloon aortic
v. ▸ percutaneous balloon mitral
v. ▸ percutaneous balloon pulmonic
v. ▸ percutaneous mitral
v. ▸ percutaneous mitral balloon (PMB)
v. ▸ percutaneous transluminal balloon
v., pulmonary

v. ▸ single balloon
v., tricuspid
v. ▸ triple balloon
valvulotomy
v., aortic
v., bicuspid
v., mitral
v., pulmonary
v., tricuspid
VAMC prognostic score
VAMP (vincristine, amethopterin, 6-mercaptopurine, and prednisone)
VAMP (vincristine, methotrexate, 6-mercaptopurine, and prednisone) therapy
van (Van)
v. Creveld syndrome, Ellis-
V. de Graaff generator
V. de Graaff machine
v. den Bergh test
v. Gieson stain
V. Gorder's operation
V. Hoorn's maneuver
V. Lint akinesia
V. Lint block
V. Lint conjunctival flap
V. Lint technique
V. Millingen's graft
V. Slyke test
Vanderput graft, Tanner-
vandersandi, Trombicula
Vanghetti's prosthesis
Vanguard deep therapy unit ▸ Picker
vanillylmandelic acid
vanishing lung
Vanzetti's sign
vapor
v., anesthetic
v. bath
v. density
v. lamp, cold quartz mercury
v. lamp, mercury
v. laser, Metalase copper
v. massage
v., oxygen
v. permeable
vaporization
v. and excisional conization, laser
v., carbon dioxide (CO_2) laser
v., laser
v. of lesion, laser
v. of prostate (PVP) ▸ photoselective
v. of prostate tissue ▸ transurethral

vaporize(s)
v. abnormal cells
v. cancerous tumors
v. cavity
v., cut coagulate or
v. fibroid tumor
v. plaque blockage
v., skin
v. tissue
v. water in herniated disk
vaporized
v. hemorrhoidal tissue
v. plaque
v. plaques, laser
v. tissue, laser
vaporizer
v., cold air
v., cool mist
v., steam
vaporizing
v. breast tumor
v. corneal cells
v. creases
v. diseased tissue
VAPP (vaccine associated paralytic polio)
Vaquez
V. disease
V. disease, Osler-
V. -Osler disease
var. (variant/variety)
v. aureus, Micrococcus pyogenes
v. canina, Centrocestus cuspidatus
v. capitis, Pediculus humanus
v. ceylonensia, Escherichia dispar
v. corporis, Pediculus humanus
v. madampensis, Escherichia dispar
v. vestimentorum, Pediculus humanus
vara
v., coxa
v. luxans,coxa
v., tibia
variabilis, Dermacentor
variability
v., baseline
v., beat-to-beat
v., cardiac
v., color
v., heart rate
v., interobserver
v., muscle tension
v., normal
v., nuclear

v. of fetal heart rate, baseline
v., range of normal
v., sensory
variable(s)
v. agammaglobulinemia, common
v. alopecia
v. amplitude
v. appearance
v., autonomic
v., basic
v., biological
v. component
v. coupling
v. deceleration
v., demographic
v. disorders
v. effects of cocaine
v. filter
v. findings
v. frequency, controlled
v. frontocentral beta rhythm
v. immunodeficiency
v., impedance
v., physiological
v. positive airway pressure
v., psychological
v., psychosocial
v. rate
v. threshold angina
variance
v., analysis of
v., ball
v. ▸ multivariate analysis of
variant(s) (see also var.)
v., alpha
v. angina
v. angina pectoris
v. angina, Prinzmetal's
v., chronic and dilute
v., chronic lymphocytic leukemia
v., compatible with petit mal
v., compatible with psychomotor
v. Creutzfeldt-Jakob disease (vCJD)
v. discharge, petit mal
v. discharge, psychomotor
v., gene
v., neurotropic
v., normal
v. of migraine
v. pattern, psychomotor
v., petit mal
v., physiological
v., psychomotor
v. rhythm, fast alpha

variant(s)—*continued*
  v., seizure
  v., slow alpha
  v., urticarial
variation(s)
  v., alpha beta
  v., bacterial genetic
  v., biological
  v., circadian
  v., coefficient of
  v., conative negative
  v. (CNV), contingent negative
  v., daily
  v., diurnal
  v., diurnal and matutinal
  v., epidemiological
  v., human
  v. in electrical activity
  v. in pattern of excretion ▸
    significant
  v. in rate of change
  v., intrathoracic pressure
  v., negative
  v. of patterns
  v., random
variceal
  v. hemorrhage ▸ recurrent
  v. lesion
  v. sclerosing
  v. sclerotherapy
varicella
  v. gangrenosa
  v. immunity
  v. inoculata
  v. pneumonia
  v., pustular
  v. pustulosa
  v., vaccination
  v. virus infection
  v. -zoster
  v. -zoster immune globulin (VZIG)
  v. -zoster immunoglobulin (VZIG)
  v. -zoster virus (VZV)
varicelliform eruption
varicelliform eruption, Kaposi's
varices
  v., bleeding esophageal
  v. ▸ downhill esophageal
  v. ▸ endoscopic sclerosis of
    bleeding esophageal
  v., esophageal
  v., esophagus without
  v., gastric
  v., intra-abdominal
  v., prostatic

  v., sclerosing of esophageal
varicocele, ovarian
varicocele, utero-ovarian
varicose
  v. aneurysm
  v. ophthalmia
  v. ulcers
  v. vein stripping and ligation
  v. veins
  v. veins, bulging
  v. veins ▸ secondary
  v. veins stripped and ligated
  v. veins, vaginal
varicosity(-ies)
  v. in lower extremities, tortuous
  v. in omentum
  v. of leg
  v. of lower extremities
  v. ▸ saphenous vein
  v., superficial
  v., tortuous
varied gain control ▸ time-
varied nervous symptoms
variegata, parakeratosis
variegata porphyria
variegatum, Amblyomma
variety (*see also* var.)
  v. ▸ bronchogenic carcinoma, small
    cell
  v., oat cell
  v. of abuse patterns
  v. of small cells
variola virus
varioliformis, acne
variolosa, orchitis
variolosa, purpura
variotii, Paecilomyces
various
  v. body functions
  v. brain wave components,
    production of
  v. disciplines
  v. psychiatric conditions
  v. stimuli
varipalpus, Aedes
varium, Fusobacterium
varius, Paragordius
varix (varices)
  v., aneurysmal
  v., arterial
  v., cirsoid
  v., esophageal
  v. of trachea
varolii, pons
varum, genu

varus [*valgus*]
  v. cubitus
  v. deformity
  v. deformity, metatarsus primus
  v., hallux
  v., metatarsus
  v., pes
  v. strain
  v. stress test
  v. stress tests ▸ valgus-
  v., talipes
vary [*very*]
varying
  v. amplitude
  v. degrees of electrode polarization
  v. degrees of paralysis
  v. degrees of syncope
  v. flow rates
  v. mental deficiency
  v. voltages
vas
  v. aberrans
  v. aberrans of Roth
  v. afferens glomeruli
  v. anastomoticum
  v. capillare
  v. collaterale
  v. deferens
  v. deferens, ampulla of
  v. deferens, twisting of
  v. efferens glomeruli
  v. epididymidis
  v. lymphaticum profundum
  v. lymphaticum superficiale
  v. lymphocapillare
  v. prominens ductus cochlearis
  v. sinusoideum
  v. spirale
vasa
  v. aberrantis hepatis
  v. afferentia
  v. afferentia lymphoglandulae
  v. afferentia nodi lymphatici
  v. auris internae
  v. brevia
  v. efferentia
  v. efferentia lymphoglandulae
  v. efferentia nodi lymphatici
  v. intestinitenuis
  v. lymphatica
  v. nervorum
  v. nutritia
  v. praevia
  v. propria of Jungbluth
  v. recta

v. sanguinea integumenti communis
v. sanguinea retinae
v. vasorum
v. vasorum, aortic
v. vorticosa
Vascu-Flo carotid shunt
vascular (Vascular)
v. abnormality
v. abnormality, cervicothoracic
v. abnormality ▸ intracranial
v. access in hemodialysis
v. anastomosis
v. anastomosis ▸ laser-assisted
v. angiography
v. angiography (IVA) ▸ intraoperative
v. anomalies, unruptured
v. anomaly
v. assessment
v. atrophy
v. bed
v. birth mark
v. bleeding disorder
v. bundle
v. calcification
v. calcifications ▸ aortoiliac
v. catheter
v. catheter ▸ indwelling
v. cecal fold
v. cells
V. Center, Retinal
v. changes ▸ retinal
v. channels
v. cirrhosis
v. claudication
v. clip
v. collapse, peripheral
v. compromise
v. compromise, acute
v. congestion
v. congestion, bilateral
v. constriction
v. crisis, hypertensive
v. deafness
v. dementia
v. dementia stroke
v. destruction ▸ plasmatic
v. dilatation
v. dilation system ▸ Simpson-Robert
v. disease
v. disease, arteriosclerotic
v. disease, arteriosclerotic peripheral

v. disease, atherosclerotic
v. disease, brain stem
v. disease, calcific atherosclerotic
v. disease, collagen
v. disease ▸ digestive system
v. disease (HVD), hypertensive
v. disease, hypertensive pulmonary
v. disease in diabetic heart
v. disease ▸ ischemic
v. disease ▸ mild atherosclerotic
v. disease, obliterative
v. disease, occlusive
v. disease of legs
v. disease (PVD), peripheral
v. disease ▸ premature
v. disease ▸ pulmonary
v. disease ▸ severe renal
v. disorder
v. disorder, pulmonary
v. disorder ▸ systemic
v. disorder ▸ upper extremity
v. ectasia
v. endothelial growth factor (VEGF)
v. endothelial growth factor (VEGF) therapy
v. engorgement
v. evaluation ▸ intracranial
v. examination
v. extravasation
v. failure
v. flow headaches
v. funnel
v. gene transfer
v. goiter
v. graft
v. graft, albumin-coated
v. graft ▸ Gore-Tex
v. graft ▸ Hancock
v. graft infection
v. graft ▸ Ionescu-Shiley
v. graft prosthesis
v. graft prosthesis, Milliknit
v. graft ▸ Shiley Tetraflex
v. graft ▸ Velex woven Dacron
v. graft ▸ Vitagraft
v. grafting
v. granulation tissue
v. groove
v. headache
v. headache, bicranial
v. headache, cocaine-related
v. headache, hemicranial
v. headache syndrome
v. heart disease
v. hyperplasia, pulmonary

v. hypertension
v. hypertension, renal
v. hypertension ▸ systemic
V. Imager (DVI), Digital
V. Imager (DVI) Multicenter, Digital
v. imaging
v. imaging, digital
v. impedance
v. implications, peripheral
v. in origin
v. incident
v. infection, nosocomial
v. inflammation
v. injection, conjunctival
v. injury
v. injury ▸ femoral
v. instability
v. insufficiency
v. insult
v. intermediate tissue
v. intervention, directional
v. invasion
v. invasive technique
v. involvement
v. irregularity
v. keratitis
v. laboratory assessment ▸ noninvasive
v. laboratory ▸ peripheral
v. layer of choroid of eye
v. lesion
v. lesion disease ▸ retina
v. lesion, renal
v. loop
v. lung shunt
v. malformation
v. malformation, aneurysm or
v. malformation ▸ intracranial
v. markings
v. markings, pulmonary
v. murmur
v. necrosis
v. neoplasm
v. neoplasm, benign
v. nephritis
v. nerve
v. obstruction
v. obstruction ▸ pulmonary
v. obstructive disease ▸ pulmonary
v. occluding agent ▸ fluid
v. occlusion
v. occlusion ▸ inferior mesenteric
v. occlusion ▸ mesenteric
v. occlusion ▸ recurrent mesenteric

vascular—*continued*
- v. occlusion ▸ superior mesenteric
- v. occlusion ▸ venous mesenteric
- v. occlusions ▸ treatable
- v. organ
- v. organ transplants
- v. pain
- v. pattern
- v. pattern, submucosal
- v. pedicle
- v. peripheral resistance
- v. permeability
- v. permeability ▸ pulmonary
- v. phenomena
- v. pigmented tunic
- v. plexus
- v. poor tissue
- v. pressure ▸ pulmonary
- v. proliferation
- v. prominence, central
- v. prosthesis
- v. prosthesis, DeBakey Vasculour II
- v. prosthesis, insertion of
- v. prosthesis ▸ knitted
- v. prosthesis, Medi-graft
- v. prosthesis, Wesolowski Weavenit
- v. pulsations, pulmonary
- v. reactivity ▸ pulmonary
- v. reconstruction
- v. reconstruction ▸ bifurcated vein graft for
- v. redistribution
- v. redistribution ▸ pulmonary
- v. reflex
- v. renal sclerosis
- v. reperfusion
- v. reserve, coronary
- v. reserve ▸ impaired coronary
- v. resistance
- v. resistance, coronary
- v. resistance, decreasing peripheral
- v. resistance index
- v. resistance index ▸ pulmonary
- v. resistance index ▸ systemic
- v. resistance, peripheral
- v. resistance, pulmonary
- v. resistance, renal
- v. resistance, systemic
- v. resistance (TPVR) ▸ total pulmonary
- v. response
- v. rich tissue
- v. ring

- v. ring division
- v. sclerosis
- v. screening
- v. sensation
- v. sheath
- v. shunt ▸ Pruitt
- v. skin ulcer
- v. sling
- v. smooth muscle cells
- v. smooth muscle contraction
- v. spasm
- v. stenosis
- v. stent ▸ Medtronic interventional
- v. stiffness
- v. stimulant
- v. structure
- v. structures, congested
- v. studies
- v. study ▸ mini-invasive
- v. styptic
- v. supply, renal
- v. supply, splenic
- v. swelling
- v. system
- v. system of brain
- v. system, radiation injury of
- v. test, ultrasound
- v. thrombi
- v. thrombosis
- v. tissue
- v. tone and elasticity
- v. tonic
- v. trauma
- v. tumor
- v. tumor, malignant
- v. turgor, coronary
- v. zone

vascularis, corona
vascularity, peripheral
vascularity, pulmonary
vascularization, corneal
vascularized bone graft
vasculature
- v., central pulmonary
- v., cerebral
- v., choroidal
- v., coronary
- v. engorged
- v. free of emboli ▸ pulmonary
- v., hilar
- v., prominence of pulmonary
- v., pulmonary
- v., pulmonary arterial
- v., renal
- v., retinal

vasculitis
- v., allergic
- v., cerebral
- v., eosinophilic granulomatous
- v. ▸ Henoch-Schönlein
- v., hypersensitivity
- v., leukocytoblastic
- v., leukocytoclastic
- v., livedo
- v., necrotizing
- v., nodular
- v., noninflammatory toxic
- v., pulmonary
- v., retinal
- v. ▸ segmented hyalinizing
- v. ▸ small vessel
- v. ▸ systemic necrotizing

vasculocardiac syndrome of hyperserotonemia
vasculogenic impotence
vasculonebulous keratitis
vasculopathy
- v., allograft
- v., cardiac allograft
- v., cerebral
- v., graft
- v., hypertensive

vasculosa lentis, tunica
vasculosa oculi, tunica
vasculospastic activity, reflex
Vasculour II vascular prosthesis, DeBakey
vasectomy reversal
vasectomy, sterilization
Vaseline
- V. dressing
- V. gauze
- V. wick dressing

vasoactive drug
vasoactive intestinal peptide (VIP)
vasoconstriction
- v. action
- v., arteriolar
- v., block
- v., cerebral
- v., cold-induced
- v., hypoxic pulmonary
- v. of coronary arteries
- v. or vasodilation of vessels
- v., pulmonary

vasoconstrictor
- v. center
- v. nerve
- v. peptide
- v. tone, sympathetic

vasodepressor
　v. cardioinhibitory syncope
　v. material
　v. substance
　v. syncope
vasodilatation, bilateral
vasodilating agent
vasodilating therapy
vasodilation
　v. and hypotension ▸ increased
　　peripheral
　v., coronary
　v., decreased
　v. of vessel, vasoconstriction or
　v., reflex
　v., temporary
　v., visceral
vasodilator(s)
　v. administration
　v. agent
　v. center
　v., coronary
　v. drug
　v. increase cardiac output
　v. medication
　v. nerves
　v., oral
　v., peripheral
　v. reserve
　v. reserve, coronary
　v. therapy
　v., topical coronary
vasodilatory capacity ▸ metabolic
vasoexcitor material
vasofactive cells
vasoformative cells
vasogenic edema
vasogenic shock
vasography test
vasomotion, coronary
vasomotor
　v. activity
　v. angina
　v. ataxia
　v. center
　v. changes in upper extremities
　v. epilepsy
　v. headache
　v. instability
　v. nerves
　v. nerves, derangement of
　v. paralysis
　v. rhinitis
　v. stimulant
　v. symptoms

　v. syncope
　v. syndrome, Friedmann's
　v. system, unstable
　v. wave
vasomotoria, angina pectoris
vaso-occlusive disease, carotid
vasopacemaker insertion
vasopressor deficiency
vasopressor reflexes
vasorum, aortic vasa
vasorum, vasa
vasosensory nerve
vasospasm
　v., arterial
　v., coronary
　v., coronary artery
　v. in fingers
　v., intracranial
　v., refractory ergonovine-induced
vasospastic
　v. angina
　v. disorder
　v. drug
　v. reaction ▸ prolonged
vasotonic angina
vasovagal
　v. attack
　v. episode
　v. hypotension
　v. pacemaker study (VPS)
　v. reaction
　v. reflex
　v. syncope
　v. syndrome
vastus
　v. intermedius muscle
　v. lateralis muscle
　v. lateralis, musculus
　v. medialis muscle
　v. medialis, reefing of
Vater, ampulla of
Vater, papilla of
vault
　v., cartilaginous
　v., cecal
　v., cranial
　v. of palate
　v. of skull
　v. repair, anteroposterior (AP)
　　vaginal
　v., vaginal
VBAC (vaginal birth after cesarean)
VC (vital capacity)
V/C ratio
VC (vital capacity), timed

VC (vital capacity), total
VCE (vaginal, cervical, endocervical)
　Pap (Papanicolaou) smears
VCE (vaginal, cervical, endocervical)
　Pap smears ▸ Richart and
VCF (vaginal contraceptive film)
VCG (vectorcardiogram)
vCJD (variant Creutzfeldt-Jakob
　disease)
VCUG (vesicoureterogram)
VCUG (voiding cystourethrogram)
VD (venereal disease)
VDC (Venereal Disease Clinic)
VDG (venereal disease—gonorrhea)
VDG (ventricular diastolic gallop)
VDH (valvular disease of heart)
VDP (vincristine, daunorubicin,
　prednisone)
VDRL (Venereal Disease Research
　Laboratories)
　VDRL, nonreactive
　VDRL, positive
　VDRL, reactive
　VDRL Test
VDRS (Verdun Depression Rating
　Scale)
VDS (venereal disease—syphilis)
VDT (video display terminal)
VDT (video display terminal) screen
　glare
Veau-Wardill palatoplasty
vector
　v., biological
　v. -borne disease
　v. electrocardiogram (ECG)
　v., initial
　v., instantaneous
　v. loop
　v. loop, atrial
　v., manifest
　v., maximum QRS
　v. ▸ mean manifest
　v., mechanical
　v. of disease
　v., P
　v., primary
　v., QRS
　v., spatial
　v., ST
　v. T
　v. transmission
　v. transmission, environmental
　v., viral
vectorcardiogram (VCG)
　v., spatial

vectorcardiogram—*continued*
- v. study
- v. study, spatial

vectorcardiography, spatial

vécu, déjà

VEE (Venezuelan equine encephalomyelitis) virus

vegan-vegetarian diet

vegetable(s)
- v., cruciferous
- v. exchange
- v. laxative, natural
- v. matter, intrabronchial
- v. milk
- v. oils, polyunsaturated
- v. parasite

vegetal bronchitis

vegetans, pemphigus

vegetarian
- v. diet
- v. diet ‣ demi-
- v. diet ‣ lacto-ovo
- v. diet, low fat
- v. diet ‣ pesco
- v. diet ‣ pollo-
- v. diet ‣ semi-
- v. diet ‣ vegan-

vegetating salpingitis, chronic

vegetation(s)
- v., aortic valve
- v., endocardial
- v., leaflet
- v., prosthetic
- v. ‣ prosthetic valve
- v. ‣ pulmonary valve
- v. ‣ tricuspid valve
- v., valve
- v. ‣ ventricular septal defect
- v., verrucous

vegetative
- v. and restless
- v. disturbance
- v. endocarditis
- v. lesion
- v. life
- v. nervous system
- v. neurosis
- v. process
- v. state
- v. state ‣ near-
- v. state, patient in
- v. state ‣ permanent
- v. state, persistent
- v. symptoms

VEGF (vascular endothelial growth factor)

VEGF (vascular endothelial growth factor) therapy

vehicle(s)
- v. crash ‣ injurious motor
- v., fecally contaminated
- v. injury, motor

vehicular accident

vehicular spread

veil, Sattler's

veiled puff

Veillonella
- V. alcalescens
- V. discoides
- V. orbiculus
- V. parvula
- V. reniformis
- V. vulvovaginitidis

veils, Jackson's

vein(s)
- v., accessory hemiazygos
- v., accessory saphenous
- v., accessory vertebral
- v., accompanying
- v. aldosterone, adrenal
- v., allantoic
- v., allogeneic
- v. allograft, CryoVein saphenous
- v., allografts, artery and
- v. aneurysm ‣ portal
- v., angular
- v., anomalous
- v., anomalous pulmonary
- v., anonymous
- v., antebrachial cephalic
- v., antecubital
- v., anterior auricular
- v., anterior cardiac
- v., anterior cerebral
- v., anterior horizontal jugular
- v., anterior intercostal
- v., anterior jugular
- v., anterior labial
- v., anterior scrotal
- v., anterior temporal diploic
- v., anterior tibial
- v., anterior vertebral
- v., appendicular
- v., aqueous
- v., arciform
- v., arcuate
- v., ascending lumbar
- v., Ascher's
- v. assay ‣ renin

- v., autogenous
- v., axillary
- v., azygos
- v., basal
- v., basilic
- v., basivertebral
- v., beveled
- v., Boyd perforating
- v., brachial
- v., brachiocephalic
- v., Breschet's
- v., bridging
- v., bronchial
- v., Browning's
- v., bulging varicose
- v., Burow's
- v. bypass, aortocoronary
- v. bypass, aortocoronary saphenous
- v. bypass ‣ end-to-side
- v. bypass graft
- v. bypass graft angiography ‣ saphenous
- v. (HUV) bypass graft ‣ human umbilical
- v. bypass ‣ renal artery reverse saphenous
- v. bypass, saphenous
- v. bypass ‣ side-to-side
- v. cannulation, internal jugular
- v. cannulation, subclavian
- v., cardiac
- v., cardinal
- v. catheter, umbilical
- v. catheterization, hepatic
- v., central
- v., central retinal
- v., cephalic
- v., cerebral
- v., ciliary
- v., cilioretinal
- v. clotting ‣ leg
- v., colic
- v. collapsed, jugular
- v., common anterior facial
- v., common femoral
- v., common iliac
- v., condylar emissary
- v., conjunctival
- v., coronary
- v., costoaxillary
- v. cutdown
- v., cystic
- v., deep cervical
- v., deep circumflex iliac

v., deep facial
v., deep femoral
v., deep lingual
v., deep middle cerebral
v., deep temporal
v. dialysis catheter, right subclavian
v., diploic
v. disorder
v. distended, neck
v. distended, retinal
v. distention (JVD) ▸ jugular
v. distention, neck
v., dorsal interosseous metacarpal
v., dorsal lingual
v., dorsal metacarpal
v., dorsal metatarsal
v., dorsispinal
v., duodenal
v., emissary
v., emulgent
v., endophlebitis of retinal
v. engorged, neck
v. engorgement, neck
v. engorgement of
v. engorgement, retinal
v. entry
v., episcleral
v., eradicate refluxing
v. ▸ eradication of abnormal
v. eraser
v., erasing of
v., esophageal
v., ethmoidal
v. expansion
v., external carotid
v., external iliac
v., external jugular
v., external mammary
v., external nasal
v., external palatine
v., external pudendal
v., facial
v., femoral
v., femoropopliteal
v., fibular
v. filled with contrast material
v., flat jugular
v., frontal
v., frontal diploic
v., Galen's
v., genicular
v. graft (VG)
v. graft (VG) ▸ autogenous
v. graft, bypass

v. graft for vascular reconstruction
   ▸ bifurcated
v. graft, Impra
v. graft myringoplasty (VGM)
v. graft ▸ popliteal tibial bypass
v. graft ▸ reversed saphenous
v. graft ring marker
v. graft ▸ saphenous
v. graft stenosis ▸ saphenous
v. graft, three
v., great cardiac
v., great cerebral
v., great saphenous
v., greater saphenous
v. harvesting ▸ endoscopic
v., hemiazygos
v., hepatic
v. (HPV) ▸ hepatic portal
v., highest intercostal
v. ▸ human umbilical
v., hypogastric
v., hypophyseoportal
v., ileal
v., ileocolic
v., iliac
v., iliolumbar
v., incompetent
v., incompetent perforating
v., inferior anastomotic
v., inferior cerebellar
v., inferior cerebral
v., inferior epigastric
v., inferior gluteal
v., inferior hemorrhoidal
v., inferior labial
v., inferior laryngeal
v., inferior mesenteric
v., inferior ophthalmic
v., inferior palpebral
v., inferior phrenic
v., inferior rectal
v., inferior thyroid
v., inflamed
v., inflammation of
v., innominate
v., intercapitular
v., intercostal
v., interlobar
v., internal auditory
v., internal cerebral
v., internal iliac
v., internal jugular
v., internal mammary
v., internal pudendal
v., internal thoracic

v., interventricular
v., intervertebral
v., intrarenal
v. isolated, superior pulmonary
v., jejunal
v., jugular
v., Kohlrausch's
v., Krukenberg's
v., Kuhnt's postcentral
v., Labbé's
v., lacrimal
v., lateral circumflex femoral
v., lateral sacral
v., lateral thoracic
v., left azygos
v., left brachiocephalic
v., left colic
v., left coronary
v., left gastric
v., left gastroepiploic
v., left inferior pulmonary
v. ▸ left internal jugular
v., left ovarian
v., left pulmonary
v. (LSV), left subclavian
v., left superior intercostal
v., left superior pulmonary
v., left suprarenal
v., left testicular
v., left umbilical
v., leg
v., lesser superior azygos
v., levoatriocardinal
v. ligated and retracted mesially
v. ligated and transected
v. ligation and avulsion
v. ligation, femoral
v. ligation, high saphenous
v., lingual
v., lumen of
v., main renal
v., Marshall oblique
v., masseteric
v., mastoid emissary
v., maxillary
v., medial circumflex femoral
v., median antebrachial
v., median basilic
v., median cephalic
v., median cubital
v., mediastinal
v., meningeal
v., middle cardiac
v., middle colic
v., middle hemorrhoidal

vein(s)—*continued*

v., middle meningeal
v., middle sacral
v., middle temporal
v., middle thyroid
v., muscular
v., musculophrenic
v., nasofrontal
v. ▸ nest of
v., nicking of retinal
v., obliteration of
v. obstruction, central retinal
v. obstruction ▸ saphenous
v., obturator
v., occipital
v., occipital diploic
v., occipital emissary
v. occlusion, branch retinal
v. occlusion ▸ femoral
v. occlusion ▸ retinal
v., oesophageal
v. of abdomen, subcutaneous
v. of aqueduct of vestibule
v. of bulb of penis
v. of bulb of vestibule
v. of canaliculus of cochlea
v. of clitoris, deep
v. of clitoris ▸ deep dorsal
v. of clitoris ▸ superficial dorsal
v. of cochlear canal
v. of elbow, median
v. of face, transverse
v. of foot ▸ common digital
v. of foot ▸ dorsal digital
v. of foot ▸ dorsal interosseous
v. of foot, intercapitular
v. of forearm, median
v. of Galen aneurysm
v. of hand, intercapitular
v. of hand, intercostal
v. of heart, small
v. of hepatic lobules ▸ central
v. of hypoglossal nerve ▸
    accompanying
v. of kidney
v. of kidney, arcuate
v. of kidney, interlobar
v. of kidney, stellate
v. of labyrinth
v. of left atrium ▸ oblique
v. of left ventricle ▸ posterior
v. of liver, central
v. of liver, interlobular
v. of Marshall
v. of modiolus, spiral

v. of neck, median
v. of neck, transverse
v. of penis, cavernous
v. of penis, deep
v. of penis ▸ deep dorsal
v. of penis ▸ superficial dorsal
v. of pterygoid canal
v. of Rosenthal, ascending
v. of Santorini, parietal
v. of Sappey
v. of septum pellucidum
v. of Soemmering, arterial
v. of Soemmering ▸ external radial
v. of suprarenal gland ▸ central
v. of sylvian fossa
v. of Thebesius
v. of thigh, deep
v. of tongue,deep
v. of tongue, dorsal
v. of Trolard
v. of vertebral column ▸ external
v. of Vieussens
v., omphalomesenteric
v. on abdomen ▸ large
v. I and II ▸ lumbar
v., ophthalmomeningeal
v., ovarian
v., palmar digital
v., palmar metacarpal
v., palpebral
v., pancreatic
v., pancreaticoduodenal
v., paraumbilical/parumbilical
v., paraventricular
v., parietal emissary
v., parotid
v., patency of
v., perforating
v., pericallosal artery and
v., pericardiac
v., pericardiacophrenic
v., peroneal
v., persistent cilioretinal
v., pharyngeal
v. phenomenon ▸ Gartner
v., plantar digital
v., plantar metatarsal
v., plasma, peripheral
v., popliteal
v. (PV) ▸ portal
v., postcardinal
v., posterior auricular
v., posterior conjunctival
v., posterior facial
v. (IV-XI) ▸ posterior intercostal

v., posterior labial
v., posterior parotid
v., posterior scrotal
v., posterior temporal diploic
v., posterior tibial
v., precardinal
v., prepyloric
v., previously marked
v., primary head
v. ▸ profunda femoris
v., pulmonary
v., pulsating neck
v., pyloric
v., radial
v., red spider
v., renal
v. renin activity, renal
v. renin concentration, renal
v. renin ratio ▸ renal
v. renin, renal
v., retinal
v., retromandibular
v., Retzius'
v. ▸ reverse saphenous
v., right brachiocephalic
v., right colic
v., right gastric
v., right gastroepiploic
v., right inferior pulmonary
v., right internal jugular
v., right ovarian
v., right pulmonary
v. (RSV), right subclavian
v., right superior intercostal
v., right superior pulmonary
v., right suprarenal
v., right testicular
v., Rosenthal's
v., Ruysch's
v., salvatella
v., saphenous
v., Sappey's
v. ▸ sausaging of
v. sclerotherapy
v. ▸ secondary varicose
v., severed jugular
v., short gastric
v., sigmoid
v., small cardiac
v., small saphenous
v., smallest cardiac
v., spermatic
v., spider
v., spider burst
v., spinal

v., splenic
v., stenosis of
v., Stensen's
v., sternocleidomastoid
v. stone
v. ▸ stretching or damage to deep
v., striate
v. stripped and ligated ▸ varicose
v. stripper
v. stripping
v. stripping and ligation ▸ varicose
v., stylomastoid
v., subcardinal
v., subclavian
v., subcostal
v., sublingual
v., sublobular
v., submental
v., sunken
v., superficial
v., superficial circumflex iliac
v., superficial epigastric
v., superficial middle cerebral
v., superficial temporal
v., superficial vertebral
v., superior anastomotic
v., superior cerebellar
v., superior cerebral
v., superior epigastric
v., superior gluteal
v., superior hemorrhoidal
v., superior labial
v., superior laryngeal
v., superior mesenteric
v., superior ophthalmic
v., superior palpebral
v., superior phrenic
v., superior rectal
v., superior thyroid
v., supracardinal
v., supraorbital
v., suprascapular
v., supratrochlear
v. surgery ▸ endoscopic
v. ▸ swollen underlying
v., sylvian
v., temporomandibular articular
v., terminal
v., thalamostriate
v., thebesian
v. ▸ thin walled
v., thoracoacromial
v., thoracoepigastric
v. III and IV ▸ lumbar
v. thrombophlebitis, migratory deep

v., thrombosed
v. thrombosis, deep
v. thrombosis ▸ iliac
v. thrombosis, iliofemoral deep
v. thrombosis, mesenteric
v. thrombosis (PVT) ▸ portal
v. thrombosis, renal
v. thrombosis, transient cerebral
v., thymic
v. tissue, small button of
v., tortuous
v., trabecular
v., tracheal
v. transplant, right pulmonary
v., transplanted
v., transverse cervical
v., transverse facial
v., trauma to
v. treatment ▸ leg
v. treatment ▸ spider
v., tributaries, renal
v., turgescence of neck
v., tympanic
v., ulnar
v., ulnar cutaneous
v., umbilical
v., uterine
v. vaginal varicose
v. valve failure
v. valve malfunction
v., varicose
v. varicosity ▸ saphenous
v., ventricular
v., vertebral
v., vesalian
v., vesical
v., vestibular
v., vidian
v., vitelline
v., vorticose
v. walls, weakened

Veit
V. maneuver, Mauriceau-Smellie-
V. method, Smellie-
V. operation, Porro-
vejdovskii, Paraspirillum
velamenta cerebri
velamentous placenta
Velcro rale
veldt sickness
Velex woven Dacron vascular graft
Veley head rest
Veley head rest, Light-
veli
v., frenulum

v. palatini muscle, levator
v. palatini muscle, tensor
v. palatini, nerve of tensor
vellus hair
velocardiofacial syndrome
velocity
v., aortic jet
v., conduction
v., coronary blood flow
v., ejection
v. electron beams, high-
v. encoded cine-magnetic resonance imaging
v., end diastolic
v., flow
v. image ▸ phase encoded
v. index (AVI) ▸ air
v. indices ▸ end-systolic force
v. ▸ instantaneous spectral peak
v. interrogation, deep Doppler
v. ▸ left ventricular (LV) outflow tract
v. length relation ▸ force
v., maximal
v., mean
v. measurement, pulse wave
v. (MNCV) ▸ motor nerve conduction
v. of blood flow
v. of circumferential fiber shortening
v. of light
v. of movement of electroencephalogram (EEG) paper
v. of nerve, maximum conduction
v. ▸ peak A
v. ▸ peak E
v. ▸ peak systolic
v., posterior wall
v. probe, Doppler
v. profile, aortic valve
v. ratio ▸ systolic
v., shortening
v. study ▸ nerve conduction
v. study, saccadic
v. tests ▸ nerve conduction
v. ▸ time-averaged peak
v. ▸ tracheal mucus
v. ▸ translesional spectral flow
v., upstroke
v. ▸ ventricular conduction
v. volume relation ▸ force
velopharyngeal
v. closure

velopharyngeal—*continued*
- v. insufficiency
- v. portal

velour collar graft
velour graft ▸ Microvel double
Velpeau('s)
- V. axillary view
- V. bandage
- V. cast
- V. deformity
- V. dressing
- V. hernia
- V. sling
- V. sling-dressing
- V. tendon transfer

Velter's operation ▸ Duverger and
velum
- v., anterior medullary
- v., levator muscle of palatine
- v., medullary
- v., palatine
- v. palatini ▸ levator muscle of
- v. palatini ▸ tensor muscle of
- v. palatinum

velvet syndrome, blue
vena
- v. cava
- v. cava anomaly
- v. cava clip
- v. cava filter ▸ Greenfield
- v. cava (IVC) ▸ inferior
- v. cava occlusion ▸ inferior
- v. cava pressure (IVCP) ▸ inferior
- v. cava, retraction of
- v. cava (SVC) ▸ superior
- v. cava syndrome
- v. cava (SVC) syndrome ▸ superior
- v. cava (TIVC) ▸ thoracic inferior
- v. cavagram
- v. caval compression
- v. caval obstruction
- v. caval (IVC) obstruction ▸ inferior
- v. caval shunt ▸ Marion-Clatworthy side-to-end
- v. caval tumor
- v. centralis retinae
- v. puncture

Venable-Stuck nail
venacavography, inferior
venae
- v. cavae, foramen
- v. jugularis, bulbus
- v. vorticosae

veneer(s)
- v., composite

- v. crown, full
- v. crown, partial
- v., dental
- v., etched porcelain
- v., porcelain

veneered crown
venenata
- v., cheilitis
- v., dermatitis
- v., Rhus
- v., stomatitis

venenatum, erythema
venenosum, Physostigma
venerea, lues
venerea, urethritis
venereal (Venereal)
- v. bubo
- v. condylomata
- v. disease (VD)
- V. Disease Clinic (VDC)
- V. Disease Research Laboratories (VDRL)
- V. Disease Research Laboratories (VDRL) Test
- v. disease—gonorrhea (VDG)
- v. disease—syphilis (VDS)
- v. granuloma
- v. infection
- v. lymphogranuloma
- v. wart
- v. warts, recurring

venereum
- v. antigen ▸ lymphogranuloma
- v., granuloma
- v., lymphogranuloma
- v., lymphopathia
- v. psittacosis infection, lymphogranuloma
- v. virus, lymphogranuloma

veneris, mons
Venezuelan
- V. equine encephalitis (VEE)
- V. equine encephalomyelitis (VEE)
- V. equine encephalomyelitis (VEE) virus
- V. hemorrhagic fever

venezuelensis, Borrelia
venipuncture needle
venipuncture site
venoarterial shunting
venocapillary congestion
venogram
- v., portal
- v., renal
- v., splenic

- v. studies

venography
- v., contrast
- v., limb
- v., peripheral
- v., portal
- v., renal
- v., selective
- v., splenoportal

venolobar syndrome
venom
- v., allergic to insect
- v., anthropod
- v., bee
- v., black widow spider
- v., scorpion
- v., snake
- v., spider

veno-occlusive disease of liver
veno-occlusive disease ▸ pulmonary
venorespiratory reflex
venosum
- v., angioma
- v., cor
- v. racemosum, angioma

venosus
- v. atrial septal defect ▸ sinus
- v. defect ▸ sinus
- v., ductus
- v., pulsus
- v. sclerae, sinus
- v., sinus
- v. vaginalis, plexus

venous
- v. access device-related bacteremia
- v. access, portal
- v. admixture
- v. air embolism
- v. alveolar air
- v. anastomosis ▸ portopulmonary
- v. aneurysm
- v. angiocardiography
- v. aortography
- v. arch ▸ jugular
- v. arch of foot, dorsal
- v. arches, digital
- v. arches of kidney
- v. bifurcation
- v. bleeding
- v. blood
- v. blood circulation
- v. blood ▸ mixed
- v. blood pressure, elevated
- v. blood pressure, monitoring

v. blood, red
v. blood samples
v. bloodstream
v. bulging
v. cannulation
v. capacitance bed
v. capillary
v. catechol spillover ▸ jugular
v. catheter
v. catheter (CVC), central
v. catheter, indwelling
v. catheter infection, central
v. catheter, subclavian
v., central
v. channel
v. circulation
v. circulation ▸ poor
v. claudication
v. collateral
v. collateral circulation, hepatofugal
v. congestion
v. congestion, passive
v. congestion, pulmonary
v. connection anomaly ▸ pulmonary
v. connection, partial anomalous
   pulmonary
v. connection ▸ pulmonary
v. connection ▸ total anomalous
   pulmonary
v. cord, palpable
v. cutdown
v. digital angiogram
v. disease
v. distention
v. distention, cervical
v. distention (JVD) ▸ jugular
v. Doppler study
v. drainage (dr'ge)
v. drainage ▸ partial anomalous
   pulmonary
v. drainage (dr'ge) ▸ pulmonary
v. drainage (dr'ge) ▸ total
   anomalous pulmonary
v. embolism
v. endothelium
v. engorgement
v. enlargement
v. flow measurement
v. flow (PVF) ▸ portal
v. gas (HPVG) ▸ hepatic portal
v. graft
v. grooves
v. heart
v. hematocrit

v. hematocrit ratio ▸ body
   hematocrit/
v. hematocrit (HCT), repeat
v. hemorrhage
v. hum
v. hum, cervical
v. hyperemia
v. hypertension
v. hypertension ▸ systemic
v. incompetence
v. insufficiency
v. insufficiency, chronic
v. insufficiency, deep
v. intravasation
v. lake
v. lines, central
v. magnetic resonance (MR)
   angiography ▸ selective
v. major vessel
v. markings, superficial
v. membranes
v. mesenteric vascular occlusion
v., mixed
v. murmur
v. needle
v. obstruction
v. obstruction, extrahepatic
v. obstruction, suprahepatic
v. occlusion plethysmography
v. oxygen (O$_2$), mixed
v. oxygen (O$_2$) saturation ▸ mixed
v. phase
v. plethysmography
v. plethysmography, dynamic
v. plexus
v. pressure
v. pressure (CVP) ▸ central
v. pressure, coronary
v. pressure, downstream
v. pressure gradient support
   stockings
v. pressure ▸ increased
v. pressure ▸ increased central
v. pressure ▸ jugular
v. pressure (MVP) ▸ mean
v. pressure monitoring, central
v. pressure (PVP) ▸ portal
v. pulse
v. pulse, atrial
v. pulse, centripetal
v. pulse, CV wave of jugular
v. pulse ▸ f wave of jugular
v. pulse (JVP) ▸ jugular
v. pulse tracing
v. pulse tracing ▸ jugular

v. pulse, ventricular
v. pulse ▸ y depression of jugular
v. pulse ▸ y descent of jugular
v. pump
v. pump ▸ muscular
v. puncture
v. renin assay, renal
v. return
v. return, anomalous pulmonary
v. return anomaly ▸ pediatric
v. return anomaly ▸ pulmonary
v. return curve
v. return (PAPVR), partial
   anomalous pulmonary
v. return ▸ pulmonary
v. return, resistance to
v. return ▸ systemic
v. return to heart
v. return to heart, decreased
v. return ▸ total anomalous
   pulmonary
v. runoff
v. saturation
v. sclerosis
v. sheath
v. shunt
v. shunt, Denver peritoneal
v. shunt, initial
v. shunt, peritoneal
v. shunt, portal to systemic
v. sinus of sclera
v. sinus thrombosis
v. smooth muscle
v. spasm
v. spread
v. stasis
v. stasis changes
v. stasis retinopathy
v. stasis ulcer
v. structure
v. system
v. thrombectomy
v. thromboembolism
v. thrombosis
v. thrombosis, central splanchnic
v. thrombosis (DVT) ▸ deep
v. thrombosis ▸ femoral
v. thrombosis ▸ mesenteric
v. transplantation
v. transplantation, cryopreserved
v. troughing
v. ulcer
v. valvular insufficiency
v. volume changes
v. wave

venous—*continued*
  v. web
venovenous hemofiltration,
  continuous
vent (Vent)
  v. -dependent quadriplegic
  v. -dependent quadriplegic, cervical
  V. implant, Core-
Ventak defibrillator
ventilate feelings
ventilate middle ear
ventilation
  v. agent
  v. (APRV) ▸ airway pressure
    release
  v., alveolar
  v. alveolar minute
  v., artificial
  v., assisted
  v., cessation of pulmonary
  v., compression and
  v., continuous flow
  v., continuous mandatory
  v., control mode
  v., control of
  v., controlled
  v., dead space
  v. defect on lung scan
  v. device
  v., distribution of
  v. equivalent
  v., failure of
  v., forced
  v. ▸ forced mandatory intermittent
  v. ▸ high frequency
  v. ▸ high frequency jet
  v. ▸ high frequency positive
    pressure
  v. imaging ▸ xenon lung
  v., impaired
  v. impairment, pulmonary
  v., inadequate
  v., initiate pulmonary
  v. ▸ intermittent mandatory
  v. (INPAV) ▸ intermittent negative-
    pressure assisted
  v. (IPPV) ▸ intermittent positive-
    pressure
  v. ▸ inverse ratio
  v., long-term mechanical
  v., mask
  v., maximal
  v. (MVV) ▸ maximal voluntary
  v. (MVV) ▸ maximum voluntary
  v., mechanical

v., minute
v. ▸ mouth-to-mouth
v. of feelings ▸ encourage
v. (PLV) ▸ partial liquid
v. per minute, alveolar
v. perfusion
v. perfusion defect
v. /perfusion imaging
v. -perfusion lung scan
v. /perfusion lung scanning
v. /perfusion mismatch
v. /perfusion ratio
v. /perfusion relation
v. /perfusion scan
v. (PPV) ▸ positive pressure
v. ▸ pressure-controlled inverse
  ratio
v. ▸ pressure support
v. ▸ pressure-regulated volume
  control
v., pulmonary
v. rate (MVR) ▸ maximal
v. ratio (VR)
v. scan
v. scintigraphy
v. ▸ split lung
v. studies, pulmonary
v. study
v. ▸ synchronized intermittent
  mandatory
v. test ▸ walking
v. threshold
v. ▸ time-cycled
v. ▸ ultrahigh frequency
v. ▸ volume cycled decelerating
  flow
ventilator
  v. -associated pneumonia
  v., Bourns infant
  v. breathing ▸ sign mechanism for
  v., cuirass
  v. dependency
  v. dependent
  v. dependent quadriplegia
  v. ▸ high frequency jet
  v. ▸ high frequency oscillation
  v. -induced pneumopericardium
  v. -induced pneumothorax
  v. management
  v., mechanical
  v., patient on
  v. pop-off
  v., pressure
  v. ▸ pressure cycled
  v. tank

v. time
v., volume
v. weaning
ventilatory
  v. assistance
  v. assistance ▸ continuous
    mechanical
  v. assistance, total
  v. capacity
  v. capacity (MSVC) ▸ maximal
    sustainable
  v. care
  v. defect
  v. defect, obstructive
  v. defect, restrictive
  v. equivalent
  v. failure
  v. movement
  v. support
  v. support ▸ hypotensive and
  v. support in respiratory distress
  v. threshold
ventral
  v. aorta
  v. aspect
  v. column
  v. cornu
  v. epidural abscess
  v. gray column
  v. gray columns of spinal cord
  v. hernia
  v. horn cell
  v. horns of spinal cord
  v. mesentery
  v. nerve root
  v. nerve root rhizotomy
  v. pancreas
  v. portion of pons
  v. root
  v. sacrococcygeal muscle
  v. septal defect
  v. surface
  v. surface of wrist
ventricle(s)
  v., air expressed from
  v. anomaly, double inlet
  v., anterior papillary muscle of left
  v. ▸ apical thickening of left
  v., auxiliary
  v., cerebral
  v., cholesteatoma of lateral
  v., choroid plexus of
  v., contraction of
  v., contraction right
  v., damaged left

v. dilated
v. dilated and hypertrophied
v., double-inlet
v., double-inlet left
v., double-outlet left
v., double-outlet right
v., Duncan's
v., electrical stimulation of
v. ▸ enlarged left
v., excision ischemic portion of
v., floor of third
v., fluid-filled
v., fourth
v., Galen's
v., glial membrane of fourth
v. heart ▸ one-
v., horns of lateral
v., hyperdynamic
v., hypokinesia of left
v. ▸ hypoplasia of right
v., inferior horn of lateral
v., ischemic contracture of left
v., ischemic left
v., Krause's
v., lateral
v. (LV), left
v. malposition ▸ double-outlet left
v. malposition ▸ double-outlet right
v. malposition, single-
v., Morgagni's
v. of Arantius
v. of brain, fourth
v. of brain, third
v. of cerebrum, first
v. of cerebrum, fourth
v. of cerebrum, lateral
v. of cerebrum, second
v. of cerebrum, third
v. of cord
v. of heart, aortic
v. (LV) of heart, left
v. (RV) of heart, right
v. of larynx
v. of myelon
v. of spinal cord, terminal
v. of Sylvius
v. ▸ papillary muscle of the left
v., posterior papillary muscle of left
v., posterior vein of left
v., puncture of
v., recharging of
v. (RV), right
v., septal papillary muscle of right
v. septal wall, posterior
v. ▸ severe impairment of

v., single
v., sixth
v., suicide
v. syndrome, slit
v., temporal horn of lateral
v., terminal
v., Verga's
v., Vieussen's
Ventricor pacemaker
Ventricor pacemaker, Cordis
ventricosus
v., Haemodipsus
v., Pediculoides
v., Pyemotes
ventricular
v. activation time
v. actuation ▸ direct mechanical
v. afterload
v. aneurysm
v. aneurysm, congenital left
v. aneurysm ▸ left
v. aneurysm ▸ true
v. angiography
v. angiography, left
v. apex electrogram ▸ right
v. apex ▸ left
v. apex ▸ right
v. aqueduct
v. arrhythmia
v. arrhythmia ablation
v. arrhythmia ▸ life-threatening
v. arrhythmia ▸ malignant
v. arrhythmias, asymptomatic
v. arrhythmias ▸ peri-infarctional
v. assist device (AVAD), acute
v. assist device (LVAD) ▸ left
v. assist device (VAD),
    permanently implanted
v. assist device ▸ right
v. assist system ▸ implantable left
v. asynchronous pacemaker
v. asystole
v. bands
v. beat ▸ premature
v. beats, ectopic
v. bigeminy
v. biopsy
v. block
v. blood expelled ▸ total
v. bradycardia
v. bypass pump ▸ left
v. canal
v. capture
v. capture threshold
v. catheter, Raimondi

v. chamber
v. chamber compliance ▸ left
v. chambers dilated
v. complex
v. complex ▸ multiform premature
v. complex ▸ pleomorphic
    premature
v. complex ▸ polymorphic
    premature
v. complex ▸ premature
v. complex ▸ R-on-T premature
v. complex trigger hypothesis ▸
    premature
v. compliance ▸ diminished left
v. conduction
v. conduction, aberrant
v. conduction defect ▸ right
v. conduction system
v. conduction velocity
v. conductive rate
v. contour
v. contractility
v. contractility ▸ left
v. contraction
v. contraction, automatic
v. contraction ▸ escape
v. contraction, escaped
v. contraction, focal ectopic
v. contraction ▸ normal
v. contraction, right
v. contractions, focal ectopic
v. contractions (PVC), ▸ premature
v. contractions (PVC) with coupling
    ▸ premature
v. couplet with fusion
v. couplets
v. decompensation, left
v. decompensation, right
v. defect
v. defibrillation
v. demand-inhibited pacemaker
v. demand-triggered pacemaker
v. depolarization abnormality
v. depression
v. diameter ▸ left
v. diastole
v. diastolic collapse ▸ right
v. diastolic gallop (VDG)
v. diastolic phase index ▸ left
v. diastolic pressure
v. diastolic pressure (LVDP) ▸ left
v. diastolic pressure ▸ right
v. diastolic relaxation ▸ left
v. dilatation
v. dilatation, bilateral

ventricular—*continued*

v. dimension ▸ right
v. disease, left
v. disease, right
v. distensibility
v. drive
v. dysfunction
v. (LV) dysfunction, advanced left
v. dysfunction, asymptomatic left
v. (LV) dysfunction, left
v. dysfunction ▸ overt left
v. dyskinesis ▸ left
v. dysplasia ▸ arrhythmogenic right
v. dysplasia ▸ right
v. dysrhythmias
v. dysynchrony
v. ectopia
v. ectopia, recurrent
v. ectopic activity
v. ectopic beats
v. ectopic systole
v. ectopy
v. effective refractory period
v. ejection
v. ejection fraction ▸ global left
v. ejection fraction, left
v. ejection fraction, right
v. ejection time (LVET) ▸ left
v. ejection time (RVET) ▸ right
v. elastance ▸ maximum
v. end-diastolic dimension ▸ left
v. end-diastolic pressure (LVEDP)
    ▸ left
v. end-diastolic pressure (RVEDP)
    ▸ right
v. end-diastolic volume
v. end-diastolic volume (LVEDV) ▸
    left
v. end-diastolic volume (RVEDV) ▸
    right
v. endoaneurysmorrhaphy
v. end-systolic dimension ▸ left
v. end-systolic pressure volume
    relation
v. end-systolic stress ▸ left
v. end-systolic volume
v. enlargement
v. enlargement (LVE) ▸ left
v. enlargement (RVE) ▸ right
v. escape
v. evoked response ▸ paced
v. extra stimulus ▸ double
v. extrasystole
v. failure ▸ acute left
v. failure, left

v. failure, right
v. fibrillation (VF)
v. fibrillation ▸ chaotic activity of
v. fibrillation ▸ idiopathic
v. fibrillation, primary
v. fibrillation, risk of
v. filling
v. filling pressure ▸ left
v. filling pressures
v. filling, rapid
v. filling, reduced
v. fistula, coronary artery right
v. fluid
v. fluid pressure (VFP)
v. flutter
v. fold
v. forces ▸ left
v. fullness, borderline left
v. fullness, borderline right
v. function
v. function and cineangiography
v. function, assessing
v. function curve
v. function, impaired
v. function ▸ impaired left
v. function ▸ left
v. function, right
v. function study ▸ nuclear
v. gallop
v. ganglion
v. geometry
v. gradient
v. heart failure, acute left
v. heart failure, acute right
v. heart failure, left
v. heart failure, right
v. heave
v. heave ▸ right
v. hemodynamic abnormalities ▸
    left
v. horn
v. hypertrophy
v. hypertrophy, combined
v. hypertrophy, concentric left
v. hypertrophy (LVH), left
v. hypertrophy ▸ marked left
v. hypertrophy (RVH), right
v. hypoplasia ▸ right
v. infarction, right
v. inflow obstruction ▸ right
v. inflow tract obstruction ▸ left
v. inhibited pacemaker ▸ atrial
    synchronous
v. inhibited pacemaker ▸ atrial
    triggered

v. inhibited pulse generator
v. injection, left
v. injection, right
v. internal diastolic diameter ▸ left
v. internal diastolic dimension ▸ left
v. inversion
v. lead
v. lead ▸ insulation failure
v. lead pace
v. -left atrial crossover dynamics ▸
    left
v. lift
v. loop
v. mapping
v. mass ▸ left
v. mean (LVM) ▸ left
v. mean (RVM) ▸ right
v. milk spots
v. muscle compliance ▸ left
v. muscle disease ▸ left
v. muscle ▸ excessive stretching of
v. muscle mass
v. musculature
v. myocardial fibrosis ▸ interstitial
    left
v. myocardium
v. myocardium ▸ left
v. myocardium ▸ patchy fibrosis of
v. myxoma
v. myxoma ▸ right
v. needle, Hoen's
v. node reentry tachycardia ▸ atrial
v. outflow obstruction ▸ right
v. outflow tract
v. outflow tract ▸ left
v. outflow tract obstruction ▸ left
v. outflow tract ▸ right
v. outflow tract tachycardia ▸ right
v. outflow tract velocity ▸ left
v. output ▸ left
v. paced rhythm
v. pacemaker ▸ Medtronic
    Activitrax rate responsive
    unipolar
v. pacemaker ▸ P wave triggered
v. pacing
v. pacing ▸ incremental
v. pacing system, malfunction of
    permanent demand
v. pacing systems, permanent
    demand
v. pacing ▸ trains of
v. papillary muscle
v. parasystole
v. patch aneurysm

v. pathways, fascicular
v. perforation
v. performance
v. plateau
v. ponderance
v. posterior wall excursion ▸ left
v. posterior wall thickness ▸ left
v. power
v. power ▸ left
v. preexcitation
v. preload
v. premature beat (VPB)
v. premature complex
v. premature contraction
v. premature depolarization
    contractions (VPDC)
v. preponderance
v. pressure ▸ end-diastolic left
v. pressure (LVP) ▸ left
v. pressure ▸ mean diastolic left
v. pressure (MRVP) ▸ mean right
v. pressure ▸ mean systolic left
v. pressure ▸ systolic left
v. pressure volume curve ▸ left
v. pressure volume loop
v. programmed stimulation
v. prominence
v. pulse amplitude
v. pulse width
v. puncture
v. puncture ▸ apical left
v. puncture ▸ left
v. rate
v. reciprocating tachycardia ▸ atrial
v. reduction ▸ left
v. reduction surgery ▸ left
v. reentry
v. rejection fraction ▸ global left
v. rejection, left
v. relaxation
v. remodeling
v. response
v. response, controlled
v. response, patient's
v. response, rapid
v. rhythm
v. rhythm, accelerated
v. -right atrial communication
    murmur ▸ left
v. rupture
v. salient
v. segment
v. sensing conduction
v. sensitivity
v. septal defect (VSD)

v. septal defect ▸ perimembranous
v. septal defect shunt
v. septal defect ▸ subcristal
v. septal defect vegetation
v. septal rupture
v. septum
v. shunt, atrial
v. standstill
v. strain, left
v. strain pattern
v. stroke volume (LVSV) ▸ left
v. stroke work (VSW)
v. stroke work (LVSW) ▸ left
v. study, left
v. study, right
v. suppressed pacemaker
v. synchronous pulse generator
v. system, dilatation of
v. system, dilated
v. system, distention of
v. system of brain
v. systole
v. systole (PVS) ▸ premature
v. systolic performance ▸ left
v. systolic pressure (LVSP) ▸ left
v. systolic pressure ▸ right
v. systolic tension
v. systolic time interval ▸ right
v. tachyarrhythmia
v. tachyarrhythmias
v. tachyarrhythmias ▸ life-
    threatening
v. tachycardia (V tach)
v. tachycardia, bidirectional
v. tachycardia ▸ bursts of
v. tachycardia cycle length
v. tachycardia ▸ exercise-induced
v. tachycardia ▸ idiopathic
v. tachycardia ▸ inducible
    polymorphic
v. tachycardia ▸ malignant
v. tachycardia ▸ monomorphic
v. tachycardia ▸ nonsustained
v. tachycardia ▸ parasystolic
v. tachycardia (PVT) ▸
    paroxysmal
v. tachycardia ▸ polymorphic
v. tachycardia ▸ polymorphous
v. tachycardia ▸ primary
v. tachycardia ▸ rapid non-
    sustained
v. tachycardia, recurring
v. tachycardia ▸ repetitive
    monomorphic

v. tachycardia ▸ repetitive
    paroxsymal
v. tachycardia ▸ salvo of
v. tachycardia ▸ spontaneous
    reentrant sustained
v. tachycardia ▸ sustained
v. tachycardia ▸ sustained
    monomorphic
v. tachycardia with torsades de
    pointes
v. tap
v. tension ▸ left
v. thrombus
v. trigeminy
v. -triggered pacemaker
v. tunnel murmur, aortic left
v. tunnel murmur, left
v. undersensing
v. valve, narrowed atrial
v. veins
v. venous pulse
v. volume
v. wall
v. wall, left
v. wall motion
v. wall motion abnormality ▸ left
v. wall motion, left
v. wall motion, right
v. wall, right
v. wall shortening
v. wall stress
v. wall stress ▸ left
v. wall, thickness of
v. wall thinning
v. waves
v. weakness ▸ left
v. work index (LVWI) ▸ left
v. work (LVW) ▸ left
ventricularis, sacculus
ventriculectomy ▸ partial left
ventriculoarterial
    v. concordance
    v. coupling
    v. discordance
ventriculoatrial
    v. conduction
    v. conduction ▸ retrograde
    v. interval
    v. shunt
    v. shunt, Pudenz's
ventriculocaval shunt
ventriculocisternal shunt
ventriculocisternostomy by tube
ventriculofugal artery

ventriculofugal artery
▸ telencephalic
ventriculogram
v., abnormal contraction on
v., dynamic left
v. (RNV) ▸ radionuclide
v. study
ventriculography
v., biplane
v., cardiac
v., cerebral
v., contrast
v., digital subtraction
v. ▸ equilibrium multigated radionuclide
v., exercise
v. ▸ exercise digital subtraction
v., left
v. ▸ pacing digital
v. ▸ quantitative left
v., radionuclide
v. ▸ rest exercise equilibrium radionuclide
v. ▸ tomographic radionuclide
ventriculojugular shunt
ventriculoperitoneal
v. shunt
v. shunt, emergency
v. shunt, Silastic
ventriculoradial dysplasia
ventriculotomy ▸ encircling endocardial
ventriculotomy ▸ partial encircling endocardial
ventriculus
v. cordis
v. dexter cordis
v. sinister cordis
Ventritex Cadence implantable cardioverter defibrillator
ventrolateral mass
ventrolateral sclerosis
ventroposterolateral nucleus of thalamus
ventroposterolateral (VPL) thalamic electrode
ventrosuspension procedure
Venturi wave
Venturi's meter spirometer
venula
v. macularis inferior
v. macularis superior
v. medialis retinae
v. nasalis retinae inferior
v. nasalis retinae superior

v. temporalis retinae inferior
v. temporalis retinae superior
venule(s)
v., dilated
v. engorgement
v. of retina, inferior nasal
v. of retina, inferior temporal
v. of retina, medial
v. of retina, superior nasal
v. of retina, superior temporal
v., pulmonary
venustum, Simulium
VEP (visual evoked potential)
VER (visual evoked response)
vera
v., decidua
v., polycoria
v., polycythemia
v., polycythemia rubra
veracious [voracious]
Veraguth's fold
veratrin contracture
verbal (Verbal)
v. ability
v. abuse
v. agraphia
v. amnesia
v. aphasia
v. command, abstract
v. communication ▸ impaired
v. concept formation ability
v. conceptual memory organization
v. cueing
v. cueing, constant
v. cueing for ADL (activities of daily living)
v. cueing, patient uses quad cane with
v. dexterity
v. discussion
v. encouragement
v. expression
v. expression of language
v. fantasy
v. fluency
v. IQ (intelligence quotient)
v. language deficits, auditory
v. learning
V. Learning Test, Rey Auditory
v. memory
v. memory and attention
v. memory, auditory
v. memory ▸ short-term
v. memory test
v. order (VO)

v. order (KVO) ▸ constant
v. outbursts ▸ displays
v. paraphasia
v. reasoning
v. reassurance
v. relaxation
v. response
v. scale (VS)
v. sentence construction
v. skills
v. skipping
v. stand-off
v. stimuli
v. tic
v. tics ▸ involuntary
v. warning
verbalis, asemia
verbalizable material
verbalization, inappropriate
verbalization of feelings
verbalizes slowly, patient
verbalizing, patient
verbally
v. facile ▸ voluble and
v. ▸ patient responded
v., respond
Verdun Depression Rating Scale (VDRS)
Verdun Target Symptom Rating Scale (VTSRS)
vergae, cavum
Verga's lacrimal groove
Verga's ventricle
verge, anal
verge, rectal
vergens, strabismus deorsum
vergens, strabismus sursum
Verhoeff's operation
Verhoeff's suture
veridical dream
verification film
verified
v. by x-ray, reduction
v., diagnosis
v., fields
v. with beam films, fields
vermian agenesis
vermicular
v. appendage
v. colic
v. movements
v. pulse
vermicularis
v., Ascaris
v., Enterobius

v., Oxyuris
vermiform appendix
vermiform appendix, removal of
vermilion
   v. border
   v. laceration
   v. lip line ▸ red
   v. margin
   v. surface of lip
verminous
   v. aneurysm
   v. apoplexy
   v. bronchitis
   v. cachexia
   v. colic
vermis
   v., cerebellar
   v. cerebelli
   v. incision
   v., nodule of
verna, Amanita
vernal
   v. catarrh
   v. conjunctivitis
   v. edema
   v. edema of lung
Verneuil disease, Kümmell-
Verneuil's neuroma
vernix caseosa
Vernon-David operation
veronii, Aeromonas
Verres' needle
verruca
   v. acuminata
   v. plana juvenilis
   v. plantaris
   v. vulgaris
verrucarum, Phlebotomus
verruciformis, epidermodysplasia
verrucoid surfaced lesion,
   hyperkeratotic
verrucosa
   v., Amoeba
   v., arteritis
   v., dermatitis
   v., Phialophora
verrucose hyperplasia
verrucosum, Trichophyton
verrucosus, nevus
verrucous
   v. carcinoma
   v. carditis
   v. dermatitis
   v. endocarditis
   v. endocarditis, atypical

   v. endocarditis, nonbacterial
   v. lesion
   v. penile shaft
   v. vegetations
verruga peruana
Versatex cardiac pacemaker
Versenia pestis
versicolor
   v., Aspergillus
   v., pityriasis
   v., tinea
version
   v., bipolar
   v., Braxton Hicks
   v., cephalic
   v., deorsum◊
   v., dextro◊
   v., external
   v., Hicks
   v., internal
   v., levo◊
   v., pelvic
   v., podalic
   v., Potter's
   v., sursum◊
   v., Wigand's
   v., Wright's
Verstraeten's bruit
versus (vs.)
   v. -host disease (GVHD) ▸ graft-
   v. -host (GVH) ▸ graft-
   v. -host reaction (GVHR) ▸ graft-
   v. nurture controversy ▸ nature
   v. quantity of life ▸ quality
   v. sebaceous cyst ▸ dermoid
   v. total admissions ▸ total
     infections
vertebra(-ae)
   v., alignment of
   v., atlas
   v. bones, cervical
   v. bones, coccygeal
   v. bones, dorsal
   v. bones, lumbar
   v. bones, sacral
   v. bones, thoracic
   v., bony
   v. (C1-C7), cervical
   v., coccygeal
   v., collapse of
   v., compressed
   v. ▸ compression fracture in
   v. (atlas), C-1
   v. (axis), C-2
   v., damaged cervical

   v., decalcified lumbar
   v., displaced
   v., dorsal
   v., fused
   v., fusion of
   v., lateral mass of
   v. (L1-L5), lumbar
   v., misaligned
   v. of spine ▸ collapsed
   v. of spine ▸ fracture
   v. pediculus areus
   v. plana
   v. prominens reflex
   v., radix arcus
   v., sacral
   v. (T1-T2 or D1-D12), thoracic
   v., wedging of
vertebral
   v. angiography
   v. arch
   v. arch, pedicle of
   v. arches, paired
   v. arteries of intracerebral
     vessels
   v. arteriogram
   v. arteriography
   v. artery
   v. artery aneurysm ▸ thrombosed
     giant
   v. artery bypass graft
   v. arthritis
   v. basilar insufficiency
   v. bodies ▸ decalcified sections
     of
   v. bodies, thoracic
   v. body
   v. body disc surface
   v. body height
   v. bones ▸ progressive crushing
     of
   v. border abnormality
   v. canal
   v. -carotid anastomosis
   v. column
   v. column, external veins of
   v. column ▸ osteoporotic thinning
     of
   v. column ▸ thoracic
   v. compression fracture
   v. density, relative
   v. discs
   v. endplate abnormality
   v. endplates
   v. epiphysitis
   v. foramen

vertebral—*continued*
v. fracture
v. fractures, bony
v. fractures ▸ frequency of
v. ganglion
v. hemangioma
v. injury
v. interspace
v. manipulation
v. metastases
v. nerve
v. nerve, sinu◊
v. notch
v. notch, inferior
v. notch, superior
v. osteomyelitis
v. percussion tenderness
v. plexus
v. prominence
v. region
v. ribs
v. spine
v. subluxation
v. surface of body
v. vein
v. vein, accessory
v. vein, anterior
v. vein, superficial
vertebralis, theca
vertebrate blood systems ▸ cardiac-related
vertebrobasilar
v. arterial insufficiency
v. artery
v. insufficiency
v. ischemia
v. migraine
v. occlusive disease
v. system
vertebrocostal ribs
vertebromammary diameter
vertebroplasty
v., percutaneous
v. procedure
v. treatment
vertebrosternal ribs
vertex [*vortex*]
v. alopecia
v., amplitude maximal in proximity of
v. cranii
v. cranii ossei
v. delivery
v. delivery, spontaneous
v. delivery, vaginal

v. floating
v. headaches
v. height, sitting
v. of urinary bladder
v. placement
v. presentation
v. roentgenogram, submental
v. runs
v., scalp
v. sharp transients
v. sharp waves
vertical [*vertigo*]
v. alignment of body
v. axis
v. banded gastroplasty
v. banded gastroplasty, Mason
v. compression
v. diameter
v. divergence (DVD), dissociated
v. elastic
v. eye movements
v. forces
v. gaze palsy
v. groove
v. heart
v. hemianopia
v. incision
v. long axis view
v. mattress suture
v. meridian
v. meridian of cornea
v. muscle of tongue
v. nystagmus
v. opening
v. oscillations of eyeballs, rhythmic
v. overlap
v. parallax
v. pattern on breast self-exam
v. plane
v. pleural pressure gradients
v. ray
v. ridging of nails
v. sternotomy
v. strabismus
v. talus foot deformity, congenital
v. tube
v. uterine incision
verticality, visual
vertically ridged fingernails
Verticillium graphii
verticosubmental projection
vertiginous
v. attack
v. episodes, acute disabling

v. patient
vertigo [*vertical*]
v. ▸ abrupt attack of
v., acute
v. and imbalance
v. and syncope
v. and tinnitus ▸ deafness,
v. and unsteadiness ▸ patient has
v. attack ▸ sudden
v. (BPPV) ▸ benign paroxysmal positional
v. (BPV), benign positional
v., central
v., cervical
v., chronic
v., chronic post-traumatic
v. ▸ disabling positioning
v., encephalic
v., epileptic
v., episodes of
v., episodic
v., episodic positioning
v., essential
v. ▸ frequent attacks of disabling
v., hysterical
v., idiopathic
v. ▸ initial attack of
v. ▸ intermittent attacks of severe
v., laryngeal
v. ▸ migraine-associated
v., mild
v., momentary
v., nausea and anxiety
v., neurasthenic
v., paralyzing
v., paroxysmal
v. ▸ paroxysmal positional
v., patient has
v. ▸ periodic positional
v., persistent
v., positioning
v. ▸ post-traumatic
v., postural
v., prolonged
v. ▸ recalcitrant benign paroxysmal positional
v., recurrent
v., rotary
v., rotatory
v., severe incapacitating
v., stomachal
v., symptomatic
v., syncope and hypotension
v. syndrome

v., transient
v., traumatic
v., vestibular
Verwey's operation
very [*vary*]
    v. late antigen
    v. vocal ▸ patient
vesalian bone
vesalian vein
Vesely-Street nail
vesicae
    v., ectopia
    v., endometriosis
    v., sphincter
    v. urinariae, apex
    v., uvula
vesical [*vesicle*]
    v. artery
    v. calculi
    v. calculus
    v. center
    v. fold, transverse
    v. hematuria
    v. hernia
    v. mucosa
    v. neck
    v. neck contracture
    v. plexus
    v. prostatism
    v. reflex
    v. schistosomiasis
    v. tenesmus
    v. trabeculation
    v. vein
vesicalis transversa, plica
vesicatoria, Cantharis
vesicle(s) [*vesical*]
    v., Baer's
    v., chorionic
    v. fluid
    v., graafian
    v., herpes virus
    v., inflammation of seminal
    v., intermediary
    v., intraepithelial
    v., Malpighi's
    v., Naboth's
    v., ocular
    v., ophthalmic
    v., optic
    v., prostatic
    v., pulmonary
    v., secretory
    v., seminal
    v., spermatic

vesicocervical fistula
vesicocolic fistula
vesicocutaneous fistula
vesicointestinal reflex
vesicoprostatic calculus
vesicoprostatic plexus
vesicospinal center
vesicoureteral reflux
vesicoureterogram (VCUG)
vesicourethral orifice
vesicouterine
    v. deflection
    v. fistula
    v. ligament
    v. peritoneum
    v. peritoneum reflected
    v. pouch
vesicovaginal
    v. fascia
    v. fistula
    v. fistula, Latzko repair for
    v. injuries
vesicula ophthalmica
vesicular
    v. appendages
    v. breath sounds
    v. bronchiolitis
    v. bronchitis
    v. emphysema
    v. follicle
    v. keratitis
    v. murmur
    v. nuclei
    v. rales
    v. resonance
    v. respiration
    v. stomatitis virus
    v. supporting tissue
vesiculation [*fasciculation*]
vesiculation of eyelids
vesiculitis, seminal
vesiculocavernous respiration
vesiculogram, seminal
vessel(s)
    v., aberrant
    v., abnormal blood
    v. ▸ abnormal expansion of
        blood
    v., afferent
    v., alveolar
    v. anastomosis
    v., anastomosis of retinal and
        choroidal
    v. anatomy, coronary

v. angiography, total absence of
    circulation on four
v., angioneurotic edema of
v. angioplasty, bootstrap two-
v. angioplasty, brachiocephalic
v. angioplasty ▸ tibioperoneal
v., angioplasty-related
v., anomaly opticociliary
v., arterial
v. arteriogram, four
v., arteriosclerosis of eye
v. ▸ atherosclerosis of intra-
    cerebral
v., atherosclerotic blood
v., ballooning-out of blood
v. ▸ basilar of intracerebral
v., bifurcation of
v., bleeding
v. bleeding blood
v. bleeding ▸ small blood
v. blockage, blood
v. blockage ▸ eye
v., blocked
v. ▸ blocked eye
v., blood
v., bouquet
v., capacitance
v., capillary blood
v., cardinal
v., carotid
v. cells ▸ tumor blood
v., cerebral
v. circulation, small
v. ▸ clipping of blood
v., clogged
v., closed
v. closure
v. clot, blood
v., collateral
v., collateral blood
v., conductance
v., constricted blood
v., constriction of blood
v. ▸ constriction or spasm of
    blood
v., coronary
v., coronary blood
v., coronary resistance
v. coronary stenosis ▸ single
v., corrected transposition of
    great
v., cut blood
v., deterioration of blood
v. development, blood
v., dilated blood

vessel(s)—*continued*

v., dilation of blood
v. dilator ▸ blood
v. disease
v. disease, blood
v. disease, brain blood
v. disease ▸ large
v. disease ▸ single
v. disease ▸ small
v. disease ▸ three
v. disease, triple
v., diseased
v. disorder, blood
v. ▸ dissection of blood
v., efferent
v. elasticity, blood
v. elasticity ▸ impaired blood
v. ▸ endarterectomy in peripheral
v., engorged blood
v., engorgement of
v., engorgement of pulmonary
v. enlargement compensatory
v., excision of portion of blood
v. ▸ expanding blood
v. exposed, hilar
v. ▸ extra-alveolar
v., fatty plaque in blood
v., feeder
v., femoral
v. function, blood
v., gastroepiploic
v., ghost
v. graft, blood
v. ▸ grafted blood
v., great
v. growth ▸ blood
v. growth, stimulate new
v., heart and great
v., hemangioma of meningeal
v., hemangiomatosis of meningeal
v. hematocrit, large
v., hemorrhoidal
v., hyaloid
v. in cornea, ghost
v. in vital organs ▸ occlude blood
v., inadequate blood flow ▸ small
v., incision into blood
v. ▸ infarct-related
v. inflammation, blood
v., inflammation of
v., injury to meningeal
v., intercostal
v., interlacing blood
v., internal spermatic
v. ▸ intramyocardial prearteriolar

v. invasion, blood
v. ▸ invasive growth of blood
v., large blood
v. ▸ leaking retinal
v. ligated, intercostal
v., ligation of meningeal
v. loops ▸ maxi-
v. lumen
v., lymph
v., lymphatic
v., major blockage carotid
v., major blood
v., major obstruction carotid
v. ▸ malformation of blood
v. ▸ malformation of brain
v., mammary
v. ▸ medial calcification of cerebral
v. ▸ medial hypertrophy of
pulmonary
v. membranes, choroidal new
v., meningeal
v., mesenteric blood
v., microscopic blood
v., minor
v., minuscule blood
v., narrowed blood
v. ▸ narrowing of blood
v., native
v. necrosis
v. ▸ neurohumoral control of
pulmonary
v., nutrient
v. occluded, blood
v. ▸ occluded carotid
v. ▸ occluded coronary
v. occlusion, angioplasty-related
v. occlusion, branch
v. occlusion ▸ retinal
v. occlusion system
v. of brain
v. of brain, thrombosis of
v. of extremity cannulated
v. of heart ▸ multiple thrombi in
v. of heart ▸ revascularization of
blood
v. of lung ▸ pressure in blood
v. of papilla, anomalous
v. of the brain cover ▸ small blood
v. patency, epicardial
v., patent
v., penetrating wounds of great
v. perfused with fresh blood,
extremity
v., peripheral
v. problem, blood

v. ▸ problem in Raynaud's disease ▸
blood
v., prominence of pulmonary
v. prosthesis, Dacron
v. pruning, branch
v., pumpkin
v., reclogged blood
v., reconstruction of blood
v. ▸ recruitable collateral
v. ▸ renal blood
v., repair of blood
v., resistance
v., retinal
v., retinal blood
v., rupture of blood
v., ruptured brain blood
v., scarred
v. seal bleeding blood
v. sealed off, blood
v. ▸ severe spasm of blood
v., small blood
v., small caliber
v., smaller coronary
v. spasm, catheter-related
peripheral
v., spasm of blood
v. spasms
v., spastic blood
v., spinal canal
v., splanchnic
v. ▸ stented coronary
v., superficial blood
v., surface
v., surface blood
v., suture of blood
v., swollen blood
v. ▸ tearing of blood
v. technique, bootstrap two-
v., thin-walled blood
v., thoracic
v., tortuosity of
v., tortuous
v. ▸ transplanted blood
v., transposition of great
v., tumor of blood
v., turgescent
v., umbilical blood
v., uterine
v., uterine blood
v., vascular congestion of
interstitial
v. vasculitis ▸ small
v. ▸ vasoconstriction or vasodilation
of
v., venous major

v. ▸ vertebral arteries of intracerebral
v., viable
v., visualization of blood
v. wall
v. wall, congenital weakness in
v. wall, distal
v., wall of blood
v. wall open, bracing
v. walls, blood
v. walls dilated, blood
v. walls ▸ fatty plaques in
v. walls ▸ weakness in blood
v. washed out, extremity
v. ▸ weakened blood
v., widening blood
v. with reduced elasticity, blood

vest
v. hernia repair ▸ pants-over-
v., patient restrained with
v. restraint

vestibular
v. adenitis
v. and balance rehabilitation therapy
v. aqueduct
v. ataxia
v. canal
v. cecum of cochlear duct
v. compensation
v. disease
v. disease, acute
v. dysfunction
v. exercise
v. fold
v. function
v. function, caloric testing of
v. function ▸ loss of
v. ganglion
v. gland
v. hypofunction
v. labyrinth
v. laryngitis
v. lesion
v. migraine
v. nerve
v. nerve section ▸ translabyrinthine
v. neuronitis
v. neuronitis ▸ acute
v. nuclei
v. nuclei ▸ paired
v. nystagmus
v. ocular reflex
v. pupillary reaction
v. receptors

v. region
v. rehabilitation program
v. saccule
v. schwannoma
v. screen
v. stimuli
v. suppressants
v. system
v. test
v. trough
v. veins
v. vertigo
v. window

vestibularis, sacculus
vestibule
v. and cochlea, dilated
v., aqueduct of
v. cancer, nasal
v., Gibson's
v., nasal
v. of ear
v. of larynx
v. of mouth
v. of nose
v. of vagina
v. of vagina, fossa of
v., Sibson's
v., urogenital
v., vein of aqueduct of
v., vein of bulb of

vestibuli
v., aqueductus
v., fenestra
v. of cochlea, scala
v., scala
v. vaginae, fossa

vestibulocochlear nerve
vestibulopathy
v., chronic
v., peripheral
v., recurrent
v., relapsing

vestibulum
v. auris
v. glottidis
v. laryngis
v. nasi
v. oris

vestige, branchial
vestigial
v. fold
v. muscle
v. nodule
v. notochord

vestimenti, pediculosis

vestimentorum, pediculosis
vestimentorum, Pediculus humanus var.
vet counseling, Vietnam era
Veterans Affairs Medical Center
veterinary medicine
veto activity
vexabilis, Xenopsylla
vexans, Aedes
vexans, Cercosporalla
vexator, Phlebotomus
VF (visual field)
V-5, Lead
V-4, Lead
VFP (ventricular fluid pressure)
VG (vein graft)
VGM (vein graft myringoplasty)
VI (vision impaired)
VI (volume index)
Vi agglutination
Vi strain
viability
v. assessment, cell
v., myocardial
v. of human islets ▸ functional
v., organ
v. scintigraphy ▸ myocardial

viable [*friable*]
v. bacteria
v. colostomy
v. female infant
v. fetus
v. flaps
v. heart
v. infant
v. male infant
v. myocardium
v. offspring
v. organ
v. tissue
v. tissue, pad of
v. treatment
v. tumor
v. vessels

vials, glass
vials, transport
vibrating pulse
vibrating reed electrometer
vibration(s)
v., airborne
v. and position sensation ▸ impaired discriminatory
v., chest percussion and
v. disease
v., double

vibration(s)—*continued*
- v., eardrum
- v., low frequency
- v., molecular
- v. seconds
- v. ‣ sound wave
- v., tissue

vibrational angioplasty

vibratory
- v., discriminatory and postural sensation
- v. massage
- v. nystagmus
- v. sense
- v. sensibility
- v. treatments

vibrio (Vibrio)(s)
- v. abortion
- V. alginolyticus
- V. bulbulus
- v., Celebes
- V. cholerae
- V. cholerae-asiaticae
- V. coli
- V. comma
- V. comma, gram-negative
- V. danubicus
- v., El Tor
- V. faecalis
- V. fetus
- V. finkleri
- V. ghinda
- v. infections
- V. jejuni
- V. massauah
- V. metschnikovii
- V. niger
- v., nonagglutinating
- v. organism
- v., paracholera
- V. parahemolyticus
- v., pathogenic
- V. phosphorescens
- V. proteus
- V. septicus
- V. tyrogenus
- V. vulnificus

vibrioides, Caulobacter

vibrion septique

vibrocardiography study

vibrocardiography technique

vicarious
- v. excretion
- v. hemoptysis

- v. hemorrhage
- v. hyperplasia
- v. hypertrophy
- v. liability
- v. menstruation
- v. respiration
- v. traumatization

vicarius, Oeciacus

vicina, Musca domestica

vicious cicatrix

vicious circle

vicissitudes of superego ‣ maturational

Vicq d'Azyr, bundle of

Vicryl suture

Vicryl suture material

victim(s)('s)
- v., acquaintance rape
- v., AIDS (acquired immune deficiency syndrome)
- v., burn
- v., cancer
- v., cardiac arrest
- v., choking
- v., cocaine-related heart attack
- v., conscious
- v., crash
- v., domestic violence
- v., drug
- v., fibromyalgia
- v., heart attack
- v., high risk potential
- v., ice
- v., irradiated
- v. mouth, tight seal over
- v. ‣ nerve death in stroke
- v. of drowning
- v. of frostbite
- v. of incest
- v., patient near-drowning
- v., plaque
- v., potential stroke
- v., rape
- v., sexual abuse
- v., shock
- v. situation ‣ multiple
- v., sleep apnea
- v., trauma, crime
- v., unconscious
- v. ‣ unconscious choking

victimization, childhood

Victoreen dosimeter

video
- v. arthroscopy
- v. -assisted thoracic surgery

- v. -assisted thorascopic thymectomy
- v. densitometry
- v. display camera
- v. display terminal (VDT)
- v. display terminal (VDT) glare screen
- v. gambling
- v. image
- v. imaging
- v. laseroscopy
- v. loop
- v. monitor
- v. otoscopic ear canal inspection
- v. pill ‣ wireless
- v. stroboscopy
- v. system
- v. terminal use

videoscope surgery, balloon

videoscopic surgery

videotape recorder

videotape study

vidian
- v. artery
- v. canal
- v. nerve
- v. nerve, deep
- v. neuralgia
- v. veins

Vi-drape

Vienna total artificial heart

Vietnam
- V. era vet counseling
- V. syndrome
- V. syndrome, post-

Vieussens(')
- V. annulus
- V. ‣ circle of
- V., loop of
- V. ‣ valve of
- V., veins of
- V. ventricle

view(s)
- v., anteroposterior (AP)
- v., AP (anteroposterior) and lateral
- v., apical lordotic
- v., Arcelin's
- v., axillary
- v. body, prepare family to
- v., Caldwell x-ray
- v., caudocranial hemiaxial
- v., Chamberlain-Towne x-ray
- v., Chausse's
- v., color enhanced

v., comparison
v., coned-down
v., craniocaudad
v., cross-sectional
v., dorsal
v. echocardiogram ‣ apical five chamber
v. echocardiogram ‣ apical four chamber
v. echocardiogram ‣ apical two chamber
v. echocardiogram ‣ long-axis parasternal
v. echocardiogram ‣ parasternal long-axis
v. echocardiogram ‣ parasternal short-axis
v., field of
v., five chamber
v., four chamber
v., frog-leg
v., gently brought into
v., Granger x-ray
v., hemiaxial
v. ‣ horizontal long-axis
v. ‣ ice-pick
v. ‣ laid back
v., lateral
v., Laws x-ray
v. ‣ long axial oblique
v., long axis
v., lordotic
v., Low-Beer
v., Mayer x-ray
v., Mayer's
v., mediolateral
v. MRI (magnetic resonance imaging) scan, side-
v., notch
v., oblique
v., oblique spot
v. of cervical spine, dens
v., orthogonal
v., Owen's
v., PA (posteroanterior)
v., panoramic
v., pantomographic
v., parasternal
v. ‣ parasternal long-axis
v. ‣ parasternal short-axis
v., plain
v., plantar
v., posterior
v. projection, blowout
v. ‣ right anterior oblique (RAO)

v., sagittal
v., Schuller's
v., scottie dog
v., scout
v., short-axis
v. ‣ short-axis parasternal
v. ‣ sitting up
v., skyline
v., spot
v., Stenver x-ray
v., stereo
v., stereo x-ray
v., subcostal
v., supine mediolateral
v., suprasternal
v., swimmer's
v., tangential
v., three-dimensional
v., Towne's
v., tunnel
v. ‣ two chamber
v., Velpeau axillary
v. ‣ vertical long-axis
v., Waters' x-ray
v. ‣ weeping willow
viewer self-imaging screen
viewing
v. a near object
v., fiberoptic
v. instrument
v. of body
v., prepare body for
v., wide angle
vigil, coma
vigilance response
Vignal's cells
vigorous
v. activity
v. exercise
v. exercise program
v. exercise ‣ prolonged
v. inflight exercise program
v. lifestyle
v. maternal exercise
v. movement
v. past activity
v. physical activity
v. pulmonary toilet
v. walking
v. warm-up
vigorously, area scraped
vilification ‣ violation and
Villafranca operation, Suarez-
villosa nigra, lingua
villosa, pericarditis

villose (*see* **villous**)
villosum, carcinoma
villosum, cor
villotubular adenoma
villous/villose
v. adenoma
v. arthritis, chronic
v. atrophy, subtotal
v. duct cancer
v. folds of stomach
v. placenta
v. structures
v. tumor
villus(-i)
v., amniotic
v., anchoring
v., arachnoid
v. biopsy (CVB), chorionic
v., chorionic
v. hairs to thicken and grow
v., intestinal
v., jejunal
v., placental
v., pleural
v. sampling (CVS) ‣ chorionic
v., synovial
Vim needle
Vim-Silverman needle
vinaceus, Actinomyces
vinca alkaloid
Vincent('s)
V. angina
V. angina, Plaut-
V. gingivitis
V. infection
V. organisms
V. stomatitis
V. tonsillitis
vincenti, Borrelia
vincenti, Spirochaeta
vincristine
v., amethopterin, 6-mercaptopurine and prednisone (VAMP)
v., daunorubicin, prednisone (VDP)
v., methotrexate, 6-mercaptopurine, and prednisone (VMMP) therapy
v., prednisone (CVP) ‣ Cytoxan,
Vineberg procedure
Vineberg's operation
vinegar douche
Vinethene and ether
Vinke tong skull traction
Vinke tong traction

Vinson
- V. applicator, Plummer-
- V. dilator, Plummer-
- V. radium applicator, Plummer-
- V. syndrome, Plummer-

violacea, taenia
violaceous macules
violaceous nodules
violaceum, Chromobacterium
violaceum, Trichophyton
violence
- v., alcohol-related
- v., cocaine-related
- v., domestic
- v., drug-related
- v., family
- v., family conflict and
- v., hands-off
- v., human
- v. immune deficiency syndrome (AVIDS) ‣ acquired
- v., impulse
- v., irrational
- v., marital
- v., media
- v., patient has potential for
- v. ‣ physical harm or
- v. ‣ self-directed
- v. ‣ self-directed potential for
- v., sexual
- v. ‣ threats of physical
- v. to others ‣ potential for
- v. victim, domestic
- v., workplace

violent
- v. aggression
- v. and aggressive behavior
- v. and irregular jerking motions
- v. attack
- v. behavior
- v. behavior, aggressive or
- v. behavior, alternatives to
- v. crime
- v. ‣ hyperactive and
- v. involuntary contraction of voluntary muscles
- v. obsessional urges
- v. outbursts
- v. pain
- v. patients, treatment of acute drug reactions in
- v. personality, alter
- v. reaction
- v. relationship
- v. repetitive movement

- v. schizophrenic behavior
- v. shaking
- v. spinning sensation

violet
- v., aniline gentian
- v., area painted with gentian
- v., area swabbed with gentian
- v., cresyl
- v., gentian
- v. treatment, gentian
- v. vision

VIP (vasoactive intestinal peptide)
viral [vital]
- v. agent
- v. antigenic structure
- v. antigens
- v. asthenia ‣ post-
- v. bronchiolitis
- v. bronchitis
- v. bronchopneumonia
- v. capsid antigen
- v. cardiomyopathy
- v. conjunctivitis
- v. cultures
- v. cure
- v. destruction of nerves
- v. diagnosis
- v. diarrhea
- v. disease
- v. disease attacks
- v. disease, contagious
- v. dysentery
- v. encephalitis
- v. encephalitis ‣ West Nile-like
- v. encephalomyelitis
- v. enteritis
- v. etiology
- v. exanthem
- v. fringent
- v. gastroenteritis
- v. gene
- v. genome
- v. glycoproteins
- v. hematodepressive disease
- v. hemorrhagic fever
- v. hepatitis
- v. hepatitis, acute
- v. hepatitis ‣ confirmed transmission of
- v. hepatitis ‣ food-borne transmission of
- v. hepatitis ‣ hemodialysis transmission of
- v. hepatitis, hospital-acquired

- v. hepatitis ‣ inoculation transmission of
- v. hepatitis ‣ intrafamily transmission of
- v. hepatitis ‣ intrainstitutional transmission of
- v. hepatitis ‣ maternal-neonatal transmission of
- v. hepatitis ‣ oral transmission of
- v. hepatitis panel
- v. hepatitis ‣ sexual transmission of
- v. hepatitis ‣ transfusion transmission of
- v. hepatitis ‣ water-borne transmission of
- v. illness
- v. infection
- v. infection, acute
- v. infection, benign
- v. infection, congenital
- v. infection, gastrointestinal
- v. inflammation
- v. inflammation of nerves
- v. inhibitor
- v. inner ear infection
- v. isolation
- v. labyrinthitis
- v. -like infection
- v. lode ‣ heterogeneity of
- v. lode testing
- v. meningitis
- v. meningoencephalitis
- v. mononeuritis
- v. multiplication
- v. myocarditis
- v. neurolabyrinthitis
- v. neutralization
- v. nucleoprotein
- v. oncogenesis theory
- v. particles
- v. pericarditis
- v. pharyngitis
- v. pneumonia
- v. producing common organisms
- v. rebound
- v. replication
- v. replication ‣ stimulate
- v. respiratory infection
- v. sepsis
- v. shedding
- v. shedding, asymptomatic
- v. shedding time
- v. strains, major
- v. syndrome ‣ upper respiratory

v. titers
v. transmission
v. vector
v. warts
virality studies
Virchow('s)
    V. cells
    V. granulations
    V. node
    V. triad
viremia
    v., chronic
    v., hepatitis
    v., persistent
virgaurea, Solidago
virgin silk
virginal abdomen
virginal introitus
virginiae, Branchiostoma
virginiana, Hamamelis
viridans
    v., Aerococcus
    v. endocarditis
    v., gram-positive Streptococcus
    v., icterus
    v. streptococcus
    v., Streptococcus
viridis, Cellfalcicula
viridis, Euglena
viridula, Stipa
virile reflex
virilis, urethra
virilism, congenital adrenal
virility [*fertility*]
virilizing adrenal hyperplasia,
    congenital
virilizing tumor
virological efficacy ▸ potential
    clinical
virosa, Cicuta
virtual
    v. cautery
    v. colonoscopy
    v. radiation fields
    v. stimulation
virulent
    v. disease
    v. organism
    v. strain
virus(es) (Virus)
    v. A, hepatitis
    v., acute laryngotracheo-bronchitis
    v., adeno◊
    v., adeno-associated
    v., altered

v., animal
v., animatum
v. (HIV) antibodies, human
    immunodeficiency
v. antigen, Gross
v., arbor
v., arthropod-borne
v. (HIV) associated dementia ▸
    human immunodeficiency
v. (HIV) associated motor cognitive
    disorder ▸ human
    immunodeficiency
v., Astroviridae
v., attenuated
v., Australian X disease
v., auto-inoculated
v., avian leukosis
v., B
v. B, hepatitis
v., bacterial
v. ▸ blood products contaminated
    by AIDS (acquired immune
    deficiency syndrome)
v., blood-borne
v. bronchopneumonia
v., Brunhilde
v., bushy stunt
v., C (Coxsackie)
v., CA (croup-associated)
v., Cache Valley
v., Calciviridae
v., California
v., California encephalitis
v., cancer-inducing
v. carrier, potential
v., CCA (chimpanzee coryza
    agent)
v., CELO (chicken-embryo-lethal-
    orphan)
v., chickenpox
v. (CEBV) ▸ chronic Epstein-Barr
v., CMID (cytomegalic inclusion
    disease)
v., Coe
v., cold
v., Colorado tick fever
v., Columbia SK
v., common cold
v. conduit ▸ respiratory syncytial
v., contagious
v. contaminated nasal secretions
v., corona◊
v., Coronaviridae
v., coryza
v., Coxsackie (C)

v., Coxsackie A
v., Coxsackie B
v., Coxsackie C
v., croup-associated (CA)
v., cytomegalic inclusion disease
    (CMID)
v. (CMV) ▸ cytomegalo◊
v., deadly
v., deadly flu
v., defective
v., dengue
v., dermotropic
v. diarrhea
v., DNA (deoxyribonucleic acid)
v. ▸ drug-resistant
v., eastern equine encephalitis
    (EEE)
v., eastern equine
    encephalomyelitis (EEE)
v., EB (Epstein-Barr)
v., Ebola
v., ECBO (enteric cytopathic bovine
    orphan)
v., ECHO (enteric cytopathic human
    orphan)
v., ECHO 28
v., ECMO (enteric cytopathic
    monkey orphan)
v., ECSO (enteric cytopathic swine
    orphan)
v., EEE (eastern equine
    encephalitis)
v., EEE (eastern equine
    encephalomyelitis)
V. -8 (HHV-8) ▸ Human Herpes
v., EMC (encephalomyocarditis)
v., encephalomyelitis
v., encephalomyocarditis (EMC)
v. (HIV) encephalopathy ▸ human
    immunodeficiency
v. encephalopathy, transmissible
    spongiform
v., enteric
v., enteric cytopathic bovine orphan
    (ECBO)
v., enteric cytopathic human orphan
    (ECHO)
v. ▸ enteric cytopathic human
    orphan (ECHO) 28
v., enteric cytopathic monkey
    orphan (ECMO)
v., enteric cytopathic swine orphan
    (ECSO)
v., enteric orphan
v., epidemic keratoconjunctivitis

virus(es)—*continued*

v. (EBV) ▸ Epstein-Barr
v. (EEV) ▸ equine encephalomyelitis
v., error-prone
v., exanthematous disease
v., exposure to
v., FA
v., fatal
v., feline ataxia
v. ▸ fifth disease
v., Filoviridae
v., filterable
v. fixé
v., fixed
v., flu
v. 40 (SV40) ▸ simian
v., free extracellular
v. ▸ genetically engineered
v., genital herpes
v., Graffi
v., granulosis
v., Gross
v., Guama
v., Guanarito
v., Guaroa
v., Hantaan
v., helper
v., hemorrhagic
v., hepatitis
v. (HAV), hepatitis A
v. (HBV), hepatitis B
v. ▸ hepatitis C
v. (HDV) ▸ hepatitis D
v. ▸ hepatitis E
v. ▸ hepatitis G
v., herpangina
v., herpes◊
v. ▸ herpes family of
v., herpes simplex
v. ▸ herpes zoster
v., herpes-like
v., herpes-type
v. hominis, herpes◊
v. (HIV), human immuno-deficiency
v. (HIV-2), human immunodeficiency
v. (HPV), human papilloma
V. (HTLV), Human T Cell Lymphotropic
v. IH, hepatitis
v., Ilheus
v. inactivating agent
v., inclusion conjunctivitis

v. -induced
v. -infected tumor cells
v. infection, acquired immune deficiency syndrome (AIDS)
v. infection, chickenpox
v. infection ▸ chronic hepatitis B
v. infection, Coxsackie
v. infection, ECHO
v. infection, herpes◊
v. infection ▸ varicella
v., infectious wart
v., influenza
v. injected therapy
v., insect
v., invading
v. isolated from patients
v. IV immune globulin ▸ respiratory syncytial
v., Japanese B encephalitis
v., JH
v., Junin
v., K
v. (KSHV) ▸ Kaposi's sarcoma herpes
v., keratoconjunctivitis
v., Kumba
v., Kyasanur Forest disease
v., lactic dehydrogenase (LDH)
v., Lansing
v., Lassa
v., latent
v., LCM (lymphocytic choriomeningitis)
v., Leon
v., leukemia
v., lifelong carriers of
v., live
v., louping ill
v., Lunyo
v. ▸ lymphadenopathy associated
v., lymphocytic choriomeningitis (LCM)
v., lymphogranuloma venereum
v., lytic
v., mammary tumor
v., Marburg
v., masked
v., Mayaro
v., measles
v. medication, anti-
v., Mengo
v., MM
v., modified
v., Moloney leukemogenic
v., Moloney sarcoma

v., monkey
v., mononucleosis
v., Mossuril
v., mother infected with acquired immune deficiency syndrome (AIDS)
v., M-25
v. ▸ multiple sclerosis
v., mumps
v. ▸ murine encephalomyelitis
v., murine leukemia
v., murine sarcoma
v., Murray Valley encephalitis
v. ▸ mutant cold
v., myxo◊
v., neurotropic
v. neutralization
v. neutralizing
v. neutralizing capacity
v. (NDV) ▸ Newcastle disease
v., nononcogenic
v., nonreversible
v., Norwalk
v. of right eye ▸ herpes
v., oncogenic
v. 1, parainfluenza
v., O'nyong-nyong
v., oral
v., origin of
v., ornithosis
v., Oropouche
v., orphan
v., Orthomyxoviridae
v. outbreak, Ebola
v., panleukopenia
v., papilloma/papilloma◊
v., pappataci fever
v., parainfluenza
v., paramyxo◊
v., Paramyxoviridae
v., parrot
v. particles
v., patient has natural immunity to hepatitis B
v., pharyngoconjunctival fever
v., Picornaviridae
v., plant
v. pneumonia ▸ influenza
v., pneumonitis
v., polio◊
v., poliomyelitis
v., polyoma/polyoma◊
v., Powassan
v., pox/pox◊
v., psittacosis

v., rabbit fibroma
v. rabbit myxoma
v., rabies
v., respiratory
v. (RSV), respiratory syncytial
v., Reston
v., rhino◊
v., Rift Valley fever
v., RNA (ribonucleic acid)
v., Rous sarcoma
v. (RAV) ▸ Rous-associated
v., RS (respiratory syncytial)
v., rubella
v., SA
v., Sabia
v., salivary gland
v., Schwartz's leukemia
v. screening
v., Semliki Forest
v., Sendai
v. (HIV) seroconversion ▸ human
   immunodeficiency
v., ▸ serotype A, B and C
V. -7 (HHV-7) ▸ Human Herpes
v. SH, hepatitis
v., Simbu
v., simian
v. (SIV) ▸ simian immuno-
   deficiency
v., Sindbis
v., slow
v., slow growing
v., smallpox
v. ▸ South American Junin
v., St. Louis encephalitis
v. strain
v., street
v., Sydney
v., syncytial
v. syndrome, Epstein-Barr (EB)
v., synthesis of
v., synthetic
v., temperate
v., teratogenic
v., Teschen
v. testing, acquired immune
   deficiency syndrome (AIDS)
v. testing, AIDS (auto-immune
   disease syndrome)
v., Theiler's
v., tick-borne
v. ▸ tick-borne encephalitis
v. to unborn child ▸ transmit
v., tobacco mosaic
v., toga◊

v., Togaviridae
v., trachoma
v. transmission, AIDS
v., tumor
v., Turlock
v. 2, parainfluenza
v. (HA1) ▸ type 1 hemadsorption
v. type ▸ simian T cell lymphotropic
v. (HA2) ▸ type 2 hemadsorption
v., U (Uppsala)
v., Uganda S
v., unorganized
v., Uruma
v. vaccine ▸ influenza
v. vaccine, live-
v. vaccine ▸ split
v., vaccinia
v. vaccinicum
v., vacuolating
v. (VZV), varicella-zoster
v., variola
v., Venezuelan equine
   encephalomyelitis (VEE)
v. vesicles, herpes
v., vesicular stomatitis
v., weakened
v., WEE (western equine
   encephalitis)
v., WEE (western equine
   encephalomyelitis)
v., Wesselsbron
v., West Nile-like
v., western equine encephalitis
   (WEE)
v., western equine
   encephalomyelitis (WEE)
v., Willowbrook
v., Wyeomyia
v., Yaba
v. ▸ yellow fever
v., Zika
**VISC (vitreous infusion suction
   cutter)**
viscera
v., abdominal
v. packed inferiorly
v., pelvic
v. surrounded by hematoma ▸
   pelvic
v., thoracic
visceral
v. angiitis
v. angiography
v. aortography
v. aortography, selective

v. arches
v. arteriography
v. arteritis ▸ localized
v. artery
v. brain
v. carcinoma
v. distention
v. disturbance
v. epilepsy
v. fat
v. herpes simplex
v. heterotaxy
v. larva migrans
v. leishmaniasis
v. manipulation
v. muscle
v. nervous system
v. organs
v. pain
v. peel
v. peel, thick
v. pericardiectomy
v. pericardium
v. peritoneum
v. pleura
v. pleura incised
v. pleural layer
v. pleurisy
v. reflex
v. sense
v. vasodilation
visceroatrial heterotaxy syndrome
visceroatrial situs
**viscerobronchial cardiovascular
   anomaly**
viscerocardiac reflex
visceromotor manifestations
visceromotor reflex
viscerosensory reflex
viscerosomatic pain
viscerotrophic reflex
viscerum, situs inversus
Vischer's lumboiliac incision
viscid dark green bile
viscid mucus
viscolactis, Alcaligenes
viscosa, Pseudomonas
viscosimeter, Ostwald
viscosimeter, Stormer
viscosity
v. absolute
v. and elasticity ▸ sputum
v. barium and air, high
v., blood
v. cement, Zimmer low

viscosity—*continued*
- v., dynamic
- v., kinematic
- v., plasma
- v., serum

viscous
- v. bile, black
- v. bile, dark green
- v. blood
- v. silicone gel

viscus organs, hollow

viscus, perforated

vise
- v., hemodynamic
- v. -like pain
- v., torque

visible
- v. calculi
- v. chromatin
- v. stones

vision(s)
- v., abrupt change in
- v., achromatic
- v., acuity of color
- v. aids ▸ low
- v., arthroscopic
- v., binocular
- v., blurred
- v., blurred or fuzzy
- v., blurring of
- v., blurring or dimming of
- v. capability
- v. center of field of
- v., central
- v., central field of
- v. change
- v. change in aging
- v. check, peripheral
- v., chromatic
- v., clouded
- v., cloudy
- v., color
- v., complete loss of
- v. control
- v., corrected
- v. correction
- v. correction ▸ laser
- v. correction surgery
- v., day
- v., daylight
- v., declining
- v., decreased
- v., decreased, right
- v. defect

- v. deficiency
- v. deficiency, color
- v., degeneration of
- v., depressed
- v. deteriorate with aging ▸ color
- v., deterioration in
- v. deviant, color
- v., dichromatic
- v., diminished
- v., diminishing
- v., diminution of
- v., dimmed
- v., dimming of
- v. ▸ dimness or loss of
- v., direct
- v. ▸ disabling double
- v. disorder
- v., distance
- v. distorted
- v. distortions
- v. disturbance
- v., disturbance of
- v. ▸ dizziness with double
- v., double
- v., enhanced
- v., enhancing poor
- v., facial
- v., failing
- v., false
- v., faulty
- v., field of
- v., finger
- v., finger-counting test of
- v., floaters in
- v., foggy
- v., foveal
- v. from anemia ▸ blurred
- v. from diabetes ▸ blurred
- v. from myasthenia gravis ▸ double
- v. function
- v. glasses, single
- v., gradual blurring of
- v., half
- v., hallucinatory
- v., halo
- v., haploscopic
- v., hazy
- v. impaired (VI)
- v. impairment
- v. impairment ▸ low
- v. improving lenses
- v. in one eye, blurred
- v. in one eye, dimmed

- v. in one eye ▸ double
- v., indirect
- v., infant
- v., intact
- v., intermittent double
- v. internal urethrotomy (DVIU), direct
- v., iridescent
- v., left eye (VOS)
- v., lens system, angled-
- v., limited peripheral
- v. loss, central
- v., loss of
- v. ▸ loss of peripheral
- v. loss ▸ permanent
- v. loss ▸ progressive
- v. loss ▸ severe
- v. loss ▸ sudden
- v. loss ▸ temporary
- v., low
- v. measured, peripheral
- v., mismatched
- v., monocular
- v., multiple
- v. (Nv) ▸ naked
- v. ▸ narrowed field of
- v., nasal field of
- v., near
- v., night
- v., normal color
- v. null
- v., obscure
- v. of each eye (VOU)
- v. of retina, central
- v., oscillating
- v., painful
- v., partial
- v., partial loss of
- v. ▸ patient sees
- v., peripheral
- v., permanent loss of
- v., photopic
- v., Pick's
- v., poor color
- v. problem
- v. problem ▸ sudden
- v., progressive impairment of
- v., pseudoscopic
- v., rainbow
- v. rating
- v., reduced
- v. ▸ reduced distance
- v. rehabilitation
- v. rehabilitation ▸ low
- v. ▸ residual functional

v., right eye (VOD)
v., rod
v., scoterythrous
v., scotopic
v. screening
v. screening, preschool
v. services ▸ low
v., shaft
v., side
v., solid
v. ▸ specks in
v., sports
v. ▸ spotty loss of
v., stereoscopic
v., sudden change in
v. ▸ sudden dimness of
v. ▸ sudden dimness or loss of
v. ▸ sudden dizziness, weakness or change in
v. ▸ sudden loss of
v. syndrome, computer
v. system, object
v. system, spatial
v., temporal field of
v. test, Allen
v. test, color
v. test, near
v. therapy
v. therapy ▸ low
v. -threatening cataracts
v., toddler
v., total loss of
v. training ▸ low
v. ▸ transient loss of
v., triple
v., tunnel
v., tunnel-like
v., 20/20
v., twilight
v. with eye redness ▸ double
v. with headache ▸ double
v., word

visit(s)
v., antenatal
v., daily
v., home health
v., office follow-up
v., outpatient
v., postoperative office
v., postsurgical office
v., prenatal office
v., preoperative
v. ▸ stress of overlapping
v. to physician ▸ frequent
v., trial

visitation
v., limited
v., pastoral
v. privileges
v. skills

visiting (Visiting)
v. hours
V. Nurse (VN)
V. Nurse Association (VNA)
v. nurse service
V. Registered Nurse (VRN)

Visna provirus
visnaga, Ammi
Visscher-Bowman test
visual (Visual)
v. acuity (VA)
v. acuity, central
v. acuity, decreased
v. acuity (DVA) ▸ distance
v. acuity left eye
v. acuity (NVA) ▸ near
v. acuity right eye
v. acuity screening
v. acuity test
v. agnosia
v. aid
v. amnesia
v. analogue scale
v. analysis
v. and perceptual losses
v. angle
v. aphasia
v. apparition
v. area
v. association areas
v. attention
v., auditory and olfactory hallucinations ▸ vivid
v. axis
v. blind spots
v. blurring
v. capacity
v. capacity ▸ retraining
v. cells
v. centers
v. centers of brain
v. constructural task, spatial-
v. contact, constant
v. control center
v. cortex
v. cue
v. cut
v. decoordination
v. defect
v. deficits

v. delusions
v. detail analysis
v. detection level
v. dimness
v. discriminatory acuity
v. disorder
v. distortion
v. disturbance
v. disturbance ▸ chronic
v. disturbance ▸ nausea, vomiting and
v. efficiency
v. effort
v. evoked potential (VEP)
v. evoked response
v. examination, direct
v. exploration
v. feedback
v. feedback of myoelectric output
v. field (VF)
v. field ▸ abnormal
v. field, confrontation of
v. field cut
v. field defect
v. field deficit
v. field examination
v. field floaters
v. field loss
v. field machine, computerized
v. field, narrowing of
v. field test
v. field, tubular
v. fixation
v. floaters
v. function
v. function, disturbance of
v. habits
v., half-field
v. hallucinations
v. hearing
v. hearing loss
v. illusions
v. image
v. imagery
v. imagery exercise
v. imagery ▸ vivid
v. images and hallucinations ▸ distorted
v. impairment
v. impairment, age-related
v. impairment ▸ permanent
v. impulse
v. information
v. inspection
v. interpretation

visual—*continued*
- v. line
- v. loss
- v. loss ▸ severe
- v. memory
- v. motility
- v. -motor coordination
- v. -motor deficit
- v. -motor function
- v. motor recognition
- v. -motor skills
- v. -motor task
- v. or auditory stimulation
- v. pathway
- v. perception
- v. perception ▸ distorted
- v. perceptual deficit
- v. power
- v. purple
- v. recovery
- V. Retention Test, Benton
- v. scanning
- v. screening
- v. signals
- v. signals, auditory and
- v. spatial ability test
- v. spatial skills
- v. spikes
- v. stimulation
- v. stimulation, patterned
- v. strands
- v. symptoms, transient
- v. system
- v. -tactile stimulation ▸ audio-
- v. therapy
- v. thinking
- v. type
- v. verticality
- v. word center

visualization
- v. and concentration ▸ motivation,
- v. and imagery ▸ meditation,
- v. and relaxation methods
- v., behavioral
- v., direct
- v., double contrast
- v., fluoroscopic
- v. ▸ imagery and
- v., laryngoscopic
- v. of blood vessels
- v., poor

visualize, power to

visualized
- v., appendix
- v., gallbladder

- v. kidney, non-
- v., orifices adequately

visualizing gallbladder, poorly
visually handicapped
visually impaired
Visudyne therapy
Vitagraft arteriovenous shunt
Vitagraft vascular graft
vital [*viral*]
- v. body function
- v. brain centers
- v. capacity (VC)
- v. capacity analysis ▸ forced
- v. capacity (FVC) ▸ forced
- v. capacity (FIVC) ▸ forced inspiratory
- v. capacity (FVC) ▸ functional
- v. capacity (MVC) ▸ maximal
- v. capacity (VC) ▸ measurement of
- v. capacity ▸ normal
- v. capacity ratio ▸ forced
- v. capacity (VC) ▸ slow
- v. capacity (VC) ▸ timed
- v. capacity (VC) ▸ total
- v. centers
- v. energy
- v. forces
- v. functions
- v. functions artificially maintained
- v. functions, monitor
- v. health information
- v. information
- v. microscopic air sacs
- v. needs
- v. node
- v. organ donation
- v. organ donor
- v. organ donor candidate
- v. organ ▸ occlude blood vessel in
- v. organ recovery
- v. organs
- v. organs, total system failure of
- v. processes, body's
- v. rays
- v. resistance
- v. rhythms
- v. sign check
- v. signs (VS)
- v. signs normal
- v. signs ▸ orthostatic
- v. signs stable
- v. staining
- v. statistics
- v. tissues

vitalis, turgor
vitality, loss of
vitality, spiritual
Vitallium
- V. cap prosthesis, McKeever
- V. hip prosthesis
- V. implant
- V. implant material
- V. mechanical knee prosthesis ▸ Walldius
- V. Moore self-locking prosthesis

vitam, intra
vitamin(s) (Vitamin)
- v. and minerals ▸ malabsorption of
- v., antioxidant
- v. B-12 deficiency
- v. concentrate
- v. D milk
- v. D resistant rickets
- v. deficiency
- v. deficiency, alcohol-related
- v., fat soluble
- v., high potency
- V. K (ketamine)
- v. levels
- v., megadose of
- v. overdose
- v. preparation
- v. pretreatment, antioxidant
- v. supplement
- v. supplementation
- v., therapeutic
- v. therapy
- v. therapy ▸ megadose
- v. toxicity
- v., water soluble

Vitatron pacemaker
vitelliform macular degeneration
vitelline
- v. circulation
- v. duct
- v. duct cyst
- v. duct, patent
- v. vein

vitiligo, symmetric
vitium cordis
vitrectomy
- v. and scleral buckle
- v. procedure
- v. surgery

vitreoretinopathy ▸ familial exudative
vitreous
- v., abscess of

v. -block glaucoma
v., blood filled
v. body
v. cavity
v. chamber
v., cholesterol in
v. collapse
v., coloboma of
v. detachment
v. detachment (PVD) ▸ posterior
v., embryonic
v. face
v. floater
v. floaters, stringy
v. fluff
v. fluid
v. fluid, preserved
v. fluid ▸ shrinkage of
v. fluorophotometry
v. gel
v. hemorrhage
v. herniation
v. humor
v. infusion suction cutter (VISC)
v. jelly
v., liquefaction of
v. membrane
v., micelles in
v. opacity
v. penetration
v. (PHPV), persistent hyperplastic primary
v., primary
v., primary persistent hyperplastic
v. pulling and separation
v. retraction, massive
v., sagging
v., secondary
v. space
v. strands
v. stroma
v. table
v., tertiary
vitreum, corpus
vitreum, stroma
vitrinus, Trichostrongylus
vitro
v. activity ▸ in
v., analogous in
v. fertilization (IVF) ▸ in
v. fertilization services ▸ in
v. fetal anomalies ▸ pneumococcus in
v., in
v. reconstruction ▸ in

v. sensitivity testing ▸ in
v. splicing, in
v. studies, in
v. synergism, in
v. technique, in
v. test, in
vittata, Epicauta
vitticeps, Trypanosoma
vitulorum, Ascaris
Vitus' dance, St.
Vivalith-10 pacemaker
vivax minuta, Plasmodium
vivax, Plasmodium
vive skin testing
viverrini, Opisthorchis
vivid
v. acute symptoms
v. dreams
v. hallucinations
v. visual imagery
vivo
v. adhesive platelet, in
v. binding ▸ in
v., ex
v. exposure, in
v., fixation in
v. gene transfer ▸ ex
v. gene transfer ▸ in
v., in
v. microdialysis study ▸ in
v. stereologic assessment ▸ in
v. studies, in
Vivosil implant
Vivosil implant material
VLDL (very low density lipoprotein)
vlistow repair
VMA (vanillylmandelic acid)
VN (Visiting Nurse)
VNA (Visiting Nurse Association)
VNS (vagus nerve stimulator)
VO (verbal order)
vocal [*focal, local*]
v. cord
v. cord activity
v. cord cancer
v. cord dysfunction
v. cord, false
v. cord, nodule
v. cord, opposing
v. cord paralysis
v. cord paralyzed
v. cord polyp
v. cord ▸ senile bowing of
v. cord ▸ squamous cell carcinoma of

v. cord stripping
v. cord, true
v. cords, bowed
v. cords, larynx with
v. cords with ease ▸ bronchoscope inserted through
v. fold
v. fold, false
v. fremitus
v. muscle
v. obstructive problems
v. paralysis
v. ▸ patient very
v. process
v. resonance
v. system
v. tic disorder ▸ chronic motor or
vocalis, chorditis
vocalis, plica
vocalization, inappropriate
vocational
v. adjustment assessment
v. aspirations
v. aspirations ▸ shifting
v. counseling
v. counselor
v. evaluation
v. functioning
v. guidance
v. potential
v. rehabilitation
v. rehabilitation counselor
v. screening
v. skills
v. therapist
VOD (vision, right eye)
Vogt's
V. cataract
V. cornea
V. degeneration
V. disease
V. -Koyanagi syndrome
V. -Spielmeyer disease
V. syndrome
V. syndrome, Stock-Spielmeyer-
voice(s)
v. -activated computer
v. -activated unit
v., amphoric
v. box
v. box ▸ inflammation of
v., breathy
v. button, Panje
v., cavernous
v. change from aging

voice(s)—*continued*
  v. change from antihistamine
  v. change from anxiety
  v. change from cancer
  v. controlled surgical robot
  v., conversational
  v., deep
  v. disorder
  v. disorder, chronic
  v. disorder ▸ neurologic
  v., distorted
  v. disturbance
  v., double
  v., esophageal
  v., eunuchoid
  v., hallucinatory
  v., hearing
  v., hoarse
  v., husky
  v., loss of
  v. ▸ patient hears
  v. pitch, monotonous
  v. prosthesis, duckbill
  v. prosthesis ▸ ultra low
    resistance
  v. (sv) ▸ shouted
  v., spoken
  v. therapy
  v. tremors
  v. (wv) ▸ whispered
void ▸ immediate intense need to
void, patient unable to
voided
  v. specimen
  v. specimen, clean-
  v. urine
voiding
  v., bladder emptied on
  v. cystogram
  v. cystogram, triple
  v. cystography
  v. cystography, triple
  v. cystourethrogram (VCUG)
  v. cystourethrography
  v. cystourethrography,
    radionuclide
  v., difficulty
  v. disorder
  v. dysfunction
  v. dysfunction ▸ postpartum
  v., induced reflex
  v., night
  v., nighttime
  v. schedule, strict
  v., spontaneous

  v., voluntary
voix de polichinelle
volar
  v. angulation
  v. antebrachial region
  v. artery
  v. aspect
  v. carpal ligament
  v. displacement
  v. flap
  v. interosseous muscles
  v. ligament
  v. pad
  v. plate fracture
  v. plate injury
  v. region of hand
  v. regions of fingers
  v. splint
  v. surface
volatile
  v. alkali
  v. mood swing
  v. substance
Volhard's nephritis
volition versus consciousness,
    passive
volitional
  v. collapse
  v. control
  v. intent
  v. movement
  v. tremor
Volk conoid ophthalmic lens
Volkmann('s)
  V. canal
  V. contracture
  V. deformity
  V. disease
  V. ischemic paralysis
  V. subluxation
  V. syndrome
Vollmer's test
volt(s)
  v. (BeV), billion electron
  v. (eV), electron
  v. (keV), kilo electron
  v. (MeV) ▸ mega electron
  v., million electron
  v. ohmmeter
voltage(s)
  v., AC (alternating current)
  v. activity
  v. activity, high
  v. activity, low
  v. activity, medium

  v. amplifier
  v. arrhythmic slow waves ▸ high
  v. asymmetry
  v., bilateral reduction in
  v. brain waves, high
  v. brain waves, low
  v. bursts, high
  v. changes
  v. -dependent block
  v. -dependent calcium channel
  v. differences
  v. diphasic slow wave ▸ high
  v., direct current (DC)
  v. discharge, paroxysmal high
  v. electroencephalogram (EEG) ▸
    low
  v. electrophoresis, high
  v., excessive
  v., extremely low
  v. fast activity, high
  v. fast activity, low
  v. fast electroencephalogram
    (EEG) ▸ low
  v. firing, high
  v. foci, low
  v. gain
  v., generalized low
  v., generalized reduced
  v., high
  v., input
  v., irregular low
  v., lateralized reduction of
  v., localized moderate decrease
    in
  v., localized reduction of
  v., low
  v., mega◊
  v., moderate
  v., operating
  v., output
  v. pattern, high
  v., periodic bursts of high
  v. production
  v., progressive increase in
  v., QRS
  v., ratio of input signal
  v., ratio of output signal
  v. record, low
  v., ripple
  v. ▸ root-mean-square
  v. slow wave activity ▸ high
  v. slow wave, medium
  v. slow waves ▸ paroxysmal
    high
  v. slowing

v. slowing, medium
v. suppression
v., symmetrical reduction in
v. transformer, high
v., transmembrane
v. unit
v., varying
v. waking activity, low
v. waves, large
v. waves, low
v. waves, slow high
v., zero frequency
volubilis, Leptothrix
voluble and verbally facile
volume
v. ▸ adequacy of intravascular
v., adequate blood
v., air
v. analysis ▸ pressure
v. and dose, treatment
v. and elasticity ▸ bladder
v. and frequency of diarrhea
v. and tension
v. -assured pressure support
v., atomic
v. ▸ augmentation of intrathoracic
    blood
v. averaging
v., blood
v., body
v. capacity (TVC) ▸ total
v., cardiac
v., cell
v., central blood
v. -challenge test
v. changes, blood
v. changes, venous
v., circulating blood
v., circulation
v. compensator
v., compressible
v., conductance stroke
v. control ventilation ▸ pressure-
    regulated
v., corpuscular
v., corrected blood
v. curve, flow
v. curve ▸ left ventricular
    pressure
v. curve, pressure
v. cycled decelerating flow
    ventilation
v. cycled respirator
v., decreased respiratory
v., decreased stroke

v. deficiency
v. deficit ▸ fluid
v. depletion
v. diagram ▸ pressure
v. distribution, blood
v., effective circulating blood
v. element (voxel)
v., end-diastolic
v. ▸ end-systolic
v. excess ▸ fluid
v. expander ▸ Hespan plasma
v. expander, plasma
v. expanders
v. expansion, intravascular
v. (ERV) ▸ expiratory reserve
v., extracellular
v., extracellular fluid
v. filtered
v., fluid
v. (FEV) ▸ forced expiratory
v., functional extracellular fluid
v. ▸ high lung
v. in one second ▸ forced
    expiratory
v. in radiation therapy, treatment
v. index (VI)
v. index ▸ end-diastolic
v. index ▸ end-systolic
v. index (SVI) ▸ stroke
v., initial target
v. (IRV) ▸ inspiratory reserve
v., interarterial
v., intracellular fluid
v., intrathoracic gas
v., intravascular
v., irradiated
v. (LVEDV) ▸ left ventricular end-
    diastolic
v. (LVSV) ▸ left ventricular
    stroke
v. load hypertrophy
v. loading
v. localization, target
v. loop, flow
v. loop ▸ ventricular pressure
v., low residual urine
v., lung
v. ▸ mandatory minute
v. (MEFV) ▸ maximal expiratory
    flow
v. (MCV) ▸ mean corpuscular
v. measurements, blood
v. (MV) ▸ minute
v., molar
v., normal assay

v. of air, average
v. of air inspired
v. of air, reduction in
v. of distribution of bilirubin
v. of fluid
v. of heart ▸ stroke
v. of packed red cells
v. overload
v. overload, fluid
v. oxygen (O₂) consumption
v., packed cell
v. per volume (v/v)
v. percent
v., placental residual blood
v., plasma
v., postvoiding residual
v., predicted blood
v. pressure (VP)
v. ▸ presystolic pressure and
v. profile, cell
v., prostate
v. (PBV) ▸ pulmonary blood
v. reabsorbed
v. recorder, pulse
v. recording ▸ pulse
v., red blood cell (RBC)
v., red cell
v., reduce circulating
v. ▸ reduction in plasma
v. reduction surgery ▸ lung
v., regional cerebral blood
v. regulation
v. relation ▸ diastolic pressure
v. relation ▸ end-systolic
    pressure
v. relation ▸ force velocity
v. relation ▸ pressure
v. relation ▸ ventricular end-systolic
    pressure
v. ▸ relative cardiac
v. repletion
v., residual
v. (RV), respiratory
v. (RMV) ▸ respiratory minute
v. ▸ restriction of lung
v. (RVEDV) ▸ right ventricular end-
    diastolic
v. rotation, mediastinal
v. rotation therapy ▸ mediastinum
v. rotation therapy ▸ small
v. stiffness
v., stroke
v. studies, blood
v. test, blood
v. thickness index

volume—*continued*
v., thoracic
v., thoracic gas
v., tidal
v. time curve
v. to total lung capacity (RV/TLC)
   ratio ▸ residual
v., total
v., total air
v., total blood
v. ▸ total lung
v. ▸ trapped gas
v. treated in external irradiation
v., treatment
v., urinary
v. ventilator
v., ventricular
v. ▸ ventricular end-diastolic
v., ventricular end-systolic
volumetric
v. acquisition, continuous
v. aspect of lungs
v. graduation
v. infusion pump, IVAC
v. pump, McGaw
v. solution
volumic ejection
voluminous hernia
voluntary
v. active euthanasia
v. activity
v. activity, no
v. admission
v. basis
v. contraction
v. contraction of muscle, full
v. control
v. control and strength
v. control, individual
v. control of autonomic functions ▸
   biofeedback
v. control of bleeding
v. control of internal state
v. control of pain
v. control of physiological state
v. control of psychological state
v. control of tension headaches
v. dehydration
v. dislocation
v. effort
v. euthanasia
v. guarding
v. heart rate changes ▸ large
   magnitude
v. heart rate control

v. hyperpnea
v. movement
v. movement, binocular
v. movement ▸ impairment of
v. movement ▸ incoordination
   of all
v. movement, loss of power of
v. muscle
v. muscle movement, absence of
v. muscles, activity of
v. muscles, clonic spasm of
v. muscles, tonic spasm of
v. muscles ▸ violent involuntary
   contraction of
v. muscular action
v. muscular movements
v. pelvic muscle
v. relaxation of masseter muscle
v. self-starvation
v. starvation
v. subluxation
v. testing program
v. tremors
v. ventilation (MVV) ▸ maximum
v. voiding
volunteer blood donor
volunteer, hospice
volutin granules
Volutrol apparatus
volvulus
v., gastric
v. neonatorum
v., Onchocerca
v., sigmoid
vomer bone
vomerine
v. groove
v. ridge
v. spur
vomeronasal cartilage
vomica, nux
vomit, blood in
vomited large quantities of blood ▸
patient
vomited undigested food particles ▸
patient
vomiting
v. ▸ abdominal pain, nausea and
v. after presedation ▸ nausea and
v. and dehydration
v. and diarrhea
v. and diarrhea ▸ nausea,
v. and headache
v. and lethargy ▸ nausea,
v. and nystagmus ▸ nausea,

v. and retching
v. and visual disturbance ▸
   nausea,
v. blood
v. blood, patient
v. center
v., cerebral
v., chemotherapy-induced
v. ▸ chills, nausea and
v., copious
v., cyclic
v. ▸ diarrhea with
v. disease ▸ winter
v., dry
v., ejectile
v., fecal
v., forceful
v. from appendicitis
v., hysterical
v., intentional
v., intermittent
v. (N and V) ▸ nausea and
v., nervous
v. of pregnancy
v. or confusion ▸ persistent
   headache,
v. ▸ pain in abdomen with
v., patient
v., patient retching and
v., periodic
v., pernicious
v., persistent
v., postoperative
v. ▸ post-tussive
v. ▸ problem with central nervous
   system from
v., projectile
v., psychogenic
v., recurrent
v. reflex
v., self-induced
v., severe or persistent
v. ▸ severe postchemotherapy
v. sickness
v. sickness, Jamaican
v., stercoraceous
v. ▸ stomach pain and
v. syndrome (CVS) ▸ cyclic
v. up blood
v. with nausea
v. without nausea
vomitoria, Calliphora
vomitoria, Musca
vomitus
v., aerosolized

v., bloody
v., ejectile
v., fecal
v. or gastric aspirant
v., projectile
von (Von)
  v. Behring's fluid
  v. Bekhterev-Strümpell
    spondylitis
  V. Bergmann's hernia
  V. Brunn's nests in bladder
    carcinoma
  V. Fernwald's sign
  v. Gierke's disease
  v. Gies' joint
  v. Graefe's cautery
  v. Graefe's disease
  v. Graefe's operation
  v. Graefe's sign
  v. Hippel disease, Lindau-
  v. Hippel-Lindau syndrome
  v. Jaksch's anemia
  v. Kossa staining
  v. Langenbeck's bipedicle
    mucoperiosteal flap
  v. Mering reflex
  v. Monakow's fibers
  v. Poehl's test
  v. Recklinghausen's disease
  v. Rokitansky's disease
  v. Saal medullary pin
  v. Willebrand's disease
  v. Willebrand's factor
V-1, Lead
VOO pacemaker, atrial
voodoo death
Voorhees' bag
voracious [*veracious*]
voracious appetite
vortex [*cortex*] [*vertex*]
vorticosa, vasa
vorticosae, venae
vorticose vein
VOS (vision, left eye)
Vossius' lenticular ring
VOU (vision of each eye)
voulu, déjà
voxel (volume element)
voxel gray scale
voyeur exhibitionist type
VP (volume pressure)
VPB (ventricular premature beat)
VPC (ventricular premature
   contraction)

VPDC (ventricular premature
   depolarization contractions)
VPL (ventroposterolateral) thalamic
   electrode
VPS (vasovagal pacemaker study)
V/Q quotient
VR (ventilation ratio)
VRI (viral respiratory infection)
VRN (Visiting Registered Nurse)
VS (vs)
  VS (venisection)
  VS (verbal scale)
  vs. (versus)
  VS (vital signs)
  vs. acquired syndrome,
    congenital
VSD (ventricular septal defect)
V-shaped
  V. arch
  V. incision
  V. scar
V-6, Lead
VSW (ventricular stroke work)
V-3, Lead
VTSRS (Verdun Target Symptom
   Rating Scale)
V-2, Lead
vu, déjà
vu, jamais
vulcanite dental plate
vulcanite stomatitis
vulgaris
  v., acne
  v., Cellvibrio
  v., Ephedra
  v., gram-negative Proteus
  v., impetigo
  v., lupus
  v., lupus erythematosus (LE)
  v., pemphigus
  v., Proteus
  v., Sideromonas
  v., verruca
vulnerability
  v., emotional
  v. ▸ extreme narcissistic sensitivity
    and
  v. in self-esteem
  v., individual
  v., inherited
  v. ▸ polysubstance abuse
  v. ▸ signs of
  v. thesis, characterological
vulnerable
  v., biologically

v. cells, cancer
v., emotionally
v., genetically
v. period
v. phase
v. to blockage
v. to injury
v. to injury ▸ grafted skin
v. to stress ▸ unduly
vulnificus, Vibrio
Vulpian's atrophy
vulva(e)
  v., cancer of
  v., chlorosis
  v., elephantiasis of
  v., focal herpes of
  v., fused
  v., kraurosis
  v., lesion of
  v., leukoplakia
  v., noma
  v., pruritus
  v., synechia
vulvar
  v. adenoid cystic adenocarcinoma
  v. carcinoma
  v. carcinoma, invasive
  v. condylomata
  v. condylomata, giant
  v. cyst
  v. intraepithelial neoplasia
  v. irritation
  v. itching
  v. lesions
  v. neoplasia
  v. pain, chronic
  v. regrowth
vulvectomy
  v., en bloc
  v., radical
  v., scalpel
  v., skinning
vulvitis
  v. blenorrhagica
  v., chronic
  v., creamy
  v., diabetic
  v., diphtheric
  v., diphtheritic
  v., eczematiform
  v., follicular
  v., herpes
  v., intertriginous
  v., leukoplakic
  v., monilial

vulvitis—*continued*
    v., phlegmonous
    v., plasma cell
    v., pseudoleukoplakic
    v., secondary
    v., ulcerative
vulvorectal fistula
vulvovaginectomy, partial skinning
vulvovaginitidis, Veillonella
vulvovaginitis, candida
v/v (volume per volume)
V-Y advancement flap
VZIG (varicella-zoster immune globulin)
VZV (varicella-zoster virus)

W

w (watt)
w (wave)
w hernia
W rays
W waveform
Waaler test, Rose-
Waardenburg's syndrome
WACH (wedge adjustable cushioned
   heel) shoe
Wachtel phenomenon, Katz-
Wada('s)
   W. hingeless heart valve prosthesis
   W. test
   W. valve prosthesis
wadding, sterile sheet
waddling gait
Wade-Fite-Faraco stain
Wadsworth-Todd cautery
wafers implanted, chemo
Wagener-Barker classification ▸
   Keith-
Wagener's retinitis
Wagner('s)
   W. disease
   W. operation
   W. reduction technique
wagon wheel fracture
Wagstaffe's fracture
wailing ▸ weeping, whining and
WAIS (Wechsler Adult Intelligence
   Scale)
WAIS (Wechsler Adult Intelligence
   Scale) Test
waist
   w., cardiac
   w. -hip ratio (WHR)
   w. of heart
   w. -to-hip ratio
wait
waiting
   w. list
   w. list, patient on
   w. recipients
   w., watchful
waiver and consent, informed
WAK (wearable artificial kidney)

wake (Wake)
   w. after sleep onset (WASO)
   w. cycle, biological sleep-
   w. cycle, daily sleep-
   w. cycle ▸ phase-shift disruption of
     24-hour sleep-
   w. cycle, sleep-
   w. disorders, sleep-
   w. pattern change, sleep-
   w. pattern, sleep-
   w. patterns ▸ erratic sleep-
   w. record
   w. response
   w. schedule disorder ▸ sleep-
   w. shift, sleep-
   w. time
   W. -Ups (amphetamines)
wakefield, Shigella
wakeful state
wakefulness
   w., abnormal
   w., full
   w. ▸ persistent disorder of initiating
   w., relaxed
   w., restoration of
   w. ▸ transient disorder of initiating
   w. ▸ transient disorder of
     maintaining
waking
   w. activity, low voltage
   w. activity, normal
   w. activity, slow
   w. anxiety
   w. by rhythm
   w. electroencephalogram (EEG) ▸
     normal
   w. electroencephalogram (EEG)
     pattern ▸ normal
   w. hours
   w. phobia
   w., score sleep stages and
   w., sleep-
   w. state
   w. subject
Waldenström disease ▸ Legg-Calvé-
Waldenström's macroglobulinemia

Waldeyer('s)
   W. fluid
   W. ring
   W. sulcus
Waldhauer's operation
Waldhausen subclavian flap
   technique
walk(s)
   w. alone, patient
   w., alteration in normal
   w. -in laser clinic
   w. -in medical center
   w., inability to
   w. ▸ loss of ability to
   w., mall
   w., patient unable to
   w. ▸ progressive inability to
   w., thermal
   w. -through angina
   w., unsteady
walker (Walker)
   w., ambulate with
   w. applied to cast
   W. deformity, Dandy-
   w., Linde
   W. -Murdoch wrist sign
   w., nonweight bearing ▸ patient
     ambulating with
   w., patient ambulating with
   w., patient transfers with
   w., patient uses
   W. pin
   w. placement
   w., platform
   W. syndrome, Dandy-
   w. ▸ weighted cane of
   w. with wheels
walking
   w. aids
   w. and jogging
   w. assistance device
   w., assistance with
   w. brace, Cook
   w., brisk
   w. button
   w. caliper
   w. cast

W

walking—*continued*
w. cast, short leg
w., crutch
w., difficulty
w., exercise
w., fitness
w. ▸ fitness pole
w. foot exercise ▸ sand
w. for fitness
w. ▸ health benefits of
w. heel
w. heel, Bush
w. heel, Stryker
w. heel, Telson hinged
w. ▸ heel-to-toe
w., level
w. ▸ mobility, muscle strength and
w., moderate
w. ▸ pain on
w. patterns
w. pneumonia
w. program
w. programs, mall
w. ▸ progressive difficulty in
w., race
w. shoes
w., sleep
w. ▸ sudden trouble
w., tandem
w. technique, proper exercise
w. therapy ▸ treadmill
w. time ▸ maximum
w. time ▸ pain-free
w., uncontrollable
w., unsteadiness while
w. ventilation test
w., vigorous
w. water
w. without support

wall(s)
w., abdominal
w. active drug, cell
w. adhesion, chest
w. akinesia, anterior
w., alveolar
w. amplitude
w. aneurysm, anterior
w., anterior
w., anterior chest
w., aortic
w., arterial
w., artery
w., atrial
w., atrophic vaginal
w., ballooning-out of artery

w. balloons out ▸ arterial
w., barium adherent to esophageal
w., bladder
w., blood vessel
w., bony
w., bowel
w., bronchial
w. cancer, pharyngeal
w., capillary
w., chest
w. closure, abdominal
w., colon
w., colonic
w., congenital weakness in vessel
w., cyst
w. defect, muscle
w. deformity, chest
w., dehiscence, abdominal
w., depressed chest
w. dilated, blood vessel
w. disease, chest
w. disorder, chest
w., distal vessel
w. dyskinesis, anterior
w. ▸ elastic recoil of arterial
w., esophageal
w. excision portion of chest
w. excursion, left ventricular posterior
w. excursion, posterior
w. fascia, abdominal
w. ▸ fatty plaques in vessel
w., fibromuscular
w. ▸ fibrosis of anteroseptal
w. flap, chest
w., gallbladder
w., gingival
w. ▸ hematoma of chest
w. hemorrhages, bowel
w. ▸ hyalinization of alveolar
w. hypokinesis, cardiac
w. infarct, posterior
w. infarction (AWI) ▸ anterior
w. infarction (PWI), posterior
w., inferior
w., inferobasal
w., inflammation of bladder
w., inherent weakness in arterial
w., inner artery
w., inner surface of abdominal
w., integrity, arterial
w., interior chest
w., intestinal
w. ischemia, anterior
w. ischemia, inferior

w. ischemia, lateral
w., ischemic heart
w., jugular
w., lateral
w., lateral membranous
w., left lateral chest
w., left ventricular
w. lesion, posterior vaginal
w. lesion, ring-
w., malformation of chest
w. manipulation, chest
w., mastoid
w. mattress suture ▸ through-the-
w., medial
w., membranous
w. metastases, chest
w. ▸ microscopic invasion of duodenal
w. motion
w. motion abnormality
w. motion abnormality ▸ left ventricular
w. motion abnormality ▸ regional
w. motion analysis
w. motion, left ventricular
w. motion ▸ paradoxic
w. motion ▸ regional
w. motion, right ventricular
w. motion score
w. motion score index
w. motion ▸ segmental
w. motion ▸ septal
w. motion study
w. motion study ▸ floating
w. motion ▸ ventricular
w., mucosal
w., muscle
w., muscular
w. musculature, abdominal
w. myocardial infarction (AWMI) ▸ anterior
w. myocardial infarction (IWMI) ▸ inferior
w. myocardial infarction (IWMI) ▸ old inferior
w., myometrial
w., nasopharyngeal
w. of arteries, degeneration of
w. of arteries, hardening of
w. of bladder ▸ hemorrhage into
w. of bladder, muscular
w. of blood vessel
w. of cavity
w. of cavity, incision through
w. of gallbladder, calcified

w. of intestines ▸ spasms in
w. of orbit, medial
w. of organ
w. of organism, cell
w. of stomach ▸ muscular
w. of urinary bladder
w. open, bracing vessel
w., outer cell
w., outer layer of alveolar
w. pain, chest
w., patulous urethral
w., pelvic
w. perforation
w. perforation ▸ intestinal
w. permeability, artery
w., posterior
w. ▸ posterior pharyngeal
w. ▸ posterior ventricle septal
w., posteroseptal
w., prolapsed vaginal
w., pulpal
w. push-up exercise
w. radiation, abdominal
w., relaxed anterior
w., right anterior chest
w., right ventricular
w. roof, tegmental
w. ▸ sagging abdominal
w. ▸ scarring of anteroseptal
w. shortening indices
w. shortening ▸ ventricular
w. sling ▸ vaginal
w., small intestinal
w. spasm, chest
w. ▸ spasm of intestinal
w. stent
w. stoma, abdominal
w., stomach
w. stress
w. stress, circumferential
w. stress ▸ left ventricular
w. stress ▸ meridional
w. stress ▸ ventricular
w. structure
w. surface, abdominal
w., suture attached to arterial
w. ▸ swelling of airway
w. syndrome, anterior chest
w. synthesis, cell
w., tegmental
w. tension
w. tension, myocardial
w., thickened arterial
w. thickened, bladder
w. ▸ thickened heart

w. thickening
w. thickening, cardiac
w. thickening ▸ heart
w. ▸ thickening of capillary
w. ▸ thickening of muscle
w. thickness
w. thickness ▸ left ventricular
  posterior
w. thickness, myocardial
w. ▸ thickness of ventricular
w. thickness ▸ relative
w. thickness—diastole, posterior
w. thickness—systole, posterior
w. thin and trabeculated ▸ bladder
w., thin septal
w. thinning ▸ ventricular
w., thoracic
w. tissues ▸ swelling of
w. trabeculated, bladder
w., tracheal
w., transthoracic biopsy chest
w., urethral
w., using bolus adjacent to chest
w., uterine
w., vaginal
w. velocity, normal mean posterior
w. velocity, posterior
w., ventricular
w., vessel
w. ▸ weakened tissue
w., weakened vein
w., weakness in abdominal
w., weakness in arterial
w. ▸ weakness in blood

Walldius prosthesis
**Walldius Vitallium mechanical knee
  prosthesis**
walled
  w. blebs, thin-
  w. blood vessels, thin-
  w. cyst of liver ▸ thin-
  w., thick
  w. uterus, smooth
  w. veins ▸ thin

Wallenberg's syndrome
wallerian degeneration
wallerian law
wallet card ▸ medical alert
Walter's bromide test
Walthard's cell
Walthard's inclusions
Walther's
  W. canal
  W. duct
  W. ganglion

Wampole's test
wander aimlessly, eyes
wandering
  w., aimless
  w. cell
  w. cell, irregular
  w. cell, primitive
  w. cell, resting
  w. eye
  w. goiter
  w. heart
  w. histiocytes
  w. impulsion
  w., increased
  w. kidney
  w., night
  w. ovary
  w. pacemaker
  w. pain
  w. pneumonia
wane, symptoms wax and
waned
  w. ▸ left motor function waxed and
  w. ▸ mental status waxed and
  w. ▸ right motor function waxed and
Wangensteen('s)
  W. awl
  W. carrier
  W. colostomy
  W. drainage (dr'ge)
  W. graft, Braun-
  W. suction
  W. tube
waning
  w. chest pain, waxing and
  w., rhythmic waxing and
  w., waxing and
Wanscher's mask
war (War)
  w. nephritis
  w. neurosis
  w. on drugs
  W. syndrome ▸ Gulf
ward (Ward)
  w. clerk
  w. environment
  W. -Mayo vaginal hysterectomy
  w. milieu
  w. off infection ▸ drugs to
  W. operation, Grant-
  w., patient disrupting
  w. ▸ restrictive long-term
  w., specialized
  W. syndrome ▸ Romano-
  W. vaginal hysterectomy, Mayo-

Wardill palatoplasty, Veau-
Ware test, Balke-
warfare
- w., biological
- w., chemical
- w., germ

warfarin sodium
warfarin therapy
warm (Warm)
- w. agglutinin
- w. baths ▸ healing power of
- w. breast ▸ red and
- w. joint
- w. moist heat
- w. nodule
- w. sitz baths ▸ daily
- w., skin tone pink and
- w. soaks
- W. Springs brace
- w. to the same (COWS) ▸ cold to the opposite,
- w. -up and cool-down
- w. -up exercises
- w. -up period
- w. -up phenomenon
- w. -up routine
- w. -up, vigorous
- w. weather rash

warmer
- w., Armstrong
- w., blood
- w., bottle
- w., infant placed in

warming blanket
warmth
- w. and redness
- w. at incision site
- w., sensation of

warning (Warning)
- w. arrhythmias
- w., drug abuse
- w. label
- W. Network (DAWN), Drug Abuse
- w. sign, acute
- w. sign identification
- w. sign, important
- w. sign management
- w. signals of cancer
- w. signs
- w. signs, early
- w. signs of drug abuse
- w. signs of eye disease
- w. signs of hearing loss
- w. signs of heart attack
- w. signs of mental problems

- w. signs of oral cancer
- w. signs of serious illness
- w. signs of sexually transmitted disease
- w. signs of smoking-related problems
- w. signs of stress
- w. signs of suicide attempt
- w. signs of transient ischemic attack (TIA)
- w. signs, stroke
- w. stimulus
- w. system, faulty
- w., verbal

warpage, corneal
Warren's
- W. incision
- W. operation
- W. shunt

warrior cells
warrior white cells, cancer patients'
wart(s)
- w., anogenital
- w., common
- w., electrodesiccation of
- w. ▸ excision benign
- w. ▸ excisional biopsy perianal
- w., genital
- w., Hassall-Henle
- w., juvenile
- w. -like growth
- w., mucocutaneous
- w., necrogenic
- w. ▸ paring of
- w., periungual
- w., pitch
- w., plane
- w., plantar
- w., rectal
- w., recurring venereal
- w., removal
- w., seborrheic
- w., senile
- w., telangiectatic
- w., venereal
- w., viral
- w. virus, infectious

Wartenberg's sign
Wartenberg's syndrome
Warthin's
- W. cell
- W. sign
- W. tumor

Warwick urethroplasty, Turner-
wash, mouth◊

wash, saline mouth◊
washcloth, disposable
washed
- w., lining brushed and
- w. out, extremity vessels
- w. out ▸ feeling
- w. out, remnants of lens
- w., prepped and infiltrated
- w. red cells
- w. spores

washing(s)
- w. and brushings
- w., brain◊
- w., bronchial
- w., bronchoalveolar
- w., bronchopulmonary
- w., culture of nasal
- w., gastric
- w. in critical care areas ▸ hand-
- w. in nursery ▸ hand-
- w., lung
- w., nasal
- w., nasopharyngeal
- w., postoperative pelvic
- w., segmental
- w. soda
- w., sperm
- w. taken for examination ▸ multiple
- w. technique ▸ hand-
- w., throat
- w., urinary

Washington strut ▸ George
washout
- w., helium
- w., kidney
- w. myocardial perfusion image ▸ stress
- w. period
- w. phase
- w. phenomenon
- w. pyelography
- w. study
- w. test
- w. test ▸ single breath nitrogen
- w., thallium

WASO (wake after sleep onset)
Wassermann
- W. -positive pulmonary infiltrate
- W. reaction
- W. test
- W. test, cardiolipin

wastage, fetal
wastage, severe muscular
waste(s)
- w., body's toxic

w. ▸ diffusion of metabolic
w. disposal, environmental
w. dumps, chemical
w., elimination of
w., hazardous
w., medical
w., nuclear
w. product lactic acid ▸ metabolic
w. products
w. products, excretes
w., radioactive
w., solid
w., toxic
wasted muscles
wasting
w. and fasciculations ▸ muscle
w. disease
w. disease, brain
w. disease, childhood muscle-
w. disease (CWD) ▸ chronic
w. disease, muscle
w. diuretic ▸ potassium-
w., muscle
w. of muscles ▸ weakness and
w. of skeletal muscle
w., potassium
w., salt
w. syndrome
w., tissue
watch
w. test
w. tick
w., wellness
watchful waiting
Water('s) (water)(s)
W. (amphetamines)
w. aerobics
w. aerobics for arthritis
w., bag of
w. balance
w. balance, chronic disordered
w. balance ▸ disordered
w. balance of body, salt and
w. balance ▸ severe disordered
w. balance (DWB) ▸ syndrome of
   disordered
w. bed
w. blackout ▸ shallow
w., bladder distended with
w., body
w., boiling
w. -borne illness outbreak
w. -borne infection
w. -borne transmission of viral
   hepatitis

w. -bottle heart
w. brain
w. brash
w. bulging, bag of
w. cancer
w. cesarean section (CS)
w. choke
w. -clear cell
w., cold
w., contaminated
w., contaminated drinking
w., contaminated tap
w. contamination, ground
w. content, total sodium and
w. cooler, dual use
w. cystoscopy
w., deionized
w. density
w. density area
w. (D/W) ▸ dextrose in
w., distilled
w. drinking behavior ▸ unusual
w. drinking ▸ massive
w. equivalent
w. exercise
w., extracellular
w. extraction
w. ▸ extravascular lung
w. feedings, glucose and
w. ▸ filtered tap
w. (D-5-W/D$_5$W) ▸ 5% dextrose in
w., fluoridated
w. fluoridation
w. gurgle test
w. -hammer pulse
w., hot
w. imbalance, salt and
w. immersion
w. implant, salt
w. in herniated disk, vaporize
w. ingestion
w. intake
w., interstitial
w. intoxication
w., intracellular
w. load test
w. loss, evaporative
w. loss, transepidermal
w. mattress
w. on the knee
W. operation
w. phobia
w., plasma
W. position
w. pressure, tissue

W. projection
w. provides gentle resistance
w., pure
w. -purification system
w., radioactive
w. -resistant sunscreen
w. -retaining laxative
w. retention
w. retention ▸ salt and
w., ruptured bag of
w. seal chest tube
w. seal drainage bottle
w. seal drainage, closed chest
w. seal drainage system
w. seal drainage system, closed
w. -seeking behavior
w. -silk reflex
w. siphon
w. siphonage test
w. soluble
w. soluble dye
w. soluble vitamin
w. solution, salt
w. stool, rice
w. study
w., tap
w., tepid
w. test, T
w. therapist
w. therapy
w., total body
w. -trap stomach
w., tritiated
w. vacuole
W. view
W. view roentgenogram
w. walking
w. -wheel murmur
W. x-ray view
watered-silk retina
waterfall appearance
waterfall stomach
Waterhouse-Friderichsen syndrome
watering of eyes ▸ excessive
watering-can scrotum
waterproof sunscreen
watershed
w. infarct
w. infarction
w. region
Waterston
W. anastomosis, Cooley
   modification of
W. extrapericardial anastomosis
W. shunt

watertight seal
waterwheel sound
watery
 w. and bloody diarrhea
 w. blisters
 w. bowel movements
 w. diarrhea
 w. discharge
 w. exudate
 w. eyes
 w. eyes ▸ itchy-
 w. fluid
 w. fluid in pleural cavity
 w., itchy eyes
 w., profuse diarrhea
 w. stools
 w. stools, loose
Watkins' operation
Watkins-Wertheim operation
Watson('s)
 W. -Jones operation
 W. method
 W. operation, Spencer-
 W. reagent
 W. -Schwartz test
 W. test
watsoni, Amphistoma
Watsonius watsoni
watt second (ws)
wave(s) (w)
 w., a
 w. ablation, continuous
 w., abnormal brain
 w. abnormalities, S-T and T
 w. abnormality, spike
 w. activity and emotions ▸ brain
 w. activity ▸ deficiency of slow brain
 w. activity ▸ excessive fast EEG brain
 w. activity ▸ high voltage slow
 w. activity, slow
 w., alpha
 w., alpha brain
 w., alpha-theta
 w. alternans ▸ T
 w. alternans ▸ U
 w., amplitude of
 w., amplitude of electroencephalogram (EEG)
 w. amplitude ▸ R
 w. and complexes ▸ electroencephalogram (EEG)
 w. -and-spike
 w., aperiodic
 w., arterial

w., atrial
w., atrial repolarization
w., atypical repetitive spike-and-slow
w., atypical spike
w. axis ▸ P
w., beta
w., bifid P
w. biofeedback, brain
w., biphasic
w., brain
w., burst of arch-shaped
w. bursts, spike and
w., C
w. carrier, sine
w., catacrotic
w., catadicrotic
w. changes compatible with ischemia, ST-T
w. changes, nonspecific ST-T
w. changes, T
w., complex electrical
w. complex, multiple spike-and-slow
w. complex, polyspike-and-slow
w. complex, sharp-and-slow
w. complex, slow
w. complex, slow spike-and-
w. complex, spike-and-
w. complex, spike-and-slow
w. complexes, sequence of spike-and-slow
w. component, P
w. components, brain
w. components, production of various brain
w., conducted P
w., continuous
w., contraction
w. coupling ▸ shock
w. cycle ▸ sound
w. deceleration time ▸ transmitral E
w. definition ▸ shock
w., delta
w., depressed T
w. diathermy, short
w. diathermy, ultrashort
w., dicrotic
w., diphasic
w., diphasic P
w., diphasic T
w. discharges, abnormal brain
w. discharges, frontoparietal spike-and-

w. discharges, six per second spike-and-
w. discharges, spike-and-
w., distortion of electroencephalogram (EEG)
w. Doppler echocardiogram, continuous
w. Doppler echocardiography, continuous
w. Doppler echocardiography ▸ pulsed
w. Doppler imaging, continuous
w. Doppler mapping ▸ pulsed
w. Doppler ultrasound, continuous
w., duration of
w., E
w., early diastolic
w., EEG (electroencephalogram)
w. EEG (electroencephalogram) activity ▸ suppress specific seizure
w., EEG (electroencephalogram) delta
w. ▸ electrically generated shock
w., electrocardiogram (ECG/EKG)
w., electroencephalogram
w. electroencephalogram (EEG) activity ▸ suppress specific seizure
w., electromagnetic
w., Erb's
w., exaggerated positive
w., excitation
w., expectancy
w., F
w., fast
w., fibrillary
w., fibrillatory
w. ▸ flipped T
w., fluid
w. ▸ flutter-fibrillation
w., focal delta
w., focal slow
w. foci, occipital slow
w. foci, slow
w. focus, anterior temporal slow
w. focus, central slow
w. focus, frontal slow
w. focus, midtemporal slow
w. focus, occipital slow
w. focus, parietal slow
w. focus, slow
w. focusing ▸ shock
w. formation, polymorphous
w., frequencies of

w. frequencies, rhythmic
w. frequencies, slow brain
w. frequency
w. frequency range, brain
w. function, abnormal brain
w. gating ▸ R
w. generator, slow
w. ▸ giant a
w. ▸ giant v
w., H
w., high frequency sound
w., high voltage arrhythmic slow
w., high voltage brain
w. ▸ inaudible sound
w., independent slow
w. index, brain
w., individual
w. interval
w. inversion, T
w. inversion ▸ U
w., inverted
w., inverted T
w. irradiation, long
w., irregular extremely slow
w., ischemic sylvian
w., isoelectric T
w., J
w., joule
w., K complex
w., kappa
w., lambda
w., lambdoid
w., large voltage
w., larval spike-and-slow
w. laser ablation, continuous
w. laser, continuous
w., light
w. -like pattern
w. lithotripsy (ESWL),
  extracorporeal shock-
w., lithotripter shock
w., longitudinal
w., low voltage
w., low voltage brain
w., M
w., medium voltage slow
w., millisecond (msec) slow
w., millivoltage (mv) slow
w., monophasic
w., msec (millisecond) slow
w., multiple spike
w., mv (millivoltage) slow
w. myocardial infarction ▸ non-Q-
w. myocardial infarction ▸ Q
w., negative P

w., normal P
w., notched
w., occasional late filling
w. of alpha frequency
w. of cardiac apex pulse ▸ SF
w. of drowsiness, slow
w. of high frequency ▸ square
w. of inconstant period ▸ sequence
  of
w. of increasing amplitude
w. of jugular venous pulse
w. of jugular venous pulse ▸ F
w. of Öhnell, X
w. of opposite phases
w. of pain
w. of youth, slow
w., oscillation
w., overflow
w., P
w., papillary
w., paravertex
w., paroxysmal high voltage slow
w., paroxysmal slow
w. pattern, brain
w. pattern, recorded brain
w. pattern ▸ sine-
w. pattern, slow
w. pattern, spike-and-
w. patterns, brain
w. ▸ peaked P
w., percussion
w., peridicrotic
w., period of the
w., peristaltic
w., persistent
w., phantom spike-and-
w. phenomenon, spike-and-slow
w. ▸ photo-acoustic shock
w., phrenic
w., point of maximum amplitude of
w., polarity EEG
  (electroencephalogram)
w. ▸ polymorphic slow
w., polyphasic
w., positive
w., positive sharp
w., posterotemporal slow
w. ▸ postextrasystolic T
w. ▸ precordial A
w., predicrotic
w., pre-excitation
w., pressure
w. pressure measurement ▸ shock
w. progression ▸ poor R
w. progression ▸ R

w. ▸ propagation of R
w. ▸ pseudonormalization of T
w., pulse
w. pulse ▸ square
w. pulse ▸ tidal
w., Q
w., QRS
w., QS
w., R
w., radio
w., radiofrequency
w., random
w. ratio ▸ E:A
w., recoil
w., reflection of sound
w. reflection ▸ shock
w., regression ▸ Q
w., regularly repeated
  electroencephalogram (EEG)
w., regurgitant
w., repetitive
w., repetitive sharp-and-slow
w., respiratory
w. response ▸ square
w., responses, brain
w. ▸ retrograde P
w., RF
w. rhythm ▸ spike-and-slow
w., rhythmic
w., S
w., sawtooth
w., scattered slow
w., seismic
w., sequence of
w., sharp
w., sharp peaks of component
w., sharp-and-slow
w., shift in frequency of sound
w., shock
w., short
w. (SSSDW) ▸ significant sharp,
  spike or delta
w., sine
w., sinusoidal
w., six hertz spike-and-slow
w. sleep, fast
w. sleep (SWS), slow
w., slow
w., slow brain
w., slow high voltage
w., slow spike-and-
w., sonic
w., sound
w. speed mechanism
w., spike

wave(s) (w)—*continued*
- w., spike and sharp
- w. spike, parietal area left
- w. spike, parietal area right
- w. spike, parietal area sharp
- w., spike-and-
- w., spike-and-slow
- w., sporadic slow
- w., ST
- w. stimulation, square
- w., stimulus
- w. stimulus ▸ square
- w., ST-T
- w., supersonic
- w., suppression of seizure specific brain
- w., T
- w. techniques, sound-
- w. technology, sound-
- w. therapy, short
- w., theta
- w., three hertz spike-and-slow
- w., tidal
- w. to A wave ▸ E
- w., total pattern of
- w. transient, central sharp
- w. transients and eye blinks, slow
- w., transients, slow
- w., transmits sound
- w., transverse
- w., Traube-Hering
- w. treatment ▸ shock
- w., tricrotic
- w. triggered ventricular pacemaker ▸ P
- w., triphasic
- w., TU
- w. tube ▸ Z-
- w., U
- w., ultrashort
- w., ultrasonic
- w., ultrasound
- w., unequal development of electroencephalogram
- w., V (vertex)
- w., vasomotor
- w. velocity measurement, pulse
- w., venous
- w., ventricular
- w., Venturi
- w. vibrations ▸ sound
- w., x
- w., y
- w. ▸ y descent

waveform
- w., abnormal
- w., alteration in
- w. analysis
- w. analysis, Doppler
- w., complex
- w., instrumental elevation in
- w., pressure
- w. pulmonary pressure
- w. quasi-sinusoidal biphasic
- w., rectangular
- w., sharp transient
- w., spectral
- w., stimulus
- w., W

wavefront scanning device
wavefront-guided LASIK (laser-assisted in situ keratomileusis) surgery
wavelength
- w., Compton
- w. data
- w., deBroglie
- w., effective
- w., energy
- w., equivalent
- w., minimum
- w. of rhythmic activity

wavy
- w. fiber
- w. respiration
- w. skin

wax
- w. and wane, symptoms
- w. bite
- w., bone
- w. build-up, ear
- w. build-up ▸ excessive
- w. cast
- w. depilatories
- w., Horsley's
- w., Horsley's bone
- w. in ear canals
- w. in ears
- w. -like rigidity
- w. -like rigidity ▸ impacted
- w. -like secretion
- w. matrix technique
- w. pattern

waxed
- w. and waned, left motor function
- w. and waned, mental status
- w. and waned, right motor function

waxing
- w. and waning

- w. and waning chest pain
- w. and waning, rhythmic

waxy
- w. cast
- w. deposit
- w. deposit in brains
- w. exudate ▸ hard
- w. finger
- w. flexibility
- w. kidney
- w. sunscreen
- w. tissue

Way (way)
- W. (LSD), Four-
- w. irrigating catheter, three-
- w., non-addictive
- w. of thinking, bizarre
- w. ▸ patient a perfectionist in self-defeating

WBC
- WBC (white blood cells)
- WBC (white blood count)
- WBC (white blood count) ▸ elevated
- WBC (white blood count) ▸ reduced
- WBC (white blood count) ▸ weekly

W/D (well developed)
weak [*week*]
- w. and debilitated ▸ exhausted,
- w. and flabby abdominal muscles
- w. and nauseated ▸ patient
- w. and rapid pulse
- w. and thready ▸ pulse
- w. and/or listless
- w. arm movement
- w. contact
- w. cry, infant had
- w., emaciated condition
- w. foot
- w., hypotensive and unresponsive ▸ patient
- w. muscles
- w. muscles in neck
- w. or interrupted urine stream
- w., patient
- w., patient physically
- w. pedal pulses
- w. pulse
- w. ▸ somnolent, lethargic and
- w. tendon
- w. urinary system

weaken, supportive structures
weakened
- w. area, reinforce
- w. artery

weather-related migraine headache
Weavenit
    W. patch graft
    W. valve prosthesis
    W. vascular prosthesis,
       Wesolowski
weaver's bottom
web(s)
    w., esophageal
    w., laryngeal
    w. of fingers
    w. ▸ pulmonary arterial
    w. space
    w., subsynaptic
    w., terminal
    w., thenar
    w., venous
webbed fingers
webbed toes
webbing of neck
Weber('s)
    W. -Christian disease
    W. -Christian syndrome
    W. -Dimitri disease, Sturge-
    W. disease ▸ Rendu-Osler-
    W. douche
    W. fractions
    W. implant
    W. paradox
    W. sign
    W. syndrome
    W. syndrome, Sturge-
    W. syndrome ▸ Sutton-Rendu-
       Osler-
    W. test
Webster operation, Baldy-
Webster's operation
Wechsel sponge
Wechsler
    W. Adult Intelligence Scale (WAIS)
    W. Adult Intelligence Scale (WAIS)
       Test
    W. -Bellevue Test
    W. Intelligence Scale for Children
       (WISC)
    W. Intelligence Scale for Children
       (WISC) Test
    W. Memory Scale (WMS)
Wedge(s) (wedge)
    W. (LSD)
    w. adjustable cushioned heel
       (WACH) shoe
    w. angiography ▸ pulmonary
    w., arterial
    w. arteriogram

w., ball
w., bed
w. biopsy
w. biopsy of breast, excision and
w. colon resection
w. excision
w. excisional biopsy
w. heel
w. mean pressure (PWMP) ▸
    pulmonary
w. mean (PWM) ▸ pulmonary
w., mediastinal
w. of skin
w. of tissue
w. position, pulmonary
w. pressure (WP)
w. pressure, capillary
w. pressure ▸ mean pulmonary
    artery
w. pressure, monitor pulmonary
    capillary
w. pressure (PWP) ▸ pulmonary
w. pressure ▸ pulmonary artery
w., pulmonary
w., pulmonary angiography
w., pulmonary artery
w. (PCW), pulmonary capillary
w. resection
w. resection ▸ infundibular
w. section ▸ nail
w. section pattern on breast self-
    exam
w. -shaped
w. -shaped appearance
w. -shaped area
w. -shaped cut into bone
w. -shaped density
w. -shaped piece of tissue
w., sole
w. -type osteotomy, opening
wedged fetal head
wedging of vertebra
WEE (western equine encephalitis)
    virus
WEE (western equine
    encephalomyelitis) virus
Weed
    W. (marijuana)
    W. juice (hashish)
    W. (phencyclidine) ▸ Killer
    W. oil (hashish)
week [*weak*]
    w., gestational
    w. (tiwk), three times a
Weekend Family Program

Weeker's operation
weekly
    w. blood count
    w. injections ▸ patient to receive
    w. intervals
    w. outpatient basis
    w. WBC (white blood count)
Weeks(')
    W. bacillus, Koch-
    W. conjunctivitis, Koch-
    W. haemophilus, Koch-
    W. operation
weeping
    w. dermatitis
    w. dermatophytosis
    w. eczema
    w. of uterus
    w. or rage ▸ senseless laughter,
    w., senseless
    w. sinew
    w. sores
    w. threshold
    w., whining and wailing
    w. willow view
weevil disease ▸ wheat
Wegener's disease
Wegener's pulmonary
    granulomatosis
Weichselbaum's diplococcus
Weigert's hematoxylin stain
Weigert's stain
weighing, daily
weight (Weight) (wt) [*wait*]
    w., atomic
    w., average
    w. bearing
    w. bearing activity
    w. bearing as tolerated
    w. bearing brace, ischial
    w. bearing, complete
    w. bearing exercises
    w. bearing exercises, full
    w. bearing exercises, regular
    w. bearing, full
    w. bearing, gradual
    w. bearing joint
    w. bearing, non◇
    w. bearing, partial
    w. bearing ▸ reduced
    w. bearing, strenuous activity ▸
       repetitive
    w. bearing with crutches
    w., birth
    w., body
    w. change

w. conscious
w. control
w. control counseling
w. control diet
w. control ▸ long-term
w. control ▸ nutrition and
w. control, permanent
w. control program
w. cycle
w., desirable
w. dextran, low molecular
w., dry
w. /electrolyte monitoring
w., elevation of body
w. ▸ ever-present effects of
w., excess
w., fat-free dry
w., fat-free wet
w. fluctuated
w. fluctuation
w. fluctuations ▸ diurnal
w. ▸ full body
w. gain
w. gain and bloating
w. gain, body
w. gain diet
w. gain, diurnal weight
w. gain ▸ easy
w. gain, episodic
w. gain, erratic
w. gain, excessive
w. gain, gradual
w. gain in aging
w. gain, infant
w. gain, maternal
w. gain ▸ postmenopause
w. gain, rapid
w. gain, significant
w. gain, subsequent
w. gain, sudden
w., goal
w. (GMW) ▸ gram-molecular
w., high birth
w., high molecular
w., ideal body
w. inability to control
w., increased
w. infant (LBWI), low birth
w. level
w., lose excess
w. loss
w. loss ▸ abdomen showed
  evidence of
w. loss and exercise
w. loss attempt

w. loss, body
w. loss diet
w. loss, enhancing
w. loss, excessive
w. loss ▸ exercise-induced
w. loss from anxiety
w. loss from cancer
w. loss from depression
w. loss from diabetes
w. loss from pernicious anemia
w. loss, infant
w. loss medication
w. loss method
w., loss of appetite and
w. loss products
w. loss program
w. loss, rapid
w. loss, significant
w. loss, sudden
w. loss surgery
w. loss, unexplained
w. loss ▸ weakness, anorexia,
w. (LBW), low birth
w., low molecular
w. ▸ maintain stable
w. maintenance
w. management
w., molecular
w., normal birth
w., normal body
w., optimal
w. pattern
w., peak
w., per-unit
w., pre-pregnancy
w. problem
w. problems ▸ age-related
w. ratio, body-
w. reduction
w. reduction diet
w. reduction ▸ exercise and
w. reduction program
w. reduction surgery
w. -related health problems
w. shifting
w., significant gain in
w., significant loss in
w., stabilizes
w., stable
w., total body
w., toxic
w. training
w. training exercise
W. Watcher's diet

weighted
  w. ankle cuffs
  w. cane or walker
  w. image ▸ T1-T2
  w. image ▸ T2
  w. MRI (magnetic resonance
    imaging) ▸ diffusion
  w. speculum
  w. squat exercise
  w. utensils
  w. wrist bracelets
Weil('s)
  W. disease
  W. -Felix reaction
  W. reaction, Felix-
  W. syndrome
Weill sign
Weill-Marchesani syndrome
Weinberg's test
Weir
  W. excisions
  W. Mitchell's disease
  W. Mitchell's treatment
Weiss(')
  W. procedure
  W. reflex
  W. sign, Chvostek-
  W. syndrome, Mallory-
  W. tear, Mallory-
Weissmann's bundle
Welander disease, Kugelberg-
welchii
  w., Bacillus
  w., Clostridium
  w., gram-positive Clostridium
welder('s)
  w. conjunctivitis
  w. keratoconjunctivitis
  w. lung, arc
Welin's technique
well (Well)
  w. aerated and crepitant, lungs
  w. aerated, lungs
  w. aerated, sinuses
  w., alive and
  w. articulated, speech
  w., atrial
  w. -balanced diet
  w. -being, cognitive aspect of
  w. -being, emotional
  w. -being, enhanced
  w. -being, euphoric sense of
  w. -being, feeling of
  w. -being, general
  w. -being, health and

well—*continued*
- w. -being index ▸ general
- W. -Being Index ▸ Quality of
- w. -being ▸ individual
- w. -being, patient's
- w. -being ▸ periods of
- w. -being, physical
- w. -being, sense of
- w. compensated
- w. controlled, diabetes
- w. controlled, pain
- w. counter, gamma
- w. -defined
- w. -defined margin
- w. -demarcated margin
- w. demonstrated
- w. -developed (W/D), patient
- w. differentiated
- w. differentiated adenocarcinoma of uterus
- w. differentiated carcinoma
- w. differentiated hepatocellular carcinoma
- w. differentiated squamous cell tumor
- w. healed
- w. healed previous excisional scars
- w. healed scar
- w. hydrated, patient
- w. (L/W), living and
- w. monitored patient
- w. -nourished (W/N), patient
- w. outlined, cytoplasmic borders
- w. outlined discs
- w., patient tolerated diagnostic procedures
- w., patient tolerated procedure
- w., pericardial
- w. suspended vaginal cuff
- w. technique, atrial
- w., wound healing

wellness
- w., health
- w. program
- w. screening
- w. watch

welt from aspirin

wen cyst

Wenckebach('s)
- W. atrioventricular block
- W. biopsy, AV
- W. block
- W. cycle
- W. disease
- W. heart block

- W. period
- W. periodicity block
- W. phenomena
- W. sign
- W. with 2:1 block

went full term, patient

Wepman Aphasia Screening Test ▸ Halstead-

Werdnig-Hoffman disease

Werdnig-Hoffman syndrome

Wermer's syndrome

werneckii, Cladosporium

Werner's disease

Werner's syndrome

Wernicke('s)
- W. aphasia
- W. area
- W. area, damage to
- W. center
- W. disease
- W. disease, Posadas-
- W. encephalopathy
- W. encephalopathy symptoms
- W. -Korsakoff syndrome
- W. -Mann hemiplegia
- W. pupillary reaction
- W. sign
- W. syndrome

Wertheim('s)
- W. hysterectomy, Ries-
- W. operation
- W. operation, Ries-
- W. operation, Schauta-
- W. operation, Watkins-
- W. procedure, radical
- W. radical hysterectomy
- W. -Schauta operation

Wesolowski Weavenit vascular prosthesis

Wesselsbron virus

West('s)
- W. Nile encephalitis
- W. Nile fever
- W. Nile virus
- W. Nile-like fever
- W. Nile-like viral encephalitis
- W. Nile-like virus
- W. operation

Westberg space

Westcott's test

Westergren method

Westergren's sedimentation rate (SR)

westermani, Distoma

westermani, Paragonimus

Westermark sign

Western
- W. Blot Analysis
- W. Blot Test
- W. equine encephalitis (WEE)
- W. equine encephalitis (WEE) virus
- W. equine encephalomyelitis (WEE)
- W. equine encephalomyelitis (WEE) virus
- W. medical ethics

Westminster drug-free protocol

Westphal('s)
- W. nucleus, Edinger-
- W. -Piltz reflex
- W. pupillary reflex
- W. sign
- W. -Strümpell disease
- W. zone

wet
- w. age-related macular degeneration (ARMD)
- w. brain
- w. brain syndrome
- w. cough
- w. disinfection
- w. dream
- w. eye
- w. field cautery
- w. film
- w. lung
- w. lung syndrome
- w. lung, traumatic
- w. macular degeneration
- w. mount of cervical discharge
- w. nesting on plates
- w. pasteurization
- w. pleurisy
- w. rale
- w. reading of x-rays
- w. smear
- w. swallow
- w. weight, fat-free

wetting, bed

Wetzel grid

Weve's electrode

Weve's operation

WH (well healed)

Wharton's
- W. duct
- W. gelatin
- W. jelly
- W. operation

wheal(s) [*wheel*]
- w. and flare
- w. and plaques

w. -flare reaction

wheat
w. fly, Hessian
w. germ
w. germ agglutinin
w. weevil disease

Wheatstone bridge

wheel(s) (Wheels) [*wheal*]
w., entropy
w. fracture, wagon
w., heat
w. injury, steering
w. lounger
W., Meals On
w. murmur ▸ mill
w. rigidity, cog◊
w., thermal
w., walker with

wheelchair
w. access
w. accessible
w. accommodations
w. artifact
w. bound
w. carrier
w. cushion
w., customized
w. lift
w. mobility
w. mobility, patient needs minimal
assistance for
w., motorized
w. obstacle course
w. pad
w., patient propels
w., pivot transfer to
w. propulsion
w. ramp

Wheeler's
W. implant
W. implant material
W. operation

wheeze(s) [*sneeze, squeeze*]
w., asthmatic
w., asthmatoid
w., diffuse
w., expiratory
w., intermittent
w., monophonic
w., rales or
w., respiratory
w., year-round

wheezing
w. and dyspnea with exertion
w., asthmatic

w., bronchial
w., coughing and/or
w., expiratory
w. in lungs
w., inspiratory
w. on inspiration
w., patient
w. sounds, characteristic
w. while breathing

whenever necessary (prn)

whettle bones

wh/fe (white female) ▸ patient

whiff test

while walking, unsteadiness

whining and crying

whining and wailing ▸ weeping,

whiplash
w. injury
w. injury, pain in back from
w. injury, patient has
w. injury to neck
w. pain

whipping, systolic

Whipple procedure

Whipple's disease

whirlpool
w. bath
w. exercises
w. therapy
w. therapy ▸ sterile
w. treatment, cold or ice
w. treatment ▸ sterile

whirl (*same as* whorl)

whisper test

whispered bronchophony

whispered voice (wv)

whispering pectoriloquy

whispering resonance

whistle
w. test
w. -tip catheter
w. -tip drain

whistling in nose while breathing

whistling rales

Whitacre's operation

White(s) (white)
W. (amphetamines)
W. (cocaine)
w. atrophy
w. blood cell (WBC) count
w. blood cell transfusions
w. blood cell transplant
w. blood cells, aggregation of
w. blood cells, donor's

w. blood cells per high power field
(WBC/hpf)
w. blood cells, separate
w. blood corpuscle
w. blood count (WBC)
w. blood count (WBC) ▸ reduced
w. blood count suppression
w. blood count, transient
depression
w., brain pale
W. bypass tract ▸ Wolff-Parkinson-
w. cell
w. cell casts
w. cell count
w. cell precursors, red and
w. cell protection
w. cells, cancer patients' warrior
w. cells depleted
w. cells float to top of container
w. cells ▸ infection-fighting
w. cells taken off top of solution
w. centers, oval lesions with small
w., cheesy discharge
W. (opioid), China
w. clot syndrome
W. clotting time method ▸ Lee-
w. coat angina
w. coat effect
w. coat hypertension
w. coat phenomenon
w. coat phobia
w. coat syndrome
w. column, anterior
w. commissure, anterior
w. commissure of spinal cord
w. corpuscle
w. crystalline powder
w. diarrhea
w. epithelium
w. epithelium, punctation, and
mosaicism
w. female (wh/fe)
w. female (wh/fe) ▸ patient
w. fibrous tissue
w. graft
w. -graft reaction
w. knuckle sobriety
w. lead
W. Lightning (LSD)
w. line, Sergent's
w. lung
w., lungs pink
w. male (wh/m)
w. male (wh/m) ▸ patient
w. matter

White(s)—*continued*
- w. matter echogenicity of periventricular
- w. matter loss due to aging
- w. matter of brain
- W. method, Lee-
- w. muscle
- w., of Arnold ▸ reticular substance,
- w. of eyes ▸ yellowing of
- w. or pale nails from anemia
- w. or pale nails from cirrhosis
- w. out
- w. patches from anemia
- w. patches from diabetes
- w. patches on mucosa of stomach ▸ small, flat,
- w. plaques
- w. pneumonia
- w. pulp, rudimentary
- W. reentrant tachycardia ▸ Wolff-Parkinson-
- w. scar of ovary
- W. sign, McGinn-
- w. softening
- w. spot
- w. sputum
- w. substance
- w. substance of cerebellum, arborescent
- w. substance of Schwann
- w. substance of spinal cord
- w. swelling
- W. syndrome, Bland-Garland-
- W. (WPW) syndrome, Wolff-Parkinson-
- w. thrombus
- w. tongue
- w. tonsillitis

whitening, teeth

whitish
- w. coating back of tongue
- w. discharge
- w. plaques
- w. plaques, thickened
- w. vaginal discharge ▸ itchy,

whitlow
- w., herpetic
- w., melanotic
- w., thecal

Whitman's frame

Whitman's operation

Whitmore's bacillus

whitmori
- w., Actinobacillus
- w., Bacillus

- w., Malleomyces

Whitnall ligament

wh/m (white male)

wh/m (white male) ▸ patient

WHO (World Health Organization)

whole [*hole*]
- w. abdomen radiation therapy
- w. abdominal treatment in radiation therapy
- w. blood
- w. blood cardioplegia
- w. blood folate
- w. blood hematocrit
- w. blood ▸ patient admitted and transfused with
- w. blood ▸ tonometered
- w. blood transfusion
- w. body
- w. body counter
- w. body counting
- w. body hematocrit
- w. body, hyperthermia
- w. body irradiation
- w. body, musculature of
- w. body scanner
- w., body symptom
- w. bone transplant graft
- w. brain death
- w. brain irradiation
- w. brain radiation
- w. brain radiation therapy
- w. brain versus local brain radiation therapy
- w. cell pertussis vaccine ▸ diphtheria, tetanus toxoids and
- w. common disorder of body
- w. complement
- w. milk
- w. organ transplant
- w. pelvis radiation
- w. person, effects of pain on the
- w. saliva
- w. skull irradiation

whoop, systolic

whooping cough

whooshing
- w. murmur
- w. noise
- w. sound

whorl(s) (*same as* whirl)
- w., bone
- w., keratin
- w., lens
- w. motion
- w. of spindle-shaped cells

whorled cells

whorled pattern

WHR (waist-hip ratio)

Wiberg classification

Wicherkiewicz' operation

wick dressing, Vaseline

wick, gauze

Wickersheimer's fluid

Wickersheimer's medium

wicket rhythm

Wickwitz esophageal stricture

Widal('s)
- W. reaction
- W. reaction, Gruber-
- W. syndrome, Hayem-

wide (Wide)
- w. -angle glaucoma
- w. -angle monoplane ultrasound scanner, Biosound
- w. -angle viewing
- w. -based gait
- w. biopsy
- w. broad based scars
- w. clinics, city-
- w. complex rhythm
- w. excision
- w. excision mastectomy
- w. -field eyepiece
- w. -field laryngectomy
- w. -field lesion
- w. intervertebral spaces
- w. local excision
- w. mesenteric resection
- w. practice, hospital-
- w. QRS tachycardia ▸ regular,
- W. Range Achievement Test
- w. -ranging mood swings
- w. resection
- w. skin incision
- w. stare
- w., tortuous aorta

widely patent ▸ coronary arteries

widely patent, orifices

Widen operation, Palmer-

widened, incision

widening
- w., aneurysmal
- w. blood vessels
- w., decrease in mediastinal
- w., fusiform aneurysmal
- w., mediastinal
- w. of abdominal aorta ▸ fusiform
- w. of aorta, aneurysmal
- w. of carina
- w. of interspace

w. of mediastinum
w. of QRS complex
w. of superior mediastinum
w. of suture lines
widespread
w. allergic skin reaction
w. anoxic changes
w. bony metastases
w. bony osteolytic lesions
w. carcinoma
w. dermatosis
w. disturbance
w. ecchymoses and hematomas
w. extramedullary hematopoiesis
w. glomerulosclerosis and
  arteriosclerosis
w. metastases
w. metastases, multiple
w. muscle aching and stiffness
w. osseous metastases
w. pain
w., pain chronic and
Widmark's conjunctivitis
widow spider venom, black
Widowitz sign
widow's hump
width
w. at half maximum (FWHM) ▸ full
w., atrial pulse
w., band-
w., pulse
w. ▸ ventricular pulse
Wiedemann's syndrome
Wiener's operation
wife, bereaved husband/
wife syndrome, battered
Wigand's maneuver
Wigand's version
Wigby-Taylor position
Wiggers-Starling principle ▸ Frank-
  Straub-
Wiktor stent
wild limb jerks
wild mint
Wildermuth's ear
Wilder's sign
Wilde's incision
wildly, arms flail
wildly ▸ legs flail
Wilke boot brace
will ▸ exercise of
will, living
Willebrand('s)
W. disease, von
W. factor, von

W. -Jürgens syndrome
Williams('s)
W. exercise
W. flexion exercises
W. operation
W. pelvimeter
W. position
W. -Richardson operation
W. sign
W. tracheal tone
williamsii, Iodamoeba
Williamson's sign
Willis('s)
W., circle of
W., nerve of
W. operation, Kirkaldy-
W. pancreas
W. ▸ sclerosis circle of
Willock respiratory jacket
willow fracture
willow view ▸ weeping
Willowbrook virus
Wills test
Willy Meyer radical mastectomy
Wilmer's operation
Wilms'
W. operation
W. tumor
W. tumor, adult
Wilson('s)
W. block
W. central terminal
W. chamber
W. cloud chamber
W. disease
W. disease, Kimmelstiel-
W. leads
W. -McKeever operation
W. muscle
W. operation
W. plate
W. syndrome
W. syndrome, Foville-
W. syndrome, Kimmelstiel-
W. syndrome, Mikity-
W. test
WIMP (weakly interacting massive
  particle)
window
w., acoustic
w., antral
w., aortic
w., aorticopulmonary
w., core
w. crown

w., cycle length
w. defect ▸ oval
w., imaging
w. in cast
w. ▸ intact round
w., nasoantral
w. niche, oval
w. niche, round
w. operation
w., oval
w., pericardial
w., pleuropericardial
w. ▸ pulmonary parenchymal
w. reflex, oval
w. reflex, round
w. replaced in cast
w., round
w., skin
w., tachycardia
w. technique, Rebuck skin
w., therapeutic
w., vestibular
Windowpanes (LSD)
windpipe, fractured
windsock aneurysm
windsock sign
wine hemangioma, port
wine stain, port
wineglass appearance
wing
w., bite-
w. cells
w. of scapula
w. scaler
w. shadow, bat
w., sphenoid
w. sutures
w. x-rays, bite-
winged
w. incisor
w. scapula
w. shunt
Winkelman's disease
winking
w., blinking or squinting of eyes ▸
  increased
w., jaw
w. reflex, opticofacial
w. spasm
w. syndrome, jaw-
winogradskii, Leptothrix
Winslow('s)
W. ▸ epiploic foramen of
W., foramen of
W. ligament

Winslow('s)—*continued*
  W. pancreas
  W. stars
Winter('s) (winter)
  W. arch bar
  w. blues
  w. bronchitis
  w. cough
  w. depression
  w. dysentery
  W. elevation torque technique,
    George
  w. exercise
  w. itch
  w. melancholy
  w. syndrome
  W. technique
  w. vomiting disease
winthemi, Margaropus
Wintrich sign
Wintrobe('s)
  W. indices
  W. sedimentation rate (SR)
  W. test
wire(s)
  w. appliance, Johnson twin
  w., arch
  w., atrial pacing
  w., Bunnell pull-out
  w., central core
  w., Compere fixation
  w., continuous loop
  w., control
  w. crimped
  w., cutting
  w., delivery
  w. effect, copper
  w. effect ▸ silver
  w. electrode
  w. electrodes, fine
  w. fixation, tantalum
  w., flow
  w., hyperflexed
  w., ideal arch
  w. implant, iridium
  w., interdental
  w., intraoral
  w., Ivy
  w., Killip
  w. (K-wire) ▸ Kirschner
  w., ligature
  w. localization
  w. -loop lesion
  w. -loop strut
  w. -loop test

w., Lunderquist guide
w., magnet
w. mesh implant
w. mesh implant material
w., monofilament stainless steel
w., multifilament
w., myocardial cell, chicken
w. osteotomy plane
w., pacing electrode
w. passed, guide
w. piston prosthesis ▸ Schuknecht
  Teflon
w., Risdon's
w., subcuticular
w. sutures
w. sutures, pull-out
w. sutures, sternal
w., tantalum
w. template
w., Thiersch
wired
  w., fractured fragments
  w., jaw
  w. together, teeth
wireless endoscopy capsule
wireless video pill
wiring
  w. of retinal arteries ▸ silver
  w. of sternum
  w., sternal
wiry pulse
WISC (Wechsler Intelligence Scale
  for Children) Test
wisdom teeth
wise movement ▸ jerky step-
Wiskott-Aldrich syndrome
witch's milk
withdraw life sustaining procedures
withdrawal
  w., abrupt
  w., acute treatment for
  w., adjustment disorder with
  w., adjustment reaction with
  w., alcohol
  w., alcohol intake
  w. ▸ alleviate symptoms of nicotine
  w., amphetamine
  w. ▸ amphetamine or similarly
    acting sympathomimetic
  w., asocial
  w., barbiturate
  w., Big H (heroin)
  w. bleeding
  w. bleeding, estrogen
  w., blood

w., caffeine
w., clinical manifestations of
w., cocaine
w., drug
w. delirium, alcohol
w. delirium, anxiolytic
w. delirium, hypnotic
w. delirium, sedative
w. disorder ▸ sensitivity, shyness,
  social
w. disorders
w., emotional
w., features associated with drug
w. feeding tube
w. from cannabinoids
w. from depressants
w. from family, friends or school
  activities
w. from hallucinogens
w. from inhalants
w. from multiple drugs
w. from opioids
w. from phencyclidines
w. from stimulants
w., gradual
w. hallucinosis, alcohol
w. headache
w., heroin (Big H)
w. insomnia, drug
w. ▸ isolation and
w., isolation, depression and fatigue
w., LSD (lysergic acid diethylamide)
w., medically supervised
w. medication, acute
w. ▸ minimizing discomfort of
w., narcotic
w., nicotine
w. of fluid
w. of life-saving treatment
w. of purulent matter
w., opiate
w., opioid
w., pacing
w., peak
w., physiological
w., postoperative
w., psychoactive substance
w., psychological state during
w. reaction
w. reaction, painful
w. reaction, severe
w. scale ▸ narcotic
w., schizoid
w. seizure, alcohol
w. seizures

w. sickness
w. ▸ signs of
w., social
w., subacute treatment on
w. symptomatology ▸ opiate
w. symptoms
w. symptoms, acute
w. symptoms, cigarette
w. symptoms, control
w. symptoms, differential diagnosis of alcohol
w. symptoms, experiencing
w. symptoms ▸ opiate
w. symptoms ▸ patient experiencing
w. symptoms, physical
w. symptoms ▸ prevent
w. symptoms ▸ severe
w. symptoms, unpleasant
w. syndrome, acute
w. syndrome, alcohol
w. syndrome, drug
w. syndrome, neonatal
w. syndrome ▸ nicotine
w. syndrome ▸ opiate
w. syndrome, protracted
w. syndrome, severe alcohol
w. test, progesterone
w., treatment of acute drug reaction
w., uncomplicated alcohol
withdrawing life support systems
withdrawn
w. behavior
w., depressed and apathetic ▸ patient
w. from activities
w. from life ▸ patient
w. from relationships
w., medications
w., patient
w. ▸ patient socially
w., scope
w., socially
w., supportive care
withdraws purposefully
withering cancer
withholding
w. and uncaring, caregiver
w. feeding tube
w. food and fluids
w. of life-saving treatment
within
w. affected area ▸ inflammation
w. body ▸ scattered radiation

w. brain substance ▸ electrode implanted
w. functional limits
w. joint ▸ accumulation of blood
w. joint, inflammation
w. normal limits (WNL)
w. normal limits (WNL) ▸ hematology
w. physiologic limits
without
w. agoraphobia ▸ panic disorder,
w. history of panic disorder ▸ agoraphobia
w. hyperactivity ▸ attention deficit disorder
w. infection, blister
w. nausea, vomiting
w. palpable lesion
w. palpable lesion ▸ calvarium
w. palpable lesion ▸ scalp
w. panic attacks ▸ agoraphobia
w. pigmentation ▸ scattered fibrosis
w. psychotic features ▸ bipolar disorder, depressed, severe,
w. psychotic features ▸ bipolar disorder, manic, severe,
w. psychotic features ▸ bipolar disorder, mixed, severe,
w. psychotic features ▸ major depression, recurrent, severe
w. psychotic features ▸ major depression, severe,
w. psychotic features ▸ major depression, single episode, severe,
w. support, walking
w. varices, esophagus
witness, autopsy
witness, disinterested
Wittek operation, Koenig-
Wittenborn Psychiatric Rating Scale (WPRS)
Wladimiroff-Mikulicz amputation
Wladimiroff's operation
WMA (World Medical Association)
WMS (Wechsler Memory Scale)
w/n (well nourished)
WNL (within normal limits)
WOC (wound, ostomy, continence) nurse
Wohlgemuth unit
Woillez' disease
Wolfe('s)
W. graft
W. -Krause graft

W. operation
wolffian
w. body
w. cyst
w. duct
Wolff-Parkinson-White (WPW)
WPW bypass tract
WPW reentrant tachycardia
WPW syndrome
Wolfring's glands
Wolf's method
Wolf's syndrome
wolhynica, Rickettsia
Wolman's xanthomatosis
woman, menopausal
womb
w. drainage, closed
w. operation, open
w., penetrated mother's
w. procedure, closed
w. stone
w. surgery, in-the-
w. surgery, open
w. syndrome ▸ haunted
w. technique, closed
women (Women)
w., alcohol abuse among
W. and Chemical Dependency
w., childless
w., crack-abusing
w. ▸ drug-abusing pregnant
w., drug-dependent
w., healthy pregnant
w., heterosexual
w. ▸ infect parturient
w., infertility in
w., lactating
w., menopausal
w. ▸ opioid-abusing
w., postmenopausal
w., postpartum
w. ▸ premenopausal diabetic
w. with alcohol abuse problems
wonder drug
Wonderland" syndrome, "Alice in
wood (Wood('s))
w. block, balsa
W. lamp
W. light examination of eye
w. pulp worker's lung
W. units
wooden resonance
wooden-shoe heart
woody edema
woody thyroiditis

Wookey's neck flap
Wookey's pharyngoesophageal (PE)
   reconstruction
wool
   w. fat, hydrous
   w. fat, refined
   w. skein test, Holmgren's
woolly hair
woolly thinking
woolsorter's disease
woolsorter's pneumonia
word(s) (Word)
   w., ability to repeat
   w. and actions, repetitive
   w. associations
   w., binary
   w. blindness
   w., brain processing of
   w. center, auditory
   w. center, visual
   w. deafness
   w. debris
   w., decimal
   w., inability to arrange
   w. ▸ inability to interpret written
   w., inability to remember spoken
   w. -list memory
   w., loss of memory for
   w., misuse of
   w. of others ▸ echoing
   w. ▸ patient uses inappropriate
   w. processing
   w. properly, inability to arrange
   w. recall test ▸ delayed
   w. recognition
   w. ▸ repetition of
   w. retrieval
   w. salad
   w., spatial
   W. test, Harvard Spondee
   W. Test, Stroop Color and
   w. vision
work (Work)
   w., acclimation to heat and
   w. activity ▸ physical
   w. addiction
   w. adjustment
   w., admission blood
   w. behavior ▸ inability to sustain
      consistent
   w. behavior ▸ irresponsible
   w. behavior ▸ sustain consistent
   w. capacity
   w. capacity, cardiovascular

W. Capacity exercise stress test ▸
   Physical
w. capacity, physical
w., clinical social
w., community service
w. ▸ deteriorating quality of
w. environment, physical
w. ▸ excessive devotion to
w. hardening program
w. hypertrophy
w. index (CWI) ▸ cardiac
w. index, contractile
w. index (LVWI) ▸ left ventricular
w. index (SWI) ▸ stroke
w. inhibition ▸ academic or
w. (LVW) ▸ left ventricular
w. (LVSW) ▸ left ventricular stroke
w. ▸ liver function blood
w. load ▸ peak
w. metabolic rate
w. pattern, compulsive
w. rehabilitation
w. -related dermatitis
w. -related emotional stress
w. -related injury
w. -related physical stress
w., root canal
w. simplification
w. site, smoke-free
w., social
w. status
w., stress of
w., stroke
w. therapeutically
w. threshold
w. -tolerance peak
w., unstructured
w. (VSW) ▸ ventricular stroke
workaholic
   w. activity
   w. lifestyle
   w. personality
worked up, patient
worker(s)('s)(s')
   w., admission
   w. anthracosis, coal
   w. cancer, dye
   w. cancer, pitch-
   w., clinical social
   w., compulsive
   w., crisis
   w., grief
   w. (HCW), health care
   w. lung, cheese
   w. lung, detergent

w. lung disease, cheese
w. lung ▸ mushroom
w. lung ▸ wood pulp
w., paraprofessional health
w. pneumoconiosis, coal
w., psychiatric social
w., social
working
   w. contact
   w. diagnosis
   w. memory
   w. muscles, cool
   w. occlusion
   w. relationship
   w. relationship, short-term
   w. side
   w. through
   w. under the influence
workout
   w., aerobic
   w., high stress
   w. ▸ low impact aerobic
   w. time
Workplace Act ▸ Drug-Free
workplace violence
workup
   w. and staging, diagnostic
   w., biochemical
   w., cardiac
   w., cord blood
   w., diagnostic
   w., epilepsy
   w., full blood
   w., gastrointestinal
   w., immunologic
   w., infertility
   w., laboratory
   w., mobile mass lab
   w. not diagnostic
   w., patient had previous
   w., patient hospitalized for
   w., preoperative laboratory
   w., presurgical laboratory
   w., routine
   w., sterility
   w., stroke
   w., thoracic medical
world (World)
   w. around him/her
   W. Health Organization (WHO)
   w., inner
   W. Inventory (EWI), Experiential
   W. Medical Association (WMA)
   w., mental
   W. Trade Center cough

worldwide, death
worm
  w. aneurysm
  w., bilharzia
  w., bladder
  w., blinding
  w., case
  w., cayor
  w., dragon
  w., eel
  w., eye
  w., flat
  w., fluke
  w., guinea
  w., heart
  w., horsehair
  w., kidney
  w., lung
  w., maw
  w., meal
  w., Medina
  w. of cerebellum
  w., palisade
  w., parasitic
  w., pork
  w., ribbon
  w., screw
  w., serpent
  w., spiny-headed
  w., stomach
  w., thorny-headed
  w., tongue
  w., trichina
worn
  w. cartilage
  w. facet joints
  w. hearing aid, body
worry cycle
worrying, excessive
worsening relapsing-remitting
  multiple sclerosis (MS)
Worst Medallion Lens
worth (Worth's)
  w., augment individual's sense of
    self-
  w., diminished self-
  w. ▸ rediscovering a sense of self-
  w., self-
  w. ▸ sense of self-
  W. stereopsis test
worthless treatment
worthlessness
  w. and helplessness ▸ feeling of
    guilt,
  w., feelings of

  w. ▸ self-perceived
wound(s) (Wound)
  w., abdominal
  w. abscess
  w., accidental
  w., active oozing from
  W. and Skin Isolation
  w. anesthetized
  w., appendix brought into surgical
  w. approximated
  w., aseptic
  w. biopsy, fasciotomy
  w., bite
  w., blowing
  w. botulism
  w. brought into apposition ▸
    margins of
  w., bullet
  w., burn
  w. care
  w. care, follow-up
  w. care, special
  w. cautery
  w. cavity
  w., chronic granulating
  w. classification, surgical
  w., clean
  w. clean and healed
  w. clean and healed, operative
  w., clean-contaminated
  w. cleanser, skin
  w. closed
  w. closed in anatomic layers
  w. closed in layers
  w. closed in layers without drainage
    (dr'ge)
  w. closed loosely
  w. closed over
  w. closed with sutures
  w. closure
  w. closure, abdominal
  w. closure, delayed
  w., closure of skin
  w., clots expressed from
  w., contaminated
  w., contused
  w., corneoscleral
  w. covered with collodion, surgical
  w. debrided
  w., decubitus
  w., deep puncture
  w., deep-penetrating
  w. dehiscence
  w., dehydration of
  w., delayed closure of accidental

  w., delayed closure of operative
  w., dirty
  w. discharge
  w. disruption
  w., disruption of operative
  w., drain brought out through stab
  w., drain placed into
  w. drain, stab
  w. drainage (dr'ge)
  w., draining
  w. dressed
  w. dressing
  w. edge
  w. edges, approximate
  w. edges debrided
  w. edges, gaping
  w. edges retracted
  w. endocervical canal, secondary
    puncture
  w. entrance
  w. evaluation
  w. evisceration
  w. examined for hemostasis
  w. excision
  w., exit
  w., exploration of
  w. exploratory, deep
  w. fever
  w., foreign object in
  w., fragment
  w., fungating
  w., gas gangrene
  w. granulating in
  w., gunshot
  w. healed by first intention
  w. healed by second intention
  w. healed per primam
  w., healing
  w. healing capability
  w. healing ▸ poor
  w. healing satisfactorily
  w. healing well
  w., incised
  w. incision, stab
  w., infected
  w. infection
  w. infection ▸ nosocomial
  w. infection, postoperative
  w. infection ▸ sternal
  w. infection, surgical
  w., inferior border of
  w. infusion ▸ continuous
  w., intraocular leaking
  w. irrigated
  w. irrigated with normal saline

wound(s)—*continued*
- w. irrigated with saline solution
- w. isolation
- w. knife
- w., lacerated
- w., lateral flank
- w., lip of
- w. loosely approximated
- w. management
- w. margins
- w. margins revised
- w. margins undermined
- w., minor
- w., minor skin
- w., multiple fragment
- w., multiple needle puncture
- w., multiple puncture
- w., needle puncture
- w., nonpenetrating
- w. of great vessels, penetrating
- w. of heart, penetrating
- w. of the abdomen, penetrating
- w. of the chest, sucking
- w. of the skin, open
- w., oozing from
- w. oozing purulent material
- w., open
- w., open fresh traumatic
- w., operative
- w., ostomy, continence (WOC) nurse
- w. packed
- w., penetrating
- w., penetrating abdominal
- w., penetrating cardiac
- w., penetrating neck
- w., perforating
- w., perforating corneal
- w., plantar puncture
- w., poisoned
- w., posterior angle of
- w., primary puncture
- w. probed, depths of
- w., probing of
- w., punctate
- w., puncture
- w., purulent
- w., pyelotomy
- w. redressed
- w., resuture disrupted operative
- w., rib spreaders enlarged
- w. secretion
- w., self-inflicted
- w., separate stab
- w. separation

- w., septic
- w., seton
- w. site
- w., spiral
- w., stab
- w., subcutaneous
- w., sucking
- w. sucking chest
- w., summer
- w., superficial
- w. superficially explored
- w., surgical
- w. surveillance, surgical
- w., sutured
- w., sutured parallel with edges of
- w., tangential
- w. tenderness
- w. tension
- w., thoracotomy
- w., tissue brought out through
- w., traumatic
- w., traumatopenic
- w., ulcerated

woven
- w. coronary artery disease
- w. Dacron graft, Cooley
- w. Dacron tube graft
- w. Dacron vascular graft ▸ Velex
- w. Teflon prosthesis

WP (wedge pressure)

W-plasty

W-plasty revision

WPRS (Wittenborn Psychiatric Rating Scale)

WPW (Wolff-Parkinson-White) syndrome

wrap
- w., Ace
- w. -around surgery
- w., cardiac muscle
- w. ▸ no-phase

wrapper's asthma ▸ meat-

wrapping aneurysm

Wreden's sign

wrenching pain

wrenching, strain or

wretch [*retch*]

Wright's
- W. plate
- W. stain
- W. version

wrinkle(s)
- w. artifact
- w. cream, anti-
- w. depth

- w., eyelid
- w., face
- w., facial
- w. ▸ laser resurfacing for facial
- w. ▸ laser treatments for
- w. line
- w., lip
- w. method
- w., premature skin
- w. removal
- w. removal ▸ laser face
- w., sags and bags
- w., smoker's

wrinkled
- w. ear in aging
- w. lid skin
- w. skin
- w. skin, dry
- w. skin fold
- w. tongue

wrinkling
- w., coarse
- w., facial
- w. of skin ▸ drying and

Wrisberg's
- W. cartilage
- W. ganglia
- W. ganglion
- W. ligament
- W. nerve
- W., nerve of

wrist
- w. and forearm, immobilize
- w. arthroplasty
- w. bone
- w. bracelets, weighted
- w., carcinomatous arthritis in
- w. clonus reflex
- w., dermatomyositis in
- w. drop
- w., first metacarpal of
- w. flexed
- w., fracture of radius at
- w. full range of motion (ROM) ▸ left
- w. full range of motion (ROM) ▸ right
- w. fusion
- w. ganglion
- w., hand flexed at
- w. ▸ hemochromatosis in
- w., immobilize forearm and
- w. injury
- w. joint
- w. joint implant, Swanson
- w. joint ▸ repetitive motion of

w. motion ▸ repetitive
w. replacement
w. rest, Chan
w. restraints
w. scars
w. sign ▸ Walker-Murdoch
w., swelling of
w., ventral surface of

write ▸ loss of ability to
write time
writhing [*rising*]
writhing patient
writing

w. difficulty
w. disorder
w. disorder ▸ developmental
expressive
w. hand
w. mirror
w. skills ▸ journal
w. specular

written

w. consent for surgery
w. expression
w. home exercise program
w. language nonfunctional
w. orders
w. treatment protocols
w. word ▸ inability to interpret

ws (watt second)
W-shaped incision
wt (weight)
wucher atrophy
wuchereri, helminthiasis
Wuchereria bancrofti
Wuchereria malayi
Wucherer's conjunctivitis
Wullstein's type tympanoplasty
w/v (weight per volume)
wv (whispered voice)
Wyatt disease, Brushfield-
Wyeomyia melanocephala
Wyeomyia virus
Wyeth's operation
Wylie's operation
Wylie's pessary

X-Y-Z

X antigen, factor
X axis
X chromosomal aberration
 X c.a., penta-
 X c.a., tetra-
 X c.a., triple-
X deficiency, Factor
x depression
X disease virus, Australian
X ▸ gamma hydroxybutyrate (GHB)
 Liquid
X, globulin
X, histiocytosis
X ▸ primary pulmonary histiocytosis
X, syndrome
X syndrome, Fragile
x wave
X wave of Öhnell
X, Y, and Z coordinates
xanthelasma
 x. around eyelids
 x., generalized
 x. palpebrarum
xanthine oxidase reaction
Xanthium pennsylvanicum
xanthochromia, presence of
xanthochromic fluid
xanthoerythrodermia perstans
xanthofibroma thecocellulare
xanthogranuloma, juvenile
xanthogranulomatous pyelonephritis
xanthoma
 x., craniohypophyseal
 x., diabetic
 x. diabeticorum
 x. disseminatum
 x., eruptive
 x. eruptivum
 x., generalized plane
 x. multiplex
 x., palmar
 x. palpebrarum
 x., planar
 x., plane
 x. planum
 x. striatum palmare
 x. tendinosum

x., tendinous
x., tuberoeruptive
x. tuberosum
x. tuberosum multiplex
x., tuberous
xanthomatosis
 x., biliary hypercholesterolemic
 x. bulbi
 x., cerebrotendinous
 x., chronic idiopathic
 x. generalisata ossium
 x. iridis
 x., primary familial
 x., Wolman's
xanthomatous granuloma
Xanthomonas hyacinthi
Xanthomonas maltophilia
X-bite
XC (excretory cystogram)
X-descent trough
Xe (xenon)
XEM (xonics electron
 mammography)
xenogeneic antigen
xenogenous siderosis
xenograft
 x., human tumor
 x., Ionescu-Shiley pericardial
 x., porcine
 x. rejection ▸ hyperacute
 x. ▸ stentless porcine
 x. transplantation
 x., valve
xenon (Xe)
 x. arc laser
 x. arc light
 x. (Xe) arch photocoagulator
 x. -enhanced computed
  tomography
 x. lung ventilation imaging
Xenophor femoral prosthesis
xenopi, Mycoplasma
Xenopsylla
 X. astia
 X. brasiliensis
 X. cheopis
 X. hawaiiensis

X. vexabilis
Xenopus laevis test
Xenopus test
xenotransplantation procedure
xeroderma
 x., follicular
 x. of Kaposi
 x. pigmentosum
xerodermic idiocy
Xeroform gauze
xerogram, suspicious area on
xerography
xeromammogram study
xeroradiography
xerosis
 x. conjunctivae
 x., conjunctival
 x., corneal
 x., Corynebacterium
 x. cutis
 x. parenchymatosus
 x. superficialis
xerotic keratitis
xerotica obliterans
xerotica obliterans, balanitis
Xiphias gladius
xiphisternal crunching sound
xiphisternal process
xiphoid (same as xyphoid)
 x. angle
 x. bone
 x. cartilage
 x. process
 x. to pubis
X-linked
 X. agammaglobulinemia
 X. dilated cardiomyopathy
 X. disorder
 X. genetic defect
 X. inheritance
 X. lymphoproliferative
 X. lymphoproliferative (XLP)
  syndrome
 X. retardation syndrome ▸ alpha
  thalassemia
xonics electron mammography
 (XEM)

x-ray(s)
- x. absorptiometry (DEXA) bone density test ▸ dual energy
- x. absorptiometry (DEXA) ▸ dual energy
- x., admission chest
- x. anatomy
- x. beam dosimetry, adjacent field
- x. beam dosimetry ▸ dual
- x. beam dosimetry, four field
- x. beam dosimetry, large field
- x. beam dosimetry, rotational
- x. beam dosimetry, single
- x. beam filtration
- x., bite-wing
- x. body scanner
- x. burn
- x., cervical
- x., chest
- x. contrast media instilled
- x. control, biopsy under
- x., diagnostic
- x. diagnostic evaluation
- x. diagnostic studies
- x. diffraction analysis
- x. dosage
- x. dosage, Kienböck's unit of
- x. evaluation
- x. examination, low dose
- x., exposure to
- x., FB (foreign body) seen on
- x. findings
- x. findings limited
- x. findings, negative
- x. findings, positive
- x. follow-up
- x., follow-up chest
- x., foreign body (FB) seen on
- x., full mouth
- x. generator
- x. ▸ high dose beams of
- x. image
- x. images ▸ three-dimensional
- x. imaging, live
- x. immunosuppressive measures
- x., inversion strain
- x. ▸ low-dose breast
- x. machine, portable
- x. magnification
- x. mammography
- x. microscope
- x. microscope, projection
- x., mobile mass
- x. on admission, chest
- x. or positrons

- x., patient given enema prior to
- x. pelvimetry
- x., periodic
- x., plain
- x., reduction verified by
- x., repeat chest
- x. ▸ Scanning Beam Digital
- x., serial chest
- x. sickness
- x., sinus
- x., spark
- x. spectrum
- x. studies
- x. tables, inadequately cleaned
- x. technician-on-call
- x. technique, low dose
- x. therapy
- x. therapy, combination high and low energy
- x. therapy, deep
- x. therapy, supervoltage
- x. tube
- x., ultra
- x. unit, AMX 110 mobile
- x. view, Caldwell
- x. view, Chamberlain-Towne
- x. view, Granger
- x. view, Laws
- x. view, Mayer
- x. view, Stenver
- x. view, Waters'
- x., wet reading of

XU (excretory urogram)
Xu (X-unit)
X-unit (Xu)
XXY syndrome
xylinum, Acetobacter
xylinus, Acetobacter
Xylocaine, infiltrated with
xylol pulse indicator
Xylose (xylose)
- X. absorption test ▸ d-
- x. concentration test
- X. tolerance test ▸ d-

xylosoxidans, Achromobacter
xylosoxidans, Alcaligenes
xyphoid (see xiphoid)
Xytron pacemaker
****

Y (yttrium)
Y and spleen pedicle, inverted
Y, and Z coordinates ▸ X,
Y axis
Y bypass ▸ Roux-en-
y depression of jugular venous pulse

y descent (Y descent)
- y. of jugular venous pulse
- y. ▸ rapid
- Y. trough
- y. wave

Y flap, V-
Y graft
Y incision, standard
Y, Roux-en-
y wave
Yaba virus
YAG (yttrium, aluminum, garnet)
Yakima, hemoglobin
yang meridian
Yasargil neurological instrument
Yasargil technique
Yates correction
yawning, sweating and lacrimation
Yb (ytterbium)
Yb (ytterbium) penetate sodium
year(s)
- y., childbearing
- y., latency
- y., menopausal
- y. molar, sixth-
- y. molar, twelfth-
- y., procreative
- y. -round wheezes
- y. survival rate ▸ one-

yearning and sadness ▸ pining,
yeast
- y. and hyphae
- y. extract, charcoal
- y. fungus
- y., genetically programmed
- y., hyphae of
- y. infection
- y. infection ▸ Candida
- y. infection ▸ chronic
- y. infection ▸ oral
- y. infection, periodic
- y. infection ▸ recurrent vaginal
- y. infection ▸ systemic
- y. infection, vaginal
- y. -like fungus
- y. organisms
- y. spores
- y., vaginal
- y. vaginitis
- y. vaginitis ▸ chronic
- y. vaginitis ▸ recurring

Yellow(s) (yellow)
- Y. (barbiturates)
- y. atheroma
- y. atrophy

y. atrophy, acute
y. atrophy, healed
y. atrophy, subacute
y. bone marrow
y. -brown serous ascites
y. cortical structures
y. elastic tissue
y. fever
y. fever immunization
y. fever, jungle
y. fever virus
Y. Jackets (barbiturates)
y. ligament
y. marrow
y. material, diffluent
y. nail syndrome
y. reaction ▸ egg
y. serous fluid
y. softening
y. spot (YS) of retina
y. sputum
y. tympanic membrane ▸ bulging
y. urine, turbid
yellowing
y. from aging ▸ tooth
y. of eyes
y. of skin
y. of whites of eyes
yellowish
y. -brown cortex ▸ laminated
y. phlegm
y. sputum
yellowness of skin
Yeo's treatment
Yerba (marijuana)
Yerkes-Bridges test
yersinia (Yersinia)
y. enterocolitica
Y. enterocolitica colitis
Y. pestis
Y. pseudotuberculosis
Yersin's serum
yet diagnosed (NYD), not
yield, ectocervical cell
yield, endocervical cell
yin meridian
ylang-ylang
yoga
y. breathing
y. derived exercises
y. exercise ▸ hatha
y., medical
y. stretches
y. treatment
yogic complete breath

yoke(s) [*yolk*]
y. of bone of cranium cerebral
y. of mandible, alveolar
y. of maxilla, alveolar
y., sphenoidal
yoked muscles
yokogawai, Metagonimus
yolk [*yoke*]
y., accessory
y., egg
y., formative
y., nutritive
y. sac
y. -sac entoderm
y. sac placenta
y. -sac tumor
y. sputum, egg
y. stalk
Yoon ring
York Heart Association (NYHA) ▸ New
Yorke-Mason incision
Youman-Parlett serologic test
young (Young)('s)
y. cadaver
Y. -Helmholtz theory
Y. operation
Y. procedure
Yount's operation
youth, slow waves of
youth/parent support group
yo-yo
y. diet
y. dieting ▸ hazards of
y. syndrome
YS (yellow spot) of retina
Y-shaped scar
y-suture
ytterbium (Yb)
ytterbium (Yb) pentetate sodium
yttrium (Y)
yttrium, aluminum, garnet (YAG)
yttrium-aluminum-garnet (Nd:YAG)
laser, neodymium:
Y-type incision
Y-type ureteropelvioplasty, Foley
yuppie flu
yuppie influenza
Yvon's coefficient
Yvon's test
****

Z coordinates ▸ X, Y, and
Z disc
Z incision
Z incision, lazy
Z line

z point pressure
Zag Man (LSD), Zig-
zag stent ▸ zig-
Zahn('s)
Z. lines
Z. ▸ pockets of
Z. ribs
Zahradnicek's operation
Zancolli's operation
Zanelli's position
Zang's space
zap surgery ▸ flap and
Zappert's chamber
zapping cataracts
Zaufal's sign
Z-cut osteotomy
zeal, therapeutic
Zeeman effect
Zeis, glands of
zeisian gland
zeisian sty
Zeiss
Z. counting cell ▸ Thoma-
Z. counting chamber ▸ Abbe-
Z. counting chamber ▸ Thoma-
Z. instruments
Z. microscope
Z. operating microscope
Z. photocoagulator
Zellweger syndrome, Fanconi-
Albertini-
Zenker('s)
Z. crystals
Z. degeneration
Z. diverticulum
Z. fixative
Z. fluid
Z. necrosis
Z. solution
Zephiran irrigation
Zephiran solution
zero (Zero)
z., absolute
z. cryogenic fluid ▸ sub-
z. degree teeth
z. end-expiratory pressure
z. end-inspiratory pressure
z. family
z. frequency
z. frequency voltages
z. isopotential axis
z., limes
z. offset, E-
z. -order kinetics
z., physiologic

zero (Zero)—*continued*
   z. potential reference electrode
zest (PMZ) ▸ postmenopausal
zeylandica, Haemadipsa
Z-flap
Z-flap incision
Ziegler('s)
   Z. cautery
   Z. operation
   Z. scale
Ziehen-Oppenheim disease
Ziehen's test
Ziehl-Neelsen method
Ziehl-Neelsen stain
Zieve's method
ZIG (zoster immune globulin)
zig-zag (Zig-Zag)
   z. lines
   z. lines ▸ shimmering
   Z. Man (LSD)
   z. stent
Zika virus
Zim carpal tunnel projection,
   Templeton and
Zimaloy femoral head prosthesis
Zimany's bilobed flap
Zimany's flap
Zimfoam finger splint
Zimfoam head halter traction
Zimmer
   Z. electrodes
   Z. equipment
   Z. low viscosity cement
   Z. method
   Z. pin
Zimmerman personality test,
   Guilford-
Zimmerman's arch
zinc
   z. flocculation test
   z. gelatin
   z. paste, Lassar's plain
   z. sulfate turbidity
   z. turbidity test
Zinn('s)
   Z., annulus of
   Z. aponeurosis
   Z. artery
   Z. cap
   Z. circle
   Z. circlet
   Z. corona
   Z. ligament
   Z. tendon
   Z. zone

   Z. zonule
zinnii, annulus
Zinsser disease, Brill-
Zinsser inconsistency
ZIP (zoster immune platelet)
zipper artifact
zipper scar
zirconium granuloma
Zollinger-Ellison syndrome
Zoll's pacemaker
zombie-like, patient
zona fasciculata
zona pellucida
zonal aberration
zonal anatomy
zonary placenta
Zondek test, Aschheim-
zone(s)
   z., benign transformation
   z., cornuradicular
   z., echo
   z., erotogenic
   z. (FZ), focal
   z., ischemia in peri-infarct
   z. (DREZ) lesion, dorsal root entry
   z., Lissauer's
   z., Looser's
   z., mature transformation
   z. of heart ▸ tendinous
   z. of hip, orbicular
   z. of inhibition
   z., pain-free
   z., parasagittal
   z. plate, Fresnel
   z., prophylactic destruction of
      transformation
   z., protective
   z., slow
   z., subcostal
   z., subendocardial
   z., subpapillary
   z. ▸ target heart rate
   z., transformation
   z. ▸ transitional cell
   z., traumatized
   z., vascular
   z., Westphal's
   z., Zinn's
zonography, stereoscopic
zonula ciliaris
zonula occludens
zonular
   z. cataract
   z. fibers
   z. perinuclear cataract, lamellar

   z. placenta
   z. space
zonule
   z., ciliary
   z. fibers
   z., hypoplasia of
   z., Zinn's
zonulolysis, enzymatic
zooepidemicus, Streptococcus
zooglea stage
zoonosis, bacteria
zoonotic disease
Zoon's erythroplasia
zoophil psychosis
zoster (shingles)
   z., herpes
   z. immune globulin (ZIG)
   z. immune globulin (VZIG),
      varicella-
   z. immune platelet (ZIP)
   z. infection, disseminated herpes
   z., intercostal
   z. of cornea, herpes
   z. of iris, herpes
   z., trigeminal
   z., varicella-
   z. virus ▸ herpes
   z. virus, varicella-
Zovickian's flap
Z-plasty
   Z. closure, multi-sided
   Z. incision
   Z. revision
   Z. scar
Z-shaped incision
Z-shaped scar
Zuckerkandl's convolution
Zueler hook plate
Zugsmith's sign
Zung Depression Scale
Zwanck's pessary
Z-wave tube
Zwislocki test, Luscher-
Zyderm collagen treatment
zygapophyseal joints
zygoma, fracture of
zygomatic
   z. arch
   z. arch fracture ▸ nondisplaced
   z. bone
   z. muscle
   z. muscle, greater
   z. muscle, lesser
   z. nerve
   z. process

z. reflex
z. region
z. suture line, frontal
zygomaticofacial nerve
zygomaticofrontal suture lines
zygomaticomaxillary fracture
zygomaticomaxillary suture
zygomaticotemporal nerve
zygomaticotemporal suture
zygomaticum, os
zygote intra-fallopian transfer (ZIFT)
zymogen cells
zymogen granules
zymogenes, Streptococcus
zymoplastic substance
zymosis gastrica
Zyrel's pacemaker
Zytron pacemaker